W9-BJC-734

# Primary Preventive Dentistry

## SIXTH EDITION

Norman O. Harris, DDS, MSD, FACD

*Professor (Retired), Department of Community Dentistry*
*University of Texas Health Science Center at San Anotnio*
*San Antonio, Texas*

Franklin García-Godoy, DDS, MS, FICD

*Editor, American Journal of Dentistry,*
*Professor and Associate Dean for Research,*
*Director, Clinical Research Center,*
*Director, Bioscience Research Center,*
*College of Dental Medicine*
*Nova Southeastern University*
*Fort Lauderdale, Florida*

PEARSON
Prentice
Hall

Upper Saddle River, New Jersey 07458

A CIP catalog record for this book can be obtained from the Library of Congress

**Publisher:** Julie Levin Alexander
**Assistant to Publisher:** Regina Bruno
**Acquisitions Editor:** Mark Cohen
**Assistant Editor:** Melissa Kerian
**Editorial Assistant:** Mary Ellen Ruitenberg
**Marketing Manager:** Nicole Benson
**Product Information Manager:** Rachele Strober
**Director of Production and Manufacturing:**
  Bruce Johnson
**Managing Production Editor:** Patrick Walsh
**Production Liaison:** Alexander Ivchenko
**Production Editor:** Patty Donovan, Pine Tree
  Composition

**Manufacturing Manager:** Ilene Sanford
**Manufacturing Buyer:** Pat Brown
**Design Director:** Cheryl Asherman
**Design Coordinator:** Maria Guglielmo Walsh
**Cover and Interior Designer:** Janice Bielawa
**Composition:** Pine Tree Composition, Inc.
**Manager of Media Production:** Amy Peltier
**New Media Project Manager:** Stephen Hartner
**Printing and Binding:** Banta Book Group
**Cover Printer:** Phoenix Color Corp.

Pearson Education, Ltd., *London*
Pearson Education Australia Pty. Limited, *Sydney*
Pearson Education Singapore Pte. Ltd.
Pearson Education North Asia Ltd., *Hong Kong*
Pearson Education Canada, Ltd., *Toronto*
Pearson Educación de Mexico, S.A. de C.V.
Pearson Education—Japan, *Tokyo*
Pearson Education Malaysia, Pte. Ltd.
Pearson Education, Upper Saddle River, New Jersey

10  9  8  7  6  5
ISBN 0-13-091891-1

# CONTENTS

Preface        vii
Acknowledgments        ix
Contributors        xi

1    Introduction to Primary Preventive Dentistry        1
     *Norman O. Harris*

2    The Development and Structure of Dental Plaque (A Bacterial
         Biofilm), Calculus, and other Tooth-Adherent Organic
         Materials        23
     *Max A. Listgarten*
     *Jonathan Korostoff*

3    The Developing Carious Lesion        45
     *Norman O. Harris*
     *Adriana Segura*

4    The Role of Dental Plaque in the Etiology and Progress
         of Periodontal Disease        73
     *Donald E. Willmann*
     *Norman O. Harris*

5    Toothbrushes and Toothbrushing Methods        93
     *Samuel L. Yankell*
     *Ulrich P. Saxer*

6    Dentifrices, Mouthrinses, and Chewing Gums        119
     *Stuart L. Fischman*
     *Samuel L. Yankell*

7   Oral-Health Self-Care Supplemental Measures to Complement
    Toothbrushing    145
    *Terri S.I. Tilliss*
    *Janis G. Keating*

8   Water Fluoridation    181
    *Elaine M. Neenan*
    *Michael W. Easley*
    *Michael Ruiz, Research Assistant*

9   Topical Fluoride Therapy    241
    *Kevin J. Donly*
    *George K. Stookey*

10  Pit-and-Fissure Sealants    285
    *Franklin Garcia-Godoy*
    *Norman O. Harris*
    *Denise Muesch Helm*

11  Oral Biologic Defenses in Tooth Demineralization
    and Remineralization    319
    *Norman O. Harris*
    *John Hicks*

12  Caries Risk Assessment and Caries Activity Testing    337
    *Svante Twetman*
    *Franklin Garcia-Godoy*

13  Periodontal Disease Prevention: Facts, Risk Assessment,
    and Evaluation    367
    *Norman O. Harris*
    *Donald E. Willmann*

14  Sugar and Other Sweeteners    399
    *Peter E. Cleaton-Jones*
    *Connie Mobley*

15  Nutrition, Diet, and Oral Conditions    419
    *Carole A. Palmer*
    *Linda D. Boyd*

16  Understanding Human Motivation for Behavior Change    449
    *Mary Kaye Sawyer-Morse*
    *Alexandra Evans*

17  Dental Public-Health Programs    467
    *Mark D. Macek*
    *Harold S. Goodman*

18  Preventive Oral-Health in Early Childhood    501
    *Stephen J. Goepferd*
    *Franklin Garcia-Godoy*

19  Oral-Health Promotion in Schools    521
    *Alice M. Horowitz*
    *Norman O. Harris*

20  Preventive Oral-Health Care for Compromised
    Individuals    559
    *Roseann Mulligan*
    *Stephen Sobel*

21  Geriatric Dental Care    589
    *Janet A. Yellowitz*
    *Michael S. Strayer*

22  Primary Preventive Dentistry in a Hospital Setting    605
    *Norman O. Harris*
    *Jeffery L. Hicks*

23  Rationale, Guidelines, and Procedures for Prevention
    of the Plaque Diseases    645
    *Norman O. Harris*
    *Marsha A. Cunningham-Ford*

Glossary    685
Index    695

# PREFACE

This is the sixth edition of the text, *Primary Preventive Dentistry*. The successive editions since 1982 have provided an excellent example of the fact that the useful lifetime of much knowledge is finite. At the time of the first edition even such dental essentials as mechanical and chemical plaque control, access to dental care and dental insurance were only being slowly accepted. Now, a new wave of dental visionaries is coming on the world stage to speak with confidence about future vaccines, genetic engineering and therapeutic stem cells. These are exceedingly important basic science subjects to all health professions and are only now creeping into the general dental lexicon and application.

Like in past editions, the information in the text and supporting references has been greatly upgraded, although every effort has been made to retain original citations from past landmark research. An increased emphasis has been given to school programs because of the increasing number of school based health clinics (SBHC) that are being developed to care for children. Risk assessment is highlighted in the text as a necessity for determining at the time of an initial/annual clinical examination whether a patient's treatment is to be preventive or restorative. Remineralization of incipient caries, an old idea, but a relatively new weapon in the dentists' arsenal, offers a new preventive strategy for those seeking to maintain intact teeth for a lifetime.

Throughout this approximate last quarter-century of metamorphosis, the format of the book has remained constant. It is written in a style that is user-friendly, whether the user is a dental or dental-hygienist student, a dental assistant, a private- or public-health practitioner, a health educator, or a school nurse. The book and suggested learning strategies have been successfully used for class-paced study; they have been used for remedial programs; and they have been used for remote self-paced learning as well as for scheduled continuing education courses.

Each chapter commences with a series of objectives—subject matter that the authors consider essential. Key words and concepts are *italicized* in each chapter to help focus on information deemed important. Throughout the text, there are embedded clusters of true-and-false questions, as well as answers and fill-in-the-blank questions at the end of the chapter. These are included for student self-evaluation.

Following the class presentation of the subject matter it is recommended that about an hour-or-so should be spent outside the classroom to review the chapter. As each question

is encountered for which the answer is not completely understood, a check mark should be made before reading on. At the end of the chapter, the marked questions should be again reviewed and the answers learned at the 100% level—not just memorized.

Prentice Hall has, with this sixth edition, established a website for the book that permits a student to take a "mock examination" at the end of each chapter. A personal or institutional computer is a requisite for Prentice Hall to respond to new true-or-false, essay, and to fill-in-the-blank type of questions. The true-or-false questions will be computer marked and returned immediately to the students e-mail address. The essay and fill-in-the blank questions will *not* be marked because of the variety of possible correct answers submitted, but will be immediately returned to the student along with the "school answers" for comparison. This exchange between the student and the Prentice Hall website is strictly between two computers. ***No student records will be kept at the website***. The goal of the program is to provide the learner with a means of self-evaluation of his/her level of attainment. Student participation in this voluntary, non-jeopardizing, website program can result in a huge step towards achieving long-term mastery learning. The questions in the question bank are also available to teachers who might desire to use them for their own purposes

Since curriculum time allocations vary from institution-to-institution, the chapters do not need to be scheduled in a given sequence, being free standing for the indexed subject matter. The 23 chapters include the theory and practice of preventive dentistry in private and public health environments. One chapter discusses plaque formation, while two chapters each emphasize the importance of caries and periodontal disease and disease prevention. To aid in combating these two plaque diseases, there are chapters on dentifrices, toothbrushing and auxiliary tooth cleaning devices used in accomplishing mechanical and chemical plaque control. Sugars, diets, and human motivation are included to facilitate better counseling of patients. A chapter is devoted to the use of pit-and-fissure sealants. Chapters on public health point out the responsibilities of a public health dentist, as well as two chapters on the oral health advantages of fluoride—water fluoridation, and topical applications—both of which are prime preventive tools of a public health dentist as well as for the private practitioner. Different age and health status groups are also considered in separate chapters—pedodontic, geriodontic, handicapped, and hospitalized individuals. Finally, there is a chapter on how to use risk assessment to integrate prevention into the total treatment plan.

In summary, the authors have contributed the chapters of updated information, the editors have established the learning system, while Prentice Hall has provided a website for worldwide user self-evaluation.

# ACKNOWLEDGMENTS

For a multiauthored and multi-edition book text, there is a need for a lot of credit to go around. Lest we forget, the authors of the first edition established the foundation, from which the several later editions in preventive dentistry have been upgraded. Approximately 60 authors and authoresses have contributed of their knowledge and time through their writings from the first to the present sixth edition. These authors and authoresses have come from research laboratories, state and national public health agencies and teaching institutions in the United States and overseas. Authors from Canada, Korea, England, South Africa, Switzerland and Sweden are represented in the latter group. A spin-off Spanish edition of the fifth edition of the text has been published reflecting this multinational approach to the book. Manufacturers and dental-supply houses have contributed photos and information on their products, while journal publishers have given permission for use of copyright material. Teachers using the book, and students learning from the book, have both made suggestions that have enhanced the value of the texts.

Very few texts would be published without the help of a publisher. For this publication by Prentice Hall, there is Melissa Kerian who kept us on schedule, Amy Peltier who has lent her computer expertise, and Mark Cohen, the book editor, who harmoniously kept everyone staying the course. To those many other known and unknown individuals who helped develop this edition of the primary dental prevention text, the editors desire to voice heartfelt appreciation. Of a more personal nature, both editors wish to thank their wives, Katherine Garcia-Godoy and Grace Harris for their continuing support and encouragement.

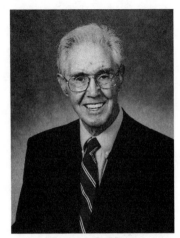

Norman O. Harris
DDS, MSD, FACD

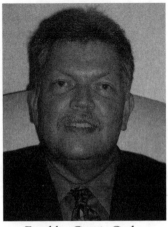

Franklin García-Godoy
DDS MS, FICD

# CONTRIBUTORS

**Linda D. Boyd, MS, RDH, R**
Assistant Professor
Department of Periodontology
Oregon Health Sciences University
School of Dentistry
Portland, OR

**Peter E. Cleaton-Jones, BDS, MB, BCH**
Professor of Experimental Odontology
Director, Dental Research Institute
Director, Medical Research Council
University of Witwatersrand
Witwatersrand, South Africa

**Marsha A Cunningham-Ford, RDH, BS, MS**
Associate Professor
Department of Preventive Dentistry
    and Community Dentistry
University of Iowa,
Iowa City, IA

**Kevin J. Donly, DDS, MS**
Professor
Director Postdoctoral Pediatric Dentistry
Department of Pediatric Dentistry
University of Texas Dental School
    at San Antonio
San Antonio, TX

**Michael Easley, DDS, MPH, FACD**
Associate Professor
Department of Health Promotion and
Administration
Eastern Kentucky University
Richmond, KY

**Alexandra E. Evans, PHD**
Assistant Professor
Department of Health Promotion, Education
    and Behavior
University of South Columbia, SC

**Stuart Fischman, DMD, FACD, FICD**
Professor Emeritus
School of Dental Medicine
State University of New York at Buffalo
Buffalo, NY

**Franklin García-Godoy, DDS, MS, FICD**
Associate Dean for Research
Professor of Restorative Dentistry
Professor of Pediatric Dentistry
Nova Southeastern University
Fort Lauderdale, FL

**Stephen J Goepferd. DDS, MS**
Professor
Department of Pediatric Dentistry
College of Dentistry
University of Iowa
Iowa City, IA

**Harold S. Goodman, DMD, MPH**
Associate Professor
Department of Pediatric Dentistry
Baltimore College of Dental Surgery,
Dental School
University of Maryland
Baltimore, MD

**Norman O. Harris, DDS, MSD, FACD**
Professor (Retired)
Department of Community Dentistry
Department of Dental Hygiene
University of Texas Dental School
at San Antonio
San Antonio, TX

Denise Muesch Helm, RDH MA
Assistant Professor
Northern Arizona University
Department of Dental Hygiene
Flagstaff, AZ

**Jeffery L. Hicks, DDS**
Associate Professor
General Dentistry
University of Texas Dental School
at San Antonio
San Antonio, TX

**M. John Hicks, DDS, MS, PhD, MD**
Associate Professor of Pathology and Director
of Surgical and Ultrastructure Pathology
Department of Pathology
Texas Children's Hospital Houston and Baylor
College of Medicine
Houston, TX

**Alice M. Horowitz, PhD**
Senior Scientist
National Institute of Dental and Craniofacial
Research
National Institutes of Health
Bethesda, MD

**Janis G. Keating, RDH**
Professional Educator
Phillips Oral Healthcare, Inc.
Littleton, CO

**Jonathan Korostoff, DMD, PhD**
Assistant Professor
Department of Periodontics
University of Pennsylvania
Philadelphia, PA

**Max A. Listgarten, DDS**
Professor Emeritus
University of Pennsylvania,
Philadelphia, PA
Visiting Professor, University of California
in San Francisco
Foster City, CA

**Mark D. Macek, DDS, DrPH**
Assistant Professor
Department of Oral Health Care Delivery
and Director of Community Programs
Baltimore College of Dental Surgery, Dental
School
University of Maryland
Baltimore, MD

**Connie Mobley, PhD**
Associate Professor
Department of Community Dentistry
University of Texas Dental School
at San Antonio
San Antonio, TX

**Mary Kaye Sawyer-Morse, PhD**
Associate Professor, Nutrition
University of the Incarnate Word
San Antonio, TX

**Roseann Mulligan, DDS, MS**
Associate Professor and Chairman
Department of Dental Medicine and Public
Health
Section of Geriatric and Special
Care Dentistry
School of Dentistry
University of Southern California
Los Angeles, CA

**Elaine M. Neenan, MS, DDS, MPH**
Associate Dean, External Affairs
School of Dentistry
University of Texas Dental School
San Antonio, TX

**Carole A. Palmer, EdD, RD**
Professor and Head
Division of Nutrition and Oral Health
Promotion
Department of General Dentistry
School of Dental Medicine
Tufts University
Boston, MA

**Ulrich P. Saxer, DDS, PhD**
Professor and Head of Prophylaxis School
Lecturer in Periodontology
University of Zurick
Zurick, Switzerland

**Adriana Segura Donly, DDS, MS**
Associate Professor
Department of Pediatric Dentistry
University of Texas Dental School
    at San Antonio
San Antonio, TX

**Stephen Sobel, DDS**
Associate Professor of Clinical Dentistry
School of Dentistry
University of Southern California
Los Angeles, CA

**George K. Stookey, MSD, PhD**
Distinguished Professor
Indiana University School of Dentistry
Indianapolis, IN

**Michael S. Strayer**
Associate Professor
Section of Primary Care
College of Dentisitry
Ohio State University
Columbus, OH

**Terri S. I. Tillis, RDH, MS, MA**
Professor
Dental Hygiene Department
School of Dentistry
University of Colorado Health
    Science Center
Denver, CO

**Svante Twetman, DDS, PhD, Odont Dr**
Professor
Department of Pediatric Dentistry
Faculty of Odontology
University of Lund
Malmo, Sweden

**Donald E. Willmann, DDS, MS**
Associate Professor
Department of Periodontics
University of Texas Dental School
    at San Antonio
Dental School
San Antonio, TX

**Dr. Samuel L. Yankell, PhD, RDH**
Research Professor in Periodontics
School of Dental Medicine
University of Pennsylvania
Philadelphia, PA

**Janet A. Yellowitz, DMD, MPH**
Associate Professor
Department of Oral Health Care Delivery
Baltimore College of Dental Surgery, Dental
School
University of Maryland
Baltimore, MD

## Reviewers

**Chris French Beatty, RDH, Ph.D.**
Associate Professor
Department of Dental Hygiene
Texas Woman's University
Denton, TX

**Margaret Bloy, CDA, RDH, MS**
Coordinator
Dental Assisting Program
Middlesex Community College
Lowell, MA

**Janet Hillis, RDH, MA**
Chair
Dental Hygiene
Iowa Western Community College
Council Bluffs, IA

**William Johnson, DMD, MPH**
Director
Dental Auxiliary Programs
Chattanooga State Technical Community College
Chattanooga, TN

**Vickie Jones, RDH**
Instructor
Department of Dental Hygiene
Northeast Mississippi Community College
Booneville, MS

**Shawn Moeller, RDH**
Associate Professor
Dental Hygiene
Salt Lake Community College
Salt Lake City, UT

**Barbara Ringle, RDH, M.Ed.**
Assistant Professor
Dental Hygiene Program
Cuyahoga Community College
Cleveland, OH

**Katharine R. Stilley, RDH, MS**
Assistant Professor
Department of Dental Hygiene
University of Mississippi Medical Center
Jackson, MS

**Pamela Wade, RDH, BS, MS, CFCS**
Instructor
Department of Dental Hygiene
Tyler Junior College
Tyler, TX

# CHAPTER 1

# Introduction to Primary Preventive Dentistry

*Norman O. Harris*

## OBJECTIVES

*At the end of this chapter, it will be possible to*

1. Define the following key terms: health, primary prevention, secondary prevention, and tertiary prevention. Also, provide one specific example of each.
2. Name three convenient categories that aid in classifying dental disease and in planning oral-disease prevention and treatment programs.
3. Name four strategies and two administrative means for reducing the prevalence of dental caries and/or periodontal disease.
4. Cite two early actions that are essential for arresting the progression of the plaque diseases once primary preventive measures have failed.
5. Explain why the planned application of preventive-dentistry concepts and practices, including use of sealants and fluoride therapy, when coupled with early detection and immediate treatment of the plaque diseases, can result in a zero or near-zero annual extraction rate.

# INTRODUCTION

In the year 2000, in the Executive Summary of the Surgeon Generals Report[a] on the "Oral Health in America," some of the major challenges facing American dentistry were listed.[1,2] It is appropriate to abstract a number of these problem areas in order to better understand the role that prevention can play in their solution.

1. Tobacco: This is a major societal health problem with very strong relationships to dentistry. Smoking has a very devastating relationship to periodontal disease and oral and pharyngeal cancer, while the use of chewing tobacco is associated with oral cancer as well as root decay (see Chapter 23).

2. The statistics of dental need:

**Children**

a. Dental caries is the most common chronic childhood disease.

b. Over 50% of 5- to 9-year-olds have at least one cavity or filling; by age 17, the percentage has increased to 78%.

c. As a part of childhood, children have many injuries to the head, face, and neck.

d. Twenty-five % of the children have not seen a dentist before entering kindergarten.

e. More than 51 million school hours are lost each year to dental-related illness.

**Adults**

a. Most adults show signs of periodontal or gingival diseases. Severe periodontal disease [measured as 6 millimeters of periodontal attachment loss (pockets)] affects about 14% of adults aged 45 to 54.

b. Employed adults lose more than 164 million hours of work each year because of dental disease and dental visits.

c. A little less than two-thirds of adults report having visited a dentist in the past 12 months.

**Older adults**

a. Twenty-three % of 65- to 74-year-olds have severe periodontal disease (characterized by 6 millimeters or more of periodontal attachment loss). At all ages, men are more likely than women to have more severe disease.

b. About 30% of adults 65 years and older are edentulous, compared to 46% 20 years ago.

c. Oral and pharyngeal cancers are diagnosed in about 30,000 Americans annually. Nine thousand die from these diseases each year. Prognosis is poor.

d. At any given time, 5% of Americans aged 65 and older (currently some 1.65 million people) are living in long-term care facilities where dental care is problematic.

[a]United States Public Health Service.

Throughout the entire Surgeon General's report, there is major emphasis on the great disparity *between those who get dental care and those that do not* have access to a dental facility.[3,4] These are the people who are poor,[5,6] are mentally handicapped,[7] those that are disabled,[8] children,[9–12] the aged,[13] and those without dental insurance. There are others living in underserved geographical areas,[14] and still others who do not have access to dental care because of disease,[15] culture, or race.[16] To address these problems a national program and guidelines of dental care is needed that will include these dentally neglected groups. The questions then become, "What kind of a national program should it be? Is it possible to take care of *so many* people with *so few* dental health professionals?"

It is the goal of the dental profession to help individuals achieve and maintain maximum oral health throughout their lives. Success in attaining this objective is highlighted by the decline of caries throughout the Western world,[17] and the dramatic reduction of tooth loss among adults in the United States. This progress has been mainly attributed to the use of *water fluoridation* and *fluoride-containing products*—toothpastes and mouthrinses—and the growing acceptance and practice of primary preventive care.[18] Yet, dental caries remains a major public-health problem.

Untold millions of research hours and money have been invested in reaching our present capability to control the ravages of the *plaque diseases*. Effective strategies that can markedly reduce the number of carious teeth and better control of periodontal disease are now available. *They only need to be used.*

All health professions emphasize that patients should seek entry into well-planned preventive programs. For dentistry, lack of prevention results in more restorations, periodontal treatment, extractions, and dentures. The changeover in priority from treatment to prevention will require active leadership and health promotion by the dental profession, consumer advocates, public health educators, and health-policy planners. Public-health delivery systems, such as the military, national and state public-health services, and industrial organizations that provide benefits to their personnel, have usually been in the forefront of such change because of the economic advantages accruing to the provider and health benefits to the recipients. For example, in 1989, a report by Malvitz and Broderick[19] recounted the results following the change of focus toward a maximum emphasis on prevention for dental services by the Indian Health Service in the Oklahoma City area. The total number of visits increased by 10%, yet the number of dental personnel remained constant. The percentage of *preventive services increased*, along with a *decrease* of restorative procedures.

## Benefits of Primary Preventive Dentistry to the Patient

For the patient who thinks in terms of economic benefits and enjoyment of life, prevention pays. Many studies document the *prevalence* of dental disease, but behind these numbers there is little mention of the adverse affects on humans caused by dental neglect. One study points out that 51% of dentate patients have been affected in some way by their oral health, and in 8% of the cases, the impact was sufficient to have reduced their quality of life.[20] If preventive programs are started early by the patient (or, preferably, by the parents of young children) long-range freedom from the plaque diseases is possible—a sound cost–benefit investment. After all, the teeth are needed over a lifetime for eating. Speech is greatly improved by the presence of teeth. A pleasant smile enhances personality expression. Teeth also contribute to good nutrition for all ages. At rare times, teeth have even provided a means of self-defense. On the other hand, the *absence* of teeth or presence of broken-down teeth often results in a loss of self-esteem, minimizes employment possibilities and often curtails social interaction.

## Benefits to the Dentist

Possibly the first benefit of preventive dentistry is the fulfillment of the moral commitment to the Hippocratic Oath that was taken by health professionals at graduation "to render help to those in need, and to do no harm." Through ethics and training, the dentist should derive a deep sense of satisfaction by helping people maintain their oral structures in a state of maximum function, comfort, and aesthetics. A well-balanced practice that actively seeks to prevent disease but is also able to care for those individuals where prevention has failed should prosper. Patients can be outstanding public relations advocates if they are convinced that their dentist and staff are truly interested in preventing disease.

If for no other reason, a dentist should consider prevention to avoid possible *legal problems*. A now strongly supported law for medicine, but to a lesser extent for dentistry, requires that prior to treatment, all options—preventive as well as treatment—should be explained to secure *informed patient consent*. This discussion should include a comparison of health benefits and hazards, as well as the economic and the oral-health benefits of prevention. Long-term patients, the lawyers and the court system are taking a more unsympathetic attitude toward practitioners who have permitted a disease to progress over many years without having taken some accepted primary preventive actions to have slowed, or halted its progress. Patients no longer tolerate supervised professional neglect.[21]

## What is Primary Prevention?

When discussing primary prevention, we must first define a few key words. Health is what we want to preserve, and it is defined as *a state of complete physical, mental, and social well-being, and not merely the absence of disease or infirmity*. For instance, some individuals may actually be in excellent health but believe, for some reason

logical to them, that they have oral cancer. Such individuals do not have an optimum mental well-being and will continue to worry until they are somehow convinced otherwise that they are indeed healthy. Another person may be functionally healthy, although facially disfigured, and as such be socially shunned throughout life.[22] Thus, health can at times be what the patient thinks and not the actual condition of the body. Even the terminology "preventive dentistry" has different connotations to different people. As a result, preventive dentistry can be arbitrarily classified into three different levels.

1. *Primary* prevention employs strategies and agents to *forestall* the onset of disease, to *reverse* the progress of the disease, or to *arrest* the disease process before secondary preventive treatment becomes necessary.

2. *Secondary prevention* employs routine treatment methods to *terminate* a disease process and/or to *restore* tissues to as near normal as possible.

3. *Tertiary prevention* employs measures necessary to *replace* lost tissues and to *rehabilitate* patients to the point that physical capabilities and/or mental attitudes are as near normal as possible after the failure of secondary prevention (Figure 1–1).

---

### Question 1

Which of the following statements, if any, are correct?

A. The absence of a disease or infirmity is a good sign of physical health but not necessarily of mental and social well-being.

B. A professional football player who looks well, has no physical infirmities, but continually worries about his $10 million contract, can be considered in excellent health.

C. An amalgam restoration that is placed in a carious occlusal pit of a molar is an

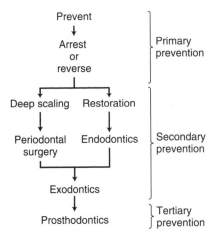

FIGURE 1-1 From natural teeth to denture teeth in three not-so-easy stages. (*Source:* Dr. Norman O. Harris, University of Texas Dental School at San Antonio.)

excellent example of tertiary prevention.

D. The avoidance of an etiologic factor for a specific disease—sucrose for instance to reduce caries—is an example of primary prevention.

E. Preventive dentistry, in its broadest sense, embodies primary, secondary, and tertiary prevention.

In going from primary to tertiary prevention, the cost of health care increases exponentially, and patient satisfaction decreases proportionately. An excellent example of the comparative cost of these two levels of care was the treatment of an individual with poliomyelitis. It has only been a few years ago that the cost of the polio vaccine was only a few dollars. The use of the polio vaccine to prevent the onset of the disease was *highly* effective. But, for someone not adequately immunized, the cost of treatment for poliomyelitis and subsequent rehabilitation approximated $50,000 or more for the first 7 weeks of hospitalization and outpatient care.[23] Yet, the individual receiving the

$50,000 worth of tertiary preventive treatment and the attendant disability was certainly not as happy as the one who benefited from only a few dollars' worth of primary preventive care. The payoff of the worldwide drive to eliminate polio promises to have this disease follow smallpox into oblivion. Another appropriate example is the fluoridation of drinking water. This costs approximately $0.50 per year per individual, yet it reduces the incidence of dental caries in the community by 20 to 40%. If this primary-preventive measure is not available, the necessary restorative dentistry (secondary prevention) can cost approximately 100 times more, or about $50.00 per restoration.[18] Finally, if restorative dentistry fails, as it often does, prosthetic devices must be constructed at an even greater cost. This great disparity between the lower cost of prevention and the much higher cost of treatment must be seriously considered *if* the United States is to develop an affordable national health program in which dentistry is represented.

This text emphasizes primary prevention, and specifically focuses on primary prevention as it applies to the control of dental caries and periodontal disease. On the other hand, it must be recognized that primary prevention often fails for many reasons. When such failure occurs, *two actions* are essential to contain the damage: (1) *early identification* of the disease (diagnosis) and (2) *immediate treatment* of the disease.

## Categories of Oral Disease

For planning purposes, dental diseases and abnormalities can be conveniently grouped into three categories: (1) dental caries and periodontal disease, *both* of which are acquired conditions, (2) acquired oral conditions *other than* dental caries and periodontal disease (opportunistic infections, oral cancer, HIV/AIDS), and (3) craniofacial disorders which would include a wide variety of conditions ranging from heredity to accidents.[24,25] For instance, the or-

dinary seat belt and the air bags in a car exemplify how a simple preventive measure can greatly reduce the facial injuries of car accidents. Looming in the not-too-far distant future is the very real possibility that many acquired health problems will be corrected or ameliorated for total populations by use of vaccines, genetic engineering, or specifically targeted drugs ("magic bullets").

The treatment of caries and periodontal disease (and their sequelae) accounts for most of the estimated $60 billion U.S. dental bill for the year 2000.[26] *Both* caries and periodontal disease are caused by the presence of a pathogenic dental plaque on the surfaces of the teeth and hence are known as the *plaque diseases*. Any major reduction in the *incidence* of caries and periodontal disease will release resources for the investigation and treatment of conditions included in the acquired and craniofacial category.

The ideal, or *long-range* planning objectives for coping with both dental caries and periodontal disease should be the development of a preventive delivery system and methods to eventually attain a zero or near-zero *disease incidence* for the target population. However, a more realistic and feasible *shorter-term goal* is the attainment of a zero or near-zero rate of *tooth loss* from these diseases by integrated preventive *and* treatment procedures. Because of the varied etiology of the second and third categories, that is, other acquired conditions and craniofacial malformations and diseases, the planning for the control of each of these problem areas must be individually addressed and placed within the priorities of any overall health plan.

---

### Question 2

Which of the following statements, if any, are correct?

A. A disfiguring facial deformity resulting from an automobile accident can be considered an acquired craniofacial problem.

B. The broad concept of preventive dentistry places major emphasis on primary preventive care but also considers the equal need for secondary and tertiary preventive care.

C. Because dental caries and periodontal disease are infectious diseases (true), they are acquired conditions.

D. The ideal or long-range objective for dentistry is an eventual zero annual extraction rate; the more realistic, and much more encompassing *short-range objective* is to totally prevent the onset of any pathology requiring extraction.

E. Acquired conditions (*other than* caries or periodontal disease) and hereditary diseases account for the great proportion of income derived by the dental profession.

---

## Strategies to Prevent the Plaque Diseases

Before providing an overview of methods used to implement primary prevention programs, it is important to point out that both dental caries and periodontal disease are *transmissible diseases*. If a child is considered at high risk for caries, one of the parents[27]—usually the mother—can usually be identified as high risk; if a child has periodontal problems, usually one of the parents is also afflicted. Any infectious (acquired) disease can only begin if the challenge organisms are in sufficient numbers to overwhelm the combined manmade and body defenses and repair capabilities. For this reason, all strategies to prevent, arrest, or reverse the ravages of the plaque diseases are based on (1) reducing the number of challenging oral pathogens, (2) building up the tooth resistance and maintaining a healthy gingiva, and (3) enhancing the repair processes.

In general, periodontal disease is a disease that involves the soft tissue and bone surrounding the affected teeth. Caries involves

the demineralization and eventual *cavitation* of the enamel and often of the root surface. If the *incipient* lesions (earliest *visible* sign of disease) of caries and periodontal disease are recognized at the time of the initial/annual dental examination, they can often be reversed with primary preventive strategies. For caries, the *visible* incipient lesion is a *white spot*, which appears on the surface of the enamel as a result of subsurface acid-induced demineralization. For periodontal disease, the *visible* incipient lesion is *gingivitis*—an inflammation of the gingiva that is in contact with the bacterial plaque. Not all "white spots" go on to become caries, nor do all cases of gingivitis go on to become periodontal disease. In both cases, i.e., caries and periodontal disease, it should be noted *that if dental plaque did not exist, or if the adverse effects of its microbial inhabitants could be negated, the decrease in the incidence of the plaque diseases would be very dramatic. Based on these facts, it is understandable why plaque control is so important in any oral-health program.*

To control the *plaque diseases* with *available* methods and techniques, strong emphasis has been directed to four general strategies to reduce caries and two administrative requirements:

**General Strategies**
1. Mechanical (toothbrush, dental floss, irrigator, or rinse)
2. Chemical plaque control. Use of *fluorides* to inhibit *demineralization* and to enhance *remineralization;* use of antimicrobial agents to supress cariogenic bacteria.
3. Sugar discipline.
4. Use of pit and fissure sealants, when indicated, on posterior occlusal surfaces.

**Administrative**
5. Education and health promotion.
6. Establish access to dental facilities where diagnostic, restorative, and preventive services are rendered, and where planned recalls based on risk are routine.

A brief summary of each of these primary preventive procedures will serve as an introduction for the more detailed information presented in later chapters.

Plaque Control

Dental plaque is composed of *salivary proteins* that adhere to the teeth, plus *bacteria and endproducts* of bacterial metabolism. Both cariogenic and periodontopathogens accumulate in the plaque located along the gingival margin, interproximally, and in the pits and fissures. Plaque collects more profusely in these specific areas because none of these locations is optimally exposed to the normal self-cleansing action of the saliva, the abrasive action of foods, nor the muscular action of the cheeks and tongue. Plaque decreases in thickness as the incisal or occlusal surface is approached. Little plaque is found on the occlusal surface except in the pits and fissures. As would be expected, plaque forms more profusely on malposed teeth or on teeth with orthodontic appliances, where access for cleaning is often difficult.

In the *gingival sulcus* between the gingiva and the tooth, little or no plaque normally accumulates *until* gingival inflammation begins, at which time the bacterial population increases in quantity and complexity. This is the beginning of *gingivitis* that, if continued, may eventually result in an *irreversible periodontitis.*

It is important to differentiate between the *supragingival* and the *subgingival* plaques. The *supragingival* plaque can be seen above the gingival margin on all tooth surfaces; the *subgingival* plaque is found in the sulcus and pocket below the gingival margin, where it is not visible. The supragingival plaque harbors specific bacteria that can cause supragingival (coronal) caries. The subgingival plaque microbiota is mainly responsible for periodontal problems. The bacterial populations of each of these plaques differ qualitatively and quantitatively in health and disease.[28] The pathogenicity of each of the plaques can vary independently of the other. For example, it is possible

to have periodontal disease with or without caries, to have neither, or to have a shifting status of caries or periodontal disease, or both.

The pathogenicity of the subgingival plaque is becoming an increasing concern. Not only does it cause periodontal disease, which is a lifelong debilitating disease of the tooth supporting tissues, but it is now believed that there is a causal relationship between periodontitis[29] and such diverse conditions as, cardiovascular disease,[30] diabetis mellitus,[31] chronic respiratory disease,[32] and immune function.[33] There is also the possibility in some cases that this is a bi-directional association where the oral problem begins with a systemic condition, instead of vice versa.

In many cases, plaque is difficult for a patient to identify. This problem can be overcome, at least in the case of the supragingival plaque, by the use of *disclosing* agents, which are harmless dyes such as the red-staining agent, FD&C Red. The dyes may be in solution and painted on the teeth with a cotton applicator, or they may be tablets which are chewed, swished around the mouth, and then expectorated. Once *disclosed*, most of the supragingival plaque and food debris can be easily removed by the daily use of a toothbrush, floss, and an *irrigator* (Figure 1–2). Plaque can also be removed at planned intervals by the dental hygienist or a dentist as part of an oral *prophylaxis*. This is a procedure that has as its objective the mechanical removal of all soft and hard deposits, followed by a polishing of the tooth surfaces. However, because daily removal of the plaque is more effective, it is the individual—not the hygienist or the dentist—who is vital for preserving lifelong intact teeth.

One site where neither the dentist nor an individual can successfully remove plaque is in the depth of pits and fissures of *occlusal* surfaces where the orifices are too small for the toothbrush bristle to penetrate (see Chapter 10). The flow of saliva or the muscular action of the cheeks and tongue also have little influence over the eventual development of caries in these

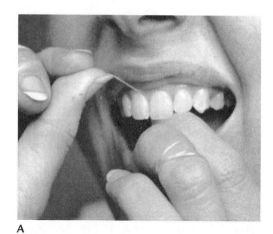

A

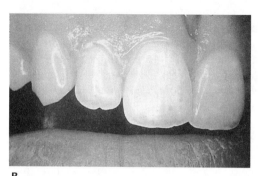

B

FIGURE 1–2    **A.** Flossing gets down under the gingiva and **B.** cleans the space between the teeth as well. (*Source:* Dr. Norman O. Harris, University of Texas Dental School at San Antonio.)

areas. Not coincidentally, the occlusal surface is where the *greatest percentage* of caries lesions occur. *For this reason, it is recommended that all occlusal surfaces with deep convoluted fissures be sealed with a pit-and-fissure sealant.*

As soon as the plaque is removed from any surface of the tooth, it *immediately* begins to reform. This should not be unexpected, since by definition, dental plaque is composed of salivary residue, bacteria, and their end-products, all of which are always present in the mouth. Thus, a good plaque-control program must be continuous. It must be a daily commitment over a lifetime.

## Question 3

Which of the following statements, if any, are correct?

A. Four general areas that form the basis for strategies for the primary prevention of dental diseases are (1) plaque control, (2) fluoride use, (3) sealants, and (4) restorations.

B. Plaque is found only on the smooth enamel surfaces of the tooth.

C. Plaque removal requires the use of instrumentation by a dentist or a dental hygienist.

D. Good flossing and toothbrushing techniques can completely remove the supragingival plaque from all five tooth surfaces.

E. The daily self-care removal of plaque by an individual is more productive than a semiannual removal by the dental hygienist.

Not only does the daily removal of dental plaque reduce the probability of dental caries; equally important, it also reduces the possibility of the onset of gingivitis. This occurs when the metabolic end-products of the *periodontopathogens* that are contained in the plaque irritate the adjacent gingival tissues, producing an inflammation (i.e., gingivitis). If the inflammation continues, bleeding (hemorrhage) can be expected following even minimal pressure ("pink toothbrush"). This gingivitis can be arrested and reversed (cured) in the early stages by proper brushing, flossing, and irrigation, especially if accompanied with professional guidance.

Plaque concentrates mineralizing ions such as calcium, phosphate, magnesium, fluoride and carbonates from the saliva to provide the chemical environment for the precipitation and formation of *calculus*, a concretion that adheres firmly to the teeth. If the plaque is not removed by flossing and brushing before the cal-

culus begins to form, the resultant mineralized mass provides a greater surface area for an even more damaging plaque accumulation. This *additional* mass of *periodontopathic* plaque covering the rough porous surface causes the stagnation of even more bacteria and is responsible for the damage to the periodontal tissues. Also, the hard, irregular calculus deposits pressing against the soft tissues serves to *exacerbate* the inflammation caused by the bacteria alone. The daily removal of plaque can successfully abort or markedly retard the build-up of calculus. Once the calculus forms, the brushing and flossing usually used for plaque control does *not* remove the deposits. At this time, the dental hygienist or dentist must intercede to remove the calculus by instrumentation.

To this point, only mechanical plaque control (i.e., use of a toothbrush, dental floss, and an irrigator) has been highlighted. Rapidly growing in importance as a supplement to mechanical plaque control (but not as a replacement), is *chemical plaque control*. This approach utilizes mouthrinses containing antimicrobial agents that effectively help control the plaque bacteria involved in causing *both* caries and gingivitis. For helping to control gingivitis, a popular and economical over-the-counter product is Listerine; the most effective *prescription* rinse is *chlorhexidine*. Many studies indicate that chlorhexidine is as effective in suppressing cariogenic organisms as it is effective in controlling gingivitis and periodontitis.[34,35]

### Fluorides

The use of fluorides has provided exceptionally meaningful reductions in the incidence of dental caries. Because of water fluoridation, fluoride dentifrices, and mouthrinses, dental caries is declining throughout the industrialized world. Historically, the injection of fluoride into water supplies in the mid-20th century resulted in a decrement of approximately 60 to 70% in caries. Since that time, fluoride has been introduced into proprietary products such

as dentifrices and mouthrinses. As a result, the caries decrement *directly attributable* to water fluoride over the past years has declined. Yet, the placement of fluoride into communal water supplies *still* results in an estimated 20 to 40% reduction in coronal caries, and a similar 20 to 40% decrease in root caries[36] (Figure 1–3).

Approximately 126 million individuals in the United States consume fluoridated water through *communal water* supplies and another 9 million are drinking *naturally* fluoridated water. It is estimated that 65% of the U.S. population, therefore, is receiving fluoride through drinking water.[37] Many times during the past years, it has not been possible to fluoridate city water supplies because of political, technical, or financial considerations. In such cases, it is still

possible to receive the *systemic* benefits of fluoride by using *dietary supplements* in the form of fluoride tablets, drops, lozenges, and vitamin preparations. Some countries permit fluorides to be added to table salt.[38] Elsewhere, ongoing research studies are being conducted to determine the anticariogenic effect of fluoride when placed in milk,[39,40] and even sugar.[41]

It is also possible to apply fluoride directly *to the surface* of the teeth by use of cotton pledgets, and/or by use of fluoride-containing dentifrices, gels, varnishes or mouth rinses. Such applications to the surface of the teeth are referred to as *topical applications*. The extent of caries control achieved through topical applications is directly related to the number of times the fluoride is applied and the length of time the fluoride is maintained in contact with the teeth. Research data also indicate that it is better to apply *lower* concentrations of fluoride to the teeth *more often* than to apply higher concentrations at longer intervals.

Fluorides and chlorhexidine are the most effective agents used by the profession to combat the plaque diseases. The fluorides help prevent demineralization and enhance remineralization, while chlorhexidine severely suppresses the mutans streptococci that cause the demineralization. Chlorhexidine also helps suppress bacteria causing the inflammation of periodontal disease.

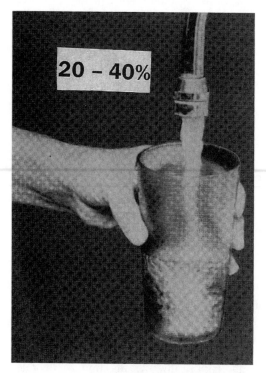

FIGURE 1–3 Water fluoridation reduces cavities in the population by 20 to 40%. (*Source:* Dr. Norman O. Harris, University of Texas Dental School at San Antonio.)

---

### Question 4

Which of the following statements, if any, are correct?

A. Prophylaxes and chlorhexidine are effective in the partial control of *both* caries and gingivitis.

B. Even after calculus becomes attached to the tooth, it can still be removed by good home self-care plaque control programs.

C. The addition of fluoride to communal water supplies is now accompanied by a 20 to 40% decrease in caries incidence.

Neither the action of topically applied nor of systemic (ingested) fluoride in preventing dental caries is completely understood. It is believed that fluoride has several key actions: (1) it may enter the dental plaque and affect the bacteria by depressing their production of acid and thus reduce the possibility of demineralization of the teeth; (2) it reacts with the mineral elements on the surface of the tooth to make the enamel less soluble to the acid end-products of bacterial metabolism; and (3) it facilitates the remineralization (repair) of teeth that have been demineralized by acid end-products. The latter is probably the most important of these three effects.

The natural source of minerals such as calcium and phosphate, fluoride and others needed for this remineralization is the *saliva*.

## Sugar and Diet

The development of dental caries depends on four interrelated factors: (1) diet, (2) inherent factors of host resistance, (3) the number of challenge bacteria located in the dental plaque, and (4) *time* (Figure 1–4). Without bacteria, no caries can develop. For the bacteria in the plaque to live, they must have the same amino acids, carbohydrates, fatty acids, vitamins, and minerals that are required for all living organisms. Because these nutrients are also required by the cells of the body, the food that is ingested by the host or that which later appears in the saliva in a metabolized form, provides adequate nutrients for bacterial survival and reproduction. With three *well-balanced* meals per day, however, the usual plaque bacteria proba-

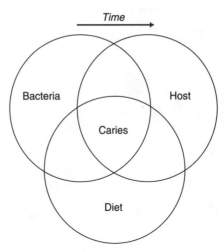

FIGURE 1–4   Caries is a *multifactorial* disease caused by bacteria, a supporting host diet of refined carbohydrates, decreased host resistance, and time for the cavity to develop. (*Source:* Dr. Norman O. Harris, University of Texas Dental School at San Antonio.)

bly would not release a sufficient quantity of metabolic acids to cause caries development (Figure 1–5a). But, as soon as *sugar and sugar products* are included in the diet of the host, bacterial acid production markedly increases in

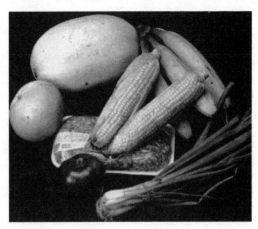

FIGURE 1–5a   This balanced meal does not provide the bacteria with enough energy to produce acids.

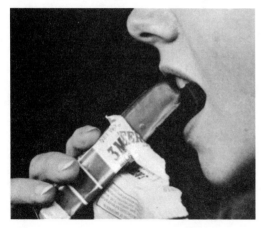

FIGURE 1–5b    Snacks such as this expose teeth to bacterial acids.

the plaque. This release of acid end-products is the major cause of the initiation and progression of caries.[42] Of even greater importance *than* the *total intake* of refined carbohydrates is the *frequency* of intake and the *consistency* of the sugar-containing foods.[43] The continuous snacking of refined carbohydrates that characterizes modern living results in the teeth being constantly exposed to bacterial acids (Figure 1–5b). For example, the prolonged adherence of sugar products to the teeth, such as that experienced after eating *taffies* and *hard candies*, results in prolonged production of the plaque acids that are in direct contact with the tooth surface. Thus, if caries incidence is to be reduced, all three factors—*total intake* of sugar, *consistency* of the cariogenic foods, and especially *frequency* of intake should be considered.

Possibly one of the most promising means of reducing caries incidence in the United States has been the wide-scale acceptance of sugar substitutes such as NutraSweet, Sweet'n Low, and Splenda. In the Nordic countries, there is considerable enthusiasm for use of xylitol—a sugar alcohol. Xylitol has been found to inhibit decay, reduce the amount of plaque and plaque acid, inhibit growth and metabolism of streptococci,[44] reduce decay in animal studies, and contribute to remineralization. It is considered

noncariogenic and cariostatic.[45] All the Nordic dental associations recommend its use. Since the 1970s, one of the favorite ways to take advantage of xylitols unique anticaries property, has been to use it to sweeten chewing gum, a product that is a popular item among school children.[46]

Two other dental uses of xylitol chewing gum have come out in Scandinavia:

1. Chlorhexidine can dramatically suppress the number of mutans streptococcus in the saliva. However, after discontinuing use of the product, there is a rapid repopulation of the bacteria. This repopulation can be arrested or greatly slowed by the use of xylitol chewing gum.[47]

2. Previously it was mentioned that a child's flora often reflected that of the mother. To help minimize this mother-child transmission of cariogenic bacteria, mothers have been urged to chew xylitol gum.[48]

This creditable background of xylitol has prompted Anasavice to ask, "Are chlorhexidine, fluoride, fluoride varnishes, and xylitol chewing gum under ustilized preventive therapies?"[49]

### Pit and Fissure Sealants

Approximately 90% of all the carious lesions in the mouth occur on the occlusal surfaces of the posterior teeth.[50] These surfaces represent only 12% of the total number of tooth surfaces, so that occlusal surfaces with their deep pits and fissures are approximately *eight times as vulnerable* as all the other smooth surfaces. The availability of sealants offers an alternative to a restoration. With the use of sealants, a thin layer of a plastic, called Bis-GMA, is flowed into the deep occlusal pits and fissures of teeth not having open carious lesions. This action effectively isolates these areas from the oral environment (Figure 1–6). Since no cavity preparation is necessary, no pain or discomfort accompanies sealant placement. Following the

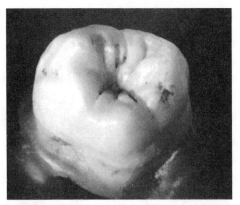

A

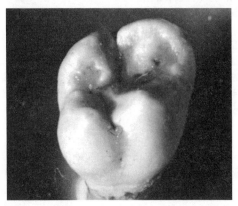

B

FIGURE 1-6    Molar **A.** without and **B.** with a clear plastic sealant to protect the deep occlusal fissures. (*Source:* Dr. Norman O. Harris, University of Texas Dental School at San Antonio.)

With these performances, the average life of the sealant approximates the 10 years projected for an amalgam.[53] It should be emphasized that sealant placement should be followed by a topical fluoride application to the teeth, because *fluorides are most effective in protecting the smooth surfaces and least effective on the occlusal surfaces, a situation that is the reverse of the results expected of the sealants.*

### Question 5

Which of the following statements, if any, are correct?

A. Using fluoride to remineralize incipient lesions, one can expect the reminerlized lesion to be more resistant to future demineralization than incipient lesions before remineralization.

B. The calcium and phosphate that is lost from the tooth in demineralization can be replaced during remineralization.

C. The development of dental caries depends on four essential factors: (1) diet; (2) inherent factors of host resistance; (3) bacteria; and (4) time.

D. Refined carbohydrates alone provide sufficient nutrition for cariogenic bacteria.

E. Sealant longevity closely coincides with the longevity of amalgam restorations.

### Public Dental Health Education

If the profession of dentistry can control caries effectively through plaque control, systemic (ingested) and topical (local application) use of fluorides, dietary control, and the use of plastic sealants, two important questions need to be asked.

1. Why do we not have a more effective dental caries–control program in the United States?

2. If daily toothbrushing, flossing of teeth, and irrigation removes plaque and food residue,

placement of the sealant in the deep fissures, the newly created fossae can be effectively cleaned with a toothbrush.

As long as the sealants are retained, no bacteria or bacterial acids can affect the sealed areas. If they are not retained, no damage to the teeth results from a retreatment. The lost sealant can be easily replaced. One 10-year study demonstrated a 57% retention of the original sealants.[51] In another study, approximately 95% retention occurred over 2 years.[52]

why are these simple procedures not used effectively to control both caries and periodontal disease?

Probably the best answer to these questions is that people must first *know* what they need to do as well as *how* it is to be done. Unfortunately, the public has relatively little information about the tremendous potential of primary preventive dentistry for reducing their adverse exposures to the plaque diseases. Without this information, *it is difficult to convince people that they can greatly control their own dental destiny.* Many individuals think of dentistry as a treatment-oriented profession that specializes in periodontal treatment, restorations, endodontics, exodontics, and prosthetics. An expanded public education and promotion program is essential to ensure the success of any preventive dentistry program in which an individual or a community is asked to participate.

In dentistry, a one-on-one relationship between the patient and the health professional is still a basic approach to patient education and motivation. This approach makes the task impossible because there are 250 million people in the United States and only approximately 165,000 practicing dentists, plus 120,000 dental hygienists and 175,000 assistants.[54,55] The main thrust of public dental-health education and oral-health promotion is provided by the various dentrifice manufacturers advocating the daily toothbrushing routine and biannual visits to the dentist for a checkup. The effectiveness of this approach was underlined by the long-running advertisement for the first marketed, stannous fluoride containing, Crest toothpaste, "Look Mom, no cavities."

Knowing facts and applying the information are two separate processes. The application of knowledge by an individual requires a personal commitment; it is at this point of personal commitment that most primary preventive-dentistry programs fail. *If* people embraced the daily use of mechanical and chemical plaque control regimens, the risk of caries and gingivi-

tis would be minimized. *If* people would exercise reasonable sugar discipline the possibility of caries development would be further reduced. *If* individuals rejected the use of cigarettes as well as smokeless ("spit") tobacco, oral and pharyngeal cancer and periodontitis would be much less prevalent. Clearly, education, motivation, and behavior modification are a necessary part of enjoying good oral and general health.

A sound, well-planned program of dental-health education and promotion is lacking in the curriculum of the great majority of primary and secondary schools. Few people can discuss the advantages and disadvantages of water fluoridation and the topical application of fluorides. Few have any detailed information about the dental plaque and the disease-inducing potentialities of this bacterial film.[b] Few people know why sugar is cariogenic. Even fewer people know that gingivitis can be *cured*, but that if allowed to progress, there is the possibility of a life long future of periodontal disease treatment and maintenance. Finally, the public has not been adequately informed that the timely use of sealants and remineralization therapy provides a hope of possessing a full intact dentition for life. Even though the Internet has greatly expanded the delivery of health education, there is always the question of the quality of information (or misinformation) that is disseminated.[56]

Ideally, school-based and public-education programs should exist to help people to *help themselves* in applying primary preventive procedures. The same programs should also teach all individuals to *recognize the presence of oral disease.* With proper instruction that can be provided by *schoolteachers.* The general public can be taught to understand that they must

---

[b]Biofilm = A collection (film) of living organisms attached to a solid base, such as algae to the bottom of a swimming pool, or dental plaque to a tooth. Both terms are used in the book, but dental plaque is preferred because of public familiarity and understanding of "dental plaque."

assume major responsibility for their own oral health (see Chapter 19). Only the individual can seek immediate treatment when pain or disease occurs. Public dental-health education might benefit if there was a consumer organization such as an American Oral Health Association that could promote oral health education, much like the American Cancer Society and the American Heart Association.

### Access to Comprehensive Dental Care

This factor is probably the most important of all preventive options. Without the benefit of a routine periodic dental examination, it is difficult for individuals to realize that they are vulnerable to oral disease. The first indication of a dental problem is pain, which is the wrong starting point for prevention. An example of the benefits of combining prevention with the advantages of early identification, prevention and treatment is seen in the New Zealand school-dental-nurse program. In the New Zealand School Dental Service, a dental nurse visits every primary and secondary school in the country at approximately 6-month intervals. At that time, all children receive a dental examination. If necessary, the dental nurse applies fluoride varnish to achieve remineralization of incipient caries, removes visible calculus, or when indicated, refers the child to a dentist for more complex treatment requirements.[57]

As a result of this program, the average rate of extractions dropped from 19 per 100 students in 1960, to 2 per 1,000 in 1979. From 1973 until 1992, the average decayed, missing, or filled permanent teeth (DMFT) for 12- to 14-year-old children plummeted from 10.7 to 1.88 per child. Approximately 96% of all New Zealand schoolchildren are enrolled in this program. Unfortunately, relatively few comprehensive primary-preventive dentistry school programs are being conducted in the United States school systems. However, there are more than 1,400 School Based Dental Health Clinics (SBDHC) now in operation in the United States (see Chapter 19).

### Prognostic and Diagnostic Tests

Several methods for preventing the onset or progress of caries and periodontal disease have been discussed. Because it is impossible to apply vigorously *all* the preventive procedures to *all* the people *all* the time, it would be desirable to have some tests to indicate the extent of caries and periodontal disease *risk* of an individual at any given time. This need is highlighted by the fact that an estimated 60% of all carious lesions in schoolchildren *occur in 20%* of the students.[58] It would save much time to be able to identify this 20% group of high-risk students without having to examine an entire school population. Although no tests are 100% correlated with the extent of caries activity or periodontal disease, several test procedures are sufficiently well correlated with either condition to be of interest. To be successful, such screening tests should be simple to accomplish, valid, economical, require a minimum of equipment, be easy to evaluate, and be compatible with mass-handling techniques.

Laboratory methods exist for counting the number of bacteria in the saliva. If the caries-causing mutans streptococci or lactobacilli counts are high, the individual from whom the sample was derived can be presumed to have a higher risk for dental caries, whereas a low count permits the opposite assumption.[59] A second general method for estimating caries susceptibility is by use of a refined-carbohydrate dietary analysis to (1) evaluate the patient's overall diet with special attention to food preferences and amounts consumed and (2) to determine if the intake of refined carbohydrates is excessive in quantity or frequency (see Appendix 23–2). A well-balanced diet is assumed to *raise host resistance* to all disease processes, whereas a frequent and excessive intake of refined carbohydrates (i.e., sugar) has been associated with a high risk of caries development.

The dietary analysis is very effective when used as a guide for patient education.

The onset of *gingivitis* is much more visible than the early demineralization that occurs in caries. The sign of impending periodontal disease is an inflammation of the gingiva that can be localized at one site, or generalized around all the teeth. Red, bleeding, swollen, and a sore gingiva are readily apparent to dentist and patient alike.

### Remineralization of Teeth

Both demineralization and remineralization occur *daily* following the cyclic ebb-and-flow of the caries process during and after eating meals and snacks. An eventual caries lesion develops *over a period of time* when the rate of acid-induced demineralization of teeth exceeds the capability of the saliva to remineralize the damaged enamel components. A negative mineral balance at the enamel–plaque interface, if continually repeated, results in an incipient lesion that eventually can become an overt lesion. It often requires months, or even years, for the overt lesion to develop.[60,61] During this time, under proper conditions, remineralization can reverse the progress of the caries front, with the mineral components coming from the saliva. There is a physiological precedent for such a mineralization. Immediately after eruption of the teeth the outer layer of the enamel is not completely mineralized; the maturation (mineralization) of this outer layer requires approximately 1 year, during which time the tooth is continuously bathed in the saliva.

The point at which a developing caries lesion is no longer reversible is considered to be when *cavitation* occurs; clinical experience indicates that as long as the lesion is incipient (i.e., with *no* cavitation), remineralization is possible.[62] The need to exploit this possibility to the benefit of all patients was emphasized by Koulourides's statement many years ago that "there is a wide gap between current practices of many dental clinicians and the potential application of present scientific knowledge to arrest and reverse incipient carious lesions."[63]

The outstanding electron microscope research contributions of Silverstone several decades ago clearly demonstrated that demineralized tooth structure could be remineralized.[64] No longer was a simple interproximal x-ray radiolucency a signal to place an interproximal restoration. Several reports from Scandinavia now indicate that even when the caries front of an incipient lesion extends *past* the dentinoenamel junction, it can be remineralized. Foster (England) has recommended "... that operative intervention (be) considered for approximal lesions which extend *deeper* that 0.5 mm into the dentine, while *preventive treatment and re-assessment* may be considered for *shallower lesions*."[65] Missing at the present time is an accurate predictive test for caries that would permit the targeting of individuals who would be candidates for remineralization therapy (see Chapter 23).

The conditions for optimum remineralization are the same as for preventing the initiation of a lesion: (1) plaque control to reduce the number of cariogenic bacteria, (2) a strict self-imposed sugar discipline to minimize the number of acidogenic episodes, (3) the use of sealants to interdict bacterial entry into deep pits and fissures, and (4) the use of topical and/or systemic fluoride to inhibit demineralization and to potentiate the remineralization process. Thus, with the same primary preventive dentistry routines using fluoride, an individual can *simultaneously* protect the tooth into the future by prevention, as well as to compensate for limited past damage through reversal strategies.

> ### Question 6
> Which of the following statements, if any, are correct?
>
> A. Sealants are most effective in preventing smooth-surface caries, whereas fluorides are most effective in preventing caries in the deep occlusal pits and fissures.
>
> B. There are enough dentists and dental auxiliaries in the United States to provide approximately 1 hour per year of

educational lectures to each of the 250 million citizens of the United States.

C. Caries activity indicators (tests) are indicative of a patient's vulnerability at the time of the test.

D. Plaque control, sugar restriction, and topical-fluoride therapy not only are effective in preventing demineralization, but they also can enhance remineralization.

E. The process of natural mineralization (maturation) of enamel during the first year after eruption is a precedent for man-initiated remineralization (repair) of incipient lesions.

## SUMMARY

Each year more than $60 billion is spent in the United States for dental care, mainly for the treatment of dental caries and periodontal disease or their sequelae. Yet, strategies now exist that with patient knowledge and cooperation, could greatly aid in preventing, arresting, or reversing the onset of caries or periodontal disease. The six general approaches to the control of both caries and periodontal disease involve (1) plaque control, (2) water fluoridation and use of fluoride products for self-care and for professionally initiated remineralization procedures, (3) placement, when indicated, of pit and fissure sealants, and (4) sugar discipline. Supporting these measures are (5) public and private enterprise financed media distributed programs extolling the benefits of oral health and proprietory products for family prevention; and (6) access to a dental facility where diagnosis, comprehensive preventive, restorative treatment, and planned recall and maintenance[c] programs are available. The zeal and thoroughness with which these preventive measures should be prescribed and used are indicated by the information obtained from the clinical and roentgenographic oral examination, dietary analysis, patient history, and laboratory tests.

*If* at the time of the clinical and roentgenographic examinations, emphasis was placed on searching out the incipient lesions ("white spots") and early periodontal disease (gingivitis), preventive strategies could be applied that would result in a reversal or control of either/or both of the plaque diseases. It is essential that both the profession and the public realize that biologic "repair" of incipient lesions, and "cure" of gingivitis is a preferred alternative to restorations or periodontal treatment.

Even if these primary preventive dentistry procedures fail, tooth loss can still be avoided. In practice, the early identification and expeditious treatment of caries and periodontal disease greatly minimizes the loss of teeth. When such routine diagnostic and treatment services are linked with a dynamic preventive-dentistry program that includes an annual dental examination and recall program based on risk assessment, tooth loss can realistically be expected to be reduced to zero or near-zero.

This introductory chapter has briefly pointed out some of the problems of dentistry and the means by which the dental profession can make primary preventive dentistry its hallmark. The remaining chapters provide the detailed background that can make this challenge become a reality.

---

[c]There is a trend to consolidate the two terms, "recall" and "maintenance", into the word, "recare".

# ANSWERS AND EXPLANATIONS

1. A, D, and E—correct.

   B—incorrect. With salaries now escalating, maybe the poor fellow has something to worry about; the true answer is that continued worry is not healthy.

   C—incorrect. An amalgam restoration is an excellent example of secondary prevention, not tertiary.

2. A, B, and C—correct.

   D—incorrect. It is easier to reduce the extraction rate to zero or near-zero by the combined application of treatment and preventive procedures, than to reduce the incidence of disease by preventive procedures alone.

   E—incorrect. The major income of a dentist is derived from treatment of the plaque diseases and their sequelae.

3. E—correct.

   A—incorrect. Restorations are not a primary preventive-dentistry option; rather they are the mainstay of secondary prevention.

   B—incorrect. Plaque is found in the pits and fissures of the occlusal surfaces.

   C—incorrect. Plaque can be removed by use of toothbrush and floss; it is calculus removal that requires instrumentation.

   D—incorrect. It is not possible to remove oral debris from deep pits and fissures.

4. A and C—correct.

   B—incorrect. Once calculus has formed, professional intervention is required for its removal.

   D—incorrect. It is vice versa—the more often that fluoride is applied topically (dentifrices), the more effective it is.

   E—incorrect. Remember, brushing with a fluoride dentifrice constitutes a topical application.

5. A, B, C, and E—correct.

   D—incorrect. Bacteria require carbohydrates, fats, proteins, minerals, and water to exist; they need the carbohydrates for their energy needs, which, in turn, results in their acid production and cariogenicity.

6. C, D, and E—correct.

   A—incorrect. Just the opposite. The sealants are used to seal off the convoluted pits and fissures of the occlusal surfaces.

   B—incorrect. The only means to promote preventive dentistry to a *total* population is by the use of the schools and the popular media.

## Self-evaluation Questions

1. Health is defined as _____.

2. If primary prevention fails, the two sequential actions necessary to minimize progression of a disease process are _____ and _____.

3. For planning purposes, oral diseases and abnormalities can be grouped into three general categories: (1) _____, (2) _____, and (3) _____.

4. Five strategies used to attain primary prevention in caries control are: (1) _____ (2) _____, (3) _____, (4) _____, and (5) _____.

5. Of the six general methods for caries control, the two that are also valuable in periodontal disease control are (1) _____ and (2) _____.

6. Plaque control in a home environment requires essential items or devices: (1) _____ and (2) _____ and (3) an irrigator.

7. Caries development depends on four interrelated factors: (1) _____, (2) _____, (3) _____ and (4) time.

8. Fluoride is most effective in preventing caries on (smooth)(occlusal) surfaces of the teeth, whereas plastic sealants are most effective in preventing caries on (smooth)(occlusal) surfaces of the teeth.

9. "Biologic repair" of a tooth results from a positive mineral balance at the enamel surface; the process of replacing the ions lost in demineralization is known as _____.

10. Name three American sugar substitutes and one foreign anticariogenic sugar alcohol used for sweetening: _____, _____, _____ and _____.

## REFERENCES

1. U.S. Surgeon General's Report: Part II. (2000). What is the status of oral health in America, 35–39.
2. Evans, C. A., & Kleinman, D. V. (2000). The Surgeon General's report on America's oral health: Opportunities for the dental profession. *JADA*, 31:1721–28.
3. Milgrom P., & Reisine, S. (2000). Oral health in the United States: The post-fluoride generation. *Annu Rev Public Health*, 21:403–36.
4. Watt, R., & Sheiham, A. (1999). Inequalities in oral health: A review of the evidence and recommendations for action. *Br Dent J*, 187:6–12.
5. Locker, D. (2000). Deprivation and oral health. *Community Dent Oral Epidemiology*, 28:161–9.
6. Marcias, E. P., & Morales, L. S. (2001). Crossing the border for health care. *J Health Care Poor Underserved*, 12:77–87.
7. Waldman, H. B., & Permah, S. P. (2001). Community-based dental services for patients with special needs. *NY State Dent J*, 67:39–42.

8. Waldman, H. B., & Perlman, S. P. (2000). Providing general dentistry for people with disabilities; a demographic review. *Gen Dent*, 48:566–9.

9. Cho, I. (2000). Disparity in our nation's health: Improved access to oral health care for children. *NY State Dent J*, 66:34–7

10. Mouradian, W. E., Wehr, E., & Crall, J. J. (2000). Disparities in children's oral health and access to dental care. *JAMA*, 284:2625.

11. Gilcrist, J. A., Brumley, D. E., & Blackford, J. U. (2001). Community status and children's dental health. *JADA*, 132:216–22.

12. Newacheck, P. W., Hughes, D. C., Hung, W. R., Wong, S., & Stoddard, J. J. (2000). The unmet needs of America's children. *Pediatrics*, 105:989–97.

13. Warren, J. J., Cowen, H. J., Watkins, C. M., & Hand, J. S. (2000). Dental caries prevalence and dental care utilization among the very old. *JADA*, 131:1571–9.

14. Stearns, S. C., Slifkin, R. T., & Edin, H. M. (2000). Access to care for rural Medicare beneficiaries. *J Rural Health*, 16:131–42.

15. Hicks, M. J., Flaitz, C. M., Carter, A. B., Cron, S. G., Rossman, S. N., Simon, C. L., Demmler, G. J., & Kline, M. W. (2000). Dental caries in HIV-infected children: a longitudinal study. *Pediatr Dent*, 22:359–64.

16. Gilbert, G. H., Foerster, U., Dolan, T. A., Duncan, R. P., & Ringelburg, M. L. (2000). Twenty-four month coronal caries incidence: The role of dental care and race. *Car Res*. 34:367–79.

17. Report of the Ad Hoc Subcommittee to Coordinate Environmental Health and Related Programs. Review of Fluoride Benefits and Risks. Washington DC: U.S. Department of Health and Human Services, U.S. Public Health Service: 1991.

18. Blair, K. P. (1992). Fluoridation in the 1990s. *J Am Coll Dent*, 59:3.

19. Malvitz, D. M., & Broderick, E. B. (1989). Assessment of a dental disease prevention program after three years. *J Publ Health Dent*, 49:54–57.

20. Nuttal, N. M., Steele, J. G., Pine, C. M., White, D., & Pitts, N. B. (2001). The impact of oral health on people in the UK in 1998. *Brit Dent J*, 190:121–6.

21. Sfikas, P. M. (1998). Informed consent and the law. *JADA*, 129:1471–73.

22. Clarke, A., & Cooper, C. (2001). Psychological rehabilitation after disfiguring injury or disease; investigating the training needs of specialist nurses. *J Adv Nurs*, 1:18–26.

23. Personal communication, Easter Seal Foundation. San Antonio, TX; 1997.

24. Mouradian, W. E. (1995). Who decides? Patients, parents or gatekeeper: Pediatric decisions in the craniofacial setting. *Cleft Palate Craniofac J*, 32:510–14.

25. Haug, R. H., & Foss J. (2000). Maxillofacial injuries in the pediatric patient. *Oral Surg Oral Med Oral Path and Oral Radiol Endod*, 90:126–34.

26. Health Care Financing Administration (HCFA), National Health Expenditures Projections: 1998-2000. Office of the Actuary. http//www.hcfa.gov/stats/NHE-Proj, April 25.

27. Caufield, P. W., & Griffen, A. L. (2000). Dental caries: An infection and transmissible disease. *Pediatr Cln North Am*, 47:1001–19.

28. Ximenez-Frvie, L. A., Hoffagee, A. D., & Socransky, S. S. (2000) Comparison of the microbiota of supra- and subgingival plaque in health and periodontitis. *J Clin Peridonol* 27:648–57.

29. Fowler, E. D., Breault, L. G., & Cuenin, M. F. (2001). Periodontal disease and its associations with systemic disease. *Mil Med* 166:85–89.

30. [No author listed] (2000). Parameter on systemic conditions affected by periodontal disease. *J. Periodontol*, 21:880–3.

31. Tomar, S. L., & Lester, A. (2000). Dental and other health care visits among U.S. adults with diabetes. *Diabetes Care*, 223:1505–10.

32. Scannapeco, F. A., HO, F. W. (2001). Potential association between chronic respiratory disease; analysis of National Health and Nutrition Examination Survey III. *J Periodontol*, 92:183–89.

33. MacFarlane, G. D., Herzberg, M. C. Wolff, L. F., & Hardie, N. A. (1992). Refractory periodon-titis associated with abnormal leucocyte phagocytosis and cigarette smoking. *J. Periodontol*, 63:908–13.

34. Luoma, H. (1992). Chlorhexidine solutions, gels and varnishes in caries prevention. *Proc Finn Dent Soc*, 88:147–53.

35. Twetman, S., & Petersson, L. G. (1999). Interdental caries incidence and progression in rela-tion to mutans streptococci suppression after chlorhexidine-thymol varnish treatment in school children. *Acta Odontol Scand*, 57:144–8.

36. Newbrun, E. (1992). Current regulations and recommendations concerning water fluoridation, fluoride supplements and topical fluoride agents. *J Dent Res*, 67:1255–1265.

37. Letter: FL-139, May 1992. Department of Health and Human Services. U.S. Public Health Service, Centers for Disease Control and Prevention: May 1992.

38. Fabian, V., Obry-Musset, A. M., Meddin, G., & Cohen, P. M. (1996). Caries prevalence and salt fluoridion among 9-year-old school children in Strasbourg, France. *Community Dent Oral Epidemiol*, 24:408–11,

39. Twetman, S., Nederfors, T., & Petersson, L. C. (1998). Fluoride concentrations in whole saliva and separate gland secretions in school children after intake of fluoridated milk. *Car Res*, 32:412–16.

40. Marino, R. (1995). Should we use milk fluoridation? A review. *Bull Pan Am Health Organ*, 29:287–98.

41. Bratthall, D., & Barnes, D. E. (1995). Adding fluoride to sugar—a new avenue to reduce dental caries, or a "dead end"? *Adv Dent Res*, 9:3–5.

42. Rosan, B., & Lamont, R. J. (2000). Dental plaque formation. *Microbes Infect*, 2:1599–605.

43. Gustafsson, B. E., Qensel, C. E., Lanke, L. S., Lunqrist, D., Grahnen, H., Bonow, B. E., & Krasse, B. (1954). The Vipehold dental caries study. *Acta Odont Scand*, 11:232–264.

44. Scheie, A. A., & Fejerskov, O. B. (1998). Xylitol in caries prevention: what is the evidence for clinical efficacy. *Oral Dis*, 4:226–30.

45. Tanzer, J. M. (1995). Xylitol chewing fums and dental caries. *Internat Dent J*, 45:65–86.

46. Honkala, S., Honkala, E., Tynjala, K., & Kanas, L. (1999). The use of xylitol chewing gum among Finnish schoolchildren. *Acta Odontolog Scand*, 57:306–9.

47. Hildebrandt, G. H., & Sparks, B. S. (2000). Maintaining mutans streptococci suppression with xylitol chewing gum. *JADA*, 131:909–16.

48. Isokanges, P., Soderling, E., Pienihekkinen, K., & Alanen, P. (2000). Occurrence of dental decay in children after maternal consumption of xylitol chewing gum, a follow-up from 0 to 5 years of age. *J Dent Res*, 29:1885–9.

49. Anasavice, K. J. (1998). Chlorhexidine, fluoride varnish, and xylitol chewing gum: underuti-lized preventive therapies? *Gen Dent*, 1:34–8, 40.

50. Mertz-Fairhurst, E. J. (1992). Pit and fissure sealants; a global lack of scientific transfer? [Editor-ial in] *J Dent Res*, 71:1543–4.

51. Simonson, R. J. Retention and effectiveness of a single application of white sealant after 10 years (1987). *JADA*, 115:31–6.

52. Mertz-Fairhurst, E. J., Shuster, G. S., & Fairhurst, C. W. (1986). Arresting caries with sealants: results of a clinical study. *JADA*, 112:194–323.

53. Qvist, J., Qvist, V., & Mjor, I. A. (1990). Placement and longevity of amalgam restorations in Denmark. *J Dent Res* [Spec Issue], 69:237 (Abst. 1018).

54. Personal communication, American Dental Association, Chicago, 1997.

55. Personal communication, American Dental Hygienists Association, Chicago 1997.

56. Best, H. A., & Bedi, R. (2001). Is the current access to health care information helping or hin-dering effective decision-making for dentists and patients? Guidelines for dental practice. *Prim Dental Care*, 8:77–80.

57. MacKenzie, F. M., & Peterson, M. (1994). The New Zealand School Dental Service. In Harris, N. O., & Christen, A. G., Eds. *Primary preventive dentistry*, (4th ed.) Norwalk, CT: Appleton & Lange, 601–5.

58. Miller, A. J., & Brunelle, J. (1983). A summary of the NIDR Community Caries Prevention Demonstration Program. *JADA*, 107:265–9.

59. Krasse, B. (1984). Can microbiological knowledge be applied in dental practice for the treatment and prevention of dental caries? *J Can Dent Assoc*, 50:221–23.

60. Backer-Dirks, O. (1961). Longitudinal dental caries study in children 9–15 years of age. *Arch Oral Biol (Supp.)*, 6:94;108–27.

61. Foster, L. Y. (1998). Three years in vivo investigating to determine the progression of approximal primary carious lesions extending into dentine. *Br Dent J*, 185:353–7.

62. Elderton, R. J. (1993). Overtreatment with restorative dentistry: when to intervene. *J Internat Dent*, 43:20–4.

63. Koulourides, T. I. (1977). To what extent is the incipient lesion of dental caries reversible? In Rowe N. H., Ed. Proceedings of Symposium on Incipient Lesions in Enamel. Ann Arbor, MI; University of Michigan School of Dentistry; November 11–12:51–68.

64. Silverstone, L. M. (1984). Significance of remineraliztion in caries prevention. *J Can Dent Assoc*, 50:156–166.

65. Foster, L. V. (1998). Three year in vivo investigation to determine the progression of approximal primary carious lesions extending into dentine. *Br Dent J*, 185:353–57.

# CHAPTER 2

# The Development and Structure of Dental Plaque (A Bacterial Biofilm), Calculus, and Other Tooth-adherent Organic Materials

*Max A. Listgarten*
*Jonathan Korostoff*

## OBJECTIVES

*At the end of this chapter it will be possible to*

1. Differentiate between organic coatings of *endogenous* and *exogenous (acquired)* origin.
2. Explain why dental plaque is not unique among naturally occurring microbial layers.
3. Discuss some of the mechanisms proposed to explain *bacterial adhesion* to the *acquired pellicle*.
4. Distinguish between *primary* and *secondary* bacterial colonizers in dental plaque, and cite examples of each.
5. Identify the prime sites of calculus formation, explain how calculus forms, and detail the differences between *supragingival* and *subgingival* calculus.
6. Explain the basis for the involvement of the acquired pellicle, bacterial dental plaque, and dental calculus in caries and the inflammatory periodontal diseases.

# INTRODUCTION

The dental profession has to deal with two of the most widespread of all human maladies, dental caries (tooth decay), and inflammatory diseases of the periodontium (i.e., the supporting tissues of the teeth), gingivitis, and periodontitis (Figure 2–1). These conditions are known to have a bacterial etiology. Unlike some other infectious diseases, these diseases are not caused by a single pathogenic microorganism. Dental caries and inflammatory periodontal diseases result from the accumulation of many different bacteria that form *dental plaque*,[1,2] a naturally acquired bacterial biofilm that develops on the teeth (Figure 2–2). Some bacterial species in dental plaque may be of greater relevance to caries and periodontal diseases than others. Dental plaque *cannot* be removed by rinsing alone but can be removed by mechanical debridement. The *proportions* of different bacteria in plaque from a healthy mouth are different from those in plaque associated with caries, and both are different from the dental plaque of an individual with inflammatory periodontal disease.[3,4]

If the role of dental plaque in caries and inflammatory periodontal diseases is to be understood,[5,6] the logical place to start is by examining how dental plaque forms and, as will be discussed in later chapters, how changes in the proportions of different plaque bacteria lead to oral disease.

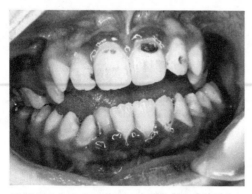

FIGURE 2–1   A 13-year-old female with dental caries on facial surface of the maxillary incisors and swollen, discolored gingival tissues around the mandibular incisors, characteristic of chronic gingivitis. (Courtesy of Dr. WK Grigsby, University of Iowa College of Dentistry.)

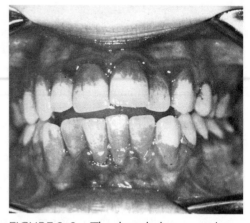

FIGURE 2–2   The dental plaque on these teeth has been stained with a discoloring solution and rinsed. Note the presence of plaque interproximally and adjacent to the gingiva, but relatively absent closer to the incisal edge. (Courtesy of Dr. WK Grigsby, University of Iowa College of Dentistry.)

## Dental Plaque as One of Many Microbial Biofilms

Most natural surfaces have their own coating of microorganisms or biofilm adapted to its individual habitat. The features of dental plaque formation are by no means unique and merely reflect a single instance of a widespread and ancient natural phenomenon. One of the first known examples of life are mineralized bacteria or algae[7,8] found on rocks from the Precambrian era. These are quite similar to dental calculus. The physicochemical and biochemical interactions that underlie bacterial adhesion elsewhere in nature are the same as those observed in plaque formation.[9–11] For example, all living cells, including bacterial cells, have a *net negative surface charge*. The cells can, therefore, be attracted to oppositely charged surfaces on such items as rocks in a stream, skin, or teeth. As with plaque bacteria, organisms in other environments can produce extracellular coatings or slime layers, or a variety of surface fibrils or appendages extending from their cell walls that mediate their attachment to the substrate.[9,12]

In response to environmental conditions and interactions with other members of the microbial community, biofilm bacteria behave differently from planktonic (liquid-phase) cells. This has significant clinical implications. Current research indicates that bacteria growing in biofilms are more resistant to the effects of host defense mechanisms and exogenous antimicrobial agents when compared to the same cells in a liquid suspension.[13,14,15] Thus, it becomes of paramount importance to mechanically disturb the biofilm when utilizing antimicrobial therapy.

## Bacterial Colonization of the Mouth

Microorganisms initially colonize the mouth during birth, being naturally acquired from the *mother*. Thereafter, bacteria are acquired from the atmosphere, food, human contact, and even from animal contacts (e.g., pets). The bacteria subsequently colonize interfaces between saliva and both oral soft (e.g., gingiva, tongue, cheeks, and alimentary tract) and hard tissues (e.g., erupted teeth). Mucosal surfaces of the tongue and tonsils may serve as reservoirs for dental plaque-forming organisms, including those related to disease.[16]

With increasing age and improper toothbrushing, gingival recession may occur and result in the exposure of root cementum and dentin. These surfaces, like enamel, may become colonized by oral bacteria that can trigger dental caries.

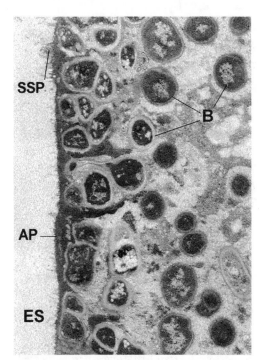

FIGURE 2-3  This transmission electron micrograph demonstrates remnants of the subsurface pellicle (SSP) and the acquired pellicle (AP) between the enamel (ES) surface and the bacterial cells (B) of the dental plaque. (Courtesy of Dr. MA Listgarten, University of Pennsylvania School of Dental Medicine.)

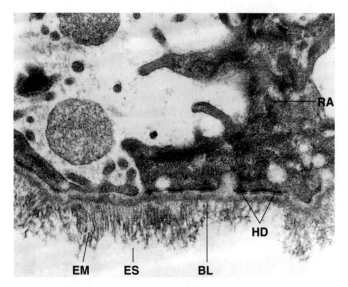

**FIGURE 2–4**   Junction of reduced enamel epithelium and enamel. The reduced ameloblasts (RA) are attached to the enamel by hemidesmosomes (HD) and a basal lamina (BL). EM, enamel matrix remnants form a subsurface pellicle; ES, enamel space. ×45,000. (Courtesy of Dr. MA Listgarten, University of Pennsylvania School of Dental Medicine.)

Prior to eruption, the enamel is lined by remnants of the enamel-forming organ, namely the *reduced enamel epithelium and the basal lamina* that connects it to the enamel surface. The basal lamina is also continuous with organic material that fills the microscopic voids in the superficial enamel. This subsurface material appears as a fringe attached to the basal lamina and is composed of residual enamel matrix proteins (Figures 2–3, 2–4). It is referred to as a *subsurface pellicle*. Because it originates from local cells during tooth formation, it is considered to be of *endogenous* origin. When the tooth emerges into the oral cavity, the remnants of the reduced enamel epithelium are worn off or digested by salivary and bacterial enzymes. The underlying enamel becomes exposed to saliva and the oral microbiota. Salivary components become adsorbed to exposed enamel *within seconds*, forming a microscopic coating over the exposed tooth surface. This thin coating can subsequently become colonized by oral bacteria. Because this coating originates from salivary proteins rather than the dental organ, it is considered to be of *exogenous* origin. Thus, the tooth surface is almost always coated by a variety of structures that are either of endogenous origin (i.e., derived from cells of the dental organ) or of exogenous origin (i.e., acquired following eruption of the teeth into the oral cavity).[17]

## The Acquired Pellicle

The coating of salivary origin that forms on exposed tooth surfaces is called the *acquired pellicle*.[18,19] It is acellular and consists primarily of glycoproteins[a] derived from saliva (Figure 2–3). The pellicle also occupies the millions of microscopic voids in the erupted tooth caused by chemical and mechanical interactions of the tooth surface with the oral environment. Collectively these organic fringe-like projections form a *subsurface pellicle*, which is of *exogenous* or acquired origin. Oral fluids and small molecules can slowly diffuse through the acquired pellicle into the superficial enamel. If the pellicle is displaced, for example by a prophylaxis, it

[a]A glycoprotein is a protein molecule that includes an attached carbohydrate component.

begins to reform immediately.[20,21] It takes about a week for the pellicle to develop its condensed, mature structure which may also incorporate bacterial products.[22–24]

An acquired pellicle also forms on artificial surfaces, including dental restorations and dentures. These organic coatings are similar to the pellicles on natural teeth and may be colonized by bacteria.[25–27] Colonization of the acquired pellicle can be beneficial for the bacteria because the pellicle components can serve as nutrients.[28] For example, proline-rich salivary proteins may be degraded by bacterial collagenases,[29] releasing peptides, free amino acids, and salivary mucins that may enhance the growth of dental plaque organisms, such as actinomycetes and spirochetes.[30]

The carbohydrate components of certain pellicle glycoproteins may serve as receptors for bacterial-binding proteins such as *adhesins*, thereby contributing to bacterial adhesion to the tooth.[31–33] There is competition for the binding sites on the pellicle, not only by receptors on bacteria, but also from *host proteins*, including immunoglobulins (i.e., antibodies), proteins of the complement system, and the enzyme *lysozyme*. These host proteins originate from saliva and gingival sulcus fluid.[34,35] Once a pellicle site is occupied by one of the competing entities, occupancy by another is inhibited.[36] Not only does competition arise for occupancy of binding sites, but an antagonistic relationship often exists between different types of bacteria competing for the binding sites. For example, it has been shown that some streptococci synthesize and release *bacteriocins*, which can inhibit some strains of *Actinomyces*[37] and *Actinobacillus* species.[38]

## Dental Plaque Formation

All bacteria that initiate plaque formation come in contact with the organically coated tooth surface fortuitously. Forces exist that tend to allow bacteria to accumulate on teeth or to remove them. Shifts in these forces determine whether more or less plaque accumulates at a given site on a tooth. Many factors influence the build-up of plaque,[39] ranging from simple factors, such as mechanical displacement, stagnation (i.e., colonization in a sheltered or undisturbed environment), and availability of nutrients, to complex factors, including interactions between the microbes and the host's inflammatory-immune systems. Bacteria tend to be removed from the teeth during mastication of foods, by the tongue, toothbrushing, and other oral-hygiene activities. For this reason, bacteria tend to accumulate on teeth in sheltered, undisturbed environments (sites at risk), such as the occlusal fissures, the surfaces apical to the contact between adjacent teeth, and in the gingival sulcus.

### Question 1

Which of the following statements, if any, are true?

A. The acquired pellicle is a layer of cells on the *external surface* of the clinical crown of the tooth.

B. Salivary glycoproteins are a major source of organic materials *in* the acquired pellicle.

C. Bacteria produce enzymes that may degrade some of the acquired pellicle components such as proteins.

D. It usually takes *several days* before the acquired pellicle is reformed after a prophylaxis.

E. The presence of immunoglobulins in the acquired pellicle guarantees that the acquired pellicle will remain free from bacterial colonization.

Therefore, it is no coincidence that the major plaque-based diseases, caries and inflammatory periodontal diseases, arise at these sites where plaque is most abundant and stagnant. Initial plaque formation may take as long as 2

hours.[40] Binding sites and individual strain affinity for a given surface vary considerably.[41,42] Colonization begins as a series of isolated colonies, often confined to microscopic tooth surface irregularities.[23] With the aid of nutrients from saliva and host food, the colonizing bacteria begin to multiply. About 2 days are then required for the plaque to double in mass, during which time, the bacterial colonies have been coalescing.[43] The most dramatic change in bacterial numbers occurs during the first 4 or 5 days of plaque formation.[44,45] After approximately 21 days, bacterial replication slows so that plaque accumulation becomes relatively stable.[46] The increasing thickness of the plaque limits the diffusion of oxygen to the entrapped original, oxygen-tolerant populations. As a result, the organisms that survive in the deeper aspects of the developing plaque are either *facultative* or *obligate anaerobes*.[b]

The forming bacterial colonies are rapidly covered by saliva.[47] When seen with the scanning electron microscope, growing colonies protrude from the surface of the plaque as *domes*, giving the appearance of a cluster of igloos beneath newly fallen snow (Figure 2–5). In individuals with poor oral hygiene, superficial dental plaque may incorporate food debris and mammalian cells such as desquamated epithelial cells and leukocytes. This debris is called *materia alba* (literally, "white matter"). Unlike plaque, it is usually removed easily by rinsing with water.[18] At times, the plaque demonstrates staining, with the discoloration being caused by sources including tea, heavy metal salts, drugs, and chromogenic bacteria.

## Molecular Mechanisms of Bacterial Adhesion

The initial bacterial attachment to the acquired pellicle (Figure 2–6A) is thought to in-

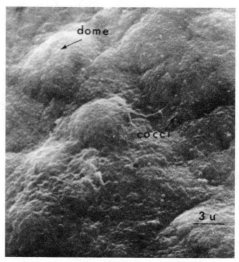

FIGURE 2–5   Scanning electronmicrograph of dome formation in the plaque. (From Brady, J. M. *J Periodontol*, 1973, 44:416–428.)

volve physicochemical interactions (e.g., electrostatic forces and hydrophobic bonding)[48–51] between molecules or portions of molecules, such as the side chains of the amino acids phenylalanine and leucine. It has been suggested that the hydrophobicity of some streptococci, a major plaque group, is caused by cell wall–associated molecules including *glucosyltransferase*, an enzyme that converts the glucose portion of the sugar, sucrose, into extracellular polysaccharide. Some glucosyltransferases have been designated as *hydrophobins*.[52]

Another molecular mechanism of bacterial adhesion is *calcium bridging*[53–55] which links *negatively* charged bacterial cell surfaces to the *negatively* charged acquired pellicle (Figure 2–6B) via interposed positively charged, divalent calcium ions from the saliva. Calcium bridging may only be important in early plaque formation, because recently formed plaque is readily disrupted by exposure to a calcium-complexing (*chelating*) agent, such as ethylenediaminetetraacetic acid (EDTA).[56]

[b] Facultative anaerobes can exist in an environment with or without oxygen; obligate anaerobes cannot exist in an environment with oxygen.

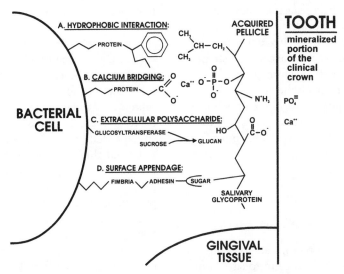

**FIGURE 2-6**    This diagram illustrates some of the possible molecular mechanisms mediating bacterial attachment to teeth during dental plaque formation. **A.** A side chain of a phenylalanine component of a bacterial protein interacts via hydrophobic bonding with a side chain of a leucine component of a salivary glycoprotein in the acquired pellicle. **B.** The negatively charged carboxyl group of a bacterial protein is attracted to a positively charged calcium ion (i.e., electrostatic attraction), which in turn is attracted to a negatively charged phosphate group of a salivary phosphoprotein in the acquired pellicle. **C.** The host's dietary sucrose is converted by the bacterial enzyme, glucosyltransferase, to the extracellular polysaccharide, glucan, which has many hydrophobic groups and can interact with amino acid side-chain groups, such as serine, tyrosine, and threonine. **D.** The fimbrial surface appendage extends from the bacterial cell to permit the terminal adhesin portion to bind to a sugar component of a salivary glycoprotein in the acquired pellicle.

Some of the streptococci in plaque use the enzyme glucosyltransferase to synthesize extracellular polysaccharides (ECP). Among these are "sticky" *glucans* that, through hydrogen bonding, are thought to contribute to the mediation of bacterial adhesion (Figure 2–6C).[57] Once the bacteria adhere, they are often "entombed" as additional glucan is produced.[58]

Bacteria also exhibit external cell surface proteins termed *adhesins*,[33,59] that have lectin-like[c] activity as they can bind to carbohydrate components of glycoproteins.[32,60] These molecules, which some researchers have suggested may be located on bacterial surface appendages, such as fimbriae[61] (Figure 2–6D), are believed to facilitate colonization of the acquired pellicle.[62] Fimbria-associated adhesins probably mediate bacterial adhesion via ionic or hydrogen-bonding interactions. Adhesins and fimbriae may function together to promote bacterial attachment to pellicle-coated surfaces.[63] For example, *pilin*, a structural protein that constitutes the bulk of some fimbriae, is hydrophobic because of its amino-acid content.[64] These fibrillar surface appendages extend from the bac-

[c]Lectins are plant proteins with receptor sites that bind specific sugars.

terial surface and *may reduce* or *mask* the repelling effect of the net negative surface charges. Carbohydrate-binding adhesins have been shown to link actinomycetes to streptococci in early dental-plaque formation.[65,66]

While some or all of the above-described mechanisms may play a role in the attachment of bacteria to one another and to the tooth surface, the nature of the actual linking molecules in plaque, or between plaque and tooth surface coatings is not known.

## Bacteria in the Dental Plaque

Plaque bacteria vary in number and proportions from time to time and from site to site within the mouth of any one individual. The diversity is even greater between individuals,[67] between races,[68] and between supra- and subgingival plaques.[69] The only abundant bacteria found almost universally in the mouths of humans and animals are streptococci and actinomycetes.

The bacteria colonize the teeth in a reasonably *predictable* sequence. The first to adhere are *primary colonizers*, sometimes referred to as pioneer species. These are *microorganisms* that are able to stick directly to the acquired pellicle. Those that arrive later are *secondary colonizers*. They may be able to colonize an existing bacterial layer, but they are unable to act as primary colonizers. Generally speaking, the primary colonizers are not pathogenic. If the plaque is allowed to remain undisturbed, it eventually becomes populated with secondary colonizers that are the likely etiologic agents of caries, gingivitis, and periodontitis, the destructive form of inflammatory periodontal disease.

The earliest colonizers are overwhelmingly *cocci* (i.e., spherical cells),[1,69,70] especially streptococci, which constitute 47 to 85% of the cultivable cells found during the first 4 hours after professional tooth cleaning.[71] These tend to be followed by short rods and filamentous bacteria. Because of stagnation, the most abundant colonization is on the proximal surfaces, in the

fissures of teeth, and in the gingival sulcus region.[72]

Cocci are probably the first to adhere because they are small and round and, therefore, have a smaller energy barrier to overcome than other bacterial forms.[73] The first or primary colonizers tend to be *aerobic* (i.e., oxygen-tolerant) bacteria including *Neisseria and Rothia*. The streptococci, the Gram-positive facultative rods, and the actinomycetes are the main organisms in both early fissure and approximal plaque.[73–75] As plaque oxygen levels fall, the proportions of Gram-negative rods, for example fusobacteria, and Gram-negative cocci such as *Veillonella* tend to increase.

Of the early colonizers, *Streptococcus sanguis* often appears first,[76] followed by *S. mutans*. Both depend on a sheltered environment for growth and the presence of extracellular carbohydrate (e.g., sucrose). Sucrose is used to synthesize *intracellular* polysaccharides that serve as an internal source of energy, as well as external polysaccharide coats.[77,78] The polysaccharide coating helps protect the cell from the *osmotic* effects of sucrose. In addition, it reduces the inhibitory effect of toxic metabolic *end products*, such as lactic acid, on bacterial survival.

Whereas nonmotile cells, including streptococci and actinomycetes, come into contact with the tooth randomly, motile cells such as the spirochetes are likely to be attracted by *chemotactic* factors (e.g., nutrients). Surface receptors probably provide a means of attachment for secondary colonizers *onto the initial bacterial layer*.[79] Bacteria that cannot adhere easily to the tooth initially via organic coatings can probably attach by strong lectin-like, cell-to-cell interactions with *similar* or *dissimilar bacteria* that are already attached (i.e., the primary colonizers).[33,80,81]

Gram-negative, *anaerobic* (e.g., oxygen-intolerant) species predominate in the *subgingival* plaque during the later phases of plaque development,[82] but they may also be present in early plaque, for example, *Treponema, Porphyromonas, Prevotella,* and *Fusobacterium* species.

There is evidence that oxygen does not penetrate more than 0.1 mm into the dental plaque,[83,84] a fact that may explain the presence of anaerobic bacteria in early plaque.

## Dental-Plaque Matrix

A great variety of factors affect the colonization of the teeth by bacteria. Dental plaque consists of different species of bacteria that are not uniformly distributed, since different species colonize the tooth surface at different times and under different circumstances. The newly formed supragingival biofilm frequently exhibits "palisades" (i.e., columnar microcolonies of cells) of firmly attached cocci, rods, or filaments. The organisms are positioned perpendicular to the tooth surface,[1,69,85] the result

of competitive colonization. The bacterial cells in the biofilm are surrounded by an *intercellular plaque matrix* (Figure 2–7).[56] The matrix is composed of both organic and inorganic components that *originate primarily from the bacteria*. Polysaccharides derived from bacterial metabolism of carbohydrates are a major constituent of the matrix while salivary and serum proteins/glycoproteins represent minor components. The bacteria in the subgingival biofilm consist of several motile species that do not form distinctive microcolonies. They tend to be located on the surface of the adherent bacterial layer and are separated by an abundant intercellular matrix. Some bacteria on the surface of the biofilm aggregate into distinctive structures that include arrangements of cocci ("corncob" configurations) and rods ("test-tube brush"

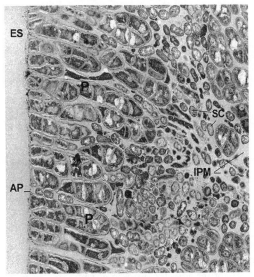

FIGURE 2–7  An electron micrograph showing palisades (P) of bacteria perpendicular to the enamel surface (ES), bacterial cells that are probably secondary colonizers (SC), the intercellular plaque matrix (IPM), and the acquired pellicle (AP). (Courtesy of Dr. MA Listgarten, University of Pennsylvania School of Dental Medicine.)

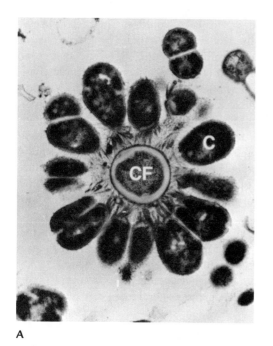

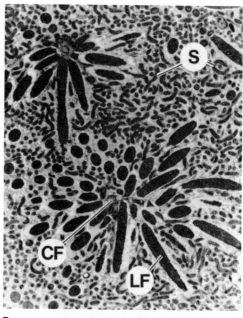

A                                                              B

FIGURE 2-8   **A.** Cross section of "corn cob" from 2-month-old plaque. A coarse fibrillar material attaches the cocci (C) to the central filament (CF). Original magnification × 22,500. (From Listqarten, M. A., Mayo, H. E., Tremblay, R. *J Periodontol,* 1975; 46:10-26.) **B.** Coarse "test-tube brush" formations consisting of central filament (CF) surrounded by large, peritrichously flagellated filamentous bacteria (LF). Background consists of a spirochete-rich microbiota (S). Original magnification × 4,300. (From Listgarten M. A. *J Periodontol.* 1976; 47, 1–18.)

configurations)[1,2,69,86] radially arranged around a central filament (Figure 2–8).

## Dental-Plaque Metabolism

For metabolism to occur, a source of energy is required. For the caries-related *S. mutans* and many other acid-forming organisms, this energy source can be *sucrose.*[87] Almost immediately following exposure of these microorganisms to sucrose, they produce (1) acid, (2) intracellular polysaccharides (ICP), that provide a reserve source of energy for each bacterium, much like glycogen does for human cells,[88] and (3) extracellular polysaccharides including glucans

(dextran)[89] and fructans (levan).[90] Glucans can be viscid substances that help anchor the bacteria to the pellicle, as well as stabilize the plaque mass. Fructans can act as an energy source for any bacteria having the enzyme levanase.[91,92] Quantitatively, the glucans constitute up to approximately 20% of plaque dry weight, levans about 10%, and bacteria the remaining 70 to 80%. As mentioned previously, the glucans and fructans are major contributors to the *intercellular plaque matrix.*[92]

Plaque organisms grow under adverse environmental conditions. These include pH, temperature, ionic strength, oxygen tension, nutrient levels, and antagonistic elements, such as competing organisms and the host inflamma-

tory-immune response. To cope with this hostile environment, the plaque organisms must find a safe haven in relation to their neighbors and the oral environment. Such a favorable location is termed an *ecologic niche*.[5] Normally, once the niches are established, the bacteria of the resident microbiota coexist with the host and the surrounding microcosm. This symbiosis results in a resistance to colonization by subsequent *nonindigenous* organisms. In this manner, the resident microbiota can protect the host against infection by major primary pathogens, e.g., *Corynebacterium diphtheria* and *Streptococcus pyogenes*.

With dietary sugars entering the plaque, *anaerobic glycolysis* results in acid production (*acidogenesis*) and accumulation of acid in the plaque.[5] If no acid-consuming organisms (e.g., *Veillonella*) are available to utilize the acids, the plaque pH drops rapidly from 7.0 to below 4.5. This drop is important because *enamel begins to demineralize between pH 5.0 and 5.5*. One possible outcome of the drop in pH may be the dissolution of the mineralized tooth surface adjacent to the plaque, resulting in carious *cavitation* of the tooth.[77] This process provides the bacteria access to the inorganic elements (e.g., calcium and phosphate) needed for their nutritional requirements. By adhering to the tooth surface via an organic layer of salivary origin, dental plaque bacteria can gain access to a supply of organic nutrients, a widespread phenomenon.[47] The same search for nutrients may explain the extension of bacteria from the supragingival plaque into the gingival sulcus.[93,94] To prevent or reduce subgingival colonization, the host tissues defend against the bacterial challenge with antibacterial strategies, such as the passage of antibodies and the emigration of polymorphonuclear neutrophils from the adjacent connective tissue into the gingival sulcus. The continued metabolic activity of plaque in the subgingival environment initiates the inflammatory response of the gingival tissues (gingivitis)[95] and also may eventu-

ally lead to progressive destruction of the periodontium (periodontitis)[96].

Until supragingival plaque mineralizes as dental calculus, it can be removed by toothbrushing and flossing.[97] As the plaque matures, it becomes more resistant to removal with a toothbrush. In one study, at 24, 48, and 72 hours after formation, 5.5, 7.8, and 14.0 $g/cm^2$ of pressure, respectively, were required to dislodge the plaque—almost three times as much pressure to remove it on the third day as on the first.[98] Once dental calculus is formed, professional instrumentation is *necessary* for its removal.

---

### Question 3

Which of the following statements, if any, are correct?

A. Dental plaques typically exhibit uniform structures, composition, and properties.

B. The intercellular dental plaque matrix is probably formed by a combination of host *materials,* such as salivary proteins, *and* bacterial metabolites.

C. The term "corn-cob" configuration, describes one of several possible aggregates between different kinds of bacterial cells in the dental plaque matrix.

D. The acid dissolution of tooth mineral supplies calcium for both bacterial nutrition and for calcium binding.

E. Gingival inflammation is generally caused by bacteria that reside in dental plaque adjacent to the tooth.

---

### Dental Calculus

A last stage in the maturation of some dental plaques is characterized by the appearance of mineralization in the deeper portions of the plaque to form dental calculus[99]. The term

*calculus* is derived from the Latin word meaning pebble or stone. The lay term, *tartar*, refers to an accumulated sediment or crust on the sides of a wine cask. Some people do not form calculus, others form only moderate amounts, and still others form heavy amounts.

Calculus itself is not harmful. However, a layer of unmineralized, viable, metabolically active bacteria that are closely associated with the external calculus surface is potentially pathogenic. Calculus *cannot* be removed by brushing or flossing. It is often difficult to remove all the calculus, even professionally, without damaging the tooth, especially the softer root cementum. However, calculus needs to be removed because its presence makes routine oral hygiene more difficult or even impossible by forming calculus *spurs* (Figure 2–9). These structures may contribute to plaque accumulation and stagnation. Calculus removal is also a prerequisite to regenerate lost or damaged periodontal tissues following treatment.

In addition to local factors, behavioral and systemic conditions may affect calculus formation. For example, smoking causes an accelerated formation of calculus.[100] Children afflicted with asthma or cystic fibrosis form calculus at approximately twice the rate of other children.[101] Similarly, non-ambulatory, mentally handicapped individuals, tube-fed over long periods, may develop heavy calculus within 30 days, despite the fact that no food passes through the mouth.[102] Conversely, medications such as beta-blockers, diuretics, and anticholinergics can result in significantly reduced levels of calculus. The authors of the latter study concluded that either the medications were excreted directly into the saliva, affecting the rate of crystallization, or altered the composition of the saliva and thus indirectly affected calculus formation.[103]

Calculus formation is related to the fact that saliva is saturated with respect to calcium and phosphate ions.[104] Precipitation of these elements leads to mineralization of dental plaque giving rise to calculus. The crystals in calculus include hydroxyapatite, brushite, and whitlockite, all of which have different proportions of calcium and phosphate in combination with other ions, such as magnesium, zinc, fluoride, and carbonate. *Supragingival calculus* forms on the tooth *coronal* to the gingival margin, and frequently develops opposite the duct orifices of the major salivary glands. It is often found where saliva pools on the lingual surfaces of the mandibular incisors (Figure 2–10), and can form in the fissures of teeth. Subgingival calculus forms from calcium phosphate and organic materials derived from serum, which contribute to mineralization of subgingival plaque.

One of the means by which formation and growth of calculus may be studied is by ligating thin plastic strips around the teeth and then removing the strips at various intervals.[105]

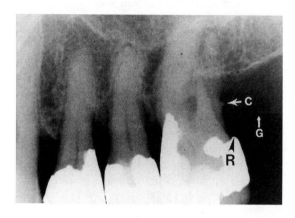

FIGURE 2–9  Radiograph demonstrating a "spur"- shaped deposit of calculus (C) on the distal side of the maxillary left first molar apical to the overhanging metallic restoration (R). The arrow (G) marks the coronal level of the gingival tissues indicating that this is a subgingival deposit of calculus. (Courtesy of Dr. WK Grigsby University of Iowa College of Dentistry.)

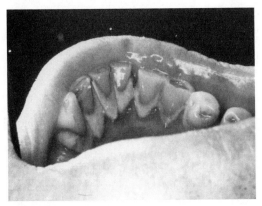

FIGURE 2-10    Deposits of supragingival calculus on the lingual surface of incisors and canines that could not be removed by brushing. (Courtesy of Dr. WK Grigsby, University of Iowa College of Dentistry.)

formation.[107] Calculus formation is not restricted to one bacterial species, or even to those growing at neutral or slightly acidic pHs. This is evidenced by the fact that caries-related streptococci may mineralize.[108] Not all plaques mineralize, but a plaque that is destined to mineralize begins to do so within a few days of its initial formation, even though this early change is not detectable at a clinical level. Mineralization usually begins in the *intercellular plaque matrix* but eventually occurs *within* the bacterial cells (Figure 2–11). Bacterial phospholipids and other cell-wall constituents may act as initiators of mineralization,[109] in which case mineralization may begin *in the cell wall* and subsequently extend to the rest of the cell and into the surrounding matrix (Figure 2–12).

Within 12 hours after placement, x-ray diffraction studies demonstrate mineral elements in the forming plaque. By 3 to 4 days, the concentration of calcium and phosphate is significantly higher in the plaque of those with heavy calculus formation than in the plaque of those with no calculus formation.

Subgingival calculus is about 60% mineralized, whereas supragingival calculus is only about 30% mineralized.[106] Because it is harder, thinner, and more closely adapted to tooth surface imperfections, subgingival calculus can be more difficult to remove than supragingival calculus. The two types of calculus may differ in color. Supragingival calculus, which derives its mineral content from saliva, usually appears as a yellow to white mass with a chalky consistency. Subgingival calculus, which derives its mineral from the inflammatory exudate in the sulcus and periodontal pocket, appears gray to black in color and has a flint-like consistency. The dark coloration may be caused by bacterial degradation of components of the hemorrhagic exudate that accompanies gingival inflammation.

Alkaline conditions in dental plaque may be an important predisposing factor for calculus

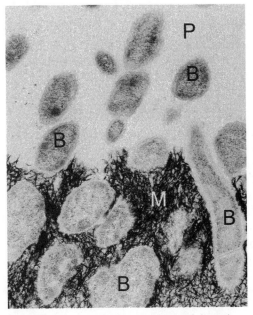

FIGURE 2-11    Typical pattern of dental plaque mineralization in which the initial mineralization occurs in the interbacterial plaque matrix (M), with bacterial cells (B) becoming mineralized secondarily, × 40,000. (Courtesy of Dr. MA Listgarten, University of Pennsylvania School of Dental Medicine.)

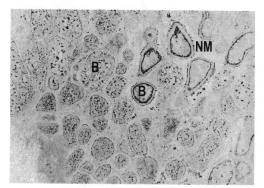

FIGURE 2-12 Atypical pattern of dental plaque mineralization in which bacterial cells (B) act as foci of initial mineralization, with the matrix (NM), becoming mineralized secondarily, ×25,000. (Courtesy of Dr. MA Listgarten, University of Pennsylvania School of Dental Medicine.)

Calculus may also form on the tooth surfaces of germfree animals.[110] This type of calculus consists of an organic matrix of nonmicrobial origin which becomes mineralized.

### Attachment of Calculus to the Teeth

At the tooth interface with calculus, the enamel or root cementum are never perfectly smooth and invariably contain a variety of surface imperfections. These normal irregularities such as the *perikymata*[d] and the point of origin of *Sharpey's fibers*[e] on the cementum appear to aid calculus attachment. Other defects in the enamel and cementum, including areas of demineralization and cemental tears,[111] may also contribute to a stronger calculus attachment to the tooth. Electron micrographs indicate a very

close relationship between the matrix of the tooth surface and the matrix of calculus; the crystalline structures of both are also very similar.[112]

### Inhibiting Calculus Formation

Several agents are currently available to reduce calculus formation, including dentifrices that contain pyrophosphate, or metal ions such as zinc.[113,114] One dentifrice contains two soluble phosphates, *tetrasodium pyrophosphate* and *disodium dihydrogen pyrophosphate*, in addition to fluoride.[114,115] The pyrophosphate ion not only serves as a structural analog of the orthophosphate ion, disrupting the formation of calcium phosphate crystals, but also inhibits some bacterial growth at concentrations significantly lower than the levels found in dentifrices.

---

### Question 4

Which of the following statements, if any, are correct?

A. Intracellular polysaccharides are a source of energy available to bacteria, but levans are available only to the synthesizing bacteria.

B. An operational definition of calculus might be that it is "a mineralized dental plaque that cannot be removed from the tooth by brushing or flossing."

C. The flow of saliva over the tooth surfaces near the major salivary gland ducts keeps those teeth free of calculus deposits.

D. Subgingival calculus is usually more densely mineralized than supragingival calculus.

E. Calculus formation usually begins in the bacterial cell wall and extends to the intercellular matrix.

---

[d]Perikymata are the numerous, small, transverse ridges on the exposed surface of the enamel of the permanent teeth.

[e]The tooth is anchored by connective tissue fibers that extend between the cementum and the bone; the ends embedded in the cementum and bone are known as Sharpey's fibers.

# SUMMARY

Bacteria in dental plaque are the direct cause of the most widespread of all human diseases—dental caries and inflammatory periodontal diseases. These diseases, however, are not classical infections. They arise because of complex changes in plaque ecology and are affected by many factors in the host's protective responses. To understand the role of dental plaque in disease and how to prevent or control the plaque-associated diseases, it is essential to understand the nature of dental plaque. Plaque forms initially on the organic layer coating the erupted tooth. This organic layer originates from salivary products that are deposited on the teeth, forming an acquired pellicle to which bacteria adhere. Adhesion is mediated by a variety of bonding mechanisms, including physicochemical and electrostatic interactions, and stereo-chemical interactions between bacterial adhesins and receptors in the acquired pellicle and bacterial surfaces. The earliest of the primary bacterial colonizers are mainly Gram-positive facultative cocci. They are followed by a variety of Gram-positive and Gram-negative species—the secondary colonizers. Caries-related bacterial species have a greater ability than others to adapt to excess sugars and their metabolites. Supragingival plaque is associated with caries and gingivitis, whereas subgingival plaque is associated with gingivitis and periodontitis. With higher pH (i.e., less acidity), some plaques mineralize to form supra- and subgingival dental calculus. In calculus formation, mineralization of dental plaque generally begins in the extracellular matrix and eventually spreads to include the bacteria. Rarely, mineralization may begin within the walls of bacterial cells and spread to the extracellular matrix. Calculus is generally covered by actively metabolizing bacteria, which can cause caries, gingivitis, and periodontitis. Regular toothbrushing and flossing can remove dental plaque and control its formation. Once dental plaque mineralizes to form calculus, professional instrumentation is necessary for its removal. Notwithstanding the contribution of calculus to inflammatory periodontal diseases, it is stagnation of pathogenic bacteria at critical sites that leads to both dental caries and periodontal diseases. Later chapters deal with the wide range of methods, mechanical and chemical, increasingly used to control plaque and calculus formation. All of these methods have the aim of preventing, arresting, or reversing the progression of dental caries and periodontal tissue inflammation.

# ANSWERS AND EXPLANATIONS

1. B and C—correct.

    A—Incorrect. The acquired pellicle is "acellular," i.e., cell-free.

    D—Incorrect. The acquired pellicle begins to reform immediately and is reestablished within several hours.

    E—Incorrect. Even though some binding sites are occupied by immunoglobulins, many more are occupied by bacteria.

2. A, B, D, and E—correct.

   C—Incorrect. Like charges (i.e., negative to negative or positive to positive) repel; unlike charges attract.

3. B, C, D, and E—correct.

   A—Incorrect. So many factors affect plaque formation that composition, structure, and properties are greatly varied.

4. B and D—correct.

   A—Incorrect. It should be the reverse, with intracellular polysaccharides available to the synthesizing bacteria, and levans to the surrounding bacteria with the enzyme levanase.

   C—Incorrect. The presence of high concentrations of calcium and phosphate ions at the duct openings results in more, not less, calculus formation.

   E—Incorrect. Calculus *usually* begins in the intercellular matrix, and spreads to engulf the cells.

## SELF-EVALUATION QUESTIONS

1. The presence of a preponderance of cocci is a sign of (early)(late) plaque formation.

2. Following prophylaxis, it takes about _____ (hours)(days) for the acquired pellicle to completely reform.

3. Two of the host's *defensive proteins that* compete with bacteria for receptor sites on the acquired pellicle are _____ and _____.

4. It takes approximately _____ (hours) (days) for the initial plaque to form and about _____ days to double in mass. Once formed, the growth is rapid for about _____ days and finally stabilizes in mass around the _____ day.

5. Given the choice of (water)(a toothbrush) or a (prophylaxis); which one is required to remove each of the following: (1) materia alba, (2) plaque, or (3) calculus?

6. Bacteria can attach to the acquired pellicle via _____ bonding, by calcium _____, via attachment to the sticky _____, and by surface proteins called _____.

7. The three places on the teeth where bacterial colonization is most abundant are _____, _____, and _____.

8. "Corn-cob" configurations are caused by (cocci) (rods) radially attached to a central rod, whereas the "_____" configuration is caused by rods radially attached to a central rod.

9. Between the cells of the plaque is the (extracellular polysaccharide)(intracellular polysaccharide) containing _____ and levans that serve as energy sources for the bacteria.

10. The "safe haven" where a bacterial colony can exist in the plaque environment is known as a(n) _____.

11. Calculus is mainly made up of calcified _____.

12. One condition causing accelerated calculus formation is _____. Reduced formation is seen after use of _____ (drugs).

13. *Supragingival* calculus derives its minerals from the _____; whereas *subgingival* calculus derives them from the _____.

## REFERENCES

1. Listgarten, M. A. (1976). Structure of the microbial flora associated with periodontal health and disease in man. A light and electron microscopic study. *J Periodontol*, 47:1–17.
2. Listgarten, M. A. (1999). Formation of dental plaque and other oral biofilms. In Newman, H. N., & Wilson, M., Eds. *Dental plaque revisited—Oral biofilms in health and disease*. BioLine, Cardiff: 187–210.
3. Wolinsky, L. E. (1994). Caries and cariology. In Nisengard, R. J., & Newman, M. G., Eds. *Oral microbiology and immunology* (2nd ed.). Philadelphia: Saunders, 341–59.
4. Nisengard, R. J., Newman, M. G., & Zambon, J. J. (1994). Periodontal disease. In: Nisengard, R. J., Newman, M. G., Ed. (1994). *Oral microbiology and immunology* (2nd ed.). Philadelphia: Saunders, 360–84.
5. Marsh, P. D. (1999). Microbiologic aspects of dental plaque and dental caries. *Dent Clin N Amer*, 43:599–614.
6. Chen, C. (2001). Periodontitis as a biofilm infection (2001). *J Calif Dent Assoc*, 29:362–67.
7. Schopf, J. W. (1974). The development and diversification of Precambrian life. *Orig Life*, 5:119–35.
8. Schopf, J. W. (1975). The age of microscopic life. *Endeavor*, 34:51–58.
9. Costerton, J. W., Cheng, K. J., Geesey, G. G., Ladd, T. I., Nickel, J. C., Dasgupta, M., & Marrie, T. J. (1987). Bacterial biofilms in nature and disease. *Ann Rev Microbiol*, 41:435–64.
10. Costerton, J. W., Lewandowski, Z., Caldwell, D. E., Korber, D. R., & Lappin-Scott, H. M. (1995). Microbial biofilms. *Ann Rev Microbiol*, 49:711–45.
11. Costerton, J. W., Cook, G., & Lamont, R. (1999). The community architecture of biofilms: Dynamic structures and mechanisms. In Newman, H. N., & Wilson, M., Eds. *Dental plaque revisited—Oral biofilms in health and disease*. Cardiff: BioLine, 5–14.
12. Newman, H. N. (1974). Microbial films in nature. *Microbios*, 9:247–57.
13. Gilbert, P., Das, J., & Foley, I. (1997). Biofilm susceptibility to antimicrobials. *Adv Dent Res*, 11:160–67.
14. Bowden, G. H. W., & Hamilton, I. R. (1998). Survival of oral bacteria. *Crit Rev Oral Biol Med*, 9:54–85.
15. Socransky, S. S., & Haffajee, A. D. (2002). Dental biofilms: Difficult therapeutic targets. *Periodontol 2000*, 28:12–55

16. Van der Velden, U., Van Winkelhoff, A. J., & Abbas de Graf, J. (1986). The habitat of peri-odontopathic microorganisms. *J Clin Periodontol*, 13:243–48.

17. Listgarten, M. A. (1976). Structure of surface coatings of teeth. A review. *J Periodontol*, 47:139–47.

18. Ericson, T. (1967). Adsorption to hydroxyapatite of proteins and conjugated proteins from human saliva. *Caries Res*, 1:52–58.

19. Meckel, A. R. (1965). The formation of biological films. *Swed Dent J*, 10:585–99.

20. Leach, S. A., Critchley, P., Kolendo, A. B., & Saxton, C. A. (1967). Salivary glycoproteins as components of the enamel integuments. *Caries Res*, 1:104–11.

21. Mayhall, C. W. (1970). Concerning the composition and source of the acquired enamel pellicle on human teeth. *Arch Oral Biol*, 15:1327–41.

22. Hardie, J. M., & Bowden, G. H. (1976). The microbial flora of dental plaque: Bacterial succession and isolation considerations. In Stiles, H. M., Loesche, W. J., & O'Brien, T. C., Eds. *Proceedings Microbial Aspects of Dental Caries. Microbiol Abstr*, 1 (Spec Suppl):63–87.

23. Lie, T., & Gusberti, F. (1979). Replica study of plaque formation on human tooth surfaces. *Acta Odontol Scand*, 79:65–72.

24. Baier, R. E. (1977). On the formation of biological films. *Swed Dent J*, 1:261–71.

25. Tullberg, A. (1986). An experimental study of the adhesion of bacterial layers to some restorative dental materials. *Scand J Dent Res*, 94:164–73.

26. Kawai, K., Urano. (2001). Adherence of plaque components to different restorative materials. *Operative Dentistry*, 26:396–400.

27. Quirynen, M., De Soete, & van Steenberghe, D. (2002). Infectious risks for oral implants: A review of the literature. *Clin Oral Implant Res*, 13:1–19.

28. Leach, S. A., & Critchley, P. (1966). Bacterial degradation of glycoprotein sugars in human saliva. *Nature*, 209:506.

29. Hay, D. I., & Oppenheim, I. G. (1974). The isolation from human parotid saliva of a further group of proline-rich proteins. *Arch Oral Biol*, 19:627–32.

30. Glenister, D. A., Salamon, K. E., & Smith, K. et al. Enhanced growth of complex communities of dental plaque bacteria in mucin-limited continuous culture. *Microbiol Ecol Hlth Dis*, 1:31–38.

31. Gibbons, R. J., & van Houte, J. (1975). Bacterial adherence in oral microbial ecology. *Ann Rev Microbiol*, 29:19–44.

32. Weerkamp, A. H., van der Mei, H. C., Engelen, D. P., et al. (1984). Adhesion receptors (adhesins) of oral streptococci. In ten Cate, J. M., Leach, S. A., & Arends, J., Eds. *Bacterial adhesion and preventive dentistry*. Oxford: IRL Press, 85–97.

33. Rosan, B. R., & Lamont, R. J. (2000). Dental plaque formation. *Microbes and Infection*, 2:1599–1607.

34. Kraus, F. W., Orstavik, D., Hurst, D. C., & Cook, C. H. (1973). The acquired pellicle: Variability and subject dependence of specific proteins. *J Oral Pathol Med*, 2:165–173.

35. Orstavik, D., & Kraus, F. W. (1973). The acquired pellicle: Immunofluorescent demonstration of specific proteins. *J Oral Pathol Med*, 2:68–76.

36. Williams, R. C., & Gibbons, R. J. (1975). Inhibition of streptococcal attachment to receptors or human buccal epithelial cells by antigenically similar salivary glycoproteins. *Infect Immun*, 11:711–18.

37. Rogers, A. H., van der Hoeven, J. S., & Mikx, F. (1978). Inhibition of *Actinomyces viscosus* by bacteriocin producing strains of *Streptococcus mutans* in the dental plaque of gnotobiotic rats. *Arch Oral Biol*, 23:477–83.

38. Hammond, B. F., Lillard, S. E., & Stevens, R. H. (1987). A bacteriocin of *Actinobacillus actinomycetemcomitans*. *Infect Immun*, 55:686–91.

39. Christersson, L. A., Grossi, S. G., Dunford, R. G., Nachtei, E. E., & Genco, R. J. (1992). Dental plaque and calculus: Risk indicators for their formation. *J Dent Res*, 71:1425–30.

40. Baier, R. E., & Glantz, P-0. (1979). Characterization of oral *in vivo* film formed on different types of solid surfaces. *Acta Odontol Scand*, 36:289–301.

41. Liljemark, W. F., & Schauer, S. V. (1977). Competitive binding among oral streptococci to hydroxyapatite. *J Dent Res*, 56:156–65.

42. Kuramitsu, H., & Ingersoll, L. (1977). Molecular basis for the different sucrose-dependent adherence properties of *Streptococcus mutans and Streptococcus sanguis*. *Infect Immun*, 17:330–37.

43. Tanzer, J. M., & Johnson, M. C. (1976). Gradients for growth within intact *Streptococcus mutans* plaque *in vitro* demonstrated by autoradiography. *Arch Oral Biol*, 21:555–59.

44. Bjorn, H., & Carlsson, J. (1964). Observations on a dental plaque morphogenesis. *Odontol Rev*, 15:23–28.

45. Furuichi, Y., Lindhe, J., Ramberg, P., & Volpe, A. R. (1992). Patterns of de novo plaque formation in the human dentition. *J Clin Periodontol*, 19:423–33.

46. Howell, A. Jr., Risso, A., & Paul, F. (1965). Cultivable bacteria in developing and mature human dental calculus. *Arch Oral Biol*, 10:307–313.

47. Rudney, J. D. (2000). Saliva and dental plaque. *Adv Dent Res*, 14:29–39.

48. Newman, H. N. (1974). Diet, attrition, plaque and dental disease. *Br Dent J*, 136:491–97.

49. Leach, S. A. (1979). On the nature of interactions associated with aggregation phenomena in the mouth. *J Dent*, 7:149–60.

50. Rosenberg, M., Judes, H., & Weiss, E. (1983). Cell surface hydrophobicity of dental plaque microorganisms. *Infect Immun*, 42:831–34.

51. Busscher, H. J., & van der Mei, H. C. (1997). Physico-chemical interactions in initial microbial adhesion and relevance for biofilm formation. *Adv Dent Res*, 11:24–32.

52. Doyle, R. J., Rosenberg, M., & Drake, D. (1990). Hydrophobicity of oral bacteria. In Doyle, R. J., Rosenberg, M., Eds. *Microbial Cell Surface Hydrophobicity*. Washington, DC: American Society for Microbiology, 387–419.

53. Edgar, W. M. (1979). Studies of the role of calcium in plaque formation and cohesion. *J Dent*, 7:174–79.

54. Matsukubo, T., Katow, T., & Takazoe. (1978). Significance of Ca-binding activity of early plaque bacteria. *Bull Tokyo Dent Coll*, 19:53–57.

55. Rose, R. K., Dibdin, G. H., & Shellis, R. P. (1993). A quantitative study of calcium binding and aggregation in selected oral bacteria. *J Dent Res*, 72:78–84.

56. Newman, M. N., & Britton, A. B. (1974). Dental plaque ultrastructure as revealed by freeze-etching. *J Periodontol*, 45:478–88.

57. Germaine, G. R., Harlander, S. K., Leung, W-L.S., & Schachtele, C. F. (1977). *Streptococcus mutans* dextran-sucrase: Functioning of primer dextran and endogenous dextransucrase in water-soluble and water-insoluble glucan synthesis. *Infect Immun*, 16:637–48.

58. Gibbons, R. J., & van Houte, J. (1980). Bacterial adherence and the formation of dental plaque. Receptors and recognition. In Beachey, E. H., Ed. *Bacterial adherence*. London. Chapman and Hall, Ltd., 6:63–104.

59. Ofek, I., & Perry, A. (1985). Molecular basis of bacterial adherence to tissues. In Mergenhagen, S. E., & Rosan, B., Eds. *Molecular basis of oral microbial adhesion*. Washington, DC: American Society for Microbiology, 7–13.

60. Gibbons, R. J. (1984). Adherent interactions which may affect microbial ecology in the mouth. *J Dent Res*, 63:378–85.

61. Clark, W. B., Wheeler, T. T., Lane, M. D., & Cisar, J. O. (1986). Actinomyces adsorption mediated by type-I fimbriae. *J Dent Res*, 65:1166–68.

62. Kolenbrander, P. E., & London, J. (1992). Ecological significance of coaggregation among oral bacteria. *Adv Microb Ecol*, 12:183–217.

63. Handley, P. S., McNab, R., & Jenkinson, H. F. (1999). Adhesive surface structures on oral bacteria. In Newman, H. N., & Wilson, M., Eds. *Dental plaque revisited—oral biofilms in health and disease*. Cardiff: BioLine, 145–70.

64. Irwin, R. T. (1990). Hydrophobicity of proteins and bacterial fimbriae. In Doyle, R. J., & Rosenberg, M., Eds. *Microbial cell surface hydrophobicity*. Washington, DC: American Society of Microbiology, 137–77.

65. Cisar, J. O., Brennan, M. J., & Sandberg, A. L. (1985). Lectin-specific interaction of *Actinomyces* fimbriae with oral streptococci. In Mergenhagen, S. E., & Rosan, B., Eds. *Molecular basis of oral microbial adhesion*. Washington, DC: American Society for Microbiology, 159–63.

66. Kolenbrander, P. E., & Andersen, R. N. (1985). Use of co-aggregation-defective mutants to study the relationship of cell-to-cell interactions and oral microbial ecology. In Mergenhagen, S. E., & Rosan, B., Eds. *Molecular basis of oral microbial adhesion*. Washington, DC: American Society for Microbiology, 164–66.

67. Rosenberg, E. S., Evian, C. I., & Listgarten, M. A. (1981). The composition of the subgingival microbiota after periodontal therapy. *J Periodontol*, 52:435–41.

68. Cao, C. F., Aeppli, D. M., Liljemark, W. F., Bloomquist, C. G., Brandt, C. L., & Wolff, L. F. (1990). Comparison of plaque microflora between Chinese and Caucasian population groups. *J Clin Periodontol*, 17:115–18.

69. Listgarten, M. A., Mayo, H. E., & Tremblay, R. (1975). Development of dental plaque on epoxy resin crowns in man. A light and electron microscopic study. *J Periodontol*, 46:10–26.

70. Lie, T. (1978). Ultrastructural study of early plaque formation. *J Periodont Res*, 13:391–409.

71. Kolenbrander, P. E., & London, J. (1993). Adhere today, here tomorrow: Oral bacterial adherence. *J Bacteriol*, 175:3247–52.

72. Theilade, J., Fejerskov, O., Hørsted, M. (1976). A transmission electron microscopic study of 7-day-old bacterial plaque in human tooth fissures. *Arch Oral Biol*, 21:587–98.

73. Newman, H. N. (1980). Retention of bacteria on oral surfaces. In Bitton, G., & Marshall, K. C., Eds. *Adsorption of Microorganisms to Surfaces*. New York: Wiley-Intersciences, 207–51.

74. Hardie, J. M., & Bowden, G. H. (1974). The normal microbial flora of the mouth. In Skinner, F. A., & Carr, J. G., Eds. *The normal microbial flora of man*. London: Academic Press, 47–83.

75. Socransky, S. S. (1977). Microbiology of periodontal disease—present status and future considerations. *J Periodontol*, 48:497–504.

76. van Houte, J., Gibbons, R. J., & Banghart, S. B. (1970). Adherence as a determinant of the presence of *Streptococcus salivarius* and *Streptococcus sanguis* on the human tooth surface. *Arch Oral Biol*, 15:1025–34.

77. Donoghue, H. D., & Newman, H. N. (1976). Effect of glucose and sucrose on survival in batch culture of *Streptococcus mutans* C67-1 and a non-cariogenic mutant, C67-25. *Infect Immun*, 13:16–21.

78. Kilian, M., & Rölla, G. (1976). Initial colonization of teeth in monkeys as related to diet. *Infect Immun*, 14:1022–27.

79. Weerkamp, A. H. (1985). Coaggregation of *Streptococcus salivarius* with Gram-negative oral bacteria: Mechanism and ecological significance. In Mergenhagen, S. E., & Rosan, B., Eds. *Molecular basis of oral microbial adhesion*. Washington, DC: American Society for Microbiology, 177–83.

80. Ciardi, J. E., McCray, G. F. A., Kolenbrander, P. E., & Lau, A. (1987). Cell-to-cell interaction of *Streptococcus sanguis* and *Propionibacterium acnes* on saliva-coated hydroxyapatite. *Infect Immun*, 55:1441–46.

81. Lamont, R. J., & Rosan, B. (1990). Adherence of mutans streptococci to other oral bacteria. *Infect Immun*, 58:1738–43.

82. Shah, H. N., & Gharbia, S. E. (1991). Microbial factors in the aetiology of chronic inflammatory periodontal disease. In Newman, H. N., & Williams, D. N., Eds. *Inflammation and immunology in chronic inflammatory periodontal disease*. Northwood, England: Science Reviews Limited, 1–32.

83. Van der Hoeven, J. S., de Jong, M. H., & Kolenbrander, P. D. (1985). *In vivo* studies of microbial adherence in dental plaque. In Mergenhagen, S. E., & Rosan, B., Eds. *Molecular basis of oral microbial adhesion*. Washington, DC: American Society for Microbiology, 220–27.

84. Globerman, D. Y., & Kleinberg, I. (1979). Intra-oral $pO_2$ and its relation to bacterial accumulation on the oral tissues. In Kleinberg, I., Ellison, S. A., Mandel, I. D., Eds. *Proceedings: Saliva and dental caries* (A special supplement for *Microbiol Abst*). New York: Information Retrieval, 275–92.

85. Newman, H. N. (1973). The organic films on enamel surfaces. 2. The dental plaque. *Br Dent J*, 135:106–11.

86. Kolenbrander, P. E. (1991). Coaggregation: Adherence in the human oral microbial ecosystem. In Dworkin, M., Ed. *Microbial cell-cell interactions*. Washington, DC: American Society for Microbiology, 316.

87. Simmonds, R. S., Tompkins, G. R., & Goerge, R. J. (2000). Dental caries and the microbial ecology of dental plaque: a review of recent advances. *New Zealand Dent J*, 96:44–49

88. Mattingly, S. J., Daneo-Moor, L., & Shockman, G. D. (1977). Factors regulating cell wall thickening and intracellular iodophilic polysaccharide storage in *Streptococcus mutans*. *Infect Immun*, 16:967–73.

89. Critchley, P., Wood, J. M., Saxton, C. A., & Leach, S. A. (1967). The polymerization of dietary sugars by dental plaque. *Caries Res*, 112–29.

90. McDougall, W. F. (1964). Studies on the dental plaque. IV. Levans and the dental plaque. *Aust Dent J*, 9:1–5.

91. Da Costa, T., & Gibbons, R. J. Hydrolysis of levan by human plaque streptococci. *Arch Oral Biol*, 13:609–17.

92. Manly, R. S., & Richardson, D. T. (1968). Metabolism of levan by oral samples. *J Dent Res*, 47:1080–86.

93. Newman, H. N. (1972). Structure of approximal human dental plaque as observed by scanning electron microscopy. *Arch Oral Biol*, 17:1445–53.

94. Soames, J. V., & Davies, R. M. (1975). The structure of subgingival plaque in a beagle dog. *J Periodont Res*, 9:333–41.

95. Löe, H., Theilade, E., & Jensen, S. B. (1965). Experimental gingivitis in man. *J Periodontol*, 36:177–87.

96. Kinane, D. F. (2001). Causation and pathogenesis of periodontal disease. *Periodontol 2000*, 25:8–20.

97. Petersilka, G. J., Ehmke, B., & Flemmig, T. F. (2002). Antimicrobial effects of mechanical Debridement. *Periodontol 2000*, 28:56–71.

98. Mehrotra, K. K., Kapoor, K. K., Pradhan, B. P., & Bhushan, A. (1983). Assessment of plaque tenacity on enamel surface. *J Periodont Res*, 18:386–92.

99. White, D. J. (1997). Dental calculus: Recent insights into occurrence, formation, prevention, removal and oral health effects of supragingival and subgingival deposits. *Eur J Oral Sci*, 105:508–22.

100. Feldman, R. S., Bravacos, J. S., & Rose, C. L. (1983). Association between smoking different tobacco products and periodontal disease indexes. *J Periodontol*, 54:481–88.

101. Wotman, S., Mercadante, J., Mandel, I. D., Goldman, R. S., & Denning, C. (1973). The occurrence of calculus in normal children, children with cystic fibrosis, and children with asthma. *J Periodontol*, 44:278–80.

102. Klein, F. K., & Dicks, J. L. (1984). Evaluation of accumulation of calculus in tube-fed mentally handicapped patients. *J Am Dent Assoc*, 108:352–54.

103. Turesky, S., Breur, M., & Coffman, G. (1992). The effect of certain systemic medications on oral calculus formation. *J Periodontol*, 63:871–75.

104. Ten Cate, J. M. (1988). *Recent advances in the study of dental calculus*. Oxford: IRL Press, 143–259.

105. McDougall, W. A. (1985). Analytical transmission electron microscopy of the distribution of elements in human supragingival dental calculus. *Arch Oral Biol*, 30:603–608.

106. Galil, K. A., & Gwinnett, A. J. (1975). Human tooth-fissure contents and their progressive mineralization. *Arch Oral Biol*, 2:559–62.

107. Turesky, S., Renstrup, G., & Glickman, I. (1961). Histologic and histochemical observations regarding early calculus formation in children and adults. *J Periodontol*, 32:7–14, 69–100.

108. Sundberg, M., & Friskopp, J. (1985). Crystallograph of supragingival human dental calculus. *Scand J Dent Res*, 93:30–38.

109. Schroeder, H. E. (1969). *Formation and inhibition of dental calculus*. Bern, Switzerland: Hans Huber Publishers, 559–62.

110. Listgarten, M. A., & Heneghan, J. B. (1973). Observations on the periodontium and acquired pellicle of adult gernfree dogs. *J Periodontol*, 44:85–91.

111. Moskow, B. S. (1969). Calculus attachment in cemental separations. *J Periodontol*, 4:1125–130.

112. Selvig, K. A. (1970). Attachment of plaque and calculus to tooth surfaces. *J Periodontol Res*, 5:8–18.

113. Zacherl, W. A., Pfeiffer, H. J., & Swancar, J. R. (1985). The effect of soluble pyrophosphates on dental calculus in adults. *J Am Dent Assoc*, 110:737–38.

114. Ciancio, S. G. (1995). Chemical agents: Plaque control, calculus reduction and treatment of dentinal hypersensitivity. *Periodontol 2000*, 8:75–86.

115. Drake, D. R., Chung, J., Grigsby, W., & Wu-Yuan, C. (1992). Synergistic effect of pyrophosphate and sodium dodecyl sulfate on periodontal pathogens. *J Periodontol*, 63:696–700.

# The Developing Carious Lesion

*Norman O. Harris*
*Adriana Segura*

## OBJECTIVES

*At the end of this chapter, it will be possible to*

1. Name the four general types of carious lesions that are found on the different surfaces of the teeth.
2. Describe the histologic characteristics of enamel and dentin that facilitate fluid flow throughout a tooth.
3. Describe the four zones of an incipient caries lesion.
4. Describe the conduits (pores) that directly conduct acid from the bacterial plaque to the body of the lesion.
5. Name the two bacteria most often implicated in the caries process, and indicate when each is present in the greatest numbers during the caries process.
6. Describe the series of events in a cariogenic plaque and subsurface lesion from the time of bacterial exposure to sugar until the pH returns to a resting state.
7. Discuss the characteristics of root caries and explain the differences and similarities to coronal caries.
8. List measures to prevent and to remineralize root and coronal caries.
9. Explain why so much time is taken by the profession in treating secondary caries.
10. Explain the relationship between pH and calcium and phosphorus saturation in caries development.
11. Discuss the protective relationship of calcium fluoride to hydroxyapatite and fluorhydroxyapatite during an acidogenic attack.

## Understanding Caries: Concepts

Every day there is a *normal, but minute, demineralization* of the hard tooth structures caused by bacterial acid production, as well as consuming acid foods such as fruit juices, vinegar, and soft drinks—even from the abrasion of toothbrushing.[1,2] So long as the demineralization is limited, the body's *remineralization* capabilities can replace the lost minerals from elements such as calcium, phosphate, fluoride and other elements that are found in the saliva. The *physiologic demineralization* does not become pathologic until the demineralization outstrips the remineralization over an indefinite period of time that leads to the onset of *cavitation*. A favorable balance between de- and remineralization is necessary to maintain the homeostasis needed for a lifetime of intact tooth retention.

When a cavity occurs, it can be defined as a localized, post-eruptive pathological process involving bacterial acid demineralization of hard tooth tissue, which if continued without a compensatory remineralization, results in the formation of a cavity.

The history of dental caries is as long as history itself. Probably one of the oldest and most whimsical theories of caries and toothache was that of the *tooth worm* which allegedly lived in the center of the tooth.[3] Many early barber-surgeons reported sighting the "worm," but none seemed to be able to capture the creature, nor could explain how it got into the tooth in the first place. In the late 1700s the worm theory was largely replaced by the *vital theory*, a theory that postulated that inflammation arising from *within* a defective tooth eventually caused a surface lesion. Robertson in 1835-England, and probably one of the first preventive-oriented dentists believed and published, that food impaction and fermentation might be the cause.[4] By the end of the 19th century, others in Europe began to indict bacteria as the culprit.

In 1890 W. D. Miller, an American dentist teaching in Germany, published his *chemicoparasitic theory* of caries which (with many modifications) is still accepted in concept today.[5] As a result of his experimentation, Miller believed that the extraction of the "lime salts" from the teeth was a result of bacterial acidogenesis and was the first step in dental decay. Miller's work however, failed to identify dental plaque as the source of the bacteria and the bacterial acids. The chemicoparasitic theory became more cogent when taken in conjunction with the finding of other contemporary dental researchers, including G. V. Black (the "Grand Old Man of Dentistry") who described the "gelatinous microbic plaque" as the source of the acids.[6]

Caries lesions occur in four general areas of the tooth: (1) *pit and fissure* caries, which are found mainly on the occlusal surfaces of posterior teeth as well as in lingual pits of the maxillary incisors and buccal surfaces of lower molars; (2) *smooth-surface* caries, that arise on intact smooth enamel surfaces other than at the location of the pits and fissures; (3) *root-surface* caries, which might involve any surface of the root; and (4) *secondary* or *recurrent* caries that occur on the tooth surface adjacent to an existing restoration. Smooth-surface caries can be further divided into caries affecting

the *buccal* and *lingual* tooth surfaces, and *approximal* caries, affecting the contact area of adjoining tooth surfaces (i.e., mesial or distal surfaces).

Dental caries is a *multifactorial* disease process, often represented by the three interlocking circles and an arrow depicting the passage of *time* (Chapter 1, Figure 1–4). For caries to develop, three conditions must occur simultaneously: (1) there must be a susceptible tooth and host; (2) cariogenic microorganisms must be present in quantity; and (3) there must be excessive consumption of refined carbohydrates. When exposed to a suitable substrate (usually *sugar or sugar-laden snacks or desserts*), cariogenic bacteria present in the plaque produce acid. If this occurs over a sufficiently long period of *time*, a caries lesion develops. Each of these main factors includes a number of secondary factors and can be introduced to either protect or further damage the tooth. For example, fluoride incorporated into dental enamel increases tooth resistance (see Chapter 8 and 9). Conversely, a reduction in the saliva flow (*xerostomia*) greatly increases the caries risk.

## Embryology and Histology of Enamel

Before discussing the carious process further, it is *necessary* to briefly review the embryology and histology of enamel. Without this review it is very difficult to understand how de- and remineralization can occur in such a highly mineralized tissue as enamel.

The enamel is made up of billions of crystals that in turn make up millions of individual rods. The enamel rods, when viewed in cross section with an electron microscope, appear *not* as rods, but as *keyhole-shaped structures*, approximately 6 to 8 microns in diameter, with the enlarged portion of the keyhole called the *head* and the narrow portion the *tail*. With this configuration, each head fits between two tails. The tail is *always* positioned toward the *apex*. In the head of the rod the long axes of the *crystals*, called the *C axis*, are parallel to the enamel rod. However, as the periphery of the rod is approached, the crystals assume an angle to the more central crystals; in fact, in the tail this angle may be around 30°. (Figure 3–1).

Each rod that extends from the dentoenamel junction (DEJ) to the tooth surface is completed start-to-finish by *one* ameloblast. The final enamel is approximately 95% inorganic, and 5% organic material and water. This 5% porosity forms a network of channels for fluid diffusion of ions and small molecules that are dispersed throughout the entire *enamel cap*.[a] The space available for this diffusion is found between the rods and even between the crystals. To further extend this intra enamel network throughout the enamel, there are morphologic structures in the enamel with a high protein content, such as the striae of Retzius, enamel lamellae, enamel tufts, pores, and enamel spindles. These several diffusion channels probably serve two very important purposes in preserving the teeth: (1) their teleological purpose was possibly to *permit physiological remineralization* throughout life, and (2) the voids and protein content in the enamel probably *cushion intense biting pressures* to help prevent fractures. Unfortunately, these same channels of diffusion also serve another purpose, viz., the conducting of plaque acids into the enamel interior to *cause demineralization*.

---

[a] If an intact tooth was stripped of its pulp chamber, dentin and cementum, the only remaining structure is the enamel cap.

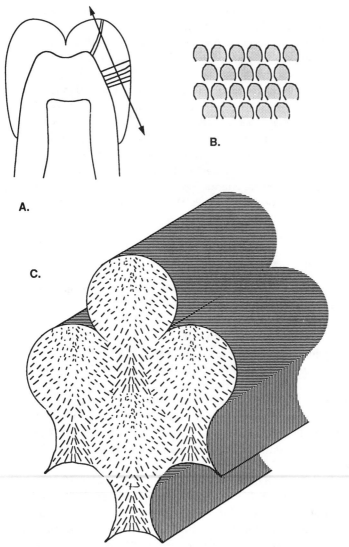

FIGURE 3–1    Enamel structure. **A.** The orientation of the enamel rods from the dentoenamel junction to the tooth surface. **B.** An arcade of rods seen at the section indicated by the line in A.
**C.** The keyhole morphology of the rods. Shading differences represent different orientations of the crystals. (Courtesy of MWJ Dodds, University of Texas Dental School, San Antonio.)

This brief summary also points out the *exquisite genetic control* exercised over the rapidly changing and complex tissue building that marks the development of enamel. The following review begins at the time when odontoblasts and ameloblasts are lined up opposite each other along the *future* dentino-enamel junction.

The initial event of the *secretory* stage occurs with an odontoblastic deposition of the first few microns of *predentin*. This is followed by the initiation of the secretory phase of the ameloblast. The first secreted enamel proteins do *not* accumulate as a layer, but instead, penetrates *into* the developing predentin and subjacent odontoblasts.[7] The microenvironment of the ameloblast at this time, is mainly one of proteins

and water.[8] As the ameloblast retreats towards the future surface of the tooth, it uses these proteins to form an acellular and avascular matrix template upon which the future hydroxyapatite crystals are to be positioned.[9,10] This requires a very rigid *genetic control* over the sequence of events that will extend through matrix formation, crystal nucleation, and crystal growth; as well as rod formation (elongation, widening, and maturation).

The matrix is highly heterogenous because of the involvement of protein contributions from many different genes—amelogens, enamelin, ameloblastin, tuftelin, and various enzymes.[b] Possible functions of these proteins are nucleation (tuftelin), mineral ion binding, (amelogenin, enamelin), and crystal growth (amelogenin, enameling, ameloblastin).[11] If there is a failure of initiation or integration of action of any of these proteins, a dysplastic tissue can result, for example, amelogenesis imperfecta that is caused by a defect in the amelogen gene.[12] It should be emphasized that the ameloblast does *not* complete the matrix template from the dentino-enamel junction to the exterior of the tooth before enamel formation begins. Instead, while the ameloblast is *matrix-building* on the lateral sides, at the same time the Tomes process at the *basal end* of the cell is modulating the enamel-building from the time of initial secretion to the pre-eruption maturation stages.[13] This is a continuous process as the ameloblast moves outward. In an early *supersaturated* environment of high calcium and phosphorus initiated by the ameloblast, *octacalcium phosphate* is laid down as a *precursor* to the *hydroxyapatite* crystal.[14] The early hydroxyapatite crystals are small and of poor crystalinity. As the ameloblast moves outward, the rod increases in length and thickness. Towards the end of the secretory stage, the matrix is *almost* completely *degraded*. Accompanying this event, there is a massive crystal growth.[15] The maturing enamel growth is now approaching the pre-eruptive state. The hydroxyapatite crystals are unusually large, uniform in size, and regularity positioned.[11] The enamel that was originally a soft product is now the hardest and most durable produced in the human body.

There are still a few more points about the life span of the amazing ameloblast. As the tooth approaches eruption, the columnar configuration of the ameloblasts flattens to form the *reduced enamel epithelium* that covers (and protects) the yet immature enamel. After eruption, the reduced enamel epithelium disappears and is succeeded by the *acquired (also called salivary) pellicle* that, in turn, is covered by the *dental plaque* (Chapter 2). Even at this time, the crystals of the rod are not yet fully mineralized. For the first year after eruption into the mouth, the rods undergo a post-eruptive maturation, with the additional tooth minerals being derived from the saliva. This temporary hypomineralization of the enamel with its greater porosity, in part explains why newly erupted teeth are more susceptible to caries than teeth that have been present in the mouth for some time.[16]

---

[b]At this point in time, it is not necessary to memorize the names and functions of genes. Just remember that the tooth morphology depends on genetic guidance.

## Physical and Microscopic Features of Incipient Caries

The development of a carious lesion occurs in three distinct stages. The earliest stage is the *incipient* lesion, which is accompanied by histologic changes of the enamel; the second stage includes the progress of the demineralization front toward the dentino-enamel junction and/or into the dentin; while the final phase of caries development is the development of the *overt*, or *frank*, lesion, which is characterized by actual *cavitation*. If the time between the onset of the incipient lesion in one or more teeth, and the development of cavitation is rapid and extensive, the condition is referred to as *rampant* dental caries. Usually rampant caries occurs following either the excessive and frequent intake of sucrose, or the presence of a severe *xerostomia* (i.e., dry mouth) or both. From a preventive dentistry standpoint, the early identification of the incipient lesion is extremely important, because it is during this stage that the carious process *can be arrested or reversed*. The overt lesion can *only* be treated by operative intervention.

Clinically, it is often difficult to recognize and diagnose the early lesion, and for this reason it is important to be familiar with its features from etiologic and histologic standpoints.[17] The incipient lesion is macroscopically evidenced on the tooth surface by the appearance of an area of *opacity*—the *white spot* lesion. At this earliest clinically visible stage, the subsurface demineralization at the microscopic level is well established with a number of recognizable zones. Probably a most important fact is that the surface of the enamel appears relatively intact (although the electron microscope shows a surface that is more porous than sound enamel). On the buccal and lingual surface of a tooth, the white spot may be localized, or it can extend along the entire gingival area of the tooth, or multiple teeth where food tends to lodge. *Interproximally*, the incipient le-

sion is usually first detected on a *bite wing x-ray*. It usually starts as a small lucency immediately *gingival* to the *contact point* and then gradually expands to a small kidney shape, with the indentation of the kidney contour directed coronally.[18] In fissure caries, the initial lesion comparable to the "white spot," usually occurs *bilaterally* on the two surfaces *at the orifice* of the fissure and eventually coalesces at the base[19] (Figure 3–2). Occasionally lesion formation begins along the wall of the fissure or at the base, either unilaterally or bilaterally.[20]

During the early stages the incipient lesion is not a surface lesion in which loss of outer enamel can be detected. Instead, the mature surface layer of 10 to 100 microns remains intact. If an explorer is used, the surface enamel

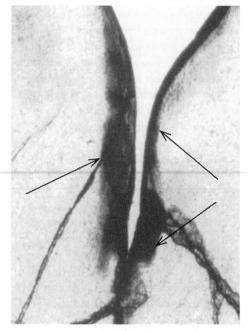

FIGURE 3–2    Incipient caries in an occlusal fissure. The bilaterality of the lesion is evident in the microradiograph. (Courtesy of JS Wefel, University of Iowa College of Dentistry.)

feels hard and provides no indication of demineralization. However, microscopic pores extend through the mature surface layer to the point where subsurface demineralization occurs; the main body of the lesion is located and enlarges from this point.

The incipient lesion has been extensively studied and best described by Silverstone.[18] Many of the observations of the incipient lesion have been based on the use of a polarizing microscope, which permits precise measurements of the amount of space—called *pore space*—that exists in normal enamel and to a greater extent in enamel defects. Thus as demineralization progresses, *more* pore space occurs; conversely, as remineralization occurs, *less* pore space is present.

In the incipient lesion as described by Silverstone, four zones are *usually* present. Starting *from the tooth surface*, the four zones are the (1) *surface* zone, (2) *body of the lesion*, (3) *dark zone*, and (4) the *translucent* zone. (Figure 3–3)

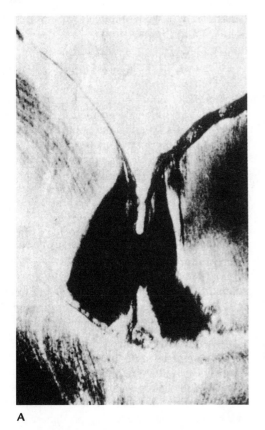
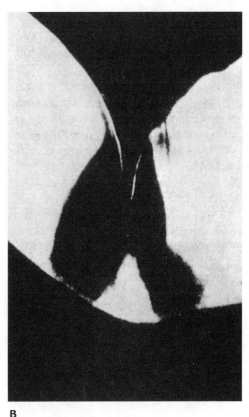

**A**    **B**

FIGURE 3–3    **A** and **B.** The bilaterality of caries development. Note coalescence of two lateral carious areas at base of fissure. (From Konig, K.G. Dental morphology in relation to caries resistance with special reference to fissures as susceptible areas. *J Dent Res.* 1963. 42:461–476.)

## Pore Spaces of the Different Zones

The translucent zone, the *deepest* zone is seen in approximately 50% of the carious lesions examined.[18] In this zone, which is the *advancing front* of the lesion, slight demineralization occurs, with a 1% pore space, compared with 0.1% for intact enamel. In contrast, the dark zone occurs in approximately 95% of carious lesions and has a pore volume of 2 to 4%. When teeth showing no dark zone are placed in a remineralizing solution, the dark zone becomes visible in its expected position between the translucent zone and the body of the lesion.[21] On the basis of this phenomenon, it is suggested that *this dark zone is the site where remineralization can occur* and that a wider dark zone indicates a greater amount, or a longer period, of remineralization.

Peripheral to the dark zone lies the main body of the lesion. In this zone, pore volume ranges from approximately 5% on the fringes of the lesion to about 25% in the center.[18] Despite this considerable amount of demineralization, the remaining crystals still maintain their basic orientation on the protein matrix. Finally, the surface zone has a near-normal pore space of approximately 1%. It is the surface zone and the dark zone that are the remineralization zones of the incipient lesion.

## Direct Connection of the Bacterial Plaque to the Body of the Lesion

Demineralization of the surface enamel produces a ragged profile when seen with the electron microscope (Figure 3–4). Small pores, or microchannels, have been observed by electron microscopy in the *surface zone* of incipient lesions. The initial attack may be on the rod ends, between the rods, or both.[22] There is a *widening* of the areas between adjacent rods.[23] When conditions are optimum, this ragged interface between surface and subsurface can be remineralized (repaired), either by the body defenses (calcium and phosphate and other ions

from the saliva), or by man-made strategies (fluoride therapy and sugar discipline).

*Figure 3–4 is an outstanding electron micrograph to aid in visually understanding caries initiation and progression beyond the details provided by Silverstone.* For orientation, in the upper-left corner of the illustration, there is the bacterial plaque (B); immediately below is the salivary pellicle (SP), followed by the enamel (EN). The lighter area labeled CM leads *directly* from the bacterial plaque to the area that is, or will be, the expanding body of the lesion. In turn, the body of the lesion opens into many interrod spaces that continue uninterrupted to the dentino-enamel junction (DEJ). It is along these inter-rod spaces that the bacterial plaque fluids diffuse (Figures 3–5 A and B).

En route to the DEJ, the stria of Retzius allows lateral acid access out of the inter-rod space into the center of the intact or damaged rods and crystals. Once at the DEJ, any fluid flow whether causing de- or remineralization, can trichotomize[c] either along the hypomineralized DEJ, or into the dentinal tubules to the pulp chamber (Figure 3–6). The speed of progression of the caries front depends on such factors as ion concentration, pH, saliva flow, and buffering actions—all of which are continually changing. In summarizing, there is a trail of interconnecting channels for diffusion of fluids transiting from the bacterial plaque to the pulp chamber. Any chemical changes in the *plaque* can be soon reflected *throughout* the enamel and dentin as part of the incipient lesion.

These ultrastructural enamel defects—the pores—allow the exit of plaque acids direct to the subsurface region. The initial acid attack preferentially dissolves the magnesium and carbonate ions and is later followed by a removal of the less soluble calcium, phosphate, and other ions that are part of the crystal.

---

[c]trichotomize = go in one of three directions—along the DEJ in either direction, or into the dentinal tubules.

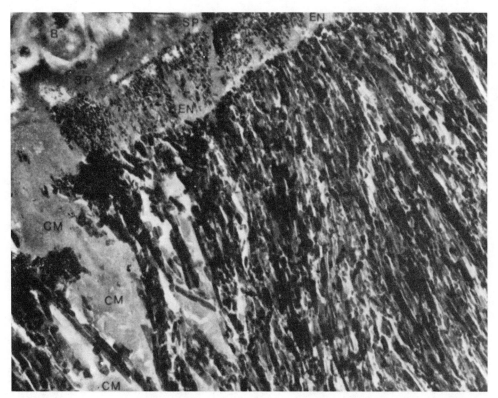

FIGURE 3-4    From a mesial brown spot on a lower second molar. An 0.8 um defect filled with organic material (CM) extends from the plague (upper left, B), through the enamel (EN) as the surface zone, and continues into the larger area of the demineralized subsurface body of the lesion. On either side of the body of the lesion are areas with disoriented crystals that constitute the (demineralizing) translucent zones. (From Frank RM, Brendel A. Ultrastructure of the approximal dental plaque and the underlying normal and carious enamel. ArchOral Biol. 1996:11:909. Permission granted by Pergaron Press, Ltd., Oxford, England.) Teaching comment: This electron micrograph is very important to understanding the route of ions from the plaque of the tooth to the interior and vice versa, in de-and remineralization, respectively of an incipient lesion.

Eventually the undermined surface zone collapses. Concurrent with this change, the more soluble proteins are lost from the subsurface matrix. Once cavitation occurs, the zones of the incipient lesion become less clearly defined because of mineral loss and the presence of bacteria, bacterial end products, plaque, and residual substrate, which may support further lesion development. The lesion is *no longer* an incipient lesion; it is now an *overt caries lesion* requiring operative intervention.

## Question 1

Which of the following statements, if any, are correct?

A. All the following structures are involved in the passage of fluids in the enamel:

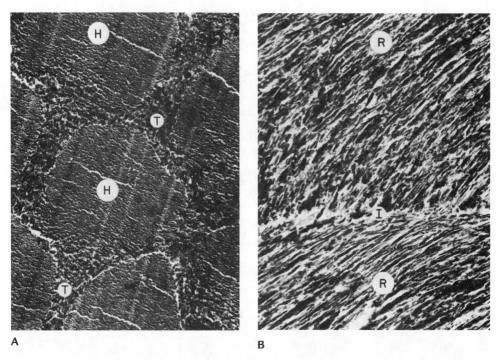

**A**                                                    **B**

FIGURE 3–5   **A.** Electron micrograph of rod cut perpendicular to long axis, showing head (H) and tail (T) relationship. **B.** Electron micrograph of parallel to long axis showing two rods (R) and interrod area (I). Original magnification ×5000. (From Meckel AH, Griebstein WJ, Neal RJ. Structure of mature human dental enamel as observed by electron microscopy. *Arch Oral Biol.* 1965; 10:775–783.)

interrod space, intercrystalline matrix, pores, and striae of Retzius.

B. The head of the enamel rod is always oriented toward the incisal or occlusal surfaces in both the maxillary and mandibular teeth.

C. A rampant caries attack implies a previous incipient lesion for each overt lesion that develops.

D. The incipient lesion usually starts incisal to the contact point in interproximal caries and at the base of the fissure in occlusal caries.

E. The dark and the translucent zones are the centers of remineralization when "biologic repair" of the tooth is occurring.

## Know your Enemy, the Cariogenic Bacteria

Following Miller's works in the 1890s, it was not until 1954 that fundamental *experimental evidence proved* that bacteria were the agents of acid production. Orland and colleagues[24] demonstrated that *gnotobiotic*[d] rats did not develop caries when fed a cariogenic diet; they did develop caries when acidogenic bacteria, plus a *cariogenic diet were introduced* into the previous germ-free environment. The *transmissible* nature of caries in animals was later demonstrated by the experiments of Keyes[25] who showed that previously gnotobiotic, caries-inactive hamsters developed caries after contact with caries-active animals.

[d]Gnotobiotic = germ-free environments.

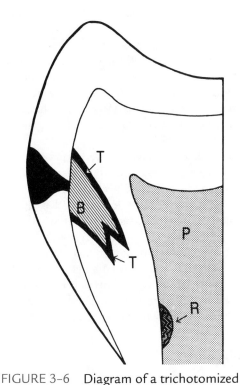

FIGURE 3-6   Diagram of a trichotomized lesion, due to diffusion of acids in both directions under the enamel, and directly into the body of the lesion in the dentin.
T = translucent zone, B = body of the lesion, R = reactionary dentin, P = pulp. (Silverstone LM, Hicks MJ. The structure and ultrastructure of the carious lesion in human dentin. *Gerodontics*, 1985, 1:185–93.)

## Mutans Streptococci and Caries

For caries to develop, acidogenic (acid-producing) bacteria *must* be present, and a means *must* exist to prevent the acid from being washed away from the point where caries is to develop. Dental plaque fulfills both of these functions. It helps protect the bacterial colonies in a cocoon of (a gel-like) *glucan* from being flushed, neutralized, or effected by antimicrobials in the saliva or introduced by humans.

Of the 300-or-more species of microorganisms inhabiting the plaque, the great majority are not directly involved in the caries process. Two bacterial genera are of special interest in cariogenesis: (1) the *mutans streptococci*[e] and (2) the *lactobacillti*.[26,27] The mutans streptococci (MS) are a group of bacterial species previously considered to be serotypes of the single species, *Streptococcus mutans*.[26] These bacteria are characterized by their ability to produce *extracellular glucans* from sucrose and by their acid production in animal and human studies. *Streptococcus mutans* received its name in 1924 when J. K. Clarke in England isolated organisms from human carious lesions. He noted that they were more oval than round and assumed them to be a mutant form of a streptococcus.[28]

Mutans streptococci are now considered to be the major pathogenic bacterial species involved in the caries process. Innumerable surveys have indicated an association between the number of S. *mutans* and dental caries.[29–31] The counts have been repeated worldwide for over more than five decades for all ages—in the United States,[32] Sweden,[33] Latvia,[34] Finland,[35] and China[36]—with high MS bacterial counts being overwhelmingly correlated to the number of teeth with caries or restorations.

Mutans streptococci are usually found in relatively large numbers in the plaque occurring immediately over developing smooth-surface lesions. In one longitudinal study, specific sites were periodically sampled for the presence of MS, and the teeth later examined for caries. Teeth destined to become carious exhibited a significant increase in the proportions of MS from 6 to 24 months *before* the eventual diagnosis of caries.[37] Similarly, dental plaques isolated from sites overlying white spot lesions were characterized by a significantly higher proportion of MS than plaques sampled from sound enamel sites.[38] Increased numbers of MS

---

[e]Originally, it was believed that Streptococci mutans was the only species of streptococci that caused caries; however, when it was found that other streptococci were also involved, they were all grouped under the umbrella designation of mutans streptococci. In the older references, the original terminology will be maintained.

in the saliva also parallel the development of the smooth-surface lesion. In another study, MS counts from the saliva of 200 children indicated that 93% with detectable caries were positive for MS, whereas uninfected children were almost always caries-free.[39]

Certain physiological characteristics of the MS favor their reputation as a prime agent in caries. These traits include the ability to *adhere* to tooth surfaces, production of abundant insoluble *extracellular* polysaccharides (glucan) from sucrose, *rapid* production of lactic acid from a number of sugar substrates, acid tolerance, and the production of *intracellular* polysaccharide (energy) stores. These features help the MS survive in an unfriendly environment due to periods of very low availability of substrate (i.e., between meals and snacks). As a general rule, the cariogenic bacteria metabolize sugars to produce the energy required for their growth and reproduction. The by-products of this metabolism are acids, which are released into the plaque fluid. The damage caused by MS is mainly caused by *lactic acid*, although other acids, such as butyric and propionic, are present within the plaque.[40]

### Lactobacilli and Caries

Lactobacilli (LB) are cariogenic, acidogenic, and aciduric. Indeed, from the early 1920s until the 1950s, LB was considered *the* essential bacteria causing caries. It was not until 1954 when the gnotobiotic[f] studies of Orland demonstrated that if rodents living in a germ-free environment were infected with a lactic acid-producing *enterococci* (but *no* LB), they still developed caries.[24] This was the first time that it was *known* that LB were not requisite for caries development. Often, the number of lactobacilli isolated from either saliva or plaque was too low in number to be considered capable of producing the range of pH values re-

---

[f]Gnotobiotic = In this use, the animals were raised in a *sterile* environment.

quired for caries initiation.[41] However, once a caries lesion develops, the stability of the immediate plaque population changes rapidly. The low pH environment of LB often eliminates, or at least suppresses the continuity of colonization of MS.[42] This, despite the fact that some organisms such as MS probably have genetic defensive mechanisms to minimize the effects of a low pH.[43]

This phenomenon of a lowering pH resulting in MS being displaced by LB, is seen following irradiation for head and neck cancer, when extensive, multiple, caries lesions develop rapidly because of the destruction of the salivary glands.[44] During the *initial* phases of the developing carious lesions, large numbers of MS are involved, only to *decrease* later in number as the LB population *increases*. This is believed to be caused by LB creating a sufficiently low pH to establish a monopoly of the environment.

### Adherence

Continuous *adherence* to the solid tooth surface by *S. mutans* is necessary both before and after initial colonization. The first bacteria must establish a foothold on the tooth surface (acquired pellicle) and then maintain their positions while other bacteria continue to colonize in other protected areas offered by the interproximal spaces, along the gingiva, or in the pits and fissures. Otherwise they would be swept away by the saliva.

Mutans streptococci are able to attach to the tooth surface by either of two mechanisms:[26,27,45] (1) attachment to the acquired pellicle through extracellular proteins (*adhesins*) located on the fimbriae (fuzzy coat) of these organisms; and (2) sucrose-*dependent* mechanisms, in which bacteria *require* the presence of sucrose to produce sticky *extracellular polysaccharides* (*glucans*), that allows attachment and accumulation of additional waves of bacterial colonization.[46]

Sucrose is a disaccharide, consisting of one glucose and one fructose unit (moieties). One

of the key enzymes in the conversion of the glucose moiety of sucrose to glucan is *glucosyl-transferase*. At times the enzyme may be altered, resulting in the production of a *soluble* glucan that does not support adherence. These mutant strains that form *soluble* glucan are usually noncariogenic.[47]

The effect of sucrose restriction on glucan production is seen in several clinical situations. Children who consume little or no sucrose because of sucrase or fructase enzyme deficiencies have a less cariogenic plaque. Similarly, patients receiving long-term nourishment via stomach tube have less plaque and fewer MS.[48] Individuals restricting their sucrose intake have a decreased proportion of MS in their plaque, but the MS increases when sucrose is reintroduced into the diet.[49] Dietary restriction of sugar has also been shown to reduce the acidogenicity of dental plaque.[50,51]

## Ecology of Caries Development

Several studies support the possibility that the initial colonizers can help to determine the eventual pathogenicity of the plaque.[37] Once a species of bacteria has established its *ecologic niche*,[g] other bacteria introduced at a later date appear to have a more difficult task in colonizing. Once established, a niche can be long-lasting. For instance, children with the highest number of MS for deciduous teeth usually experience a higher attack rate for the later permanent teeth.[52]

Mutans streptcoccoi require a *solid surface*— the tooth surface—for successful colonization. During the first year of life *before* eruption of the primary teeth, very few MS are found in the mouth.[53] When teething begins at approximately 8 months, MS often rapidly colonizes the plaque of newly erupting teeth.[54] It has been shown that an important source of infec-

tion of infants by MS is from the *caregivers (usually the mother)* by the mouth-to-mouth transmission, such as via kissing, or by sharing a spoon during feeding.[55] Mothers with the highest MS counts often have infants with similarly high caries lesion counts.[56] Since early infection by MS is associated with high decay rates,[57] it has been strongly suggested that an effective means of preventing caries in young children would be to reduce the number of MS in the parents' and siblings' mouths before a child's birth.

Because no entrenched competition from other organisms occurs on eruption, the first bacterial colonizers probably have little difficulty in establishing their ecologic niches on the acquired pellicle and in the saliva. Once the teeth erupt, many of these oral reservoirs of bacteria participate in the formation of the plaque. Each firmly established niche can act as a "seeding" area for other areas of the mouth. Mutans streptcoocci decrease in number as teeth are lost throughout life and practically disappear following full-mouth extraction.[58] After dentures are inserted, *S. mutans* reappear, only to disappear again when the dentures are removed for an extended period.

---

> ### Question 2
> Which of the following statements, if any, are correct?
> A. Streptococcus mutans can be expected in increased numbers at the site of an incipient lesion.
> B. Lactobacilli are usually found even earlier than mutans streptococci at the incipient lesion site.
> C. Soluble glucans foster better bacterial adherence than insoluble glucans.
> D. Caregivers can be a child's worst dental friend.
> E. The mutans streptococci require a solid surface on which to colonize.

---

[g]An area in the plaque where specific species of bacteria are relatively safe from host protective function of saliva and from other antagonistic bacteria.

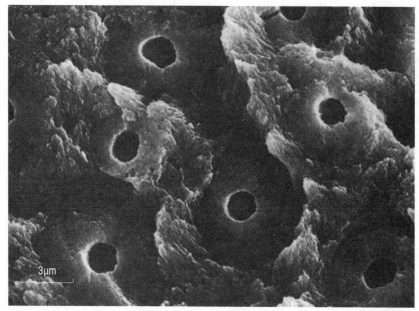

FIGURE 3–7A    Scanning electron micrograph of dentinal tubules. The tubules are approximately 1.5 um in diameter and surrounded by a highly mineralized collar of peritubular dentin. The matrix between the tubules and peritubular dendentin is the intertubular matrix and consists of bundles of collagen fibrils running in a plane at right-angles to the long axis of the tubules. Mineral crystals are also found aligned along the collagen fibril. (Silverstone, L. M. & Hicks, M. J. The structure and ultrastructure of the carious lesion in the human dentin. *Gerodontics* 1985;1:185–93.)

## Coronal Dentin Caries

It is now desirable to revisit the embryology of the tooth,[59] starting at the dentoenamel junction (DEJ) when the ameloblasts and the odontoblasts were lined up at the future DEJ. The objective of the ameloblasts was the future surface of the tooth, while the objective of the odontoblasts was the future border of the dental pulp. During the period of tooth formation, each day the odontoblast laid down a trailing odontoblastic process and a concentric increment layer of *predentin*. Each succeeding day the predentin became a calcified layer of dentin forming a tubule around the odontoblastic process, the lining of which is a hypercalcified layer called the *peritubular dentin*. These tubules extended from the DEJ to the dental pulp, in fact a few extended into the enamel as *enamel spindles*.

Between the tubules there is *intertubular* dentin (also called mantle dentin).[60] The tubules contain fluid that originates from the pulp chamber. There is intertubular communication and fluid transport, via *secondary tubules* and smaller sized *canaliculi*. All tubules act as channels for the *convection*[h] flow of fluids that flow *outward* from the pulp.[61] Dentinal fluid is con-

[h]The fluid entering the tooth from the surface is said to *diffuse* inward; fluids arising from the pulp are said to be *convection fluids*.

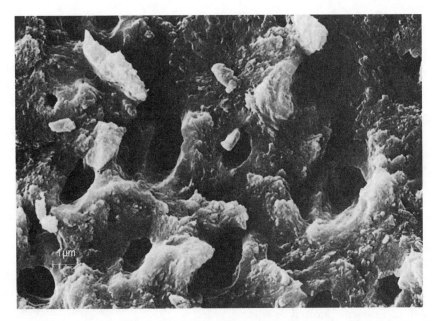

FIGURE 3-7B   Scanning electron micrograph showing the zone of demineralization in the body of a lesion in dentin caries. This region is bacteria-free and shows evidence of acid dissolution, especially in the peritubular denin. The sclerosed tubular contents of the translucent zone have also been lost as a result of dissolution. (Silverstone, L. M. & Hicks, M. J. The structure and ultrastructure of the carious lesion in human dentin. *Gerodontics* 1985:1:185–93.)

stantly pumped into tubules by the forces of mastication, with a return of the fluid to the pulp upon release of the pressure.[62] When there are infection products (caries) arriving in the tubules, more fluid is forced into the tubule.[63,64] The pulp fluid also contains important calcium, phosphate and secretory immunoglobulin A.[64,65]

Upon the approach of enamel caries to the DEJ, many of the odontoblastic processes underlying the carious enamel interrod areas of the enamel will lose their vitality. These tubules become *dead tracts* and may begin to partially or wholly calcify The complete calcification results in a hard calcified group of tubules, called *sclerotic dentin* that acts as a protective barrier to the advancing caries. At the same time, the odontoblasts located on the periphery of the pulp are triggered to begin laying down increments of amorphous *reparative dentin* to further protect the pulp.

In summary, the millions of diffusion and convection channels in the enamel and dentin respectively, permit a movement of fluid from the tooth surface to the pulp.[66,67] The intertubular secondary canals and the canaliculi provide permeability within the dentin, whilst the DEJ provides the same lateral fluid (acid) mobility that can undermine the enamel and aid in its collapse to form an overt caries lesion. It should be pointed out that even with a visible x-ray lucency that extends into the dentin, if the originating surface zone has not broken down into an overt cavity, the entire pre-caries lesion, even in deep dentin can on the basis of in vitro studies, theoretically (and slowly), be remineralized.[68]

## Root Caries

A general demographic shift is continually occurring in America, with each successive generation living longer. This provides a longer time for more gingival recession and more root caries. In addition, Seniors are consuming an increasing number of medicines that are known to reduce saliva and cause root caries.[69] Katz and colleagues estimated that individuals going into their 30s have about 1 out of 100 surfaces with recession and root caries; when they leave their 50s, about 1 out of 5 exposed surfaces is involved. The roots of the mandibular molars and the mandibular incisors are at the greatest, and the least risk, respectively.[70]

The Third National Health and Nutrition Examination Survey found that the percentage of persons with at least one decayed or filled root surface increased from 20.8% in the 35- to 44-year age group, to 55.9% in those aged 75 years and older.[71] A Canadian study concluded that "the increase in the prevalence of root decay with age may not be due to aging per se, but instead, may be the result of neglect of oral health during the years of growing older." Older adults with continual good oral health still had low rates of root decay.[72] In a study of 5000 subjects in Finland, it was found that men had from 1.1 to 2.5 times more root caries than women. The greatest difference was in the group 60 to 69 years of age.[73]

A number of risk factors have been defined for root caries development, including age, gender, fluoride exposure, systemic illness, medications, oral hygiene, and diet.[74] In terms of the microbiology of root caries, despite early indications of a strong association between Actinomyces species and progressive root lesions,[75,76] more recent studies indicate that plaque and salivary concentrations of the mutans streptococci are correlated positively with the presence of root surface caries.[77,78]

Root caries differs from coronal caries in several aspects. A critical difference is that the tissues affected—enamel vs. cementum—are fundamentally dissimilar. Enamel is much more highly mineralized than cementum or dentin. Because of the *lower mineral* content and *higher organic content* of the cementum–dentin complex, root caries may progress *both* by *acid demineralization of the inorganic structure* and by *proteolysis of the organic component*.[79] These tissue variations determine the differences in the rate of lesion formation, histologic and visual appearance, as well as in the potential for and rate of remineralization.[80] Clinically, the lesion is initially noncavitated. The carious material is soft and has a yellowish-brown coloration. The lesion can eventually assume any outline and may involve multiple root surfaces (Figure 3–8). When cavitation is evident, lesions tend to spread laterally, have a depth of approximately 0.5 to 1.0 mm, and are of a dark-brown appearance.[81] The lesions appear immediately *below* the cemento–enamel junction, undermining but *not* involving the enamel (Figure 3–8).

Root caries differ from coronal caries in that *bacterial invasion* of cementum and dentin occurs *early*. At times, the invasion features columns of organisms between spikes of relatively intact cementum. At other times, a complete loss of cementum exposes the dentin. Like enamel caries, root caries is amenable to remineralization and/or arrest.[80] Arrested root caries lesions demonstrate three physical characteristics: (1) an *outer* barrier of hypermineralized surface dentin; (2) a sclerotic *inner* barrier between carious and sound dentin; and (3) mineralization occurring *within* the dentinal tubules.[82] Clinically, such remineralized lesions may appear dark and hard; under tactile examination by the explorer, arrested lesions are easily distinguished from active lesions by their smooth, hard, and glassy feel compared to the leathery feel of active root caries.

## Prevention of Root Caries

The best prevention for root caries in the elderly population *is the prevention of periodontal disease in middle-age or earlier*. However, since ex post

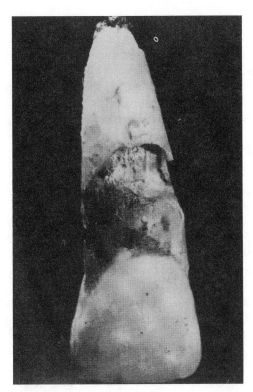

FIGURE 3-8 Root caries. The darker staining of the coronal half of the root indicates considerable gingival recession, which is a prerequisite to lesion development.

facto[i] remedial treatment is not possible, earlier preventive dentistry care needs to be practiced. The strategies include: (1) daily *mechanical and chemical plaque control* (2) *severe restriction of refined carbohydrates*; and (3) routine professional dental attendance for preventive office identification of risks and counseling on self-care needs. For instance, for those at high risk, a *prescription* dentifrice with a high-fluoride content, Prevident, with 5,000 parts fluoride per million, has been found to significantly increase the electrical resistance[j] of a tooth surface.[83] Frequent pro-

fessional examinations based on an individual's risk should be routine. All extensive periodontal surgery for pocket elimination should place an individual in a higher root caries risk category for life.[84,85] In later chapters, the use of the antimicrobial mouth rinse, *chlorhexidine*, will be introduced as a very effective mutans streptococci control agent. With professional guidance and patient cooperation, biological repair of a root caries lesion can be achieved in many cases—a desirable option in view of the difficulty and lack of success in restoring root caries via operative procedures.

### Secondary, or Recurrent, Caries

Secondary caries start with small imperfections or restoration overhangs that exist between the tooth and the margins of a restoration.[86] Also, some tooth-colored fillings have a higher affinity for plaque.[87] Bacteria are able to colonize and multiply at these vulnerable sites, sheltered from the protective effects of saliva and self-care efforts. Eventually, a lesion develops between the cavity margin and the restoration.

The diagnosis of these lesions is difficult.[88] In one study, extracted teeth were cut so that the section included both a clinically *sound amalgam margin* and one defined as *"ditched."* The prevalence of recurrent lesions in both sound and ditched restorations was close to 50%, although it is unknown whether these lesions were truly recurrent or due to residual caries left during a previous cavity preparation.[89] The magnitude of the problem of secondary decay is illustrated by studies indicating that the median survival time of restorations ranges from *5 to 10 years*.[90] Replacement of defective restorations account for inserting several-times-more than needed restorations over a life time.[91] Reducing this problem can

---

[i]Ex post facto = After the fact, meaning the it is not possible to correct some events of the past.

[j]Several devices are on the market that are modified versions of the common volt-ohm meter. The patient holds

one electrode, while the explorer serves as the second electrode. When the explorer is placed on the suspect area, the resistance of the tooth is measured. A high resistance is associated with no caries, and little resistance is associated with caries probability.

best come from preventing the number of primary lesions (primary prevention). Some future relief may be forthcoming from the use of materials that bond directly to the tooth tissue, eliminating the gap between tooth and filling, or from restorative materials that slowly release fluoride, such as glass ionomers and newer fluoride-releasing composites and amalgams.[92,93]

---

### Question 3

Which of the following statements, if any, are correct?

A. The critical pH for enamel demineralization ranges between 6.0 to 5.5.

B. There cannot be secondary caries, without having had a previous incipient lesion at the same site.

C. Once the incipient lesions become overt, all the lesion zones disappear.

D. Root caries is not necessarily a part of the aging process but is usually a sign of periodontal disease and/or previous periodontal neglect.

E. A dentist usually inserts more restorations as a result of secondary caries than for primary caries.

---

*Measuring Plaque pH, the Stephan Curve*

Every time a person eats a food, there is a continuous pH change in the plaque. In many studies, pH microelectrodes have been inserted in bridges and telemonitored to determine these changes. For sugar and sugary snacks, an almost immediate drop in pH occurs, followed by a longer recovery period. This drop and recovery curve has been termed the *Stephan Curve* after Dr. Robert Stephan, an officer in the United States Public Health Service who first reported on the continuous changes in pH that followed eating and drinking different foods and drinking different beverages.[94] Plaque pH responses to simple sugar rinses by caries-free and caries active individuals exhibited different drops in pH and different lengths of time to return to normal. Thus, different individuals have different capabilities to buffer acid production. (Figure 3–9). Similar pH studies have been accomplished that identify foods that are not hazardous to the teeth, and vice versa, those that are accompanied by a drop past the "critical pH" of pH 5.5 to 5.0. These lists are of considerable value when counseling patients.[95]

*The Relationship of Saturation to pH*

The concentration of calcium and phosphate ions in the *plaque fluid* bathing the tooth at the plaque–tooth interface is extremely important, because these are the same elements that compose the hydroxyapatite crystal. *If the fluid adjacent to the tooth is supersaturated with calcium and phosphate ions at a given pH, the enamel cannot undergo demineralization.*

The saliva in contact with the teeth is normally supersaturated with respect to the calcium and phosphate in enamel.[15] The bacterial plaque can concentrate these ions to an even greater extent. For instance, both calcium and phosphate are threefold times greater than in the saliva.[96] This increased concentration is of practical importance because calcium and phosphate levels tend to be inversely related to the caries score.[47] It is also of great importance because it is the *plaque fluid that determines the eventual caries status.*

As the pH drops in an acid attack, the level of supersaturation also drops, and the risk of demineralization increases. There is no exact pH at which the demineralization begins, only a general range of 5.5 to 5.0. The range is rather large because demineralization is a function of both pH and duration of exposure of the enamel surface to the acid environment. Different plaques have different initial pHs, buffering potentials, and concentrations of calcium and phosphate in different parts of the mouth. A change in any of these variables results in a different level of supersaturation in the tooth environment.

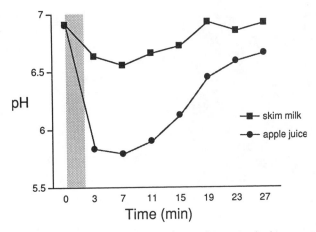

FIGURE 3-9    Stephan curves. These curves show the typical plaque pH response to an oral glucose rinse (indicated by the screened area). There is an immediate fall in the pH, followed by a gradual return to resting values after about 40 minutes. Each curve represents the mean of 12 subjects; the pH was measured by sampling method (see Chap. 15) and therefore is an average value for the whole mouth plaque pH. In individual sites away from the salivary buffers, the pH values may fall close to 4.0. The upper curve was obtained from reconstituted skim milk and the lower one from an apple-flavored drink, showing a large difference in the acidogenicity of these two drinks. (Courtesy of MWJ Dodds, University of Texas Dental School, San Antonio.)

*De- and Remineralization of Teeth, Principles*

Throughout this book, there will continue to be many references to de- and remineralization of teeth, both as a pathologic and as a therapeutic process. The demineralization is caused by *plaque acids* causing the dissolution of the tooth minerals making up the basic calcium, phosphate, and hydroxyl crystals of the enamel, dentin and cementum. Remineralization on the other hand, requires the *availability of the same ions, preferably with fluoride as a catalyst* to reconstruct the missing or damaged rods—a process that ten Cate aptly calls, *non-restorative repair.*[97]

There are many calcium and phosphate compounds in the body that vary in formulae and with changes in pH. However, at this time, for the sake of simplicity, the crystals and fluoride compound of most dental interest in the de- and remineralization process are hydroxyapatite (HAP), fluorhydroxyapatite (FHA), and calcium fluoride ($CaF_2$).

The long-term exposure of teeth to *low concentrations* of fluoride (as found in fluoridated water) results in the gradual incorporation of fluoride into the existing hydroxyapatite (HAP) crystals to form fluorhydroxyapatite (FHA) that is more resistant to acid damage. Conversely, a *higher* concentration of fluoride (as occurs in topical applications, use of fluoride dentifrices, gels, and varnishes, etc.), results in the formation of *surface globules* of calcium fluoride (as seen in electron microscope images). A subsequent coating of these globules by phosphates and proteins of the saliva renders these globules more insoluble.[98] As a matter of terminology, when the fluoride is incorporated into HAP to form FHA, it is said to be firmly bound; whereas, loosely bound fluoride is in the form of calcium fluoride that is *adsorbed onto* the surface of HAP and FHA crystals.[99]

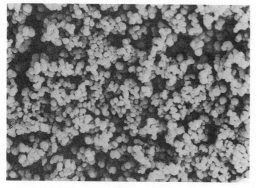

FIGURE 3-10 Electron micrograph. Loosely bound calcium flouride globules on the surface of the enamel following an application of sodium flouride. These reaction products following the flouride application will be dissolved in two or three weeks into the saliva. Each time an application of flouride dentifrice or mouth rinse occurs, this pattern of globule distribution is repeated, with the extent depending on the specific flouride and concentration. (Courtesy, Dr. M.J. Hicks, Texas Childrens Hospital, Houston, TX. Magnification 5000X)

## The Relationship Between HAP, FHA and $CaF_2$

Following an attack by plaque acid(s), the $CaF_2$ dissolves first, followed in sequence by the HAP, and finally, the FHA (with its fluoride substitutions). As the attack continues, the dissociated ions *increase the saturation level of the immediate fluid sufficiently to slow crystal dissolution, and eventually arrest* further solution of the crystals. As the pH begins to return to normal, crystals begin to *re-form* from the complex *pool* of dissolved ions—some as HAP, some as FHA (with many of the fluoride ions coming from the previous $CaF_2$, and finally the precipitation of newly adsorbed $CaF_2$. Any deficiencies are subsequently replaced in time by calcium, phosphate, and fluoride from sources such as the saliva, water, and toothpastes. In observing the above process, one must marvel at the body

defense system that in the absence of a cellular or humeral surveillance of the enamel, can use a chemical system to maintain homeostasis— one in which $CaF_2$ *provides a reservoir for fluoride that is immediately available when and where it is needed.*[100] The only time the system breaks down is when the attacks are too frequent and too prolonged.

### Depth of Remineralization

There is little controversy about the success of surface remineralization procedures involving topical procedures, and of using commercial fluoride products such a dentifrices, gels, and varnish to compensate for the daily wear and tear of demineralization (Chapter 9). In the New Zealand School System, they consider x-ray lucencies of incipient lesions that extend midway through the enamel as candidates for remineralization. ten Cate, in an *in vitro* study, found that both the inner enamel and dentin could be remineralized, but very slow. Only the *outer part* of the enamel appeared to be responsive to fluoride diffusion and remineralization.[97] At deeper levels, remineralization could be achieved, but only very slowly. In Scandinavia, the literature reflects the belief that remineralization is a reasonable objective even for lesions reaching to the dentin. The test for remineralization in these cases is that there is no demonstrable caries progress for 2 to 3 years. However, the important fact is that there are no reported studies that indicate whether deep remineralization is or is not successful.

### Methods of Varnish Application

In the United States, topical administration of fluorides is usually via cotton applicators, gel trays, and less frequently by using varnish. (Chapter 9). In Europe, varnishes appear preferable because of the longer exposure to fluoride following application. Since varnishes *do* seal dental tubules involved in hypersensitivity,[101] there is a possibility that they also temporarily seal pores as seen in Figure 3–7.

temporarily seal pores as seen in Figure 3–7. Once sealed, there could be little or no acid penetration into the "white spot."

At least three commercial varnishes are available in North America—Duraphat (Colgate-Palmolive, NY), Duraflor (Pharmascience, Montreal), and Fluor Protector (Ivoclar, Viyadent, Amherst, NY). The U.S. Food and Drug Administration (FDA) has cleared varnishes for applying fluoride varnish—but only as medical devices to be used as cavity liners and desensitizing agents, not for caries control. Semiannual applications are the most accepted time interval.[102] Supporting this time interval was Seppa's study in Finland where increasing the application interval from two, to four times per year *did not* increase the effectiveness of Duraphat, even in high-risk children.[103]

Varnishes have proved to be effective. One study of 142 2- to 3-year-old children was conducted to determine the anticaries effectiveness of Duraphat. At the end of 9 months, 37.8% of the originally active occlusal, lingual, and buccal lesions of the *control* group became inactive, 3.6% had progressed, and 36.9% did not change. For the *Duraphat group*, 81.2% became inactive, 2.4% progressed, and 8.2% did change (P > .0001). The author concluded that the use of varnish was easy, safe and efficient; that it was possibly a non-invasive alternative for the treatment of decay in children.[104]

The application of the varnish is preceded by a prophylaxis, flushing, isolating the target teeth, drying, and applying the varnish with a small brush—techniques that are well known and practiced by the *dental hygienist*.

---

## Question 4

Which of the following questions, if any, are correct?

A. After examining the Stephan Curve recorded for several foods, it is possible to determine which foods and snacks are hazardous to tooth health.

B. As the pH of the plaque fluid falls, it is necessary to have an increasing amount (saturation) of calcium and phosphate in the plaque fluid to prevent the dissolution of the tooth mineral.

C. As the pH drops past the critical pH for enamel dissolution, the dissolving crystals gradually increase the immediate concentration (saturation) of tooth minerals that gradually slow, and possibly arrest the further solution of the rod crystals.

D. It requires a lower critical pH to dissolve a crystal that is in the fluid environment of dissolving $CaF_2$.

E. The many studies of "deep remineralization" provide adequate scientific (evidence based) verification that it is a valid means to manage incipient lesions where the body of the lesion has progressed past the mid point in the enamel.

---

## SUMMARY

Dental caries is a multifactorial disease involving an interaction of bacteria, diet, host resistance, and time. Cavitation can only occur when demineralization outstrips the body's defensive capability for remineralizations over a period of time. The embryology and histology of the enamel are favorable for either the de- or the remineralization of the enamel. The residual matrix and spacial relationships of rod-to-rod and crystalite-to-crystalite, as well as the less-calcified structures as the incremental lines of Retzius, lamellae, and tufts, allow fluids to diffuse throughout the

enamel. Like the wick of an oil lamp, this network is available for the in-and-out movement of tooth-mineral ions and plaque acids. Even when there has been a penetration of the enamel cap by an incipient lesion, this is a pre-caries lesion that can often be remineralized without the need for a restoration. Possibly months or years will elapse before cavitation, or there may even be a natural remineralization that entirely reverses the caries progression. There are several acidogenic bacteria that are causal for caries production, with mutans streptococci and lactobacilli being the most studied. Silverstone opened up the possibility of a new nonrestorative repair era when he described the de- and remineralizing zones of an incipient lesion. If those in the dental care profession and research can bring remineralization to fruition, millions of teeth can be saved from the dentist's drill. The polarizing and the electron microscopes allow us to see the details of how the plaque acids can easily flow into the body of the lesion and beyond. To increase tooth resistance and, at the same time, the probability of remineralizing any known or unknown incipient lesions, *mechanical plaque control* strategies consisting of tooth brushing, flossing, and irrigation are used to *remove the plaque. Chemical plaque control* stratagems involve the use of antimicrobials *to kill or suppress* the cariogenic bacteria; and fluoride in the forms of water fluoridation, office topical applications, or the use of fluoride rinses or dentifrices are used to *improve tooth resistance*. There are now the means to greatly reduce the toll of dental caries; yet needed is access to examination and treatment systems based on early identification and treatment of risk factors before they become treatment requirements. Throughout this book, emphasis will be placed on the various strategies now available for preventing or limiting demineralization, or of enhancing remineralization.

# ANSWERS AND EXPLANATIONS

1. A, B, and C—correct.

    D—incorrect. The interproximal starting point is apical to the contact point; for the pit-and-fissure lesion, it usually begins bilaterally at the orifice of the fissure.

    E—incorrect. The dark and the surface zones are the centers for remineralization; the body of the lesion and the translucent zones are centers for demineralization.

2. A, D, and E—correct.

    B—incorrect. The MS usually precede the lactobacilli.

    C—incorrect. The bacteria-producing soluble glucans often are noncariogenic because of adherence problems; the insoluble glucans are usually produced by the cariogenic bacteria and facilitate adherence.

3. B, D, and E—correct.

    A—incorrect. The critical pH for enamel demineralization is from 5.5 to 5.0.

    C—incorrect. The same zones are present but are less clearly defined because of the presence of bacteria, plaque, and debris.

4. A, B, C and D—correct.

   E—incorrect. No studies to date indicate that "deep remineralization" by use of fluoride therapy is or is not an appropriate method of caries control. There is a theoretical basis, much research, and a plethora of hope and enthusiasm for this approach to nonrestorative "repair" of teeth. (What sugar hath rendered asunder, humankind is now laboring to correct!)

## Self-evaluation Questions

1. In 1890, Miller proposed the _____ theory for caries, which is still (with many modifications) a basis for our present concept of the dental caries.

2. The beginning and end-points of a carious lesion are the _____ (initial) lesion, which can be arrested or reversed by remineralization therapy, and the _____ (end point) lesion, which must be restored.

3. The four zones of an incipient lesion seen with the polarizing microscope (starting from the tooth surface) are the _____, _____, _____, and the _____ zones.

4. The zone of the incipient lesion that is the best indicator of remineralization is the _____ zone; the two zones of demineralization are the _____ and the _____ zones.

5. As the pH drops in the environment of the HAP, the sa _____n of calcium and phosphate in the environment must increase in order to protect the crystals. The presence of _____ (element) will also help to protect the crystal at a lower pH.

6. The critical pH for enamel demineralization is within the generally accepted range of pH _____ to _____.

7. The diagramming of the drop and recovery of pH on a graph is often referred to as the _____ curve for the investigator who first published on the phenomenon.

8. Two possible sources of the calcium and phosphate accounting for the hypermineralized surface of root caries are _____ and _____.

9. The four major types (location) of caries are: _____, _____, _____, and _____.

10. Two causes for rampant caries are _____ (dietary "food") and _____ (dry mouth).

11. The pore space in both the translucent and surface zones is 1 percent; dark zone approximately _____ percent, and the body of the lesion ranges up to _____ percent.

# REFERENCES

1. Kim, J. W., Jang, K. T., Lee, S. H., et al. (2001). *In vivo* rehardening of enamel eroded by cola drink. *J Dent Child*, 68:122–24.
2. Aftin, T., Buchalla, W., Gollner, M., & Hellwig, E. (2000). Use of variable remineralization periods to improve the abrasion resistance of previously eroded enamel. *Caries Res*, 34:48–52.
3. Ring, M. E., Ed. (1985). *Dentistry: An illustrated history*. New York: Harry N. Abrams, Inc.
4. A practical treatise on the diseases of the teeth, in which the origine and nature of decay are explained: and a means of prevention pointed out. Ed. William Robertson. Longman, Rees, Brown, Green and Longman. Paternosterrow, and J. Belcha and Son, Birmingham. 1835.
5. Miller, W. D. (1973). *The microorganisms of the human mouth*. Philadelphia: SS White Dental Manufacturing Company; 1890. Reprinted Basel, Switzerland: Karger.
6. Black, G. V. (1898). Dr. Black's conclusions reviewed again. *Dental Cosmos*, 40:440–51.
7. Smith, O. E., & Nanci, A. (1995). Overview of morphological changes in enamel organ cells associated with major events in amelogenesis. *Int J Dev Biol*, 39:153–61.
8. Diekwisch, T. G. (1998). Subunit compartments of secretion of secretory enamel matrix. *Connect Tissue Res*, 38:101–11; discussion 139–45.
9. Wen, H. B., Finchan, A. G., & Moradian-Oldak, J. (2001). Progressive accretion of amelogenin molecules during nanospheres assembly revealed by atomic force microscopy. *Matrix Biol*, 20:387–99.
10. Moradian-Oldak, J. (2001). Amelogenins: Assembly, processing and control of crystal morphology. *Matrix Biol*, 20:293–305.
11. Robinson, E., Brooks, S. J., Shore, R. C., & Kirkham, J. (1998). The developing enamel matrix: nature and function. *Eur J Oral Sci*, 106:282–91.
12. Simoner, J. P., & Hu, J. C. (2001). Dental enamel formtion and its impact on clinical dentistry. *J Dent Educ*, 65:896–905.
13. Smith, C. E. (1998). Cellular and chemical events during enamel maturation. *Crit Rev Oral Biol Med*, 9:128–61.
14. Robinson, C., Kirkham, J., Brooks, S. J., Borass, W. A., & Shore, R. C. (1995). The chemistry of enamel development. *Int J Dev Biol*, 39:145–52.
15. Moradian-Oldak, J., Leung, W., Tan, J., & Fincham, A. G. (1998). Effect of apatite crystals on the activity of amelogen degrading enzymes in vitro. *Conn Tissue Res*, 39:131–40.
16. Crabb, H. S. M. (1976). The porous outer enamel of unerupted human premolars. *Caries Res*, 10:1–7.
17. Dodds, M. W. J. (1993). Dilemmas in caries diagnosis—applications to current practice, and need for research. *J Dent Educ*, 57:433–38.
18. Silverstone, L. M. (1973). The structure of carious enamel, including the early lesion. *Oral Sci Rev*, 3:100–60.
19. König, K. G. (1963). Dental morphology in relation to caries resistance with special reference to fissures as susceptible sites. *J Dent Res*, 42:461–76.
20. Juhl, M. (1983). Localization of carious lesions in occlusal pits and fissures of human premolars. *Scand J Dent Res*, 91:251–55.
21. Silverstone, I. M. (1977). Remineralization phenomena. *Caries Res*, 11 (Suppl 1):59–84.
22. Johnson, N. W. (1967). Some aspects of the ultrastructure of early human enamel caries seen with the electron microscope. *Arch Oral Biol*, 12:1505–21.
23. Haikel, Y., Frank, R. M., & Voegel, J. C. (1983). Scanning electron microscopy of the human enamel surface layer of incipient enamel lesions. *Caries Res*, 17:1–13.

24. Orland, F. J., Blayney, J. R., Harrison, R. W., Reynzers, J. A., Trexler, P. C., Wagner, M., Gordon, H. A., & Luckey, T. D. (1954). Use of germ-free animal technic in the study of experimental dental caries. I. Basic observations on rats reared free of all microorganisms. *J Dent Res*, 33:147–74.

25. Keyes, P. H. (1960). The infections and transmissible nature of experimental dental caries—findings and implications. *Arch Oral Biol*, 1:304–20.

26. Loesche, W. J. (1986). Role of Streptococcus mutans in human dental decay. *Microbiol Rev*, 50:353–80.

27. Tanzer, J. M. (1989). On changing the cariogenic chemistry of coronal plaque. *J Dent Res*, 68 (Special Issue): 1576–87.

28. Clarke, J. K. (1924). On the bacterial factor in the aetiology of dental caries. *Br J Exp Pathol*, 5:141–47.

29. Twetman, S., & Frostnec, N. (1991). Salivary mutans streptomutans and caries prevalence in 8-year-old Swedish schoolchildren. *Swed Dent J*, 15:145–51.

30. Keene, H. J., & Shklair, I. L. (1975). Relationship of Streptococcus mutans carrier status to the development of carious lesions in initially caries free recruits. *J Dent Res*, 53:1295.

31. Loesche, W. J., Rowan, J., Straffon, L. H., et al. (1975). Association of Streptococcus mutans with human dental decay. *Infect Immun*, 11:1252–60.

32. Thibodeau, E. A., & O'Sullivan, D. M. (1999). Salivary mutans streptococci and caries development in the primary and mixed dentitions of children. *Community Dent Oral Epidemiol*, 27:406–12.

33. Fure, S. (1998). Five-year incidence of caries, salivary and microbial conditions in 60-, 70-, and 80-year-old Swedish individuals. *Caries Res*, 32:166–74.

34. Kohler, B., Bjarnason, S., Care, R., et al. (1995). Mutans streptococci and dental caries prevalence in a group of Latvian preschool children. *Eur J Oral Sci*, 103:264–6.

35. Alaluusua, S., Kleemola-Jujala, E., Gronroos, L., & Evalahti, M. (1990). Salivary caries-related tests as predictors of future caries increment in teenagers. A three-year longitudinal study. *Oral Microbiol*, 5:77–81.

36. Shi, S., Liang, Q., Hayashi, Y., Yakushiji, M., & Achida, Y. (1998). The relationship between caries activity and the status of dental caries—application of the Dentocult SM method. *Chin J Dent Res*, 1:52–55.

37. Loesche, W. J., Eklund, S., Earnest, R., & Burt B. (1984). Longitudinal investigation of bacteriology of human fissure decay: Epidemiological studies in molars shortly after eruption. *Infect Immun*, 46:765–72.

38. Van Houte, J., Sansone, C., Joshipura, K., & Kent, R. (1991). *In vitro* acidogenic potential and mutans streptococci on human smooth-surface plaque associated with initial caries lesions and sound enamel. *J Dent Res*, 70:497–502.

39. Edelstein, B., & Tinanoff, N. (1989). Screening preschool children for dental caries using a microbial test. *Pediatr Dent*, 11:129–32.

40. Geddes, D. A. M. (1975). Acids produced by human dental plaque metabolism *in situ*. Caries Res, 9:98–109.

41. Gibbons, R. J. (1964). Bacteriology of dental caries. *J Dent Res*, 43:1021–28.

42. Burne, R. A. (1998). Oral streptococci . . . Products of their environment. *J Dent Res*, 77:445–52.

43. Quivey, R. G., Kuhnert, W. L., & Hahan, K. (2001). Genetics of acid adaption in oral streptococci. *Crit Rev Oral Biol Med*, 12:301–14.

44. Brown, L. R., Dreizen, S., & Handler, S. (1976). Effects of elected caries regimens on microbial changes following radiation-induced xerostomia in cancer patients. In Stiles, H. M., Loesche,

W. J., & O'Brien, T. C., Eds. Proceedings: Microbial Aspects of Dental Caries. Washington, DC: Information Retrieval, 275–290.

45. Gibbons, R. J. (1989). Bacterial adhesion to oral tissues: A model for infectious diseases. *J Dent Res*, 668:750–760.

46. Jenkinson, H. F. (1994). Adherence and accumulation of oral streptococci. *Trends Microbiol*, 2:209–12.

47. Murchison, H., Larrimore, S., & Curtiss, R. (1985). *In vitro* inhibition of adherence of *Streptococcus mutans* strains by nonadherent mutants of *S. mutans 6715*. *Infect Immun*, 50:826–32.

48. Littleton, N. W., McCabe, R. M., & Carter, C. H. (1967). Studies of oral health in persons nourished by stomach tube. II. Acidogenic properties and selected bacterial components of plaque material. *Arch Oral Biol*, 12:601–9.

49. De Stoppelar, S. D., van Houte, J. S., & Backer-Dirks, O. (1970). The effect of carbohydrate restriction on the presence of *Streptococcus mutans*, *Streptococcus sanguis* and iodophilic polysaccharide-producing bacteria in human dental plaque. *Caries Res*, 4:114–23.

50. Dodds, M. W. J., & Edgar, W. M. (1986). Effects of dietary sucrose levels on pH fall and acid–anion profile in human dental plaque after a starch mouthrinse. *Arch Oral Biol*, 31:509–12.

51. Sgan-Cohen, H. D., Newbrun, E., Huber, R., Tenebaum, G., & Sela, M. N. (1988). The effect of previous diet on plaque pH response to different foods. *J Dent Res*, 67:1434–37.

52. Zickert, I., Emilson, C-G, & Krasse, B. (1982). Effect of caries preventive measures in children highly infected with the bacterium Streptococcus mutans. *Arch Oral Biol*, 27:861–68.

53. Carlsson, J., Grahnen, H., & Jonsson, G. (1975). Lactobacilli and streptococci in the mouth of children. *Caries Res*, 9:333–9.

54. Suhonen, J. (1992). Mutans streptococci and their specific oral target: New implications to prevent dental caries. *Schweiz Monafsschr Zahnmed*, 102:286–91.

55. Alalluusia, S. (1991). Transmission of mutans streptocci. *Proc Finn Dent Soc*, 87:443–7.

56. Köhler, B., & Bratthall, D. (1978). Intrafamilial levels of Streptococcus mutans and some aspects of the bacterial transmission. *Scand J Dent Res*, 86:35–42.

57. Zickert, I., Emilson, C-G, & Krasse, B. (1983). Correlation of level and duration of Streptococcus mutans infection with incidence of dental caries. *Infect Immun*, 39:982–85.

58. Carlsson, J., Soderholm, G., & Almfedt, I. (1969). Prevalence of Streptococcus sanguis and Streptococcus mutans in the mouth of persons wearing full-dentures. *Arch Oral Biol*, 14:243–49.

59. Avery, J. K. (2000). *Essentials of oral histology and embryology: A clinical approach* (2nd ed.) St Louis, MO: Mosby, Inc., 94–106.

60. Silverstone, L. M., & Hicks, M. J. (1985). The structure and ultra structure of the carious lesion in human dentin. *Gerodontics*, 1:185–93.

61. Pashley, D. H., & Matthews, W. G. (1993). The affects of outward forced convective flow on inward diffusion in human dentine in vitro. *Arch Oral Biol*, 38:577–82.

62. Ciucchi, B., Bouillaguet, S., Holz, J., & Pashley, D. (1995). Dentinal fluid dynamics in human teeth, in vivo. *J Endod*, 21:919–4.

63. Heyeraas, K. J., & Berggreen, E. (1999). Insterstitial fluid pressure in normal and inflamed puls. *Crit Rev Oral Biol Med*, 10:328–36.

64. Hahn, C. L., & Overton, B. (1997). The effects of immunoglobulins on the convective permeability of human dentine *in vitro*. *Arch Oal Biol Med*, 42:835–43.

65. Pashley, D. H. (1996). Dynamics of the pulpo-dentin complex. *Crit Rev Oral Biol Med*, 7:104–33.

66. Pashley, D. H. (1992). Dentin permeability and dentine sensitivity. *Proc Finn Dent Soc*, 88: Suppl. 1;31:13–7.

67. Pashley, D. H. (1991). Clinical correlations of dentin structure and function. *J Prosthet Dent,* 66:777–81.
68. ten Cate, J. M. (2001). Remineralization of caries lesions extending into dentin. *J Dent Res,* 80:1407–11.
69. Tugnait, A., & Clerehugh, V. (2001). Gingival recession—its significance and management. *J Dent,* 29:381–94.
70. Katz, R. V., Hazen, S. P., Chilton, N. W., & Mumm, R. D. Jr. (1982). Prevalence and intraoral distribution of root caries in an adult population. *Caries Res,* 16:265–71.
71. Winn, D. M., Brunelle, J. A., Selwitz, R. H., Oblakowski, R. J., Kingmon, A. & Brown, L. J. (1996). Coronal and root caries in the dentition of adults in the United States, 1988–1991 *J Dent Res,* 75:642–51.
72. Locker, D., Slade, G. D., & Leake, J. L. (1989). Prevalence of and factors associated with root decay in older adults in Canada. *J Dent Res,* 68:768–72.
73. Vehkalahti, M. M., & Paunlo, I. K. (1988). Occurrence of root caries in relation to dental health behavior. *J Dent Res,* 67:911–14.
74. Banting, D. W. (1986). Epidemiology of root caries. *Gerodontology,* 5:5–11.
75. Jordan, H. V., & Hammond, B. F. (1972). Filamentous bacteria isolated from human root surface caries. *Arch Oral Biol,* 17:1333–42.
76. Sumney, D., & Jordan, H. (1974). Characterization of bacteria isolated from human root surface carious lesions. *J Dent Res,* 63:343–51.
77. Van Houte, J., Jordan, H. V., Laraway, R., Kent, R., Sopark, P. M., & DePaula P. F. (1990). Association of the microbial flora of dental plaque and saliva with human root-surface caries. *J Dent Res,* 69:1463–68.
78. Bowden, G. H. W. (1990). Microbiology of root surface caries in humans. *J Dent Res,* 69:1205–10.
79. Dung, S. Z. (1999). Effects of mutans streptococci, Actinomyces species and Porphyromona gingivalis on collagen degenerations. *Chung Hua I, Hsueh Tsa Chihi* (Taipai). 62:764–74.
80. Mellberg, J. R. (1986). Demineralization and remineralization of root surface caries. *Gerodontology,* 5:25–31.
81. Nyvad, B., & Fejerskov, O. (1986). Active root surface caries converted into inactive caries as a response to oral hygiene. *Scand J Dent Res,* 94:281–84.
82. Schüpbach, P., Lutz, F., & Guggenheim, B. (1992). Human root caries: Histopathology of arrested lesions. *Caries Res,* 26:153–64.
83. Baysan, A., Lynch, E., Ellwood, R., Petterson, L., & Borsboom, P. (2001) Reversal of primary root caries using dentifrices containing 5,000 and 1,100 ppm. Fluoride. *Caries Res,* 35:41–46.
84. Van der Reijden, W. A., Delemijn-Kippuw, N., Stijne-van Nes, A. M., deSoet, J. J., & van Vinkelhoff, A. J. (2001). Mutans streptococci in subgingival plaque of treated and untreated patients with periodontitis. *J Clin Periodontol* 28:686–91.
85. Reikeer, J., van der Velden, U., Barendeqt, D. S., & Loos, B. G. (2000). Root caries in patient with periodontal follow-up care. Prevalence and risk factors. *Ned Tijschr Tandheelkd,* 107:402–5.
86. Wallman, C., & Krasse, B. (1992). Mutans streptococci on margins of fillings and crowns. *J Dent,* 20:163–66.
87. Lindquist, B., & Emlson, C. G. (1990). Distribution and prevalence of mutans streptococci in the human dentition. *J Dent Res,* 69:1160–66.
88. Kidd, E. A. M. (1990). Caries diagnosis within restored teeth. *Adv Dent Res,* 4:10–13.
89. Kidd, E. A. M., & O'Hara, J. W. (1990). The caries status of occlusal amalgam restorations with marginal defects. *J Dent Res,* 69:1275–77.
90. Elderton, R. J. (1983). Longitudinal study of dental treatment in the General Dental Service in Scotland. *Br Dent J,* 155:91–96.
91. Elderton, R. J. (1990). Clinical studies concerning re-restoration of teeth. *Adv Dent Res,* 4:4–9.

92. Skartveit, L., Wefel, J. S., & Ekstrand, J. (1991). Effect of fluoride amalgams on artificial recurrent enamel and root caries. *Scand J Dent Res*, 99:287–94.

93. Dijkman, G. E. H. M., de Vries, J., Lodding, A., & Arenda, J. (1993). Long-term fluoride release of visible light-activated composites *in vitro*: A correlation with in situ demineralization data. *Caries Res*, 27:117–23.

94. Stephan, R. M. (1910). Changes in hydrogen–ion concentration on tooth surfaces and in carious lesions. *JADA*, 27:718–23.

95. Dodds, M. W. J., & Edgar, W. M. (1998). The relationship between plaque pH, plaque acid anion profiles and oral carbohydrate retention after ingestion of several 'reference foods' by human subjects. *J Dent Res*, 67:861–65.

96. ten Cate, J. M. (1992). Saliva a physiological medium. *Ned Tijdschr Tandheelkr*, 99:82–4.

97. ten Cate, J. M. (2001). Remineralization of caries lesions extending into dentin. *J Dent Res*, 80:1407–11.

98. Ogaard, B. (1999). The cariostatic mechanism of fluoride. *Comp Contin Educ Dent*, 20 (1 Suppl):10–17.

99. ten Cate, J. M., & Loveren, van Cor (1999). Fluoride mechanisms. *Dent Clinics Nor Amer*, 43:713–42.

100. Rosin-Grget, K., & Lincir, J. (2001). Current concept on the anticaries fluoride mechanism of the action. *Coll Antropol*, 25:703–12.

101. Gaffar, A. (1998). Treating hypersensitivity with fluoride varnishes. *Comp Cont Edu Dent*, 19:1088–90.

102. Beltran-Aguilar, E. D., Goldstein, J. W., & Lockwood, S. A. (2000). Fluoride varnishes. A review of their clinical use, cariostatic mechanisms, efficacy and safety. *JADA*, 131:589–96.

103. Seppa, L. (1991). Studies of fluoride varnishes in Finland. *Proc Finn Dent Soc*, 87:541–47.

104. Autio-Gold, J. T., & Courts, F. (2000). Assessing the effect of fluoride varnish on early enamel carious lesions in the primary dentition. *JADA*, 132:1247–53.

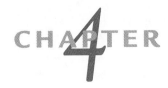

# CHAPTER 4

# The Role of Dental Plaque in the Etiology and Progress of Periodontal Disease

*Donald E. Willmann*
*Norman O. Harris*

## OBJECTIVES

*At the end of this chapter it will be possible to:*

1. Name and describe the functions of the five components of the periodontium.
2. Give the boundaries of the normal gingival sulcus.
3. Differentiate between gingivitis and periodontitis and explain the role of the junctional epithelial attachment in making the correct diagnosis.
4. Describe characteristic microflora associated with periodontal health, gingivitis, and periodontitis.
5. Explain how periodontal disease progresses starting with a healthy periodontium and ending with advanced periodontitis.
6. Describe the role of the host defenses involved in periodontal disease.
7. Briefly discuss the value of identifying a genetic factor that would permit predicting the level of risk for periodontal disease.

# INTRODUCTION

Periodontal disease is a biofilm[a] (dental plaque) induced disease.[1] In its mildest form, periodontal disease is characterized by slight inflammatory changes of the surface tissues surrounding the teeth; in its severest form, there is a massive loss of tooth-supporting structures and subsequent tooth loss[2,3] (Figure 4–1A and B).

When early periodontal disease is limited to the surface tissues (i.e., the gingiva), it is referred to as *gingivitis*. Gingivitis is a common clinical finding, and it affects nearly everyone at some time during a lifetime. Gingivitis can usually be cured by use of *primary* preventive measures.

Periodontal disease that affects the deeper tooth-supporting structures is referred to as *periodontitis*. Damage done by periodontitis is usually *not* reversible with primary preventive measures, but primary preventive procedures play an essential role in the *control* of periodontitis.[4]

Periodontal diseases are widespread and worldwide. It is now the consensus that *periodontal disease* is an umbrella term designating several clinically similar diseases with probable different modifiers. Periodontitis has been estimated to affect the majority of adults in the United States, with *advanced* periodontitis affecting 5 to 20% of the overall population.[5] Periodontitis is age-related, but this statement can be misleading because it implies that periodontal disease is directly related to the aging process. Instead, studies have shown that the periodontal health of seniors is more closely related to personal oral hygiene habits than age per se.

Periodontal disease is a multifactorial disease with the primary etiology being bacteria, but with the subsequent tissue damage being amplified by associated factors such as *medical conditions,*[6-9] *environmental* factors,[10,11] and *genetic background*.[12-14] Prime examples of these associated factors that can affect the progress of periodontal disease are: (1) the close relationship between the severity of periodontal disease and the severity of Type 2 diabetes mellitus;[15,16] (2) the relationship between periodontal disease and exposure to tobacco and tobacco products—cigarettes, spit (chewing) tobacco, and the environmental exposure of nonsmokers to cigarette smoke.[17,18] and (3) the relationship between genetically influenced inflammatory mediators and periodontitis.[19-21] To these can be added two more: calculus, and the term idiopathic—meaning that it is not known.

At one time, it was believed that the systemic disease—periodontal disease relationship was *unidirectional* and that periodontitis could adversely affect a systemic disease, but not vice versa. It is clear today, however, that the presence of some systemic diseases can also affect the dental status of some patients. This complex relationship between periodontitis and systemic diseases has been referred to as *bidirectional synergism*.[22,23]

---

[a]The terms "biofilm" and "plaque" will be used interchangeably throughout the book.

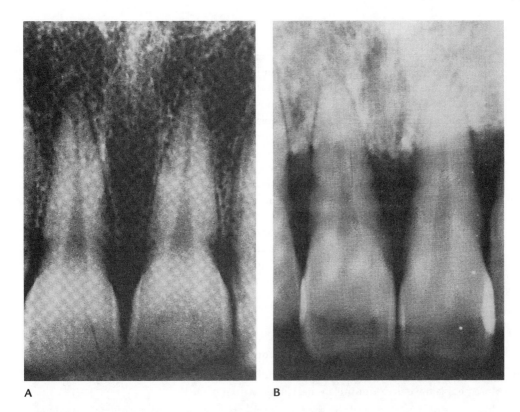

A                                                      B

FIGURE 4-1    **A.** X-ray film of two central incisors showing only slight interproximal bone loss. **B.** A much greater bone loss is seen in advanced periodontal disease. (Courtesy of Dr. O Langland, University of Texas Dental School at San Antonio.)

The prevalence of periodontal diseases in the United States may increase in the future because (1) longer life spans are increasing the *time* that teeth are at risk, and (2) people are taking better care of their teeth, thus maintaining their teeth longer and thereby increasing the *number* of teeth at risk. On the other hand, the prevalence of periodontal disease in the United States may *decrease* because access to information about periodontal disease has exploded making more people aware enough to employ preventive measures. Either way improvements in the early diagnosis and the early treatment rendered are needed since some people will not have access to the manpower intensive periodontal care needed for the repeated monitoring and treatment for what is a lifelong disease.[24]

Possibly science will help supply the answer. The successful completion of the Human Genome Project to decode the DNA molecule offers the tantalizing possibility of developing genetic approaches to prevention, diagnosis, prognosis, more effective and nonsurgical care of periodontal disease—or even to the development of a vaccine.

Roy Page, a noted periodontal research scientist, has sounded an optimistic evaluation of our present status of prevention and control of periodontal disease: ". . . there has been a convergence of basic and clinical research to produce a logarithmic increase in the rate of progress. Scientific consensus has been reached in many areas. . . . The microbial etiology is accepted and the identity of the major pathogenic bacterial species are known . . . the immuno-inflammatory pathways activated by bacteria that underlie destruction of the alveolar bone and the connective tissues of the periodontium are reasonably well understood. The evidence shows that these pathways are held in common *by all forms* of periodontitis. . . ."[25]

In spite of many scientific advances, there are problems for practicing dentists. It is not possible to *predict* periodontal disease risk accurately.[26,27] The presence of periodontal pockets is *not* an indicator of the actual activity of disease at the time of examination. Thus, there are from 3 to 5% of periodontal patients who have frequent episodes of rapid disease progression that cannot be identified until an *ex post facto* examination confirms that the damage has already occurred.[28,29] This may sound discouraging, but it should be noted that genetic research is being accomplished to find a marker that will help predict periods of disease activity and may then lead to more effective treatment.[30]

---

### Question 1

Which of the following statements, if any, are correct?

A. Periodontitis can be cured; gingivitis cannot usually be cured.

B. More people have periodontitis in their lifetime than gingivitis.

C. Most cases of periodontitis look similar clinically but probably have different etiologies and modifiers.

D. Currently, it is not possible to predict future prevalence or severity or periodontal disease.

E. Bidirectional synergism is believed to link some systemic diseases with periodontal disease.

---

### The Periodontium

There are five anatomical structures that function to support the teeth in the jaws: (1) *alveolar bone*, (2) *cementum*, and (3) *periodontal ligament*, which serve to *anchor* the teeth in the alveolar sockets of the maxilla and mandible, and (4) the dentogingival junction (epithelial attachment), which acts as a seal to protect the anchoring components from the hostile oral environment, and (5) the free marginal gingiva, which protects the dentogingival junction and underlying structures. Collectively these five structures comprise the *periodontium*.

A network of collagen fibers makes up the periodontal ligament. The periodontal ligament suspends the tooth in the alveolar socket with one end of each fiber embedded in the alveolar bone and the other end of each fiber embedded in the cementum of the tooth root. The principal fibers of the periodontal ligament have different orientations and functions at various levels on the tooth root (Figure 4–2). The *apical* fibers are generally parallel to the long axis of the tooth and help *cushion* the tooth from occlusal forces. Those at the *midpoint* on the root are *oblique* to the tooth surface, with the cemental origin *apical* to the

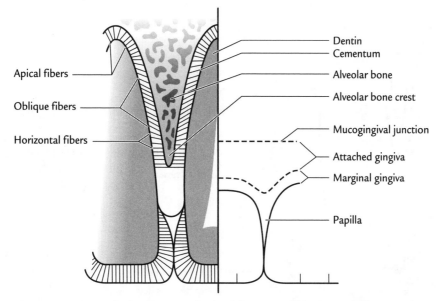

Apical fibers

Oblique fibers

Horizontal fibers

Dentin
Cementum
Alveolar bone
Alveolar bone crest
Mucogingival junction
Attached gingiva
Marginal gingiva
Papilla

FIGURE 4–2    Periodontium: Apical, oblique, and horizontal fibers make up the *periodontal ligament,* which connects the cementum of the tooth to the alveolar bone. Marginal gingiva follows the contour of the tooth. Dentogingival junction is shown in Figure 4–3.

bony insertion; those of the cervical area are nearly *horizontal*. The oblique fibers act as a *sling* to help resist downward pressures while the horizontal fibers resist lateral forces. In addition, a network of blood vessels within the periodontal ligament serve as a *hydraulic cushion* to protect the bone and periodontal fibers from excessive occlusal forces.

The dentogingival junction is at the apical termination of the gingival sulcular epithelium where it attaches to the enamel. This biologic seal functions to anchor the sulcular epithelium to the tooth surface and to protect the underlying periodontal fibers from the hostile oral environment (Figure 4-3).

The *free* margin of the gingival is a narrow coronal extension of the *attached gingival* ending up as the interproximatl papilla between the teeth. It is attached by collegen fibers to the cementum and periosteum of the alveolar bone. The free margin tightly *encircles, but is*

*not attached* to the cervical area of the tooth. Thus, a *potential* space exists between the free margin of the gingival and the tooth. This narrow crevice is called the *gingival sulcus* (or crevice)[b], and the epithelial lining of the sulcus is termed *sulcular* (or *crevicular*) epithelium (Figure 4–3B).

At the base of the gingival sulcus is the junctional epithelium. This very special epithelium is actually attached to the enamel, forming a seal between the soft tissue and the tooth surface. This biologic seal functions not only to anchor the soft tissues to the tooth surface but also to protect the underlying periodontal fibers from the hostile oral environment (Figure 4–3C).

The *junctional epithelium* forming the dentogingival attachment is one of the most crucial structures in the practice of periodontics

[b]The terms *sulcus* and *crevice* can be used interchangeably.

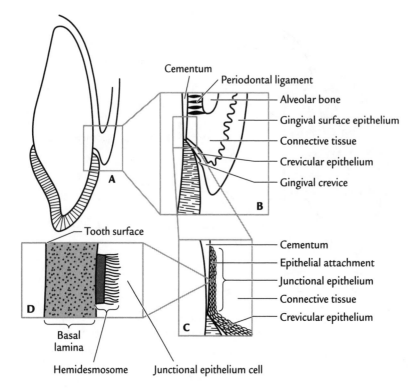

Cementum
Periodontal ligament
Alveolar bone
Gingival surface epithelium
Connective tissue
Crevicular epithelium
Gingival crevice

Tooth surface

Cementum
Epithelial attachment
Junctional epithelium
Connective tissue
Crevicular epithelium

Basal lamina

Hemidesmosome

Junctional epithelium cell

FIGURE 4-3

Dentogingival junction: The junction between the tooth and gingival soft tissues **A.** and **B.** occurs where a few layers of junctional epithelial cells **C.** are joined to the tooth by an attachment mechanism that consists of hemidesmosomes located in each cell and a basal lamina between the cell body and the tooth **D.**

(Figure 4–3D). The junctional epithelial cells (JEC) are joined to the tooth surface by hemidesmosomes, and they consist of a few layers of epithelial cells that *initially* extend a short distance along the *enamel* surface at the cementoenamel junction[31] (Study 4–3). Any inflammation, especially chronic inflammation such as in the periodontitis, can result in an apical migration of the JE cells, first over the cementoenamel junction, and then apically onto the cementum.

This apical migration of junctional epithelium is of critical importance. For each millimeter of apical migration of the attachment, there is also an accompanying loss of one millimeter of periodontal fibers attached between the cementum and bone. As the junctional epithelium migrates apically in more advanced disease, there can be loss of alveolar bone and an exposure of the cementum to which the fibers were originally attached. The migration

also causes a deepening of the sulcus to form a *periodontal pocket*. This apical migration of the junctional epithelium and consequent loss of attachment is the hallmark sign of periodontitis.

## The Supracrestal Collagen Fiber Apparatus

The marginal gingiva is held firmly against the tooth by a complex arrangement of collagen fibers. These fibers, which are arranged in bundles, are divided into groups according to their orientation and insertion into the periodontal tissues. Some fibers encircle the tooth and are called *circumferential* fibers. These are attached to other collagen fibers much like in Figure 4–4. Other groups of fibers are inserted into cementum and extend into the crest and periosteum of the alveolar bone and are known as *dento-periosteal* fibers. Still another group of fibers, called

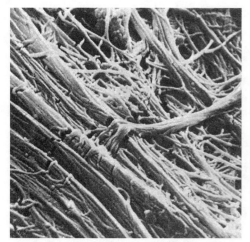

**FIGURE 4-4**   Electron scanning microscopic view of collagen bundles in the periodontal ligament space. Note narrow bundle crossing thick bundle at right angle. (From Svejda J, Skach M. The periodontium of the human teeth in the scanning electron microscope (stereoscan). *J. Periodont.* 1973;44:478–484.)

*transseptal fibers*, extend from the cementum of one tooth, over the alveolar crest of interproximal bone, and into the cementum of the adjacent teeth (Figure 4–5). Together, all these fibers serve to maintain the close, tight contact of the free marginal gingiva against the tooth.

Surrounding the teeth and covering the marginal alveolar bone, the soft tissue is keratinized and is referred to as the *attached gingiva;* on the palatal side it can simply be referred to as *palatal mucosa*. The attached gingiva extends to the *muco-gingival junction* where the mucosa and the attached gingiva meet (Figure 4–2B).

## The Gingival Sulcus

As previously discussed, the gingival sulcus is a potential space between the free margin of the gingiva and the tooth (Figure 4–3B and C). The gingival sulcus, that is *normally* 2 to 3 millimeters in depth, is bounded on the outer side by a thin *sulcular epithelium* and on the inner side by the *tooth;* the orifice of this sulcus opens into the oral cavity. As already discussed, the *apical* termination of the sulcus is the junctional epithelium (epithelial attachment).

In a longitudinal section of the free gingiva (Figure 4–3A), the tissues encountered in going from the sulcus to the oral vestibule or palate are (1) sulcular epithelium, (2) connective tissue, and (3) attached gingiva surface epithelium. The sulcular and attached gingiva merge at the crest of the free gingival margin (Figure 4-3B). In the interposed connective tissue there are plexi of blood vessels, lymphatics, and nerves supplying both surfaces (Figure 4–3B and C). It should be noted that immediately beneath the sulcular epithelium in the connective tissues, the entire resources of the host cellular and humoral defense system are available via the vascular system to help minimize the noxious effects of plaque bacteria.

When gingival inflammation is present, fluid flows from the depths of the gingival sulcus. This *gingival crevicular fluid (GCF)* is a transudate derived from blood vessels in the connective tissue adjacent to the sulcus, and an increase in GCF flow is one of the first detectable signs of impending gingivitis. An increase in GCF flow is present prior to the development of the overt signs of inflammation, and the flow rate is primarily dependent on the severity of inflammation.[32] Following a cessation of all attempts at oral hygiene, an increase of gingival crevicular flow can be observed as early as the ninth day.[33]

The flow of GCF has been measured and the total flow of fluid has been estimated to replace the fluid in the crevice approximately 40 times an hour.[34] Gingival crevicular fluid serves several protective functions. It can help clear bacteria from the gingival sulcus, as well as serve as the vehicle for leukocytes, complement, antibodies, and assorted enzymes that help protect the enamel *and* the periodontium from bacterial attack. GCF serves as one of the first lines of *host defense* against the bacteria that cause peri-

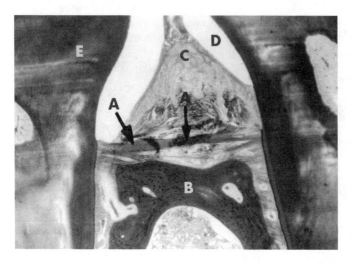

FIGURE 4–5    Cross-sectional view of interdental papillae showing **A.** transseptal fibers, **B.** alveolar crest, **C.** dental papillae, **D.** enamel space, and **E.** dentin. (Courtesy of Dr. Don Willmann, University of Texas Dental School at San Antonio.)

odontal disease and the bacteria that cause caries. The presence of an increasing flow of GCF has been related to the presence and *increasing severity* of gingivitis but *not* to the severity of periodontitis.

---

**Question 2**

Which of the following statements, if any, are correct?

A. The periodontium consists of the following four components: alveolar bone, dentogingival junction, dentin, and periodontal ligament.

B. All the principal fibers of the periodontal ligament are parallel to the long axis of the tooth.

C. The gingival crevicular fluid is a filtrate of the saliva.

D. A predictable increase in the flow of gingival sulcular fluid can be expected to parallel the severity of gingivitis but not the severity of periodontitis.

E. The circumferential fibers of the supracrestal fiber apparatus are attached to the alveolar bone.

---

## The Developing Gingival Lesion

When a phase microscope is used to view a sample of crevicular fluid from a healthy, tightly adapted marginal gingival, only a relatively few forms of bacteria can be seen in the sulcus. They include mainly non-motile coccal forms, with the only bacterial movement being confined to a *few* vibrio moving erratically about the field.

The microscopic view of the flora from a diseased gingival sulcus, is markedly different and includes *many* motile bacteria. Although it is not possible to use these phase-scope evaluations to quantitate the numbers and types of bacteria present, the contrasting differences in microbial activity seen at the two ends of the spectrum of periodontal health and disease may permit subjective evaluations to be made (Figure 4–6).

Since the free margin of the gingiva constitutes the first line of defense for the periodontium, it is usually the initial site of gingival disease. If plaque is allowed to accumulate on a tooth surface adjacent to the gingiva, inflammation of the free margin results. In a healthy mouth following cessation of oral hygiene measures, this change takes only *9 to 21* days before gingivitis can be observed clinically.

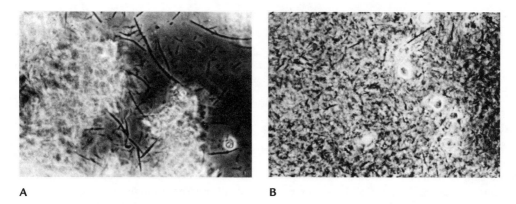

A                                    B

FIGURE 4-6    **A.** Few plaque organisms (dark figures) from a relatively healthy crevice as seen with a phase microscope. **B.** Great increase in number of organisms seen in moderate-to-severe marginal gingivitis.

With gingivitis, the extent of the gingival involvement parallels the extent of the plaque build-up. Early gingival clinical changes include alterations in color, contour changes from knife-edge-to-rolled, and a consistency change from firm-to-spongy. In addition with gingivitis, the free margin often bleeds on gentle manipulation such as from toothbrushing or probing. In the early stages, the developing inflammatory process can be completely reversed (i.e., cured) by professional intercession and personal home oral hygiene (Figure 4–7).

Not all gingival pathology is caused solely by bacterial plaque. Systemic conditions such as pregnancy or other hormonal changes cause the tissues to react more readily to the bacterial insult. There can also be gingival changes caused by inherited diseases such as hereditary fibromatoses, and by the use of certain drugs such as phenytoin that is commonly used to

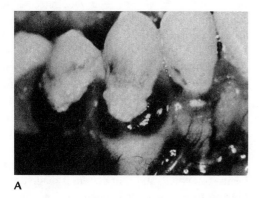
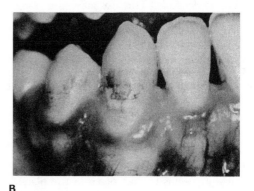

A                                    B

FIGURE 4-7    **A.** A severe gingivitis with calculus, food debris and abysmally poor self care. Note the rolled and edematous gingival. **B.** After a few days of diligent use of a brush, floss and irrigation. (Courtesy of Dr. Donald Willmann, University of Texas Dental School at San Antonio, TX.)

control epilepsy.[35,36] Control of these latter conditions can be shared medical-dental responsibilities.

## Periodontal Microflora

Historically, two hypotheses have guided most thinking about periodontal microflora; the *nonspecific* plaque hypothesis and the *specific* plaque hypothesis. The nonspecific plaque hypothesis simply related periodontal disease to the overall amount of plaque present—the more plaque, the more disease. The specific plaque hypothesis attributed the various manifestations of the periodontal plaque diseases to "specific" (although not necessary known) bacteria.

Periodontitis appears to conform to the specific hypothesis because certain bacterial species have been associated (but not always) with most destructive periodontal diseases.[12] Much evidence incriminates certain microorganisms, or combinations of organisms as etiological factors.[13] For example, the microbial species that appear to be associated with the most common variety of periodontitis (chronic periodontitis) are *Actinobacillus actinomycetemcomitans* (AA), *Porphyromonas gingivalis*, *Prevotella intermedia*, *Bacteroides forsythus*, *Fusobacterium species*, *Campylobacter rectus*, and *Treponema denticola*. This list may seem long, but keep in mind that 300 to 500 different species of bacteria are estimated to inhabit the oral cavity.[37,38] Despite this presumptive evidence of etiology, none of the suspected organisms has yet been successfully implanted into a test animal to duplicate the original disease followed by recovery of the same organism from the test animal as required by Koch's postulates.

As the health status of the marginal gingiva deteriorates from health to gingivitis, a proportional shift begins to take place in the plaque bacteria, going first *from* aerobic, nonmotile Gram-positive cocci and rods,[39–41] to facultative bacteria *to* anaerobic, Gram-negative, motile species. This major shift in the plaque

bacteria foreshadows the onset of pathology—in this case, gingivitis. Microscopic examination reveals an increase in numbers of both motile rods and spirochetes, with the latter two comprising approximately 20% of the microorganisms.[39,41,42]

## The Plaque of the Deepening Pocket

All periodontitis is preceded by gingivitis, but not all untreated gingivitis progresses to periodontitis. For example, Ronderos completed a study of the indigenous people of the Amazon rain forest and found that most individuals had a loss of epithelial attachment. In spite of poor oral hygiene and extensive gingival inflammation, they did *not* have severe periodontal destruction.[43]

A diagnosis of gingivitis implies that the actual level of the junctional epithelial attachment has *not* migrated apically but is still on the enamel or on the cementoenamel junction. A diagnosis of periodontitis implies that the junctional epithelium has migrated apically 2, 3, or more millimeters *from its original* level at the cementoenamel junction (CEJ). This migration creates a deeper gingival sulcus that is the *periodontal pocket*. The formation of the periodontal pocket with its relatively inaccessible subgingival plaque creates the need for periodontal treatment.

As the pocket deepens, subgingival plaque acquires new characteristics that differentiate it from the supragingival plaque. In the *supra*gingival plaque, the bacteria and the interbacterial matrix are well confined to the enamel. This biofilm can easily be removed by a dental prophylaxis. In the subgingival plaque, a two-compartment subgingival plaque system begins to evolve, and that system is made up of (1) the tooth-associated subgingival plaque (a biofilm on the cementum), and (2) a more fluid environment referred to as the epithelium-associated plaque that bathes the cemen-

tum. This fluid consists of purulent fluids (pus), food debris, body defense cells, and saliva—all confined under low-oxygen tension without circulation within the pocket.[44] Bacteroides and spirochetes are consistent inhabitants of this more fluid environment. The Gram-negative organisms that extend deep into the pocket are believed to be the plaque inhabitants responsible for the continued damage and migration of the epithelial attachment.

The tooth-associated subgingival plaque is initially an apical extension of the supragingival plaque into the deepening crevicular area. The bacterial population may still include some mutans streptococci although their numbers decrease as the distance increases below the gingiva.[45] However, the fact that they are there probably accounts for the root caries that often accompanies periodontal diseases. Subgingival calculus complicates disease control by sheltering the plaque bacteria from routine plaque control measures.

## Cellular Defense of the Body

The body has three key functions of immunological defense: (1) to protect it from outside invaders (antigens); (2) to destroy or neutralize the antigens that do penetrate the epithelial defenses, and, (3) to repair any damage caused by the antigen-antibody reactions. To accomplish this task, the body uses a cellular immunity and a humoral immunity. The cells responsible for the cellular defense are the granular cells that consist of the granulocytes (basophils, eosinophils and polymorphonuclear neutrophils), the monocytes (macrophages) plus those of lymphoid origin, the T and the B lymphocytes.

During the cellular response to a periodontal infection, there is first a chemotactic signal from an inflamed gingival site that initiates the cellular immune response.[46,47] This signal could possibly arise from the epithelial cells under

bacterial attack. For example, in laboratory studies, it was demonstrated that the gingival epithelial cells can cause an increase in the secretion of potent neutrophil chemotactic IL-8 following *Actinobacillus actinomycetemcomitans* challenge.[48] The defense cells then arrive at the inflamed site in a definite sequence. Initially, during the *acute* phase of inflammation, large numbers of polymorphonuclear neutrophils (PMNs, polys) enter the connective tissue underlying the sulcus. The acute phase may last from a few days to a few weeks. However, if the inflammation continues to the *subacute* stage, there is a decrease of PMNs that are replaced by lymphocytes. This stage lasts a few weeks to a few months. Finally, if healing does not occur, the lymphocytes are largely replaced by plasma cells, macrophages and mast cells. The inflammation is now in the *chronic* stage.

The above-cellular immune response can be linked to predictable histopathologic events. Within 2 to 4 days of plaque accumulation, the microscopic picture of the connective tissue is one of early inflammation. *Vasculitis* is present and extra vascular PMNs begin to appear in large numbers in the connective tissue. Edema is present because of fluid permeation through the capillary walls. After 4 to 7 days the vasculitis becomes *clinically apparent* with the appearance of the *four cardinal signs of inflammation*—heat, redness, swelling, and pain.

The heat and the change of color of the marginal gingival to red is caused by the increased blood flow to the area. The gingival swelling is caused by the edema which in turn is caused by leakage from the dilated capillaries. The fluid pressure of edema on nerve endings can cause an acute soreness. When the pain and swelling of the gingivitis is sufficiently painful, altered eating habits can result.

If the gingivitis is treated at this point by professional and home care, there can be a *complete* return of the gingiva to normal. The shallow sulcus is soon cleared of killed bacteria and dead cells by the gingival crevicular fluid,

while the saliva flushes and neutralizes residual oral debris.

The development of a chronic stage, especially with pocket formation is accompanied by a different series of reactions. The bacteria possess enzymes that can be lethal to the defense cells,[49] and the defense cells contain potent weaponry in the form of enzymes to destroy the bacteria. Thus, there are cellular or humoral reactions, dying cells and dying bacteria in the inflamed area that contribute to the "battlefield debris" while the destruction of the nearby epithelial cells, fibroblasts, and bone are the "collateral damage." Also, the macrophage alone has its own repertoire of bacterial killing agents such as oxygen and nitrogen, as well as hypochlorite (bleach).[50] Other products of an activated macrophage include numerous proteins that affect coagulation, and multiplication of cells that generate new tissue and repair damaged tissue.[51] This bacteria-epithelial-and-defense cell carnage is *continuously* taking place in the small pocket area. The low-oxygen tension and low circulation within the pocket aid in *perpetuating* the pathogenicity of the involved inflamed periodontal site.

Because of its complexity, a discussion of the *humoral* defense of the periodontal site is beyond the scope of this book. But growing evidence points to the immune system playing an important role in the pathogenesis of periodontitis. One genetic factor, interleukin-1 should be mentioned because it has received attention as a marker that can help predict the risk for periodontal disease.[52] Interleukin-1 is a pro-inflammatory cytokine that is a key regulator of the host responses to microbial infection and a major modulator of the extracellular matrix catabolism and bone resorption.[53] There are other cytokines involved in tissue destruction such as IL-8, IL-10, and IL-11.[54]

Since interleukin-1[c] is a genetic factor, it may serve as a marker for a lifetime risk factor.

A great advantage of such a marker is that it would help identify higher-risk individuals early in the periodontal disease process.[55] Since bacteria are an *essential* ingredient of periodontal disease, a positive genetic marker would serve to focus immediate attention on the daily requirement for meticulous mechanical and chemical plaque control to negate the effect of the plaque bacteria. For a clinical practice it would greatly aid in developing the periodontal treatment plan and recall schedules.[56]

There is already a test for interleukin-1 that is now being marketed. Thus, this genetic marker is currently being used to help predict the future course of the disease.[57]

---

**Question 3**

Which of the following statements, if any, are correct?

A. It takes 9 to 21 days after ceasing toothbrushing and flossing before a gingivitis develops.

B. *Actinobacillus actinomycetemcomitans* is the correct spelling for the bacterium often designated as *AA*. (Better learn the correct spelling since it will confront you often.)

C. When the junctional epithelium is positioned on the enamel, the diagnosis would be either that of a healthy periodontium, or at worst, gingivitis.

D. More motile organisms would be expected on the tooth-associated biofilm than in the epithelium-associated plaque.

E. A specific genetic marker for a disease could predict the probability of specific disease at any time after birth.

---

### Terminal Events

To complete this brief introduction to the periodontal disease process, a few of the concluding events need to be mentioned. As the chronic

---

[c]Interleukin Genetics, Inc., Waltham, MA. 02452

inflammation continues, the junctional epithelium slowly migrates onto the cemento-enamel junction and continues apically onto the cementum. Bone and soft tissue continue to be lost (Figure 4–1B). The periodontal pocket continues to deepen, making the control of disease even more difficult. Eventually, this continuing loss of tooth support results in a loosening of the tooth. This destruction of hard and soft tissues can continue until little or no support remains for the tooth. Extraction then becomes necessary, at which time all components of the periodontium are lost.

### Enter Primary Preventive Dentistry

The most important strategy for preventing periodontal disease is avoidance by exercising prevention from the earliest age (Figure 4–8). In principal, prevention requires the daily removal of plaque from the teeth with a toothbrush, dental floss, and with the use of an irrigator to flush away debris. *Mechanical plaque control* can be supplemented with the use of *chemical plaque control* measures as an adjunct. This may involve the use of chlorhexidine or essential-oil mouthrinses as an easy way to help aid in bacterial plaque control. Fluoride mouthrinses can be used to aid in preventing root caries, as well as coronal caries.

Patients who note "bleeding gums" should be encouraged to consult a dentist. A thorough prophylaxis, including removal of plaque-retention factors such as calculus and overhanging restorations, plus more diligent home care, usually suffices to accomplish a quick cure for gingivitis. Recall appointments should be on a schedule that is reasonable to limit future pathogenic plaque build-up.

For patients with periodontitis, there is a focus on removing biofilm from the cementum and a focus on disruption of the subgingival microbial flora. With some irrigation units, special tips permit patients to irrigate shallow pockets, which aids in flushing out the toxins from the epithelial-related plaque.[58] Thorough debridement of tooth surfaces is also necessary. This can be accomplished by either using curets or ultrasonic instrumentation. In some patients with *shallow pockets*, the selective use of microbrushes, or air abrasive techniques can also be used to clean the biofilm from the cementum.[59,60]

Some periodontal patients have such advanced tissue destruction and deep pockets that periodontal surgery becomes necessary. But no matter how complex the surgical procedures nor how intensive the therapy used to treat patients, primary preventive measures play a critical role in helping to *maintain disease control* once periodontal health has been reestablished.

A major challenge in primary preventive dentistry is to increase public awareness that home-care programs can maintain excellent oral health. An effective supragingival plaque-control program and a biannual professional examination routine that is established *early* in

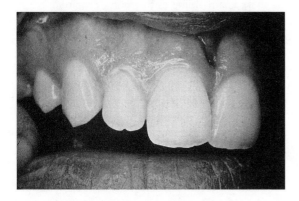

FIGURE 4–8 "Good periodontal health. This is what we want to keep." (Courtesy of Dr. Donald Willmann, University of Texas Dental School at San Antonio, TX.)

life minimizes the conditions leading to the development of periodontal disease.

It was long believed that once the subgingival plaque was permanently organized, supragingival plaque control activities had no effect on the subgingival plaque. However, more recent evidence has demonstrated that meticulous supragingival plaque control measures can indeed delay the initiation and organization of the subgingival plaque.[61–63]

This introduction to the periodontal diseases will be continued in Chapter 13.

## Question 4

Which of the following statements, if any, are correct?

A. A chemotactic signal is necessary to initiate an immune response.

B. The objective for both supra- and subgingival plaque control is to routinely disrupt, remove and delay the re-population of the plaque by pathogenic microbes.

C. The supra- and the subgingival plaques are completely independent of each other.

D. The tooth-associated subgingival plaque is on the cementum; the fluid epithelium-associated plaque is not.

E. There is biofilm that can be removed from enamel, and also biofilm that can be removed from the cementum.

# SUMMARY

Periodontitis is a disease involving pathology of one or more of the four components of the periodontium—the epithelial attachment, alveolar bone, cementum, and periodontal ligament. The term "periodontal disease" is an umbrella term for several clinically similar types of diseases due to different bacteria and different modifying factors. Gingivitis, by definition, becomes periodontitis when the epithelial attachment migrates apically from the cemento-enamel junction. Periodontitis is caused by a combination of bacterial species. The bacteria associated with healthy gingiva are usually composed of aerobic, nonmotile, Gram-positive cocci. In contrast, the microorganisms for the subgingival plaque that are associated with disease usually are anaerobic, Gram-negative motile rods and treponema. The supragingival biofilm is on the enamel, the tooth-associated subgingival plaque is on the cementum. In the area separating the supra- from the subgingival plaque there is a melding of bacteria of the two biofilms. To combat the bacterial challenge, when there is a site of inflammation, the body recognizes chemotactic signals that bring both cellular and humoral elements to the inflamed areas. In the treatment of patients with periodontal disease, it is not possible to *predict* speed of development and severity of the disease with complete accuracy. Estimating of these variables can be made by study of clinical signs of inflammation and past disease behavior. Much research is being accomplished to tap the great potential of genetics to identify etiologic bacteria, to aid in diagnosis, and to enhance treatment. The Human Genome Project, a worldwide effort that decoded the DNA molecule is expected to enhance these efforts in the future. Studies of interleukin-1

(IL-1), a cytokine, have indicated that laboratory evaluation of this cytokine can help identify those individuals at higher risk for developing severe periodontal diseases. IL-1 has also been found to be related to bleeding on probing (which is an accepted method of determining the severity of periodontitis). Since IL-1 is a lifetime genetic factor, one test for this factor may suffice to assign risk for a lifetime. This test may also be used in developing treatment plans for individual patients.[64] Since bacteria are essential for periodontitis, a positive (high blood level) of interleukin-1 should alert the dentist and the patient of the importance of carrying out daily mechanical and chemical plaque control.

## ANSWERS AND EXPLANATIONS

1. C, D, E—correct.

    A—incorrect With proper treatment, gingiva affected by gingivitis can be restored to normal. With periodontitis, the apical migration of the epithelial attachment cannot usually be returned to its original position on the enamel.

    B—incorrect. Most people have gingivitis at some time in their lives, but not everyone acquires periodontitis.

2. D—correct

    A—incorrect. Dentin is wrong; cementum would have been right.

    B—incorrect. The oblique fibers and the horizontal fibers are not parallel to the long axis of the tooth—only the apical fibers are parallel.

    C—incorrect. GCF is a filtrate of blood, not of the saliva.

    E—incorrect. The circumferential fibers are intertwined with the various fiber bundles of the supragingival crest.

3. A, B, C, E—correct.

    D—incorrect. The greatest number of *motile* organisms are in the fluid of the epithelial-associated plaque; the bacteria making up the biofilm on the cementum are more permanently fixed.

4. A, B, D, E—correct.

    C—incorrect. Scrupulous supragingival plaque control aids in subgingival plaque control.

## SELF-EVALUATION QUESTIONS

1. The four components of the periodontium are _____, _____, _____, and _____.

2. Bacteria are the etiological factor for periodontal diseases; however three important amplifying factors of bacterial pathogenicity are _____, _____, and _____.

3. A widespread systemic disease that is closely associated with periodontal diseases is _____.

4. For every millimeter of attachment loss, there is an approximate one millimeter loss of _____ and _____.

5. The two components of the subgingival plaque are the _____ -associated plaque and the _____ -associated plaque.

6. The three functions of the immune defenses are _____, _____ and _____.

7. When a chemotactic signal is received, the defense cells arrive in the following order: _____ in the acute phase; _____ in the subacute phase and _____ in the chronic stage.

8. Total body defense following a chemotactic signal involves both cellular immunity and _____ immunity.

9. The four cardinal signs of inflammation are _____, _____, _____, and _____.

10. One immune factor has been of interest to the periodontist because of its possible clinical use to predict severity of the periodontal diseases. Name it: _____.

## REFERENCES

1. Socransky, S. S., & Haffajee, A. D. (1992). The bacterial etiology of destructive periodontal disease. J Periodontol, 63:322–31.
2. The American Academy of Periodontology. (1999). The pathogenesis of periodontal diseases. (Position paper) J Periodontol, 70:457–70.
3. Williams, R. C. (1990). Periodontal disease. N Engl J Med, 322:373–76.
4. Greenstein, G. (1992). Periodontal response to mechanical non-surgical therapy: A review. J Periodontol, 63:118–30.
5. Position paper. (1996). Epidermiology of periodontal disease. J Periodontol, 67:935–45.
6. Kiane, D. F., & Marshall, G. J. (2001). Periodontal manifestations of systemic disease. Aust Dent J, 46:2–12.
7. Cichon, P., Crawford, L., Grimm, W. D. (1998). Early onset periodontitis associated with Down's syndrome—clinical intervention study. Ann Periodontol, 3:370–80.
8. Nuabe, Y., Ogawa, T., Kamoi, H., Kiyonobu, K., Sato, S., Kamoi., K., & Deguchi, S. (1998). Phagocytic function of salivary PMN after smoking or secondary smoking. Ann Periodontol, 3:370–80
9. Janson, L., Lavstedt, S., Frithiof, L., & Theobold, H. (2000). Relation between oral health and mortality in cardiovascular diseases. J Clin Periodont, 28:762–8.

10. Hashim, R., Thomson, W. M., & Pack, A. R. (2001) Smoking in adolescence as a predictor of early loss of periodontal attachment. *Comm Dent Oral Epidemiol, 29*:130–5.

11. Wilson, T. G. Jr. (1998). Effects of smoking on the periodontium. *Quintessence Int, 29*:265–66.

12. Michalowicz, B. S., Diehl, S. R., Gunsolley, J. C., Sparks, B. S., Brooks, B. S., Koetge, T. E., Califano, J. V., Burmeister, J. A., & Schenkein, H. A. (2000). Evidence of a substantial genetic basis of risk of adult periodontitis. *J Periodontol, 71*:1699–1707.

13. Kornman, K. S., Knobelman, C., & Wang, N-Y. (2000). Is periodontitis genetic? The answer may be yes! *Mass Dent Soc, 49*:2–6.

14. Salvi, G. E., Lawrence, H. P., Offenbacher, S., & Beck, J. D. (1997). Influence of risk factors on the pathogenesis of periodontitis. *Periodontol 2000, 14*:173–201.

15. Taylor, G. W., Loesche, W. J., & Terpenning, M. S. (2000). Impact of oral diseases on systemic health in the elderly: diabetes mellitus and aspiration pneumonia. *J Public Health Dent, 60*:313–20.

16. Stewart, J. E., Wager, K. H., Friedlander, A. H., & Zadek, N. H. (2001). The effect of periodontal treatment on glycemic control in patients with type 2 diabetes mellitus. *J Clin Periodontol, 28*:306–10.

17. Tonetti, M. S. (1998). Cigarette smoking and periodontal diseases; etiology and management of disease. *Ann Periodontol, 25*:88–101.

18. Arbes, S. J. Jr, Agerstsdottier, H., Slade, G. D. (2001). Environmental tobacco smoke and periodontal disease in the United States. *Amer J Public Health, 91*:253–7.

19. Lerner, U. H., Modeer, T., Krekmanova, L., Claesson, R., & Rasmussen, L. (1998). Gingival crevicular fluid from patients with periodontitis contains bone resorbing activity. *Eur J Oral Sci, 106*:778–87.

20. Genco, R. J. (1992). Host responses in periodontal diseases: Current concepts. *J Periodontol, 63*(4 suppl):338–55.

21. Page, R. (1991). The role of inflammatory mediators in the pathogenesis of periodontal disease. *J Periodontal Res, 26*:230–42.

22. Fowler, E. B., Brealt, L. G., & Cuenin, M. F. (2001). Periodontal disease and its association with systemic disease. *Mil Med, 166*:85–9.

23. Brandtzaeg, P. (2001). Inflammatory bowel disease: Clinics and pathology. Do inflammatory bowel disease and periodontal disease have similar immunopathogeneses? *Acta Odontol Scand, 59*:235–43.

24. Oral Health in America: A report of the Surgeon General. Executive Summary. Year 2000. Department of Health and Human Services, U.S. Public Health Service, Washington, D.C.

25. Page, R. C. (1999). Milestones in periodontal research and the remaining critical issues. *J Periodontal Research, 34*:331–9.

26. Pearlman, B. (2000). Prognosis: The dilemma of modern periodontics. *Ann R Australas Coll Dent Surg, 15*:141–43.

27. Socransky, S. S., & Haffajee, A. D. (1997). The nature of periodontal diseases. *Ann Periodontol, 2*:3–10.

28. Page, R. C. (1998). A new paradigm. *J Dent Edu, 62*:812–20.

29. Hart, T. C., & Kornman, K. S. (1997). Genetic factors in the pathogenesis of periodontitis. *J Periodontol, 14*:141–43.

30. Cattabriga, M., Rotundo, R., Muzzi, L., Nieri, M., Verrocchi, G., Cairo, F., & Pine Prato, G. (2001). Retrospective evaluation of the influence of the interleukin-1 genotype on radiographic bone levels in treated periodontal patients over 10 years. *J. Periodontol, 72*:767–73.

31. Hormia, M., Owaribe, K., & Virt, I. (2001). The dento-epithelial junction cell adhesion by Type I hemidesmosomes in the absence of true basal lamina. *J Periodontol, 72*:788–97.

32. Griffiths, G. S., Sterne, J. A., Wilton, J. M., Eaton, K. A, & Johnson, N. W. (1992). Associations between volume and flow rate of gingival crevicular fluid and clinical assessments of gingival inflammation in a population of British male adolescents. *J Clin Periodontol, 19*:464–70.

33. Weidlich, P., Lopez de Souza, M. A., & Opperman, R. V. (2001). Evaluation of the dentogingival area during early plaque formation. *J Periodontol*, 72:901–10.

34. Position paper. (2000). The role of controlled drug delivery for periodontitis. *J Periodontol*, 71:125–140.

35. Bhowmick, S. K., Giduani, V. K., & Retting, K. R. (2001). Hereditary gingival fibromatosis and growth retardation. *Endocr Prac*, 7:383–7.

36. Majola, M. P., McFadyen, M. L., Connolly, C., et al. (2000). Factors influencing phenytoin-induced gingival enlargement. *J Clin Periodontol*, 27:506–12.

37. Socransky, S. S., & Haffajee, A. D. (1991). Microbial mechanisms in the pathogenesis of destructive periodontal diseases: A critical assessment. *J Periodontol Res*, 26:195–212.

38. Paster, B. J., Boches, S. K., Galvin, J. L., Paster, B. J., Boches, J. L., Ericson, R. E., Lau, C. N., Levarios, V. A., Sahasrabudhe, A., & Dewhirst, F. E. (2001). Bacterial diversity in human subgingival plaque. *J Bacteriol*, 183:3770–83.

39. Friedman, M. T., Barber, P. M., Mardan, N. J., & Newman, H. N. (1992). The "plaque-free zone" in health and disease: A scanning electron microscope study. *J Periodontol*, 63:890–6.

40. Periodontal Literature Review (1996). Chicago: The American Academy of Periodontology, 68–72.

41. Loe, H., Theilade, E., & Borglum, J. S. (1965). Experimental gingivitis in man. *J Periodontol*, 36:177–187.

42. Moore, W. E. C., & Moore, L. V. H. (1994). The bacteria of periodontal diseases. *Periodontol 2000*, 5:66–77.

43. Ronderas, M., Pihlstrom, B. L., & Hodges, J. S. (2001). Periodontal disease among indigenous people in the Amazon rain forest. *J Clin Periodontol*, 28:995–1003.

44. Sanz, M., & Newman, M. G. (1988). Dental plaque and calculus. In Newman, M. G., & Nisengard, R., Eds. *Oral microbiology and immunology* (367–380). Philadelphia: WB Saunders.

45. Berghton, D., Lynch, E., & Heath, M. R. (1993). A microbiological study of primary root caries lesions with different treatment needs. *J Dent Res*, 72:623–29.

46. Boch, J. A., Wara-aswapati, N., & Auron, P. E. (2000). Interleukin 1. Signal transduction—current concepts and revalence to periodontitis. *J Dent Res*, 80:400–407.

47. Flood, P. M., Washington, O., Stevens, D. P., & Ptak, W. (1992). Immunological signals which control T cell responses. *J Endod*, 18:435–39.

48. Huang, G. T., Haake, S. K., & Park, N. H. (1998). Gingival epithelial cells increase interleukin-8 secretion in response to *Actinobacillus actinomycetemcomitans* challenge. *J Periodontol*, 69:1105–10.

49. Guthmiller, J. M., Lally, E. T., & Korostoff, J. (2001). Beyond the specific plaque hypothesis: are highly leukotoxic strains of *Actinobacillus actinomycetemcomitans* a paradigm of periodontal pathogenesis? *Crit Rev Oral Biol Med*, 12:116–24.

50. Widmann, F. K., & Itatani, C. A., Eds. (1998). *An Introduction to Clinical Immunology and Serology*. Philadelphia: F.A. Davis Company. 473.

51. Gustafasson, A., Asman, B., & Bergstrom, K. (2001). Increased release of IL-B from monocytes for patients with chronic periodontitis. *J Dent Res*, 80: Spec Iss. (Abs. #0075).

52. McGuire, M. K., & Nunn, M. E. (1999). Prognosis versus actual outcome. IV. The effectiveness of clinical parameters and IL-1 genotype in accurately predicting prognoses and tooth survival. *J Periodontol*, 70:49–56.

53. Kornman, K. S., Crane, A., Wang, H-Y, diGiovine, F. S., Newman, M. G., Pink, F. W., Wilson, T. G. Jr., Higginbottom, F. L. & Duff, G. W. (1997). The interleukin-1 genotype as a severity factor in adult periodontal disease. *J Clin Periodontol*, 24:72–77.

54. Seymour, G. J., & Gemmell, E. (2001). Cytokines in periodontal disease: where to from here. *Acta Odonto Scan*, 59:167–73.

55. Schenkein, H. A. (1998). Inheritance as a determinant of susceptibility for periodontitis. *J Dent Edu*, 62:840–51.
56. McDevitt, M. J., & Wang Y-H, K. (2000). Interleukin-1 genetic association with periodontitis in clinical practice. *J Periodontol*, 71:156–62.
57. Bowers, J. E. (1999). Genetic testing. One part of periodontal risk assessment. *Pract Hygiene*, 27:627–39.
58. Cutler, C. W., Stanford, T. W., Abraham, C., Cederberg, R. A., Boardman, T. J. & Ross, C. (2000). Clinical benefits of oral irrigation for periodontitis are related to reduction of pro-inflammatory cytokine levels and plaque. *J Clin Periodontol*, 27:134–43.
59. Casey, H. M., & Daly, C. G. (2001). Subgingival debridement of root surfaces with a micro-brush: macroscopic and ultrastructural assessment. *J Clin Periodontol*, 28:820–27
60. Petersilk, G. J., Steinman, D., & Haberlein, T. F. (2001). Subgingival plaque removal by a novel low abrasive polishing powder. *J Dent Res*, 80: Spec Iss. (Abstr 180).
61. Dahlen, G., Lindhe, J., Sato, K., Hanamura, H., & Okamoto, H. (1992). The effect of supragingival plaque control on the subgingival microbiota in subjects with periodontal disease. *J Clin Periodontol*, 19:802–809.
62. Katsanoulas, T., Renee, I., & Attstrom, R. The effect of supragingival plaque control on the composition of the subgingival flora in periodontal pockets. *J Clin Periodontol*, 19:760–5.
63. Corbet, E. F., & Davies, W. I. (1993). The role of supragingival plaque in the control of progressive periodontal disease: A review. *J Clin Periodontol*, 20:307–13.
64. Bowers, J. E. (1999). Genetic testing. One part of periodontal risk assessment. *Pract Hygiene*, 27:627–39.

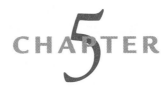

# CHAPTER 5

# Toothbrushes and Toothbrushing Methods

*Samuel L. Yankell*
*Ulrich P. Saxer*

## OBJECTIVES

*At the end of this chapter it will be possible to:*

1. Give a brief history of the toothbrush, describe its parts in detail, and explain why there is no one "ideal" brush.
2. Compare natural and nylon bristles for their uniformity of length, diameter, and durability.
3. Discuss the wide range of head and handle designs and explain why there are many "new" manual and powered toothbrush products being marketed.
4. Compare and contrast laboratory and clinical evaluations of toothbrush effectiveness.
5. Compare manual and powered toothbrushes for effectiveness and safety.
6. Compare the ADA process for evaluating "standard" and "new" manual toothbrushes.
7. Discuss modifications of toothbrushing methods applicable to special patient care, patients using prostheses, and those under orthodontic care.
8. Discuss interproximal access of different toothbrushes and their possible role in oral-disease treatment and prevention.

# INTRODUCTION

After teeth have been completely cleaned by the dental professional or by the individual, soft microbial dental plaque continually reforms on the tooth surfaces. With time, plaque is the primary agent in the development of caries, periodontal disease, and calculus—the three conditions for which individuals most often seek professional services. If plaque, particularly at interproximal and gingival areas, is completely removed with home-care procedures, these dental-disease conditions can be prevented. Unfortunately, the majority of the population is unable, uninstructed, or unwilling or does not realize the need to spend the time to remove plaque from all tooth surfaces, and/or the product(s) used are not adequate to remove plaque at critical sites. Plaque deposits can be removed either mechanically or chemically. The focus of this chapter is the mechanical removal of plaque, using toothbrushes and toothbrushing techniques. The following two chapters emphasize the use of products and auxiliary aids with toothbrushes in removing plaque and the maintenance of healthy teeth and gingival tissues.

## The Manual Toothbrush

### History

Hirschfeld, in his 1939 landmark textbook on the toothbrush and oral care, included an in-depth review of the history of toothbrushing.[1] The exact origin of mechanical devices for cleaning teeth is unknown. Ancient peoples chewed twigs from plants with high aromatic properties. Chewing these twigs freshened the breath and spread out fibers at the tips of the twig for cleaning the tooth and gum surfaces. The Arabs before Islam used a piece of the root of the arak tree because its fibers stood out like bristles; this device was called a siwak. After several uses, the bristle fibers became soft, and a new "brush" was created by stripping off the end and making new bristle fibers. In the seventh-century, Mohammed made rules for oral hygiene, and so it became a religious obligation. To this day the siwak, composed from aromatic types of wood, is still used. Chew sticks not only help to physically clean teeth but also, because they contain antibacterial oils and tannins, may help prevent or remove plaque.[2]

The Chinese are credited for inventing the toothbrush comprising a handle with bristles during the Tang dynasty (618–907 A.D.). They used hog bristles similar to those in some contemporary models. In 1780, in England, William Addis manufactured what was termed "the first modern toothbrush."[3,4] This instrument had a bone handle and holes for placement of natural hog bristles, which were held in place by wire. In the early 1900s, celluloid began to replace the bone handle, a changeover that was hastened by World War I when bone and hog bristles were in short supply. As a result of the blockade of high-quality natural hog bristles from China and Russia during World War II, nylon bristles were used instead. Initially, nylon bristles were copies of natural bristles in length and thickness. They were stiffer than natural bristles of similar diameter. They did not have the hollow stem of natural bristles and, accordingly, did not absorb water. Compared to natural bristles, nylon filaments have the additional advantages that they can be prepared in various uniform diameters and shapes, and can be end-rounded to be more gentle on gingival tissues during the brushing procedure. In 1924, an American dentist reported on 37 different manual toothbrushes with regard to handle shape, head design, bris-

tle type, length, and width. Individual dentists disagreed then, and still do today, on what type of toothbrush was best. The primary toothbrush shapes marketed in the 1940s through 1980s in the United States had flat, multitufted toothbrush-head shapes. Since the 1990s new manual toothbrushes have been introduced with new shapes, sizes, colors, and claimed advantages. By varying the length and the angle of the filaments in the brush head, brushing with these newly designed products has been documented to improve plaque removal since the bristle filaments can be directed into the sulcus or interproximal areas.[3-12] New unconventional toothbrushes with two or more heads or segments of filaments in angular relationship have shown improved plaque removal. One new brush with three heads can be used to simultaneously clean the buccal, occlusal, and lingual surfaces.[13-15] The proliferation of brushes can be attributed, in part, to advances in manufacturing, for example, the attachment of bristles into the handle using molding techniques rather than stapling to allow a wider flexibility in toothbrush designs and bristle angulations. In addition, toothbrush bristles are now available in a variety of colors, textures and shapes.

There also has been an increase in both the quality and number of laboratory and clinical research studies on toothbrushes. The International Association of Dental Research and American Association of Dental Research are major meetings for both academic and industry scientists to present their latest research. In the 1991 and 1992 key-word indexes of the abstracts accepted for presentation at these meetings, toothbrushes were not included as a topic. In 1993 the number of abstracts were ranked as dentifrices > mouthrinses > toothbrushes. Since then, through 2001, the number of dentifrice abstracts has shown marked increases or decreases, with a peak of over 90 abstracts in 1998. Mouthrinse abstracts have shown essentially a leveling-off or a slight decrease in number since 1991. Toothbrush abstracts have con-

tinued to demonstrate a consistent increase, and at the 2001 AADR meeting, exceeded dentifrices and mouthrinses.

With the scientific reports about toothbrush contamination after oral or medical bacterial/viral infections, dental professionals recommend replacing toothbrushes at 3- to 4-month intervals, so repeat purchasing of toothbrush products is done more frequently. The increase in toothbrush sales may be an additional driving force for the marketing of new designs and variety of toothbrushes. Toothbrush pricing has reached new highs with the introduction of "high-tech" manual toothbrush designs and stronger claims, yet the cost per individual product is generally less than the cost for a "family-size" tube of toothpaste or mouthrinse. Toothbrush shipping costs are less, breakage is minimal and the shelf-life (stability) is longer than for other product categories thus, the potential profitability of toothbrushes to the manufacturers may be greater than for dentifrice or mouthrinse products.

---

### Question 1

Which of the following statements, if any, are correct?

A. The toothbrush became commercially available in the United States just before the Civil War; the celluloid handle became popular during World War I; and nylon bristles appeared just before World War I.

B. While toothbrush-head designs have changed considerably in the past decade, toothbrush bristles shapes have remained essentially the same.

C. The cross section of the average toothbrush in the United States, prior to the 1990s, had a flat head and a flat bristle profile.

D. Nylon bristles are more firm or stiffer than natural bristles with the same diameter.

E. In the 1990s toothbrushes have been the subject of a steadily increasing number of laboratory and clinical research studies.

### Manual Toothbrush Designs

Manual toothbrushes vary in size, shape, texture, and design more than any other category of dental products.[5] A manual toothbrush consists of a head with bristles and a handle (Figure 5–1). When the bristles are bunched together, they are known as tufts. The head is arbitrarily divided into the toe, which is at the extreme end of the head, and the heel, which is closest to the handle. A constriction, termed the shank, usually occurs between the handle and the head. Many toothbrushes are manufactured in different sizes—large, medium, and small (or compact)—to adapt better to the oral anatomy of different individuals.[5,7] Toothbrushes also differ in their defined hardness or texture, usually being classified as hard, medium, soft or extra soft. Descriptions and measurements of selected U.S. toothbrushes are shown in Table 5–1.

Much of the early data comparing the efficacy of various toothbrush designs is contradictory because of (1) the lack of quantitative methods used to measure cleaning (plaque removal), (2) the many sizes and shapes of toothbrushes used, and (3) the lack of standardized toothbrushing procedures used in the studies. More recently, toothbrush heads have been altered to vary bristle lengths and placement in attempts to better reach interproximal areas. Handles have also been ergonomically designed to accommodate multiple dexterity levels. As described in the introduction, the change from the old flat toothbrush to multilevel designs was possible because of new bristle technology and manufacturing procedures.

### Profiles

When viewed from the side, toothbrushes have four basic lateral profiles: concave, convex, flat, and multileveled (rippled or scalloped). The concave shape can be useful for improved cleaning of facial surfaces, whereas convex shapes appear more useful for improved cleaning of lingual surfaces.[5] Lateral and cross-section profiles and the overhead appearance of selected toothbrushes commercially available in the United States are shown in Figures 5–2, 5–3 and 5–4. In laboratory and clinical studies, toothbrushes with multilevel profiles were consistently more effective than flat toothbrushes, especially when interproximal efficacy was monitored.[6,8,11,16,17]

### Bristle Shapes

Recently, new toothbrush bristle shapes and textures have been fabricated, as shown in Figure 5–5. Toothbrush products utilizing these bristles in multiple diameters, textures, and bristle trims have been developed, and laboratory studies have documented improved efficacy of toothbrushes with tapered, feathered and diamond-shaped bristles, compared to toothbrushes with standard round bristles.[18–20]

#### End-rounding

Originally, individual toothbrush bristles were cut bluntly and often had sharp end configurations. In 1948, Bass reported that these bristle tips could damage the soft tissues and that rounded, tapered, or smooth bristle tips were less abrasive.[21] Although Bass's research was not performed according to strict research protocol, his findings have remained undisputed

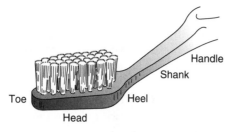

FIGURE 5–1    Parts of a toothbrush.

**TABLE 5-1** Description and Measurements of Selected U.S. Toothbrushes

| Name | Manufacturer | Top | Bottom | Number of Tufts | Head Length (cm) | Head Width (cm) | Bristle Length (cm) | Handle Length (in) |
|---|---|---|---|---|---|---|---|---|
| Aquafresh Flex | SmithKline Beecham | Oval | Oval | 43 | 3.1 | 1.1/0.5 | 1.1 | 6.2 |
| Colgate Plus | Colgate-Palmolive | Oval | Oval | 47 | 3.3 | 1.1/0.5 | 1.1 | 5.9 |
| Colgate Total | Colgate-Palmolive | Oval | Flat | 57 | 2.7 | 1.5 | 1.1/0.9 | 6.3 |
| Colgate Wave | Colgate-Palmolive | Oval | Oval | 43 | 2.9 | 1.1/0.6 | 1.2/0.9 | 6.2 |
| Crest Complete | Procter & Gamble | Flat | Flat | 38 | 2.9 | 1.0/0.5 | 1.1/0.8 | 6.2 |
| GUM 4 1 1 | J.O. Butler Co. | Oval | Flat | 42 | 2.9 | 0.8/0.4 | 1.1/0.9 | 6.2 |
| Lactona M-39 | Lactona Corp. | Oval | Flat | 43 | 3.3 | 1.3 | 1.2 | 6.3 |
| Mentadent | Chesebrough-Pond's | Oval | Flat | 56 | 3.0 | 1.5/0.4 | 1.1/0.8 | 6.2 |
| Oral-B CrossAction | Oral-B Laboratories | Oval | Flat | 31 | 3.3 | 1.0 | 1.2/1.0 | 6.6 |
| Oral-B P-35 | Oral-B Laboratories | Flat | Flat | 39 | 2.4 | 0.8 | 1.1 | 6.0 |
| Oral-B P-40 | Oral-B Laboratories | Flat | Flat | 47 | 2.8 | 1.0 | 1.1 | 5.8 |
| Oral-B P-60 | Oral-B Laboratories | Flat | Flat | 55 | 3.2 | 1.0 | 1.1 | 5.6 |
| Pepsodent | Chesebrough-Pond's | Oval | Flat | 50 | 3.6 | 1.1 | 1.1 | 6.3 |
| Pycopay Softex | Block Drug Company | Flat | Flat | 51 | 3.3 | 1.2 | 1.1 | 6.5 |
| Reach Advanced Design | Johnson & Johnson | Oval | Oval | 46 | 2.9 | 1.2/0.5 | 1.1/1.0 | 6.2 |
| Reach Plaque Sweeper | Johnson & Johnson | Oval | Oval | 43 | 3.0 | 1.1/0.6 | 1.2/0.9 | 6.2 |
| Reach Tooth & Gum Care | Johnson & Johnson | Flat | Flat | 42 | 2.9 | 1.2/0.4 | 1.2/1.0 | 6.2 |

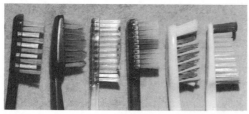

FIGURE 5–2    Lateral profiles of selected toothbrushes: Aquafresh Flex; Colgate Plus; Colgate Total; Colgate Wave; Crest Complete; Mentadent; Oral-B Advantage; Oral-B P-40; Reach Advanced Design; Reach Plaque Sweeper; Reach Tooth & Gum Care.

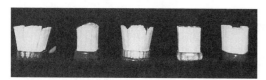

FIGURE 5–3    Cross-sectional profiles of four toothbrushes: Butler GUM; Colgate Total; Oral-B; Reach.

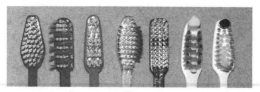

FIGURE 5–4    Overhead appearance of selected toothbrushes, from left to right: Reach Advanced Design; Aquafresh; Colgate Plus; Crest Complete; Jordan V.

for more than 40 years. Indeed, advertisers still recommend end-rounded tips for safety and to promote toothbrush sales. When toothbrushes are examined under low magnification, most bristles labeled as "rounded" do in fact appear smooth or end-rounded. However, at higher magnification, as shown in Figure 5–6, many of these "rounded" bristles take on different configurations.[5] During use, bristles become smoother and more end-rounded. With continued use, the bristles of the tuft expand and spread out.[22] Bristle wear has been shown to vary directly with the toothbrushing load and amount of dentifrice and inversely with bristle diameter.[23] In a recent study, there were no significant differences in plaque or gingivitis indices in a group in which toothbrushes were replaced on a monthly basis compared to the second group using their same toothbrush over the 3 month period. The toothbrushes used for 3 months exhibited a significant increase in the wear index compared to the baseline values.[24] A 1988 scanning-electron microscope study[25] compared end-rounding of bristles from eight marketed types. Based on statistical analysis of 30 toothbrushes of each type, acceptability varied from 22 to 88%, indicating to these authors that some brushes are not sufficiently rounded and are likely to produce gingival damage. In addition, they have abrasive potential on dentin and cementum.

A 1992 study[26] compared a ripple design with a flat-profile brush using a stereoscopic microscope with fiberoptic lighting. Close to

Hexagonal                Rectangular                Feathered

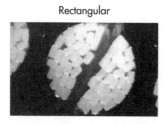

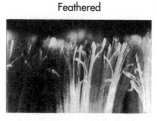

FIGURE 5–5    New shapes and textures of Tynex nylon toothbrush filaments. (Courtesy of DuPont Filaments.)

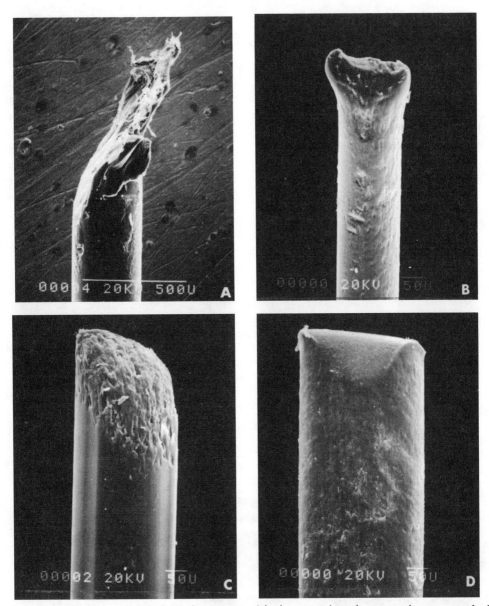

FIGURE 5-6    Toothbrush bristle ends as seen with the scanning electron microscope. **A.** A coarse-cut toothbrush bristle end, probably the result of an incomplete single-blade cut during the manufacturing process. These sharp projections can reduce the bristles' overall cleaning efficiency and damage oral tissues (SEM 85×). **B.** A slightly enlarged, bulbous nylon bristle end, resulting from a double-blade or scissor cut during the manufacturing process (SEM 170×). **C.** A tapered or round-end nylon bristle produced by heat or a mechanical polishing process (SEM 170×). **D.** The scrubbing, mechanical action of a toothbrush wear machine has nicely rounded off this bristle removed from a brush that was originally coarse cut. (SEM 170×). (Courtesy of KK Park, BA Matis, AG Christen, Indiana University Dental School.)

90% of the bristles of the ripple brush were end-rounded, whereas the flat brush had an average of 52% rounded bristles. Apparently, the degree of end-rounding depends on a manufacturer's specifications and not on toothbrush design.

In a study conducted in 2001 on 31 different toothbrushes, only 4 products had more than 50% of the filaments rounded; in 19 products, end-rounding was 12 to 40% and only 0 to 7% in 8 brands. The authors concluded that a large percentage of marketed toothbrushes do not meet acceptable end-rounding criteria.[27] If bristles are cut, frayed, or are hollow they can harbor bacteria, viruses, and other potential periopathogens, especially if no dentifrice is used, and they can transfer these into and around the mouth.[28]

### Handle Designs

Many of the new toothbrushes in the United States have a styled-handle design. Modifications, such as triangular extrusions or indentations along the sides for a better grasp, a "thumb position" on the back of the handle for more comfort, and various angle bends to permit better access into and around the mouth, have been introduced. Four toothbrush-handle designs are shown in Figure 5–7. Several brushes have recently been marketed with an "angled" design, stated to be like a dental instrument. As shown in Figure 5–8, these toothbrushes are similar to a dental professional's mirror. Brushes are also available, as depicted in Figure 5–9, with a handle on the same plane as the bristle tips, as are dental instruments used for caries evaluations and prophylaxes. With both the offset and angled-offset designs, points of bristle contact are in line with the longitudinal axis of the handle during brushing. Handle design and length may provide comfort and compliance during toothbrush use and these factors have recently been documented to improve the quality of tooth brushing. This is particularly true of toothbrushes for children, whose dexterity may not be highly developed.[8,9]

### Texture

Nylon bristles have a uniform diameter and a wide range of predictable textures. Texture is defined as bristle resistance to pressure and is also referred to as firmness, stiffness, and hardness. The firmness or texture of a bristle is related to its (1) composition, (2) diameter, (3) length, and (4) number of individual bristles per tuft. In the manufacturing process, the di-

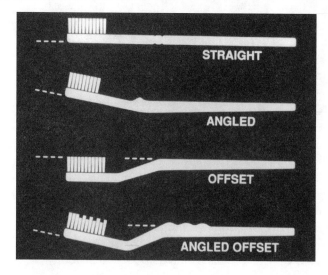

STRAIGHT

ANGLED

OFFSET

ANGLED OFFSET

FIGURE 5-7   Four basic shapes of toothbrush handles. (*J Clin Dent.*)

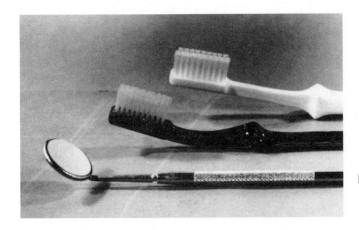

FIGURE 5–8    Similarity of angled toothbrushes and a dental mirror.

ameter of nylon bristles can be well controlled. Because the majority of toothbrushes contain bristles 10- to 12-millimeters long, the diameter of the bristle becomes the critical determinant of texture. The usual range of diameters for adult toothbrush bristles is from 0.007 to 0.015 inches. Factors such as temperature, uptake of water (hydration), and toothbrush-use frequency affect texture.

Texture labeling is not standardized. Individual manufacturers label their brushes according to their testing criteria. Thus one manufacturer's "soft" grade may be stiffer than another manufacturer's "medium" grade. The International Organization for Standardization (ISO) has formulated testing procedures that permit manufacturers to label their brushes in a consistent manner.[29] The American Dental Association is a member of ISO.

### Nylon Versus Natural Bristles

The nylon bristle is superior to the natural (hog) bristle in several aspects. Nylon bristles flex as many as 10 times more often than natural bristles before breaking; they do not split or abrade and are easier to clean. The configurations and hardness of nylon bristles can be standardized within specified and reproducible tolerances. Natural bristle diameters, since they are tapered, vary greatly in each filament. This can lead to wide variations in the resulting texture of the marketed toothbrush. As a result of the advantages of nylon, as well as its ease and

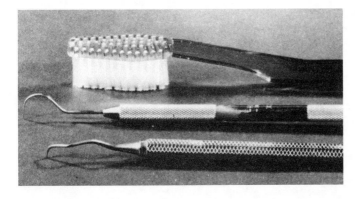

FIGURE 5–9    Similarity of two dental instruments and a toothbrush with the head on the same plane as the handle.

economy of production, relatively few natural bristle toothbrushes are marketed.

## Actions

Bristle actions caused by different brushing motions are illustrated in a 1992 publication[7] that measured and quantified three-dimensional individual movements during brushing. Data frames were filmed to create a computer-generated reanimation of brushing motions in order to design new toothbrush bristle conformations. These authors concluded that an individual's brushing techniques do not vary and are inadequate; therefore bristle configurations in newly designed toothbrushes could be developed to be adaptable to any brushing style

## Powered Toothbrushes

### Introduction

Powered toothbrushes were first advertised in *Harper's Weekly* in February 1886,[30] but only became a factor in the U.S. marketplace beginning in the 1960s with the introduction of Broxadent. With the commercial success of this product, battery-powered products were introduced with the advantage of being portable and available at a lower cost. Unfortunately, problems with these battery-powered products included short "working times" and mechanical breakdowns. The enthusiasm for the powered toothbrush declined and was recommended mainly for the handicapped.

In the 1980s, the category of powered toothbrushes was revitalized with the introduction of the InterPlak product. This "second generation" powered toothbrush had a uniquely rotating head and was powered by long-life/rechargeable batteries. Increased efficacy compared to manual toothbrushes was consistently demonstrated in published studies.[4,8,9, 31–33]

Since then, sonic-powered toothbrushes of a "third" generation have been developed and shown to remove more plaque in comparison to manual toothbrushes, especially in long-term studies. Two primary types of head designs are now used: the rotating, oscillating type with a small, round molar-crown-size brush head and three oscillating brushes with either vibrating or rotational sonic movements.[34–37] Plaque removal by these brushes appears equally effective; periodontal therapeutic effects were demonstrated in pockets of ≤ 5 mm. "Generations" of powered toothbrushes are presented in Table 5–2.

Most recently, powered toothbrushes have been introduced that are battery-powered or disposable after "running down," and are

TABLE 5-2 **Overview of Powered Toothbrushes**

| "Generation" | Description | Examples |
|---|---|---|
| Initial | Powered by electricity | Broxodent |
| | Battery-powered, inexpensive | Many brand names |
| Second | Vibrating, reciprocal, rotating, head movements | Braun Oral-B Plaque Remover |
| | Premium-priced | Interplak |
| | Rechargeable | Philips Jordan |
| | Pressure-sensor heads | Rotadent |
| | Brushing timer | |
| Third | "Sonic" | Rowenta Dentasonic |
| | Premium-priced | Sonicare |
| | Rechargeable | Waterpik SenSonic |

priced, in the United States below $20.00. Published studies have been found on two of these brushes.[38–39]

In most developed countries, the number of powered toothbrush products sold has increased dramatically in recent years. In Switzerland, the regular use of powered toothbrushes increased from 10 to 30% in the last decade. In epidemiological studies, it has been documented that populations are exhibiting increased gingival abrasion and recession. This has been associated with the increased use of oscillating powered toothbrushes. In comparison to these oscillating toothbrushes, sonic toothbrushes have been shown to do little harm to the gingiva. Also sonic brushes of this type can be used up to 6 or 12 months because the bristles show minimal overt signs of use and do not splay.[40–44]

### Bristle/Designs

The heads of most powered or mechanical toothbrushes are smaller than manual toothbrushes and are usually removable to allow for replacements (Figure 5–10). The head follows three basic patterns when the motor is started: (1) reciprocating, a back-and-forth movement; (2) arcuate, an up-and-down movement; and (3) elliptical, a combination of the reciprocating and arcuate motions. Powered toothbrushes are consistently superior to manual toothbrushes in plaque removal and gingivitis effi-

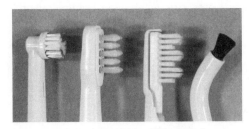

FIGURE 5–10    Toothbrush heads from four powered toothbrushes: Braun; Interplak; Sonicare; Rota-dent.

cacy.[9,31,45] Differences are most significant when tested against manual toothbrushes.

### Motivation

Motivation to improve oral hygiene appears to be a key factor for patients to purchase powered toothbrushes.[31,46] In a survey by the ADA, of the 139 respondents who owned powered toothbrushes, 21.6% used them regularly, and 25.2% used them occasionally.[47] This survey does not indicate the toothbrushing frequency of the remaining 53%. A published study on the use of powered toothbrushes found that when consumers first purchased the electric brush they increased their frequency of brushing. The effectiveness is especially improved when the users are given instructions and controlled during the first 6-month period. More recently,[48] a survey conducted 6 months after subjects completed a clinical efficacy study indicated that most subjects were not using their powered device twice a day. With the development of the second and third generation of powered toothbrushes, it appears that long-term use is increasing; however, recent publications on this have not been definitive.

Weinstein et al.[49] analyzed the failures of motivation. One of the important aspects is to accept each patient as an individual, and the dental hygienist and dentist should be able to listen to the patient. Oral hygiene can be instructed only when we are informed about a patient's attitudes, and he or she has to demonstrate their oral hygiene. The procedure in brushing for any method used should have a definite sequence. Health professionals should take time and not expect the patient to change more than one thing from session to session. It is important to have a preventive program for each patient, and this starts with the charting. After the first steps we should follow the program to obtain the goals with the patient. The patients' progress should be evaluated from session to session and from year to year. Dental professionals should also accept failures and

have an alternative plan to implement in case of failure.

## Efficiency / Safety Evaluations

Toothbrushing devices have been developed that accurately standardize all of the above factors, in addition to length and number of toothbrushing strokes over simulated anterior or posterior teeth. Published testing methods are now available to evaluate both safety and efficacy of manual and powered toothbrushes (Table 5–3). Differences between products can be determined and, in several areas, are predictive of clinical results. For example, three laboratory methods have been predictive of clinical plaque removal when plaque assessments focusing on interproximal areas were used. Significant clinical differences between toothbrush designs have also been documented.[8,9,17] Interproximal access efficacy has been directly related to increasing brushing pressures and inversely correlated with bristle texture (the "softer" the texture, the higher the interproximal efficacy).[50,51]

Clinical advantages of various toothbrush-head configurations for removing dental plaque and debris (cleaning efficacy) have been difficult to substantiate. This is attributed to the wide variations among individuals in tooth-

brushing times, motions, pressures, and in the shape and number of teeth present. Published studies on the clinical superiority of one newly designed manual or powered toothbrush versus another have been inconsistent. It is clear, however, that these new products are more effective than standard manual brushes.[8,9]

## The American Dental Association (ADA) Acceptance Program

The American Dental Association (ADA) has established guidelines to enable manufacturers to obtain an acceptable rating and use the ADA Seal of Acceptance. In 1996, the Council on Scientific Affairs of the American Dental Association proposed new guidelines for the Seal of Acceptance.[52] These guidelines require laboratory documentation of acceptable end-roundedness, good manufacturing procedures (GMPs), and equivalency in clinical plaque and gingivitis efficacy compared with a control toothbrush provided by the ADA.

Manual toothbrushes with a standard design, acceptable laboratory data, and GMPs do not require clinical testing. For manual toothbrushes with new designs and for mechanical brushes, the guidelines require only equivalency in plaque and gingivitis reduction compared with a toothbrush provided by the ADA. The clinical protocol is summarized in Table 5–4. The statement to be used in the labeling of products accepted by the ADA is: "(Product Name) is accepted as an effective cleansing device that has been shown to remove plaque and reduce gingivitis when used as directed in a program of good oral hygiene to supplement regular professional care."

As listed on the American Dental Association's website (www.ADA.org), more than 140 manual toothbrushes have been awarded the ADA Seal of Approval (August 2001).

The ADA has developed criteria for acceptance of powered toothbrushes based on both safety and efficacy. These are: (1) laboratory evidence of electric safety, that is, no electric

---

TABLE 5-3 **Toothbrush Laboratory Testing Procedures**

Abrasion

Depth of deposit removal

Distal surface cleaning

Gingival margin cleaning

Interproximal Access Efficacy

Polishing

Smooth surface (area) deposit removal

Stain removal

Subgingival access efficacy

TABLE 5-4 **Summary of the American Dental Association Acceptance Program Clinical Study Protocol for Mechanical and Newly Designed Manual Toothbrushes**

1. Minimum of 28 healthy adult subjects assigned to
   a. A toothbrush provided by the ADA
   b. The test brush
2. Single-blind design (investigators not aware of product assignment)
3. Measurements at baseline, 15 days and 30 days
   a. Safety
   b. Plaque
   c. Gingivitis
4. Appropriate statistical analysis of data

shock hazard; (2) clinical evidence of both hard- and soft-tissue safety under unsupervised conditions; (3) clinical evidence of plaque and gingivitis efficacy compared to a toothbrush already accepted and provided by the ADA; and (4) evidence of proper labeling and advertising claims that may mention plaque reduction but not improvement of any existing oral disease.[52] The required statement for labeling and commercial claims on powered toothbrushes accepted by the ADA is the same as for manual toothbrushes. As of August 2001, 10 powered toothbrushes have been awarded the ADA Seal of Acceptance. Five of these products are distributed by Water Pik Technologies.

**Question 2**

Which of the following statements, if any, are correct?

A. Using laboratory tests, the relative effectiveness of different toothbrushes can be compared and specific brushes identified as effective for removal of plaque.

B. Interproximal access decreases as the textures of the bristles increases.

C. Interproximal access is better with vertical brushing procedures, compared

with a horizontal motion of the brush head.

D. Standard manual toothbrushes can remove plaque as effectively as the newly designed powered toothbrushes.

E. An interproximal plaque index is used to measure interproximal toothbrush cleaning efficiency.

## Toothbrushing Methods

The objectives of toothbrushing are to (1) remove plaque and disturb reformation; (2) clean teeth of food, debris, and stain; (3) stimulate the gingival tissues; and (4) apply dentifrice with specific ingredients to address caries, periodontal disease or sensitivity.

During the last 50 years many toothbrushing methods have been introduced, and most are identified by an individual's name, such as Bass, Stillman, Charters, or by a term indicating a primary action to be followed, such as roll or scrub. No one method shows consistently better results in removing plaque than scrubbing. Most studies with manual toothbrushes and the different instructed methods show more gingival abrasion than with powered sonic toothbrushes. Most people brushing with an instructed professional method are not aware that they are brushing in a specific way. Thus it may be more effective to instruct patients to improve their own method. This can be achieved by using a plaque disclosant to stain plaque or identify areas that are missed during tooth brushing. Then the patient can be taught how to clean the sites properly and on the next visit be rechecked. The proposed adaptation has to be recorded in the patient's chart and rechecked at the beginning of the next session, as not all patients can remember all the instructions. Additionally, professionals should never argue with a patient but instead should encourage and help.

Various toothbrushing methods will be briefly described here. For more details see the

original papers or this chapter in the previous textbook edition. The toothbrushing methods most emphasized are horizontal scrub, Fones, Leonard, Stillman, Charters, Bass, rolling stroke (press roll), and Smith-Bell. All of these techniques are applicable to the cleaning of the facial, lingual, and to some extent to occlusal surfaces; all are relatively ineffective in cleaning interproximal areas; and only the Bass technique is effective in cleaning the sulcus. The brush motions used in each of these techniques are summarized in Table 5-5.

### Natural Methods of Brushing

The most natural brushing methods used by patients are a reciprocating horizontal scrub technique,[53] a rotary motion (Fones's technique),[54] or a simple up-and-down motion over the maxillary and mandibular teeth (Leonard's technique).[55] Patients managing effective toothbrushing with these methods without causing traumatic problems or disease should not alter their brushing methods just for the sake of change.[56]

---

### TABLE 5-5 Brush Motions Used in Toothbrushing Methods

I. Horizontal reciprocating scrub

II. Vibratory

    Bass (sulcular technique)

    Stillman

    Charters

III. Vertical sweeping

    Rolling stroke (press roll)

    Modified Stillman

    Modified Charters

    Modified Bass

    Leonard

    Smith-Bell (physiologic technique)

IV. Rotary

    Fones

---

Stillman's method was originally developed to provide gingival stimulation.[57] The toothbrush is positioned with the bristles inclined at a 45-degree angle to the apex of the tooth, with part of the brush resting on the gingiva and the other part on the tooth (Figure 5-11). A vibratory motion is used with a slight pressure to stimulate the gingiva. The brush is lifted and then replaced in the same area, and pulsing is repeated.

Charters advocated a pressure–vibratory technique to clean interproximal areas.[58] The toothbrush should be placed at a 90-degree angle to the long axis of the teeth so that the bristles are gently forced between the teeth but do not rest on the gums. The brush is moved in several small rotary motions so that the sides of the bristles are in contact with the gum margin. After two or three such motions, the brush is removed and replaced in the same area and the motions are repeated.

It is important to note that the Bass technique was the first to focus on the removal of plaque and debris from the gingival sulcus by the combined use of a soft toothbrush and dental floss. The method is effective for removing plaque adjacent to and directly beneath the gingival margins as part of the self-care regimen for controlling periodontal disease and caries. In the Bass technique, the toothbrush is positioned in the gingival sulcus at a 45-degree angle to the tooth apex. The bristles are then gently pressed to enter the sulcus. A vibratory action, described as a back-and-forth horizontal

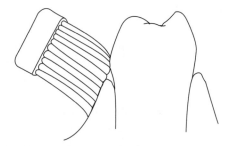

FIGURE 5-11 Stillman technique seen diagrammatically.

jiggle, causes a pulsing of the bristles to clean the sulci[59] (Figure 5–12). Ten strokes are advised for each area.

In the rolling-stroke method, the toothbrush bristles are positioned parallel to and against the attached gingiva, with the toothbrush head level with the occlusal plane. The wrist is then turned to flex the toothbrush bristles first against the gingiva and then the facial surface. A sweeping motion is continued until the occlusal or incisal surface is reached (Figure 5–13). The toothbrush bristles are at right angles to the tooth surface as the brush passes over the crown. The press roll action is repeated at least five times before proceeding to the next site.[60]

### Modified Brushing Methods

In attempts to enhance brushing of the entire facial and lingual tooth surfaces, the original techniques have been modified. Some modifications like the Bass method may induce a more pronounced gingival trauma with standard brushes.[61] New toothbrush designs such as multilevel and cross-section bristles that have been tested are not only more effective but can be also less harmful.[62]

The following considerations are important when teaching patients a particular toothbrushing technique: (1) the patient's oral health status, including number of teeth, their

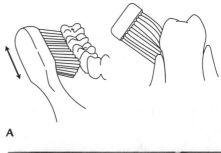

**A**

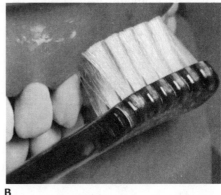

**B**

FIGURE 5-12    Bass technique: **A.** graphically; **B.** pictorially.

alignment, patient's mouth size, presence of removable prostheses, orthodontic appliances, periodontal pockets, and gingival condition; (2) the patient's systemic health status, including muscular and joint diseases, and mental retardation; (3) the patient's age; (4) the pa-

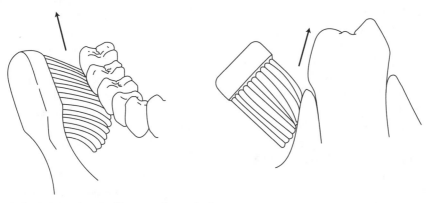

FIGURE 5-13    Rolling stroke technique.

tient's interest and motivation; (5) the patient's manual dexterity; and (6) the ease and effectiveness with which the professional can explain and demonstrate proper toothbrushing procedures.

## Recommended Powered Toothbrushing Methods

Most powered toothbrush manufacturers do not recommend a specific brushing method, however, the electric brushes should be used in a specified manner. The Swiss Dental Society, in 2001 developed an instruction manual.[63] Instructions for brushes with a sweeping and /or oscillating rotary motion are as follows:

1. The brushes are positioned on the tooth surfaces in a 45- or 90-degree angle to the incisal plane. Only when positioned should the brush be switched to "on." The mouth should be almost closed.
2. The brush should be moved slowly over and around each tooth for 3 to 5 seconds, making sure that the bristles clean the crevices between the teeth.
3. The brush head can be lifted distally and mesially into the interproximal areas to reach the interdental area; the brush always remains on a single tooth.
4. After a period of approximately 5 seconds, the brush is moved to the next tooth surface and repositioned.
5. Experienced individuals can use the brush also in a perpendicular angle to the teeth and gums, but the applied force has to be gentle. In this way, each tooth in the upper and lower arch is cleaned on the buccal and lingual surfaces.
6. It is best to divide the mouth into four quadrants (upper-right, upper-left, lower-right, and lower-left) and to start brushing on a tooth in the upper rear and then clean one surface after the other very systematically.
7. It is an easy way, gives good control for the individual, and does not omit any tooth surface. This method takes more time, because at a single time interval, only one tooth surface can be cleaned.

## Toothbrushing Time and Frequency

For many years the dental professional advised patients to brush their teeth after every meal. The ADA has modified this position by use of the statement that patients should brush "regularly." Research has indicated that if plaque is completely removed every other day, there will be no deleterious effects in the oral cavity.[64] On the other hand, because few individuals completely remove plaque, daily brushing is still extremely important to maximize sulcular cleaning as a periodontal disease control measure, as well as to afford an opportunity to use fluoride dentifrices more often in caries control. Where periodontal pockets exist, even more frequent oral hygiene procedures are indicated.

Studies have been conducted in which patients were asked to brush exactly as they did at home and then covertly monitored to determine the length of time of brushing. In the last two decades, the average brushing time was shown to have increased from about 20 to 30 seconds, to 60 seconds,[65,66] and to 80 seconds in a 1995 study.[67] In all of these studies, the individuals claimed that they usually brushed for 2 or 3 minutes. These results demonstrate that people greatly overestimate their efforts or else are telling their professionals what the individuals believe or would like the professionals to hear.

Thorough toothbrushing requires a different amount of time for each individual, depending on such factors as the innate tendency to accumulate plaque and debris; the psychomotor skills; and the adequacy of clearance of foods, bacteria, and debris by the saliva. Only after patients have repeatedly brushed their teeth under the supervision of a dental professional can the adequacy of cleaning in a given time be

determined. Often a compromise is made by suggesting 5 to 10 strokes in each area or by advocating the use of a timer. This amount of time, which might be adequate for the average person, may not be sufficient for patients in most need of maximum plaque-control programs. To ensure continued commitment to a personal oral-hygiene program, the benefits of proper oral care must be explained and demonstrated to patients.[9]

## Toothbrushing Procedures

### Occlusal Surfaces

The occlusal surfaces may be cleaned by either (1) short vibratory strokes, with pressure being maintained to accomplish as deep a penetration of the pits and fissures as possible; or (2) a rapid back-and-forth vibrating motion to force the bristles into the pits and fissures, followed by a sweeping motion to expel the dislodged debris. Long, sweeping, horizontal strokes are contraindicated, because the toothbrush bristles have minimum contact in the deeper and more critical fissures (Figure 5–14). The orifices of the pits and fissures are too narrow for

bristle penetration and, whatever the technique, are inaccessible for adequate cleaning. This helps explain why more than 60% of all carious lesions in the mouth are found on the occlusal surface, even though most individuals attempt to brush this surface.

### The Anterior Lingual Areas

Access to the lingual surfaces of the mandible and maxilla is difficult. Brushing in these areas can be facilitated by cutting off all tufts on a brush, except the first four or five rows in the toe. This modified brush has unimpeded access to the gingival sulci and lingual fossae areas (Figure 5–15). In the lower arch, the heel of the brush can be used for the same purpose.

### Brushing Sequence

A routine brushing pattern should be established to avoid exclusion of any area. One systematic pattern is to teach children to begin by cleaning the occlusal surfaces of the maxillary arches, starting with the molars, and then the same on the mandibular arches. For children it is most important to brush the pit and fissures. The use of a three-dimensional brush can be recommended as long as children are not able

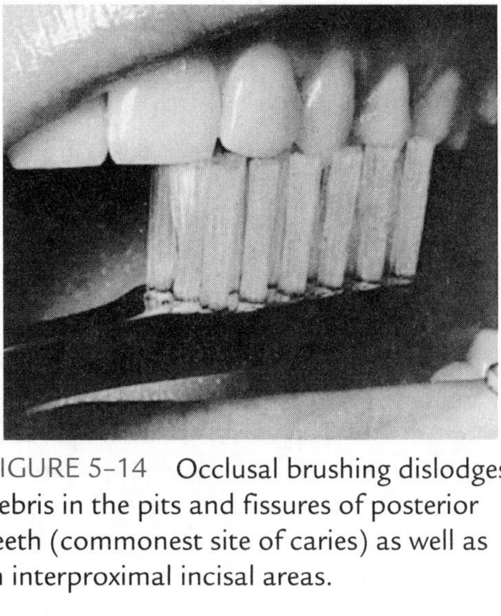

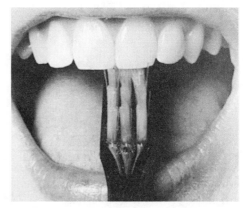

**FIGURE 5–14**  Occlusal brushing dislodges debris in the pits and fissures of posterior teeth (commonest site of caries) as well as in interproximal incisal areas.

**FIGURE 5–15**  Vertical position of the toothbrush for the often constricted lingual area.

to brush the more difficult buccal and lingual surfaces.[68] Such toothbrushes that hug the teeth and clean the buccal, lingual, and occlusal surfaces simultaneously are easier for children to use, as the brush guides itself from tooth to tooth. Studies show that children favor such toothbrushes.

Adult patients are taught to begin with the distal surface of the most posterior tooth and to continue brushing the occlusal and incisal surfaces around the arch until the last molar on the other side of the arch has been reached. The lower arch is then brushed in a similar manner.

Patients tend to apportion more time and effort on the facial areas of the anterior teeth.[69] Often, right-handed people do not brush the right side of the arch as well as the left side; left-handed people similarly neglect the left side over the right side.

### Clinical Assessments of Toothbrushing

Whatever techniques are recommended, the main purpose of tooth brushing is to remove dental plaque from the teeth, including the gingival crevice, with the minimum amount of damage to the teeth and surrounding structures. Disclosing agents provide the means of evaluating the thoroughness of cleaning the teeth.[56,70] The most widely marketed red disclosing products contain FD&C Red #28.

Disclosing agents may be in either a liquid or tablet form. The chewable tablet or the liquid disclosant should be swished around in the mouth for 15 to 30 seconds and then expectorated. Home use of disclosants by the patient should be encouraged to permit self-evaluation of the effectiveness of plaque-control programs. Clinical assessments should be made for evidence of improper tooth brushing. Minor damage that may be noted includes abrasion to the soft tissues (scuffing, bruising, and punctate lesions) or damage to the tooth surface.

Toothbrush abrasion, or the wearing away of tooth substances, occurs from the use of highly abrasive dentifrices, too-firm brush bristles, in-correct brushing methods, and excessive pressure during brushing. Common abrasion locations are on the surfaces of the teeth displaced facially and on the cervical areas of exposed root surfaces. Because enamel is harder than cementum, tooth damage usually occurs as a V-shaped, horizontal notch immediately apical to the cementoenamel junction. Further progress of the abrasion can be minimized by use of soft-bristle brushes, changes in brush angulation, pulsing instead of stroking, the use of less abrasive dentifrices, and less pressure during brushing.

### Toothbrush Replacement

Toothbrush wear (splayed, bent, or broken bristles) is influenced more by brushing methods than by the length of time or number of brushings per day.[71] The average "life" of a manual toothbrush is approximately 3 months. This estimate can vary greatly, however, because of differences in brushing habits. It is also sound advice for patients to have several toothbrushes and to rotate their daily use, to assure drying between brushings. If toothbrushes need to be replaced more frequently than every three months, the patient's brushing technique should be checked. Even if the brushing technique is acceptable or has been corrected, toothbrushes should still be replaced frequently. Indeed, after every oral or contagious medical illness, it is imperative that patients be made aware of the importance of having a new toothbrush.

## Special Needs

### Tongue Brushing

Malodor from the mouth most often has its origin on the tongue. Therefore, for persons expiring mouth odor, tongue brushing is important. Tongue cleaning is also indicated for patients harboring a coated tongue. A coated tongue is a bacterial reservoir but could also be a locus for intraoral transmission of organisms during

toothbrushing, through infection or reinfection of periodontally treated pockets. This is another reason that Quirynen et al. introduced the full-mouth disinfection concept in periodontal patients to prevent recolonization of bacteria.[28]

The brushing of the tongue and palate helps reduce the debris, plaque, and number of oral microorganisms. The papillae on the tongue provide an area especially conducive to bacterial and debris retention. Tongue cleansing can be accomplished by placing the side of the toothbrush near the middle of the tongue, with the bristles pointed toward the throat. The brush is swept forward, and this motion is repeated six to eight times in each area. The palate should also be cleansed with a sweeping motion. A dentifrice should be used with this brushing of soft tissues to improve cleansing action.[72]

## Abutment Teeth and Orthodontic Appliances

Abutment teeth, implants, fixed bridgework and fixed orthodontic appliances require special emphasis on sulcular brushing to prevent gingivitis. Thorough cleansing between orthodontic appliances and gingiva will prevent dental caries. A pre-teen or teenager, as well as patients with extensive reconstruction bridgework, are prone to dental diseases but are also more motivated; therefore, a rigid, preventive program is required. A powered brush and auxiliary aids are suggested.

The effectiveness of a new toothbrush design in orthodontic patients has been documented in different publications. At the end of a 4-month study, a three-sided manual toothbrush significantly decreased gingivitis and was more effective in plaque removal compared to a flat multitufted toothbrush.[73] Powered toothbrushes have been documented to provide superior efficacy in orthodontic patients compared to results in patients using manual toothbrushes.[9]

## Dentures and Removable Orthodontic Appliances

Patients with full dentures can meet their oral hygiene needs with a soft nylon brush for the oral tissues and a denture brush that cleans all areas of the denture. The denture brush with a nonabrasive cleaner should reach into the recessed alveolar ridge area of the denture to ensure maximum cleansing. The oral tissues should be brushed at least once a day using a gentle vibration and long, straight strokes from the posterior to anterior mouth regions.[70]

Patients with removable partial dentures and removable orthodontic appliances need at least three toothbrushes, one for the natural teeth, another for the appliance, and a third for clasps. Brushing clasps, wires, and other metal parts can wear out a regular toothbrush. A clasp brush—2 or 3 inches long, narrow, and tapered—can be obtained as a third brush. Special care is needed to carefully clean all plaque from the clasps as a preventive measure for the supporting teeth.

## Handicapped Patients

Some handicapped patients are able to brush their own teeth and can often do so with support and encouragement from dental personnel and the use of special toothbrushes. A manual brush with an enlarged handle, elastic cuff, or small strap attached to the brush or a long-handled holder for patients who cannot raise their arms or do not have hands, permits the patient to brush.[74] The elastic cuff is fitted around the hand and holds the toothbrush in the patient's palm. Patients who are unable to reach their mouths for brushing can, at times, attach the brush in a stationary upright position by using a clamp.[75] The patients bend over to position the brush in the mouth. The National Foundation of Dentistry for the Handicapped is developing a preventive program to encourage toothbrushing to the beat of music. A brush wheel, which can be used in between the teeth and moved through the dentiton without using the hands

might be helpful for tetraplegics. The results are almost comparable with handbrushes.[76,77] Mentally retarded patients can often brush using a soft toothbrush with the plastic handle bent for better grasping. A horizontal scrub is often the best that these patients can manage. A three-headed toothbrush or a powered toothbrush assisted by a caregiver can be useful.[37]

## Special Uses for Powered Toothbrushes

Powered toothbrushes can be beneficial for parental brushing of children's teeth; for children and adults who are physically handicapped, mentally retarded, aged, arthritic, or otherwise with poor dexterity; and for those patients who are poorly motivated. These brushes are especially recommended for patients who require a larger handle, because powered models are easier to grasp.

### Question 3

Which of the following statements, if any, are correct?

A. A meticulous, once-every-other-day program may be as effective as daily morning and evening brushings.

B. The high incidence of caries that occurs on the occlusal surface is usually traceable to inadequate brushing.

C. Toothbrush replacement every 3 months is as important as proper brushing techniques.

D. For a person with a partial denture, the toothbrush used for the natural teeth is not adequate for cleaning the clasps.

E. It is necessary for handicapped persons to have others aid in brushing their teeth.

## SUMMARY

Toothbrushing alone cleans buccal and lingual tooth surfaces. No single toothbrushing technique adequately cleans occlusal pits and fissures. No toothbrushing procedure removes all interproximal and subgingival plaque, especially around malposed teeth and fixed prostheses. Interproximal cleaning aids are necessary to complete the tooth-cleaning process. No one toothbrush design has been demonstrated to be most effective for all patients in long-term studies. Dental professionals should be familiar with various toothbrush products, primarily from their own use experience, and have examples of toothbrushes demonstrating various degrees of splaying or bending. These should be demonstrated when prevention methods are being discussed with their patients.

Although manufacturers are advertising variations in bristle shape, bristle size, and number of filaments, no accepted criteria exist for product labeling. The American Dental Association does not yet consider one toothbrush design superior to another but is developing clinical-testing guidelines associated with both plaque and gingivitis reductions. Thoroughness and frequency of brushing are probably more important than a specific toothbrushing method and toothbrushing products. Any method that is taught should be effective, not damaging to the hard or soft tissues, routinely used and should not cause excessive tooth wear. In initiating effective toothbrushing, it is necessary to (1) select the appropriate toothbrush(es) suitable for the patient; (2) instill in individuals the goals of toothbrushing and the need for good oral physiotherapy; (3) teach a technique or combination of brushing methods needed to meet special needs; and (4) assess thorough and effective toothbrushing as a part of the total oral hygiene program

# ANSWERS AND EXPLANATIONS

1. A, C, D, and E—correct.

   B—incorrect. Toothbrush bristles have also undergone major changes in shape and design.

2. A, B, C, and E—correct.

   D—incorrect. The standard manual toothbrush is not as effective as the new powered toothbrushes.

3. C and D—correct.

   A—incorrect. It is true that one good cleaning would do the job, but so few people do a good job that several cleanings might be equal to one good try. However, either answer could be correct.

   B—incorrect. No matter how well the occlusal surface is brushed, the deep pits and fissures cannot be adequately cleaned with a brush.

   E—incorrect. Handicapped persons can often manage brushing with slightly modified oral-hygiene aids or with specially developed brushing devices.

## Self-evaluation Questions

1. Three general reasons that people do not spend adequate time for personal oral-health care are _____, _____, and _____.

2. Wadsworth introduced the toothbrush into the United States just before the _____ War.

3. The constricted part of the toothbrush between the handle and the head is the _____. The end of the head is arbitrarily termed the _____; the part closest to the handle is called the _____.

4. Four lateral profiles of brushes sold in the United States are _____, _____, _____, and _____.

5. The American Dental Association Council on _____ (name) continually accomplishes scientific evaluations of devices used in dentistry. To support standardization of professional devices, the ADA is a member of the International _____, which has as its objective the establishment of consistency of labeling.

6. Two synonyms for hardness of bristles and toothbrushes are _____, and _____. Firmness of bristles is caused by three general characteristics of bristles; they are _____, _____, and _____. A medium-texture bristle has a diameter of approximately _____ in.

7. Gingival abrasion can occur with manual toothbrushes because of _____, _____, or _____.

8. Three basic motions of electric toothbrush heads are _____, _____, and _____.

9. Three groups of people who can especially benefit from use of electric tooth-brushes are _____, _____, and _____.

10. Four objectives of toothbrushing are _____, _____, _____, and _____. The three natural methods of toothbrushing are _____, _____, and _____. The motion of the brush in blank no. 1 in the previous sentence is _____; in blank no. 2 is _____; and in blank no. 3 is _____.

## ACKNOWLEDGMENTS

The authors express their sincere appreciation to Jenifer B. She for assistance in the translations, P. Heller and her staff at library of the University of Pennsylvania School of Dental Medicine for their valuable cooperation, and to Jessica and Claire Yankell for their computer expertise.

## REFERENCES

1. Hirschfeld, I. (1939). *The toothbrush: Its use and abuse*. Brooklyn, NY: Dental Items of Interest Publishing Co., 1–591.
2. Hattab, F. N. (1997). Meswak: The natural toothbrush. *J Clin Dent*, 8:125–29.
3. Golding, P. S. (1982). The development of the toothbrush. A short history of tooth cleansing. *Dent Health* (London), 21:25–27.
4. Smith, C. (2000). Toothbrush technology - Even the Pharaohs brushed their teeth. *J Dent Technol*, 17:26, 27.
5. Yankell, S. L., & Emling, R. C. (1978). Understanding dental products: What you should know and what your patient should know. *U Pa Cont Dent Educ*, 1:1–43.
6. Volpe, A. R., Emling, R. C., & Yankell, S. L. (1992). The toothbrush—A new dimension in design, engineering and clinical evaluation. *J Clin Dent*, 3: S29–S32.
7. Mintel, T. E., & Crawford, J. (1992). The search for a superior toothbrush design technology. *J Clin Dent*, 3:C1–C4.
8. Saxer, U. P., & Yankell, S. L. (1997). Impact of improved toothbrushes on dental diseases. I. *Quintessence Int*, 28:513–25.
9. Saxer, U. P., & Yankell, S. L. (1997). Impact of improved toothbrushes on dental diseases. II. *Quintessence Int*, 28:573–93.
10. Benson, B. J., Henyon, G., & Grossman, E. (1993). Clinical plaque removal efficacy of three toothbrushes. *J Clin Dent*, 4:21–25.
11. Volpenhein, D. W., Handel, S. E., Hughes, T. J., & Wild, J. (1996). A comparative evaluation of the in vitro penetration performance of the improved Crest Complete toothbrush versus the current Crest Complete toothbrush, the Colgate Precision toothbrush and the Oral-B P40 toothbrush. *J Clin Dent*, 7:21–25.
12. Garcia-Godoy, F. (2000). A new toothbrush design. *Am J Dent*, 13:4A.
13. Chava, V. K. (2000). An evaluation of the efficacy of a curved bristle and conventional tooth-brush. A comparative study. *J Periodontol*, 71:785–89.
14. Yankell, S. L., Emling, R. C., Shi, X., & Perez, B. (1996). A six-month evaluation of the Den-trust toothbrush. *J Clin Dent*, 7:106–109.

62. Imfeld, T., Sener, B., & Simonovic, I. (2000). In vitro-untersuchen der mechanischen wirkung von handelsublichen handzahnbursten. *Acta Med Dent Helv*, 5:27–37

63. Imfeld, T., & Saxer, U. P. (2001). Anleitung zur Zahnreinigung mit elektrishen zahnbursten Swiss Dent Soc, 1–813.

64. Lang, K. P., Cumming, B. R., & Löe, H. (1973). Tooth brushing frequency as it relates to plaque development and gingival health. *J Periodontol*, 44:396–405.

65. Emling, R. C., Flickinger, K. C., Cohen, D. W., & Yankell, S. L. (1981). A comparison of estimated versus actual brushing time. *Pharm Therap Dent*, 6:93–98.

66. Saxer, U. P., Emling, R., & Yankell, S. L. (1983). Actual vs. estimated tooth brushing time and toothbrush used. *Caries Res*, 17:179–80.

67. Saxer, U. P., Barbakow, J., & Yankell, S. L. (1998). New studies on estimated and actual toothbrushing times and dentifrice use. *J Clin Dent*, 9:49–51.

68. Zimmer, S. (2001). Neuartige Handzahnbürsten: Marketing-gag oder zahnmedizinischer fortschritt? *Quintessenz Team-Journal* 31:187–192.

69. Tsamtsouris, A. (1978). Effectiveness of tooth brushing. *J Pedodontics*, 2:296–303.

70. Wilkins, E. M. (1994). *Clinical practice of the dental hygienist* (7th ed.) Philadelphia: Lea & Febiger, 1–893.

71. Craig, T. T., & Montague, J. L. (1976). Family oral health survey. *JADA*, 92:326–32.

72. Christen, A. G., & Swanson, B. Z., Jr. (1978). Oral hygiene: A history of tongue scraping and brushing. *JADA*, 96:215–19.

73. Yankell, S. L., Greco, M. R., Lucash, D. A., & Emling, R. C. (1997). Four-month assessment of the Dentrust and Oral-B P35 toothbrushes in orthodontic patients. *J Clin Dent*, 8: 95–99.

74. Fuller, L., & Dunn, M. J. (1966). An occupational therapist's role in oral hygiene for the handicapped. *Am J Occup Therap*, 20:35–36.

75. Birch, R. H., & Mumford, J. M. (1963). Electric tooth brushing. *Dent Practice*, 13:182–86.

76. Marthaler, T. M., Menghini, G., Bultmann, H., & Ingold, R. (1987). Beeinflussunng der gingivalen verhaltnisse durch den gebrauch einer zahnburste oder eines kauradchens. *Schweiz Monatsschr Zahnmed*, 97:591–94.

77. Kozlovsky, A., Dreiangel, A., & Perlmutter, S. (1991). The chewing wheel device: plaque removing efficiency and use in oral hygiene programs. *Quint Int*, 22:727–30.

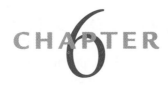

# CHAPTER 6

# Dentifrices, Mouthrinses, and Chewing Gums

*Stuart L. Fischman*
*Samuel L. Yankell*

## OBJECTIVES

*At the end of this chapter, it will be possible to:*

1. Differentiate between a *cosmetic* and a *therapeutic* dentifrice, mouthrinse, or chewing gum.
2. Explain the three phases of research necessary when applying to investigate a new drug (IND)—the process that precedes receiving a new drug application (NDA), which is necessary to market a new product with a therapeutic claim.
3. Discuss how approval or nonapproval of a new product by the Food and Drug Administration (FDA) differs from acceptance or rejection by the American Dental Association (ADA).
4. Explain the various reasons that the same abrasive material in toothpaste can cause differing levels of abrasion on tooth structure.
5. Name the usual dentifrice ingredients and their percentages in a dentifrice.
6. Name the agents used in dentifrices to produce anticaries, anticalculus, whitening, and antihypersensitivity effects.
7. Name the active ingredients in typical antiplaque and antigingivitis mouth rinses: one sold over the counter, the other as a prescription item.

# INTRODUCTION

Dentifrices and mouthrinses are the major products for routinely administering effective *cosmetic* and *therapeutic* agents in the mouth. These products are the most widely used by consumers, generating the largest sales of all dental products. Chewing gums are a new category of products with cosmetic claims and the ability to deliver therapeutic compounds.

Dentifrices and mouthrinses differ considerably. Dentifrices are complex and difficult to formulate. Tremendous innovations have occurred in the past 20 years in the appearance and packaging of dentifrices. The contemporary consumer is faced with many alternatives in *appearance* (pastes, clear gels, stripes) and *packaging* (conventional tubes, stand-up tubes, pumps), as well as products marketed specifically for children. In addition, numerous claims are made for dentifrices. They are said to *prevent* calculus and caries, to whiten teeth, to eliminate hypersensitivity, and to reduce plaque and gingivitis.

Because the public routinely uses them one to three times per day, dentifrices are the most beneficial dental products. Some of this benefit may be lost if a person rinses immediately after brushing because rinsing *decreases* the concentration or reservoir of the active agent(s) in the oral cavity.

Mouthrinses are available in liquid form, the traditional method for stabilizing and delivering many pharmaceutically active agents. Mouthrinses are considered by consumers to have primarily cosmetic benefits (i.e., breath fresheners) and are therefore not used as frequently or routinely as dentifrices in the daily oral-hygiene regimen. Two categories of mouthrinses have been recognized by the American Dental Association (ADA) as effective against *plaque* and *gingivitis* (see ADA website www.ada.org). One category contains the *essential oils* as the active ingredients. Products in this category include Listerine and its generic equivalents containing the original *essential oils*. To date, more than 200 generic versions have been reviewed and accepted by the ADA. These products are sold over the counter. The other category of products contains *chlorhexidine* as the active agent. Currently marketed products are Peridex and Prevident. The Food and Drug Administration (FDA), has approved chlorhexidine-containing products *only* as prescription products.

Chewing gums have the potential to be used by the consumer for periods of 5 to 20 minutes several times a day, until the flavor of the product dissipates. This would enable delivery of a cosmetic or therapeutic agent for a *longer time* than dentifrices or mouthrinses. In addition to prolonged delivery of an agent, chewing gums *stimulate salivary flow*, which can provide a buffer effect and also ensure removal of debris from occlusal and interproximal sites. To assure safety and avoid harmful gastrointestinal effects, active agents delivered by chewing gums must be *safe for swallowing* at the dose delivered in one use or contained in the entire product sold in one package.

## Monitoring the Safety and Effectiveness of Therapeutic Dental Products

Caution is needed before introducing a new therapeutic product to the market. Some of the concerns surrounding new products are: Will the active agent disrupt the "normal" bacterial balance of the mouth? Should the search for an ideal agent focus on depressing or eliminating specific disease-related organisms or a broad spectrum of organisms? Should a product be used to preserve a disease-free state while risking the possibility of developing drug resistance? Regardless of the apparent effectiveness of any new product in the laboratory or in controlled clinical studies, public *safety* with unsupervised, widespread availability and use by consumers *is paramount.*

The process by which oral-care agents are evaluated and regulated in the United States has been reviewed by Trummel.[1] Safety and efficacy standards apply not only to prescription medications but *also* to over-the-counter (OTC) drugs. There are three levels of regulation of oral chemotherapeutic agents. The government level includes the *Food and Drug Administration (FDA)* and the *United States Pharmacopoeia Convention.* The *professional or voluntary level* includes the Council on Scientific Affairs (CSA) of the *American Dental Association (ADA).* The *third* level of review includes *consumer advocacy organizations,* advertising standards review panels, and the Federal Trade Commission. In addition, each of the major television networks has its own in-house review committee.

The FDA conducts an ongoing review of all OTC products. One aim of regulation is to protect the patient–consumer from *useless* or *harmful* products. All approval or disapproval decisions by the FDA have the *force of law.*

The stages of FDA approval include preclinical research and development (animal testing, laboratory testing, and toxicity evaluation) followed by clinical research conducted with an approved *investigational new drug (IND)* application. The IND usually includes *three* phases: In phase 1, the study *is limited in scope* and uses only a few subjects to determine the safe dose for humans. For dental products, this usually involves ingestion or exaggerated (three or four times per day) topical applications or both. Phase 2 *involves more subjects* to demonstrate the initial clinical efficacy of the drug and define a dose range for both safety and efficacy. Phase 3 generally includes *double-blind, controlled trials* with "final" formulas to demonstrate long-term safety and efficacy. These range from 3 to 6 months for plaque and gingivitis studies to 2 or 3 years for caries studies. After the company receives an *approved new drug application* (NDA), marketing may begin, but post-marketing surveillance of the product is *mandatory.*

Over the years, the FDA has requested manufacturers of OTC products to submit a *listing* of the active and inactive ingredients in their products as a basis for helping to codify regulations governing OTC sales. Among the many recommendations of the FDA advisory panel[2] that provide for better control of OTC oral therapeutic products is the stipulation that all inactive ingredients be listed on the label by quantity in descending order. Active ingredients, as well as inactive agents, should be in no higher concentrations than necessary for the intended purpose. The panel also recommended that the indicated objective of the active agent(s) must be on the label and that the inclusion of the name of an active agent(s) without stating the proposed benefits would be considered misleading. Proof must exist to substantiate any claim for a specific therapeutic benefit. For example, dentifrices that have not been subjected to laboratory or clinical trials and do not have the ADA Seal of Acceptance, but only list the inclusion of "decay-fighting fluorides" in their products, *cannot claim* that the dentifrice is anticariogenic, *only* that it contains fluoride. It is possible that the fluoride in the untested dentifrice might not be com-

patible with other dentifrice ingredients, or the fluoride may not be released in active ionic form and therefore be totally ineffective.

Recommendations also apply to *packaging* and *labeling* guidelines to regulate advertising. For example, the recommendations suggest that all containers for OTC therapeutic dentifrices, rinses, and gels containing fluoride have a label to identify the product, e.g., "anticaries dentifrice"; its use, e.g., "aids in the prevention of dental caries"; a *warning*, e.g., "Do not swallow. Developing teeth of children under 6 years of age may become permanently discolored if excessive amounts of fluoride are repeatedly swallowed"; and directions for use, e.g., "Adults and children 6 years of age or older should brush teeth thoroughly at least twice daily, or as directed by a dentist or physician."

In April 1997, the FDA issued a labeling requirement for fluoride toothpaste. This states, "Keep out of reach of children under 6 years of age. If you accidentally swallow more than used for brushing, seek professional help or contact a poison control center immediately." This recommendation may be an exaggerated response, as most experts believe that neither an adult nor a child could absorb enough fluoride to cause a serious problem.

After years of ignoring claims of antigingivitis efficacy for various OTC dentifrices and rinses, in 1988 the FDA advised manufacturers of such products that they must either cease making such claims or substantiate them. In 1990, the FDA published its call for data stating:

> The Food and Drug Administration is announcing a call for data for ingredients containing products bearing antiplaque and antiplaque related *claims*, such as "for the reduction or prevention of plaque, tartar, calculus, film, sticky deposits, bacterial buildup and gingivitis." The agency will review the submitted data to determine whether these products are generally regarded as safe and effective and not misbranded for the label uses. This notice also describes the

Attorney General's enforcement of policy governing the marketing of over-the-counter (OTC) drug products bearing antiplaque and antiplaque related claims during the pendency of this review. This request is part of the ongoing review of OTC drug products conducted by the FDA.[3]

In addition to the FDA's regulation of OTC products, the American Dental Association's Council on Scientific Affairs (CSA) continually reviews dental products. The Council is directed to study, evaluate, and disseminate information with regard to dental therapeutic agents, their adjuncts, and dental cosmetic agents that are offered to the public or to the profession.[1] The most important activity of the CSA in meeting this charge is its acceptance program. Unlike the IND process, submission by a manufacturer to the ADA program is *voluntary*. Also, unlike the FDA review process, the primary review responsibilities are conducted by consulting dental professionals who are appointed by the CSA but are not employees of the ADA. If the product is *safe* and *effective*, the *Seal of Acceptance* is granted and *can be used by the manufacturer* in marketing the product. The Seal provides *assurance* to dental professionals and to the public. In addition to the traditional "print media," this information is available at the ADA website, www.ada.org.

The council recognized that plaque control might best be demonstrated by clinically significant reduction of gingivitis. In 1986, the council issued "Guidelines for Acceptance of Chemotherapeutic Products for the Control of Supragingival Dental Plaque and Gingivitis."[4] The Guidelines for Acceptance are presented in Table 6–1.

The purpose of the separate and independent actions of the FDA and the ADA is to ensure the effectiveness and safety of OTC products and to prevent mislabeling and thus misleading information. *The ADA and FDA differ in their acceptance criteria, which places the responsibility for selecting an effective product on the dental professional.*

**TABLE 6–1** American Dental Association Guidelines for Acceptance of Chemotherapeutic Products for the Control of Supragingival Dental Plaque and Gingivitis

The 1986 American Dental Association Guidelines require the following clinical study efficacy criteria:

- Two independent studies should be conducted.
- The study populations should represent typical product users.
- The test product should be used in a normal regimen and compared to a placebo.
- The study design should be either parallel or crossover.
- Each study should be at least 6 months in duration.
- The plaque and gingivitis scoring procedure should be conducted at baseline, after 6 months, and at an intermediate period of time.
- Microbiologic profile should demonstrate that pathogenic or opportunistic microorganisms do not develop over the course of the study.

---

### Question 1

Which of the following statements, if any, are correct?

A. The Food and Drug Administration (FDA) and the American Dental Association (ADA) have both recognized essential oils and chlorhexidine as antiplaque/antigingivitis agents.

B. The decisions of both the Food and Drug Administration and of the American Dental Association to approve a product have the force of law.

C. To receive the ADA's Seal of Acceptance an antiplaque product must prevent or reduce the severity of some disease caused by the plaque.

D. The sales of both therapeutic and over-the-counter dental products are regulated by the FDA.

E. A manufacturer must secure the ADA's Seal of Acceptance before marketing a dental product.

## Dentifrices

According to the dictionary, the term dentifrice is derived from dens (tooth) and fricare (to rub). A simple, contemporary definition of a dentifrice is a mixture used on the tooth in conjunction with a toothbrush. The historic aspects of dentifrice use has been reviewed by Fischman.[5]

Dentifrices are marketed as toothpowders, toothpastes, and gels. All are sold as either cosmetic or therapeutic products. If the purpose of a dentifrice is therapeutic, it must reduce some disease-related process in the mouth. Usually the actual or alleged therapeutic effect is to reduce caries incidence, gingivitis, or tooth sensitivity. The sales appeal of a product, however, is strongly linked to its flavor and foaming action.

In 1970, the dentifrice market amounted to an estimated $355 million; by 1988 it had increased to $1 billion; in 1996 to $1.5 billion; in 2000 to $1.9 billion; and the estimated market for 2005 is $2.2 billion (Figure 6–1).

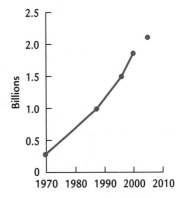

**FIGURE 6–1** Showing the rapid sevenfold increase in toothpaste sales over the past 30 years, and projected increase till 2005.

## Packaging

The development of the toothbrush in 1857 provided the stimulus to market commercial dentifrices. Toothpowders were popular because boxes and cans from which they could be dispensed already existed. The formulas consisted of little more than water, soap, and flavor.

Toothpastes began to appear on the market following the development of lead tubes for packaging. The change to plastic packaging during World War II simultaneously:

- Eliminated the possibility of the user ingesting lead,
- Reduced the possibility of incompatibility of the tube and paste components,
- Aided the expelling of the paste by squeezing,
- Permitted an easier and more economic production of tubes, and
- Provided a good surface for the printing of decorative designs and information.

A drawback with the initial use of plastic tubes was the permeability and subsequent loss of flavors though the packaging. This has been resolved with the use of new plastic materials and the use of laminated or layered packaging materials.

In 1984, Colgate introduced the pump dispenser to the market. Separate color compartments used to dispense "striped" products were introduced in Stripe dentifrice by Lever Brothers and are now used in Aquafresh (Smith, Kline, Beecham) and Colgate Total Stripe (Colgate-Palmolive Co.). Cheseborough-Pond's introduced a dual-chamber pump dispenser to keep the peroxide and baking soda components of their dentifrice, Mentadent, separate until immediately prior to use when they are delivered together on the toothbrush.

## Dentifrice Ingredients

Dentifrices were originally developed to provide a cosmetic effect and deliver a pleasant taste. They are effective in removing extrinsic stains, those that occur on the surface of the tooth. These stains, which are often the end-products of bacterial metabolism, range in color from green to yellow to black. Stains may also result from foods, coffee, tea, cola-containing drinks, and red wines. OTC dentifrices do not remove intrinsic stains, which are a result of altered amelogenesis, such as the white-to-brown color changes seen in fluorosis or the grayish-blue appearance of enamel following administration of tetracycline. Dentifrices, and other OTC products, are also ineffective in altering the yellowing color of teeth seen with physiologic aging and in altering the hues of tooth color produced by differing shades of dentin. Therefore, they can only claim to "make your teeth their whitest or brightest"; they cannot state, "Makes your teeth whiter or tooth color lighter."

Toothpastes contain several or all of the ingredients listed in Table 6–2. Gel dentifrices are also marketed. Gels contain the same components as toothpastes, except that gels have a higher proportion of the thickening agents. Both tooth gels and toothpastes are equally effective in plaque removal and in delivering active ingredients.

## Abrasives

The degree of dentifrice abrasiveness depends on the inherent hardness of the abrasive, size of

TABLE 6–2 **Toothpaste Constituents**

| Ingredient | Percentage |
|---|---|
| Abrasives | 20–40 |
| Water | 20–40 |
| Humectants | 20–40 |
| Foaming agent (soap or detergent) | 1–2 |
| Binding agent, up to | 2 |
| Flavoring agent, up to | 2 |
| Sweetening agent, up to | 2 |
| Therapeutic agent, up to | 5 |
| Coloring or preservative, less than | 1 |

the abrasive particle, and the *shape* of the particle. Several other variables can affect the abrasive potential of the dentifrice: the brushing technique, the pressure on the brush, the hardness of the bristles, the direction of the strokes, and the number of strokes. The abrasive *tested alone* can differ from the same abrasive *tested as part* of a dentifrice formula. The salivary characteristics of individuals may also affect dentifrice abrasiveness.

Calcium carbonate and calcium phosphates were previously the most common abrasives used. These agents often reacted adversely with fluorides. Chalk (calcium carbonate) and baking soda (sodium bicarbonate) are also common dentifrice abrasives. New silicas, silicon oxides, and aluminum oxides are being introduced into dentifrice formulas, with additional efficacy claims.[6-9]

### Abrasiveness Testing

Standard laboratory testing uses a machine with several brushes. The *length* of the reciprocating stroke, *number* of strokes, and *pressure* of the brush can be adjusted. Depending on the experimental objectives, enamel, dentin, or cementum is brushed, and the amount of calcium or phosphorus in the resultant slurry is analyzed. A more accurate method has been developed in which extracted teeth are irradiated to activate some of the tooth phosphorus to *radioactive phosphorus*. After brushing root surfaces of sound canines and molars, the amount of radioactive phosphorus removed may be more accurately assessed than with classical chemical analyses. Results are referenced against the amount of tooth substance removed by the use of the control-abrasive, calcium pyrophosphate.[10]

Abrasives usually do not damage enamel, but they may dull the tooth luster. To compensate for this, *polishing agents* are added to the dentifrice formulation. These polishing agents are usually small-sized particles of aluminum, calcium, tin, magnesium, or zirconium compounds. Typically, the manufacturer *blends the*

*abrasives* and the *polishing agents* to form an *abrasive system.* Agents, such as chalk or silica, may have both polishing and abrasive effects. *Smaller* particles (1 mm) have a polishing action, and *larger* particles (20 mm) have an abrasive action.[11]

In selecting a dentifrice, the abrasiveness and polishing characteristics should meet individual needs. For instance, up to 20% of the population does not accumulate visible stain when engaged in their own style of personal oral hygiene.[12] For these individuals, a dentifrice with high polishing and low abrasion should be recommended. For the average individual, an additional amount of abrasive is needed to control accumulating stain. The stains on neglected teeth may be green, orange, or black stains of chromogenic bacterial origin, or yellow and brown stains from smoking. As the abrasive level increases, greater care must be taken to perfect brushing techniques that do not cause *self-inflicted injury* to the teeth or soft tissues. Such injuries can result from excessive pressure, hard bristles, and prolonged brushing.

When toothbrushing is done without toothpaste, there is little possibility of abrasion. When damage does occur, it usually appears as a V-shaped notch in the *cementum immediately below the cementoenamel junction* (Figure 6–2). This area is vulnerable, because enamel is about *20 times harder* than dentin or cementum. More serious defects usually occur in older individuals who maintain a very high level of oral hygiene.

### Humectants

Toothpaste consisting only of a toothpowder and water results in a product with several undesirable properties. Over time, the solids in the paste tend to settle out of solution and the water evaporates. This may result in caking of the remaining dentifrice. Until the 1930s, most toothpaste had a short shelf-life because of this problem. Once the tube was opened, the first expelled paste was too liquid, but the last paste in the tube was either impossible to

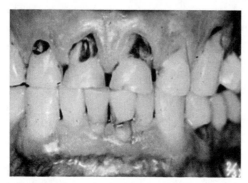

FIGURE 6-2   V-Shaped notches in central incisors resulting from use of a dentifrice with a harsh abrasive system. (Courtesy of Dr. B Baker, University of Texas Dental School, San Antonio.)

expel or too hard to use. To solve this problem, *humectants were added to maintain the moisture.* Commonly used humectants are sorbitol, mannitol, and propylene glycol. These humectants are nontoxic, but mold or bacterial growth can occur in their presence. For this reason, *preservatives* such as sodium benzoate are added.

Humectants help maintain the consistency of toothpaste, but despite their presence, the solids tend to settle out of the paste. To *counteract* this, *thickening or binding agents* are added to the formula. Gums, such as gum tragacanth, were first used. These were followed by colloids derived from seaweed, such as carrageenan. These, in turn, were replaced by synthetic celluloses. These celluloses in *low* concentrations are also often used as humectants; in *higher* concentrations they function as gelling agents in the formulation of gel dentifrices. At *high* concentrations (> 40%), humectants also act as preservatives.

## Soaps and Detergents

Because toothpastes were originally manufactured to keep the teeth clean, soap was the logical cleansing agent. As the toothbrush bristles dislodge food debris and plaque, the foaming or sudsing action of the soap aids in the removal of the loosened material. Soaps have several disadvantages: they can be irritating to the mucous membrane, their flavor is difficult to mask and often causes nausea, and many times soaps are incompatible with other ingredients, such as calcium.

When detergents appeared on the market, soaps largely disappeared from dentifrices. Today, *sodium lauryl sulfate (SLS) is the most widely used detergent.* It is *stable,* possesses some *antibacterial* properties, and has a *low surface tension,* which facilitates the flow of the dentifrice over the teeth. SLS is active at a neutral pH, has a flavor that is easy to mask, and is compatible with the current dentifrice ingredients. Barkvoll has suggested that patients who suffer from various oral mucosal diseases should avoid the use of dentifrices containing SLS.[13] Low SLS dentifrices have been marketed, which claim to be associated with a lower incidence of oral ulcers.

### Flavoring and Sweetening Agents

*Flavor,* along with *smell, color,* and *consistency* of a product, are important characteristics that lead to *public acceptance of a dentifrice.* If dentifrices did not possess these characteristics, they would probably be poorly accepted. For taste acceptance, the flavor must be pleasant, provide an immediate taste sensation, and be relatively long-lasting. Usually synthetic flavors are blended to provide the desired taste. Spearmint, peppermint, wintergreen, cinnamon, and other flavors give toothpaste a pleasant taste, aroma, and refreshing aftertaste. Some manufacturers use essential oils such as thymol, menthol, etc., which may provide a "medicinal" taste to the product. In addition, these oils may impart antibacterial effects, as will be discussed later in this chapter. It is difficult to formulate a flavor that is universally acceptable, because people have different color and taste preferences.

## Question 2

Which of the following statements, if any, are correct?

A. Gel dentifrices are the same as regular dentifrices, except that they contain a greater proportion of thickening agent.

B. The abrasiveness of an abrasive agent depends on the inherent hardness of an abrasive, the size of the abrasive particles, and the shape of the abrasive particles.

C. The V-shaped damage to the tooth from using an excessively abrasive dentifrice occurs apical to the cemento-enamel junction.

D. Synthetic celluloses are now used as thickening agents for toothpastes and gels.

E. If sodium lauryl sulfate is added to the dentifrice formula, foaming can be expected when brushing.

## Sweetening Agents

In early toothpaste formulations, sugar, honey, and other sweeteners were used. Because these materials can be broken down in the mouth to produce acids and lower plaque pH, they may increase caries. They have been replaced with saccharin, cyclamate, sorbitol, and mannitol as primary *noncariogenic* sweetening agents. Sorbitol and mannitol serve a *dual role* as sweetening agents and humectants. Glycerin, which also serves as a humectant, adds to the sweet taste. A new sweetener in some dentifrices is *xylitol*. In laboratory studies, it is not metabolized by bacteria to produce acid. In human studies, where it was placed in chewing gums and food, xylitol was noncariogenic. In addition, it demonstrated an anticaries capability by *facilitating* the *remineralization* of incipient carious lesions.

## Baking-Soda Dentifrices

Baking soda (sodium bicarbonate) has had a *long history of use as an oral-hygiene aid*. Church and Dwight, a manufacturer of baking soda, and also the manufacturer of the original baking-soda toothpaste, has stated "two out of three dentists and hygienists recommend brushing with baking soda for healthier teeth and gums." In a series of papers published in 1998, antiplaque, gingivitis reduction, stain-removal, and odor-reducing efficacy were *documented* for sodium bicarbonate–containing dentifrices.[6]

Some dentists have also suggested the mixture of baking soda with peroxide as an alternative to the use of commercial dentifrices. Anecdotally, many patients attribute benefit to the routine use of these products. It was inevitable that these products would be incorporated into toothpastes. Selected examples of currently marketed baking soda dentifrices are presented in Appendix 6–1. All contain hydrated silica that is compatible with fluoride. No dentifrice containing baking soda as the *sole* active ingredient has received the ADA Seal of Acceptance. It was only *after fluoride* was added to the formulations, and after required laboratory, animal, and clinical studies were completed, that several baking soda–fluoride dentifrices were accepted as effective in caries control. These baking-soda dentifrices actually contain only a small amount of baking soda, in addition to the standard fluoride-compatible abrasives.

## Essential-Oil Dentifrices

The essential-oil ingredients found in Listerine mouthrinse (see below) are also available in a dentifrice formulation. The clinical and laboratory data suggest a benefit to gingival health and plaque reduction.[14,15] This product does *not* carry the ADA Seal of Acceptance.

## Therapeutic Dentifrices

The most commonly used therapeutic agent added to dentifrices is *fluoride*, which aids in

the control of caries. In 1960, the Council on Dental Therapeutics of the American Dental Association, based on several studies that indicated its effectiveness, classified Crest toothpaste with stannous fluoride as a *caries prophylactic dentifrice*. For the first time, a therapeutic dentifrice was awarded the Seal of *Provisional* Acceptance. In 1964, on the basis of further new and favorable data,[16] the classification was upgraded to *full* acceptance.

The original level of fluoride in OTC dentifrices and gels was restricted to 1,000 to 1,100 ppm fluoride and a total of no more than 120 mg of fluoride in the tube, with a requirement that the package include a safety closure. Therapeutic toothpastes, dispensed on prescription, could contain up to 260 mg of fluoride in a tube.

The following fluorides are generally recognized as effective and safe for OTC sales: 0.22% sodium fluoride (NaF) at a level of 1,100 ppm, 0.76% sodium monofluorophosphate (MFP) at a level of 1,000 ppm, and 0.4% stannous fluoride (SnF$_2$) at a level of 1,000 ppm. Fluoride levels were increased to 1,500 ppm sodium monofluorophosphate in "Extra Strength Aim," marketed OTC. In published studies,[17,18] this product was 10% more effective than an 1,100 ppm NaF dentifrice. A recently introduced *prescription dentifrice*, Colgate Prevident 5,000, contains 5,000-ppm fluoride.

One baking soda–peroxide–fluoride dentifrice (Mentadent) is unique in its packaging. Mentadent contains a combination of 0.75% stable *peroxide gel* in conjunction with *baking soda*, and *1,100 ppm sodium fluoride*. The materials are packaged in a two-chamber pump to permit the baking soda and peroxide components to be mixed with the fluoride at the time of delivery. The product has been demonstrated to be safe,[19] and the low level of hydrogen peroxide does not present problems alleged to result from higher levels of peroxide in early animal studies.[20]

Multiple clinical studies of fluoride dentifrices containing NaF, MFP, or SnF$_2$ in the presence of compatible abrasives and stable formulations have been submitted to and been accepted by the ADA. The Association, therefore, awards the Seal of Acceptance to fluoride dentifrices based solely on laboratory data if they comply with previously submitted clinical data.[21]

The fluoride dentifrices currently accepted by the Council on Scientific Affairs of the American Dental Association are available at the ADA web site, www.ada.org. *Not all fluoride-containing dentifrices have demonstrated anticaries activity.* The level of active fluoride must be adequate and must be maintained over the shelf-life of the dentifrice. The Seal of Acceptance of the American Dental Association is one assurance of an active product. Fluoride dentifrices are discussed more extensively in Chapter 9.

### Control of Plaque and Gingivitis

Most intriguing is the concept of *chemical plaque control*, in which chemical compounds are used to *supplement* the usual brushing, flossing, and use of auxiliary aids employed in mechanical plaque control. Antiplaque agents can act directly on the plaque bacteria or can disrupt different components of plaque to permit easier and more complete removal during toothbrushing and flossing. This opportunity to use chemistry to enhance oral hygiene procedures is important because manual plaque-control methods are difficult to teach and monitor, tedious to perform, time-consuming, impossible to accomplish by some physically and mentally handicapped persons, and not used by nonmotivated individuals.

The present chemical plaque-control agents should *not* be considered a panacea because they have not been proven to be a total substitute for routine oral-hygiene measures. *Excessive emphasis on chemical control may encourage some patients to deemphasize proven oral-hygiene methods.*

At the present time, an agent (or agents) analogous to fluoride in controlling caries is

being sought to control plaque and gingivitis and to prevent periodontitis. The properties of an ideal form of such an agent are listed in Table 6–3. Although many OTC products are being marketed with plaque-gingivitis claims, only *two* dentifrices are currently marketed with *ADA-accepted* claims (see ADA website, www.ada.org). Both contain *triclosan* and will be discussed further in this chapter.

### Stannous Salts

Stannous fluoride ($SnF_2$), specifically the stannous ion, has reported activity against caries, plaque, and gingivitis.[22] While $SnF_2$ has a long record as an anticaries agent, long-term stability in dentifrices and mouthrinses has been questioned since clinical antimicrobial activity has only been demonstrated in anhydrous products.[22] The development and subsequent laboratory and clinical efficacy of a stabilized $SnF_2$ dentifrice has been reported.[23,24] This dentifrice

---

TABLE 6-3 **Properties of an Ideal Agent to Control Gingivitis**

High immediate antimicrobial activity

Broad-spectrum efficacy against bacteria and yeasts

Chemical stability in formulations and in the oral cavity

Substantivity (ability to stick) to oral tissues, and be released over time in an active form

Toxicologic and ecological safety

    No topical adverse reactions (staining, burning)

    No taste or aftertaste problems

    No inhibition of taste perception

    No systemic toxicity

        No change in oral or gastrointestinal flora

        Neither carcinogenic nor teratogenic

No adverse reactions

Compatibility with dentifrice or mouthwash formulations

---

has been marketed in the United States by Procter & Gamble as Crest Gum Care. Clinical studies have been performed versus essential-oil mouthrinses, baking-soda/peroxide dentifrices, and triclosan-containing dentifrices with pyrophosphate/copolymer/zinc citrate. Superior efficacy has been shown for Crest Gum Care in antimicrobial, plaque acidogenicity, gingivitis or gingival bleeding, and calculus control.[25,26] However, long-term studies with this $SnF_2$ dentifrice demonstrated an increase in extrinsic stain attributed to the stannous ion.

### Triclosan

Triclosan is a broad-spectrum antibacterial agent, marketed by its manufacturer, Ciba-Geigy, for use in oral products under the trade name Irgacare. It is effective against a wide variety of bacteria and is widely used as an antibacterial agent in OTC consumer products in the United States, including deodorant soaps and antibacterial skin scrubs. It has also been shown to be a useful antibacterial agent in oral products. A review of the available pharmacological and toxicological information concluded, "Triclosan can be considered safe for use in dentifrice and mouth rinse products."[27]

Many dentifrices and mouthrinses containing triclosan are marketed in Europe. In the United States, one dentifrice, developed by Colgate-Palmolive, contains triclosan, a patented copolymer, 'Gantrez', and fluoride. This product, Colgate Total, has undergone extensive safety[27] and clinical-efficacy testing.[28,29,30] and was approved in 1997 by the FDA as the first dentifrice to help prevent *gingivitis, plaque, and caries*. Colgate Total also has received the American Dental Association's Seal of Acceptance as an "effective decay preventive dentifrice, and to help prevent and reduce gingivitis when used as directed in a conscientiously applied program of oral hygiene and regular professional care. It has also been shown to help reduce the formation of plaque and tartar above the gum line. Its effect on pe-

riodontitis has not been determined." Two other "Colgate Totals" have been accepted; "Fresh Stripe" and a new formula making all of the above claims plus whitening. Recently, a 2-year study on Total has documented long-term anticaries efficacy.[31] Research on a triclosan-pyrophosphate combination in a dentifrice has demonstrated plaque *regrowth inhibition* and *anticalculus activity*.[32,33]

A Unilever product containing zinc citrate and triclosan has also received attention. Clinical evaluation has shown this to be effective in reducing plaque formation and in preventing gingivitis. A summary of the zinc citrate–triclosan studies has been published.[34] This product is not currently marketed in the United States.

### Anticalculus Dentifrices

Calculus-control dentifrice formulations are designed to *interrupt the process of mineralization of plaque to calculus*. Plaque has a bacterial matrix that mineralizes due to the *super saturation* of saliva with calcium and phosphate ions. Crystal growth inhibitors may be added to dentifrices to provide a reduction in calculus formation.

In the late 1970s, anticalculus dentifrices began to appear on the market without any evidence of effectiveness.[35] In 1985, Procter & Gamble supplemented their existent Crest anticariogenic toothpaste with a similar anticaries formula that also contained a combination of *tetra sodium phosphate and disodium dihydrogen pyrophosphate*. The soluble pyrophosphates are crystal growth inhibitors, which retard the formation of calculus.[36] This combination has been demonstrated in clinical studies to significantly reduce the amount of calculus formed, compared with a control dentifrice. The dentifrice is marketed as Crest Tartar Control. The formula received the American Dental Association's Seal of Acceptance, but only as a caries control product and only because of its fluoride content. Other similar anticalculus products that are now on the market all contain NaF.

A recent addition to the list of available products is a dentifrice with both a whitening and an anticalculus claim.[37] The product, "Colgate Tartar Control Plus Whitening Fluoride Toothpaste" contains tetrasodium pyrophosphate, sodium tripolyphosphate, a copolymer, and NaF.

Rølla and Saxegaard[38] have noted the possibility of "crystal poisons," such as pyrophosphates and phosphonates, inhibiting remineralization. Such inhibition might adversely affect the anticaries effect of the fluoride in this type of calculus control dentifrice. Zinc citrate trihydrate is used to inhibit calculus formation in the tartar control versions of both Aim and Close-Up. Clinical studies[39] have shown that *zinc citrate does not affect the caries inhibition of fluoride*.

Despite favorable anticalculus data, the ADA seal *has not been awarded* to products with only an anticalculus claim, because the ADA considers calculus inhibition as a cosmetic, not a therapeutic effect. With an anticalculus agent, two simultaneous beneficial effects—caries control and calculus inhibition—are available with one brushing operation. The currently marketed ADA accepted anticaries products that also inhibit calculus formation might be found at the ADA web site, www.ada.org (see Appendix 6–2).

---

**Question 3**

Which of the following statements, if any, are true?

A. Baking soda, peroxide, and fluoride are incompatible in a dentifrice.

B. The present consensus is that chemical-plaque control is only a supplement to mechanical-plaque control.

C. Stannous fluoride is both an anticaries and an antigingivitis agent.

D. Triclosan is an effective antibacterial agent.

E. Crest Tartar Control toothpaste has received the American Dental Association's Seal of Acceptance as a therapeutic anticalculus product.

## Antihypersensitivity Products

Many people experience pain when exposed areas of the root, especially at the cemento-enamel junction, are *subjected to heat or cold*. To address this issue the ADA has formed the Ad Hoc Committee on Dentinal Sensitivity. Several OTC dentifrices have been accepted with the active agents such as *potassium nitrate*, *strontium chloride*, and *sodium citrate*.[40] Currently accepted products may be found on the ADA web site, www.ada.org (see Appendix 6–2). Potassium citrate has also been accepted by the British Department of Health.

The American Dental Association's Council on Dental Therapeutics has approved a dentifrice (Sensodyne F) with a combination of active ingredients, demonstrating both antihypersensitivity and caries-preventive benefits. This is another example of a therapeutic dentifrice directed simultaneously at solving two problems, caries and hypersensitivity, with the same brushing operation.

## Whiteners

Considerable controversy surrounds the use of stain removers and tooth whiteners. Products are being marketed for professional use or for use by the patient at home. Many claims for efficacy and safety are under review by agencies and government panels. The ADA website should be consulted for a list of currently accepted products. Cosmetic benefits of dentifrices remain important to patients.

Surveys reveal a growing U.S. market share for dentifrices claiming "whitening" or "stain control." These dentifrices control stain via *physical methods* (abrasives) and *chemical mechanisms* (surface active agents or bleaching/oxidizing agents). Although the public perceives these as more abrasive than ordinary toothpastes, their abrasiveness is usually intermediate among the products tested.

Dentifrices marketed with tooth-whitener claims are available as a toothpaste or gel, or are used in a two- or three-step treatment "process." These products usually contain *hydrogen peroxide* or *carbamide peroxide* as their bleaching or whitening ingredient. Carbamide peroxide breaks down to form urea and hydrogen peroxide. Hydrogen peroxide, in turn, forms a free radical containing *oxygen*, which is the active bleaching molecule. Home-bleaching products may contain other chemicals to aid in the delivery of the *bleaching* agent. Glycerin or propylene glycol is commonly added to thicken the solution and prolong contact with the tooth surface. In the two- or three-step products, agents can be delivered to teeth via a custom-made tray or by toothbrushing.

There is concern that regular use of the peroxides or their breakdown products may enable overgrowth of undesirable organisms, including yeasts, possibly leading to "black hairy tongue." In addition, peroxides may damage the pulp or the soft tissues of the mouth. Delayed wound healing is also a concern, as is the possible mutagenic effect of strong oxygenating agents. The Food and Drug Administration has sent a regulatory letter to producers of those commercial tooth-whitening agents containing peroxides to inform them that these products are classified as drugs. The letter asked for information about possible side effects, such as delayed wound healing, periodontal harm, and mutagenic potential. The American Dental Association's Council on Scientific Affairs has issued "Guidelines for the Acceptance of Peroxide Containing Oral Hygiene Products."[41]

A dentifrice (Crest Extra Whitening) has been introduced which uses a stain specific soft tissue technology.[42] This product, which contains NaF, claims calculus control activity as well as stain removal and an anticaries benefit.

## Mouthrinses

Freshening bad breath has been the traditional purpose of mouthrinses. The 1992 market for such products was estimated at $635 million. Sales increased to $739 million in 2000. In addition to the traditional cosmetic use, therapeutic mouthrinses are now available.

The claimed active ingredients of mouthrinses include *quaternary ammonium compounds, boric and benzoic acids, and phenolic compounds*. As with dentifrices, commercial sales of cosmetic rinses have been related to taste, color, smell, and the pleasant sensation that follows use. The pleasant sensation is often enhanced by the addition of astringents. Commonly used astringents are alum, zinc stearate, zinc citrate, and acetic or citric acids. Zinc sulfate has been added to mouth rinses as a claimed antiplaque ingredient.

Alcohol in mouthrinses is used as a *solvent, a taste enhancer*, and an agent providing an *aftertaste*. The alcohol content of commercial rinses, ranging *up to 27%*, may constitute a danger for children, especially those from 2 to 3 years of age. According to the National Poison Center Network, 5 to 10 ounces of a mouthrinse containing *alcohol can be lethal for a child* weighing 26 pounds. Between 1987 and 1991, the nation's poison-control centers logged more than 10,000 reports of children younger than 6 years old drinking mouthrinses containing alcohol; *3 died* and another 40 had life-threatening conditions or suffered permanent injuries.[43] The American Academy of Pediatrics has recommended that OTC liquid preparations be *limited to 5% ethanol*, that safety closures be required, and that the packaged volume be kept to a "reasonable minimum to prevent the potential for lethal ingestion."[44]

The Council on Scientific Affairs of the American Dental Association requires child-resistant caps on all alcohol-containing mouth rinses that bear the Seal of Acceptance.[43] The council also requires manufacturers of ADA-accepted mouthrinses that contain more than 5% alcohol to include the following statement on the label: "Warning: Keep out of reach of children. Do not swallow. Contains alcohol. Use only as directed." The attorneys general of 29 states have petitioned the U.S. Consumer Products Safety Commission to require child safety caps on bottles of mouthwash that contain more than 5% alcohol.

Research from the National Cancer Institute (NCI) has *linked* alcohol and mouthwash to *mouth and throat cancers*.[45] After taking into account participants' smoking and drinking habits, it was found that cancer patients were more likely than the control group to have rinsed regularly with a high-alcohol (25% or more) mouthwash. The researchers concluded that alcohol may or may not cause cancer in and of itself but may promote the disease by dissolving and dispersing other cancer-causing substances within the mouth and throat. The ADA has stated, "According to a statement from the NCI, it is premature to make recommendations about any alcohol-containing mouthwashes. In the meantime, the Association suggests that patients continue to use the therapeutic mouthrinses accepted by the ADA . . . and recommended by their dentists."[46]

## Cosmetic Mouthrinses

### Halitosis

Oral malodor has been a neglected research area. Indeed, the first scientific symposium on halitosis research was not held until 1991. Further research and education is needed in this important area because many practicing dental professionals still believe that bad breath usually comes from the stomach. Identifying the cause of halitosis and developing an appropriate treatment plan can be difficult.[47] Published studies by Spouge[48] and by Tonzetich[49] have demonstrated that oral malodor *usually derives from the mouth* itself and may be reduced fol-

lowing oral hygiene. To motivate improvement in oral hygiene, dental professionals should advise patients that bad breath might result from microbial putrefaction within the mouth. Rosenberg[50] notes, "Bad breath is a cause of concern, embarrassment, and frustration on the part of the general public. Oral malodor, whether real or perceived, can lead to social isolation, divorce proceedings, and even 'contemplation of suicide.' "

A body of science currently exists to permit the *quantitative assessment of bad breath*, which should be able to verify product claims for treating this important symptom. Many rinses have breath-freshening claims. Many claim breath freshening, but the effect is caused by flavors and has no effect after 3 to 5 hours. In diagnosing and treating complaints of bad breath, the clinician should consider psychological as well as physical factors.[51]

### Xerostomia Mouth Rinses

Many people experience dry mouth (*xerostomia*) traceable to *several possible causes*, such as damage to the salivary glands following radiation therapy for head and neck cancer, Sjögren's syndrome, and use of tranquilizing drugs, especially the tricyclic antidepressants. In such cases the mucous membrane is continually dry and uncomfortable. To ameliorate the dryness, artificial salivas have been developed, which are used *ad libitum* by the patient to moisten the mucous membrane.

Because xerostomia is correlated with an *increased caries incidence*, the rinses usually contain *fluoride* as well as chemical compounds in concentrations that closely parallel those of saliva. The rinses that contain fluoride may, in reality, be *remineralizing solutions*. Several artificial salivas have been accepted by the ADA; among which are Salivart and Xero-Lube. For a current listing, consult the ADA website, www.ada.org. Several moisturizing agents are also available to xerostomia patients.[52]

### Therapeutic Mouth Rinse Agents

#### Chlorhexidine

*The FDA has approved prescription plaque-control rinses containing 0.12% chlorhexidine.* Peridex (Omni Oral Pharmaceuticals) has received the ADA seal and Prevident (Colgate) is also marketed. Directions call for a twice daily, 30-second rinse with 1 oz of such solutions.

Chlorhexidine has proved to be one of the most effective antiplaque agents to date.[53] Chlorhexidine is a cationic compound that binds to the hydroxyapatite of tooth enamel, to the pellicle, to plaque bacteria, to the extracellular polysaccharide of the plaque,[54] and especially to the mucous membrane.[55] The chlorhexidine adsorbed to the hydroxyapatite is believed to inhibit bacterial colonization.[56] After binding, the agent is *slowly released in active form over 12 to 24 hours.*[57] This ability of the oral tissues to adsorb an active agent and to permit its slow release in active form over a prolonged period is known as *substantivity*. As the substantivity of an antiplaque agent decreases, the frequency of use needs to be increased.

Chlorhexidine has not proved beneficial as the *sole* method of treating periodontitis with deep pockets. Following root planing, prophylaxis, or periodontal surgery, chlorhexidine irrigation may be effective in helping to control inflammation and subgingival plaque.[58]

In some countries, such as the United States, chlorhexidine products are available only by prescription. In others, such as the United Kingdom, they are available over the counter. Although chlorhexidine is quite effective, it is not active against all relevant anaerobes. A high minimal concentration is necessary for efficacy. Some side effects are associated with chlorhexidine use, of which stain is the most common.[59] Occasionally *altered taste* sensation is reported.[60] *Increased calculus* formation,[61] *superficial desquamation of*

*tissue*, and *hypersensitivity* have also been noted.[62,63] Chlorhexidine is inactivated by most dentifrice surfactants and, therefore it is not included in dentifrices. Also, because of this inactivation, it is *critical for dental professionals* to alert patients not to use chlorhexidine mouthrinses within 30 minutes before or after regular toothbrushing.

Although chlorhexidine may be more effective than any other current antiplaque agent and has a definite role in preventive and control dental procedures, it is not a "magic bullet." Its *side effects* and inadequate activity range somewhat limit its use.

## Essential Oils

Listerine antiseptic was the first OTC antiplaque and antigingivitis mouth rinse to be approved by the ADA.[64] Patients are advised to rinse twice daily with 20 mL of Listerine for 30 seconds, in addition to their usual oral-hygiene regimen. Listerine has been used as a mouthrinse for more than 110 years. The active ingredients are *thymol, menthol, eucalyptol, and methyl salicylate*, termed *essential oils*. The original formula contains *26.9% alcohol*. A flavor variation of the product, Cool Mint Listerine Antiseptic, which also has received the ADA seal, contains 21.6% alcohol. Microorganisms *do not* develop a resistance to the antibacterial effects of essential oils, such as clove oil (eugenol) and thyme oil (thymol).[65] In long-term clinical trials, Listerine has been shown to *reduce* both plaque accumulation and severity of gingivitis by up to 34%.[66] Microbial sampling of plaque in these trials has demonstrated no undesirable shifts in the composition of the microbial flora.

Based on laboratory testing, more than 200 generic versions of original Listerine have also been granted the ADA seal and are marketed under numerous trade names. These may be found at the ADA website, www.ada.org.

A recent study evaluated the comparative efficacy of Listerine and an antiplaque/antigingivitis dentifrice (Colgate Total).[67] When used in conjunction with a fluoride dentifrice and usual oral hygiene, Listerine was reported to provide a greater benefit in reducing plaque than did Colgate Total.

As with chlorhexidine, rinsing with an essential oil mouth rinse *per se* is unlikely to be effective in treating periodontitis because the solution does not reach the depths of the periodontal pockets. Irrigation studies, using irrigator tips designed to deliver solutions subgingivally, suggest that Listerine and Peridex may have some value as adjuncts to mechanical therapy.

For the dental professional, it *may be important* for patients to use a mouthrinse prior to aerosol-generating procedures. Unless an effective dry-field technique is used, the bacterial aerosol generated by a high-speed turbine in a 30-second period is roughly equivalent to the patient sneezing in the dentist's face.[68] A study by Wyler and coworkers[69] found that even a preliminary water rinse temporarily reduced the bacterial aerosol population by 61%, brushing alone by 85%, and an antibacterial mouthrinse by 97%. Fine and coworkers,[70] using a simulated office visit model, showed that *preprocedural* use of an antimicrobial mouth rinse (Listerine) resulted in a 93.6% reduction in the number of viable bacteria in a dental aerosol produced by ultrasonic scaling. The effect of this reduction on actual disease transmission has not been determined.[71]

## Fluoride Rinses

The active agents in over-the-counter fluoride mouthrinse products are sodium fluoride (NaF) or acidulated phosphofluorides (APF) at concentrations of 0.05 and 0.44%, respectively. The dose directions are 10 ml of product to be used *once daily*.

Published long-term clinical studies have consistently shown anticaries effectiveness *equal or superior* to fluoride dentifrices. The ADA website, www.ada.org, currently lists seven nonprescription fluoride-containing

mouthrinses that have received the Seal of Acceptance for anticaries effectiveness.

---

### Question 4

Which of the following statements, if any, are correct?

A. Xersostomia mouthrinses are usually formulated to prevent demineralization and promote remineralization.

B. The ADA has awarded its Seal of Acceptance to a whitener-containing carbamide peroxide.

C. The agent in cosmetic mouthrinses that poses the greatest danger to 2- to 4-year-old children is alcohol.

D. Chlorhexidine mouthrinses are most effective when used immediately after brushing.

E. Fluoride-containing mouthrinses are not as effective as fluoride-containing dentifrices for anticaries activity.

---

### Chewing Gum

Because gum chewing is pleasurable, people normally chew for longer periods of time than they spend brushing their teeth. Likewise, gum may complement toothbrushing by reaching many of the tooth surfaces commonly missed during brushing. The average American fails to contact approximately 40% of tooth surfaces during toothbrushing, especially the posterior teeth and lingual surfaces. Regular toothbrushing removes only about 35 to 40% of dental plaque present on tooth surfaces. In addition, chewing gum is especially advantageous during the course of the day when toothbrushing is not possible or convenient.

Beneficial effects of gum chewing include *increased saliva* production resulting in the mechanical removal of dental plaque and debris. Studies have shown that chewing sugared or sugar-free gum is an effective means of reducing plaque accumulation and that gum chewing can also effectively reduce established plaque on many tooth surfaces (see Appendix 6–3).

Since 1997, three major review articles devoted solely to chewing gum and potential oral health benefits have been published.[72–74] The interest of researchers in effective gum additives coupled with the acceptance and use of chewing-gum products by the general public makes this a new and potentially important category to be considered by dental professionals. In 1999, the worldwide chewing-gum market was estimated to be 560,000 tons per year, or approximately 5 billion U.S. dollars.[74]

During gum chewing, salivary flow rates increase, especially in the first few minutes, because of *both mechanical and gustatory stimulation.* Increased salivary stimulation can continue for periods of *5 to 20 minutes,* usually until the flavor(s) in the product dissipates. However, even with unflavored chewing gum, saliva flow, as evidenced by swallowing rates, increase over baseline.[75] The beneficial effects of additional saliva in the mouth include increased *buffer capacity* and *mineral super saturation,* both of which help regulate or increase plaque pH, and increase plaque calcium levels (pCa).[76] In addition, increased saliva flow can assist in loosening and removing debris from occlusal or interproximal sites, and can be beneficial to xerostomia patients.

The focus of chewing gum research to date has been on "sugar-free" products,[77] which contain polyol sweeteners such *as sorbitol or xylitol.* These sweeteners are not broken down by plaque or oral microorganisms to produce acid. Plaque pH studies have documented reduction of plaque acidity and maintenance of plaque neutrality both during and, with xylitol, for periods of 2 to 3 weeks following, gum chewing.[73] In addition, gums containing xylitol have shown *anticaries* activity in several *long-term studies.*[73] Chewing a *sorbitol-based chewing gum* after meals significantly *reduced dental caries* incidence in a three-year study.[78]

Studies[79] have shown that a commercial chewing gum containing 5% sodium bicarbon-

ate (Arm and Hammer Dental Care) is capable of removing significant amounts of plaque and reducing gingivitis when used as an adjunct to regular toothbrushing. Stain removal is also of interest to the consumer. Studies simulating a realistic situation (twice-daily brushing and unsupervised use of a baking soda chewing gum) demonstrated *reduction in stain* after four weeks.[79]

Consumers have relied on chewing-gum products for "fresh breath." A recent report on reducing volatile sulfur compounds associated with oral malodor and organoleptic scores indicates that the products tested are effective primarily as masking agents (flavor) and for the mechanical role in cleaning tooth surfaces. Reduced malodor levels were obtained during initial use of the products, but decreased to baseline levels at the three-hour assessment times.[80]

Reynolds[81] has proposed the introduction of *casein phosphopeptide* to chewing gum as a mechanism to *remineralize* early carious lesions. In situ studies appear promising.[82] Trident Advantage, with Recaldent, makes use of this technology.

An overview of selected agents added to chewing gums is presented in Appendix 6–3. Compounds such as chlorhexidine and fluorides would appear to be useful when delivered using chewing gum as the vehicle, since there would be a minimum of potentially interfering agents in the gum product (compared to abrasives in dentifrices and water and alcohol vehicles in mouthrinses), as well as a sustained time of release and availability in the oral cavity. In addition, the active agents would be available at occlusal sites, which are prime areas for plaque growth and pit and fissure decay. Neither of these agents is available in the United States. Since chewing-gum products are often in the mouth several times a day, the concentration of ingredients released (especially fluoride) *must be safe for swallowing.*

---

### Question 5

Which of the following statements, if any, are correct?

A. Saliva flow rates increase while using chewing gum.

B. An increased saliva flow would help dilute any acids in the plaque.

C. Xylitol and sorbitol flavoring of chewing gum is ideal because both are anticariogenic.

D. A chewing gum with 5% sodium bicarbonate has been demonstrated to reduce stain and reduce gingivitis.

E. Casein phosphopeptide appears to be a promising agent in chewing gum for enhancing remineralization.

---

## SUMMARY

The self-use of dentifrices and mouthrinses is proving to be an important preventive dentistry measure.

Dentifrices, mouthrinses, and chewing gums can be categorized as either cosmetic or therapeutic. Cosmetic products have traditionally been used to remove debris, provide a pleasant "mouth feel," and temporarily reduce halitosis. To improve on their marketability, flavors, stripes, sprinkles, and colors have been added to dentifrices and mouthrinses. Recently, other ingredients have also been added to temporarily depress the oral bacterial population or to prevent or moderate some disease process in the mouth.

The widespread use of therapeutic fluoride dentifrices and mouthrinses is credited with helping to reduce the worldwide prevalence of dental decay. All products carrying the ADA Seal also contain fluoride.

Other agents are now being used to target other oral-health problems.

The Food and Drug Administration has developed rigid guidelines for testing the safety and efficacy of products prior to their introduction on the market. Part of the function of the regulatory process is to differentiate between products whose potential risks are sufficiently low to allow them to be sold over the counter and those whose possible hazards justify restriction to prescription use.

While the ADA considers antiplaque, anticalculus, and breath-freshening claims as cosmetic, they will review data and allow manufacturers to make these statements, if coupled with a disease related activity (e.g., prevents gingivitis or caries). Toothpastes containing potassium nitrate, strontium chloride, and sodium citrate have antihypersensitivity properties; other toothpastes with tetrasodium phosphate and disodium dihydrogen pyrophosphate retard the formation of calculus. Chlorhexidine is a highly effective antiplaque, antigingivitis agent, accepted by the ADA, but with significant side effects and may only be dispensed on prescription. Listerine, containing essential oils, has been popular for over a century, and has demonstrated the same properties but without the side effects of chlorhexidine. More than 200 generic versions of Listerine, containing essential oils, have been accepted by the ADA for plaque and gingivitis claims.

Chewing gum products are a new dental category in which manufacturers are making claims for cosmetic and therapeutic effectiveness. At this time, neither the ADA nor the FDA has approved any chewing gum products for dental therapeutic claims.

## ANSWERS AND EXPLANATIONS

1. A, C, and D—Correct

    B—incorrect. The rulings by the FDA have the force of law; the rulings by the ADA are advisory to the profession and public.

    E—incorrect. All actions to secure the Seal of Approval are voluntary. The manufacturer is not committed to apply for it, or to use it in advertising. However, to use it for marketing purposes is to the advantage of any manufacturer having received it.

2. A, B, C, D, and E—correct.

3. B, C, and D—correct.

    A—incorrect. Under some circumstances, it is possible they are incompatible. However, the fact that there is now a dentifrice called Mentadent is proof that peroxide, baking soda, and fluoride can be compatible.

    E—incorrect. Remember, the ADA awards the Seal of Acceptance for therapeutic products, and not for cosmetic agents. Calculus is considered a cosmetic blight.

4. A, C—correct.

   B—incorrect. This is another example of the ADA policy of not awarding the Seal of Acceptance for a cosmetic product.

   D—incorrect. Since chlorhexidine is inactivated by most dentifrice surfactants, a period of about 30 minutes should elapse between toothbrushing and chlorhexidine mouthrinsing.

   E—incorrect. The fluoride mouthrinses are probably better than fluoride dentifrices, possibly because they allow better access to caries-prone interproximal locations.

5. A, B, C, D, and E—correct.

## Self-evaluation Questions

1. Name at least four tooth and gum conditions for which formulas have been developed to help prevent or control: _____, _____, _____ and _____.

2. The _____ is the name of the award given by the ADA to dental manufacturers who have prepared a therapeutic product that is safe and efficient.

3. There are three levels of concern for the safety and efficiency of prescription and over-the-counter dental products. The government level includes the Food and Drug administration and the _____; the second level is voluntary professional oversight assumed voluntarily by the _____, while the third level is by _____ advocates.

4. The two mouthrinses granted the Seal of Acceptance by the ADA as antiplaque and antigingivitis are _____ and _____.

5. Two factors that can decrease or enhance the abrasiveness of a toothpaste are: _____ and _____.

6. The difference between an abrasive and a polishing agent is _____; when the two are mixed together, they constitute an _____.

7. The three fluoride compounds most used in fluoride dentifrices are _____, _____, and _____.

8. Three properties of a dentifrice or a mouthrinse that do not contribute to the therapeutic or cosmetic effects, but must be considered because of marketing necessities are _____, _____, and _____.

9. The agent added to a toothpaste formula to preserve the moisture is called a _____.

10. A toothpaste formula where the effective agent is solely baking soda is a (cosmetic)(therapeutic) dentifrice.

# REFERENCES

1. Trummel C. (1994). Regulation of oral chemotherapeutic products in the United States. *J Dent Res*, 73:704–708.

2. Department of Health, Education, and Welfare, Food and Drug Administration (1980). Establishment of a monograph on anticaries drug product for over-the-counter human use; proposed rulemaking. *Federal Register*. March 28, Part IV.

3. Over-the-counter dental and oral health care drug products for antiplaque use; safety and efficacy review. *Federal Register*. September 9, 1990; 55:38560–38562.

4. American Dental Association, Council on Dental Therapeutics (1986). Guidelines for acceptance of chemotherapeutic products for the control of supragingival dental plaque and gingivitis. *JADA*, 112:529–532.

5. Fischman, S. (1997). The history of oral hygiene products: How far have we come in 6000 years? *Periodontology 2000*, 15:7–14.

6. Hefferrren, J. J. (1998). Historical view of dentifrice functionality methods. *J Clin Dent*, 9:53–56.

7. White, D. J. (2001). Development of an improved whitening dentifrice based upon "stain-specific soft silica" technology. *J Clin Dent*, 12:25–29.

8. White, D. J. (2002). A new and improved "dual action" whitening dentifrice technology-sodium hexametaphosphate. *J Clin Dent*, 13:1–5.

9. Volpe, A. R., Petrone, M. E., Principe, M., & DeVizio, W. (In press). The efficacy of a dentifrice with caries, plaque, gingivitis, tooth whitening and oral malodor benefits. *J Clin Dent*, 13:55–58.

10. Hefferren, J. J. (1976). A laboratory method for assessment of dentifrice abrasivity. *J Dent Res*, 55:563–753.

11. Adams, D., Addy, M., and Absi, E. (1992). Abrasive and chemical effects of dentifrices. In Embery G., & Rolla, G., Eds. *Clinical and biological aspects of dentifrices*. Oxford: Oxford University Press, 345–55.

12. Kitchen, P. C., & Robinson, H. B. G. (1948). How abrasive need a dentifrice be? *J Dent Res*, 27:501–6.

13. Barkvoll, P. (1992). Considerations concerning the sodium lauryl sulphate content of dentifrices. In Embery, G., & Rolla, G., Eds. *Clinical and biological aspects of dentifrices*. Oxford: Oxford University Press, 171–180.

14. Coelho, J., Kohut, B., Mankodi, S., Parikh, R., & Wu, M. (2000). Essential oils in an antiplaque and antigingivitis dentifrice: a six-month study. *Amer J Dent*, 13, Special Issue, C5–C10.

15. Fischman, S., & Coelho, J. (2001). A review of efficacy studies of an antiplaque/antigingivitis essential oil-containing dentifrice. *J Pract Hygiene*, 10:29–33.

16. American Dental Association (1964). Council on Dental Therapeutics. American dental reclassification of Crest toothpaste. *JADA*, 69:195–96.

17. Conti, A. J., Lotzkar, S., & Daley, R., Cancro, L., Marks, R. G., & McNeal, D. R. (1988). A three year clinical trial to compare efficacy of dentifrices containing 1.14 per cent and 0.76 per cent sodium monofluorophosphate, *Community Dent Oral Epidemiol*, 16, 135–138.

18. Fogels, H. R., Meade, J. J., Griffith, J., Miragliuolo, R., & Cancro, L. P. (1988). A clinical investigation of a high-level fluoride dentifrice, *J Dent Child*, 55, 210–15.

19. Fischman, S., Truelove, R., Hart, R., & Cancro, L. P. (1992). The laboratory and clinical safety evaluation of a dentifrice containing hydrogen peroxide and baking soda. *J Clin Dent*, 3:104–10.

20. Marshall, M., Kuhn, J., Fischman, S., Torry, C., & Cancro, L. (1992). Carcinogenicity bioassay of a $H_2O_2$ containing dentifrice. *J Dent Res*, 1992;71:195.

21. American Dental Association. (1984). Clinical uses of fluorides: A state-of-the-art conference on the uses of fluorides in clinical dentistry. *JADA*, 109:472–74.

22. Tinanoff, N. (1995). Progress regarding the use of stannous fluoride in clinical dentistry. *J Clin Dent*, 6:37–40.

23. White, D. J. (1995). A return to stannous fluoride dentifrices. *J Clin Dent*, 6:29–36.

24. White, D. J. (1997). Recent advances in clinical research on toothpastes and mouthwashes. Clinical efficacy of commercial products for gingivitis, tartar control and antimicrobial activity. *J Clin Dent*, 8:37–38.

25. Beiswanger, B. B., Doyle, P. M., Jackson, R. D., Mallatt, M. E., Bollmer, B. W., Crisanti, M. M., Quay, C. B., Lanzalaco, A. C., Lakacovic, M. F., Majeti, S., & McClanahan, S. F. (1995). The clinical effect of dentifrices containing stabilized stannous fluoride on plaque formation and gingivitis—a six-month study with ad libitum brushing. *J Clin Dent*, 6 Spec Iss:46–53.

26. Perlich, M. A., Baca, L. A., Bollmer, B. W., Lanzaloco, A. C., McClanahan, S. F., Sewak, L. K., Beiswanger, B. B., Eichald, M. A., Hull, J. R., Jackson, R. D., & Mau, M. S. (1995). The clinical effect of a stabilized stannous fluoride dentifrice on plaque formation, gingivitis and gingival bleeding: a six-month study. *J Clin Dent*, 6 Spec Iss:54–8.

27. DeSalva, S., King, B., & Lin, Y. (1989). Triclosan: A safety profile. *Am J Dent*, 2:185–96.

28. Volpe, A., Petrone, M., DeVizio, W., & Davies, R. M. (1993). A review of plaque, gingivitis, calculus, and caries clinical efficacy studies with a dentifrice containing triclosan and PVM/MA copolymer. *J Clin Dent*, 4:31–41.

29. Volpe, A. R., Petrone, M. E., DeVizio, W., Davies, R. M., & Proskin, H. M. (1996). A review of plaque, gingivitis, calculus and caries clinical efficacy studies with a fluoride dentifrice containing triclosan and PVM/MA copolymer. *J Clin Dent*, 7:S1–S14.

30. Proskin, H. M., Kingman, A., Naleway, C., & Wozniak, W. T. (1995). Comparative attributes for the description of the relative efficacy of therapeutic agents: General concepts and definitions, and application to the American Dental Association guidelines for the comparison of the clinical anticaries efficacy of fluoride dentifrices. *J Clin Dent*, 6:176–84.

31. Mann, J., Vered, Y., Babayof, I., Sintas, J., Petrone, M. E., Volpe, A. R., & Proskin H. M. (2001). The comparative anticaries efficacy of a dentifrice containing 0.3% Triclosan and 2.0% copolymer in a 0.243% sodium fluoride/silica base and a dentifrice containing 0.243% sodium fluoride/silica base: A two-year coronal caries clinical trial on adults in Israel. *J Clin Dent*, 12:71–76.

32. McClanahan, S. F., Bollmer, B. W., Court, L. K., McClary, J. M., Majeti, S., Crisanti, M. M., Beiswanger, B. B., & Mau, M. S. (2000). Plaque regrowth effects of a Triclosan/pyrophosphate dentifrice in a 4-day non-brushing model. *J Clin Dent*, 11:107–13.

33. Fairbrother, K. J., Kowolik, M. J., Curzon, M. E. J., Müller, I., McKeown, S., Hill, C. M., Hannigan, C., Bartizek, R. D., & White, D. J. (1997). The comparative clinical efficacy of pyrophosphate/Triclosan, copolymer/Triclosan and zinc citrate/Triclosan dentifrices for the reduction of supragingival calculus formation. *J Clin Dent*, 8:62–66.

34. Fischman S. (1993). Self-care: practical periodontal care in today's practice. *Int Dent J*, 43:179–83.

35. *Therapeutics* (38th ed.). Chicago: American Dental Association, 1979:345–46.

36. Zacherl, W. A., Pfeiffer, H. J., & Swancar, J. R. (1985). The effect of soluble pyrophosphates on dental calculus in adults. *JADA*, 110:737–38.

37. Volpe, A., Manhold, J., Lobene, R., & Yankell, S. (2000). "Influences of directed research and clinical observation on the development of a tartar control whitening dentifrice." *J Clin Dent*, 11:63–67.

38. Rølla, B., & Saxegaard, E. (1990). Critical evaluation of the composition and use of topical fluorides, with emphasis on the role of calcium fluoride in caries inhibition. *J Dent Res*, 60:780–85.

39. Stephen, K. W., Creanor, S. L., Russell, C. K., Huntington, E., & Downie, C. F. A. (1988). A three-year oral health dose-response study of sodium monofluorophosphate dentifrices with and without zinc citrate: Anti-caries results. *Community Dent Oral Epidemiol*, 16:321–25.

40. American Dental Association, Council on Scientific Affairs, Products of Excellence. ADA Seal Program. April 1, 1997.

41. American Dental Association, Council on Dental Therapeutics (1994). Guidelines for the acceptance of peroxide-containing oral hygiene products. *JADA*, 125:1140–42.

42. White, D. J. (2001). "Development of an improved whitening dentifrice based upon stain specific soft silica technology." *J Clin Dent*, 12:25–33.

43. American Dental Association (1993). CDT acts on mouthrinses. *JADA*, 124:26.

44. American Academy of Pediatrics, Committee on Drugs (1984). Ethanol in liquid preparations intended for children. *Pediatrics*, 73:405.

45. Winn, D. M., Blot, W. J., McLaughlin, J. K., Austin, D. F., Greenberg, R. S., Prestin-Martin, S., Schoenberg, J. B., & Fraumeni, J. F. Jr. (1991). Mouthwash use and oral conditions in the risk of oral and pharyngeal cancer. *Cancer Res*, 51:3044–47.

46. Ciancio, S. (1993). Alcohol in mouthrinse: Lack of association with cancer. *Biological Therapies in Dentistry*, 9:1–2.

47. McDowell, J., & Kassebaum, D. (1993). Diagnosing and treating halitosis. *JADA*, 124:55–64.

48. Spouge, J. (1964). Halitosis: A review of its causes and treatment. *Dent Pract Dent Rec*, 14:307–17.

49. Tonzetich, J. (1977). Production and origin of oral malodor, a review of mechanisms and methods of analysis. *J Periodontol*, 48:13–20.

50. Rosenberg, M. (1992). Halitosis—the need for further research and education. *J Dent Res*, 71:424.

51. Eli, I., Baht, R., Koriat, H., & Rosenberg, M. (2001). Self-perception of breath odor. *JADA*, 132:621–26.

52. Haveman, C. W., & Redding, S. W. (1998). Dental management and treatment of xerostomic patients. *Texas Dent J*, 115:43–56.

53. Addy, M. (1986). Chlorhexidine compared with other locally delivered antimicrobials. A short review. *J Clin Periodontol*, 13:957–64.

54. Turesky, S., Warner, V., Lin, P. S., & Saloway, B. (1977). Prolongation of antibacterial activity of chlorhexidine adsorbed to teeth. *J Periodontol*, 48:646–49.

55. Rølla, G., Löe, H., & Schiott, C. R. (1970). The affinity of chlorhexidine for hydroxyapatite and salivary mucins. *J Periodont Res*, 5:90–95.

56. Yankell, S. L., Moreno, O. M., Saffir, A. J., Lowary, R. L., & Gold, W. (1982). Effects of chlorhexidine and four antimicrobial compounds on plaque gingivitis and staining in beagle dogs. *J Dent Res*, 61:1089–93.

57. Axelson, P., & Lindhe, J. (1987). Efficacy of mouthrinses in inhibiting dental plaque and gingivitis in man. *J Clin Periodontol*, 14:205–12.

58. Wieder, S. G., Newman, H. N., & Strahan, J. D. (1983). Stannous fluoride and subgingival chlorhexidine irrigation in the control of plaque and chronic periodontitis. *J Clin Periodontol*, 10:172–81.

59. Eriksen, H., & Gjermo, P. (1973). Incidence of stained tooth surfaces in students using chlorhexidine-containing dentifrices. *Scand J Dent Res*, 81:533–37.

60. Flotra, L., Gjermo, P., Rølla, G., & Waerhaug, J. (1971). Side effects of chlorhexidine mouth washes. *Scand J Dent Res*, 79:119–25.

61. Löe, H., Mandell, M., Derry, A., & Schiott, C. (1971). The effect of mouthrinses and topical application of chlorhexidine on calculus formation in man, *J Periodontol Res*, 6:312–14.

62. Moghadam, B. K. H., Drisko, C. L., & Gier R. E. (1991). Chlorhexidine mouthwash-induced fixed drug eruption. *Oral Surg, Oral Medicine, Oral Path*, 71:431–34.

63. Skoglund, L. A., & Holst, E. (1982). Desquamative mucosal reactions due to chlorhexidine gluconate. *Int J Oral Surg*, 11:380–82.

64. American Dental Association (1988). Council on Dental Therapeutics accepts Listerine. *JADA*, 117:515–17.

65. Meeker, H. G., & Linke, H. A. B. (1988). The antibacterial action of eugenol, thyme oil, and related essential oils used in dentistry. *Comp Cont Educ Dent*, 9:32–40.

66. Menaker, L., Weatherford, T. W., Pitts, G., Ross, N. M., & Lamm, R. (1979). The effects of Listerine antiseptic on dental plaque. *Ala J Med Sci*, 16:71–77.

67. Charles, C., Sharma, N., Galustians, H., McGuire, A., & Vincent, J. (2001). Comparative efficacy of an antiseptic mouthrinse and an antiplaque/antigingivitis dentifrice, A six-month trial. *JADA*, 132:670–75.

68. Miller, R. L., & Micik, R. E. (1978). Air pollution and its control in the dental office. *Dent Clin North Am*, 22:453–76.

69. Wyler, D., Miller, R., & Micik, R. (1990). Efficacy of self-administered preoperative oral hygiene procedures in reducing the concentration of bacteria in aerosols generated during dental procedures. *J Dent Res*, 50:509.

70. Fine, D., Yip, J., Furgang, D., Barnett, M. L., Olshan, A. M., & Vincent, J. (1993). Reducing bacteria in dental aerosols: Pre-procedural use of an antiseptic mouthrinse. *JADA*, 124:56–58.

71. Molinari, J., & Molinari, G. (1992). Is mouthrinsing before dental procedures worthwhile? *JADA*, 123:75–80.

72. Itthagarun, A., & Wei, S. H. (1997). Chewing gum and saliva in oral health. *J Clin Dent*, 8:159–62.

73. Edgar, W. M. (1998). Sugar substitutes, chewing gum and dental caries—a review. *Brit Dent J*, 184:29–32.

74. Imfeld, T. (1999). Chewing gum—facts and fiction: a review of gum chewing and oral health. *Crit Rev Oral Biol Med*, 10:405–19.

75. Yankell, S. L., & Emling, R. C. (1999). Clinical effects on plaque pH, pCa and swallowing rates from chewing a flavored or unflavored chewing gum. *J Clin Dent*, 10:86–88.

76. Koparol, E., Ertugrul, F., & Sabah, E. (2000). Effect of gum chewing on plaque acidogenicity. *J Clin Pediatric Dent*, 24:129–32.

77. Edgar, W. M. (1999). "A role for sugar free gum in oral health." *J Clin Dent*, 10:89–93.

78. Beiswanger, B. B., Boneta, A. E., Mau, M. S., Katz, B. P., Proskin, H. M., & Stookey, G. K. (1998). The effect of chewing sugar-free gum after meals on clinical caries incidence. *JADA*, 129:1623–26.

79. *Compend Contin Educ Dent*, Spec Iss 7, 2001, 22 no. 7-A:1–52.

80. Reingewirtz, Y., Girault, O., Reingewirtz, N., Senger, B., & Tanenbaum, H. (1999). Mechanical effects and volatile sulfur compound-reducing effects of chewing gums: comparison between test and base gums and a control group. *Quintessence Int*, 30:319–23.

81. Reynolds, E. C., Black, C. L., Cai, F., Cross, K. J., Eakins, D., Huq, N. L., Morgan, M. V., Nowicki, A., Perich, J. W., Riley, P. F., Shen, P., Talbo, G., & Webber, F. (1999). Advances in enamel remineralization: casein phosphopeptide-amorphous calcium phosphate. *J Clin Dent*, 10:86–88.

82. Shen, P., Cai, F., Nowicki, A., Vincent, J., & Reynolds, E. C. (2001). Remineralization of enamel subsurface lesions by sugar-free chewing gum containing casein phosphopeptide-amorphous calcium phosphate. Accepted for publication. *J Dent Res*, 80:2066–70.

# APPENDICES OF SELECTED DENTIFRICES AND CATEGORIES

### APPENDIX 6–1  Baking Soda Dentifrice Products

| Product | Supplier | Fluoride | Abrasive |
|---|---|---|---|
| Aim | Chesebrough-Pond's | MFP | Hydrated silica |
| Close Up | Chesebrough-Pond's | NaF | Hydrated silica |
| Colgate | Colgate-Palmolive | NaF | Hydrated silica |
| Crest | Procter & Gamble | NaF | Hydrated silica |
| Dental Care | Arm & Hammer | NaF | Sodium bicarbonate, hydrated silica |
| Mentadent | Chesebrough-Pond's | NaF | Hydrated silica |
| Pepsodent | Chesebrough-Pond's | NaF | Hydrated silica |

### APPENDIX 6–2  Specialty Toothpastes Awarded the American Dental Association Seal of Acceptance*

| | Company and Product |
|---|---|
| Tartar Control | Colgate-Palmolive Company |
| | Colgate Tartar Control Baking Soda and Peroxide |
| | Colgate Tartar Control Gel |
| | Colgate Tartar Control Toothpaste |
| | GlaxoSmithKlein Consumer Healthcare |
| | Aquafresh All with Tartar Control Toothpaste |
| | Procter & Gamble Company |
| | Crest Multicare Toothpaste |
| | Crest Tartar Protection Fluoride Gel |
| | Crest Tartar Protection Fluoride Toothpaste |
| Sensitivity Control | Butler Company, John O. |
| | Protect Sensitive Teeth Gel Toothpaste |
| | Del Laboratories, Inc. |
| | Orajel Sensitive Pain Relieving Toothpaste for Adults |
| | Procter & Gamble |
| | Crest Sensitivity Protection Fluoride Toothpaste |

(continued)

## APPENDIX 6-2 *Continued*

| | Company and Product |
|---|---|
| Whitener | Den-Mat Corporation |
| |     Rembrandt Whitening Toothpaste, Original and Mint Flavor |
| | Colgate-Palmolive Company |
| |     Colgate Total Plus Whitening Toothpaste |
| |     Colgate Tartar Control Plus Whitening Gel |
| | GlaxoSmithKline Consumer Healthcare |
| |     Aquafresh Whitening Toothpaste |
| | Procter & Gamble Co. |
| |     Crest Extra Whitening with Tartar Protection Toothpaste |
| |     Crest Multicare Whitening Toothpaste |

*Because new products are continually coming on the market, it is recommended that the American Dental Association website (www.ada.org) be consulted for the latest information on toothpastes and other dental products.

## APPENDIX 6-3 **Examples of Agents Added to Chewing Gums**[*]

| Agent | Purpose/Claim | U.S. Example(s) |
|---|---|---|
| Aspirin | Pain relief | Aspergum |
| Caffeine | Increase alertness | Stay Alert |
| Calcium carbonate | Neutralize stomach acid | Chooz |
| Casein Phosphopeptide | Remineralize and Strengthen teeth | |
| Amorphous calcium | | |
| Phosphate | | Trident Advantage |
| Chlorhexidine | Antiplaque, antigingivitis | none in U.S. |
| Dimenhydrinate | Motion sickness | none in U.S. |
| Fluoride | Anticaries | none in U.S. |
| Sodium bicarbonate | Freshen breath | Dental Care |
| | Whiten teeth | Trident Advantage |
| | Reduce plaque | |

*Because new products are continually coming on the market, it is recommended that the American Dental Association website (www.ada.org) be consulted for the latest information on toothpastes and other dental products.

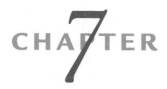

CHAPTER 7

# Oral Health Self-Care Supplemental Measures to Complement Toothbrushing

*Terri S. I. Tilliss*
*Janis G. Keating*

## OBJECTIVES

*At the end of this chapter, it will be possible to*

1. Explain the reasons why supplemental oral health self-care is needed to complement toothbrushing.
2. Identify factors, in addition to oral conditions, that influence selection of supplemental oral hygiene devices and techniques.
3. State the purposes, indications, contraindications, techniques, advantages, and limitations of the following oral hygiene devices:
   · Dental floss,
   · Dental floss holder,
   · Dental floss threader,
   · Wooden or plastic triangular stick,
   · Toothpicks and holder,
   · Interproximal brush or devices,
   · Tongue cleaners,
   · Others: yarn, rubber or plastic tip, gauze, automated interproximal devices.
4. Justify the purpose and explain techniques for the use of mouthrinses and oral irrigators.
5. Describe proper oral hygiene self-care for dental implants.
6. Explain proper oral hygiene self-care for removable partial and full dentures.

# INTRODUCTION

Supplemental plaque removal measures beyond toothbrushing are necessary in order to thoroughly remove plaque.[1,2,3] Although toothbrushing can be effective at removing the plaque residing on buccal and lingual aspects of teeth, it is generally ineffective for interproximal surfaces.[4,5] There are numerous intraoral sites and conditions better served by plaque removal methods and devices other than toothbrushing. Examples of these sites include, fixed prostheses, crown margins, furcations of multirooted teeth, orthodontic appliances, the tongue, implants, and dentures.

Interproximal aspects of teeth are not very accessible for the removal of plaque by the toothbrush.[1] These sites have consistently been shown to harbor high amounts of plaque.[6–8] Regular interproximal plaque removal is recommended for the following reasons:

- Incomplete plaque removal can increase the rate and growth of new plaque.[9]
- Allowing plaque to remain on some tooth surfaces can facilitate development of a complex microflora on other cleaned surfaces.[10,11]
- Individuals who clean interproximally on a daily basis have less plaque and calculus.[12]
- Interproximal plaque removal is beneficial for preventing gingival and periodontal infections as well as for reducing or eliminating diseases in these soft tissues.[1,13,14]
- There is interproximal site predilection for gingivitis, periodontitis, and caries.[1,15,16]
- Prevention of dental caries can be facilitated by effective daily interproximal plaque removal.[17]

The dentition or periodontal tissues can be altered as a result of disease, repair, or from architectural tissue changes following therapy. When this occurs, a device and/or technique must be introduced to accommodate these changes. It has been shown that supragingival plaque removal influences subgingival plaque composition, however, plaque removal efforts should extend as far subgingivally as possible.[10,11,18]

To determine the most appropriate products and practices for interproximal plaque removal the *Process of Care Model* is useful (Figure 7–1). This treatment model is de-

| Phases | Activities |
| --- | --- |
| Assessment | Systematic data collection of general and oral health status |
| Diagnosis | Data are analyzed in order to formulate a diagnosis |
| Planning | The evidence-based plan is derived and prioritized based upon mutually congruent goals |
| Implementation | Preventive procedures to promote/maintain oral health and therapeutic procedures to control disease in order to achieve oral health goals |
| Evaluation | Attainment of oral health goals is mutually analyzed and new care plan components determined as necessary |

FIGURE 7–1    Phases of the Process of Care Model.

scribed in detail in the textbook, *Dental Hygiene Theory and Practice*.[19] The oral health professional must carefully assess numerous oral health and disease risk factors. These include current oral self-care practices, and past and current oral health status. The importance of this *assessment* phase cannot be overemphasized. During the *diagnosis* and *planning* phases, the risk factors and the appropriate oral self-care products and procedures to address these risks are jointly determined with the individual. The oral health professional can then apply theory-based educational and motivational strategies during the *implementation* phase to facilitate behavioral change. Ensuring that such behavioral changes are consistent with the lifestyle of the individual will increase the potential for long-term compliance of oral self-care practices. The *evaluation* phase focuses upon outcomes to determine whether modifications to the oral hygiene strategies are indicated. Continuation or change of an oral hygiene regimen is based upon the evaluation of tissue health. The evaluation process is continuous over the lifespan as the dentition and soft tissues may become altered with time.

A personalized oral hygiene regimen will best meet the needs of the individual. When employing an interproximal cleaning technique, a systematic approach following prescribed techniques will enhance plaque removal without causing soft tissue damage. The oral hygiene self-care recommendations, which have been agreed upon by the individual and the oral health care provider, are documented in the dental chart and modified as necessary at subsequent re-care visits. This type of documentation allows for continuity of care.

## Oral Health Self-Care

Self-care includes all activities and decisions of an individual to prevent, diagnose, or treat personal ill health. This concept as applied to care of the oral cavity is referred to as oral self-care or oral health self-care, replacing earlier terms such as personal plaque control, home care, and oral physiotherapy. One primary purpose of oral health self-care is to prevent or arrest periodontal disease and caries by reducing plaque accumulation.[5] Less than optimal oral self-care is regarded as a major risk factor for periodontal disease. In order to determine the most appropriate self-care practices for each individual, a variety of factors must be assessed:

- Presence of gingival inflammation and bleeding,
- Alterations of the interdental gingival architecture caused by tooth alignment, spacing, recession, and lack of attached tissue,
- Malalignment of teeth and tooth morphology,
- Configuration of embrasure spaces,
- Extent and location of plaque and calculus accumulation,
- Caries experience and susceptibility,
- Evidence and risk factors for periodontal diseases,
- Trauma from improper use of oral-hygiene devices,
- Current oral self-care practices and level of manual dexterity/mental capacity,
- Compliance potential, and
- Presence, configuration, and condition of restorations.

There is no universally accepted oral hygiene device. The appropriate oral hygiene regimen is determined according to the dictates of the oral condition, personal preferences, dex-

terity, and lifestyle.[16] Adequate instruction in the use of any recommended device must be provided.

## Additional Considerations: Plaque and Caries

Utilizing an *evidence-based* approach to understand oral disease, several conclusions can be drawn. Little data supports the theory that interproximal plaque removal alone reduces the incidence of caries. One reason for this is that the ubiquitous use of fluoride makes it difficult to separate out the benefits of fluoride from that of interproximal plaque removal. One study did demonstrate that interproximal caries could be prevented when daily interproximal flossing is performed by an oral health professional.[17] However, other studies of supervised self-performed interproximal cleaning were unable to demonstrate a caries reduction.[20–23] There are several studies documenting the correlation between the general level of mechanical plaque removal and the incidence of caries.[24–26] It appears that only a very high level of personal mechanical plaque removal impacts the caries rate. This level is difficult for the average person to sustain.[27] Consequently, fluorides and dietary carbohydrate control should be emphasized, in addition to interproximal plaque removal for optimal effect on the caries rate.

## Plaque and Gingivitis

It has been shown that removing plaque once every 48 hours is sufficient to reduce microbial plaque accumulations that are mature enough to induce gingival inflammation.[6,28] For those with existing inflammation or periodontitis, every 48 hours is not frequent enough.[1] Under these conditions it has been shown that colonization and maturation of plaque occurs more rapidly in the presence of, than in the absence of inflammation.[4,6,29,30]

## Frequency of Plaque Removal

The preceding information describing the relationship between plaque and caries and plaque and gingivitis, suggests that the optimal frequency for mechanical plaque removal is not precisely known. Based on the one study correlating caries with daily flossing,[17] it seems advisable to remove interproximal plaque at least once every 24 hours for caries prevention. Likewise, the evidence-based approach suggests that those with an existing gingivitis or periodontitis should remove interproximal plaque on a daily basis. However, those with healthy gingiva may be able to practice interproximal plaque removal only once every 48 hours. Therefore, with more daily attempts at plaque removal, it is more likely that the additive efforts will maximize the removal of plaque. Since the ideal frequency of interproximal plaque removal has not been shown, individual factors such as the amount of inflammation, caries susceptibility, plaque removal efficiency, and accumulation and virulence of plaque must be considered in the recommendation.

Interestingly, although 94% of oral health professionals and researchers attending a symposium on mechanical plaque removal believed interproximal cleaning was an essential component of a successful oral self-care program, only 51% believed it was needed on a daily basis. Only 77% percent felt that interproximal cleaning should be advised for the whole dentate population rather than just for those deemed susceptible to periodontal disease and caries.[31] Determining the risk factors that increase one's susceptibility to caries and periodontal diseases could identify which individuals are in need of consistent interproximal cleaning, and at what frequency.

Supervised oral self-care practice sessions promote proper utilization of oral hygiene devices by providing an opportunity to monitor technique. Adjustment of technique can maximize plaque removal while minimizing tissue damage. After such instruction and reinforce-

ment, success in oral health measures ultimately rests with the individual. Principles of learning and motivation should be applied to encourage compliance (see Chapter 16).

---

### Question 1

Which of the following statements, if any, are correct?

A. Supplemental plaque removal is useful for individuals with orthodontic appliances.

B. Plaque allowed to remain on interproximal surfaces will not impact plaque accumulations on clean surfaces.

C. The Process of Care Model begins with the evaluation phase.

D. Self-care as it relates to health includes all activities and decisions individuals make about their health.

E. A large body of research supports the theory that interproximal plaque removal alone reduces the incidence of caries.

---

## Dental Floss

Dental floss is best indicated for plaque and debris removal from Type I embrasures where the papilla fills the interproximal space and the teeth are in contact. For Type II and III embrasures, devices other than floss may be more effective in removing plaque[32,33] (Figure 7–2). Effective use of dental floss accomplishes the following objectives.

1. Removes plaque and debris that adheres to the teeth, restorations, orthodontic appliances,[34] fixed prostheses and pontics,[35] gingiva in the interproximal embrasures,[36] and around implants.[37,38]

2. Aids the clinician in identifying the presence of interproximal calculus deposits, overhanging restorations, or interproximal carious lesions.

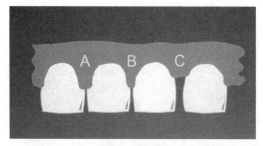

FIGURE 7–2    Embrasure Types. **A.** Type I—papilla fills interproximal space. **B.** Type II—slight to moderate recession of papilla. **C.** Type III—extensive recession or complete loss of papilla.

3. May arrest or prevent interproximal carious lesions.[17]

4. Reduces gingival bleeding.[1,39]

5. May be used as a vehicle for the application of polishing or chemotherapeutic agents to interproximal and subgingival areas.[39]

Not all interproximal contact areas, whether natural or restored, have the same configuration. Consequently, several types of floss are available to accommodate these differences. These vary from thin unwaxed varieties, to thicker waxed tapes and include variable thickness floss (Figure 7–3). Clinical trials have shown no significant differences in the cleansing ability between waxed and unwaxed floss.[1] Wax residue has not been found on tooth surfaces cleaned with waxed floss.[40]

Unwaxed floss is frequently recommended because it is thin and slips easily through tight contact areas. However, unwaxed floss can fray and tear when contacting rotated teeth, heavy calculus deposits, or defective and overhanging restorations. Frequent floss breakage may discourage continued use. For these conditions, waxed, lightly waxed, or shred-resistant floss are recommended.

Waxed dental tape, unlike round dental floss, is broad and flat, and may be effective in

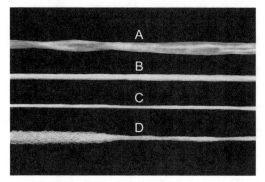

FIGURE 7–3     Varieties of Floss. **A.** Dental tape. **B.** Waxed. **C.** Unwaxed. **D.** Variable thickness floss.

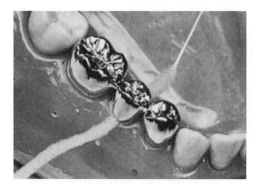

FIGURE 7–4     Variable thickness floss with stiff end used to clean under the pontic and at interproximals of abutments of a fixed partial denture. (Courtesy of Dr. Linda S. Scheirton, Creighton University, Omaha, NB.)

an interproximal space without tight contact points. Additional types of floss, such as those made of polytetrafluoroethylene (PTFE, teflon-like), are stronger and more shred-resistant. They have been shown to be preferred by those who have tight contacts or rough proximal tooth surfaces.[41] Other varieties, such as tufted floss increments alternated with standard floss, and floss which stretches for insertion are alternatives.

Some brands of dental floss and tape are colored and flavored. In addition to increased appeal, color provides a visual contrast to plaque and oral debris, thus enabling one to see what is being removed, possibly increasing the motivation to floss. One study indicated a user preference for waxed over unwaxed floss and mint-flavored waxed floss over plain waxed floss.[42] Flosses impregnated with a variety of agents have been introduced; examples of these include floss treated with baking soda, fluoride, herbal extracts, antimicrobial agents, or abrasives for whitening. Fluoride-impregnated floss has been *marketed* but lacks efficacy data for affecting the caries rate.

One type of variable-thickness floss has a stiff end to allow for threading under bridges, beneath tight contact areas, under pontics,

through exposed furcations, and around orthodontic wires (Figure 7–4). This floss combines a section of unwaxed floss with an area of thicker nylon meshwork to clean larger surface areas. Variable thickness floss may be recommended for use in cleaning implant abutments, areas with open contacts, wide embrasures, or sites where recession and bone loss permit access to furcations. It can also be used to remove plaque from the distal aspect of the most distal tooth in all quadrants.

When recommending a type of floss, the specific oral conditions, patient preference, and ability are all factors that need to be considered. A limitation of flossing is the inability to conform to a concave interproximal surface such as the mesial of maxillary premolars. Other interproximal devices will clean those surfaces more effectively (Figure 7–5).

Dental Flossing Methods

Two frequently used flossing methods are the spool method and the circle, or loop, method. Both facilitate control of the floss and ease of

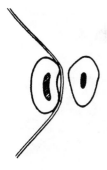

FIGURE 7–5    Dental floss is not as effective in cleaning teeth with inter-proximal root concavities since it does not contact the surfaces of the concavity. (Courtesy of Dr. Linda S. Scheirton, Creighton University, Omaha, NB.)

handling. The spool method is particularly suited for teenagers and adults who have acquired the necessary neuromuscular coordination required to use floss. The loop method is suited for children as well as adults with less nimble hands or physical limitations caused by conditions such as poor muscular coordination or arthritis. Flossing is a complex skill, so until children develop adequate dexterity, usually around the age of 10 to 12 years, an adult should perform flossing on the child. Younger children whose teeth still exhibit primate spaces (no interproximal contact) will not require flossing.

When using the spool method, a piece of floss approximately 18 inches long is utilized. The bulk of the floss is lightly wound around the middle finger. Space should be left between wraps to avoid impairing circulation to the fingers (Figure 7–6A). The rest of the floss is similarly wound around the same finger of the opposite hand. This finger can wind, or "take up," the floss as it becomes soiled or frayed to permit access to an unused portion. The last three fingers are clenched and the hands are moved apart, pulling the floss taut, thus leaving the thumb and index finger of each hand free (Figure 7–6B). The floss is then secured with the index finger and thumb of each hand by grasping a section three quarters

to 1 inch long between the hands (Figure 7–6C).

For the loop method, the ends of the 18-inch piece of floss are tied in a knot. All of the fingers, but not the thumbs of the two hands are placed close to one another within the loop (Figure 7–7). Whether using the spool or the loop method of flossing, the same basic procedures are followed. The thumb and index finger of each hand are used in various combinations to guide the floss between the teeth.

When inserting, floss, it is gently eased between the teeth with a seesaw motion at the contact point. The gentle seesaw motion flattens the floss, making it possible to ease through the contact point and prevent snapping it through, thus avoiding trauma to the sulcular gingiva (Figure 7–8A). Once past the contact point, the floss is adapted to each interproximal surface by creating a C-shape. The floss is then directed apically into the sulcus and back to the contact area (up-and-down against the side of the tooth) several times or until the tooth surface is clean (Figure 7-8B). The procedure is repeated on the adjacent tooth in the proximal area, using care to prevent damage to the papilla while readapting to the adjacent tooth. A clean, unused portion should be used for each interproximal area.

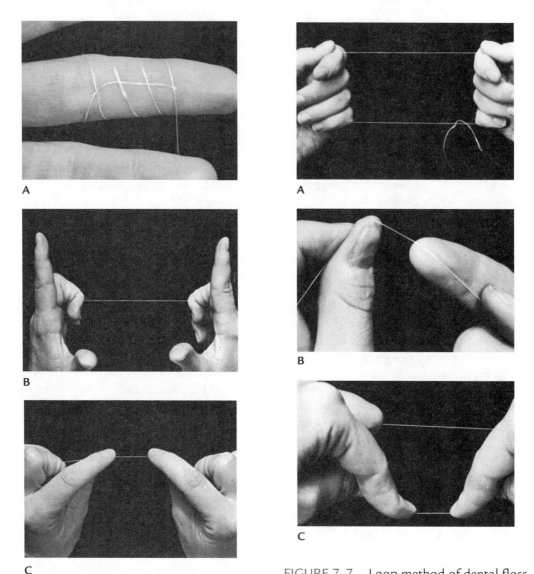

A

B

C

FIGURE 7-6    Spool method for dental flossing. **A.** Floss is lightly wound and spaced around the middle finger of each hand. **B.** The last three fingers are clenched, pulling the floss taut and leaving the index finger and thumb of each hand free. **C.** The floss is held with the index finger and thumb of each hand by grasping a section three quarters to 1 in. long between the hands. (Courtesy of Dr. Linda S. Scheirton, Creighton University, Omaha, NB.)

A

B

C

FIGURE 7-7    Loop method of dental flossing. **A.** All fingers except the thumbs are placed within the loop for easy maneuverability. **B.** For the mandibular teeth, the floss is guided with the two index fingers. **C.** For the maxillary teeth, the floss is guided with two thumbs or one thumb and one index finger. (Courtesy of Dr. Linda S. Scheirton, Creighton University, Omaha, NB.)

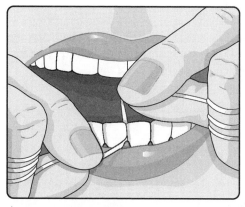

**A**

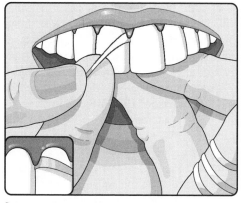

**B**

FIGURE 7–8    **A.** To insert, the floss is gently eased between the teeth, while sawing it back and forth at the contact point. **B.** the floss is directed into the sulcus and back to the contact area several times or until the tooth surface is clean. (Courtesy of John O. Butler Co., Chicago, IL.)

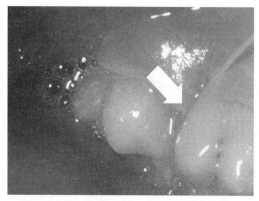

FIGURE 7–9    Improper dental floss technique with potential for gingival "floss-cuts." (Floss should adapt to interproximal surface in a C-shape.)

ing method. Incorrect flossing can often be detected through clinical observation of the gingiva and the technique (Figure 7–9). Signs that suggest incorrect use of dental floss include gingival cuts, soft tissue clefting, and cervical wear on interproximal root surfaces. (Figures 7–10, 7–11) If flossing trauma is evident, further instruction should be given until the individual has become adept. Proper instruction and prac-

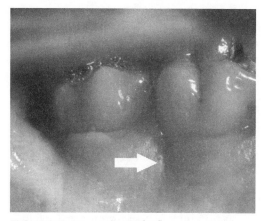

FIGURE 7–10    Gingival "floss-cuts" created by failure to adapt floss to interproximal surface in a C-shape.

In general, flossing is best performed by cleaning each tooth in succession, including the distal surface of the last tooth in each quadrant. The individual should be assisted with problem areas and encouraged to utilize whichever method produces the best results.

Criteria for evaluation are based on the efficacy of plaque removal and safety of the floss-

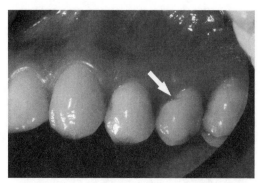

FIGURE 7-11   Groove created on mesial aspect of tooth (arrow) caused by movement of floss in bucco-lingual (horizontal) rather than apical-occlusal (vertical) direction.

tice allows most motivated adults to master either the spool or loop method of flossing. In certain circumstances, the use of a floss holder, floss threader, variable-thickness floss, or pre-cut floss strands with a stiff end may be more effective.

It is important to note that a flossing habit has traditionally been difficult for people to embrace. In reality, only a very small proportion of individuals practice daily flossing. Findings have ranged from 10 to 21% of population.[43–48] Floss may be superior to other interproximal cleaning methods, but for those who have not or will not adopt a flossing behavior another interproximal device may be more effective than no interproximal cleaning.[49] A less effective device used on a regular basis is superior to sporadic use of a more effective device. Participation of the individual in selecting an interproximal cleaning device and regimen is crucial to improving and/or enhancing compliance. Sometimes individuals agree to adopt a behavior because this is what the clinician wants to hear. Axelsson has referred to this as "a hasty affirmative in a moment of suddenly inspired courage."[43]

### Dental Floss Holder

The floss holder is a device that eliminates the need for placing fingers in the mouth. It is recommended for individuals with:

- Physical disabilities,
- Poor manual dexterity,[50]
- Large hands,
- Limited mouth opening,
- A strong gag reflex, and/or
- Low motivation for traditional flossing.[50]

The floss holder may also be helpful when one person is assisting another with flossing. Limited scientific data comparing finger-manipulated flossing to the use of a floss holder shows no difference in plaque removal.[47] Studies have found that, when compared, a significant majority of individuals preferred the floss holder over finger-manipulated flossing.[47,51,52] It should be emphasized that effective initial education and reinforcement are necessary for proper use of the floss holder. Use of the floss holder may aid in developing a flossing habit and should be considered when individuals experience difficulty with manual flossing.[53]

A variety of different floss-holder designs are available (Figure 7–12). Most commonly, they consist of a yoke-like device with a 3/4- to 1-inch space between the two prongs of the yoke.

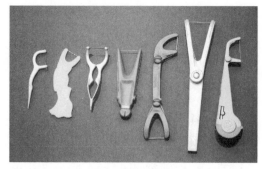

FIGURE 7-12   A variety of floss holders. The first three depicted in photograph are pre-threaded for one-time use. The last floss holder exhibits a floss-reservoir in handle.

The floss is secured tightly between the two prongs and the handle is grasped to guide the floss during use. The width and length of the handle are important features to consider when recommending the use of a floss holder to those with limited gripping abilities.[54] Most floss holders require that floss be strung around various parts of the holder prior to each use. This assembly mechanism allows for re-threading of the floss whenever the working portion becomes soiled or begins to fray. Some devices have a floss reservoir in the handle. This improvement allows for ease of threading and advancing the floss while maintaining the proper tautness. Several brands of pre-threaded, one-time-use floss holders are available; they require minimal dexterity, a factor that may help improve compliance.

When using a holder, the floss is inserted interproximally, using the same technique employed for finger-manipulated flossing. Once through the contact point, the floss and holder are pushed distally to clean the mesial surface of a tooth or pulled mesially to clean the distal surface (Figure 7–13). This pulling or pushing motion creates conformity to the tooth convexities, thus allowing the floss to slide apically into the sulcus. The floss is then activated in the same manner as with finger-manipulated flossing, by moving the floss in the direction of the long axis of the tooth.

Strict attention should be given to achieving the desired floss tension when assembling the floss holder. To ensure tautness, the prongs can be forced together while securing the floss. The most persistent problems with the yoke-like devices are the difficulties in loading and threading the floss, maintaining tension of the floss between the prongs and decreased ability to adapt the floss into a C-shape around the proximal surface. Any device recommended should allow for ease of threading, maintenance of proper tautness, and easy manipulation by the user.

Automated floss holders have been introduced but have not shown an advantage over manual flossing.[55] However, those with large diameter handles may be especially helpful for patients with limited manual dexterity and inability to grip a smaller diameter (Figure 7–14).

### Dental Floss Threader

A floss threader is a plastic loop into which a length of floss is inserted, similar to threading a needle. The threader is used to carry the floss interproximally in the following circumstances:

- Through embrasure areas under contact points that are too tight for floss insertion,

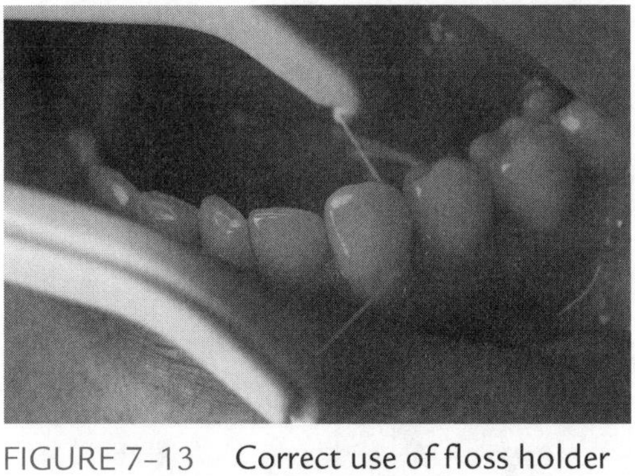

FIGURE 7–13    Correct use of floss holder on mesial aspect of tooth. Note that floss is taut, pulled mesially to adapt in C-shape, and extended subgingivally.

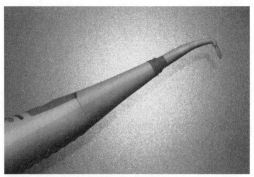

FIGURE 7–14    Automated floss holder. Note large diameter handle for easier grasping.

- Between the proximal surface and gingiva of abutment teeth of fixed prostheses,
- Under pontics,
- Around orthodontic appliances, and
- Under teeth that are splinted together.

Care should be taken to prevent trauma by *not* forcing the stiff end of the floss threader into the gingival tissues. When cleaning under a fixed partial denture, the floss threader is inserted from the facial and pulled completely through to the lingual aspect until the floss is against the abutment or pontic (Figure 7–15A). The floss may then be disengaged from the threader. The floss is adapted to one abutment tooth surface in the area of the embrasure (Figure 7–15B) and moved in the direction of the long axis of the tooth to remove plaque from the proximal surface. It is impor-

tant to glide the floss through the space between the pontic and the gingiva in order to clean the underside of the pontic (Figure 7–15C). After cleaning the underside of the pontic, it is necessary to slide the floss to the opposite proximal surface (Figure 7–15D). Removal of the floss from between the abutment and pontic is accomplished by pulling it out from the facial aspect.

## Question 2

Which of the following statements, if any, are correct?

A. Waxed dental floss is better for removing interproximal dental plaque than unwaxed.

B. A major problem encountered with the dental floss holder is maintaining tautness of the floss.

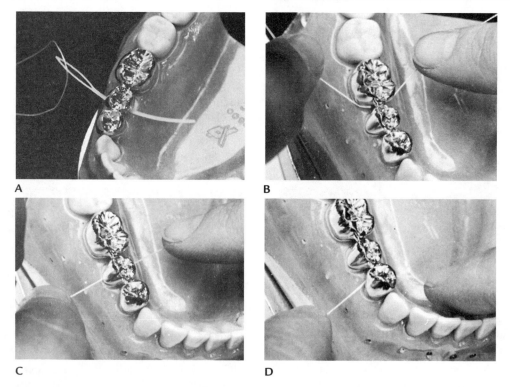

FIGURE 7–15    Use of a dental floss threader. **A.** Floss threader inserted under pontic. **B.** Floss adaption to mesial of abutment. **C.** Floss underneath pontic. **D.** Floss adaption to distal of abutment. (Courtesy of Dr. Linda S. Scheirton, Creighton University, Omaha, NB.)

C. The spool method of using interdental floss is the preferable technique for introducing children to flossing.

D. Individuals indicate a preference for the floss holder, but it is not as effective as flossing with the spool or loop methods.

E. Only about 70% (plus or minus 5%) of the people who routinely brush, floss.

### Wooden or Plastic Triangular Sticks

Interproximal cleaning can be facilitated using sticks made of wood or plastic (Figure 7–16). Balsa and birchwood are most common since they are pliable. A reduction in inflammation and bleeding sites has been demonstrated utilizing wooden or plastic sticks to reduce plaque accumulations.[14,56] They can be used for Type I, II, or III embrasures, but are best suited where the papilla does not completely fill the embrasure space.[43] These sticks are triangular in cross section to slide easily between teeth and to reduce potential tissue trauma. The stick is inserted interproximally from the buccal aspect with the flat surface, the base of the triangle, resting on the gingiva. The tip of the stick is angled coronally and is moved in a bucco-lingual direction (Figure 7–17). Wooden sticks have an advantage over plastic in that the pointed end can be softened in the mouth by moistening it with saliva. A softer stick can be more easily adapted to the interproximal surface. The stick should be discarded if the wood becomes splayed as splinters could be forced into the gingival tissues. Plastic sticks can be thoroughly washed and reused.

Triangular wood sticks have been shown to reduce bleeding sites and to do so better than rinsing with chlorhexidine.[56] In oral hygiene studies of participants exhibiting bleeding papillae, it was found that plaque removal with wooden triangular sticks effectively reduced inflammation more in the coronal regions of the interproximal pocket than in the apical regions.[56] It has also been suggested that by depressing the papilla, wood sticks can extend 2 to 3 millimeters into the sulcus, thus enhancing subgingival plaque removal.[43] A resurgence in the popularity of wood sticks has prompted recent marketing of design variations from the traditional triangular woodsticks. One such model is a fabric coated or "flocked" plastic stick (Figure 7–16).

### Toothpicks

A comprehensive history of toothpick use suggests that toothpicks are one of the earliest and

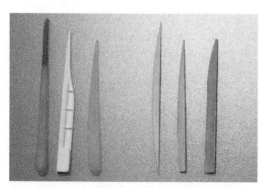

FIGURE 7-16   Variety of wooden and plastic triangular sticks. Plastic—three sticks depicted at left. Note flocked design of first plastic stick. Wooden—three sticks depicted at right. Note balsa wood composition of last wooden stick (others are birch).

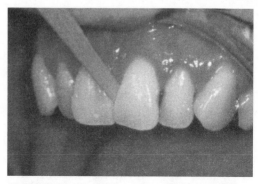

FIGURE 7-17   Placement of balsa wood triangular stick interproximally. (Note: base of triangular stick rests at gingival aspect.)

The toothpick may date back to the days of the cavepeople, who probably used sticks to pick food from between the teeth.[57,58] The nobility and the affluent used elaborate toothpick kits of metal, ivory, and carved wood; the less affluent whittled sticks for the same purpose.

Toothpicks are utilized along the sulcus and in the interproximal surface to dislodge food debris and plaque. Consistent use of the toothpick can result in firm, resilient tissue. Outcomes are generally similar to triangular wood sticks, although one study showed superior benefits of the triangular wood stick.[59] Toothpicks are generally considered easier to manipulate than floss and indeed are used more than floss for oral hygiene.[60] A drawback with toothpick utilization is the possibility of contributing to recession, blunting the papillae, or causing even more severe damage with improper use. Recommended use of the toothpick is described with the toothpick holder and is an important aspect of oral hygiene self-care instruction.

### Toothpick Holder

Although a toothpick may be manipulated by hand, the toothpick holder is a handle designed to increase effective application of the traditional toothpick by holding it securely at the proper angle. It also serves as an extension of the fingers in hard-to-reach areas. In particular, toothpicks in a handle have been suggested for cleaning the lingual embrasures of the posterior teeth.[61]

Plaque removal is achieved by tracing the gingival margin around each tooth or furcation area, and in each interproximal area with moderate pressure. Interproximally, the toothpick is moved back and forth between the buccal and lingual aspects to remove plaque and stimulate gingival tissues (Figure 7–18).

A variety of toothpick holders are available commercially (Figure 7–19). The toothpick is inserted into an adjustable plastic contra-angled handle, with the excess wood end broken off by snapping the toothpick in a downward

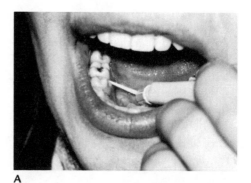

A

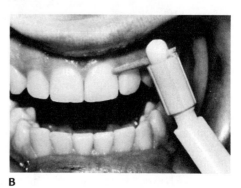

B

FIGURE 7–18

Use of a toothpick holder. **A.** Tip is placed perpendicular to the long axis of the tooth to clean along gingival margins. **B.** Tip is placed at less than a 45° angle on the tooth to clean along marginal gingiva. Frayed tip is used to burnish or brush the tooth surface. (Courtesy of Marquis Dental Manufacturing Company, Aurora, CO.)

direction. This leaves a stem to prevent the tip from disengaging from the holder. The toothpick can be positioned acutely on one end to access lingual surfaces and obtusely at the other end to adapt to buccal surfaces. The use of the toothpick holder is indicated in the following circumstances:

- Plaque removal along the gingival margin and within the gingival sulci or periodontal pockets,

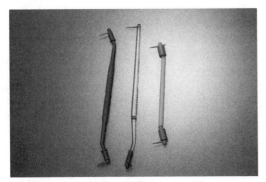

FIGURE 7–19    A variety of toothpick holders.

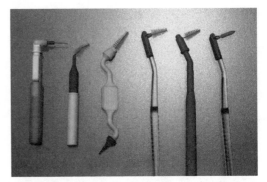

FIGURE 7–20    A variety of interproximal brush devices.

- Cleaning of concave proximal surfaces (Figure 7–5C),
- Cleaning of accessible furcation areas,
- Cleaning around orthodontic appliances and fixed prostheses,
- Application of chemotherapeutic agents (such as burnishing fluoride into the tooth to treat hypersensitivity or delivering chlorhexidine into the gingival sulcus).

When using a toothpick to remove plaque, it may be pre-moistened with saliva to soften the wood, just as with the wood stick. When applied to the gingival margin, the blunt tip is placed perpendicular to the long axis of the teeth. As previously mentioned, care should be taken to avoid subgingival insertion or vigorous interproximal use because of potential damage to the gingiva or teeth.

### Interproximal and Uni-tufted Brushes

Small interproximal brushes which are attached to a handle come in a variety of designs. Some of the designs have a nonreplaceable brush; the entire device is discarded when the brush is worn (Figure 7–20). Interproximal brushes can be utilized to clean spaces between teeth and around furcations, orthodontic bands, and fixed prosthetic appliances with spaces that are large enough to easily receive

the device (Figures 7–21, 7–22). They may also be used to apply chemotherapeutic agents into interproximal areas as well as furcations. Foam tips initially developed for use with implants are an ideal mechanism for delivery of medicaments interproximally or at furcations. Interproximal brushes are preferable to the use of dental floss for cleaning between teeth where the papilla does not fill the embrasure space or where root concavities are present[2,32] (Figure 7–5B). The brushes are tapered or cylindrical in shape and are available in a variety of sizes (Figure 7–23). The core of the brush that holds the bristles is made of plastic, wire, or nylon-coated wire.

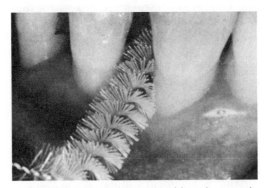

FIGURE 7–21    Interproximal brush moved in a bucco-lingual direction between teeth.

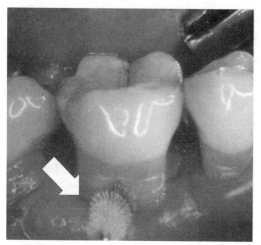

FIGURE 7-22 Interproximal brush directed into furcation.

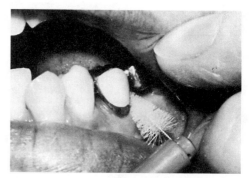

FIGURE 7-24 Interproximal brush inserted between abutment and pontic of fixed partial denture at angle approximating the gingival contour. Brush can be inserted under pontic if space allows. (Courtesy of Dr. Linda S. Scheirton, Creighton Universary, Omaha, NB.)

When determining the appropriate size of interproximal brushes, the diameter of the bristles should be slightly larger than the space to be cleaned. The brush can be moistened, and then inserted into the area at an angle approximating the normal gingival contour (Figure 7–24). A bucco-lingual movement is used to remove plaque and debris. Caution should be exercised to prevent damage to the tooth or soft tissues from the firm wire or plastic core of the brush. Implant abutments are easily cleaned with interdental brushes however, extreme caution should be exercised to prevent scratching of the titanium surface.[38] **Only plastic coated wires are recommended.** Foam brushes can also be utilized for this purpose.

The uni-tufted brush, also known as the single-tufted brush, is efficient for removing plaque in numerous sites (Figure 7–25). These include the following:

* Mesial and distal surfaces of teeth adjacent to edentulous spaces, including the distal of the last molar in each quadrant,

* Furcations and fluted root surfaces (mesial aspect of maxillary first premolars and mandibular first molars) that have been exposed because of gingival recession or periodontal surgery,

* Wide open embrasures where papillae have been lost,

* Around dental appliances, including implants and orthodontic wires and brackets.

One study demonstrated the advantages of combining the use of the uni-tufted brush with

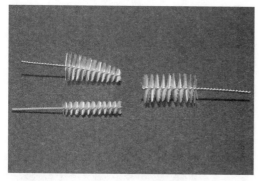

FIGURE 7-23 Replaceable interproximal brush inserts in 3 varying sizes.

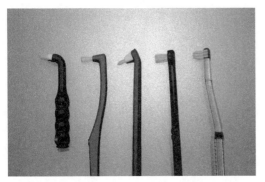

FIGURE 7–25    A variety of uni-tufted brushes.

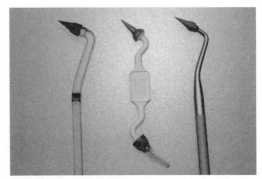

FIGURE 7–26    A variety of rubber or plastic tip devices.

the toothpick.[62] The end of the tuft is directed into the interproximal area by combining a rotating motion with intermittent pressure. The uni-tuft brush has also been suggested for application of chemotherapeutic agents. By softening in very hot or boiling water, handles of some uni-tufted brushes can be bent in order to allow easier access to the posterior buccal and lingual interproximal areas.

### Other Interproximal Devices

#### Rubber or Plastic Tip

These devices consist of a conical, flexible rubber or plastic tip attached to a handle or to the end of a toothbrush (Figure 7–26). Primarily utilized for gingival massage, they can be used to remove plaque and debris from exposed furcation areas, open embrasures, and along the gingival margin. In one study, no differences were found in plaque or gingival index scores when comparing the rubber tip, dental floss, and interproximal brushes.[63] However, practitioners do not generally view rubber or plastic tips as effective plaque removal devices. Additional research is warranted. The lack of consistent evidence underscores the value of selecting a device that the educator is enthusiastic about in order to enhance compliance and

have the greatest likelihood of success for an individual.

The tip is placed at a 90-degree angle to the long axis of the tooth and traced with moderate pressure along the gingival margin (Figure 7–27). In an open embrasure area, the tip is moved in and out in a bucco-lingual direction. The use of a tip attached to an angled shank rather than a toothbrush handle may allow for

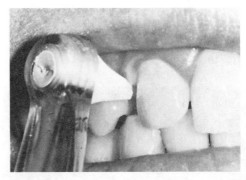

FIGURE 7–27    Use of interdental tip stimulator to remove plaque. The tip is placed at a 90° angle to the long axis of the tooth and traced along the gingival margin or moved in a buccolingual direction in an open embrasure area. (Courtesy of John O. Butler Co., Chicago, IL.)

greater ease of access and adaptation. To prevent damage to the soft tissues, care should be taken to avoid inserting the tip subgingivally. Another design is made of elastomeric flanges and adds texture to the rubber tip allowing for a potential increase in plaque removal ability (Figure 7–28).

When used to massage the gingiva the rubber tip stimulates the tissue leading to increased keratinization.[64,65] However, since the keratinization occurs in the oral rather than the sulcular gingiva, improved gingival health probably results from removal of bacterial plaque rather than from the stimulation.[66] Some practitioners also recommend the rubber tip following periodontal surgery to aid in tissue re-contouring.

### Knitting Yarn

In areas where the papillae have receded and the embrasure is open, white knitting yarn (no dyes) can be used in place of floss for proximal cleaning. Wool yarns should be avoided because of the possibility of tissue irritation. The rationale for use of yarn is that the increased thickness and texture can enhance plaque removal. When access is limited, a floss threader may be used to insert the yarn into the embrasure (Figure 7–29). Once the yarn has been drawn through the embrasure, the technique is the same as for dental

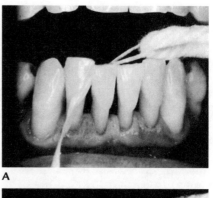

**A**

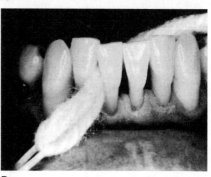

**B**

FIGURE 7-29    Use of knitting yarn in wide open embrasure. **A.** Yarn is looped through dental floss and inserted through the contact point. **B.** Yarn is drawn through the embrasure. (Courtesy of Dr. Linda S. Scheirton, Creighton University, Omaha, NB.)

floss, taking care not to traumatize the tissue. The inconvenience of acquiring yarn, which is not a common household item, may affect compliance.

### Gauze Strip

A gauze strip can be used for cleaning the proximal surfaces of teeth adjacent to edentulous areas, teeth that are widely spaced, or implant abutments. To prepare the strip, a 2-inch-wide gauze bandage is unfolded and refolded lengthwise. The lengthwise edge of the gauze is positioned with the fold toward the gingiva and the ends folded inward to avoid gingival irritation

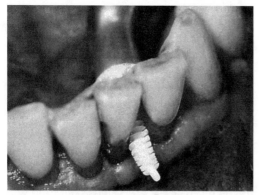

FIGURE 7-28    Rubber tip device with textured elastomeric flanges.

(Figure 7–30). The gauze is adapted by wrapping it around the exposed proximal surface to the facial and lingual line angles of the tooth. A bucco-lingual "shoeshine" stroke is used to loosen and remove plaque and debris. Gauze strips are recommended to clean the most distal surface of the most distal tooth in the mouth. It is particularly beneficial for the distal abutment tooth for partial dentures, an area where plaque accumulation is frequently abundant and thick.

*Automated Interproximal Cleaners*

Automated interproximal cleaning devices have been developed to help improve individual compliance with cleaning the proximal surfaces of teeth. One such device is a nylon filament tip that moves at 10,000 linear strokes per minute (Figure 7–31). When compared to manual flossing, research demonstrates that the device is able to reduce plaque levels and bleeding, and improve gingival parameters equal to that achieved with manual flossing.[67]

Several powered toothbrushes have attachments that are designed with a small number of bristles to remove plaque at the interproximal areas, around furcations, prosthetic abutments,

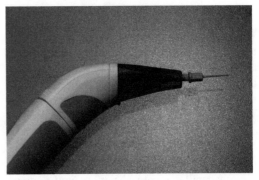

FIGURE 7–31    Automated interproximal cleaner.

and implants. One such device uses a uni-tuft of microfine filaments that move in an orbital motion. Another uses several bristle tufts that are 0.006 millimeters diameter with end-rounded bristles that oscillate when activated. One study found this automated oscillating interproximal brush to be safe and effective in removing plaque from the interproximal area.[68]

---

### Question 3

Which of the following statements, if any, are correct?

A. Utilization of wood or plastic sticks does reduce plaque accumulations and does clear food debris from the mouth.

B. Incorrect use of a toothpick may cause gingival recession or damage to the papillary tissues.

C. The diameter of an uni-tufted brush should be slightly smaller than the embrasure space to be cleaned.

D. When utilizing a gauze strip to clean in interproximal surface the fold should be positioned toward the gingival margin.

E. A rubber tip aids in removing oral debris and plaque from the gingival sulcus, but the keritinization it stimulates, is on the oral side of the gingival margin.

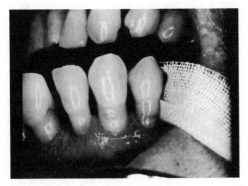

FIGURE 7–30    A 6-in. length of 1-in. gauze bandage folded in half with the folded edge adjacent to the gingiva for adaptation. (Courtesy of Dr. Linda S. Scheirton, Creighton University, Omaha, NB.)

## Tongue Cleaners

Tongue cleaning has been practiced since antiquity.[69] Studies on tongue debridement have renewed interest in this supplemental measure to further reduce bacterial plaque beyond toothbrushing and interproximal cleaning.[70,71] The large papillary surface area of the tongue dorsum favors the accumulation of oral microorganisms and oral debris. Anatomically, the shorter fungiform papillae and the longer filiform papillae create elevations and depressions that may entrap debris and harbor microorganisms, making the tongue an ideal location for bacterial growth. Oral debris from these sites may contribute to plaque formation in other areas of the mouth.[72] Reduction of this debris by mechanical tongue debridement can affect plaque accumulation, and oral malodor.[73]

Various designs of tongue cleaners are available (Figure 7–32). A soft-bristled toothbrush can also be used after the standard toothbrushing regimen. When using a tongue cleaner, the device is placed on the dorsal surface of the tongue close to the base of the tongue and pulled forward, pressing lightly against the surface of the tongue (Figures 7–33, 7–34). This process is repeated to cover the entire surface area of the tongue. Smokers or those with coated, deeply fissured tongues, or with elongated papillae (hairy tongue) will find that tongue debridement is especially beneficial in reducing oral bacteria.

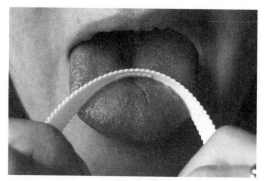

FIGURE 7-33   Plastic tongue cleaning device used by pressing against tongue in an arc. Note serrations that provide a scraping action.

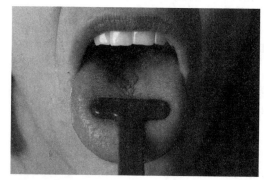

FIGURE 7-34   Plastic tongue cleaning device used by pressing in a posterior to interior direction.

### Oral Malodor and the Tongue

Oral malodor, another term for bad breath or halitosis, can have a systemic origin or may originate in the oral cavity. A thorough physical examination can rule out a systemic disorder. Usually odors in the oral cavity occur when sulfur-containing proteins and peptides are hydrolyzed by Gram-negative bacteria in an alkaline environment.[74] Odiferous sulfur-containing end products created by this process include hydrogen sulfide, methylmercaptans, and dimethyl sulfide. A shift from a predominantly gram posi-

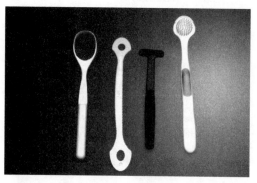

FIGURE 7-32   A variety of tongue cleaners.

tive *to* a gram negative and anaerobic bacterial population is associated with odor production. Local factors such as reduced salivary flow, and/or a rise in oral pH may affect this shift. Inconsistent or ineffective interproximal plaque removal can provide a niche for gram negative bacteria to degrade sulfur-containing amino acids resulting in malodor.[72] The presence of periodontal disease may also be a contributing factor since the inflammatory process creates substrates that stimulate bacterial growth.[75] Also, the putrefaction process and its concomitant odor occurs more rapidly when bacterial accumulations on the tongue are high. Active periodontal disease, exhibiting deeper pockets, contributes to malodor. Thus, for some people, management of periodontal disease is an important aspect in the control of malodor.

Treatment considerations can include instruction in consistent tongue brushing or scraping since the dorsoposterior surface of the tongue seems to be a common site for production of volatile sulfur compounds. Additionally, the intraoral use of chlorine dioxide rinse, which oxidizes the malodorous sulfides has been shown to effectively reduce malodor.[72]

## Rinsing

Vigorous rinsing of the mouth will aid in the removal of food debris and loosely adherent plaque. Although water rinsing does not remove attached plaque, it may help return the mouth to a neutral pH following the acid production that results from ingesting fermentable carbohydrates. Rinsing or use of an irrigator is also helpful for individuals with orthodontic appliances.

For maximum effectiveness, a technique should be adopted whereby fluid is forced through the interproximal areas of clenched teeth with as much pressure as possible in order to loosen and clear debris. Use of the lip, tongue, and cheek muscles aids in forcing the fluid back and forth between the teeth prior to expectoration.

Rinsing has a limited impact supragingivally and is not efficient in subgingival penetration. It has no impact in reducing clinical parameters associated with gingival inflammation. However, the use of a therapeutic agent enhances the effect of rinsing. Antimicrobial rinsing has been utilized as part of a full mouth disinfection approach to improve oral tissue health.[76,77] See Chapter 6 for a detailed discussion of the impact of chemotherapeutics.

## Irrigation Devices

Irrigation devices are a means of irrigating specific areas of the mouth whereas rinsing is a means of flushing the entire mouth. A home-irrigation device that is used for self-care provides a steady or pulsating stream of fluid, although the pulsating stream is preferable (Figure 7–35). Irrigation can result in the disruption of loosely attached or unattached supra- and subgingival plaque. The action is twofold. Loosely attached microflora are disrupted when the pulsating fluid makes initial contact. There is a secondary flushing action as the irrigant is deflected from the tooth surface. The microflora is disrupted both qualitatively and quantitatively.[78]

It has been demonstrated that irrigation with water or a nontherapeutic placebo can improve gingivitis or early periodontitis, when combined with toothbrushing.[79-83] Supragingival water irrigation alone, without toothbrushing, is not effective and is inferior to toothbrushing.[84-87] Home irrigation is not indicated for those who brush effectively and have no gingival inflammation. Individuals with inconsistent or ineffective interproximal cleaning, fixed orthodontic appliances, crowns, fixed partial dentures, and implants however, may benefit from a home irrigation self-care regimen.[86,88] Oral irrigation may also be helpful for individuals who have jaws temporarily wired together for stabilization following surgery or head and neck trauma. Irrigation has been shown to reduce proinflammatory cytokines involved in

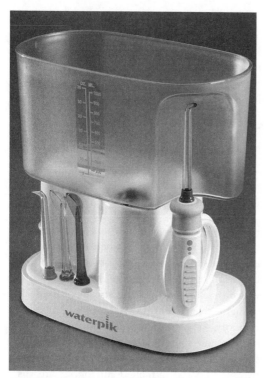

FIGURE 7–35 Oral irrigator for home use. Note standard tip and additional hygiene accessories. (Courtesy of Waterpik Technologies.)

the bone destructive process when periodontal diseases are present.[89]

The standard tip is designed for supragingival use. The tip is directed perpendicular to the tooth at or near the gingival margin. The cannula-type tip is directed into the gingival sulcus and allows a focused lavage adding to the depth of penetration.[90] Rubber-tipped cannulas can be angled into the sulcus about 2 millimeters. Home subgingival irrigation has been used to deliver medicaments further into the gingival sulcus.[81,91] Several studies demonstrated additional reductions in gingivitis and bleeding when using an antimicrobial agent in an oral irrigator with a cannula-type tip.[82, 92–94] Use of the cannula-type tip should be limited to individuals with adequate skill and dexterity.

Antimicrobial agents used as the irrigant have shown clinical and microbiologic improvements in those with gingivitis.[83,95,96] The failure to reach the base of the pocket may explain why supragingival irrigation is more effective against gingivitis than periodontitis. Investigations have compared supragingival irrigation with water to rinsing with chlorhexidine. Some studies show no difference[97] while others found chlorhexidine rinse more effective in plaque removal than water irrigation alone.[82,86]

The potential for supragingival irrigation to induce bacteremias has been studied, but does not appear hazardous to healthy patients[98] since toothbrushing,[99] creates a similar level of bacteremia. Oral irrigators used inappropriately by those with poor oral hygiene have induced bacteremias, but the relationship to bacterial endocarditis is unclear.[98] There is less risk of bacterial endocarditis from irrigation of a healthy mouth than when irrigating an inflamed mouth because of differences in microbial load.[98, 99]

## Implant Maintenance

Meticulous oral hygiene self-care is essential in maintaining dental implants. Plaque and calculus accumulate more rapidly, in larger amounts and adhere more easily to the implant abutment than to natural teeth.[100] The epithelial barrier and connective tissue attachment mechanism is not as strong around an implant when compared to a natural tooth. This weaker attachment allows for a more rapid bacterial invasion of the biologic seal which can contribute to the destruction of osseous integration. Effective plaque removal is a critical factor in the maintenance of a healthy biologic seal and to prevent implant failure.[101] There is a positive correlation between the amount of plaque and subsequent gingivitis and bone loss around implants.[102]

The loss of natural teeth resulting in the placement of implants is often caused by a his-

tory of poor oral hygiene resulting in dental disease. A commitment to meticulous daily oral hygiene self-care is critical for those with implants. Cleaning the abutment posts, bars, and prosthetic superstructures, presents a challenge that can be even more demanding than cleaning natural teeth. As with natural teeth, a combination of devices is usually needed to remove plaque from all surfaces. The goal of implant maintenance is to regularly remove soft deposits without altering the surface of the implants. Damage to titanium implants can increase corrosion and affect the molecular interaction between the implant surface and host tissue.[103] A scratched surface may lead to increased plaque accumulation.[104] The subsequent bacterial invasion can progress rapidly to peri-implantitis and potential implant failure.

An effective brushing technique should be the first component of an implant oral hygiene self-care regimen. A soft, manual toothbrush can be used. A sonic powered toothbrush has been shown to be better than a manual toothbrush in reducing plaque and bleeding scores around implants.[105] Some individuals may prefer a powered rotary brush with a tapered brushhead design. Neither type of powered brush was found to damage the implant surface and both were effective in areas where access is difficult.[105,106] Whatever brush is used, a demonstration of the adaptation of the brush to the abutment posts and pontics should be provided. The dentifrice used should meet American Dental Association standards to ensure that it is not abrasive.

To aid in plaque removal from abutment posts there are a variety of other devices that can be utilized (Figure 7–36). A tapered or cylindrical shaped interproximal brush or unitufted brush can be used with an in-and-out motion to clean the abutment posts. (Figure 7–36B, 7–36C) The interproximal brush must have a nylon-coated wire rather than the standard metal wire to prevent scratching the implant with the tip of the interproximal brush.

Foam tips are an alternative choice for cleaning the interproximal surface of an implant. To help control bacteria, the foam tip, interproximal brush, or either of the powered brushes may be dipped into an antimicrobial solution such as chlorhexidine gluconate (0.12%). Alternately, a cotton swab can be used to apply the agent.

Any type of floss, tape, or yarn can be used for circumferential plaque removal around abutment posts. In some cases, traditional floss with a floss threader, variable thickness floss or gauze can be placed in a 360-degree loop around the abutment post and moved with a shoeshine motion in the direction of the long axis of the tooth. Alternately, floss products designed specifically for use with implants can be used (Figure 7–36A). Ribbon floss is a wide, woven, sometimes braided, gauze-like version of floss, which provides increased texture to enhance plaque removal. One product has a hook on the end of the floss ribbon to allow for wrapping the floss around an entire post by inserting from the facial aspect, thus eliminating insertion from both facial and lingual surfaces. Yarn and shoelaces can also be used. Placing a small amount of nonabrasive toothpaste on the flossing product can polish the posts.

Oral irrigators can be used for cleaning around abutments, however, the water spray should be used on the lowest setting and should not be directed subgingivally. Daily subgingival irrigation with 0.06% chlorhexidine has shown beneficial effects on gingival, plaque, bleeding, and calculus indices while rinsing with 0.12% chlorhexidine affected gingival and bleeding indices only.[107] The substantivity effect is not as strong for implants as for natural teeth but would be better facilitated by subgingival irrigation than rinsing.

A critical factor in successful implant maintenance as with all oral health self-care is to recommend only the minimal number of cleaning devices needed for effective plaque removal. With proper instruction, the motivated individual can successfully maintain implants.

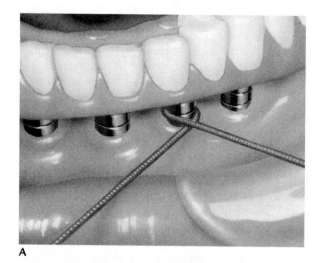

**A**

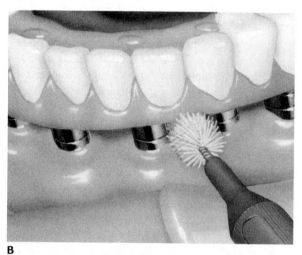

**B**

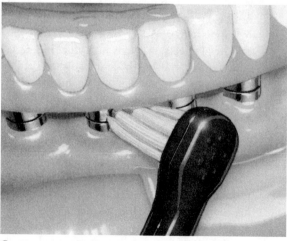

**C**

FIGURE 7–36   Cleaning implants:
**A.** Circumferential placement of Post-care braided nylon cord. **B.** Interproximal brush. **C.** End-tuft brush. (Courtesy of John O. Butler Co., Chicago, IL.)

## Denture Maintenance

Instructions should be provided for the proper care and cleaning of both the dentures and the underlying tissues. According to one survey, only 40% of dentures worn by the elderly are adequately cleaned.[108]

Care of the soft tissues on which a denture rests includes removing the denture overnight or for a substantial time each day, cleaning and massaging the tissues under the denture daily,[109,110] and performing regular oral self-examinations to observe and report any irritation or chronic changes in appearance of the tissues. Failure to remove the denture may result in oral malodor, excessive alveolar ridge resorption, diseased or irritated oral tissues, or the development of epulis fissuratum.

Cleaning and massaging of the soft tissues can be performed simultaneously by brushing with a soft-bristled toothbrush or by massaging with the thumb or forefinger wrapped in a clean facecloth. Deposits that form on dentures include pellicle, plaque, calculus, oral debris (e.g., desquamated epithelial cells), stain and food debris. The microscopic porous surface of a denture attracts dental deposits.

Consistent, effective cleaning of dentures not only serves to enhance the sense of oral cleanliness, but also serves to prevent oral malodor, denture stomatitis, and other tissue irritations. Mucosal irritation may impair eating, which can have a negative nutritional impact on a frail, elderly individual. The incidence of denture stomatitis varies from 20 to 40% of the denture population and occurs most commonly in females. Frequently, denture wearers are only aware of the aesthetic benefits to be derived from maintaining cleanliness. It is incumbent upon the oral health professional to stress the numerous health benefits of denture cleaning.

Bacterial and fungal organisms can colonize the porous denture surface. For candidial infections the denture should be soaked in a nystatin antifungal suspension while simultaneously treating the oral tissues with the same medication. Daily thorough cleansing of the denture is recommended because dentures harbor the bacteria involved in the creation of the volatile sulfur compounds that contribute to oral malodor.[110,111] Commonly practiced cleaning methods include immersion, brushing, or a combination of both.

### Immersion Cleaners

Immersing the denture in a cleaning solution has the advantage of reaching all parts of a denture, while with brushing, areas of the denture may be missed. Consequently a combination may result in a more thoroughly cleaned denture. When selecting an immersion cleaner, the type of denture material must be considered. Alcohol or essential oils found in commercial mouthwashes are not compatible with denture acrylic, which may become dry or lose color from prolonged contact with these substances.

Hypochlorite solutions diluted 1:10 with tap water act as antifungal and antibacterial agents.[112] Adding a teaspoon of calcium-chelating dishwasher detergent (e.g., Calgonite®) may help to control calculus or stains. Care must be taken to not immerse appliances with metallic components in hypochlorite solutions since the metallic surface may corrode.[112] It is imperative that individuals be instructed to thoroughly rinse the bleach off before placement on the oral tissues. Acetic acid (vinegar) can be used for immersion, will kill some organisms, and is less caustic to soft tissues if not thoroughly rinsed.

Commercial alkaline peroxide powders and tablets are available. These typically contain an alkaline for oxidizing, perborate or carbonate for effervescing, and a chelating agent (EDTA).[106] When dissolved in water, these agents decompose and release oxygen bubbles, which mechanically loosen plaque debris on the denture surface. The alkaline substances and detergent enhance the mechanical effect of the bubbles. A 99% bacterial kill has been reported with these commercial products, and

their effects are enhanced at 122° F.[113] Enzyme proteolytic agents have been used but appear inferior to alkaline peroxides.[114]

## Cleaning the Denture

Brushing in conjunction with an abrasive agent or brushing a denture before and after it has soaked in an immersion cleaner, can be utilized to aid in the removal of deposits. Incorrect use of an abrasive agent (poor technique and/or too much pressure) can damage the denture. A brush with medium or soft end-rounded bristles, if used properly, should not abrade denture materials. A denture brush provides access to all surfaces of a denture (Figure 7–37). The dental professional should assess the level of manual dexterity when providing instruction in denture brushing.

Nonabrasive agents such as soap or baking soda, or a commercial dentifrice may be safely used in conjunction with a brush. Other agents may be harmful to denture materials. The denture delivery appointment is an excellent time to explain and demonstrate how to care for the new denture.

Ultrasonic or sonic devices are available for home denture cleaning. They utilize a cleaning solution in conjunction with agitation produced by ultrasonic (inaudible, high frequency) or sonic (audible) sound waves to remove debris and stains. Studies verify the efficacy of the ultrasonic cleaner; they are more effective than brushing with water.[115,116] Use of these devices may be particularly helpful for individuals with limited dexterity or for the personal-care staff at long-term care facilities. Whichever method is used, the denture should be thoroughly rinsed under running, tepid water before reinsertion into the mouth in order to remove any substances that could irritate soft tissue.

Instruction in the recommended method of self-care of their denture and of the tissues upon which it rests is critical to successful denture

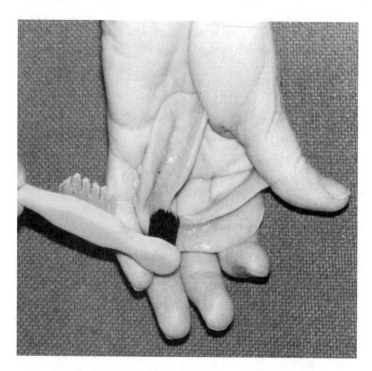

FIGURE 7–37  Brushing the alveolar surface of a full denture with a denture brush. Note the firm hold to prevent the denture slipping out of the hand.

maintenance. It is the responsibility of the dental professional to ensure an understanding of both the "why" and "how" of denture maintenance and the potential consequences of poor denture self-care. Explaining the procedure, demonstrating the correct method, and then requesting a return demonstration are all instructional methods to improve compliance. Written instructions and recommendations should be provided for easy reference and referral.

### Question 4

Which of the following statements, if any, are correct?

A. Implants accumulate dental plaque and thus can contribute to the development of periodontal disease.

B. Plaque removal from an implant can best be accomplished with a pipe cleaner.

C. The stream of solution from an irrigating device should be directed apically to clean the sulcus around implants.

D. Immersion cleaning of dentures is usually more effective than brushing because immersion ensures the cleaning agent reaches all areas of the denture.

E. After providing education on auxiliary methods of oral hygiene, instructions should be given on the use of several methods to solve the patient's problem.

## SUMMARY

In addition to oral conditions, several factors affect the appropriate selection and use of supplemental oral hygiene devices. The dexterity and motivation for performing oral hygiene procedures, and the preferences for specific devices should be assessed when recommending supplemental oral hygiene devices and techniques. When a device is introduced, it is essential that the proper application in all areas of the mouth be demonstrated and that the potential for damage with improper use is understood.

Despite adequate dexterity and ability, attainment of optimal oral health requires motivation and daily compliance in performing oral care. To enhance compliance and skill development, the number of recommended oral hygiene devices should be limited. Studies examining compliance and effectiveness indicate that development of proper skills and a willingness to use supplemental oral hygiene devices is facilitated when the number of devices is limited to no more than two.[117,118] Personal preferences for particular oral hygiene devices should also be considered. Although a specific device may be favored by the oral health professional, it will be ineffective if not used. If an individual has shown a preference for a specific device, its use should be encouraged. For example, if an individual uses a toothpick but presents with inadequate oral hygiene as evidenced by disclosed plaque and/or tissue inflammation the oral health professional might consider one of the following:

· Instruction to enhance the effectiveness with the toothpick,
· Introduction of a toothpick holder to facilitate access and manipulation of the toothpick,

· Use of the wooden or triangular interdental stick because of its similarity to the toothpick.

A wide variety of interproximal plaque removal devices are available. The oral health professional will need to stay informed of the research describing new devices, as it becomes available. Devices with evidenced based significance should be considered. Clinical experience and expertise should not be discounted, however, since these are also important components of evidence-based decision making.[119,120] It is incumbent upon the oral health professional to consistently investigate evidence and apply clinical judgment.

# ANSWERS AND EXPLANATIONS

1. A and D—correct.

    B—incorrect. Studies show incomplete plaque removal increases rate and growth of new plaque.

    C—incorrect. Motivational factors are considered during the planning phase. The evaluation phase focus is on patient outcomes and whether the oral hygiene self-care regimen needs to be adjusted.

    E—Incorrect. Only when rigorous interproximal cleaning was performed by an oral hygiene professional was there a reduction in caries incidence; there is very little evidence to support that theory.

2. B and E—correct.

    A—incorrect. Waxed and unwaxed floss have both been shown to be equally effective in removing plaque from the interproximal surface, without leaving a waxy residue. There is no evidence to indicate that one type of floss is better than the other.

    C—incorrect. The circle (or loop) method is best for children who do not yet have the dexterity needed for the spool method.

    D—incorrect. There is no study to date that shows one method is more effective than the other. Patient preference on the other hand, favors the use of floss holders.

3. A, B, D, and E—correct

    C—incorrect. It should be slightly larger so as to effectively scrub against the surface disrupting and removing bacterial plaque.

4. A and D—correct.

    B—incorrect. Circumferential plaque removal from an implant is best accomplished with a soft material that can be wrapped around its circumference: floss, tape, or yarn. Metal wire in a pipe cleaner could scratch the implant.

    C—Incorrect. The stream of solution from an irrigating device should be at a right angle to the long axis of the tooth; otherwise bacteria can be forced into the blood supply to the area.

E—Incorrect. It is best to restrict the recommendation to one or two options, which will enhance compliance potential.

## Self-evaluation Questions

1. The tooth surface least accessible to the toothbrush is the (interproximal) (buccal) (lingual) surface.

2. The (waxed) (unwaxed) floss frays and breaks more frequently on contact with calculus and restoration overhangs. The spool method of flossing requires (more) (less) psychomotor coordination than is required for the circle method. When using floss for the loop method, approximately _____ inches are needed, of which only about _____ inch(es) is/are held between the fingers to insert the floss between the teeth. A new segment of floss (is) (is not) used to clean each interdental space. If floss is forced too deeply into the sulcus, it can cause _____ in the gingiva, whereas if it is whipsawed buccolingually with too much force, it causes _____ of the cementum. If a periodontal condition exists, there is/are usually (one best) (several satisfactory) device(s) for plaque removal from areas with difficult access.

3. Four indications for the use of a dental floss holder in lieu of regular finger flossing are _____, _____, _____, and _____.

4. Three indications for the use of a floss threader are _____, _____, and _____.

5. Research (has) (has not) proved the value of the toothpick in maintaining oral health.

6. Irrigation devices have been used (successfully) (unsuccessfuly) to deliver medicaments further into the gingival sulcus.

7. Scratching the titanium implant while removing plaque can cause a more rapid buildup of _____ and hence pose a greater risk of gingivitis and periodontitis.

8. The wrapping of floss around an implant post for plaque removal is accomplished using a _____ _____ motion.

9. One study indicates that as few as _____% of the dentures worn by the elderly are adequately cleaned. Failure to maintain clean dentures can result in denture _____ _____ (overgrowth of tissue), a condition which is seen in 60 to 70% of denture wearers.

10. Four objectives that may be attained by proper use of dental floss are: _____, _____, _____, and _____.

11. Two auxiliary cleaning aids that can be used to safely and effectively clean under a fixed partial denture are _____ and _____.

# REFERENCES

1. Kinane, D. F. (1998). The role of interdental cleaning in effective plaque control: Need for interdental cleaning in primary and secondary prevention. Lang, N. P., Löe, H., & Attström, R., Eds. In Proceedings of the European Workshop on Mechanical Plaque Control: Quintessence, Berlin, 156–68.

2. Kiger, R. D., Nylund, K., & Feller, R. P. (1991). A comparison of proximal plaque removal using floss and interdental brushes. *J Clin Periodontol*, 18:681–84.

3. Löe, H. (2000). Oral hygiene in the prevention of caries and periodontal disease. *Int Dent J*, 50:129–39.

4. Brecx, M., Theilade, J., & Attström, R. (1980). Influence of optimal and excluded oral hygiene on early formation of dental plaque on plastic films. A quantitative and descriptive light and electron microscopic study. *J Clin Periodontol*, 7:361–73.

5. Mayfield, L., Attström, R., & Soderhelm, A. (1998). Cost-effectivnesss of mechanical plaque control. Lang, N. P., Löe, H., and Attström, R. Eds. In Proceedings of the European Workshop on Mechanical Plaque Control: Quintessence, Berlin, 177–89.

6. Lang, N. P., Cumming, B. R., & Löe, H. (1973). Toothbrushing frequency as it relates to plaque development and gingival health. *J Perioiodontol*, 44:396–05.

7. Lang, N. P., Cumming, B. R., & Loe, H. A. (1977). Oral hygiene and gingival health in Danish dental students and faculty. *Comm Dent & Oral Epidemiol*, 5:237–42.

8. Furuichi, Y., Lindhe, J., Ramberg, P., & Volpe, A. R. (1992). Patterns of *de novo* plaque formation in the human dentition. *J Clin Perio*, 19:423, 433.

9. DeLaRosa, M. R., Guerra, J. Z., Johnston, D. A., & Radike, A. W. (1979). Plaque growth and removal with daily toothbrushing. *J Periodontol*, 50:661–64.

10. Dahlen, G., Lindhe, J., Sato, K., Hanamura, H., & Okamoto, H. (1992). The effect of supragingival plaque control on the subgingival microbiota in subjects with periodontal disease. *J Clin Periodontol*, 19:802–9.

11. Katsanoulas, T., Renee, I., & Attström, R. (1992). The effect of supragingival plaque control on the composition of subgingival flora in periodontal pockets. *J Clin Periodontol*, 19:760–65.

12. Lang, N. P., Farghaly, M. M., & Ronis, D. L. (1994). The relation of preventive dental behaviors to periodontal health status. *J Clin Periodontol*, 21:194–98.

13. Graves, R. C., Disney, J. A., & Stamm, J. W. (1989). Comparative effectiveness of flossing and brushing in reducing interproximal bleeding. *J Periodontol*, 60:243–47.

14. Bowsma, O., Caton, J., Polson, A., & Espeland, M. (1988). Effect of personal oral hygiene bleeding interdental gingiva. *J Periodontol*, 59:80–86.

15. Addy, M., & Adriaens, P. (1998). Epidemiology and etiology of periodontal diseases and the role of plaque control in dental caries. Long, N. P., Löe, H., and Attström, R. Eds. In Proceedings of the European Workshop on Mechanical Plaque Control, 98–101.

16. Egelberg, J., & Claffey, N. (1998). Role of mechanical dental plaque removal in prevention and therapy of caries and periodontal diseases. Lang, N. P., Löe, H., & Attström, R., Eds. In Proceedings of the European Workshop on Mechanical Plaque Control, 169–72.

17. Wright, G. Z., Banting, D. W., & Feasby, W. H. (1979). The Dorchester dental flossing study: Final report. *Clin Prev Dent*, 1:23–26.

18. Corbet, E. F., & Davies, W. I. R. (1973). The role of supragingival plaque in the control of progressive periodontal disease. A review. *J Clin Periodontol*, 20:307–13.

19. Darby, M. L., & Walsh, M. M. (1995). *Dental hygiene theory & practice*. Philadelphia: WB Saunders.

20. Agerbaek, N., Melsen, B., Lind, O. P., Glavind, L., & Kristiansen, B. (1979). Effect of regular small group instruction per se on oral health status of Danish school children. *Comm Dent Oral Epidemiol*, 7:17–20.
21. Silverstein, S., Gold, D., Heilbron, D., Nelms, D., & Wycoff, S. Effect of supervised deplaquing on dental caries, gingivitis and plaque. *J Dent Res*, 56(A85): Abstract 169.
22. Granath, L. E., Rootzlen, H., Liljegven, E., Holst, K., & Kohler, L. (1978). Variation in caries prevalence related to combinations of dietary and oral hygiene habits and cleaning fluoride tablets in 4-year-old children. *Caries Res*, 12:83–92.
23. Horowitz, A. M., Suomi, J. D., Peterson, J. K., Voglesong, R. H., & Mathews, B. L. (1980). Effects of supervised daily plaque removal by children after three years. *Comm Dent Oral Epidemiol*, 8:171–76.
24. Axelsson, P., & Lindhe, J. (1981). Effect of controlled oral hygiene procedures on caries and periodontal disease in adults—results after 6 years. *J Clin Periodontol*, 8:239–48.
25. Wendt, L. K., Hallonsten, A. L., Koch, G., & Birkhead, D. (1994). Oral hygiene in relation to caries development and immigrant status in infants and toddlers. *Scand J Dent Res*, 102:269–73.
26. Nyvad, B., & Frjerskov, O. (1986). Active root surface caries converted into inactive caries as a response to oral hygiene. *Scand J Dent Res*, 94:281–84.
27. Straub, A. M., Salvi, G. E., & Lang, N. P. (1998). Supragingival plaque formation in the human dentition. Long, N. P., Löe, H., & Attström, R., Eds. In Proceedings of the European Workshop on Mechanical Plaque Control, 72–84.
28. Kelner, R. M., Wohl, B. R., Deasy, M. J., & Formicola, A. J. (1974). Gingival inflammation as related to frequency of plaque removal. *J Periodontol*, 45:301–3.
29. Saxton, C. A. (1973). Scanning electron microscope study of the formation of dental plaque. *Caries Res*, 7:102–19.
30. Ramberg, P., Lindhe, J., & Eneroth, L. (1994). The influence of gingival inflammation on de novo plaque formation. *J Clin Periodont*, 21:51–66.
31. Lang, N. P., Attström, R., & Löe, R., Eds. (1998). Proceedings of the 2nd European Workshop on Mechanical Plaque Control. Quintessence, Berlin, 259–61.
32. Bergenholz, A., & Olsson, A. (1984). Efficacy of plaque removal using interdental brushes and waxed dental floss. *Scan J Dent Res*, 92:198–203.
33. American Academy of Periodontology (1989). Proceedings of the World Workshop in Clinical Periodontics. Consensus report. Discussion Session II, 11–33.
34. Newman, H. N. (1991). Beyond floss. Interdental cleaning devices. *JADA*, 122:14–17.
35. Tolboe, H., Isidor, F., & Budtz-Jorgensen, E., et al. (1987). Influence of oral hygiene on the mucosal conditions beneath bridge pontics. *Scand J Dent Res*, 95:475–82.
36. Schwab, C. (1989). Flossing compliance. *Dent Hygiene News*, 2:5.
37. Jensen, R. L., & Jensen, J. H. (1991). Peri-implant maintenance. *Northwest Dent*, 70:14–23.
38. Steele, D. L., & Orton, G. S. (1992). Dental implants: Clinical procedures and homecare considerations. *J Pract Hyg*, June/July:9–12.
39. Kinane, D. F., Jenkins, W. M., and Peterson, A. J. (1992). Comparative efficacy of the standard flossing procedure and a new floss applicator in reducing interproximal bleeding: A short term study. *J Periodontol*, 63:757–60.
40. Perry, D. A., & Pattison, G. (1986). An investigation of wax residue on tooth surfaces after the use of waxed dental floss. *Dent Hygiene*, 60:16–19.
41. Ciancio, S. G., Shilby, O., & Farber, G. A. (1992). Clinical evaluation of the effect of two types of dental floss on plaque and gingival health. *Clin Prevent Dent*, 14:14–18.
42. Beaumont, R. H. (1990). Patient preference for waxed or unwaxed floss. *J Periodontol*, 61:123–25.

43. Axelsson, P. (1998). Needs-related plaque control measures based on risk prediction. Lang, N. P., Löe, H., & Attström, R. (Eds.). In Proceedings of the European workshop on mechanical plaque control. Quintessence, Berlin, 190–247.

44. Kuusela, S., Honkala, E., Kannas, Tynjala, J., & Wold, B. (1997). Oral hygiene habits of 11-year-old schoolchildren in 22 European countries and Canada in 1993/1994. *J Dent Res*, 76:1602–9.

45. MacGregor, I., Regis, D., & Balding J. (1997). Self-concept and dental health behaviors in adolescents. *J Clin Periodontol*, 24:335–9.

46. Honkala, E., Kannas, L., & Riise, J. (1991). Oral health habits of schoolchildren in 11 European countries. *Int Dent J*, 15:253–58.

47. Spolsky, V. W., Perry, D. A., Meng, Z., & Kissel, P. (1993). Evaluating the efficacy of a new flossing aid. *J Clin Periodontol*, 20:490–97.

48. Rimondini, L., Zolfanelli, B., Bernardi, F., & Bez, C. (2001). Self-preventive oral behavior in an Italian university student population. *J Clin Periodontol*, 28:207–11.

49. Bergenholtz, A., & Brithon, J. (1980). Plaque removal by dental floss or toothpicks. An intra-individual comparative study. *J Clin Periodontol*, 7:516–24.

50. Pucher, J., Jayaprakash, P., Aftyka, T., Sigman L., & Van Swol, R. (1995). Clinical evaluation of a new flossing device. *Quint Int*, 24:273–78.

51. Kleber, C. J., & Putt, M. S. (1988). Evaluation of a floss-holding device compared to hand-held floss for interproximal plaque, gingivitis, and patient acceptance. *Clin Prevent Dent*, 10:6–14.

52. Carter-Hanson, C., Gadbury-Amyot, C., & Killoy, W. (1996). Comparison of the plaque removal efficacy of a new flossing aid. *J Clin Periodontol*, 23:873–78.

53. Kleber, C. J., & Putt, M. S. (1990). Formation of flossing habit using a floss-holding device. *J Dent Hygiene*, Mar/Apr:140–43.

54. Mulligan, R., & Wilson, S. (1984). Design characteristics of floss-holding devices for persons with upper extremity disabilities. *Spec Care Dent*, 4:168–72.

55. Isaacs, R. L., Beiswanger, B. B., Crawford, I. L., Mau, M. S., Proskin, H., & Warren, R. R. (1999). Assessing the efficacy and safety of an electric interdental device. *JADA*, 130:104–8.

56. Caton, J., Bouwsma, O., Polson, A., & Espland, M. (1989). Effects of personal oral hygiene and subgingival scaling on bleeding interdental gingiva. *J Periodontol*, 60:84–90.

57. Bahn, P. G. (1989). Early teething troubles. *Nature*, 337:693.

58. Mandel, I. D. (1990). Why pick on teeth. *JADA*, 121:129–32.

59. Bergenholtz, A., Bjornes, A., & Vikstrom, B. (1974). The plaque-removing ability of some common interdental aids. An intra-individual study. *J Clin Periodontol*, 1:160–65.

60. Axelsson, P., Kocher, T., & Vivien, N. (1997). Adverse effects of toothpastes on teeth, gingiva, and oral mucosa. Lang, N. P., Karring, T., & Lindhe, J., Eds. In Proceedings of the 2nd European Workshop on Periodontology Chemicals in Periodontics: Quintessence, Berlin, 258–61.

61. Axelsson, P. (1993). New ideas and advancing technology in prevention and nonsurgical treatment of periodontal disease. *Int Dent J*, 43:223–38.

62. Gjermo, P., & Flotra, L. (1970). The effect of different methods of interdental cleaning. *J Periodontol Res*, 5:230–36.

63. Mauriello, S., Bader, J., George, M., & Klute, P. (1987). Effectiveness of three interproximal cleaning devices. *Clin Prev Dent*, 9:18–22.

64. Cantor, M. T., & Stahl, S. S. (1965). The effects of various interdental stimulators upon the keratinization of the interdental col. *Periodontics*, 3:243–47.

65. Glickman, I., Petralis, R., & Marks, R. (1965). The effect of powered toothbrushing and interdental stimulation upon microscopic inflammation and surface keratinization of the interdental gingiva. *J Periodontol*, 36:108–11.

66. Carranza, F. A., & Newman, M. G. (1996). *Clinical periodontology*. Philadelphia: WB Saunders, 503.

67. Anderson, N. A., Barnes, C. M., Russell, C. M., & Winchester, K. R. (1995). A clinical comparison of the efficacy of an electromechanical flossing device or manual flossing in affecting interproximal gingival bleeding and plaque accumulation. *J Clin Dent*, 6:105–7.

68. Danser, M. M., & Timmerman, M. F. (2001). Approximal brush head used in a power toothbrush. *J Dent Res*, 80 (Spec Iss.)(743):Abst 1734.

69. Gillette, W. A., & Van House, R. L. (1980). Ill effects of improper oral hygiene procedures. *JADA*, 101:476–80.

70. Ralph, W. J. (1988). Oral hygiene—why neglect the tongue? *Aust Dent J*, 33:224–25.

71. Rosenberg, M. (1996). Clinical assessment of bad breath: Current concepts. *JADA*, 127:475–82.

72. Richter, J. L. (1996). Diagnosis and treatment of halitosis. *Comp Cont Edu*, 17:370–86.

73. McDowell, J., & Kassebaum, D. K. (1993). Diagnosing and treating halitosis. *JADA*, 129:55–64.

74. Kleinberg, I., & Westbay, G. (1990). Oral malodor. *Crit Rev Oral Med*, 1:247–59.

75. Kostek, J. C., Preti, G., Zelson, P. R., Brauner, L., & Baehni, P. (1984). Oral odors in early experimental gingivitis. *J Periodontol Res*, 19:303–12.

76. Bray, K. K., & Wilder, R. S. (1999). Full mouth disinfection: A new approach to non-surgical periodontal therapy. *Access*, Sept/Oct, 57–60.

77. DeSoetes, M., Mongardi, C., Pauwels, M., Haffajee, A., Socransky, S., VanSteenberghe, D., & Quirynen, M. (2001). One-stage full-mouth disinfection. Long-term microbiological results analyzed by checkerboard DNA hybridization. *J Periodontol*, 72:374–82.

78. Cobb, C. M. (1988). Ultrastructural examination of lumen periodontal pockets following the use of an oral irrigation device. *J Periodontol*, 59:155–63.

79. Newman, M. G., Cattabriga, M., Etienne, D., Flemming, T., Sanz, M., Kronman, K. S., Doherty, F., Moore, D. J., & Ross, C. (1994). Effectiveness of adjunctive irrigation in early periodontis. Multi-center evaluation. *J Periodontol*, 65:224–29.

80. Flemming, T. F., Newman, M. G., & Doherty, F. (1990). Supragingival irrigation with 0.06% chlorhexidine in naturally occurring gingivitis. I. 6-month clinical observations. *J Periodontol*, 61:112–17.

81. Jolkovsky, D. L., Waki, M. Y., & Newman, M. G. (1990). Clinical and microbiological effects of subgingival and gingival marginal irrigation with chlorhexidine gluconate. *J Periodontol*, 61:112–17.

82. Brownstein, C. N., Briggs, S., & Schweitzer, K. L. (1990). Irrigation with chlorhexidine to resolve naturally occurring gingivitis. A methodologic study. *J Clin Peridontol*, 17:588–93.

83. Ciancio, S. G., Mather, M. L., Zambon, J. J., & Reynolds, H. S. (1989). Effect of a chemotherapeutic agent delivered by an oral irrigation device on plaque, gingivitis, and subgingival microflora. *J Periodontol*, 60:310–15.

84. Hugoson, A. (1978). Effect of the Water Pik device on plaque accumulation and development of gingivitis. *J Clin Periodontol*, 5:95–104.

85. Southard, G. L., Parson, L. G., & Thomas, L. G. (1987). Effect of sanguinaria on development of plaque and gingivitis when supragingivally delivered as a manual rinse or under pressure in an oral irrigator. *J Clin Periodontol*, 14:377–80.

86. Lang, N. P., & Raber, K. (1981). Use of oral irrigators as vehicles for the application of antimicrobial agents in chemical plaque control. *J Clin Periodontol*, 8:177–88.

87. Lang, N. P., & Ramseir-Grossman, K. (1981). Optimal dosage of chlorhexidine digluconate in chemical plaque control when applied by an oral irrigator. *J Clin Periodontol*, 8:189–202.

88. Aziz-Gandour, I. A., & Newman, H. N. (1986). The effects of a simplified oral hygiene regime plus supragingival irrigation with chlorhexidine or metronidazole on chronic inflammatory periodontal disease. *J Clin Periodontol*, 13:228–36.

89. Cutler, C. W., Stanford, T. W., Abraham, C., Cederberg, R. A., Broadman, T. J., & Ross, C. (2000). Clinical benefits of oral irrigation for periodontics are related to reduction of pro-inflammatory cytokine levels and plaque. *J Clin Periodontol*, 27:134–43.

90. American Academy of Periodontology, Committee on Research Science and Therapy (1995). The role of supra- and subgingival irrigation in the treatment of periodontal diseases. American Academy of Periodontology, 11–33.

91. Lofthus, J. E., Waki, M., Jolkovsky, D., Otomo-Corgel, J., Newman, M. G., Flemming, T., & Nachnani, S. (1991). Bacteremia following subgingival irrigation and scaling and root planing. *J Periodontol*, 62:602–7.

92. Grossman, E., Meckel, A. H., Isaacs, T. I., Ferretti, G. A., Sturzenberger, O. P., Bollmer, B. W., Moore, D. J., Lijana, R. C., & Manhart, M. D. (1989). A clinical comparison of antibacterial mouthrinses: Effects of chlorhexidine, phenolics, and sanguinarine on dental plaque and gingivitis. *J Periodontology*, 60:435–40.

93. Chaves, E. S., Kornman, K. S., Manwell, M. A., Jones, A. A., Newbold, D. A., & Wood, R. C. (1994). Mechanism of irrigation effects on gingivitis. *J Periodontol*, 65:1016–21.

94. Lyle, D. (2000). The role of pharmacotherapeutics in the reduction of plaque and gingivitis. *J Prac Hygiene*, 9:46–49.

95. Parsons, L. G., Thomas, L., & Southard, G. (1987). Effect of sanguinaria extract on established plaque and gingivitis when supragingivally delivered as a manual rinse under pressure under oral irrigator. *J Clin Periodontol*, 14:381–85.

96. Walsh, T. F., Glenwright, H. D., & Hull, P. S. (1992). Clinical effects of pulsed oral irrigation with 0.2% chlorhexidine digluconate in patients with adult periodontitis. *J Clin Periodontol*, 19:245–48.

97. Newman, M. G., Flemmig, T. F., & Nachnani, S. (1990). Irrigation with 0.06% chlorhexidine in naturally occurring gingivitis. II. 6-month microbiological observations. *J Periodontol*, 61:427–33.

98. Dajani, A. S., Tanbert, K. A., Wilson, W., Bolger, A. F., Bayer, A., Ferrier, P., Gewitz, M. A., Shulman, S. T., Nouri, S., Newburger, J. W., Hutto, C., Pallasch, T. J., Gage, T. W., Levinson, M. E., Peter, G., & Zuccaro, G. Jr. (1997). Prevention of bacterial endocarditis: Recommendations of the American Heart Association. *JAMA*, 277:1794–1801.

99. Pallasch, T. J., & Slots, J. (2000). Antibiotic prophylaxis and the medically compromised patient. *J.Periodontol*, 1996;10:107–38.

100. Van Steeberghe, D. (1990). Periodontal aspects of osseointegrated oral implants modum Branemark. *Dent Clin North Amer*, 32:355–70.

101. Bapoo-Mohamed, K. (1996). Post-insertion peri-implant tissue assessment: A longitudinal study. *J Oral Implantol*, 22:225–31.

102. Lekholm, R., Adell, R., Lindhe, J., Branemark, P. I., Eriksson, B., Rockler, B., Lindvall, A. M., & Yoneyama, T. (1986). Marginal tissue reactions of osseointegrated titanium fixtures: A cross-sectional study. *Int J Maxillofac Surg*, 15:53–61.

103. Baier, R. E., Meenaghan, M. A., Hartman, L. C., Wirth, J. E., Flynn, H. E., Meyer, A. E., Natiella, J. R., & Carter, J. M. (1988). Implant surface characteristics and tissue interaction. *J Oral Implantol*, 13:594.

104. Dmytryk, J., Fox, S., & Moriarty, J. (1990). The effects of scaling titanium implant surfaces with metal and plastic instruments on cell attachment. *J Periodontol*, 61:491–96.

105. Wolf, L., Kim, A., Nunn, M., & Bakdash, B. (1998). Effectiveness of a sonic toothbrush in maintenance of dental implants. *J Clin Periodontol*, 25:821–28.

106. Thomson-Neal, D., Evans, G., & Meffert, R. M. (1989). A SEM evaluation of various prophylactic modalities on different implants with titanium-sprayed surfaces. *Int J Periodont Restor Dent*, 9:301–11.

107. Felo, A., Shibly, O., Cidnero, S. G., Lauciella, F. R., & Ho, A. (1997). Effects of subgingival chlorhexidine irrigation on peri-implant maintenance. *Amer J Dent*, 10:107–10.

108. Hoad-Reddick, G., Grant, A. A., & Griffith, C. S. (1990). Investigation into the cleanliness of dentures in an elderly population. *J Prosthet Dent*, 64:48–52.

109. Zarb, G. A., Bolender, C. L., Hickey, J. C., & Carlsson, G. E. (1990). *Bouher's prosthetic treatment for edentulous patients* (10th ed.) Mosby, St. Louis.

110. Shay, K. (2000). Denture hygiene: A review and update. *J Contemp Dent Prac*, 1:2.

111. Chan, E. C. S., Iogovas, I., Silbo, R., Bilyk, M., Barolet, R., Amsel, R. Wooley, C., & Klitorinos, A. (1991). Comparison of two popular methods for removal and killing of bacteria from dentures. *J Can Dent Assoc*, 57:937–39.

112. Jaggar, D. C., & Harrison, A. (1995). Denture cleansing—the best approach. *Br Dent J*, 178:413–17.

113. McCabe, J. F., Murray, I. F., & Kelly, P. J. (1995). The efficacy of denture cleaners. *Eur J Prosthodont Restor Dent*, 3:203–7.

114. Nakamoto, K., Tamanoto, M., & Hamada, T. (1991). Evaluation of denture cleaners with and without enzymes against Candida albicans. *J Prosthet Dent*, 66:792–95.

115. Gwinnett, A. J., & Coputo, L. (1983). The effectiveness of ultrasonic denture cleaning: A scanning electron microscope study. *J Prosthet Dent*, 50:20–25.

116. Shay, K., Renner, R. P., & Truhlar, M. R. (1997). Oropharyngeal candidosis in the older patient. *J Amer Geriatr Soc*, 45:863–70.

117. Heasman, P. A., Jacobs, D. J., & Chapple, I. L. (1989). An evaluation of the effectiveness and patient compliance with plaque control methods in the prevention of periodontal disease. *Clin Prevent Dent*, 11:24–28.

118. Johansson, L. A., Oster, B., & Hamp, S. E. (1984). Evaluation of cause-related periodontal therapy and compliance with maintenance care recommendations. *J Clin Periodontol*, 15:689–99.

119. Jahn, C. A. (2000). Automated oral hygiene self-care devices: Making evidence-based choices to improve client outcomes. *J Dent Hygiene*, 2:171–86.

120. Abt, E. (1999). Evidence-based dentistry: An overview of a new approach to dental practice. *Gen Dent*, Jul–Aug, 369–73.

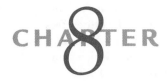

# CHAPTER 8

# Water Fluoridation

*M. Elaine Neenan*
*Mike Easley*
*Michael Ruiz, Research Assistant*

## OBJECTIVES

*At the end of this chapter, it will be possible to*

1. Define water fluoridation and the rationale for using water systems to provide for primary prevention of dental caries.
2. List and describe the four historical periods in the evolution and development of community water fluoridation.
3. Discuss the benefits and efficacy/effectiveness of water fluoridation.
4. Describe the cariostatic mechanisms of fluoride, including the pre- and post-eruptive effects.
5. Define the impact of multiple sources of fluoride on the decline of dental caries and the role of water fluoridation.
6. Discuss fluorosis, fluoride supplementation, and the need to monitor exposure to fluoride.
7. Describe the effect on caries prevalence when water fluoridation is discontinued in a community.
8. Describe the economic aspects of water fluoridation.
9. State the optimal fluoride concentration range, in parts per million (ppm), for maximum caries protection with minimal risk of fluorosis.
10. List the chemicals used for water fluoridation and briefly describe the technical aspects of fluoridation, including monitoring and surveillance of water fluoridation in the United States.
11. Discuss the Safe Drinking Water Act and the EPA standards for natural fluoride levels.

12. Discuss the safety of fluoridation in terms of impact on health.
13. Define the role of dental-health professionals in continuing to educate the public about water fluoridation.
14. Discuss the mechanisms in which community water fluoridation may be enacted in the United States.
15. Summarize the readiness assessment factors for initiating a fluoridation campaign.
16. Discuss Sandman's principles of risk perception, the principles of risk communication and the myths related to risk communication.
17. Summarize the techniques used by opponents of water fluoridation and elaborate on the means to overcome these objections.
18. Summarize the current status of water fluoridation as it relates to Healthy People 2010, the National Health Objectives.

# INTRODUCTION

Community water fluoridation (hereafter known as fluoridation) is defined as the upward *adjustment of the natural fluoride level* in a community's water supply to prevent dental caries. It is a population-based method of primary prevention that uses piped water systems to deliver low-dose fluoride over frequent intervals. Through water fluoridation, the preventive benefits accrue to consumers, *regardless of age or socioeconomic status*. Fluoridation has been cited as one of the *top-ten* public-health achievements of the century. Extensive research over the past half-century has consistently confirmed the efficacy, safety, and cost-effectiveness of fluoridation. Fluoridation, a major contributor to the documented decline in dental caries in the 1950s to 1980s, has continued to be efficacious in caries reduction during the past 20 years in which *multiple sources of fluoride* (especially fluoride-containing dentifrices) have played a role in caries reduction. Continued monitoring of fluoride exposure, especially from adjunctive sources like fluoride-containing dentifrices, is important in achieving the appropriate balance between *maximum caries preventive benefit and minimal risk of fluorosis*. Enactment of fluoridation can occur at the state level but more often has been implemented at the local level through *administrative action* or a *vote* of the electorate. Initiating a fluoridation campaign requires that an assessment be done to determine community readiness. External forces, including public opinion, the political climate, role of the media, voter turnout, knowledge, skills, and savvy of campaign committee, etc., impact the ability to garner majority support for this issue. While fluoridation is sound public policy, the practice of fluoridating community water supplies has been challenged by vocal opponents since its inception. Consequently, communities often become embroiled in major campaigns attracting significant media attention. Dental-health professionals need to remain informed about fluoridation and keep abreast of the literature and latest research. They also need to provide accurate information to their patients and remain prepared to address any concerns and/or fears. Equally as impor-

tant, they need to be able to assess the forces that affect public attitudes, evaluate the policy process, and understand the strategies employed by the opposition. This chapter reviews the history, as well as the efficacy, cariostatic mechanisms of action, safety, cost-effectiveness, and engineering aspects of fluoridation. Additionally, strategies used by opponents of fluoridation are discussed along with the principles of risk communication.

## Definition and Background

The American Dental Association officially defines water fluoridation as "the adjustment of the natural fluoride concentration of fluoride-deficient water supplies *to the recommended level* for optimal dental health."[1] For all practical purposes, fluoridation can be considered a 20th century adaptation of a naturally occurring process since *virtually all sources of community drinking water in the United States* contain some natural fluoride.[1] Fluoridation is classified as a primary public-health intervention for dental-disease prevention because everyone benefits just by drinking fluoridated water.

Fluoridation can also be thought of as a form of *nutritional supplementation* in which fluoride is added to the drinking water. Nutritional supplementation is frequently used to prevent diseases with the addition of: vitamin C to fruit juices to prevent scurvy; vitamin D to milk and breads to prevent rickets; iodine to table salt to prevent goiter; folic acid to grains, cereals, and pastas to prevent birth defects (including spina bifida); and other vitamins and minerals to breakfast cereals to promote normal growth and development.[2-3]

The treatment of water for public consumption is a primary public-health activity that has been used by public-health agencies to prevent diseases since the 1840s. Water treatment prevents diseases such as: amoebic dysentery, cholera, enteropathogenic diarrhea (*E. coli*), giardiasis, hepatitis A, leptospirosis, paratyphoid fever, schistosomiasis, typhoid fever, and many other diseases including dental caries.[2-3]

Fluoridation is an example of an ideal public-health intervention in that: (a) it is socially equitable and *does not discriminate* against any group; (b) consumers receive *continuous protection* with no conscious effort on their part to participate when they drink optimally fluoridated water; (c) it works without requiring individuals to gather in a central location as with other disease-prevention programs, such as immunizations; (d) it does *not require the costly services of health professionals* to deliver; (e) there are *no daily-dosage schedules* to remember; (f) there are no bad-tasting oral medications to be taken; and (g) *no painful inoculations* have to be endured in order to receive the benefits.[2-3]

Extensive scientific documentation over the past half-century, including several comprehensive reviews has established and consistently reaffirmed the *safety and efficacy* of community-water fluoridation. Based on the preponderance of scientific evidence, every U.S. Surgeon General since 1950 has advocated the adoption of water fluoridation by communities. Dr. Luther Terry, U.S. Surgeon General, 1961 to 1965, described water fluoridation as one of the four great advances in public health, calling it one of the *"four horsemen of public health,"* along with *chlorination, pasteurization,* and *immunization.* Dr. C Everett Koop, U.S. Surgeon General, 1981 to 1989 stated the following: "Fluoridation is the single most important commitment that a community can make to the oral health of its children and to future generations."[4] In 1992, Dr. Antonia Novello, the U.S. Surgeon General at that time, stated that "the optimum standard for the success of any prevention strategy should be measured by its ability to *prevent or minimize disease, ease of implementation, high benefit-to-cost ratio,* and *safety.* Community water fluoridation to prevent

tooth decay clearly meets this standard."[5] Most recently, U.S. Surgeon General David Satcher stated: "community water fluoridation remains one of the great achievements of public health in the twentieth century" and "an inexpensive means of improving oral health that *benefits all residents* of a community, young and old, rich and poor alike."[6] In the first-ever report released in May 2000, on oral health in the United States, "Oral Health in America: A Report of the Surgeon General," Dr. Satcher noted that ". . . . one of my highest priorities as Surgeon General is *reducing the disparities in health* that persist among our various populations. Fluoridation holds great potential to contribute toward elimination of these disparities."[7]

Fluoridation is a population-based method of primary prevention designed to serve as the *cornerstone* for the prevention of dental caries, one of the most prevalent childhood diseases. It was initiated on *January 25, 1945* when Grand Rapids, Michigan fluoridated its public-water supply. Since then, more than 14,300 community-water systems serving nearly 10,500 American communities have fluoridated their water systems.[8] This includes *47 of the 50 largest U S. cities* where fluoridation is either actively practiced or where it is in the process of being implemented following approval by governmental/legislative bodies or voters. See companion website table.[a]

## History of Community Water Fluoridation

The history of community water fluoridation in the United States can be traced back to the early years of the 20th century and may be categorized into four separate periods or phases.[3,9–12] The *four* periods are: (1) clinical discovery phase; (2) epidemiological phase; (3) demonstration phase; and (4) technology transfer phase.

The first period, the *clinical discovery phase*, 1901 to 1933, was characterized by the pursuit of knowledge relative to the cause of developmental enamel defects present in dental enamel of people living in certain western areas of the United States. *Dr. Frederick McKay*, a Colorado Springs, Colorado, dentist, noticed that some of his patients presented with an enamel defect that occurred during tooth formation and appeared to be undermineralized or *hypomineralized*.[13] Local dental practitioners noted that the defects, which became known by local residents as *"Colorado Brown Stain,"* varied in degree of *hypomineralization* of the teeth with the most severe form consisting of a brown stain and pitting (*mottling*) of the enamel.[13] Dr. McKay notified the dental profession about his findings through publication of his observations in *Dental Cosmos*, the premier national dental journal of the times. After reporting his findings, Dr. McKay sought the consultation of Dr. G. V. Black, a noted researcher, and subsequently began to examine children in various nearby communities in order to determine the extent of the condition in the population. Not only was McKay able to demonstrate that what he now termed "mottled enamel" was confined to specific geographic areas, but he also hypothesized that it was directly related to *something in* the drinking water in these areas.[3,13]

Around the same time period (early 1930s), *H. V. Churchill*, a *chemist* with the Aluminum Company of America (ALCOA), demonstrated an association between high levels of naturally occurring fluoride in the drinking water and mottled teeth.[13–14] Subsequently, researchers Smith and Smith submitted a report, demonstrating a *causal relationship* between fluoride and mottling which was identified in the scientific literature as *dental fluorosis*.[13–14]

Drs. McKay and Black also observed a corollary finding: *People who had dental fluorosis also experienced less dental decay.* The search for ad-

[a]On Feb. 11, 2003, California's largest water agency— Metro Water District of Sonata, California—approved a measure to add fluoride to its water supply. This involves 26 cities and water districts, the largest being San Diego.

ditional information about the role of fluoride in the cause of dental fluorosis and the prevention of dental caries led to what is known as the second period, the *epidemiological phase* (1933 to 1945). During this phase, *a major epidemiological study*, known as "Dean's 21-City Study," was conducted by *Dr. H. Trendley Dean* with assistance from colleagues at the U. S. Public Health Service's National Institutes of Health. In this study, teams of researchers examined the teeth of children who lived in 21 different communities with varying levels of naturally occurring fluoride in the drinking water.[13–14] Dean and his team documented *the number of carious lesions and fluorosed teeth* observed in each of the 21 communities and *compared the findings with the fluoride concentration* in the respective water supplies. The findings from "Dean's 21-City Study," showed that: (1) the more fluoride in the water, the fewer dental caries in children, constituting an *inverse relationship* between the level of natural fluoride in the water and the prevalence of dental caries; and (2) higher levels of fluoride were associated with fluorosis of the teeth, meaning that there was a *direct relationship* between the level of natural fluoride in the water and the prevalence of dental fluorosis.[13] Dean's

results showed that both a decreased risk of dental caries and a decreased risk of dental fluorosis were attained with water fluoride levels of approximately *1 part per million (ppm) of fluoride.*[13] At this level, substantial reductions (*up to 60%) in dental caries* were exhibited with approximately 10% of the population exhibiting *very mild* dental fluorosis, which the investigators considered to be acceptable and cosmetically inconsequential.[13] The unattractive form of *fluorosis* (often called *mottling*) that was associated with higher levels of fluoride did not occur at the 1 ppm level. Consequently, 1 ppm became the benchmark level used by the U.S. Public Health Service in establishing the optimal range, *0.7 to 1.2 ppm* required to maximize the benefits of dental caries reduction and minimize the risk for dental fluorosis.[15–16] (Optimal levels discussed in subsequent section) (see Figure 8–1, Dean's Index/caries/fluorosis curve).

The third period, known as the *demonstration phase*, began in January 1945, and was characterized by a series of clinical trials that compared the dental and medical results following the deliberate addition of fluoride to the drinking water in four cities.[13–14] These four cities were also paired with four "control cities," in which the same study criteria were

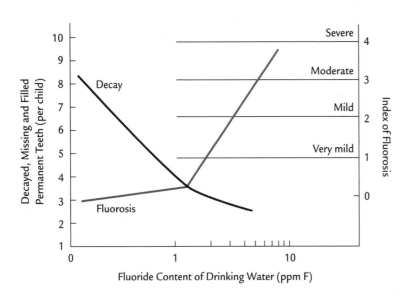

FIGURE 8–1   As the fluoride content of water increases beyond 1 ppm, the index of fluorosis escalates more rapidly than the decayed, missing, filled permanent (DMF) decreases. (From Horowitz HS. *An Update for Dental Practice.* New York: American Academy of Pedodontics, MedCom, Inc., 1976.)

observed in communities with negligible levels of naturally occurring fluoride. Fluoride was added to the public water supply of *Grand Rapids, Michigan,* in order to test the hypothesis that an upward adjustment of the natural fluoride level to a concentration of 1.0 ppm would prevent dental caries in the population. Grand Rapids was the *first city* in the world to fluoridate its drinking water as a dental health promotion/disease prevention measure; after *13 to 14 years, a 55% reduction* in the rates of decayed, missing, and filled teeth (dmft) for children 12 to 14 years of age was observed. Three other experimental cities, Evanston, Illinois; Newburgh, New York; and Brantford, Ontario participated in similar controlled fluoridation studies, achieving similar reductions in dental caries rates (48 to 70%) after 13 to 15 years[7,13–14] (Table 8–1, Demonstration Phase).

The *demonstration phase* lasted until about 1954 when the benefits of the optimal adjustment of fluoride levels in drinking water became so apparent that many U.S. cities began fluoridation programs for their citizens. Thus the *demonstration phase* overlapped slightly with the fourth period in the history of community water fluoridation, the *technology transfer phase*.

The *technology transfer phase* began about 1950 when planning for the implementation of fluoridation began in earnest in many large U.S. Cities. Continuing to this day, the technology transfer phase is characterized by the establishment of a set of national health goals, which includes fluoridation. The **Year 2010 Health Objectives for the Nation** call for the implementation of water fluoridation in *all American communities that have communal water sources where implementation is technologically feasible. The target goal for fluoridation is: 75% of the population on community-water systems should live in communities with fluoridated water by the year 2010.*[17]

In 1992, when the last *Fluoridation Census* was published, approximately *135 million Americans* were consuming fluoridated water while an *additional 10 million* were drinking water with optimal levels of *naturally occurring fluoride,* equating to 57% of the entire population or 62% of those who are served by *centralized piped-water systems.*[7–8] (see Table 8–2.) As of 2000, the percentage of the population receiving optimally fluoridated water through public water systems has risen to 65.8% and 26 states achieved the Healthy People 2000 goal of 75% of the population served by community water fluoridation[8] (see Figure 8–2). From 1992 to 2000, 28 cities adopted fluoridation, with an estimated 8,295,552 million people added to the Fluoridation Census.[18] In the *November 2000* presidential election, 23 U.S cities/counties voted on fluoridation ordinances/as either referenda or initiatives.[19] Of the 23 cities, 9

### TABLE 8-1  Classic Fluoridation Studies

| Demonstration Phase | | |
| --- | --- | --- |
| Fluoridated Cities | Year | Percent Decrease In DMF Teeth Per Child Since Implementing Water Fluoridation |
| Grand Rapids, Michigan | 1959 | 55.5% |
| Newburgh, New York | 1960 | 70.1% |
| Evanston, Illinois | 1959 | 48.4% |
| Brantford, Ontario | 1959 | 56.7% |

*Note:* All four communities began fluoridating in 1945–1946.

*Sources:* Ripa and Clark, *Primary Preventive Dentistry,* 5th edition, Chapter 8; 1999; Burt/Eklund, Dentistry, *Dental Practice and the Community,* 4th edition, 1992

TABLE 8-2  U.S. Population Served by Waterborne Fluoride Fluoridation Census, 1992*

| Fluoridation Type | U.S. Population | Number of Water Systems | Number of Communities |
|---|---|---|---|
| Adjusted | 134.6 million | 10,567 | 8,572 |
| Natural | 10.0 million | 3,784 | 1,924 |
| Total | 144.6 million | 14,351 | 10,496 |

* = Fluoridation Census has not been published since 1992

*Source:* Oral Health in America: A Report of the Surgeon General, Dept of HHS/NIDCR, NIH Pub # 00-4713, Sept 2000).

cities with a total population of *3,957,079 approved fluoridation* while 14 cities with a total population of *366,347 rejected fluoridation* at the polls. While the actual numbers of cities rejecting fluoridation exceeded those approving the measure during this election, the population voting to benefit from fluoridation exceeded the population denying themselves the benefits by ten-fold.

The *technology transfer phase* has extended fluoridation *worldwide*, with Singapore implementing fluoridation in 1958, serving 100% of the population.[20] The Republic of Ireland became the first country to actually legislate

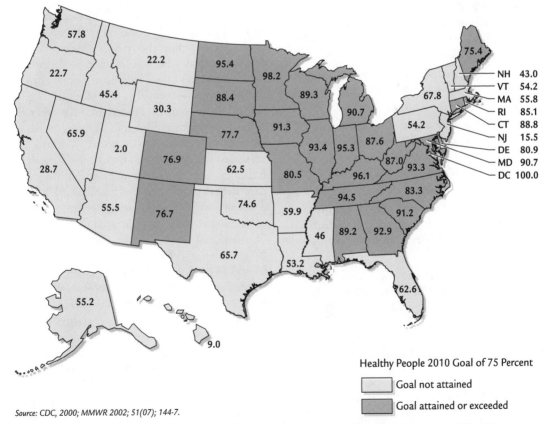

NH   43.0
VT   54.2
MA   55.8
RI   85.1
CT   88.8
NJ   15.5
DE   80.9
MD   90.7
DC  100.0

Healthy People 2010 Goal of 75 Percent

☐ Goal not attained

■ Goal attained or exceeded

*Source: CDC, 2000; MMWR 2002; 51(07); 144-7.*

FIGURE 8-2   Percentage of U.S. Population by State Served by Fluoridated Public Water Supply, 2000. (*Source:* CDC, 2000; *MMWR 2002;* 51(07); 144-7.)

mandatory nationwide fluoridation in 1960. Israel initiated its mandatory universal fluoridation program in 1981. Currently, a national fluoridation effort is underway in Chile in conjunction with the Pan American Health Organization. Advocated by the World Health Organization, fluoridation benefits over 360 million people in 60 countries worldwide.[1,21]

Because of its 56-year history of effectiveness in reducing the prevalence of dental caries in the United States, water fluoridation was recently cited as one of the top-10 public-health achievements of the 20th century by the U. S. Centers for Disease Control and Prevention.[22]

---

### Question 1

Which if any of the following statements, is/are correct?

A. Virtually all sources of water for community water systems in the United States contain some natural fluoride.

B. Fluoridation does not involve adding anything to the water supply that is not already there.

C. The history of the water fluoridation story in the United States began with the investigation of "Colorado brown stain" by Dr. Frederick McKay and Dr. G. V. Black

D. H. Trendley Dean of the U.S. Public Health Service established the relationship between fluoride and dental fluorosis.

E. The optimal concentration of fluoride in drinking water for dental therapeutic purposes, is between 2.0 and 4.0 ppm.

---

### Benefits and Efficacy/Effectiveness of Fluoridation

Over the past 56 years, numerous studies have been conducted on the *effectiveness of fluorides* and fluoridation in *preventing dental caries and*

*decreasing caries rates.* When Grand Rapids, Michigan, decided to fluoridate its water supply in 1945, a long-term study of schoolchildren was initiated to determine the effectiveness of fluoridation in decreasing dental caries rates; the study found that after 11 years of fluoridation, dental caries rates declined by 50 to 63%.[1,13,23] Corroborative studies in the same era conducted in New York (Newburgh-Kingston) and Illinois (Evanston-Oak Park) reported reductions in caries rates from 57 to 70%.[1,13] "Of 73 studies published between 1956 and 1979, the most frequently reported caries reduction was 50 to 60% and it was generally acknowledged that fluoridating a community's water supply would *reduce dental decay by half.*"[13]

While children and adolescents are the major beneficiaries of fluoridation, adults can also benefit. The impact of fluoride on the teeth of adults has become more important as adults are retaining their teeth longer than in previous decades because of improved dental-health practices and availability of preventive interventions, especially fluoridation. With aging, teeth remain susceptible to coronal caries, and more of the root surfaces become exposed to the oral environment, resulting in increased susceptibility to root caries. Research indicates that "*root caries* manifests as a significant dental problem as early as ages 35 to 44, doubling in the 45- to 54-year age group, and redoubling in the 55- to 66-year group."[13,24] Results of a national survey of root caries found that 67% of men and 61% of women between ages 65 and 84+ had root-surface lesions.[13,25]

Studies in adults have consistently reported less coronal and root caries in the teeth of adults residing in communities with higher levels of water-borne fluoride.[9] Results of one study of young adults aged 20 to 34 years, showed 25% less coronal caries (decayed, filled surfaces) in those who resided in fluoridated (adjusted or natural) communities compared with those who had no exposure to fluoridated water.[13,26] Similar findings were noted in a

study of older adults, mean ages 40 and 43 where residents of communities with 1.6 ppm fluoride in the water had 28% fewer coronal caries and 17% fewer root caries than residents of communities with 0.2 ppm fluoride.[13,24] Newbrun has estimated that the reduction in caries attributable to water fluoridation for adults, *aged 20 to 44*, is between *20 to 30%* for *coronal caries* and 20 to 40% for *root caries*.[13,27]

During the early periods of fluoridation, the primary source of fluoride was the drinking water; consequently, the reductions in dental caries rates attributed to water fluoridation were significant. Decades later, an epidemiological study of more than 39,000 children aged 5 thru 17 years was conducted in 1986/1987 by the National Institute of Dental Research (NIDR).[13,28,29] This study determined that younger children who had lived all their lives in optimally fluoridated communities experienced 39% fewer carious lesions and fillings when compared with those children who had lived in communities that were not fluoridated.[13,28,29] Other reports showed similar levels of reduction in decay rates.

In 1992, Newbrun estimated that fluoridation prevents *30 to 39%* of dental caries in the *primary* dentition, 11 to 38% in the *mixed* dentition, and 35% in the *permanent* dentition.[27] The decline in percentages of caries reduction has been found in both fluoridated and nonfluoridated communities, with children who had always been exposed to community water fluoridation demonstrating mean DMFS scores ranging from 18 to 40% lower than those who had never lived in fluoridated communities.[18,27,30,31] Water fluoridation has played a dominant role in the decline in caries even though the absolute differences in caries prevalence that once were observed between fluoridated and nonfluoridated communities appears to be diminishing.[28] The recently released York review (published in 2000) of 26 studies on fluoridation effectiveness, found that fluoridation of drinking water supplies reduces caries prevalence in variable ranges with a median of

14.6% reduction in rates as measured by the change in dmft/DMFT scores and the proportion of caries-free children.[32] The report also attempted to address the *impact of fluoride-containing toothpaste* on the effectiveness of fluoridation.[33] The authors of the review acknowledged that the effectiveness estimates could be biased because of inadequate adjustment for the impact of potential confounding variables.[32] Dental scientists contend that the failure to adjust for confounding variables in the review made it difficult to interpret the findings. The use of a median range of reduction in caries by the authors was considered misleading and inappropriate for establishing fluoridation effectiveness. Nonetheless, it is clear from studies cited previously that there has been a worldwide decline in dental-caries rates even though certain population groups are still disproportionately affected by dental caries. The decline in dental-caries rates has been attributed to the widespread use of multiple fluorides from various sources: community *water supplies*, *supplements*, *fluoride rinses gels*, and *varnishes*, and *dentifrices*.[13,34–36]

The reduction in the absolute measurable benefits of water fluoridation has been attributed to the *dilution* and *diffusion* effects.[13] *Dilution* results from the increased availability of fluoride from multiple sources, *diluting the impact of any one source of fluoride,* including water.[9,29,36–37] According to Ripa, *"dilution is the apparent reduction in the measurable water fluoridation benefits resulting from the ubiquitous availability of fluoride from other sources in both the fluoridated and the fluoride deficient comparison community."*[13] Today, the most universally available source of fluoride in the United States is fluoride-containing dentifrice (toothpaste).[13,35] All *fluoride-containing dentifrices* have *very high levels of fluoride (1,100 to 1,500 ppm)* and are a significant source of fluoride overexposure and fluorosis. Moreover, they are not meant to be swallowed, especially during the years when the crowns of teeth are forming. Nearly four decades ago, the American Dental

Association (ADA) gave its seal of approval to Crest toothpaste, the only fluoride dentifrice available at that time. However, by 1980, 98% of the available dentifrices contained fluoride.[13,38]

In separate studies, Brunelle and Carlos in 1990 and Murray in 1992 found greater percentages of caries-free children and lower caries-prevalence rates in fluoridated communities where other sources of fluoride were also available. After adjusting for other sources of fluoride, they found a 25% difference in dental-caries prevalence. The findings of these two studies led the researchers to conclude that *water fluoridation remains an important contributor* to caries prevention.[9,29]

The other major modifying factor regarding the effectiveness of fluoridation, the *diffusion* effect, results from the consumption of commercial foods and beverages that were processed in a fluoridated community and transported to fluoride-deficient communities,[13,39] making fluoride available to consumers in the fluoride-deficient community.[13,39] Ripa described *diffusion* as *"the extension of benefits of community water fluoridation to residents of fluoride-deficient communities."*[13] *Diffusion* has also been called the *"halo effect."* The differences in caries prevalence rates between fluoridated and nonfluoridated communities are diminishing.[13,40] According to Ripa, "the weaker association reported by contemporary studies between exposure to fluoridated drinking water and caries experience, therefore, is not due to a lessening of the effects of waterborne fluoride, but is actually caused by the extension of those effects, through a process of 'diffusion,' of fluoride into fluoride-deficient areas."[13] Increased traveling to fluoridated communities impacts the effect of diffusion as well. Also, residents who live in a fluoride-deficient community and work on a *military base* in the same community may be exposed to fluoridated water since most military bases are fluoridated.

As described above, the decline in dental-caries rates was greatest (up to 65 to 70%) in the earlier years (1940s, 1950s, 1960s) of fluo-

ridation when water was the primary source of fluoride and the availability of other sources of fluoride was limited. The caries-inhibition effectiveness of fluoride in water resulted in a parallel rush to develop other sources of fluorides: (1) adjunctive *systemic fluorides*, such as tablets, drops, lozenges, and vitamins with fluoride, which are meant to be swallowed and are prescription items intended to be dispensed to the public by licensed health professionals; and (2) topical fluorides, which are intended only for topical application and are not meant to be swallowed.[13,34] Some *topical fluorides* are used by professionals in the dental office while others are used in public-health programs and in schools. Additionally, over-the-counter (OTC) products are used by consumers.[13,34] As more cities adopted fluoridation and the ingestion of dietary fluoride supplements increased in fluoride-deficient communities, consumer use of fluoride-containing products such as toothpastes, mouthrinses, and gels also increased. As a result, exposure to fluoride from numerous sources has become more widespread, with benefits accruing at varying levels. At the same time, it is becoming more *difficult to accurately determine the level of reduction* in caries rates attributed to fluoridated water alone versus other sources. Most researchers now believe that the *"dilution"* and *"diffusion"* effects are responsible for the decline in dental caries rates in nonfluoridated, and to a lesser degree, in fluoridated communities.[9]

## Mechanisms of Action

Systemic fluorides are beneficial in decay prevention in that they are ingested and incorporated directly into the hydroxyapatite crystalline structure of the developing tooth. The smaller fluoride ions replace hydroxyl ions in the crystalline structure of the tooth, producing a less-soluble apatite crystal[13,41] Over the past several decades, the caries-preventive properties of fluoride have been attributed primarily

to its *pre-eruptive effects* on the developing teeth. But systemic fluorides also provide a topical effect resulting in marked *post-eruptive benefits*. Saliva, which contains fluoride from ingestion, is continually available at the tooth surface and becomes concentrated in dental plaque where it inhibits acid-producing cariogenic bacteria from demineralized tooth enamel. Fluoride accomplishes this by interfering with the enzymatic activity of the bacteria and by controlling intracellular pH, thus reducing bacterial acid production and thereby reducing dissolution of tooth enamel.[1,22,42–48] According to Bowen, fluoride concentration in the plaque is 50 to 100 times higher than in the whole saliva.[13,49]

Fluoride also interacts with calcium and phosphate ions from saliva and adsorbs to the tooth surface, thereby enhancing remineralization.[50] Recent research shows that remineralization represents the primary mechanism by which fluoride works, occurring after tooth eruption, and making the topical effect important in caries reduction for people of all ages.

In summary, systemic fluoride has been found to reduce dental decay by three mechanisms: (1) the conversion of hydroxyapatite into fluorapatite which reduces the solubility of tooth enamel in acid and makes it more resistant to decay; (2) reduction of acid production by dental-plaque organisms; and (3) the remineralization of tooth enamel that has been demineralized by acids produced by decay causing bacteria.[1]

---

**Question 2**

Which of the following statements, if any, is/are correct?

A. Fluoridation prevents an estimated 20 to 30% of coronal caries in adults and an estimated 20 to 40% of root caries.

B. *Dilution* is the "apparent reduction in measurable water fluoridation benefits resulting from the ubiquitous availabil-

ity of fluoride from other sources" such as fluoride-containing dentifrice, fluoride mouthrinses, and professionally-applied topical fluorides.

C. *Diffusion* is the "extension of the benefits of community water fluoridation to residents of fluoride-deficient communities" such as occurs when residents of nonfluoridated communities work in fluoridated communities, when, children from nonfluoridated communities attend school in fluoridated communities, and when people from nonfluoridated communities consume certain foods processed in fluoridated communities.

D. All fluoride-containing dentifrices have very low levels of fluoride and do not contribute to fluoride overexposure and fluorosis.

E. Fluoride reduces (1) acid production in the plaque which (2) reduces the amount of demineralization, which (3) allows the tooth to more easily "repair" itself by remineralization.

---

### Dental Fluorosis

Dental fluorosis has been described as a series of conditions occurring in those teeth that have been exposed to excessive sources of fluoride ingested during enamel formation. Dental fluorosis can present in a number of ways, from a barely discernable white lacy appearance to a more severe form that could be classified as a developmental defect of the enamel.[13] Fluorosis, regardless of severity, *cannot occur once enamel formation is complete and the teeth have erupted; therefore older children and adults are not at risk for dental fluorosis*.[1,51–52] Dental fluorosis occurs when children consume excessive levels of fluoride in various ways, such as when drinking water from private wells or community-water systems with higher-than-optimum levels of naturally occurring fluoride. However, the

greatest likelihood of exposure to excess fluoride in children results from: (1) *inadvertent ingestion of toothpaste* containing very high concentrations of fluoride and (2) taking of inappropriately prescribed dietary fluoride supplements.[1,53] The degree of fluorosis depends on the total dose of fluoride, as well as on the timing and duration of fluoride exposure.[54]

In 1942, H. Trendley Dean developed a *system of classification for dental fluorosis.* He established a series of categories that ranged from questionable (white flecks or spots or "snow-capping"), to very mild (small opaque paper-white areas or streaks known as veining, covering less than 25% of the tooth surface, to mild (opaque white areas covering less than 25% of the tooth surface), to moderate (marked wear on occlusal/incisal surfaces, may include brown stains), to severe (mottling and brown staining affecting all tooth surfaces).[13] Dean's fluorosis index continues to be widely used today.[1,55] However, not all enamel opacities are caused by fluorosis; some are caused by other chemical agents such as *strontium* or pharmaceutical agents such as *tetracycline*. Idiopathic opacities also exist for which the cause(s) is/are currently unknown.[13,56] According to a survey conducted by the National Institute of Dental Research in 1986 to 1987, the majority of fluorosis cases identified *were classified as being very mild or mild.* The minor forms of fluorosis (questionable, very mild, or mild fluorosis) are not considered to be abnormal, nor are they considered to constitute an adverse health effect. However, both researchers and practitioners should continue to monitor and assess the risk of dental fluorosis in order to ensure that the more severe forms of fluorosis do not occur. In 1936, Trendley Dean estimated that approximately *10%* of children who drank optimally fluoridated water would develop *very mild dental fluorosis*.[57] More recent studies have shown that dental fluorosis attributed to fluoridation is around *13%*.[1,58]

As previously mentioned, questionable, very mild, and mild fluorosis usually result from very

young children swallowing too much fluoride-containing toothpaste or from the inappropriate supplementation with prescription fluoride products such as (1) when physicians and dentists independently prescribe fluoride supplements, or (2) when physicians and dentists prescribe fluoride supplements without checking the fluoride content of the child's water supply so that, in either case, a child gets a "double" dose of fluoride on a daily basis. Monitoring total fluoride intake is complicated considering the availability of multiple sources of fluoride. Also, fluoride from tablets/drops is ingested and absorbed at one time of day as opposed to fluoride in water where the ingestion and absorption of low-dose fluoride is distributed throughout the day. These factors have been considered in the establishment of fluoride dosage schedules where in recent years, the dosages have been lowered, particularly in the first 6 months of life. The *Dietary Fluoride Supplement Schedule* approved by the American Dental Association, the American Academy of Pediatrics, and the American Academy of Pediatric Dentistry should be followed when prescribing fluoride supplements[7] (see Table 8–3, fluoride supplements). Fluoride ingestion should be reduced during the ages of tooth development, particularly under the age of three. Parents need to assist in attainment of this goal *by supervising small children* during toothbrushing to ensure that their children do not swallow the toothpaste.

Antifluoridation groups frequently and inappropriately exhibit photographs of children and/or adults having severe *fluorosis* in which pitting or mottling of the enamel and brown stains are evident and attribute these manifestations directly to water fluoridation, often describing dental fluorosis as a major risk factor for people of all ages. In making dental-health decisions, patients depend upon the dental professional team to assist them in evaluating the risks versus the benefits of a given procedure or public health measure. To do this, dentists and dental hygienists need to stay current regarding

TABLE 8-3 **Dietary Fluoride Supplement Schedule, 1994**

| Age | Fluoride ion level in drinking water (ppm)[*] | | |
|---|---|---|---|
|  | <0.3 ppm | 0.3–0.6 ppm | >0.6 ppm |
| Birth–6 months | None | None | None |
| 6 months–3 years | 0.25 mg/day[**] | None | None |
| 3–6 years | 0.50 mg/day | 0.25 mg/day | None |
| 6–16 years | 1.0 mg/day | .50 mg/day | None |

[*] 1.0 part per million (ppm)= 1 milligram/liter (mg/L)
[**] 2.2 mg sodium fluoride contains 1 mg fluoride ion.

*Source:* Fluoridation Facts, American Dental Association, 1999.

the scientific literature and to use this knowledge as a basis for educating themselves and their patients. The risk of developing *very mild fluorosis versus* the benefit of decreased dental caries and attendant treatment costs should be communicated to patients who express concern.

### Discontinuation of Water Fluoridation

Opposition to fluoridation, as well as governmental action, has resulted in the discontinuance of this public-health measure in various locales. Interestingly enough, the *cessation* or *discontinuation* of fluoridation has resulted in the implementation of several studies to determine the impact of such reversals on dental health. Results have consistently shown that dental-caries rates *increase dramatically* when fluoridation is discontinued. In 1960, the city of Antigo, Wisconsin, discontinued fluoridation after having fluoridation for 11 years. Six years later, when Antigo elementary school children were found to have substantial increases in caries rates, ranging from *41 to 70 percent, fluoridation was reinstated.*[13,59] Similar findings occurred in Scotland upon cessation of fluoridation where in the town of Wick, caries rates increased by *40% in primary teeth and by 27% in permanent teeth.* This dramatic increase in dental-caries rates occurred *despite* fluoride toothpaste being readily available and na-

tional-caries rates in Scotland continuing to decline.[13,60] Moreover, 5 years after fluoridation was discontinued in the town of Stranraer, caries rates increased to levels approaching those found in the nonfluoridated town of Annan. In Stranraer, restorative dental treatment costs for decay alone rose by *115%.*[1,13,61]

Similar results can occur if a city changes its water source from one that is optimally fluoridated to one that is fluoride-deficient. The impact would be equivalent to discontinuation of fluoridation. In a Public Health Service Report on risks and benefits of fluoride, it stated that "one way to demonstrate the effectiveness of a therapeutic agent, such as fluoride, is to observe if the benefits are lost when the agent is removed."[13,62] Clearly, these studies serve to demonstrate that the discontinuation of community water fluoridation has resulted in the significant loss of dental caries preventive benefits.[1,63]

### Cost of Water Fluoridation

Water fluoridation provides significant cost savings for a community and has been described as "one of the most cost-effective preventive dental programs available."[13,64] Estimates of the cost of water fluoridation will vary depending upon the factors included in the calculations.[13,65] The size and complexity of the water system, including the number of systems,

the number of wells, whether or not the systems use a dry feeder or solution (wet) feeder system, purchase of equipment and installation, purchase of fluoride, labor, and maintenance, as well as the number of service connections and size of the population all factor into the cost of fluoridation.[13,64–66]

*"The cost of water fluoridation is usually expressed as the annual cost per person of the population being served."*[13] An inverse relationship exists between the cost per person and the population of a community. Consequently, the cost per person is lower in larger communities and higher in smaller communities where the actual cost of fluoridation may approach that of other methods of caries prevention.[65] Fluoridation also eliminates or diminishes additional costs incurred through other forms of fluoride administration, such as costs incurred when accessing professionals in order to obtain provider-prescribed fluoride products, compliance irregularities, and the lower effectiveness of other forms of fluoride distribution. Fluoridation is the most cost-efficient and cost-effective method of dental caries prevention for almost all communities[7] (see Table 8–4, cost/benefit).

Another way to look at cost-saving benefits is to determine the beneficiaries of dental-treatment cost savings. Employers who pay prepaid dental-care fringe benefits for their employees save on costs. Hidden production or service costs caused by dentally-related missed workdays by employees are also minimized through fluoridation. Taxpayers who support public programs would also benefit from dental-treatment cost savings. In fact, skyrocketing dental Medicaid expenditures in California (a state with a low percentage of the population having access to fluoridation) provided the impetus for the enactment of a statewide mandatory fluoridation bill there in 1995.[67–68] As will be discussed later, recent studies comparing dental Medicaid expenditures in Louisiana and Texas also demonstrated that treatment costs were significantly higher in nonfluoridated

communities than they were in fluoridated communities. Patients can also be expected to benefit from lower health-care bills, lower dental-care costs, and lower insurance premiums because of lower costs incurred by providers for uncompensated care.[2]

With the availability of baseline levels of dental-caries rates and treatment costs, two different types of analyses can be done to determine (1) the *effectiveness* of fluoridation as a *dental-caries preventive measure (cost-effectiveness analysis)* as well as (2) associated cost savings (a *cost-benefit analysis.*)[13] Ripa has stated that "the *greater the initial caries prevalence* and treatment costs, the *greater the potential benefits* to be realized by the introduction of fluoridation."[13] The national average recurring cost of water fluoridation has been estimated at $0.50 per person per year while the national average cost of one simple restoration is $62.[7,66] If one were to multiply the approximate average life expectancy of a U.S. resident (75 years) by the annual per capita cost of fluoridation ($0.50), it appears evident that the $37.50 total for a *lifetime of protection* through fluoridation would more than offset the cost of just one simple restoration for one tooth.[3,13,69] Additionally, for every carious lesion initially prevented, the need for repeated restorations and treatment of *recurrent* carious lesions is reduced over a lifetime.[13,70] Different studies have shown that the replacement rates for amalgam restorations caused by recurrent decay varies between 38 and 50%; the savings to be realized from prevention are substantial.[13,71,72] The national average benefit-to-cost ratio for fluoridation is: 80:1; (MMWR/CDC) on average, *for every $1 dollar spent on fluoridation, $80 is saved in treatment costs.*[3,66]

Three recent studies further demonstrate the substantial cost-benefits generated through community water fluoridation. Brown and colleagues, in a comprehensive study for the Texas Department of Health were able to demonstrate cost-savings for the publicly funded Texas Health Steps Program (Texas EPSDT-Medicaid Program) when comparing program costs for

TABLE 8-4 Estimated Annual Per Capita Costs & Effectiveness For Community Level Fluoride-Based Dental Caries Prevention Modalities

| Method | Cost ($) | | Range/% Reduction in Dental Caries | Beneficiaries |
|---|---|---|---|---|
| | Range | Mean | | |
| **Community-Based** | | | | |
| Community Water Fluoridation | | | 30–39%/primary dentition[*] | All Ages |
| | | | 11–38%/mixed dentition[*] | |
| | | | 35% permanent dentition[*] | |
| <10,000 persons (small systems) | 0.60–5.42 | $3.00 | | All Ages |
| 10,000 – 50,000 persons (medium systems) | 0.18–0.75 | $0.98 | | All Ages |
| >50,000 persons (large systems) | 0.12–0.21 | $0.68 | | All Ages |
| *National weighted average* | | $0.50 | | All Ages |
| School Based | | | | |
| Fluoride Supplements | 0.81–5.40 | $2.53 | 20–28% | School Children[**] |
| School-Based Fluoride Mouthrinse | 0.52–1.78 | $1.00 | 20–50% (5–18yrs)[***] | School Children |

*Source:* Benefits and Risks. Department of Health and Human Services Report of the AD Hoc Subcommittee on Fluoride. PHS February 1991; Burt B. J Public Health Dent, 1989, and SG Report/Garcia

[*] Newbrun, E. Effectiveness of water fluoridation. J. Public Health Dent 1989; 49 (5 Spec No):279–89.

[**] Most community supplement programs are school-based; implementation dependent upon nurses and/or teacher willingness and availability. (*Oral Health in America: A Report of the Surgeon General*, Dept of HHS/NIDCR, NIH Pub # 00-4713, Sept 2000)

[***] While recommended for school children, 5–18 years, implementation beyond the elementary school grades may be rare as older children may be reluctant to participate. *Oral Health in America: A Report of the Surgeon General*, Dept of HHS/NIDCR, NIH Pub # 00-4713, Sept 2000)

clients from fluoridated communities with those from non-fluoridated communities.[73] Similarly, Barsley and colleagues were able to demonstrate that the costs for hospital-based treatment of acute dental conditions to Louisiana's publicly funded Medicaid Program were much less for residents of fluoridated communities than for residents of nonfluoridated communities.[74,75] Finally, Wright and colleagues established conclusively that fluoridation remains an extremely cost-effective public-health program in New Zealand in their comprehensive 1999 report for the New Zealand Ministry of Health.[76]

---

### Question 3

Which of the following statements, if any is/are correct?

A. Dental fluorosis occurs when an excessive amount of fluoride is ingested during the period of enamel formation *only*.

B. Dental fluorosis does not occur once enamel formation is complete and the teeth have erupted, therefore older children and adults are not at risk for dental fluorosis.

C. Discontinuation of fluoridation has no impact on dental caries rates.

D. The national cost-benefit ratio attributed to water fluoridation is 95:1.

E. The national average cost to fluoridate a public water system in the U.S. is approximately $0.50 per person per year.

---

### Optimal Fluoride Levels

The U.S. Public Health Service established an optimal standard for fluoride in the drinking water in the United States based upon the *annual average of maximum daily air temperature*. As a result, the optimal level is actually a range, 0.7 to 1.2 ppm (see Table 8–5, optimal levels), which assumes greater water consumption in hotter climates and less water consump-

**TABLE 8–5  Recommended Optimal Fluoride Level**

| Annual Average of Maximum Daily Air Temperature (°F)[a] | Optimal Fluoride Level (ppm) |
|---|---|
| 40.0–53.7 | 1.2 |
| 53.8–58.3 | 1.1 |
| 58.4–63.8 | 1.0 |
| 63.9–70.6 | 0.9 |
| 70.7–79.2 | 0.8 |
| 79.3–90.5 | 0.7 |

[a]Based on average annual temperature over a minimum of 5 years.

*Source:* Centers for Disease Control, National Center for Prevention Services. Dental Disease Prevention Activity, 1991.

tion in colder climates.[14] Consequently, *the higher the average temperature in a community, the lower the recommended water fluoride level.*

However, determining daily fluoride intake is impacted by other factors such as consumer use of home distillation and reverse-osmosis water-treatment systems which can remove significant amounts of fluoride from the water supply.[13,77–80] The consumption of bottled water and other beverages, such as soft drinks and fruit juices, complicate the matter since fluoride levels in these beverages varies greatly.[13,78,80–81] Additionally, determination of fluoride intake may be altered by the widespread use of air conditioning in homes, automobiles, and workplaces such that some people from warmer climates no longer require the higher volumes of liquid. For these reasons, Burt has cautioned that temperature guidelines used in establishing the optimal range need to be periodically monitored in order to determine the need for revision.[14] Hong Kong has adjusted its water fluoride level since initiating fluoridation to achieve its goal of maximizing the benefits of caries reduction while minimizing the risk of fluorosis in an environment of

increased fluoride exposure.[82] In a 1994 report issued by the World Health Organization, it was recommended that some regions, especially tropical and subtropical areas, revise the optimal range to establish appropriate higher and lower limits.[82]

## Safety of Water Fluoridation

The issue of safety relative to adding fluoride to the water supply has often been raised in fluoridation campaigns by opponents who attribute nearly every disease known to mankind to fluoridation. It is common practice for fluoridation opponents to distribute pictures of children alleged to have crippling skeletal fluorosis and attribute the malady to fluoridation. Skeletal fluorosis occurs in India and other areas that have *extremely high natural fluoride levels*, ranging *from 20 to 80 ppm*.[83] Decades ago, five documented cases of skeletal fluorosis were found in the United States, (in rural areas with well water in which the natural fluoride level was found to be very high).[1,83] At the time, public health authorities resolved the problem by installing *defluoridation* equipment and since then, there has not been a documented case of skeletal fluorosis in the United States other than about 25 cases occurring from occupational exposures.[1] Because of fluoride's affinity for bones and teeth, its impact on bone health is often called into question by anti-fluoridationists. By implementing water fluoridation at the recommended level (0.7 to 1.2 ppm), there is no evidence of anyone developing skeletal fluorosis.[1] Currently, in the United States, naturally occurring fluoride levels vary widely from less than 0.1 ppm to greater than 13 ppm. The variation in fluoride levels in public water systems is amenable to adjustment: (a) upward to achieve dentally therapeutic levels in community water supplies that are fluoride deficient through fluoridation or (b) downward to attain the maximum concentration of fluoride allowable by *defluoridation*.[13] However, instances of *defluoridation* are rare (discussed in later section).

In general, safety concerns about fluoridation relate to a number of factors, including: toxicity of fluoride, total fluoride intake, fluoride absorption, the impact on human health, the effect on the environment, water quality, and the engineering aspects. Over the past 56 years, numerous studies have been conducted in communities where the natural fluoride level is either higher than or equivalent to the recommended level for dental-caries prevention, as well as in communities where the fluoride level has been adjusted to the optimal level; results have repeatedly and convincingly confirmed the safety of fluoride in the water supply.[84–86]

Since the late 1970s, allegations against fluoridation have focused on cancer. The possibility of a cancer risk associated with fluoridation of public-water supplies was raised in a 1977 self-published paper about 20 U.S. cities.[87–88] The analyses purported to show that fluoridation of drinking water in 10 of the cities caused a 10% increase in cancer mortality in those cities compared with 10 other cities that did not have fluoridation. According to the authors, before fluoridation, the average cancer death rates were increasing in a similar manner in both groups of cities but immediately after the start of fluoridation, the rates diverged with higher cancer mortality rates seen in the fluoridated group vs. the nonfluoridated group.[87–88] The immediate divergence in rates failed to factor in the latency period for cancer (usually over 5 years, and for some cancers, as long as 20 to 30 years).[89–90] Manifestation of a divergence in cancer mortality rates would require 5 to 10 years between exposure and death from cancer. Since the divergence in crude cancer mortality occurred at the exact same time that fluoridation was introduced, it is inaccurate and disingenuous to attribute the divergence to fluoridation.[89–90] Also, average crude death rates were used in the study, ignoring the differences and changes in age, race, and sex composition, widely recognized risk factors known to affect the death rates from specific types of cancer.[89–90] Subsequent analyses of the same set of

data by National Cancer Institute investigators, using internationally accepted epidemiological methods and controlling for confounding variables, concluded that there was *no evidence* that fluoridation caused cancer in the 10 fluoridated cities.[91] Follow-up studies, including studies in populations with high levels of naturally occurring fluoride in water in the U.S. and various other countries also failed to show a positive relationship between fluoridation and cancer.[92-98] Results of studies of fluoridation and cancer were reported by the Royal College of Physicians in Britain in 1976 in which they concluded: "there is no evidence that fluoride increases the incidence or mortality of cancer in any organ." Subsequently, British researchers, Drs. Doll and Kinlen, reported in the *Lancet* that "none of the evidence provided any reason to support that fluoridation is associated with an increase in cancer mortality, let alone causes it."[99]

In 1990 two separate studies by the National Toxicology Program (NTP) of the National Institute of Environmental Health Sciences and Procter and Gamble were conducted to assess the carcinogenicity of sodium fluoride in which rats and mice were deliberately fed excessive amounts of fluoride (75 to 125 ppm). One group, male rats, showed "equivocal" evidence of carcinogenicity, where "equivocal" is defined by the NTP as a marginal increase in osteosarcomas that may be chemically related, but in which there is insufficient evidence to prove or disprove that a relationship exists.[1,100-102] Subsequently, the U.S. Public Health Service established a Subcommittee on Fluoride to review the studies. The Subcommittee on Fluoride determined that the two animal studies failed to establish an association between fluoride and cancer. The NTP Report prompted a comprehensive "Review of fluoride: benefits and risks" by the U.S. Public Health Service in 1991 in which it concluded that fluoride in water is not carcinogenic. Other comprehensive reviews came to the same conclusion.[1,84,86,97,103-104]

Additionally, scientists at the National Cancer Institute examined more than 2.2 million death records and 125,000 cancer case records in counties using fluoridated water and concluded that there was no indication of a cancer risk associated with fluoridated drinking water.[1]

In a report prepared in 1993 by the National Academy of Science, National Research Council at the request of Environmental Protection Agency (EPA), a review of the literature focused on toxicity and health risks of fluoride. This report stated that the "currently allowable fluoride levels in drinking water do not pose a risk for health problems such as cancer, kidney failure or bone disease" and that the EPA's primary standard of 4 ppm for naturally occurring fluoride would provide an adequate margin of safety against adverse health effects.[1,86,105-106]

*The Safe Drinking Water Act*, enacted by Congress in 1986, established *primary* and *secondary standards* for *natural fluoride levels* in public drinking water in the United States. The legislation set the *primary standard* (the maximum concentration of fluoride allowed in public drinking water systems) at *4.0 ppm* and further stated that *natural* water sources exceeding this level *must* be defluoridated,[13,14,107] although no communities have defluoridated under this provision. A *secondary standard* of 2.0 ppm for a *natural* source was also established as the *recommended* maximum. Under this *secondary standard*, when the water exceeds 2.0 ppm, community residents are *informed* of the greater risk for dental fluorosis.[13,107]

Whereas the EPA is responsible for monitoring public-water systems in the United States, it requires that public-water systems not exceed fluoride levels of 4 ppm; public water systems with natural levels exceeding the limit are expected to *defluoridate* in accordance with the primary standard. *Defluoridation* is infrequently implemented in the United States primarily because of the lack of demand on the part of the public living in high natural fluoride areas of the country.[13] *Defluoridation* also has budgetary implications in that the cost of defluoridation

for a community having high natural fluoride levels is approximately *10 times greater* than the cost of fluoridating a water supply in a community with deficient natural fluoride levels.[13] Also, some communities may be forced to find alternative water supplies in the event of forced closure of existing water supplies having natural fluoride levels exceeding the *primary standard*. Finding alternative water supplies poses a major challenge for many communities in the United States. Compliance with EPA standards in geographical areas having high natural fluoride levels may be greatly affected by these factors.[13,14]

When fluoride is ingested, it is rapidly absorbed from the stomach and small intestine into the systemic circulation, where about half becomes bound to the hard tissues (the bones and unerupted teeth) and the rest is eliminated via efficient urinary excretion. Since the major site of fluoride accumulation in the body is the bone, almost no fluoride is present in the soft tissues.[13] As stated by Ripa in the previous edition of this textbook: "fluoride can be deposited in the (1) *adsorbed layer* of the bone, (2) the *crystal structure*, and (3) the *bone matrix*.[13,49,108–109] The fluoride in the adsorbed layer is in equilibrium with the blood and can be rapidly raised or lowered, depending on ingestion patterns and the efficiency of kidney function."[13] It is known that "blood plasma fluoride levels begin to rise about 10 minutes after ingestion and reach *maximal levels within 60 minutes*, subsequently returning to pre-ingestion levels after 11 to 15 hours."[13,110] In crystal formation, the fluoride ion is thought to be involved in an ionic exchange with the hydroxyl ion and is incorporated into the crystals of the bone, where it is more slowly removed, most likely through the osteoclastic action seen in remodeling."[13] Fluoride that is not stored in bone is rapidly excreted through the kidneys, where the rate is highest the first hour, then begins to fall for the next 3 hours, after which there is a low, continuous plateau.[13] With the consumption of fluoridated water, the excretion rate is more constant because of a more continuous intake of fluoride.[13]

Because of the role of the kidneys in fluoride excretion, concerns have been raised by anti-fluoridationists about the safety of fluoridation in patients with impaired kidney function or who have kidney failure requiring dialysis. Impact on kidney function was addressed by the National Research Council in which it concluded that the "ingestion of fluoride at currently recommended concentrations is not likely to produce kidney toxicity in humans."[86] The standard of care relative to the treatment of kidney failure patients on hemodialysis machines who are exposed to large quantities of water, calls for the removal of all minerals, including fluoride, from water used in dialysis.[1,111–112] This requirement for removal of minerals (including fluoride) *only applies to the dialysate* used during the dialysis process and *does not apply to minerals ingested* through drinking water. In other words, renal dialysis patients and patients with chronic kidney disease can continue to ingest water with optimal fluoride levels. Additionally, numerous studies of people with long-term exposure to drinking water with fluoride concentrations, some as high as 8 ppm, showed no increase in kidney disease.[112]

Concerns about the accumulation of fluoride in the body[113–115] relate primarily to people's concerns about the effect of fluoridation on bone mineral density and whether or not there is increased risk for osteoporosis and fractures. The results of several ecological studies over a 20 year period from 1980–2000, comparing fracture rates in fluoridated and non-fluoridated communities were mixed, from increased rates in hip,[116–118] proximal humerus and distal forearm fractures[119] to no effect on fracture risk[120–123] to decreased risk of hip fracture.[124,125] Since ecological studies use community-wide data, confounding variables associated with rates of fracture including age, sex, estrogen use, smoking, and body weight cannot be controlled. To address these deficiencies and the limitations of ecological study design, a multi-

center prospective study on risk fractures for osteoporosis and fractures was done by Phipps et al. in which investigators assessed bone mass, risk factors, development of incident nonspinal fractures, ascertainment of prevalent and incident vertebral fractures, and exposure to fluoridated water in 7,129 women 65 years and older.[126] The conclusions of this study reported in October 2000 were as follows: (1) "long term exposure to fluoridation does not increase the risk of osteoporotic fracture among older women and may reduce the risk of fracture of the hip and vertebrae in older white women" and (2) "our results support the safety of fluoridation as a public health measure for the prevention of dental caries".[126]

Interestingly enough, sodium fluoride has been used to treat established osteoporosis for over 30 years.[127] Data on the use of high-dose sodium fluoride (75 mg daily) for the treatment of vertebral osteoporosis suggests that the incidence of hip fracture may be increased and bone density may be diminished while the use of low-dose sodium fluoride (25–50 mg daily) therapy appears to have a protective effect against spine fractures but no apparent effect on hip or wrist fracture risk.[128]

According to the National Institute of Dental and Craniofacial Research (NIDCR), "no credible scientific evidence supports an association between fluoridated water and conditions such as cancer, bone fracture, Down's syndrome, or heart disease as claimed by some opponents of water fluoridation."[129]

Most recently, the York Review examined studies relative to the safety of fluoridation and concluded that there was no evidence of any adverse health affect caused by community water fluoridation.[32]

## Engineering Aspects: Chemicals and Technical Systems Used

Water-treatment chemicals are used for a number of reasons including: disinfection, absorption, algae control, decolorization, oxidation, metal coagulation, water softening, filtration, pH control, iron control, coagulation, corrosion control, chlorination, and fluoridation.[13,130–131] Primarily, three chemicals are used for water fluoridation in the United States and are required by the states to meet the American Water Works Association (AWWA) standards for the specific chemical: *sodium fluoride, sodium silicofluoride*, and *hydrofluosilicic acid*.[48] Sodium fluoride (granular or powder) and sodium silicofluoride (granular) are used in distribution systems that use "dry" compounds, while hydrofluosilicic acid, a liquid, is used in solution or "wet" systems. Sodium fluoride was the first compound used in controlled water-fluoridation programs and is still widely used in smaller community-water systems (usually those serving fewer than 5,000 people).[13,130–131] *Sodium silicofluoride* is substantially less expensive than *sodium fluoride* and tends to be used in community-water systems serving between 5,000 and 50,000 people. Today, the most frequently used compound for water fluoridation in the United States is *hydrofluosilicic acid*, because of its low cost and ease of handling; it is used primarily in larger communities with water-distribution systems serving 50,000 or more people and represents approximately 57% of all fluoridation systems in the United States.[130,132] Opponents of fluoridation often attempt to distinguish between *sodium fluoride* and the hexafluorosilicates, *sodium silicofluoride* and *hydrofluosilicic acid* in terms of availability of the fluoride ion. Fluoridation opponents disparage the hexafluorosilicates as "junk dumped into the drinking water" that "contaminates the water with a harmful residue." However, according to the Environmental Protection Agency (EPA), no hexafluorosilicate remains in drinking water at equilibrium, which is readily achieved.[133] This means that there is no difference in the source of fluoride ions from the three chemicals used in fluoridation as the detractors would have one believe.[133] In response to anti-fluoridationist claims, Newbrun stated that "the use of fluorosilicates is a good exam-

ple of successful recycling which benefits both the environment and the consumer."[134]

Determination of the appropriate compound to use in fluoridation depends largely upon the type of distribution system used by the individual water plant. According to Reeves, National Fluoridation Engineer at the U.S. Centers for Disease Control, the most common methods by which fluoride is added to water supplies in the United States are: (1) the *volumetric dry feeder* system which delivers a predetermined quantity of fluoride chemical (either sodium fluoride or sodium silicofluoride) in a given time interval. However, sodium fluoride is not recommended for volumetric dry feeders because of its higher cost which is nearly two and a half times that of sodium silicofluoride; (2) the *acid-feed* system, in which a small metering pump is used to add *hydrofluosilicic acid* to the water-supply system; and (3) *the saturator feed* system, which is unique to water fluoridation, uses an upflow saturator to provide saturated solutions of sodium fluoride in constant strengths of 4% and is pumped into the water system via a small metering pump.[130–131] Additionally, the Venturi fluoridation system is used by the U.S. Indian Health Service in some extremely small rural communities.

## Monitoring and Surveillance of Fluoridation

The process of adding fluoride to drinking water supplies to the level recommended for achieving the maximum dental therapeutic benefits is technically simple, uncomplicated, and similar to the processes used when dealing with chlorine and other water-treatment chemicals.[13,130] All three types of fluoride chemicals used in the water fluoridation process are certified as to their purity and safety when used appropriately. Interestingly, there are 48 additional chemicals approved by the U.S. Environmental Protection Agency and certified as safe for addition to drinking water by the American Water Works Association and NSF

International (National Sanitation Foundation). Contrary to popular perception, fluoride does not affect the taste, odor, color, or turbidity of the water at the levels used for water fluoridation.[13,130–131]

In order for fluoridation to be implemented, a number of factors should be taken into consideration. Of prime importance is the *compatibility* of the fluoride chemical to be used with the existing water-treatment and distribution system.[13,130–131] Other factors impacting the technical engineering aspects of fluoridation include: (a) source of water—underground or surface water, (b) size of the water plant; (c) number and types of point sources of water (one treatment plant or many treatment plants with water coming from wells, reservoirs, rivers, aqueducts, or desalination plants); (d) number of injection points (where fluoride is introduced into the water); (e) fluoride chemical costs, including transportation; (f) modification of existing plant vs. construction of a new plant; (g) need for training of water-plant operators; and (h) type of monitoring and surveillance system to be used.[7,13,130–131]

Modern water-plant design ensures that excessive amounts of fluoride are prevented from entering the water supply. Properly designed fluoridation systems prevent the addition of excess fluoride to the water system in several ways: (1) only a limited amount of fluoride is maintained in the hoppers (or day tanks), (2) positive controls have been installed for feeding fluoride from the hoppers into the dissolving tanks, and (3) metering pumps are installed so that they are electrically connected to the water pump in a manner that ensures that if one fails, both stop operating and no fluoride is added to the system.[13,130–131]

Maintaining a constant level of fluoride in the water supply is the responsibility of the water-plant operators. Variation in the adjusted water fluoride levels has occurred in water plants where the operators are not properly trained and/or the operator turnover is high.[50–56] Variability in water fluoride concen-

tration may also occur if a water plant fails to provide adequate and appropriate storage facilities, if there is malfunctioning of feed equipment, or if proper water-analysis equipment is lacking, all of which are readily avoidable with proper planning and implementation. Most of the variances in fluoride concentrations that have occurred are due to poor monitoring at water treatment facilities and have resulted in fluoride levels *below* the recommended level (*hypofluoridation*).[13,135] For this reason, communities that have implemented fluoridation must continue to monitor the fluoride levels in order to ensure that the full benefits of fluoridation will accrue in a community. *Hyperfluoridation* occurs when an excess amount of fluoride is added to the drinking water over several days, usually secondary to an overfeed from malfunctioning equipment and/or maintenance errors.[13,136–137] Over the past 56 years there have been seven instances of *hyperfluoridation* which resulted in outbreaks of acute fluoride poisoning in the United States, all of which could have easily been prevented.[13,138] Thus, when a community decides to fluoridate its public-water supplies, it also must assume the responsibility for monitoring the equipment, training the water-plant operators, and implementing performance reviews to ensure that the process is in place to protect the public from an overfeed. The Centers for Disease Control and Prevention offers weeklong water-plant operators training programs designed to assist plant operators in sustaining and monitoring their fluoridation systems.[131]

## Question 4

Which of the following statements, if any is/are true?

A. Numerous studies over the past several years have consistently demonstrated the safety of water fluoridation.

B. The National Cancer Institute has reviewed the literature on fluoridation and has concluded that there is sub-stantial credible evidence associating fluoridation with cancer and has recommended that fluoridation be halted worldwide immediately.

C. Sodium fluoride is the most frequently used chemical for water fluoridation in the United States.

D. Monitoring of fluoride levels at water treatment plants is essential to prevent both hypofluoridation and hyperfluoridation.

E. Fluoride does not affect the taste, color, odor, or turbidity of the water at the levels used for fluoridation.

### Other Fluoride Vehicles

Many countries without centralized water distribution systems have chosen to add fluoride to table salt, a process known as *"salt fluoridation,"* in order to provide primary dental caries preventive benefits to their populations; approximately 40 million people use fluoridated salt.[82] Using salt as a vehicle of fluoride supplementation is similar to the concept of iodine supplementation and is a relatively inexpensive method of fluoride delivery. Like water fluoridation, *salt fluoridation* results in small amounts of fluoride being released from plasma throughout the day.[139–140] In order to achieve dental-caries reductions at levels comparable to water fluoridation, the level of fluoride supplementation of refined salt should be at least 200 mg F/kg as NaF or Ca $CaF_2$.[141–142] *Salt fluoridation* requires centralized salt production, as well as monitoring.[82] Since the consumption of high quantities of sodium is a risk factor for hypertension, the use of fluoridated salt is not recommended for those at risk.[82,143] Countries utilizing *salt fluoridation* extensively include Switzerland, France, Costa Rica, Jamaica, and Germany.[144,145] It has also been introduced in Mexico, Spain, Columbia, Brazil, and Hungary where its use has been found to be appropriate.[82,139,142,146–148]

Also, *"milk fluoridation,"* the addition of 5 mg of fluoride to 1 litre of milk has been introduced as a vehicle of school-based fluoride delivery in some countries (Bulgaria, Chile, China, the Russian Federation, and the United Kingdom).[82] While encouraging results have been reported with *milk fluoridation*, no widespread clinical trials have been reported.[82] Additional studies are required to adequately assess *milk fluoridation* as a viable caries prevention strategy. According to the WHO Report, "the distribution of fluoridated milk can be more complicated than that of fluoride supplements (tablets or drops)."[82] As a result, the existence of an established distribution system that includes provisions for pasteurization and refrigeration is a limiting factor in *milk fluoridation* programs.[82]

*Fluoride mouthrinses* were developed in the 1960s as a *school-based* public-health measure designed to provide access to fluoride without requiring a visit to the dentist office. *School-based weekly fluoride rinse programs* using 0.2% sodium fluoride have been shown to be effective in preventing coronal caries in school children who are at risk for dental caries. Estimates of dental caries reductions observed prior to the establishment of efficacy, range from 20 to 50%. Since the establishment of efficacy for fluoride mouthrinses, the level of caries reduction appears to be less than originally observed. Additionally, the cost-effectiveness of fluoride mouthrinse programs appears to be diminished because of the declining prevalence of dental caries in general.[7,149]

Implementation requires that children enrolled in the program participate consistently over time to receive maximum benefit. However, many children as they get older (middle/high school years) decline to participate, believing that fluoride rinsing is a program for younger children. Significant coordination and monitoring in the schools, parental consent, tracking children as they move from elementary school to middle and high school, and commitment on the part of school officials

is required for caries-reduction outcomes. According to the Centers for Disease Control, 3.25 million schoolchildren were participating in fluoride-rinse programs in 1988.[7]

## Enactment of Water Fluoridation as Public Policy

In May 2001, Partnership for Prevention, a nonprofit, nonpartisan organization issued a report, *Priorities in Prevention: Oral Health,* in which it stated that "oral health is not solely dependent on individual behaviors." This report identified prevention opportunities for policy makers and business/community leaders with community water fluoridation topping the list of oral-health strategies that work.[150]

Fluoridation is not legislated at the federal level in the United States. However, legislation may be introduced in state legislatures, although very few of these measures have been enacted at the state level in recent years. Statewide *fluoridation laws* were enacted primarily in the late 1960s and require fluoridation in ten states: California, Connecticut, Delaware, Georgia, Illinois, Minnesota, Nebraska, Nevada, Ohio, and South Dakota. Moreover, the District of Columbia and the U.S. Commonwealth of Puerto Rico also legislated jurisdiction-wide mandatory fluoridation. In addition, Kentucky mandates fluoridation of all public water systems serving 1,500 persons or more by *administrative regulation* under the authority of its state health commissioner (see Table 8–6, statewide fl). Legislation requiring fluoridation failed in two states in 1989 along with anti-fluoridation bills that failed in five states. Anti-fluoridation bills failed in four states in 1990 as well (ADA, 1991).

Successful adoption by legislatures of mandated statewide fluoridation laws in recent history include Nevada and Delaware. California passed legislation in 1995, mandating fluoridation in communities having 10,000 or more service connections, pending availability of funds. Around the same time period, a bill was

TABLE 8-6 **United States Statewide/Geopolitical Enabling Legislation/Regulation Fluoridation**

| State | Date | Status |
|---|---|---|
| Connecticut | 1965 | Required (> 200,000 population) |
| Kentucky | 1966 | By Administrative Regulation (>1,500 population) |
| Illinois | 1967 | Fully enforced |
| Minnesota | 1967 | Fully enforced (Municipal System) |
| Ohio | 1969 | Required (>5,000 population); vigorously enforced |
| South Dakota | 1969 | Enforced |
| Georgia | 1973 | Funded by state |
| Nebraska | 1973 | Referendum required |
| California | 1995 | Not funded; required, i.e., system must fluoridate if funding available (<10,000 service connections) which approximates >25,000 population |
| Delaware* | 1998 | Fully enforced; fully funds fluoridation |
| Nevada | 2000 | Applies to Las Vegas and Clark County only |
| District of Columbia | 1952 | *Required/jurisdiction-wide* |
| *Commonwealth of Puerto Rico*** | *1998* | *Required/jurisdiction-wide* |

*Delaware initially passed statewide legislation in 1968 but it was not enacted/not enforced

**Puerto Rico initially passed legislation in 1952 but it was not enacted/not enforced

introduced in Oregon, requiring that communities fluoridate; if they failed to comply, they would be required to reimburse the health department for dental-treatment bills.[151–152] Economics appears to have been the driving force and the common denominator in these state legislative initiatives. For some states, especially those in which a small percentage of the population has access to fluoridated water and/or those states with high dental-caries rates and high Medicaid costs, mandatory statewide fluoridation laws could be a viable strategy. Equally important, however, is the political will to implement fluoridation at the local level as "mandatory" state laws often have local option provisions.

From a public-policy perspective, fluoridation is more often perceived as a local issue that is enacted either by *governmental administrative action* (ordinance that is voted upon by a city council or city/county commission) or by a vote of the public. Interestingly enough, the

local health official often has both the power and authority under city/county charter to order the fluoridation of public water systems but rarely invoke such power. Generally speaking, a vote of the public is referred to as a *voter initiative* if the vote is to implement fluoridation or as a *voter referendum*, if the vote is to confirm, alter, or eliminate an existing mandatory fluoridation law. Frequently, a *voter initiative* is often referred to as an *initiative referendum*. *Voter initiative* and a *voter referendum* have been used interchangeably. Consequently, it is important to review the city charter to ascertain the correct mechanism to be pursued in a community.

In some cases, public officials seek to avoid controversy by opting to put an ordinance on the ballot; in other cases, a referendum vote can be forced by a signature petition. A forced petition referendum usually requires a percentage of signatures, usually 10 to 20% (varies according to city or county charter provisions or

state constitutional requirements) of registered voters who voted in the previous election. In the final analysis, implementation of fluoridation in the United States is now achieved primarily by *governmental administrative decision* or by a *vote of the electorate*.

## Fluoridation Actions

In the 1950s to 1960s, "*initiative referenda*" represented the majority of fluoridation actions in the United States; of the 1,009 *initiative referenda*, fluoridation was adopted in 411 communities and defeated in 598 communities.[68] In the 1980s, two out of every three fluoridation *initiative referenda* were defeated, while gains were achieved by 77% (199/258) of communities utilizing the governmental *administrative mechanism*. In the late 1980s and early 1990s: city council/commission *administrative action* authorized fluoridation in 318 communities while 32 *initiative referenda* were held in which 19 were won and 13 were lost, indicating an improvement in *initiative referenda* success compared to previous decades. In 1994, 47 U.S. communities authorized fluoridation: 46 were city council or commission actions and one was an "*initiative referenda*" action.[68,153] Of the 46 communities, authorizing fluoridation by administrative action, 36 had populations less than 10,000 while the remaining 10 communities had populations greater than 10,000. Greater successes in terms of numbers of communities have been achieved through the governmental administrative decision process but they are concentrated in the smaller communities.[154-157]

As previously stated, 23 U.S cities/counties voted on fluoridation ordinances in the November 2000 presidential election. Of the 23 cities, 9 cities with a total population of 3,829,185 approved fluoridation while 14 cities with a total population of 381,888 rejected fluoridation at the polls (see Table 8–7 and Table 8–8). Further analysis of this data shows that in general, the *initiative/referenda* wins occurred in larger popula-

TABLE 8-7  **Fluoridation Referenda Wins, November 2000 Election**

| City | Population |
| --- | --- |
| Gilbert, AZ | 109,697 |
| Sunnyvale, CA | 131,760 |
| Leavenworth, KS | 35,420 |
| North Attlboro, MA | 16,796 |
| Clark County, NV | 1,375,765 |
| Las Vegas, NV | 478,434 |
| Abilene, TX | 115,930 |
| San Antonio, TX | 1,144,646 |
| Salt Lake City, UT | 181,743 |
| Davis County, UT | 238,994 |
| Total: | 3,829,185 |

*Source:* U.S. Census Bureau, 2000

TABLE 8-8  **Fluoridation Ballot Defeats, November 2000 Election**

| City | Population |
| --- | --- |
| Ozark, MO | 9,665 |
| Pequannock, NJ | 13,888 |
| Ithaca, NY | 29,287 |
| Wooster, OH | 24,811 |
| Logan, UT | 42,670 |
| Hyrum, UT | 6,316 |
| Nibley, UT | 2,045 |
| Providence, UT | 4,377 |
| River Heights, UT | 1,496 |
| Smithfield, UT | 7,261 |
| Brattleboro, VT | 8,289 |
| Spokane, WA | 195,629 |
| Wenatchee, WA | 27,856 |
| Shawano, WI | 8,298 |
| Total: | 381,888 |

*Source:* U.S. Census Bureau, 2000

tion centers (except North Attleboro, MA, and Leavenworth, KS) while the *initiative/referenda* losses tended to occur in the smaller communities, except Spokane, WA.[19,158]

## Readiness Assessment for Initiating a Fluoridation Campaign

In order for the United States to achieve the goal of 75% fluoridation by the year 2010, the obstacles that affect the legal framework in which fluoridation is implemented must be carefully analyzed. An assessment of a number of factors that impact the implementation of fluoridation in the United States is essential to developing targeted educational strategies and defining the fluoridation campaign message. Some of the major factors include: demographic trend data, external forces, public opinion, political climate, media influence, voter turnout/apathy, lack of public awareness of the benefits of fluoridation, perception of benefits vs. risks of fluoridation, and lack of political campaign skills among health professionals.

## Demographics

According to projections, the United States will need to add approximately 30 million people, served by more than 1,000 water systems to the *Fluoridation Census* in order to get within striking range of the Year 2010 Goal.[7] Between 1990 and 1998, the greatest population growth occurred in metropolitan areas in the West (mountain and pacific states) and South (south atlantic, east south central, and west south central states) regions of the United States.[158] The 15 largest nonfluoridated cities in the United States have a total population approximating 5 million people; 12 of the largest nonfluoridated cities are located in the West and South regions where metropolitan population gains ranged from 13.1% in the South to 13.8% in the West.[158] At the same time, nonmetropolitan population gains ranged from 7.5% in the South to 16.1% in the West.[158] As previously stated, 7 of the largest nonfluoridated cities are

in California where fluoridation legislation passed in 1995. A significant percentage of the needed fluoridation census gains will have to come from our nation's cities which continue to be the population magnets and represent approximately 80% percent of the total population in the United States.[159] Achieving fluoridation, whether by city council/commission action or by *voter initiative or voter referendum*, is more difficult in our urban centers where massive resources and protracted major grassroots, culturally relevant campaigns are generally required. While suburbanites tend to vote, inner-city residents often tend not to vote. The implications of urbanization/suburbanization will have an impact on efforts to fluoridate many of the nonfluoridated cities.

The diversity of the U.S. population presents a challenge to the preventive health educational and political efforts because each racial and ethnic group has unique attitudes, beliefs, and expectations about preventive health outcomes that need to be considered. While racial and ethnic minorities are not as likely to vote as whites, efforts should be made to provide accurate information to the entire community, as well as to encourage broader participation in the voting process by all voters. Additionally, the ability to communicate in a language other than English may also be important in a local campaign effort. In 1990, nearly 32 million (14% of the nation's population 5 years and over) said that they spoke a language other than English at home, compared with 23 million (11%) a decade earlier.[68] Over half of those who said they spoke a language other than English at home reported speaking Spanish.[68] America is also aging. More and more people in their 50s and 60s have surviving parents, aunts, and uncles and four-generation families are common. Those aged 65 years and older comprised 17% of the adult population but cast 22% of the ballots while those aged 18 to 24 comprised 14% of the voting age population, but accounted for only 6% of voters.[160] Older populations have higher rates of edentu-

lousness and are less likely to visit the dentist.[66] As noted, the elderly do vote and they also tend to view fluoridation as a benefit primarily directed at children and therefore may be less likely to be supportive. Framing fluoridation solely as a childrens' health issue is problematic for campaign organizers.

The likelihood of voting increases with education as well as age and income, resulting in certain groups making up a disproportionate share of voters. According to the Census Bureau, 84% of all adults, ages 25 and older, had completed high school while only 26% had completed a bachelor's degree.[161] Homeowners were about twice as likely as renters to vote (53% vs. 27%).[162,163] One in three children born in America live in poverty.[164] The poor are also less likely to have dental insurance or to obtain preventive care. And while the economically disadvantaged stand to benefit the most from fluoridation, they often do not vote. Geographic mobility of the population, often related to the job market, can also impact fluoridation success at the polls. People who have lived in fluoridated communities are often surprised to find that their new community is not fluoridated and are even more surprised by the controversy generated when fluoridation is placed on the public agenda. Having lived in a fluoridated area previously, it is speculated that new residents to a nonfluoridated community would generally tend to favor fluoridation.[165]

## External Forces/Public Opinion/Political Climate

Over the past two decades, there has been a move towards federal decentralization, that is transferring power, control, and funding from the federal government back to the states to administer programs. States are faced with problems associated with many of the social issues that are likely to have significant budgetary implications. As a result of statutes requiring balanced budgets, governors have been forced to control costs. Rapid increases in Med-

icaid costs alone have strained many state budgets, causing greater scrutiny of expenditures. Dental Medicaid expenditures were among those examined by the state of California and viewed by some as the impetus for passing fluoridation legislation in 1995.[68]

Fluoridation campaign committees need to research their local city or county charter to ascertain the mechanisms/processes by which their community can fluoridate as well as the provisions and timeframes, taking into account early voting and/or extended voting periods which impact the campaign. Fluoridation campaign committees also must analyze the economic climate, as well as the results of recent local issue elections, including the impact of negative campaigns, in order to assess the mood of the electorate. The opposition, its strength and credibility must also be assessed; underestimating the energy, tenacity, and ingenuity of the opposition are major causes of fluoridation ordinance failures. Research, including an assessment of external forces, such as in a SWOT analysis (strengths, weaknesses, opportunities, and threats) is critical to the development of a strategic campaign plan. Fluoridation committees also need to determine if community leaders and elected officials have the political will to shepherd a fluoridation measure through the enactment of an ordinance, either by administrative action or a vote of the electorate.

In his book, *Rational Lives: Norms and Values in Politics and Society*, Dennis Chong noted that individuals make decisions across both social and economic realms and that "our preferences inevitably reflect the costs and benefits of the available options and the influence of psychological dispositions formed over the life span."[166] Knowing the public stance on a particular issue is also important. In a 1990 National Health Interview Survey (NHIS) of 41,104 adults regarding public knowledge of the purpose of fluoridation, 62% correctly identified the purpose.[66] Knowledge of the purpose of fluoridation was highest among persons aged 35 to 54 years of age (68 to 70%) while

younger (18 to 24) and older (≥ 75) persons had less understanding, at 49% and 40%, respectively.[66] Other findings showed that persons with higher educational attainment levels were more than twice as likely as those with less than a high school education to correctly identify the purpose of fluoridation (76% vs. 36%).[66] When presented with conflicting information regarding benefits and risks of fluoridation, discernment and the ability of the electorate to make informed decisions may be compromised. Additionally, the dynamics inherent in plebiscites (fears, anxieties, discontentment, anger, resistance to authority, and resentment of professionals) can derail the decision-making process.[167] Direct democracy poses a significant challenge for proponents of any issue because they must "settle the public's mind on all aspects of a question and they must bear the burden of restraint."[167] Securing majority support for any issue placed before the voters requires a very high level of initial support in order to achieve a successful result on election day because support erodes over the duration of a campaign.[165,167]

Intensive and ongoing efforts to educate the public about fluoridation should be implemented prior to initiation of a political campaign and sustained through the decision making process and continued thereafter. It took 25 years to enhance public knowledge and change attitudes about smoking in the United States; to sustain the gains, the education must continue. Similarly, just because communicable diseases are rare today, it doesn't follow that immunization programs should receive less emphasis. Public-health professionals have learned the hard way that eliminating public-health programs, such as immunization, is quickly followed by a rapid reappearance of previously rare diseases. They also recognize that once diseases are under control, the most difficult task is to educate the public about the need to continue successful programs in order to prevent return of the disease. Similarly, fluoridation education should continue.

In a telephone survey conducted by Research!America in May 2000, 85% of Americans responded that oral health is *very important* to their overall health.[150,168] A 1998 national Gallup poll of consumers' opinions about water fluoridation showed that 70% supported fluoridation,[1,169,170] however, a local poll may be necessary to provide local elected officials with public opinion data in order for them to enter the fluoridation fray. Public opinion polls may be essential in determining a community's willingness to adopt fluoridation; they can also provide crucial information relative to crafting a clear fluoridation message. Knowing who votes is also important. Additionally, it should be pointed out that not all voters are wealthy, or are better educated suburbanites, and not all nonvoters are poor, less educated inner city dwellers. According to a national survey, there are 5 different groups of nonvoters: "doers", "unpluggeds", "irritables", "don't knows", and "alienateds."[171] A common strategy used in campaigns is to focus on consistent voters and elderly voters while neglecting the nonvoters, including, in some cases, the inner city voter.[171] Limited resources mean many campaigns limit their focus to groups of expected voters, a practice that is contrary to the principle of inclusiveness, and generally ill-advised, especially with controversial issues.

Perhaps the most crucial parameters for assessing fluoridation success are *timing, readiness,* and *organization.* There are numerous examples of communities throughout the United States where timing, readiness, and organization have played a role in the success or failure of a fluoridation ballot measure; many communities have held more than one fluoridation *initiative/ referendum* to obtain passage. Professional campaign managers, particularly those with experience running issues campaigns, can assist local fluoridation committees in evaluating the TIMING options and in establishing a timeline. Fluoridation campaigns also require financial resources to get the message out. Fundraising can be a major stumbling block for many com-

munities and needs to be considered early on in the campaign.

## Public Perception of Risks vs. Benefits of Fluoridation

A mandatory law that passed in both houses of the California state legislature[67] and was signed into law by the governor in 1995, requires communities to fluoridate but it also placed the cost at the local level where it could be interpreted as an *"unfunded mandate."* Many *unfunded mandates* are seen by the electorate to be designed to help the poor at the expense of the working middle class. *Unfunded mandates* generally are viewed as being coercive (not voluntary) and as being controlled by society rather than by the individual, and as such, may be thought to raise the level of public outrage (discussed in later section). According to Sandman (1990), the public's perception of risk is based on the level of outrage felt with respect to a given potential or perceived hazard while the scientific/public health community views risk in terms of the degree of actual hazard. These differing perspectives are exploited by fluoridation opponents who seek to increase the perception of hazard.[172] In Sandman's risk perception analysis of fluoridation (see Table 8–9), 13 variables were examined in which an overall negative score of 7 was assigned.[68,172] Only 4 variables were considered to be positive with respect to mitigating public outrage. On the negative side, fluoridation was summarized as being: "coercive when done by administrative action; industrial or man-made (artificial); dreaded because of alleged association with cancer; unknowable due to the scientific controversy that results when experts appear to disagree; controlled when the public is excluded from the decision making process; not trustworthy with respect to the source of information

### TABLE 8-9 Public Perception of Fluoridation Risks

| Risk Perception Variables | Risk Perception Score |
|---|---|
| Voluntary vs. *Coerced* | (−) |
| Natural vs. *Industrial/Man-made* | (−) |
| *Familiar* vs. Unfamiliar/Exotic | (+) |
| *Non-memorable* vs. Memorable | (+) |
| Not Dreaded vs. *Dreaded* | (−) |
| *Diffuse* vs. Static/Focused | (+) |
| Knowable vs. *Unknowable* | (−) |
| Control by individual vs. *Control by society* | (−−) |
| *Fair* vs. Unfair | (+) |
| Morally irrelevant vs. Morally relevant | (+/−) |
| Trustworthy vs. *Not trustworthy* | (−−) |
| Open sources vs. *Secret sources* | (−−) |
| Courtesy/Caring vs. *Arrogance* | (−) |
| *Overall fluoridation risk perception score* | −7 |

+ indicates that the italicized variable reduces public outrage about fluoridation

− indicates that the italicized variable increases public outrage about fluoridation

[*Sources:* Sandman 1990 and Centers for Disease Control (Park, Smith, Malvitz, Furman)]

and mechanisms of accountability; as having closed or secret sources, giving the impression that information is being withheld; and is viewed as being arrogant, as evidenced by contempt for the public's perception."[173] The challenge for fluoridation advocates is to effectively communicate risk/benefit information, using strategies targeted at reducing the outrage towards fluoridation.[172,173] (These strategies are discussed in a later section.)

---

### Question 5

Which of the following statements, if any is/are true?

A. Many countries without centralized water distribution systems use *salt fluoridation,* a process whereby fluoride is added to table salt, in order to provide primary dental caries preventive benefits to their populations.

B. An objective of the U.S. Public Health Service is to have 75% of United States citizens consuming fluoridated water by 2010.

C. The likelihood of voting decreases with education as well as age and income, resulting in certain groups making up a disproportionate share of voters.

D. The public's perception of risk is based on the level of outrage felt with respect to a given potential or perceived hazard while the scientific/public health community views risk in terms of the degree of actual hazard.

E. From a public-policy perspective, fluoridation is more often perceived as a federal or national issue that is mandated by legislation.

---

### Role of Media in Forming Public Opinion and Public Policy

According to a recent report, 93% of persons surveyed said that they regularly watched local news, while 48% reported having watched television network news and 50% reported having read a newspaper, the previous night; 18% listened regularly to talk radio.[174] Over the past decade, there has been increased interest on the part of scholars, political scientists, sociologists, pollsters, politicians, and journalists in tracking the role of mass media on public policy, public opinion, and voting behaviors.[174] Reporting on health issues has not been immune to the confluence of forces where the media often resort to generating controversy in order to increase readership and/or listening/viewing audience. Also, manufacturing of the news seems to be a trend on the rise in the United States, raising questions of accountability. A 1995 U.S. News poll found that the public appears wary of both the mainstream media and talk radio.[174]

Older, wealthier, and more educated consumers are more likely to read a newspaper. More often than not, fluoridation is explored more thoroughly in the print media, yet readership is declining all over the country, as newspapers merge or shut down operations. While the print media have often editorialized in favor of fluoridation at the time of a public vote, it often comes too late, as doubt has been solidified in the minds of the public. In some cases, however, the media have taken a proactive role in enacting fluoridation[175]; this occurred in Phoenix, Arizona, in 1989 and consequently, 1 million people were added to the fluoridation census.

A busier consumer often turns to the TV for a quick capsule view of what is happening locally, around the state, nationally, and internationally.[176] Consequently, messages are transmitted via 1- to 2-minute sound bites where the negative perspective is more amenable to the world of sound bites than the positive perspective. Converting detailed data to sound bites is a challenge for proponents of a complex public-policy issue, who are held to a veracity standard. In other words, it is far easier to convey opposition to public policy than it is to

convey support. Additionally, the visual impact of this medium can be used either for or against a public policy issue and must be considered in a media campaign strategy. In a network's attempt to be fair and get the viewers attention, mixed messages are often conveyed through use of a news clip that portrays a highly negative visual image coupled with a verbal message that is positive and educational. Mixed messages can create doubt and sometimes apathy and/or cynicism.

Radio, and especially talk radio is not a mass medium to the extent that television is. Over the past decade, the number of radio talk shows has escalated dramatically, with nearly 10% of radio stations having a talk format, serving as a vehicle for the listening public to participate in the political debate.[174] Radio talk shows or "talk radio" are a powerful force in U.S. politics today, in part because of the end of the Fairness Doctrine as well as to changing technology.[174] In 1985, the Federal Communications Commission (FCC) ruled that the Fairness Doctrine, requiring that broadcasters provide a reasonable opportunity for the presentation of opposing views on controversial public issues, was no longer needed.[174] The FCC's ruling was upheld by a Federal Appeals court in 1989.[174] With the end of the Fairness Doctrine, neither radio program hosts nor stations have an obligation to provide balance or present competing views.[174] Consequently, talk radio is an important vehicle for the public to obtain information on a given topic, including fluoridation. If only one viewpoint is expressed on fluoridation, the impact on public opinion could be significant given that talk radio listeners tend to be more politically active.

The use of the satellite dish has enabled stations to receive broadcast quality from anywhere in the country at a relatively low cost; it has also fostered national syndication, allowing local hosts to have access to an instant network.[174] This has been demonstrated in various local efforts to bring fluoridation to the forefront of various communities' agendas. Talk radio hosts connect the listeners with spokespersons from around the country, sometimes establishing a platform for anti-science perspectives that are repeated over and over, yet, have not been substantiated or subjected to evidence-based review. It is not unheard of to encounter talk radio in which a majority of the callers tend to be the solid "aginer voting block" that votes against any issue brought forward by local, state, or federal government. National syndication however, cannot guarantee listenership in today's high-speed world where competition for large audiences in major markets is fierce.[174] Radio is an important medium for disseminating information and should be factored into educational and political media strategies.

Talk radio can be considered an intimate medium in which the caller is usually anonymous and the discussion is spontaneous.[174] According to a report released in 1996 by the Annenberg Public Policy Center: (a) 18% of adults in the United States listen to at least one political call-in radio show twice a week or more; and (b) political talk-show listeners are more likely to consume all news media (other than TV news) and to be more politically savvy and involved, regardless of ideology.[174]

According to a recent nationwide poll of talk radio programs, three-fourths of the talk radio audience is younger than age 60 and listeners tend to have higher incomes and be better educated, with 39% holding college degrees, compared with 21% of Americans overall. Also, 9 of every 10 political talk-radio listeners are registered to vote, compared with 6 of 10 Americans in general.[174]

As public-policy issues, including fluoridation, surface in a given community, they are subjected to media review. The role of mass media in framing critical issues and influencing public policy as well as their impact on how public opinion and values are formed is important to American democracy. Understanding and working with the media in educating the public about public policy issues, including fluoridation is critical to an informed electorate.

Recent advances in technology, such as the information superhighway, have provided yet another powerful communication tool—the *World Wide Web (internet)*. The proliferation of websites has exploded in the past few years and with it, the instantaneous dissemination of information and opinions on every topic imaginable. The internet has been embraced by the public as a means of ready access to information. There are a number of health-related websites, including those dealing with water fluoridation. If one searches the internet using various search engines, a significant quantity of information can be found. One search engine turned up 24,100 matches while another had 2,500 matches for "fluoridation." The downside of internet use as a source of valid information is that much of the health information available on the web is opinion-based and has not gone through a rigorous scientific review process, putting the onus on the public for discerning truth from fiction regarding the information presented. Another problem associated with fluoridation information on the internet is the paucity of information from credible re-search-based entities and recognized professional organizations. Unfortunately, the public is subjected via the internet to predominately negative information from biased opposition groups, rather than being provided objective, science-based information about the safety, efficacy, and cost-effectiveness of fluoridation.

### Voter Turnout/Voter Apathy

Knowledge of voter participation is important because *fluoridation is the only public-health issue that is regularly voted on in a community*. Many Americans have opted out of the political decision-making process because of business/time constraints, apathy, and other factors.[177] In the November 2000 presidential election, only 51.21% of eligible voters (voting age population—all persons of age 18 or over) actually cast votes compared to 63.06% in 1960. Historically, voter turnout has been higher in presidential election years than in federal election "off years" where voter turnout went from 47.27% in 1962 to 36.4% in 1998 (see Figure 8–3). Since 1990, nearly three-quarters of the

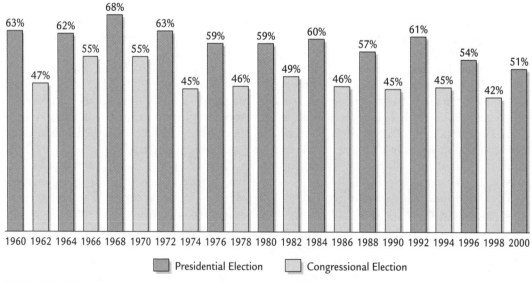

*Source:* Census Bureau, 2000

FIGURE 8–3   Voter Turnout Presidential & Congressional Elections: 1960–2000. (*Source:* Census Bureau, 2000.)

growth in the voting-age population occurred in the 45- to 64-year-old age group, representing approximately 3 of 10 of the voting-age population.[178] According to the Census Bureau, the most likely voters tend to be: white, women, older, married, those with more education, those having higher incomes, those who are employed, and those who are homeowners and/or longtime residents. Interestingly enough, people living in the West are the least likely to register to vote but those who do register to vote are most likely to vote (see Figure 8–4, map/voting/US).

Voter turnout at the local level has followed the same pattern as seen at the state and national levels, with percentages dipping into the teens.[68] Low voter turnouts and special elections have traditionally spelled disaster for fluoridation, especially in larger cities where the "aginer factor" (a constant block of voters who vote against any government initiative or government involved proposal) is sure to vote in an *initiative/referendum*. Supporters of fluoridation, seeking a vote of the electorate, should consider placing an ordinance for fluoridation on a regularly called ballot that is expected to have higher voter turnouts. Mayoral or county commissioners elections (or even gubernatorial or presidential elections if election laws allow for local issues) generally have voter-turnout rates that are greater than those observed in a special election. In cases where local governing

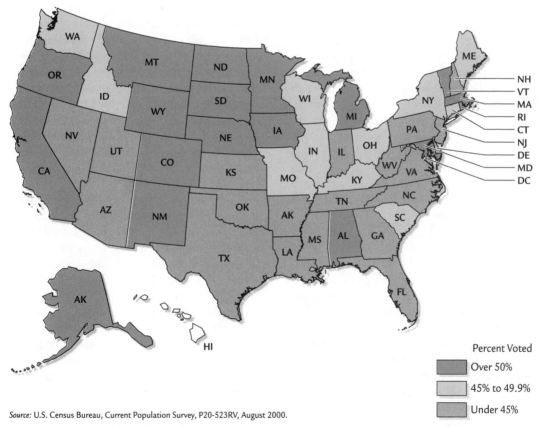

Percent Voted
Over 50%
45% to 49.9%
Under 45%

*Source:* U.S. Census Bureau, Current Population Survey, P20-523RV, August 2000.

FIGURE 8–4   Voting Percentages in the United States by State, 1998. (*Source:* U.S. Census Bureau, *Current Population Survey*, P20-523RV, August 2000.)

authorities decide to call a public vote on fluoridation in order to let the voters decide, they often opt to have a special election or vote to place it on any other election other than the mayoral or county commissioners election, in order to avoid taking a position on fluoridation that might affect their election or reelection status.[68]

Because of low voter turnout, the prevailing wisdom among proponents of fluoridation suggests that referenda be avoided, but this is contrary to Sandman's (1990) warning that decisions that are perceived as being coercive or as not allowing for individual control/freedom of choice, are more likely to increase the level of outrage, and therefore decrease acceptability. In view of the skepticism of the electorate and taking Sandman's risk perception principles into consideration, it may be necessary to consider the full range of options for implementing fluoridation in communities where city council/commission action are not possible.[68] Perhaps the initiative process or changes in the jurisdictional charter should be considered as part of a comprehensive political strategy. Some jurisdictions, however, may not allow citizens the right to petition. Additionally, in many U.S. communities today, voting periods have been extended. The impact of these factors on an *initiative/referenda* campaign can be substantial in terms of organization, resources, and sustaining get-out-the-vote (GOTV) efforts.[68]

Negative campaigning has also contributed to public disillusionment with policy issues as well as to voter apathy. Political advertisements have not been subject to the same scrutiny as other forms of campaigning, although some networks are taking on the challenge of analyzing such advertisements. Engendering fear and anger among the electorate is the basis of negative campaigning. Fluoridation is one of those issues that lends itself very well to negative campaigning because people's fears and/or anger are exploited by the opposition. Unfortunately, the electorate doesn't necessarily have to agree with those opposed to fluoridation for the issue to fail at the polls. Instead, the voters often react to the vicious negative campaigning and tune out altogether, opting out by voting the issue down or failing to vote at all (no-shows) in hopes that the "controversy" will go away. Even if the voters question the claims of the anti-fluoridation faction, they may be encouraged to vote against fluoridation just because they have a scintilla of doubt about which side is right and opt to "wait and see" until all "questions" have been answered.

Mistrust of government and erosion of public confidence in the government's ability to solve problems, anger at being left out of the process, anger at tax increases, fear of the future because of loss of economic security, fear of employment layoffs, anger and fear caused by declining incomes and benefits, fear of crime, fear of loss of individual rights and freedom, and a sense that the government is ineffective, have had the effect of simultaneously immobilizing a large sector of the population while mobilizing a negatively motivated electorate.[68] Anger and fear are the two most powerful factors motivating people to act and both take front-and-center stage in a fluoridation campaign. They are also the emotions capitalized upon by the anti-fluoridationists to defeat fluoridation and they are the basis of Sandman's risk perception principles.

Skepticism on the part of the public resulting from programmatic failures in public health (e.g., swine-flu vaccine) combined with a distrust of established scientific methods and confusion over recommended health practices that seem to change weekly, tend to fuel the flames, angering and frustrating the public.[179] Public knowledge and attitudes toward fluoridation demonstrate the need for health professionals to continually advocate for fluoridation in order to preserve the successes already achieved.[176,180-183] Fluoridation campaigns that are not sufficiently broad-based with multiple constituencies involved in the decision-making process are likely to encounter problems when political decisions have to be made.[154,184-188]

Fluoridation committees composed of health professionals alone are not enough to realize a fluoridation win on a ballot measure, or for that matter, in governmental body actions.

## Political Skills and Knowledge of Fluoridation Committees

Even though fluoridation is the only health issue that is often voted on (plebiscite), it is taught as a public-health intervention, not as a political issue. Health professionals are frequently called upon to be involved in fluoridation efforts, yet they often lack political experience, skills in mediation and conflict resolution, or media expertise to deal with the issues raised in a campaign. Knowledge and experience in managing an actual political campaign, including marketing the pro-fluoride message, fundraising, organizing phone banks and get-out-the-vote (GOTV) efforts, such as block-walking, are not normally taught in the curricula of the health disciplines, and certainly not in U.S. dental schools.[68] Physicians and dentists are often co-opted into reacting negatively, by withdrawing and disappearing and by being defensive and condescending when confronted with a potential voter who disagrees with the premise that fluoridation is the best caries preventive method that a community can adopt.[68] Sometimes, health professionals fail to get involved in fluoridation efforts because they don't feel confident that they can cite evidence-based rebuttals to the broad, all-inclusive laundry list of allegations and objections to fluoridation.[2,189-192] Familiarity with Sandman's risk perception principles (see Table 8–9) as they relate to fluoridation and knowing how to decrease the level of outrage are critical skills that every health professional should have but are not taught. Health professional students are taught to deliver care to individuals not to communities. Even in public health programs, students do not learn these skills, creating a leadership gap as it relates to advocating for fluoridation. In the final analysis, the desired outcome is more dependent upon political skills than on knowledge of fluoridation.[68]

> ## Question 6
>
> Which of the following statements, if any is/are true?
>
> A. Newspapers usually are helpful in screening misinformation contained in letters to the editor and by columnists
>
> B. The Federal Communications Commission (FCC) ruled in 1985 that the Fairness Doctrine is necessary because it requires that broadcasters provide a reasonable opportunity for the presentation of opposing views on controversial public issues.
>
> C. Talk-radio programs are good forums for serious debates on controversial subjects because they present all sides of an issue equally.
>
> D. Converting detailed data to sound bites is a challenge for proponents of a complex public-policy issue because they are held to a veracity standard.
>
> E. Internet use is a good source of valid health information because the internet site guarantees that all the information provided has gone through a rigorous scientific review process and therefore the public need not be concerned about discerning truth from fiction regarding the information presented.

## Why Dentists and Dental Hygienists Should Be Involved in Promoting Community-Water Fluoridation

The third of the five major ethical principles included in the American Dental Association's *Principles of Ethics and Code of Professional Conduct* is the *Principle of Beneficence* that expressly states ". . . that professionals have the duty to act for the benefit of others." Directly related to this specific ethical principle is a designated

Code of Professional Responsibility regarding Community Service, that further states that ". . . dentists have an obligation to use their skills, knowledge, and experience for the improvement of the dental health of the public and they are encouraged to be leaders in their community . . . ."[193] Furthermore, the fourth principle is the Principle of Justice emphasizing that "the dentist has a duty to treat people fairly." In concert with this principle is the designated *Code of Professional Responsibility* that states, "in its broadest sense, this principle expresses the concept that the dental profession should actively seek allies throughout society on specific activities that will help improve access to care for all," [*including access to known preventive measures like community-water fluoridation*].[b] The American Dental Association's ethical standards are but one reason that community-water fluoridation, clearly the gold standard of community-based programs for the prevention of dental caries, should be actively supported by practicing dentists and dental hygienists. Similarly, the *American Dental Hygienists Association's Code of Ethics* states that "ethics compel us to engage in health promotion/disease prevention activities"[194]—advocating for water fluoridation meets this criteria.

The obligation to promote scientifically justified community-based programs, such as community-water fluoridation, also stems from a dentist's/dental hygienist's obligation to serve the community in exchange for the community's contribution to the dentist's/dental hygienist's privilege of practicing dentistry/dental hygiene. First, the privilege of practicing dentistry/dental hygiene has been granted to dentists/dental hygienists by the public, through their state legislators, in the form of a statewide dental practice act managed by a state dental-

licensing board. The privilege of practicing dentistry/dental hygiene has been allocated to dentists/dental hygienists because of society's recognition of the need for having qualified practitioners to serve the public's oral-health needs. Society retains the right to maintain, modify, or cancel these privileges at any point that they feel that the dentists/dental hygienists of their state are not meeting society's needs. By assisting communities to authorize and implement community-water fluoridation, dentists/dental hygienists demonstrate in one small way, their desire to meet their many obligations to society.

## Opposition to Community-Water Fluoridation

While fluoridation is generally not considered controversial among the scientific community, it persists as a political lightening rod, an issue to be avoided at all costs by the political community. Pasteurization, immunization, and chlorination all faced opposition initially which subsequently subsided.[195] However, since Grand Rapids, Michigan, began fluoridating its public-water supply in January 1945, there has been a relentless effort by a small but determined opposition to undermine the efforts of health professionals and civic leaders to implement fluoridation around the world. Interestingly enough, "pure-water committees" seem to spring up wherever there appears to be a fluoridation measure on the public agenda. Such committees define pure water as fluoride-free; forty-eight other chemicals frequently used in water treatment are excluded from their definition of pure water. Invoking "the pure water/fluoride-free zone" is a clever tactic designed to push emotional buttons against fluoridation. On the other hand, fluoridation proponents assume that the misinformation disseminated by the opponents will be easily refuted and/or readily dismissed since the facts favoring fluoridation are mistakenly thought to be clear and convincing. However, such a miscalcula-

---

[b]Bracketed phrase added. Brackets enclose a phrase added by authors to further illustrate the relationship of the dentist's obligation to promote community-water fluoridation to the ADA's Code of Ethics and Code of Professional Conduct.

tion may be the basis for underestimating the power of the highly motivated opposition who believe that fluoridation is a prime example of government intrusion.[68]

## Techniques Employed by Opponents of Fluoridation

Bernhardt & Sprague compiled a list of techniques frequently used by the opposition in attempting to stop the process of fluoridation.[196] Several additional techniques have been categorized and included in the following summary of various techniques employed by opponents of fluoridation.

1. *Neutralizing Politicians*: Once the fluoridation legislation/ordinance has been introduced, opponents attempt to convince state and local elected officials to remain neutral, rather than make the appropriate health policy decision to fluoridate the water supply. Opponents often attempt to give the impression that there is "scientific" legitimacy for their positions by quoting "alternative medicine" websites or using pseudo-scientific spokespersons in hearings, correspondence, and distributed propaganda. Anti-fluoridationists try to convince the elected officials to refer the issue to public vote, usually, a special election where there is inadequate time for proponents to organize effectively, rather than to decide the issue through the normal legislative/administrative process. This strategy is favorable to fluoridation opponents who are often more adept at running a scare campaign focused on negative claims about fluoridation than they are at convincing skeptical legislators/city/county officials to agree with their views without verification.

The opposition often resorts to massive letter-writing and phone-calling campaigns designed to give the impression that "everyone is against fluoridation," when in fact the vast majority of citizens may very well be supportive of fluoridation. The strategy also involves bombarding the print media with letters-to-the-editors to foster the notion that there is widespread disapproval of fluoridation. Swamping legislators and/or city leaders with reams of propaganda falsely claiming "evidence of harm," without substantiation or of interference with their "freedom of choice," even though legitimate research results universally refute claims of harm and the courts have repeatedly held that fluoridation interferes with no ones' constitutional freedoms, is part of the overall strategy.

Co-opting legislators and/or city leaders is another strategy designed to neutralize public officials. Overestimating the extent of the opposition often results in leaders taking the path of least resistance and concluding that it is safer to have the electorate make the decision rather than enter the fray. By arousing serious doubts about safety, antifluoride zealots give local elected officials an expedient excuse to delay favorable administrative action. Thus, not only has the legislative/city/county official been neutralized, the antifluoridationists have gained more time to inundate the public with negative propaganda designed to create fear and doubt among the public and alter public perception of fluoridation.

2. *Use of the Big Lie*: Anti-fluoridationists repeatedly allege that fluoride causes cancer, kidney disease, heart disease, genetic damage, osteoporosis, Down's syndrome, AIDS, Alzheimer's disease, nymphomania, violent behavior, crime, and practically every other malady known to man—a veritable laundry list of unproved allegations. Nonetheless, these laundry lists are repeated so frequently in anti-fluoride pamphlets, letters-to-the-editor, and phone calls to talk-radio shows, that the public may actually begin to believe the unsubstantiated claims. In order to lend some aura of legitimacy to the unproved claims, pseudo-scientists frequently appear as the authors of such letters. In the fall of 2000, a leading anti-fluoridationist spokesman announced to radio listeners in San Antonio, Texas, that fluoridation was directly responsible for 35,000 deaths each year in the United States. If there were any truth to this big lie, fluoridation would cease simultaneously

all over the United States and around the world. Yet, while this big lie is clearly off the charts, some questioned why anyone would make such a serious allegation if it weren't true, or possibly true. Public skepticism often results from such a scenario.

The appearance of an allegation in print (such as in the letters to the editor section of local newspapers) is often believed by the public to be evidence of the allegation's validity. The public incorrectly assumes that the "authorities" (in this case print media editors) would not allow allegations to be printed if they were untrue. Thus, the media often become unwitting pawns of the anti-fluoridationists, unless the newspapers are large enough and sophisticated enough to have employed qualified and responsible science editors to eliminate from publication those letters that are scientifically unsound and which constitute a potential for harm to the public.

3. The use of *Half-Truths*, where an out-of-context statement is used to imply a cause-and-effect relationship with some negative result alleged to have been caused by fluoridation: For example, fluoridation opponents claim that "fluoride is poison, so don't let them put it in our water." This statement ignores the principle that toxicity is related to dose of a substance and not to mere exposure to the substance itself. Chlorine, vitamin D, table salt, iodine, antibiotics, even water, serve as excellent examples of substances that are harmful in the wrong amounts but beneficial in the correct amounts.

Another example is: "fluoride causes dental fluorosis or mottling." By itself, this claim fails to take into account either the source of the fluoride, the amount of fluoride, the mechanism of fluoride exposure, or the time of exposure as related to the dental age of the person exposed. When this claim is made, opponents disingenuously equate fluoridation with the severe form of fluorosis, not the milder forms, even though they know their information is a misrepresentation of the facts. Community-water fluoridation is not responsible for causing the severe dental fluorosis depicted in the photos displayed by the anti-fluoridationists. As stated previously, approximately 13% of children who drink optimally fluoridated water will develop very mild fluorosis. Dental fluorosis as seen in the United States manifests primarily as the milder forms and has been mostly attributed to the inappropriate ingestion of large amounts of fluoride-containing dentifrice by young children who were not properly supervised during toothbrushing and to improper supplementation of fluoride through careless prescriptive practices. Anti-fluoridationists frequently adopt the intellectually dishonest practice of showing photographs of teeth with tetracycline staining or of extremely rare cases of severe dental fluorosis that have occurred in other countries because of extensive industrial pollution or long-term ingestion of extremely high naturally-occurring fluoride levels from noncommunal water sources. They then falsely claim that this will be the result for anyone, including adults, who might drink fluoridated water. As stated previously, adults are not at risk for dental fluorosis.

Another half-truth espoused frequently in the 1980s was: "The majority of AIDS victims come from fluoridated cities." This half-truth was frequently made in misguided attempts to persuade San Francisco's public into stopping fluoridation in that city. This claim continued to be made, even after the discovery of the virus that causes AIDS. While most AIDS patients coincidentally reside in major metropolitan areas and most major metropolitan areas are fluoridated (47 of the 50 largest cities in the United States), the anti-fluoridationists logic never did explain the high incidence of AIDS in Los Angeles, San Diego, or Newark (New Jersey), all not fluoridated at the time of the claim. This same anti-fluoridationist apparently changed his mind and claimed during his unsuccessful 1992 third-party campaign for the U.S. presidency, that AIDS is caused by the

AIDS drug AZT, implying that there is a plot by medical professionals, drug companies, and the government to infect certain groups with AIDS.

4. Utilization of *Innuendo:* A frequently used fluorophobic tome is, that "while one glass of fluoridated water will not kill anyone, it is the glass after glass of fluoridated water, as with cigarette after cigarette, that takes its toll in human health and life." This technique uses a guilt-by-association ploy, attempting to link the known health risks of cigarette smoking (for which there is substantial scientific evidence) to alleged risks from drinking fluoridated water (for which there is no scientific evidence).

Another oft-used claim by fluoridation opponents is that "insufficient research has been carried out to prove absolute safety, and therefore consumers and government officials are urged to wait until all doubt about the safety of fluoridation has been 'scientifically' resolved." This argument could be used indefinitely in that it is impossible to ever prove absolute safety for all time for anything. Unqualified acceptance of this argument would mean that literally all technologic advancements achieved in the age of science would have to be eliminated. Thousands of studies and untold risk-benefit analyses have shown that fluoridation is safe and effective for the entire population.

5. *Quoting of Inaccurate Statements and the Use of Statements Taken Out of Context:* The best way to illustrate this common technique of anti-fluoridationists is to refer to two frequently used anti-fluoridation publications, the *Lifesavers* (Sic) *Guide to Fluoridation* (a pamphlet)[197] and *Fluoride: the Aging Factor.*[198] (a book). Both use essentially the same "scientific references," both are distributed frequently in campaigns, opposing fluoridation, and both documents were marketed by their author as "scientific documents." The one-sheet pamphlet claimed over 250 references. Subsequently, a group of 20 scientists and public health officials from around the United States

did a systematic review, tracking down the original references in order to evaluate their validity as used by the author. The project took two years and resulted in the production of a 184-page monograph, entitled *Abuse of the Scientific Literature in an Anti-fluoridation Pamphlet.*[199] In the monograph, the 20 scientists documented that the information in the *Lifesavers (Sic) Guide to Fluoridation*[197] pamphlet was primarily fabricated pseudo-science for which no scientific evidence was available. Some of the findings of this protracted review included: (a) of the 250 references, only—48 were from reputable scientific journals; (b) 116 of the 250 references had no relevance to community water fluoridation whatsoever; (c) many of the references actually supported fluoridation with the works of respected scientists selectively quoted, misquoted, and misrepresented in order to make them appear to discourage the use of fluorides.[198]

6. *Quoting of Experts:* Some of the quoted experts have legitimate academic or professional credentials, although not necessarily in disciplines qualified to serve as experts in health research specific to fluorides. Moreover, anti-fluoridationists occasionally find a credentialed individual to speak against mainstream science. The statements by these marginalized individuals, while of questionable authority, are often exploited by the opposition.

Some nationally known figures who may have opposed fluoridation early in their professional life prior to the accumulation of overwhelming scientific evidence in its favor, often have their earlier statements quoted by anti-fluoridationists despite having publicly changed their position to one of support for fluoridation. As an example, the opposition repeatedly claim that Nobel Laureate and physician Hugo Theorell "condemns" fluoridation when, in fact, he publicly changed his position to one of support as far back as 1967. The public is further confused when anti-fluoride zealots utilize the services of "alternative medicine" spokespersons

to "prove" that the medical community is divided in its position on fluoridation. Unable to discriminate between legitimate scientists and purveyors of unproven therapies, some in the public see the dispute as a conflict between competing health care philosophies and ideologies.

7. *The Conspiracy Gambit:*[196] Because alleged conspiracies are difficult to disprove, they are a favorite of the health-conspiracy theorists. The alleged "conspirators" often include the American Medical Association, the American Dental Association, the American Council on Science and Health, the equipment and chemical supply companies, the Communist Party, both the aluminum and phosphate fertilizer industries, toothpaste manufacturers, or any other organization appearing to be threatening to the anti-fluoridationists. Highest on their list of conspirators is the "government" (including the Public Health Service, the Environmental Protection Agency, the prestigious National Institutes of Health, the world-renowned Centers for Disease Control, and the Food & Drug Administration). Conspiracies generate a tremendous amount of anger among those susceptible to conspiracy propaganda, a factor that negatively impacts fluoridation efforts.

8. *The use of Scare Words:*[196] Anti-fluoridationists frequently play on the current phobias and concerns of the public by describing fluoridation in ecologically-linked or environmentally-loaded terms or phrases such as, "pollutant, toxic waste product, chemical by-product, dumped in the water, or forced down our throats." Fluoride is also frequently linked by fluorophobics with words like "poison, genetic damage, cancer, AIDS, or artificial"—words that certainly conjure up fear by the public when linked to something to which they think they will be unwittingly exposed. Fear is a major factor that negatively impacts fluoridation efforts.

9. *The Debate Ploy:*[196,200] The opponents of fluoridation often try to entice unsuspecting media commentators, government officials, or program planners into holding a debate on the "pros and cons" of fluoridation. Proponents of fluoride are then often trapped into consenting to public debates. Jarvis has published a list of reasons for not debating the anti-science health viewpoint: (a) the purpose of the debate is to win the audience, not to discover truth. Science is not decided by debating in a public forum, but by careful experimentation, confirmation of findings through independently conducted experiments, submission of all findings to qualified colleagues and peers for critical analysis, and publication of findings in reputable peer-reviewed journals. In a debate, even though the proponents may win the debate, they are just as likely to lose the audience. (b) In media circles, there is a saying that "everyone is the same size on television." In other words, debates give the illusion that a scientific controversy exists when, in reality, this is not the case. Public debates also promote the illusion that there are equal numbers of "scientists" on each side of the issue. The vision of "dueling PhD's or dueling doctors" encourages the public to reject fluoridation until the "experts on both sides can agree." (c) An opponent of fluoridation, utilizing the laundry list approach, can present more misinformation in 5 minutes than can be refuted in 5 hours, thus fostering confusion on the part of the public. Proponents are never provided enough time to adequately refute the opponents' charges, because complete refutations, by their nature, take much longer than the sound-bite length charges of the anti-fluoridationists. (d) Public exposure favors the opponent, enabling him or her to gain name recognition for the viewpoint they are promoting. By sharing the platform with respected scientists who are there to defend fluoridation, equal status and credibility is granted. Anti-fluoride groups often "attach" themselves to other organizations' events in order to draw attention to their cause. (e) It is difficult to compete in a debate without ap-

pearing to discredit the opponents personally. When a fluoridation proponent is refuting a negative statement made by the anti-fluoridation spokesperson who is spreading misinformation, the proponent has to be able to separate the anti-science message from the anti-science messenger, an extremely difficult task. Moreover, the debate format often favors the maverick viewpoint as the perceived underdog, as in a David vs. Goliath showdown, generating sympathy for the anti-fluoridation perspective. One of the strategies used by anti-fluoridationists in a debate setting is to intimidate the proponent(s) by threatening to file a lawsuit for defamation of character. This strategy is very unsettling for an untrained proponent who often loses focus, confidence, and becomes ineffective as a debater. When such a threat is made in a debate, it is hard to remember that few lawsuits have actually been filed and none of these lawsuits have been successfully prosecuted by any of the anti-fluoridationists.

Five additional anti-fluoridationist techniques not cited by Bernhardt & Sprague in their paper because they have appeared since its publication include the use of contrived organizations, subversion of the media, commandeering established organizations, misuse of electronic publishing, and commandeering meetings.[2]

(1) The *use of contrived organizations* is most disturbing:[2] The opponents often form their own pseudo-scientific organizations having names that sound like legitimate scientific entities, but which are in reality, front organizations for the anti-fluoridationist movement.

(2) *Subversion of the media:*[2] The job of the media is to present all sides of an issue. Often the media appear to be more interested in publicizing a controversy than in accurately representing an issue.[2] Many campaign committees have encountered a popular media philosophy "if it bleeds, it leads". Moreover, it is often more profitable for the media to do a story on the "dangers" of fluoridation which can be sensationalized than to do one on the many scientifically sound, but emotionally unexciting, reasons for supporting fluoridation. Also, the anti-establishment and anti-science viewpoint tends to be more flamboyant and interesting to a media seeking to portray readily understandable examples of John Q. Public fighting city hall. It is important to remember that scientific rebuttals to flamboyant anti-fluoridation claims are often, by their nature, dry, unemotional, complex, difficult to explain in lay terms, hard for the public to grasp conceptually, and difficult for the media to interpret and report.

(3) *Commandeering Established Organizations:*[2] In several instances, anti-fluoridationists have commandeered established organizations in an attempt to gain access to the organization's credibility for the anti-fluoride cause.[2] Two recent examples involve the Pennsylvania Sierra Club and one of the collective bargaining units for the U.S. Environmental Protection Agency. In August 1997, a member of the Pennsylvania Chapter of the Sierra Club held a press conference in Harrisburg in which she claimed that the Sierra Club called for a ban on fluoridation in that state.[2,201] Within a few days, the officers of the Chapter issued an official statement rebuking the member's action and stating that the press conference was held "without the knowledge or authorization of any Pennsylvania Sierra Club officer."[2,202]

The U.S. Environmental Protection Agency (EPA) has over 18,000 employees represented mostly by four collective bargaining units. The smallest of these bargaining units was Local 2050 of the National Federation of Federal Employees (NFFE), a union that variously claimed to represent about 900, 1000, 1100, and finally 1550 EPA employees, but whose dues-paying membership was apparently much less.[2]

About 20 dissident members of the union held a meeting on July 2, 1997, where a minority of them voted to oppose California's mandatory fluoridation law.[2] A subsequent press conference falsely claimed that all union members unanimously approved the resolution and subsequent mass mailings of propaganda leaflets from two of the union's anti-fluoride activists falsely implied that the USEPA opposed fluoridation.[2,203]

(4) *Misuse of Electronic Publishing:*[2] Numerous anti-fluoridation websites have been established in order to promote the anti-fluoride political agenda and to recruit converts to their movement.[2] In addition, many "alternative medicine" websites have included anti-fluoridation sections as part of their marketing effort, along with information that: opposes traditional scientific medical practice, attacks orthodox medical practice, including such widely accepted public-health practices as immunization programs. Many of these anti-fluoridation web sites contain "articles," letters, endorsements, or references to purveyors of "alternative" or "complementary medicine." Some also contain links to websites operated by practitioners and marketers of non-scientific therapies.

(5) *Commandeering Meetings:*[2] Often, anti-fluoridation spokespersons attempt to insert themselves into the agenda of scheduled meetings or hearings in order to gain a forum from which to disseminate their anti-fluoridation message.[2] It is not uncommon for anti-fluoridationists to attempt to utilize question and answer periods in public meetings to espouse the "pitfalls" of fluoridation rather than to ask questions of scheduled speakers. Town meetings, allegedly scheduled to provide opportunities for proponents and opponents to present their cases, often serve as a convenient forum from which anti-fluoridation spokespersons try to dominate the available time.

**Question 7**

Which of the following statements is correct, if any?

A. Pseudo-science can prevail over science when the electorate is not familiar with either side of the subject being debated.

B. Fear is often used by fluoridation opponents to create doubt about the safety and benefits of fluoridation.

C. Support by practicing dentists and dental hygienists for community water fluoridation is incongruent with American Dental Association's ethical standards.

D. The use of half-truths to imply a cause-and-effect relationship such as "fluoride is a poison, so don't let them put it in our water" is a common technique employed by fluoridation opponents.

E. In a debate, one speaker's truth is no more authoritative than the second speaker's misinformation in a highly technical discussion.

## Risk Communication

Community water fluoridation, while long accepted by qualified scientists and credible professional organizations as a safe, effective, efficient, economic, socially equitable, and environmentally sound public-health activity, has endured attacks from a small, but highly vocal, group of tenacious antagonists throughout its 56-year history. These attacks have served to raise questions among some members of the public, have sometimes served as a convenient excuse for elected officials to avoid making decisions to fluoridate individual community water systems, and have accommodated some in the media where the issue is often exploited so as to appear to be a rift among "experts" on both sides of the issue, creating doubt among the public about the issue. Most communities

successfully work through the "controversy," usually a result of hard work by health professionals and sustained objectivity on the part of community leaders and elected officials. Often misinformation is broadly disseminated, adversely influencing community sentiment such that other measures become necessary to counter the mass phobia sometimes generated during the legislative, campaign or administrative process.

Risk communication is a recent addition to the armamentarium of health professionals promoting fluoridation in their communities. It serves as a mechanism by which to counter some of the negative community sentiment generated during attempts to fluoridate communities. Sandman has classified this intense negative feeling about what is perceived by some to be a health risk as *outrage*.[172] According to Sandman, the public defines risk in terms of "levels of outrage". The scientific and health community, who define risk in terms of "hazard, are often too slow to recognize the disparity between actual risk (hazard) as calculated by the scientific community and perceived risk (outrage) as echoed by the public.[172] According to Sandman, the public pays far too little attention to hazard, while most experts pay absolutely no attention to outrage.[172] A public whose level of outrage has been heightened by a well-orchestrated anti-fluoridation campaign, will be less receptive to educational campaigns by proponents of fluoride until the level of outrage is reduced. Pertinent risk information cannot be communicated when the level of outrage is high because the intended recipients of the information cannot collate the complex explanations while frightened by the fluoridation message and/or angry at the fluoridation messenger.

Scholars of risk perception have defined more than 20 factors that affect the public's level of outrage. A few of Sandman's favorite factors are presented as follows (see Sandman/Table 8–9).

- **Voluntariness:** A voluntary risk is much more acceptable to people than a risk felt by the public to have been coerced because a voluntary risk generates little or no outrage.[204] Voluntariness helps explain why antifluoridation propagandists will offer organized voluntary fluoride supplement programs as an acceptable (to them) alternative to "coerced" community water fluoridation.[204]

- **Control:** When disease prevention and exposure mitigation are in the hands of individuals (fluoride supplements), the risk (though not the hazard) is perceived by them to be much lower than when the same programs are controlled by a government agency (municipal water system and health department).

- **Fairness:** People who feel that they are enduring greater risks than their neighbors, especially if they feel that they are without access to greater benefits, are naturally outraged, more so if the rationale for increasing their risk appears to have been decided through the political process rather than through science.[204] Even though fluoridation benefits people of all ages, older Americans often assume that it only benefits children and frequently complain that they are being put at risk without accruing any benefits themselves.

- **Process:** Sometimes the process by which fluoridation is approved becomes the principle focus of the public's outrage, particularly when the agency or group promoting fluoridation portrays itself as arrogant rather than concerned, dishonest rather than trustworthy, and manipulative rather than collaborative.[204]

- **Morality:** American society has evolved in its thinking about pollution to feel that it is not just harmful, it is morally evil.[204] Fluoridation opponents often attempt to portray fluoridation as a form of pollution and claim

that fluoride chemicals are products marketed by the chemical industry as beneficial (fluoridation) in order to avoid paying the costs to dispose of these chemicals. When fluoridation proponents start talking about cost-risk tradeoffs in this kind of political climate, they often appear to be callously advocating a morally relevant risk.

- **Familiarity:** Exotic, high-tech facilities and processes (computer-monitored water treatment plants that add fluoride and other chemicals) provoke more outrage than do familiar risks (fluoride-containing toothpaste as part of home dental care).[204]

- **Memorability:** A memorable accident (especially one involving chemicals or radiation, like Love Canal (New York), Bhopal (India), Times Beach (Missouri), Three-Mile Island (Pennsylvania), or Chernobyl (Ukraine), makes the potential risk easier to imagine and therefore, perceived to be more risky.[204] A strategy used by fluoridation opponents is to attempt to engender fear among the public by emphasizing the statistically minute potential of overfluoridation or hyperfluoridation as if it were a likely catastrophic event.

- **Dread:** Illnesses like cancer, AIDS, Alzheimer's disease, or end stage renal disease are more dreaded than dental caries.[204] Fluoridation opponents help incite fear among the public by falsely claiming that fluoridation causes these dreaded diseases or makes them incurable, while at the same time attempting to minimize fluoridation's strong preventive effect on dental caries.

- **Diffusion in Time and Space:** Hazard-A (rampant dental caries) ultimately could result in the deaths of 50 or more anonymous people a year across the country, while Hazard-B (a poorly monitored and poorly operated fluoridation system) resulted in one very well publicized death recently (despite 56 years of safe, effective fluoridation efforts that daily benefited tens of millions of people).[204]

## Myths and Actions Related to Risk Communication

Some of those involved in community organization for fluoridation promotion fail to properly consider the role of outrage in the community decision-making process. They assume that the public will trust them and that by merely presenting the scientific data, the public will be "won over." By ignoring the role of outrage, they miss the opportunity to succeed through use of a collaborative effort in community education and community decision-making. Chess and others have categorized a number of *myths* and actions *related to risk communication*.[205] Ten of them include:

- **Myth 1:** Because the fluoridation referendum is so close, we don't have enough time and resources to have a risk communication program.[205]

- **Action 1:** Train fluoridation proponents to communicate more effectively. Plan projects such that there is time to involve the public in priority setting and decision-making.[205]

- **Myth 2:** Telling the public about a potential risk related to fluoridation is more likely to unduly alarm people than keeping quiet.[205]

- **Action 2:** Fluoridation proponents can decrease the potential for alarm by giving the public a chance to express their concerns and by appropriately responding to these concerns.[205]

- **Myth 3:** Communication is less important than education. If people knew the true risks related to fluoridation, they would accept them.[205]

- **Action 3:** Pay as much attention to your process for dealing with people and their fears of fluoridation as you do to explaining the scientific data.[205]

- **Myth 4:** We shouldn't go to the public until we can provide answers or solutions to all their perceived fears about fluoridation.[205]

- **Action 4:** Provide information about fluoridation and discuss concerns about risk man-

agement options. Involve the community in the development of strategies for which they have a stake.[205]

- **Myth 5:** These issues and this scientific data regarding fluoridation are too difficult for the public to understand.[205]

- **Action 5:** Separate public disagreement with your fluoridation promotion practices from misunderstanding of the highly technical issues related to fluoridation.[205]

- **Myth 6:** One of the easiest myths for dental professionals to embrace is that technical decisions should be left in the hands of technical people.[205]

- **Action 6:** Provide the public with information about fluoridation. Listen to community concerns about fluoridation. Involve people with diverse backgrounds on the fluoridation committee so that much thought and discussion goes into developing fluoridation policies and strategies.[205]

- **Myth 7:** I am just a dentist/dental hygienist, risk communication is not my job.[205]

- **Action 7:** As a public servant, whether the fluoridation promoter works for a health department or has a private dental/dental hygiene practice, you have a responsibility to the public. Learn to integrate risk communication into your efforts and help others from the fluoridation committee do the same.[205]

- **Myth 8:** If we give them an inch, they will take a mile.[205]

- **Action 8:** If you listen to people when they are asking for inches, they are less likely to demand miles. Avoid the battleground that could result from attempts to stifle discussion about all aspects of fluoridation. Do not attempt to stifle discussion of issues about which fluoridation proponents are uncomfortable. Involve the public early and often.[205]

- **Myth 9:** If we listen to the public complain about risks from fluoridation, we will devote scarce resources to issues that are not really a great threat to the public's health.[205]

- **Action 9:** Listen carefully and early to avoid controversy and the potential for disproportionate attention to lesser issues.[205]

- **Myth 10:** Activist anti-fluoride groups are responsible for stirring up unwarranted concerns.[205]

- **Action 10:** Anti-fluoride activists help to focus public anger. Work hard to gain the public's trust early, so that you can work with responsible public groups to promote the adoption of responsible public policy regarding fluoridation.[205]

Covello and Allen[206,207] have developed a list of *Ten Deadly Sins of Communication*. They are fairly self-explanatory and follow: (1) appearing unprepared; (2) handling questions improperly; (3) apologizing for yourself or your organization; (4) not knowing knowable information; (5) unprofessional use of audiovisual aids; (6) seeming to be off schedule; (7) not involving participants; (8) not establishing rapport; (9) appearing disorganized; and (10) providing the wrong content.

It remains obvious that the mere dissemination of information to the public, without any attempts to communicate the complexities and uncertainties of risk, does not necessarily ensure that the public will understand or accept community water fluoridation. Well-managed risk-communication efforts will help ensure that the public is provided with messages that are constructively formulated, transmitted, and received, and that they will be more likely to result in positive thoughts and an acceptance of fluoridation. In the words of Baruch Fischhoff, "If we have not gotten our message across, then we ought to assume that the fault is not with our receivers."[208]

## Principles of Risk Communication

The *principles of risk communication*, if practiced universally, can go a long way towards increasing the speed with which the public accepts community water fluoridation as a local policy

option. Covello and Allen[208] have developed *Seven Cardinal Principles of Risk Communication*, all designed to help fluoridation promoters accomplish their goals.

1. **Accept and involve the public as a partner.** Your goal is to produce a public informed about the advantages of fluoridation, not to defuse public concerns or replace actions.

2. **Plan carefully and evaluate your efforts.** Different goals, audiences, and media require different approaches and different actions.

3. **Listen to the public's specific concerns.** People often care more about trust, credibility, competence, fairness, and empathy than about statistics and details.

4. **Be honest, frank, and open.** Trust and credibility are difficult to obtain and, once lost, are almost impossible to regain.

5. **Work with other credible sources.** Conflicts and disagreements among organizations make communication with the public much more difficult.

6. **Meet the needs of the media.** The media are usually more interested in controversy than risk, simplicity than complexity, danger than safety. Help them understand the differences.

7. **Speak clearly and with compassion.** Never let your efforts prevent your acknowledging the tragedy of an illness, injury, or death, or even their potential. Acknowledge and empathize with people's fears. People can understand risk information, but they may still not agree with you. Some people will never be satisfied with your answers.

## SUMMARY

Water fluoridation is the prime example of community-based caries prevention where the benefits accrue to all individuals consuming drinking water that is optimally fluoridated without regard to socioeconomic status. Fluoridation remains a safe, effective, efficient, economical, environmentally sound, and socially equitable public health measure to prevent dental caries.[2] It also fulfills all of the requirements of an excellent public policy.[2] Based upon extensive scientific evidence, regarding the safety and effectiveness of fluoridation, numerous national and international organizations and agencies have advocated for the adoption of fluoridation as a means of reducing dental caries in a community. Despite some minor opposition that sporadically delayed fluoridation's implementation in some locales, substantial progress has been made toward achieving the long-term goal of universal fluoridation in the United States. While the opposition to fluoridation has been fairly disorganized and generally not too effective, recent opposition from "alternative medicine" zealots and purveyors of unproved health modalities suggests that the public, elected officials, and the media may be both confused and unduly influenced in the future by such open support of anti-fluoridation efforts. Open opposition to fluoridation gives the "alternative medicine" promoters a convenient public forum with which to stress their "philosophical" differences from traditional science-based health care. The dental profession should educate the public, using risk-communication principles as a standard business practice to assist patients in obtaining accurate information about fluoridation.

What needs to be kept in perspective is the tremendous success that health professionals have had in bringing community water fluoridation, one of the greatest public-health achievements of the 20th century, to more and more Americans each year. The Surgeon General of the United States has included a fluoridation objective in his *Year 2010 Health Objectives for the Nation.*[7,209] By the year 2010, 75% of the population on community-water systems should live in communities with fluoridated water according to one of the document's goals. Given the substantial growth in population in the U.S. since the last official fluoridation census was published in 1992 where over 62% of the population on community-water systems were benefiting from fluoridation, and the addition of millions of people because of recent successful fluoridation campaigns in Los Angeles, San Diego, Las Vegas, San Antonio, and Salt Lake City, the gap between those who have access to fluoridated water and those who do not have access to this public-health measure is beginning to be acknowledged by policy makers, community leaders, and health professionals (see Figure 8–5, Fluoridation Growth).

As health professionals, we must realize "oral health is not solely dependent on individual behaviors," that attainment of optimal oral health requires a partnership between the dental health profession and both the patient and their community. "Universal access to fluoride requires a community's commitment to water fluoridation"

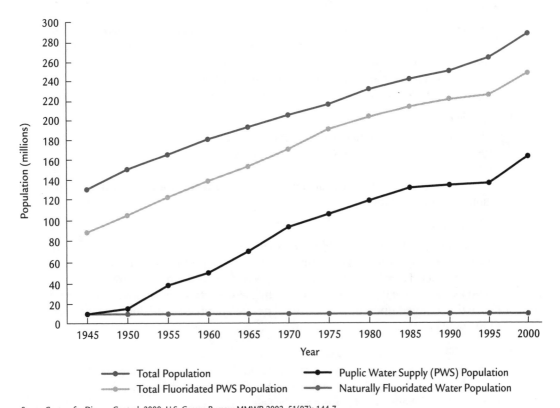

*Source:* Centers for Disease Control, 2000; U.S. Census Bureau; MMWR 2002, 51(07); 144-7.

FIGURE 8–5    Fluoridation Growth, by Population, United States, 1945–2000. (*Source:* Centers for Disease Control, 2000; U.S. Census Bureau; *MMWR 2002*, 51(07);144–7.)

and the dental profession must provide the leadership, technical expertise and guidance to policy makers as well as to the public to bring fluoridation to fruition. Every dental office, dental health department, community dental health program, and dental school should have copies of the American Dental Association's monograph, *Fluoridation Facts* in its libraries in order to be adequately briefed on the issue.

## ANSWERS AND EXPLANATIONS

1. A, B, C, D—correct.

   E—incorrect. The recommended optimal range of fluoride concentrations in drinking water is .7 to 1.2 ppm depending on mean annual temperature.

2. A, B, C, E—correct.

   D—incorrect. All fluoride-containing dentifrices have very high levels of fluoride (1,100 to 1,500 ppm) and are a significant source of fluoride overexposure and fluorosis.

3. A, B, E—correct.

   C—incorrect. Discontinuation of fluoridation has a significant deleterious impact on dental-caries rates; several studies have consistently shown that dental-caries rates increase dramatically when fluoridation is discontinued.

   D—incorrect. The national cost-benefit ratio has been demonstrated to be 80:1 where for every $1 dollar spent on fluoridation, $80 is saved in treatment costs.

4. A, D, E—correct.

   B—incorrect. No credible scientific evidence has associated water fluoridation with cancer, and the National Cancer Institute has not recommended the cessation of fluoridation.

   C—incorrect. Hydrofluosilicic acid is the most frequently used chemical for community water fluoridation.

5. A, B, D—correct.

   C—incorrect. The likelihood of voting *increases* with education as well as age and income, resulting in certain groups making up a disproportionate share of voters.

   E—incorrect. From a public-policy perspective, fluoridation is more often perceived as a *local issue* that is enacted either by *governmental administrative action* (ordinance that is voted upon by a city council or city/county commission) or by a vote of the public.

6. D—correct.

   A—incorrect. First, newspapers usually do not have experts in all technical areas; secondly, they try to publish an equal number from each side of an issue to be fair, to encourage debate—and to promote the sale of the paper.

   B—incorrect. In 1985, the Federal Communications Commission (FCC) ruled that the Fairness Doctrine, requiring that broadcasters provide a reasonable oppor-

tunity for the presentation of opposing views on controversial public issues is *no longer needed*. With the end of the Fairness Doctrine, neither radio program hosts nor stations have an obligation to provide balance or present competing views.

C—incorrect for the same reasons as A.

E—incorrect. The downside of internet use as a source of valid information is that much of the health information available on the web is opinion-based and has not gone through a rigorous scientific review process, putting the onus on the public for discerning truth from fiction regarding the information presented.

7. A, B, D, E—correct.

C—incorrect. The third of the five major ethical principles included in the American Dental Association's *Principles of Ethics and Code of Professional Conduct* is the *Principle of Beneficence* that expressly states ". . . that professionals have the duty to act for the benefit of others." Directly related to this specific ethical principle is a designated Code of Professional Responsibility regarding Community Service, that further states that ". . . dentists have an obligation to use their skills, knowledge, and experience for the improvement of the dental health of the public and they are encouraged to be leaders in their community. Support by practicing dentists and dental hygienists for community water fluoridation *is congruent* with the American Dental Association's ethical standards.

## Self-Evaluation Questions

1. The first person to demonstrate the relationship between dental caries and water fluoride levels in the United States was _____ (U.S. Public Health Officer).

2. The apparent reduction in measurable water fluoridation benefits resulting from the ubiquitous availability of fluoride from other sources in both fluoridated and fluoride-deficient comparison communities is known as _____.

3. The extension of the benefits of community water fluoridation to residents of fluoride-deficient communities due to the transport of food and beverages commercially prepared with fluoridated water is known as _____; it is called the _____ effect.

4. A _____ **analysis** is used to relate the dollar cost of water fluoridation to the treatment costs saved.

5. The major posteruptive effect of fluoride from community water supplies is its reduction of _____ and enhancement of _____.

6. Other community-based methods of providing fluoride to communities where water fluoridation is not feasible include _____ and _____.

7. _____ communication is a new tool to be used by dental and public health professionals in order to assist communities in choosing to fluoridate their community water systems.

8. Jarvis recommends that dental and public health professionals not get involved in a _____ with antifluoridationists because the primary goal of such an activity is to win the audience rather than to discover scientific truths.

9. _____ has stated that the use of sodium silicofluoride and hydrofluosilicic acid for fluoridating community water systems serves as an excellent example of beneficial recycling, where both industry and the public benefit.

10. _____ state(s) (plus the District of Columbia and Puerto Rico) currently mandate(s) statewide fluoridation through legislation, while state(s) have/has mandated statewide fluoridation through administrative regulation.

11. Every recent _____ of the U.S. Public Health Service has recognized the value of community water fluoridation and has promoted its adoption as good public policy.

12. The level of risk as perceived by the public (perceived risk) is often defined by community organizers as _____ while the level of risk as determined by science-based experts (actual risk) is often defined by community organizers as _____

13. A _____ is an election which has been designed to affirm, change, or cancel previously established legislation, while a voter _____ is an election that was petitioned by voters to establish a law requiring something (for example requiring fluoridation or banning fluoridation).

14. In the final analysis, winning a fluoridation campaign depends more upon _____ than on knowledge of fluoridation.

15. Radio talk shows or "talk radio" are a powerful force in U.S. politics today, in part because of the end of the _____ as well as changing technology.

# REFERENCES

1. American Dental Association Council on Access, Prevention and Interprofessional Relations (1999). *Fluoridation Facts*.
2. Easley, M. (2000). Opposition to community water fluoridation and connections to the "alternative medicine" movement. *Sci Rev Altern Med*, 5(1):24–31.
3. Easley, M. W. (1995). Celebrating 50 years of fluoridation: a public health success story. *Br Dent J*, January 21:72–5.
4. U.S. Department of Health and Human Services, Public Health Service (1983). *Surgeon General statement on community water fluoridation (Dr. C. Everett Koop)*. Washington, DC: February 8.
5. U.S. Department of Health and Human Services, Public Health Service (1995). *Surgeon General statement on community water fluoridation (Dr. Antonio Novello)*. Washington, DC: December 14.
6. National Institute of Dental and Craniofacial Research, National Institutes of Health (2000). *First-ever Surgeon General's Report on Oral Health Finds Profound Disparities in Nation's Population*. Bethseda, MD: March 25.

7. U.S. Department of Health and Human Services (2000). *Oral Health in America: a report of the surgeon general*. Rockville, MD: U.S. Department of Health and Human Services, National Institute of Dental and Craniofacial Research, National Institutes of Health.

8. U.S. Department of Health and Human Services, Centers for Disease Control, *Fluoridation Census*, September 1993 and Supplement; Atlanta.

9. Ripa, L. W. (1999). Water Fluoridation (Chapter 8). In: Harris, N.O., & Garcia-Godoy, F., eds. *Primary Preventive Dentistry, 5th ed.* Stamford, Connecticut: Appleton and Lange, 658 pp.

10. McClure, F. J. (1970). *Water fluoridation. The search and the victory*. Washington, DC: U.S. Government Printing Office.

11. Murray, J. J., Rugg-Gunn, A. J., & Jenkins, G. N. (1991). *Fluorides in caries prevention* (3rd ed.) Oxford: Butterworth-Heinemann, Ltd.

12. Leske, G. S. (1983). Water fluoridation. In Mellberg, J. R., & Ripa, L. W., Eds. *Fluoride in preventive dentistry*. Chicago: Quintessence Publishing Co., p. 290.

13. Harris, N. O., & Garcia-Godoy, F. (1999). *Primary Preventive Dentistry, 5th ed.* Stamford, Connecticut: Appleton and Lange, 658 pp.

14. Burt, B. A., & Eklund, S. A. (1992). *Dentistry, dental practice, and the community (4th ed.)* Philadelphia, PA: W.B. Saunders Company.

15. Dean, H. T. (1938). Endemic fluorosis and its relation to dental caries. *Public Health Reports*, 53(33):1443–52.

16. Dean, H. T., Arnold, F. A., & Elvove, E. (1942). Domestic water and dental caries. *Public Health Reports*, 57(32):1155–79.

17. U.S. Department of Health and Human Services (1998). *Healthy People 2010 Objectives: Draft for public comment* (Oral Health Section). Washington, DC: U.S. Government Printing Office, September 15.

18. Personal communications (e-mail) from Dr. Mark Greer; November 13, 2000.

19. Personal communications (e-mail) from Teran Gall, CDA; November 13, 2000.

20. Loh, T. (1996). Thirty-eight years of water fluoridation—the Singapore scenario. *Community Dent Health*, 13(Suppl 2):47–50.

21. British Fluoridation Society (1998). *Optimal water fluoridation: status worldwide*. Liverpool, May.

22. U.S. Centers for Disease Control & Prevention (1999). Ten great public health achievements: United States, 1900–1999. *MMWR*, 48(12):241–43.

23. Arnold, F. A. Jr., Likins, R. C., Russell, A. L., & Scott, D. B. (1962). Fifteenth year of the Grand Rapids fluoridation study. *J Am Dent Assoc*, 65:780–85.

24. Stamm, J. W., Banting, D. W., & Imrey, P. B. (1990). Adult root caries survey of two similar communities with contrasting natural water fluoride levels. *J Am Dent Assoc*, 120:143–49.

25. National Institutes of Health (1987). *Oral health of United States adults. The national survey of oral health in U.S. employed adults and seniors: 1985–1986. National findings*. NIH Pub. No. 87-2868. U.S. Department of Health and Human Services: August.

26. Grembowski, D., Fiset, L., & Spadafora, A. (1992). How fluoridation affects adult dental caries. *J Am Dent Assoc*, 123:49–54.

27. Newbrun, E. (1989). Effectiveness of water fluoridation. *J Public Health Dent*, 49(Special Issue):279–89.

28. Newbrun, E. (1992). Current regulations and recommendations concerning water fluoridation, fluoride supplements, and topical fluoride agents. *J Dent Res*, 67:1255–65.

29. Brunelle, J. A., & Carlos, J. P. (1990). Recent trends in dental caries in U.S. children and the effect of water fluoridation. *I Dent Res*, 69(Special Issue):723–27.

30. Kaminsky, L. S., Mahoney, M. C., Leach, J., Melius, J., & Miller, M. J. (1990). Fluoride benefits and risks of exposure. *Crit Rev Oral Biol Med*, 1:261–81.

31. Barnard, P. D., & Sivaneswaran, S. (1990). Oral health of Tamworth schoolchildren 24 years after fluoridation. *J Dent Res*, 69(Div. Abstr.): 934. Abstr. 9.

32. McDonagh, M. Whiting, P., Bradley, M., Cooper, J., Sutton, A., Chestnutt, I., Misso, K., Wilson, P., Treasure, E., & Kleijnen, J. (2000). *A systematic review of public water fluoridation*. University of York: NHS Centre for Reviews and Dissemination.

33. Morris, J., & White, D. (2000). The York Review of Water Fluoridation-key points for the busy practitioner. *Dent Update*, December, 474–5.

34. Burt, B. A. (1985), Fluoride: How much of a good thing? *J Public Health Dent*, 5:37–38.

35. Horowitz, H. S. (1991). Appropriate uses of fluoride: Considerations for the '90s. *J Public Health Dent*, 51:20–22.

36. Rozler, R. G. (1995). The effectiveness of community water fluoridation: Beyond dummy variables for fluoride exposure. *I Public Health Dent*, 55:195.

37. Horowitz, H. S. (1996). The effectiveness of community water fluoridation in the United States. *J Public Health Dent*, 56(5 Spec No):253–8.

38. Stookey, G. K. (1994). Review of fluorosis risk of self-applied topical fluorides: Dentifrices, mouthrinses and gels. *Community Dent Oral Epidemiol*, 22:181–86.

39. Clovis, J., & Hargreaves, J. A. (1988). Fluoride intake from beverage consumption. *Community Dent Oral Epidemiol*, 16:11–15.

40. Slade, G. D., Davies, M. J., Spencer, A. J., & Stewart, J. F. (1995). Associations between exposure to fluoridated drinking water and dental caries experience among children in two Australian states. *J Public Health Dent*, 55:218–28.

41. Moreno, E. C. (1983). Role of Ca-P-F in caries prevention: Chemical aspects. *Int Dent J*, 43:71–80.

42. Newbrun, E. (1986). *Fluorides and dental caries (3rd ed.)* Springfield, IL: Charles C. Thomas, publisher, p. 289.

43. Lambrou, D., Larsen, M., Fejerskov, O., & Tachos, B. (1981). The effect of fluoride in saliva on remineralization of dental enamel in humans. *Caries Res*, 15:341–5.

44. Backer-Dirks, O., Kunzel, W., & Carlos, J. P. (1978). Caries-preventive water fluoridation. In Progress in caries prevention. Ericsson Y, Ed. *Caries Res*, 12(Suppl 1):7–14.

45. Silverstone, L. M. (1993). Remineralization and enamel caries: new concepts. *Dental Update*, May: 261–73.

46. Featherstone, J. D. (1987). The mechanism of dental decay. *Nutrition Today*, 22(3): 10–16.

47. Fejerskov, O., Thylstrup, A., & Larsen, M. J. (1981). Rational use of fluorides in caries prevention. *Acta Odontol Scan*, 39:241–9.

48. Silverstone, L. M., Wefel, J. S., Zimmerman, B. F., Clarkson, B. H., & Featherstone, M. J. (1981). Remineralization of natural and artificial lesions in human dental enamel in vitro. *Caries Res*, 15:138–57.

49. Bowen, W. H., & Geddes, D. A. M. (1990). Summary of Session III: Fluoride in saliva and dental plaque. *J Dent Res*, 69(Special Issue):637.

50. Beltran, E. D., & Burt, B. A. (1988). The pre- and post-eruptive effects of fluoride in the caries decline. *J Public Health Dent*, 48:233–40.

51. Whitford, G. M. (1996). The metabolism and toxicity of fluoride (2nd rev. ed.) *Monographs in Oral Science*, Vol. 16. Basel, Switzerland: Karger.

52. Horowitz, H. S. (1986). Indexes for measuring dental fluorosis. *J Public Health Dentistry*, 46(4):179–83.

53. Pendrys, D. G. (2000). Risk of enamel fluorosis in nonfluoridated and optimally fluoridated populations: considerations for the dental professional. *J Am Dent Assoc*, 131:746–55.

54. Den Besten, P. K. (1999). Mechanism and timing of fluoride effects on developing enamel. *J Public Health Dent*, 59(4):247–51.

55. Dean, H. T. (1942). The investigation of physiological effects by the epidemiological method. In Moulton, F. R., Ed. Fluorine and dental health. *American Association for the Advancement of Science*, Publication No. 19. Washington DC: 23–31.

56. Cutress, T. W., & Suckling, G. W. (1990). Differential diagnosis of dental fluorosis. *J Dent Res*, 69(Special Issue):714–720. Discussion 721.

57. Dean, H. T. (1936). Chronic endemic dental fluorosis. *J Am Med Assoc*, 107(16):1269–73.

58. Lewis, D. W., & Banting, D. W. (1994). Water Fluoridation: current effectiveness and dental fluorosis. *Community Dent Oral Epidemiol*, 22:153–8.

59. Lemke, C. W., Doherty, J. M., & Arra, M. C. (1970). Controlled fluoridation: The dental effects of discontinuation in Antigo, Wisconsin. *J Am Dent Assoc*, 80:782–86.

60. Stephen, K. W., McCall, D. R., & Tullis, J. I. (1987). Caries prevalence in Northern Scotland before and 5 years after water defluoridation. *Brit Dent J*, 163:324–26.

61. Attwood, D., & Blinkhorn, A. S. (1991). Dental health in schoolchildren 5 years after water fluoridation ceased in south-west Scotland. *Int Dent J*, 41(1):43–8.

62. U.S. Public Health Service (1991). *Report of the Ad Hoc Subcommittee on Fluoride of the Committee to Coordinate Environmental Health and Related Programs. Review of Fluoride Benefits and Risks.* Washington, DC: U.S. Dept. of Health and Human Services.

63. Way, R. M. (1964). The effect on dental caries of a change from a naturally fluoridated to a fluoride-free communal water. *J Dent Child*, 31:151–7.

64. White, B. A., Antezak-Bouckoms, A. A., & Weinstein, M. C. (1989). Issues in the economic evaluation of community water fluoridation. *J Dent Educ*, 53:646–57.

65. Ringelberg, M. L., Allen, S. J., & Jackson Brown, L. (1992). Cost of fluoridation: 44 Florida communities. *J Public Health Dent*, 52:75–80

66. U.S. Department of Health and Human Services, Centers for Disease Control (1992). Morbidity and mortality weekly report: a framework for assessing the effectiveness of disease and injury prevention. *MMWR*, 41:1–7.

67. Speier and Brown, Assembly Members, and Maddy, California Legislature, 1995–96, Regular Session Senator, Assembly Bill No. 733, February 22, 1995.

68. Neenan, M. E. (1996). Obstacles to extending fluoridation in the United States. *Community Dental Health*, 13(Suppl 2):10–20.

69. Blair, K. P. (1992). Fluoridation in the 1990s. *J Am Coll Dent*, 59:3.

70. Mjor, I. A. (1989). Amalgam and composite resin restorations: Longevity and reasons for replacement. In Anusavice, K. J., Ed. *Quality Evaluations of Dental Restorations*. Chicago: Quintessence Publishing Co. pp. 61–72.

71. MacInnis, W. A., Ismail, A., Brogan, H., & Kavanagh, M. (1990). Placement and replacement of restorations in a military population. *J Dent Res*, 69(Special Issue):179. Abstr. 564.

72. Qvist, J., Qvist, V., & Mjor, I. A. (1990). Placement and longevity of amalgam restorations in Denmark. *J Dent Res*, 69(Special Issue):236. Abstr. 1018.

73. Brown, J. P. (2000). *Water fluoridation costs in Texas: Texas Health Steps (EPSDT-Medicaid)*, May.

74. Barsley, R. Sutherland J., & McFarland L. (1999). Water Fluoridation and the Costs of Medicaid Treatment for Dental Decay, Louisiana, 1995–1996. *MMWR*, 48(34):753–757.

75. U. S. Public Health Service, Centers for Disease Control. Water fluoridation and costs of medicaid treatment for dental decay—Louisiana, 1995–1996 (1999) *MMWR*, 48(34):753–757.

76. Wright, J., Bates, M., Cutress, T., & Lee, M. (1999). The cost-effectiveness of fluoridating water supplies in New Zealand: a report for the New Zealand Ministry of Health. Porirua, *New Zealand: Institute of Environmental Science and Research*, Nov., 1–31.

77. Robinson, S. N., Davies, E. H., & Williams, B. (1991). Domestic water treatment appliances and the fluoride ion. *Brit Dent J*, 171:91–93.

78. Levy, S. M. (1994). Review of fluoride exposures and ingestion. *Community Dent Oral Epidemiol*, 22:173–80.

79. Brown, M. D., & Aaron, G. (1991). The effect of point-of-use conditioning systems on community fluoridated water. *Pediatr Dent*, 13(1):35–8.

80. Levy, S. M., Kiritsy, M. C., & Warren, J. J. (1995). Sources of fluoride intake in children. *J Public Health Dent*, 55(1):39–52.

81. Kiritsy, M. C., Levy, S. M., Warren, J. J., Guha-Chowdhury, N., Heilman, J. R., & Marshall T. (1996). Assessing fluoride concentrations of juices and juice-flavored drinks. *J Am Dent Assoc*, 127:895–902.

82. World Health Organization (1994). *Fluorides and oral health*. Geneva: World Health Organization (Technical Report Series 846).

83. Institute of Medicine, Food and Nutrition Board (In press). *Dietary reference intakes for calcium, phosphorous, magnesium, vitamin D and fluoride. Report of the Standing Committee on the Scientific Evaluation of Dietary Reference Intakes*. Washington, DC: National Academy Press.

84. U.S. Department of Health and Human Services, Public Health Service (1991). *Review of fluoride: benefits and risks. Report of the Ad Hoc Subcommittee on Fluoride*. Washington, DC: February.

85. *Fluoride, teeth and health* (1976). Royal College of Physicians. Pitman Medical, London.

86. National Research Council (1993). *Health effects of ingested fluoride. Report of the Subcommittee on Health Effects of Ingested Fluoride*. Washington, DC: National Academy Press.

87. Yiamouyiannis, J. A., & Burk, D. (1975). A definite link between fluoridation and cancer death rate. *Nat Health Fed Bul*, 21:9.

88. Yiamouyiannis, J. A., & Burk, D. (1977). Fluoridation and cancer: age-dependence of cancer mortality related to artificial fluoridation. *Fluoride*, 10(3):102–23.

89. Hoover, R. N., McKay, F. W., & Fraumeni, J. F. (1976). Fluoridated drinking water and the occurrence of cancer. *J Natl Cancer Inst*, 57(4):757–68.

90. Erickson, J. D. (1978). Mortality in selected cities with fluoridated and non-fluoridated water supplies. *New Eng J Med*, 298(20):1112–6.

91. Hoover, R. N., DeVesa, S. S., Cantor, K., & Fraumeni, J. F. (1990). Fluoridation of drinking water and subsequent cancer incidence and mortality. *Report to the Director of the National Cancer Institute*, June.

92. Chilvers, C. (1983). Cancer mortality and fluoridation of water supplies in 35 U.S. cities. *Int J Epidemiol*, 12(4):397–404.

93. Kinlen, L. (1975). Cancer incidence in relation to fluoride level in water supplies. *Br Dent J*, 138:221–4.

94. Chilvers, C., & Conway, D. (1985). Cancer mortality in England in relation to levels of naturally occurring fluoride in water supplies. *J Epidemiol Comm Health*, 39:44–7.

95. Cook-Mozaffari, P. C., Bulusu, L., & Doll, R. (1981). Fluoridation of water supplies and cancer mortality I: a search for an effect in the UK on risk of death from cancer. *J Epidemiol Comm Health*, 35:227–32.

96. Richards, G. A., & Ford, J. M. (1979). Cancer mortality in selected New South Wales localities with fluoridated and non-fluoridated water supplies. *Med J Aust*, 2:521–3.

97. International Agency for Research on Cancer (1982). *IARC monographs on the evaluation of the carcinogenic risk of chemicals to humans*, Vol. 27. Switzerland.

98. Clemmesen, J. (1983). The alleged association between artificial fluoridation of water supplies and cancer: a review. *Bulletin of the World Health Organization*, 61(5):871–83.

99. Doll, R., & Kinlen, L. (1977). Fluoridation of water and cancer: mortality in the USA. *Lancet i*, 1300–02.

100. Bucher, J. R., Hejtmancik, M. R., Toft, J. D. II, Persing, R. L., Eustis, S. L., & Haseman, J. K. (1991). Results and conclusions of the National Toxicology Program's rodent carcinogenicity studies with sodium fluoride. *Int J Cancer*, 48:733–7.

101. Maurer, J. K., Cheng, M. C., Boysen, B. G., & Anderson, R. L. (1990). Two-year carcinogenicity study of sodium fluoride in rats. *J Natl Cancer Inst*, 82:1118–26.

102. U.S. Department of Health and Human Services, NIH, National Toxicology Program (1991). *Toxicology and carcinogenesis studies of sodium fluoride (CASNo. 7681-49-4) in F344/N rats and B6C3Fl mice (Drinking Water Studies)*. Publication No 91-2848. Technical Report 393. Washington, D.C.: U.S. Department of Health and Human Services, Public Health Service.

103. Knox, E. G. (1985). *Fluoridation of water and cancer: a review of the epidemiological evidence. Report of the Working Party*. London: Her Majesty's Stationary Office.

104. Safe Drinking Water Committee, National Research Council (1977). Drinking water and health. *National Academy of Sciences*. Washington, DC.

105. 62 Fed. Reg. 64297 (Dec. 5, 1997).

106. National Research Council, Committee on Toxicology (1993). *Health Effects of Ingested Fluoride*. Washington, DC: National Academy Press.

107. Corbin, S. B. (1992). Fluoridation Symposium. Policy options for fluoride use. *J Am Coll Dent*, 59:18–23.

108. Hodge, H. C. (1956). Fluoride metabolism: its significance in water fluoridation. *J Am Dent Assoc*, 52:301–14.

109. Whitford, G. M. (1990). The physiological and toxicological characteristics of fluoride. *J Dent Res*, 69(Spec Iss):539–49.

110. Trautner, K., & Siebert, G. (1986). An experimental study of bio-availability of fluoride from dietary sources in man. *Arch Oral Biol*, 31:223–28.

111. U.S. Department of Health and Human Services, Public Health Service (1980). *Surgeon General's advisory: treatment of water for use in dialysis: artificial kidney treatments*. Washington, DC: Government Printing Office 872-021, June.

112. Centers for Disease Control (1980). Fluoride in a dialysis unit-Maryland. *MMWR*, 29(12):134–6.

113. Leone, N. C., Shimkin, M. B., Arnold, F. A. Stevenson, C. A., Zimmermann, E. R., Geiser, P. B., & Lieberman, J. E. (1954). Medical aspects of excessive fluoride in a water supply. *Public Health Rep*, 69(10):925–36.

114. Geever, E. F., Leone, N. C., Geiser, P., & Lieberman, J. (1958). Pathologic studies in man after prolonged ingestion of fluoride in drinking water I: necropsy findings in a community with a water level of 2.5 ppm. *J Am Dent Assoc*, 56:499–507.

115. Schlesinger, E. R., Overton, D. E., Chase, H. C., & Cantwell, K. T. (1956). Newburgh-Kingston caries-fluorine study XIII: pediatric findings after ten years. *J Am Dent Assoc*, 52:296–306

116. Jacobsen, S. J., O'Fallon, W. M., & Melton, L. J. (1993). Hip fracture incidence before and after the fluoridation of the public water supply, Rochester, Minnesota. *Am J Public Health*, 83(5):689–93.

117. Danielson, C., Lyon, J. L., Eggen, M., & Good Gough, G. K. (1992). Hip fractures and fluoridation in Utah's elderly population. *J Am Med Assoc*, Aug 12, 268(6):746–8.

118. Jacobsen, S. J., Goldberg, J., Cooper, C., & Lockwood, S. A. (1992). The association between water fluoridation and hip fracture among white women and men aged 65 years and older: a national ecologic study. *Ann Epidemiol*, 2(5):617–26.

119. Karagas, M. R., Baron, J. A., Barrett, J. A., & Jacobsen, S. J. (1996). Patterns of fracture among the United States elderly: geographic and fluoride effects. *Ann Epidemiol*, 6(3):209–16.

120. Madans, J., Kleinman, J. C., & Corroni-Huntley, J. (1983). The relationship between hip fracture and water fluoridation: an analysis of national data. *Am J Public Health*, Mar; 73(3):296–8.

121. Avorn, J., Niessen, L. C. (1986). Relationship between long bone fractures and water fluoridation. *Geriodontics*, 2:175–79.

122. Arnala, I., Alhava, E. M., Kivivuori, R., & Kauranen, P. (1986). Hip fracture incidence not affected by fluoridation. Osteofluorosis studied in Finland. *Acta Orthop Scand*, Aug; 57(4):344–8.

123. Cooper, C., Wickham, C., Lacey, R. F., & Barker, D. J. (1990). Water fluoride concentration and fracture of the proximal femur. *J Epidemiol Community Health*, Mar; 44(1):17–9.

124. Simonen, O., et al. (1985). Does fluoridation of drinking water prevent bone fragility and osteoporosis? *Lancet*, Aug 24; 2(8452):432–4.

125. Jacobsen, S. J., Goldberg, J., Miles, T. P., Brody, J. A., Stiers, W., & Rimm, A. A. (1990). Regional variation in the incidence of hip fracture: U.S. white women aged 65 years and older. *Am Med Assoc*, 264(4):500–2.

126. Phipps, K. R., Orwoll, E. S., Mason, J. D., & Cauley, J. A. (2000). Community water fluoridation, bone mineral density, and fractures: prospective study of effects in older women. *Brit Med J*, 321:860–4.

127. Kanis, J. A. (1993). Treatment of symptomatic osteoporosis with fluoride. *Am J Med*, 95(Suppl 5A):53S–61S.

128. Hillier, S., Cooper, C., Kellingray, S., Russell, G., Hughes, H., & Coggon, D. (2000). Fluoride in drinking water and risk of hip fracture in the UK: a case-control study. *Lancet*, 355:265–9

129. U.S. Public Health Service, Department of Health and Human Services (June 2000). *National Institute of Dental and Craniofacial Research Statement on Water Fluoridation*.

130. Reeves, T. G. (1996). Technical aspects of water fluoridation in the United States and an overview of fluoridation engineering world-wide. *Community Dent Health*, 13(Suppl 2):21–26.

131. U.S. Department of Health and Human Services (Sept. 1986). U.S. Public Health Service Centers for Disease Control Water Fluoridation. *A Manual for Engineers and Technicians*.

132. Hinman, A. R., Sterritt, G. R., & Reeves, T. G. (1996). The U.S. experience with fluoridation. *Community Dent Health*, 13(Suppl 2):5–9.

133. Urbansky, E. T., & Schock, M. R. (2000). Can fluoridation affect lead (II) in potable water? Hexafluorosilicate and fluoride equilibria in aqueous. *Intern J Environ Studies*, 57:597–637.

134. Personal communication (email) from Dr. Ernest Newbrum in response to query by Eleanor Nadler, Chair of the San Diego Coalition for Fluoridation, January 16, 2000.

135. Shannon, I. L. (1978). The fluoride concentration in drinking water of fluoridating communities in Texas. *Tex Dent J*, 96(6):10–12.

136. Leland, D. E., Powell, K. E., & Anderson, R. S. (1980). A fluoride overfeed incident at Harbor Springs, Michigan. *J Am Water Works Assoc*, 72:238–43.

137. Petersen, L. R., Deniš, D., Brown, D., Hadler, J. L., Helgerson, S. D. (1998). Community health effects of a municipal water supply hyperfluoridation accident. *Am J Public Health*, 78: 711–13.

138. Gessner, B. D., Beller, M., Middaugh, J. P., & Whitford, G. M. (1994). Acute fluoride poisoning from a public water system. *N Engl J Med*, 330:95–99.

139. Bergmann, K. E., & Bergmann, R. L. (1995). Salt fluoridation and general health. *Adv Dent Res*, 9:138–43.

140. Pakhomov, G. N., Ivanova, K., Moller, I. J., & Vrabcheva, M. (1995). Dental caries-reducing effects of a milk fluoridation project in Bulgaria. *J Public Health Dent*, 55(4):234–7.

141. Mejia, R., Espinal, F., Velez, H., & Aguirre, M. (1976). Estudio sobre la fluoruracion de la sal. VIII Resultados obtenidos de 1964 a 1972. *Boll Of Sanit Panam*, 80:67–80.

142. Kunzel, W. (1993). Systemic use of fluoride—other methods: salt, sugar, milk, etc. *Caries Res*, 27(Suppl 1):16–22.

143. Intersalt Cooperative Research Group (1988). Intersalt: an international study of electrolyte excretion and blood pressure. Results for 24 hour urinary and potassium excretion. *Br Med J*, 297:319–28.

144. Steiner, M., Menghini, G., & Marthaler, T. M. (1989). The caries incidence in schoolchildren in the Canton of Glarus 13 years after the introduction of highly fluoridated salt. *Schweiz Monatss Zahnmed*, 99: 897–901.

145. Murray, J. J., Ed. *Appropriate use of fluorides for human health*. Geneva: World Health Organization, 1986.

146. Toth, K. (1976). A study of 8 years domestic salt fluoridation for prevention of caries. *Community Dent Oral Epidemiol*, 4:106–10.

147. Restrepo, D. (1967). Salt fluoridation: an alternative measure to water fluoridation. *Int Dent J*, 17:4–9.

148. Marthaler, T. M., Mejía, R., & Viñes, J. J. (1978). Caries-preventive salt fluoridation. *Caries Res*, 12(Suppl 1):15–21

149. Klein, S. P., Bohannan, H. M., Bell, R. M., Disney, J. A., Foch, C. B., & Graves, R. C. (1985). The cost and effectiveness of school-based preventive dental care. *Am J Public Health*, Apr, 75(4):382–91.

150. Partnership for Prevention (2001). Oral health: Common and preventable ailments. *Priorities in Prevention*, May:1–8.

151. Committee on Health and Human Services, 68th Oregon Legislative Assembly. *Regular Session, Senate Bill 973 (filed at the request of Task Force on Access to Oral Health Services, Oregon Dental Hygienists Association)*. Salem, Oregon: Oregon Legislative Assembly, 1995.

152. Carter, Brown, Eighmey, Gordly, Johnston, and Shibley (Representatives), and Bradbury, Hamby, and McCoy (Senators). *68th Oregon Legislative Assembly Regular Session, House Bill 3312 (filed at request Oregon Dental Association)*. Salem, Oregon: Oregon Legislative Assembly, 1995.

153. Association of State and Territorial Dental Directors/ADA, May 1995, personal communication.

154. U.S. Government Printing Office. *National Summary of Fluoridation Referenda Reported Between November 1950 and December 31, 1967*. 1968.

155. Faine, R. C., Collins, J. J., Daniel, J., Isman, B., Boriskin, J., Young, K. L., Fitzgerald, C. M. (1981). The 1980 Fluoridation Campaigns: A Discussion of Results. *J Public Health Dent*, 41(3):138–42.

156. Jones, R. B., Mormann, D. N., & Durtsche, T. B. (1989). Fluoridation referendum in La Crosse, Wisconsin: contributing factors to success. *Am J Public Health*, 79:1405–07.

157. Easley, M. W. (1990). The status of community water fluoridation in the United States. *Public Health Rep*, 105:348–53.

158. U.S. Census Bureau. General Population Data, Census 2000.

159. U.S. Census Bureau, Department of Commerce (July 2000). Population trends in metropolitan areas and central cities. *Current Population Reports*, Series P25–1133.

160. U.S. Census Bureau, Department of Commerce. *Voting age population*. Census Bureau Press Release, CB92-24. Census and You, March 1992. Washington, DC: U.S. Department of Commerce.

161. U.S. Census Bureau, Department of Commerce (Dec. 2000). Educational attainment in the United States (Update). *Current Population Reports*, Series P20–536.

162. U.S. Census Bureau, Department of Commerce (1992). Voting age and registration in the election November 1992. *Current Population Reports*, January, Series P-20.

163. U.S. Department of Commerce, Bureau of the Census (1992). Housing characteristics of recent movers: 1989. *Current Housing Reports*, February, Series H121/91-2.

164. U.S. Department of Commerce, Bureau of the Census (1992). *Poverty in the United States: 1992*. Series P60–185. Census and You, November 1992. Washington, DC: U.S. Department of Commerce.

165. *A poll of likely voters in San Antonio, Texas*. Hill Research Consultants. August 11, 2000.

166. Chong, D. (2000). *Rational lives: Norms and values in politics and society*. University of Chicago Press.

167. Bonham, G. (1993). Direct Democracy: Lessons from fluoridation. *Can J Public Health*, 84(2):82–83.

168. Harris Interactive, Inc. for Research!America (2000). May 2000 Omnibus Survey. New York, NY: *Harris Interactive, Inc.*

169. Scott, D. B. (1996). The dawn of a new era. *J Public Health Dent*, 56(5 Spec No):235–8.

170. Gallup Organization, Inc. (1991). *A Gallup study of parents' behavior, knowledge and attitudes toward fluoride*. Princeton, NJ: Gallup Organization, Inc.

171. Doppelt, J. C., & Shearer, E. (1999). *Nonvoters: America's No-Shows*. Thousand Oaks, CA: Sage Publications, p. 246.

172. Sandman, P. M. (1990). *Hazard Versus Outrage: Public Perception of Fluoridation Risks*. Environmental Committee Research Program, Cook College, Rutgers University, New Brunswick, NJ, April.

173. Park, B., Smith, K., Malvitz, D., & Furman, L. (1990). Hazard vs. outrage: Public perception of fluoridation risks. *J Public Health Dent*, 50:7–44.

174. Cappella, J. N., Turow, J., & Jamieson, K. H. (1996). *Call-in talk radio: background, content, audiences, portrayal in mainstream media*. Annenburg Public Policy Center's Report Series, August 7:1–68.

175. Smith, K. G., & Christen, K. A. (1990). A fluoridation campaign: the Phoenix experience. *J Public Health Dent*, 50:319–22.

176. Isman, R. (1983). Public views on fluoridation and other preventive dental practices. *Community Dent Oral Epidemiol*, 11:217–23.

177. U.S. Census Bureau, Department of Commerce (July 1998). Voting and registration in the election of November 1996. *Current Population Reports*, Series P20–504.

178. U.S. Census Bureau, Department of Commerce. (Aug 2000). Voting and registration in the election of November 1998. *Current Population Reports*, Series P20–523RV.

179. Evans, C. A., & Pickles, T. (1978). Statewide Antifluoridation Initiatives: A New Challenge to Health Workers. *Am J Public Health*, 68(1):59–62.

180. Lemke, C. W., Doherty, J. M., & Arra, M. C. (1970). Controlled fluoridation: the dental effects of discontinuation in Antigo, Wisconsin. *J Am Dent Assoc*, 80:782–6.

181. Glasard, P. H., & Frazier, P. J. (Nov. 19, 1985). *Future teachers' knowledge and opinions about methods to prevent oral diseases. Presented at American Public Health Association annual meeting*. Washington, DC.

182. Kay, E. J., & Blinkhorn, A. S. (1989). A study of mothers' attitudes towards the prevention of caries with particular references to fluoridation and vaccination. *Community Dent Health*, 6(4):357–63.

183. Lennon, M. A. (1993). Promoting water fluoridation. *Community Dent Health*, 10:57–63.

184. Dolinsky, H. B., et al. (1981). A Health Systems Agency and a Fluoridation Campaign. *J Public Health Policy*, 2(2):158–63.

185. McGuire, K. M. (1981). Strategies for a fluoridation campaign. *J Michigan Dent Assoc*, 63:681–86.

186. Borinskin, J. M., & Fine, J. I. (1993). Fluoridation election victory: a case study for dentistry in effective political action. *J Am Dent Assoc*, 102:486–91.

187. Barrett, S. (1983). Winning a Campaign for Fluoridation. *CDAJ*, 11(1): 61–6.

188. Clark, D. C., & Hann, H. J. (1989). A Win for Fluoridation in Squamish, British Colombia. *J Public Health Dent*, 49(3):170–1.

189. Elwell, K. R., & Easlick, K. (1960). *Classification and appraisal of objections to fluoridation*. Ann Arbor, Michigan: The University of Michigan.

190. Watson, M. L. (1985). The Opposition to Fluoride Programs: Report of a Survey. *J Public Health Dent*, 45(3):142–48.

191. Easley, M. W. (1984). The antifluoridation movement. *Health Matrix*, 2:74–77.

192. Easley, M. W. (1985). The new antifluoridationists: who are they and how do they operate? *J Public Health Dent*, 45; 133–41.

193. American Dental Association, Principles of Ethics and Code of Professional Conduct (1998). Chicago: *The Association*, iii.

194. American Dental Hygienists' Association, Code of Ethics (1995). Chicago: ADHA.

195. Newbrun, E. (1996). The fluoridation war: a scientific dispute or a religious argument? *J Public Health Dent*, 56(5 Spec Iss):246–52.

196. Bernhardt, M., & Sprague, B. (1980). The poisonmongers. In Barrett S, Rovin S, Eds. *The tooth robbers* (pp. 1–8). Philadelphia: GF Stickley.

197. Yiamouyiannis, J. (1983). *Lifesavers guide to fluoridation*. Delaware, OH: Safewater Foundation.

198. Yiamouyiannis, J. (1983). *Fluoride: The aging factor*. Delaware, OH: Health Action Press.

199. Wulf, C. A., Hughes, K. F., Smith, K. G., & Easley, M. W., Eds. (1999). *Abuse of the scientific literature in an antifluoridation pamphlet* (2nd ed.). Atlanta: Centers for Disease Control & Prevention, xxxv.

200. Jarvis, W. (1983). Should we debate quacks? *CCAHF (California Council Against Health Fraud) Newsletter*. July–Aug, 6:7.

201. Shearer, D. (1997). Sierra club to take on water fluoridation. *Pittsburgh Post-Gazette*, August 13, p. C1.

202. Coleman, P. (1997). Not authorized. Letter to the Editor. *Pittsburgh Post-Gazette*, August 24, p. B3.

203. Citizens for Safe Drinking Water. *EPA scientists take stand against fluoridation (Press Release)*. July 2, 1997.

204. Hance, B., Chess, C., & Sandman, P. (1990). *Industry risk communication manual*. Boca Raton, FL: CRC Press/Lewis Publishers, 1990.

205. Chess, C., Hance, B., & Sandman, P. (1988). *Improving dialogue with communities: a risk communication manual for government*. Trenton, NJ: Division of Science and Research, New Jersey Department of Environmental Protection, 1988.

206. Covello, V. (1989). Issues and problems in using risk comparisons for communicating right-to-know information on chemical risks. *Environmental Science and Technology, 23*(12):1444–9.

207. Covello, V., & Allen, F. (1988). *Seven cardinal rules of risk communication*. Washington, DC: U.S. Environmental Protection Agency, Office of Policy Analysis.

208. Fischoff, B., Lichtenstein, S., Slovic, P., & Keeney, D. (1981). *Acceptable risk*. Cambridge, MA: Cambridge University Press, 1981.

209. U.S. Public Health Service (2000). *Healthy people 2010* (Vol. 2, 2nd ed.): Objectives for improving health (Part B, focus areas 15–28). Washington, DC: U.S. Government Printing Office, November, 664.

# CHAPTER 9

# Topical Fluoride Therapy

*Kevin J. Donly*
*George K. Stookey*

## OBJECTIVES

*At the end of this chapter, it will be possible to*

1. Indicate the only three fluoride compounds accepted for professional applications to control caries and indicate their relative effectiveness.
2. Discuss the possible chemical reactions associated with the topical application of sodium fluoride (NaF), stannous fluoride (SnF$_2$), and acidulated phosphate fluoride (APF).
3. Relate what percentages of NaF and SnF$_2$ are available for office and home use (as solutions or as gels).
4. Describe how a liquid or gel topical application of fluoride is applied to the teeth. Emphasize particularly those parts of the technique that are especially important with regard to safety and efficacy.
5. Nearly all dentifrices on the market contain fluoride. Indicate why the early dentifrices did not produce the expected caries decrements.
6. State the expected decrease in caries formation following use of dentifrices and mouthrinses containing fluoride.
7. Describe fluoridated varnishes and fluoride-releasing dental restorative materials and the potential of these materials to inhibit demineralization and enhance remineralization.

# INTRODUCTION

When communal-water supplies are available, water fluoridation clearly represents the most *effective, efficient,* and *economical* of all known measures for the prevention of dental caries although similar results have been observed with fluoridated salt in many countries. Unfortunately, fluoridated water is available to only about two-thirds of the population. Thus it is obvious that additional measures are needed for the dental profession to provide greater protection against caries to as many segments of the population as possible.

The term *topical fluoride therapy* refers to the use of systems containing relatively large concentrations of fluoride that are applied locally, or topically, to erupted tooth surfaces to prevent the formation of dental caries. Thus this term encompasses the use of fluoride rinses, dentifrices, pastes, gels, and solutions that are applied in various manners.

## Mechanism of Action

Studies of the use of professional topical fluoride applications for the control of dental caries began in the early 1940s. Since that time, it has been generally accepted that the fluoride content of enamel is *inversely* related to the prevalence of dental caries.

Using *in vivo* enamel-sampling techniques and improved analytic methods investigators have been better able to quantitate this relationship. For example, Keene and coworkers[1] explored this relationship in young naval recruits 17 to 22 years of age; their observations are summarized in Table 9–1. These data suggest that the presence of *elevated* levels of fluoride in surface enamel is associated with minimal caries experience.

A much more extensive investigation of this relationship was reported by DePaola and coworkers.[2] These investigators similarly examined 1,447 subjects, 12 to 16 years of age, who were lifetime residents of selected fluoridated and nonfluoridated communities; again the inverse relationship between enamel fluoride content and caries prevalence is apparent.

At the time of tooth eruption, the enamel is not yet completely calcified and undergoes a *post-eruptive period,* approximately 2 years in length, during which enamel calcification continues. Throughout this period, called the period of enamel *maturation,* fluoride, as well as other elements, continues to accumulate in the more superficial portions of enamel. This fluoride is derived from the *saliva* as well as from the exposure of the teeth to fluoride-containing *water* and *food.* Following the period of enamel maturation, relatively little additional fluoride is incorporated from such sources into the enamel surface.[3] Thus, most of the fluoride that is incorporated into the developing enamel occurs during the *pre-eruptive* period of enamel formation and the *post-eruptive* period of enamel maturation.

TABLE 9–1  **Relationship Between Surface Enamel Fluoride Content and Caries Prevalence in Young Adults[a]**

| Number of Subjects | Caries Prevalence (DMFT) | Enamel Fluoride Content (ppm) |
|---|---|---|
| 47 | 0 | 3459 |
| 31 | 5–11 | 2229 |
| 29 | 12–26 | 1944 |

[a]Calculated from data presented by Keene, et al.[1]

The continued deposition of fluoride into enamel during the later stages of enamel formation, and especially during the period of enamel maturation, results in a concentration gradient of fluoride in enamel. Invariably the *highest* concentration of fluoride occurs at the very outermost portion of the enamel surface, with the fluoride content *decreasing* as one progresses inward *toward the dentin*.[4,5] This decrease in fluoride concentration is extremely rapid in the outermost *5 to 10 microns* of enamel and is much less pronounced thereafter. This characteristic fluoride concentration gradient has been observed in unerupted teeth as well as in erupted teeth and in both the permanent and deciduous dentition, regardless of the amount of previous exposure to fluoride.

The presence of elevated concentrations of fluoride in surface enamel serves to make the tooth surface more resistant to the development of dental caries. Fluoride ions, when substituted into the *hydroxyapatite crystal*, fit more perfectly into the crystal than do *hydroxyl ions*. This fact coupled with the greater bonding potential of fluoride serves to make the apatite crystals more compact and more stable. Such crystals are thereby *more resistant* to the *acid dissolution*[6,7] that occurs during caries initiation. This effect is even more apparent as *the pH* of the enamel environment *decreases* due to the momentary loss of minute quantities of fluoride from the dissolving enamel and its nearly simultaneous *reprecipitation* as a fluorhydroxyapatite.[8]

Most of the initial studies concerning topical fluoride applications were conducted with sodium fluoride. It was recognized at that time that prolonged exposure of the teeth to low concentrations of fluoride in the dental office was not practical. To overcome this problem, two approaches were explored: *increasing the fluoride concentration and decreasing the pH of the application solution*.

Although the ability of sodium fluoride to increase the resistance of enamel to acid dissolution had been reported on several occasions,

it had also been reported that lowering the pH of the sodium fluoride solution greatly increased its protection against enamel decalcification. Five clinical caries studies were conducted to evaluate the effectiveness of *acidulated sodium fluoride* topical solutions. The fluoride solutions were acidulated in various manners (e.g., acetic acid, acid phthalate) and used with varying conditions, but in no instance was a statistically significant caries-preventive effect observed. Thus, the use of acidulated sodium fluoride systems was abandoned, at least *temporarily*.

On the other hand, the observed results of increasing concentrations of fluoride were very encouraging, particularly when multiple applications were used. Although it was initially postulated that the effectiveness of topically applied sodium fluoride was due to the formation of a fluorhydroxyapatite,[9,10] subsequent investigations indicated that the primary reaction product involved the transformation of surface hydroxyapatite *to calcium fluoride*.[11–16]

$$Ca_{10}(PO_4)_6(OH)_2 + 20F^- \rightleftharpoons$$
hydroxyapatite

$$10CaF_2 + 6HPO_4^= + 2(OH)^-$$
calcium fluoride

## Question 1

Which of the following statements, if any, are correct?

A. The maturation of enamel is an occurrence that continues at a linear rate from eruption into adulthood.

B. The fluoride content is highest at the outer surface of the enamel and decreases at a linear rate toward the dentin.

C. As a result of acid-induced demineralization followed by remineralization in the presence of fluoride, hydroxyapatite can become fluorhydroxyapatite.

D. The enamel is relatively more protected by neutral pH fluoride solutions than acidulated solutions.

E. With higher concentrations of fluoride, the main reaction product is fluorhydroxyapatite.

The preceding reaction involves the breakdown of the apatite crystal into its components followed by the reaction of fluoride and calcium ions to form calcium fluoride with a net *loss* of phosphate ions from treated enamel. Newer fluoride systems incorporate a means of preventing such phosphate loss.

The early investigators of the reaction between soluble fluoride and enamel observed that the nature of the reaction products was markedly influenced by a number of factors, including fluoride *concentration*, the *pH* of the solution, and the length of *exposure*. For example, the use of *acidic fluoride* solutions greatly favored the formation of *calcium fluoride*.[11] *Neutral sodium fluoride* solutions with fluoride concentrations of *100 ppm or less* resulted primarily in the formation of *fluorapatite*, whereas higher fluoride concentrations resulted in the formation of *calcium fluoride*.[15] Because topical applications of sodium fluoride involve the use of 2.0% solutions (slightly over 9,000 ppm), it follows that the use of these solutions essentially involves the formation of *calcium fluoride*.[14]

The second fluoride compound developed[17,18] for topical use in the dental office during the 1950s was *stannous fluoride* ($SnF_2$). Compared with that of sodium fluoride, the reaction of $SnF_2$ with enamel is unique in that *both* the cation (stannous) and the anion (fluoride) react chemically with enamel components. This reaction is commonly depicted as follows:

$$Ca_{10}(PO_4)_6(OH)_2 + 19nF_2 \longrightarrow$$

hydroxyapatite        stannous fluoride

$$10CaF_2 + 6Sn_3F_3PO_4 + SnO \cdot H_2O$$

calcium        stannous        hydrated
fluoride       fluorophosphate   tin oxide

Note from the equation that the formation of *stannous fluorophosphate* prevents, at least temporarily, the *phosphate* loss typical of sodium fluoride applications. Incidentally, the exact nature of the tin-containing reaction products varies depending on reaction conditions, including pH, concentration, and length of exposure (or reaction time).[19,20]

A third topical fluoride system for professional use was developed during the 1960s and is widely known as APF, *acidulated phosphate fluoride*. This system was developed by Brudevold and coworkers[21,22] in an effort to achieve greater amounts of fluorhydroxyapatite and lesser amounts of calcium fluoride formation. These investigators reviewed the various chemical reactions of fluoride with enamel (hydroxyapatite) and concluded that (1) if the pH of the fluoride system was made acidic to enhance the rate of reaction of fluoride with hydroxyapatite and (2) if phosphoric acid was used as the acidulant to increase the concentration of phosphate present at the reaction site, it should be possible to obtain greater amounts of fluoride deposited in surface enamel as *fluorhydroxyapatite* with minimal formation of *calcium fluoride* and minimal loss of *enamel phosphate*. On the basis of this chemical reasoning, APF systems were developed and shown to be effective for caries prevention.

Subsequent independent studies of the reactions of APF with enamel indicated, however, that the original chemical objectives were only partially achieved. The major reaction product of APF with enamel is also *calcium fluoride*,[12,23,24] although a greater amount of fluorhydroxyapatite is formed than with the previous topical fluoride systems. The chemical reaction of APF with enamel may be written as follows:

$$Ca_{10}(PO_4)_6(OH)_2 + F^- \longrightarrow$$

hydroxyapatite        stannous fluoride

$$CaF_2 + Ca_{10}(PO_4)_6(OH)_{2x}F_x$$

calcium        fluorhydroxyapatite
fluoride

It is obvious from the preceding discussion that the primary chemical reaction product with *all* three types of topical fluoride systems (i.e., NaF, SnF$_2$, and APF) is the formation of *calcium fluoride* on the enamel surface.

The initial deposition of calcium fluoride on the treated tooth surfaces is by *no means* permanent; a relatively rapid loss of fluoride occurs within the first *24 hours*,[25] with some continued loss occurring during the *next 15 days*.[26–29] The rate of loss varies between patients and is influenced by the nature of the fluoride treatment.[30,31] Nevertheless, it is known that *each individual professionally-applied fluoride treatment results in an *increase* in the permanently-bound fluoride content of the outermost layers of the enamel with a subsequent decrease in the susceptibility of the enamel for caries initiation and progression.

The role of the calcium fluoride deposits on the enamel surface following professional fluoride applications in providing the observed cariostatic benefits has been the subject of numerous investigations. It is known that the *most desirable form of fluoride* in enamel for caries prevention is *fluorhydroxyapatite* and that the most efficient means of forming this reaction product occurs with *prolonged exposure* of the enamel to *low* concentrations of fluoride. It is also known that *calcium fluoride* may serve as a fluoride *source for enamel remineralization*,[32,33] and that calcium fluoride dissolves much more slowly in the oral environment than in an aqueous solution due to the presence of a phos-

phate or protein-rich coating of the globular deposits of calcium fluoride on the enamel surface.[34] As a result of this continued research, there is a growing body of convincing evidence suggesting that the deposits of calcium fluoride serve as an important *fluoride reservoir* and that these phosphate-coated globules are dissolved in the presence of plaque acids providing an available *source of both fluoride and phosphate* to facilitate the remineralization of decalcified areas.[35]

Regardless of the mechanism of action of professionally applied topical fluoride treatments, the results of clinical trials clearly indicate that the *benefits are related to the number of treatments*. Table 9–2 summarizes a clinical study[36] in which schoolchildren were given a dental prophylaxis and a topical application of 8 percent SnF$_2$ at 6-month intervals throughout a 3-year period. Dental-caries examinations were performed initially and each year thereafter. It is apparent from these data that the caries-preventive benefits *increased* in relation to the number of treatments. Similar observations have been noted with the other two fluoride systems used for professional applications. The original sodium fluoride topical application procedure developed by Knutson[37] specified a series of four treatment during a 2-week period. Mellberg[38] and coworkers[39] have also indicated the need for repeated topical applications of APF to obtain maximal benefits. Thus, it follows that maximal patient benefits can *only* be obtained with repeated topical applica-

TABLE 9–2  **Clinical Reductions in Incremental Caries as a Function of the Number of Topical Fluoride Applications**[a]

| Study Period (Years) | Total Number of Topical Applications | Caries Reduction (%) | |
|---|---|---|---|
| | | DMF Teeth | DMF Surfaces |
| 1 | 2 | 2.8 | 12.6 |
| 2 | 4 | 29.2 | 34.1 |
| 3 | 6 | 47.4 | 51.5 |

[a]Calculated from data presented by Beiswanger, et al.[36]

tions regardless of the nature of the fluoride system used.

It was noted earlier that the reaction of $SnF_2$ with enamel resulted in the formation of tin-containing compounds. Although much less is known regarding the precise nature and ultimate fate of these compounds, it appears that they contribute significantly to the cariostatic activity of $SnF_2$. The tin reaction products formed on sound enamel surfaces appear to be leached from the enamel in a manner similar to that for calcium fluoride.[40] The greatest accumulation of stannous complexes *occurs in circumscribed areas of enamel defects*; typically such areas are *hypo*mineralized and are frequently the result of decalcification associated with the initiation of the caries process. Extremely high concentrations of tin, about 20,000 ppm, have been reported in these locations.[41] Clinically, these areas, which have been described as frank carious areas, *become pigmented* (presumably because of the presence of the tin complexes) and appear to be more calcified following the application of $SnF_2$. This pigmentation has thus been suggested as being indicative of the arrest of carious lesions and is typically retained for 6 to 12 months or longer, implying that these stannous reaction products are of considerably *greater* significance than those formed on sound enamel.

At reduced concentrations of *0.10 to 0.15% fluoride*, all of the foregoing fluoride compounds have also been approved for use in dentifrices and gels intended for personal use, and sodium fluoride at a concentration of *0.05%* has also been approved for use in *mouthrinses sold over-the-counter*. In general, it is recognized that the mechanism of action of these fluoride compounds is *similar* at all the concentrations utilized for both professional and home-use products.

One additional fluoride compound, *sodium monofluorophosphate*, has been approved for use in dentifrices; this compound has the empirical formula $Na_2PO_3F$ and is commonly known as MFP. Though evaluated in one study as an agent for topical fluoride application in the dental office, its use in this manner has received little consideration. Although the mechanism of action of MFP is thought to involve a chemical reaction with surface enamel, the precise nature of this reaction is *poorly understood*. Some investigators have suggested that the fluorophosphate moiety, $PO_3F^5$, may undergo an exchange reaction with phosphate ions in the apatite structure but the presence of $PO_3F^5$ in enamel has never been demonstrated, and such a reaction mechanism appears unlikely. Others have suggested that the $PO_3F^5$ complex is enzymatically dissociated by phosphatases present in saliva and dental plaque into $PO_3^2$ and $F^2$, with the ionic fluoride reacting with hydroxyapatite in a manner similar to that described earlier. The fact that the treatment of enamel with MFP results in less fluoride deposition and less protection against enamel decalcification than is observed with simple inorganic fluoride compounds such as sodium fluoride, while yet imparting nearly comparable cariostatic activity, is indicative of a more complex mechanism of action.

For the most part, the foregoing discussion of the chemical reactions of concentrated fluoride solutions with enamel suggests that the reactions occur on the *outer enamel surface* and serve to make that surface more resistant to demineralization. It is apparent that this process is particularly predominant in newly erupted teeth that are undergoing continued enamel maturation (calcification) for the first 2 years following eruption into the oral cavity. In such instances, some of the applied fluoride readily penetrates the relatively permeable enamel surface to *depths of 20 to 30 millimeters* and readily reacts with the calcifying apatite to form a fluorhydroxyapatite. Furthermore, the dissolution of the calcium fluoride deposited on the enamel surface provides additional fluoride ions, which become incorporated in maturing enamel.

It has become increasingly apparent, however, during the last decade that very little fluo-

ride deposition *lasting more than 24 hours* occurs when fluoride is applied to sound, *fully maturated enamel.* This situation apparently occurs regardless of the nature of the fluoride compound, the concentration of fluoride, or the manner of application. Thus, there appears to be *no* preventive benefits from the application of fluoride to maturated, sound enamel.

As noted in Chapter 3, the caries process begins with a demineralization of the *apatite adjacent to the crystal sheaths.* This permits the diffusion of weak acids into the subsurface enamel, and because the subsurface enamel has a lower fluoride content and is less resistant to acid demineralization, it *is preferentially* dissolved, forming an *incipient, subsurface lesion.* As this process continues, it becomes clinically apparent as a so-called *"white spot"* that, in reality, is a rather extensive subsurface lesion covered by a relatively intact enamel surface. Thus, enamel surfaces that clinically appear to be sound or free of demineralization frequently have areas that have been slightly decalcified with *minute subsurface lesions* that are not yet detectable clinically. This situation is particularly likely to exist in patients with clinical evidence of *caries activity on other teeth.*

It now appears that the predominant mechanism of action of fluoride involves its ability to *facilitate the remineralization* of these demineralized areas. Topically applied fluoride clearly *diffuses* into these demineralized areas and reacts with calcium and phosphate to form fluorhydroxyapatite in the remineralization process. It is also noteworthy that such remineralized enamel is *more resistant* to subsequent demineralization than was the original enamel. This process has been shown to occur with all forms and concentrations of fluoride, including concentrations as low as 1 ppm such as is found in optimally fluoridated drinking water. Studies conducted in our laboratories, however, have clearly shown that the amount of fluoride deposition in subsurface lesions following a topical fluoride application is much greater than that occurring following the use of lesser con-

centrations of fluoride provided by fluoride rinses or dentifrices. As a result, topical fluoride applications appear to be an *effective means of inducing the remineralization of incipient lesions.*

## Question 2

Which of the following statements, if any, are correct?

A. On demineralization, more phosphate is lost from the hydroxyapatite crystal in the presence of sodium fluoride than when stannous fluoride is present.

B. Calcium fluoride deposits on the tooth surface serve as a fluoride reservoir.

C. As the number of treatments with topical fluoride increases, so does the caries-preventive benefit.

D. Stannous fluoride is deposited in greatest concentration where the enamel is least perfectly mineralized.

E. The use of MFP results in less cariostatic action than other neutral fluorides, even though a higher concentration is usually found on the tooth surface.

## Effects of Fluoride on Plaque and Bacterial Metabolism

Thus far, we have assumed that the cariostatic effects of fluoride are mediated through a chemical reaction between this ion and the outermost portion of the enamel surface. The preponderance of data supports this view. A growing body of information suggests, however, that the caries-preventive action of fluoride may also include an *inhibitory effect on the oral flora involved in the initiation of caries.* The ability of fluoride to *inhibit glycolysis* by interfering with the enzyme *enolase* has long been known; concentrations of fluoride as low as 50 ppm have been shown to interfere with bacterial metabolism. Moreover, fluoride may *accumulate in dental plaque in concentrations above 100 ppm.* Although the fluoride normally present in

plaque is largely bound (and thus unavailable for antibacterial action), it *dissociates* to ionic fluoride when the pH of plaque decreases (i.e., when acids are formed). Thus, when the carious process starts and acids are formed, plaque fluoride in ionic form may serve to *interfere* with further acid production by plaque microorganisms. In addition, it may react with the underlying layer of dissolving enamel, *promoting its remineralization as fluorhydroxyapatite*. The end result of this process is a "physiologic" *restoration* of the initial lesion (by remineralization of enamel) and the formation of a *more resistant* enamel surface. The ability of fluoride to promote the reprecipitation of calcium phosphate solutions in apatitic forms has been repeatedly demonstrated.

In addition to these possible effects of fluoride, several investigators have reported that the presence of tin, especially as provided by stannous fluoride, is associated with significant *antibacterial activity*, which has been reported to *decrease both* the amount of *dental plaque* and *gingivitis* in both animals[42] and adult humans.[43] Existing evidence suggests that these antibacterial effects of fluoride and tin may also contribute to the observed cariostatic activity of topically applied fluorides.

## Topical Fluoride Applications

The use of concentrated fluoride solutions applied topically to the dentition for the prevention of dental caries has been studied extensively during the past 50 years, although few studies have been conducted since the 1970s. This procedure results in a significant *increase* in the resistance of the exposed tooth surfaces to the development of dental caries and, as a result, has become a standard procedure in most dental offices.

At present, three different fluoride systems have been adequately evaluated and approved for use in this manner in the United States. These three systems are *2% sodium fluoride, 8%*

*stannous fluoride, and acidulated phosphate fluoride systems containing 1.23% fluoride.*

### Available Forms

When topical fluoride applications became available to the profession, the fluoride compounds (sodium fluoride and stannous fluoride) were obtained in powder or crystalline form, and aqueous solutions were prepared immediately prior to use. Subsequently it was realized that sodium fluoride solutions were stable if stored in plastic containers, and this compound became available in liquid and gel, as well as powder, form. With continued research of different types of agents and recognition by the dental profession of their inherent disadvantages with regard to patient acceptance and stability, as well as the need to use professional time more efficiently, the trend has been toward the use of ready-to-use, stable, flavored preparations in gel form.

### Sodium Fluoride (NaF)

This material is available in powder, gel, and liquid form. The compound is recommended for use in a 2% concentration, which may be *prepared* by dissolving 0.2 g of powder in 10 mL of distilled water. The prepared solution or gel has a basic pH and is stable if stored in plastic containers. Ready-to-use 2% solutions and gels of NaF are commercially available; because of the relative *absence of taste considerations* with this compound, these solutions generally contain little flavoring or sweetening agents.

### Stannous Fluoride (SnF₂)

This compound is available in powder form either in bulk containers or preweighed capsules. The recommended and approved concentration is 8%, which is obtained by dissolving 0.8 g of the powder in 10 mL of distilled water. Stannous fluoride solutions are quite acidic, with a pH of about 2.4 to 2.8. Aqueous solutions of $SnF_2$ are not stable because of the formation of stannous hydroxide and, subse-

quently, stannic oxide, which is visible as a white precipitate. As a result, solutions of this compound must be prepared immediately prior to use. As will be noted later, $SnF_2$ solutions have a bitter, metallic taste. To eliminate the need to prepare this solution from the powder and to improve patient acceptance, a stable, flavored solution can be prepared with glycerine and sorbitol to retard hydrolysis of the $SnF_2$ and with any of a variety of compatible flavoring agents. Ready-to-use solutions or gels with the proper $SnF_2$ concentration, however, are *not* commercially available.

### Acidulated Phosphate Fluoride (APF)

This treatment system is available as either a *solution or gel*, both of which are stable and ready to use. Both forms contain 1.23% fluoride, generally obtained by the use of 2.0% sodium fluoride and 0.34% hydrofluoric acid. Phosphate is usually provided as orthophosphoric acid in a concentration of 0.98%. The pH of true APF systems should be about 3.5. Gel preparations feature a greater variation in composition, particularly with regard to the source and concentration of phosphate. In addition, the gel preparations generally contain thickening (binders), flavoring, and coloring agents.

Another form of acidulated phosphate fluoride for topical applications, namely *thixotropic* gels, is also available. The term thixotropic denotes a solution that sets in a gel-like state but is not a true gel. On the application of pressure, thixotropic gels behave like solutions; it has been suggested that these preparations are more easily forced into the interproximal spaces than conventional gels. The active fluoride system in thixotropic gels is *identical* to conventional APF solutions. Although the initial thixotropic gels exhibited somewhat poorer biologic activity in in vitro studies, subsequent formulations were at least equivalent to conventional APF systems. Even though few clinical efficacy studies have been reported,[44] the collective data

were considered adequate evidence of activity; these preparations have been *approved by the American Dental Association*.

Within the past few years, a foam form of APF has become available. Laboratory studies indicate that the amount of fluoride uptake in enamel following applications using the foam is *comparable* to that observed with conventional APF gels and solutions. The primary advantage of foam preparations is that appreciably less material is used for a treatment and therefore lesser amounts are likely to be inadvertently swallowed by young children during the professional application.

### Application Procedure

In essence, two procedures are available for administering topical fluoride treatments. One procedure, in brief, involves the isolation of teeth and continuously painting the solution onto the tooth surfaces. The second, and *currently* more popular, procedure involves the use of fluoride gels applied with a *disposable tray*.

Until recently it was assumed that it was necessary to administer a thorough dental prophylaxis prior to the topical application of fluoride. This hypothesis was supported by the results of an early study that suggested that topically applied sodium fluoride was more effective if a prophylaxis preceded the treatment.[45] The results of four clinical trials,[46-49] have indicated that a prophylaxis immediately prior to the topical application of fluoride is *not necessary*. In these studies, the children were given topical applications of APF in the conventional manner except that three different procedures were used to clean the teeth immediately prior to each treatment; these procedures were either a dental prophylaxis, toothbrushing and flossing, or no cleaning procedure. The results indicated that the cariostatic activity of the APF treatment was *not* influenced by the different preapplication procedures. Thus, the administration of a dental prophylaxis prior to the topical ap-

plication of fluoride must be considered *optional*; it should be performed if there is a *general need* for a prophylaxis, but it need not be performed as a prerequisite for topical fluoride applications.

Figures 9–1 through 9–6 illustrate the major steps recommended for applying topical fluoride solutions. The essential armamentarium for the application of concentrated fluoride solutions consists of cut cotton rolls, suitable cotton-roll holders, cotton applicators, and treatment solution. If a prophylaxis is performed, the patient is allowed to rinse thoroughly, and then the cotton rolls and holders are positioned so as to isolate the area to be treated. It is a common practice when using fluoride solutions to isolate *both* right or left quadrants at one time so as to be able to treat one-half of the mouth simultaneously. The isolated teeth are then dried with compressed air, and the fluoride solution is applied using cotton applicators. Care should be taken to be certain that all tooth surfaces are treated. The application is performed by merely swabbing or "painting" the various tooth surfaces with a cotton applicator thoroughly moistened with the fluoride solution. The swabbing procedure is repeated *continuously and methodically* with repeated

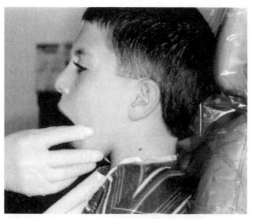

FIGURE 9–1 It is advisible to seat the patient in an upright position to help minimize the flow of topical solution down the child's throat.

"loading" of the cotton applicator so as to keep the tooth surfaces moist throughout the treatment period. At the conclusion of this period, the cotton rolls and holders are removed, the patient is allowed to expectorate, and the process is repeated for the remaining quadrants.

It should be stressed that various precautions should be routinely taken to *minimize* the amount of fluoride that is inadvertently swallowed by the patient during the application procedure. A number of reports[50–56] have shown that 10 to 30 mg of fluoride may be *inadvertently* swallowed during the application procedure, and it has been suggested that the ingestion of these quantities of fluoride by young children may contribute to the development of dental fluorosis in those teeth that are unerupted and in the developmental stage. Precautions that should be undertaken include (1) using only the *required* amount of the fluoride solution or gel to perform the treatment adequately; (2) positioning the patient in an *upright* position; (3) using efficient *saliva aspiration* or suctioning apparatus; and (4) requiring the patient *to expectorate thoroughly on completion* of the fluoride application. The use of these procedures has been shown to reduce the amount of inadvertently swallowed fluoride to *less than 2 mg*, which may be expected to be of little consequence.[57]

After the topical application is completed, the patient is advised not to rinse, drink, or eat for 30 minutes. The necessity of the latter procedure has not been substantiated; the fact that it has been followed in most of the prior clinical studies serves as the primary basis for this recommendation. This recommendation is also supported, however, by a 1986 study[58] that measured the amount of fluoride deposition in incipient lesions (subsurface enamel demineralization) in patients who either were, or were not, permitted to rinse, eat, or drink during this 30-minute posttreatment period. It was found that *significantly greater fluoride deposition occurred when the patients were not permitted to rinse, eat, or drink following the fluoride treatment.*

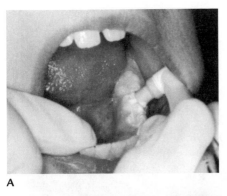

**A**

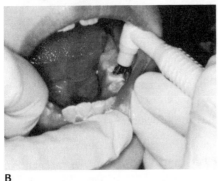

**B**

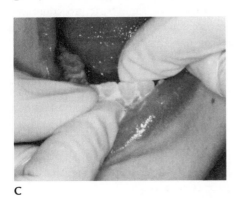

**C**

FIGURE 9-2    If desired, the topical application may be preceded by a thorough prophylaxis. The smooth tooth surfaces are cleaned with a prophylactic paste applied with a prophy cup, **A**, following the gross removal of heavy exogenous deposits (calculus) with hand instruments. A prophy brush is similarly used on the occlusal surfaces, **B**, while unwaxed dental floss is used to draw the paste interproximally to clean the proximal surfaces, **C**.

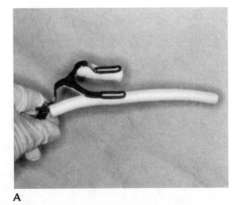

**A**

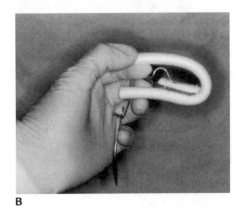

**B**

FIGURE 9-3    A 6-inch and 4-inch roll are placed in a Garmer holder in such a manner that, **A**, the lingual roll extends across the midline to isolate an area beyond the central incisors, and **B**, the long buccal roll is bent so as to isolate both the upper and lower vestibules.

Whichever fluoride system is used for topical fluoride applications, the teeth should be exposed to the fluoride for *4 minutes* for maximal cariostatic benefits. This treatment time has consistently been recommended for both sodium fluoride and APF. Some confusion has arisen, however, with regard to stannous fluoride, because shorter application periods of 15 to 30 seconds with stannous fluoride have been reported to result in significant cariostatic ben-

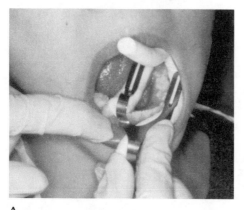
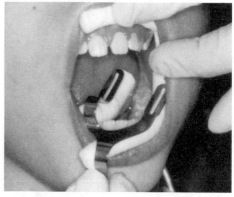

A                                          B

FIGURE 9-4    The cotton-roll holder is placed in the mouth, thereby isolating both an upper and lower quadrant from the retromolar to a point beyond the central incisors.

efits. Nevertheless, the collective results of these and subsequent clinical investigations indicate that maximum caries protection is achieved only with the use of the *longer* exposure period. Thus, although reduced exposure periods of 30 to 60 seconds might be appropriate as a fluoride maintenance or preventive measure in patients with very little caries activity, the use of the longer, 4-minute application should be *required* for patients with existing or potential caries activity.

### Application Procedure—Fluoride Gels

A slightly different technique is commonly suggested for providing treatments with fluoride gels. Although these preparations may be applied by using the same basic procedure as described for solutions, the use of *plastic trays* has been suggested as a more convenient procedure. As with the use of topical fluoride solutions, the treatment may be preceded by a prophylaxis if indicated by existing oral conditions. With the so-called tray application technique,

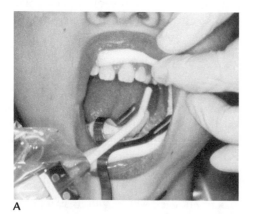

A

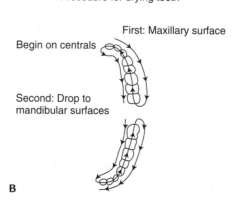

Procedure for drying teeth

First: Maxillary surface

Begin on centrals

Second: Drop to
mandibular surfaces

B

FIGURE 9-5    The isolated teeth are, **A**, dried with an air syringe in a systematic manner, **B**, so as to avoid missing any tooth surface.

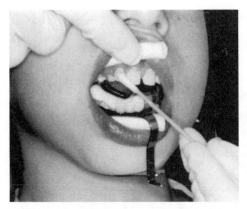

FIGURE 9-6    Using the same application pattern as in Figure 9-5B, fluoride solution is applied with a cotton applicator, with continual reapplications to maintain all tooth surfaces moist with the solution for a 4-minute period.

the armamentarium consists simply of a *suitable tray and the fluoride gel.*

Many different types of trays are available; selection of a tray adequate for the individual patient is an important part of the technique. Most manufacturers of trays offer sizes to fit patients of different ages. An adequate tray should *cover all the patient's dentition;* it should also have enough depth to reach beyond the neck of the teeth and contact the alveolar mucosa to prevent saliva from diluting the fluoride gel. Some of the trays used in the past did not meet these requirements. Some were made of vinyl and frequently either did not reach the mucosa or impinged on the tissue, thus forcing the dentist to cut the flanges of the tray. Currently, disposable *soft styrofoam trays* are available and seem to be adequate. These trays can be bent to insert in the mouth and are soft enough to produce no discomfort when they reach the soft tissues. With these trays, as well as with some of the previous types of trays, it is possible to *treat both arches simultaneously.*

If a prophylaxis is given, the patient is permitted to rinse, and the teeth of the arch to be treated are dried with compressed air. A ribbon of gel is placed in the trough portion of the tray and the tray seated over the entire arch. The method used must ensure that the gel reaches *all* of the teeth and flows interproximally. If, for instance, a soft pliable tray is used, the tray is pressed or molded against the tooth surfaces, and the patient may also be instructed to bite gently against the tray. Some of the early trays contained a sponge-like material that "squeezed" the gel against the teeth when the patient was asked to bite lightly or simulate a chewing motion after the trays were inserted. It is recommended that the trays be kept in place for a *4-minute treatment period* for optimal fluoride uptake, although some systems recommend a 1-minute application time. As noted previously, the patient is advised not to eat, drink, or rinse for 30 minutes following the treatment.[58] Figure 9–7 illustrates the tray technique of fluoride gel application.

> **Question 3**
>
> Which of the following statements, if any, are correct?
> A. Assuming that less than 1 ppm of fluoride is in the saliva (true), the dental plaque may have 100 times this level.
> B. Stannous fluoride is quite stable when stored in aqueous phase.
> C. A thixotropic gel looks like a gel, acts like a gel, and is a gel.
> D. After a topical application of fluoride, a patient should not eat or drink for a half-hour.
> E. A liquid topical solution should be maintained on the teeth for the same time as a gel tray treatment: 4 minutes.

### Application Frequency

As previously mentioned, although a single, topical application is accepted as not being able to impart maximal caries protection, considerable confusion has arisen regarding the preferred frequency for administering topical fluoride treatments. Much of this confusion is

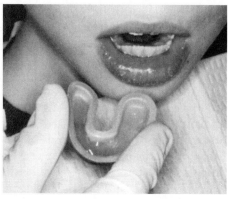
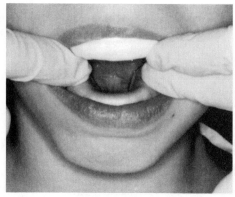

**A**                                                    **B**

FIGURE 9-7    Appropriate sized soft styrofoam trays are used to avoid pinching the soft tissues. A ribbon of gel is dispensed into the trough of the tray. Enough gel should be used to cover all tooth surfaces, but care should be used to avoid an excess which will flow into the mouth. (Experience will teach the operator how much gel to use.) The patient is shown the loaded mandibular tray, **A**, which is ready for insertion, **B**. The maxillary tray is inserted after the mandibular is in place. The patient is then asked to bite together so as to be more comfortable and, at the same time, to force the gel against the teeth. The use of thixotropic gels facilitates the wetting of all tooth surfaces. The trays should be maintained in place for 4 minutes.

caused by the absence of controlled, clinical evaluations of this variable, particularly with the most commonly used agent, acidulated phosphate fluoride.

The original Knutson technique[37] for the topical application of sodium fluoride consisted of a series of four applications provided at approximately 1-week intervals with only the first application preceded by a prophylaxis. It was further suggested that this series of applications be administered at ages 3, 7, 10, and 13 years, with these ages selected, or varied, in accordance with the eruption pattern of the teeth.[59] The objective of the timing was to provide protective benefits to "the permanent teeth during the period of changing dentition." Because this treatment sequence did not coincide with the common patient-recall pattern in the dental office, Galagan and Knutson[60] explored the possible use of longer intervals of 3 or 6 months between the individual applications constituting each treatment series. The results of their

work indicated that although significant benefits were obtained with single applications provided at 3- or 6-month intervals, maximal benefits were obtained only with a series of treatments. Nevertheless, the administration of single applications of sodium fluoride at 3- to 6-month intervals became a common practice, because these intervals were more convenient to the dentist and his or her normal recall system.

When stannous fluoride and acidulated phosphate fluoride were subsequently developed and evaluated, apparently little if any attempt was made to determine the optimal treatment frequency. Instead, the treatments were administered as single applications provided at 6- or 12-month intervals, which were convenient to the normal office schedules. Because these treatment intervals resulted in significant cariostatic benefits, the procedure that was ultimately approved and recommended involved this application frequency.

In view of this background, it seems that the frequency of topical applications should be *dictated by the conditions and needs presented by each patient and not by the convenience of the dental office.* This conclusion is supported by the data cited earlier that a series of applications is required to impart maximal caries resistance to the tooth surface.

Thus, it is recommended that new patients, regardless of age, with active caries be given an initial series of four topical fluoride applications within a period of 2 to 4 weeks. If desired, the initial application may be preceded by a thorough prophylaxis, the remaining three applications constituting the initial treatment series should be *preceded by toothbrushing* to remove plaque and oral debris. It should be obvious that this series of treatments may be very conveniently combined with the plaque control, dietary counseling, and initial restorative programs that the dentist has devised for these patients. Following this initial series of treatments, the patient should be given single, topical applications at intervals of 3, 6, or 12 months, *depending on his or her caries status.* Patients with *little* evidence of existing or anticipated caries should be given single applications every 12 months as a preventive measure.

Special effort should be made by the dentist to schedule topical fluoride applications so as to provide the treatment to newly erupted teeth within 12 months after eruption, and preferably *as close to eruption as possible.* As noted earlier, an approximate 2-year enamel maturation period occurs immediately following tooth eruption. As illustrated in Table 9–3, the preventive benefits of fluoride are invariably much greater on *newly erupted teeth* than on previously erupted teeth. This finding is apparent regardless of the fluoride system used and is presumably due to the greater reactivity, permeability, and ease of formation of fluorhydroxyapatite in enamel still undergoing calcification (or maturation).

Although it is important to expose newly erupted teeth to topical fluoride, it may be more appropriate to utilize a fluoride varnish for newly erupted primary teeth. Children at this young age may swallow too much of a topical fluoride gel and may have precooperative behavior making it difficult to use typical topical fluoride gels or foams.

### Efficacy of Topical Fluoride Therapy

Well over 100 human clinical studies demonstrate that topical fluoride therapy contributes significantly to the partial control of dental caries. Unfortunately, the practitioner is frequently concerned, and sometimes confused, about which procedure or agent should be employed in a given situation to provide a maximal degree of dental caries protection for the patient. Such concern and confusion is under-

TABLE 9–3  **Comparative Effectiveness of Topical Fluoride Applications on Previously Erupted and Newly Erupted Teeth**

| Clinical Investigation | Topical Agent | Caries Reduction (%) | |
| --- | --- | --- | --- |
| | | Previously Erupted Teeth | Newly Erupted Teeth |
| Averill (1967)[59] | NaF | 22.9 | 37.1 |
| Horowitz (1969)[61] | $SnF_2$ | 20.7 | 61.3 |
| Muhler (1960)[62] | $SnF_2$ | 44.2 | 84.0 |
| Szwejda (1972)[63] | $SnF_2$ | 20.4 | 44.4 |
| Szwejda (1972)[63] | APF | 22.5 | 63.0 |

standable when it is realized that dental caries investigators themselves frequently do not agree on these matters.

The results of the numerous clinical investigations with various topical fluoride agents and treatment procedures have been the subject of several reviews.[64-76] Therefore no attempt is made to repeat these reviews here.

As noted earlier, three different types of fluoride systems (i.e., NaF, SnF$_2$, and APF) have been evaluated and approved as safe and effective for topical fluoride applications *by both the American Dental Association (ADA)[77] and the Food and Drug Administration (FDA).[78]* To determine which of these systems may be the most effective, it would be desirable to compare the results of independent clinical studies in which all three systems have been tested when used in the recommended manner. Unfortunately, such data are not available, and alternative procedures must be sought.

Different approaches have been taken to estimate the magnitude of the cariostatic benefits that may be expected from topical applications of the different approved fluoride systems. One approach is simply to list all of the pertinent clinical trials and then determine the arithmetic mean of the reported caries reduction. This approach has been utilized by several investigators,[69-71] and the results observed for children residing in a nonfluoridated community are summarized in Table 9–4. Another approach is to utilize an empirically based procedure with existing clinical data to predict the efficacy of different systems;[79] these data are also shown in Table 9–4. Whatever the approach, *study designs varied in a number of ways,* such as the number and frequency of topical applications and the study duration. These variations serve to confound estimates of cariostatic efficacy. Nevertheless, it is apparent from Table 9–4 that all three types of topical fluoride systems result in *appreciable cariostatic benefits* of comparable magnitude with percentage reductions ranging from 27 to 36%. Furthermore, the data suggest that fluoride applied in gel form may be slightly less effective than solutions.

Considerably less information is available to document the efficacy of topical fluoride applications in adults. A total of 14 clinical trials were conducted in adults during the period 1944 through 1974, but the studies utilized a wide variety of experimental conditions, including the type of topical fluoride system, frequency of applications, and duration of the test period.[80-93] Although most of the methods resulted in a significant cariostatic benefit, the magnitude of this effect varied considerably, as might be expected. Furthermore, none of these studies used the application frequency suggested earlier for children.

It is generally recognized by dental scientists, however, that the dental caries process is fundamentally the *same in both children and adults,* although the rate of progression in young and middle-aged adults is frequently

TABLE 9–4  **Comparative Effectiveness of Different Topical Fluoride Systems (Average Percentage Reduction in Caries Incidence)**

| Fluoride System (%) | Form Used | Ripa[69] 1981 | Mellberg & Ripa[70] 1983 | Stookey[71] 1987 | Clark, et al[79] 1985 |
|---|---|---|---|---|---|
| NaF (2.0) | Solution | 29 | 29 | 27 | NA |
| SnF$_2$ (8.0) | Solution | 32 | 32 | 36 | NA |
| APF (1.2) | Solution | 28 | 28 | 36 | 38 |
| APF (1.2) | Gel | 19 | 19 | 25 | 26 |

TABLE 9-5  **Clinical Effectiveness of Varying Concentrations of Topically Applied Stannous Fluoride**

| SnF$_2$ Concentration (%) | Number of Subjects | Caries Reduction (%) | |
| | | DMFT | DMFS |
| --- | --- | --- | --- |
| 8 | 135 | 54.7 | 57.2 |
| 4 | 140 | 44.1 | 43.5 |
| 0.4 | 138 | 29.0 | 27.4 |

(From Mercer and Muhler, 1972.[94])

much slower because of a variety of factors, including more efficient oral hygiene and fewer between-meal snacks. Conversely, in older adults the rate of progression may increase because of medications that *reduce salivary flow.* It is commonly assumed, therefore, that topical fluoride applications are effective for coronal caries prevention *regardless of the age of the patient.* Root caries will be discussed later. Once again the frequency of application should be dictated by the needs of the patient; in the presence of frank or incipient caries activity, an initial series of applications should be followed by *maintenance applications* at 3, 6, or 12 months, depending on patient needs (i.e., evidence and extent of caries activity). Similarly, the choice of the fluoride system (NaF, APF, SnF$_2$) may be at the discretion of the dentist because there appears to be little, if any, difference in their efficacy.

On occasion it has been suggested that present topical fluoride treatment systems involve the use of excessive concentrations of fluoride. For example, some have suggested that the use of 0.4% rather than 8% stannous fluoride is adequate to obtain maximal benefits from topical applications of this compound. The basis for such suggestions invariably rests with the results of *in vitro* studies, quite commonly enamel-solubility studies, in which maximal effects are achieved with lesser concentrations of fluoride. Unfortunately, *in vitro* data do not necessarily predict clinical effects, and the results of a clinical investigation[94] clearly contradict these suggestions. As shown in Table 9–5,

the use of lower concentrations of stannous fluoride resulted in smaller caries-preventive benefits in children. Thus, until considerably more clinical data to the contrary become available, there is no legitimate basis for using concentrations of fluoride for topical applications *other than those that have been adequately evaluated clinically* and approved by review groups.

The relative superiority of acidulated phosphate fluoride gel or solution systems is a frequent topic for research. Five clinical trials directly investigated this question, and the results are summarized in Table 9–6. Four of these studies[63,95-97] involved single annual applications; another one[44] involved semiannual treatments. These data suggest that the two forms are quite comparable, particularly when applied semiannually. In practice the gels are greatly preferred due to their ease of application and reduced chair time when trays are used.

TABLE 9-6  **Comparative Effectiveness of Topically Applied APF Gels and Solutions**

| Clinical Trial | Reduction in Caries Incidence | |
| | APF Solution (%) | APF Gel (%) |
| --- | --- | --- |
| Ingraham & Williams[95] | 11 | 41 |
| Cons, et al[96] | 0 | 22 |
| Horowitz & Doyle[97] | 28 | 24 |
| Szwejda[63] | 28 | 4 |
| Cobb, et al[44] | 34 | 35 |

### Question 4

Which of the following statements, if any, are correct?

A. The semiannual application of fluoride to the teeth has proved to be the most effective time interval to reduce caries incidence.

B. There are no documented studies in which sodium fluoride, stannous fluoride, and acidulated phosphate fluoride have been tested in the same study.

C. Stannous fluoride is better than acidulated fluoride and sodium fluoride in nonfluoridated areas.

D. Both stannous fluoride and acidulated fluoride are effective on children, but neither is effective on adults.

E. A liquid topical of a 0.4% solution of stannous fluoride is as effective as an 8% solution.

## Root Surface Caries

As noted elsewhere, the increased retention of the teeth during adulthood because of various caries-preventive measures and the increase in life expectancy in many countries has resulted in an increased prevalence of root surface caries in adults. According to the 1985 to 1986 United States Public Health Service (USPHS) survey of adults,[98] about one-half of U.S. adults are afflicted with root surface caries by age 50, with an average prevalence of about three lesions by age 70. Interestingly, a study conducted at the University of Iowa[99] has indicated that adults over age 65 can expect an incidence of about 0.9 newly decayed, missing, or filled (DMF) coronal surfaces per year as well as about 0.6 new DMF root surfaces per year. Thus, this form of caries has received increased attention of dental scientists during the past decade, with investigations covering both its *cause* and *measures for prevention*.

Quite clearly, fluoride is very effective for the prevention of root surface caries as evi-denced by a limited number of clinical trials and numerous *in vitro* as well as *in situ* studies. For example, the results of several epidemiologic studies have demonstrated that the presence of *fluoridated drinking water* throughout the lifetime of an individual prevents the development of root surface caries.[100–103] The magnitude of this effect is consistently *greater than 50%*. Furthermore, it has been observed[104] that the use of a NaF dentifrice results in a significant decrease in root surface caries of *more than 65%*.

Much less information is available, however, to document the effect of topical fluoride applications on the prevention of root caries and particularly the relative efficacy of different fluoride systems. Nyvad and Fejerskov[105] reported the arrestment of root surface caries following the topical application of 2% NaF and the daily use of a fluoride dentifrice. Wallace and coworkers[106] reported a 70% reduction in the incidence of root surface caries following semiannual applications of an APF gel during a 4-year study period. To obtain some perspective on the potential efficacy of different topical fluoride systems[107,108] we have utilized an established animal root caries model. The results of this investigation are summarized in Table 9–7. From these data it is apparent that all three approved topical fluoride systems decreased the formation of root caries by 63 *to* 76% in this preclinical model. In the absence of the results of similar clinical data and with the recognition that the application of 8% $SnF_2$ imparts a brown pigmentation to exposed dentin, it seems appropriate to recommend the topical use of *2% NaF* for the prevention of root caries.

## Recommendations—Topical Fluoride Treatments

On the basis of the foregoing discussion, it is apparent that although periodic topical applications of any of the three approved agents provide protection against dental caries, maximal patient benefits may be expected only through

TABLE 9-7  **Effect of Professional Topical Fluoride Systems on Root Caries in Hamsters**

| Topical Fluoride System | Root Caries Score | Percent Reduction |
|---|---|---|
| Control (H$_2$O) | 8.2 | — |
| SnF$_2$ (0.4%) + APF (0.3%) | 4.9 ⎤ [a] | 40.2 |
| APF (1.2%) | 3.0 ⎦ ⎤ | 63.4 |
| NaF (2.0%) | 2.3 ⎟ | 72.0 |
| SnF$_2$ (8.0%) | 2.0 ⎦ | 75.6 |

[a]Values within brackets do not differ significantly.
(From Stookey GK, et al., 1989.[108])

the use of selected procedures. These recommended procedures include the following:

- Accepting the relative inefficiency of single, topical applications of fluoride solutions, patients with existing evidence of caries activity, whatever their age, should be given an *initial series of topical fluoride treatments followed by quarterly, semiannual, or annual treatments* as required to maintain cariostasis. The initial series of treatments should consist of four applications administered during a 2- to 4-week period, with the first treatment preceded by a thorough prophylaxis if indicated.

- Whatever fluoride system is selected, the application period (i.e., the time the teeth are kept in contact with the fluoride system) should be 4 minutes in all patients with existing caries activity. Shorter treatment periods may be permissible in the performance of treatments to *maintain* cariostasis.

### Fluoride Varnishes

Fluoride-containing varnishes have more recently become available in the United States and are being recommended for providing topical fluoride treatments, particularly for very young children. Most varnishes contain 5.0% *sodium fluoride* (2.26% fluoride) and a typical application requires only 0.3 to 0.5 mL of the varnish, which contains 3 to 6 mg of fluoride. The application procedure involves cleaning

the tooth surfaces by toothbrushing, painting the varnish on the teeth, and drying. The *varnish is retained for 24 to 48 hours* during which time fluoride is released for reaction with the underlying enamel. It is recommended that the applications be repeated at 4- to 6-month intervals.

The efficacy of fluoride varnishes for caries prevention has been repeatedly demonstrated in Europe, where they have been in common use for many years, and the results of these studies have been summarized in recent reviews.[76,109,110] These studies have consistently demonstrated a significant reduction in the incidence of dental caries and also have indicated that the magnitude of the benefit is related to the frequency of application, particularly in children at high risk for caries. Promising research has been conducted in the United States, specifically aimed at using fluoride varnishes as a preventive agent for children *at high risk for early childhood caries.*[111]

Little information is available to compare the effectiveness of fluoride varnishes with professionally applied topical fluoride solutions or gels. The results of a clinical study[112] conducted in children in India comparing the efficacy of a fluoride varnish with topical applications of an APF gel indicated that while both treatments resulted in a significant reduction in caries, the *fluoride varnish was more effective.* Seppa and coworkers[113] recently reported the results of a clinical trial comparing semiannual applications of the sodium fluoride varnish with simi-

lar applications of an APF gel in 12- and 13-year-old children with high past caries experience, and observed *no* significant differences between the two treatment regimens. In the absence of additional clinical data it appears that these *two treatment procedures are at least equivalent.*

### Initiation of Therapy

Practitioners frequently wonder when they should recommend and initiate a topical fluoride application program. All too frequently the tendency is to defer such treatments until the child is 8 to 10 years of age and a majority of the permanent dentition has already erupted.

As discussed earlier, it is well established that the enamel surface of a newly erupted tooth is not completely calcified and therefore that the period when the tooth is most susceptible to carious attack is the first few months after eruption. Furthermore, it has been shown that topical fluoride treatments are effective for both the deciduous and permanent dentitions. Thus, it follows that topical fluoride therapy should be initiated *when the child reaches about 2 years of age,* when most of the deciduous dentition should have erupted. The treatment regimen should be maintained at least on a semiannual basis throughout the period of increased caries susceptibility, which *persists for about 2 years after eruption* of the permanent second molars (i.e., until the child is about 15 years of age).

It should be added that the susceptibility of the dentition to dental caries *does not end at age 15.* It is probable, however, that the gradual *decrease in caries susceptibility with increasing age* will permit a less frequent topical application program to maintain cariostasis in many patients, and annual fluoride treatments may suffice.

### Problems and Disadvantages

Some clinical situations may alter the selection of the treatment agent. For example, the use of stannous fluoride may be contraindicated for aesthetic reasons in specific instances. The reaction of tin ions with enamel, particularly carious enamel, results in the formation of *tin phosphates,* some of which are brown in color. Thus, the use of this agent produces a temporary brownish pigmentation of carious tooth structure. This stain may exaggerate existing aesthetic problems when the patient has carious lesions in the anterior teeth that will not be restored. Stannous fluoride, however, has not been found to discolor composite restorative materials.

Another problem frequently raised, particularly by pedodontists, concerns the strong, unpleasant, metallic taste of stannous fluoride. Although experienced practitioners can handle this problem, there is no question that flavored, APF preparations are much *better accepted by children.* Experimental, flavored, stannous fluoride preparations that diminish, but by no means eliminate, the taste problem have been evaluated clinically but are not yet commercially available.[36] Until the taste problem of stannous fluoride is solved, most pedodontists agree that the *agent of choice* for children is APF.

Acidulated phosphate fluoride systems have the disadvantage of possibly etching ceramic or porcelain surfaces. As a result, porcelain veneer facings and similar restorations should be *protected with cocoa butter, vaseline, or isolation* prior to applying APF. Alternatively, sodium fluoride may be used instead of APF.

Without doubt, the tendency in many dental offices is to use a specific topical fluoride system and treatment regimen for every patient. It should be emphasized, however, that the specific needs of the patient should be ascertained initially and a specific treatment program developed to fulfill those needs. For example, the use of a series of four or more topical fluoride applications within a 4-week period followed by repeated single applications at 3- to 6-month intervals should be considered for a patient with a severe caries problem. Likewise,

a reduced topical application time of 30 seconds as opposed to 4 minutes may be adequate to maintain a patient with little or no current caries activity. In other words, the practitioner should be familiar with the indications and contraindications for using various approaches and select the treatment system and conditions that best meet the needs of the patient.

## Fluoride-Containing Prophylactic Pastes

Fluoride-containing prophylactic pastes have been available and widely used in dental offices for more than 40 years to clean and polish accessible tooth surfaces and restorations. Because these pastes contain abrasives, which are harder than enamel, in order to clean and polish efficiently, inevitably a *small amount of the enamel surface will be removed by abrasion during the prophylaxis*. The actual amount of enamel removed during a prophylaxis is very small and has been shown[114,115] to involve the loss of surface enamel to a depth of about 0.1 to 1.0 microns during a 10-second polishing. Since it has been noted that the greatest concentrations of fluoride in enamel occur in the outermost surface layers, it follows that the loss of even this small amount of surface enamel during a prophylaxis results in the exposure of an enamel surface having a *lower concentration* of fluoride than was present prior to the prophylaxis.[116,117]

When fluoride-containing prophylactic pastes first became available in the 1950s it was thought that the use of the preparations to perform a routine dental prophylaxis would result in a significant reduction in the subsequent development of dental caries and a number of clinical trials were conducted to determine the magnitude of this benefit. The results of these investigations, considered collectively, indicated that the use of these pastes resulted in a very modest increase in the resistance of the tooth surfaces to the development of dental caries, but the magnitude of this effect was not statistically significant. As a result, fluoride-containing prophylactic pastes have *never been accepted* as therapeutic agents by review agencies such as the ADA or the FDA. However, they are *commonly recommended* for use during a prophylaxis in order to at least replace the fluoride lost from the enamel surface by abrasion during the procedure. Should the clinician use fluoride-containing phophylaxis pastes? In summary, the following recommendations are proposed:

- When a simple prophylaxis is administered, which will not be followed by a topical fluoride application, fluoride-containing prophylactic pastes should be used to replenish the fluoride lost during the procedure.

- When a topical fluoride application is given to a caries-susceptible patient and a prophylaxis is deemed to be necessary, it is advisable to administer the preceding prophylaxis with a fluoride-containing paste. Although no definitive proof of the additive benefits of both procedures exists as yet, an increased benefit has been shown in some studies. Even when doubt exists, it is preferable to give the patient the possible benefit of any increased protection.

---

**Question 5**

Which of the following statements, if any, are correct?

A. The first active programs for topical fluoride therapy should be initiated following the eruption of the first permanent molar.

B. After age 15, the need for topical applications of fluoride ceases.

C. A prophylaxis increases the effectiveness of the topical application of fluorides.

D. From 0.1 to 1.0 mm of enamel is removed during a prophylaxis.

E. The use of a fluoride-containing prophylactic paste results in a significant reduction in caries formation.

## Dentifrices

Through the years dentifrices have been defined as preparations intended for use with a toothbrush to clean the accessible tooth surfaces. They have been prepared in a variety of forms, including pastes, powders, and liquids. The history of dentifrices dates back several centuries. The earliest writings concerning measures to achieve oral cleanliness refer to the use of toothpicks, chewsticks, and sponges; suggested dentifrice ingredients were dried animal parts, herbs, honey, and minerals.

Materials actually detrimental to oral health were used for many years; these materials included excessively abrasive materials, lead ores, and sulfuric and acetic acids. With the appreciation for the need of safe and efficient dentifrices came the research and development that have led to the dentifrices available today and the development of a major industry. In the United States alone, dentifrice sales approached $1.5 billion during 1995, and major manufacturers have invested millions of dollars, particularly during the past three decades, to improve these products further and to expand their capacities to promote oral health. Without question the dental profession and the scientific community, as well as the general population, have profited immeasurably, both directly and indirectly, from the efforts of the dentifrice industry.

As a result, the functions of present-day dentifrices have been considerably expanded to include the following: (1) cleaning accessible tooth surfaces, (2) polishing accessible tooth surfaces, (3) decreasing the incidence of dental caries, (4) promoting gingival health, and (5) providing a sensation of oral cleanliness, including the control of mouth odors. These functions should be accomplished in a safe manner without undue abrasion to the oral hard tissue, particularly dentin, and without irritation to the oral soft tissues.

This chapter makes no attempt to review the components and functions of dentifrices. For information on these topics, as well as a review of the early attempts to develop therapeutic dentifrices using agents other than fluoride, the reader is referred to several excellent reviews[118–123] (see also Chapter 6).

### Fluoride Dentifrices

At present fluoride is by far the *most effective dentifrice* additive for caries prevention. The initial studies with fluoride-containing dentifrices were only modestly encouraging. The results of two clinical trials indicated a significant beneficial effect with formulations containing fluorapatites and rock phosphates. However, studies using products containing sodium fluoride at concentrations of 0.01 to 0.15 percent failed to indicate any beneficial effect.[118] In retrospect, these and later failures were probably largely caused by the use of an *incompatible abrasive system* (i.e., calcium carbonate) in the formulations. In the 40-year period since the initial clinical trials with fluoride-containing dentifrices, the results of more than 140 controlled clinical studies have been published. For a review of many of these studies, the reader is referred to a recent report.[123]

In 1954, the first report was published concerning the use of a dentifrice containing stannous fluoride (0.4%); this study indicated a significant beneficial effect attributable to this agent.[124] Since then the results of more than 60 clinical investigations with stannous fluoride-containing dentifrices have been reported; the vast majority of this work has been performed with formulations containing *calcium pyrophosphate* as the abrasive agent, although insoluble sodium metaphosphate and hydrated silica have also been used.

Without doubt, the most extensive documentation of the cariostatic benefits of fluoride dentifrices was generated with the original stannous fluoride–calcium pyrophosphate formulation (i.e., Crest) with supportive information using this fluoride compound with other abrasive systems. The results of these investigations not only indicated that the normal home use of the stannous fluoride dentifrice resulted

in a significant decrease in the incidence of dental caries in children but that *similar benefits were derived by adults.* Furthermore, these effects were found to be additive to those provided by communal fluoridation and by topical fluoride treatments. As a result of these findings, the Council on Dental Therapeutics of the ADA first awarded complete acceptance to a fluoride dentifrice, specifically the stannous fluoride–calcium pyrophosphate formulation *(Crest)*, in 1964.

Primarily because of the identification of a formal mechanism by the ADA to recognize dentifrices on the basis of clinical documentation of a cariostatic activity, much effort was devoted by dentifrice manufacturers to the development and documentation of effective formulations during the past four decades. A number of effective products subsequently became available.

During the 1960s, a number of reports of clinical trials indicated that the use of *sodium monofluorophosphate* (MFP), $Na_2PO_3F$, in a dentifrice likewise contributed significantly to the control of dental caries. The first product, *Colgate MFP*, used insoluble sodium metaphosphate as the abrasive system, and this formulation was shown to reduce the incidence of caries in children by as much as 34%. On the basis of these studies, this dentifrice was *approved as safe and effective by the FDA in 1967 and accepted by the ADA in 1969.*

An interesting and unique characteristic of MFP is its compatibility with a *wide variety of dentifrice abrasive systems.* In contrast to other fluoride compounds, such as sodium fluoride and stannous fluoride, which are almost completely dissociated in aqueous solution to yield fluoride ions that readily react with available cations, the fluoride in MFP remains largely complexed as $PO_3F^5$ in solution. This fluoride complex is compatible with a wide variety of abrasive systems and therefore may be readily incorporated into a variety of different dentifrice formulations while continuing to provide cariostatic activity.

Additional studies with dentifrices containing sodium fluoride have indicated that this agent also effectively contributes to the control of dental caries in children. The first of the sodium fluoride dentifrices to be substantiated in this regard included sodium metaphosphate as the abrasive agent. On the basis of three favorable clinical trials, this product (Durenamel) was given *provisional acceptance* by the ADA Council on Dental Therapeutics; however, this product is *no longer available.* Another sodium fluoride dentifrice has been the subject of several clinical trials. This formulation (Gleem) contains calcium pyrophosphate as the abrasive agent and has been found to exert a significant beneficial effect on the incidence of dental caries in children in both low-fluoride and optimal fluoride areas.

In 1981, the formulation of Crest was changed by replacing stannous fluoride with sodium fluoride and using hydrated silica in place of calcium pyrophosphate as the abrasive system. Interestingly, these changes and the resultant increase in the amount of available and biologically active fluoride in the product resulted in the revised formulation being significantly more effective than the formulation originally approved.[125,126] Since that time, many additional products containing sodium fluoride have been approved by the ADA. One reason for the increased use of sodium fluoride is that it is the preferred agent for use *in tartar-control formulations containing soluble pyrophosphates.* Furthermore, as noted later in this section, there is evidence that sodium fluoride formulated in a highly compatible abrasive system may be a superior anticaries agent. In terms of fluoride concentration, most dentifrices currently marketed in the United States contain *1,000 ppm fluoride, with two exceptions.* The Crest family of products contain a hydrated silica abrasive system which is less dense than other conventionally used abrasive systems. Because dentifrice is dispensed by the consumer on the basis of volume, not weight, the concentration of fluoride *was increased to 1,100 ppm* so

that the dose delivered would be comparable to nonsilica-based products. On the other hand, *Extra Strength Aim, which contains 1,500 ppm* fluoride from sodium monofluorophosphate, has an elevated fluoride content in an attempt to enhance its anticaries efficacy. Several controlled clinical trials have shown that, in dentifrices employing silica-abrasive systems and sodium monofluorophosphate as the fluoride source, 1,500 ppm of fluoride is *statistically significantly more effective than 1,000 ppm*, with a margin of superiority of about 15%.[127–129]

The potential role of fluoride dentifrices in the etiology of dental fluorosis needs to be mentioned. Several reports have indicated an *increasing prevalence of fluorosis in the United States.*[130–132] A national survey of U.S. children conducted between 1986 and 1987 indicated that about 22% displayed some evidence of dental fluorosis; however, it is important to note that, in terms of severity, *a majority had either very mild or mild fluorosis, and only about 1% were classified as moderate or severe.*[133,134] Certainly a number of sources of fluoride may be responsible, individually or collectively, for causing fluorosis. In evaluating the role fluoride toothpastes may play, however, the practitioner should consider several important factors. First, for fluorosis to occur, excessive levels of fluoride must be ingested *during the time of enamel formation.*[135] For practical purposes, the *anterior teeth* are of most concern aesthetically, and these are *only susceptible to becoming fluorotic during the first 3 years of life*[136] *and particularly during the period of 15 to 20 months of age.*[137] Of course, the risk of toothpaste ingestion is increased in younger children, and some studies have shown that very young children may ingest enough toothpaste to be at risk of dental fluorosis.[138] In fact, one study found that children who brush with a fluoride toothpaste *before 2 years of age have an elevenfold greater risk of developing fluorosis than children who begin brushing later.*[139] These considerations have prompted the ADA to recommend that *children under age 3 should be advised to use only a "pea-*

*sized" quantity of a fluoride dentifrice for brushing and that this quantity be gradually increased with age so that not until age 6 is the child using a "full-strip" of dentifrice on the brush head.* In making recommendations, the practitioner must consider what other sources of fluoride the child may be ingesting, such as fluoride or fluoride–vitamin supplements, fluoridated communal-water supplies, and infant formula prepared with fluoridated water.[139]

Not infrequently, the practitioner is asked if all fluoride dentifrices provide the same amount of caries-preventive benefits. In an attempt to answer this question, a review[123] examined the results of all published studies involving fluoride dentifrices. It was concluded on the basis of a considerable body of information that the use of *sodium fluoride with highly compatible abrasive systems, such as hydrated silica or acrylic particles, is the most effective dentifrice system for caries prevention at this time.*

Subsequent literature reviews compared all available clinical data regarding the relative efficacy of compatible sodium fluoride dentifrices and those containing sodium monofluorophosphate.[140–142] Using different statistical procedures, these reviews concluded that sodium fluoride was significantly more effective than sodium monofluorophosphate. Based on a meta-analysis, Johnson[143] concluded that the magnitude of this difference was 7%. It is interesting that many fluoride dentifrices marketed outside the United States contain mixtures of sodium fluoride and sodium monofluorophosphate with a total fluoride content of 1,500 ppm. Clinical efficacy data of these latter systems have also been reviewed recently[140,141] with the conclusion that they are numerically less effective than an equivalent concentration of bioavailable sodium fluoride.

It is significant that the extensive research with fluoride dentifrices has resulted in the regular use of these products by a major segment of our population. In terms of total dentifrice sales, nearly 95% consists of the *accepted or approved formulations.* For an updated listing of

fluoride-containing dentifrices receiving acceptance by the ADA, *the reader is referred to the ADA website at http://www.ada.org.* The widespread acceptance and use of these products by the general public has been considered one of the primary factors contributing to the apparent decrease in the prevalence of dental caries observed in the United States.[144,145]

In general, it should be apparent from this brief review that the use of approved fluoride dentifrices results in a significant decrease in the incidence of dental caries. In view of this, the use of such preparations should be routinely recommended.

---

### Question 6

Which of the following statements, if any, are correct?

A. The use of fluoride dentifrices have yielded equivocal results as caries control agents when used as the sole method of fluoride application.

B. Fluoride dentifrices appear to reduce caries in a range of approximately 20 to 45%.

C. The safety of a new dentifrice containing new fluoride compounds must be approved by the FDA before it is accepted by the ADA.

D. In 1981, Crest changed the fluoride in its formula from sodium fluoride to stannous fluoride.

E. Despite the fact that several dentifrices contain fluoride, approximately 40% of the population prefers nonfluoride-containing brands.

---

## Multiple Fluoride Therapy

From the prior discussions of various measures to apply fluoride to erupted teeth, it is apparent that *no* single fluoride treatment provides *total protection* against dental caries. Recognition of

this fact led early investigators to evaluate the use of combinations of fluoride measures.

Multiple fluoride therapy is a term that has been used to describe these fluoride combination programs. As originally developed, this program included the application of fluoride in the dental office in the form of both a fluoride-containing prophylactic paste and a topically applied fluoride solution and the home use of an approved fluoride dentifrice. In addition, some form of systemic fluoride ingestion, preferably communal-water fluoridation, was included.

The only published reports of clinical investigations that attempted to assess the total effect of this type of multiple fluoride therapy on dental caries involved the use of stannous fluoride topical systems.[146–151] In each of these studies, the topical fluoride treatments were administered semiannually; the results are summarized in Table 9–8. The results of these investigations indicate that the combination of *topical fluoride applications and home use of a fluoride dentifrice resulted in about 59% fewer carious lesions.*

The fact that the magnitude of this benefit is somewhat less than that of the components evaluated individually indicates that the caries-protection effects of the individual components (i.e., prophylactic paste, topical solution, and dentifrice) are only partially additive. Nevertheless, it is important to note that the combination of stannous fluoride treatments not only reduced the incidence of caries by more than 50% in both children and young adults but did so in both the *presence and absence of communal fluoridation.* If one accepts a 50% caries reduction attributable to water fluoridation and another 50% reduction of the remaining caries from the use of multiple fluoride treatments, it is apparent that the use of multiple fluoride therapy, including communal fluoridation, results in an *overall reduction in caries of about 75%.*

During the past few years, clinical investigators have explored combinations of fluoride

TABLE 9-8 **Results of Clinical Studies Using Multiple Fluoride Therapy Involving SnF$_2$-Containing Prophylactic Paste, Topical Fluoride, and Dentifrice**

| Clinical Investigation | Study Population | Fluoride in Water | Study Duration | Caries Reduction (%) |
|---|---|---|---|---|
| Gish & Muhler[145] | Children | Yes | 3 years | 55 |
| Bixler & Muhler[144] | Children | No | 3 years | 58 |
| Muhler, et al[146] | Adults | Yes | 30 months | 64 |
| Scola & Ostrom[148] | Adults | No | 2 years | 58[a] |
| Scola[149] | Adults | No | 2 years | 56[a] |
| Obersztyn, et al[147] | Adults | No | 1 year | 60 |

[a]Average reduction for multiple similar groups.

treatments using agents other than stannous fluoride with variable success. For example, Beiswanger and coworkers[152] reported that additive benefits were observed with topical applications of acidulated phosphate fluoride and the home use of a stannous fluoride dentifrice. Neither Downer and associates[153] nor Mainwaring and Naylor,[154] however, were able to demonstrate additive benefits from the combined use of a sodium monofluorophosphate dentifrice and topical application of acidulated phosphate fluoride.

The available data relating to multiple fluoride therapy thus suggest additive benefits from the use of either stannous fluoride or acidulated phosphate fluoride in the dental office and the home use of dentifrices containing fluoride. This does not necessarily mean that other combinations of fluoride treatments may not provide additive benefits but merely that they have not yet been evaluated; hopefully the results of future investigations will clarify this matter. In the meantime, the dental practitioner is strongly advised to use *combinations of fluoride treatments to provide maximal caries protection for patients.*

### Fluoride Rinses

In 1960, reports began to appear indicating that the regular use of neutral sodium fluoride solutions decreased the incidence of caries. In an attempt to identify topical fluoride measures

especially appropriate for use *in dental public health programs*, this approach was studied extensively during the subsequent 15 years. Whereas these studies employed a wide variety of experimental conditions, a number of investigations involved either the daily use of solutions containing 200 to 225 ppm or the weekly use of solutions containing about 900 ppm fluoride. The majority of these studies were conducted *in schools* with supervised use of the rinse throughout the school year.

The results of these investigations have been summarized on several occasions and will not be repeated here.[77,121,155–158] In general, both types of fluoride rinses resulted in significant caries reduction of about *30 to 35%.* On the basis of these findings, the simplicity of administration, and the lack of need for professional dental supervision, weekly fluoride-rinse programs in schools are becoming increasingly popular and are being aggressively promoted by dental public-health agencies. Fluoride rinses were approved as safe and effective by the FDA in *1974*[78] and by the Council of Dental Therapeutics of the ADA in *1975.*[157] A "Guide to the Use of Fluoride" was published in the September 1986 issue of the *Journal of the American Dental Association.* The composition and recommended use of approved products is shown in Table 9–9.

Nearly all of the early investigations using fluoride rinses involved children residing in

TABLE 9-9 **Composition and Usage of Approved Fluoride Rinses**

| Source of Fluoride | Fluoride Content | | Recommended Usage |
|---|---|---|---|
| | Percent | ppm | |
| NaF | 0.20 | 900 | Weekly |
| NaF | 0.02 | 100 | Twice daily |
| NaF | 0.05 | 225 | Daily |
| APF | 0.02 | 200 | Daily |
| $SnF_2$ | 0.10 | 243 | Daily |

areas in which the drinking water was deficient in fluoride. As a result, the approvals given to fluoride rinses were related to their use in non-fluoridated communities. Reports[61,122,159,160] indicated, however, significant benefits from fluoride rinses used in the presence of an optimal concentration of fluoride in the drinking water. Three additional reports have appeared relative to the use of fluoride rinses in children residing in fluoridated communities. The results of all three studies indicate that *cariostatic benefits provided by fluoride rinses are additive to those derived from communal fluoridation.*[161–163] In view of these collective observations there appears to be *no reason* to restrict the use of fluoride rinses to nonfluoridated communities.

The approval of fluoride rinses by the FDA and the ADA's Council on Dental Therapeutics for use in public health programs opened the door for the home use of these products as a component of multiple fluoride preventive programs. Although the approved preparations were intended to be available strictly by prescription, a *0.05% neutral sodium fluoride* rinse (Fluorigard) was subsequently introduced for over-the-counter (OTC) sale. Ultimately, approval was given to fluoride rinses distributed OTC for home use, although some restrictions were required. These restrictions included the distribution of quantities containing *no more than 300 mg fluoride in a single container, a cautionary label to avoid swallowing, and an indication that the preparations should not be used by* children younger than 6 years of age. At present there are several fluoride rinses distributed in this manner; these products contain about 225 ppm fluoride and are intended *for daily usage.*

The question of additivity of the effects of fluoride rinses to those obtained using fluoride with other vehicles has received contradictory answers. Ashley and associates[164] found a modest additivity of benefits from the supervised daily rinsing in school with an acidulated phosphate fluoride rinse coupled with supervised brushing in school plus normal home use of a sodium monofluorophosphate dentifrice. A similar observation was reported by Triol and coworkers.[165] On the other hand, Blinkhorn and coworkers[166] failed to observe any indication of additive caries protection between the similar supervised daily use of a neutral 0.05% sodium fluoride and the home use of this same dentifrice. Likewise, Ringelberg and associates[167] failed to find additivity between a daily sodium fluoride rinse and home use of a stannous fluoride dentifrice. Similarly, Horowitz and coworkers,[168] in a study involving the supervised weekly use of a sodium fluoride rinse and daily fluoride tablets plus the home use of approved fluoride dentifrices, observed a caries reduction comparable in magnitude to that reported earlier by these investigators with fluoride tablets or rinses used individually.

Additive effects can also be inferred from the numerous school fluoride rinse studies in which caries reductions from 30 to 35% were observed. Because the majority of these children in both the control and experimental groups used fluoride-containing dentifrices, it follows that the benefits observed in those studies were obtained above those provided by the fluoride dentifrices. The same conclusion can be reached from the data reported by Birkeland and coworkers[155] in Norway, a country where *over 90% of the children use fluoride dentifrices.* After 10 years of a mouthrinsing program, these authors found a caries reduction of *over 50% and reduction in the need for restoration of more than 70%.*

It can thus be concluded that fluoride rinses have a place as a component of a preventive program *along with*, but not as substitutes for, other modalities of fluoride use. Their main use is for patients with a high risk of contracting caries. Although existing evidence may lead some to doubt whether additional benefits for the patients accrue from the use of rinses, it is preferable in these instances to give the patients the benefit of the doubt. Examples of patients for whom fluoride rinses should be recommended include:

- Patients who, because of the use of medication, surgery, radiotherapy, and so on, have reduced salivation and increased caries formation.
- Patients with orthodontic appliances or removable prostheses, which act as traps for plaque accumulation.
- Patients unable to achieve acceptable oral hygiene.
- Patients with extensive oral rehabilitation and multiple restorative margins, which represent sites of high caries risk.
- Patients needing fluoride in their home care but cannot tolerate a custom-fitted tray.
- Patients with gingival recession and susceptibility to root caries.
- Patients with rampant caries, at least as long as the high caries activity persists.

As a general rule, *daily rinses* should be recommended rather than a weekly regimen; not only does the daily procedure appear to be slightly more effective, but, as a practical consideration, it is easier for patients to remember and comply with a daily procedure. In all these instances, it is important to remember that the rinses should *not be used in place of any of the other modalities* of fluoride use but as part of a comprehensive, preventive program that should also comprise plaque control, frequent fluoride topical applications, the home use of a fluoride dentifrice, diet control, and testing to determine if and when the oral environment is no longer conducive to caries. For children living in nonfluoridated areas, the prescription of fluoride supplements may also be considered.

## Fluoride Gels for Home Use

During the past 15 years, a number of fluoride gels have become available as additional measures that may be used to help achieve caries control. These procedures contain 0.4% stannous fluoride (*1,000 ppm fluoride*) or 1.0% sodium fluoride (*5,000 ppm*) and are formulated in a nonaqueous gel base that *does not contain an abrasive system*. Their recommended manner of usage involves toothbrushing with gel (similar to using a dentifrice), allowing the gel to remain in the oral cavity for 1 minute, and then expectorating thoroughly.

Even though no controlled clinical trials have been conducted of these products used in this manner, a number of them have been approved by the ADA's Council on Dental Therapeutics as an additional caries-preventive measure for use in patients with rampant caries. The basis for the approval of these products has been the numerous prior clinical caries studies using dentifrices containing the same amount of stannous fluoride coupled with analytic data demonstrating the stability of these preparations.

From a practical point of view, the recommended use of fluoride gels is generally similar to that cited earlier for fluoride rinses. In other words, they may be considered as an *alternative* to the use of fluoride rinses and an *adjunct* to the use of professional, topical fluoride applications and fluoride dentifrices as a collective means of achieving caries control in patients who are especially prone to caries formation. Like fluoride rinses, the use of these gels is generally restricted to the period required to achieve caries control. Compared with fluoride rinses, however, fluoride gels appear to have an *advantage in terms of patient compliance*. Because these preparations are only distributed to patients by their dentists, it is commonly thought that patients are more likely to use them in

compliance with the recommendations of their dentist.

It should be stressed that fluoride gels should *not be used in place of fluoride dentifrices*. Because the gels contain *no abrasive system* to control the deposition of pellicle, their use in place of a dentifrice results in the accumulation of stained pellicle in the majority of patients within a few weeks. Nevertheless, the proper use of these preparations in combination with professional topical fluoride applications and the home use of fluoride dentifrices may be expected to help achieve caries control in caries-active patients.

---

### Question 7

Which of the following statements, if any, are correct?

A. If a 20% reduction in caries occurs from water fluoridation and then another 25% from topical fluoride therapy, the total reduction is 45%.

B. Fluoride rinses are of little value in fluoridated areas.

C. A fluoride-rinse container should not contain more than 300 mg of fluoride.

D. A school rinse program can be expected to produce caries reduction on the order of 30%.

E. It is more practical to have people use a daily rinse than a weekly rinse.

---

### Fluoride-Releasing Dental Restorative Materials

Fluoride-releasing dental restorative materials may provide an additional benefit in preventive dentistry. Although not currently available in the United States, a fluoride-releasing amalgam has demonstrated *recurrent caries inhibition* at enamel and dentin restoration margins.[169] Likewise, both chemical-cured and light-cured *glass ionomer cements* have demonstrated caries inhibition at enamel and dentin restoration margins.[170–173] Fluoride-releasing *resin composites* have also consistently demonstrated recur-

rent caries inhibition at enamel margins, yet there are *conflicting results whether caries inhibition occurs at dentin margins*.[170,171,173,174] Preliminary studies indicate that glass ionomer cement and fluoride-releasing resin composite have synergistic effects with fluoride rinses and fluoridated dentifrices, in the *remineralization of incipient enamel caries*.[175–178] The materials may act as a fluoride delivery system. Upon exposure to additional external fluoride, the material surface *undergoes an increase in fluoride*. This fluoride is subsequently released and has demonstrated demineralization inhibition and even remineralization at adjacent tooth structure. Further clinical research to evaluate these fluoride-releasing restorative materials may provide more information for clinical recommendations.

---

### Question 8

Which of the following statements is incorrect?

A. Fluoride-releasing dental restorative materials can effectively inhibit adjacent enamel demineralization.

B. Fluoride-releasing dental restorative materials have been shown to effectively inhibit enamel demineralization on adjacent interproximal tooth surfaces.

C. Glass ionomer cements and fluoride-releasing resin composites have similar effectiveness of adjacent demineralization inhibition.

D. Glass ionomer cements and resin composites can uptake fluoride at the surface, following exposure to topical fluorides, and subsequently release the fluoride.

---

## Toxicology of Fluoride

The handling of fluorides is carefully regulated in industry by *occupational safety health legislation* and in the marketplace by *the FDA*. Com-

mercial dental fluoride products and professional practices can be toxic and even lethal when used inappropriately. The lethal dose for an adult is somewhere between 2.5 and 10 g, with the *average lethal dose being 4 to 5 g*. The use of the "average lethal dose" is a very imprecise designation that makes it difficult to predict the outcome of an accidental swallowing of an excess of fluoride. To correct this problem, a body-weight based, *probable toxic dose* (PTD) standard has been recommended as a more practical approach to making treatment decisions. With it, the urgency for first aid and more definitive emergency treatment can be determined rapidly. The PTD approach, first

reported by Bayless and Tinanoff, bases the level and urgency of treatment on the *number of multiples of 5 mg/kg* of fluoride ingested (Table 9–10).

If the amount ingested is *less than 5 mg/kg*, the office use of available calcium, aluminum, or magnesium products as first aid antidotes should suffice. If the amount is *over 5 mg/kg*, first aid measures should be *expeditiously* applied, *followed by hospital observation* for possible further care. Finally, if the amount of fluoride ingested approaches or *exceeds 15 mg/kg*, the immediate first aid treatment should be followed by a *most urgent action to move the patient swiftly into a hospital emergency room where cardiac monitoring, elec-*

---

**TABLE 9–10 Emergency Treatment for Fluoride Overdose**

| Milligram Fluoride Ion per Kilogram Body Weight[a] | Treatment |
|---|---|
| Less than 5 mg/kg | 1. Give calcium orally (milk) to relieve GI symptoms. Observe for a few hours. |
| | 2. Induced vomiting not necessary. |
| More than 5 mg/kg | 1. Empty stomach by inducing vomiting with emetic. For patients with depressed gag reflex caused by age (<6 months old), Down syndrome, or severe mental retardation, induced vomiting is contraindicated and endotracheal intubation should be performed before gastric lavage. |
| | 2. Give orally soluble calcium in any form (for example, milk, 5% calcium gluconate, or calcium lactate solution). |
| | 3. Admit to hospital, and observe for a few hours. |
| More than 15 mg/kg | 1. Admit to hospital immediately. |
| | 2. Induce vomiting. |
| | 3. Begin cardiac monitoring and be prepared for cardiac arrhythmias. Observe for peaking T waves and prolonged QT intervals. |
| | 4. Slowly administer intravenously 10 mL of 10% calcium gluconate solution. Additional doses may be given if clinical signs of tetany or QT interval prolongation develops. Electrolytes, especially calcium and potassium, should be monitored and corrected as necessary. |
| | 5. Adequate urine output should be maintained using diuretics if necessary. |
| | 6. General supportive measures for shock. |

[a]Average weight per age: 1–2 years = 10 kg; 2–4 years = 15 kg; 4–6 years = 20 kg; 6–8 years = 23 kg.
(From Bayless JM, Tinanoff N. Diagnosis and treatment of acute fluoride toxicity. *J Am Dent Assoc.* 1985, 110:209–211.)

*trolyte evaluation, and shock support is available. Ingestion of 15 mg/kg fluoride can be lethal.*

## Fluoride Toxicity

Fluoride acts in four general ways: (1) when a concentrated fluoride salt contacts moist skin or mucous membrane, hydrofluoric acid forms, causing a *chemical burn*; (2) it is a general *protoplasmic poison* that acts to inhibit enzyme systems; (3) it *binds calcium* needed for nerve action; and (4) *hyperkalemia occurs, contributing to cardiotoxicity.*

When dry fluoride powder contacts the mucous membrane or the moist skin, a reddened lesion occurs, and later the area becomes swollen and pale; still later, ulceration and necrosis may occur. In past years, skin burns of this type were common for many water engineers who emptied drums of fluoride agents into the hoppers feeding water supplies. Federal and state occupational safety acts have greatly reduced this danger.

Following excessive ingestion of fluoride, nausea and vomiting can occur. The vomiting is usually caused by the formation of hydrofluoric acid in the acid environment of the stomach, *causing damage to the lining cells of the stomach wall*. Local or general signs of *muscle tetany* ensue caused by the drop in blood calcium. This can be accompanied by abdominal *cramping* and pain. Finally, as the hypocalcemia and hyperkalemia intensify, the severity of the condition *becomes ominous with the onset of the three C's that can portend death—coma, convulsions, and cardiac arrhythmias.* Generally, death from ingestion of excessive fluoride occurs within 4 hours; *if the individual survives for 4 hours, the prognosis is guarded to good.*

## Emergency Treatment

Four actions are salient in treating fluoride poisoning: (1) *immediate treatment*, (2) *induced vomiting*, (3) protection of the stomach by binding fluoride with *orally administered calcium or aluminum preparations*, and (4) maintenance of blood calcium levels *with intravenous calcium.* Urgent and decisive treatment is mandatory once the PTD of 15 mg/kg has been approached or exceeded. The speed of initiating proper treatment can be critical to a person's chance for survival.[179] The blood level reaches its maximum from 0.5 to 1 hour after the fluoride is ingested. *By that time it can be too late.*

If an excessive amount of sodium fluoride is ingested, *first aid treatment can be initiated.* Milk, or better yet, milk and eggs should be given, for two reasons: (1) As demulcents, they help protect the mucous membrane of the upper-GI tract from chemical burns; and (2) they provide the calcium that acts as a binder for the fluoride. Lime water (calcium hydroxide) or Maalox (an aluminum preparation), can be drunk to accomplish the same purpose. Plenty of fluid, *preferably milk*[a] should be ingested to help dilute the fluoride compound in the stomach. *Vomiting is beneficial* and often occurs spontaneously; it also can be induced by *digital stimulus* to the base of the tongue or with syrup of ipecac, if available. When vomiting does occur, the majority of the ingested fluoride is often expelled. Preferably, the patient should be taken *directly to the emergency room of a hospital.* Otherwise the closest emergency medical service unit or physician capable of dealing with fluoride toxicity is the alternative. Once in a well-equipped medical facility, several options are possible, such as *gastric lavage, blood dialysis, or oral intravenous calcium gluconate to maintain the blood calcium levels. Every effort should be made to rid the body rapidly of the fluoride or to negate its toxicity before a refractory hyperkalemia and cardiac fibrillation become a greater problem than the fluoride intoxication.*[180]

## Chronic Fluoride Exposure

At high levels of industrial fluoride exposure, as experienced by cryolite and bauxite workers

U.S. population, and alternative methods for the provision of systemic fluoride leave much to be desired. Thus, additional measures are obviously needed for providing greater protection against caries to as many segments of the population as possible.

The term topical fluoride therapy refers to the use of systems containing relatively large concentrations of fluoride that are applied locally, or topically, to erupted tooth surfaces to prevent the formation of dental caries. This term encompasses the use of fluoride rinses, dentifrices, pastes, gels, and solutions that are applied in various manners. Among dental practitioners, however, this term is generally considered to refer to professional topical fluoride treatments performed in the dental office.

prior to the era of occupational safety regulations, the combined intake of fluoride through inhalation, ingestion, and water consumption often resulted in a daily dose of over 20 mg. This exceedingly high level of continual intake for 10 to 20 years resulted in a *severe skeletal fluorosis* characterized by *osteosclerosis, calcification of the tendons, and the appearance of multiple exostoses*. This same crippling bone fluorosis can also occur from long-term consumption of naturally fluoridated waters found *in some parts of the world, which contain 14 ppm or more of fluoride*. Other factors that increase the severity of bone fluorosis are high temperatures with a concomitant increase in drinking episodes, an elevated intake of fluoride in food, nutritional diseases, and low-calcium diets. *No* cases of skeletal fluorosis have been reported in the United States where water fluoridation concentrations were under 3.9 ppm.[181]

Despite all precautions, there is a potential for signs and symptoms of fluoride toxicity in dental office and home use of topical fluoride. The most probable cause is in *children in the 15- to 30-month age bracket* having an excess of dentifrice placed on the toothbrush and then swallowing the fluoride-laden saliva. In most cases, this results in a very mild, often unnoticeable change in the enamel of erupting teeth around age 6. A more serious toxicity can arise in the dental office from the mishandling and ingestion of fluoride salts used for professional purposes. To be prepared for such an unlikely emergency, the professional staff should be prepared for instituting possible emergency procedures.

## Home Security of Fluoride Products

The *lack of home storage security* of OTC and prescription fluoride products poses hazards to consumers. As presently packaged, the fluoride content of OTC fluoride products *can exceed the PTD for children*.[182] That the danger at home is real is attested by two *deaths of children after swallowing fluoride tablets*: one in Austria, and the other in Australia.[183] In one year (1986–1987), 13 cases of fluoride poisoning were reported to the North Carolina Poison Center. It was noted by the poison center that *no health-care providers who contacted the center were familiar with the treatment of the GI symptoms induced by fluoride poisoning*.[184] Clearly, parents need to be educated about the hazards of fluoride-containing dental products. Dentifrices, mouthrinses, and fluoride supplements need to be securely stored. Equally, health professionals need to be educated about the emergency treatment protocol following excessive intake of fluoride.

In a larger study, the American Association of Poison Control Centers reported that the number of fluoride-related calls had increased from 3,856 cases in 1984 to 7,794 in 1989. Of these, the number seeking clinical treatment was 366 in 1984 and 668 in 1989. In each of these years, young children were involved in 90% of the calls.[185]

### Question 9

Which of the following statements, if any, are correct?

A. The ingestion of 360 mg of fluoride by a 90-kg, 21-year-old adult is not as dangerous as the ingestion of 280 mg of fluoride by a 40-kg, 15-year-old adolescent.

B. Hypocalcemia and hyperkalemia are signs of an impending cardiotoxicity.

C. If a patient has ingested an excessive amount of fluoride, the occurrence of nausea and vomiting is a favorable sign.

D. The frequent topical applications of fluoride to the teeth at age 6 is believed to be the cause of fluorosis.

E. The ingestion of 15 mg/K of fluoride requires that the patient be under appropriate emergency medical care before 30 minutes has elapsed.

## SUMMARY

A number of different aspects of topical fluoride therapy have been reviewed in the foregoing material. Without doubt, the use of topical fluoride therapy contributes significantly to the control of dental caries; however, one cannot expect to control dental caries completely through the use of fluorides alone. Furthermore, because no single fluoride treatment procedure provides the maximal degree of caries protection possible with fluoride, the use of multiple fluoride therapy is advocated. In particular, the dentist should identify the needs of each patient and institute a multiple fluoride treatment program designed specifically to fulfill those needs.

## ANSWERS AND EXPLANATIONS

1. C—correct.

   A—incorrect. Enamel maturation is very rapid the first month, slows down over the next year or so, and then remains relatively stable.

   B—incorrect. Fluoride content decreases very rapidly in the first 10 mm and then more slowly, until the dentinoenamel junction is reached.

   D—incorrect. As the pH falls, the fluoride becomes more effective in protecting the enamel; at a neutral pH no protection is needed.

   E—incorrect. The main reaction product is calcium fluoride.

2. A, B, C, and D—correct.

   E—incorrect. There is a lesser concentration on the tooth with MFP and about the same cariostatic action as for other inorganic fluorides.

3. A, D, and E—correct.

   B—incorrect. Stannous fluoride in water goes to a hydroxide and then a white oxide.

   C—incorrect. Thixotropic gel looks like a gel, acts like a gel, but is not a gel.

4. B—correct.

> A—incorrect. A series of applications within a short period appears best.
> C—incorrect. There appears to be little, if any, difference in their efficacy.
> D—incorrect. The first part is correct; the second part is incorrect; both are effective, but the amount of difference between the $SnF_2$ and APF is debatable.
> E—incorrect. In the critical field studies, the 8 % solution wins easily.

5. D—correct.

> A—incorrect. Topical fluoride therapy should be started as soon as possible after the eruption of the first deciduous tooth.
> B—incorrect. Fluoride is a lifelong adjunct for dental health.
> C—incorrect. Recent studies have shown that it is not necessary to give a prophylaxis prior to a fluoride application.
> E—incorrect. The use of these products did not result in significant reductions in caries.

6. A, B, and C—correct.

> D—incorrect. Vice versa. Crest started with $SnF_2$ but now has NaF.
> E—incorrect. People use the fluoride dentifrices—up to 90%.

7. A, C, D, and E—correct.

> B—incorrect. The effects of fluoride are additive; the more often it is applied, the better.

8. A, B, and D—correct.

> C—incorrect. Glass ionomer cements have greater adjacent demineralization inhibition.

9. B, C, and E—correct.

> A—incorrect. First the age of the individual is not pertinent; what is critical is the mg/K. In this case, the first individual has had 3 mg/K (360/90), whereas the second individual has ingested 7 mg/K, 280/40—a potentially lethal dose.
> D—incorrect. Fluoride ingestion at age 6 or later will not cause fluorosis since pre-eruptive enamel formation is essentially completed.

## Self-evaluation Questions

1. There is an (inverse) (direct) relationship between the amount of fluoride (F) in the surface of the enamel and the number of caries. It requires about _____ (time) for the enamel surface to mature following eruption. The greatest amount of F in the enamel is located in the outer _____ (distance) of the enamel.

2. The reaction of elevated concentrations of fluoride with hydroxyapatite (HA) is accompanied by the formation of _____ (on the surface) (in the apatite crystal) and a loss of _____ (one of the key elements of HA). This element is not lost when $SnF_2$ is one of the reactants, in which case, the compound _____ (name)

is formed. Along with this compound, _____ (another F compound) is formed on the surface.

3. The calcium fluoride ($CaF_2$) formed on the surface of the tooth with neutral sodium fluoride, APF, or $SnF_2$, is lost relatively rapidly for _____ (time) and almost completely lost in _____ (time). During this period, the calcium fluoride (is) (is not) protective. Along with the formation—then loss—of $CaF_2$, there is a slow change in the apatite crystal from _____ (apatite) to _____ (name of crystalline form), which is more permanent. Because studies indicate that the $CaF_2$ is leached from the tooth, the long-term benefit must be from the _____ (crystalline form). Thus, if the build-up of the crystalline form is slow, (multiple) (single) applications of fluoride probably provide the best long-term prevention.

4. Fluoride accumulates to a greater extent in demineralized areas (true); two fluoride compounds with a low pH that de-mineralize enamel (and thus increase F uptake) are _____ and _____. Two times when the tooth is not optimally mineralized are just after _____ (event) of the tooth and just after bacterial _____ (event) of enamel; in either event, fluoride aids in the mineralization or remineralization process.

5. The three different solutions of fluoride used in office applied topical applications are NaF, _____ %; APF, _____ %; and $SnF_2$, _____ %. The APF is made acidic by adding two acids, _____ and _____ to a _____ _____ %.

6. The three "C's" indicating impending death from fluoride intoxication are _____, _____, and _____.

## REFERENCES

1. Keene, H. J., Mellberg, J. R., & Nicholson, C. R. (1973). History of fluoride, dental fluorosis, and concentrations of fluoride in surface layer of enamel of caries-free naval recruits. *J Public Health Dent*, 33:142–48.
2. DePaola, P. F., Brudevold, F., Aasenden, R., Moreno, E. C., Englander, H., Bakhos, Y., Bookstein, F., and Warram B. (1975). A pilot study of the relationship between caries experience and surface enamel fluoride in man. *Arch Oral Biol*, 20: 859–64.
3. Weatherall, J. A., Hallsworth, A. S., & Robinson, C. (1973). The effect of tooth wear on the distribution of fluoride in the enamel surface of human teeth. *Arch Oral Biol*, 18:1175–89.
4. Aasenden, R., Moreno, E. C., & Brudevold, F. (1973). Fluoride levels in the surface enamel of different types of human teeth. *Arch Oral Biol*, 18:1403–10.
5. Brudevold, F. (1975). Fluoride therapy. In Bernier, J. L., & Muhler, J. C., Eds. *Improving dental practice through preventive measures*, 3rd ed. St. Louis: Mosby, 1975.
6. Isaac, S., Brudevold, F., Smith F. A., & Gardner, D. E. (1958). Solubility rate and natural fluoride content of surface and subsurface enamel. *J Dent Res*, 37:254–63.
7. Thylstrup, A. (1979). A scanning electron microscopical study of normal and fluorotic enamel demineralized by EDTA. *Acta Odont Scand*, 37:127–35.

8. Brudevold, F., & McCann, H. G. (1968). Enamel solubility tests and their significance in regard to dental caries. *Ann NY Acad Sci*, 153:20.

9. Bibby, B. G. (1944). Use of fluorine in the prevention of dental caries. I. Rationale and approach. *J Am Dent Assoc*, 31:228–36.

10. Phillips, R. W., & Muhler, J. C. (1947). Solubility of enamel as affected by fluorides of varying pH. *J Dent Res*, 26:109–17.

11. Fischer, R. B., & Muhler, J. C. (1952). The effect of sodium fluoride upon the surface structure of powdered dental enamel. *J Dent Res*, 31:751–55.

12. Frazier, P. D., & Engen, D. W. (1966). X-ray diffraction study of the reaction of acidulated fluoride with powdered enamel. *J Dent Res*, 45:1144–48.

13. Gerould, C. H. (1945). Electron microscope study of the mechanisms of fluoride deposition in teeth. *J Dent Res*, 24:223–33.

14. Joost-Larsen, M., & Fejerskov, O. (1978). Structural studies on calcium fluoride formation and uptake of fluoride in surface enamel in vitro. *Scand J Dent Res*, 86:337–45.

15. McCann, H. G., & Bullock, F. A. (1955). Reactions of fluoride ion with powdered enamel and dentin. *J Dent Res*, 34:59–67.

16. Scott, D. B., Picard, R. G., & Wyckoff, W. G. (1950). Studies of the action of sodium fluoride on human enamel by electron microscopy and electron diffraction. *Public Health Rep*, 65:43–56.

17. Muhler, J. C., & Van Huysen, G. (1947). Solubility of enamel protected by sodium fluoride and other compounds. *J Dent Res*, 26:119–27.

18. Muhler, J. C., Boyd, T. M., & Van Huysen, G. (1950). Effects of fluorides and other compounds on the solubility of enamel, dentin, and tricalcium phosphate in dilute acids. *J Dent Res*, 29:182–93.

19. Jordan, T. H., Wei, S. H. Y., Bromberger, S. H., & King, J. C. (1971). $Sn_3F_3PO_4$: The products of the reaction between stannous fluoride and hydroxyapatite. *Arch Oral Biol*, 16:241–46.

20. Wei, S. H. Y., & Forbes, W. C. (1974). Electron microprobe investigations of stannous fluoride reactions with enamel surfaces. *J Dent Res*, 53:51–56.

21. Brudevold, F., Savory, A., Gardner, D. E. Spinelli, M., & Speirs, R. (1963). A study of acidulated fluoride solutions. *Arch Oral Biol*, 8:167–77.

22. Wellock, W. D., & Brudevold, F. (1963). A study of acidulated fluoride solutions. II. The caries inhibition effect of single annual topical applications of an acidic fluoride and phosphate solution, a two year experience. *Arch Oral Biol*, 8:179–82.

23. DeShazer, D. O., & Swartz, C. J. (1967). The formation of calcium fluoride on the surface of fluorhydroxyapatite after treatment with acidic fluoride-phosphate solution. *Arch Oral Biol*, 12:1071–75.

24. Wei, S. H. Y., & Forbes, W. C. (1968). X-ray diffraction and analysis of the reactions between intact and powdered enamel and several fluoride solutions. *J Dent Res*, 47:471–77.

25. Mellberg, J. R., Laakso, P. V., & Nicholson, C. R. (1966). The acquisition and loss of fluoride by topically fluoridated human tooth enamel. *Arch Oral Biol*, 11:1213–20.

26. Bruun, C. (1973). Uptake and retention of fluoride by intact enamel in vivo after application of neutral sodium fluoride. *Scand J Dent Res*, 81:92–100.

27. Lovelock, D. J. (1973). The loss of topically applied fluoride from the surface of human enamel in vitro using [18]F. *Arch Oral Biol*, 18:27–29.

28. Mellberg, J. R. (1973). Topical fluoride controversy symposium. Enamel fluoride uptake from topical fluoride agents and its relationship to caries inhibition. *J Am Soc Prev Dent*, 3:53–54.

29. Rinderer, L., Schait, A., & Muhlemann, H. R. (1965). Loss of fluoride from dental enamel after topical fluoridation. Preliminary report. *Helv Odont Acta*, 9:148–50.

30. Ahrens, G. (1976). Effect of fluoride tablets on uptake and loss of fluoride in superficial enamel in vivo. *Caries Res*, 10:85–95.

31. Wei, S. H. Y., & Schulz, E. M. Jr. (1975). In vivo microsampling of enamel fluoride concentrations after topical treatments. *Caries Res*, 9:50–58.

32. Kanauya, Y., Spooner, P., Fox, J. L., Higuchi, W. I., & Muhammad, N. A. (1983). Mechanistic studies on the bioavailability of calcium fluoride for re-mineralization of dental enamel. *Int J Pharmacol*, 16:171–79.

33. Chandler, S., Chiao, C. C., & Fuerstenau, D. W. (1982). Transformation of calcium fluoride for caries prevention. *J Dent Res*, 61:403–7.

34. Rolla, G. (1988). On the role of calcium fluoride in the cariostatic mechanism of fluoride. *Acta Odontol Scand*, 46:341–45.

35. Ten Cate, J. M. (1997). Review on fluoride, with special emphasis on calcium fluoride mechanisms in caries prevention. *Eur J Oral Sci*, 105:461–65.

36. Beiswanger, B. B., Mercer, V. H., Billings, R. J., & Stookey, G. K. (1980). A clinical caries evaluation of a stannous fluoride prophylactic paste and topical solution. *J Dent Res*, 59:1386–91.

37. Knutson, J. W. (1948). Sodium fluoride solution: Technique for applications to the teeth. *J Am Dent Assoc*, 36:37–39.

38. Mellberg, J. R. (1977). Enamel fluoride and its anticaries effects. *J Prev Dent*, 4:8–20.

39. Mellberg, J. R., Nicholson, C. R., Miller, B. G., & Englander, H. R. (1970). Acquisition of fluoride in vivo by enamel from repeated topical sodium fluoride applications in a fluoridated area: Final report. *J Dent Res*, 49:1473–77.

40. Puttnam, N. A., & Bradshaw, F. (1964). X-ray fluorescence studies on the effect of stannous fluoride on human teeth. *Adv Fluorine Res Dent Caries Prev: (ORCA)*, 3:145–50.

41. Hoermann, K. C., Klima, J. E., Birks, L. S., et al. (1966). Tin and fluoride uptake in human enamel in situ: Electron probe and chemical microanalysis. *J Am Dent Assoc*, 73:1301–5.

42. McDonald, J. L., Schemehorn, B. R., & Stookey, G. K. (1978). Influence of fluoride upon plaque and gingivitis in the beagle dog. *J Dent Res*, 57:899–902.

43. Beiswanger, B. B., McClanahan, S. F., Bartizek, R. D., Lanzalaco, A. C., Bacca, L. A., & White, D. J. (1997). The comparative efficacy of stabilized stannous fluoride dentifrice, peroxide/baking soda dentifrice and essential oil mouthrinse for the prevention of gingivitis. *J Clin Dent*, 8:46–53.

44. Cobb, H. B., Rozier, R. G., & Bawden, J. W. (1980). A clinical study of the caries preventive effects of an APF solution and an APF thixotropic gel. *Pediatr Dent*, 2:263–66.

45. Knutson, J. W., Armstrong, W. D., & Feldman, F. M. (1947). Effect of topically applied sodium fluoride on dental caries experience. IV. Report of findings with two, four, and six applications. *Public Health Rep*, 62:425–30.

46. Houpt, M., Koenigsberg, S., & Shey, Z. (1983). The effect of prior toothcleaning on the efficacy of topical fluoride treatment. Two-year results. *Clin Prev Dent*, 5(4):8–10.

47. Katz, R. V., Meskin, L. H., Jensen, M. E., & Keller, D. (1984). Topical fluoride and prophylaxis: A 30-month clinical trial. *J Dent Res*, 63(Prog. & Abstracts). Abstr. 771.

48. Ripa, L. W., Leske, G. S., Sposato, A., & Varma, A. (1983). Effect of prior toothcleaning on biannual professional APF topical fluoride gel-tray treatments. Results after two years. *Clin Prev Dent*, 5(4):3–7.

49. Bijella, M. F. T. B., Bijella, V. T., Lopes, E. S., & Bostos, J. R. (1985). Comparison of dental prophylaxis and toothbrushing prior to topical APF applications. *Community Dent Oral Epidemiol*, 13:208–11.

50. Ekstrand, J., & Koch, G. (1980). Systemic fluoride absorption following fluoride gel application. *J Dent Res*, 59:1067.

51. Ekstrand, J., Koch, G., Lindgren, L. E., & Petersson, L. G. (1981). Pharmacokinetics of fluoride gels in children and adults. *Caries Res*, 15:213–20.

52. LeCompte, E. J., & Whitford, G. M. (1982). Pharmacokinetics of fluoride from APF gel and fluoride tablets in children. *J Dent Res*, 61:469–72.

53. LeCompte, E. J., & Doyle, T. E. (1982). Oral fluoride retention following various topical application techniques in children. *J Dent Res*, 61:1397–1400.

54. LeCompte, E. J., & Rubenstein, L. K. (1984). Oral fluoride rentention with thixotropic and APF gels and foam-lined and unlined trays. *J Dent Res*, 63:69–70.

55. McCall, D. R., Watkins, T. R., Stephan, K. W., Collins, W. J., & Smalls, M. J. (1983). Fluoride ingestion following APF gel application. *Br Dent J*, 155:333–36.

56. Pourbaix, S., & Desager, J. P. (1983). Fluoride absorption: A comparative study of 1% and 2% fluoride gels. *J Biol Buccale*, 11:103–8.

57. LeCompte, E. J., & Doyle, T. E. (1985). Effects of suctioning devices on oral fluoride retention. *J Am Dent Assoc*, 110:357–60.

58. Stookey, G. K., Schemehorn, B. R., Drook, C. A., & Cheetham, B. L. (1986). The effect of rinsing with water immediately after a professional fluoride gel application on fluoride uptake in demineralized enamel: An *in vivo* study. *Pediatr Dent*, 8(3):153–57.

59. Averill, H. M., Averill, J. E., & Ritz, A. G. (1967). A two-year comparison of three topical fluoride agents. *J Am Dent Assoc*, 74:996–1001.

60. Galagan, D. F., & Knutson, J. W. (1948). Effect of topically applied sodium fluoride on dental caries experience. VI. Experiments with sodium fluoride and calcium chloride. Widely spaced applications. Use of different solution concentrations. *Public Health Rep*, 63:1215–21.

61. Horowitz, H. S., & Heifetz, S. B. (1969). Evaluation of topical fluoride applications of stannous fluoride to teeth of children born and reared in a fluoridated community: Final report. *J Dent Child*, 36:355–61.

62. Muhler, J. C. (1960). The anticariogenic effectiveness of a single application of stannous fluoride in children residing in an optimal communal fluoride area. II. Results at the end of 30 months. *J Am Dent Assoc*, 61:431–38.

63. Szwejda, L. F. (1972). Fluorides in community programs: A study of four years of various fluorides applied topically to the teeth of children in fluoridated communities. *J Public Health Dent*, 32:25–33.

64. Brudevold, F., & Nanjoks, R. (1978). Caries preventive fluoride treatment of the individual. *Caries Res*, 12(Suppl. 1):52–64.

65. Forrester, D. J. (1971). A review of currently available topical fluoride agents. *J Dent Child*, 38:52–58.

66. Horowitz, H. S., & Heifetz, S. B. (1970). The current status of topical fluorides in preventive dentistry. *J Am Dent Assoc*, 81:166–77.

67. Forrester, D. J., & Shulz, E. M., Eds. (1974). International Workshop of Fluorides and Dental Caries Reductions. Baltimore: University of Maryland.

68. Stookey, G. K. (1970). Fluoride therapy. In Bernier, J. L., & Muhler, J. C., Eds. *Improving dental practice through preventive measures* (2nd ed.) St. Louis: Mosby. pp. 92–156.

69. Ripa, L. W. (1981). Professionally (operator) applied topical fluoride therapy: A critique. *Int Dent J*, 31:105–20.

70. Mellberg, J. R., & Ripa, L. W. (1983). Professionally applied topical fluoride. In Fluoride in Preventive Dentistry. Theory and Clinical Applications. Chicago: Quintessence, 181–214.

71. Katz, S., McDonald, J. L., & Stookey, G. K. (1979). *Preventive dentistry in action*, (3rd ed.) Upper Montclair, NJ: DCP Publishing Company.

72. Ripa, L. W. (1989). Review of the anticaries effectiveness of professionally applied and self-applied topical fluoride gels. *J Public Health Dent*, 49:297–309.

73. Ripa, L. W. (1990). An evaluation of the use of professional (operator-applied) topical fluorides. *J Dent Res*, 69:786–96.

74. Wei, S. H. Y., & Yiu, C. K. Y. (1993). Evaluation of the use of topical fluoride gel. *Caries Res*, 27(Suppl. 1):29–34.

75. Johnston, D. W. (1994). Current status of professionally applied topical fluorides. *Community Dent Oral Epidemiol*, 22:159–63.

76. Horowitz, H. S., & Ismail, A. I. (1966). Topical fluorides in caries prevention. In Fejerskov, O., Ekstrand, J., & Burt, B. A., Eds. *Fluoride in dentistry*, 2nd ed. (pp. 311–27) Copenhagen: Munksgaard.

77. Council on Dental Therapeutics (1984). Fluoride compounds. In *Accepted dental therapeutics*, (4th ed.) Chicago: American Dental Association. pp. 395–420.

78. Fine, S. D. (1974). Topical fluoride preparations for reducing incidence of dental caries. Notice of status. *Federal Register*, 39:17245.

79. Clark, D. C., Hanley, J. A., Stamm, J. W., et al. (1985). An empirically based system to estimate the effectiveness of caries-preventive agents. A comparison of the effectiveness estimates of APF gels and solutions, and fluoride varnishes. *Caries Res*, 19:83–95.

80. Arnold, F. A. Jr., Dean, H. T., & Singleton, D. C. Jr. (1944). The effect on caries incidence of a single topical application of a fluoride solution to the teeth of young adult males of a military population. *J Dent Res*, 23:155–62.

81. Frank, R. (1950). Research and clinical evaluation of local applications of sodium fluoride. *Schweiz Mschr Zahnh*, 60:283–87.

82. Driak, F. (1951). Kariesprophlaxe mit besonderer Berücksichtigung der Impragnierungsmethoden. *Oester Ztschr Stomat*, 48:153–68.

83. Klinkenberg, E., & Bibby, B. G. (1950). Effect of topical applications of fluorides on dental caries in young adults. *J Dent Res*, 29:4–8.

84. Rickles, N. H., & Becks, H. (1951). The effects of an acid and a neutral solution of sodium fluoride on the incidence of dental caries in young adults. *J Dent Res*, 30:757–65.

85. Kutler, B., & Ireland, R. L. (1953). The effect of sodium fluoride application on dental caries experience in adults. *J Dent Res*, 32:458–62.

86. Carter, W. J., Jay, P., Shklair, I. L., & Daniel, L. H. The effect of topical fluoride on dental caries experience in adult females of a military population. *J Dent Res*, 34:73–76.

87. Muhler, J. C. (1957). Effect on gingiva and occurrence of pigmentation on teeth following the topical application of stannous fluoride or stannous chlorofluoride. *J Periodont*, 28:281–86.

88. Muhler, J. C. (1958). The effect of a single topical application of stannous fluoride on the incidence of dental caries in adults. *J Dent Res*, 37:415–16.

89. Protheroe, D. H. (1961). A study to determine the effect of topical application of stannous fluoride on dental caries in young adults. *Roy Can D Corps Q* 3:18–23.

90. Harris, N. O., Hester, W. R., & Muhler, J. C., & Allen, J. F. (1964). Stannous fluoride topically applied in aqueous solution in caries prevention in a military population. SAM-TDR-64-26. Brooks Air Force Base, TX: United States Air Force School of Aerospace Medicine.

91. Obersztyn, A., Kolwinski, K., Trykowski, J., & Starosciak, S. (1979). Effects of stannous fluoride and amine fluorides on caries incidence and enamel solubility in adults. *Aust Dent J*, 24:395–97.

92. Viegas, Y. (1970). The caries inhibiting effect of a single topical application of an acidic phosphate solution in young adults. A one year experience. *Rev Saude Publica*, 4:55–60.

93. Curson, I. (1973). The effect on caries increments in dental students of topically applied acidulated phosphate fluoride (APF). *J Dent*, 1:216–18.

94. Mercer, V. H., & Muhler, J. C. (1972). Comparison of single topical application of sodium fluoride and stannous fluoride. *J Dent Res*, 51:1325–30.

95. Ingraham, R. Q., & Williams, J. E. (1970). An evaluation of the utility of application and cariostatic effectiveness of phosphate-fluorides in solution and gel states. *J Tenn Dent Assoc*, 50:5–12.

96. Cons, N. C., Janerich, D. T., & Senning, R. S. (1970). Albany topical fluoride study. *J Am Dent Assoc*, 80:777–81.

97. Horowitz, H. S., & Doyle, J. (1971). The effect on dental caries of topically applied acidulated phosphate-fluoride: Results after three years. *J Am Dent Assoc*, 82:359–65.

98. U.S. Public Health Service. (Aug 1987). Oral health of United States adults. The national survey of oral health in U.S. employed adults and seniors: 1985–1986. National findings. *NIH Publ. No.* 87–2868.

99. Hand, J. S., Hunt, R. S., & Beck, J. D. (1988). Incidence of coronal and root surface caries in an older adult population. *J Pub Health Dent*, 48:14–19.

100. Burt, B. A., Ismail, A. I., & Eklund, S. A. (1986). Root caries in an optimally fluoridated and a high-fluoride community. *J Dent Res*, 65:1154–58.

101. Brustman, B. A. (1986). Impact of exposure to fluoride-adequate water on root surface caries in elderly. *Gerodontics*, 2:203–7.

102. Hunt, R. J., Eldredge, J. B., & Beck, J. D. (1989). Effect of residence in a fluoridated community on the incidence of coronal and root caries in an older adult population. *J Pub Health Dent*, 49:138–41.

103. Stamm, J. W., Banting, D. W., & Imrey, P. B. (1990). Adult root caries survey of two similar communities with contrasting natural water fluoride levels. *J Am Dent Assoc*, 120:143–49.

104. Jensen, M. E., & Kohout, F. J. (1988). The effect of a fluoridated dentifrice on root and coronal caries in an older adult population. *J Am Dent Assoc*, 117:829–32.

105. Nyvad, B., & Fejerskov, O. (1986). Active root surface caries converted into inactive caries as a response to oral hygiene. *Scand J Dent Res*, 94:281–84.

106. Wallace, M. C., Retief, D. H., & Bradley, E. L. (1993). The 48-month increment of root caries in an urban population of older adults participating in a preventive dental program. *J Pub Health Dent*, 53:133–37.

107. Stookey, G. K. (1990). Critical evaluation of the composition and use of topical fluorides. *J Dent Res*, 69:805–12.

108. Stookey, G. K., Rodlun, C. A., Warrick, J. M., & Miller, C. H. (1989). Professional topical fluoride systems vs root caries in hamsters. *J Dent Res*, 68:372, Abstr. 1521.

109. Petersson, L. G. (1993). Fluoride mouthrinses and fluoride varnishes. *Caries Res*, 27 (Suppl. 1):35–42.

110. Petterson, L. G., Arthursson, L., Ostberg, C., Jonsson, G., & Gleerup, A. (1991). Carries-inhibiting effects of different modes of Duraphat varnish reapplication: A 3-year radiographic study. *Caries Res*, 25:70–73.

111. Weinstein, P., Domoto, P., Koday, M., & Leroux, B. (1994). Results of a promising trial to prevent baby bottle tooth decay: A fluoride varnish study. *J Dent Child*, 61:338–41.

112. Shobha, T., Nandlal, B., Prabhakar, A. R., & Sudha, P. (1987). Fluoride varnish versus acidulated phosphate fluoride for school children in Manipal. *J Ind Dent Assoc*, 59:157–60.

113. Seppa, L., Leppanen, T., & Hausen, H. (1995). Fluoride varnish versus acidulated phosphate fluoride gel: A 3-year clinical trial. *Caries Res*, 29:327–30.

114. Biller, I. R., Hunter, E. L., Featherstone, M. J., & Silverstone, L. M. (1980). Enamel loss during a prophylaxis polish in vitro. *J Int Assoc Dent Child*, 11:7–12.

115. Stookey, G. K. (1978). *In vitro* estimates of enamel and dentin abrasion associated with a prophylaxis. *J Dent Res*, 57:36.

116. Vrbic, V., Brudevold, F., & McCann, H. G. (1967). Acquisition of fluoride by enamel from fluoride pumice pastes. *Helv Odont Acta*, 11:21–26.

117. Vrbic, V., & Brudevold, F. (1970). Fluoride uptake from treatment with different fluoride prophylaxis pastes and from the use of pastes containing a soluble aluminum salt followed by topical application. *Caries Res*, 4:158–67.

118. Bibby, B. G. (1945). Test of the effect of fluoride-containing dentifrices on dental caries. *J Dent Res*, 24:297–303.

119. Gershon, S. D., & Pader, M. (1972). Dentifrices, In Balsam H., & Sagarin H., Eds. *Cosmetics, science and technology* (2nd ed.) (pp. 423–531). New York: Wiley.

120. Muhler, J. C., Hine, M. K., & Day, H. G. (1954). *Preventive dentistry*. St. Louis: Mosby.

121. Volpe, A. R. (1982). Dentifrices and mouth rinses. In Caldwell, R. C., & Stallard, R. E., Eds. A *textbook of preventive dentistry*. Philadelphia: W.B. Saunders.

122. Wei, S. H. Y. (1974). The potential benefits to be derived from topical fluorides in fluoridated communities. In Forrester, D. J., & Schulz, E. M. Jr., Eds. International Workshop on Fluoride and Dental Caries Reductions. Baltimore: University of Maryland, pp. 178–251.

123. Stookey, G. K. (1983). Are all fluoride dentifrices the same? In Wei, S. H. Y., Ed. *Clinical uses of fluorides*. Philadelphia: Lea & Febiger. pp. 105–131.

124. Muhler, J. C., Radike, A. W., Nebergall, W. H., & Day, H. G. (1954). The effect of a stannous fluoride-containing dentifrice on caries reduction in children. *J Dent Res*, 33:606–12.

125. Beiswanger, B. B., Gish, C. W., & Mallatt, M. E. (1981). Effect of a sodium fluoride-silica abrasive dentifrice upon caries. *Pharmacol Ther Dent*, 6:9–16.

126. Zacherl, W. A. (1981). A three-year clinical caries evaluation of the effect of a sodium fluoride-silica abrasive dentifrice. *Pharmacol Ther Dent*, 6:1–7.

127. Fogels, H. R., Meade, J. J., Griffith, J., Miraqliuolo, R., & Cancro, L. P. (1988). A clinical investigation of a high-level fluoride dentifrice. *ASDC J Dent Child*, 55(3):210–15.

128. Conti, A. J., Lotzkar, S., Daley, R., Cancro, L., Marks, R. G., & Menkal, D. R. (1988). A 3-year clinical trial to compare efficacy of dentifrices containing 1.14% and 0.76% sodium monofluorophosphate. *Comm Dent Oral Epidemiol*, 16(3):135–38.

129. Stephen, K. W., Russell, J. I., Creanor, S. L., & Burchell, C. K. (1987). Comparison of fiber optic transillumination with clinical and radiographic caries diagnosis. *Comm Dent Oral Epidemiol*, 15(2):90–94.

130. Szpunar, S. M., & Burt, B. A. (1987). Trends in the prevalence of dental fluorosis in the United States: A review. *J Pub Health Dent*, 47:71–79.

131. Heifetz, S. B., Driscoll, W. S., Horowitz, H. S., et al. (1988). Prevalence of dental caries and dental fluorosis in areas with optimal and above-optimal water fluoride concentrations. *J Am Dent Assoc*, 116:490–95.

132. Pendrys, D. G., & Stamm, J. W. (1990). Relationship of total fluoride intake to beneficial effects and enamel fluorosis. *J Dent Res*, 69(Special Issue):529–38.

133. Brunelle, J. A. (1989). The prevalence of dental fluorosis in U.S children. *J Dent Res*, 68(Special Issue):995. Abstr.

134. U.S. Department of Health and Human Services (1989). Oral health of United States children. The national survey of dental caries in U.S. schoolchildren: 1986–1987 national and regional findings. NIH Pub. No. 89–2247.

135. Larsen, M. J., Richards, A., & Fejerskov, O. (1985). Development of dental fluorosis according to age at start of fluoride administration. *Caries Res*, 19:519–27.

136. ten Cate, A. R. (1985). *Oral histology—development, structure and function*. St. Louis: Mosby.

137. Evans, R., & Darvell, B. (1995). Refining the estimate of the critical period for susceptibility to enamel fluorosis in human maxillary central incisors. *J Pub Health Dent*, 55:238–49.

138. Beltran, E. D., & Szpunar, S. M. L. (1988). Fluoride in toothpaste for children: Suggestion for change. *Pediatr Dent*, 10:185–88.

139. Osuji, O. O., Leake, M. L., Chipman, G., Niki Loruk, G., Locker, D., & Levine, N. (1988). Risk factors for dental fluorosis in a fluoridated community. *J Dent Res*, 67:1488–92.

140. Beiswanger, B. B., & Stookey, G. K. (1989). The comparative clinical cariostatic efficacy of sodium fluoride and sodium monofluorophosphate dentifrices: A review of trials. *J Dent Child*, 56:337–47.

141. Stookey, G. K., DePaola, P. F., Featherstone, J. D. B., Fejerskov, O., Mollen, I. J., Rotberg, S., Stephen, K. W., & Wefel, J. S. (1993). A critical review of the relative anticaries efficacy of sodium fluoride and sodium monofluorophosphate dentifrices. *Caries Res*, 27:337–60.

142. Bowen, W. H. (1994). Relative efficacy of sodium fluoride and sodium monofluorophosphate as anti-caries agents in dentifrices. London: The Royal Society of Medicine Press Ltd.

143. Johnson, M. F. (1993). Comparative efficacy of NaF and MFP dentifrices in caries prevention: A meta-analytic overview. *Caries Res*, 27:328–36.

144. Glass, R. L., Scheinin, A., & Barmes, D. E. (1981). Changing caries prevalence in two cultures. *J Dent Res*, 60(Special Issue A): 361, Abstr. 202.

145. Zacherl, W. A., & Long, D. M. (1979). Reduction in caries attack rate—nonfluoridated community. *J Dent Res*, 58(Special Issue A): 227, Abstr. 535.

146. Bixler, D., & Muhler, J. C. (1966). Effect on dental caries in children in a nonfluoride area of combined use of three agents containing stannous fluoride: A prophylactic paste, a solution, and a dentifrice. II. Results at the end of 24 and 36 months. *J Am Dent Assoc*, 72:392–96.

147. Gish, C. W., & Muhler, J. C. (1965). Effect on dental caries in children in a natural fluoride area of combined use of three agents containing stannous fluoride: A prophylactic paste, a solution, and a dentifrice. *J Am Dent Assoc*, 70:914–20 (and personal communication).

148. Muhler, J. C., Spear, L. B. Jr., Bixler, D., & Stookey, G. K. (1967). The arrestment of incipient dental caries in adults after the use of three different forms of $SnF_2$ therapy: Results after 30 months. *J Am Dent Assoc*, 75:1402–6.

149. Obersztyn, A., Piotrowski, Z., Kowinski, K., & Ekler, B. (1973). Stannous fluoride in the prophylaxis of caries in adults. *Czas Stomat*, 26:1181–87.

150. Scola, F. P., & Ostrom, C. A. (1968). Clinical evaluation of stannous fluoride when used as a constituent of a compatible prophylactic paste, as a topical solution, and in a dentifrice in naval personnel. II. Report of findings after two years. *J Am Dent Assoc*, 77:594–97.

151. Scola, F. P. (1970). Self-preparation stannous fluoride prophylactic technique in preventive dentistry: Report after two years. *J Am Dent Assoc*, 81:1369–72.

152. Beiswanger, B. B., Billings, R. J., Sturzenberger, O. P., & Bollmer, B. W. (1978). Effect of an $SnF_2Ca_2P_2O_7$ dentifrice and APF topical applications. *J Dent Child*, 45:137–41.

153. Downer, M. C., Holloway, P. J., & Davies, T. G. H. (1976). Clinical testing of a topical fluoride caries prevention program. *Br Dent J*, 141:242–47.

154. Mainwaring, P. J., & Naylor, N. M. (1978). A three-year clinical study to determine the separate and combined caries-inhibitory effects of sodium monofluorophosphate toothpaste and an acidulated phosphate fluoride gel. *Caries Res*, 12:202–12.

155. Birkeland, J. M., Broch, L., & Jorkjend, J. (1977). Benefits and prognoses following 10 years of a fluoride mouthrinsing program. *Scand J Dent Res*, 85:31–37.

156. Birkeland, J. M., & Torell, P. (1978). Caries-preventive fluoride mouthrinses. *Caries Res*, 12(Suppl. 1):38–51.

157. Reports on Councils and Bureaus, Council on Dental Therapeutics, American Dental Association (1975). Council classifies fluoride mouthrinses. *J Am Dent Assoc*, 91:1250–52.

158. Torell, P., & Ericsson, Y. (1974). The potential benefits to be derived from fluoride mouthrinses. In Forrester, D. J., & Schulz, E. M. Jr, Eds. International Workshop on Fluorides and Dental Caries Reductions. Baltimore: University of Maryland, pp. 113–176.

159. Heifetz, S. B., Franchi, G. J., Mosley, G. W., MacDougall, O., & Brunelle, J. (1979). Combined anticariogenic effect of fluoride gel-trays and fluoride mouthrinsing in an optimally fluoridated community. *J Clinic Prevent Dent* 6:21–23.

160. Radike, A. W., Gish, C. W., Peterson, J. K., King, J. D., & Zegreto, V. A. (1973). Clinical evaluation of stannous fluoride as an anticaries mouthrinse. *J Am Dent Assoc*, 86:404–8.

161. Driscoll, W. S., Swango, P. A., Horowitz, A. M., & Kingman, A. (1981). Caries-preventive effects of daily and weekly fluoride mouthrinsing in an optimally fluoridated community: Findings after 18 months. *Pediatr Dent*, 3:316–20.

162. Jones, J. C., Murphy, R. F., & Edd, P. A. (1979). Using health education in a fluoride mouthrinse program: The public health hygienist's role. *Dent Hyg*, 53:469–73.

163. Kawall, K., Lewis, D. W., & Hargreaves, J. A. (1981). The effect of a fluoride mouthrinse in an optimally fluoridated community—final two year results. *J Dent Res*, 60(Special Issue A):471. Abstr. 646.

164. Ashley, F. P., Mainwaring, P. F., Emslie, R. D., & Naylor, M. N. (1977). Clinical testing of a mouthrinse and a dentifrice containing fluoride. A two-year supervised study in school children. *Br Dent J*, 143:333–38.

165. Triol, C. W., Franz, S. M., Volpe, A. R., Frankl, N., Alman, J. E., & Allard, R. L. (1980). Anticaries effect of a sodium fluoride rinse and an MFP dentifrice in a nonfluoridated water area. A thirty-month study. *Clin Prev Dent*, 2:13–15.

166. Blinkhorn, A. S., Holloway, P. J., & Davies, T. G. H. (1977). The combined effect of a fluoride mouthrinse and dentifrice in the control of dental caries. *J Dent Res*, 56(Special Issue D):D111.

167. Ringelberg, M. L., Webster, D. B., Dixon, D. O., & Lezotte, D. C. (1979). The caries-preventive effect of amine fluorides and inorganic fluorides in a mouthrinse or dentifrice after 30 months of use. *J Am Dent Assoc*, 98:202–8.

168. Horowitz, H. S., Heifetz, S. B., Meyers, R. J., Driscoll, W. S., & Korts, D. C. (1979). Evaluation of a combination of self-administered fluoride procedures for the control of dental caries in a nonfluoride area: Findings after four years. *J Am Dent Assoc*, 98:219–23.

169. Skartveit, L., Wefel, J. S., & Ekstrand, J. (1991). Effect of fluoride amalgams on artificial recurrent enamel and root caries. *Scand J Dent Res*, 99:287–94.

170. Donly, K. J. (1995). Enamel and dentin demineralization inhibition of fluoride-releasing materials. *Am J Dent*, 7:275–78.

171. Erickson, R. L., & Glasspoole, E. A. (1995). Model investigations of caries inhibition by fluoride-releasing dental materials. *Adv Dent Res*, 9:315–23.

172. ten Cate, J. M., & van Duinen, R. N. B. (1995). Hyper-mineralization of dentinal lesions adjacent to glass-ionomer cement restorations. *J Dent Res*, 74:1266–71.

173. Donly, K. J., Segura, A., Kanellis, M., & Erickson, R. L. (1999). Clinical performance and caries inhibition of resin-modified glass ionomer cement and amalgam restorations. *JADA* 130:1459–66.

174. Rawls, H. R. (1991). Preventive dental materials: sustained delivery of fluoride and other therapeutic agents. *Adv Dent Res*, 5:50–6.

175. Jones, D. W., Jackson, G., Suttow, E. J., Hall, A. C., & Johnson, J. (1988). Fluoride release and fluoride uptake by glass ionomer materials (abstract 672). *J Dent Res*, 67(A):197.

176. Marinelli, C. B., Donly, K. J., Wefel, J. S., Jakobsen, J. R., & Denehy, G. E. (1997). An in vitro comparison of three fluoride regimens on enamel remineralization. *Caries Res*, 31:418–22.

177. Bynum, A. M., & Donly, K. J. (1999). Enamel de/remineralization on teeth adjacent to fluoride releasing materials without dentifrice exposure. *ASDC J Dent Child*, 66:89–92.

178. Donly, K. J., Segura, A., Wefel, J. S., & Hogan, M. M. (1999). Evaluating the effects of fluoride-releasing dental materials on adjacent interproximal caries. *JADA*, 130:817–25.

179. Heifetz, S. B., & Horowitz, H. S. (1986). The amounts of fluoride in current fluoride therapies; safety considerations for children. *J Dent Child*, 77:876–82.

180. Melvor, M. E. (1987). Delayed fatal hyperkalemia in a patient with acute fluoride intoxication. *Ann Emerg Med*, 16:1165–67.

181. Department of Health and Human Services (1991). U.S. Public Health Service. Report of the Ad Hoc Subcommittee to Coordinate Environmental Health and Related Programs. Review of Fluoride Benefits and Risks. Washington, DC: U.S. Department of Health and Human Services.

182. Whitford, G. M. (1987). Fluoride in dental products: Safety considerations. *J Dent Res*, 66:1056–60.

183. Newbrun, E. (1992). Current regulations and recommendations concerning water fluoridation, fluoride supplements, and topical fluoride agents. *J Dent Res*, 67:1255–65.

184. Keels, M. A., Osterhout, S., & Vann, W. F. Jr. (1988). Incidence and nature of accidental fluoride ingestions. *J Dent Res*, 67(Special Issue):335. Abstr. 1778.

185. Whitford, G. M. (1992). Acute and chronic fluoride toxicity. *J Dent Res*, 71:1249–54.

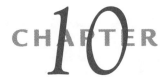

# CHAPTER 10

# Pit-and-Fissure Sealants

*Franklin García-Godoy*
*Norman O. Harris*
*Denise Muesch Helm*

## OBJECTIVES

*At the end of this chapter, it will be possible to*

1. Explain how sealants can provide a primary preventive means of reducing the need for operative treatment as 77% of the children 12 to 17 years old in the United States have dental caries in their permanent teeth.[1]
2. Discuss the history of sealant development through the 20th century.
3. List the criteria for selecting teeth for sealant placement and the four essentials in attaining maximum retention of sealants.
4. Describe the several steps preliminary to, during, and after the placement of a sealant—including surface cleanliness, dry fields, details of the application procedure, and remedial measures following the excess application of sealant.
5. Explain the rationale for adding fluorides to sealants.
6. Compare the advantages and disadvantages of light-cured and self-cured sealants.
7. Discuss the advantages of protecting the occlusal surfaces of teeth with sealants.
8. Cite five reasons given for the underuse of sealants by practitioners and analyze the validity of the reasons.

# INTRODUCTION

Fluorides are highly effective in reducing the number of carious lesions occurring on the *smooth surfaces* of enamel and cementum. Unfortunately, fluorides are *not* equally effective in protecting the occlusal pits and fissures, where the majority of carious lesions occur.[2] Considering the fact that the occlusal surfaces constitute only 12% of the total number of tooth surfaces, it means that the *pits and fissures are approximately eight times as vulnerable as the smooth surfaces.* The placement of sealants is a highly effective means of preventing these.[3]

Historically several agents have been tried to protect deep pits and fissures on occlusal surfaces.

- In 1895, Wilson reported the placement of *dental cement* in pits and fissures to prevent caries.[2] In 1929, Bödecker[4] suggested that deep fissures could be broadened with a large round bur to make the occlusal areas more self-cleansing, a procedure that is called *enameloplasty.*[5] Two major disadvantages, however, accompany enameloplasty. First, it requires a dentist, which immediately limits its use. Second, in modifying a deep fissure by this method, it is often necessary to remove more sound tooth structure than would be required to insert a small restoration.

- In 1923 and again in 1936, Hyatt[6] advocated the early insertion of small restorations in deep pits and fissures before carious lesions had the opportunity to develop. He termed this procedure *prophylactic odontotomy.* Again, this operation is more of a treatment procedure than a preventive approach, because it requires a dentist for the cutting of tooth structure.

- Several methods have been unsuccessfully used in an attempt either to seal or to make the fissures more resistant to caries. These attempts have included the use of topically applied zinc chloride and potassium ferrocyanide[7] and the use of ammoniacal silver nitrate;[8] they have also included the use of copper amalgam packed into the fissures.[9]

- Fluorides that protect the smooth surfaces of the teeth are less effective in protecting the occlusal surfaces.[10] Following the use of fluorides, there is a large reduction of incidence in smooth-surface caries but a smaller reduction in occlusal pit-and-fissure caries. This results in an *increased proportion* in the ratio of occlusal to interproximal lesions, even though the total number may be less.

- A final course of action to deal with pit-and-fissure caries is one that is often used: *do nothing; wait and watch.* This option avoids the need to cut good tooth structure until a definite carious lesion is identified. It also results in many teeth being lost when individuals do not return for periodic exams. This approach, although frequently used is a violation of the ethical principle of beneficence and patient autonomy.

In the late 1960s and early 1970s, another option became available—the use of pit-and-fissure sealants.[11] With this option, a liquid resin is flowed over the occlusal surface of the tooth where it penetrates the deep fissures to fill areas that cannot be

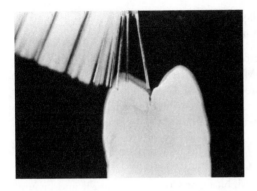

FIGURE 10–1    One of the reasons that 50% of the carious lesions occur on the occlusal surface. Note that the toothbrush bristle has a greater diameter than the width of the fissure. (Courtesy of Dr. J. McCune, Johnson & Johnson.)

cleaned with the toothbrush (Figure 10–1).[12] The hardened sealant presents a barrier between the tooth and the hostile oral environment. Concurrently, there is a significant reduction of Streptococcus mutans on the treated tooth surface.[13] Pits and fissures serve as reservoirs for mutans streptococci, sealing the niche thereby reduces the oral count.

## Criteria for Selecting Teeth for Sealant Placement

Following are the criteria for selecting teeth for sealing. Because no harm can occur from sealing, when in doubt, seal *and monitor*.

- A deep occlusal fissure, fossa, or incisal lingual pit is present.

### A sealant is contraindicated if:

- Patient behavior does not permit use of adequate dry-field techniques throughout the procedure.
- An open carious lesion exists.
- Caries exist on other surfaces of the same tooth in which restoring will disrupt an intact sealant.
- A large occlusal restoration is already present.

### A sealant is *probably indicated if:*

- The fossa selected for sealant placement is well isolated from another fossa with a restoration.
- The area selected is confined to a fully erupted fossa, even though the distal fossa is

impossible to seal due to inadequate eruption.

- An intact occlusal surface is present where the *contralateral tooth* surface is carious or restored; this is because teeth on opposite sides of the mouth are usually equally prone to caries.
- An *incipient* lesion exists in the pit-and-fissure.
- Sealant material can be flowed over a conservative class I composite or amalgam to improve the marginal integrity, and into the remaining pits and fissures to achieve a *de facto* extension for prevention.

## Other Considerations in Tooth Selection

All teeth meeting the previous criteria should be sealed and resealed as needed. Where the cost–benefit is critical and priorities must be established, such as occurs in many public health programs, ages 3 and 4 years are the most important times for sealing the eligible deciduous teeth; ages 6 to 7 years for the first permanent molars;[14] and ages 11 to 13 years for the second

permanent molars and premolars.[15] Currently, 77% of the children 12-to-17-years-old in the United States have dental caries in their permanent teeth.[1] Many school days would be saved, and better dental health would be achieved in School Dental Health Clinic programs by combining sealant placement and regular fluoride exposure.[16]

*The disease susceptibility of the tooth should be considered when selecting teeth for sealants, not the age of the individual.* Sealants appear to be equally retained on occlusal surfaces in primary, as well as permanent teeth.[3] Sealants should be placed on the teeth of adults if there is evidence of existing or impending caries susceptibility, as would occur following excessive intake of sugar or as a result of a drug- or radiation-induced xerostomia. They should also be used in areas where fluoride levels in community water is optimized, as well as in non-fluoridated areas.[17]

The following are two good illustrations of this philosophy. After a 3-year study, Ripa and colleagues[18] concluded that the time the teeth had been in the mouth (some for 7 to 10 years) had no effect on the vulnerability of occlusal surfaces to caries attack. Also, the incidence of occlusal caries in young Navy[19] and Air Force[20] recruits (who are usually in their late teens or early 20s) is relatively high.

## Background of Sealants

Buonocore first described the fundamental principles of placing sealants in the late 1960s.[10,21] He describes a method to bond polymethylmethacrylate (PMMA) to human enamel conditioned with phosphoric acid. Practical use of this concept however, was not realized until the development of bisphenol A-glycidyl methacrylate (Bis-GMA), urethane dimethacrylates (UDMA) and trithylene glycol dimethacrylates (TEGDMA) resins that possess better physical properties than PMMA. The first successful use of resin sealants was reported by Buonocore in the 1960s.[22]

## Bisphenol A–Glycidyl Methylacrylate Sealants

Bisphenol A–glycidyl methylacrylate (Bis-GMA) is now the sealant of choice. It is a mixture of Bis-GMA and methyl methacrylate.[23] Products currently accepted by the American Dental Association (ADA) include:[24]

- Baritone L3, Type II **Confi-Dental Products Co.**
- Alpha-Dent Chemical Cure Pit and Fissure Sealant **Dental Technologies, Inc.**
- Alpha-Dent Light Cure Pit and Fissure Sealant **Dental Technologies, Inc.**
- Prisma-Shield Compules Tips VLC Tinted Pit & Fissure Sealant **Dentsply L.D. Caulk Division**
- Prisma-Shield VLC Filled Pit & Fissure Sealant **Dentsply L.D. Caulk Division**
- Helioseal F, Type II **Ivoclar-Vivadent, Inc.**
- Helioseal, Type II **Ivoclar-Vivadent, Inc.**
- Seal-Rite Low Viscosity, Type II **Pulpdent Corp.**
- Seal-Rite, Type II **Pulpdent Corp.**

The ADA National Standard sets aside specific criteria of pit-and-fissure sealants stating; Specification No. 39 established the following requirements:

- That the working time for type I sealants is not less than 45 seconds;
- That the setting time is within 30 seconds of the manufacturer's instruction and does not exceed three minutes;
- That the curing time for type II sealants is not more the 60 seconds;
- That the depth of cure for type II sealant is not less than 0.75 millimeter;
- That the uncured film thickness is not more than 0.1 millimeter;
- That sealants meet the bicompatibility requirements of American Nation a Standard/American Dental Association

Document No. 41 for Recommended Standard Practices for Biological Evaluation of Dental Materials.[25]

Sealant products accepted by the American Dental Association carried the statement: "[Product name] has been shown to be acceptable as an agent for sealing off an anatomically deficient region of the tooth to supplement the regular professional care in a program of preventive dentistry."[26]

Nuva-Seal was the first successful commercial sealant to be placed on the market, in 1972. Since then more effective second- and third-generation sealants have become available see Table 10–1. The first sealant clinical trials used cyanoacrylate-based materials. Dimethacrylate-based products replaced these. The primary difference between sealants is their method of polymerization. First-generation sealants were initiated by ultraviolet light, second-generation sealants are autopolymer-

TABLE 10–1  **A Comparison of Retention of First- and Second-Generation Sealants from Several Studies**

| Generation | Sealant Product | Months after Placement | | | | | | | | |
|---|---|---|---|---|---|---|---|---|---|---|
| | | 6 | 12 | 24 | 36 | 48 | 60 | 72 | 84 | ⇒15 years |
| First | Nuva-Seal | | 87 | 73 | 59 | 42 | | | | |
| **Nuva-Seal**[b] | | | 84 | 58 | 60 | | 35 | 37 | 35 | |
| Total | | | 85 | 65 | 60 | 42 | 35 | 37 | 35 | |
| Second | Concise | | 100 | | | | | | | |
| Concise | | | 96 | 95 | 94 | | | | | |
| Delton | | | 95 | | | | | | | |
| Delton | | | 92 | | 80 | | | | | |
| Delton | | | 96 | | | | | | | |
| Delton | | | | | 80 | | | | | |
| **Delton**[b] | | | 95 | 84 | 80 | | 72 | 68 | 65 | |
| Nuva-Cote | | 100 | 100 | | | | | | | |
| Oralin | | | 98 | | 78 | | | | | |
| Oralin | | | 97 | | 95 | | | | | |
| Prisma-Shield | | 94 | 95 | | | | | | | |
| Prisma-Shield | | | 94 | | | | | | | |
| Concise | | | | | | | | | | 63[1] |
| Concise | | | | | | | | | | 78[2] (caries free surfaces) |
| Total | | 97 | 95 | 89 | 84 | | 72 | 68 | 65 | |

[a]Bold lettering is from a study by Mertz-Fairhurst.[108]
[b]Direct 7-year comparison of first- and second-generation sealants.
[1]From Simonsen.[190]
[2]From Wendt et al.[191]

ized, and third-generation sealants use visible light.

Some sealants contain *fillers*, which makes it desirable to classify the commercial products into *filled* and *unfilled* sealants. The *filled* sealants contain microscopic glass beads, quartz particles, and other fillers used in composite resins. The fillers are coated with products such as *silane*, to facilitate their combination with the Bis-GMA resin. The fillers make the sealant more *resistant to abrasion and wear*. Because they are more resistant to abrasion the occlusion should be checked and the sealant height may need to be adjusted after placement. In contrast, unfilled sealants wear quicker but usually do not need occlusal adjustment.

## Fluoride-Releasing Sealants

The addition of fluoride to sealants was considered about 20 years ago,[27] and it was probably attempted based on the fact that the incidence and severity of secondary caries *was* reduced around fluoride-releasing materials such as the silicate cements used for anterior restorations.[28,29] Because fluoride uptake increases the enamel's resistance to caries,[30] the use of a fluoridated resin-based sealant may provide an additional anticariogenic effect if the fluoride released from its matrix is incorporated into the adjacent enamel.

Fluoride-releasing sealants have shown antibacterial properties[31–33] as well as a greater artificial caries resistance compared to a nonfluoridated sealant.[34–36] A recent *in vitro* study showed that pit-and-fissure sealants containing fluoride provided a caries-inhibiting effect with a significant reduction in lesion depth in the surface enamel adjacent and a reduction in the frequency of wall lesion.[37] Moreover, the fluoridated sealant laboratory bond strength to enamel,[38] and clinical performance,[39,40] is similar to that of nonfluoridated sealants.[41,42] In a recent study, it was shown that teeth sealed with Teethmate F fluoridated sealant revealed high amounts of enamel fluoride uptake in

vitro and in vivo to a depth ranging from 10 to 20 µm from the surface.[43] The residual fluoride was also observed within the sealing material. This agrees with another study showing the high amount of fluoride released from Teethmate F-1.[44]

The addition of fluoride to the sealants will greatly increase their value in the preventive and restorative use as mentioned above. Fluoride is added to sealants by two methods. The first is by adding a soluble fluoride to the unpolymerized resin. The fluoride can be expected to leach out over a period of time into the adjacent enamel. Eventually the fluoride content of the sealant should be exhausted, but the content of the enamel greatly increased.

The second method of incorporating fluoride is by the addition of an organic fluoride compound that is chemically bound to the resin to form an ion exchange resin. As such, when fluoride is low in the saliva, fluoride would be released. Vice versa, when the fluoride in the environment is high, it should bind to the resin to form—at least theoretically—a continuous reservoir for fluoride release and recharge.[45] See Table 10–2 on page 292 for a list of current available sealant materials.

## Polymerization of the Sealants

The liquid resin is called the *monomer*. When the catalyst acts on the monomer, repeating chemical bonds begin to form, increasing in number and complexity as the hardening process (*polymerization*) proceeds. Finally, the resultant hard product is known as a polymer. Two methods have been employed to catalyze polymerization: (1) light curing by use of a visible blue light (synonyms: photocure, photoactivation, light activation) and (2) self-curing, in which a monomer and a catalyst are mixed together (synonyms: cold cure, autopolymerization, and chemical activation).

The two original Caulk products, Nuva-Seal and Nuva-Cote, were the only sealants in the United States requiring ultraviolet light for ac-

tivation. Both have been *replaced* by other light-cured sealants that require *visible blue light*. In the manufacture of these latter products, a catalyst, such as *camphoroquinone*, which is sensitive to visible blue-light frequencies, is placed in the monomer at the time of manufacture. Later, when the monomer is exposed to the visible blue light, polymerization is initiated.

With the autopolymerizing sealants, the catalyst is incorporated with the monomer; in addition, another bottle contains an *initiator*— usually *benzoyl peroxide*. When the monomer and the initiator are mixed, *polymerization begins*.

### Light-Cured Versus Self-Cured Sealants

The main advantage of the light-cured sealant is that the operator can initiate polymerization at *any suitable time*. Polymerization time is shorter with the light-cured products than with the self-curing sealants. The light-cured process does require the purchase of a light source, which adds to the expense of the procedure. This light, however, is the same one that is used for polymerization of composite restorations, making it available in all dental offices. When using a light-cured sealant in the office, it is prudent to store the product away from bright office lighting, which can sometimes initiate polymerization.

Conversely, the self-curing resins do not require an expensive light source. They do, however, have the great disadvantage that once mixing has commenced, if some minor problem is experienced in the operating field, the operator must either continue mixing or stop and make a new mix. For the autopolymerizing resin, the time allowed for sealant manipulation and placement *must not be exceeded*, even though the material might still appear liquid. Once the hardening begins, *it occurs very rapidly, and any manipulation of the material during this critical time jeopardizes retention*.

The light-cured sealants have a higher compressive strength and a smoother surface;[46] which is probably caused by air being introduced into the self-cure resins during mixing[47] Despite these differences, both the photocured and the autopolymerizing products appear to be equal in retention.[43,48–50]

### The High-Intensity Light Source

The light-emitting device consists of a high-intensity *white light*, a blue filter to produce the *desired blue color*, usually between 400 to 500 nm, and a light-conducting rod. Some other systems consist of a blue light produced by light-emitting diodes (LED) (Figure 10–2). Most have timers for automatically switching off the lights after a predetermined time interval. In use, the end of the rod is held only a few millimeters above the sealant during the first 10 seconds, after which it can be rested on the

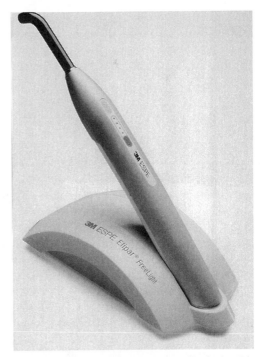

FIGURE 10–2    Light emitting diode (LED) curing unit for direct, intraoral exposure.

TABLE 10–2 Sealant Products Available

| Manufacture | Product Name | Application Method | Curing Method | Color | Filler Content | Contains Fluoride | ADA Seal |
|---|---|---|---|---|---|---|---|
| Bisco Inc | Sealant G-9200S | Brush on | Light-cure | White | Glass & fumed silica 52% by weight | No | No |
| Confi-Dental. Products Co | Baritone L3, Type II Sealants | Syringe Brush on | Light-cure Chemical Cure | | | No | Yes |
| Den-Mat Corp | Flo-Restore | Syringe | Light-cure | A2,A3,B1,B2, B3,C2,C3, Opaquer | Barium glass & fumed silica 40% by weight | Yes | No |
| Dental Technologies, Inc. | Alpha-Dent Chemical Cure | | Chemical Cure | | | | Yes |
| | Alpha-Dent Light Cure | | Light Cure | | | | Yes |
| Dentsply Ash | Delton Plus Pit & Fissure Sealant | Syringe | Light-cure | Opaque | Glass ionomer 38% by weight | Yes | No |
| Dentsply Caulk | FluorShield | Brush on | Light-cure | Tooth colored or Opaque white | Glass 50% by weight | Yes | No |
| | Prisma-Shield Compules Tips VLC Tinted Pit & Fissure Sealant | | | | | | Yes |
| | Prisma-Shield VLC | | | | Filled | | Yes |

| Manufacturer | Product | Delivery | Cure | Color | Filler | | |
|---|---|---|---|---|---|---|---|
| Heraeus Kilzer | Estiseal LC | Syringe | Light-cure | Yellow tint transparent & opaque white | Silica 32% by weight | No | No |
| Ivoclar North America | Helioseal F Type II Cartridge | Brush on | Light-cure | Opaque | Fluorosilicate glass & fumed silica 42% by weight | Yes | No |
| J. Morita USA | Helioseal, Type II | Syringe | Light-cure | Changes color | | No | Yes |
| | Teeth mate, F1 | Syringe | Light-cure | Opaque, Natural | Unfilled | Yes | No |
| Pulpdent Corp. | Seal-Rite Type II | Syringe | Light-cure | Tooth-colored | Glass filler in methacrylate resins 34% by weight | Yes | Yes |
| | Seal-Rite Low Viscosity, Type II | Syringe | Light-cure | Off-white | Glass filler in methacrylate resins 7.7% by weight | Yes | Yes |
| Sds Kerr | Guardian Seal | Syringe | Light-cure | Opaque | Filled 30% by weight | Yes | No |
| Ultradent Products | UltraSeal XT Plus | Syringe | Light-cure | Opaque white, tinted translucent, A2 | Fluoride glass ionomer 60% by weight | Yes | No |
| 3M Dental Products | Clinpro Sealant | Syringe | Light-cure | Changes color | Unfilled | Yes | No |

hardened surface of the partially polymerized sealant. The time required for polymerization is *set by the manufacturer* and is usually around *20 to 30* seconds. The *depth* of cure is influenced by the *intensity of light*, which can differ greatly with different products and length of exposure. Often it is desirable to set the automatic light timer for longer than the manufacturer's instructions.[51] Even after cessation of light exposure, a final, slow polymerization can *continue* over a 24-hour period.[52]

It is not known whether long-term exposure to the intense light can damage the eye. Staring at the lighted operating field is uncomfortable and does produce afterimages. This problem is circumvented by the use of a round, 4-inch dark-yellow disk, which fits over the light housing. The disk filters out the intense blue light in the 400- to 500-nanometers range as well as being sufficiently dark to subdue other light frequencies.

---

**Question 1**

Which of the following statements, if any, are correct?

A. In an area with fluoridated water, a *lower incidence* of caries can be expected, along with a *lower proportion* of occlusal to smooth-surface lesions.

B. Sealants should *never* be flowed over incipient caries.

C. Bis-GMA are the initials used to specify the chemical family of resins containing bisphenol A-glycidyl methyl-acrylate.

D. A monomer can polymerize, but a polymer cannot monomerize.

E. Sealants are contraindicated for adults.

---

### Requisites for Sealant Retention

For sealant retention the surface of the tooth must (1) have a *maximum surface area*, (2) have *deep, irregular pits and fissures*, (3) be *clean*, and (4) be *absolutely dry* at the time of sealant placement and uncontaminated with saliva residue. *These are the four commandments for successful sealant placement, and they cannot be violated.*

### Increasing the Surface Area

Sealants do not bond directly to the teeth. Instead, they are retained mainly by *adhesive forces.*[53] To increase the surface area, which in turn increases the adhesive potential, *tooth conditioners* (also called *etchants*), which are composed of a 30 to 50% concentration of phosphoric acid, are placed on the occlusal surface prior to the placement of the sealant.[54] The etchant may be either in *liquid* or *gel* form. The former is easier to apply and easier to remove. Both are equal in abetting retention.[55,56] If any etched areas on the tooth surface are not covered by the sealant or if the sealant is not retained, the normal appearance of the enamel returns to the tooth within 1 hour to a few weeks *due to a remineralization* from constituents

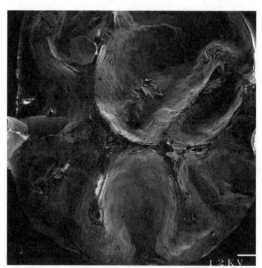

FIGURE 10–3    An electron scanning microscope view of the deep pits and fissures of the occlusal surface of a molar. (Courtesy of Dr. A. J. Gwinnett, State University of New York, Stony Brook.)

in the saliva.[57] The etchant should be carefully applied to avoid contact with the soft tissues. If not confined to the occlusal surface, the acid may produce a mild inflammatory response. It also produces a sharp acid taste that is often objectionable.

## Pit-and-Fissure Depth

Deep, irregular pits and fissures offer a much more favorable surface contour for sealant retention compared with broad, shallow fossae (Figure 10–3). The deeper fissures protect the resin sealant from the shear forces occurring as a result of masticatory movements. Of parallel importance is the possibility of caries development increasing as the *fissure depth and slope* of the inclined planes increases.[58,59] Thus, *as the potential for caries increases, so does the potential for sealant retention.*

## Surface Cleanliness

The need and method for cleaning the tooth surface prior to sealant placement are controversial. Usually the acid etching alone is sufficient for surface cleaning. This is attested to by the fact that two of the most cited and most effective sealant longevity studies by Simonsen[60] and Mertz-Fairhurst[61] were accomplished without use of a prior prophylaxis. Recently, however, it was shown that cleaning teeth with the newer prophylaxis pastes with or without fluoride (NuPro, Topex) did not affect the bond strength of sealants,[62] composites,[63] or orthodontic brackets.

Other methods used to clean the tooth surface prior to placing the sealant included, air-polishing, hydrogen peroxide, and enameloplasty.[63–65] The use of an air-polisher has proven to thoroughly clean and removes residual debris from pits and fissures.[65–68] Hydrogen peroxide has the disadvantage that it produces a precipitate on the enamel surface.[68] Enameloplasty, achieved by bur or air abrasion has

proven effective. Yet, no significant differences were observed in comparison with either etching or bur preparation of the fissures on the penetration to the base of the sealant. However, the use of enameloplasty, even if equal or slightly superior would have very serious ramifications. The laws of most states require a dentist to use air abrasion and/or to cut a tooth, a requirement that would severely curtail hygienists and assistants participation in office and school preventive dentistry programs.[69]

Whatever the cleaning preferences—either by acid etching or other methods—all heavy stains, deposits, debris, and plaque should be removed from the occlusal surface before applying the sealant.

## Preparing the Tooth for Sealant Application

The preliminary steps for the light-activated and the autopolymerized resins are similar up to the time of application of the resin to the teeth. After the selected teeth are isolated, they are thoroughly dried for approximately *10 seconds*. The 10-second drying period can be mentally estimated by counting off the seconds—1,000, 2,000—until 10,000 has been reached. The liquid etchant is then placed on the tooth with a small resin sponge or cotton pledget held with cotton pliers. Traditionally, the etching solution is gently daubed, *not rubbed*, on the surface for *1 minute* for permanent teeth and for *1½ minutes* for deciduous teeth.[70,71] Other clinical studies, however, have shown that acid etching the enamel of both primary and permanent teeth for only 20 seconds produced similar sealant[70] and composite[72] retention as those etched for 1 and 1½ minutes. Currently, *20 to 30 seconds* enamel-etching time is recommended. Alternatively, acid gels are applied with a supplied syringe and left undisturbed. Another 15 seconds of etching is indicated for fluorosed teeth to compensate for the greater acid resistance of

the enamel. The etching period should be timed with a *clock*. At the end of the etching period, the aspirator tip is positioned with the bevel interposed *between the cotton roll and the tooth*. For 10 seconds the water from the syringe is flowed over the occlusal surface and thence into the aspirator tip. Again, this 10-second period can be mentally counted. Care should be exercised to ensure that the aspirator tip is close enough to the tooth to prevent any water from reaching the cotton rolls, yet not so close that it diverts the stream of water directly into the aspirator (see Figure 10–5).

Following the water flush, the tooth surface is dried for *10 seconds*. The air supply needs to be absolutely dry. The dried tooth surface should have a white, dull, frosty appearance. This is because the etching will remove approximately 5 to 10 μm of the original surface,[73] although at times interrod penetrations of up to 100 μm may occur.[74] The etching *does not always* involve the interrod areas; sometimes the central portion of the rod is etched, and the periphery is unaffected. The pattern on any one tooth is unpredictable.[75] In any event, the surface area is greatly increased by the acid etch.

---

**Question 2**

Which of the following statements, if any, are correct?

A. Autopolymerizing sealants and light-cured sealants have approximately the same record for longevity.

B. A 40% phosphoric acid etchant should be satisfactory for both etching and cleaning the average tooth surface prior to sealant placement.

C. Fossae with deep inclined planes tend to have more carious fissures; fossae with deep inclined planes tend to retain sealants better.

D. In studies in which a rubber dam was used to maintain a dry field for sealant

placement, the retention of sealants was greater than when cotton rolls were used.

E. In placing a sealant, 10 seconds are devoted to each of the drying and etching phases and 1 minute to the flushing of the etchant from the tooth.

---

## Dryness

The teeth *must* be dry at the time of sealant placement because sealants are hydrophobic. The presence of saliva on the tooth is even more detrimental than water because its organic components interpose a barrier between the tooth and the sealant. Whenever the teeth are dried with an air syringe, the air stream should be *checked* to ensure that it is not moisture-laden. Otherwise, sufficient moisture sprayed on the tooth will prevent adhesion of the sealant to the enamel. A check for moisture can be accomplished by directing the air stream onto a cool mouth mirror; any fogging indicates the presence of moisture. Possibly the omission of this simple step accounts for the inter-operator variability in the retention of fissure sealants.

A dry field can be maintained in several ways, including use of a *rubber dam*, employment of *cotton rolls*, and the placement of *bibulous pads* over the opening of the parotid duct. The rubber dam provides an ideal way to maintain dryness for an extended time. Because a rubber dam is usually employed in accomplishing quadrant dentistry, sealant placement for the quadrant should also be accomplished during the operation. Under most operating conditions, however, it is not feasible to apply the dam to the different quadrants of the mouth; instead it is necessary to employ cotton rolls, combined with the use of an effective *high-volume, low-vacuum aspirator*. Under such routine operating conditions, cotton rolls, with and without the use of bibulous pads, can usu-

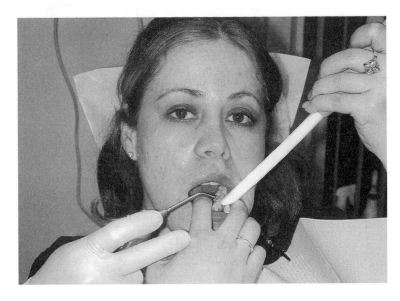

FIGURE 10-4    Four-handed dentistry with no assistant. The patient holds the cotton rolls with the index and third finger, thumb under chin. Patient also holds aspirator with other hand when it is not being used by operator.

ally be employed as effectively as the dam for the relatively short time needed for the procedure. *The two most successful sealant studies have used cotton rolls for isolation.*[60,61] In one study in which retention was tested using a rubber dam versus cotton rolls, the sealant retention was approximately *equal.*[76] Others have shown excellent sealant retention after 3 years[77] and after 10 to 20 years.[60,78]

In programs with *high patient volume* where cotton rolls are used, it is best to have two individuals involved—the *operator,* whose main task is to prepare the tooth and to apply the sealant, and the *assistant,* whose task is to maintain dryness. An operator working alone, however, can maintain a maximum dry field for the time needed to place the sealants, although it is not recommended, particularly for young children or those that are difficult to manage. For the maxilla, there should be little problem with the placement of *cotton rolls* in the buccal vestibule and, if desirable, the placement of a *bibulous pad* over the parotid duct. For the mandible, a 5-inch segment of a 6-inch cotton roll should be looped around the last molar and then held in place by the patient using the index and third fingers of the opposite hand

from the side being worked on (Figure 10–4). With aid from the patient and with appropriate aspiration techniques, the cotton rolls can usually be kept dry throughout the entire procedure. Cotton roll holders may be used, but they can be cumbersome when using the aspirator or when attempting to manipulate or remove a roll. If a cotton roll does become *slightly* moist, many times another short cotton roll can be placed on top of the moist segment and held in place for the duration of the procedure. In the event that it becomes necessary to replace a wet cotton roll, it is essential that *no* saliva contacts the etched tooth surface; if there is *any* doubt, it is necessary to repeat all procedures up to the time the dry field was compromised. This includes a 15-second etch to remove any residual saliva, in lieu of the original 1-minute etch.

Another promising dry-field isolating device that can be used for single operator use, especially when used with cotton rolls, is by using ejector moisture-control systems.[a] In one study comparing the Vac-Ejector versus the cotton

[a]Whaledent International, New York, NY

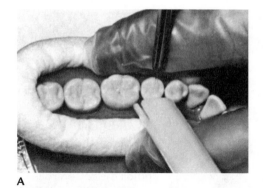

**A**

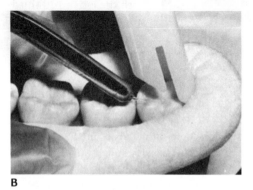

**B**

FIGURE 10-5    Showing position of aspirator tip between the bicuspid and cotton roll during flushing, **A,** and between water flow and cotton roll looped around second molar, **B.** *Complete* dryness of the cotton rolls can be maintained with this technique.

roll for maintaining dryness, the two were found to be equally effective.[79]

### Application of the Sealant

With either the light-cured or autopolymerized sealants, the material should first be placed in the fissures where there is the maximum depth. At times penetration of the fissure is negated by the presence of debris, air entrapment, narrow orifices, and excessive viscosity of the sealant.[80] The sealant should not only fill the fissures but should have some *bulk over the fissure*. After the fissures are adequately covered,

the material is then brought to a knife edge approximately *halfway* up the inclined plane.

Following polymerization, the sealants should be examined carefully *before* discontinuing the dry field. If any voids are evident, additional sealant can be added *without* the need for any additional etching. The hardened sealant has an oil residue on the surface. This is unreacted monomer that can be either wiped off with a gauze sponge or can be left. If a sealant requires repair at any time after the dry field is discontinued, it is prudent to repeat the same etching and drying procedures as initially used. Because all the commercial sealants—both the light-cured and self-cured—are of the same Bis-GMA chemical family, *they easily bond to one another*.[81]

### Occlusal and Interproximal Discrepancies

At times an excess of sealant may be inadvertently flowed into a fossa or into the adjoining interproximal spaces. To remedy the first problem, the occlusion should be checked visually or, if indicated, with articulating paper. Usually *any minor* discrepancies in occlusion are rapidly removed by normal chewing action. If the premature contact of the occlusal contact is unacceptable, a large, *no. 8. round cutting* bur may be used to rapidly create a broad resin fossa.

The integrity of the interproximal spaces can be checked with the use of dental floss. If any sealant is present, the use of scalers may be required to accomplish removal. These corrective actions are rarely needed once proficiency of placement is attained.

---

### Question 3

Which of the following statements, if any, are correct?

A. The etchant *predictably* attacks the center of the enamel prism, leaving the periphery intact.

B. When the data of a study indicate that 65% of the original sealants are retained for 7 years, it is the same as saying that an average of 5% is lost each year.

C. Bis-GMA products by different manufacturers are incompatible with one another.

D. An etched area that is not rapidly sealed will retain its rough, porous surface *indefinitely.*

E. The cleansing and etching of the occlusal surface with phospohoric acid is accomplished by *rubbing* the surface during the etching process.

## Evaluating Retention of Sealants

The finished sealant should be checked for retention without using undue force. In the event that the sealant does not adhere, the placement procedures should be repeated, with only about 15 seconds of etching needed to remove the residual saliva before again flushing, drying, and applying the sealant. If *two* attempts are unsuccessful, the sealant application should be postponed until remineralization occurs.

Resin sealants are retained better on recently erupted teeth than in teeth with a more mature surface; they are retained better on first molars than on second molars. They are better retained on mandibular than on maxillary teeth. This latter finding is possibly caused by the lower teeth being more accessible, direct sight is also possible; also, gravity aids the flow of the sealant into the fissures.[41]

Teeth that have been sealed and then have lost the sealant have had fewer lesions than control teeth.[82] This is possibly due to the presence of tags that are *retained in the enamel* after the bulk of the sealant has been sheared from the tooth surface. When the resin sealant flows over the prepared surface, it penetrates the finger-like depressions created by the etching solution. These projections of resin into the etched areas are called *tags*.[83] (Figure 10–6). The tags are essential for retention. Scanning electron microscopic studies of sealants that have not been retained have demonstrated large areas devoid of tags or incomplete tags, usually caused by saliva contamination. If a sealant is forcefully separated from the tooth by masticatory pressures, many of these tags are *retained* in the etched depressions.

The number of retained sealants decreases at a *curvolinear rate*.[41] Over the first 3 months, the rapid loss of sealants is probably caused by *faulty technique* in placement. The fallout rate then begins to plateau, with the ensuing sealant losses probably being due to abnormal *masticatory stresses*. After a year or so, the sealants become very difficult to see or to discern tactilely, especially if they are abraded to the point that they fill only the fissures. In research studies this lack of visibility often leads to *underestimating* the effectiveness of the sealants that remain but cannot be identified. Because the most rapid falloff of sealants occurs in the early stages, an initial 3-month recall following placement should be routine for determining if sealants have been lost. If so, the teeth should be resealed. Teeth successfully sealed for 6 to 7 years are likely to remain sealed.[83]

In a review of the literature, longest-term study reported that at the follow-up examination of the first molars, 20-years after sealant had been applied, 65% showed *complete* retention and 27% partial retention *without* caries. At a 15-year follow-up of the same sealants the second molars demonstrated the corresponding figures 65% and 30%, respectively. This study showed that pit-and-fissure sealants applied during childhood have a *long-lasting, caries preventive effect.*[60,77] Mertz-Fairhurst[83] cited studies in which 90 to 100% of the original sealants were retained over a 1-year period (Table 10–1). One 10-year study using 3M Concise Sealant had a 57% complete retention and a 21% partial retention of sealant, *all with no caries.* Another study, using Delton, registered 68% retention after 6 years.[108] (Figure 10–7).

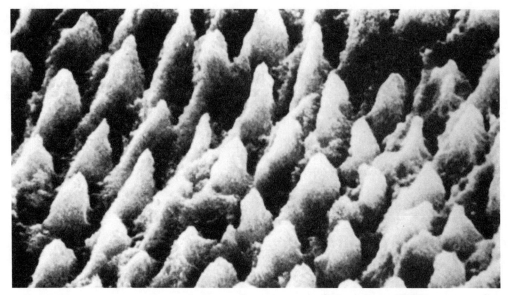

FIGURE 10-6 Tags, 30 μm. Sealant was flowed over etched surface, allowed to polylmerize, and tooth surface subsequently dissolved away in acid. (Courtesy, Silverstone LM, Dogon IL. *The Acid Etch Technique*. St. Paul, MN: North Central Publishing Co, 1975.)

These are studies in which the sealant was placed and then observed at periodic intervals; there was no resealing when a sealant was lost. *Where resealing is accomplished as needed at recall appointments, a higher and more continuous level of protection is achieved.* More recent studies report 82% of the sealants placed are retained for 5 years.[70]

### Colored Versus Clear Sealants

Both clear and colored sealants are available. They vary from translucent to white, yellow, and pink. Some manufacturers sell both clear and colored sealants in either the light-curing or autopolymerizing form. The selection of a colored versus a clear sealant is a matter of individual preference. The colored products permit a *more precise placement* of the sealant, with the visual assurance that the periphery extends halfway up the inclined planes. *Retention can be more accurately monitored* by both the patient and the operator placing the sealant. On the other hand, a clear sealant may be considered more *esthetically* acceptable.

Some clinicians prefer the clear sealants because they are more discrete than white. Others prefer the white sealants as they are easier to monitor at recall appointments. On the other hand, some clinicians seem to prefer the clear sealants because it is possible to see under the sealant if a carious lesion is active or advancing. However, no clinical study has comprehensively compared these issues. Recently, some pit-and-fissure sealants have been introduced that will change color as they are being light-polymerized. This property has not been fully investigated and seems to be only of relative advantage to the dental personnel applying the sealant.

### Placement of Sealants Over Carious Areas

Sealing over a carious lesion is important because of the professionals' concern about the possibility of caries progression under the

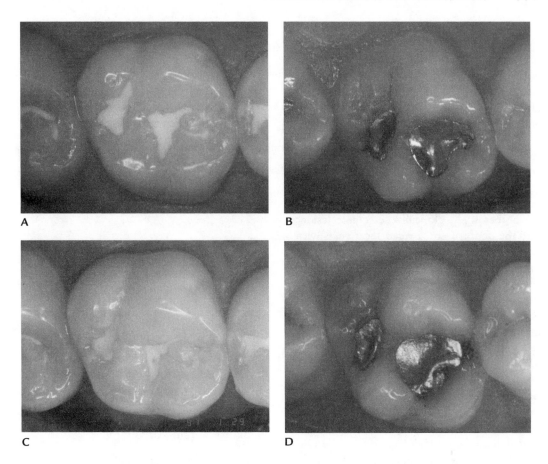

FIGURE 10–7    **A:** 5-year sealant: Five years after placement of a white pit-and-fissure sealant in the matched pair to the control subject. Sealant and control subjects were matched on age, sex, caries history and other factors. **B:** 5-year control: This matched pair to the sealed patient. This subject did not receive sealant. The first permanent molar has already been restored with two amalgam restorations in the previous 5-year period. **C:** 15-year sealant: 15 years after the single application of a white pit-and-fissure sealant. This is the same tooth as seen in Figure 1, 5-year sealant, but 10 years later. As can be seen, the sealant has served its purpose even though there has been some loss in the peripheral fissures. (Courtesy of Dr. Richard J. Simonsen, D.)

sealant sites. In teeth that have been examined *in vivo* and later subjected to histologic examination following extraction for orthodontic reasons, it has been found that areas of incipient or overt caries often occur under many fissures, which *cannot* be detected with the explorer.[85] In some studies, sealants have been purposely placed over small, overt lesions.[83,86] When compared with control teeth, many of the sealed carious teeth have been diagnosed as sound 3 and 5 years later.[87] Handelman has indicated that sealants can be considered a viable modality for *arrest* of pit-and-fissure caries.[88] In other studies of sealed lesions, the number of

bacteria recovered from the sealed area decreased rapidly.[33,34,86–89] This decrease in bacterial population is probably due to the integrity of the seal of the resin to the etched tooth surface[90] seal that does not permit the movement of fluids or tracer isotopes between the sealant and the tooth.[91]

Sealants have been placed over more extensive lesions in which carious dentin is involved.[92] Even with these larger lesions, there is a decrease in the bacterial population and arrest of the carious process as a function of time. In another study, clinically detectable lesions into the dentin were covered for 5 years with Nuva-Seal. After that time the bacterial cultures were essentially negative, and an apparent 83% *reversal* from a caries-active to a caries-inactive state was achieved.[86] Jordan and Suzuki[93] sealed small lesions in 300 teeth. During clinical and x-ray observations over a 5-year period, they found *no change in size of the carious lesion*, so long as the sealant remained intact. More recently, Mertz-Fairhurst and colleagues[94] demonstrated that sealed lesions became *inactive* bacteriologically, with the residual carious material suggesting decay cessation. This ability to arrest incipient and early lesions is highlighted by the statement in the 1979 publication of the ADA's Council on Dental Therapeutics: "Studies indicate that there is an apparent reduction in microorganisms in infected dentin covered with sealant. . . . These studies appear to substantiate that there is no hazard in sealing carious lesions." The statements end with the *cautionary* note: "However, additional long-term studies are required before this procedure can be evaluated as an alternative to traditional restorative procedures.[95] When sealing incipient lesions, care should be taken to monitor their retention at subsequent recall/annual dental examinations. In addition, there have been reports of sealants being used to achieve penetration of incipient smooth-surface lesions ("white spots") of facial surfaces."[96]

---

## Question 4

Which of the following statements, if any, are correct?

A. Tags can be easily determined by their rough feel when checking the *surface* of a sealant with an explorer.

B. Teeth that lose a sealant are more susceptible to caries than ones that retain a sealant but less caries-prone than a control tooth that was never sealed.

C. The falloff of sealants is *linear* as a function of time.

D. A study in which the periodic resealing of fissures occurs would be expected to have a *lesser* caries rate than a long-term study in which the same annual falloff is experienced, but where no resealing is accomplished.

E. Following placement of a sealant over a fissure with an undetectable carious lesion, the size of the subsurface lesion gradually *increases*.

---

### Sealants Versus Amalgams

Comparing sealants and amalgams is not an equitable comparison because sealants are used to *prevent* occlusal lesions, and amalgam is used to *treat* occlusal lesions that could have been prevented. Yet, the comparison is necessary. One of the major obstacles to more extensive use of sealants has been the belief that amalgams, and not sealants, should be placed in anatomically defective fissures; this belief stems from *misinformation* that amalgams can be placed in less time, and that once placed, they are a permanent restoration. Several studies have addressed these suppositions. For instance, sealants require approximately 6 to 9 minutes to place initially, amalgams 13 to 15 minutes.[97,98]

Many studies on *amalgam* restorations have indicated a *longevity* from only a few years to an

average life span of 10 years.[99–102] Equally perturbing is the fact that in one large study of schoolchildren, 16.2% of all surfaces filled with amalgam had marginal leakage and *needed replacement*.[103] The life span of an amalgam is shorter with younger children than with adults.[104] To emphasize the problem of replacement of older restorations, a recent questionnaire study from 91 dentists in Iceland was conducted to determine the cause for replacement of 8,395 restorations. The reason given for the replacement of composites, amalgams, glass-ionomers, and for resin modified glass ionomers was failed restorations (47.2%), primary caries (45.3%) and non-carious defects (7.5%). For every restoration inserted for an overt lesion, there was a need for one to be reinserted previously![105]

The retention data from the earlier sealant studies were discouraging. In recent years, using later-generation sealants, along with the *greater care in technique* used for their insertion, much longer retention periods have been reported. In five long-term studies from 3 to 7 years, the average sealant loss per year ranged from 1.3 to 7%.[106] If the yearly loss of these studies is extrapolated, the average life of these sealants compares favorably or exceeds that of amalgam.[107] When properly placed, sealants are no longer a temporary expedient for prevention; instead, they are the *only effective predictable* clinical procedure available for preventing occlusal caries.

The most frequent cause for sealant replacement is *loss of material*, which mainly occurs during the first 6 months; the most likely cause for amalgam replacement is *marginal decay*,[108] with 4 to 8 years being the average life span.[103] To replace the sealant, only resealing is necessary. No damage occurs to the tooth. Amalgam replacement usually requires cutting more tooth structure with each replacement. Even if longevity merits were equal, the sealant has the advantage of being painless to apply and aesthetic, as well as emphasizing the *highest objectives* of the dental profession—*prevention and sound teeth*.

## Options for Protecting the Occlusal Surfaces

The use of sealants has spawned an entirely different concept of conservation of occlusal tooth structure in the management of deep pits and fissures before, or early in caries involvement. The *preventive dentistry restoration* embodies the concepts of both prophylactic odontotomy insertion of a restoration and *covering the restoration and the connecting fissure system with a resin based sealant*. Pain and apprehension are slight, and aesthetics and tooth conservation are maximized.[108] Several options are now available to protect the occlusal surfaces, with the selection depending *on risk and professional's judgment*.[109] The first level of protection is simply to place a conventional sealant over the occlusal fissure system. This sealing preempts future pit-and-fissure caries, as well as arrests incipient or reverses small overt lesions.

The second option reported by Simonsen in 1978,[110] advocated the use of the *smallest* bur to remove the carious material from the bottom of a pit or fissure and then using an appropriate instrument to tease *either sealant or composite* into the cavity preparation. This he termed a preventive dentistry restoration. Following insertion of the restoration, sealant was placed *over* the polymerized material as well as flowed *over the remaining fissure system*. Aside from protecting the fissures from future caries, it also protects the composite or inserted sealant from abrasion.[111]

The third option is use of glass-ionomers material for sealants, which is controversial. Due to their fluoride release and cariostatic effect, glass-ionomers have been used in place of traditional materials, as a pit-and-fissure sealant, however, resin sealants have shown much higher bond strength to enamel than glass-ionomers. Clinical trials[112,113] have shown

poor retention over periods as short as 6 to 12 months. Though, in vitro studies have suggested that etching previous to application enhances the bonding of glass-ionomer sealant in fissure enamel.[114–116] One study showed that a conventional silver-reinforced glass-ionomer had superior clinical performance compared to a conventional resin sealant.[117]

Resin-reinforced glass-ionomer cements have been investigated for their effectiveness as pit-and-fissure sealants. The 1-year results revealed that although clinically the glass-ionomer wears at a faster rate than a conventional resin sealant, in the scanning electron microscopic evaluation the material could be seen at the deep recesses of the pits-and-fissures with no carious lesion present.[113] A recent study showed that after 3 years the glass-ionomer sealant was completely lost in almost 90% of the teeth compared to less than 10% of the resin sealed teeth; the relative risk of a tooth sealed with glass-ionomer over that of a tooth sealed with resin was higher. Also, the glass-ionomer sealant had poorer retention and less caries protective effect.[118]

Glass-ionomer does not carry the ADA seal of approval as sealant material. The readers should decide their personal philosophy based on the evidence.

A fourth option reported by García-Godoy in 1986 involves the use of a glass-ionomer cement as the *preventive glass-ionomer restoration* (PGIR).[119] The glass-ionomer cement (conventional or resin-modified) is placed only in the cavity preparation. (Figure 10–8). The occlusal surface is then etched with a gel etchant avoiding, if possible, etching the glass-ionomer. Etching the glass-ionomer may remove some of the glass particles weakening the material. The conventional resin sealant is placed *over the glass-ionomer and the entire occlusal fissure system.* In the event sealant is lost, the fluoride content of the glass-ionomer *helps prevent* future primary and *secondary* caries formation. The same technique has successfully protected

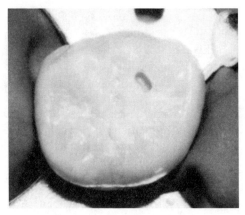

FIGURE 10–8 Preventive glass ionomer restoration (PGIR). Cavity preparation for reception of glass-ionomer cement. (Courtesy of Dr. Franklin García-Godoy, University of Texas Dental School, San Antonio.)

the marginal integrity of very small amalgam restoration, as well as providing a protection to the entire fissure system.

Each of these options requires a judgment decision by the clinician. That decision can well be based on the criterion that if an overt lesion cannot be *visualized*, it should be sealed; if it can be visualized, the smallest possible preventive dentistry restoration should be used along with its required sealant "topping." Mertz-Fairhurst and associates[120] have pointed out that the first option could provide the preferred model for conservative treatment of *incipient* and *small overt*, pit-and-fissure caries. It could also serve as an interim treatment for larger lesions. These options would be especially valuable in areas of the world with insufficient professional dental personnel and where preventive dental auxiliaries have been trained to place sealants. In all cases, the preventive dental filling should be considered as an alternative to the traditional class I amalgam with its accompanying extension for prevention that often includes the entire fissure system.

## The Sealant as Part of a Total Preventive Package

The sealant is used to protect the occlusal surfaces. A major effort should be made to incorporate the use of sealants along with other primary preventive dentistry procedures, such as plaque control, fluoride therapy, and sugar discipline. Whenever a sealant is placed, a topical application of fluoride should follow if at all possible. In this manner the whole tooth can be protected. Ripa and colleagues[121] completed a 2-year study for children in second and third grades assessing the effectiveness of a 0.2% fluoride mouthrinse used alone compared with a rinse plus sealants. Twenty-four occlusal lesions developed in the 51 rinse subjects, and *only* 3 in the 84 subjects receiving the rinse plus sealants. The conclusion was that caries could be *almost completely eliminated* by the *combined* use of these two preventive procedures. In many public-health programs, however, it is not possible to institute full-scale prevention programs, either because of apathy or lack of time and money. In such cases, there is some consolation in knowing that at least the *most vulnerable* of all tooth surfaces (the occlusal) is being protected.

## Manpower

The *cost* of sealant placement *increases* directly with the level of professional education of the operator. Dentists, hygienists, assistants, and other auxiliaries can be trained to place sealants.[122–124] In view of the cost-effectiveness, dental auxiliaries should be considered as the logical individuals to place sealants. This is important if manpower is to be increased.

Often auxiliaries who have received sealant instruction, either through continuing-education courses or as part of a curriculum, are stymied either because of state laws interdicting their placing sealants or by the nature and philosophy of the practice of the employing dentist.[125] Only fourteen states allow hygienists to practice under less restrictive or unsupervised practice models in which they can initiate treatment based on assessment of patient, treat the patient, and maintain a provider–patient relationship without the participation of the patients' dentist of record. For example, Maine and New Hampshire have a separate supervision for settings outside of the dental office public-health supervision, which is less restrictive than general supervision. New Mexico allows for a collaborative-practice agreement between dentists and hygienists in outside settings. Yet, in states such as Georgia and Illinois, hygienists are required to practice under direct supervision. This means the dentist must be present in the office while the care is being provided.[126]

In a Swedish study, 77 *dental assistants* working in 12 dental clinics sealed 3,218 first and second molars with a 5-year retention rate of between 74 and 94%.[127] Because many dentists consider the placement of sealants to be a relatively simple procedure, few are returning for continuing-education programs to learn the exacting and precise process necessary to ensure maximum sealant retention. Even when the dental professionals desire to participate in such continuing education, a survey found relatively few courses available.[128]

## Economics

Bear in mind that not every tooth receiving a sealant would necessarily become carious; hence the cost of preventing a single carious lesion is greater than the cost of a single sealant application. For instance, Leverett and colleagues calculated that five sealants would need to be placed on sound teeth to prevent one lesion over a 5-year period,[129] and Rock and Anderson estimated one tooth for every three sealant applications are prevented from becoming carious.[130] Sealants would be most cost-effective if they could be placed in only those pits

and fissures that are destined to become carious. Unfortunately, we do not have a caries predictor test of such exactitude, but, the use of vision plus an economic, portable electronic device that objectively measures conductance (or resistance) would greatly aid in evaluating occlusal risk.[131] Without such a device, it is necessary to rely on professional judgment, based on the severity of the caries activity indicators: number of "sticky" fissures, level of plaque index, number of incipient and overt lesions, and microbiologic test indications.

In an office setting, it is estimated that it costs 1.6 times more to treat a tooth than to seal.[55] The Task Force on Community Preventive Services, an independent, non-federal group formed to evaluated oral-health interventions, was charged with determining interventions that promote and improve oral health. The Task Force examined six public-health programs cost of placing pit-and-fissure sealants revealing a mean cost of $39.10 per person.[132] However, even these numbers are misleading. For instance, what is the value of an intact tooth to its owner? How much does it cost for a dentist and assistant to restore a tooth, compared to the cost of sealing a tooth? Later in life, what is the cost of bridges and dentures that had their genesis when children were at high risk with little access to dental care?

## Use of Pit-and-Fissure Sealants

By the mid-1980s most of the answers were available as to the need and *effectiveness* of Bis-GMA sealants to reduce the incidence of occlusal caries, and the *techniques* of placement of pit-and-fissure sealants were known.[133] The *safety* of their placement has been demonstrated by many studies showing that even when placed over incipient and minimally overt caries sites, there was no progression *as long as the sealant remained intact*.[134] Finally, several clinical studies have pointed out that

sealants could be *applied by properly trained auxiliaries*, thus providing a more economical source of manpower for private and military practices as well as for large school and public health programs.

Bis-GMA sealant usage has been strongly supported by the ADA "as a safe and effective means for caries control."[25] The United States Public Health Service, in a request for a proposal for a school pit-and-fissure study, stated *"This combination of preventive techniques (combined use of fluoride and sealants) is expected to essentially eliminate caries in teeth erupting after the initiation of the study."*[135] Despite the support from the two largest organizations most interested in the dental health of the nation, the rank-and-file of the dental profession *have not accepted sealants as a routine method for prevention*.

In spite of all the knowledge of the properties and successes of the sealants usage has lagged, with about 10% of the posterior teeth of children demonstrating the presence of sealants.[136] For example, a 1994 examination of 117,000 children in North Carolina between the ages of 6 and 17 found that approximately 12% had sealants,[137] while the percentage for 927,000 in Tennessee was 10%.[138] Other states demonstrate similar sealant usage. One study revealed that 88 children did have sealants while 508 did not have needed sealants.[139] For recruits entering the U.S. Air Force, sealants were found on 13.1% of the teeth while there was a need for 47.5% more. In the latter case, it was noted that a third of these personnel had occlusal caries that might have been prevented by the sealants.[20]

Many barriers exist in meeting the Healthy People 2010 Objective for sealants. In 2001, the State of Alabama was planning how to meet national dental objectives, when 50% of U.S. children are expected to have dental sealants on at least one permanent molar by the age of 14 years.[140] (Currently, 22% of the children between 12 to 14 years have at least one sealant claim.) A final assessment of the

2010 prospects and the current State's demographics concluded that racial and gender disparities, difficulty in accessing care, the non-availability of Medicaid-participating dentists in a country, and a lower payment/claim ratio may make the national sealant objective difficult to achieve.[140] It should be mentioned that in many surveys, children from lower socioeconomic groups had greater sealant needs than those from more affluent neighborhoods.

On the other hand, other countries have had marked success with increasing the number of teeth sealed. A study involving 68,704 children living in Lanarkshire, Scotland found approximately 10% of the occlusal surfaces were sealed.[141] Five years later, in England the percentage of children *having sealants dramatically increased* between 20 to 50% in several areas.[142]

The placement of sealants is making slow progress. The 1998-99 Ohio State survey of 3rd-grade students in School Based/School Link programs found that in addition to oral-health benefits, "Providing sealant programs in all eligible, high-risk schools could reduce or eliminate racial and economic disparities in the prevalence of dental sealants".[143] Yet, there are problems in examining the number of sealants *versus* the *need* for sealants.

## Dentist Involvement

Pit-and-fissure sealants are underused in private practice and public health. There are many complex reasons for such under use, but efforts should be undertaken to increase sealant use.[3] Increasing sealant use is dependent, in part, on dentists' acceptance and understanding of the preventive technique. In a mail survey in Minnesota, 95% of 375 dentists reported the use of sealants, varying from 1 to 25 per week. Possibly, the incongruity of numbers stems from the fact that although the majority of dentists use sealants, the *frequency* of use is *low*.[144]

Reasons for this apathy have ranged from alleged concerns of sealing over carious lesions, lack of technical skill, short longevity of sealants, and the need for more research—all problems that have been adequately addressed in the literature.[133] Probably the most important factor now restricting the placement of sealants is the lack of an adequate insurance fee schedule.[145] Another is that most dentists are treatment-oriented. This fact is amplified by an explanation by Galarneau and Brodeur that "A dentists lack of comfort with withholding treatment may stop him/her from offering preventive care and cause him to follow a restoration-oriented practice."[146] Another factor is that dentists rarely explain the oral-health advantages of sealants over dental restorations.[147]

In attempting to alter the attitudes of dentist on sealant use, several studies have been conducted to measure *changes in knowledge and attitudes* following continuing-education courses. The follow-up indicated that there had been an increase in *knowledge* but little change in *attitudes* concerning sealant use.[148] In Colorado, pediatric dentists, who are continually involved in treating children, placed more sealants than general dentists—again, probably a manifestation of attitudes.[145]

Regardless of increased rhetoric about prevention, the concepts and actions of prevention are *not* being fully implemented in dental schools.[149] Dental school faculties need to be educated about the effectiveness and methods of applying sealants.[150,151] Possibly the development of a model curriculum for teaching pit-and-fissure sealant usage would help.[152] The dental community must develop a consensus about the value and economic effect of preventive measures.[150]

Other barriers to effective delivery of sealants include (1) state-board restrictions on auxiliary placement of sealants, (2) lack of consumer knowledge of the effectiveness of sealants, and, resultantly, a lack of demand for the product.[122] *The economics and education of the profession and of the public are the prime requisites for expanded sealant acceptance.*[153]

### Question 5

Which of the following statements, if any, are correct?

A. The longevity expectation for a properly placed amalgam restoration is approximately twice that of a properly placed sealant.

B. Sealants should be placed only on permanent teeth of children up to age 16.

C. Sealants are found on approximately 54% of U.S. children.

D. Following the graduation of students presently in dental schools, a large increase in the use of sealants can be expected.

E. Caries does not progress under a properly sealed composite or amalgam.

## Other Pit-and-Fissure Initiatives

The findings of the following studies must be considered an *important extension* of the present use of pit-and-fissure sealants, which are used to prevent the development of incipient lesions and to arrest minimal overt lesions. If professional judgment dictates, conservative sealed amalgams or composites could be used to maintain *marginal integrity, extend the longevity of the restorative materials, and for achieving a de facto extension for prevention without the need to remove sound tooth structure to extend the restoration over the entire fissure system.* These two uses of resins for prevention and restorations without major operative considerations should be of great value in developing countries where professional manpower is at a minimum and the demand for dental care is great.

Probably the most important recent research on the use of Bis-GMA sealants and carious lesions were described by Mertz-Fairhurst and coworkers.[87,154] In the 10-year study,[154] patients with paired permanent molars or premolars with *obvious clinical and radiographic class I lesions* were selected. The carious lesions extended halfway into the dentin or to the nearest pulp horn. The randomized placement of restorations for each of the tooth pairs consisted of two of the following: (1) a *classic* amalgam restoration, complete with extension for prevention of all connecting fissures (79 subjects); (2) a *conservative* amalgam restoration involving only the carious site with a sealant "topping," the latter which was extended into the entire pit-and-fissure system (77 subjects); and (3) with each one of the amalgam restorations, a paired composite restoration placed over the carious tissue with a "topping" of sealant that included all the pits and fissures (156 subjects). In the preparation for the composite, *no attempt was made to remove the carious tissue*. A 1-millimeter wide, 40- to 60-degree bevel was made in the sound enamel surrounding the lesion. The area was washed, dried, and a bonding agent was placed on the bevel. Hand instruments were used to place the composite, after which rotary instruments were used to shape the occlusal anatomy. Following this step, the occlusal surface was treated as for the placement of the average sealant—dry, etch, rinse, and dry before placing the resin over the composite and the entire fissure system.

The conclusions of this study after 10 years were: (1) *both* the sealed composites and the sealed amalgam restorations exhibited *superior clinical performance and longevity* compared to the unsealed amalgam restorations; (2) bonded and sealed composite restorations placed over the frank cavitated lesions *arrested the clinical progress of these lesions for the 10 years of the study*.[154]

## SUMMARY

The majority of all carious lesions that occur in the mouth occur on the occlusal surfaces. Which teeth will become carious cannot be predicted; however, if the surface is sealed with a pit-and-fissure sealant, no caries will develop as long as the sealant remains in place. Recent studies indicate an approximate 90% retention rate of sealants 1-year after placement. Even when sealants are eventually lost, most studies indicate that the caries incidence for teeth that have lost sealants is less than that of control surfaces that had never been sealed. Research data also indicate that many incipient and small overt lesions are arrested when sealed. Not one report has shown that caries developed in pits or fissures when under an intact sealant. Sealants are easy to apply, but the application of sealants is an extremely sensitive technique. The surfaces that are to receive the sealant *must be completely isolated from the saliva during the entire procedure, and etching, flushing, and drying procedures must be timed to ensure adequate preparation of the surface for the sealant.* Sealants are comparable to amalgam restorations for longevity and do not require the cutting of tooth structure. Sealants do not cost as much to place as amalgams. Despite their advantages, the use of sealants has not been embraced by all dentists, even though endorsed by the ADA and the U.S. Public Health Service. Even when small overt pit-and-fissure lesions exist, they can be dealt with conservatively by use of preventive dentistry restorations. What now appears to be required is that the dental schools *teach* sealants as an effective intervention, that the dental professional *use* them, that the hygienists and the auxiliary personnel be permitted to *apply* them, and the public *demand* them.

## ANSWERS AND EXPLANATIONS

1. C and D—correct.

   A—incorrect. Because the fluorides protect the smooth surface, there will be a greater proportion of pit-and-fissure lesions.

   B—incorrect. By definition, an incipient lesion has not been invaded by bacteria; thus the use of a sealant is an ideal preventive measure.

   E—incorrect. Remember, it is the caries susceptibility of the teeth that is important—not the age of the individual.

2. A, B, and C—correct.

   D—incorrect. All the major, successful, long-term retention studies have used cotton-roll isolation; in the one study of rubber dam versus cotton rolls, the rolls were equal to, or better than, the dam.

   E—incorrect. Ten seconds are used for the drying and flushing procedures, and 20 to 30 seconds for the etching.

3. A and B—correct.

C—incorrect. Bis-GMA plastics are of the same chemical family and will bond to each other regardless of manufacturer.

D—incorrect. Remineralization from saliva constituents occurs rapidly in a period of hours to days.

E—incorrect. Cleansing and etching do occur; however, rubbing tends to obliterate the delicate etching pattern and reduce retention potential.

4. B and D—correct.

A—incorrect. The tags of the sealant cannot be felt with the explorer; they extend into the enamel from the underneath side of the plastic.

C—incorrect. The curvolinear falloff is greatest at 3 months, less at 6 months, after which it gradually plateaus.

E—incorrect. The literature is unanimous that caries does not progress under an intact sealant.

5. C and E—correct.

A—incorrect. There is little difference between the longevity of a well-placed amalgam compared with a well-placed sealant.

B—incorrect. If a tooth is susceptible to caries, it should be sealed, whatever the patient's age.

D—incorrect. All signs indicate that the teaching of sealant placement is greatly neglected in dental schools.

## Self-evaluation Questions

1. Approximately _____ % of all carious lesions occur on the occlusal surfaces; the continual use of fluorides (increases) (decreases) this percentage.

2. Four different methods used prior to the advent of polyurethane, cyanoacrylate, and Bis-GMA sealants, were _____, _____, _____, and _____.

3. One condition that *indicates the use of a sealant is* _____; *four conditions that con-traindicate* the use of sealants are _____, _____, _____, and _____; three conditions that *probably indicate* the use of sealants are _____, _____, and _____.

4. Two photoactivated, and two chemically activated sealants that have been accepted, or provisionally accepted, by the ADA are (photoactivated) _____, _____, and (chemically activated) _____ and _____.

5. The liquid resin in a sealant kit is known as the _____; when it is catalyzed the hardening process is known as _____. The catalyst used for the polymerization of chemically activated sealants is _____ and for visible photoactivation, _____.

6. Two advantages to light-cured sealants are _____ and _____; and two advantages of autopolymerized sealants are _____ and _____.

7. _____ forces, not chemical bonding, causes retention of the sealant to the tooth; the four commandments to ensure maximum retention are _____, _____, _____, and _____.

8. Three methods by which a dry field can be established are _____, _____, and _____.

9. The placement of sealants is extremely technique-sensitive; after selection of the tooth for sealant placement, it should be dried for _____ (time); then etched for _____ (time), followed by a water flush of _____ (time), and finally, dried for _____ (time) before placing the sealant.

10. Excessively high sealants that interfere with occlusion can be reduced by use of a number _____ (cutting) (finishing) bur.

11. The falloff of sealants is (linear) (curvilinear); long-term studies where 65% of the sealants are retained after 7 years indicate an average yearly loss of _____ %. After 10 years, _____ _____ % would be retained. This contracts to an average life expectancy of an amalgam of approximately _____ (years).

12. To protect the total tooth, the application of a sealant should be followed by an application of _____.

13. To ensure that sealant placement techniques have been perfected in dental and dental hygiene schools, it should be necessary for _____ (state dental-regulating agency) to require a demonstration of proficiency for all candidates prior to state licensure.

14. The three key components of a light source of polymerizing sealants are _____, _____, and _____ (which results in the blue color).

15. The three basic options for a preventive dentistry restoration are _____, _____, and _____.

## REFERENCES

1. National Center for Health Statistics (NCHS) (1996). Third National Health and Nutrition Examination Survey (NHANES III) reference manuals and reports. Hyattsville (MD): NCHS, U.S. Department of Health and Human Services, Public Health Service, Centers for Disease Control and Prevention.
2. Wilson, I. P. (1985). Preventive dentistry. *Dent Dig*, 1:70–72.
3. NIH Consensus Development Conferences Statement (1983). Dental sealant in the prevention of tooth decay, Dec 5–7, 4(11):1–18.
4. Bödecker, C. F. (1929) The eradication of enamel fissures. *Dent Items Int*, 51:859–66.

5. Sturdevant, C. M., Barton, R. E., Sockwell, C. L., & Strickland, W. D. (1985). *The art and science of operative dentistry*. 2nd ed. St. Louis; C. V. Mosby, 97.

6. Hyatt, T. P. (1936). Prophylactic odontotomy: The ideal procedure in dentistry for children. *Dent Cosmos*, 78:353–370.

7. Ast, D. B., Bushel, A., & Chase, C. C. (1950). A clinical study of caries prophylaxis and zinc chloride and potassium ferrocyanide. *J Am Dent Assoc*, 41:437–42.

8. Klein, H., & Knutson, J. W. (1942). Studies on dental caries. XIII. Effect of ammoniacal silver nitrate on caries in the first permanent molar. *J Am Dent Assoc*, 29:1420–26.

9. Miller, J. (1951). Clinical investigations in preventive dentistry. *Br Dent J*, 91:92–95.

10. Backer-Dirks, O., Houwink, B., & Kwant, G. W. (1961). The results of 6½ years of artificial fluoridation of drinking water in the Netherlands. The Tiel-Culemborg experiment. *Arch Oral Biol*, 5:284–300.

11. Buonocore, M. G. (1971). Caries prevention in pits and fissures sealed with an adhesive resin polymerized by ultraviolet light: A two-year study of a single adhesive application. *J Am Dent Assoc*, 82:1090–93.

12. Gillings, B., & Buonocore, M. (1961). Thickness of enamel at the base of pits and fissures in human molars and bicuspids. *J Dent Res*, 40:119–33.

13. Mass, E., Eli, I., Lev-Dor-Samovici, B., & Weiss, E. I. (1999). Continuous effect of pit-and-fissure sealing on S. mutans present *in situ*. *Pediatric Dent*, 21:164–68.

14. Vehkalati, M. M., Solavaaral, L., & Rytomaa, I. (1991). An eight-year follow-up of the occlusal surfaces of first permanent molars. *J Dent Res*, 70:1064–67.

15. Simonsen, R. J. (1984). Pit-and-fissure sealant in individual patient care programs. *J Dent Educ*, 48(Suppl. 2):42–44.

16. U.S. Department of Health and Human Service (2002). Healthy People 2010. Volume 2/21 Oral Health. Centers for Disease Control and Prevention. Available at: http://www.health.gov/healthypeople/, Accessed Summer 2002.

17. Bohannan, H. M. (1983). Caries distribution and the case for sealants. *J Public Health Dent*, 33:200–4.

18. Ripa, L. W., Leske, G. S., & Varma, A. O. (1988). Ten to 13-year-old children examined annually for three years to determine caries activity in the proximal and occlusal surfaces of first permanent molars. *J Public Health Dent*, 48:8–13.

19. Arthur, J. S., & Swango, P. (1987). The incidence of pit-and-fissure caries in a young Navy population: Implication for expanding sealant use. *J Public Health Dent*, 47:33. Abstr.

20. Foreman, F. J. (1994). Sealant prevalence and indication in a young military population. *JADA*, 184:182–84.

21. Buonocore, M. G. (1955). A simple method of increasing the retention of acrylic filling materials to enamel surfaces. *J Dent Res*, 34:849–53.

22. van-Dijken, J. W. (1994). A 6-year evaluation of a direct composite resin inlay/onlay system and glass ionomer cement-composite resin sandwich restorations *Acta-Odontol-Scand*, Dec, 52(6):368–76.

23. Bowen, R. L. Dental filling material comprising vinyl silane treated fused silica and a binder consisting of the reaction product of bis-phenol and glycidyl acrylate. U.S. Patent #3,006,112. November 1962.

24. The ADA Seal of Acceptance, Professional Products. Available at: http://www.ada.org/prof/prac/seal/sealsrch.asp. Retrieved 1-11-02.

25. American National Standards Institute and American Dental Association. American Nation Standard/American Dental Association specification no 39. For pit and fissure sealant. Chicago: American Dental Association Council on Scientific Affairs;1992 (reaffirmed 1999) Available at: www://ada.org/prof/prac.stands/Specification%20No.%20391.pdf. Accessed 1/11/2003.

26. Council on Dental Materials (1983). Instruments and Equipment. Pit and fissure sealants. *J Am Dent Assoc*, 107:465.

27. Mills, R. W., & Ball, I. A. (1993). A clinical trial to evaluate the retention of a silver cement-ionomer cement used as a fissure sealant. *Oper Dent*, 18:148–54.

28. Swartz, M. L., Phillips, R. W., Norman, R. D., et al. (1976). Addition of fluoride to pit-and-fissure sealants: A feasibility study. *J Dent Res*, 55:757–71.

29. Hicks, M. J., Flaitz, C. M., & Silverstone, L. M. (1986). Secondary caries formation in vitro around glass ionomer restorations. *Quint Int*, 17:527–31.

30. Forsten, L. (1977). Fluoride release from glass ionomer cement. *Scand J Dent Res*, 85:503–4.

31. Bjerga, J. M., & Crall, J. J. (1984). Enamel fluoride uptake and caries-like lesion inhibition *in vitro*. *J Dent Res*, 63:239 (Abstr. 618).

32. Kozai, K., Suzuki, J., Okada, M., & Nagasaka N. (2000). In vitro study of antibacterial and antiadhesive activities of fluoride-containing light-cured fissure sealants and a glass ionomer liner/base against oral bacteria. *ASDC J Dent Child*, 67:117–22.

33. Carlsson, A., Patersson, M., & Twetman, S. (1997). 2 year clinical performance of a fluoride-containing fissure sealant in young schoolchildren at caries risk. *Am J Dent*, 10:3:115–19.

34. Loyola-Rodríguez, J. P., & García-Godoy, F. (1996). Antibacterial activity of fluoride release sealants on mutans streptococci. *J Clin Pediatr Dent*, 20:109–12.

35. Hicks, J. M., & Flaitz, C. M. (1992). Caries-like lesion formation around fluoride-releasing sealant and glass ionomer restorations. *Am J Dent*, 5:329–34.

36. Jensen, M. E., Wefel, J. S., Triolo, P. T., Hammesfahr, P. D. (1990). Effects of a fluoride-releasing fissure sealant on artificial enamel caries. *Am J Dent*, 3:75–78.

37. Hicks, M. J., Flaitz, C. M., & García-Godoy, F. (2000). Fluoride-releasing sealant and caries-like enamel lesion formation in vitro. *J Clin Pediatr Dent*, 24:215–9.

38. Marcushamer, M., Neuman, E., & García-Godoy, F. (1997). Fluoridated and unfluoridated sealants show similar shear strength. *Pediatr Dent*, 19:289–90.

39. Koch, M. J., García-Godoy, F., Mayer, T., & Staehle, H. J. (1997). Clinical evaluation of Helioseal-F sealant. *Clin Oral Invest*, 1:199–202.

40. Jensen, O. E., Billings, R. J., & Featherstone, D. B. (1990). Clinical evaluation of FluroShield pit-and-fissure sealant. *Clin Prev Dent*, 12:24–27.

41. García-Godoy, F. (1986). Retention of a light-cured fissure sealant (Helioseal) in a tropical environment. *Clin Prev Dent*, 8:11–13.

42. Lugidakis, N. A., & Oulis, K. I. (1999). A comparison of Fluroshield with Delton fissure sealant four year results. *Pediatr Dent*, 21:7 429–31.

43. Shinji, H., Uchimura, N., Ishida, M., Motokawa, W., Miyazaki, K., & García-Godoy, F. (1998). Enamel fluoride uptake from a fluoride releasing sealant. *Am J Dent*, 11:58–60.

44. García-Godoy, F., Abarzúa, I., de Goes, M. F., & Chan, D. C. N. (1997). Fluoride release from fissure sealants. *J Clin Pediatr Dent*, 22:45–49.

45. Morphis, T. L., Toumba, K. J., & Lygidakis, N. A. (2000). Fluoride pit-and-fissure sealants: A review. *Int J Pediatr Dent*, 15:90–8.

46. Blankenau, R. J., Kelsey, W. P., Cavel, W. T., & Blankenau, P. (1983). Wavelength and intensity of seven systems for visible light curing composite resins: A comparison study. *JADA*, 106:471–74.

47. Council on Dental Materials, Instruments, and Equipment (1985). Visible light-cured composites and activating units. 110:100–103.

48. Houpt, M., Fuks, A., Shapira, J., Chosack, A., & Eidelman, E. (1987). Autopolymerized versus light-polymerized fissure sealant. *J Am Dent Assoc*, 115:55–56.

49. Waren, D. P., Infante, N. B., Rice, H. C. et al. (2001). Effect of topical fluoride on retention of pit-and-fissure sealants. *J Dent Hyg*, 71:21–4.

50. Gandini, M., Vertuan, V., & Davis, J. M. (1991). A comparative study between visible-light-activated and autopolymerizing sealants in relation to retention. *ASDC J Dent Child* 58:4 297–9.

51. Leung, R., Fan, P. L., & Johnston, W. M. (1982). Exposure time and thickness on polymerization of visible light composite. *J Dent Res*, 61:248. Abstr. 623.

52. Leung, R., Fan, P. L., & Johnston, W. M. (1983). Postirradiation polymerization of visible light-activated composite resin. *J Dent Res*, 62:363–65.

53. Buonocore, M. G. (1963). Principles of adhesive retention and adhesive restorative materials. *J Am Dent Assoc*, 67:382–91.

54. Gwinnett, A. J., & Buonocore, M. G. (1965). Adhesion and caries prevention. A preliminary report. *Br Dent J*, 119:77–80.

55. García-Godoy, F., & Gwinnett, A. J. (1987). Penetration of acid solution and high and low viscosity gels in occlusal fissures. *JADA*, 114:809–10.

56. Brown, M. R., Foreman, F. J., Burgess, J. O., & Summitt, J. B. (1988). Penetration of gel and solution etchants in occlusal fissures sealing. *J Dent Child*, 55:26–29.

57. Arana, E. M. (1974). Clinical observations of enamel after acid-etch procedure. *J Am Dent Assoc*, 89:1102–6.

58. Bossert, W. A. (1937). The relation between the shape of the occlusal surfaces of molars and the prevalence of decay. II. *J Dent Res*, 16:63–67.

59. Konig, K. G. (1963). Dental morphology in relation to caries resistance with special reference to fissures as susceptible areas. *J Dent Res*, 42:461–76.

60. Simonsen, R. J. (1987). Retention and effectiveness of a single application of white sealant after 10 years. *JADA*, 115:31–36.

61. Mertz-Fairhurst, E. J. (1984). Personal communication.

62. Bogert, T. R., & García-Godoy, F. (1992). Effect of prophylaxis agents on the shear bond strength of a fissure sealant. *Pediatr Dent*, 14:50–51.

63. García-Godoy, F., & O'Quinn, J. A. (1993). Effect of prophylaxis agents on shear bond strength of a resin composite to enamel. *Gen Dent*, 41:557–59.

64. Kanellis, M. J., Warren, J. J., & Levy, S. M. (2000). A comparison of sealant placement techniques and 12-month retention rates. *J Public Health Dent*, 60:53–6.

65. Chan, D. C., Summitt, J. B., García-Godoy, F., Hilton, T. J., & Chung, K. H. (1999). Evaluation of different methods for cleaning and preparing occlusal fissures. *Oper Dent*, 24:331–6.

66. Sol, E., Espasa, E., Boj, J. R., & Canalda, C. (2000). Effect of different prophylaxis methods on sealant adhesion. *J Clin Pediatr Dent*, 24:211–4.

67. García-Godoy, F., & Medlock, J. W. (1988). An SEM study of the effects of air-polishing on fissure surfaces. 19:465–7.

68. Titley, K. C., Torneck, C. D., & Smith, D. C. (1988). The effect of concentrated hydrogen peroxide solution on the surface morphology of human tooth enamel. *J Dent Res*, 67(Special Issue):361, Abstr. 1989.

69. Blackwood, J. A., Dilley, D. C., Roberts, M. W., & Swift, E. J. Jr. (2002). Evaluation of pumice, fissure enameloplasty and air abrasion on sealant microleakage. *Pediatr Dent*, 24:199–203.

70. Dental Sealants ADA Council of Access and Prevention and Interprofessional Relations (1997). Council on Scientific Affairs *JADA*, 128:484–88.

71. Nordenvall, K. J., Brannstrom, M., & Malgrem, O. (1980). Etching of deciduous teeth and young and old permanent teeth. A comparison between 15 and 60 seconds etching. *Am J Orthod*, 78:99–108.

72. Eidelman, E., Shapira, J., & Houpt, M. (1988). The retention of fissure sealants using twenty-second etching time: Three-year follow-up. *J Dent Child*, 55:119–20.

73. Pahlavan, A., Dennison, J. B., & Charbeneau, G. T. (1976). Penetration of restorative resins into acid-etched human enamel. *JADA*. 1976; 93:1070–76.

74. Silverstone, L. M. (1974). Fissure sealants, laboratory studies. *Caries Res*, 8:2–26.

75. Bozalis, W. B., & Marshall, G. W. (1977). Acid etching patterns of primary enamel. *J Dent Res*, 56:185.

76. Straffon, L. H., More, F. G., & Dennison, J. B. (1984). Three year clinical evaluation of sealant applied under rubber dam isolation. *J Dent Res*, 63:215. IADR Abstr. 400.

77. Wendt, L. K., Koch, G., & Birhed, D. (2001). On the retention and effectiveness of fissure sealant in permanent molars after 15-20 years: a cohort study. *Community Dent Oral Epidemiol* 29:4 302–7.

78. Wood, A. J., Saravia, M. E., & Farrington, F. H. (1989). Cotton roll isolation versus Vac-Ejector isolation. *J Dent Child*, 56:438–40.

79. Powell, K. R., & Craig, G. G. (1978). An *in vitro* investigation of the penetrating efficiency of Bis-GMA resin pit-and-fissure coatings. *J Dent Res*, 57:691–95.

80. Silverstone, L. M. (1983). Fissure sealants: The enamel-resin interface. *J Public Health Dent*, 43:205–15.

81. Myers, C. L., Rossi, F., & Cartz, L. (1974). Adhesive tag-like extensions into acid-etched tooth enamel. *J Dent Res*, 53:435–41.

82. Hinding, J. (1974). Extended cariostasis following loss of pit-and-fissure sealant from human teeth. *J Dent Child*, 41:41–43.

83. Mertz-Fairhurst, E. J. (1984). Current status of sealant retention and caries prevention. *J Dent Educ*, 48:18–26.

84. Mertz-Fairhurst, E. J., Fairhurst, C. W., Williams, J. E., Della-Giustina, V. E., Brooks, J. D. (1982). A comparative clinical study of two pit-and-fissure sealants: Six year results in August, Ga. *JADA*, 105:237–9.

85. Miller, J., & Hobson, P. (1956). Determination of the presence of caries in fissures. *Br Dent J*, 100:15–18.

86. Going, R. E., Loesche, W. J., Grainger, D. A., & Syed, S. A. (1978). The viability of organisms in carious lesions five years after covering with a fissure sealant. *JADA*, 97:455–67.

87. Mertz-Fairhurst, E. J., Richards, E. E., Williams, J. E., Smith, C. D., Mackert, J. R., Schuster, G. S., Sherrer, J. D., O'Dell, N. L., Pierce, K. L., Wenner, K. K., & Ergle, J. W. (1992). Sealed restorations: 5-year results. *Am J Dent*, 5:5–10.

88. Handelman, S. L., Washburn, F., & Wopperer, P. (1976). Two year report of sealant effect on bacteria in dental caries. *JADA*, 93:976–80.

89. Jeronimus, D. J., Till, M. J., & Sveen, O. B. (1975). Reduced viability of microorganisms under dental sealants. *J Dent Child*, 42:275–80.

90. Theilade, E., Fejerskov, O., Migasena, K., & Prachyabrued, W. (1977). Effect of fissure sealing on the microfloral in occlusal fissures of human teeth. *Arch Oral Biol*, 22:251–59.

91. Jensen, O. E., & Handelman, S. L. (1978). *In vitro* assessment of marginal leakage of six enamel sealants. *J Prosthet Dent*, 36:304–6.

92. Handleman, S. (1982). Effects of sealant placement on occlusal caries progression. *Clin Prevent Dent*, 4:11–16.

93. Jordan, R. E., & Suzuki, M. (1984). Unpublished report, quoted by Going, R.E. Sealant effect on incipient caries, enamel maturation and future caries susceptibility. *J Dent Educ*, 48(Suppl.) 2:35–41.

94. Mertz-Fairhurst, E. J., Shuster, G. S., & Fairhurst, C. W. (1986). Arresting caries by sealants: Results of a clinical study. *JADA*, 112:194–203.

95. *Accepted Dental Therapeutics*, 39th ed. American Dental Association, Chicago, Ill. 1982.

96. Micik, R. E. (Mar 1972). Fate of in vitro Caries-like Lesions Sealed within Tooth Structure. *IADR Program*, Abstr. 710.

97. Burt, B. A. (1984). Fissure sealants: Clinical and economic factors. *J Dent Educ*, 48 (Suppl.) 2:96–102.

98. Dennison, J. B., & Straffon, L. H. (1984). Clinical evaluation comparing sealant and amalgam after seven years—final report. *J Dent Res*, 1984; 63(Special Issue):215. Abstr. 401.

99. Allen, D. N. (1977). A longitudinal study of dental restorations. *Br Dent J*, 143:87–89.

100. Cecil, J. C., Cohen, M. E., Schroeder, D. C., et al. (1982). Longevity of amalgam restorations: A retrospective view. *J Dent Res*, 61:185. Abstr. 56.

101. Healey, H. J., & Phillips, R. W. (1949). A clinical study of amalgam failures. *J Dent Res*, 28:439–46.

102. Lavell, C. L. (1976). A cross-sectional, longitudinal survey into the durability of amalgam restorations. *J Dent*, 4:139–43.

103. Robinson, A. D. (1971). The life of a filling. *Br Dent J*, 130:206–8.

104. Hunter, B. (1982). The life of restorations in children and young adults. *J Dent Res*, 61:537. Abstr. 18.

105. Mjör, I. A., Shen, C., Eliasson, S. T., & Richters, S. (2002) Placement and replacement of restorations in general dental practice in Iceland. *Oper Dent*, 27:117–23.

106. Hassal, D. C., & Mellor, A. C. (2001). The sealant restoration: indications, success and clinical technique. *Br Dent J*, 191:358–62.

107. Dennison, J. B., & Straffon, L. H. (1981). Clinical evaluation comparing sealant and amalgam—4 years report. *J Dent Res*, 60(Special Issue A):520. Abstr. 843.

108. Swift, E. J. (1987). Preventive resin restorations. *JADA*, 114:819–21.

109. Shaw, L. (2000). Modern thought on fissure sealants. *Dent Update*, 27:370–4.

110. Simonsen, R. J. (1978). Preventive resin restorations. *Quintessence Int*, 9:69–76.

111. Dickinson, G., Leinfelder, K. F., & Russell, C. M. (1988). Evaluation of wear by application of a surface sealant. *J Dent Res*, 67:362. Abstr. 1999.

112. Aranda, M., & García-Godoy, F. (1995). Clinical evaluation of a glass ionomer pit-and-fissure sealant. *J Clin Pediatr Dent*, 19:273–7.

113. Ovrebo, R. C., & Raadal, M. (1990). Microleakage in fissures sealed with resin or glass ionomer cement. *Scand J Dent Res*, 98:66–69.

114. De Luca-Fraga, L. R., & Freire Pimienta, L. A. (2001). Clinical evaluation of glass-ionomer/resin-based hybrid materials used as pit-and-fissure sealants. *Quintessence Int*, 32:6 463–8.

115. Kervanto-Seppala, S., Lavonius, E., Kerosuo, E., & Pietilla, I. (2000). Can glass-ionomer sealants be cost-effective? *J Clin Dent*, 11:11–3.

116. Pereira, A. C., Pardi, V., Basting, R. T. Menighim, M. C., Pinelli, C., Ambrosano, G. M., & García-Godoy, F. (2001). Clinical evaluation of glass-ionomers used as fissure sealants: twenty four-month results. *ASDC J Dent Child*, 68:168–74.

117. Forss, H., & Halme, E. (1998). Retention of a glass ionomer cement and resin-based fissure sealant and effect on carious outcome after 7 years. *Community Dent Oral Epidemiol*, 26:21–25.

118. Poulsen, S., Beiruti, N., & Sadar, N. (2001). A comparison of retention and the effect on caries of fissure sealing with a glass-ionomer and a resin-based sealant. *Community Dent Oral Epidemiol*, 29:298–301.

119. García-Godoy, F. (1986). Preventive glass-ionomer restorations. *Quintessence Int.* 17:617–19.

120. Mertz-Fairhurst, E. J., Call-Smith, K. M., Shuster, G. S., Williams, G. E., Davis, Q. B., Smith, C. D., Bell, R. A., Sherrer, J. D., Myers, D. R., & Morse, P. K. (1987). Clinical performance of sealed composite restorations placed over caries compared with sealed and unsealed amalgam restorations. *J Am Dent Assoc*, 115:689–94.

121. Ripa, L. W., Leske, G. S., & Forte, F. (1987). The combined use of pit-and-fissure sealants and fluoride mouthrinsing in second and third grade children: Final clinical results after two years. *Pediatr Dent*, 9:118–20.

122. Harris, N. O., Lindo, F., Tossas, A., et al. (1970). The Preventive Dentistry Technician: Concept and Utilization. Monograph, Editorial UPR. University of Puerto Rico, October 1.

123. Leske, G., Cons, N., & Pollard, S. (1977). Cost effectiveness considerations of a pit-and-fissure sealant. *J Dent Res*, 56:B–71, Abstr. 77.

124. Horowitz, H. S. (1980). Pit-and-fissure sealants in private practice and public health programmes: analysis of cost-effectiveness. *International Dental Journal*, 30(2):117–26.
125. Deuben, C. J., Zullos, T. G., & Summer, W. L. (1981). Survey of expanded functions included within dental hygiene curricula. *Educ Direc*, 6:22–29.
126. Access to Care Position Paper, 2001, American Dental Hygienists' Association, available at: http://www.adha.org/profissues/access_to_care.htm. Accessed January 2003.
127. Holst, A., Braun, K., & Sullivan A. (1998). A five-year evaluation of fissure sealants applied by dental assistants. *Swed Dent J*, 22:195–201.
128. American Dental Association. Department of Educational Surveys (1991). Legal Provisions for Delegating Functions to Dental Assistants and Dental Hygienists, 1990. Chicago, April.
129. Leverett, D. H., Handelman, S. L., Brenner, C. M., et al. (1983). Use of sealants in the prevention and early treatment of carious lesions: Cost analysis. *JADA*, 106:39–42.
130. Rock, W. P., & Anderson, R. J. (1982). A review of published fissure sealant trials using multiple regression analysis. *J Dent*, 10:39–43.
131. Pereira, A. C., Verdonschot, E. H., & Huysmans, M. C. (2001). Caries detection methods: can they aid decision making for invasive sealant treatment? *Caries Res*, 35:83–89.
132. Truman, B. I., Gooch, B. F., Sulemana, I., Gift, H. C., Horowitz, A. M., Evans, C. A. Jr., Griffin, S. O., & Carande-Kulis, V. G. (2002). The task force on community preventive services. Reviews of evidence on interventions to prevent dental caries, oral and pharyngeal cancers, and sports-related craniofacial injuries. *American Journal of Preventive Medicine*, 23,1:21–54.
133. Ripa, L. W. (1993). Sealants revisited: An update of the effectiveness of pit-and-fissure sealants. *Caries Res*, 27:77–82.
134. Handelman, S. L. (1991). Therapeutic use of sealants for incipient or early carious lesions in children and young adults. *Proc Finn Dent Soc*, 87:463–75.
135. National Institute of Dental Research. RFP No., NIH-NIDR-5-82, IR. Washington, DC: National Institutes of Health, May 1982.
136. Gerlach, R. W., & Senning, J. H. (1991). Managing sealant utilization among insured populations: Report from Vermont's "Tooth Fairy" program. *ASDC J Dent Child*, 58:46–49.
137. Rozier, R. G., Spratt, C. J., Koch, C. G., & Davies, G. M. (1994). The prevalence of dental sealants in North Carolina schoolchildren. *J Pub Health Dent*, 54:177–83.
138. Gillcrist, J. A., Collier, D. R., & Wade, G. T. (1992). Dental caries and sealant prevalences in schoolchildren in Tennessee. *J Pub Health Dent*, 52:69–74.
139. Selwitz, R. H., Colley, B. J., & Rozier, R. G. (1992). Factors associated with parental acceptance of dental sealants. *J Pub Health Dent*, 52:137–45.
140. Dasanayake, A. P., Li, Y., Philip, S., Kirk, K., Bronstein, J., & Childers, N. K. (2001). Utilization of dental sealants by Alabama Medicaid children barriers in meeting the year 2010 objectives. *Pediatr Dent*, 23:401–6.
141. Chestnutt, I. G., Shafer, F., Jacobson, A. P., & Stephen, K. W. (1994). The prevalence and effectiveness of fissure sealants in Scottish adolescents (Letter). *Br Dent J*, 177:125–29.
142. Hassal, D. C., Mellor, A. C., & Blinkhorn, A. S. (1999). Prevalence and attitudes to fissure sealants in the general dental services in England. *Int J Paediatr Dent*, 9:243–51.
143. *MMWR Morb Mor Rep* 2000; Aug 31; 50:736–8. Impact of integrated school-based dental sealant programs in reducing racial and economic disparities in sealant prevalence among school children.
144. Gonzalez, C. D., Frazier, P. J., & Messer, L. B. (1988). Sealant knowledge and use by pediatric dentists. 1987, Minnesota survey. *J Dent Child*, 55:434–38.
145. Hicks, M. J., Flaitz, C. M., & Call, R. L. (1990). Comparison of pit-and-fissure sealant utilization by pediatric and general dentists in Colorado. *J Pedodont*, 14:97–102.
146. Galarneau, C., & Brodeur, J. M. (1998). Inter-dentist variability in the provision of fissure sealants. *J Can Dent Assoc*, 64:718–25.

147. Silverstone, L. M. (1982). The use of pit-and-fissure sealants in dentistry: Present status and future developments. *Pediatr Dent*, 4:16–21.

148. Lang, W. P., Farghaly, M. M., Woolfolk, M. W., Ziemiecki, T. L., & Faja, B. W. (1991). Educating dentists about fissure sealants: Effects on knowledge, attitudes and use. *J Pub Health Dent*, 51:164–69.

149. Terkla, L. G. (1981). The use of pit-and-fissure sealants in United States dental schools. In Proceedings of the Conference on Pit-and-fissure Sealants: Why Their Limited Usage. Chicago: American Dental Association, 31–36.

150. Frazier, P. L. J. (1983). Public health education and promotion for caries: The role of the dental schools. *J Public Health Dent*, 43:28–42.

151. McLeran, J. H. (1981). Current challenges and response of the College of Dentistry. *Iowa Dent Bull*, 12:21.

152. American Association of Public Health Dentistry. Recommendations for teaching pit-and-fissure sealants. *J Public Health Dent*, 48:112–14.

153. Cohen, L., BaBelle, A., & Romberg, E. (1988). The use of pit-and-fissure sealants in private practice: A national survey. *J Public Health Dent*, 48:26–35.

154. Mertz-Fairhurst, E. J., Curtis, J. W. Jr., Ergle, J. W., Rueggeberg, F. A., & Adair, S. M. (1998). Ultraconservative and cariostatic sealed restorations: Results at year 10. *JADA*, 129:55–66.

# 11

# Oral Biologic Defenses in Tooth Demineralization and Remineralization

*Norman O. Harris*
*John Hicks*

## OBJECTIVES

1. Describe at least five body defense systems that are operational in and-around the oral cavity.
2. List the names of the major salivary glands in rank order of both their daily output of unstimulated (resting) saliva and the amount of stimulated output.
3. List three means of stimulating saliva output and three methods of inhibiting saliva output.
4. Define and compare the terms sialorrhea, xerostomia, and ptyalism.
5. Describe the appearance and the implications of the contour of the Stephan Curve.
6. Describe how the fluid viscosity of the plaque affects diffusion within the plaque.
7. Describe the ultramicroscopic morphology of enamel rods, enamel crystals and the unit cell of hydroxyapatite (HAP).
8. Explain why an extracted tooth immersed in a liquid acid solution (*in vitro*) will not yield an incipient lesion, whereas, if it is immersed in a buffered gel of similar pH, the incipient lesion develops.
9. Explain why a newly erupted tooth is at high risk to develop a carious lesion.
10. Recount the key events that cause and occur in demineralization, and how the reverse events of remineralization can often repair the damage.

*[Chapter 11 is a continuation of Chapter 3. Whereas Chapter 3 emphasized the basics of the caries process, chapter 11 concentrates on the saliva and the ultramicroscopic structure of the tooth, as they affect de- and remineralization.]*

The mouth is the gateway for food and drink destined for the gastrointestinal (GI) tract. To ensure the safety of the body from the oft-unknown quality of foods being brought into the mouth, two powerful evolutionary monitoring sensory systems exist to help determine safety and quality *before* ingesting the gustatory fare—*vision and smell*. Both of these senses allow the host to reject food deemed to be undesirable. Once within the oral cavity, there is the protective umbrella of the body's immune system—*the cellular and the secretory immune systems*. The former is cell-mediated and consists of the phagocytic and lymphoid elements involved in preventing infection. The secretory system mainly protects mucous membranes with secretions of antibodies, such as sIgA (secretory immunoglobulin A).[1] Two other defense mechanisms are *taste*[2] and *tactile sense*. As an example, tactile sense allows for proprioception[a] via nerves in the oral tissues to evaluate morsel size, texture and shape of the entering food; to segregate foods that need to be chewed from food that needs to be incised; and to determine when a bolus of food is of the correct size and consistency from chewing to be safely swallowed.[3]

The defense functions of the *saliva* are part of the total body's ability to maintain *homeostasis,* i.e., the ability to resist routine daily challenges by chemical and bacterial agents, and to repair limited amounts of tissue damage typical of the wear and tear of daily life.[4] It is only when the bacterial challenge exceeds the body's defense capabilities and/or there is a lack of a person's commitment to self-care, that dental caries ensues.

The *saliva* helps modulate and augment the previously described major body defense systems in protecting oral tissues. However, in the demineraliztion and remineraliztion process of tooth structure (caries and repair), the saliva cannot be isolated from an interrelated three compartment model consisting of *saliva, plaque and teeth.*[5]

## The Saliva Compartment

The saliva is derived mainly from the major salivary glands—the parotid, submandibular, and sublingual glands. Of these, the parotid elaborates a serous (watery, mucous-poor) fluid containing eletrolytes, but is relatively low in organic substances. The parotid gland secretes the majority of the *sodium bicarbonate* that is essential in neutralizing acids produced by cariogenic bacteria in the dental plaque,[6,7] and the majority of the enzyme *amylase* that initiates intraoral digestion of carbohydrates. The submandibular gland secretes a mixed serous and mucuos fluid, while the sublingual gland has a greater proportion of mucous output than the other major glands. The minor glands—palatal, lingual, buccal, and labial salivary glands empty onto the mucus membrane in many locations—

---

[a]Proprioception = The reception of sensory nerve stimuli that locate the location of position of parts of the body. Example: While eating, a diner with every bite, provides the brain with information as to where the opposing teeth are in time to prevent a traumatic occlusion.

on the palate, under the tongue, and on the inner side of the cheeks and lips. These minor glands are mainly mucous secreting glands that lubricate these surfaces and allows for improved mastication and passage of food substance into the esophagus.[3] The minor salivary glands also contribute fluoride that bathes the teeth and enhances caries resistance.[8,9,10]

Pure saliva produced by the oral glands is sterile, until it is discharged into the mouth. When the fluids from all major and minor glands mix with each other, this secretion becomes known as *whole saliva*. Whole saliva is further altered by the presence of particles of food, tissue fluid, lysed bacteria, and sloughed epithelial cells. It becomes even more complex with the inclusions of *living cells and their metabolic products*, for example, bacteria and leucocytes, the latter derived from the gingival crevices and tonsils.

### Functions of saliva

The physical and chemical protective functions of saliva can be divided into five convenient categories—(1) lubrication, (1) flushing/rinsing, (2) chemical, (3) antimicrobial (includes antibacterial, antifungal and antiviral), and (4) maintenance of supersaturation of calcium and phosphate level batheing the enamel, helping to stymie demineralization and/or to aid remineralization of tooth structure.[11,12] To reinforce the concept expressed in (4), Peretz aptly opined that saliva can be considered similar to enamel but in a liquid phase.[13]

The salivary defensive system functions continuously, but its secretion becomes greatest and most active during foodstuff ingestion. It has the lowest flow rate during the sleep period of the daily 24-hour cycle.

### Lubrication and Flushing

A very thin microscopic layer of mucus protects the oral hard and soft tissues from the often harsh and abrasive foods, as they are being chewed and swallowed. It also protects the soft tissues from dessication and the teeth from abrasion. The moistening of food by saliva *facilitates chewing and swallowing*. Speech is enhanced by the reduced friction between the dry tongue and soft tissues. Coversely, a lack of saliva (*xerostomia*) results in a greatly increased risk of caries with its accompaniment of an extremely *annoying dry-mouth sensation*. Chewing, swallowing and speaking can all be difficult and uncomfortable with *dry-mouth syndrome* and often requires frequent ameliorating sips of water.

### Flow Rate

Providing a constant fluid flow is probably the most important defense function of the salivary glands, because it is the fluid that transports the buffering agents, the antimicrobials, and the mineral content of saliva to help control the equilibrium between the demineralization and remineralization of tooth structure. Also, the fluid output of the glands is essential for *diluting* acids, *flushing* food particles embedded around the teeth, *clearing* refined carbohydrates (acid-producing sugar substrates) and physically *removing any displaced* bacteria[12] Oral fluids in contact with food particles results in solubilizing food substances that interact with the taste buds to provide an accurate assessment of taste.[2]

The composition of saliva varies, depending on whether it is *stimulated* or *unstimulated (resting)*. During the day, submandibular glands secrete the greatest proportion of the unstimulated saliva, although the flow rate of resting saliva for *all* three glands is very low, being about one tenth that during stimulated flow. Approximately 2/3 of the *resting* saliva is derived from the submandibular glands, one-quarter is from the parotids, and about 1/20 is from the sublingual glands. The minor salivary glands secrete almost 1/10 of the total amount of saliva. The unstimulated flow rate of the salivary glands is subject to a circadian rhythm, with the highest flow in mid-afternoon and the lowest around 4:00 A.M.

Upon *moderate stimulation*, the submandibular and parotid glands secrete approximately equal amounts of saliva, whereas at full stimulation the parotid has the greatest output. When salivary flow is stimulated by chewing gum or paraffin, 1 to 2 mL of whole saliva per minute can be expected. The minimum level of stimulated salivary flow necessary to maintain hard- and soft-tissue health is unknown, but when it is *below 1 mL/minute*, there is cause for concern regarding a possible dry mouth and caries formation. Once the flow rate is below *0.7 mL/minute*, a diagnosis of xerostomia may be rendered. In the course of a single day, up to 1 liter (1 quart) of saliva is secreted into the oral cavity.

The total amount of saliva secreted varies considerably between and within individuals, depending on the environmental factors. Seasonal variations occur, with flow being lower in warm weather and higher in cold. The act of smoking increases flow rates. Flow is greater while standing than when sitting and greater when recumbent, with these postural changes paralleling changes in systemic blood pressure.

Saliva flow may be *stimulated* (1) physiologically, (2) pharmacologically (over the counter drugs, herbals and prescription medications) and by (3) many different disease states[14,15] Examples of physiologic stimulation are the simple acts of *chewing* food and gum, *gustatory stimuli* caused by *tasting* an enjoyable food, while *psychologic* stimulation for food can be evoked by anticipating the first bite of a delicious food via the sense of sight and/or smell. Saliva can also be stimulated by the use of *drugs*, such as pilocarpine. Under certain conditions, saliva flow can be abnormally high—a condition termed *sialorrhea*,(or *ptyalism*) which is often manifested by drooling. Under some conditions drug therapy can be used,[16, 10] but *sialorrhea* or *ptyalism* may be so severe as to require surgical removal (excision)of the responsible gland or *ligation* of the gland duct.[17]

Saliva flow can also be *suppressed* physiologically, pharmacologically[16] and/or by disease.

The dry mouth sensation (xerostomia) that accompanies *fear* is an example of a physiological response; pharmacologically it may follow the intake, among others, of antidepressant and antihypertensive drugs;[18,19] it occurs when there are *sialoliths* (stones) within the gland ducts resulting in obstruction of saliva flow,[19,20] or following radiation exposure of the glands during cancer therapy.

The concentration of the various saliva components secreted by the glands is closely related to the flow rate. Stimulation of the rate of flow by stimulation increases the concentration of *some* constituents and decreases it for others. Stimulation of the parotid glands causes an increase in calcium, sodium, chloride, bicarbonate and pH. The same saliva demonstrates a concomitant decrease in phosphate and potassium.

In addition to the secretion of different proportions of electrolytes, *organic* molecules are secreted that can be categorized into five major groups: amylase, mucins, phosphoproteins, glycoproteins, and immunoglobulins. Two of the families of small salivary proteins—histadine and statherin—deserve specific mention because they help control the status of calcium and phosphate in the saliva. These proteins prevent fall-out of the calcium and phosphate that maintain supersaturation in relation to HAP. They prevent a rapid drop in saliva pH and aid in its quicker recovery. In addition, they both are antifungal and help prevent mucosal infections.

---

### Question 1

Which of the following statements, if any, is correct?

A. sIgA (secretory immunoglobulin A) is a guardian of moist epithelial surfaces (mucous membranes).

B. The major salivary glands are the parotid, palatal, and the submandibular.

C. The saliva output of the major salivary glands increases in defense effectiveness at the time of chewing.

D. In the order of maximum flow rate, the parotid is first, the sublingual second, and the minor salivary glands third.

E. All the major salivary glands can be both stimulated or retarded in flow rate by physiological stimulus, drugs, or disease.

## Protective Functions of Saliva

The protective functions of saliva are from its *physical*, *chemical*, and *antimicrobial* properties.[10] Saliva is not equally distributed around the oral cavity because of differences in anatomical and orthodontic features. It also has a tendency to stay on the side it was secreted.[21] These differences mean there is an increased risk for caries formation owing to retention of refined carbohydrates at difficult-to-reach sites in the mouth.[22] Of parallel importance, a viscid saliva is not as effective in clearing food particles and snacks, as is normal saliva.

## Antibacterial Functions

The most easily understood major antibacterial function is performed by one of the glycoproteins—the mucins—that trap or *aggregate* bacteria that are eventually swallowed. The same mucins provide a thin film over the mucous membrane and teeth to serve as lubricants.

Four important antimicrobial proteins found in saliva are: lysozyme, lactoferrin, salivary peroxidase and secretory immunoblobulin A (sIgA). *In vitro*, lactoferrin strongly inhibited adherence of mutans streptococci to saliva coated hydroxyapatite (HAP) blocks.[23] Lactoferrin combines with iron and copper to *deprive* bacteria of these essential nutrients. Salivary peroxidase reacts with saliva to form the antimicrobial compound *hypothiocyanate*, which in turn inhibits the capability of the bacteria to *fully use glucose*. Lactoperoxidase strongly ad-

sorbs to hydroxyapatite as a component of the acquired pellicle, and can *influence* the qualitative and quantitative characteristics of the microbial population of dental plaque. The role of the body's cellular and immunologic defense systems in moderating the course of the plaque-induced disease needs clarification. The main access that phagocytic cells and their antibacterial products, have to the oral cavity is through the gingival crevice and the tonsils. It is difficult to conceive of the cellular immune system operating in the bacterial plaque, yet about 500 leukocytes per second are estimated as emigrating from the tissues through the gingival crevice into the oral cavity. The majority of these soon disintegrate in the saliva, a phenomenon that may be related to the fact that more intact polymorphonuclear leukocytes occur in caries-free than in caries-susceptible individuals. On a research basis, there is reason to believe that a linkage exists between normal humoral and cellular defenses, and both caries and periodontal disease. How the cells and immunoglobulins exercise this potential is unclear. The development of a successful vaccine against caries and possibly, against periodontal disease will ultimately depend on such a clarification.

## The Plaque Compartment

The plaque compartment begins with the acquired (salivary) pellicle, which is an acellular protein layer of saliva components that is adsorbed onto the surface of the enamel (Chapter 2). Upon this pellicle, the bacteria colonize. The pellicle plus the bacteria and the gel they create, constitutes a *biofilm* (dental placque). For several hours after a prophylaxis (that removes biofilm) there is a steady change in the quantity and composition of the pellicle as new proteins are added from the saliva. Glycoproteins appear to mediate the attachment sites of the subsequent colonizing plaque bacteria. Even though mucins are a minor component of the pellicle, they can be very protective *against acid diffusion*.

To understand the effect that plaque has on teeth, it is neccesary to focus on the action of acid in demineralizing teeth. To reduce the potential of demineralization, it is necessary to (1) reduce the *number* of bacteria producing the acid, (2) reduce the *amount of acid* produced by the existing bacteria, and/or (3) negate the effects of the acid produced by plaque.

## Physical Character of Plaque

A major consideration in the defense of the tooth is the physical character of plaque itself. In order for the fluid and chemical components of saliva and plaque to function, they must be able to diffuse freely (intermix) with the constituents of the plaque. This diffusion requires time, which is contingent on two important factors. (1) If the fluid content in the plaque is relatively high, incoming and exiting ions diffuse rapidly. (2) If the colloid and glucan content of the plaque is high, the diffusion is slow, thus *retaining any acid against the tooth surface longer*.

Probably the most unpredictable factor relating to the plaque diffusion is the character of the microbial population. Variations in bacterial species from one plaque to another or in different parts of the same plaque result in different diffusion patterns. In other words the bacteria and their metabolites can act as either a *barrier*, or as a *gateway* to the passage of selected anions, cations and proteins. For example, bacteria use phosphate in their metabolism—a metabolic need that is *accentuated* during periods of acidogenesis. *Thus, the bacterial need for phosphate from the plaque metabolic pool occurs at the same time that the same phosphate is required to maintain supersaturation at the plaque tooth interface.*

Not all bacteria are bad. Veillonella, when present, metabolizes lactic acid generated by mutans streptococci, lactobacilli, actinomycetes, and other acidogenic organism. Presumably this action *decreases* the amount of acid available to demineralize tooth structure.

Several studies indicate that the presence of Veillonella, indeed, decreases caries risk. Thus the varieties, metabolic characteristics and interrelationships of the plaque bacteria at any one time, are important in determining whether caries will occur.

---

### Question 2

Which of the following statements, if any, are correct?

A. All parts of the mouth are equally assessable to the flushing effect of saliva.

B. The following are anti-microbial agents found in saliva: lysozme, lactoferrin, and salivary peroxidase.

C. If a cross section of a plaque coated crown of a tooth is studied, the following structures would be seen starting with the tooth surface: the enamel surface, acquired (salivary pellicle), bacterial plaque, and finally, saliva.

D. The bacteria of the plaque cannot use the phosphate diffusing out of the pores for their own metbolism.

E. Plaque acidogenesis could probably be reduced to inoculous levels by a major commitment to sugar discipline as a part of self-care.

---

## Reducing Acid Production

Toothbrushing, flossing and irrigation ("brush, floss and flush") are ideal for personal self-care. However, there are *natural* oral defense mechanisms that exist in the body that are *not dependent on the frailities of human motivation, memories or techniques.*

1. Great numbers of bacteria in the saliva are eliminated by *flushing*, aggregation and *swallowing*.

2. The bacterial populations in the saliva and plaque are continually exposed to the *antimicrobial elements of saliva*.

Reducing the amount of acid produced by the bacteria is mainly a function of limiting the intake of refined carbohydrates (i.e., *sugar discipline*). This subject is discussed in detail in later chapters dealing with sugars, nutrition and clinical preventive dentistry. *The ingestion of refined sugars makes dental caries a self-inflicted disease.*

### Reducing the Acid Damage

The plaque pH can drop to as low as 4.0 on the Stephan Curve after a glucose mouth rinse. Damage control from acid in the plaque, is achieved by dilution, chemical buffering, and by increasing the protective ions (mainly, calcium, phosphate and fluoride) in the environs of the teeth.[24,10] The water content of the saliva and plaque aid greatly in diluting the acid and in transporting acid into the main flow of saliva where it is further diluted and swallowed. This dilutional effect is supplemented by the buffering capacity of the plaque which can be 10 times higher than for the fluoride in the saliva. This higher adsorption capacity for fluoride in the plaque also occurs to differing extents in increasing bicarbonates, phosphates and ammonia concentrations derived from the saliva. These neutralizing actions serve as a brake in the rapidity and extent to which the pH can drop during periods of acidogenesis.

Each individul has a different potential for modifying the drop and recovery of the pH represented by his/her individual Stephan Curve. As an example, if a group of individuals is given a glucose mouth rinse, each person demonstrates a different, but reproducible pH pattern. Once the pH has started to fall, the availability of statherin and other salivary buffers help to shorten the time that the pH is at its lowest and most damaging level.

### The Tooth Compartment

Coronal caries involves the enamel cap[b] and the underlying dentin. Enamel is more mineralized than bone or dentin. It is estimated that enamel is composed of approximately 96% mineral by weight with an average volume of 87%. The enamel contains millions of enamel rods that run from the dentinoenamel junction (DEJ) to the tooth surface. The rods are approximately 4 to 7 micrometers, and by 6 to 8 micrometers in cross section for primary and permanent teeth, respectively. In cross sections they resemble keyholes, more than rods. Around each rod there is an enveloping protein matrix. During formation of the crown, this organic matrix forms the template that is involved in determining crystal and rod size and orientation (Chapter 3).

The inorganic phase of enamel is based on the mineral, hydroxyapatite (HAP), made up mainly of calcium (Ca), phosphate ($PO_4$) and hydroxyl (OH) ions. It also contains trace amounts of other elements that happen to be in the bloodstream during enamel formation, in fact more than 40 elements have been identified in analysis of enamel. Each rod is made up of millions of *crystals* each which are shaped much like a carpenters hexagonal lead pencil—one that is slightly flattened on two opposite sides between the submicroscopic *crystals* there are also *submicroscopic amounts of matrix.* These enveloping protein wraps of both the enamel rods and crystals are the main channels for diffusion for demineralizing acids and remineralizing electrolytes as explained in Chapter 3.

[In order to better understand the tooth histology at increasing magnifications, this is to invite you to join the following art and photographic tour featuring the "Anatomy of a Tooth." The starting point is Figure 11–1. You will need this information throughout your career.

Illustration 11–1a is a cross section of enamel, showing how each of the tails are cradled between the heads of the adjoining rods. The drawing 11–1b provides a concept of a sin-

---

[b]If an intact tooth is stripped of all dentin and cementum, the remaining portion of the tooth is the "enamel cap".

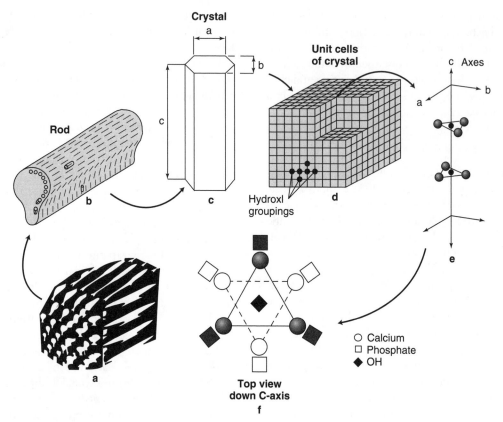

FIGURE 11-1    Enamel: From the electron microscope to the molecule. **a.** An electron microscope model of the keyhole morphology of enamel. Note that the crystals (dotted lines) within any single prism are coaxial with the prism in the head region. From Meckel, A. H., Griebstein, W. J. and Neal. R. J. *International Symposium on the Composition, Properties and Fundamental Structure of Tooth Enamel.* April 1964. Courtesy: Ed. Stack, M. V., and Fearnhead, R. W., Bristol, England: John Write and Sons, Ltd, 1965. **b.** Individual enamel rod, showing different crystal orientations in head and tail. **c.** Illustration of a crystal with labels a, b, and c axes. **d.** Theoretic presentation of unit cells that make up the crystallites. **e.** Vertical arrangement of hydroxyapatite along C axis of the unit cell. **f.** Showing how every other molecular configuration is rotated 180° as illustrated by the solid and then the dotted lines. (Courtesy of N. O. Harris, University of Texas Dental School, San Antonio.)

gle enamel rod.[c] With these two background schematics, the head and tail positioning becomes even more understandable when viewed on an electron micrograph, (Figure 11–2) that shows the rod as a crude keyhole structure.

[c]Enamel rods can be correctly called enamel prisms.

Figure 11-1c is of a single crystal portrayed as a carpenter-shaped pencil configuration. Each crystal is composed of Ca, $PO_4$ and (OH) (and other extraneous contaminants) . Each of the crystals making up the enamel rod is considered as a unit cell.(11–1d) A unit cell is the smallest subdivision of a crystalline substance that is en-

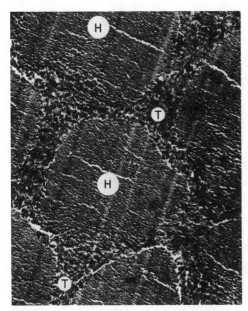

FIGURE 11-2    Same electron micrograph as 3–2a. Same caption. (A repeat) Electron micrograph of rod cut perpendicular to long axis, showing head (H) and tail (T) relationship.

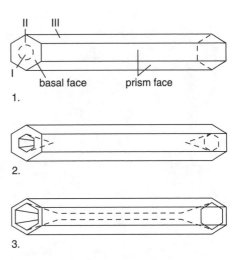

FIGURE 11-3    Dissolution of the crystal schematic: Each enamel prism is made up of parallel crystals of hydroxyapatite that have a slightly flattened hexagonal appearance. **1.** The initial etching of the crystal begins at the ends with, **2.** the formation of etchpits. **3.** These etchpits deepen along the c-axis to eventually produce a hollow core. (From Arends J. Jangerbloed WL. Ultrastructure studies of synthetic apatite crystals. *J Dent Res*, 1979 [Special Issue B]; 58:837–843.)

tirely representative of the structure of the crystal. This means that all rods of any dimensions can be constructed (or remineralized) by adding additional unit cells , much as a building can be increased in size by adding additional bricks. It is important to recognize that unit cells, unlike the bricks, have no physical meaning as such; they are just a convenient means of conceptualizing the atomic structure and relationship of crystals at the simplest level.

If one unit cell could be detached along the c-axis, it would resemble a windchimes on a string, with each successive triangular grouping being comprised of calcium, phosphate and hydroxl ions equidistant from adjacent groupings (Figure 11-1e) When looking at the arrangement from the top of the column, the center position is occupied by hydroxyl ions, surrounded by a trianglular configuration with a calcium ion at each point of the triangle. Immediately peripheral to each calcium ion is a phosphate

grouping (11–1f). Each successive triangular grouping grouping along the c-axis is rotated 180-degrees from the ones above and below, as illustrated by the solid and dotted lines in Figure 11–1f). Each of the atoms can be replaced by other atoms. For instance, a hydroxyl group can be substituted by fluoride; a calcium ion by strontium, and a phosphate by a carbonate.

Next, let us take a more detailed look at how a *crystal* dissolves starting with Figures 11–1c, and then illustrations 11–3 parts 1, 2, and 3 that show the sequence of dissolution of a crystal, which starts with a central *etch pit*. The etch pits on the basal faces are beautifully illustrated at electron microscope level, as are the images of hallowed out crystals shown in Figure 11–4, parts 1 and 4, respectively.

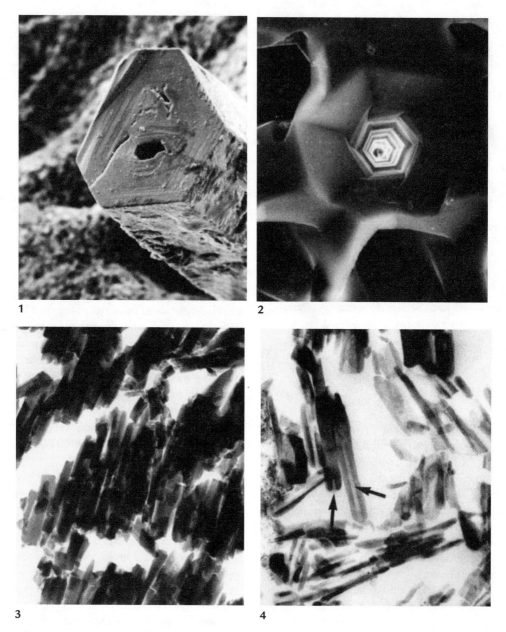

FIGURE 11-4   Dissolution of the crystal, photographic. **1.** Artificially grown apatite crystal with etchpit on basal face, original magnifiction × 500. **2.** A hexagonal etchpit in fluorapatite, original magnifiction × 2500. **3.** TEM picture of sound enamel crystallites, original magnification × 100,000; and **4.** TEM picture of etched enamel crystallites that are partially hollowed out, original magnification × 100,000. (Courtesy of Dr. W.L. Jongebloed, I. Molenaar and L. Arends. University of Groningen, *The Netherlands and Joel News,* Japan. 1976; 13e(2):14.)

## Demineralization

There were a few early interesting experiments by Silverstone who first focused worldwide attention to the overall subject of de- and remineralization. Several decades ago, researchers could not understand the reason why a typical cavity did not form when a tooth was directly placed in acid Instead the outer layers of the tooth would continue to dissolve, but there were no white spots. There were no incipient (subsurface) lesions. However, when Silverstone used an acidified pH *gel* (instead of an acid solution) in which to immerse the tooth, an incipient lesion *did* form with the expected four zones of enamel caries.[25-27] The surface zone had sufficient calcium and phosphate exiting from the body of the lesion to the surface zone to create a supersaturation of calcium and phosphate ions to cause a HAP precipitation *between the gel and the tooth surface*. The next study by Silverstone was to grind off the entire mature surface of the crown and again immerse the tooth in the buffered gel. The entire surface area of the tooth was recreated, showing that the outward diffusing minerals had attained sufficient saturation to precipitate and form the exterior of the enamel. This was interesting, but he carried the study one or two steps further towards practical application.

When a tooth with a carefully *preserved pellicle* was subjected to the same gel immersion treatment, there was the same build-up of mature enamel and closing of the *pores between the tooth surface and the pellicle*. He reasoned that the pellicle acted as a template to maintain the contour of the remineralized area. This demonstrated for the first time that *the pellicle served as a protective layer*.

When using saliva as the remineralization solution, the ability to remineralize tooth sections in vitro varies with the saliva from *different individuals*, but occurs consistently with the saliva of each individual, indictating that some people have a greater capacity for remineralization (*host resistance*) than others.

Fluoride has a major influence on both demineralization and remineralization.[28] Fortunately,

only small concentrations of fluoride are needed to inhibit demineralization or to enhance remineralization. As little as 0.1 ppm fluoride can reduce the amount of enamel dissolution *in vitro*. The presence of fluoride at the remineralizing site can accelerate rehardening by a factor of up to fivefold. In the mouth, the fluoride can come from four sources (1) transitory contact with fluoridated drinking water; (2) the continual low fluoride ouput of the salivary glands; (3) the bound fluoride occurring in the plaque which is released when the pH drops to around 5.5; or, (4) from the fluoride contained in the mature enamel layer following demineralization.

### Question 3

Which of the following statements, if any, is correct?

A. The enamel is a solid piece of hydroxyapatite.

B. The crystal of a rod is the first component of the enamel cap to dissolve; it is also the first to be reconstituted in remineralization..

C. A protein matrix envelops each crystal as well as each rod.

D. The central configuration of the unit cell is made up of calcium and phosphate, the OH is at the corners of the triangle.

E. It requires more acid of the same pH to dissolve a crystal than to dissolve the rod.

## Remineralization

Remineralization is the *repair* of enamel rod structure following acidogenic episodes. When teeth erupt, they are anatomically complete, but crystallographically incomplete and immature. Following eruption, the missing ions are supplied from the saliva, a process termed *post-eruptive maturation*, Throughout life, minerals from the saliva are used to repair acid-damaged tooth structure. This repair process can range from an almost immediate replacement of daily ion losses from the enamel surface, to a slow repair (under proper conditions) of more extensive

subsurface (white spot) lesions. Without specific knowledge of the caries process, a lay person is likely to envision the development of a caries lesion as a continuous process, accompanied by an ever-increasing loss of tooth mineral until the stage is reached when a clinically discernible cavity is present. Fortunately, this conception is incorrect. The process of demineralization is *not irreversible or inevitably progressive*. If damage has not progressed beyond a still yet to be defined point, lost mineral *can be replaced*.

Considerable clinical evidence exists for remineralization. Head, a physician and a dentist, pointed out in 1912 that teeth underwent cycles of softening and hardening.[29] By 1933, Boedecker[30] advocated the use of Andreasen's method of remineralizing "soft" teeth and "white spots." Andreasen's remineralizing powder consisted of tartaric acid, gelatin, calcium phosphate, calcium carbonate, magnesium carbonate, sodium bicarbonate and sodium chloride. Boedecker commented as follows: "The purpose that this powder is to fulfill, is to go into solution in the saliva and in this state, permeate and recalcify the porous area in the enamel . . . and after the remineralizing powder has been used for 6 weeks, decay around fillings will come to a standstill."

Muhler, in several clinical studies of the anticaries effectiveness of stannous fluoride, often found that the experimental subjects had more sound teeth later in the study than at the initial examination.[31] Invariably, the number of these reversals was greater in the stannous fluoride treatment groups than in the controls. Von der Fehr and colleagues were able to induce white spots with sucrose mouth rinses and reversed the process with fluoride rinses.[32] Backer-Dirks,[33] in a long-term study, noted that over 50 percent of the interproximal lesions seen at the initial examination did not progress, indicating an arrestment phenomenon due to remineralization. Additional support for remineralization is derived from the frequent observations of teeth that are acid-etched prior to placement of pit-and-fissure sealants. For those etched areas not covered with the resin, the chalky white appearance disap-

pears over a period of a few days and the enamel regains its initial translucent, glossy appearance.

Except under unusual circumstances, such as occur following the destruction of the salivary glands during cancer radiotherapy or diseases of the glands, deviations from remineralizing conditions in the mouth are transient. For example, the local pH may be lowered to where enamel demineralization occurs during the ingestion of acid foods or from the production of acid by the plaque bacteria following the ingestion of refined carbohydrates. If the insults are *brief* and *widely* separated in time, remineralizing conditions can be restored in the intervening periods and the slight damage repaired. On the other hand, frequent or protracted periods of acidogenesis, with insufficient time intervals for remineralization, ultimately lead to the development of overt caries.

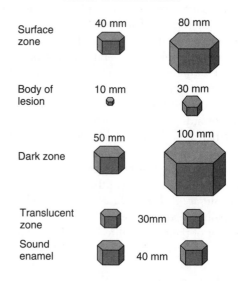

FIGURE 11-5    Illustration of the relative crystal diameters in sound enamel (bottom) and in the four histological zones of the enamel lesions (right). (Courtesy of Silverstone LM. The significance of remineraliztion in caries prevention. *J Can Dent Assn.* 1984; 50: 157–184.)

Crystal Size in Demineralization and Remineralization

Siverstone, when he published the article, "The significance of remineralization in caries prevention." opened up a new area of conservative dentistry—an era that ten Cate calls "noninvasive restorative care." In his review of remineralization. Silverstone pointed out that crystal sizes differ predictably in each of the zones of the incipient lesion and in remineralized caries areas.[34] In the incipient carious lesions, the crystals in the two zones of demineralization—the body of the lesion and the *translucent zone*—were smaller than in sound enamel. (Figure 11–5). The crystals in the two zones of *remineralization*—the dark and the surface zones—were equal to, or greater in size than those found in normal enamel. Predictably, when a remineralizing solution with fluoride is used to remineralize the subsurface lesion, the crystal sizes are greater than for normal sound enamel.

## Question 4

Which of the following statements, if any, are correct?

A. The concept of remineralization dates from the last quarter of the 20th century.

B. The crystals of the body of the lesion are larger than those of the dark zone.

C. An incipient lesion with a low pH and a low saliva calcium and phophate concentration is more likely to remineralize than one with a high saliva pH and is supersaturated with calcium and phosphate.

D. The anti-caries benefits of saliva during the Stephan Curve both slows demineralization and accelerates remineralization.

E. A remineralized rod in the presence of fluoride is a more acid resistant rod than one originally made up of hydroxyapatite.

# SUMMARY

It has been emphasized that oral disease, in fact, all disease occurs when the challenge posed by pathogens exceed the body's capability for defense and repair. In the case of dental caries, the defense and self-repair mechanisms of the body operate continuously in the saliva, in the plaque, and in the enamel cap. Aside from the host's usual humoral and cellular defense functions to destroy pathogens, the oral cavity is protected by the senses of smell and vision, taste and tactile sensation, the body's immunological defenses, and the saliva. Demineralization is dependent on two major factors—pH of the plaque, and saturation of the tooth minerals. If the saturation is high and the pH high, demineralization will not occur. If both the pH and the saturation are low, the risk of caries is high. The output of resting saliva is moderate to low throughout the day; it is only through the period of the Stephan Curve that the maximum stimulated saliva protection occurs.

Bacterial acidogenesis in the dental plaque causes the plaque pH to fall and recover is a manner predicted by the Stephan Curve. If the maximum drop in pH is below the 5.5 to 5.0 range, demineralization occurs with the extent dependent on calcium and phosphate saturation level as well as the *duration* and *frequency* of the acid attacks. The increased secretions of haptins and statherin slow the drop in pH. An increased

amount of salivary buffering minimizes the affect of the acidogenic end-products of the plaque bacteria. The increased flow of saliva, with its high fluid content, enhances the removal of cariogenic residues. As the pH drops, supersaturation of calcium and phosphate ions decline along the plaque-tooth interface. Ions, such as magnesium and carbonate that are adsorbed onto the tooth, dissolve preferentially and add to the buffering capacity of the local environment. When undersaturation occurs, somewhere between pH 5.5 and 5.0, calcium fluoride, HAP and FHA begin to dissolve in successive order. These dissolving crystals add to the saturation along the dissolving plaque-tooth interface, thus slowing and eventually arresting tooth demineralization. At that time, remineralization takes over. Ions necessary for mineral repair are again available from the inorganic components of the plaque that participate in the remineralization process and are ready for combating the next acidogenic cycle.

## ANSWERS AND EXPLANATIONS

1. A, C, and E—correct.

   B—incorrect. The *palatal* glands are minor salivary glands. The correct answer should have included the submandibular gland, not the palatal gland.

   D—incorrect. The order should be: parotid, submaxillary, and sublingual glands.

2. B, C, and E—correct.

   A—incorrect. There can be teeth that overlap, the palate can be malformed and/or an abnormally large tongue can block saliva flow to some parts of the oral cavity. This problem of difficult-to-reach areas is best solved by a counseling session with a dental hygienist.

   D—Bacteria need phosphate for energy; there is no way to tell the $PO_4$ from one source compared to another.

3. B and C—correct.

   A—incorrect. The enamel cap is porous with over 10% of the spacing being between the rods and crystals—also in areas such as the hypomineralization of the DEJ, stria of Retzius, spindles and tufts.

   D—incorrect. The central core of the HAP crystal is made up of mainly hydroxyl ions, but can include exchanged elements.

   E—It requires much less acid to dissolve an individual crystal than a rod. (Just remember the rod is made up of crystals, not vice versa.)

4. D and E—correct.

   A—incorrect. Remineralization is mentioned in *Dental Cosmos* (an early dental journal) prior to the turn of the 20th Century and became of interest to researchers in the mid 20th century. If is rarely used in private or public health practice in the United States. (Now routinely used in New Zealand and Scandinavia public health school programs).

B—incorrect. The crystals in the two zones of recrystalization—the surface and the dark zones are the larger.

C—incorrect. The higher the pH and saturation of the saliva the greater the chance for remineralization.

## Self-evaluation Questions

1. The ability of the brain to continually monitor the location and action of a body part is known as _____.

2. The parotid gland produces the most amylase (enzyme to break down carbohydrates) and _____. (neutralizing agent).

3. The ability of the body to balance the factors causing disease, and the events promoting body health is known as maintaining _____.

4. The quantity and quality associated with Stephan's Curve in (resting)(stimulated) saliva is usually seen at the time of (eating)(fasting between meals). Circle correct responses.

5. Sialorrhea is best treated with (a saliva stimulant) (an antisialogogue).[d] Circle correct response.

6. A desalivated animal (glands removed) or a person with excised glands would have a problem with _____.

7. A pellicle acts to slow the transit of acid from the plaque to the subsurface _____.

8. The glycoprotein of the saliva that serves to lubricate the oral tissues (to reduce friction and abrasion) and to aggregate bacteria for swallowing is _____.

9. It was _____ (name of individual) who gave the major impetus to the modern basic concepts of de- and remineralization.

## REFERENCES

1. Proctor, G. B., & Carpenter, G. H. (2001). Chewing stimulates secretion of human salivary secretory immunoglobulin A. *J Dent Res*, 80:909–13.
2. Matsuo, R. (2000). Role of saliva in the maintenance of taste sensitivity. *Rev Oral Biol Med*, 11:216–29.
3. Pedersen, A. M., Bardow, A., Jensen, S. B., & Nauntofte, B. (2002). Saliva and gastrointestinal functions of taste, mastication, swallowing and digestion. *Oral Dis.*, 8:117–29.

[d] Antisialogogue = an antidote to sialorrhea.

4. Tandler, B., Gresick, E. W., Nagoto, T., & Philliss, C. J. (2001). Secretion by striated ducts of mammalian major glands: a review of ultrastructural, functional and evolutionary pespective. *Anat. Rec*, 264:125–45.

5. Tanaka, M., Matsunaga, K., & Kadoma, Y. (2000). Correlation in inorganic content between saliva and plaque fluid. *J Med Dent Sci*, 47:55–9.

6. Park, K., Hurley, P. T., Roussa, E., et al. (2002). Expansion of sodium bicarbonate cotransporter in human parotid glands. *Arch Oral Biol*, 47:1–9.

7. Bardow, A., Madson, J., & Nautofte, B. (2000). The bicarbonate concentration in human saliva does not exceed the plasma level under normal physiological conditions. *Clin Investig*, 42:45–53.

8. Feruson, D. B. (1999). The flow rate and composition of human labial gland saliva. *Arch Oral Biol*, 44 Suppl 1511–4.

9. Boros, I., Kesler, P., & Zelles, T. (1999). Study of saliva secretion and the salivary fluoride concentration of the human minor labial glands by a new method. *Arch Oral Biol*, 44: Suppl 1:511–14.

10. Lagerof, F., & Oliveby A. (1994). Caries-protective factors in saliva. *Adv Dent Res*, 8:229–38.

11. Dowd, F. J. (1995). Saliva and dental caries. *Dent Clin North America*, 43:579–6.

12. Lageroff, F. (1998). Saliva: natural protection against caries. *Rev Belge Med Dent*, 337–481.

13. Peretz, B., Sarnat, H., & Moss, S. J. (1990). Caries protective aspects of saliva and enamel. *NY State Dental J*, 56:257.

14. Sreebny, L. M. (2000). Saliva in health and disease: an appraisal and update. *Int Dent J*, 14:48–56.

15. Chausau, S., Becker, A., Chausau, G., & Sharpiro, J. (2002). Stimulated parotid saliva flow rates in patients with Down syndrome. *Spec Care Dentist*, 103:378–83.

16. Bothwell, J., Clarke, K., Dooley, J., Gordon, K. E., Anderson, A., Wood, E. P., Camfield, C. S., & Camfield, P. R. (2002). Botulinum toxin as a treatment for excessive drooling in children. 27:18.

17. Bardow, A., Myvad, B., & Nontofte, B. (2001). Relation between medication intake to dry mouth, salivary flow rate and composition and the rate of tooth demineralization in situ. *Arch Oral Biol*, 47:413–23.

18. Bergdhal, M., & Bergdhal, J. (2000). Low unstimulated salivary flow and subjective oral dryness; association with medication, anxiety, depression and stress. *J Dent Res*, 27:18.

19. Salerno, S., Cannizzaro, F., Lo Castro, A., Loinbardo, F., Barress, B., Speciale, R., & Lagalla, R. (2002). Interventional treatment of sialoliths in main salivary glands. *Radiol Med (Torino)*, 13:378–83.

20. Stern, Y., Feinmesser, R., Collins, M., Shotts, S. R., & Cotton, R. T. (2002). Bilateral submandibular gland excision and parotid duct ligation for treatment of sialorrhea in children: long term results. *Arch Otolaryngol Head and Neck Surg*, 128:801–3.

21. McDonnell, S. T., & Hector, M. P. (2001). The distribution of stimulated saliva in children. *Int J Paedriatric Dent*, 11:417–23.

22. Weatherell, J. A., Strong, M., Robinson, C., Nakagaki, H., & Ralph, J. P. (1989). Retention of glucose in oral fluid at different sites in the mouth. *Car Res*. 23:399–405.

23. Oho, T., Mitoma, M., & Koya, T. (2002). Functional domain of bovine milk lactoferrin which inhibits the adherence of Streptococcus mutans cells to a salivary film. *Inf Immun*, 70:5279–82.

24. Edgar, W. M., Higham, S. M., & Manning, R. H. (1994). Saliva stimulation and caries prevention. *Adv Dent Res*, 8:239–45.

25. Silverstone, L. M. (1988). Remineraliztion and enamel caries: new concepts. *Dent Update*, 19:683–711.

26. Silverstone, L. M., Featherstone, M. J., & Hichs, M. J. (1988). Dynamic factors affecting lesion initiation and progression in human dental enamel. Part I. The dynamic nature of enamel caries. *Quintessence Int*, 19:683–711.

27. Silverstone, L. M., Featherstone, M. J., & Hicks, M. J. (1994). Dynamic factors affecting lesion initiation and progression in human dental enamel. Part II. Surface morphology of sound enamel and caries-like lesions of enamel. *Quintessence Int*, 19:333–85.

28. Tenouvo, J. (1997). Salivary parameters of relevance for assessing caries activity in individuals and populations. *Community Dent Oral Epidemiol*, 25:82–86.

29. Head, J. A. (1912). A study of saliva and its action on tooth enamel in reference to its hardening and softening. *JAMA*, 19:333–85.

30. Bodecker, C. F. (1933). Dental erosion, its possible cause and treatment. *Dental Cosmos*, 75:1056–63.

31. Muhler, J. C. (1961). A practical method of reducing dental caries in children not receiving the established benefits of communal fluoridation. *J Dent Child*, 28:5–12.

32. von der Fehr, F. R., Loe, H., & Theilade, F. (1970). Experimental caries in man. *Caries Res*, 4:131–48.

33. Backer-Dirks, O. (1970). Posteruptive changes in dental enamel. *J Dent Res*, 4:131–48.

34. Silverstone, L. M. (1984). The significance of remineralization in caries prevention. *J Can Dent Assn*, 50:157–67.

# CHAPTER 12

# Caries Risk Assessment and Caries Activity Testing

*Svante Twetman*
*Franklin García-Godoy*

## OBJECTIVES

*At the end of this chapter, it will be possible to*

1. State the purpose of caries activity tests.
2. Indicate the limitations and advantages of caries activity tests.
3. Identify the two bacteria most often measured in caries activity tests to determine the magnitude of the bacterial challenge to the teeth.
4. Understand terms used in caries-prediction tests.
5. Explain the general approach of caries-risk assessment.
6. List the background data of importance for caries activity.
7. Perform a clinical examination for evaluation of caries activity.
8. Name caries activity tests used in the dental office.
9. Cite new methods available to assess caries risk.

## INTRODUCTION

*Dental caries can be defined as a carbohydrate-modified transmissible local infection with saliva as a critical regulator.*[1] The diagnosis is most often based on a clinical examination. Terms like primary and secondary caries, initial and cavitated lesions, white spot lesions, arrested caries, and root caries are often used in an effort to describe the activity and severity of the disease. Although these observations certainly are important,

337

the modern dentistry diagnosis should be extended with identification and evaluation of factors *related* to, or the *causative agents of, the disease*. The multifactorial etiology of dental caries today is relatively well known and the disease is therefore not only a treatable, but in most aspects also a *preventable, infection*. Evaluation of etiologic factors can be made before clinical signs occur as well as in cases with already existing lesions or fillings. Subsequently, measures can be taken to reduce risk factors considered to create problems in the future. This chapter deals with different methods to determine caries risk and caries activity, focusing on the prevention of the disease. The presentation is focused on the description of clinical tests and methods that can be incorporated in the daily work and concentrated on the individual patient; therefore, the community approach is less discussed. For a more thorough discussion of the background of caries, the reader should refer to appropriate textbooks and overview papers cited in the references at the end of this chapter. To be able to discuss clinical implications, however, it might be helpful to take a closer look at the events leading to demineralization.

## Caries—A Transmissible Local Infection

It is generally recognized that certain strains of *mutans streptococci*[a] and *lactobacilli* are highly cariogenic (reviewed by van Houte[1]). The former group plays an active role in the early stages of lesion formation while the latter is linked to the *progression of the cavity*. Evidence suggesting a microbial three-step event in caries development exists (Figure 12–1).[2]

The first step is the *primary infection* with mutans streptococci; the second is a local accumulation of mutans streptococci and other aciduric microorganisms to *pathogenic levels* in the dental plaque—a microbial shift that is an ecologic consequence of local acid conditions; the third step is the *demineralization and cavitation* of the enamel. Consequently, three levels of prevention—linked to the steps—could be defined, each with its own profile and characteristic.

- *Primary prevention* (step 1)—to prevent the intrafamily transmission of mutans strepto-

cocci and delay the establishment in infants, toddlers, and young children.

- *Secondary prevention* (step 2)—to prevent, arrest, or reverse the microbial shift before any clinical manifestations of the disease occur.

- *Tertiary prevention* (step 3)—focuses on limiting (stopping) the progression of the caries process by initiating remineralization therapy of the existing lesions.

### First Step—Transmission and Establishment of Mutans Streptococci

Before the eruption of the first primary teeth, *no* mutans streptococci can be harbored permanently in the oral cavity because the bacteria need a *nonshedding surface* (i.e., a tooth) to colonize. From several studies it has been suggested that the transmission of mutans streptococci in most cases occurs vertical within the family. *The main source is the mother of the child*[3] but recent studies using DNA fingerprinting suggest that the child may also be infected by fathers and other caretakers from outside the family.[4] The most common routes of infection are close contacts and everyday nursing items such as pacifiers, baby bottles, and spoons

[a]The term mutans streptococci includes several species of streptococci which historically were often collectively referred to as *Streptococcus mutans*.

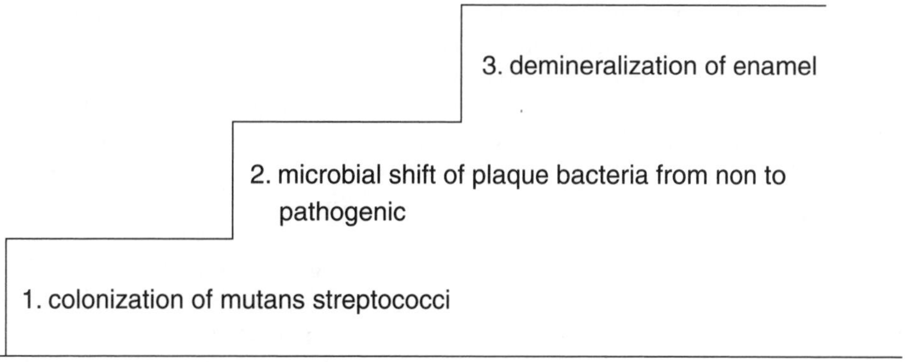

3. demineralization of enamel

2. microbial shift of plaque bacteria from non to pathogenic

1. colonization of mutans streptococci

FIGURE 12-1    Enamel demineralization – caries – can be described as a three-step event.

(Figure 12–2). The colonization and establishment of mutans streptococci is highly facilitated by a frequent and sucrose-rich *diet of the parent as well as the child*. The higher the counts in mothers, the more frequent and the earlier risk for colonization in their children.[5-7] There are also a variety of other factors, such as salivary immunoglobulins and agglutinins, presence of competing bacteria, tooth anatomy, and pH, that might influence the colonization. Furthermore, the earlier the establishment and the more mutans streptococci present in children, the more caries is likely to develop in the primary and permanent dentition.[8,9]

The prevalence of mutans streptococci infection increases with age and the number of erupted teeth. Among toddlers, approximately 5 to 10% of a population harbor the bacterium and a rapid increase in prevalence up to around 50 to 60% in the late preschool ages has been observed.[b,10,11] In fact, it has been suggested that children are most susceptible for mutans streptococci colonization between *19 and 31 months of age, a so-called "window of infectivity."*[12,13] This is mainly explained by a combination of frequent and close maternal contacts, cessation of lactation with its protective antibodies, and an immature immune response of the child as well as an individual susceptibility. Approximately 80% of all adolescents and adults are positive for mutans streptococci, so the oral cavity can be regarded as a natural habitat for the bacteria.

### Second Step—Microbial Shift

Once a mutans streptococci- and lactobacilli-containing microflora is established in the oral cavity, there is a *risk* for future caries development. It is however a general misunderstanding that the disease is an inevitable result of the colonization. Instead, it is more common to harbor mutans streptococci without subsequent decay. A crucial process develops *if*, and *when*, the caries associated microorganisms turn path-

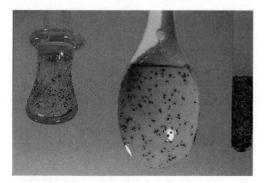

FIGURE 12-2    Common routes of mutans streptococci transmission: an infected dummy and spoon.

[b]These data are representative for Sweden and the percentages may be different in other countries.

ogenic and this in turn is regulated and modified by local environment. Early in life, and especially in connection to nocturnal and nightly nursing bottle meals, the microbial shift is often *concomitant* with colonization while at later ages, the shift might occur at any time due to a disturbed homeostasis of the oral ecology.

Once established, the "normal" content of mutans streptococci and lactobacilli constitute less than 1% of the total microbial community in saliva and dental plaque. *During long-term acidic conditions, however, aciduric bacterial strains will be favored.* Lactobacilli are the most acid-tolerating of the species in the dental plaque and are able to maintain their metabolic activity down to pH 3.0.[14] Mutans streptococci are also highly aciduric and can grow at pH 5.0 and continue acid production to under pH 4.5.[15] Common reasons for the prolonged acid conditions are increased frequency of sugar intake, reduced oral clearance due to low saliva secretion or impaired buffer capacity, and plaque accumulation due to insufficient oral hygiene or interference by fixed orthodontic appliances. Consequently, the proportion of the extremely acid-tolerating mutans streptococci and lactobacilli will increase on the expense of nonmutans streptococci and other bacteria. The higher the proportion of acidogenic and aciduric microorganisms in plaque, the more acid is produced and a negative trend has been started. For example, the proportion of mutans streptococci in plaque associated with nursing bottle caries can be up to 30 percent of the total viable counts.[16] It is important, however, to point out that the microbial shift is a *local* event and it does not happen at the same time in the whole oral cavity. The shift is most likely to occur in fissures and interdental areas that are well-known predilection sites for caries. They are also the sites of greatest plaque accumulation. Furthermore, it should be stressed that microbial shifts *can be reversed* by temporary means (i.e., drugs, antibacterial agents) and permanent changes (i.e., diet alteration, sugar restriction) in the

local environment. By using selective antibacterial measures, the cariogenic flora can be suppressed and a noncariogenic flora can be reestablished (reviewed by Emilson[17]). However, if the causative factors of the local shift remain unchanged, a recolonization back to pathogenic level is sooner or later likely to occur.[18] It should also be mentioned that the range of bacteria potentially involved in enamel demineralization has widened in recent years. There is evidence suggesting that Actinomyces species and "low pH," non–mutans streptococci under selected environmental conditions can contribute to caries in the absence of mutans streptococci.[1,19] In rare occasions, these organisms resembling *S. anginosus*, *S. mitis*, *S. gordonii*, and *S. oralis*, are thought to be responsible for the establishment of an initial low-pH environment.

### Third Step—Demineralization of Enamel

At food intake, the accumulated plaque is fed with carbohydrates, which rapidly will be converted to organic acids, mainly *lactic acid*, through the metabolism of acidogenic bacteria.[20] This will further trigger the acidic milieu and a result in a local pH drop of the plaque fluids. During this drop, protons are diffusing into the enamel with calcium and phosphates leaving the tooth and a demineralization of the hard tissue occurs. From the time of the local microbial shift on a clinically sound enamel surface, an "incubation" period of approximately 6 to 9 *weeks* can be expected before the first visual signs of enamel demineralization ("white spots") on a smooth surface can be observed. In everyday practice, this is not an uncommon side effect associated with fixed orthodontic appliances.[21] Interdentally, however, it takes up to 9 *months* or more before the enamel lesion is visible as radiolucency on a bitewing radiograph.[22] This is a serious concern in modern dentistry that puts high demands on the diagnostic process. There is an evident risk that patients, who in fact have undergone a

**TABLE 12-1. Caries Risk and Caries Activity**

| From ⇒ | to | means |
|--------|-----|-------|
| Sound ⇒ | carious | caries-risk assessment: before onset of disease |
| Carious ⇒ | more decay | caries activity assessment: before progression of lesion |

bacterial shift, still are clinically uneventful when examined and not given the appropriate preventive care.

In normal cases, after carbohydrate (sugar) intake the acid production diminishes when the bacterial substrate is consumed or washed away by saliva dilution. The pH will return to normal and a period of "repair" (remineralization) will again occur. This process is facilitated if fluorides are present locally. *The balance between net loss and net gain of mineral is crucial whether progression or regression of a lesion will occur.* It is important to stress that this is not a continuous process in either direction and that caries-active and caries-inactive periods will follow each other through the lifespan. A "white spot" enamel lesion *without cavitation* can be completely repaired through remineralization while a lesion that has reached the dentin, irrespective of enamel surface breakdown, has usually passed the "point of no return." Although it is unlikely that such a lesion can be totally repaired by aggressive remineralization therapy, a conservative attitude toward operative treatment is recommended favoring "watchful-waiting" and close monitoring during the preventive treatment period. Several clinical studies have demonstrated an extreme slow progression rate, if any, of enamel and dentine lesions subjected to effective and continuous prevention.[23,24] For example, the progression rate in enamel was found to be much slower than through the outer half of the dentin that, in turn, exhibited a median survival time of 3.1 years in a cohort of children that was followed prospectively from 11 to 22 years of age.[25]

## Caries Risk and Caries Activity

It is well known that certain individuals develop much more caries than others. The object of *caries prediction*[c] *and caries risk assessment*[d] is *to improve oral health* in children, adolescents, and adults and to utilize resources in a cost-effective way. Risk is defined as the *probability that a harmful (or unwanted) event will occur.* From the material presented above, it might be useful to separate caries risk assessment from attempts to determine the *caries activity.* By definition, a caries risk assessment is a procedure to *predict future caries development* before the clinical onset of the disease, thus limited to steps 1 and 2; while a caries activity test preferably should estimate the actual state of disease activity (progression/regression), as found in step 3 (Table 12–1).

The caries-risk assessment is performed in order to introduce causal measures before irreversible lesions have become established, while the caries activity test is carried out in order to decide and monitor correct and efficient treatment of a patient. When applied on populations, the caries-risk procedure is termed "caries prediction." As recently expressed by Hausen,[26] "clinicians assess risk, researchers predict." For the clinician it might be useful in this aspect to distinguish between *risk factors and risk indicators* (risk markers). A risk factor plays an essen-

[c]Prediction is a clinical decision about the outcome of a disease process based on available information and professional experience.

[d]Risk assessment is a professional judgement of an individual's future risk of disease based on the best information available.

tial role in the etiology and occurrence of the disease, while a risk indicator is a factor or circumstance that is indirectly associated with the disease.[27] Risk factors are the life-style and biochemical determinants to which the tooth is directly exposed and which contribute to the development or progression of the lesion (plaque, saliva, diet, etc.). Examples on risk indicators are socioeconomic factors (socially deprived, low education level, poor economy, self-esteem), factors related to general health (diseases, handicap), and epidemiologic factors (living in a high-caries area or country, high past-caries experience). Caries-risk assessment as well as caries-activity evaluation are based on defined and selected risk factors and risk indicators that are evaluated and put together to an individual profile.

## Terms Used in Prediction

To study the validity[e] of a caries diagnostic test and whether or not it is useful for caries prediction, the relation to caries incidence[f] must be established. It must be immediately pointed out that a close association in cross-sectional studies between en etiologic factor or its measure in a test on one hand and caries on the other does not necessarily mean that it also is a powerful predictor of the disease. The predictive ability of caries tests or risk indicators must therefore be evaluated in longitudinal studies. The results are generally expressed in terms of *sensitivity, specificity,* and *prognostic values*. The proportion of diseased subjects whose test (or risk factor) is positive is termed sensitivity. Similarly, the proportion of non-diseased subjects whose test (or risk factor) is negative is called specificity. The predictive values are per-

haps of higher interest for the clinician, and a higher predictive value indicates a more valid test. The positive predictive value (PV1) denotes the probability of an individual to develop the disease, while the negative predictive value (PV2) gives the probability to stay healthy. All the above measures should be looked at as pairs. For instance, knowing the sensitivity of a caries test has a limited meaning if one does not know the respective specificity of the test. More recently, *odds–ratio values*, referring to the chance of an event versus the chance of a nonevent, have been introduced in prediction models. The odds–ratio provides information on the chance that the disease will occur given a specific condition. It must, however, be understood that all values above are highly dependent on a number of factors that must be defined and considered to be able to understand the predictive power:[28]

- The level of caries prevalence and incidence in the study population or study group
- The methods used for data collection and especially the criteria for caries scoring
- The validity of the test method
- The number of tests and/or the combinations of tests applied
- The patient's access to preventive and restorative care
- Age of the participants

For instance, the predictive value of a mutans streptococci saliva sample is dependent on the disease level. It is fairly easy to understand that it is harder to predict the eruption of a rare disease compared with a common one. When a test is applied to a population with a high prevalence of disease compared to a population with a lower prevalence, the positive predictive value will increase and the negative predictive value will decrease. The definition of caries activity (disease) is of course very important. Were only new lesions or also progression of previous lesions considered? Is a certain number of new cavities within the dentin or a single

---

[e]Validity means sufficiently supported by actual fact, sound, good or effective means.

[f]Caries incidence is the number of lesions that occur over a given period of time. Thus, two examinations are required to determine incidence; one before and one at the end of a selected period.

early enamel lesion regarded as disease? The selected cutoff points for positive tests and disease and the motivation why they were chosen must be considered. Furthermore, *restorative treatment and preventive efforts conducted in predictive investigations may obscure the predictive power of the tested model.* Environmental factors, such as the natural content of fluoride in the drinking water, can interfere with the predictive process.[11] The predictive power may also be influenced by age. It is generally believed that caries risk assessments are more accurate in preschoolers compared with older age groups and adults. For instance, Swedish investigators demonstrated in a prospective study that mutans streptococci colonization, immigrant background, consumption of candy and mothers' level of education were significant predictors for caries before 3.5 years of age.[29] When all these variables were present at 1 year of age, the probability for caries development was 87%. Thus, one can state that predictive values are valid *only* for the population studied and for the *given time* when the investigation was conducted. This does not mean that such studies lack merit—on the contrary—considerable experience has been gathered within the field and forms the base for many national oral health care programs.

The number of false responses following a test should naturally be as few as possible. For caries, however, the occurrence of *false-positive* answers are less crucial as long as they only result in an intensified prevention program and not in unneeded restorations. *False-negative* results, on the other hand, can seriously jeopardize dental health due to neglected treatment.

## General Approach of Caries Risk Assessment

As discussed earlier, a risk-assessment strategy can be applied on three different levels, each with somewhat different aims: (1) *for populations*, (2) *for groups*, and (3) *for the individual*. For preventive strategies today, it is important

to distinguish populations with contrasting prevalence of the disease. On a national level, it seems important to evaluate the actual "challenge" to the teeth and data can be obtained through caries tests in epidemiologic investigations. Such findings evaluated in combination with, for example, sugar-consumption figures, are of highest relevance for oral-health planners. Based on such data, the community can implement preventive programs or dispense health care resources in a cost-effective way. The same approach can be applied to groups for which the current prognostic value can be established. For the individual, caries activity tests can map etiologic factors for caries and serve as a measure of compliance to a given treatment. However, before describing the methods used in the risk assessment procedure, it is valuable to discuss historically why the risk approach has gained so much attention during the recent decades.[30]

*In communities with a high prevalence of caries, the need for a risk approach is limited.* This was the situation in most industrialized Western countries a few decades ago. A whole population strategy with general preventive measures given to everyone, such as water fluoridation and fluoride supplements, were highly cost-effective since the vast majority of the population benefited from these programs. Hence, caries declined rapidly and the polarized distribution of today became evident.[31] A large and increasing proportion of the population became caries-free, while others still exhibited a high caries activity. In order to limit the costs for dental health care in a period of economic recession and limited resources, the efforts were then directed to the relative minority of individuals that developed oral diseases.

Consequently, a risk approach was instituted and caries-risk assessment became a part of dental practice. After caries-risk assessment, the persons with the highest need for treatment were provided intensive targeted actions with individualized recalls. Low-risk individuals did not receive further attention with recall periods

extended up to 24 months. Epidemiologic and analytic surveys, however, soon identified certain subgroups of individuals with a high prevalence and incidence within the skewed caries distribution.[32] Common examples are ethnic and cultural groups, immigrants (especially refugees), and inhabitants of low-socioeconomic areas. Furthermore, medically compromised individuals could also constitute such a group. In these groups and subgroups, screening procedures of children at various ages in school have been proven rational and cost-effective. However, in comparison with whole population strategies, the general effects of the individualized approach are less evaluated and documented. Therefore, *a balanced mix of a risk selection strategy and collective measures seem to be the "state of the art" in many communities today.* It should be emphasized that in an extreme low-caries population where practically no persons develop caries, a risk assessment would be of little use. It has also been claimed that the risk selection procedure, after proper education, can be *delegated to auxiliary personnel,* which may reduce the cost for the patient and the society.[33]

---

## Question 1

Which of the following statements, if any, are correct?

A. Caries can be defined as a carbohydrate-modified transmissible local infection.

B. A caries *risk factor* incidence test requires only *one* dental examination.

C. Sensitivity of a caries activity test denotes the probability for caries development.

D. A risk-assessment strategy is most important in communities with high-caries prevalence.

E. For preventive care, a false-positive caries-activity test would probably be more advantageous to the patient than a false-negative test.

---

## Community and Group Approach of Caries Risk Assessment

Since the prevalence of caries in many countries shows a skewed distribution, the interest of finding methods for prediction of individuals or groups of patients at risk within the community has become widespread. *The methods used for this identification are predominantly based on past dental caries, oral hygiene, dietary variables, microbial and salivary factors, and social variables.*[34,35] It has been proposed that both the sensitivity and specificity must be at least 80% to be useful in caries-predictive models or when added, exceed 150%.[36] In practice, this means that every fifth individual with a true high risk would remain undetected and not receive intensified prevention. Correspondingly, every fifth individual with a true low risk would receive treatment with no or little effect. Furthermore, it is thought that a risk model should select not more than 20 to 30% of a population believed to be at risk to be manageable. With such precautions, the sensitivity of the bacterial tests and past caries experience, single or combined, are commonly reported within the range of 60 to 80%. On the other hand, the prediction of patients at low risk seems more reliable than those at high risk with a specificity around 80 to 90%. This means that it appears to be more relevant to select patients with low risk for future caries development than predicting those at risk.

Due to the complex and multifactorial etiology of dental caries, it is generally thought that a multivariate approach rather than the use of single variables improves the predictive ability. Biochemical variables have been combined with sociodemographic and dental behavior data.[37,38] However, results from recent studies using such multivariate methods have been unexpectedly poor.[35,39] The accuracy proved to be much lower than anticipated considering the power of the individual predictors. In fact, the highly complicated relationship has raised the question whether prediction of caries with reasonable, simple, and inexpensive methods

will ever be a reality. While the prediction of caries risk using currently available methods is useful in certain communities with a skewed caries distribution and in groups of individuals with medium and high caries levels, its value in a low caries community can be questioned. The clinical value of caries *prediction models*, therefore, may differ from population to population and from children to adults, as recently reviewed by Powell.[40]

The number and the degree of sophistication of predictive methods are of course limiting factors in the population because of practicalities and costs. Therefore, few and strong variables have to be advocated on the population level while a higher degree of combinations can be utilized in smaller groups and for the individual. An example of a very simple community protocol for risk selection is given in Table 12–2. The concept can—and should—of course be altered

depending on local conditions and the age of the target group. The past caries experience is thought to be the most powerful single indicator of future caries development in children.[39] It can however be argued that it does not precede the disease but rather is a result of an already existing—or treated—disease and represents an accumulation of long-term disease experience. Thus, considerable interest has been focused on anticipated risk factors and risk indicators, i.e., simple chairside methods for saliva evaluation, directly dependent on the state of oral microbiology at a given time, which will be discussed below.

## Ages of Interest for Caries Risk Assessment

Data on the time when caries-risk assessment is most cost-effective in childhood are sparse. *It is well known, however, that all newly erupted teeth are more or less deficient in mineral content and thus more susceptible for caries than after some years of posteruptive maturation.*[41] Moreover, the eruption of teeth constitutes a caries risk *per se*, since new surfaces become available for the disease. Therefore, in this aspect it might be possible to define certain *risk ages* of utmost importance of risk assessment procedures.

An early dental examination and diagnosis must be regarded as extremely important for efficient preventive intervention. Recent studies have unveiled that approximately 75% of all cavities found in 2-year-old children were located in the upper incisors and that 90% of those exhibiting caries in the upper front also developed cavities in the primary molars.[42,43] Furthermore, the primary molars are caries-prone between 4 and 6 years of age,[44] and the eruption of the first permanent molars constitute a well-known occlusal risk. Finally, the early teenage period (12 to 16 years) offers a high number of newly erupted surfaces susceptible for decay. Based on recent epidemiologic data on caries incidence, the "key ages" as suggested in Table 12–3 might be considered for caries-risk assessment.

---

TABLE 12-2 **Example of a Simple Risk Evaluation Protocol for Schoolchildren Suggested for Large-scale Use on Community Level**[a]

| Oral Risk Factors | Yes | No |
|---|---|---|
| New lesions | ❏ | ❏ |
| Progression of previous lesions | ❏ | ❏ |
| Bleeding on probing >20% | ❏ | ❏ |
| **Medical Risk Factors** | | |
| Chronic disease | ❏ | ❏ |
| Handicap | ❏ | ❏ |
| **Family Risk Factors** | | |
| >5 in-between meals/day | ❏ | ❏ |
| Dental fear | ❏ | ❏ |
| Cooperation problem | ❏ | ❏ |

**Evaluation:**   Oral risk factor(s) present = 1
Medical risk factor(s) present = 1
Family risk factor(s) present = 1

**Estimated Risk:**
Low = 0; Moderate = 1; High = 2–3

---

[a]The protocol is based on relatively few and nonlaboratory risk factors.

TABLE 12-3 **Risk Ages to Be Considered for Caries-risk Assessment**

| Age | Where? | Why? |
| --- | --- | --- |
| 1 yr | At child-health centers | To prevent nursing-bottle caries, early diagnosis |
| 3 yrs | At the dental clinic | To prevent caries in primary molars |
| 6–7 yrs | At the dental clinic | To prevent caries in first permanent molars |
| 12–13 yrs | Screening in school | To prevent caries in second molars and premolars; part of health education |

## Individual Approach of Caries Activity

For an appropriate assessment of caries activity, facts from the case history, clinical and radiographic examinations, dietary history, and supplementary laboratory tests must be taken into account.[45] An individual approach has been suggested and described by Bratthall and Tynelius-Bratthall.[46] According to their method, biochemical and demographic parameters should be combined with a *clinical judgment* ("gut feeling") of the dental professional to elicit proper results. First, determine which particular factors are involved. Next, find out *why* these factors are present. Finally, try to change the situation by targeted actions against identified factors. Some examples are given in Table 12–4 to illustrate this concept.

When reviewing the findings of an individual, the trading of multiple pros and cons becomes very complex to evaluate. For example, think about two caries-free children with contrasting levels of mutans streptococci in their saliva. If each has the same diet, it is very likely that the child with the high counts will develop more caries than the one with low counts. However, if the child with low counts eats candy frequently and the one with high counts has a very restricted sugar intake, which one now has the greatest chance of developing caries? The question becomes harder to answer even though most professionals probably would have an opinion. Imagine in the next step that the first child with low bacterial counts and frequent sugar intake is supplemented with fluoride and the other is opposing the use of fluoride; who will, under such circumstances, develop the most caries? Is the buffer capacity contrasting? In this way, by adding several aggravating and counteracting risk factors and risk indicators, there are thousands of possible combinations to consider. To be able to handle this, it is important to realize that a risk value, such as high mutans streptococci levels, indicates a certain "pressure" on the teeth. With a proper diet and optimal fluoride administration, the risk can be controlled. When several risk values are disclosed, a very strong pressure is evident and more counteracting factors are needed to balance the situation. Suggested cutoff values for commonly used risk factors in pediatric dentistry are listed in Table 12–5. It can be recommended to use interactive software tool that are developed as an aid for the clinician in the caries predictive process. Such an example is the educational "Cariogram."[g,47] Graphically, the PC-program maps the interaction between caries related factors, a process known as cariography (Figure 12–3). Background data and clinical findings, with their varying impact on caries, are entered into a computer and the factors are weighed against each other forming a "risk profile" of the patient. The program can be adjusted for local conditions such as socioeconomic status and fluoride content in the piped water. The

[g]Copyright © Prof. D. Bratthall.

TABLE 12-4 **Some Reasons for Caries Risk Factors**[a]

| Risk Factors | Why? (Examples) |
| --- | --- |
| Large amount of plaque | The patient |
| | · does not know how to clean the teeth |
| | · is not interested or motivated; personal problems |
| | · is handicapped, making brushing difficult |
| | · has unfavorable tooth anatomy, crowded teeth |
| | · has previous fillings with overhangs |
| High proportion of cariogenic bacteria | The patient has |
| | · a sugar-rich diet, favoring aciduric bacteria |
| | · many retention sites, margins of fillings |
| | · bacteria transferred from relatives |
| | · genetic factors of importance |
| High frequency of sucrose | The patient |
| | · is not informed about cariogenicity of diet has a work, economic, medical, cultural, social situation that makes frequent sweet intakes easy or necessary |
| Reduced saliva flow/low-buffer capacity | The patient |
| | · has constitutionally low saliva secretion |
| | · is stressed |
| | · takes medicines which affect saliva |
| | · exhibits seasonal variations |
| Fluorides not available/decreased remineralization | The patient |
| | · lives in a low-fluoride area |
| | · does not use fluoridated toothpaste |
| | · is opposing fluoride supplement |

[a]Adapted from Bratthall and Tynelius-Bratthall[42]

*chance,* expressed as percentage, for a person *to avoid new decay* is thereafter presented graphically on the screen. The program also provides an individualized suggestion on suitable preventive activities when needed. The Cariogram concept has recently been evaluated in a prospective study in which the assessed risk at baseline in a group of 10 to 11-year-old schoolchildren was compared with the actual caries increment after 2 years.[48] Although the general caries incidence was low in the study popula-

tion, the Cariogram was the most powerful explanatory variable. For example, children in the highest risk group (0 to 20% chance to avoid caries) had 50 times higher risk (odds ratio) than the children in the lowest risk group (81 to 100% chance to avoid caries).

We will now focus and comment on the clinical implication of caries-risk assessment of the individual, covering background data (case history), clinical examination, and caries activity tests.

**TABLE 12-5** Risk Factors and Risk Indicators Commonly Used for an Individual Assessment of Caries Risk[a]

| Variables | Method | Dimension | Suggested Cutoff Point |
| --- | --- | --- | --- |
| **Case History** | | | |
| Misuse of sugar | Interview | Frequency | Every day |
| Juice/soft drinks | Interview | Frequency | >3 per day |
| Nocturnal meals | Interview | Frequency | Present |
| Fluoride exposure | Interview | Frequency | Absent |
| Socioeconomic level | Interview | Profession/education | Low |
| Immigrant background | Interview | Parent generation | Mother, 1st |
| **Clinical Examination** | | | |
| Caries experience | Clinical exam | DMFS/defs | >2–4 |
| Incipient lesions | Clinical exam | Frequency > | >2–4 |
| Oral hygiene | Clinical exam | VPI | >50% |
| Gingivitis | Clinical exam | GBI | >20% |
| **Saliva Tests** | | | |
| Mutans streptococci | Dentocult SM | score 0–3 | ≥ 2 |
| Lactobacilli | Dentocult LB | score 0–4 | ≥ 3 |
| Buffer capacity | Dentobuff | pH; color | ≤ 4.0; yellow |
| Saliva secretion rate | Sialomethry | mL/min | <0.5 (stim) |

[a]Variables and suggested cutoff points might be adjusted for age.
DMFS = decayed, missing, filled surfaces (permanent dentition); defs = decayed, extracted, filled surfaces (primary dentition); VPI = visible plaque index; GBI = gingival bleeding index.

## Background Data of Importance for Caries Activity

The background factors that *directly or indirectly* can be of importance for the disease usually belong to one or more of the following groups:

- General diseases
- Medication
- Social/family situation
- Dietary habits/feeding
- Oral-hygiene routines, fluoride support

When interviewing the patient for the case history, questions should be asked to clarify these points. There are few general diseases that directly affect the teeth, although there are several that *indirectly* influence the carious process. In fact, and especially regarding chil-

dren, being ill with medication in combination with anxious and sometimes overprotective parents constitutes a greater caries risk than

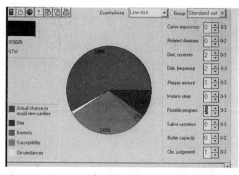

FIGURE 12-3    The Cariogram—an educational interactive PC-program for caries risk evaluation.

the disease itself. Several drugs contain a high content of fermentable carbohydrates and have a low pH. Furthermore, the depressing influence on saliva secretion exerted by various medicines is a well-documented risk.[49] A troubled family or social situation might be reflected by factors such as stress (decreased saliva secretion), lack of interest in hygiene (poor plaque control), and low income (cariogenic diet). The topic of diet and caries is vast and needs its own textbook to be adequately covered, but it can be stated that the diet clearly affects the teeth in a direct (in the form of erosion) and indirect (through tooth formation, saliva secretion, and bacterial activity) way. In developing a risk profile, the diet should always be considered. An interview or a "3-day record" of all food and snack intakes are common methods used to obtain information about the diet of a patient.

## Clinical Examination for Evaluation of Caries Activity

One aim of the clinical examination is to get a quantitative estimation of the caries problem up to the present and another aim is to reveal if the disease is ongoing or if observed lesions or fillings reflect a past disease activity. A few important points for estimating caries activity are discussed below.

For the individual patient, it is important to collect data in a standardized and systematic way. As stated earlier, the past caries prevalence is always important, but one is not necessarily at risk in spite of 30 previous fillings. It is very useful to try to look "behind" the recorded decayed, missing, or filled primary or permanent teeth (dmft/DMFT) values as indicated in Table 12–6. First, one should consider if there are more or fewer fillings or extractions than

TABLE 12-6 **Examples of Clinical Findings for Evaluating Caries Activity**

| Clinical Finding | High Activity | Low Activity |
| --- | --- | --- |
| Number of Teeth | Less than normal | Normal |
| Reason for extraction | Caries/perio treatment | Orthodontic treatment |
| When were teeth extracted | Recently | In the past |
| Number of Fillings | More than normal | Less than normal |
| When were fillings made | Recently | Long time ago |
| Frequency | >2 fillings each year | Very rare, occasionally |
| Filling material | Composites | Gold, glass ionomers |
| Number of Enamel Lesions and Cavities | More than expected | None |
| | Appeared recently | Old, neglected |
| Localization | Smooth or lingual | Predilection sites only |
| | Surfaces, lower incisors | Fissures |
| Surface, color | Soft, light | Hard, dark |
| X-rays | Progression into dentin | Regression, still within enamel |
| Oral Hygiene | Poor | Acceptable |
| Aggravating Factors | Crowded teeth | Spaced arches |
| | Deep fissures | Shallow fissures |
| | Marginal overhangs | Perfect adaptation |
| | Orthodontic appliances | Removable appliances |

considered normal for a particular age group. The patients should then be asked questions such as "*Why* and *when* were the teeth extracted (caries, periodontal disease, orthodontics), or were the restorations placed long ago or recently?" Check the number, extension, and appearance of the lesions, cavities, and fillings. The texture and localization of lesions might provide important hints for caries activity (Figure 12–4). For example, presence of early enamel lesions ("white spots") on newly erupted teeth indicates an active demineralization process. The evaluation will provide the examiner with information on the extent of the problem and if caries seems to be a past or present problem. In the next step, local aggravating factors such as crowded arches, deep fissures, imperfect fillings and exposed root surfaces are evaluated. The morphology of the enamel must always be checked. Although the present evidence supporting an inherited susceptibility to dental caries is limited, altered enamel development, such as increased porosity and decreased mineral content are directly linked to an increased caries risk.[50] Finally, the

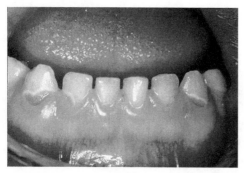

FIGURE 12–4  Caries in a disturbed homeostasis. At the clinical examination, inspect carefully the appearance of the lesion. An active lesion, as in the figure, is often soft light in color, or surrounded by enamel with early whitish demineralization. An arrested lesion is usually darker with a harder surface.

estimation of the oral hygiene standard with a disclosing solution can be recommended. It should be emphasized that visible plaque on the labial surfaces of maxillary incisors of a young child is a serious sign of caries risk.[51]

## Caries-Activity Tests for the Dental Office

It is well known that dental caries has a multifactorial and complex etiology, and unfortunately, there is no single test available that can fully explain or predict the disease. The term "caries-activity test" may furthermore be misleading since, at best, information can only be obtained on selected factors of importance for the process. Ideally, laboratory tests should be simple, inexpensive, rapid, and accurately reflect the three overlapping circles presented by Keyes[52] in 1962: (1) the bacterial challenge, (2) the sugar content of the diet, and (3) tooth and host resistance (susceptibility) with remineralization potential. In the light of these requirements and circles, the following set-up of tests might be suggested:

- *Bacterial challenge*—determination of mutans streptococci as an indicator of relative risk.
- *Diet*—determination of lactobacilli as an indicator of sugar content in diet.
- *Remineralization potential*—salivary flow rate and buffer capacity as an indicator of potential biologic repair.
- *Host suspectibility*—caries experience as an indicator of past activity.

After sampling, the clinician can choose between sending the tests to a fully equipped microbiologic laboratory or to use commercial test kits that can be processed within the dental office. In both cases, the results will be available after a few days. The simplified testing methods now available can be characterized as semiquantitative, although they are generally considered to significantly correspond with conventional agar plate techniques.[53,54] The most

common sources for sampling are saliva and dental plaque. *The saliva test gives an overall estimation whether or not the patient is colonized and reflects the number of colonized surfaces and the prevalence in plaque.*[55] It does not however indicate where the bacteria are harbored, which is important to understand since the cariogenic microorganisms colonize the dentition in a milieu-regulated, localized way.[56] The plaque sample can therefore be used for a detailed "mapping" of the patient's dentition with special references to selected sites. This approach enables an assessment of not only *at-risk individuals* but also *at-risk teeth* and even *risk surfaces*. Salivary tests are generally more practical than tests based on plaque since the collection is less demanding. In addition to the diagnostic value of saliva and plaque tests, the didactic properties as an individualized patient-motivating tool in caries prevention are today widely acknowledged (Figure 12–5).[57–59]

## When Should Tests Be Used?

This issue has been lively debated through the last decades. It is, of course, not realistic or even justified by cost-effective means to test all patients living in a low-caries society each time they are recalled or with certain regularity. A simple answer is that a test should be performed each time there is a need for extra information on factors of importance for caries—quantita-

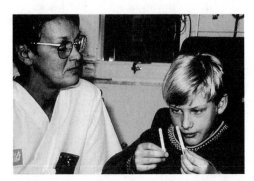

FIGURE 12–5    Saliva tests are useful as didactic and motivating tools in caries prevention.

tive as well as qualitative.[46] Thus, selected tests could be justified in several clinical situations to:

- Clarify the reasons behind an ongoing disease and formulate and motivate the preventive strategy to the patient
- Determine the effect of a causal treatment at follow-up visits
- Predict caries development (i.e., make a prognosis) at check-up visits

For the selected subjects, repeated tests are preferred compared to single in order to establish the normal values of the patient and be able to monitor any deviation from the "norm," indicating an altered oral environment. For example, if the unstimulated secretion rate suddenly decreases, this is a sign of an altered ecologic environment with increased caries risk and should be followed by a closer check-up of the medical and psychosocial conditions and drug intake.

## Mutans Streptococci Counts

As already mentioned, mutans streptococci are strongly associated with the initiation of dental caries.[1,60,61] They have several cariogenic properties that are enhanced in the presence of sucrose. The most important are the ability to:

- Colonize and grow on nonshedding surfaces
- Produce acids, acidogenic
- Withstand low pH, aciduric
- Form and store extra- and intracellular polysaccharides
- Tolerate high-sucrose concentrations

The human dentition is the natural habitat for mutans streptococci (Figure 12–6). They have a localized way of growing which means that in one individual's mouth, some teeth may harbor bacteria while others do not. The levels of mutans streptococci in saliva and on the tooth surfaces (plaque) reflect the number of colonized sites in the mouth.[62] The *higher the*

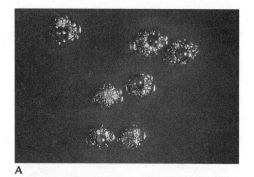

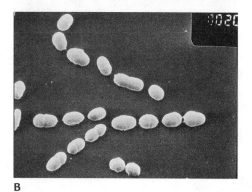

FIGURE 12–6   Close-up of mutans streptococci, cultivated on MSB-agar **(A)** and as appearing in a scanning electron microscope **(B)**.

*mutans streptococci count on the teeth, the more caries.*[63] A number of different strains can be found in humans and the prevalence seems to vary by age and population. The most common inhabitants in humans worldwide are *Streptococcus mutans* and *Streptococcus sobrinus*.[64] About 10 to 30% of a population have low levels of the bacterium, while 10 to 50% are highly colonized.

The quantitative evaluation of mutans streptococci in saliva and plaque is performed at the laboratory on agar plates with a selective media, the mitis-salivarius-bacitracin agar.[65] A serial dilution of the sample is performed and aliquots are placed on the agar surface with a pipette. After 4 days of anaerobic incubation,

the number of colony forming units (CFU)[h] are counted. The bacteria have a significant morphologic appearance and it is possible to distinguish between various strains. Variations of this technique have been suggested to adopt and facilitate use in the dental office, i.e., direct impressions on a wooden spatula on an elevated agar.[66] However, the short storing duration of the plates in combination with demanding incubation requirements make the plate counts best suited for the research laboratory.

### Strip Mutans Method for Mutans Streptococci Counts

Several simple chairside methods have been developed in recent years for the estimation of mutans streptococci levels in saliva.[67,68] These simplified methods, however, are not only used in the modern dental office but also in dental research as described in numerous papers. The most common method today is the *Strip mutans* technique (Dentocult-SM)[i] developed by Jensen and Bratthall.[69] This method utilizes the ability of mutans streptococci to grow on a hard surface in a selective mitis salivarius broth containing 20% sucrose. The kit includes a specially prepared rounded plastic strip for the sampling. The surface of the strip is slightly roughened on one side to promote bacterial adherence. Fifteen minutes prior to the sampling, a 5-mg bacitracin tablet is added to the broth. As the bacitracin can be added just before use, the shelf-life of the test is prolonged compared to agar plates. After 2 minutes of paraffin-chewing, the plastic strip is rotated a couple of times on the dorsum of the tongue and then withdrawn *through lightly closed lips*, hereby coated with a defined amount of saliva film. The strip is then immediately attached to a cap

[h]Colony-forming units (CFUs) denote the number of visual bacterial colonies that are formed following incubation, not the actual number of bacterial cells. Each colony can consist of many single bacteria.
[i]Available from Orion Diagnostica, Helsinki, Finland.

that is screwed to a glass vial, and incubated at 37°C for 48 hours.

The mutans streptococci colonies will appear on the strip as small blue dots but the color can vary from dark blue to pale blue. The density of the colonies is evaluated against a chart provided by the manufacturer (Figure 12–7) and scored 0 to 3, where the scores 2 and 3 correspond to approximately $1 \times 10^5$ CFU and $>1 \times 10^6$ CFU/mL saliva, respectively. When dry, the strips can also be evaluated and divided into groups with the aid of a special device in a stereo microscope with 6–25 × magnification.[70] The strip mutans technique has been proven reliable to use and significantly related to conventional techniques. Sometimes, gas-forming or other nonmutans bacteria can grow in the broth (grayish), but not on the strip. Furthermore, large mutans streptococci colonies may be found on the bottom of the tube. They normally fall from the smooth side of the strip, but usually this will not affect the scoring. A useful advantage with this method is that the strips can be stored for years in a plastic foil for future comparisons.[71]

A further modification of the Strip mutans technique has recently been developed for *site-specific* microbial plaque diagnosis.[72] The sampling of selected sites is carried out either with a wooden toothpick[73] or a small saline-wetted brush[74] and transferred straight across the plastic strip on an elevated pad, thus enabling four sites to be sampled on each strip. After the cultivation procedure as described above, the CFUs are counted and scored on the predetermined area in a microscope or by aid of a chart (Figure 12–8). This method is especially useful for monitoring the outcome of a site-specific antibacterial treatment.[75]

### Lactobacilli Counts

Lactobacilli constitute an acidogenic and aciduric group of microorganisms associated with dental caries.[76] The bacteria need retentive sites for the colonization of tooth surfaces, such as fissures, fillings, gaps, overhangs, etc. Lactobacilli are often found in the deep parts of the caries lesion. Thus, they are considered as secondary invaders and responsible for the *progression of already established lesions.*[14]

*Lactobacilli levels are highly influenced by the intake of dietary carbohydrates, thus reflecting the amount of bacterial substrate and indicating an acid environment within the oral cavity.* The prevalence of lactobacilli is lower compared

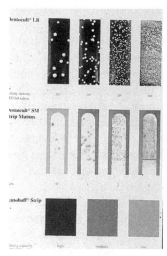

FIGURE 12–7   A chart for evaluating chairside saliva tests as indicated. Four classes are used for bacterial enumeration while three levels are used for buffering capacity.

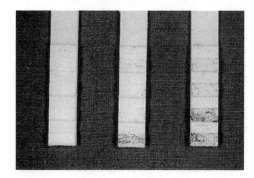

FIGURE 12–8   A specially designed strip for site-specific enumeration of mutans streptococci in plaque.

with mutans streptococci. Approximately 50% of a population exhibits low values while 10 to 20% have high counts.[77] It could however be noted that reports from Scandinavia suggest a decreasing prevalence of lactobacilli in children[78] in spite of unchanged or even increased sugar consumption, and this may partly be explained by diminishing numbers of retentive sites (cavities and restorations) in the young population. The proportion of lactobacilli in the plaque is normally low (<1%), and the presence in saliva and plaque are determined using a selective medium (Rogosa SL-agar[79]) with conventional culturing methods at the laboratory.

*Dip Slide Method for Lactobacilli Counts*

The number of salivary lactobacilli can be estimated with the aid of the Dentocult-LB[h] method,[80] consisting of a plastic device covered with selective agar. Paraffin-stimulated saliva is collected in a cup or a tube. The saliva is poured over both sides of the slide, and the excess allowed dropping off. The slide is then inserted in a plastic container and incubated at 37°C for 4 days. After incubation, the lactobacilli appear as small whitish dots and the number on the agar surface is estimated by comparison with a chart supplied by the manufacturer (see Figure 12–7). As an alternative, the slide can be incubated in room temperature for 7 days. However, this may lead to an increased recovery of yeasts, which may jeopardize the evaluation of the slide.[81] The results of the test can be shown directly to the patient but the slides cannot be stored for longer periods, unless they are stored in a computer with the use of a video camera.

General Comments on Bacterial Values

Most selective media underestimate the real number of targeted bacterial strains. This does not impair the value of the sample as long as the levels are within those of clinical relevance. It is highly advisable not to regard the test results as exact bacterial numbers but rather as *ranges* of bacterial counts. Furthermore, it must be emphasized that counts obtained with different methods cannot be directly compared with each other. There is no apparent association between mutans streptococci and lactobacilli counts although a tendency to high levels of *both* species often can be seen in caries-active patients.[82] This fact emphasizes the assumption that the tests measure two separate stages of the caries process in the oral milieu and cannot be substituted by each other.

*It is recommended not to have a "fixed" position to threshold values regarded as a caries risk.* The risk level for one factor depends on the influence of other factors. One million mutans streptococci per ml of saliva may, under certain conditions, lead to cavity formation, but with a proper diet and fluoride administration, the risk will be considerably lower. For example, a certain level of bacteria or saliva secretion rate does not mean the same for an individual living in a fluoridated area compared with an individual from a low fluoridated or nonfluoridated area.[83,84]

A common question is to what extent must the sampling for the use of the tests be standardized. It is well known that a number of factors such as antibiotics, diet, smoking, toothbrushing, saliva secretion, and retentive sites can affect the number of bacteria in the oral cavity.[28] A normal variation over time of both lactobacilli, mutans streptococci, buffer capacity, and saliva flow rate should always be expected.[85] Studies have shown that *pronounced natural variations are rare in the short-term perspective.*[55,71] The highest bacterial counts in saliva are usually found in the morning before toothbrushing. During daytime, the levels seem to be fairly stable if no particular measures are taken. In epidemiologic surveys, a strict and well-defined collection procedure is of course crucial while such precautions are somewhat limiting for the daily routine work. For the individual patient, the results must be evaluated

in the light of practicalities—they represent the *challenge at the time they were taken.* However, check if the patient is taking or recently had (within 1 month) an antibiotic medication and, if possible, try to avoid sampling just after toothbrushing or eating.

---

## Question 2

Which of the following statements, if any, are correct?

A. A valid test can be both accurate and reliable.

B. Presence of mutans streptococci in the oral cavity always implies a caries risk.

C. A useful caries predictor should have a strong and stable association to caries prevalence.

D. A better correlation usually exists between low-bacterial counts and low-caries risk than between high counts and high risk.

E. Lactobacilli, being highly aciduric, are linked to the initiation of the enamel lesion.

---

Saliva Flow Rate

An appropriate flow of saliva is essential for the maintenance of oral health. It is evident that the oral bacteria are subjected to several important salivary functions, which affect their colonization, survival, and metabolism. The most important mechanisms by which saliva can affect caries are:

• Mechanical cleansing of debris and plaque bacteria

• Antibacterial activity against the oral microflora, i.e., lysis and aggregation

• Buffering and neutralization of plaque acids

• Enhancement of remineralization

The salivary flow from both major and minor glands is controlled by parasympathetic (water,

electrolytes) and sympathetic (proteins) stimuli. The water fraction is most important for the clearance process while the antimicrobial activity resides mainly in the protein fraction.

*Salivary flow rate is considered as a "key" parameter in caries-risk assessment.*[86] Although there is no linear association between salivary flow rate and caries activity, it is important to evaluate whether the secretion is normal or impaired. Absence of saliva, xerostomia, or hyposalivation can result in an extremely increased caries risk. A decreased flow rate is a common side effect to a large number of medicines and radiation therapy.[87] For the individual, a regular and longitudinal followup of the flow rate is of higher clinical value than a single measurement to be able to identify reduction and alterations over time.[85]

*Measurement of Saliva Flow Rate*

When measuring the flow rate, one can either sample unstimulated or stimulated whole saliva. In addition, saliva from separated secretions, parotid or submandibular/sublingual, can be collected. Stimulated whole saliva samples are *most often* used for routine work. The stimulation can be done by paraffin chewing or by adding droplets of a sour liquid (3% citric acid) on the back of the tongue. The amount of saliva obtained is *divided by the collection time* and the secretion is expressed as ml/minute or mL/5min.

For adult patients, a normal stimulated secretion rate is around *1.0 to 1.5 mL/minute*. Values below 0.7 ml/minute should be considered as low and indicate a caries risk.[88] Women generally have somewhat lower stimulated and unstimulated secretion rates than men. In children, the levels highly depend on age and cooperation, but the corresponding levels in preschoolers for stimulated and unstimulated secretions are around 0.5 and 0.3 mL/minute, respectively.

For collection of unstimulated (resting) saliva, the patient is seated in an upright re-

laxed position with the head bent forward. The subject lets the saliva passively drip into a graduated tube for 5 to 15 minutes. An unstimulated secretion of less than 0.1 mL/minute is considered as a risk value. In cases of hyposalivation, the saliva is often viscous and "foamy" and the secreted volume is difficult to determine. A gravitation method is therefore advocated. The test tube is weighed before and after sampling and 1 gram corresponds to approximately one milliliter of saliva.

---

## Question 3

Which of the following statements, if any, are correct?

A. An average collection of 7.5 mL of stimulated whole saliva over 5 minutes is considered abnormally low.

B. A lactobacilli test reflects the carbohydrate intake and retentive sites in the oral cavity.

C. A saliva sample provides accurate information on where in the mouth cariogenic bacteria are harbored.

D. Caries-risk assessment for the individual gathers data from case history, clinical examination, and laboratory tests.

E. A person with a mutans streptococci score of 3 (high counts) cannot stay caries-free and demineralization will inevitably occur.

---

### Buffering Capacity of Saliva

The buffering capacity of saliva is important for the maintenance of normal pH levels in saliva and plaque. A low secretion might indicate a low buffering effect and a weak inverse relationship to caries has been noted by several investigators.[89,90] Both the saliva secretion rate and buffer capacity differ however at different parts of the mouth. The composition and acidogenicity of plaque may be affected differently when situated close to a salivary duct or hidden

deep down in a fissure. Nevertheless, unfavorable values of buffer capacity and salivary flow rate should be considered as risk factors for the individual. The tests commonly used are based on the titration technique with the final pH determined by a dye color change.

### Dentobuff Method for Measurement of Buffer Capacity

A simple chairside method to measure the buffer capacity of saliva, the Dentobuff strip[j], has been developed by Ericsson and Bratthall.[91] A small amount of acid is impregnated on a pH indicator strip. One droplet of stimulated saliva is placed on the testing pad of the strip in a flat position to dissolve the acid. After exactly 5 minutes, the color of the strip is compared with a provided chart, indicating the final pH. The method reflects mainly the bicarbonate buffer system and identifies saliva with low (yellow), intermediate (green), and normal (blue) buffer capacity (see Figure 12–7). It is important that the test is read after exactly 5 minutes as color will change with time and thus give misleading results. The yellow color indicates a final pH of 4 or less, meaning that the saliva was unable to raise the pH. This result should be considered as a risk value.

### Collecting Bacterial and Saliva Samples

To obtain information from *all* the chairside methods the following procedure is recommended.

- Prepare the chairside kits and inform the patient.
- Start the sampling with the patient in an upright position. Ask the patient to chew paraffin and swallow the saliva after 1 minute. Then start a timer for the secretion rate and instruct the patient to spit frequently into a graded test tube.

[j]Orion Diagnostica, Espoo, Finland

- Stop spitting after 5 minutes and take the Strip mutants test on the tongue.
- Measure the amount of saliva and calculate secretion rate.
- Take a droplet of the saliva with a pipette on the Dentobuff strip. Set timer for 5 minutes.
- Pour the remaining saliva on both sides of the Dentocult LB agar and let excess drip off.
- Incubate mutans streptococci and lacto-bacilli tests.
- Evaluate buffer strip after 5 minutes, mutans streptococci after 2 days, and lactobacilli after 4 days.

### What Is the Next Step?

The effectiveness of caries risk and caries activity tests has been evaluated in various populations over the past decades with more or less encouraging findings.[40,92,93] The risk or activity approach *per se* is not a controversial issue but rather by which means this assessment should be done. Even though the multifactorial models are proven as useful in one country or society, it might be less useful in others.[94] Another important fact is that risk assessment programs must be evaluated continuously since the value can vary over time. A striking example can be taken from lactobacilli tests when used as a didactic tool to reduce sugar-consumption in schoolchildren. Two decades ago, this program reduced caries increment with 50%[57] while it was of only limited value when recently reevaluated within the same community.[95]

For the individual, the identification of factors responsible for caries risk and caries activity should form the basis for targeted action against the etiological factors involved. Knowledge of risk factors gives the patient an opportunity to reflect over his or her situation and an option to take a personal responsibility for the future oral health. It may be argued that there is a weak scientific support for the fact that gained knowledge is an efficient tool to change

a nonhealthy dental behavior.[96] This may be true for a non-specific general message and therefore it seems even more important to individualize the information, as disclosed by the tests. Both the therapist and the patient can be made aware on the main problem and focus on one strategy rather then the whole concept. In that aspect, the tests are also a matter of quality care and a guidance simply to do the right thing at the right costs. As previously stated, the relative importance of one risk factor may differ from one patient or group of patients to another. For example, it has been shown that the main risk factor for white-spot lesions during treatment with fixed orthodontic appliances was poor oral hygiene,[97] and therefore, it may not be meaningful or cost-effective to focus on diet. Similarly, as the level of metabolic control seem to be a stronger predictor for caries than mutans streptococci in children with Type 1 diabetes,[98] the focus should be on diet rather than antibacterial measures. In many cases, however, more than one risk factor or risk indicator are strongly involved. A common question is then whether or not it is meaningful to change or improve only one of them. Yes, it is of absolute importance since the balance in the oral environment between demineralization and remineralization is equivocal and in many cases, also a minor improvement may help the patient over the threshold level and to be on track. Moreover, after a successful management of one etiological factor, the self-esteem and motivation may grow to proceed with the next factor.

The other way around is probably of even greater importance. There is consensus in literature on the high specificity of caries risk and activity assessments to select individuals at low risk for future caries. This is a very positive message to communicate and the patient may have an option to extend the recall intervals. Thereby, resources can be redirected and money saved for the patient and for the society. At the end of the day, it is a matter of philosophy and quality—the teeth are, with very few

exceptions, healthy when they erupt and it's a challenge for the dental profession to guide and assist their patients to keep them that way in a cost-efficient way.

## Other Suggested Caries Activity Tests

In order to predict caries risk or determine the disease activity, a variety of other methods have been suggested. A few of these are briefly described and commented on below.

### Snyder Test

In this test, suggested by Snyder,[99] sampled saliva is inoculated into a glucose agar and acid formation is determined by a color indicator. The procedure reflects the total number and the acidogenicity of the salivary bacteria and can be used as an alternative to the lactobacilli test.[53]

### Viscosity of Saliva

The viscosity of saliva is an important factor for the subjective perception of dry mouth and hyposalivation. Today, however, there are no methods of clinical significance in use to estimate the viscosity and furthermore, its relation to caries incidence is not clear. Measurement of oral mucosal friction by the aid of a rheologic device has been developed and may, in the light of the widespread use of xerogenic drugs, grow in importance for elderly patients.[100]

### Dip-Slide Measurement of Salivary Yeast

In general, the presence of an oral yeast infection can be considered as a reflection of the host response and indicative of a medically compromised patient. A high number of salivary yeasts are often found in patients with hyposalivation. Moreover, fungi are aciduric and their presence might be a reflection of an acidic environment and caries activity.[101] A dip-slide system for measuring oral yeast (*Candida albicans*) infection, ORICULT-N,[k] (Figure 12–7)

has been developed and is commercially available.[102]

### Plaque-forming Rate

General plaque has been suggested as a caries predictor.[103] The speed of plaque development can be estimated by the plaque-forming-rate index (PFRI).[104] Twenty-four hours after professional tooth cleaning, plaque reaccumulation rate is assessed on a scale from 1 to 5 on 6 measuring points per tooth. No oral hygiene measures are carried out during the 24-hour period. Although used in several clinical studies with a positive relationship to caries incidence, the method has not gained a widespread clinical acceptance.

### Plaque pH Measurement—Acid Formation by Dental Plaque

Plaque pH can be directly measured intraorally by using either glass or antimony electrodes.[105] Caries-active subjects exhibit lower resting pH and final pH following sucrose rinses compared to caries-free persons. Telemetric monitoring, however, seems more useful in evaluating pH changes after intake of various foods than in determining caries activity.[106] Consequently, the technique is more often used in research laboratories at universities rather than in the everyday dental office.

### Future Methods

A serious concern with the culturing methods of today is the time span from sampling until the results are available for the professionals and their patients. Furthermore, sampling must be planned to fit weekends and other activities. It is not likely that the current available tests can be significantly improved, especially if they are to be suitable for chairside use or aimed for field conditions. New tests, measuring for example bacterial adhesion and bacteria-binding saliva ligands as genetically determining factors for caries, might be developed. Existing immunologic methods like enzyme-linked immunosorbent assay (ELISA) kits will probably

[k]Orion Diagnostica, Espoo, Finland

be transferred from the specialized laboratory to the dental clinic in coming years. A call for faster and more accurate techniques will certainly stimulate the development of new and improved products. Moreover, improved knowledge of lifestyle-factors such as oral hygiene and sugar consumption pattern obtained through qualitative studies can add precision to the caries risk evaluation process.

### Question 4

Which of the following statements, if any, are correct?

A. Salivary mutans streptococci levels are influenced by antibiotic medication.

B. A high-buffer capacity is often found in patients with a low-secretion rate.

C. Microbiologic caries activity tests can be used as didactic and motivating tools in caries prevention.

D. Past caries experience is found to be the most valuable single predictor in many caries risk studies.

E. The predictive ability of a test depends on the prevalence of the disease in the population.

## SUMMARY

Caries is a *transmissible* local infection and aciduric microorganisms, like *mutans streptococci* and *lactobacilli,* are the prime pathogens. This chapter has reviewed the ecologic events leading to caries development: (1) early establishment of mutans streptococci, (2) microbial shift and, (3) enamel demineralization. This process can be *prevented, arrested, or reversed* with the knowledge of factors such as the microbial challenge, intake of refined carbohydrates, and the body's capacity of self-repair.

*Caries-risk assessment* strategies can be applied for populations, larger or smaller groups, or individuals. There is no single test that can accurately reflect the complex etiology of caries. Although tests of mutans streptococci and lactobacilli show strong correlation with caries in cross-sectional and longitudinal surveys, they are generally of limited value for risk-screening purposes in communities with a low prevalence of caries. In groups of individuals with higher caries incidence such as medically compromised patients, inhabitants of low socioeconomic areas, and low fluoride areas, the predictive power and the value of the microbial tests are increased. Negative or very low counts of mutans streptococci and lactobacilli are highly predictive for subjects at low risk of getting caries. The past caries prevalence is the most powerful single predictor on a population basis.

For the individual patient, a *risk assessment* is performed by compiling data of importance for caries development from the case history, clinical examination, and chairside tests. Microbiologic tests should be regarded as monitors of the oral ecology and repeated samplings may indicate deviations from the normality of the individual. Any increase in the challenge factors or decrease in defense and repair factors at any time should be considered as a warning sign. This knowledge should form the basis for an individualized and targeted preventive oral health care program.

Chairside tests covering bacterial challenge, diet, and remineralization potential of saliva are described. The simplified methods can be characterized as semiquantitative

although they significantly correspond to conventional laboratory methods. Furthermore, the chairside methods have been proven useful as a didactic tool in patient education and motivation.

Many diagnostic criteria of caries activity that are used today represent historic events. The chairside microbiologic tests improve quality and add a possibility of early risk assessment and diagnosis. We hope that this chapter has given the reader inspiration to incorporate caries activity tests in their daily work, for the benefit of their patients.

## ANSWERS AND EXPLANATIONS

1. A and E—correct.

    B—incorrect. Two examinations are necessary to determine the number of carious lesions occurring over a given amount of time.

    C—incorrect. Sensitivity is the percentage of subjects with a positive test who develop the disease.

    D—incorrect. Caries-risk assessment is recommended in a low caries population with a skewed distribution.

2. A, B, C, and D—correct.

    E—incorrect. Lactobacilli are more commonly associated with cavitation and progression of existing lesions.

3. B and D—correct.

    A—incorrect. The stimulated secretion rate of whole saliva is 1.5 mL/minute, which is normal.

    C—incorrect. Plaque samples disclose where the bacteria are harbored.

    E—incorrect. Score 3 (corresponding to $10^6$ CFUs) indicates caries risk but not necessarily demineralization.

4. A, C, D, and E—correct.

    B—incorrect. A low buffering capacity is often found in patients with a low stimulated secretion rate.

### Self-evaluation Questions

1. If an epidemiologic clinical caries survey is being conducted, the number of decayed teeth (d; D) present at that time constitutes a caries _____ study; if the same patients are reexamined 1 year later, the number of new decayed teeth constitutes a caries _____ study.

2. The two most common mutans streptococci strains in humans are *Streptococcus* _____ and *Streptococcus* _____.

3. An incipient enamel lesion can be seen with the unaided eye. (True, False)

4. Usually, mutans streptococci are established during childhood, between ages _____ and _____, but may increase in numbers during the following years.

5. Studies have shown a family pattern concerning mutans streptococci, meaning that bacteria often are transferred from _____ to children, but other sources may also be found.

6. Chairside bacterial test results in saliva should be regarded as _____ rather than exact bacterial numbers.

7. A risk factor plays an essential role in the _____ of the disease while a closely associated variable that is not causative is called a _____.

8. With the decreasing prevalence of caries seen over the last decades in the industrialized world, one could expect a greater number of (false-negatives) (false-positives) to be diagnosed.

9. A microbial shift in dental plaque can occur when _____ microorganism(s) are favored.

10. The positive predictive value (PV+) is probably of highest interest for the clinician since the _____ for an individual with a positive test to develop the disease is denoted.

## Useful Dental Websites for Caries Activity Information

- World Health Organization (WHO): Oral Health Country Profile Project http//www.whocollab.odont.mah.se/index.html

- International Health Care Foundation (IHCF): Caries-risk assessment; saliva interactive site, WWW-based management of dental prevention; Cariogram; other dental web sites of interest http://www.ihcf.li

- Malmö University, Faculty of Odontology: continuously updated list of references on caries risk assessment, mutans streptococci and lactobacilli. http://www.db.mah.se/car/data/riskbasic.html

- NIH Consensus Development Conference on Diagnosis and Management of Dental Caries Throughout Life: complete version of papers on caries diagnosis and caries risk. http://nidcr.nih.gov/news/consensus.asp

- Orion Diagnostics, Turku, Finland: manufacturer of kits for saliva diagnosis http://www.oriondiagnostica.fi

# REFERENCES

1. van Houte, J. (1994). Role of microorganisms in caries etiology. *J Dent Res*, 1994; 73:672–81.
2. Marsh, P. D. (1994). Microbial ecology of dental plaque and its significance in health and disease. *Adv Dent Res*, 8:263–271.
3. Köhler, B., Andreen, I., & Jonsson, B. (1984). The effect of caries-preventive measures in mothers on dental caries and the presence of the oral bacteria *Streptococcus mutans* and lactobacilli in their children. *Archs Oral Biol*, 29:879–83.
4. Emanuelsson, I. R. (2001). Mutans streptococci—in families and on tooth sites. Studies on the distribution, acquisition and persistence using DNA fingerprinting. *Swed Dent J*, Suppl, 148:1–66.
5. Berkowitz, R. J., Turner, J., & Green, P. (1981). Maternal salivary levels of *Streptococcus mutans* and primary oral infection of infants. *Archs Oral Biol*, 26:147–49.
6. Köhler, B., Bratthall, D., & Krasse, B. (1983). Preventive measures in mothers influence the establishment of bacterium *Streptococcus mutans* in their infants. *Archs Oral Biol*, 28:225–31.
7. Brown, J., Junner, C., & Liew, V. (1985). A study of *Streptococcus mutans* levels in both infants with bottle caries and their mothers. *Austr Dent J*, 30:96–98.
8. Alaluusua, S., Kleemola-Kujala, E., Nyström, M., Evalähti, M., & Grönros, L. (1987). Caries in primary teeth and salivary *Streptococcus mutans* and lactobacilli levels as indicators of caries in permanent teeth. *Pediatr Dent*, 9:126–130.
9. Köhler, B., Andreen, I., & Jonsson, B. (1988). The earlier the colonization by mutans streptococci, the higher the caries prevalence at 4 years of age. *Oral Immunol Microbiol*, 3:14–17.
10. Grindefjord, M., Dahllöf, G., Wikner, S., Höjer, M., & Modéer T. (1991). Prevalence of mutans streptococci in one-year-old children. *Oral Microbiol Immunol*, 6:280–83.
11. Twetman, S., Petersson, L. G. (1996). Prediction of caries in pre-school children in relation to fluoride exposure. *Eur J Oral Sci*, 104:523–28.
12. Caufield, P. W., Cutter, G. R., & Dasanayake, A. P. (1993). Initial acquisition of mutans streptococci by infants: Evidence for a discrete window of infectivity. *J Dent Res*, 72:37–45.
13. Brambilla, E., Felloni, A., Gagliani, M., Malerba, A., Garcia-Godoy, F., & Strohmenger, L. (1998). Caries prevention during pregnancy. Results of a 32-month study. *J Am Dent Assoc*, 129;871–77.
14. van Houte, J. (1980). Bacterial specificity in the etiology of dental caries. *Int Dent J*, 30:305–26.
15. van Ruyven, F. O., Lingstrom, P., van Houte, J., & Kent, R. (2000). Relationship among mutans streptococci, "low-pH" bacteria, and iodophilic polysaccharide-producing bacteria in dental plaque and early enamel caries in humans. *J Dent Res*, 79; 778–84.
16. Berkowitz, R. J., Turner, J., & Hughes, C. (1984). Microbial characteristics of human dental caries associated with prolonged bottle feeding. *Arch Oral Biol*, 29:949–51.
17. Emilson, C. G. (1994). Potential efficacy of chlorhexidine against mutans streptococci and human dental caries. *J Dent Res*, 73:682–91.
18. Emilson, C. G., Lindquist, B., & Wennerholm, K. (1987). Recolonization of human tooth surfaces by *Streptococcus mutans* after suppression by chlorhexidine treatment. *J Dent Res*, 66:1503–8.
19. Bowden, G. H. (1997). Does assessment of microbial composition of plaque/saliva allow for diagnosis of disease activity of individuals? *Community Dent Oral Epidemiol*, 25:76–81.
20. Geddes, D. A. M. (1975) Acids produced by human dental plaque metabolism in situ. *Caries Res*, 9:98–109.
21. Ögaard, B., Rölla, G., & Arends J. (1988). Orthodontic appliances and enamel demineralization. 1. Lesion development. *Am J Orthod*, 94:68–73.

22. Lang, K. P., Hotz, P. R., Gusberti, F., & Joss, A. (1987). Longitudinal, clinical and microbiological study on the relationship between infection with *Streptococcus mutans* and the development of caries in humans. *Oral Microbiol Immunol,* 2:39–47.

23. Pitts, N. B. (1983). Monitoring of caries progression in permanent and primary posterior approximal enamel by bitewing radiography. *Community Dent Oral Epidemiol,* 11:228–35.

24. Shwartz, M., Gröndahl, H. G., Pliskin, J. S., & Boffa, J. (1984). A longitudinal analysis from bitewing radiographs of the rate of progression of approximal carious lesions through human dental enamel. *Archs Oral Biol,* 29:529–36.

25. Mejàre, I., Källestål, C., & Stenlund, H. (1999). Incidence and progression of approximal caries from 11 to 22 years of age: A prospective radiographic study. *Caries Res,* 33:93–100.

26. Hausen, H. (1997). Caries prediction—state of the art. *Community Dent Oral Epidemiol,* 25:87–96.

27. Rothman, K. J. (1986). *Modern epidemiology.* Boston: Little, Brown and Co.

28. Bratthall, D., & Carlsson, J. (1986). Current status of caries activity tests. In Thylstrup, A., & Fejerskov, O., Eds. *Textbook of cariology* (pp. 149–265). Copenhagen: Munksgaard.

29. Grindefjord, M., Dahllöf, G., Nilsson, B., & Modeer, T. (1996). Stepwise prediction of dental caries in children up to 3.5 years of age. *Caries Res,* 30:343–8.

30. Rose, G. (1985). Sick individuals and sick populations. *Int J Epidemiol,* 14:32–38.

31. Petersson, H. G., & Bratthall, D. (1996). The caries decline: A review of reviews. *Eur J Oral Sci,* 104:436–43.

32. van Houte, J. (1993). Microbiological predictors of caries risk. *Adv Dent Res,* 7:87–96.

33. Disney, J. A., Abernathy, J. R., Graves, R. C., Mavriello, S. M., Bohannan, H. M., & Zach, D. D. (1992). Comparative effectiveness of visual/tactile and simplified screening examinations in caries risk assessment. *Community Dent Oral Epidemiol,* 20:326–32.

34. Demers, M., Brodeur, J. M., Simpard, P. L., Mourton, C., Veilleux, G., & Franchette, S. (1990). Caries predictors suitable for mass-screening in children. A literature review. *Community Dent Oral Epidemiol,* 7:11–21.

35. Stamm, J. W., Disney, J. A., Beck, J. D., Weintraub, J. A., & Stewart, P. W. (1993). The University of North Carolina caries risk assessment study: Final results and some alternative modeling approaches. In Bowen, W. H., Tabak, L. A., Eds. *Cariology for the nineties* (pp. 209–234). Rochester, NY: University of Rochester Press.

36. Kingman, A. (1990). Statistical issues in risk models for caries. In Bader, J. D., Ed. *Risk assessment in dentistry* (pp. 193–200). Chapel Hill, NC: University of North Carolina Dental Ecology.

37. Disney, J. A., Graves, R. C., Stamm, J. W., et al. (1992). The University of North Carolina Caries Risk Assessment Study: Further developments in caries risk prediction. *Community Dent Oral Epidemiol,* 20:64–75.

38. Leverett, D. H., Proskin, H. M., Featherstone, J. D., et al. (1993). Caries risk assessment in a longitudinal discrimination study. *J Dent Res,* 72:538–43.

39. Hausen, H., Seppä, L., & Fejerskov, O. (1994). Can caries be predicted? In Thylstrup A, Fejerskov O, eds. *Textbook of clinical cariology* (2nd ed.) (pp. 393–411). Copenhagen: Munksgaard.

40. Powell, L. V. (1998). Caries prediction: a review of the literature. *Community Dent Oral Epidemiol,* 26:361–71.

41. Backer Dirks, O. (1966). Posteruptive changes in dental enamel. *J Dent Res,* 45:503–511.

42. Wendt, L. K., Hallonsten, A. L., & Koch, G. (1991). Dental caries in one- and two-year-old children living in Sweden. *Swed Dent J,* 15:1–6.

43. Grindefjord, M., Dahllöf, G., & Modéer T. (1995). Caries development in children from 2.5 to 3.5 years of age. A longitudinal study. *Caries Res,* 29:449–54.

44. Hinds, K., & Gregory, J. R. (1995). National diet and nutrition survey: Children aged 1.5 to 4.5 years. Vol. 2. *Report of the dental survey.* London: The Stationery Office Books.

45. Newbrun, E. (1993). Problems in caries diagnosis. *Int Dent J,* 43:133–42.

46. Bratthall, D., & Tynelius-Bratthall, G. (1994). Diagnosis as basis of causal treatment: Tools and tests for evaluation of caries and periodontal diseases. In Illig, V. *Professional prevention in dentistry. Advances in dentistry 1* (pp. 29–68). Munich: Williams & Wilkins.

47. Bratthall, D. (1996). Dental caries: Intervened-interrupted-interpreted. Concluding remarks and cariography. *Eur J Oral Sci,* 104:486–91.

48. Hänsel Petersson, G., Twetman, S., & Bratthall, D. (2002) Evaluation of a computer program for caries risk assessment in schoolchildren. *Caries Res.* 36: 327–340.

49. Sreebney, L. M., & Schwartz, S. S. (1986). A reference guide to drugs and dry mouth. *Gerodontology,* 5:75–99.

50. Schuler, C. F. (2001). Inherited risk for susceptibility to dental caries. *J Dent Educ,* 65:1038–45.

51. Alalusuua, S., & Malmivirta, R. (1994). Early plaque accumulation—a sign for caries risk in young children. *Community Dent Oral Epidemiol,* 22:273–76.

52. Keyes, P. H. (1962). Recent advances in dental caries research. Bacteriology. *Int Dent J,* 12:443–64.

53. Birkhed, D., Edwardsson, S., & Andersson, H. (1981). Comparison among a dip-slide test (Dentocult), plate count and Snyder test for estimating number of lactobacilli in human saliva. *J Dent Res,* 60:1832–41.

54. Bratthall, D., & Carlsson, P. (1989). Clinical microbiology of saliva. In Tenovuo, J., Ed. *Human saliva: Clinical chemistry and microbiology* (pp. 203–241). Boca Raton, FL: CRC Press.

55. Togelius, J., Kristoffersson, K., Andersson, H., & Bratthall, D. (1984). *Streptococcus mutans* in saliva: Intraindividual variations and relation to the number of colonized sites. *Acta Odontol Scand,* 42:157.

56. Lindquist, B., Emilson, C. G. (1990). Distribution and prevalence of mutans streptococci in the human dentition. *J Dent Res,* 69:1160–66.

57. Crossner, C. G., & Unell, L. (1986). Salivary diagnostic counts as a diagnostic and didactic tool in caries prevention. *Community Dent Oral Epidemiol,* 14:156–60.

58. Larmas, M. (1992). Saliva and dental caries: Diagnostic tests for normal dental practice. *Int Dent J,* 42:199–208.

59. Twetman, S., Ståhl, B., & Nederfors, T. (1994). Use of Strip mutans test in the assessment of caries risk in a group of preschool children. *Int J Paediatr Dent,* 4:245–50.

60. MacPherson, L. M. D., MacFarlane, T. W., & Stephen, K. W. (1990). An intra-oral appliance study of the plaque microflora associated with early enamel demineralization. *J Dent Res,* 69:1712–16.

61. Thibodeau, E. A., & O'Sullivan, D. M. (1995). Salivary mutans streptococci and incidence of caries in preschool children. *Caries Res,* 29:148–53.

62. Lindquist, B., Emilson, C. G., & Wennerholm, K. (1989). Relationship between mutans streptococci in saliva and their colonization of tooth surfaces. *Oral Microbiol Immunol,* 4:71–76.

63. Kristoffersson, K., Gröndahl, H. G., & Bratthall, D. (1985). The more *Streptococcus mutans,* the more caries on approximal surfaces. *J Dent Res,* 64:58–61.

64. Coykendall, A. L., & Gustafson, K. B. (1986). Taxonomy of *Streptococcus mutans.* In Hamada S. et al., Proceedings of an International Conference on Cellular, Molecular and Clinical Aspects of *Streptococcus mutans.* Amsterdam, New York, Oxford: Elsevier, 157.

65. Gold, O., Jordan, H. V., & van Houte, J. (1973). A selective medium for *Streptococcus mutans.* *Archs Oral Biol,* 18:1357–64.

66. Köhler, B., & Bratthall, D. (1979). Practical method to facilitate estimation of *Streptococcus mutans* levels in saliva. *J Clin Microbiol,* 9:594–98.

67. Matsukubo, T., Ohta, K., Maki, Y., Takeuchi, M., & Takazoe I. (1981). A semiquantitative determination of *Streptococcus mutans* using its adherent ability in selective medium. *Caries Res,* 15:40–45.

68. Jordan, H. V., Laraway, R., Snirch, R., & Marmel, M. (1987). A simplified diagnostic system for cultural detection and enumeration of *Streptococcus mutans*. *J Dent Res*, 66:57–61.
69. Jensen, B., & Bratthall, D. (1989). A new method for the estimation of mutans streptococci in saliva. *J Dent Res*, 68:468–71.
70. Twetman, S., & Frostner, N. (1991). Salivary mutans streptococci and caries prevalence in 8-year-old Swedish schoolchildren. *Swed Dent J*, 15:145–51.
71. El-Nadef, M. A. I., & Bratthall, D. (1991). Individual variations in count of mutans streptococci measured by "Strip mutans" method. *Scand J Dent Res*, 99:8–12.
72. Bratthall, D., Hoszek, A., & Zhao, X. (1997). Evaluation of a simplified method for site-specific determination of mutans streptococci levels. *Swed Dent J*, 20:215–20.
73. Wallman, C., & Krasse, B. (1993). A simple method for monitoring mutans streptococci in margins of restorations. *J Dent*, 21:216–19.
74. Twetman, S. (1995). Eine einfache methode Methode zur Überprüfung der Wirkung der topikalen Behandlung mit einem antibakteriellem Lack. *ZWR*, 104:381–83.
75. Twetman, S., & Petersson, L. G. (1997). Effect of different chlorhexidine varnish regimens on mutans streptococci levels in interdental plaque and saliva. *Caries Res*, 31:189–93.
76. Crossner, C. G. (1981). Salivary lactobacillus counts in the prediction of caries activity. *Community Dent Oral Epidemiol*, 9:182–90.
77. Klock, B., & Krasse, B. (1977). Microbial and salivary conditions in 9–12 year old children. *Scand J Dent Res*, 85:56–63.
78. Nylander, A., Kumlin, I., Martinsson, M., & Twetman, S. (2000). Decreasing prevalence of salivary lactobacilli in Swedish schoolchildren 1987–1998. *Eur J Oral Sci*, 108:255–58.
79. Rogosa, M., Mitchell, J. A., & Wieseman, R. F. (1951). A selective medium for the isolation and enumeration of oral lactobacilli. *J Dent Res*, 30:682–89.
80. Larmas, M. (1975). A new dip-slide method for the counting of salivary lactobacilli. *Proc Finn Dent Soc*, 71:31–35.
81. Crossner, C. G., & Hagberg, C. (1977). A clinical and microbiological evaluation of the Dentocult dip-slide test. *Swed Dent J*, 1:85–94.
82. Zickert, I., Emilson, C. G., & Krasse, B. (1985). Prediction of caries incidence based on salivary S. mutans and lactobacilli counts. *J Dent Res*, 64:347.
83. Twetman, S., Mathiasson, A., Varela, J., & Bratthall, D. (1990). Mutans streptococci in saliva and dental caries in children living in a high and a low fluoride area. *Oral Microbiol Immunol*, 6:169–71.
84. Twetman, S., Petersson, L. G., & Pakhomov, G. N. (1996). Caries incidence in relation to salivary mutans streptococci and fluoride varnish applications in preschool children from low- and optimal-fluoride areas. *Caries Res*, 30:347–53.
85. Tukia-Kulmala, H., & Tenovuo, J. (1993). Intra- and inter-individual variation in salivary flow rate, buffer effect, lactobacilli, and mutans streptococci among 11- to 12-year-old schoolchildren. *Acta Odontol Scand*, 51:31–37.
86. Tenovuo, J. (1997). Salivary parameters of relevance for assessing caries activity in individuals and populations. *Community Dent Oral Epidemiol*, 25:82–86.
87. Sreebny, L. M., & Valdini, A. (1987). Xerostomia. A neglected symptom. *Arch Intern Med*, 147:1333–37.
88. Heintze, U., Birkhed, D., & Björn, H. (1983). Secretion rate and buffer effect of resting and stimulated whole saliva as a function of age and sex. *Swed Dent J*, 7:227–38.
89. Ericsson, Y. (1959). Clinical investigations on the salivary buffering action. *Acta Odontol Scand*, 17:131–65.
90. Alaluusua, S., Kleemoja-Kujala, E., Grönros, L., & Evälahti, M. (1990). Salivary caries tests as predictors of future caries increment in teenagers. A three-year longitudinal study. *Oral Microbiol Immunol*, 5:77–81.

91. Ericson, D., & Bratthall, D. (1989). A simplified method to estimate the salivary buffer capacity. *Scand J Dent Res*, 97:405–407.

92. van Palenstein Helderman, W. H., Mikx, F. H., Van't Hof, M. A., Trvin G, & Kalsbeek, H. (2001). The value of salivary bacterial counts as a supplement to past caries experience as caries predictor in children. *Caries Res*, 109:312–15.

93. Pienihäkkinen, K., & Jokela, J. (2002). Clinical outcomes of risk-based caries prevention in pre-school aged children. *Community Dent Oral Epidemiol*, 30:143–50.

94. Zero, D., Fontano, M., & Lennon, A. (2001). Clinical applications and outcomes of using indicators of risk in caries management. *J Dent Educ*, 65:1126–32.

95. Nylander, A., Kumlin, I., Martinsson, M., & Twetman, S. (2001). Effect of a school-based preventing program with salivary lactobacillus counts as a sugar-motivating tool on caries increment in adolescents. *Acta Odontol Scand*, 59:88–92.

96. Kay, E. J., & Locker, D. (1996). Is dental health education effective? A systematic review of current evidence. *Community Dent Oral Epidemiol*, 24:231–35.

97. Øgaard, B., Larsson, E., & Birkhed, D. (2002). Prediction of white spot lesion development during orthodontic treatment. *Caries Res*, 36:174–222.

98. Twetman, S., Johansson, I., Birkhed, D., & Nederfors, T. (2002). Caries incidence in young type 1 diabetes mellitus patients in relation to metabolic control and caries-associated risk factors. *Caries Res*, 36:31–35.

99. Snyder, M. (1951). Laboratory methods in the clinical evaluation of caries activity. *J Am Dent Assoc*, 42:400–13.

100. Nederfors, T., Henriksson, V., Ericson, T., & Dahlöf, C. (1993). Oral mucosal friction and subjective perception of dry mouth in relation to salivary secretion. *Scand J Dent Res*, 101:44–48.

101. Pienihäkkinen, K. (1988). Salivary lactobacilli and yeasts in relation to caries increment. *Acta Odontol Scand*, 46:57–62.

102. Parvinen, T., & Larmas, M. (1981). The relation of stimulated salivary flow rate and pH to lactobacillus and yeast concentrations in saliva. *J Dent Res*, 60:1929–35.

103. Wendt, L. K., Hallonsten, A. L., Koch, G, Birkhed, D. (1994). Oral hygiene in relation to caries development and immigrant status in infants and toddlers. *Scand J Dent Res*, 102:269–73.

104. Axelsson, P. (1991). A four-point scale for selection of caries risk patients, based on salivary S. *mutans* levels and plaque formation rate index. In Johnson N., Ed. *Rick markers for oral diseases*, Vol. 1 (pp. 158–70). London: Cambridge University Press.

105. Neff, D. (1967). Acid production from different carbohydrate sources in human plaque in situ. *Caries Res*, 1:78–87.

106. Lingström, P., & Birkhed, D. (1993). Plaque pH and oral retention after consumption of starchy snack products at normal and low secretion rate. *Acta Odontol Scand*, 51:379–88.

# CHAPTER 13

# Periodontal Disease Prevention: Facts, Risk Assessment, and Evaluation

*Norman O. Harris*
*Donald E. Willmann*

## OBJECTIVES

*At the end of this chapter, it will be possible to:*

1. Cite the one main sign that delineates gingivitis from periodontitis.
2. Explain the rationale for the latest classification of the periodontal diseases.
3. Explain the purpose of O'Leary's Index, Silness and Löe's Plaque Index, and Löe and Silness's Gingival Index.
4. Describe how manual periodontal probes are used, and contrast them to constant-force electronic probes.
5. Explain how pocket depth and attachment loss are measured and how gingival recession measurements are related to both.
6. Clarify the differences between the Community Periodontal Index of Treatment Needs (CPITN) and the Periodontal Screening and Recording System (PSR).
7. Discuss the value of the gingival crevicular fluid and how the flow is quantitated.
8. Explain why smoking constitutes a high-risk habit that jeopardizes the prevention, treatment and maintenance of the periodontal diseases.

# INTRODUCTION

In 1875, Riggs' disease,[a] (later known as pyorrhea[b] alveolaris[1,2] and still later as periodontal disease) was easy to diagnose. If pus could be expelled from the gingival crevice by exerting finger pressure over the root, from the apex towards the crown, the correct diagnosis was pyorrhea alveolaris.[3] This diagnosis could be confirmed by placing a drop or two of guaiacum on the exudate producing a deep blue color.[4] At the time it was estimated that 95% of all people over 25 were "more or less affected."[5] Of interest is the fact that systemic conditions were suspect as possibly associated with, or as causal agents of pyorrhea alveolaris—such conditions as gastric dyspepsia, phthisis,[c] adenoids, nasal catarrh, constipation, general congestion due to intemperance, malnutrition, and cold feet or other extremities that indicate poor circulation.[3]

Throughout the first half of the 20th century, pyorrhea alvolaris and receding gums remained the popular terms for the disease by both the profession and lay persons. The cause of pyorrhea alveolaris at the time was attributed to the presence of calculus.[6] Both the long-time terminology and the well-established calculus etiology was to again change. Periodontal disease was to supercede the designation of pyorrhea alveolaris while the accepted etiology of calculus[6] was dropped in favor of a nonspecific plaque hypothesis. According to the nonspecific hypothesis, periodontal disease was caused by a mixed overgrowth of known and unknown organisms in the dental plaque.[7,8] It was still assumed that once a patient was "infected with periodontal disease," the process became more severe with time; in other words, periodontal disease was considered a pathologic penalty for aging. The public still continued to recognize periodontal disease as an inflammatory disease characterized by *periododontal pockets* accompanied with a *silent bone loss*.

By the mid-20th century, the "non" of the nonspecific hypothesis was dropped in favor of a new, "specific bacterial hypothesis" that now postulated that gingivitis and periodontitis were caused by specific as well as still-unknown bacterial species indigent to the plaque.[8] At the same time, a consensus began to emerge that the one-time single periodontal disease was instead, a series of different, but related diseases categorized as (1) gingivitis and (2) adult, prepubertal, juvenile, rapidly progressive, and refractory periodontitis. With this change, calculus rebounded into a secondary etiological role, where its porous surface was, and still is, believed to serve both as a *habitat* for plaque bacteria and their end products and as an *irritant* to the marginal gingival tissues.[9–11] The presence of subgingival calculus contributes to the progression and chronicity of periodontal disease.[9,12]

The relationship between the different periodontal diseases was not, and is not yet well understood. This was underscored by the past classification system that was based on a narrative description that related to the patient's age at the time of onset,

---

[a]Riggs' disease: Named after a Boston Dentist. Dr. Riggs extracted the first tooth ever to be extracted under general anesthesia. His patient was Dr. Horace Wells, the dentist given credit for the discovery of nitrous oxide as a anesthetic.
[b]Pyorrhea = pus.
[c]Phthisis = asthma.

rapidity of disease progression, response to therapy, and severity of the disease—and not to definite causal agents like for caries, where mutans streptococci and lactobacilli are the prime cariogenic pathogens.[13]

There are still major voids of knowledge about the specific periodontal pathogens, or those that might be indicted in the future as synergistic or causal to the periodontal disease process. Plaque samples from individuals with periodontitis can demonstrate approximately 350 microbial species in the dental plaque and about 150 species in the supragingival plaque, tongue,and other oral structures.[14] Yet, singularly or in combination, a very strong case can now be made for implicating among others, *Actinobacillus actinomycetemcomitans* (Aa), *Porphyromonas gingivalis* (Pg), *Bacteroides forsythus*, *Prevotella intermedia* (Pi), *Eikenella corrodens*, *Fusobacterium nucleatum*, *Campybacterrectus* and *Treponema* (spirochetes).[15–18]

Routine laboratory, and more sophisticated DNA probe analyses (described later) can be accomplished to identify suspect bacteria. Such positive identifications aid the clinician in selecting drugs to suppress the organisms found in the different periodontal diseases.

In 1998, the profession experienced another nomenclature change. This *new classification system* eliminated the groupings based on age of onset, rapidity of onset, etc., and replaced it with a classsification *that attempts to identify the local and systemic causes of gingivitis and periodontitis.* For instance, bacteria in the plaque cause periodontal disease, but the action of any of the same bacteria may be *modified* by systemic factors such as the endocrines, blood dyscrasias, ingested medication, etc. The full classification with sub groupings and examples is contained in Appendix 13-1.[19] This new classification system will be incorporated into future Dental and Dental Hygienist National Board Examinations.

## Facts about Gingivitis and Periodontitis

Although bacteria are the causative factor of the periodontal diseases, there are powerful influencing factors that can modify the course of the diseases such as (1) *smoking,* (2) *genetic differences,* (3) baseline severity of disease, (4) Presence of *P. gingivalis, P. intermedia,* and *B. forsythus,* and *Actinobacillus actinomycetemcomitans,* and (5) *individual compliance* with established standards for oral self-care.[20,21] Of interest to married couples is the fact that spouses and children of an adult periodontitis patient might be at a relatively high risk of developing a periodontal breakdown.[22] Another strong risk indicator is the observed relationship of several *systemic* diseases to gingivitis and periodontitis. Among these are diabetes mellitus,[23] Down's syndrome,[24] and more rarely diagnosed conditions such as Haim–Munk syndrome and Papillon–Le Fevre syndromes.[25] Also noticed has been a greater frequency of cardiovascular accidents and nonhemorrhagic strokes among individuals with periodontitis.[26,27]

Both gingivitis and periodontitis affect the tissues of the periodontium. By *definition,* a plaque-induced gingivitis is an inflammation of the marginal gingiva *without any loss of the epithelial attachment.* Once there is a loss of the epithelial attachment, again by *definition,* periodontitis begins. The term periodontitis can be defined as (1) an inflammation of the marginal gingival *with* (2) a loss of the epithelial attachment, *plus* (3) irreversible damage to any of the other three remaining components of the periodontium, i.e., the cementum, alveolar bone,

and the periodontal ligament that connects the latter two structures.

---

### Question 1

Which of the following statements, if any, are correct?

A. One of the highly suspect bacteria associated with periodontitis has been abbreviated Aa; the correct full spelling of the bacteria is *Actinobacillus actinomycetemcomitans*.

B. The last "official" change of periodontal disease classification in 1998 should make it easier to determine the etiology (or cofactors) to the periodontal diseases.

C. Three powerful nonbacterial factors that influence the course of periodontal disease are genetic differences, smoking and adequate daily self-care.

D. Three systemic diseases that are associated with periodontitis are cardiac disease, diabetes mellitus and most viral diseases.

E. It is possible to have a 4-millimeter deep pocket with a slow apical migration of the epithelial attachment, and yet have a gingivitis.

---

With good oral hygiene practices, a plaque-induced gingivitis of bacterial origin can be *cured*, i.e., the free margin of the gingiva can be returned to its original histology. On the other hand, because of the irreversible changes that occur to the components of the periodontium in periodontitis, it is usually not possible for the affected tissues to return to normal. Once periodontal treatment is completed, any further preventive and/or treatment therapy is considered as *maintenance* (and not a cure) and is intended to sustain the status quo of the tooth as much as possible throughout a lifetime. The recognition of the early signs and symptoms of gingivitis and/or periodontitis and beginning

immediate treatment is crucial to the arrest and control of disease progression. This gatekeeper function can best be served by the *general dentist*.[28]

There is abundant evidence that the microbial population of the *supra*gingival plaque is associated with gingivitis, and the *sub*gingival plaque with periodontitis.

In the earliest stages of gingivitis, there is an infiltration of body defense cells beneath the crevicular epithelium. If the gingivitis is not arrested at an early time, the color of the marginal gingiva changes from a pale *pink-to-red*; the contour of the marginal gingival becomes *edematous*, and there is *bleeding* on probing or during toothbrushing ("pink toothbrush"). Any gingival bleeding at *any age* and at any time is not normal and should be viewed with concern by both the clinician and the patient. Yet, because gingival bleeding is considered such a commonly occurring entity, dentists and patients alike often fail to recognize early inflammatory gingival changes, *even though this is the time that complete recovery (cure) is possible*. Patients are often not informed of the presence of periodontal disease until the opportunity for cure or early arrest is past. In one study, only 48% of the patients with diagnosed advanced periodontitis had been informed of their condition by their dentist. Only 12% of those with gingivitis and 20% of the patients with early periodontitis had been made aware of their conditions.[29,30] These data support the fact that one of the complaints about periodontal disease diagnoses, is that they often occur too late to be really helpful.[28] This finding has both *ethical and legal* overtones.[31,32]

Marginal gingivitis is extremely common among *all* age groups, and is *not* necessarily related to aging per se. Many Senior citizens enjoy excellent periodontal health into old age.[33] On the other hand, many advanced cases of periodontitis seen in aging are the result of lifelong neglect of self-care.

Unfortunately, many periodontal cases can be traced back to youth. For example, in Reykjavik, Iceland, gingival bleeding was found in

16% of 230 6-year old children.[34] In a military population of 1,334 soldiers, 40.3% were found to have gingivitis, while 35.7% of the subjects had pocket depths of 3 to 5 millimeters (considered as possible early periodontitis).[35] Bhat reported 34% of 14- to 17-year-old youths had supragingival, and 23% had subgingival calculus.[36] It is of concern that so many children and young persons are not under professional care.[37] Children or adolescents with gingivitis, subgingival calculus, or early signs of alveolar bone loss should be considered as high periodontitis–risk individuals and should be entered into a monitored preventive program as early as possible. These repeated findings of gingivitis that occur at relatively early ages, are a harbinger for the periodontal disease that becomes the leading cause of tooth loss after the third decade.[38]

### Noninvasive Treatment Guidelines for Gingivitis

Gingivitis of plaque origin is a *preventable and curable* periodontal disease. The *objective of professional and home self-care is to eliminate or severely reduce the etiologic organisms in the dental plaque and to prevent or reverse gingival inflammation.* This effort can be abetted by a thorough prophylaxis, supplemented at home by use of the *toothbrush, dental floss* and an *irrigation device.* Generally, an electric toothbrush is more effective than a manual brush (see Chapters 5, 6, 7). This "brush, floss, and flush" routine can be enhanced by the daily use of a fluoride toothpaste, over-the-counter products with *essential oils,* such as Listerine, or dentist prescribed *chlorhexidine* mouthrinses.

The daily self-care routine should be habituated from early childhood to prevent challenge organisms from significantly populating, or repopulating the plaque. In the event that these empirical measures fail, a differential diagnosis should be considered to determine if one of the plaque modified etiologies for gingivitis listed in Appendix 13–1 is the primary cause.[19] If so, a medical referral may be in order.

### Noninvasive Primary Preventive Care for Periodontitis

Once a patient develops *periodontitis,* therapy usually includes additional measures to those recommended for gingivitis. As the probing depth increases, it becomes more difficult to eliminate the bacteria of the subgingival plaque. In addition to routine calculus removal at the time of the prophylaxis, *scaling* and *root planing* needs to be accomplished.[39] Many clinicians advocate irrigating the deeper pockets. The depth of penetration of irrigation solutions into the pocket depends on the tip design of the irrigator, the fluid pressure, and the calculus present that might divert the irrigant stream.[40] Chlorhexidine,[41] stannous fluoride,[42,43] and Listerine[44] are but a few of the solutions that have been used. Research to find more effective antimicrobial agents is a continuing quest.[45] The *dental hygienist is probably the key person to deliver the subgingival irrigation therapy.*[46] *as well as to instruct the patient on how to accomplish the task at home.*[47] (See Figure 13–1.)

The mouthrinses used in a self-care programs do not penetrate deeply enough into the periodontal pockets. However, when irrigation is accomplished in the office, a greater penetration of the pocket can be attained by placing the therapeutic irrigating solution in the fluid container of the ultrasonic scaler.[48] To complete the treatment, often a slow-delivery medication is placed in the pocket, or antibiotic therapy can be initiated to eliminate microbes that have invaded the sulcular tissues.[49] Once a maximum treatment success has been achieved, an every-3-month monitoring is *mandatory.*

### Invasive Procedures Required to Access the Subgingival Pocket

As the pocket continues to deepen it becomes more difficult to apply noninvasive preventive procedures. To solve this problem, the periodontist can sometimes perform *flap surgery,* a surgical procedure that removes a circumferential portion part of the marginal gingiva and

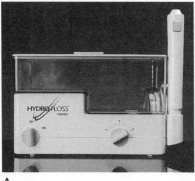

A

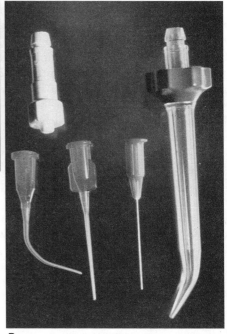

FIGURE 13-1   **A.** An irrigator is an outstanding device to use a *plentiful* amount of water to flush debris still remaining after brushing and flossing ("brush and flush"). **B.** An irrigator with the use of an accessory nozzles can utilize a limited amount of antimicrobial solution to carefully irrigate periodontal pockets. (Courtesy of Hydro Floss, Inc., Birmingham, AL, 35244.)

B

exposes the root. Following the operation, the previous inaccessible subgingival pocket area becomes more accessible to apply routine dental hygiene procedures. It should be emphasized that this surgery is *not* a cure—it only provides a reprieve to help arrest a disease that has been out of control.

### Advanced Periodontal Surgery

On the basis of studies, it is estimated that approximately 5 to 20% of adults have severe periodontal disease while the majority have mild-to-moderate periodontitis.[50] In the advanced stage of periodontal disease there is a dramatic loss of the epithelial attachment with a concurrent loss of supporting alveolar bone that can severely compromise the support of a tooth. A discussion of advanced surgical techniques is beyond the scope of this book; however, there are surgical procedures that can often be used to repair damage caused by periodontitis.

In an effort to compensate for losses of bone and tissue, *guided regenerative techniques*[d] have been introduced in the past several years with a divided emphasis on *bone* as well as *soft-tissue* regeneration. This is accomplished by use of bone grafts and bone stimulants, as well as plastic surgery procedures to reshape soft tissues. At times when the bony support is minimal, prosthetic devices interlinking several teeth are constructed to act as a splint to prevent any one or more teeth being subjected to excessive lateral tooth movement upon mastication.

Following surgical interventions to manage moderate and severe stages of periodontitis, the preventive actions that must be taken *still require meticulous mechanical ("brush, floss, and*

---

[d]Periodontal regeneration means healing after periodontal surgery—a healing that results in a partial or complete restoration of the tooth supporting tissues, namely cementum, alveolar bone and periodontal ligament. *Ann Periodontology*, 1997; 2:215–22.

*flush"*) *and chemical plaque control* (*antimicrobial mouthrinses*). Chlorhexidine is probably the antimicrobial mouth rinse of choice to protect the integrity of the restored tissues and to help suppress the transmission of periodontopathogens from other soft and hard tissue locations in the mouth.

### What Is Peri-implantitis?

To improve esthetics and function following the extraction of a tooth, the void can usually be filled by either a bridge or an implant. For a bridge, it is necessary to prepare two intact teeth as anchor teeth. This can involve a considerable loss of tooth structure. On the other hand, an *implant* can be "implanted" between the two adjacent teeth to function much as a normal tooth.

An implant consists of noncorrosive metallic "root" that is inserted into a cylindrical preparation in the alveolar bone. (Figure 13–2). After bone healing, a prepared crown is cemented to the prepared portion of the implant that remains above the mucosa. This allows the implant to serve the *same function* as

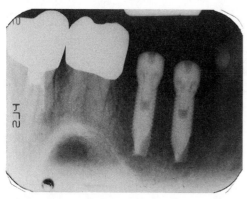

FIGURE 13-2 Two bicuspid crowns will be placed on the implants once the bone wound has healed. At that time they will serve the same functions as natural teeth. (Dr. Donald Willmann, University of Texas Dental School at San Antonio, TX.)

other natural teeth. Unfortunately, the implant is also exposed to the same bacterial flora as are all the other normal teeth—teeth that develop gingivitis and periodontitis. The same primary-preventive procedures are necessary for survival of an implant as for the other teeth of the mouth; neglect of self-care results in the same gingival infection and sequela as for periodontitis. The same destructive bacteria are involved as in periodontitis. The failure and removal of an implant parallels the terminal extraction of a natural tooth from periodontal disease(s). In other words, the same problems and the nearly same solutions apply to an implant with *peri-implantitis* as for a natural tooth with periodontitis.

---

### Question 2

Which of the following statements, if any, are correct?

A. A case of gingivitis can be cured (cured = gingival tissues returned to orignal histology).

B. A case of periodontitis can be cured. (cured = gingival tissues returned to original histology).

C. The mechanical part of self-care consists of use of a toothbrush, floss, and an irrigator ("brush, floss, and flush").

D. Mouthrinses are effective in the irrigation of deep pockets to treat periodontitis.

E. An implant between two teeth requires abuttment teeth for support.

---

## Epidemiology and Risk Assessment

### Periodontal Disease Indicators

Two objectives have been established for this chapter: (1) To provide some *basic facts* about gingivitis and periodontitis, highlighting the role of preventive dentistry—which has been done, and (2) to now explain how some

*evidence*-based tests[e] and indices can be used to assess risk, severity, and prevalence of the periodontal diseases. Some of these indicators were developed to *screen populations* to determine the *prevalence* and *severity* of periodontal conditions, while others were developed to evaluate the periodontal *health of individuals in a private practice*. Others serve both purposes, but *no single index is appropriate for all types of studies*.

Those tests and indices used to evaluate the various stages of gingivitis and periodontitis usually include one or more of the following: (1) pocket depth; (2) amount and location of dental plaque; (3) extent of gingival inflammation; (4) calculus deposits; (5) bacterial identification; (6) evidence of epithelial attachment loss; and (7) smoking habits.

The bleeding index is a most positive indicator of *existing gingivitis*, while a smoking history is probably the most reliable *predictor* of periodontal disease.

## Measuring Dental Plaque

### O'Leary's Plaque Record (Index)

The relationship between plaque and gingivitis was first established by Löe et al. in 1965.[51] Seven years later, O'Leary developed one of the first useful and widely used indices to identify the location and extent of plaque. O'Leary's index is useful for monitoring patients' plaque control performance, is easy to accomplish, is economical, and is reproducible.[52] Only a mouth mirror and explorer are necessary. The completed chart indicates the locations where plaque accumulates and where improved brushing and flossing techniques are required.

The steps for manually recording and interpreting the O'Leary Index are as follows.

1. The smooth surfaces of the teeth in the mouth are divided at the anatomic line an-gles into four sections—mesial, buccal, distal, and lingual (Figure 13–3).

2. All missing teeth are crossed out, and the total number of remaining teeth are determined. For plaque control purposes, the pontic(s) of a fixed bridge and implants should be scored in a manner similar to that of natural teeth.

3. The patient is first asked to rinse vigorously with water to dislodge any loose food debris.

4. The plaque is then disclosed by applying a *disclosing solution* to all teeth, making sure that the dentogingival junction is covered with the agent. As an alternative, a disclosing *tablet* can be chewed and the colored saliva swished around the mouth.

5. The mouth is again rinsed vigorously with water. The operator then uses the explorer or tip of a periodontal probe to confirm the presence of disclosed accumulations of plaque at the dentogingival junction. If the plaque on a tooth surface is in contact with the gingival margin or papillae, the entire tooth surface space is filled in with a red pencil to increase visibility and to enhance the form's impact on the patient. Areas having stained pellicle alone should *not* be scored as having plaque.

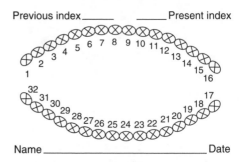

**Plaque control score**

Previous index_____      _____Present index

Name_____ Date

FIGURE 13-3  The chart used for O'Leary's Plaque Index.

[e]Evidence-developed indicator = a sign or test that has a scientific background linking the indicator to the disease.

The total number of scored tooth surfaces is then counted; the sum is then divided by the number of available teeth (including pontics and implants), and multiplied by 100 in order to establish the plaque score as a percentage. This baseline plaque score should be compared with future recall scores to objectively *monitor* a patient's progress.

O'Leary and colleagues[52] have stated that a suitable goal in teaching personal self-care is to reduce the plaque index to *10% or less*. It is suggested that no periodontal surgery or fixed prostheses should be started until this goal has been reached. If surgical or prosthetic intervention is not contemplated, an initial reduction to 15% is probably more realistic for most individuals.

Several record forms are available that are modifications of O'Leary's original presentation (Appendix 23–1). With the introduction of the chairside computer recording of dental examinations, these computer generated plaque index records will eventually become part of the "paperless" dental office.

### The Plaque Index of Silness and Löe

The plaque index of Silness and Löe provides a modication of O'Leary's index. It too is visual and required only a mouth mirror. A deficiency of the O'Leary index is that it requires that the surfaces of every tooth be examined for plaque but that there was no gradations between a great amount of plaque and no plaque.

The index of Silness and Löe also requires that the four surfaces of designated teeth be visually examined and a score recorded, viz., the maxillary right first molar, maxillary right lateral incisor, and the left first bicuspid; the the mandible, the mandibular left first molar, the left lateral incisor and the right first bicuspid—a total of six teeth. For each of the surfaces of these teeth a score of 0 to 3 is given that matches the severity of the listings in Table 13–1. In this way, the average amount of plaque for each tooth can be determine by dividing by 4; the scores for all six teeth be di-

TABLE 13-1 **The Criteria of the Plaque Index of Silness and Löe**

| Score | Criteria |
|-------|----------|
| 0 | No plaque in gingival areas. |
| 1 | Film or plaque at free gingival margin, detectable only by removal with perioprobe or by disclosing solution. |
| 2 | Moderate accumulation of plaque, visible to the eye within the crevice, on the marginal gingiva or the adjacent tooth surface, or both. |
| 3 | Heavy accumulation of soft matter on the gingival margin of the tooth surface. Soft debris fills the interdental region. |

vided by 6 to get the average for the mouth. The highest scores can be expected to occur on the interproximal surfaces.

The index has the advantage of providing more data on the self-care habits of the patient, as well as taking less time to evaluate than to record entire dentitions—a fact that is important in large-scale epidemiology studies. The data from the Silness and Löe index can also be used to compare with other indexes, for instance to evaluate the amount of plaque against the gingival bleeding index of Löe and Silness (described later) throughout the months of pregnancy.[53]

### Oral-Hygiene Index and Simplified Oral-Hygiene Index

One of the most popular indicators for determining oral hygiene status in epidemiology studies is the Oral Hygiene Index (OHI). It was developed in 1960 by Greene and Vermillion[54] and modified 4 years later as the OHI-S.[55] The simplified (S) version provides much the same information, as did the earlier version, but can be accomplished much more rapidly. It is very useful for large-scale epidemiology surveys but is not generally believed to be sensitive enough to accurately evaluate the oral hygiene status of

an individual patient. The OHI has two components: the oral debris score and the calculus score. The term oral debris includes "plaque, materia alba, and food remnants." With the OHI-S, soft and hard deposits are evaluated only on the facial or lingual surfaces of six selected teeth. They are the *buccal* surfaces of the upper *first molars of both sides*, the *labial* surfaces of the *upper right and lower left central* incisors, and the *lingual surfaces of both lower first molars*. The criteria for the OHI-S scores are shown in Table 13–2. The total OHI-S score can be divided by the number of surfaces examined to calculate the average oral hygiene score.

### Gingival Bleeding Index of Löe and Silness

One of the most commonly used indexes to determine the prevalence and severity of gingival inflammation is the Gingival Index of Loe and Silness.[56] With the Löe and Silness index it is possible by its coding from 0 to 3 to record bleeding tendencies, color and contour changes of the gingival, alterations in the consistency of tissue and the presence of ulcerations (Table 13–3).

Like the Silness and Löe plaque index, only six teeth are selected. Data can be computed for individual teeth, or for all the six. The evaluation, coding, and recording are quite rapid and useful in larger-scale epidemiology studies.

**TABLE 13-3 The Criteria for the Löe-Silness Gingival Bleeding Index**

| Score | Criteria |
|-------|----------|
| 0 | Normal gingiva. |
| 1 | Mild inflammation—slight change in color, slight edema, *no* bleeding on probing. |
| 2 | Moderate inflammation—redness, edema and glazing, *bleeding on probing.* |
| 3 | Severe inflammation, marked redness and edema, ulceration, *tendency toward spontaneous bleeding.* |

As a part of a full-scale periodontal examination of a patient, it is desirable to determine gingival bleeding by probing of the marginal gingiva. This procedure *must* be carefully controlled to avoid *false positives and iatrogenic damage to the periodontium.*[58] *In the test for gingival bleeding, the probe should be run along the soft tissue wall at the orifice of the periodontal sulcus or periodontal pocket.* Probing at the bottom of the pocket is a *poor indicator.*[59] The basic objective of a bleeding index is *not* to determine the sulcus[f] depth, *not* to evaluate the extent of loss of the epithelial attachment, *not* to determine bone loss, but *only* to evaluate whether there is, or is *not,* gingival bleeding. When all teeth are included, the data can be used as an epidemiology instrument or for a patient's clinical record.

**TABLE 13-2 Criteria for the Oral Hygiene Index Scoring**

| Score | Criteria |
|-------|----------|
| 0 | No debris or stain present. |
| 1 | Soft debris covering not more than one third of the tooth surface. |
| 2 | Soft debris covering more than one third but not more than two thirds of the tooth surface. |
| 3 | Soft debris covering more than two thirds of the tooth surface. |

### Question 3

Which of the following statements, if any, are correct?

A. Two dental plaque indices are those of O'Leary and Silness and Löe.

B. A plaque score of 10% for the O'Leary plaque index is considered marginally satisfactory.

---

[f]Sulcus and crevice are often used interchangeably. For example, gingival sulcus and gingival crevice.

C. Gingival bleeding when there is no loss of epithelial attachment is a positive sign of gingivitis.

D. The Löe–Silness index is oriented towards monitoring gingival health.

E. Bleeding during toothbrushing ("pink toothbrush") can only be diagnosed by a dentist as a gingivitis.

## Periodontal Probes

As illustrated in Figure 13–4, there are several variations of periodontal probes. Each has circumferential markings on the probing tip to aid in determining sulcular depth; others also have color-coding to further facilitate accurate measurements. The probe is used for four main purposes: (1) the measurement of *pocket depth*, (2) the measurement of epithelial *attachment loss*, (3) *induction* of gingival and/or papillary bleeding, and (4) the detection of *subgingival calculus* as part of the periodontal examination. The probe may be of metal, or of a hard polymer.[60] The probing tip is approximately 0.5 millimeter in diameter. Its tactile *reproducibility* and *accuracy* depends much upon the experience of the operator.

There is always a need for caution in probing, especially in the presence of inflammation. Probing inflamed gingival tissue sites with its fragile capillaries risks inducing a *bacteremia*. For individuals at risk of infective *endocarditis*, both a clinical and radiographic assessment is indicated prior to a decision to probe. Prophylactic antibiotic coverage may be indicated.[62] (See Figure 13–5.)

A new era of periodontal probing was ushered in by the coupling of the computer and the constant force electronic probes (Figure 13–6).[g] One example of the electronic probe is the Florida probe,[e] which has been routinely used since 1955 in the University of Florida's Disease Research Center.[63,64] In one well-controlled study, the Florida probe was shown to be extremely accurate and reproducible. The minimum probing error was found to be around *0.2 millimeter*.[65,66] In contrast, the resolution of the standard manual probe is *1 millimeter*. When using a constant-force probe, as soon as the *resistance* at the bottom of the sulcus reaches a preset level such as 15 to 20 grams, the depth of the sulcus is *automatically* entered into the computer record form (Appendix 13–2). (For comparison, a force of 25 grams is just below the threshold of pain when a probe is inserted under the fingernail; (see Figure 13–7).

Another electronic probe is the Toronto probe that uses air pressure to extend and re-

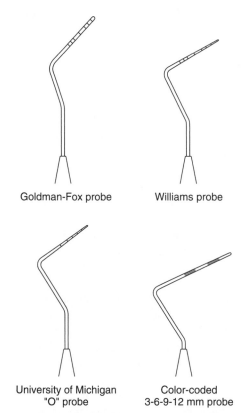

Goldman-Fox probe            Williams probe

University of Michigan            Color-coded
"O" probe                  3-6-9-12 mm probe

FIGURE 13-4    Different types of calibrated periodontal probes useful in assessing the depth and configuration of periodontal pockets.

[g]Available from Computerized Probe, Inc., Florida Probe Computerized Systems, Oklahoma City, OK.

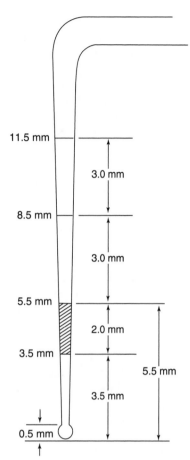

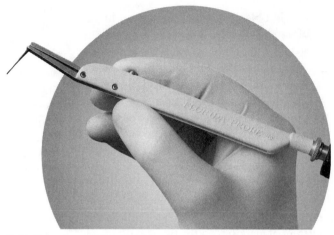

FIGURE 13-6    The Florida Probe. Note the slim barrel and the ease with which it fits within the hand. The tips are removable and sterilizable. (Courtesy Florida Probe Corporation, Gainesville, FL.)

FIGURE 13-5    Diagram of WHO periodontal probe. It has a ball-tip end to avoid false assessment by over-measurement and for easier detection of subgingival calculus. The color-coded part from 3.5 to 5.5 mm greatly facilitates rapid assessment of periodontal pocket depth. (From WHO Technical Report Series 621, 1978.)

tract the measuring tip; this action helps control the probing force. An Alabama probe automatically detects the cementoenamel junction and measures the clinical attachment levels to the bottom of the pocket within a 0.2 millimeters tolerance level.[67]

Because of the accuracy of the electronic probes, the time needed to identify periodontal disease activity (attachment loss) between recall intervals can be shortened. Printouts can be made that permit comparisons between different examinations. As can be noted in Appendix 13–2, the same computer software can be used to record the main periodontal disease indicators—pocket depth, gingival recession, plaque, bleeding, and tooth mobility. This is accomplished partially by using red, yellow, and green or other computer color designations for the various entries.

A unique convenience is that as pocket and bleeding sites are seen on the monitor and entered in the record, the information can be called out in a computer-generated male or fe-

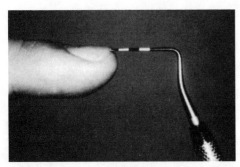

FIGURE 13-7    Practical test for establishing 20 to 25 g periodontal probing pressure. The periodontal probe is placed underneath the fingernail where the sensitivity approximates that of the bottom of a periodontal pocket. The correct amount of force should not cause pain to the patient on probing. (Dr. Arden Christen, Indiana University School of Dentistry, Indianapolis, IN.)

male voice—not that of the dentist. Additional color-coded copies of the completed patient's record can be printed out for patient records and patient information, as well as for insurance filing.

## Periodontal Probing

As previously mentioned, two of the main purposes of periodontal probing are to determine *pocket depth*, and to measure the amount of *attachment loss*. Both have one requirement in common, namely a careful step-by-step circumferential probing around each tooth.[68] To determine pocket depth; the probe is inserted into the mesial proximal sulcus. It is aligned as vertically as possible, but with a slight angle away from the midpoint of the tooth bucco-lingually because of the contact point. Without being withdrawn, the probe is then "walked" along the facial surface of the crevice until the distal proximal contact area is reached. The probe is then withdrawn and reinserted from the lingual surface and "walked" back to the proximal surface. As the probing proceeds, a record is made of the distance from the deepest site of the pocket to the crest of the free gingival margin on each of the four surfaces. A more detailed second probing might be indicated where the initial sulcular depth has been found to be of concern.[69] Other patterns of probing are acceptable. The main objective is to include all surfaces and all problem areas. Probing depth can be influenced by various factors, such as the type of probe, angulation of the probe to the tooth, pressure used in probing, and inflammation of the free gingival margin—all create possibilities for error in measuring pocket depth or attachment loss. In fact, the probing depth *seldom* corresponds to the exact microscopic (histologic) depth of a normal sulcus or pocket depth. However, the clinical pocket depth does reflect the relative level of the actual pocket depth. It does provide the clinician with a useful *reproducible* estimate of the location of the most coronal insertion of the fibers of the periodontal ligament between the alveolar bone and the cementum. (See Figure 13–8.)

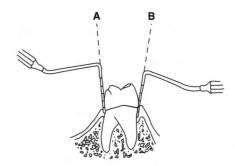

FIGURE 13-8    Examples of probing. **A.** Shallow sulcus on lingual side; **B.** deeper sulcus (pocket) on bucal surface. (Dr. Arden Christen, Indiana University School of Dentistry, Indianapolis, IN.)

The measurement of *epithelial attachment loss* involves the same format of probing as for determining *pocket depth*. The main *difference* is the *reference point from which* the measurement is recorded. For pocket depth, it is from the depth of the pocket *to the crest* of the free marginal gingiva. For calculating attachment loss, the measurement is made from the depth of the pocket on each surface *to a fixed site*, such as the cementoenamel junction or occlusal plane.[70] Two measurements *separated in time* but at the same site are necessary to estimate the amount of apical migration (if any) of the epithelial attachment. Sites that show a 2-millimeter loss of attachment between two sequential recall examinations should be considered as active.

The dividing line between gingivitis and periodontitis in a practice is objective and reproducible. It is based on the consistent finding that a normal gingival sulcus depth is approximately 3 millimeters in depth. If a probing depth of three millimeters is encountered with no bleeding and no loss of epithelial attachment, the periodontium is considered in good health. A probing depth of 4 to 6 millimeters is considered in the gray area between periodontal health and disease.[71] If bleeding is encountered, the problem may be *either* gingivitis or periodontitis, depending on the examiner's evaluation of epithelial attachment loss. When a patient is in this gray zone, frequent monitoring and scrupulous oral hygiene is required. On the other hand, a loss of greater than 6 millimeters usually constitutes an advanced periodontitis.[71] A patient with a pocket depth measurements of 6 to 9 millimeters can usually expect surgical treatment, careful monitoring and a lifetime necessity of maximum self-care. In extreme cases, pocket depths of up to 12 millimeters have been recorded before a tooth has been exfoliated or extracted. As the probing depth increases beyond 3 millimeters, *professional judgment* becomes an increasingly major factor in determining whether preventive measures alone, or whether a combination of noninvasive preventive and invasive treatment strategies are necessary.

### Gingival Recession

At this point, the term *gingival recession* should be introduced. As the attachment loss continues, the free gingival margin may recede apically along with the epithelial attachment as well as the underlying alveolar bone. In such a case, the pocket depth may be near normal (as measured from the crest of the free gingival margin), while the attachment loss increases (as measured from the cementoenamel junction).

With a receding free marginal gingiva, there is a loss of supporting alveolar bone. There is also a loss of the vertical height of the *attached* gingiva. For every millimeter of attachment loss, there is a corresponding loss of attached gingiva. If for instance, it is assumed that there were 12 millimeters of attached gingiva[h] at the time of periodontal normalcy, but after 20 years, the attachment loss is 6 millimeters, then there is only approximately 6 millimeters of attached gingiva (original 12 mm minus 6 mm epithelial attachment loss = 6 mm present attached gingiva).

---

### Question 4

Which of the following statements, if any, are correct?

A. If one is probing an infected area (meaning, periodontal pocket) and perforates a few capillaries, it can set off a bacteremia which can be dangerous to a cardiovascular patient.

B. The rapidity of apical migration of the epithelial attachment can only be determined by measurements made at two appropriately separated times.

---

[h]The attached gingiva is attached to the side of the alveolus, and extends from the base of the marginal gingival to the mucobuccal fold.

C. The computer linked periodontal probe is reproducible in replicate pocket depth measurements within a range of 1 millimeter; whereas, the manual probe has an equal or better record of reproducibility for pocket depth measurements.

D. The probing for pocket depth is the same as for probing for epithelial attachment loss; the only difference is the reference point from which measurements are made.

E. There is an inverse relationship between the depth of a periodontal pocket and the vertical height of the attached gingival, i.e., the deeper the pocket, the lessening of the height of the attached gingiva.

## Community Periodontal Index of Treatment Needs (CPITN)

The previous plaque, oral debris and bleeding indices were epidemiological instruments that could be *visually* accomplished for events occurring *above* the gingival margin. The next two widely used epidemiology indices, the Community Periodontal Index of Treatment Needs (CPITN) and the Periodontal Recording System (PSR) require probing to evaluate the periodontal health (or otherwise) that occurs below the gingival margin.

The Federation Dentaire Internationale (FDI) in collaboration with the Oral Health Unit of the World Health Organization (WHO) developed the Community Periodontal Index of Treatment Needs (CPITN)[72] to attain more uniform worldwide epidemiology data. In this screening index, the periodontal treatment needs are recorded for six segments (sextants). The segments are the anterior and two posterior sets of maxillary and mandibular teeth. The system excludes the third molars, except where the third molars are functioning

TABLE 13-4  **Criteria Used in Recording the Community Periodontal Index of Treatment Needs (CPITN)**

| Score | Criteria |
|---|---|
| 0 | Healthy sextant. |
| 1 | Bleeding after gentle probing of the pockets (25-g force). |
| 2 | Supra- or subgingival calculus or other plaque retentions. |
| 3 | One or more 4- to 5-mm deep pockets. |
| 4 | One or more 6 mm or deeper pockets. |

in the place of the second molars. A sextant must have at least two functional teeth. The *highest* (worst) of the coded conditions in Table 13–4 is recorded for *each sextant*.

A special color-coded black banded probe from 3.5 to 5.5 mm and circular rings at 8.5 and 11.5 facilitates uniformity of scores in the world-wide accomplishment of the CPITN.[72] If the black band cannot be seen above the marginal gingival following insertion, a code 4 is recorded. Other possibilities with lesser periodontal involvement are code 3 if the marginal gingival falls within the range of the black band, code 2 if there is supra- or subgingival calculus, code 1 if gingival bleeding on gentle pressure, and code 0 if there is no sign of disease. There is no rule specifying the number of separate probing to be made.[72]

## Periodontal Screening and Recording System (PSR)

This system of screening was introduced by the American Dental Association (ADA)[i] and the American Academy of Periodontology in 1992. It was developed to encourage dentists to screen individual patients 18 years of age and older for undetected periodontal disease. Only 5 minutes is needed to accomplish the screen-

[i]Additional information can be secured from http://www.ada.org/prof/prac/issues/pubs/psr/

ing (probing). The same probe and the same scoring of 0 to 4 basis is used as with the CPITN. The highest recording of "4" indicates a probing depth of over 5.5 millimeters for at least *one tooth* in the sextant. A weight force of no more than 20 to 25 g is considered sufficient to detect pathology without causing pain (see Figure 13–5). The *major difference* between the CPITN and the PSR is that with the latter, a *guideline for treatment* is suggested to match the level of treatment needs with the level of disease severity (Appendices 13–3 and 13–4).

### Identification of Periodontopathogens by DNA Analysis

The DNA analysis, (sometimes called "probe analysis") is an accurate diagnostic method for identifying bacteria.[74-76] It does not depend on the presence of living bacteria, and thus requires no special packaging before being sent to the laboratory. The test is based on the fact that the two molecular strands of DNA of a bacterium are always complementary (as in a human) and can be separated. One single control strand of the DNA from an unknown bacterial species *taken from the patient's* subgingival plaque is matched with a complementary strand of the DNA bacteria *from a known laboratory culture*. The laboratory strand is marked with a radioisotope so that it can be quanitated if it combines with the patient's DNA complementary strand, for instance from *Actinobacillus actinomycetemcomitans* (Aa), *Porphyromonas gingivalis* (Pg), or *Prevotella intermedia* (Pi). As the number of complementary strand couplings increase, the amount of radioactivity also increases. It is the total level of radioactivity detected that forms the basis of the final report.

The American Dental Association has granted its *Seal of Acceptance* to two DNA assay systems, the DMD and the Pathotek Pathogen Detection Systems. The DMD test measures *individual levels of radioactivity* for Aa or Pg or Pi, with the results reported as negative, low, moderate, or high radioactivity for *each* of the

organisms. A color-illustrated report graphically illustrates periodontal risk levels. This report can be used for purposes of treatment, patient education and motivation. Pathotek detects all *three pathogens* and reports on their combined total level.

The DNA assay tests are simple to apply. The site at the orifice of the gingival crevice to be sampled is cleaned of supragingival plaque and a paper point is gently inserted into the sulcus and removed after 10 seconds. It is then placed in a vial that is mailed to the laboratory for analysis. Test results are generally available within 10 days after mailing or within a few days if a telephone report is desired.

### The Immune Factor

Since the majority of treatment for periodontitis centers around suppressing or eliminating the bacterial challenge of the plaque organisms, it is natural to begin to look at the body's humoral and cellular immune system for help.[77,78] Many vaccines have been developed for *other diseases;*[79] a *model animal system* has been developed for serious periodontal disease vaccine testing;[80] one promising vaccine study is now underway in England for *caries* (see Chapter 23);[81] and daily, the *function of new genes* is being announced There is no doubt that the terminology of recombinant technology, combination vaccines, genetically tailored vaccines, and preformed antibodies are but a few new terms for the dental lexicon of the future.[79]

The recent completion of the *Human Genome Project* with its decoding of desoxynucleic acid, has set the stage for a tremendous surge of knowledge about chromosomes, genes, and antibodies, and their relation to disease and abnormalities. Efforts are currently directed towards identifying markers helpful in preventing, diagnosing, predicting, and curing diseases. Drug companies are studying antibodies to which drugs can be coupled to develop perfectly targeted "magic bullets." Others are working on high priority vaccines to control

diseases such as diabetes mellitus where the successful development of such a vaccine would immediately have the effect on reducing the great number of associated periodontal cases.

A few examples of individual accomplishments can be cited. Kornman has pointed out that the *pro-inflammatory cytokine*, interleukin-1 can be used as a predictor for future severe periodontitis.[82,83] *Cytokines* are produced by various cell types such as *macrophages*, *neutrophils*, and *fibrocytes* which would be expected to be the defense and repair elements in the area(s) of inflammation.[84] Another study found that a platelet-activating factor (PAF) progressively increased as the severity of periodontitis increased.[85] There is research being accomplished targeted at adhesins, with the hope that *anti-adhesin* antibodies will negate the ability of a bacterium to adhere to a tooth surface or to soft tissue.[86,87] A dramatic clinical outcome relates to a 6-year old girl diagnosed with chronic, probably congenital neutropenia, replete with recurrent oral ulcerations and significant periodontal breakdown resembling prepubertal periodontitis. Granulocytic colony stimulating factor (G-CSF) was administered, resulting in an increase in granulocyte count. In two weeks, there was a resolution of the neutropenic-induced ulceration.[88]

Unfortunately, there is yet no uniform integrating theory for the myriad of genes involved in the majority of diseases[89]—much as the Periodic Table that made possible the ability to predict the properties of elements that were not yet discovered.

---

### Question 5

Which of the following statements, if any, are correct?

A. The CPITN is a periodontal index in which pocket measurements of all teeth in the (six) sextants are recorded.

B. The PSR suggests the level of treatment of care needed to match the severity of the periodontal findings.

C. If one strand of a bacterium's DNA from a patient's mouth matches a complementary strand of a bacterium from a known laboratory bacterium, it provides a positive identity of the patient's organism.

D. Inflammatory cytokines are released by body defense cells such as the macrophage, neutrophil and fibrocyte.

E. The worldwide effort to successfully decode the desoxynucleic acid molecule is known as the Human Genetic Project.

---

## Crevicular Fluid Assessment

### Gingival Crevicular Fluid Measurement and Analysis

The physiologic flow of gingival crevicular fluid serves (1) to flush out metabolic catabolites in the sulcus,[90] and (2) this fluid also contains protective elements of the host's humoral and cellular defense system that *continually* bathes the four smooth surfaces of the teeth. As gingivitis increases in severity, so does the flow of gingival crevicular fluid—usually proportional to severity of the gingivitis,[91] but *not* to the severity of peridontitis. Thus, the measurement of the flow rate of crevicular fluid has been proposed as a means of monitoring the degree of gingival inflammation.[92,93] Others have proposed that the level of some of the chemical constituents of saliva could also be used as markers of gingival disease status.[94]

The presence of gingival crevicular fluid (GCF) as a gingivitis indicator would have numerous advantages. The knowledge that periodontal destruction progresses through periodic but *unpredictable cycles* of acute episodes followed by periods of quiescence has stimulated investigation of the GCF components. The results from GCF analysis may provide information on the host's responses to inflammation and tissue destruction during these episodes. The flow of GCF is site-specific, sometimes affecting only one individual tooth, or even one

specific site on that one specific tooth. Gingival crevicular fluid is a conveniently sampled transudate that contains components derived from both the host tissues and the subgingival plaque.[92]

It is relatively simple to measure the rate of crevicular flow. However, the fluid is now mainly used as a research tool, with the hope of discovering some marker that signals either active or inactive status. The procedure for collecting the GCF is as follows.

1. After the gingiva has been isolated with cotton rolls, the tissue is dried with a gentle stream of air for 5 seconds.

2. A paper strip is inserted into the sulcus for 5 seconds, removed, and discarded.

3. A second strip is either placed at the entrance to the gingival sulcus(extrasulcular method) or inserted into the sulcus until a frictional bind is encountered (intrasulcular technique). (The intrasulcular method can itself irritate the crevicular epithelium and trigger the flow of crevicular fluid.)

4. The strips are allowed to remain in place for 5 seconds.

5. The amount of crevicular fluid can be quantitated by placing the strips in a gingival fluid meter measuring device called the Periotron. The extent of wetness of the paper strip produced by the gingival fluid affects the flow of a current through a moisture-sensitive sensor. The amount of current flow is displayed as a digital readout.[91,95]

It is claimed that this method provides an "early warning system" for the detection of gingivitis.

## Smoking as a Major Risk Factor for Periodontal Disease

In the United States there are an estimated 50 million smokers, and another unknown number of individuals exposed to passive smoke.[96] It is well recognized that smoking is the cause of many systemic pathologies, of which *lung cancer, cardiac disease,* and *stroke* are best known and most feared.[97] Unfortunately, lethal tobacco products—cigarette and use of smokeless ("spit") tobacco—have gone unnoticed as causal agents for disabling and disfiguring oral and pharyngeal cancer.[98] There have also been many articles published over the past five decades pointing out that tobacco is a causal agent for *periodontal disease,* an oral disease that affects millions. The enormity of this relationship is found in a statement that *smoking accounts for one-half of all periodontal cases and three-fourths of oral cancer cases* in the United States.[99]

The role of smokeless ("spit")[j] tobacco on oral morbidity and mortality has received little media attention.[100,101] For instance, in providing a balanced presentation on the oral hazards of smoking, chewing tobacco must also be associated with an increased risk of root caries as well as periodontal disease.[102,103] Men who used chewing tobacco were four times more likely than those who had never used tobacco, to have one or more decayed or filled root surfaces.

It is now beginning to emerge that probably one of the most important questions that can be asked on the patient's dental and medical history form is, *"Do you smoke or live with someone who smokes, and/or do you use smokeless tobacco?"*

Smoking is a high-risk habit and constitutes a major periodontal problem.[100,104–107] Mirbod has provided a litany of tobacco-associated lesions found in the mouth—squamous-cell carcinoma, gingivitis and periodontitis, burns and keratosis patches, black hairy tongue, palate erosions, leukoplakia and epithelial dysplasia, and tooth staining.[108] All can be visually detected early when aggressive treatment produces the best results.

---

[j]Spit tobacco: A designation of a tobacco associated with this habit.

The use of tobacco products has an adverse effect of the onset, prevention, prognosis, treatment and maintenance phases of periodontitis. Part of this negative outlook is because smoking also causes adverse changes in the body's immune response system that present major barriers to successful periodontal treatment.[107,109] Smoking is associated with alveolar bone loss, with epithelial attachment loss, gingival recession, and with periodontal pocket development.[104] In an extensive review of the literature Haber discusses many of his own studies and observations to explain how a patient's smoking history differs from a nonsmoker and its effect on periodontal disease.[110] For example:

- Tobacco users are 2.5 to 6 times more likely to develop periodontal disease than nonsmokers.[109]

- A patient's smoking history is a useful clinical indicator of *future* periodontal disease activity.[110]

- There are more current smokers who seek professional periodontal care than nonsmokers.[111,112]

- There appears to be a relationship between the *number of cigarettes smoked* and the risk of developing periodontal diseases.[109,113]

- As the number of cigarettes smoked increases, so does the severity of the periodontal disease.[110,105]

- More smokers than nonsmokers are classified as having severe adult periodontitis and severe early-onset generalized periodontitis.[114]

- Almost *100%* of 30- to 40-year-old heavy smokers have periodontitis;[113] the response of these patients to therapy is *not* as favorable as for nonsmokers.[115,98]

- Approximately 86 to 90% of refractory periodontitis (not responsive to treatment) patients are current smokers.[113]

- There is a strong association between smoking and alveolar *bone and tooth loss*.[116–118,106]

- Smoking is associated with adverse changes in the body's immune system.[104]

- The *gingival fibroblastic repair function* is altered, resulting in a thickened fibrotic gingiva.[110,119]

- Following treatment, the improvements in probing depths and epithelial attachments are still more favorable for the non-smoker.[120,115]

- There is more pocketing of the anterior segments of teeth for smokers than nonsmokers.

- It is very difficult to persuade a patient to quit smoking as part of the treatment plan.

A seminal article, by Barbour and associates, focuses on the degraded immune response of smokers with periodontitis when compared to nonsmokers. They confirm Haber's observation that there is a *neutrophilic deficiency,* but in addition point out many other functions of the immune system that are compromised—including phagocytosis, chemotaxis, immune suppression, immune surveillance, and alterations of immunoglobulin function. Each of the areas is well documented and discussed. One of the considerations of the study was to determine the effects of smoking on periodontal disease, especially how it was related to host defense mechanisms.[109] An intriguing question would be, "In view of the altered immune response, is periodonitis a predictor of susceptibility to other smoking diseases that have a later onset?"

## Smoking Cessation and Recovery

Smoking cessation is an essential component for the successful treatment of periodontal disease—there is little rationale for treating periodontitis without eliminating one of the major causes of the disease.[113] Thus, there is also the question of whether periodontal surgical treatment is indicated without a commitment by the patient to quit smoking.[113] As with other smoking diseases, cessation is only the first step of a

long healing process where the smoker often does not approach the lower risk of the non-smoker for 10 to 20 years.[97,98] Krall and coworkers estimated that the risk of tooth loss 12 years after smoking cessation was reduced by 20%.[118] However, the fact that the rate of tooth loss of ex-smokers falls between the data for current smokers and those who never smoked indicates that recovery is taking place.[118] The periodontal status and bone loss of ex-smokers also appears to be intermediate between current smokers and those who never smoked.[110,116,117]

Gingival improvement is more rapid following smoking cessation although a bit quixotic. Usually a smoker's gingiva has a glazed fibrotic appearance with rolled edges after years of smoking. *Bleeding is minimal* on brushing. It is believed that this is due to the local effect of the tobacco smoke possibly suppressing the inflammatory reaction. This *local* and *direct* effect of components in the cigarette smoke are believed to also account for a greater amount of pocketing that occurs in the anterior teeth. However, about 10 to 12 weeks after quitting smoking, there is an increase in bleeding, possibly caused by a recovery of the inflammatory response. About a year after cessation, the fibrotic, thickened anatomy of the gingiva begins to assume a more normal appearance and the periodontitis appears to stabilize. For the majority of patients, attachment loss ceases or dramatically slows.[110,119]

The present methods for prevention and treatment of gingivitis and periodontal disease emphasize the need for meticulous day-to-day oral hygiene procedures. Even so these preventive actions are not intended to, nor are they adequate to continuously replace a compromised portion of the immune system brought on by smoking. Where smoking occurs, the chemical and manual methods of plaque control still help to reduce the bacterial challenge. However, with round-the-clock impaired humoral and cellular body defenses, and with an impaired gingival fibroblastic repair capability, the entire defense and recovery process is jeopardized.[120,115]

There is a need to provide smoking cessation counseling programs as an integral part of the periodontal treatment plan. The American Cancer Society, American Heart Association, and American Lung Association[k] sponsor many "No Smoking" classes throughout the nation to facilitate smoking cessation. For *youthful* smokers and potential smokers, the emphasis should be on *smoking avoidance* and *refusal* techniques. This task can probably be best accomplished in the public-school system (see Chapter 19).

The outcome of such counseling will probably be more successful if linked with a discussion of the great amount of preventable *morbidity* and *mortality* caused by active and passive smoking and the use of smokeless tobacco. *To teach dental students* to accept this counseling responsibility, the University of Indiana Dental School has established an anti-smoking curriculum program for student teaching and patient education.[121] In addition there is an Indiana University Nicotine Dependence Program at the University Cancer Center that is operated in conjunction with the medical school and several area hospitals.[122]

---

### Question 6

Which of the following statements, if any, are correct?

A. An increasing flow of Gingival Crevicular Fluid (GFC) is indicative of an increasing severity of gingivitis, but not of peridontitis.

B. If present tobacco smoking was to cease, approximately one-half of the present need for periodontal care would also cease.

---

[k]To identify the nearest location of no-smoking classes in the United States, call 1-800-LUNG-USA.

C. Smoking of cigarettes and use of smokeless tobacco can act directly on the oral tissues, as exemplified by the presence of oral and pharyngeal cancer.

D. The smoking history of an individual can aid in predicting the possibility of future onset, as well as the eventual long-range outcome of the treatment of periodontal disease.

E. Smoking can be the cause of the earlier development of periodontitis, an increase in its severity, and reduction in the probability of a successful treatment outcome.

# SUMMARY

Two of the most important messages of the entire chapter are: (1) at the first sign of gingival bleeding, regardless of age, a dentist should be seen immediately for diagnosis, treatment, education and monitoring; and, (2) for all patients who smoke, to encourage and help facilitate their participation in an anti-smoking program.

Many indices are used to determine the prevalence and severity of gingivitis and/or periodontitis among a given population, or to determine the severity of gingivitis and/or periodontitis among individual patients. The most commonly used markers are a plaque index, gingival bleeding, loss of epithelial attachment and pocket depth. With computer software, data collection can be easily extended to include recession, suppuration, furcation involvement, tooth mobility and others. The most important detail that delineates gingivitis from periodontitis is the integrity of the epithelial attachment. As long as the pocket depth measurements approximate 3 millimeters with no bleeding and no recent loss of epithelial attachment, the periodontium can be considered in excellent health. As the pocket probing depths become greater, noninvasive preventive procedures become more difficult to apply while invasive treatment becomes more frequent and complex. Manual probes are used to determine sulcus depth; however, the constant-force electronic probes appear to be more accurate, reproducible and easier to use in recording data. Laboratory tests are often used to determine the microorganisms of the subgingival plaque. Some progress has been made, but the cause-and-effect of these bacteria is not as well understood as are the cariogenic mutans streptococci and lactobacillus. Immune studies are permitting the researchers to better understand the dynamic interaction between the pathogenic organisms and the body defenses. Possibly one of the most important harbingers of gingivitis and periodontitis is cigarette smoking and/or use of smokeless tobacco products. Many studies have found that tooth loss from periodontal disease is associated with tobacco use. Investigators have reported that current smokers have a greater prevalence of severe periodontal problems, as well as accompanying breakdowns of various components of the immune system than do individuals who have never smoked. With smoking, the challenge organisms are rarely confronted by a fully effective immune defense system.

## ANSWERS AND EXPLANATIONS

1. A, B, and C—correct.

   D—incorrect. The first two, cardiac disease and diabetes are correct; most viral diseases is incorrect.

   E—incorrect. If there is a slow apical migration of the epithelial attachment past the CEJ, it is by definition a periodontitis. Once that diagnosis is correctly made, it cannot revert to a gingivitis.

2. A and C—correct.

   B—incorrect. Once periodontitis is correctly diagnosed, there is no way to restore the tissues to their previous histolology; however, future progress can be controlled—but not cured.

   D—incorrect. Mouthrinses do not penetrate the subgingival plaque to the extent necessary to kill or to remove the periodontopathogens.

   E—incorrect. An implant is anchored in alveolar bone. It is a free-standing structure that needs no support.

3. A and C—correct.

   B—incorrect. An O'Leary Index score of 10% is considered excellent—not marginal.

   D—incorrect. The Löe-Silness Index is used to record gingival bleeding—not plaque.

   E—incorrect. Bleeding can occur as a result of either gingivitis or a periodontitis. It requires a differential diagnosis to determine which.

4. A, B, D, and E—correct.

   C—incorrect. It should be vice versa. The computer linked periodontal probe is reproducible to within 0.2 millimeter; the manual probe to within 1 millimeter.

5. B, C, and D—correct.

   A—incorrect. Only one tooth—the tooth with the worst (highest) 0 to 4 score in each sextant is recorded.

   E—incorrect. The title to the program was the Human *Genome* Project.

6. A, B, C, D, and E—correct.


## Self-Evaluation Questions

1. Two popular indices for determining the location of plaque on smooth surfaces of the teeth are the _____ Index and the _____ Index.

2. Greene and Vermillion developed the _____ Index and then truncated it for convenience in epidemiology studies.

3. The _____ is an instrument to measure the flow of gingival curricular fluid.

4. Name three devices used in self-care, of which one is a toothbrush; the other two are _____ and an _____.

5. The equivalent of periodontitis around an implant is called _____.

6. The disease of the periodontium that proceeds periodontitis is _____.

7. The device used to determine pocket depth and epithelial attachment loss is called a _____.

8. For every millimeter loss of epithelial attachment, there is a corresponding loss of the same distance of the _____ gingiva.

9. A personal habit that accounts for approximately one-half of all the periodontal diseases in the United States is _____.

10. The single delineating factor (by definition) that separates gingivitis from periodontitis is _____.

# REFERENCES

1. Chisholm, G. (1916). The etiology and treatment of pyorrhea alveolaris. *Dental Items Interest,* 38:165–7.
2. Smith, T. S. (1916). The successful scientific treatment of periodontal diseases (*Pyorrha alveolaris*). *Dental Items Interest,* 38:437–50.
3. Atkinson, C. B. (1890). Pyorrhea alveolaris. *Dental Cosmos,* 32:545–50.
4. Day (NMI). (1872). A test for pus. *Dental Cosmos,* 14.
5. Talbot, E. S. (1892). A study of the degeneracy of the jaws of the human race. *Dental Cosmos,* 34;520–1.
6. Mandel, I. D. (1995). Calculus update: prevalence, pathogenicity and prevention. *JADA,* 26, 573–80.
7. Loesch, W. J. (1997). The antimicrobial treatment of periodontal disease. *J Periodontol,* 68:246–5.
8. Russell, R. R. (1994). Control of specific plaque bacteria. *Adv Dent Res,* 8:285–90.
9. Mandel, I. D., & Gaffar, A. (1986). Calculus revisited: A review. *J Clin Periodontol,* 13:249–57.
10. Rustog, K. K., Triratana, T., Kietprajuk, C., Lindhe, J., & Valpe, A. R. (1991). The association between supragingival calculus deposits and the extent of gingival recession in a sample of Thai children and teen ages. *J Clin Dent.* (Suppl C), 3:B6–B11.
11. Schuhack, P., & Guggenheim, B. Structural and ultrastrural features of sub- and supragingival human dental calulus. *J. Dent Res,* 71:(AADR Abst)251.
12. Albandar, J. M., Kingman, A., Brown, L. J., & Löe, H. (1998). Gingival inflammation and subgingival calculus as determinants of disease progression in early-onset periodontitis. *J Clin Periodontol,* 25:231–7.

13. Barrington, E. P., & Nevins, M. (1990). Diagnosing periodontal diseases. *JADA*, 121:460–64.

14. Paster, B. J., Boches, S. K., Gavin, J. L., Ericson, R. E., Lau, C. N., Levanos, V. A., Sahasrbudhe, A., & Dewhirst, F. E. (2001). Bacterial diversity in human subgingival plaque. *J Periodontol*, 183:3770–83.

15. Slots, J., & Listgarten, M. A. (1988). Bacteroides gingivalis, Bacteroides intermedius, and Actinobacillus actinomycetemcomitans in human periodontal diseases. *J Clin Periodontol*, 15:85–93.

16. Wolff, L., Dalden, G., & Aeppli, D. (1994). Bacteria as risk markers for periodontitis. *J Periodontol*, 64:498–510.

17. Beck, J. D., Kock, G. G., Zambon, H., Genko, R. J., & Tudor, G. E. (1992). Evaluation of oral bacteria as risk indicators for periodontitis in older adults. *J Periodontol*, 63:93–9.

18. Dahlen, G. (1993). Role of suspected periodontopathogens in microbiological monitoring of periodontitis. *Adv Dent Res*, 7:163–74.

19. *Annals of Periodontology*, Volume 4, number 1, December 1998, pages 1–112.

20. Wilson, T. G. (1994). Using risk assessment to customize periodontal treatment. *J Calif Dent Assn*, 27:627–32, 634–39.

21. Machtei, E. F., Dunford, R., Housmann, E. Grossi, S. G., Powell, J., Cummins, D., & Zambon, J. J. (1997). Longitudinal study of prognostic factors in established periodontitis patients. *J. Clin Periodontol*, 24:102–9.

22. Petit, M. D., van Steenbergen, T. J., Timmerman, M. F. deGraaff, J., Velden, U. (1994). Prevalence of periodontitis and suspected periodontal pathogens in families of adult periodontitis patients. *J Clin Periodontol*, 21:76–85.

23. Taylor, G. W., Burt, B. A., Becker, M. P., Genco, R. J., Schlossman, M., Knowler, W. C., & Pettitt, D. J. (1996). Severe periodontitis and risk for poor glycemic control in patients with non-insulin-dependent diabetes mellitus. *J Periodontol*, 67:1085–93.

24. Cichon, P., Crawford, L., & Grimm, W. D. (1998). Early-onset periodontitis associated with Down's syndrome—clinical interventional study. *Ann Periodontol*, 3:370–80.

25. Hart, T. C., Hart, P. S., Michalac, M. D. et al. (2000). Haim-Munk syndrome and Papillon-LeFevre syndrome are allelic mutations of cathepsin C. *J Med Genet*, 37:88–94.

26. Hujoel, P. P., Drangsholt, M., Spiekerman, C., & DeRovern, T. A. (2000). Periodontal disease and coronary heart disease risk. *JAMA*, 284:1406–10.

27. Wu, T., Trevisan, M., Genico, R. J. et al. (2000). Periodontal disease and risk of coronary heart disease: the first national health and nutrition examination and follow-up study. *Arch Intern Med*, 160:2749–55.

28. Tibbetts, L. S., & Shanelec, D. A. (1997). Periodontal treatment alternatives. *Tex Dent J*, 114:10–15.

29. Stamm, J. W. (1986). Epidemiology of gingivitis. *J Clin Periodontol*, 13:360–70.

30. Gilbert, A. D., & Nuttal, N. M. (1999). Self-reporting of periodontal health status. *Br Dent J*, 186:241–44.

31. Thompson, K. S., Yonke, M. L., Rapley, J. W., et al. (1999). Relationship between a self-reported health questionnaire and laboratory tests at initial office visit. *J Periodontol*, 70:1153–7.

32. Gilbert, A. D., & Nuttal, N. M. (1999). Self–reporting of periodontal health status. *Brit Dent J*, 186:241–4.

33. Abdellatif, H. M., & Burt, B. A. (1987). An epidemiological investigation into the relative importance of age and oral hygiene status as determinants of periodontitis. *J Dent Res*, 66:13–8.

34. Arnlalugsson, S., & Magnusson, T. E. (1996). Prevalence of gingivitis in 6-year-olds in Reyjavik, Iceland. *Acta Odontolog Scand*, 54:247–50.

35. Querna, J. C., Rossman, J. A., & Kerns D. G. (1994). Prevalence of periodontal disease in an active duty military population as indicated by an experimental periodontal index. *Military Medicine*, 159:223–26.

36. Bhat, H. (1991). Periodontal health in 14 to 17 year old U.S. School children. *J Publ Health Dent*, 51:5–11.

37. Modeer, T., & Wondimu, B. (2000). Periodontal diseases in children and adolescents. *Dent Clin North America*, 44; 633–58.

38. Bailit, H. C., Braun, R., Maryniuk, G. A., & Camp, P. (1987). Is periodontal disease the primary cause of tooth extraction in adults? *JADA*, 114:40–5.

39. Garrett, J. S. (1983). Effects of non-surgical periodontal therapy on periodontitis in humans: a review. *J Clin Periodontol*, 10:515–23.

40. Larner, J. R., & Greenstein, G. (1993). Effect of calculus and irrigator design on the depth of subgingival irrigation. *Int. J. Periodontics Restorative Dent*, 13:188–97.

41. Corbet, E. F., Tam, J. O., Zee, K. Y., Wong, M. C., Lo, E. C., Mombelli, A. W., & Long, N. P. (1997). Therapeutic effects of supervised chlorhexidine mouthrinses on untreated gingivitis. *Oral Dis*, 3:9–18.

42. Boyd, R. L., Leggot, P., Quinn, R., Buchanan, S., Eakle, W., & Chambers, D. (1985). Clinical daily irrigation with a 0.02 percent $SnF_2$ on periodontal disease activity. *J Clin Periodontol*, 12:420–31.

43. Eaton, K. A., Rimini, E. M., Zak, E., Brookman, D. J., Hopkins, L. M., Camell, P. J., Yates, L. G., Morrice, C. A., Lall, B. A., & Newman, H. N. (1997). The effects of a 0.12% chlorhexidine-diglutconate-containing mouthrinse versus a placebo on plaque and gingival inflammation over a 3-month period. A multicenter study carried out in general dental practices. *J Clin Periodontol*, 24:189–97.

44. Brecx, M., Brownstone, E., MacDonald, L., Geksky, S., & Cheong, M. (1992). Efficacy of Listerine, Meridol and Chlorhexidine as supplements to regular tooth cleaning measures. *J. Clin Periodontol*. 19:202–7.

45. Gaffar, A., Alflitto, J., & Nabi, B. (1997). Chemical agents for the control of plaque and plaque microflora: an overview. *Eur J Oral Sci*, 105:502–7.

46. Killoy, W. J., & Saiki, S. M. (1999). A new horizon for the dental hygienists: controlled local delivery of antimicrobials. *J Dent Hyg*, 73:84–92.

47. Stein, M. (1993). A literature review: Oral irrigation therapy. The adjunctive roles of home and professional use. *Probe*, 2718–25.

48. Reynolds, M. A., Lavigne, C. K., Minah, G. E., & Suzuki, J. B. (1992). Clinical effects of simultaneous ultrasonic scaling and subgingival irrigation with chlorhexidine. Mediating influenced periodontal probing depth. *J Clin Periodontol*, 19:595–600.

49. Kornman, K. S., Newman, M. G., Moore, D., et al. (1994). The influence of supragingival plaque control on clinical and microbial outcomes following the use of antibiotics for the treatment of periodontitis. *J Periodontol*, 65:848–54.

50. Brown, L. J., Brunelle, J. A., & Kingman, A. (1996). Periodontal status in the United States. 1988–1991: prevalence, extent and demographic variation. *J Dent Res*, 75 Spec No 672–83.

51. Löe, H., Theilade, E., & Jensen, S. B. (1965). Experimental gingivitis in man. *J Periodontol*, 36:177–87.

52. O'Leary, T. J., Drake, R. B., & Naylor, J. E. (1972). The plaque control record. *J Periodontol*, 43:38.

53. Silness, J., & Löe, H. (1964). Periodontal disease in pregnancy. II. Correlation between oral hygiene and periodontal condition. *Acta Odontol Scand*, 22:121–35.

54. Greene, J. C., & Vermillion, J. R. (1960). The oral hygiene index: A method for classifying oral hygiene status. *J Am Diet Assoc*, 61:172–79.

55. Greene, J. C., & Vermillion, J. R. (1964). The simplified oral hygiene index. *J Am Diet Assoc*, 68:7–13.

56. Löe, H., & Silness, J. (1963). Periodontal disease in pregnancy. I. Prevalence and severity. *Acta Odontol Scan*, 21:533–51.

57. Muhlemann, H. R., & Son, S. (1971). Gingival sulcus bleeding—a leading symptom in initial gingivitis. *Helv Odontol Acta*, 15:107–13.

58. Greenstein, G., Caton, J., & Polson, A. M. (1981). Histological characteristics associated with bleeding after probing and visual signs of inflammation. *J Periodontol*, 52:420–5.

59. Van der Weijden, G. A., Timmerman, M. F., Nijboer, A., Van der Velden, R. (1994). Comparison of different approaches to assess bleeding on probing as indicators of gingivitis. *J Clin Periodontol*, 21:589–94.

60. Loewenthal, B. (1999). A patient-centered approach to periodontal disease detection. *J Practical Hyg*, 8:39–44.

61. World Health Organization (1978). Epidemiology, etiology and prevention of periodontal diseases. Geneva: WHO Technical Report Series, No. 621.

62. Daly, C. G., Mitchell, D. H., Highfield, J. E., Grossberg, D. E. & Stewart, D. (2001). Bacteremia due to periodontal probing: a clinical and microbiologial investigation. *J Periodontol*, 72:210–4.

63. Osborn, J., Stoltenberg, J., Huso, B., Aeppli, D. & Pihlstrom, B. (1990). Comparison of measurement variability using a standard and constant force periodontal probe. *J Clin Periodontol*, 61:497–503.

64. Goodson, J. M. (1992). Diagnosis of periodontitis by physical measurement; interpretation from episodic disease hypothesis. *J Periodontol*, 63:373–82.

65. Clark, W. B., Yang, M. C. K., & Magnusson, J. (1992). Measuring clinical attachment: Reproducibility of relative measurements with an electronic probe. *J Periodontol*, 63:831–38.

66. Yang, M. C. K., Marks, R. G., Magnusson, I., Clouser, B., & Clark, W. B. (1992). Reproducibility of an electron probe in relative attachment level measurements. *J Clin Periodontol*, 19:541–48.

67. Jeffcoat, M. K., Jeffcoat, R. I., Jens, S. C., & Captain, K. (1986). A new periodontal probe with automatic cemento-enamel junction detection. *J Clin Periodontol*, 13:276–80.

68. Hunter, F. (1994). Probe and probing. *Int Dent J*, 44:577–83.

69. Johnson, N. W. (1989). Detection of high-risk groups and individuals for periodontal diseases. *Int Dent J*, 39:33–37.

70. Karim, M., Birch, P., & McCulloch, C. A. (1990). Controlled force measurements of gingival attachment level made with the Toronto automated probe using electronic guidance. *J Clin Periodontol*, 17:594–600.

71. McLeod, D. E., Laison, P. A., & Spivey, J. D. (1997). How effective is periodontal care? *JADA*, 128:316–24.

72. Ainamo, J., Barnes, D., Beagrie, G., Cutress, T., Martin, J., & Sando-Infirri, J. (1982). Development of the World Health Organization (WHO) community periodontal index of treatment needs (CPITN). *Int Dent J*, 32:281–91.

73. Periodontal Screening and Recording (PSR) System (1993). Chicago: The American Dental Asssociation and the American Academy of Peridontology. Sponsored by Procter & Gamble.

74. Loesche, W. J., Bretz, W. A., Lopatin, D., Stott, J., Rau, C. F., Hillenburg, K. L., Killoy, W. J., Drisco, C. L., Williams, R., Weber, H. P., Clark, W., Magnuson, L., & Walker, C. (1990). Multi-center clinical evaluation of a chairside method for detecting certain periodontopathic bacteria in periodontal disease. *J Clin Periodontol*, 61:189–96.

75. Savitt, E. D., Strzempko, M. N., Vaccaro, K. K., Leppke, J. A., Raia, F. F., Savitt, E. D., & Vaccaro, K. K. (1988). Comparison of cultural methods and DNA probe analysis for the detection of Actinobacillus actinomycetemcomitans, Bacteroides gingivalis and Bacteroides intermedius in subgingival plaque samples. *J Periodontol*, 59:431–38.

76. Strzempko, M. N., Simon, S. L., French, C. K., et al. (1987). A cross reactivity study of whole genomic DNA probes for Haemophilus actinomycetemcomitans, Bacteroides intermedius and Bacteroides gingivalis. *J Dent Res*, 66:1543–46.

77. Ebersole, J. L., & Holt, S. C. (1991). Immunological procedures for diagnosis and risk assessment in periodontal diseases. In Johnson, N. W., Ed. *Risk markers for oral diseases: Periodontal diseases*, Vol. 3 (pp. 223–7). Cambridge: Cambridge University Press.

78. March, P. D. (1991). Do bacterial markers exist in subgingival plaque for predicting periodontal disease susceptibility? In Johnson, N. W., Ed. *Risk markers for oral diseases: Periodontal diseases*, Vol. 3 (pp. 365–568). Cambridge: Cambridge University Press.

79. Talwar, G. P., DiWan, M., Razvi, F., & Malhata, R. (1999). The impact of new technologies on vaccines. *Natl Med J India*, 12:274–80.

80. Persson, G. R., Engle, L. D., Moncla, B. J., & Page, R. G. (1993). Macaca nemestrina: a non-human primate model for studies of periodontal diseases. *J Periodontal Res*, 28:294–300.

81. Ma, JK-C. (1999). The caries vaccine: A growing prospect. *Dent Update*, 26:374–80.

82. Kornman, K. S., Crane, A., Wang, H. Y., et al. (1997). The interleukin-1 genotype as a severity factor in adult periodontal disease. *J Clin Periodontol*, 24:71–73.

83. Kornman, K. S., Knobleman, C., & Wang, H. Y. (2000). Is periodontitis genetic? The answer may be Yes! *J Mass Dent Soc*, 49:26–30.

84. Widmann, F. K., Itatani, C. A., Eds. (1998). Philadelphia: F. A. Davis Company. *An introduction to clinical immunology and serology* (2nd ed.), pp. 473.

85. Garito, M. L., Prihoda, T. J., & McManus, L. M. (1995). Salivary PAF levels correlate with the severity of periodontal inflammation. *J Dent Res*, 74:1048–56.

86. Macotte, H., & LaVoie, M. C. (1998). Oral microbial ecology and the role of salivary immunoglobulin A. *Microbiol Mol Biol Rev*, 62:71–109.

87. Wizermann, T. M., Adamou, J. E., & Longermann, S. (1998). Adhesins as targets for vaccine development. *Emer Infect Dis*, 5:395–403.

88. Hasturk, H., Tezcan, I., Yel, L., Ersoy, F., Samal, O., Yamalik, N., & Berker, E. (1998). A case of chronic severe neutrophilia: oral findings and consequences of short-term granulocyte stimulating factor treatment. *Aust Dent J*, 43:9–13.

89. Phillipkoski, K. (February 22, 2001). The debate over tell-tale genes. Wired news, Lyceos Network.

90. Krasse, B. (1996). Discovery! Serendipity or luck: stumbling on gingival crevicular fluid. *J Dent Res*, 50:27–30.

91. Shapiro, L., Goldman, H., & Bloom, A. (1979). Sulcular exudates flow in gingival inflammation. *J Periodontol*, 50:301–4.

92. Curtis, M. A. (1991). Markers of periodontal disease susceptibility and activity derived from gingival crevicular fluid: Specific vs non specific analyses. In Johnson, N. W., Ed. *Risk markers for oral diseases: Periodontal Diseases*, Vol. 3 (pp. 254–76). Cambridge: Cambridge University Press.

93. Golub, L. M., & Kleinberg, I. (1976). Gingival crevicular fluid: a new diagnostic aid in managing the periodontal patient. *Oral Sci Rev*, 9:49–61.

94. Page, R. C. (1992). Host response tests for diagnosing periodontal diseases. *J Periodontol*, 63: 356–66.

95. Suppipat, W., & Suppipat, N. Evaluation of an electronic device for gingival fluid quantification. *J Periodontol*, 48:388–94.

96. U. S. Department of Health and Human Services (1990). The Health Benefits of Smoking Cessation. A Report of the Surgeon General. Public Health Service, Centers for Disease Control, Center for Chronic Disease Prevention and Health. DHHS, Publication No. (CDC) 90-8416.

97. U. S. Department of Health and Human Services (1989). Reducing the Health Consequences of Smoking; 25 years of Progress. A report of the Surgeon General. Public Health Service. Office on Smoking and Health. DHHS. Publication No. (PHS) 81-50-152, 269.

98. LaCrois, A. Z., Lang, J., Scherr, P., LaCroix, A. Z., Long, J., Scherr, P., Wallace, R. B., Comoni-Huntlley, J., Berhman, L., Curb, J. D., & Hennekors, C. H. (1991). Smoking and mortality among older men and women in three communities. *New Engl J Med*, 324:1619–25.

99. Winn, D. M. (2001). Tobacco use and oral diseases. *J Dent Educ*, 65:306–12.

100. Bergstrom, J., & Eliasson, S. (1987). Noxious effect of cigarette smoking on periodontal health. *J Periodontol Res*, 2:513–17.

101. Robertson, P. B., Walsh, M., Greene, J., et al. (1990). Periodontal effects associated with the use of smokeless tobacco. *J Periodontol*, 61:438–43.

102. Tomar, S. L., & Winn, D. M. (1999). Chewing tobacco use and dental caries among U.S. men. *JADA*, 130:1601–10.

103. Robinsom, P. B., Walsh, M. M., Green, J. C. (1997). Oral Effects of smokeless tobacco use by professional baseball players. *Adv Dent Res*, 11:307–12.

104. Bergstrom, J., & Preber, H. (1994). Tobacco use as a risk factor. *J Clin Periodontol*, 65:260–67.

105. Haber, J., Wattles, J., Crowley, M., Mandell, R., Joshipura, K., & Kent, R. L. (1993). Evidence of cigarette smoking as a major risk factor for periodontis. *J Periodontol*, 64:16–23.

106. Holm, G. (1994). Smoking as an additional risk for tooth loss. *J Periodontol*, 65:545–50.

107. Zambon, J. J., Grossi, S. G., Machteri, E. E., Ho, A. W., Dunford, R., & Genco, R. J. (1996). Cigarette smoking increases the risk of subgingival infection with periodontal pathogens. *J Periodontol*, 67:1050–54.

108. Mirbod, S. M., & Ahing, S. I. (2000). Tobacco–associated lesions of the oral cavity: Part I. Nonmalignant lesions. *J Can Dent Assn*, 66:252–6.

109. Barbour, S. E., Nakashima, K., Zhang, J. B., Tangada, S., Hahn, C. L., Schenkein, H. A. & Tew, J. G. (1997). Tobacco and smoking: Environmental factors that modify the host response (immune system) and have an impact on periodontal health. *Crit Rev Oral Biol Med*, 8:437–60.

110. Haber, J. (1994). Cigarette smoking: A major risk factor for periodontitis. *Comp Cont Ed Dent*, 15:1002–13.

111. Preber, H., & Bergstrom, J. (1986). Cigarette smoking in patients referred for periodontal treatment. *Scan J Dent Res*, 94:102–8.

112. Haber, J., & Kent, R. L. (1992). Cigarette smoking in a periodontics practice. *J Clin Periodontol*, 63:100–6.

113. MacFarlane, G. D., Herzberg, M. C., & Wolff, L. (1992). Refractory periodontitis associated with abnormal polymorphonuclear leukocyte phagocytosis and cigarette smoking. *J Periodontol*, 68:908–13.

114. Schenkein, H. A., Gunsalley, J. C., Koertge, T. E., Schenkein, J. G., & Tew, J. C. (1995). Smoking and its effects on early-onset periodontitis. *JADA*, 126:1007–13.

115. Ah, M. K., Johnson, G. K., Kaldahl, W. B., Patil, K. D., & Kalkwarf, K. L. (1994). The effect of smoking on the response to periodontal surgery. *J Clin Periodontol*, 21:91–7.

116. Bergstrom, J., Eliason, S., & Preber, H. (1991). Cigarette smoking and periodontal bone loss. *J Periodontol*, 62:242–46.

117. Bolin, A., Lavstedt, S., Frithiof, L., & Henrikson, C. P. (1986). Proximal alveolar bone loss in a longitudinal radiographic investigation. IV. Smoking and some other factors influencing the progress in individuals with at least 20 remaining teeth. *Acta Odontol Scan*, 44:263–69.

118. Krall, E. A., Dawson-Hughes, B., Garvey, A. J., & Garcia, R. I. (1997). Smoking, smoking cessation, and tooth loss. *J Dent Res*, 76:1653.

119. Preber, H., & Bergstrom, J. (1985). Occurrence of gingival bleeding in smoker and non-smoker patients. *Acta Odont Scand*, 43:315–20.

120. Preber, H., Linder, L., & Bergstrom, J. (1995). Periodontol healing and periopathogenic microflora in smokers and non-smokers. *J Clin Periodontol*, 22:946–52.

121. Christen, A. G. (2001). Tobacco cessation, the dental profession, and the role of dental education. *J Dent Educ*, 65:368–74.

122. Christen, A. G. (1999). Personal communication.

# APPENDIX 13

I. Dental plaque-induced gingival disease
   A. Gingivitis associated with dental plaque only
   B. Gingival disease modified by systemic factors
      1. Associated with the endocrine system
         a. Puberty-associated gingivitis
         b. Menstrual cycle-associated gingivitis
         c. Pregnancy-associated gingivitis
         d. Diabetes mellitus-associated gingivitis
      2. Associated with blood dyscrasias
         a. Leukemia-associated gingivitis
   C. Gingival disease modified by medications
      1. Drug-influenced gingival disease
         a. Drug-influenced gingival enlargement
         b. Drug-influenced gingivitis
            1) Oral contraceptive-associated gingivitis
   D. Gingival diseases modified by malnutrition
      1. Ascorbic acid-deficiency gingivitis
II. Non-plaque-induced gingival lesions
   A. Gingival diseases of specific bacterial origin
   B. Gingival disease of viral origin
   C. Gingival disease of fungal origin
      1. Candida infections
      2. Linear gingival erythema
      3. Histoplasmosis
   D. Gingival disease of genetic origin
      1. Hereditary gingival fibromatosis
   E. Gingival manifestations of systemic conditions
   F. Allergic reactions
   G. Traumatic lesions
III. Chronic periodontitis
   A. Localized
   B. Generalized
IV. Aggressive periodontitis
   A. Localized
   B. Generalized
V. Periodontitis as a manifestation of systemic disease
   A. Associated with hematological disorders
   B. Associated with genetic disorders
VI. Necrotizing periodontal disease
   A. Necrotizing ulcerative gingivitis (NUG)
   B. Necrotizing ulcerative periodontitis (NUP)
VII. Abscesses of the periodontium
VIII. Periodontitis associated with endodontic lesions
   A. Combined periodontic-endodontic lesion

APPENDIX 13-2. **Periodontal Chart**

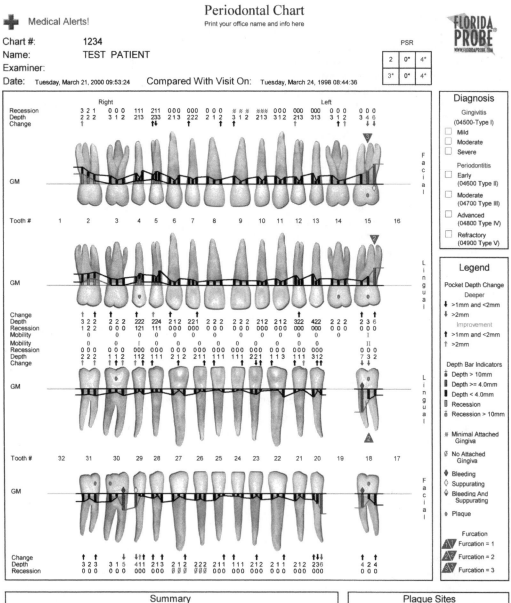

## Periodontal Chart

Print your office name and info here

✚ Medical Alerts!

Chart #: 1234
Name: TEST PATIENT
Examiner:
Date: Tuesday, March 21, 2000 09:53:24   Compared With Visit On: Tuesday, March 24, 1998 08:44:36

**Summary**

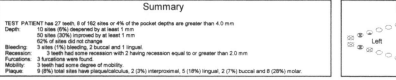

TEST PATIENT has 27 teeth, 8 of 162 sites or 4% of the pocket depths are greater than 4.0 mm
Depth: 10 sites (6%) deepened by at least 1 mm
50 sites (30%) improved by at least 1 mm
62% of sites did not change
Bleeding: 3 sites (1%) bleeding, 2 buccal and 1 lingual.
Recession: 3 teeth had some recession with 2 having recession equal to or greater than 2.0 mm
Furcations: 3 furcations were found.
Mobility: 3 teeth had some degree of mobility.
Plaque: 9 (8%) total sites have plaque/calculus, 2 (3%) interproximal, 5 (18%) lingual, 2 (7%) buccal and 8 (28%) molar.

APPENDIX 13-3  **PSR Screening Examination**

Patient Name: _____  SS# _____ - _____ - _____

Examiner: _____ Department: _____ Date: _____ / _____ / _____

The periodontal screening form is to assist in determining whether or not a periodontal consultation in needed. The dentition is divided into sextants. probing depths should be obtained from six locations on all teeth in each sextant, including: mesiofacial, midfacial, distofacial, mesiolingual, midlingual, and distolingual areas. In each sextant record the following numerical code which applies to the tooth with the highest score.

Any patient with one or more sextants coded with a **3 or higher, or with any letter codes**, deserves a periodontal consultation.

SEXTANTS

Upper right

Lower left

Assign one of the following numerical codes to each of the above sextants:

Code 0—The probing depths are *less than 3.5 mm* in the sextant. Gingival tissues are healthy with no bleeding after gentle probing. No calculus or defective restorative margins are detected.

Code 1—The probing depths are *less than 3.5 mm* in the sextant. There is bleeding upon gentle probing. No supra- or subgingival calculus and/or defective restorative margins are detected.

Code 2—The probing depths are *less than 3.5 mm* in the sextant. There is bleeding upon gentle probing. Supra- and subgingival calculus and defective restorative margins are detected.

Code 3—The probing depths are *between 3.5 and 5.5 mm* in the sextant.

Code 4—The probing depths are *greater than 5.5* in the sextant.

Letter codes denoting other periodontal abnormalities may be added to supplement numerical codes, including:

Code A—*furcation involvement*            Code B—*tooth mobility*
Code C—*mucogingival problems*           Code C— *>3.5 gingival recession*
   X—*denotes edentulous sextants*              NE—*denotes unexamined sextant*

APPENDIX 13-4 **Guidelines to Case Management Following PSR Screening Examination**

The following guidelines for patient management are suggested to assist the examiner in treatment planning and case presentations. For each numerical code a brief description of the most likely periodontal care is made. Letter codes generally indicate unique treatment needs and must be approached on a case-by-case basis.

Code 0—Generally indicates routine dental prophylaxis and semiannual recall.

Code 1—Indicates a need for oral hygiene instruction and dental prophylaxis with subgingival plaque removal and semiannual recall.

Code 2—Indicates a need for oral hygiene instruction and dental prophylaxis with subgingival plaque removal, plus removal of calculus and/or correction of plaque retentive margins, and semiannual or more frequent follow-up monitoring.

Code 3—A comprehensive periodontal examination and charting should be made of the affected sextant to determine an appropriate treatment plan. This examination and documentation should include (but not be limited to) the identification of probing depths, gingival recession, microgingival problems, and furcation involvement, as well as appropriate radiographs. If there are two or more sextants code "3's", a comprehensive full-mouth periodontal examination and charting is indicated. Following periodontal treatment, a comprehensive examination is needed to assess the results of therapy and need for further treatment.

Code 4—A comprehensive full-month periodontal examination and charting is required to determine an appropriate treatment plan. This examination and documentation should include (but not be limited to) identification of probing depths, gingival recession, mucogingival problems, and furcation invasions, as well as appropriate radiographs. It is probable that complex treatment will be required. Following periodontal treatment, a comprehensive examination is needed to assess the results of therapy and the need for further treatment.

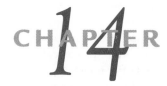

# CHAPTER 14

# Sugar and Other Sweeteners

*Peter E. Cleaton-Jones*
*Connie Mobley*

## OBJECTIVES

*At the end of this chapter it will be possible to*

1. Name the three sugars that are composed of molecules of glucose, fructose, or galactose, all of which can produce caries.
2. Define sugars, sweeteners, and sugar replacers.
3. Describe the potential impact of an excessive intake of added sugars on the quality of the human diet.
4. List three polyols that are sweeteners and cite their advantages and disadvantages in influencing caries incidence.
5. Defend the Food and Drug Administration (FDA) for either removing or attempting to remove saccharin and cyclamate from the marketplace.
6. Name a sweetener that has recently received FDA approval, and list three more that are candidates for approval.

## INTRODUCTION

To most people the term sugar refers to the common household foodstuff table sugar (sucrose). Yet sucrose is only one of many naturally occurring sugars used in the human diet. Technically the term sugar applies to two classifications of carbohydrates. Free-form monosaccharides (simple sugars) include the more common glucose, fructose, and galactose. Disaccharides (two simple sugar molecules linked together) include the most common sucrose, lactose, and maltose. Naturally occurring sugars are available in fruits, vegetables, grains, and dairy foods.

Sweeteners are added sugars that are used as ingredients to both satisfy our taste and in some cases provide added energy. Grouping sweeteners as "nutritive" or "non-nutritive" acknowledges a difference in the amount of energy provided by the sweetener. Nutritive sweeteners may be referred to as caloric and include sugars and sugar alcohols. Non-nutritive sweeteners offer no energy and can sweeten with little volume. Both the sugar alcohols and non-nutritive sweeteners can replace the sugars and are sometimes referred to as sugar substitutes, sugar replacers or alternative sweeteners.[1] Table 14–1 lists sweeteners available in the food supply and their unique characteristics.

## Sensation of Taste

It is difficult to determine whether taste is genetically linked, acquired in utero, neonatal, or influenced by visual, auditory, or taste stimuli during infancy, early childhood, or even adulthood.[2]

Taste buds are present and functioning before birth, a fact demonstrated by injecting sweetening agents into the amniotic fluid during the fourth month of pregnancy.[3] The sweetened amniotic fluid results in an increased rate of swallowing by the fetus. At birth, infants show a taste preference for sucrose, and their taste cells are more responsive to sucrose than to other sugars. Whether it is simply a pleasurable taste or a true metabolic need is not known.

Taste sensation is initiated by the arrival of a stimulus at the taste buds. Taste recognition occurs when the receptor sites of the cells of the taste buds carry, by cranial nerves, a qualitative and quantitative message to the brain. The messages are processed, and the stimulus is recognized as either sweet, sour, salty, or bitter, or some combination of these four.

## The Historic Importance of Sweeteners

The first recorded evidence of sweeteners dates to 2600 B.C. Drawings in Egyptian tombs illustrate beekeeping practices for honey production. The honey was reserved for the rich and powerful.

Cultivating sugar cane began in southeast Asia, India, and China around 100 B.C. The earliest known written reference to sugar cane occurs in a scroll dating to 375 A.D. The Arabs developed the first process for refining sugar cane into sucrose. The cultivation of sugar cane was practiced in southern Europe in the 13th century, and eventually knowledge of it spread to the New World. The cultivation of the root crop called sugar beets started more than 200 years ago.[4]

North American Indians had devised a method of bleeding the sap of the sugar maple tree long before the Pilgrims arrived in Massachusetts. The sugar in the sap of the mature sugar maple is almost exclusively sucrose.

Sweeteners made from corn starch began to appear around 1910. The lesser sweetness of the sugars derived from corn starch, mainly glucose (also referred to as dextrose), was responsible for characterizing them as substitute sweeteners. This identity imposed restrictions on their use. In the 1960s and 1970s, new chemical processes were developed which resulted in the ability to convert the glucose contained in corn starch to fructose. This conversion led to the production of a variety of high-fructose corn syrups (HFCS). Because fructose is twice as sweet as glucose, its use has increased rapidly.

The amount of HFCS used as a sweetener surpassed that of sucrose in 1985. Aspartame,

TABLE 14-1 **Sweeteners (Added Sugars) in the Food Supply, Other Names, Energy Value, and Related Details.**[1]

| Sweeteners | Kcal/g | Other Names | Details |
|---|---|---|---|
| Simple sugars—monosaccharides | | Nutritive | |
| Glucose/dextrose | 4 | Dextrin, Corn sugar | Widely used in canned foods and food processing |
| Fructose | 4 | Fruit Sugar, Levulose | Can produce laxative response from a load greater than or equal to 20 g |
| Simple sugars—disaccharides | | Nutritive | |
| Sucrose | 4 | Granulated, powdered, brown, turbinado (raw), invert sugar | Sweetens and tenderizes baked goods |
| High-fructose corn syrup | 4 | HFSC | Used in soft drinks |
| Corn syrup | 4 | Corn Sugar, corn syrup solids | Found in candy, snack foods, ice cream fruit drinks, non-dairy creamers |
| Maltose | 4 | Malt sugar or syrup | Derived from barley, found in malt flavored foods and alcoholic beverages |
| Molasses/sorghum/maple syrup | 4 | | Used in breads and on pancakes |
| Honey | 4 | Raw, comb, creamed | Produced by bees; not safe for infants |
| Lactose | 4 | Milk sugar | Used in whipped toppings and commercial baked goods |
| Polyols-monosaccharide | | Nutritive | |
| Sorbitol | 2.6 | | 50–70% as sweet as sucrose. Laxative effect for a load equal to or greater than 50 g |
| Mannitol | 1.6 | | 50–70% as sweet as sucrose. Laxative effect for a load equal to or greater than 20 g |
| Xylitol | 2.4 | | As sweet as sucrose |
| Erythritol | 0.2 | | 70% as sweet as sucrose |
| Polyols-disaccharide | | | |
| Lactitol | 2 | | 30–40% as sweet as sucrose |
| Isomalt | 2 | | 45–65% as sweet as sucrose |
| Maltitol | 3 | | 90% as sweet as sucrose |
| Polyols-polysaccharide | | Nutritive | |
| Hydrogenated starch hydrolysates | 3 | HSH, maltitol syrup | 25–50% as sweet as sucrose |
| Intense sweeteners | | Nonnutritive | |
| Saccharin | 0 | Sweet and Low | 200–700 times sweeter than sucrose. |
| Aspartame | 4 | Nutrasweet, Equal | 160–220 times sweeter than sucrose. |
| Acesulfame | 0 | Sunett | 200 times sweeter than sucrose. Used as an additive in desserts, confections and alcoholic beverages. |
| Sucralose | 0 | Splenda | 600 times sweeter than sucrose. Used as an additive in desserts, confections and nonalcoholic beverages. |

which is approximately 180 times sweeter than sucrose, is the most frequently used noncaloric sweetener. From its discovery in 1965, it is now being used by more than 100 million people worldwide.[5]

## Sucrose

Sucrose is the most commonly used tabletop sweetener. Absolute usage in a country is not known but the disappearance of sucrose from the market is the commonly used estimate but it must be understood that this estimate includes wastage which is not ingested by people. In the United States estimated usage has decreased from the high of 102 lb (46 kg) per person in 1971 to 65.8 lb (30 kg) per person in 2000[7] (Figure 14–1). For the United Kingdom the 1993 usage was 44 lb (20 kg) per person.[8] In the past, this usage was considered consumption data; however, this is a misnomer. Usage is actually the quantity of sweeteners delivered to commercial establishments to be used in various ways. It does not account for any loss caused by waste, nor does it include any additional natural sugars consumed. It has been reported that up to 31% of total sugars consumed by adolescents are hidden sugars in foods, such as in milk and fruit.[9]

Individual variation in consumption also occurs. Males generally consume more sucrose than females, and teenagers are by far the greatest consumers. Peak consumptions occur among 15- to 18-year-old males.[14] A decreased consumption rates occurs among members of large families.

## Uses of Sucrose

Sucrose has several attributes that make it desirable for the food industry. It is ideal in the following roles:

- Sweetening agent: The character of the sweet taste can be varied according to pH and temperature used to make a product, as

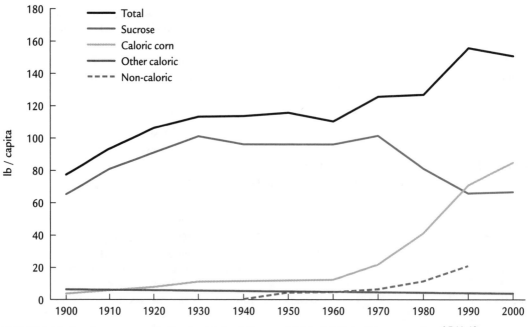

FIGURE 14–1    Sweetener use in the United States 1900–2000 in lb per capita.[6,7,11-13]

well as by its interaction with other ingredients in the formulation. The level of sweetness is important to the acceptance of certain foods.

- Flavor blender and modifier: In some foods, such as mayonnaise, sucrose is a flavor blender; in other foods, such as pickles, it reduces the acidic bite and sour taste.
- Texture and bodying agent: Sucrose gives a texture that is highly acceptable to consumers. It provides body and a distinctive "mouth feel" to food products.
- Dispersing/lubricating agent: In dry packaged mixes, sucrose is used as an agent to keep other ingredients from packing too closely. This, in turn, permits a better blending of the ingredients during food preparation.
- Caramelization/color agent: Caramelization during baking produces a brown color, which increases acceptance. It provides a desirable, characteristic flavor and aroma to the food product.
- Bulking agent: When a noncaloric sweetener that may be 200 times sweeter than sugar replaces sucrose, other ingredients must be added to replace the lost sucrose "bulk" to maintain the food's normal appearance and consistency.

Earlier in this century, home canning and baking resulted in a higher per capita consumption of sucrose than for industrially processed foods. Modern-day affluence, the desire to be liberated from the kitchen, and a higher percentage of working women are factors that have helped reverse the trend. Seventy-five percent of the sucrose manufactured between 1910 and 1930 was delivered to households. In 1950, industrial uses of sucrose surpassed that used at home.[3] The food-processing industry has greatly changed the eating habits of the average American by increasing the output of processed foods. No longer are there only three meals during the day; instead, individual food intake patterns have been extended to include a continuous morning-to-night intake of snacks and beverages, many of them containing sucrose. In a less-developed country, South Africa, home use is still 70% of total use and in the 2000/2001 season was 64 lb (29 kg) per person.[15]

Sucrose has several disadvantages that restrict its industrial use.

- The high concentration (osmolarity) used in canning often causes shrinkage and wrinkling of canned fruits. Both characteristics detract from the visual appeal of the product.
- It absorbs moisture (hygroscopic) and accordingly makes it difficult to freeze-dry food containing high concentrations of sucrose.
- It chars at high temperatures; thus, it cannot be used to sweeten items that must be fried—bacon, for instance.
- It supports bacterial growth; hence, its use in prepared food increases the potential for bacterial contamination and spoilage.

### Evaluation of the Health Aspects of Sucrose

Prior to 1958, few regulatory constraints existed on the introduction of new products into foods. If problems developed, the United States Food and Drug Administration (FDA) had to prevail on the conscience of the manufacturer to withdraw the product or to prove in court that the product was not safe. Both options were rather daunting because considerable financial interest was usually involved. In 1958, the U.S. Congress passed the Foods Additive Amendment that required preliminary marketing clearance. The act required the following information on additives: (1) chemical composition, (2) method of manufacture, (3) analytic method used for the detection of the additive, (4) proof that the additive accomplished its intended effect and that it did not occur in excess

of the amount required to achieve that effect, and (5) proof that it was safe.[16] The burden of proof in substantiating any of these factors resided in the petitioner applying for the clearance, and not with the FDA.

The Foods Additive Amendment decreed that all components added to processed foodstuffs prior to 1958 were classified as food ingredients, whereas those added thereafter were called food additives. With this act, Congress authorized a list of food ingredients which it called generally regarded as safe (GRAS). Sucrose was listed as a food ingredient and placed on the GRAS list. At that time, items on the list were considered as relatively immune from future regulatory action. With the passage of time, however, all the items listed on the original GRAS list of food ingredients have come under review.[17]

In 1986, the FDA formed a Sugars Task Force that critically reviewed all of the recent scientific literature addressing potentially adverse health effects associated with sugars consumption. They investigated the cause-and-effect relationship between the use of sugar and diabetes, cardiovascular disease, hypertension, heart disease, and obesity. The task force determined that no conclusive body of research links any of the above to sugar consumed in moderation.[14] Nutrition and Your Health: Dietary Guidelines for Americans states, "Choose beverages and foods to moderate your intake of sugar."[18]

In the United Kingdom, the Committee on Medical Aspects of Food Policy (COMA) Report noted that current consumption of sugars, particularly sucrose, played no direct role in the development of cardiovascular disease, essential hypertension, or diabetes mellitus; however, the report stated that sugars are the most important dietary factor in the cause of dental caries.[19] Others share the view, based on epidemiological evidence, that sugars are one of the essential multifactorial agents in the prevalence and progression of caries.[20,21]

It has been suggested that trends in consumption of added sugar raise concern that it may also be associated with increasing rates of obesity and inadequate intakes of essential nutrients, especially calcium. Investigators used data from the U.S. Department of Agriculture's 1994–96 Continuing Survey of Food Intakes by 15,011 individuals between 2 years and older, to identify those who consumed more than 26 teaspoons of added sugars daily. These individuals tended to be both younger and male and to frequently over consume total energy.[22]

Using these same data, Guthrie and Morton identified regular soft drinks, followed by table sugar/sweeteners and sweetened grains like cookies and cakes as the primary source of added sugar in the U.S. diet. Percent total energy from added sugars, ranged from 12% for those 65 years and older to 20% for 12- to 17-year-olds, with a mean intake for the entire population of 16%.[23] Displacement of milk in the diet by regular soft drinks in children and adolescents has been demonstrated by several researchers.[24,25]

Major sources of added sugars in the U.S. diet are: table sugar, honey, syrup, candy, jam or jelly, gelatin desserts, soft drinks, fruitades, lemonades and other fruit punches, sweetened grains like cookies and cakes, dairy desserts such as ice cream, sweetened milks and yogurts. These do not include diet or sugar-free varieties with sugar replacers or substitutes.

### Role in Caries Formation

Sugar in plaque is a contributory factor in dental caries.[26] Two animal studies and three human clinical studies have contributed to the understanding of the importance of sugar in the development of caries.

In 1955, the first animal study[27] was conducted with rodents in a gnotobiotic (germfree) environment. One group of rats was fed a caries-producing diet containing large amounts of sugar. The second group was fed the same diet, but at the same time specific microorganisms were introduced to the otherwise germfree environment. Those rats receiving the cariogenic diet alone did not develop caries; those

TABLE 14-2  Dental Caries in Germ-free Rats and Caries-free Rats Inoculated With Known Bacterial Cells (Enterococci Predominating)

| Group | Microbial State | No. of Rats | No. of Rats Developing Molar Caries |
|-------|-----------------|-------------|-------------------------------------|
| A | Germ-free | 9 | 0 |
| B | Inoculated with Entero-cocci plus others | 13 | 13 |

(Copyright by the American Dental Association. Reprinted by permission. From Orland et al., *J Am Dent Assoc.* 1955: 50.)[27]

with the cariogenic diet plus the bacteria did develop lesions (Table 14–2). Observations at that time and since have conclusively demonstrated that certain microorganisms and strains of organisms are more caries-productive than others.

In a second rodent study,[28] one group of rats was fed a caries-producing diet by means of a stomach tube, with no food coming in contact with the teeth. No caries resulted. When the same diet was fed orally and allowed to come in contact with the teeth, caries did occur (Table 14–3).

These two studies conclusively demonstrate that (1) bacteria are essential for caries development, regardless of diet, and (2) the action of the sugar in carious development is local, not systemic.

Several human studies have reported and further clarified the animal studies. Two of the most often cited occurred at Hopewood House[29] in Australia and at Vipeholm in Sweden.[30]

Hopewood House was an orphanage in Australia that accommodated up to 82 children.

From its beginning, sugar and other refined carbohydrates were excluded from the children's diet. Carbohydrates were served in the form of whole meal bread, soybeans, wheat germ, oats, rice, potatoes, and some molasses. Dairy products, fruits, raw vegetables, and nuts were prominently featured in the typical menu. As illustrated in Figure 14–2, dental surveys of these children from the ages of 5 to 11 years revealed a greatly reduced caries incidence compared with the state-school population in that age group. The children's oral hygiene was poor, with about 75% suffering from gingivitis. When the children became old enough to earn wages in the outside economy, they deviated from the original diet. A steep increase of decayed, missing, and filled teeth (DMFT) after the age of 11 years indicates that the teeth did not acquire any permanent resistance to caries (see Figure 14–2).

The Vipeholm study was conducted at a mental institution in that city located in southern Sweden. Adult patients on a nutritionally adequate diet were observed for several years and found to develop caries at a slow rate. Sub-

TABLE 14-3  Caries in Rats Fed a Decay-producing Diet Via Normal and Stomach Tube Routes

| Group | Methods of Feeding | No. of Rats | Avg. No. of Carious Molars | Avg. No. of Carious Lesions |
|-------|--------------------|-------------|----------------------------|-----------------------------|
| A | Normal | 13 | 5.0 | 6.7 |
| B | Stomach tube | 13 | 0 | 0 |

(From Kite et al. J Nutr. 1950:42.)[28]

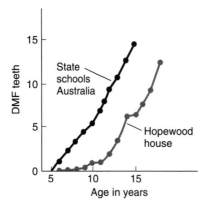

FIGURE 14-2    Plot of the mean number of DMFT versus chronologic age in state schools in Australia and in Hopewood House. (Reprinted by permission from Marthaler, *Caries Res.* 1, 1967.[21])

sequently, the patients were divided into seven groups to compare the cariogenicity accompanying various changes in frequency and consistency of carbohydrate intake. Sucrose was included in the diet as toffee, chocolate, caramel, in bread, or in liquid form. Caries increased significantly when foods containing sucrose were ingested between meals. In addition to the frequency of eating, the consistency of the sugar-containing food was very important. Sticky or adhesive forms of food that maintained high sugar levels in the mouth for a longer time were much more cariogenic than forms that were rapidly cleared.

The Vipeholm study also demonstrated that it was possible to increase the average consumption of sugar from about 30 to 330 g per day with little increase in caries, provided the additional sugar was consumed at mealtime in solution form.[30] Two points to remember about the Vipeholm study are that abnormal quantities and presentations of food were used and that, by modern standards, the study would not receive ethical clearance.

Finally, some people suffer from a condition known as hereditary fructose intolerance

(HFI). After the intake of fructose, these persons become nauseated, vomit, and sweat excessively; malaise, tremor, coma, and convulsions may develop. As a result, these individuals learn to carefully avoid foods with fructose or sucrose where fructose is one of the metabolic products. Those HFI individuals who have survived this disorder by successfully avoiding fructose or sucrose from any source are either caries-free or have very few caries.[31] The low prevalence of caries in HFI patients indicates that starchy foods alone do not produce decay, whereas sugary foods do.

What is the threshold level of sugar content above which a food is highly cariogenic? While many animal and human studies have examined the drop and recovery of plaque pH following consumption of specific foods, a truly safe level has not been established although sugar consumption of between 10 and 15 kg per person per year has been suggested.[32]

Two similar epidemiologic studies of the caries prevalence in 12-year-olds and the per capita sugar use have been done. The first, conducted in 47 countries,[33] revealed a statistically significant relationship between the availability of sugar and the number of DMFT. When daily per capita supply of sugar was less than 50 g, the DMFT index was less than 3.0 (Table 14–4). More recently, a study in 90 countries showed a statistically significant relationship between the logarithm of DMFT and sugar consumption at a slope of 0.021 per kg per person per year.[34] This significant association disappeared when only the data from the 29 industrialized countries were analyzed. This indicates that factors other than sugar consumption (i.e., oral hygiene, professional care, fluoride use), must be taken into account in explaining variation in caries prevalence.

The erroneous impression that oral hygiene and optimum fluoride exposure will protect teeth from bad dietary practices supports the oversimplified view that just removing "sugar" from the diet is an adequate approach to pre-

TABLE 14-4 **Sugar Supply and Caries Prevalence in 12-year-old Children of 47 Countries**

| DMFT Index | Sugar Supply (g/person/day) | | |
| --- | --- | --- | --- |
| | 50 | 50–120 | 120 |
| 3.0 | 21 countries | 9 countries | |
| 3.0–5.0 | | 9 countries | 1 country |
| 5.0 | | 1 country | 6 countries |

(Reprinted by permission from Sreebny Community Dent Oral Epidemiol. 1982:10.)[33]

venting caries progression. The caries promoting activity of carbohydrates and sweeteners vary based on frequency of intake as well as combined intake with other foods that may vary in protein or fat content. Processed high-starch snacks—whether gelatinized, baked, or fried—produce as much acid in dental plaque as sucrose alone but at a slower rate.[35,36] Foods containing both cooked starch and sucrose, like fried potatoes and bread, have been shown to enhance caries potential.[37] When sucrose is added to cooked starch foods the caries promoting potential is increased because the starch brings the sucrose into closer contact with the tooth surface.[38] Thus, added sugars can be part of a total diet when following guidelines that suggest that few foods or beverages containing sugars or starches be eaten between meals.[18]

Streptococcus mutans is generally regarded as the microorganism having the greatest cariogenic potential in humans. Sucrose enhances the colonization and growth of S. *mutans* in dental plaque more than other monosaccharides or disaccharides. These bacteria (1) ferment sucrose rapidly, producing acids; (2) convert sucrose to extracellular polysaccharides that facilitate the adherence of the bacteria to teeth and may function as a reserve of fermentable carbohydrate necessary for the production of acids; and (3) reduce plaque permeability that in turn decreases the rate at which saliva can neutralize or dilute acids formed in the depths of the plaque.[39]

## Question 1

Which of the following statements, if any, are correct?

A. Some sweeteners with a per-gram calorie content equal to sucrose can result in a lesser calorie intake because of their intense sweetness.

B. The *Foods Additive Amendment of 1958* established the basis for the GRAS list.

C. A *food additive* is less subject to FDA study than a *food ingredient*.

D. Approximately 50% more sugar is required in the diet of gnotobiotic (germ-free) rats to induce caries than in the diet of control rats.

E. Individuals with hereditary fructose intolerance (HFI) usually have more caries than sugar-tolerant individuals.

## Corn Sweetener Use

The large increase in the cost of sucrose in 1974 prompted a search for a less expensive alternative. The availability of high-fructose corn syrup (HFCS) with 42% fructose provided one alternative. By late 1977, a process to produce 55% fructose syrups was developed. The use of HFCS per capita in the United States has jumped from 0.7 lb (0.3 kg) in 1970 to 61.6 lb (28 kg) in 2000.[7] The wholesale list price of HFCS is approximately two-thirds that of sucrose. The caloric sweet-

ener HFCS seems to be reaching maximum use on a per capita basis, and its production is not expected to continue increasing as rapidly in the future as it did in the 1970s and early 1980s. High-fructose corn syrup use in soft drinks accounted for over 70% of its use in 1992.[40] HFCS usage outside the United States is low.

A study by Scheinin[41] determined the relative cariogenicity of fructose and sucrose. Fructose was used exclusively by one group who developed 3.8 new carious lesions, whereas the sucrose group developed 7.2 new lesions. The large decrease in caries incidence in the United States may partially be explained by the increased use of HFCS sweeteners with a concurrent decrease in sucrose.

The consumption of glucose and dextrose corn syrup has remained fairly constant in the United States over the past 60 years at 3.5 lb (1.6 kg). The three leading uses are the brewing industry, confectionary, and cereal products.[12]

## Effects of Other Sugars

Fructose, maltose, and lactose are also caloric sugars found in nature. A considerable amount of the first two sugars is contained in fruits and vegetables. Lactose in varying concentrations is present in all mammalian milk. The sweetness of these other sugars ranges from 0.2 to 1.8 times the sweetness of sucrose (Table 14–5).

The subjective evaluation of the sweetness of a substance is usually judged by taste panels. Several methods are used: (1) having the members of the panel write down in their own words a subjective perception of the sweetness, time of onset, aftertaste, or other descriptive terms; and (2) comparing the test sweetener against a reference sweetener, most likely sucrose. These two evaluations indicate quality but not intensity of the test material. For intensity, threshold detection and recognition levels are noted. For threshold detection testing, extreme dilutions of the sweetener are used. The threshold level is the lowest concentration at which sweetness

## TABLE 14–5 Relative Sweetness* of Sugar and Other Sweeteners

| Substances | Sweetness | Substances | Sweetness |
|---|---|---|---|
| Lactose | 0.2 | Aspartame | 180 |
| Galactose | 0.3 | Acesulfame K | 200 |
| Maltose | 0.3 | Stevioside | 300 |
| Sorbitol | 0.5 | Saccharin | 300 |
| Mannitol | 0.6 | Mesperidin dihydrochalcone [†] | 400 |
| Glucose | 0.7 | Naringin dihydrochalcone [†] | 500 |
| Sucrose | 1.0 | Sucralose | 600 |
| Xylitol | 1.0 | Neohesperidin dihydrochalcone [†] | 2000 |
| Glycerol | 1.0 | Thaumatin [†] | 2000 |
| Invert sugar (glucose-fructose) | 1.3 | Alitame | 2000 |
| Fructose | 1.7 | Monellin [†] | 3000 |
| Cyclamate sodium | 30.0 | Sweetener 2000 | 10,000 |
| Ammoniated glycyrrhizin [†] | 50.0 | | |

*Sucrose is assigned a value of 1.0. Sweetness depends on concentration, pH, temperature, and sensitivity of taster.

[†]Sweeteners of natural origin, which are found in various fruits, berries, roots, and leaves of plants.

can be discerned. Recognition tests are based on the lowest concentration at which a panel can recognize the specific sweetener being tested. Testing is accomplished with the sample solutions at 37°C because temperature does modify taste perception. The threshold level is much lower than the recognition level.

### The Polyols as Sweeteners

The most commonly known polyols include sorbitol, mannitol, and xylitol. These polyols are not sugars in the strictest sense. Each molecule resembles a sugar, with the exception that an alcohol grouping is attached to each carbon atom of the polyol. Often they are referred to as "sugar alcohols."

The polyols have 40 to 75% of the caloric content of sucrose. Xylitol has the same sweetness as sucrose. Polyols have similar physical characteristics to sucrose, and their substitution does not change the customary size and weight of a product. Browning or caramelization, however, does not occur with food products that have been sweetened with polyols.

### Sorbitol

Sorbitol, first isolated in 1872, is mainly used in chewing gum, toothpaste, frozen desserts, and some candy. The dental interest in sorbitol results from its use in so-called sugar-free gum, which has been claimed to be noncariogenic. This claim of noncariogenicity has not been substantiated by clinical trials, but intraoral studies have indicated that the plaque pH seldom drops below 5.7 after chewing sorbitol-sweetened gum.[42] The need for further studies is emphasized by the fact that S. mutans is known to metabolize sorbitol.

### Mannitol

Mannitol, which occurs naturally in seaweed, is also derived from the sugar mannose. This sweetener is metabolized very slowly by oral microorganisms and has virtually no cariogenic

potential.[43] Mannitol is used in toothpastes, mouth rinses, and as a dusting agent for chewing gum.

### The Polyols as Sweeteners

#### Xylitol

The polyol that has received the greatest amount of attention by the dental profession is xylitol. Xylitol is derived from birch trees, corn cobs, and oats, as well as from bananas, strawberries and certain mushrooms. As with other polyols, the appearance and texture of xylitol is similar to sucrose. Its cost is about 10 times that of sucrose. Even with a significant expansion in xylitol production, the cost cannot be reduced by much more than half.

Clinical, salivary chemistry and microbiologic evidence suggest that xylitol is the best nutritive sucrose substitute with respect to caries prevention. It has been shown to be nonacidogenic and therefore noncariogenic.[a,44] The main use of xylitol appears to be where it is used in partial substitution for other sugars. This takes advantage of its microbial action, with the food item still being competitive in price.

All of these sugar alcohols have been recognized as having a low potential of producing dental caries. Therefore, in the United States, Congress has authorized products containing less than 0.5 g of sugar and a sugar alcohol to be labeled as "reducing" or "not promoting" tooth decay.[45] This labeling went into effect in January 1998.

Regarding dental-caries prevention, the main use today of the polyols, notably sorbitol and xylitol, is in chewing gums.[46] It is believed, however, that the caries preventive effect of substituted chewing gums is the chewing process itself rather than the sugar-substitutes such as the polyols.[47]

---

[a]Noncariogenic = Does not cause caries.

### Intense Sweeteners

The need for intense sweeteners is acute. For primary preventive dentistry practices, a non-carious product that could be used in oral med-ications, mouthrinses, dentifrices, and all forms of "candy" or between-meal snacks is highly de-sirable. The American Dental Association (ADA) is encouraging the use of intense, or ar-tificial, sweeteners.

Very small amounts of intense sweeteners can be used to achieve acceptable levels of sweet-ness. Even though the cost of these sweeteners may be 100 times greater than an equal amount of sucrose, they are 90 percent more economical than sucrose because their equivalent sweetness can be 1,000 times that of sucrose.

[b]Anticariogenic = Reverses the caries process prior to cavi-tation by enhancing remineralization.

In 1977, the U.S. Senate Select Committee on Nutrition and Human Needs proposed as a dietary goal for the United States that no more than 10% of one's total daily calories be from refined sugars and other caloric sweeteners. In 1978, the average daily diet provided 18%[48] of total calories through sugar and other caloric sweeteners. In 1986, however, that percentage was estimated to be 11%[14] (Figure 14–3). Reaching closer to this goal was made possible by a reduction in sugar intake and a possible increase in the use of acceptable intense sweet-eners although evidence for the latter is lack-ing.

The most popular intense sweeteners in the United States are saccharin, aspartame, acesul-fame-K, and sucralose.

#### Saccharin

Saccharin is considered approximately 300 times sweeter than sucrose. In 1988, approximately 6 lb (3 kg) of saccharin per person (sugar-sweet-ness equivalent weight) was delivered for use as a sweetener in the United States, a drop from 10 lb (5 kg) in 1984. Because of its intense sweetness, the use of saccharin is only about 4% as costly as an equivalent sweetness derived from sucrose.[49] Saccharin is compatible with most food and drug ingredients. Its major deter-rent, a metallic aftertaste, can be recognized by most users.

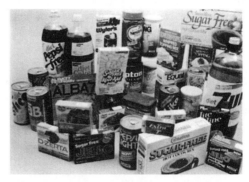

FIGURE 14–3　Sweeteners are making sig-nificant inroads into the sucrose market.

On April 15, 1977, on the basis of alleged carcinogenicity, the revocation of previous approvals for saccharin was proposed by the FDA with the recommendation that saccharin be classified as a drug, meaning it could only be sold by prescription. This decision set off a consumer furor across the nation, resulting in bills being passed in Congress to postpone the ban on saccharin for 18 months. Congress has reacted with a series of 2-year moratoriums that prohibit the FDA from banning use of saccharin in diet sodas and food while permitting more time for further research. In 1987, 1992, and 1996, 5-year moratoriums were passed by Congress. In 1992, the FDA formally withdrew its 1977 proposal to ban the use of saccharin. The agency did not address the safety of saccharin, but stated it would repropose the ban later should such action be warranted.[50]

### Aspartame

Aspartame, better known by one of its tradenames, NutraSweet, is void of an unpleasant aftertaste. It is a dipeptide of two naturally occurring amino acids, phenylalanine and aspartic acid, but it is not found in nature. It was a serendipitous discovery by James Schlatter, a chemist with G. D. Searle & Company, who produced aspartame in 1965 while working on a new antiulcer drug.[5] Aspartame has 4 Cal/g, which is characteristic of proteins; however, because it is 180 times sweeter than sucrose, the caloric intake is insignificant.

Aspartame was originally approved for use in July 1974 by the FDA as a nutritive sweetener. During the review period following the initial approval, objections were filed. In December 1975, the FDA retracted its aspartame approval pending a more detailed inspection of the manufacturer's research and public hearings. In July 1981, aspartame was reapproved for use as an artificial sweetener. In 8 years its per capita use increased to 14 lb (6 kg) (sugar-sweetness equivalent weight). More people have voluntarily consumed considerable quantities of aspartame within a few years of its in-

troduction than any other new chemical entity in history.[51] Originally, aspartame was about 30 times more expensive than saccharin; however, in 1992, the NutraSweet patent expired and the cost of the sweetener decreased substantially. In Canada the expiration of the patent precipitated a 50% drop in cost for the product. It is approved as a free-flowing sugar substitute for table use, and for use by manufacturers in over 100 products, such as cold cereals, drink mixes, instant coffee, instant tea, soft drinks, gelatins, puddings, pie fillings, toppings, dairy products, multivitamin food supplements, and other products where the "standards of identity do not preclude such use."[52] The commissioner of the FDA concluded his statement on aspartame before the Committee on Labor and Human Resources of the United States Senate by stating, "we do not have any medical or scientific evidence that undermines our confidence in the safety of aspartame."[53] Aspartame is a flavor enhancer, especially for sweetening acid flavors. It is also a flavor extender, lengthening the period of flavor for chewing gum for five to seven times as long as gums sweetened with sugar. Aspartame appears to be noncariogenic. The ADA has issued a statement supporting the approval of aspartame as a sweetener.[54] People with phenylketonuria (PKU) should avoid the intake of aspartame because of its phenylalanine content. Products sweetened with aspartame must be labeled with the statement "Phenylketonurics: Contains Phenylalanine."

### Acesulfame K

Acesulfame K is a non-caloric sweetener 200 times sweeter than sucrose, with a pleasant taste. Its sweetness is quickly perceptible and diminishes gradually without any unpleasant aftertaste. It is a derivative of acetoacetic acid. It is marketed under the tradename Sunette by the Hoechst Celanese Corporation and is classified as a noncariogenic sweetener.

This sweetener was discovered in 1967; however, it was not approved for use by the

FDA in the United States until the summer of 1988. Acesulfame has been tested in more than 90 studies and was in widespread use in 60 countries before it was approved for use in the United States. In approving the sweetener, the FDA stated that the studies it had reviewed did "not show any toxic effects that could be attributed to the sweetener."[55] It is approved for use in such items as toothpastes, mouthwashes, pharmaceuticals, dry beverage mixes, instant coffee and tea, chewing gum, gelatins, puddings, and as a tabletop sweetener. It has a synergistic action with other low-calorie sweeteners, as do most of the intense sweeteners. This means the combination of ingredients is sweeter than the sum of the individual ingredients in sweetness. It is excreted quickly and totally, unmetabolized by both animals and humans.

*Sucralose*

Sucralose is a noncaloric sweetener 600 times sweeter than sucrose that is derived from sucrose. It also exhibits synergistic effects. It is not broken down nor absorbed in the human body and therefore provides no calories. Sucralose does not promote tooth decay. More than 100 studies, including human research, support the safety of sucralose. In 1991, Canada was the first country to approve its use in foods. It was approved for use in the United States in 1998.[56]

*Cyclamate*

Cyclamate has a pleasant, sweet taste and a relative sweetness approximately 30 times greater than sucrose. It was originally included on the GRAS list. In 1960, the FDA requirements for studies were expanded to include testing for teratology and carcinogenicity. In early October 1969, there were indications of some cases of rodent bladder cancer. The FDA ruled in 1970 that cyclamate would no longer be allowed even if it were classified as a drug.

## Promising New Noncaloric Sweeteners

Many sweeteners have been submitted to the FDA for approval in the United States. Two of the more promising ones are Alitame and Sweetener 2000.

Alitame is 2000 times sweeter than sucrose. It is composed of two amino acids, L-aspartic acid and D-alanine. It is metabolized in the body; however, because of its intense sweetness, the caloric contribution to the diet is insignificant. It has a synergistic effect with other sweeteners. Alitame has a clean taste and is stable both at high temperatures and broad pH ranges.

Sweetener 2000 is 10,000 times sweeter than sucrose. Originally discovered and patented by researchers at Claude Bernard University in Lyon, France, Sweetener 2000 is exclusively licensed by the NutraSweet Company. It tastes similar to sugar and promises excellent stability in all possible applications. It could literally change the way the world thinks about sweeteners.[57]

Other sweeteners are being used in other parts of the world (Table 14–6).[58,59] Over 150 plants have been identified as possessing a sweet taste.[60]

## Current Legislation Regarding Sweetener Use

The specific use of a sweetener must be stated before it can be approved for commercial use. Will it be used as a flavoring, or will it be used as an anticaries agent? Such differences in intended use can greatly affect the cost of getting the product on the market. If it is to be used as a sweetener, then only safety, teratology, mutagenicity, and carcinogenicity are subjects of investigation. If anticariogenicity is claimed, such as is possible in the use of xylitol, a great amount of additional money must be spent in animal and human caries incidence studies before such claims can be advertised. Estimates on the time and expense of marketing an entirely new sweetener range up to 10 years and

TABLE 14-6  **Regulatory Status of Intense Sweeteners**

| Sweetener | Relative Sweetness (x sugar) | USA | Canada | Europe | Japan |
|---|---|---|---|---|---|
| Acesulfame K | 200 | A | A | A | A |
| Aspartame | 180 | A | A | A | A |
| Cyclamate | 30 | N | A | A | A |
| Saccharin | 300 | A | A | A | A |
| Sucralose | 600 | A | A | N | N |
| Thaumatin | 2000 | N | N | A | A |
| Neohesperidin dihydrochalcone | 2000 | N | N | A | A |
| Stevioside | 300 | N | N | N | A |

as high as $20 million, respectively. If the sweetener is classified as a new drug, it may require a dosage statement and package insert carrying warnings of complications, contraindications, and incompatibility with other drugs.[61]

On the other hand, public safety is paramount. Many of the original food additives were chosen from organic and inorganic compounds that were intended for fabric and paper coloration, with safety being secondary to product appeal.

### Question 3

Which of the following statements, if any, are correct?

A. The two amino acids in aspartame are phenylalanine and aspartic acid.

B. Sweetener 2000 has equivalent sweetness to saccharin but no reported aftertaste.

C. Sunette, the sweetener, is known as acesulfame K.

D. Sweetness is related to cariogenicity.

## SUMMARY

There is little doubt that the consumption of sugar is associated with the caries process, but sugar alone is not the sole determinant of whether food is cariogenic.[62] Sweetness is such a cultural characteristic, however, that behavior modification to exclude it from the diet is considered an impossibility. Also, the nonsweetening benefits of sucrose in industry would probably guarantee its continued use. In many industrial applications in the preparation and processing of food, other caloric and noncaloric sweeteners are preferable to sucrose. New sweeteners have been introduced recently that are less cariogenic and many hundred or thousand times sweeter than sucrose. Many of them are nonacidogenic and noncaloric. From a dental standpoint these new sweeteners offer the potential for a considerable decrease in caries incidence. At the present time no one sweetener dominates another from the clinical perspective of caries prevention.[43]

## ANSWERS AND EXPLANATIONS

1. A and B—correct

   C—incorrect. A food additive is considered suspect, whereas the food ingredient has a long-term record of use and apparent safety.

   D—incorrect. Without bacteria, no amount of sugar is going to produce caries in the gnotobiotic rats.

   E—incorrect. People with HFI cannot consume sucrose without adverse systemic problems and hence experience few, if any, caries.

2. A, C, D, and E—correct

   B—incorrect. It requires more sweetener to identify the product than to identify the sweet taste.

3. A and C—correct

   B—incorrect. Sweetener 2000 is 10,000 times sweeter than sucrose, whereas saccharin is 300 times the sweetness of sugar.

   D—incorrect. Cariogenicity is related to sugar, not sweetness.

### Self-evaluation Questions

1. Two synthetic caloric sweeteners are _____ and _____; two synthetic noncaloric sweeteners are _____ and _____.

2. Peanut brittle made with saccharin would be a very unusual product, mainly because the sweetener lacks the _____ (characteristic) that sucrose imparts to a product. Three other attributes of sucrose that are desirable from a commercial viewpoint are _____, _____, and _____.

3. Four properties of sucrose that make it undesirable for the preparation of some consumer products are _____, _____, _____, and _____.

4. The acronym GRAS refers to _____.

5. The Vipeholm study demonstrated that two key factors relating to cariogenicity of foods were (1) frequency of intake and (2) _____; the lesson learned at Hopewood House was _____.

6. The lowest concentration at which a substance is identified to be sweet is known as the _____ concentration; the tasting of higher concentrations to identify specific sugars is known as _____ testing.

7. The sugar alcohols are more correctly referred to as _____ (name). Three of these compounds are _____, _____, and _____.

8. The noncariogenicity of xylitol is because it is _____.

9. A sweetener that is much sweeter than sucrose is referred to as an _____ sweetener.

10. Three of the most popular sweeteners are _____, _____, and _____.

11. One sweetener that is on the market today because of congressional action is _____.

12. A new product to be accepted must include data relating to carcinogenicity, _____, and _____.

13. Aspartic acid and phenylalanine are the two molecules that make up _____ (name of sweetener).

14. The chemical name for Sunette is _____.

# REFERENCES

1. Use of nutritive and nonnutritive sweeteners—position of ADA (1998). *J Am Diet Assoc.* 98:580–87.
2. Weiffenbach, J. M. (1978). The development of sweet preference. In Shaw, J. H., & Roussos, G. G., Eds. *Proceeding: Sweeteners and dental caries*. Special Supplement. Feeding, Weight and Obesity. [Abstr.]. Washington, DC: Information Retrieval, Inc. 75–91.
3. Mandel, I. D. (1979). Dental caries. *Am Sci.* 67:680–88.
4. Institute of Food Technologists. Sugars and nutritive sweeteners in processed foods. A scientific status summary by the I.F.T. expert panel on food safety and nutrition. Chicago: Institute of Food Technologists; May 1979.
5. Homler, B. E., Deis, R. C., & Shazer, W. H. (1991). Aspartame. In Nabors, L. O., & Gelard, R. C., Eds. *Alternative sweeteners* (pp. 39–63). New York: Marcel Dekker, Inc.
6. U.S. Department of Agriculture. Sugar and Sweetener Outlook and Situation Report. No. SSSV21N4. Washington, DC: U.S. Government Printing Office; December 1996.
7. ERS Sugar & Sweetener Yearbook Data . Find at http://www.ers.usda.gov/data/; May 2001.
8. Edgar, W. M. (1993). Extrinsic and intrinsic sugars: A review of recent UK recommendations on diet and caries. *Caries Res*, 27(Suppl. 1):64–67.
9. Rugg-Gunn, A. J., Hackett, A. F., Appleton, D. R., Appleton, D. R., & Moynihon, P. J. (1986). The dietary intake of added and natural sugars in 405 English adolescents. Hum Nutr Appl. 40A:115–24.
10. Gray, F. (1971). Sweeteners consumption, utilization and supply patterns in the United States: Past trends and relationships, and prospects for target years 1980 and 2000. Dissertation. Baltimore: University of Maryland. Department of Agricultural Economics.
11. U.S. Department of Agriculture (1980). Sugar and Sweetener Outlook and Situation Report. No. SSRV5N5. Washington, DC: U.S. Government Printing Office, May.
12. U.S. Department of Agriculture. Food Consumption, Prices, and Expenditures, 1996: Annual Data, 1970–1994. Statistical Bulletin No. 928:66. Washington, DC: U.S. Government Printing Office; April 1996.
13. LMC International, Ltd. (Aug 1995). The *world sweetener market in the next decade: New demand for caloric and low calorie sweeteners*. Oxford.

14. Glinsmann, W., Irausguin, H., & Park, Y. K. (1986). Evaluation of health aspects of sugars contained in carbohydrate sweeteners: Report of Sugars Task Force, 1986. *J Nutr, 116*(11S): SI–S216.

15. South African Sugar Association (2001). Unpublished annual statistics of sugar disappearance. Durban, South Africa.

16. Ronk, R. J. (1978). Regulatory constraints on sweetener use. In Shaw, J. H., & Roussos, G. G., Eds. Proceeding: Sweeteners and Dental Caries. Special Supplement. Feeding, Weight and Obesity [Abstr.] (pp. 131–34). Washington, DC: Information Retrieval, Inc.

17. U.S. Department of Commerce, Food and Drug Administration. Evaluation of the Health Aspects of Sucrose as a Food Ingredient. No. PB 262-668. Washington, DC: U.S. Government Printing Office; 1976.

18. U.S. Department of Health and Human Services. Nutrition and Your Health: Dietary Guidelines for Americans, 5th ed. Home and Garden Bulletin No. 232. U. S. Government Printing Office; 2000.

19. Committee on Medical Aspects of Food Policy (COMA) Report. Dietary Sugars and Human Disease: Conclusions. Department of Health, Report on Health and Social Subjects No. 37. London: Her Majesty's Stationery Office; 1990.

20. Konig, K. G. (2000). Diet and oral health. *Int Dent J, 50*:162–74.

21. Depaola, D. P., Faine, M. P., & Palmer C. A. (1999). Nutrition in relation to dental medicine. In Shils, M. E., Olson, J. A., Shike, M., Ross, A. C. Eds. *Modern nutrition in health and disease.* (9th ed.) Baltimore: Williams and Wilkins, 1099–1124.

22. USDA Center for Nutrition Policy and Promotion (Oct 2000). Is intake of added sugars associated with diet quality? *Nutrition Insights.*

23. Guthrie, J. F., & Morton, J. F. (2000). Food sources of added sweeteners in the diets of Americans. *J Am Diet Assoc, 100*;43–51.

24. Morton, J. F., & Guthrie, J. F. (1998). Changes in children's total fat intakes and their food group sources of fat. *Fam Econ Nutr Rev, 11*:44–57.

25. Harnack, L., Stang, J., & Story, M. (1999). Soft drink consumption among US children and adolescents: nutritional consequences. *J Am Diet Assoc, 99*:436–41.

26. Burt, B. A. (1993). Relative consumption of sucrose and other sugars: Has it been a factor in reduced caries experience? *Caries Res, 27*(Suppl. 1):56–63.

27. Orland, F., Blaney, R., Harrison, W., et al. (1955). Experimental caries in germ-free rats inoculated with enterococci. *J Am Dent Assoc, 50*:259–72.

28. Kite, O., Shaw, J., & Sognnaes, R. (1950). The prevention of experimental tooth decay by tube-feeding. *J Nutr, 42*:89–103.

29. Marthaler, T. M. (1967). Epidemiological and clinical dental findings in relation to intake of carbohydrates. *Caries Res, 1*:222–38.

30. Gustafsson, B. E., Quensel, C. E., Lanke, L. S., et al. (1954). The Vipeholm dental caries study. The effect of different levels of carbohydrate intake on caries activity in 436 individuals observed for five years. *Acta Odont Scand, 11*:232–364.

31. Newbrun, E., Hoover, C., Mattraux, G., & Graf, H. (1980). Comparison of dietary habits and dental health of subjects with hereditary fructose intolerance and control subjects. *J Am Dent Assoc, 101*:619–26.

32. Sheiham, A. (1991). Why free sugar consumption should be below 15 kg per person per year in industrialized countries: The dental evidence. *Br Dent J, 171*:63–65.

33. Sreebny, L. M. (1982). Sugar availability, sugar consumption and dental caries. *Community Dent Oral Epidemiol, 10*:1–17.

34. Woodward, M., & Walker, A. R. P. (1994). Sugar consumption and dental caries: Evidence from 90 countries. *Br Dent J, 176*:297–302.

35. Grenby, T. H. (1991). Snack foods and dental caries. Investigations using laboratory animals. *Brit Dent J*. 171:353–61.

36. Mörmann, J. E., & Mühlemann, H. R. (1981). Oral starch degradation and its influence on acid production in human dental plaque. *Caries Res*, 15:166–75.

37. Mundorff, S. A., Featherstone, J. D. B., Bibby, B. G., Curzon, M. E. J., Eisenberg, A. D., & Espeland, M. A. (1990). Cariogenic potential of foods. 1. Caries in the rat model. *Caries Res*, 24:344–55.

38. Sgan-Cohen, H. D., Newbrun, E., Huber, R., Tenenbaum, G., & Sela, M. N. (1988). The effect of previous diet on plaque pH response to different foods. *J Dent Res*, 67:1434–37.

39. Loesche, W. J. (1986). Role of Streptococcus mutans in human dental decay. *Microbiol Rev*, 50:353–80.

40. U.S. Department of Agriculture. Sugar and Sweetener Outlook and Situation Report. No. SSRV17N4. Washington, DC: U.S. Government Printing Office; December 1992.

41. Scheinin, A. (1976). Caries control through the use of sugar substitutes. *Int Dent J*, 26:4–13.

42. Park, K. K., Shemehorn, B. R., & Stookey, G. K. (1993). Effect of time and duration of sorbitol gum chewing on plaque acidogenicity. *Pediatr Dent*, 15:197–202.

43. Imfeld, T. (1993). Efficacy of sweeteners and sugar substitutes in caries prevention. *Caries Res*, 27(Suppl. 1):50–55.

44. Mäkinen, K. K., Mäkinen, P-L., Pape, H. R. Jr., Peldyak, J., Hujoel, P., Isotupa, K. P., Sodealing, E., Isokangas, P. J., Allen, P., & Bennett, C. (1996). Conclusion and review of the "Michigan Xylitol Program" (1986–1995) for the prevention of dental caries. *Int Dent J*, 46:22–34.

45. U.S. Food and Drug Administration (1996). Health claims: Dietary sugar alcohols and dental caries. *Federal Register*, 61:43446–47.

46. Gales, M. A., & Nguyen, T. M. (2000). Sorbitol compared with xylitol in the prevention of dental caries. *Ann Pharmacother*, 34:98–100.

47. Machiulskiene, V., Nyvad, B., & Baelum, V. (2001). Caries preventive effect of sugar-substituted chewing gum. *Community Dent Oral Epidemiol*, 29:278–88.

48. Shaw, J. H. (1978). The metabolism of the polyols and their potential for greater use as sweetening agents in foods and confections. In Shaw, J. H., & Roussos, G. G., Eds. *Proceedings: Sweeteners and dental caries*. Special Supplement. Feeding, Weight and Obesity [Abstr.] (pp. 157–76). Washington, DC: Information Retrieval, Inc.

49. U.S. Department of Agriculture. Sugar and Sweetener Outlook and Situation Report. No. SSRVI7N1. Washington, DC: U.S. Government Printing Office; March 1992.

50. U.S. Food and Drug Administration (1991). Withdrawal of certain pre-1986 proposed rules: Final action. *Federal Register*, 30 December 56:67442.

51. Dews, P. B. (1987). Summary: Report of an international aspartame workshop. *Fed Chem Toxic*, 25:549–52.

52. U.S. Food and Drug Administration (1984). Aspartame, chewable multivitamin food supplement. *Federal Register*, May 30, 49:22468–69.

53. Young, F. E. Statement by FDA Commissioner before Committee on Labor and Human Resources. United States Senate; November 3, 1987.

54. American Dental Association (1981). Aspartame important as a sucrose substitute. *ADA News*, July 27, *12*(24):1.

55. U.S. Food and Drug Administration (1988). Food additives permitted for direct addition for human consumption: Acesulfame potassium. *Federal Register*, 28 July, 53:28379–83.

56. U.S. Food and Drug Administration. (April 3, 1998). Food additives permitted for direct addition for human consumption: Sucralose. *Federal Register*, 63(64):16417–33.

57. Sweetener for the 21st century? (1991). *Food Processing*, 52:54.

58. Vlitos, A. J. (March 27, 1996). A comprehensive overview of sweeteners available on the worldwide market and an analysis of how they compete in practice on price, application and legislation. Paper presented at World Sugar and Sweetener Conference, Bangkok, Thailand.

59. Newbrun, E. (1990). The potential role of alternative sweeteners in caries prevention. *Israel J Dent Sci*, 2:200–13.

60. Kinghorn, A. D., & Soejanto, D. D. (1989). Intensely sweet compounds of natural origin. *Med Res Rev*, 9:91–115.

61. Macay, D. A. M. (1979). Sucrose and sucrose substitutes: Industrial considerations. *Pharmacol Ther Dent*, 3:69–74.

62. Bowen, W. H. (1994). Food components and caries. *Adv Dent Res*, 8:215–20.

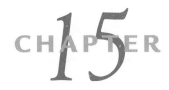

# CHAPTER 15

# Nutrition, Diet, and Oral Conditions

*Carole A. Palmer*
*Linda D. Boyd*

## OBJECTIVES

*At the end of this chapter it will be possible to*

1. Explain the underlying rationale for the Reference Daily Intakes, Food Guide Pyramid, and food labels.
2. Discuss the potential oral effects of severe malnutrition during organogenesis.
3. Discuss why foods with equal amounts of sugar are not necessarily equally cariogenic.
4. Describe how dietary patterns and food composition affects cariogenic potential.
5. Discuss the effects of food on buffering capacity.
6. Discuss the role of nutrition in periodontal disease.
7. Explain why elderly patients are at higher nutritional risk than other age groups.
8. Discuss the relevant nutritional considerations for patients who have diabetes, immunocompromising conditions, or head and neck surgery.

## INTRODUCTION

Oral health, diet, and nutritional status are closely linked (Figure 15-1). Nutrition is an essential for the growth, development, and maintenance of oral structures and tissues. During periods of rapid cellular growth, nutrient deficiencies can have an *irreversible* ef-

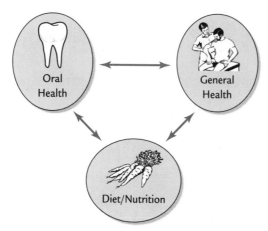

FIGURE 15–1    Relationships between Nutrition and Health.

fect on the developing oral tissues. Prior to tooth eruption, nutritional status can influence tooth enamel maturation and chemical composition as well as tooth morphology and size.[1] Early malnutrition increases a child's susceptibility to dental caries in the deciduous teeth.[2] Throughout life, nutritional deficiencies or toxicities can affect *host resistance,* healing, oral function, and oral-tissue integrity. For example, immune response to local irritants and healing of periodontal tissues may be impaired when nutritional status is compromised. Because the oral epithelium has more rapid cell turnover than most other tissues in the body, clinical signs of malnutrition are often manifest first in the oral cavity.

After tooth eruption, the effects of diet on the dentition are topical rather than systemic. Dietary factors and eating patterns can initiate exacerbate or minimize dental decay. Fermentable carbohydrates are *essential* for the implantation, colonization, and metabolism of bacteria in dental plaque. Factors such as eating frequency and retentiveness of carbohydrates influence the progression of carious lesions, while foods containing calcium and phosphorus, such as cheese, enhance remineralization. Frequent intake of *acidic foods* or beverages can cause enamel erosion. Conversely, impaired dental function may lead to poor nutritional health. Older adults with loose or missing teeth, or ill-fitting dentures often reduce their intake of foods that require chewing, such as fresh fruits, vegetables, meats, and breads.[3] When the variety of foods in a diet is reduced, there is greater risk of nutrient inadequacies. The patient who undergoes oral or periodontal surgery may require dietary guidance to prevent deleterious changes in the diet. Patients with diabetes mellitus, oral cancer, or depressed immune function may suffer from oral conditions that compromise nutritional status. The dental clinician needs to *understand* how diet and nutrition can affect oral health, and how oral conditions can affect food choices and ultimately nutritional status. This chapter provides an overview of the relationships between diet, nutrition and dental practice, and offers appropriate suggestions for patient guidance.

## Importance of Diet Assessment and Counseling in Dentistry

The modern dental practitioner is not only concerned with educating patients for the prevention of caries and periodontal disease, but also plays an important role in screening patients for other health risks. Just as a medical history and blood pressure evaluation are used to screen for underlying medical conditions, a dietary assessment and screening can help pinpoint potential nutritional problems that may affect or be affected by dental care. Because of the large number of patients seen regularly in dental practice, the *dental team* is in an excellent position to recognize areas of *nutritional risk*. The role of the dental team should be to *screen patients* for nutritional risk, provide *dietary guidance* related to oral health, and *refer patients* to nutrition professionals for treatment of other nutrition-related systemic conditions.[3]

---

### Question 1

What are appropriate nutrition interventions for dental clinicians?

A. Assess patients' nutritional status using laboratory and other biochemical assessment tools.

B. Screen patients for nutritional risk.

C. Recognize dietary problems in denture patients.

D. Provide diet guidance related to oral health.

---

## The Basis for a Healthy Diet

### Dietary Reference Intakes

Daily food intake must be sufficient to meet metabolic requirements for energy and provide the essential nutrients that the body cannot synthesize in sufficient quantities to meet physiologic needs. Since the 1940s, the *Food and Nutrition Board* (FNB) of the National Academy of Sciences has published the *Recom-*

*mended Dietary Allowances* (RDA), which were recommendations for daily nutrient intake that would support growth and maintenance of body tissues, and prevent deficiency diseases. (4-Food and Nutrition Board). Beginning in 1997, the Food and Nutrition Board began to make major changes to the format and purpose of the nutrition recommendations. *The Dietary Reference Intakes (DRI) expands and replaces the RDA*[5] by addressing the prevention of *chronic degenerative diseases* and the risk of *excess intake of nutrients.*[5]

The DRI are quantitative estimates of nutrient values to be used for planning and assessing diets for healthy people.[5] These reference values vary by *gender and life stage group.* DRI consist not only of RDA but also three other types of reference values shown in Table 15–1.

Evaluation of the true nutritional status of an individual requires a *combination* of clinical, biochemical, and anthropometric data.[5] So if an individual reports an intake of a nutrient below the RDA, more information would be necessary to determine if an actual deficiency exists. Conversely, nutrient intakes that meet the RDA over time have a low probability of being inadequate.

### Dietary Guidelines for Americans

The *Dietary Guidelines for Americans* were first published in 1980, and are revised every 5 years.[6] The guidelines are designed to complement the DRIs by making recommendations for food choices to promote health. The 2000 Dietary Guidelines for Americans contain 10 recommendations, grouped into *three areas called the ABC of good health.* They are shown in Table 15–2.[6] These *newest* guidelines place more emphasis on *physical activity* and *healthy weight* compared to previous editions. The focus on preventing obesity is caused by the increased risk it presents for many chronic and degenerative diseases, such as heart disease, stroke, diabetes, arthritis, high blood pressure, and some kinds of cancer. The recommenda-

TABLE 15-1 **Types of Daily Reference Values (DRI)**

- *Estimated Average Requirement (EAR)*

  The daily nutrient intake value estimated to meet the needs of half (50%) of all healthy people in a life stage and gender group.

- *Recommended Dietary Allowance (RDA)*

  The average daily nutrient value considered adequate to meet the nutrient needs of nearly all (97 to 98%) healthy people in a life stage and gender group.

- *Adequate Intake (AI)*

  An intake value assumed to be adequate for healthy people in each life stage and gender group when there is not enough data to determine an RDA.

- *Tolerable Upper Intake Level (UL)*

  The highest level of daily nutrient intake likely not to pose adverse health risks for almost all individuals in a life stage and gender group. The risk of adverse effects increases with intakes above the UL.

tions emphasize balance, moderation, and variety in food choices, and promote increased use of whole grains, fruits and vegetables, and decreased use of saturated fat, cholesterol, and

TABLE 15-2 **2000 Dietary Guidelines for Americans**

*Aim for fitness . . .*
- Aim for a healthy weight.
- Be physically active each day.

*Build a healthy base . . .*
- Let the Pyramid guide your food choices.
- Choose a variety of grains daily, especially whole grains.
- Choose a variety of fruits and vegetables daily.
- Keep food safe to eat.

*Choose sensibly . . .*
- Choose a diet that is low in saturated fat and cholesterol and moderate in total fat.
- Choose beverages and foods to moderate your intake of sugars.
- Choose and prepare foods with less salt.
- If you drink alcoholic beverages, do so in moderation.

salt. In addition, for the first time, the guidelines address food safety in an effort to combat food-borne illness, an important public health concern.[6]

The 2000 Dietary Guidelines for Americans define a healthy weight according to the *Body Mass Index (BMI)*. The BMI is a medical standard for defining obesity that not only is highly correlated with independent measures of body fat, but is also used to determine if a person is at increased health risk due to excess weight[7] (Table 15–3). A healthy BMI of 19 to 25 is associated with the lowest statistical health risk [8-Meisler, 1996]. Persons with BMI above 25 are considered obese, and the recommendation is to lose 1 to 2 BMI units (10 to 15 pounds) to reduce their risk for chronic disease.[7]

### Food Guide Pyramid

To help people select nutrient-rich foods and to follow the Dietary Guidelines, the *Food Guide Pyramid* was developed by the U.S. Department of Agriculture.[9] The Food Guide Pyramid displays foods in five categories based on their nutrient composition (Figure 15–2). Whole grains, such as rice, pasta, cereals, and breads, found at the broad base of the Pyramid should form the foundation of a healthful diet. They

TABLE 15-3  Body Mass Index

To use the table, find the appropriate height in the left-hand column labeled Height. Move across to a given weight. The number at the top of the column is the BMI at that height and weight. Pounds have been rounded off.

| BMI | 19 | 20 | 21 | 22 | 23 | 24 | 25 | 26 | 27 | 28 | 29 | 30 | 31 | 32 | 33 | 34 | 35 |
|---|---|---|---|---|---|---|---|---|---|---|---|---|---|---|---|---|---|
| Height (inches) | | | | | | | | Body Weight (pounds) | | | | | | | | | |
| 58 | 91 | 96 | 100 | 105 | 110 | 115 | 119 | 124 | 129 | 134 | 138 | 143 | 148 | 153 | 158 | 162 | 167 |
| 59 | 94 | 99 | 104 | 109 | 114 | 119 | 124 | 128 | 133 | 138 | 143 | 148 | 153 | 158 | 163 | 168 | 173 |
| 60 | 97 | 102 | 107 | 112 | 118 | 123 | 128 | 133 | 138 | 143 | 148 | 153 | 158 | 163 | 168 | 174 | 179 |
| 61 | 100 | 106 | 111 | 116 | 122 | 127 | 132 | 137 | 143 | 148 | 153 | 158 | 164 | 169 | 174 | 180 | 185 |
| 62 | 104 | 109 | 115 | 120 | 126 | 131 | 136 | 142 | 147 | 153 | 158 | 164 | 169 | 175 | 180 | 186 | 191 |
| 63 | 107 | 113 | 118 | 124 | 130 | 135 | 141 | 146 | 152 | 158 | 163 | 169 | 175 | 180 | 186 | 191 | 197 |
| 64 | 110 | 116 | 122 | 128 | 134 | 140 | 145 | 151 | 157 | 163 | 169 | 174 | 180 | 186 | 192 | 197 | 204 |
| 65 | 114 | 120 | 126 | 132 | 138 | 144 | 150 | 156 | 162 | 168 | 174 | 180 | 186 | 192 | 198 | 204 | 210 |
| 66 | 118 | 124 | 130 | 136 | 142 | 148 | 155 | 161 | 167 | 173 | 179 | 186 | 192 | 198 | 204 | 210 | 216 |
| 67 | 121 | 127 | 134 | 140 | 146 | 153 | 159 | 166 | 172 | 178 | 185 | 191 | 198 | 204 | 211 | 217 | 223 |
| 68 | 125 | 131 | 138 | 144 | 151 | 158 | 164 | 171 | 177 | 184 | 190 | 197 | 203 | 210 | 216 | 223 | 230 |
| 69 | 128 | 135 | 142 | 149 | 155 | 162 | 169 | 176 | 182 | 189 | 196 | 203 | 209 | 216 | 223 | 230 | 236 |
| 70 | 132 | 139 | 146 | 153 | 160 | 167 | 174 | 181 | 188 | 195 | 202 | 209 | 216 | 222 | 229 | 236 | 243 |
| 71 | 136 | 143 | 150 | 157 | 165 | 172 | 179 | 186 | 193 | 200 | 208 | 215 | 222 | 229 | 236 | 243 | 250 |
| 72 | 140 | 147 | 154 | 162 | 169 | 177 | 184 | 191 | 199 | 206 | 213 | 221 | 228 | 235 | 242 | 250 | 258 |
| 73 | 144 | 151 | 159 | 166 | 174 | 182 | 189 | 197 | 204 | 212 | 219 | 227 | 235 | 242 | 250 | 257 | 265 |
| 74 | 148 | 155 | 163 | 171 | 179 | 186 | 194 | 202 | 210 | 218 | 225 | 233 | 241 | 249 | 256 | 264 | 272 |
| 75 | 152 | 160 | 168 | 176 | 184 | 192 | 200 | 208 | 216 | 224 | 232 | 240 | 248 | 256 | 264 | 272 | 279 |
| 76 | 156 | 164 | 172 | 180 | 189 | 197 | 205 | 213 | 221 | 230 | 238 | 246 | 254 | 263 | 271 | 279 | 287 |

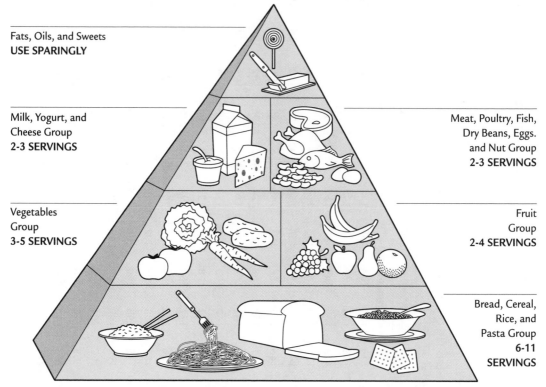

Fats, Oils, and Sweets
**USE SPARINGLY**

Milk, Yogurt, and
Cheese Group
**2-3 SERVINGS**

Meat, Poultry, Fish,
Dry Beans, Eggs.
and Nut Group
**2-3 SERVINGS**

Vegetables
Group
**3-5 SERVINGS**

Fruit
Group
**2-4 SERVINGS**

Bread, Cereal,
Rice, and
Pasta Group
**6-11
SERVINGS**

FIGURE 15-2    The Food Guide Pyramid: A Guide to Daily Food Choices is an outline of what to eat each day. Not a rigid prescription but a general guide that lets each person choose a healthful diet, the Pyramid calls for eating a variety of foods to get the needed nutrients while consuming the right amount of calories to maintain a healthy weight. (Courtesy U.S. Department of Agriculture, Human Nutrition Information Service.)

are good sources of carbohydrate (including fiber) and minerals. Fruits and vegetables form the next level of the Pyramid. The meat group contains good sources of protein, vitamins, and minerals. Meat alternates, legumes, eggs, nuts, and tofu, are included in the meat group. The dairy group is comprised primarily of good calcium sources. The small triangle at the top of the Pyramid is for the fats, oils, and sweets that provide primarily added calories and, thus, should be eaten in small amounts. No single food group is more important than another; each group provides some, but not all, of the essential nutrients.

Standardized serving sizes and the recommended number of servings for various age groups are specified. However, the caloric content of foods varies widely within a food group. The desirable number of servings from each food group depends not only upon age and sex, but also the calorie goal. For example, if 1,600 calories were the daily energy goal, an individual would choose the minimum number of servings of low-fat food choices from each group. If additional calories are needed, increased servings should come from the grain, fruit, and vegetable groups, rather than the top of the pyramid.

## Food Labels

The Nutrition Facts panel found on most processed food packages helps the consumer select foods that meet the Dietary Guidelines (Figure 15–3). The *National Labeling and Education Act of 1990* requires that comprehensive nutrition information *must* appear on the labels of most processed foods and processed meats and poultry products. In *addition*, nutrition information at point of purchase is *voluntary* for fresh fruits, vegetables, and raw fish. In accord with the mandatory food labeling regulations published by the Food and Drug Administration in 1994,[10] the nutrition panel on processed foods must include the following:

- A *standardized portion size* (designed to make nutritional comparisons of similar products easier, and reflects the serving sizes that people actually eat).

- The number of *servings per container*.

Serving sizes are now more consistent across product lines, stated in both household and metric measures, and reflect the amounts people actually eat.

The list of nutrients covers those most important to the health of today's consumers, most of whom need to worry about getting *too much* of certain items (fat, for example), rather than too few vitamins or minerals, as in the past.

The label will now tell the number of calories per gram of fat, carbohydrates and protein

New title signals that the lable contains the newly required information.

Calories from fat are now shown on the label to help consumers meet dietary guidelines that recommend people get no more than 30 percent of their calories from fat.

% Daily Value shows how a food fits into the overall daily diet.

Daily values are also something new. Some are maximums, as with fat (65 grams *or less*); others are minimums, as with carbohydrates (300 grams *or more*). The daily values on the label are based on a daily diet of 2,000 and 2,500 calories. Individuals should adjust the values to fit their own calorie intake.

## Nutrition Facts

Serving Size 1 cup (225g)
Servings Per Container 1

**Amount Per Serving**

**Calories**  225  Calories from Fat 25

| | % Daily Value* |
|---|---|
| **Total fat**  3g | **4**% |
| Saturated Fat  1.5g | **8**% |
| **Cholesterol**  10mg | **3**% |
| **Sodium**  120mg | **5**% |
| **Total Carbohydrate**  42g | **14**% |
| Dietary Fiber  0g | **8**% |
| Sugars  42g | |
| **Protein**  9g | **18**% |

| Vitamin A 2% | • | Vitamin C 2% |
|---|---|---|
| Calcium 30% | • | Iron 0% |

*Percent Daily Values are based on a 2,000 calorie diet. Your daily values may be higher or lower depending on your calorie needs:

| | | Calories: | 2,000 | 2,500 |
|---|---|---|---|---|
| Total Fat | Less than | | 65g | 80g |
| Sat Fat | Less than | | 20g | 85g |
| Cholesterol | Less than | | 300mg | 300mg |
| Sodium | Less than | | 2,400mg | 2,400mg |
| Total Carbohydrate | | | 300g | 375g |
| Dietary Fiber | | | 25g | 30g |

Calories per gram:
Fat 9 • Carbohydrate 4 • Protein 4

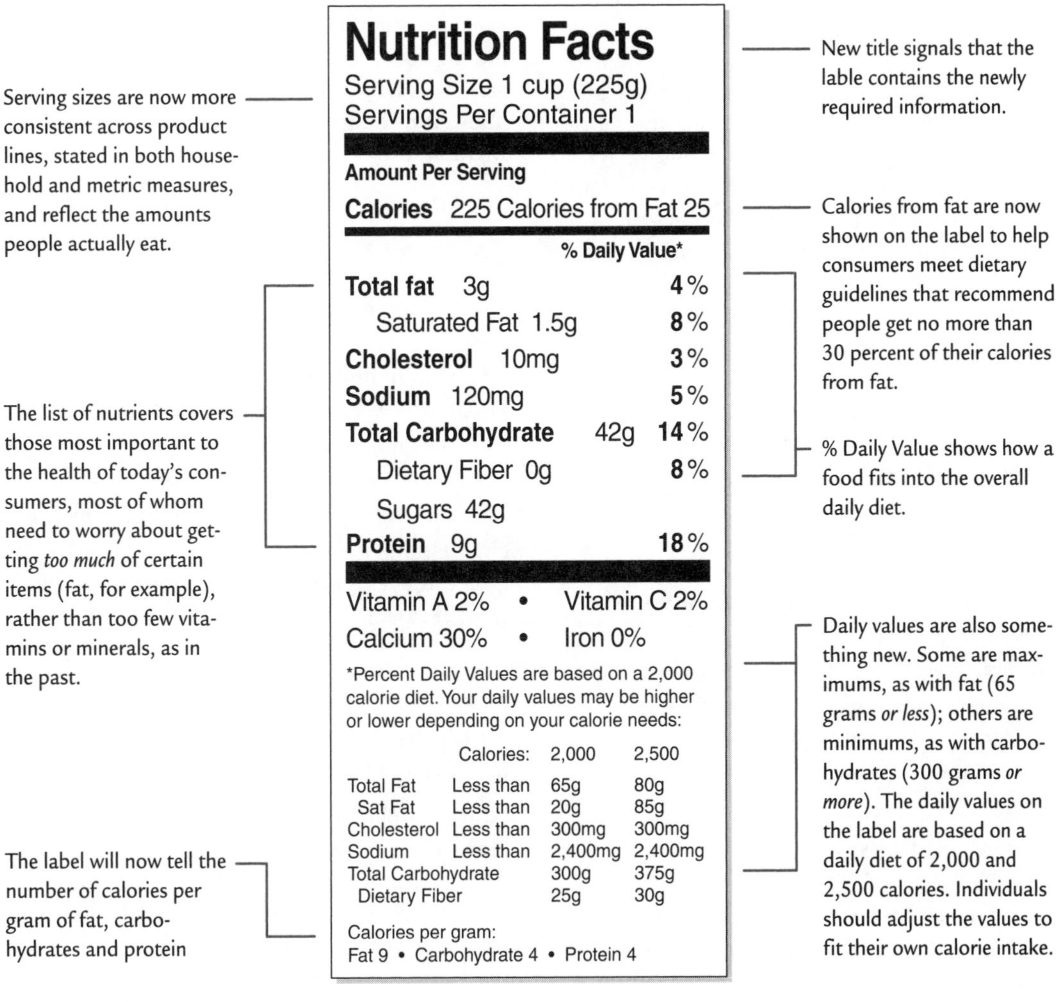

*This label is only a sample. Exact specifications are in the final rules.
*Source:* Food and Drug Administration 1992.

FIGURE 15–3    Food Label.

- The amounts of *total calories* and *calories from fat* per serving.
- The *number of grams* per serving of total fat, saturated fat, cholesterol, sodium, total carbohydrates, dietary fiber, sugars, and protein.

In addition, the nutritional contribution of *one* serving of the product must be stated as a *percentage of the Daily Values*. The Daily Values are based on the RDA for protein, vitamins, and minerals and on standards designed especially for food labels for nutrients not covered in the RDA such as fat, cholesterol, total carbohydrates, dietary fiber, and sodium. The calculations to determine the percents of Daily Values are based on a *2,000-calorie diet*. Depending on a person's age, gender, and activity level, a person may need more or less than 100% of a Daily Value. The Daily Value also helps consumers see how a food fits into an overall daily diet.

Other information, such as the amounts of polyunsaturated or monounsaturated fats or other vitamins and minerals, is optional. In addition, descriptors such as "free," "low," "high," "light," "lean," or "reduced," may be used on the label as long as a standard portion *meets defined criteria*. For example, to be labeled "low-calorie" a serving must have no more than 40 calories. To be labeled "low-fat," no more than 3 grams of fat per serving is allowed.

Health claims for the potential benefit of a nutrient or food in relation to a disease or health condition will be allowed on labels if they are supported by scientific evidence and are approved by the Food and Drug Administration (FDA). The 12 health claims currently allowed to be placed on food labels are shown in Table 15–4.[11]

---

TABLE 15–4 **Health Claims Allowed on Food Labels**

1. Calcium and osteoporosis
2. Fat and cancer
3. Saturated fat, cholesterol and coronary heart disease (CHD)
4. Dietary sugar alcohols and dental caries
5. Fiber-containing grain products, fruits, and vegetables and cancer
6. Folic acid and neural tube defects
7. Fruits and vegetables and cancer
8. Fruits, vegetables, and grain products that contain fiber and the risk for CHD
9. Sodium and hypertension
10. Soluble fiber from certain foods, such as whole oats and psyllium seed husk, and heart disease
11. Soy protein and CHD
12. Plant sterols and plant stanol esters and CHD

---

**Question 2**

The Daily Reference Intakes (DRI) are set at:

A. the minimum amount of a nutrient needed to prevent deficiency.
B. the maximum amount that will not cause toxicity.
C. the average estimated requirement for healthy people.
D. the average requirement plus a margin of safety.

---

## Nutrition in the Development and Integrity of Oral Tissues and Structures

Nutrition plays an important role in the initial growth and development or oral tissues and in their continuous integrity through the lifespan. Optimal nutrition during periods of hard and soft tissue development allow these tissues to reach their optimal potential for growth and resistance to disease. Malnutrition (either over or under-nutrition) during critical periods of *organogenesis* can have *irreversible* effects on de-

veloping tissues. Examples of this effect can be seen in the *tetracycline staining* of teeth, in dental *fluorosis,* and in the fever-induced *enamel hypoplasia* seen in the primary teeth.[12] In the dentition, malnutrition is less well documented in humans than in animals, but it appears that during the "critical periods," malnutrition can result in dentition with increased caries susceptibility.[13] Malnutrition *after* initial organ and tissue development is *usually reversible,* but can still compromise tissue regeneration and healing and increase susceptibility to oral diseases. Nutrients for which deficiencies or excesses have been directly associated with oral conditions are protein; energy; vitamins C, A, D; iodine; and fluoride.

## Protein/Calorie Malnutrition

Protein is the most abundant organic compound in the body and is required for the synthesis of virtually all body tissues and structures. Proteins account for the structure of DNA, the tensile strength of collagen, and the viscosity of saliva. Thus, aberrations in protein nutriture can have far reaching oral and systemic effects.

The normal turnover of epithelial tissue in the oral cavity requires a continual supply of nutrients. For example, *every 3 to 6 days, the basal epithelium of the gingiva undergoes renewal.*[14] Thus, any severe deficiency of protein/calorie intake will result in a decrease in mitotic activity in the crevicular epithelium, as well as elsewhere throughout the body.[15] In a comparison of periodontal involvement in patients with severe malnutrition (kwashiorkor) with that of healthy controls in South India,[16] fewer caries and more periodontal disease was found among the undernourished group. Since the oral hygiene indices of both groups were similar, it was assumed that the difference was due to nutritional factors. (It should be noted that any malnutrition of the severity of kwashiorkor represents a multi-nutrient deficiency). Impaired protein synthesis has been found if protein mal-

nutrition occurs during the developmental stage in animals.[17] In animal models, short-term fasting (4 days) resulted in a 40% reduction in collagen production.[18] In the same study, a 10% decrease in collagen synthesis was noted with a reduced dietary intake meeting 20% of requirements.[18] These findings suggest that even short-term states of undernutrition may impact collagen synthesis.

In *chronically malnourished* children, several studies have shown delays in tooth eruption patterns, and increased tooth enamel solubility, leading to increased caries susceptibility.[19–25]

The *linear hypoplasia* reported in the enamel of primary teeth of children in underprivileged populations is thought to contribute to their high prevalence of dental caries. This type of hypoplasia appears to be related to the severity of the malnutrition.[26]

With the exception of the *cleansing* and *diluting* effects of saliva, oral defense mechanisms depend on an adequate supply of proteins. The *glycoproteins* that result in aggregation of bacteria arise from the salivary glands. *Lysozyme, salivary peroxidase,* and *lactoferrin* are also *glycoproteins. Secretory IgA* (sIgA) arises mainly from the labial and buccal glands and is an immunoglobulin. The cell types involved in cellular immunity (polymorphonuclear lymphocytes and macrophages and the enzymes used in phagocytosis) also require protein for their production.[27]

Probably one of the *most deleterious* effects of protein/calorie deficiency is the depletion of the *cellular and immunocellular defenses* of both the oral and the connective sides of the barrier epithelial cells lining the gingival crevice. In general, the severity of the impaired immunologic response parallels the severity of the protein or calorie deficiency.[28]

## Minerals

Calcium, in association with vitamin D and phosphorus is essential for proper development and maintenance of mineralized tissues (teeth

and alveolar bone). A deficiency of these nutrients during critical phases of tooth development in children results in hypo-mineralization of developing teeth, and possible delayed eruption patterns.[29] Enamel hypoplasia may be seen in prematurely born very low birth-weight (VLBW) infants due to the higher needs for calcium and phosphorus in these infants.[30] In addition, VLBW infants have immature kidneys and may not metabolize adequate levels of vitamin D.[30]

Iron is of interest since iron deficiency is the *most common deficiency* in the United States. Iron deficiency anemia is manifest in the oral cavity by pallor of oral tissues, especially the tongue. The tongue may appear shiny, with blunted filiform papillae. The effects of iron deficiency on mineralized tissues are less clear. In rats, even a marginal deficiency of iron in the rat diet predisposes the rats to caries. Conversely, supplementing a caries-promoting diet with iron produced a major reduction in caries with the greatest effect shown in the neonatal period.[31] In addition, iron serves as a cofactor with ascorbic acid in collagen synthesis, as is copper.[32]

Zinc regulates *function in inflammation* by inhibiting the release of lysosomal enzymes and histamines. A zinc deficiency can inhibit collagen formation and reduce cell-mediated immunity.[33] The effect of zinc in modifying periodontal defense mechanisms has been shown in rabbits,[35] but has yet to be clearly delineated in humans.[36, 37]

### Vitamins

Vitamin A is essential for the development and continued integrity of all body organs and tissues, including the *epithelial mucosa* of the oral cavity. In vitamin-A deficiency, cell differentiation is impaired: *Mucus-secreting cells* are replaced with keratin-producing cells. The result is defective tissue formation, and impaired healing. Vitamin-A deficiency also results in impairment of *both specific and nonspecific immunoprotective mechanisms*. Deficiency can affect tissue response to bacterial infection, mucosal immunity, parasitic and viral infection, natural killer-cell activity, and phagocytosis.[38] Vitamin-A toxicity can show similar effects, with impaired healing response being the most direct affect on the oral cavity.[39] Effects include proliferation of oral epithelium, reduction of the keratin layer, thickening of the basal membrane, and increase in the granular layer. A patient who took 200,000 IU of vitamin A daily for over 6 months presented with painful gingival lesions, along with nausea, vomiting, xerostomia, and headaches. Clinical examination revealed gingival erosions, ulcerations, bleeding, swelling, loss of keratinization, color changes, and desquamation of the lips.[39] All pathologic manifestations disappeared within 2 months of the elimination of the vitamin A supplements when oral hygiene habits were unchanged.

Vitamin C (ascorbic acid) is essential to oral health. Synthesis of *hydroxyproline*, an essential component of *collagen*, requires ascorbic acid. Defects in collagen synthesis are responsible for the many manifestations of vitamin-C deficiency (*scurvy*). In the oral cavity these include spontaneous bleeding, infusions of blood into interdental papillae, loosening and exfoliation of teeth, detachment of oral epithelial tissue, and impaired wound healing.

The effects of vitamin-C deficiency are best studied in animal models, where all factors can be controlled. Acute scurvy can be produced by placing monkeys on a vitamin-C deficient diet for 12 weeks. The hydroxyproline content of the gingiva started to decline in the first four weeks and occurred at a faster rate than in skin.[40] By the end of the 8th week, the synthesis of hydroxyproline was totally impaired.[40] The results are extensive gingival pocket formation and tooth mobility due to degradation of the collagen making up periodontal ligament fibers.[25]

Although frank scurvy is rare, even marginal deficiencies may result in alterations in collagen synthesis. Thus deficient or marginal ascor-

bic acid intakes may be a conditioning factor in the development of gingivitis and one of the early manifestations of vitamin-C deficiency.[41] The most recent epidemiologic data from NHANES III (National Health and Nutrition Examination Survey) suggests that the odds of having periodontal disease are 1.2 times greater in those with low dietary vitamin-C intakes.[42] In the same study, *smokers and former smokers* with low vitamin-C intake are at 1.6 times greater risk of having periodontal disease.[42] Research findings suggest that people with marginal vitamin-C deficiency supplemented with ascorbic acid have a statistically significant increase in hydroxyproline in periodontal tissues.[43]

Ascorbic acid is essential to immune related functions, such as resistance to oral infection, via its role in leukocyte formation and subsequent *phagocytosis*.

Conversely, chronic vitamin C excess may precipitate a scurvy-like condition (rebound scurvy) upon cessation of the vitamin. Because the impact of deficient levels of vitamin C is first observed in gingival tissues, dentists and dental hygienists in clinical practice may be the first to diagnose the phenomenon.[44] The B-complex vitamins primarily function as *coenzymes in energy metabolism*. B-complex vitamins are found widely in foods, and usually together. With the exception of $B_{12}$ in the elderly and folic acid in pregnant women, deficiencies of single B vitamins are uncommon. Oral signs and symptoms of B-complex vitamin deficiencies include cracks in the corners of the mouth (cheilosis), inflammation, burning, redness, pain and swelling of the tongue.[45]

---

### Question 3

Which is *true* about vitamins and oral health?

A. Vitamin-C–deficient wounds heal as well as non-vitamin-C–deficient wounds

B. Vitamin A-toxicity does not have oral effects

C. The oral manifestations of vitamin-C deficiency are related to defects in collagen formation

D. Effects of deficiency and toxicity are best studied in humans

---

## Diet and Nutrition in Oral Conditions: Background and Counseling Strategies

### Who Needs Diet Guidance Caries Prevention

Dietary *education and guidance* are important for the prevention and control of dental caries. Patients should be carefully assessed to determine the level of prevention and nutrition guidance needed following these Institute of Medicine prevention guidelines:[46]

*Selective Prevention:* This strategy targets subset of the total population that are deemed to be at risk for caries for a variety of reasons. Examples include:

Adolescents at risk of caries because of high intake of soft drinks and snack foods.

Caries-prevention counseling for patients with xerostomia or cariogenic diet patterns.

Proactive diet suggestions for new denture wearers or those having jaw fixation.

Diet advice prior to radiation or chemotherapy.

Using current diet patterns as a basis for discussion, patients should be taught the role of diet in caries, what are cariogenic and noncariogenic eating patterns, and how to adapt current diet to lower cariogenic risk.

*Indicated Prevention:* This strategy targets individuals showing early danger signs of caries, such as extensive cervical demineralization. These individuals need the immediate aforementioned interventions as well as more detailed guidance on how to reduce cariogenicity

of their current diet. This will involve determining the factors influencing current habits, and working with the patient to develop appropriate and acceptable strategies for improvement. Patients need to be followed up on a regular basis to promote long-term change.

### Question 4

The diet assessment process in dentistry is designed to:

A. diagnose nutrient deficiencies

B. help screen patients for oral-health risk factors

C. serve as a teaching tool

D. determine patients' daily caloric intake

E. provide a therapeutic diet prescription for patients

F. be part of total preventive assessment

### Dental Caries: Role of Carbohydrates in Caries Development

Dental caries is a common plaque-dependent bacterial infection that is strongly affected by diet. Development of clinical caries is contingent upon the interaction of three local factors in the mouth: *a susceptible tooth, cariogenic bacteria, and fermentable carbohydrate* (Figure 15–4). Absence of one of these factors dramatically reduces caries risk. Mutans streptococci are the predominant oral bacteria that initiate the caries process. Newly erupted teeth with a thin enamel layer are very caries susceptible. Tooth morphology, especially the presence of deep pits and fissures, influences the likelihood that mutans streptococci will attach to and colonize the tooth's surface. Plaque bacteria ferment starches and sugars, producing organic acids. These acids demineralize dental enamel.[47]

Other dietary factors *counteract* the damaging effects of carbohydrates. The presence of protective minerals and ions such as *fluoride, calcium, and phosphorus* in *plaque and saliva,*

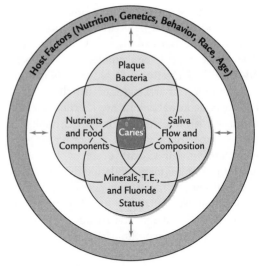

FIGURE 15–4   Factors Required for Caries Development.

promote remineralization of incipient lesions. In addition to transporting minerals, saliva contains *buffering agents, bicarbonate and phosphates,* that neutralize organic acids. Thus, the amount and composition of saliva affect the caries process. Other host factors that influence caries risk include: genetic predisposition, immune status, malnutrition during tooth formation, education level, and income status.

In the most recent national health and examination survey (NHANES III, Phase I) 94% of adults showed evidence of coronal caries and 22.5% of adults had root caries.[48] In the same survey, 25% of the children and teens aged 5 to 17 had 80% of the dental caries detected in the permanent teeth.[49] For these caries-prone children and adults, *nutrition counseling* about the damaging effects of fermentable carbohydrates on teeth is essential.

Through epidemiological and clinical studies discussed in Chapter 14, the causal relationship between sugar consumption and dental caries has been established. Animal studies suggest that an increase in the concentration of sucrose in the diet reduces dental plaque forma-

tion and increases the incidence of dental caries.[50,51] People with very low sugar intakes have low-caries scores. People in nations that have high sugar intakes have high rates of caries.[52] It is unclear if this is primarily the topical effect of sugar consumption or systemic effects on dentin formation. However, the amount of sugar consumed is not the sole dietary variable associated with caries development. Sucrose plays a more dominant role than other sugars in the development of smooth surface caries. One of sucrose's metabolic by-products, an extracellular polysaccharide called *glucan*, enables the mutans streptococci to adhere to the smooth enamel surfaces.[53] However, the amount of sucrose necessary for the implantation of mutans streptococci is very low.

Although sugar intake is high among most persons in industrialized countries, it is more difficult to demonstrate a *correlation* between caries prevalence and the amount of sugar consumed than in developing countries where sugar intake is lower. Three recent clinical trials of English, United States, and Canadian schoolchildren examined the relationship between sugar intake and dental caries. In England, 405 children with a mean age of 11.6 years were followed for 2 years. Total sugar intake (118 grams per day or 21% of total calorie intake) had the highest significant correlation with caries rates.[54] Intake of sugary foods before bedtime was highly correlated with caries incidence. In the United States, 499 children aged 11 to 15 years, living in nonfluoridated rural Michigan communities, were followed for 3 years. The average increase in decayed, missing, and filled surfaces (DMFS) over the 3 years was 3.1 in girls and 2.7 for boys. The daily average sugar intake was 142 grams, this represented 26.5% of their total energy intake. Children who obtained a higher percent of their total calories from sugars had more proximal surface caries. The average number of eating occasions and the number of sugary between-meal snacks consumed were not related to caries increment.[55]

*Fifty percent* of 232 11-year-old children in a Canadian study had *inadequate diets*. Children with superior diets tended to develop fewer caries; however, the association was not statistically significant.[56] Differences in eating patterns and intake of caries-promoting foods among the children in these studies may have been too small to result in significant differences in caries experience. Other factors contributing to the caries decline in western countries are: fluoride intake from water, the use of fluoridated dentifrices, improved plaque control, the use of dental sealants, and more frequent visits to the dentist.[57]

The use of *sugar alcohols and alternative sweeteners* in foods also has had a role in *reducing* caries. Perhaps one of the most promising sugar substitutes to be studied is *xylitol*, a sugar alcohol that has been demonstrated to be non-cariogenic as well as promoting remineralization.[58] Xylitol's ability to inhibit metabolic acid production by mutans streptococci results in minimal depression of plaque pH. Maintenance of the *plaque pH close to the saliva pH* also fosters remineralization of teeth.[59] In addition, the substitution of xylitol for fermentable sugars in the diet results in a less cariogenic bacterial flora. The importance of other non-fermentable sweeteners in caries control is detailed in Chapter 14.

Simple sugars are not the only carbohydrate that influences the development of a carious lesion. Highly refined *cooked starch-sugar combinations* such as doughnuts, cookies, potato chips, and some ready-to-eat breakfast cereals *produce a prolonged acidogenic response* when retained in interproximal spaces.[60] When starches are cooked, they are partially degraded. This allows the salivary alpha-amylase to convert starch particles retained on the tongue, oral mucosa, and teeth to *maltose*. Making maltose available to plaque bacteria extends the length of time the plaque pH will remain low and permit enamel demineralization to occur. Thus, retentive high starch foods

may be more acidogenic than high-sugar-low-starch foods that are rapidly eliminated from the mouth.[61]

## Effects of Eating Patterns and Physical Form of Foods

Other dietary factors that may hinder or enhance caries development include: the frequency of eating, the *physical form* of the carbohydrate (liquid vs. solid), *retentiveness* of a food on the tooth surface, the *sequence* in which foods are consumed (e.g., cheese eaten before a sweet food limits the pH drop), and the presence of minerals in a food.

Frequent between-meal snacking on sugar or processed starch-containing foods increases plaque formation and extends the length of time that bacterial acid production can occur. When total daily sugar intake was held constant, increasing the frequency of sugar intake for groups of rats resulted in increased number of *Streptococci mutans* in plaque and the amount of caries experienced.[62] The positive relationship between frequency of sugar intake and caries in humans was first demonstrated in the *Vipeholm* study.[63] Subjects who consumed candies *between meals* developed *more* caries than those who were fed equal amounts of sugars *with* meals. Frequent snacking between meals keeps the plaque pH low and extends the time for enamel and dentin demineralization to occur.

Bacterial fermentation can continue as long as carbohydrate adheres to the enamel and exposed dentinal tooth surfaces. Even though starchy foods vary in their cariogenic potential, the highly refined starchy foods, such as soft bread and potato chips, that are retained on tooth surfaces for prolonged periods of time, result in a lowered pH which may last *up to 60 minutes*.[64,61] High-sucrose confectionery foods deliver high levels of sugar to the oral bacteria immediately after the foods are consumed, whereas high-starch foods deliver progressively increasing concentrations of sugars over a considerably longer period of time.

The *sequence* in which foods are eaten affects how much the plaque pH falls. Sugared coffee consumed at the *end* of a meal will cause the plaque pH to remain *low for a longer time* than when an unsweetened food is eaten *following* intake of sugared coffee.[65] If peanuts are eaten before or after sugar-containing foods, the plaque pH is less depressed.[66]

Some components of foods *are protective* against dental caries. Protein, fat, phosphorus, and calcium inhibit caries in rats.[67] Aged natural cheeses have been shown to be cariostatic.[68] When cheese is eaten following a sucrose rinse, the plaque pH remains higher than when no cheese follows a sucrose rinse. In addition, enamel demineralization, measured using the intraoral cariogenicity test, is reduced. The protective effect of cheeses is attributed to *their texture* that *stimulates salivary flow,* and their protein, calcium, and phosphate content that *neutralizes plaque acids*. Fluoride found in drinking water, foods, and dentifrices increases a tooth's resistance to decay and enhances remineralization of carious lesions.

*Lipids* seem to accelerate oral clearance of food particles. Some fatty acids, linoleic and oleic, in low concentration, inhibit growth of mutans streptococcus. Lectins, proteins found in plants, appear to interfere with microbial colonization and may affect salivary function.[69]

---

### Question 5

In the diet of a patient with rampant dental caries, which is *most relevant* to the problem?

A. total amount of sucrose consumed

B. total amount of sticky sweets consumed

C. nutrient quality of the meals and snacks

D. number of meals and snacks

E. what is eaten for desert in the evening

## Measuring the Cariogenic Potential of Foods

Since it is unethical to conduct human experiments to measure the true cariogenic potential of foods, other indirect tests have been developed. These tests enable researchers to classify foods into at least three categories: protective, low, and high cariogenic potential. Currently the cariogenic potential or the ability to induce caries in humans may be assessed indirectly by measuring the ability of a test food to cause: caries formation in animals, acid production in dental plaque, or demineralization of enamel.[1]

Animal studies have been conducted using a *programmed feeding machine*. In one study, 20 common snack foods were presented to rats at specified intervals during the day.[70] After sulcal and smooth surface caries were scored in the animals, cariogenic potential indices (CPI's) were computed for each food (the sucrose group had a CPI value of one) (Table 15–5). A food with a CPI of 0.4 had low cariogenic potential. Those snack foods with high cariogenic potential had 1% or more hydrolyzable starch in combination with sucrose or other sugars.

Acid production in the mouth during bacterial fermentation of a food is predictive of the contribution of that food to the caries process. Measurement of plaque acidogenicity can be measured by determining the pH of a plaque sample taken from the mouth or *in situ*.[1] Foods that cause the plaque pH to fall below the critical demineralization level (*pH 5.5 to 5.0*) are considered acidogenic. Measurement of oral plaque pH requires placement of a wire *telemetric appliance* containing a pH microelectrode in the space where a tooth is missing in the mouth. As the test food is chewed, the pH under undisturbed plaque at the site of the indwelling electrode is continually transmitted to an external receiver. The rate of the fall and rise of the pH at an interproximal site can be recorded continuously using plaque telemetry. Foods found to have low acidogenic potential using this method include: aged cheeses, some vegetables, meats, fish, and nuts.[71]

### TABLE 15-5 Cariogenic Potential of Foods in Animal Models

| Foods | Caries Potential Index | |
|---|---|---|
| | Buccal | Sulcal |
| Raisins | 1.3 | 0.95 |
| Bananas | 1.2 | 1.17 |
| French fried (chips) | 1.2 | 0.98 |
| Granola (a breakfast cereal) | 1.1 | 0.64 |
| **Sucrose** | **1.0** | **1.0** |
| Bread | 0.82 | 0.90 |
| Grahams (digestive biscuits) | 0.66 | 0.79 |
| Cup cakes | 0.62 | 1.73 |
| Chocolate | 0.59 | 0.81 |
| Cornstarch | 0.47 | 0.76 |
| Sponge cake | 0.44 | 0.95 |
| Rye crackers | 0.36 | 0.86 |
| Saltines (savoury crackers) | 0.36 | 0.69 |
| Peanuts | 0.30 | 0.43 |
| Pretzels | 0.21 | 0.77 |
| Jello (fruit jelly) | 0.11 | 0.43 |
| Yogurt | 0.11 | 0.65 |
| Corn chips | 0.10 | 0.54 |

(Adapted from Mundorff SA, Featherstone JDB, Eisenberg AD, et al. Cariogenicity of foods: Rat study. *J Dent Res.* 64:(special issue) 1985; 294. Abstract 1071.)

To assess the ability of a food to demineralize dental enamel, an *intraoral cariogenicity test* has been developed. Bovine or human dental enamel slabs are imbedded in a prosthesis and placed in the mouth where a tooth is missing. After ingesting a test food, changes in surface microhardness or enamel porosity are determined.[72] Since each test measures a different aspect of cariogenicity, foods will be ranked differently. It is recommended that two testing methods be used to determine food acido/cariogenicity potential.[73,74] Table 15–6 shows the acidogenic potential of foods. Table 15–7 provides diet suggestions for caries prevention.

TABLE 15-6 **Acidogenic Potential of Foods**

| Non to Low Acidogenic | | Acidogenic |
|---|---|---|
| Raw vegetables: e.g. | Lower | Cooked vegetables |
|   Broccoli | | Fresh Fruits especially bananas |
|   Cauliflower | | Fruit juices, fruit drinks |
|   Cucumber | | Sweetened beverages |
|   Lettuce | | Non-dairy creamers |
|   Dill pickles | | Sweetened canned or cooked fruits |
|   Carrot | | Ice cream, sherbet, pudding, gelatin, flavored |
|   Peppers | |   yogurts |
| Meat, fish, poultry | | Potato chips, pretzels |
| Beans, peas | | Dried fruits, fruit rolls |
| Nuts, natural peanut butter | | Marshmallows |
| Milk, cheeses | | Starches: bread, rice, pasta, sweetened cereals |
| Popcorn | | Cookies, cakes, pies, pastry |
| Fats, oils, butter, margarine | | Crackers |
| Non-sugar sweeteners | | Candy, especially slowly dissolving breath |
| | Higher |   mints, cough drops |

---

### Question 6

Tooth erosion can be caused by

A. acid from vomiting
B. sugar-containing carbonated beverages
C. gastro-esophageal reflux
D. sugar-free carbonated beverages
E. all of the above

---

### Early Childhood Caries

One of the most severe forms of caries occurs in infants. Inappropriate feeding practices may result in progressive dental caries on the buccal and lingual surfaces of newly erupted primary maxillary anterior teeth of infants and toddlers. The overall prevalence of early childhood caries (also called *baby bottle tooth* decay or *nursing caries*) is estimated to be 5%.[75] How-ever, a much higher prevalence has been seen among Alaskan and Oklahoma Native American children (53%) and Navajo (72%) and Cherokee (55%) Head Start children attending Head Start programs.[76, 77]

Primary risk factors for early childhood caries include putting a child to sleep at naptime or bedtime with a bottle containing a liquid *other than plain water*, allowing an infant to breast-feed at will during the night, and extended use of the nursing bottle or sippy cup beyond 1 year of age. Results of the 1991 National Health Interview Survey show that 16.7% or 3.5 million children between 6 months and 5 years of age are put to sleep with a liquid in the bottle other than plain water.[78] Inappropriate feeding practices were reported more often by parents with *less than a high school education*, low incomes, Hispanic backgrounds, and those parents whose children had not been to a dentist in the past year.

TABLE 15-7 **Diet Suggestions for Caries Prevention**

| Food Group | Suggestions |
|---|---|
| **General** | · Limit number of eating times<br>· Avoid sticky or retentive foods |
| **Grains**/cereals<br>(6-11/day) | · Have whole grains<br>· Popcorn for snacks<br>· Avoid crackers, donuts, potato chips between meals |
| **Fruits**<br>(3-5/day)<br>Fresh, frozen, canned, juices | · Have fruits for dessert / snacks<br>· Avoid dried fruits or fruit roll-ups<br>· Don't sip slowly or often on fruit juices<br>· Avoid fruit drinks |
| **Vegetables**<br>(2-4/day)<br>Fresh, frozen, canned, juices,<br>potatoes | · All vegetables are fine<br>· Limit sweetened salad dressings<br>· Have raw vegetables for snacks |
| **Protein**<br>(2+/day)<br>Meat, fish, poultry, eggs,<br>beans (lentils etc.) tofu, nuts | · All proteins are fine:<br>· Nuts for snacks |
| **Dairy**[*]<br>**(2–3+/day)**[*]<br>Milk, cheese, ice cream, tofu,<br>cottage cheese | · Have milk in coffee, soup<br>· Cheese in sandwiches, casseroles etc.<br>· Cheese for snacks |
| **Sweets/fats**<br>Oil, margarine, butter, salad<br>dressing,<br>candy, sweet desserts, soda pop | · Avoid slowly dissolving candies<br>· Have sweets as dessert only<br>· Avoid constant sipping on sweet beverages (soda,sports drinks) |
| **Other** | · Have flavored club soda or diet soda<br>· Use sugar-free gum<br>· Have water between meals and with snacks |

[*]aim for low fat unless increased calories are indicated

Children who develop maxillary anterior caries are at increased risk of developing posterior caries in the future.[79] To prevent early childhood caries, dentists, pediatricians, and other health care professionals should ask parents about their infant feeding practices. Those parents who report inappropriate feeding practices should receive counseling. Programs serving low-income families, such as the Special Supplemental Food Program for Women, Infant, and Children (WIC), can play a major role in providing education to parents at higher risk for using inappropriate feeding practices.

### Nutrition and Periodontal Disease

Like caries, periodontal disease is an infectious disease, multifactorial in etiology, and occurs when virulence of the bacterial challenge is *greater than the host defense and repair capability*. The course of periodontal disease involves periods of progression and remission. Unlike the di-

rect causative relationship between carbohydrates and caries, nutritional factors seem to play a much more subtle role in periodontal status. Nutritional factors *can alter host susceptibility* to periodontal disease and/or modulate its progress.[80] The nutritional factors related to *preventing infection* and *enhancing wound healing* in general applies to the prevention and management of periodontal disease as well.[81] If both the challenge to and the defense and repair capabilities of the periodontal tissues are in balance, nutrition could be the deciding factor in whether health or disease results. Even when the periodontium is healthy, there is continual need for nutrients to maintain the tissues. Once inflammation is established, the need for nutrients *increases*. There is a close relationship between malnutrition and infection, with infection aggravating malnutrition and malnutrition abetting infection. Defense in the gingival crevice and connective tissue all require an adequate intake of all nutrients to ensure adequate production and function of defense and supporting cells.[82–86] With the increased needs of cellular immunity and the additional demands by the tissue cells attempting to maintain and repair damaged areas, a greater supply of all nutrients is needed. This has led to evidence showing that nutrient requirements may be higher at local sites of increased stress than in the rest of the body. Such localized challenges may result in *end-organ nutrient deficiencies*.[87, 88]

### Diet Guidelines

Whenever routine scaling, prophylaxis, and oral plaque control procedures fail to reverse gingivitis and before any treatment for periodontitis is attempted, a thorough diet evaluation and patient counseling session is indicated. The patient should be informed about the importance of systemic nutrition in the defense and repair of oral tissues. Recommendations should be made to help ensure optimal nutrition to help prevent and manage periodontal disease. These include:

- Eat a *nutritionally adequate diet* following the food pyramid guidelines.
- Increase the use of saliva-stimulating fibrous foods.
- Multivitamin/mineral supplements should be in doses *no higher* than one to two times Recommended Dietary Allowance levels.
- *Avoid fad diets* which could be deficient in nutrients.
- Avoid *single* vitamin supplements.
- *Avoid potentially detrimental megadoses* of vitamins and minerals (10× RDA or higher).

---

**Question 7**

Periodontal disease is caused by dietary deficiencies. Calcium deficiency is thought to be a contributing factor in alveolar bone loss in humans.

A. both statements are true.

B. both statements are false.

C. the first statement is true: the second is false.

D. the first statement is false the second is true.

---

### Eating Disorders

Eating disorders, especially *bulimia*, are often first diagnosed in the dental office. Patients, usually young females, present with severe erosion of the lingual tooth surfaces. The oral tissues are often red, sore, and painful. The esophagus may be inflamed, and parotid salivary glands are often swollen. Bulimia is characterized by recurrent episodes of *binge eating* (consumption of large amounts of foods at a time) followed by self-induced regurgitation (purging). The average intake of food during a binge is 3,400 calories over an hour, with some individuals ingesting as much as 50,000 calories in 24 hours.[89] Patients may also use laxatives and/or diuretics to induce malabsorption and fluid loss. The acid from stomach regurgitation

irritates the esophagus and the oropharyngeal soft tissues. The regurgitated acid in combination with xerostomia, results in rapid and extensive destruction of tooth enamel.[90]

Patients often first deny having an eating disorder. However, when confronted with the oral evidence, they often admit to the disorder. The dentist should refer the patient to an eating-disorder management program and elicit patient agreement to undergo treatment. The diagnosis of this disorder by the dentist and the realization of the dental destruction caused by the disorder, often convince patients to agree to treatment. A *multidisciplinary* approach to treatment is needed, including physicians, psychiatrists, psychologists, nutritionists, and social workers. The patient must be cautioned that for dental rehabilitation to be successful, the underlying problem (the eating disorder and its causes) must be resolved.

---

### Question 8

Oral problems that may be seen in patients with eating disorders include:

A. swollen salivary glands

B. orange-stained teeth

C. decreased salivary flow

D. decreased oral pH

E. severe enamel demineralization

---

### The Aging Patient

The aging patient is often faced with a variety of challenges that can undermine both oral health and nutritional status.[91] As a result, the elderly are considered particularly susceptible to malnutrition.[92] Compared to younger individuals, elders have a significantly decreased ability to respond to physiologic challenges. Sensory function decreases leading to *impaired taste and smell*.[93] Changes in the gastrointestinal system can affect the ability to digest, absorb and utilize food properly. Functional prob-

lems, such as arthritis or vision difficulties can affect the ability to prepare and eat food. Psychosocial problems such as loneliness, depression, lack of money, and poor access to food can all undermine good eating habits.

Problems in the oral cavity, such as xerostomia and loose teeth, have been considered major contributors to the poor eating habits of the elderly and may be a major contributor to malnutrition.[92,105,94,95] Several studies have shown that dentate status can affect eating ability[96] and subsequent diet quality.[97, 98, 99] Individuals with one or two complete dentures had a 20% decline in diet quality compared to those with at least partial dentition in one or both arches.[100] Another study showed that compared to those with 25 or more teeth, edentulous individuals consumed less fiber and carotene, fewer vegetables, and more cholesterol, saturated fat and calories.[101] Dentures can affect *taste and swallowing ability*, especially if they are maxillary dentures. The denture covers those taste buds found on the upper palate. And when the upper palate is covered, it becomes difficult to detect the location of food in the mouth. For this reason, dentures are considered to be the *major cause of choking* in adults.[102]

*Dry mouth (xerostomia)* is common in the older population, in part because of xerostomic medications commonly taken. Xerostomia makes eating more difficult and increases the cariogenic potential of the diet.[103,104] It has also been associated with burning mouth syndrome and inadequate diet.[105]

Conversely, nutrition is an important factor in oral status.[106] In a sample population of 843 elderly people, there was a significant association between low ascorbic acid levels and the prevalence of oral mucosal lesions.[107] Low calcium intake throughout life has been shown to *contribute to osteoporosis*. In turn, osteoporosis in alveolar bone is thought to be an important contributing factor to the resorption of alveolar bone that ultimately results in tooth loss.[108]

The alveolar process is composed primarily of trabecular bone, which is more labile to calcium imbalances than is cortical bone. Thus, the alveolar bone provides a potential labile source of calcium available to meet *other* tissue needs. Since the alveolar process is thought to undergo resorption *prior* to other bones; it is projected that changes detected in the alveolar process may eventually be used for early detection of osteoporosis.[109] Mandibular bone mass was correlated with total body calcium and bone mass of the radius and vertebrae in dentate and edentulous postmenopausal women with osteoporosis,[110] with the highest correlation between total body and mandibular bone mass. Thus, the mandible reflects the mineral status of the entire skeleton. Calcium intake in postmenopausal osteoporotic women was also correlated with mandibular density; supporting the hypothesis that low calcium intake may contribute to reduced bone density.[111,112] In a study of 329 healthy post-menopausal women, an inverse relationship was shown between bone mineral density and number of existing teeth, with those women who received dentures after the age of forty having the lowest bone mineral density.[113]

Older patients should be carefully screened for nutritional risk factors, and should be educated about the importance of good nutrition to general and oral health.[114, 115] If major nutritional problems are suspected the patient should be referred to a nutritionist.[116] When new dentures are provided, patients should be counseled on how to adapt their usual diet to a softer consistency for the first few days after denture insertion.

---

### Question 9

Which is true about aging?

A. Dry mouth always occurs with aging.

B. Dentures improve taste perception.

C. Taste and smell acutely tend to decrease.

D. Calcium intake is not of concern with this group.

---

### The Diabetic Patient

The *diabetic* dental patient is at *greater risk* for developing oral infections and periodontal disease than the nondiabetic patient.[117,118] The dental team needs to be aware of current approaches to diabetes management and carefully monitor the patient's health status prior to initiating dental treatment.

The nutrition care plan generally requires that patients have meals and snacks of specific nutrient composition *at regularly scheduled intervals*, coordinated with medications (insulin or oral agents) and exercise. Dietary management has changed from the high fat, low carbohydrate diets of past decades to the more liberal use of complex carbohydrates and the reductions in fat recommended today.[119,107] A well-balanced diabetic diet should be low in cariogenicity, since the use of cariogenic fermentable carbohydrates should be infrequent. Frequent use of hard candies or other foods taken to counteract hypoglycemia are an indication that the diabetes is not well controlled. Patients with uncontrolled diabetes should be referred to their physician for further management. *In the dental office, quickly assimilated carbohydrate sources such as juices, milk, and crackers, should be kept readily available in the event that a diabetic patient develops symptoms of hypoglycemia.*

### Patients with Immunocompromising Conditions (Cancer, AIDS)

Immunocompromised patients, such as those with cancer or AIDS, often have *increased* requirements for nutrients while having major

physiologic and psychosocial impediments to eating. Cancer often sets up a syndrome of weight loss and wasting in which both metabolism and nutrient losses *increase*. The cancer often causes severe anorexia, taste changes, and early satiety. The pain and discomfort of oral infections such as the herpes simplex and oral candidiasis found in AIDS and chemotherapy patients, can also impair the desire and ability to eat.[120] *Over half of all head and neck cancer patients are nutritionally compromised at initial diagnosis.*[121] Radiation therapy increases eating difficulty by causing painful oral *mucositis, dysphagia*, and severe *xerostomia*.[122]

When providing dental treatment to patients suffering from cancer or AIDS, team members need to understand the nutrition principles underlying the care, so that dental services provided can be coordinated effectively with total care. The nutrition care plan initially focuses on providing *high caloric intake in frequent small meals*. Liquid supplements may be used if optimal nutriture cannot be achieved via food alone. In more serious cases, patients may need enteral (tube) feedings or more advanced nutritional support. A high calorie diet will likely be high in sugars and total calories.[123] In these cases, the dental team should *not* caution patients to reduce the frequency of eating, since this will contradict nutritional management goals. Rather, thorough cleaning after each eating period, and use of fluoride mouth rinses and topical fluoride trays before bed should be stressed. This approach is standard protocol for immunocompromised patients as part of an aggressive preventive dental program.[124] Cancer patients should be cautioned, however, about the potential oral sequelae of an increased frequency of eating. Patients should also be cautioned to avoid the use of slowly dissolving hard candy often used to assuage the xerostomia. The most important *monitoring* tool for these patients is *weight status*. The patient should be queried at each visit about how their weight is being maintained.

Involuntary weight loss of 10 pounds or more is a warning for the need for more intensive care.

### Oral Surgery and Intermaxillary Fixation

The patient who has had oral surgery, whether therapeutic or as a result of trauma, needs special nutritional consideration (125-Kendall, 1982). An adequate diet *before surgery is needed to support adequate post-surgical response*. If food consumption will be impaired for a short period of time, the risk of nutritional deficiency is low. The risk of deficiency increases with length of eating impairment. The surgery itself can result in an anorexia, inability to chew, and increased metabolic requirements.[126] After surgery, a patient may need a *liquid diet for 1 or 2 days*, but should progress as soon as possible to a soft diet of high nutritional quality, until a normal diet can be resumed. In some cases, nutritionally complete liquid supplements may be appropriate and should be prescribed in consultation with the patient's dietitian and physician. Often patients prefer purees of normal foods over commercial liquid supplements.[127] Multivitamin/ mineral supplements may be appropriate as well.

---

### Question 10

Which of the following is/are true?

A. A well-controlled diabetic diet should be low in caries risk.

B. Patients with cancer often have increased nutrient needs.

C. Patients with immune-compromising conditions should be told to reduce the frequency of eating to reduce caries risk.

D. The oral surgery patient may require a liquid diet for 1 to 2 days after surgery but should return to a normal diet as soon as it is possible.

## SUMMARY

Nutritional status and dietary habits can affect and be affected by specific oral conditions. Comprehensive patient care requires that nutritional factors be considered in the etiology, progression, and sequelae of oral problems.[128, 129]

Dental-team members should routinely screen patients for nutritional issues, provide dentally-oriented counseling, and refer patients to dietitians for further care. The nutritional implications in dental conditions are many and complex. No longer can nutrition in dentistry be summarized as "sugar is bad, and fluoride is good."

## ANSWERS AND EXPLANATIONS

1. b, c, and d—correct.

    a—incorrect. It is not appropriate or possible for the dental team to attempt to assess actual nutritional status. This requires sophisticated laboratory testing under the supervision of a qualified medical professional.

2. d—correct.

    a—incorrect. The minimum amount of a nutrient needed to prevent deficiency is not considered an appropriate standard of adequacy

    b—incorrect. The maximum amount of a nutrient that will not cause toxicity is the UL or upper tolerable limit

    c—incorrect. The average estimated requirement for healthy people would mean that half of the population would require more. Thus it is not used as the criteria for healthy populations

3. c—correct.

    a—incorrect. Vitamin C-deficient wounds have poorer healing ability

    b—incorrect. Vitamin-C deficiency affects all epithelial tissues including those in the oral cavity

    d—incorrect. It is not ethical to conduct such studies in humans

4. b, c, and f—correct.

    a—incorrect. The diet assessment process can be used to screen patients for possible nutrition risk, but cannot be used for true nutritional assessment

    d—incorrect. Daily calorie intake cannot be determined using a diet screening tool. Patient's daily calorie intake is best assessed by a registered dietitian using an assessment tool designed for that purpose.

    e—incorrect. The dental team can use screening information to refer the patient to a registered dietitian who is qualified to provide therapeutic diets. The dental team can provide nutrition information about healthy diet and diet/oral health relationships.

5. d—correct

   a—incorrect. Sucrose is not the only cariogenic factor, and the amount is not as important as the distribution in the diet.

   b—incorrect. The amount of sticky sweets is not as relevant as the frequency of usage of these items.

   c—incorrect. The nutrient quality of the diet is only related to the caries process after tooth eruption through remineralization effects.

   e—incorrect. Dessert is only one of many contributing factors to dental caries.

6. e—correct.

   Tooth erosion can be caused by acid from vomiting, sugar-containing carbonated beverages, gastroesophageal reflux, and sugar-free carbonated beverages to name but a few factors.

7. d—correct.

   Periodontal disease is not *caused* by dietary deficiencies. However, calcium deficiency is thought to be a contributing factor to alveolar bone loss in humans.

8. a, c, d, e—correct.

   b—incorrect. Orange-stained teeth are not necessarily caused by eating disorders. The staining can come from food, beverages, or other sources.

9. c—correct.

   a—incorrect. Dry mouth is associated primarily with the use of medications and is not inevitable with aging.

   b—incorrect. Dentures can impair taste perception if they cover taste buds on the upper palate.

   d—incorrect. Calcium is important for all age groups. Calcium intake is associated with bone density in general and may be a factor in alveolar bone health as well.

10. a, b, and d—correct

    d—incorrect. Patients with immune compromising conditions should *not* be told to reduce the frequency of eating to reduce caries risk. These patients are at high risk for nutritional deficiency and must eat high calorie foods on a frequent basis throughout the day. Oral risk should be reduced by having patients rinse the mouth and clean the teeth as best they can after each eating period and use remineralizing rinses.

# REFERENCES

1. Rugg-Gunn, A. J. (1993). Nutrition, dental development and dental hypoplasia. In *Nutrition and Dental Health*. New York: Oxford University Press, 15–35.
2. Alvarez, J. O. (1995). Nutrition, tooth development, and dental caries. *Am J Clin Nutr*, 61(S):410S–416S.

3. Papas, A. S., Palmer, C. A., Rounds, M. C., Herman, J., McGandy, R. B., Hartz, S. C., Russell, R. M., DePaola, P. (1989). Longitudinal relationship between nutrition and oral health. *Ann NY Acad Sci,* 561:124–42.

4. *Food & Nutrition Board Recommended Dietary Allowances* (10th ed.) Washington, DC: National Academy Press, 1989.

5. Food and Nutrition Board (1997). *Dietary Reference Intakes: Calcium, Phosphorus, Magnesium, Vitamin D, and Fluoride.* National Institute of Medicine: Washington, DC.

6. USDA and DHHS (2001). *2000 Dietary Guidelines for Americans.* (5th ed.) Home & Garden Bulletin, No. 232. Washington, DC: US Government Printing Office.

7. American Dietetic Association (1997). Weight management—position of ADA. *Journal of the American Dietetic Association,* 97:71–74.

8. Meisler, J. G., & St. Jeor, S. (1996). Summary and recommendations from the American Health Foundation's Expert Panel on Healthy Weight. *Am J Clin Nutr,* 1996;63(suppl 1): 474S–477S.

9. US Department of Agriculture, Center for Nutrition Policy & Promotion (1996). Food Guide Pyramid *Home & Gar. Bull. No. 252.* Washington DC:U.S. Government Printing Office.

10. Food labeling: Nutrient content claims, general principles, petitions, definition of terms, definitions for fat, fatty acids, and cholesterol content of food: final rule. *Federal Register,* 58, Jan 6, 1993; 2302–2426.

11. Center for Food Safety and Applied Nutrition (2000). *Health claims.* Food and Drug Administration: Washington, DC.

12. Den Besten, P. K. (1999). Mechanism and timing of fluoride effects on developing enamel. *Journal of Public Health Dentistry,* 59(4):2226–30.

13. Navia, J. M. (1970). Evaluation of nutritional and dietary factors that modify animal caries. *J Dent Res,* 49:1213–1228.

14. Enwonwu, C. (1974). Role of biochemistry and nutrition in preventive dentistry. *J Am Soc Prev Dent,* 4:6–17.

15. DePaola, D. P., & Kuftinec, M. M. (1976). Nutrition in growth and development of oral tissues. *Dent Clin North Am,* 20:441–59.

16. Pindborg, J. J., Bhat, M., & Roed-Peterson, B. (1967). Oral changes in South India children with severe protein deficiency. *J Periodont,* 38: 218–21.

17. Menaker, L., & Navia, J. M. (1974). Effect of undernutrition during the perinatal period on caries development in the rat; Changes in whole saliva volume and protein content. *J Dent Res,* 53:592–97.

18. Spanheimer, R. Zlatev, T., Umpierrez, G., & Digitolamo, R. (1991). Collagen production in fasted and food-restricted rats: response to duration and severity of food deprivation. *J Nutr,* 121(4): 518–24.

19. Alvarez, J. O., Caceda, J., Woolley, T. W., Carley, K. W., Baiocchi, N., Caravedo, L., & Navia, J. M. (1993). A longitudinal study of dental caries in the primary teeth of children who suffered from infant malnutrition. *J Dent Res,* 72(12):1573–76.

20. Alvarez, J. O., Eguren, J. C., Caceda, J., & Navia J. (1990). The effect of nutritional status on the age distribution of dental caries in the primary teeth. *J Dent Res,* 69:1564–66.

21. Johansson, I., Saellstrom, A. K., Rajan, B. P., & Parameswaran, A. (1992). Salivary flow and dental caries in Indian children suffering from chronic malnutrition. *Caries Res,* 26(1):38–43.

22. Alvarez, J. O., & Navia, J. M. (1989). Nutritional status, tooth eruption, and dental caries: A review. *Am J Clin Nutr,* 49:417–26.

23. Rami-Reddy, V., Vijayalakshmi, P. B., Chndrassekhar-Reddy, B. K. (1986). Deciduous tooth emergence and physique of velama children of Southeastern Andrha Pradesh, India. *Acta de Odont Pediatr,* 7:1–5.

24. Delgado, H., Habicht, J. P., Yarbrough, C., Lechtig, A., Martonell, R., Malina, R. M., & Klein, R. E. (1975). Nutritional status and the timing of deciduous tooth eruption. *Am J Cliin Nutr,* 38:216–24.

25. Alvarez, J. O., Lewis, C. A., Saman, C., Caceda, J., Montalvo, J., Figueroa, M. L., Izquierdo, J., Caravedo, L., & Navia, J. M. (1988). Chronic malnutrition, dental caries, and tooth exfoliation in Peruvian children aged 3–9 years. *Am J Clin Nutr*, 48:368–72.

26. Alvarez, J. O., Carley, K., Caceda, J. et al. (1992). Infant malnutrition and dental caries: A longitudinal study in Peru. *J Dent Res*, 71(special issue): 749, Abstract 1864.

27. Vogel, R. (1985). Oral fluids: Saliva and gingival fluid. In Pollack, R. L., & Kravitz, E., *Nutrition in oral health and disease* (pp. 84–107). Philadelphia: Lea & Febiger.

28. Watson, R. R., & McMurray, D. M. (1979). Effects of malnutrition on secretory and cellular immunity In Furia, T. E. Ed. *CRS-Critical reviews of food and nutrition*. Cleveland, OH: CRS Press.

29. Dreizen, S. (1969). The mouth as an indicator of internal nutritional problems. *Pediatrician*, 16:139–46.

30. Seow, W. K., Masel, J. P., Weir, C., & Tudehope, D. I. (1989). Mineral deficiency in the pathogenesis of enamel hypoplasiz in prematurely born, very low birthweight children. *Pediat Dent*, 11(4):297–302.

31. Sintes, J., & Miller, S. (1983). Influence of dietary iron on the dental caries experience and growth of rats fed an experimental diet. *Arch Latinoam Nutr*, 33:322–28.

32. Freeland, J. H., Cousins, R. D., & Schwartz, R. (1976). Relationship of mineral status and intake to periodontal disease. *Am J Clin Nutr*, 9:745–749.

33. Solomons, N. W. (1988). Zinc and copper. In Shills, M., & Young, V., Eds. *Modern nutrition in health and disease* (pp. 238–50). Philadelphia: Lea and Febiger.

34. Pekarek, R., Sandstead, H., Jacob, R. (1976). Abnormal cellular immune responses during acquired zinc deficiency. *Am J Clin Nutr*, 29:745–49.

35. Nizel, A. E., & Papas, A. (1989). *Nutrition in clinical dentistry* (3rd. ed.) Philadelphia: WB Saunders, 201–3.

36. Frithiof, L., Lazavstedt, S., Eklund, G., Soderberg, U., Skarberg, K. O., Blomquist, J., Asman, B., & Eriksson, W. (1980). The relationship between bone loss and serum zinc levels. *Acta Med Scand*, 207:67–70.

37. Bendich, A., & Chandra, R. K. (1990). Micronutrients and immune functions. New York: *New York Academy of Sciences*.

38. DePaola, D., Faine, M., & Palmer, C., Nutrition in Relation to Dental Medicine in Shils M., Olson J, Shike M, Ross, A. C. eds. *Modern Nutrition in Health and Disease* 9th edition, Lea & Febiger, Philadelphia 1999.

39. deMenzes, A. C., Costa, I. M., & El-Guindy, M. M. (1984). Clinical Manifestations of hypervitaminosis A in human gingiva: A case report. *J Periodontol*, 8:474–76.

40. Ostergaard, E., & Löe, H. (1975). The collagen content of skin and gingival tissues in ascorbic acid deficient monkeys. *J Period Res*, 10(2):103–14.

41. Nakamoto, T., McCroskey, M., & Mallek, H. M. (1984). The role of ascorbic acid deficiency in human gingivitis—a new hypothesis. *J Theor Biol*, 108(2):163–71.

42. Nishida, M. Grossi, S. G., Dunford, R. G., Ho, A. W., Trevisan, M., & Genco, R. J. (2000). Dietary vitamin C and the risk for periodontal disease. *J Periodontology*, 71(8):1215–23.

43. Buzine, R., et al., Increase of gingival hydroxyproline and proline by improvement of ascorbic acid status in man. *Int J Vitam Nutr Res*, 1986;56(4):367–372.

44. Charbeneau, T. D., & Hurt, W. C. (1983). Gingival findings in spontaneous scurvy. A case report. *Journal of Periodontology*, 54(11):694–697.

45. DePaola, D., Faine, M., & Palmer, C. (1999). Nutrition in relation to dental medicine. In Shils, M., Olson, J., Shike, M., & Ross, A. C., Eds. *Modern nutrition in health and disease* (9th ed.), Philadelphia: Lea & Febiger.

46. National Institute of Drug Abuse (1997). *Drug abuse prevention: What works*. Washington, DC: Institute of Medicine, 10–15.

47. Navia, J. M. (1994). Carbohydrates and dental health. *Am J Clin Nutr*, 59(S):719S–727S.

48. Winn, D. M., Brunelle, J. A., Brown, L. J., Selwitz, R. H., Kaste, L. M., Oldakowski, R. J., & Kingman, A. (1996). Coronal and root caries in the dentition of adults in the United States, 1988–1991. *J Dent Res*, 75(Spec Iss):642–51.

49. Kaste, L. M., Selwitz, R. J., Oldakowski, J. A., Brunelle, J. A., Winn, D. M., & Brown, L. J. (1996). Coronal caries in primary and permanent dentition of children and adolescents 1–17 years of age: United States, 1988–1991. *J Dent Res*, 75(Spec Iss):631–41.

50. Huumonen, S., Tjaderhane, L., & Larmas, M. (1997). Greater concentration of dietary sucrose decreases dentin formation and increases the area of dentinal caries in growing rats. *J Nutr*, 127(11):2226–30.

51. Tjaderhane, L., Hietala, E. L., & Larmas, M. (1994). Reduction in dentine apposition in rat molars by a high sucrose diet. *Arch Oral Biol*, 39(6):491–195.

52. Sreebny, L. M. (1982). Sugar availability, sugar consumption, and dental caries. *Comm Dent Oral Epidemiol*, 10:1–7.

53. Tanzer, J. M. (1979). Essential dependence of smooth surface caries on, and augmentation of fissure caries by sucrose and Streptococcus mutans. *Infect Immun*, 25:526–31.

54. Rugg-Gunn, A. J., Hackett, A. F., Appleton, D. R., Jenkins, G. N., & Eastoe, J. E. (1984). Relationship between dietary habits and caries increments assessed over two years in 405 English adolescent school children. *Arch Oral Biol*, 29:983–92.

55. Burt, B. A., Eklund, S. A., Morgan, K. J., & Larkin, F. E., Guire, K. E., Brown, L. O., & Weintraub, J. A. (1988). The effects of sugar intake and frequency of ingestion on dental caries increment in a three-year longitudinal study. *J Dent Res*, 67:1422–29.

56. LaChapelle, D., Couture, C., Brodeur, J. M., & Sevigny, J. (1990). The effects of nutritional quality and frequency of consumption of sugary foods on dental caries increment. *Can J Public Health*, 81:370–75.

57. Newbrun, E. (1992). Preventing dental caries: current and prospective strategies. *J Am Dent Assoc*, 123:19–24.

58. Scheinin, A., Mäkinen, K. K., & Ylitalo, K. (1976). Turku sugar studies vs. final report on the effect of sucrose, fructose, and xylitol diets on the caries incidence in man. *Acta Odontol Scand*, 34:179–216.

59. Tanzer, J. M. (1995). Xylitol chewing gum and dental caries. *Int Dent J*, 45:65–76.

60. Pollard, M. A., Imfeld, T., Higham, S. M., Agalamanyi, E. A., Corzon, M. E., Edgar, W. M., & Borgia, M. (1996). Acidogenic potential and total salivary carbohydrate content of expectorants following the consumption of some cereal-based foods and fruits. *Caries Res*, 30:132–37.

61. Kashket, S., Zhang, J., & Van Houte, J. (1996). Accumulation of fermentable sugars and metabolic acids in food particles that become entrapped on the dentition. *J Dent Res*, 75:1885–91.

62. König, K. G., & Schmid, P. (1968). An analysis of frequency-controlled feeding of small rodents and its use in dental caries experiments. *Arch Oral Biol*, 13:13–26.

63. Gustafson, B., Quensel, E., & Lanke, L. (1954). The Vipeholm dental caries study: the effect of different carbohydrate intake on caries activity in 436 individuals observed for five years. *Acta Odontol Scand*, 11:232–64.

64. Lingstrom, P., Birkhed, D., Ruben, J., & Arends, J. (1994). Effect of frequent consumption of starchy food items on enamel and dentin demineralization and on plaque pH in situ. *J Dent Res*, 73(3):652–60.

65. Rugg-Gunn, W., Edgar, M., & Jenkins, G. N. (1981). The effect of altering the position of a sugary food in a meal upon plaque pH in human subjects. *J Dent Res*, 60:867–72.

66. Edgar, W. M., & Bowen, W. H. (1982). Effects of different eating patterns on dental caries in the rat. *Caries Res*, 16:384–88.

67. Mundorff-Shrestha, S. A., & Featherstone, J. D. B., & Eisenberg, A. D. (1994). Cariogenic potential of foods II. Relationship of food composition, plaque microbial counts, and salivary parameters to caries in the rat model. *Caries Res*, 28:106–15.

68. Jensen, M. E., Harlander, S. K., Schachtele, C. F. (1984). Evaluation of the acidogenic and antacid properties of cheeses by telemetric recording of dental plaque. In Hefferen, J. J., Koehler, H. M. and Osborn, J. C. Eds. *Food, nutrition and dental health*, Vol. V. Park Forest South, IL: Pathotox.

69. Bowen, W. H. (1994). Food components and caries. *Adv Dent Res*, 8:215–20.

70. Mundorff, S. A., Featherstone, J. D. B., & Bibby, B. G. (1990). Cariogenic potential of foods I. Caries in the rat model. *Caries Res*, 24:344–55.

71. Jensen, M. E. (1985). Dental caries: A diet-related disease. *Currents/Quarterly*, 1:18–20.

72. Koulourides, T., & Chien, M. C. (1992). The ICT *in situ* experimental model in dental research. *J Dent Res*, 71:822–27.

73. DePaola, D. (1986). Executive summary: scientific consensus conference on methods for assessment of the cariogenic potential of foods. *J Dent Res*, 65(Spec Iss):1540–43.

74. Curzon, M. E. J., & Pollard, M. A. (1996). Integration of methods for determining the acid/cariogenic potential of foods: a comparison of several different methods. *Caries Res*, 30:126–31.

75. Ripa, L. W. (1988). Nursing caries: A comprehensive review. *Pediatr Dent*, 10:268–82.

76. Kelly, M., & Bruerd, B. (1987). The prevalence of baby bottle tooth decay among two Native American populations. *J Pub Health Dent*, 47:94–97.

77. Broderick, E., Mabry, J., Robertson, D., & Thompson, J. (1989). Baby bottle tooth decay in Native American children in Head Start Centers. *Pub Health Rep*, 104:50–54.

78. Kaste, L. M., & Gift, H. C. (1995). Inappropriate infant bottle feeding. *Arch Pediatr Adolesc Med*, 149:786–91.

79. O'Sullivan, D. M., & Tinanoff, N. (1993). Maxillary anterior caries associated with increased caries risk in other primary teeth. *J Dent Res*, 72:1577–80.

80. Vogel, R., & Alvares, O. F. (1985). Nutrition and periodontal disease. In Pollack, R. L., & Kravitz, E., Eds. *Nutrition in oral health and disease*, (pp. 136–50). Philadelphia: Lea & Febiger.

81. Navia, J. M., & Menaker, L. (1976). Nutritional implications in wound healing. *Dent Clin North Am*, 20(3):549–67.

82. Alfano, M. C., Miller, S. A., & Drummond, J. F. (1975). Effect of ascorbic acid deficiency on the permeability and collagen biosynthesis of oral mucosal epithelium. *Ann NY Acad Sci*, 258:253–63.

83. Alfano, M. C., & Masi, C. W. (1978). Effect of acute folic acid deficiency on the oral mucosal permeability. *J Dent Res*, 57:312, Abstract 949.

84. Joseph, C. E., Ashrafi, S. H., Steinberg, A. D., & Waterhouse, J. P. (1982). Zinc deficiency changes in the permeability of rabbit periodontium to $^{14}$C-phenytoin and $^{14}$C-albumin. *J Periodont*, 53:251–56.

85. Alfano, M. C. (1976). Controversies, perspectives and clinical implications of nutrituion in periodontal disease. *Dent Clin North Am*, 20:519–48.

86. DePaola, D. P., & Kuftinec, M. M. (1976). Nutrition in growth and development of oral tissues. *Dent Clin North Am*, 20:441–59.

87. Malleck, H. M. (1978). An investigation of the role of ascorbic acid and iron in the etiology of gingivitis in humans. Doctoral Thesis. Cambridge, MA: *Institute Archives*, Massachusetts Institute of Technology.

88. Whitehead, N., Ryner, F., & Lindenbaum, J. (1973). Megaloblastic changes in the cervical epithelium. Association with oral contraceptive therapy and reversal with folic acid. *JAMA*, 226(12):1421–24.

89. Zachariasen, R. D. (1995). Oral manifestations of bulimia nervosa. *Women and Health*, 22(4):67–76.

90. Brown, S., & Bonifazi, D. Z. (1993). An overview of anorexia and bulimia nervosa, and the impact of eating disorders on the oral cavity. *Compendium: The Compendium of Continuing Education in Dentistry*, Dec, 14(12):1594, 1596–1602, 1604–8; quiz 1608.

91. Douglass, C. W., Jette, A. M., Fox, C. H., Tennstedt, S. L., Joshi, A., Feldman, H. A., McGuire, S. M., & McKinlay, J. B. (1993). Oral health status of the elderly in New England. *J Gerontology*, 48:M39–461.

92. Palmer, C. A. (1991). Nutrition and oral health of the elderly. In Papas, A., Niessen, L., & Chauncy, H. *Geriatric dentistry: Aging and oral health* (pp. 264–82). St. Louis: Mosby Year Book.

93. Schiffman, S. S. (1991). Taste and smell losses with age. *Contemporary Nutrition*, General Mills Nutrition Department: 16:2: 6–8.

94. Brodeur, J. M., Laurin, D., Vallee, R., & Lachapelle, D. (Nov 1993). Nutrient intake and gastrointestinal disorders related to masticatory performance in the edentulous elderly. *J Prosthetic Dentistry*, 70(5):468–73.

95. Position of the American Dietetic Association: Oral health and nutrition (1966). *J Am Diet Ass*, 96(2):184–89.

96. Slagter, A. P., Olthoff, L. W., Bosman, F., & Steen, W. H. (1992). Masticatory ability, denture quality, and oral conditions in edentulous subjects. *J Prosthetic Dentistry*, 68(2):299–307.

97. Touger-Decker, R., Schaefer, M., Flinton, R., & Steinberg, L. (1996). Effect of tooth loss and dentures on diet habits. *J Prosthet Dent*, 75:831.

98. Sebring, N. G., Guckes, A. D., Li, S., & McCarthy, G. R. (1995). Nutritional adequacy of reported intake of edentulous subjects treated with new conventional or implant-supported mandibular dentures. *J Prosthet Dent*, 74: 358–63.

99. Greksa, L. P., Parraga, I. M., & Clark, C. A. (1995). The dietary adequacy of edentulous older adults. *J Prosthet Dent*, 73:142–5.

100. Papas, A., Palmer, C., McGandy, R., Hartz, S. C., & Russell, R. M. (1987). Dietary and nutritional facctors in relation to dental caries in elderly subjects. *Gerodontics*, 3:30–37.

101. Joshipura, K., Willett, W., & Douglass, C. (1996). The impact of edentulousness on food and nutrient intake. *JADA*, April, 127:459–67.

102. Anderson, D. L. (1977). Death from improper mastication. *Int Dent J*, 27:349.

103. Dormenval, V., Budtz-Jorgensen, E., Mojon, P., Bruyere, A., & Rapin, C. H. (1995). Nutrition, general health status and oral health status in hospitalized elders. *Gerodontology*, 12(12):73–80.

104. Faine, M., Allender, D., Baab, D., Persson, R., & Lamont, R. J. (1992). Dietary and salivary factors associated with root caries. *Special Care in Dentistry*, 12(4):177–82.

105. Maresky, L. S., van der Bijl, P., & Gird, I., (March 1993). Burning mouth syndrome. Evaluation of multiple variables among 85 patients. *Oral Surgery, Oral Medicine, Oral Pathology*, 75(3): 303–7.

106. Mulligan, R. (1989). Oral health: Effect on nutrition and rehabilitation in older persons. *Top Geriatr Rehab*, 5:27–35.

107. Vaanen, M. K., Markkanen, H. A., Tuovinen, V. J., Kullaa, A. M., Karinpau, A. M., & Kumpusalo, E. A. (1993). Periodontal health related to plasma ascorbic acid. *Proc Finn Dent Soc*, 89(1–2):51–9.

108. Paganini-Hill, A. (1995). The benefits of estrogen replacement therapy on oral health. The Leisure World cohort. *Archives Intern Med*, 155(21):2325–9.

109. Whalen, J. P., & Krook, L. (1996). Periodontal disease as the early manifestation of osteoporosis (editorial). *Nutrition*, 12(1):53–4.

110. Kribbs, P. J., Chestnut, C. H., Ott, S., & Kilcoyne, R. F. (1990). Relationships between mandibular and skeletal bone in a population of normal women. *J Prosthet Dent* 63(1):86–89.

111. Kribbs, P. J. (1990). comparison of mandibular bone in normal and osteoporotic women. *J Prosthet Dent*, 63(2):218–22.

112. Houki, K., DiMuzio, M. T., & Fattore, L. (1994). Mandibular bone density and systemic osteoporosis in elderly edentulous women. *J Bone Miner Res*, 9 (suppl1):S211.

113. Krall, E. A., Dawson-Hughes, B., Papas, A., & Garcia, R. I. (1994). Tooth loss and skeletal bone density in health postmenopausal women. *Osteoporosis Int*, 4:104–9.

114. *Nutrition Interventions Manual for Professionals Caring for Older Americans* (1992). Washington DC: Nutrition Screening Initiative.

115. Saunders, M. J. (1995). Incorporating the nutrition screening initiative into the dental practice. *Special Care in Dentistry, 15*(1):26–37.

116. Pla, G. W. (1994). Oral health and nutrition. *Primary Care: Clinics in Office Practice, 21*(1):121–23.

117. Holdren, R. S., & Patton, L. L. (1993). Oral conditions associated with diabetes mellitus. *Diabetes Spectrum, 6*(1):11–17.

118. Cleary, T. J., & Hutton, J. E. (1995). An assessment of the association between functional edentulism, obesity, and NIDDM. *Diabetes Care,* 18:1007–1009.

119. The DCCT Research Group (1993). Nutrition interventions for intensive therapy in the diabetes control and complications trial. *J Am Diet Assoc,* 93:768–72.

120. Robertson, P. B., & Greenspan, J. S., Eds. (1988). *Perspectives on oral Manifestations of Aids: Diagnosis and management of HIV-associated infections.* Littleton, MA: PSG Publishing.

121. Bassett, M. R., & Dobie, R. A. (1983). Patterns of nutritional deficiency in head and neck cancer. *Otolaryngol Head Neck Surg,* 91:119–25.

122. Nikoskelainen, J. (1990). Oral infections related to radiation and immunosuppressive therapy. *J Clin Periodont, 17*(7):504–7.

123. Smith, T. J., Dwyer, J. T., & LaFrancesca, J. P. (1990). Nutrition and the cancer patient. In Osteen, R. T., Cady, B., & Rosenthal, P., Eds. *Cancer Manual* (8th ed.) (Chapter 39.8) Boston: American Cancer Society.

124. Dwyer, J. T., Efstathion, M. S., Palmer, C., & Papas, A. (1991). Nutritional support in treatment of oral carcinomas. *Nutr Rev,* 49: 332–37.

125. Kendall, B. D., Fonseca, R. J., & Lee, M. (1982). Postoperative nutritional supplementation for the orthognathic surgery patient. *J Oral Maxillofac Surg,* 40:205–213.

126. Soliah, K. (1987). Clinical effects of jaw surgery and wiring on body composition: A case study. *Dietetic Currents,* volume 14. Columbus, OH: Ross Laboratories, pp.13–16.

127. Patten, J. A. (1995). Nutrition and wound healing. *Compendium of Continuing Education in Dentistry. 16*(2):200–14.

128. Lokshin, M. F. (1994). Preventive oral health care: A review for family physicians. *American Family Physician, 50*(8):1677–84, 1687.

129. Karp, W. B. (1994). Nutrition update for the dental health professional. *J Calif Dent Assoc, 22*(8):26–9.

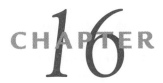

# CHAPTER 16

# Understanding Human Motivation for Behavior Change

*Mary Kaye Sawyer-Morse*
*Alexandra Evans*

## OBJECTIVES

*At the end of this chapter it will be possible to*

1. Define motivation.
2. List reasons why individuals may not be motivated to receive regular oral care.
3. Describe two different approaches to motivate individuals to change behavior.
4. Describe elements of three common behavioral health promotion theories.
5. Explain the importance of appropriate health provider communication.
6. Describe four common client-provider communication styles.
7. Describe motivational interviewing and FRAMES.

## INTRODUCTION

The mouth represents an area of the body of special importance and value. According to Horowitz and coworkers,[1] the mouth is associated with the development of (1) a healthy personality, (2) perceptions, and (3) the overall experience of pleasure. Many areas of the mouth, especially the gingival tissues, are easily accessible for self-diagnosis and primary preventive treatment. Individuals can easily detect gums that are red or bleeding. In addition, the tongue, with its highly developed neurosensory feedback system, can be useful in helping people to assess their own plaque levels and resultant

need for improved oral hygiene behavior. As a result, dental professionals should devise strategies for motivating oral self-care behavior by teaching clients how to recognize their own signs of dental distress or neglect.

In this chapter the interrelationship of motivation, education, and behavioral modification are considered—all with the objective of helping dental professionals develop more effective interpersonal skills, thereby becoming more effective health educators and counselors.[2] The task of educating the client can be greatly simplified by a knowledge of and the application of a few basic constructs of educational and health promotion and human motivation. These same constructs apply equally to either private or public health practices.

**The Problem:** Oral health is an essential component of health throughout life. Poor oral health and untreated oral diseases can have a significant effect on quality of life. The mouth is the entry point for food and the beginning of the gastrointestinal tract. The ability to chew and swallow is a critical function required to obtain essential nutrients for the body—the building blocks of good health.[3] However, millions of individuals in the United States have dental caries and periodontal disease, resulting in unnecessary pain, difficulty in chewing, swallowing, and speaking, increased medical costs, loss of self-esteem, decreased economic productivity through lost work and school days, and, in extreme cases, death.[4] The Healthy People 2010 document recognizes the importance of oral health and includes 17 specific objectives related to the overall goal: To prevent and control oral and craniofacial diseases, conditions, and injuries and improve access to related services.[5]

Regular and timely dental visits provide an opportunity for the early diagnosis, prevention, and timely treatment of oral diseases and conditions, as well as for the assessment of self-care practices. However, approximately 66% of people in the United States do not see a dentist regularly,[5] and among specific subpopulations, such as certain ethnic groups or low-income groups, the proportion not receiving regular care is even higher.[6] For example, the Medical Expenditure Panel Survey in 1996 indicated that 44% of the total population visited a dentist in the past year, while 50% of non-Hispanic whites, 30% of Hispanics, and 27% of non-Hispanic blacks had a visit. In addition, 55% of those individuals with some college education had a past-year visit compared to 24% of those with less than a high school education.[7]

The reasons individuals may not be motivated to seek regular and timely care include: high cost of dental care, lack of dental insurance, lack of providers from underserved racial and ethnic groups, fear of dental visits, habitual personal neglect, lack of knowledge, limited oral-health literacy, and negative feedback or unflattering statements about dentistry received from friends or relatives.[5] Other factors that have contributed to people losing confidence in dentists include prior negative experienced with dentists (poorly executed or ineffective treatment and unnecessary or questionable extractions or other treatments), dental treatment that did not last long enough, and lack of access to appropriate dental care. Previous painful experiences and perceived negative dentist behaviors (e.g. arrogance, sarcasm, or inconsideration) appear to be especially important to the anxious individual who is mentally preparing for dental treatment.[8] See Table 16-1. Most of these barriers can be overcome by effective client education and motivation programs and more effective interpersonal communication by the dental professional.

TABLE 16-1  **Predictors of Dental Anxiety among U.S. Adults**

| Independent Variable | $R^2$ | $R^2$ Change | F Value |
| --- | --- | --- | --- |
| Attitude towards dentists | .2115 | .2115 | <.001 |
| Check-up frequency[*] | .2723 | .0609 | <.001 |
| Satisfaction with mouth | .2908 | .0185 | <.001 |
| Average number of filled surfaces[**] | .3039 | .0181 | .002 |
| Gender[***] | .3141 | .0102 | .006 |
| Annual income | .3193 | .0052 | .036 |

[*]individuals with less frequent check-ups reported more anxiety
[**]individuals with greater numbers of filled surfaces reported less anxiety
[***]females reported greater anxiety than males

## Dental Education and Motivational Programs

In previous chapters, it is stated that primary preventive dentistry can be effectively implemented by using the following five actions: 1) plaque control, 2) reduction of sugar in the diet, 3) fluoride therapy, 4) use of pit-and-fissure sealants, and 5) client education. The successful use of any of these actions requires effective relations between dental professionals and clients to achieve and maintain a maximum level of oral health. Three major enabling factors are necessary to perform the above listed actions—appropriate skill-based education, client self-motivation, and appropriate psychomotor skills.

For any preventive dentistry program to succeed, information about what needs to be done and how it is to be accomplished must be available to both the dental professional and the client. For the client, this information (and sometimes misinformation) is often learned through school-based health programs; the dentist, media, and advertising; and from peers, friends, neighbors, or relatives. On the other hand, dental professionals learn preventive dentistry as part of the curriculum in dental and dental hygiene schools, through reading professional dental journals, by attending professional meetings and conferences, and through participation in continuing education

programs. In some cases, the gap between the information possessed by the clients and the dental professionals is great. This gap in knowledge poses a problem because people tend to seek what they already believe and avoid exposure to anything that mandates changes.

In general, the personality characteristics of dentists indicate that technical proficiency and attention to detail may be more common than strong interpersonal communication skills.[9] For this reason dental professionals may need to cultivate specific knowledge and expertise in the area of human behavior and motivation techniques. Because the skills to accomplish these tasks are not commonly taught in dental school, many dental professionals do not have adequate skills to provide information to clients appropriately.

In addition, many dental professionals are taught that providing knowledge to a client is sufficient to change the client's behavior. However, extensive research indicates that information by itself is necessary, but not sufficient. Human behavior is a product of the interaction of multiple factors such as attitude, self-efficacy, knowledge, or perceived risk and benefits. Any one factor can be powerful but none acts independently.[10] Therefore, not only do many dental professionals need to acquire or strengthen skills on how to provide information to clients, they also need to learn how to appropriately

motivate clients so that behavior change can occur. Many health behaviors theories explain health behavior and can guide effective behavior change. For further description of three common health behavior theories, see section Health Promotion Approach to Behavior Change.

## Motivation

What is motivation? Everyone is motivated to action or inaction. To not be motivated is to be dead. Some argue that humans are primarily instinctual in nature. This argument is difficult to accept because of the varied nature of human behavior. If the "instinct theory" was valid, all humans would show a uniformity of behavior across all cultures.[11] This, of course, is not the case. Others believe that behavior is learned and that our environment determines our actions. Indeed, no one should downplay the importance of environmental forces on human behavior. Motivation may be described as the interaction between the environment, personal and behavioral factors.[12] Despite the fact that human behavior is highly variable and at times unpredictable, one thing is certain: Individuals' performances or behaviors are based on the degree to which they are motivated. Motivation makes the difference.

Human motivation is complex. It is based on a blending of expectations, ideas, feelings, desires, hopes, attitudes, values, and other factors that initiate, maintain, and regulate behavior toward achieving a given goal or outcome. Other factors, such as previous adverse experiences, educational insufficiency, nonacceptance by peers, a poor self-image, and impoverished socioeconomic circumstances can significantly influence behavior. Motivation factors can change with the passage of time. Humans are strongly goal-oriented and can demonstrate a tremendous drive to achieve their personal ambitions. For some, however, a significant part of the pleasure is derived from working toward a goal; after they have "ar-

rived," their pleasure is somewhat diminished. For these individuals, getting there is not only half the fun, it is possibly all the fun. For example, some individuals periodically become intensely motivated to upgrade their oral health status. Appointments are made with the dentist, all restorative work is completed, preventive programs are developed with a great amount of client participation until all dental care has been completed, at which time the individual appears to lose interest until another sudden flurry of interest may occur at a later date.

Motivation then is seen not as a personality problem or trait but rather as a state of readiness or eagerness to change. This readiness may fluctuate from one time or situation to another and can be influenced by the dental professional.[13]

---

### Question 1

Which of the following statements, if any, are correct?

A. The layperson who is undereducated in dental health readily accepts suggested changes in preventive programs that are directed to better oral health.

B. Perceived negative dentist behaviors may deter patients from seeking necessary dental treatment.

C. Primarily, human motivation can be explained and understood as being instinctual in nature.

D. In general, providing patients with knowledge is sufficient to facilitate behavior change.

---

## Educational Approach to Behavior Change

### The Learning Process

Because information transmittal involves learning, it is desirable to turn to the teaching profession for how information is best imparted

to ensure long-term retention. Ensuring that a client adheres with a home care regimen can be the most difficult part of therapy.[14] According to Bloom's taxonomy of educational objectives, a hierarchy of six levels of learning attainment progresses from a complete lack of information to goal attainment (see Figure 16–1).[15] These successive levels are knowledge, comprehension, application, analysis, synthesis, and evaluation. Most teaching today is at the lowest knowledge stage. After mastery of this stage, the learner can only define, repeat, or name facts; it is only partial learning at best. Possible verbs used in stating cognitive outcomes of teaching programs starting with the knowledge level up to evaluation are listed in Figure 16–2. If material is only taught at the lower levels of the taxonomy, learning is incomplete.

The implication of partial learning is apparent when applied to plaque control methods. The average person knows and comprehends that brushing and flossing clean the teeth. They can even demonstrate that they can brush their teeth in some fashion. But how many people can evaluate the effectiveness of their efforts? How many can analyze where problems lie, and how many can propose innovations to their personal oral hygiene program that might make it more effective?

Teaching at the higher levels of Bloom's taxonomy is necessary to accomplish this type of learning. At each cognitive level the teaching should feature an explanation of the subject, followed in sequence by demonstration, applications, feedback, and reinforcement. The use of these sequential steps in all teaching helps to ensure a mastery of the desired topic or skill. In moving from one level of complexity to the next, the learner is exposed to an organized continuum of interrelated facts. Even after successfully mastering all levels of Bloom's hierarchy, however, it is very possible that a skill or subject area learned in an academic or clinical environment is not applied at home, in a more informal environment on a routine basis. Day-to-day application occurs only after an individual has learned sufficient information to determine that a specific benefit accrues to him or her from its use and thus has become motivated. Education involves learning; practical application involves self-motivation.[16] At this point, the knowledge needs to be incorporated into the client's existing value systems.

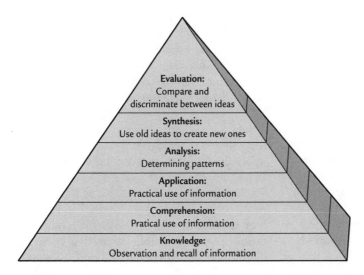

FIGURE 16–1    Bloom's Taxonomy of Educational Objectives.

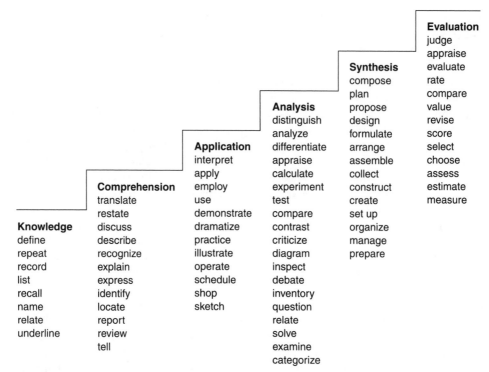

FIGURE 16-2    Some possible verbs for use in stating cognitive outcomes. (Courtesy of Marybelle Savage.)

## Incorporating Knowledge into Value Systems

Personal belief systems and values strongly influence an individual's behavior. Values are developed through the application of knowledge, which thus requires that an individual has enough facts to develop concepts and then a sufficient number of concepts to develop a value.[17] This concept is portrayed graphically in Figure 16–3. The base of the pyramid consists of facts, which are the building blocks of all learning. Sometimes great voids or even misinformation occur in this body of information. Yet, regardless of its completeness or accuracy, this substratum of information is where concepts are formed by use of one's reasoning power. Concepts, less numerous than facts, represent the organization and classification of facts into meaningful personal habits or pat-

terns. The greater number of correct facts arising from different inputs, the greater the possibility of developing correct concepts. On top of these supporting facts and concepts rest values—beliefs and bodies of knowledge important to the individual.

These values are only as strong as the supporting information. It should be noted that not all dental values are positive. For example, for individuals living under impoverished conditions who do not appreciate the value of teeth from a health or social viewpoint or where the loss of teeth is considered as normal, facts, concepts, and values are often negative. These negative perceptions can motivate nonparticipation in dental programs.[18] It has also been noted that a client's relationship with the dental professional influences their anxiety level and resulting compliance with suggested

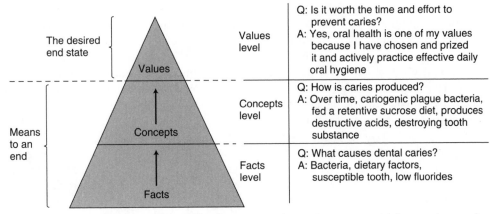

FIGURE 16-3    The interrelationship between values, concepts, and facts using oral health as a positive end value. Learning on all three levels helps individuals discern facts, make sense of them and, finally, to live by the meaning they perceive.

oral health-care practices.[8] The dental professional must carefully consider the possible myriad facts and concepts that can make up this pyramid when trying to change a client's value system—a value system that is valid to only the individual client.

Values are not neutral but are held with personal feeling.[17] When they are challenged, they frequently generate an emotional, defensive response. Making changes in one's behavior is often very difficult and involves dealing with conflict. Hayakawa[19] expands this idea when he writes, "the process of learning, which is also the process of growth, is essentially a means of resolving conflicts . . . a conflict must always be present before learning can occur . . . conflict then is a necessary accompaniment of personality development, and the progressive assimilation of disturbing stimuli is the only practical means by which a stable organization can be obtained. Without conflict, no learning results."

Therefore it is necessary that the dental professional understand that because of the client's value system, resistance is normal and permanent changes in some forms of behavior are difficult to achieve. This same resistance is met from the client in the dental office, or from

many in the community, when new health programs are proposed. For example, sugar discipline is difficult to instill because of concepts and values shaped early in childhood by the media and candy-laden shelves in the supermarkets; water fluoridation efforts have failed in some areas because of a barrage of misinformation and distorted facts, leading to strongly held values by those voting against fluoridation. Such resistance to change should not prevent the continual education and pressure for more effective oral disease control programs. In this quest, however, we must be careful how we approach the value systems of our clients or of the community. We must respect the fact that others have their own value systems tied to their own set of expectations that may be quite different from ours.

Can human values be changed? The answer is yes, but this statement must be qualified. Values are slow to form and slow to change.[17] Even if the factual information is complete and adequate, time is required for concepts to evolve and mature; even more time is required before other additional facts and concepts are acquired to support a new value. Stated another way, a dental professional should not expect dramatic and immediate changes in client be-

havior as a result of only one or two counseling sessions. Thus to attain a behavioral change, a health education program is often confronted with the imposing requirement to modify or reconstruct completely the facts and concepts making up an existing value structure. No wonder so many health education programs fail. A good example is smoking behavior. Virtually all smokers have enough facts necessary to develop the concept that the behavior, cigarette smoking, is harmful. Yet many have not accepted this concept into their own value systems to the point of behavioral change, namely of not smoking. It is also seen in caries and periodontal disease control programs in which clients are unwilling to conduct lifelong programs of plaque control.

---

### Question 2

Which of the following statements, if any, are correct?

A. Different groups of individuals presented with the same facts can develop different concepts.

B. Once facts and concepts are a part of an individual's life, values fall in place.

C. Most education results in the learner being able to attain the cognitive level of evaluation on Bloom's hierarchy.

D. The dental professional must acknowledge that values are slow to change and that resistance to changing values is normal.

---

## Health Promotion Approach to Behavior Change

An alternative way of examining human motivation draws from the health education and health promotion literature. Although many definitions for health promotion exist, one of the more common ones states that health promotion is "any combination of health education and related organizational, political, and economic interventions designed to facilitate behavioral and environmental changes conducive to health."[20]

Central to all health promotion definitions is the concept of health behavior. Positive informed changes in health behavior are usually the ultimate goals of health promotion activities. Health behavior refers to "those personal attributes such as beliefs, expectations, motives, values, perceptions, and other cognitive elements; personality characteristics, including affective and emotional states and traits; and overt behavioral patterns, actions, and habits that relate to health maintenance, to health restoration, and to health improvement."[21] Specific to the field of dental care, health behaviors include getting regular dental check-ups, regular brushing and flossing, and reducing sugar intake.

Identifying the personal attributes most significant for certain health behaviors is critical for the development of successful interventions. For example, to increase the number of individuals who obtain regular and timely dental check-ups, dental health-care providers need to be aware of the personal attributes, or the predisposing factors, that contribute to people getting regular check-ups. This information can come from two sources: empirical data and health promotion theories. Empirical data can provide us with data obtained through epidemiological studies. Health-promotion theories can explain and predict why people behave the way they do.

### Health Behavior Change Theories

Three prominent theories that will be discussed in the following sections include the Health Belief Model (HBM),[22] Social Cognitive Theory (SCT),[12] and the Transtheoretical Model (TTM).[23] These theories share the central assumptions that people are capable of forethought, planning, and rational decision making. People are goal oriented and self-regulating beings. All of these theories explicitly or implicitly recognize that people experience their

decision making and self-regulation as part of a dynamic social-learning process.[12] While the HBM mainly predicts behavior, SCT and TTM address the processes of behavior change and allow for the identification of appropriate strategies to facilitate behavior change.

Individuals' motivation is central to most health behavior theories for either prediction or behavior change purposes. As will be noted below, most of these theories include the assumption that individuals are interested in planning and controlling their actions and are not passive "lumps of clay."

### Health Belief Model

The Health Belief Model (HBM) is a commonly used theory to predict individual's behavior regarding preventive health care. Originally developed in the 1950s to explain widespread failure of people to participate in interventions to prevent tuberculosis,[24] HBM has been extended to apply to people's responses to symptoms and to their compliance with medical regimens.[22]

HBM includes five main components: *perceived susceptibility, perceived severity, perceived benefits, perceived barriers,* and *self-efficacy. Perceived susceptibility* refers to a person's subjective perception of the risk of becoming sick, while perceived severity refers to the person's feelings of the seriousness of becoming sick or leaving the illness untreated (both medical and clinical and social consequences). The combination of susceptibility and severity is often labeled *perceived threat.* Before a person will take action and change behavior, the perceived threat needs to high. For example, before a person will consider flossing every day, he or she needs to believe that not flossing will lead to periodontal disease *and* that periodontal disease can have serious negative consequences for him or her.

When an individual has a high *perceived threat,* that person will analyze the *perceived benefits and barriers* of performing a certain behavior. *Perceived benefits* refer to the beliefs re-

garding the effectiveness of the available actions in reducing the disease threat. Thus, a person who believes that flossing every day will reduce the risk of developing periodontal disease will be more likely to perform this behavior than a person who does not have this belief. Contrary to perceived benefits, *perceived barriers* (e.g. painful, difficult, upsetting, inconvenient, time-consuming) can act as impediments to engaging in the health behavior. Thus a sort of cost-benefit analysis occurs when individuals decide whether the perceived benefits override the perceived barriers. If they do, those individuals will most likely perform the behavior. If the barriers outweigh the benefits, the behavior will probably not occur. Thus, even if a person feels a high threat for periodontal disease, he or she may not change his current behavior to daily flossing when the perceived barriers for flossing every day (e.g., time-consuming, painful, inconvenient) are stronger than the benefits.

Determining their client's perceived threat, perceived benefits, and barriers can be very helpful for a dental professional who wants to encourage a client to change behaviors. By asking the right type of questions, all health professionals can obtain this information. The dental professional can then address any perceived misconceptions and, consequently, facilitate behavior change.

### Social Cognitive Theory

HBM, is a theory that focuses on psychosocial factors within the individual that can affect behavior change. Social Cognitive Theory (formerly known as Social Learning Theory) includes both individual as well as environmental influences. Thus, SCT explains human behavior in terms of a triadic, and reciprocal model, in which personal factors, environmental influences, and behavior interact continuously.[12] In addition to explaining why a person behaves in a certain manner, SCT can facilitate behavior change by providing specific learning strategies (e.g., modeling). For a more detailed descrip-

tion of the various SCT constructs, please see *Health Behavior and Education* (1997) by Glanz et al.

Reciprocal determinism is the underlying assumption of SCT. It explains that behavior, environmental factors, and individual influences are continuously interacting and each one affects the other. For example, a person who has high dental anxiety (a personal factor) and receives no reinforcement to see a dentist regularly (environmental factor) is not likely to go for preventive dental check ups. However, if this person receives positive feedback for seeing a dentist (environmental factor), and has a role model who visits a dentist every 6 months (environmental factor), her level of dental anxiety may actually decrease. As a result, she may be more likely to go see a dentist. SCT underscores the importance of avoiding simplistic "single direction of change" thinking. Behaviors do not occur in isolation and interventions should focus both on the individual and the environment.[10]

Modeling, one of the key learning strategies proposed by SCT, has been successfully used with dental clients to decrease dental fear and anxiety. A study performed by Bernstein (1982) looked at the effectiveness of different strategies to reduce fear of dentistry in adult clients who had avoided dental treatment for from 1 to 10 years. The strategies studies included participant modeling (a SCT strategy), symbolic modeling, and graduated exposure. Results suggested that even though the strategies were equally effective for the short-term, participant modeling was most effective for reducing fear for long-term period.[25]

## Stages of Change Model

Oral health care providers have sought to understand and create those conditions that would lead to beneficial and helpful behavior changes for their clients. The Transtheoretical Model (TTM), developed by two psychologists, Drs. Prochaska and DiClemente[23] is a powerful and widely accepted model for understanding how and why people change, either on their own or with the assistance of others. The model is based on the individual's state of readiness or willingness to change, which may fluctuate from one time or situation to another.

The Transtheoretical Model is composed of three main constructs, one of which is the Stages of Change. The stages of change construct describes a series of five progressive stages through which individuals pass in the course of changing a behavior. The "wheel of change" derived from the Prochaska–DiClemente model (Figure 16–4) reflects the reality that in almost any change process, it is possible for a person to go around the "wheel" or relapse several times before achieving a stable change. For example, an individual who is willing and ready to start flossing once a day may begin this practice receiving information from his dentist, then relapse after several weeks, and then start the daily flossing routine again after another dental visit. Thus, according to the Stages of Change, relapses or slips to previous behaviors is normal and a realistic occurrence.

The five stages of change as linked to the development of health behaviors, including optimal oral hygiene habits, are described below. Daily flossing will be used as the specific example to illustrate this theory.

*Precontemplation*—Individuals in this stage are not aware of the positive consequences of daily flossing and have no conscious intentions of starting to floss daily within the next 6 months.

*Contemplation*—Individuals in the Contemplation stage are aware of the positive consequences of changing their current behaviors and plan to start flossing within the next 6 months (near future).

*Preparation*—Individuals in this stage are making concrete steps to adopting oral hygiene practices. They may have bought new floss or scheduled dental appointments.

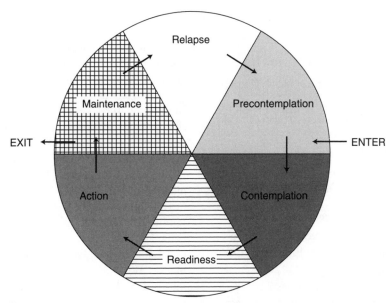

FIGURE 16-4    Prochaska and DiClemente's six stages of change (as modified by Christen, et al., 1994).

*Action*—Individuals in the Action stage are actually flossing every day but have done so less than 6 months.

*Maintenance*—Individuals have flossed daily for over 6 months.

As discussed earlier, at any time an individual may relapse to a previous stage, thus an individual in the Action stage could relapse to the Preparation or even the Contemplation stage.

Corresponding to each stage are appropriate counseling techniques. Thus, by understanding the specific stages of behavior change and the corresponding emotions that may accompany them, oral health care providers can better understand the actions, or inactions, of their clients. With a better understanding, they will be more able to meet the immediate needs of their clients and counsel them appropriately. For example, precontemplators are not ready to change their behavior and they do not want to hear threatening messages. They have a very strong preponderance of "pros" about

their current behavior and have a poor acknowledgement of the "cons." These individuals should be given balanced information about the current behavior, handled with kindness and care, and left alone. It is not reasonable to blame these individuals for being unmotivated to change their current oral hygiene practices.

Individuals who are in the contemplation stage tend to have a balance between the positive and negative feelings about their current behaviors. They are often still ambivalent about changing. Even when contemplators move into the preparation stage, when the strengths of the pros for changing behaviors have increased over the cons, they may still have positive feelings about their current behaviors that are strong.

The Stages of Change model indicates that the goal of the oral health care provider is not necessarily one of action. Because many individuals tend to be in the precontemplation or contemplation stages, it is very worthwhile to

try to "move" these individuals to the next stage.

## Approaches for Different Levels of Client Motivation and Adherence

Plaque-control measures are difficult to accomplish and require considerable time, skill, and perseverance. In fact, current measures of oral hygiene requiring fastidious removal of all supragingival plaque may be beyond the average individual.[26] Thus a blend of education, motivation, and psychomotor skills are necessary to ensure good personal oral hygiene measures. No good evidence supports the fact that mass education alters individual behavior. Instead, individualized approaches are usually necessary, and even these are not always successful.

For a dentist entrusted with the preventive care of a moderately motivated individual, the recall program should be at sufficiently frequent intervals to compensate for lapses in client self-care routines. At the same time, the educational and motivation phases of client education should be emphasized to improve the participation and effectiveness in self-care programs. In this way, the dental professional assumes the task of caring for the client to the extent that compensates for the shortcomings of the client while preparing the client to adopt a greater role in maintaining personal oral health status. Ultimately, it is the client who must assume as much responsibility for self-care as possible and to seek out the dental professional for evaluation (examination) and reinforcement when deficiencies are noted or suspected.

Once an individual becomes sufficiently motivated and changes his or her behavior, the next important issue is adherence. Adherence implies that people choose freely to undertake behavioral plans, have input to them, and have collaborative involvement in adjusting their plans.[27] What makes an individual continue to follow dental recommendations and adhere to practice oral hygiene? Although there is a paucity of literature in the area of adherence to oral hygiene practices, literature related to other health behaviors can provide some information.

Although there are some common factors, potential determinants of adherence are not consistently detected. A clinically-oriented framework by Meichenbaum and Turk (1987) may be useful for oral health-care professionals. This framework divides factors related to adherence into characteristics of the individual (e.g., knowledge, attitudes, beliefs, expectancies about health, treatment), disease (e.g., complexity, duration, side effects), the treatment regimen (e.g., complexity, duration, type, cost), relationship to the health-care-provider clinic staff (e.g., client–provider staff), and clinic organization (e.g., staff enthusiasm).[28]

This framework can be used to provide order to a list of determinants and can help identify categories of potential moderators of adherence to treatments. Thus, to improve adherence to specific regimen, oral health care professionals can use this framework to examine their clients and clinics to determine potential areas of improvement.

# Selecting Methods of Influencing Behavior Change

## Client–Provider Relationship/Communication Styles

Determining the most appropriate type of client–physician relationship is extremely important for the practicing dentist. While some health-care professionals prefer to be the expert and authority, others understand that not all clients respond well to this type of relationship. When a client does not respond well to the type of relationship practiced by the health care provider, important information may be lost. On the other hand, the positive benefits derived from good doctor–client communication include both immediate effects during the visit and long term effects following the visits and involve compliance with prescribed regimen, pain experience, physiologic changes, speed of recovery, and functional state.[29]

There are four archetypal forms of the doctor–client relationship: paternalism, consumerism, mutuality, and default. Paternalism is regarded as the more traditional and probably the most common form of the doctor–client relationship.[30] The paternalistic model provides a social control function in that the health care provider is seen as the expert and dominant, controlling figure, while the client is passive and free from social responsibilities. The physician maintains emotional detachment and acts only in his or her sphere of expertise. Although some may view this type relationship as negative, some clients may actually draw comfort and support from a doctor-father figure. The supportive nature of paternalism seems to be very important when a client is in need of extensive services and therefore is vulnerable. In times of emergency, when correct decisions must be made quickly to avoid life-threatening events, the health-care provider must take control and the paternalistic form is usually necessary.

The consumerism prototype is the opposite of paternalism. In this type of relationship, the power relationship between the client and the physician are reversed: the client or the consumer has more power or control than the physician.[10] Especially when trying to "sell" prevention to the client, the physician's role is to convince the client of the necessity of non-curative services such as regular dental checkups or daily brushing. Several authors have defined consumerism as a client challenge to unilateral decision making by physicians when reaching closure on diagnosis and treatment plans.[31] In this prototype, the health provider and client co-jointly explore the various options and planning objectives. This type of relationship appeals to higher order means of acceptance, including reasoning, nonthreatening persuasion, and rewards. The healthcare provider typically talks less, listens more, questions, reacts, and synthesizes when necessary.[32]

Compared to consumerism, the mutuality prototype offers a more moderate alternative. The client still has a great deal of power but so does the physician. In mutuality, both individuals (client and physician) bring recognized strengths and resources to the relationship. In this model, the client recognizes his or her role as part of a joint venture while the physician understands the centrality of the client in his or her care.[10]

In some cases, the client and physician remain at odds and cannot negotiate a change in the relationship due to poor fit. In this case, a total lack of control exists and the default prototype occurs.[29] Although the client and physician may still see each other during regular visits, the client may fail to make a commitment to prescribed regimens and the physician may cease to be engaged or try to educate the client.

## Motivational Interviewing in the Change Process

Motivational interviewing, introduced by Miller and Rollnick (1991) is a particular method to help people recognize and do some-

thing about their present and potential behavioral problems.[33] It is particularly useful for those clients who are reluctant to change and ambivalent about changing. This technique attempts to help resolve ambivalence and to move the individual along the path to change. Ambivalence is a state of mind in which a person has coexisting but conflicting feelings about some issue. This "I want to but I don't want to" dilemma is at the heart of the problem of all change. Ambivalence is a type of conflict within an individual that has the potential for keeping people "stuck" and creating stress. Ambivalent smokers who have been told by their periodontist that tobacco use can cause periodontal disease, might readily acknowledge that their oral health is endangered, yet may feel equally concerned about their ability to cope with stressful situations without smoking.

Oral-health-care providers must understand that ambivalence is not merely a "bad sign." It should be regarded as normal, acceptable, common, and understandable part of the change process. What is highly valued by some (e.g., having good oral health) will be of little importance to others.

Five broad clinical principles underlie motivational interviewing.[33] These principles emphasize that the clinician should: 1) express empathy (through skillful reflective listening, the clinician seeks to understand and accept the client's feelings and perspective without judging, criticizing or blaming, and realizes that ambivalence is normal); 2) develop discrepancy (help the client understand the discrepancy between their present behavior and their ability to reach their important goals; clients should discover and present their own arguments for and against change); 3) avoid argumentation (a gently persuasive/soft confrontation approach should be used—one that asserts that clients have the freedom to do as they please; avoid sending the message that "I'm the expert and I'm going to tell you how to run your life"; do not accuse clients of being "in de-

nial" or label their behavior); 4) roll with resistance (invite the client to consider new information and offer new perspectives, without being imposing); 5) support self-efficacy (it is essential to support the client's self-esteem and their general self-regard; the client is responsible for choosing and carrying out personal change and the overall message is of hope and faith to the client; "You can do it. You can succeed.").

## The FRAMES Brief Counseling Elements

Miller and Rollnick[34] have described six practical counseling elements that are active ingredients in effective and brief counseling interventions. They are summarized in the acronym "FRAMES."

- Feedback—The client is given feedback of their current status. The importance of conducting a thorough assessment provides the client an opportunity to reflect in detail upon their situation.

- Responsibility—There is an emphasis on the individual's personal responsibility for change. "It's up to you to decide what to do with this information. Nobody can decide for you, and no one can change your habit patterns if you don't want to change."

- Advice—Simple, clear advice to the client to make a change in their lifestyle is given.

- Menu—By offering clients a menu of alternative strategies for changing their problem behavior, the clinician provides a range of options, which allows clients to select strategies that match their particular needs and situations.

- Empathy—Understand another's meaning through the use of reflective listening, whether you have had similar experiences yourself. Use of warmth, respect, supportiveness, caring, concern, sympathetic understanding, commitment, and active interest to convey this element.

- Self-efficacy—Reinforcing the client's hope or optimism in their ability to make changes promotes self-efficacy. Remember that your belief in the client's ability to change is often a significant determinant of outcomes.

### Basic Philosophy

A basic philosophy of prevention is itself a value. One basic philosophy concerning preventive dentistry is that clients deserve to know the cause of their dental diseases and how they can prevent them. This is a responsibility for the health educator. Once armed with the knowledge, however, the client reserves the right to remain sick. This is a problem of self-motivation. Clients are ultimately responsible for their own dental health. In the final analysis, prevention is a shared responsibility between the practitioner and the client.

## SUMMARY

The maintenance of good oral health requires a partnership between the dental professional and the patient. No preventive program can be a success unless the patient participates in a home self-care program to supplement office care programs, with the level of success being proportionate to the amount of participation. Maximum participation can be expected when the patient knows what to do, how to do it, and above all has the motivation to adhere to recommended procedures. Educational strategies can be used to teach facts and skills, but these are useless without motivation. Motivation can be initiated by an individual based on some need or desire, or it can be facilitated by persuasion from external sources. With or without motivation, learning is best achieved in sequential steps, as described by Bloom's hierarchy of cognitive levels. As an individual accumulates facts, the facts merge into concepts and ultimately into values, which in turn engender motivation. At times motivation provides the drive to alter lifestyle to attain habit patterns necessary to maintain good oral health. The dental professional can exert a direct or indirect influence on such a change by providing appropriate behavior modeling, by taking a more active role as an authoritarian, or by participating as a nonauthoritarian in developing a program of planned change with the patient. All health education requires learning, but the successful application of all health knowledge requires motivation.

## ANSWERS AND EXPLANATIONS

1. B—correct.

   A—incorrect. The average layperson does not accept change without considerable persuasion.

   C—incorrect. Human motivation is complex in nature and best described as the interaction between the environment, personal, and behavioral factors.

   D—incorrect. Knowledge is rarely sufficient to change behavior.

2. A, D—correct.

   B—incorrect. Facts and concepts represent unorganized and organized thoughts, respectively; values represent the acceptance and personal application of facts and concepts.

   C—incorrect. Most education is directed to the initial level—facts; very little learning ends up at the evaluation level.

3. C—correct.

   A—incorrect. Most health-behavior theories attempt to explain or predict behavior.

   B—incorrect. The stages of change model suggest that behavior change does not typically follow a linear progression but rather is cyclical as an individual experiences relapse and adopts new behaviors.

   D—incorrect. Health-promotion theories *attempt* to explain or predict behavior with varying degrees of accurateness.

## SELF-EVALUATION QUESTIONS

1. Health promotion can be defined as _____.

2. An individual, through reasoning, organizes facts into _____; which in turn are the basis for a(n) _____.

3. The central assumption underlying health promotion theories is _____.

4. The five main concepts of the Health Belief Model include: _____, _____, _____, _____, _____.

5. The six cognitive levels of Bloom's hierarchy of learning are knowledge, _____, _____, _____, _____, _____, and _____.

6. The one main difference between HBM and Social Cognitive Theory is _____.

7. _____ is the underlying assumption of SCT.

8. _____ implies that an individual chooses freely to undertake behavioral plans, have input to them, and has a collaborative involvement in modifying the plan.

9. In the dentist–patient partnership, it is the _____ who must assume responsibility for home care programs, whereas the _____ must assume responsibility of identifying and correcting deficiencies that occur in a home care program.

10. In the development of optimal oral hygiene habits, patients encounter five progressive stages of change. They are: _____, _____, _____, _____, and _____.

11. In the process of applying motivational interviewing, the clinician should apply five principles, which are: ＿＿＿, ＿＿＿, ＿＿＿, ＿＿＿, and ＿＿＿.

12. The process whereby the clinician seeks to understand and accept the patient's feelings and perspectives without judgment, criticizing, or blaming is called: ＿＿＿.

# REFERENCES

1. Horowitz, L. G., Dillenberg, J., & Rattray, J. (1987). Self-care motivation: A model for primary preventive oral health behavior change. *J Sch Health*, 57:114–18.
2. Barkley, R. (1972). A rational basis for a behaviorally sound dental practice. *Successful Preventive Dental Practices*. Macomb, IL: Preventive Dentistry Press, 1972.
3. American Dietetic Association (1986). ADA reports: Position of the American Dietetic Association: Oral health and nutrition. *Am J Diet Assoc*, X96: 184–89.
4. Reisine, S., & Locker, D. (1995). Social, psychological, and economic impacts of oral conditions and treatments. In L. K. Cohen & H. C. Gift, Eds. *Disease prevention and oral health promotion: Socio-dental sciences in action* (pp. 33–71). Copenhagen: Munksgaard and la Federation Dentaire Internationale.
5. Healthy People 2010: National Health Promotion and Disease Objectives. (2000) DHHS Publication No. (PHS) Washington, DC: Public Health Service.
6. U. S. General Accounting Office (GAO) Report of Congressional Requestors. Oral Health in Low-Income Populations. (GAO/HEHS-00-72). Washington, DC: GAO, 2000.
7. Agency for Healthcare Research and Quality (AHRQ) (1996). Medical Expenditure Panel Survey (MEPS), unpublished data.
8. Doerr, P. A., Lang, W. P., Nyquist, L. V., & Ronis, D. L. (1998). Factors associated with dental anxiety. *J Am Dent Assoc*, 129:1111–18.
9. Hammer, A. L., & Macdaid, G. P. (1992). MBTI Career Report: Form G. Palo Alto, CA: Consulting Psychologists Press.
10. Glanz, K., Lewis, M. L., & Rimer, B. K., Eds. (1997). *Health behavior and health education* (2nd ed.). San Francisco: Jossey-Bass Publishers.
11. Hutchins, D. W. (1968). Motivation in preventive dentistry. Report on the *Proceedings of the Fourth Annual Preventive Dentistry Workshop*. Washington, DC: July 25–26. Columbia, MO: The Curators, University of Missouri.
12. Bandura, A. (1986) *Social foundation of thought and action*. Englewood Cliffs, NJ: Prentice-Hall.
13. Smith, T. A., Kroeger, R. F., Lyon, H. E., & Mullins, M. R. (1990). Evaluating a behavioral method to manage dental fear: a 2-year study of dental practices. *J Amer Dent Assoc, 121*(10) 525–30.
14. Van Houten, P. (1989). Motivating patients to self-care takes the staff's personal involvement. *Dent Off*, 1:8–9.
15. Bloom, B. S., Englehart, M. D., Furst, E. J., et al. (1975). *Taxonomy of educational objectives. Handbook I: Cognitive domain*. New York: D. McKay Co.
16. Savage, M. B., Johnson, R. B., & Johnson, S. R., Eds. (1971). *Assuring learning with self-instructional packages, or . . . up the up staircase*. Chapel Hill, NC: Self-Instructional Packages, Inc., 141.
17. Christen, A. (1984). The development of positive health values. *Health Values*, 8:5–12.
18. Kleinknecht, R. A., Klepac, R. K., & Alexander, L. D. (1973). Origins and characteristics of fear of dentistry. *J Am Dent Assoc*, 86:842–46.

19. Mittelman, J. S. (1988). Getting through to your patients: Psychologic motivation. *Dent Clin North Am*, 32:29–33.
20. Green, L. W., & Kreuter, M. H. (1999). *Health promotion planning: An educational and ecological approach* (3rd ed.) Mountain View, CA: Mayfield Publishing.
21. Hochbaum, G. M., Sorenson, J. R., & Lorig, K. (1992). Theory in health education practice. *Health Education Quarterly, 19*(3):295–313.
22. Becker, M. H. (1974). The Health Belief Model and personal health behavior. Health Education Monographs 1974; 2: 324–473.
23. Prochaska, J. O., & DiClemente, C. C. (1985). Common processes of self-change in smoking, weight control, and psychological distress. In Shiffman, S., & Wills, T., Eds. *Coping and substance use* (pp. 345–64). Orlando, FL: Academic Press.
24. Hochbaum, G. M. (1958). Public participation in medical screening programs: A sociopsychological study. Public Health Service Number 572.
25. Bernstein, D. A. (1982). Multiple approaches to the reduction of dental fear. *J Behav Ther and Exp Psychiat, 13*(4): 287–92.
26. Brady, W. F. (1984). Periodontal disease awareness. *J Am Dent Assoc*, 109:706–10.
27. Brawley, L. R., & Culos-Reed, S. (2000). Studying adherence to therapeutic regimens: Overview, theories, recommendations. *Controlled Clinical Trials*, 21: 156S–163S.
28. Meichenbaum, D., & Turk, D. C. (1987). *Facilitating treatment adherence: A practitioner's guidebook*. New York: Plenum.
29. Roter, D. L., & Hall, J. A. (1982). *Doctors talking to patients talking to doctors: Improving communication in medical visits*. Westport, CT: Auburn House.
30. Szasz, P. S., & Hollender, M. H. (1956). A contribution to the philosophy of medicine: The basic model of the doctor-patient relationship. *Archi Intern Med*, 97:585–92.
31. Haug, M., & Lavin, B. (1983). *Consumerism in medicine: Challenging physician authority*. Thousand Oaks, CA: Sage.
32. Iwata, B. A., & Becksfort, C. M. (1981). Behavioral research in preventive dentistry: Educational and contingency management approaches to the problem of patient compliance. *Applied Behavioral Anal*, 14:111–20.
33. Miller, W. R., & Rollnick, S. (1991). *Motivational interviewing*. New York: The Guilford Press.

# CHAPTER 17

# Dental Public-Health Programs

*Mark D. Macek and Harold S. Goodman*

## OBJECTIVES

*At the end of this chapter, it will be possible to*

1. List the core functions of public health.
2. Define dental public health and relate this definition to dental public-health programs.
3. Compare the methods of public health-care practitioners and personal health-care practitioners.
4. Describe the seven-step model for assessing oral-health-care needs and relate this model to a planning cycle for public-health programs.
5. Outline the scope of traditional dental public-health programs.
6. Describe recent changes in the United States that are relevant to dental public-health practice.
7. List the various organizations that maintain and support public health programs.
8. Describe how the Surgeon General's report on oral health in America has impacted dental public-health programs.

## INTRODUCTION

In 1994, the *Core Functions of Public Health Steering Committee*, co-chaired by Drs. Philip R. Lee (Assistant Secretary for Health) and M. Joycelyn Elders (Surgeon General of the U.S. Public Health Service), produced a consensus statement outlining the essential services of public health in the United States.[1] The new statement provided a vision for public health—*Healthy People in Healthy Communities*—and defined its mission: *Promote*

*physical and mental health and prevent disease, injury, and disability.* The consensus statement also provided broader description of the core functions of public health—*assessment, policy development,* and *assurance.*[2] According to the statement, the *purpose of public health* included: 1) preventing epidemics and the spread of disease; 2) protecting against environmental hazards; 3) preventing injuries; 4) promoting and encouraging healthy behaviors and mental health; 5) responding to disasters and assisting communities in recovery; and 6) assuring the quality and accessibility of health services. The *practice of public health* included: 1) monitoring health status to identify and solve community-health problems; 2) diagnosing and investigating health problems and health hazards in the community; 3) informing, educating, and empowering people about health issues; 4) mobilizing community partnerships and action to identify and solve health problems; 5) developing policies and plans that support individual and community health efforts; 6) enforcing laws and regulations that protect health and ensure safety; 7) linking people to needed personal-health services and assuring the provision of health care when otherwise unavailable; 8) assuring a competent public and personal health-care workforce; 9) evaluating effectiveness, accessibility, and quality of personal and population-based health services; 10) researching for new insights and innovative solutions to health problems.

In 1976, the American Dental Association adopted a definition of *dental public health,* stating that it was:

> . . . the science and art of preventing and controlling dental diseases and promoting dental health through organized community efforts. It is that form of dental practice which serves the community as a patient rather than the individual. It is concerned with the dental education of the public, with applied dental research, and with the administration of group dental care programs as well as the prevention and control of dental diseases on a community basis. . .[3].

Given this definition, *dental public-health programs* refer to organized efforts that strive to prevent and control oral and craniofacial diseases at the community level. Dental public-health programs are highly varied and include activities that cover a wide spectrum, from small-scale local projects to large-scale national and international ventures. Given that a community is the focus, dental public-health programs must satisfy the criteria of practicality, feasibility, acceptability, safety, effectiveness, and efficiency.[4,5]

## Historic Perspective

Dental disease has been a significant problem for Americans since the nation's early history.[6] Between 1862 and 1864, loss of teeth was the fourth most frequent cause for rejection of young men for draft into the Union Army during the Civil War.[7] In 1918, military draftees for World War I were rejected—because of defective and deficient teeth—at a rate that exceeded 10% in some states.[8] During the conscription period of World War II, the *U.S. War Department Mobilization Regulation* required that a recruit have a minimum of three serviceable, natural anterior and posterior teeth in opposition, per arch, to be acceptable for military service. Fifteen percent of recruits were rejected, because they could not pass these rather liberal criteria.[6] During the 1920s, the Metropolitan Life Insurance Company conducted one of the earliest epidemiological studies of the dental condition of a large, heterogeneous, adult,

civilian population.[9] Oral examinations of more than 12,000 adults revealed that, among 20- to 24-year-olds, more than half of the teeth had been affected by dental caries, and this proportion increased steadily in older age groups.

During the next several decades, the number of epidemiological surveys conducted among civilians increased dramatically.[10–15] It was not surprising that these studies reflected the high dental caries prevalence levels noted in earlier studies and conducted among military recruits. The surveys showed that dental caries was a serious health problem among young adults, and often resulted in tooth loss. The studies also showed that dental caries began early in life and affected young children.

Between 1933 and 1934, the U.S. Public Health Service (USPHS) sponsored a survey conducted among thousands of 6- to 14-year-old children in 26 states across the United States.[16] The study revealed high dental caries prevalence levels in children, as well. In 1937, the classic Hagerstown, Maryland, study,[17] which introduced the Decayed, Missing and Filled index for teeth (DMFT) and tooth surfaces (DMFS), showed moderately high caries prevalence levels among the examined children. The study also showed that children with the highest dental-caries index scores received only 2% of the treatment time rendered by dentists.

The dental-caries experience of children and the progression of the disease in adults provided the rationale for the application of dental public-health programs to address the problem. The efforts, cooperation, and interactions of a number of individuals and agencies led to one such dental public-health program, the implementation of adjusted water fluoridation.

## Fluoridation—A Monumental Public-Health Success Story

Fluoridation is the principal dental public health preventive program available in the control of dental caries in the population. During a national health conference in 1966, former Surgeon General Dr. Luther L. Terry stated, "Controlled fluoridation is one of the four great mass preventive health measures of all time. The four horsemen of health are: the pasteurization of milk, the purification of water, immunization against disease, and controlled fluoridation of water."[18] The Centers for Disease Control and Prevention recently listed fluoridation among the top ten public health triumphs of the 20th century.[19]

The historic development of fluoridation in the United States serves as an example of the contributions of individuals of varied backgrounds representing personal and public segments of the profession. For example, Dr. H. Trendley Dean, considered the "father of fluoridation," had a prominent role in the early developing story of the importance of fluoride to tooth enamel.[20] Dean was an officer in the USPHS who led extensive studies that later established that 1 part per million (ppm) of fluoride in a community water supply reduced dental-caries prevalence.[21]

As important as the contributions of Dean and the USPHS were to the subsequent implementation of community fluoridation, one should not lose sight of the roles played by Dr. Frederick McKay, a personal health-care practitioner in Colorado Springs, Colorado, and Dr. G. V. Black, a practitioner and prominent dental educator. McKay and Black conducted numerous investigations of *Colorado brown stain*, a condition indicative of excessive amounts of naturally occurring fluoride ion during tooth development, and found that dental caries was less prevalent among those afflicted.[22] In addition, one should consider the influence of an industrial chemist, H. V. Churchill, who developed the analytic method that could detect minute quantities of fluoride in water, a critical step necessary to establish the link between the level of fluoride ions in water and the dental caries experience of the population consuming the water.[23] At the same time, Smith and Smith,[24] agricultural researchers, also linked

mottled enamel with water fluoride concentrations. Following these and other studies,[25] independent researchers conducted controlled trials of the effect that fluoride ion in a community water system might have on dental caries experience in children. Beginning in 1945 and proceeding through the mid-1950s, researchers added fluoride to the water systems of four test communities (Grand Rapids, Michigan; Newburgh, New York; Evanston, Illinois; and Brantford, Ontario) and observed the dental caries experience of their residents. These trials successfully demonstrated that adjusted water fluoridation, at concentrations of 1.0 to 1.2 ppm, could dramatically reduce dental caries experience in children.[26-29]

According to the most recent national data available, approximately 162 million persons, or approximately 65.8% of the total U.S. population, drink adjusted or naturally occurring fluoridated water.[30] However, this represents a nearly 4% increase since 1992. Efforts to increase the proportion of the world population drinking fluoridated water still have been thwarted, in part, because of the continuing political activities of the anti-fluoridation movement. Supporters of this movement continue to oppose adjusted fluoridation for many reasons, the vast majority of which are equivocal.[31]

Despite the efforts of opposition groups, community-water fluoridation continues to receive widespread support from both the personal and public health-care sectors. Numerous health professional organizations, consumer and advocacy groups, and the Surgeon General continue to endorse community-water fluoridation.[32-35] Adjustment of water fluoride concentrations to optimal levels is an example of a successful dental public-health program—groups working together to prevent and control oral and craniofacial diseases in the community.

## Current Problem

Burt and Eklund[36] define a *public-health problem* as meeting two criteria: a) a condition or situation that is a widespread actual or potential cause of morbidity or mortality; and b) an existing perception the condition is a public-health problem on the part of the public, government, or public health authorities. A number of oral and craniofacial diseases and conditions represent public health problems in the United States today, and are briefly discussed below. These are the principal concerns that need to be addressed by both the personal and public healthcare sectors to improve oral health at the community level.

### Dental Caries

Dental caries is one of the most prevalent diseases in the United States. About 17% of children aged 2 to 4 years have had a carious lesion in a primary tooth during their lifetime, and the prevalence jumps to 49.7% among children aged 5 to 9 years.[37] Among permanent teeth, 26.0% of children aged 5 to 11 years have had a carious lesion and 67.3% of children aged 12 to 17 years have had a carious lesion.[37] Dental caries is also highly prevalent among U.S. adults, as approximately 94% of dentate adults aged 18 years or older have had a carious lesion during their lifetime.[38]

Dental-caries prevalence and severity also is associated with race/ethnicity and socioeconomic status (Figure 17–1). Certain minority children exhibit a higher prevalence of primary tooth decay than do their peers, as 34.2% of non-Hispanic white children aged 2 to 9 years have had a carious lesion, whereas 38.8% of non-Hispanic black children and 53.0% of Mexican-American children have had a carious lesion.[37] Among adolescents aged 12 to 17 years, lower poverty status is associated with higher mean dental-caries experience scores and a greater percentage of untreated disease.[39]

### Periodontal Diseases

Gingivitis, one of the periodontal diseases, is moderately prevalent in persons aged 13 years or older. On average, 62.9% of persons in this

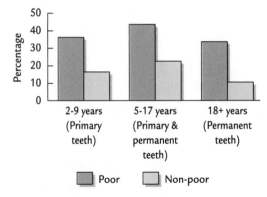

FIGURE 17-1  Disparities in prevalence of unrestored dental caries exist between poor and non-poor. (From U.S. Department of Health and Human Services. *Oral Health in America: A Report of the Surgeon General.* Bethesda, MD: U.S. Department of Health and Human Services, National Institutes of Dental and Craniofacial Research, 2000(35):63.)

age range exhibit gingival bleeding, and 12.0% of sites are involved.[40] Gingivitis, as measured by gingival bleeding, is also more prevalent among Mexican-Americans than it is among non-Hispanic blacks and non-Hispanic whites aged 30 years or older.[41] Calculus, a contributing factor in gingivitis, is present in 89.9% of persons aged 13 years or older.[40] Although most persons would not consider gingivitis a serious threat to one's health, it receives a great deal of attention in the appearance-conscious United States, given the condition's effect on esthetics and gingivitis precedes, but does not necessarily progress to periodontitis.

Periodontitis is the second of the periodontal diseases and is associated with greater morbidity than is gingivitis, and as such, is considered a more serious public-health problem. On average, 27.0% of males and 17.5% of females aged 13 years or older have at least one site with 5+mm loss of periodontal attachment.[40] This gender difference is statistically significant. The prevalence of attachment loss is also significantly higher among minority groups, as

24.9% of non-Hispanic blacks and 17.1% of non-Hispanic whites aged 13 years or older exhibit the condition.[40]

### Oral and Pharyngeal Cancer

There are approximately 30,200 cases of oral and pharyngeal cancer detected in the United States each year, and this number accounts for some 2.4% of all cancers. Of persons with oral and pharyngeal cancer, approximately 7,800 die each year. The overall 5-year survival rate for persons with oral and pharyngeal cancer is 52%, which is lower than that for cancers of the prostate, breast, bladder, larynx, cervix, colon, and rectum.[42] Persons diagnosed with oral and pharyngeal cancer at an early stage have a much better prognosis than do those diagnosed at a later stage, as the 5-year survival rate is 81.3% for early-stage diagnosis and 21.6% for advanced-stage diagnosis. Only 35% of individuals with oral and pharyngeal cancer are diagnosed at an early stage of the disease.[42]

### Craniofacial Birth Defects

Oral clefts are among the most common classes of congenital malformations in the United States. On average, there are 1.2 cases of cleft lip (with or without cleft palate) per 1,000 live births and 0.56 cases of cleft palate per 1,000 live births in the general population (Figure 17-2).[43] These defects may affect facial appearance throughout life. Cleft palate occurs more frequently in females, whereas cleft lip or cleft lip/palate occurs more frequently in males.[44-47] The oral cleft incidence rate for whites is more than 3 times the incidence rate for blacks.

### Intentional and Unintentional Injuries

It is assumed that injuries to the head, face, and teeth are relatively common, however the majority of our knowledge regarding the number of injuries comes from emergency department data and more severe injuries. The leading

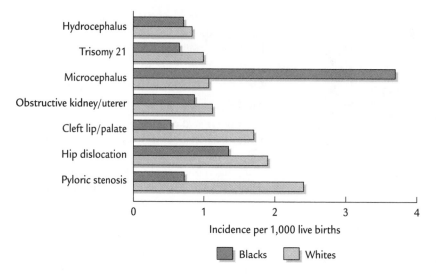

FIGURE 17–2 Incidence of selected congenital defects. (From Schulman et al., 1993.[43])

causes of such injuries include falls, assaults, sports injuries, and motor-vehicle collisions.[48–50] According to data collected in 1993 and 1994, there were approximately 20 million visits to emergency departments per year for craniofacial injuries. Falls and assaults each accounted for about 31% of visits and sports-related injuries accounted for approximately 19% of injuries.[51] Injuries resulting from bicycles and tricycles accounted for 5% of head and 19% of face injuries.[52] Overall, 24.9% of persons aged 6 to 50 years have had an injury that resulted in damage to one or more incisor teeth.[53] According to data collected in 1991, personal health-care dentists treated more than 5.9 million craniofacial injuries.[54]

## Dental Public-Health Methods

Personal oral-health-care practitioners serve the oral health needs of individual patients, and the personal health-care delivery system requires a one-on-one interaction between practitioner and individual patient. Public-health dentistry focuses on the community and, as such, does not necessarily require a one-on-one interaction between practitioner and individual patient. When a dental public-health program such as water fluoridation is successfully implemented in a community, a much broader cross section of the community benefits —much broader than could be expected by personal health-care practitioners, alone.

Knutson[55] contrasted the methods employed by personal and public healthcare practitioners. Each consisted of six, sequential steps that permit a logical progression from identification of a problem to its solution (Table 17–1). For the individual patient, a personal healthcare practitioner initiates treatment with a careful examination and history, which leads to an accurate diagnosis of the problem. Afterwards, the personal healthcare practitioner plans a course of treatment. Once treatment services have been provided, and fees paid, subsequent visits provide for evaluation and follow-up. The methods employed in public-health practice parallel those of the personal health-care practitioner, but involve the total community instead of an individual patient. Dental public-health methods are discussed in greater detail below.

TABLE 17–1 Contrast Between the Methods of Personal and Public Health Care

| Six steps of personal health care | Six steps of public health care |
| --- | --- |
| 1. Examination | 1. Survey |
| 2. Diagnosis | 2. Analysis |
| 3. Treatment planning | 3. Program planning |
| 4. Treatment | 4. Program operation |
| 5. Payment for services | 5. Financing |
| 6. Evaluation | 6. Appraisal |

(From Knutson JW. What is public health? In: *Dentistry in Public Health,* 2nd ed. Philadelphia, PA: Saunders, 1995: 20–29(55).)

Examination versus Survey

When a personal health-care practitioner begins the examination process, he or she collects subjective information from the patient and objective information, such as visual and tactile data, radiographic images, and other signs of disease. By contrast, when a public health-care practitioner assesses the extent of disease in a community, he or she must rely on descriptive information, such as existing survey data or other epidemiological assessments.

---

**Question 1**

Which of the following statements, if any, are correct?

A. As a general rule, children with the greatest oral-health treatment needs are also the children who receive priority care.

B. The overwhelming majority of Americans die with at least one carious or restored tooth.

C. The incidence of oral clefts is higher among blacks than it is among whites.

D. Core functions of public health include assessment, policy development, and assurance.

E. Dental public-health programs do not necessarily require a one-on-one interaction between practitioner and individual patient.

---

Some descriptive survey data have been collected and reported previously. At the national level, surveys such as the National Health Examination Survey, National Health and Nutrition Examination Survey, National Health Interview Survey, and surveys conducted by the National Institute of Dental and Craniofacial Research[56] have provided assessments at the community level regarding the distribution of diseases, such as dental caries and periodontitis, as well as oral health knowledge and behavioral practices. At the state level, surveys such as the Behavioral Risk Factor Surveillance System or cancer registries have provided useful descriptive information regarding oral health care utilization practices and incidence of oral and pharyngeal cancer. Selected states have also administered surveys to assess the oral-health status of their citizens (Figure 17–3).

For the dental public-health-care practitioner, the focus of the survey step is to compile all of the descriptive information that exists in a state, county, region, or local area. When descriptive data do not exist, the dental public-health-care practitioner must find a way to collect useful information. During the mid-1990s, prompted by the newly defined essential functions of public health, the Association of State and Territorial Dental Directors (ASTDD) developed a model for the collection of oral health data at state and local levels,[57] referred to as the *Seven-step Model for Assessing Oral Health Needs*. The seven steps included:

1. Identifying partners and forming an advisory committee.

2. Conducting self-assessment to determine goals and resources.

3. Planning the needs assessment.
   • Conduct inventory of available primary and secondary data

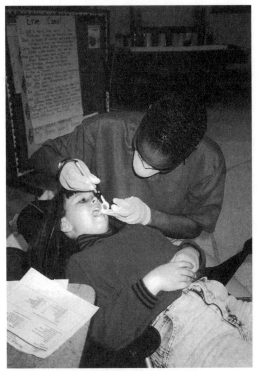

FIGURE 17-3 Surveys designed to establish the oral health needs of children frequently take place in a school setting. (Courtesy of Dr. Arthur Benito, Research Triangle Institute, North Carolina.)

- Determine need for primary data collection
- Identify resources
- Select methods
- Develop work plan
4. Collect data.
5. Organize and analyze data.
6. Report findings and utilize the data for program planning, advocacy, and education.
7. Evaluate needs assessment and return to first step, as necessary.

ASTDD intended that the collected data be used as part of a planning cycle (Figure 17–4) that would lead to the implementation of nec-

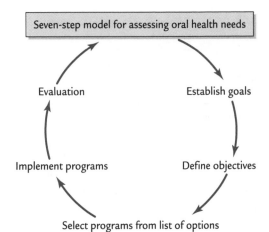

Seven-step model for assessing oral health needs

Evaluation

Establish goals

Implement programs

Define objectives

Select programs from list of options

FIGURE 17-4 Dental public-health program planning cycle.

essary dental public-health programs. Just as a personal health-care practitioner would not consider initiating treatment on a patient without subjective and objective data at hand, the public health-care practitioner would not consider initiating a dental public-health program without descriptive data regarding the needs of the community.

### Diagnosis versus Analysis

Once a personal health-care practitioner has gathered sufficient subjective and objective information from the patient, he or she uses professional judgment and experience to diagnosis a disease or condition, if one exists. Once a public health-care practitioner has collected sufficient survey data, he or she analyzes the information in order to answer specific questions. Is there a dental public health problem? If so, what is the extent of the problem? Are there appropriate solutions available to address the problem?

The analysis step helps the public health-care practitioner assess when a problem exists and helps to quantify its extent. Public health-care practitioners rely on standard statistical methods to summarize survey data findings during the analysis step. For example, state-specific

survey data may show that 45% of schoolchildren have unrestored dental caries, and that this percentage is significantly higher than would be expected at a national level. The significant difference in percentages may point to a dental public health problem in that state. In addition, survey data may show that oral and pharyngeal cancer incidence in one county is significantly higher than is the rate in a neighboring county. One would expect the first county to receive special attention or a targeted dental public health program. Without the analysis step, however, the difference between the two counties might be less obvious.

In order for a public health-care practitioner to compare analytical findings to other survey data, or transmit analytical findings to other public health-care practitioners, he or she uses standard measurement tools and descriptive guidelines, called dental indexes. A variety of dental indexes have been developed for specific oral and craniofacial diseases and conditions. Some of the more common indexes are listed below.

## Dental Indexes

An important tool used in examinations of a population group is a *dental index*, a numeric score that quantifies the magnitude of the disease measured. A number of indexes have been developed for the purpose of providing the objective measurement of the oral health status of a population group. The number of *teeth* that are decayed, missing, or filled—the DMFT index[17]—is a total score of all affected teeth and provides a dental caries experience score for an individual. A count of *tooth surfaces* that are decayed, missing, or filled is a DMFS index and provides greater precision regarding the dental caries history of an individual or population. The mean DMFT score for a population group is the total average dental caries experience at a particular time. Dental caries experience in the primary dentition is denoted by the use of *lower case letters* to represent the number of decayed, extracted, or filled primary *teeth*

and *surfaces; deft* and *defs*.[58] This index has recently been modified to *dft* and *dfs*, because of the difficulty in distinguishing a primary tooth that has been extracted from one that has been lost to the natural process of exfoliation.

The status of periodontal tissues has been evaluated using several indexes. The *Gingival Index* (GI) of Löe and Silness[59] is particularly suited for assessing changes in gingival health that might be observed during the evaluation period of an oral hygiene program. Several plaque indexes have also been developed to assess the status of oral hygiene in population groups. The *Plaque Index* (P) of Silness and Löe[60] quantifies the extent of plaque on defined areas of specific tooth surfaces. The *Oral Hygiene Index—Simplified* (OHI-S) of Greene and Vermillion[61] measures oral debris and calculus on specific tooth surfaces.

The *Periodontal Index* (PI) of Russell[62] and the *Periodontal Disease Index* (PDI) of Ramfjord[63] were once used for assessing the severity of periodontitis, but are no longer considered valid. When these indexes were developed, it was believed that gingivitis and periodontitis were on a continuum; as gingivitis became more severe, periodontitis resulted. Consequently, the PI and PDI were developed as composite indexes, assessing gingivitis and periodontitis together. Today, it is well established that gingivitis does not necessarily lead to periodontitis, and that the two diseases are unique. Although the PI and PDI are no longer used, the PDI left behind a measurement component that is valid for assessing tissue destruction. The surviving measurement component, sometimes referred to as *loss of attachment* or *LOA*, calculates the loss of periodontal attachment that has occurred adjacent to a tooth. The *Community Periodontal Index of Treatment Need* (CPITN) is not an index of periodontitis, but a measure of the necessity for periodontal treatment.[64] The CPITN has been used by nations around the world.

When public healthcare practitioners employ a dental index during the analysis step,

they must pay particular attention to the training of examiners. Consistency in the application of scoring criteria is paramount to the validity of index scores. A comparison of DMFT scores from one county to another would be of little value, for example, if the examiners in the two counties applied the scoring criteria in different ways.

### Treatment Planning versus Program Planning

Once a personal health-care practitioner has identified a disease or condition, and assessed its extent, he or she is ready to transmit the information to the patient and plan a treatment strategy. Once a public health-care practitioner has identified the existence of a dental public-health problem and assessed its extent, he or she is ready to transmit the information to concerned individuals and community partners. Together, the public health-care practitioner and partners develop a public-health program that is tailored to the needs of the community.

During the treatment planning and program planning steps, decisions must take into consideration such factors as available time, finances, knowledge, experience, attitudes, and willingness to complete the plan. Just as an individual patient must consider his or her personal circumstances when selecting treatment options, community leaders must consider community resources and priorities when selecting appropriate public health program options.

### Treatment versus Program Operation

Once the patient and personal health-care practitioner have decided on an appropriate treatment plan, treatment of the disease or condition begins. Once the community and public healthcare practitioner have decided on an appropriate program plan, the public health program is set in motion. Program operation usually includes three features, including health education, disease prevention, and provision of services.[65] Given that administrations

change, resources shift, and attitudes and motivations evolve, the program operation step is never static. Community interventions are generally more difficult to orchestrate than are plans that address an individual, because more factors must be taken into consideration at the community level.

---

### Question 2

Which of the following statements, if any, are correct?

A. *Treatment planning* requires the input of the personal healthcare practitioner and informed consent of the patient, whereas *program planning* requires the input of the public-health dentist and informed consent of involved community leaders.

B. Individual State Health Departments operate under the administrative control of the U.S. Department of Health and Human Services.

C. The *examination* step of personal health care is analogous to the *analysis* step of public health care.

D. Community-water fluoridation campaigns often fail because of political issues—not because of health department decisions.

E. The *Community Periodontal Index of Treatment Need* (CPITN) is a valid measure of periodontal tissue destruction.

---

### Payment for Services versus Financing

For the individual patient facing a treatment plan, the scope and extent of treatment services depend on personal resources and/or the existence of third-party payment plans. For the community looking forward to the initiation of a dental public-health program, the scope and extent of the program depend on the existence of available public and personal health-care funds. In most cases, public programs are

funded via the federal government or the state. Program administration and funding typically originate from state-level health departments, or county-level or local area-level health departments, when they exist.

### Evaluation versus Appraisal

When a personal health-care practitioner completes an individual patient's treatment plan, he or she evaluates the individual during periodic intervals, to assure that the oral health is maintained and any arising treatment needs are identified and met. The responsibilities of the public health-care practitioner are comparable. During the appraisal step, the public health-care practitioner first needs to assess whether the program has adequately addressed the needs of the community. As such, all public-health programs should have a measurable set of objectives against which success or failure may be appraised. If, for example, a dental public-health program were initiated to reduce the oral-cancer incidence in a county experiencing unusually high rates, then the program should contain a target incidence rate that would signify success. Once the public health-care practitioner has assessed whether an objective has been met, he or she must monitor the existence of a public health program on a regular basis. If new survey data are required, the public health-care practitioner should secure them. If the standard against which success is judged should change, the public health-care practitioner should reassess whether the program would be considered a success.

For both the personal and public health-care practitioners, the evaluation and appraisal steps represent the link between the end of a treatment plan or public-health program and the beginning of a new plan or program. As long as individual patients have treatment needs or communities have public-health problems, the six steps of the personal and public health-care practitioner can be applied.

### An Example of a Dental Public-Health Program

A *dental sealant* is a plastic material that is applied to the pit-and-fissure surfaces of the teeth by oral health-care professionals. Dental sealants function as a primary preventive agent against dental caries by obstructing the pit-and-fissure surface from bacteria. Dental sealants also may serve as a secondary preventive agent against dental caries when applied to incipient lesions. Dentists and dental hygienists apply dental sealants in private health-care facilities, however this means of providing the preventive agent is limited by access to the facilities and the personal circumstances of the patients in need.

This section of the chapter presents a dental public health problem in a fictitious community called *Yourtown* and proceeds through the six steps of the public healthcare practitioner's method, in order to illustrate how a dental sealant campaign might be employed as an effective dental public health program (Figure 17–5). Although this exercise describes a specific problem and program solution, the principles may be applied more broadly to other problems and solutions.

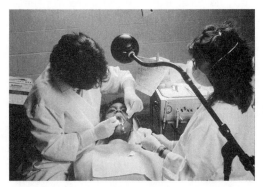

FIGURE 17–5    School-based dental sealant programs have been found to be an effective approach to reducing dental caries in pit-and-fissure tooth surfaces. (Courtesy of Ohio Division of Dental Health.)

*Survey*

The survey step of the process encompasses the seven-step model of assessing oral health needs. Dr. Sally Sealem, the county health officer in Yourtown, began the process by identifying partners and forming an advisory committee of interested parties. Dr. Sealem asked administrators from the school board to join her, as well as staff members from the health department, the director of the dental hygiene training program at Yourtown Community College, the state dental director, and the administrator of a non-profit health-care facility.

During the advisory committee's first meeting, the members discussed their resources and limitations. Dr. Sealem knew that the most cost-effective dental sealant program would involve school-aged children. The school administrators assured the health officer that a dental sealant program would be welcomed into the local schools. The administrators also said that the principals, teachers, and school nurses would be willing to coordinate communication with parents and students. Dr. Sealem also recognized that oral health-care professionals would need to participate in the program. The dental director told her that he would discuss the proposed program with the state and local dental society. He was fairly sure that the dental society would embrace the program and provide the names of a few retired practitioners who might be interested in volunteering their time to the program. The director of the training program in dental hygiene also offered the assistance of her faculty and students.

The dental director also said that there was little money in the budget for a dental sealant program. Upon hearing that the dental director's budget did not allow for a dental sealant program, the administrator of the non-profit healthcare facility said that their treatment clinic would be willing to donate some money and supplies to the program and the attendees from the health department said that they would look into the existence of grant money from private corporations, community groups, and the federal government.

Prior to the meeting, Dr. Sealem compiled demographic data for Yourtown and all of the relevant data regarding dental caries and preventive oral health programs. She discovered that the community contained approximately 10,000 school-aged children. Most of these children lived within 10 miles of their respective schools, however a few were transported via bus from neighboring rural areas. The socioeconomic status (SES) profile of the community was relatively low, with approximately 56% of children qualifying for free or reduced meals at school. Dr. Sealem also learned that Yourtown did not have access to fluoridated community water. Dr. Sealem had no data describing the dental caries prevalence or the prevalence of dental sealants in Yourtown, however she did have access to data from several national surveys.

The advisory committee recognized that survey data from Yourtown would have provided a more complete picture of the oral-health conditions in their community than the national data, but they also recognized that in order to collect such data, they would have to conduct a survey for which they had limited resources. Given the circumstances, the advisory committee ultimately decided that they would rely on the national data to draw conclusions about their community.

*Analysis*

From studies of national data,[39] Dr. Sealem knew that dental caries prevalence was higher among poor children than it was among their non-poor counterparts. She also knew that the percentage of unrestored disease was higher among the poor children. In addition, national studies showed that only 18.5% of children aged 5 to 17 years had one or more sealed teeth.[66] Given that there was a sizeable proportion of poor children in Yourtown and given that national survey data showed that poor children had greater needs, the advisory committee con-

cluded that there was good reason to initiate a dental sealant program in their community.

## Program Planning

During the program-planning stage, the advisory committee listed all of the possible ways to implement a dental-sealant program in Yourtown. Some of the options included use of a mobile dental van, visits to churches and other meeting places, expansion of services at the health department, expansion of services at the nonprofit health-care facility, and a school-based program. In deciding on the best approach, the advisory committee considered available resources and potential advantages and disadvantages of each option. Given that school administrators provided ready access to schools, and because this was where the majority of children could be found, the advisory committee decided that they would use a school-based dental-sealant program. They also decided that they would use students from the dental-hygiene training program at the community college to educate parents and teachers about the benefits of this preventive oral-health measure, and they would use the retired dentists from the community to administer the dental sealants.

In recognition of the budgetary constraints, the nonprofit health-care facility provided disposable gloves, masks, dental mirrors, and tongue blades to the program. In addition, staff members from the health department were able to procure grant funding from a local philanthropic organization and dental sealant materials from a national dental supply distributor. The advisory committee used the grant funds to purchase a portable dental chair, generator, and light source.

## Program Operation

After thorough consideration of the problem and analysis of its severity, careful planning, and procurement of funding, the school-based dental sealant program was put into operation.

In preparation for the initiation of the program, in-service training programs were conducted for all participants to affirm goals and standardize treatment protocols. The application of dental sealants to the school children progressed well, because the advisory committee had paid such careful attention during the previous stages.

## Financing

Although the advisory committee was able to solicit the necessary funds for the first year of the dental sealant program, they realized that in order for the program to have a lasting impact, they would need to procure new funding over time. The great success of the program made this step relatively easy. The advisory committee created press releases and gave them to the print media. Dr. Sealem asked the local television stations to interview her during "health spots" on the local news. The advisory committee capitalized on the popularity of the program among parents and community leaders by asking them to request additional funds from their legislative representatives for the state's health budget. Staff members at the health department wrote new grant applications and continued to solicit funds of other agencies and organizations.

## Appraisal

The advisory committee used national data to determine whether their community would be a good candidate for a dental sealant program. This approach was satisfactory for the initiation of the program, but it would not suffice during the appraisal stage. In order for the advisory committee to evaluate whether the dental sealant program had been successful in reducing dental caries experience in Yourtown, they would need new data; a baseline assessment and periodic assessments of dental-caries and dental-sealant prevalence among the school children.

The appraisal stage is arguably one of the most difficult components of a dental public

health program. It requires careful delineation of measurable goals and objectives and a detailed plan to collect evaluation data over many years. The appraisal stage must take into consideration the benefits of the program and weigh them against the cost. It must also consider alternative preventive and treatment regimens as they develop, and assess whether these new strategies might be a better option.

Enthusiasm and excitement frequently drive the first few years of a new program, however funding agencies and legislators will eventually demand that their resources are being applied to an efficient and effective program. Without a valid appraisal plan in place, the ability for an administrator such as Dr. Sealem to demonstrate efficiency and effectiveness is all but impossible.

Although this may be the most difficult component of a dental public health program, administrators have a number of resources at their disposal. Health departments typically have epidemiologists and survey researchers available for consultation. ASTDD and the Division of Oral Health at the Centers for Disease Control and Prevention also have consultants available.

## Levels of Dental Public Health Operation

There are numerous international and national organizations that have as a primary or secondary focus, the prevention and control of oral and craniofacial diseases at the community level. At the international level, the World Health Organization (WHO) has accepted the responsibility of coordinating the efforts of all member organizations in developing and improving oral and medical health programs throughout the world. WHO has several regional offices located throughout the world that aid in administering programs on a local level.

Based in Washington, D.C., the Pan American Health Organization (PAHO) is one such regional office for the Americas. Member States of PAHO include all 35 countries in the Americas and Puerto Rico is an Associate Member. France, the Netherlands, and the United Kingdom of Great Britain and Northern Ireland are Participating States, and Portugal and Spain are Observer States. The mission of PAHO is to strengthen national and local health systems and improve the health of the peoples of the Americas. It works in collaboration with Ministries of Health, other government and international agencies, nongovernmental organizations, universities, social security agencies, community groups, and many others. PAHO targets the most vulnerable groups, including mothers and children, workers, the poor, the elderly, and refugees and displaced persons. It focuses on access issues and a Pan-American approach, encouraging nations to work collaboratively on common issues.

The World Dental Federation (FDI) is an independent, professional organization for dentistry. The activities of the FDI cover all aspects of personal and public oral healthcare and take place all over the world. Among its varied responsibilities, FDI contributes to the development and dissemination of statements regarding policies, standards, and information related to oral health care. In addressing this responsibility, FDI produces the statements via its Scientific Commission or in collaboration with other professional organization throughout the world.

At the national level, the U.S. Department of Health and Human Services (DHHS) is the Cabinet-level branch of the federal government that is responsible for the planning and implementation of a broad array of health programs, from support for and protection of Americans of all ages, to aid for persons with disabilities, as well as assistance and new opportunities for those in need. In short, DHHS is responsible for public health in the United States, supporting the world's largest medical research effort, assuring the safety of foods and health care products, and fighting the ravages

of drug and alcohol abuse. Planning begins in Washington, D.C., with objectives evolving as health needs shift. For example, at one time there was a need to finance new dental and medical schools to increase the output of health professionals; more recently there has been a need for specifically focused programs to accelerate development of control measures for either caries or periodontal disease, and continually there are efforts to refine programs offering better access to, or less cost for, medical and oral healthcare. DHHS responsibilities in the United States are divided into 10 geographic regions (I to X), each one having a central office. These offices facilitate administration by providing consultation and monitoring expertise for regional and local health programs involving federal funds.

DHHS oversees 12 major organizations, each with a different influence over public health issues and dental public health programs (Figure 17–6). The *Administration for Children and Families* (ACF) is responsible for numerous programs that provide services and assistance to needy children and families, administers the new state-federal welfare program (*Temporary Assistance to Needy Families*), administers the Head Start program, provides funds to assist low-income families in paying for child care, and supports state programs to provide for foster-care and adoption assistance. The *Health Resources and Services Administration* (HRSA) helps provide health resources for medically underserved populations, supports a nationwide network of community and migrant health centers and primary care programs for the homeless and residents of public housing, works to build the health-care workforce, maintains the National Health Service Corps, works to improve child health, and provides services to persons with AIDS through the Ryan White CARE Act programs. The *Agency for Healthcare Research and Quality* (AHRQ) supports investigator-initiated research designed to improve the outcomes and quality of health care, reduce its costs, address patient safety and medical errors, and broadens

access to effective services. The *Centers for Disease Control and Prevention* (CDC) administer a health surveillance system designed to monitor and prevent outbreaks of disease. It also guards against international disease transmission, maintains national-health statistics and provides for immunization services and supports research into disease and injury prevention. The CDC's Division of Oral Health maintains and reports on national and local oral-health surveillance data, consults with states and local health departments regarding oral-health assessments and survey techniques, administers the Water Fluoridation Reporting System, and publishes policy statements regarding control of infection. The *Agency for Toxic Substances and Disease Registry* (ATSDR) works with states and other federal agencies to prevent exposure to hazardous substances from waste sites. The Substance Abuse and Mental Health Services Administration (SAMSHA) strives to improve the quality and availability of substance abuse prevention, addiction treatment, and mental health services. The *Administration on Aging* (AoA) provides and supports ombudsman services for elderly, and provides policy leadership on aging issues. The *Food and Drug Administration* (FDA) assures the safety of foods and cosmetics, and the safety and efficacy of pharmaceuticals, biological products, and medical devices, including those used in personal oral health care settings and dental public health programs. The *Centers for Medicare and Medicaid Services* (CMS), formerly *Health Care Financing Administration* (HCFA), serves the needs of Medicaid and Medicare beneficiaries. The *Indian Health Service* (IHS) oversees and supports a network of hospitals, health centers, school-based health centers, health stations, and urban Indian health centers that provide services to nearly 1.5 million Native Americans and Alaska Natives. The *National Institutes of Health* (NIH), the world's premier medical research organization, supports research projects nationwide in diseases like heart ailments, diabetes, cancer, HIV, Alzheimer's Disease, and

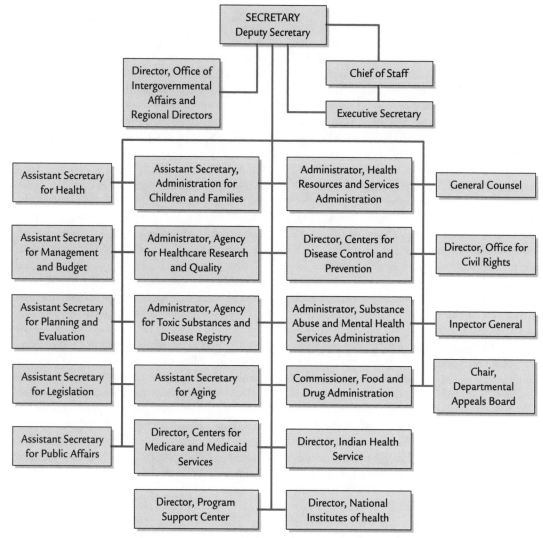

FIGURE 17-6    Organizational chart for the U.S. Department of Health and Human Services.

asthma. The *National Institute for Dental and Craniofacial Research* (NIDCR), one of the NIH institutes, supports intramural and extramural research regarding dental caries, periodontitis, oral and pharyngeal cancer, facial clefts, oral health disparities, and preventive oral health therapies. The *Program Support Center* (PSC) provides, for a fee, solution- and customer-oriented support for administrative operations, financial management and human resources

throughout DHHS, as well as other departments and federal agencies.

The USPHS encompasses the Commissioned Corps, the uniformed service of the DHHS. Dental officers in the Commissioned Corps serve the oral health treatment needs of Native Americans and Alaska Natives as part of the IHS; active duty members, dependents, and retirees of the U.S. Coast Guard; and persons incarcerated under the Federal Bureau of

Prisons. The Surgeon General leads the Commissioned Corps of the USPHS.

Each state has a health department that may or may not include an oral-health division. Of those states with an oral health focus, many divide their jurisdictional operation into regions to better administer and monitor state-administered oral-health programs. The regional programs include operation of clinics for needy populations, state prison systems, and in some cases, school systems. Consultations with communities desiring to establish or to improve community oral health, public health education programs, and fluoride initiatives receive major emphasis.

Within each state, populous counties and cities may administer community oral health treatment clinics through local health departments. These clinics usually operate in schools, economically underprivileged areas, or among population subgroups that do not otherwise have access to routine personal oral-health care. Federal, state, and local tax funds are intermixed in the delivery of care at all levels.

## Dental Public Health Programs

### Health Promotion and Health Education

Health promotion and health education are integral components of most successful dental public-health programs (Table 17–2). *Health promotion* consists of any planned combination of educational, political, regulatory, and organizational supports for actions and conditions conducive to the health of a community or group of individuals in a defined geographic location (67). Projects designed to be administered in schools, such as fluoride mouthrinse programs and dental-sealant programs, have been particularly successful, because dental caries is prevalent in children and those with the greatest needs may reside with parents/guardians who are otherwise unable to provide for their treatment needs in personal

TABLE 17-2  **Dental Public Health Program Strategies for Primary Prevention of Selected Public-Health Problems**

Dental Caries

1. Community-wide health promotion interventions, including educational, political, regulatory, and organizational

2. Fluoride use
   - Community water fluoridation
   - School-based dietary fluoride tablets
   - School-based fluoride mouthrinse

3. School-based screening and referral

Oral and Pharyngeal Cancers

1. Community-wide health promotion interventions, including educational, political, regulatory, and organizational

2. Cancer examination programs

Craniofacial Birth Defects

1. Early detection programs

Intentional and Unintentional Injuries

1. Community-wide health promotion interventions, including educational, political, regulatory, and organizational

2. Mouth protector fittings for athletic events

From U.S. Department of Health and Human Services. *Oral Health in America: A Report of the Surgeon General.* Bethesda, MD: U.S. Department of Health and Human Services, National Institutes of Dental and Craniofacial Research, 2000(35):156.

healthcare facilities. School-based health care programs are discussed elsewhere in this textbook. Health-promotion activities do not require active participation of its recipients, however. Public sanitation measures, for example, promote health among humans around the world, yet most of these persons enjoy the benefits without action or awareness. Consequently, health-promotion activities are vitally important to dental public-health programs, because they do not usually depend on recipient awareness or cooperation for success.

**Question 3**

Which of the following statements, if any, are correct?

A. The American Dental Association is under the auspices of the World Health Organization.

B. The health policies of the U.S. Department of Health and Human Services are administrated from the 10 Regional Offices of the Centers for Disease Control and Prevention.

C. Approximately 144 million persons in the United States drink fluoridated water.

D. Health promotion frequently yields more immediate effects on the public than does education of the public.

E. The Surgeon General's Report on Oral Health in America, released in 2000, was one of many such reports dedicated to dentistry.

*Health education* includes any combination of learning experiences designed to enable the voluntary adoption of behaviors or actions that are conducive to health and healthful living (Figure 17–7).[68] Whereas health-promotion activities do not require the active participation of its recipients, health education does. For this reason, dental public-health programs that rely heavily on health education are subject to the attitudes, beliefs, and other motivating factors of the recipients. In addition, although knowledge is an important element of empowerment, knowledge does not guarantee that appropriate actions or behavioral changes will follow.[69] Health-promotion activities in dental public health programs frequently include health-education components, but health-education, alone, is not sufficient to prevent oral diseases or conditions.

### Community-Water Fluoridation

Community-water fluoridation, or the addition of appropriate concentrations of fluoride com-

pounds into water systems to prevent dental caries, is a health promotion activity within a dental public health program. As beneficial as water fluoridation is in the battle against dental caries, the addition of fluoride to water is not an automatic condition, however, and frequently requires the savvy and careful coordination of dental public-health professionals, water engineers, legislators, and organized dentistry. In order to conduct a successful fluoridation campaign, one must understand political realities and recognize available resources in the community that can be used to assist in securing a favorable outcome.[70] Successful campaigns require dedicated and enthusiastic persons who are coordinated by an individual with good political skills. Support from all segments of the population, not just health professionals, is crucial. The best method to achieve fluoridation in a small community is through city council action if state laws do not require a referendum. Endorsements offered by strategic role models, such as a mayor, city council member, or other community leaders, play an important role in the process.

Coordination of activities is also important once a water fluoridation program has been initiated. Studies show that water distribution centers frequently maintain aqueous fluoride

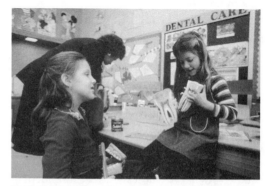

FIGURE 17–7   Classroom dental-education programs are important, but it is critical to evaluate their effect. (Courtesy of the National Institute of Dental and Craniofacial Research.)

concentrations that are lower than recommended levels.[71] In order to combat this reality, authority should rest with an administrator who is dedicated to the dental public health program and who is in a position to manage the system. Frequently, the dental director of the state health department is an ideal choice for the administrative position. When a dental director is unavailable, dental public health professionals should assign a person who has the responsibility of water fluoridation surveillance and management.

## Special Population Groups

Selected dental public-health programs include projects that focus on particular population subgroups. Certain groups, for example, because of health status, position in society, attitudinal barriers, or geographic location, do not have ready access to personal healthcare providers and must receive care in special clinics, supported by public or private funds. The oral health care needs of these groups, which include Native Americans and Alaska Natives, long-term-care populations, migrant groups, medically compromised individuals, beneficiaries of the Department of Veterans Affairs, persons with developmental disabilities, homeless individuals, the elderly, and persons with low socioeconomic status, are usually significantly greater than they are for the general population.[56,72–85] For example, medically compromised individuals and persons with Acquired Immunodeficiency Syndrome (AIDS) are frequently predisposed to rapidly progressing periodontitis and other oral problems.[86,87] Alzheimer's disease and other dementias compromise the ability of many older persons to take care of their mouths.[88, 89]

The abilities and limited experience levels of some personal oral health-care professionals, as well as the conditions within which they work may stand in the way of effective provision of care for some of these special population groups.[90–92] For example, routine treatment facilities are frequently inaccessible to a person who is homebound because of physical or mental disabilities or limitations. Dentists and auxiliaries, trained in the use of mobile treatment equipment and management of the disabled patient, are necessary in order to provide oral-health care to the homebound.[93] In this example, the removal of barriers to care is an example of an effective dental public-health program.

Dental public-health professionals in public-health agencies, local or state health departments, and academic institutions are called upon to provide consultation or initiate programs for individuals with particular diseases or conditions. Examples may include educational programs aimed toward mothers and designed to address feeding behaviors leading to early childhood caries, programs designed to produce mouth guards for high school athletes, programs designed to assess the function of removable prostheses in a geriatric population, programs designed to provide fluoride therapy to cancer patients undergoing head and neck radiation, programs designed to screen low-income children for oral diseases, or programs designed to provide information regarding oral and pharyngeal cancer prevention.

## New Strategies Needed

### Changing Disease Patterns

During the early 1900s, acute infectious diseases were more prevalent than they are today and accounted for greater morbidity and higher mortality among the general population. During the 1950s and 1960s, with the advent of immunizations and antibiotics, public health professionals began to shift their attention to chronic diseases, such as heart ailments, cancer, strokes, and diabetes. Dental public health programs have had to adapt to changing disease prevalence, as well.

One of the truly significant developments in dental public health has been the decline in dental-caries prevalence during the past 15 years.[56, 94–102] Reduced susceptibility to dental

caries, particularly among children and young adults, is altering the oral-health status of the population. NIH estimated that the United States saved approximately $100 billion in dental expenditures during the 1980s as a result of this improvement in oral health.[103] The change in dental-caries prevalence represents a major success for personal oral health preventive and treatment services and dental public health programs, but it also presents new challenges to the profession.

During the early-1900s, dental caries was highly prevalent across age groups and population sub-groups. Everyone required treatment services.[104] Today, as a result of effective prevention and improved treatment regimens, dental caries is concentrated in a substantially smaller proportion of the population. The challenge to dental public-health professionals is to concentrate on identifying high-risk individuals and expanding services for those who have not had access to care. Current trends to decrease spending for public programs as well as reduce health-care costs should favor preventive programs that are targeted to those who have higher unmet levels of oral disease.[105–106]

## Changing Public-Health Practices

Dental public-health programs should be organized to meet the needs of the population. As needs change, dental public health efforts should evolve to address these changing needs.[107] An accepted characteristic of a profession is that it shall be willing to respond to changing needs as a result of its own successful preventive and treatment activities.[108] Concern over the current ability of the public-health profession to adapt to change is addressed in an Institute of Medicine report, entitled *The Future of Public Health*.[109] The report contends that public health in the United States is disorganized, splintered, and unprepared to accommodate and address future challenges. The report goes on to state that the means to maintain and expand public health

programs and meet the demands of a changing environment is via assessment, policy development, and assurance.

Contrary to the report's recommendations, political and economic forces in the United States have served to reduce or discontinue many dental public health programs. The decline of dental public health programs at the national, state and local levels is, in part, a result of the perception that oral health is not a major concern.[110] Neighborhood, rural, migrant, and homeless health centers have suffered severe cutbacks in federal outlays for oral health care services, personnel, and scope of programs.[110] Public-health dentistry curricula in many schools of public health are experiencing major reductions or dissolution. Many community-dentistry programs in dental schools are only modest in scope, relative to the concentration of resources devoted to these programs when first initiated.

Why has the downsizing of dental public-health programs progressed with relatively few challenges? One answer may be the lack of an organized constituency or advocacy group for dental public-health issues. A partnership between the public and personal health-care dental sectors is essential if oral health concerns are to be effectively promoted. Often the aims of professional groups within dentistry tend to be compartmentalized and narrowly defined. Public dental programs may also be seen as competitive with personal healthcare practitioners. Preventive approaches are apt to be erroneously classified as public sector or personal healthcare sector programs. Yet the efforts of both should reinforce common goals. Fluoridation, for example, may be seen as an effective public health measure but the promotion of fluoride dentifrices may not be. Yet they complement each other and both are public-health measures.[111]

Cooperation between dental public-health organizations, such as, the American Association of Public Health Dentistry (AAPHD), the American Public Health Association (APHA)

Oral Health Section, and the American Dental Association (ADA) could help resolve the differing perspectives of the personal healthcare and public sectors. Cooperation could also foster an influential alliance in local and national campaigns addressing dental public health issues. Collaboration with a multitude of national and local voluntary non-dental health and educational organizations, such as, the Children's Defense Fund, American Association of Retired Persons, or the National Health Education Coalition is equally important to promote oral health as essential to overall health and to integrate oral health issues within the health, educational, and policy directives of these organizations. By working together on certain broad-based popular issues (i.e. access to health services), these separate partnerships can evolve into a coalition, such as the National Oral Health Alliance that can be recruited to actively support specific oral health issues.

In 1998, 53.8 billion dollars were spent on oral health care services, representing about 4.7% of the total health expenditures budget for that year.[112] Expenditures for oral health care services increased between 1997 and 1998 at approximately the same rate as expenditures for medical health care (5.3 versus 5.6%). Although these figures suggest that oral health-care services were adequately funded, comparisons with funding levels from earlier decades paint a different picture. In 1960, for example, 2 billion dollars were spent on oral health-care services, but this represented 7.3% of the total budget.[35] With reductions in funds to support oral health-care services, public-health program administrators will have to become more opportunistic and adaptive in order to conduct effective programs.

Other advocacy measures that can be pursued in support of dental public-health programs may be advanced through regulatory and legislative routes. An area of activity often entered with some reluctance is the political arena. Those in dental public-health programs

characteristically go about their duties quietly, content to live within the constraints imposed by citizens who, for example, vote against fluoridation. Niessen believes that there are community regulatory roles for dental public health regarding compliance with fluoridation and infection control standards.[113] If successful, efforts to educate and persuade others of the importance of these issues could pay big dividends. The preventive benefit provided to a community by initiating and/or monitoring fluoridation or a practice act that addresses infection control may be greater than the benefit attained from a lifetime of practice by a dozen dentists.

Successful public-health workers need to be opinion leaders and community decision makers regarding oral health programs and services. Gaupp expands this notion when stating that, "It is opportune for the oral health interest groups to strike out on their own by working toward a national, comprehensive, oral health bill."[114] Resource development could also be expedited if dental public-health programs attained influence in the regulatory and legislative arenas.

### National Oral-Health Objectives

The USPHS recognizes that an effective means to expand advocacy and regulatory activities and generate support for oral-health programs is via the setting of measurable and achievable, national health objectives. In 1980, the federal government established a program, entitled *Promoting Health/Preventing Disease: Objectives for the Nation, 1990*,[115] to identify and monitor a variety of health objectives, including 12 that addressed oral health and fluoridation. Although this program provided an early opportunity to promote oral health alongside other national health priorities, it did not adequately address the means by which states and localities could meet the objectives. Subsequent national-health objectives for 2000[116] built upon the previous framework, by providing strategies that would be helpful in meeting the new ob-

jectives. Toward that end, the USPHS outlined twenty-nine measurable oral health objectives and indicators in another document, entitled *Healthy Communities 2000: Model Standards*,[117] and called for periodic reports[118–200] and consortia[121] to promote the national health objectives for 2000.

In 2000, the USPHS released national health objectives for 2010, which included an oral health focus area[122] (Table 17–3). These oral health objectives differed from previous ones, in that they incorporated a "better than the best" standard for setting goals, as opposed to setting disparate goals for certain population sub-groups. For example, the best value attained for any single population subgroup in 2000 was used to determine the goal for all population sub-groups in 2010. The rationale

---

**TABLE 17-3  National Oral Health Objectives for 2010**

1  Reduce the proportion of children and adolescents who have dental caries experience in their primary and permanent teeth

2  Reduce the proportion of children, adolescents, and adults with untreated dental decay

3  Increase the proportion of adults who have never had a permanent tooth extracted because of dental caries or periodontal disease

4  Reduce the proportion of older adults who have had all their natural teeth extracted

5  Reduce periodontal diseases

6  Increase the proportion of oral and pharyngeal cancers detected at the earliest stages

7  Increase the proportion of adults who, in the past 12 months, report having had an examination to detect oral and pharyngeal cancers

8  Increase the proportion of children who have received dental sealants on their molar teeth

9  Increase the proportion of the U.S. population served by community water systems with optimally fluoridated water

10  Increase the proportion of children and adults who use the oral health care system each year

11  Increase the proportion of long-term care residents who use the oral health care system each year

12  Increase the proportion of low-income children and adolescents who receive any preventive dental service during the past year

13*  Increase the proportion of school-based health centers with an oral health component

14  Increase the proportion of local health departments and community-based health centers, including community, migrant, and homeless health centers, that have an oral health component

15  Increase the number of States and the District of Columbia that have a system for recording and referring infants and children with cleft lips, cleft palates, and other craniofacial anomalies to craniofacial anomaly rehabilitative teams

16  Increase the number of States and the District of Columbia that have an oral and craniofacial health surveillance system

17*  Increase the number of Tribal, State (including the District of Columbia), and local health agencies that serve jurisdictions of 250,000 or more persons that have in place an effective public dental health program directed by a dental professional with public health training

---

*Objective in development or to be reassessed
*(From U.S. Department of Health and Human Services. Healthy People 2010. 2nd ed. With Understanding and Improving Health and Objectives for Improving Health. 2 vols, Washington, DC: Government Printing Office, 2000(122).)*

behind this standard-setting method was to establish a single high goal for all groups, rather than to perpetuate disparities over time.

### Special Populations

During the last two decades, the United States has experienced an increase in the number of special population groups, including persons in long-term care,[74] medically compromised individuals,[78] and the homeless.[81,82] Higher unmet needs in these special population groups has been hampered by limited financial resources at the federal and state levels. The proportion of older persons in the population has also increased[123] and will continue to increase, as the "baby-boom" generation ages. The increased oral health care needs of older Americans could have dramatic effects on the oral health-care delivery system[5,124–126] and the ability to meet the national health objectives for 2010 if personal and public health-care programs are not developed to address the demand.

Limited access to oral health-care services for the special population groups also could affect the ability to meet the national-health objectives for 2010. Only a small proportion of the special population groups have personal dental-insurance coverage, and oral health-care benefits via public programs has not kept pace with changing demands.[127,128] Medicaid expenditures for oral health-care services have decreased by almost 30% since 1987, far more than any other health-care service.[112,129] In 1998, Medicaid expenditures for oral health care represented only 1.3% of the total Medicaid expenditures budget.[112]

### Other Trends Affecting Oral Health

Other trends could influence the attainment of national-health objectives, including advances in technology, personnel requirements, and professional education. Advances in implant materials, restorative methods, chemotherapeutic agents, genetics, and the identification of risk markers for disease,[130] for example, should affect personal and public healthcare

delivery systems well into the future. Advances in computer technology should lead to developments in all areas of biomedical research, innovative ways to manage and retrieve data, and the provision of health care services.

Human resources are a critical factor in any dental public health program. Changes in the distribution of oral health-care personnel certainly could impact meeting the national health objectives for 2010. Recent data have suggested that the number of dentists will decline during the next 15 to 20 years,[131] however the prediction models used to determine "appropriate" levels of personnel frequently have suffered from a lack of data and generally have been unable to account for epidemiological, social, economic, and political variability over time.[132] Consequently, whether the nation as a whole faces an undersupply of oral health care professionals remains unclear, however, unless actions are taken to address the lack of personal and public healthcare professionals in designated "dental health manpower shortage areas,"[133] it is fairly certain that these parts of the country will find it difficult meeting the national-health objectives.

The professional educational curricula is evolving continuously, as a result of budgetary constraints and redistributions in enrollment, distributions of disease, treatment and health-care delivery systems, information transfer, and demographics. Changes in the curricula generally require additional interdisciplinary research, preventive modalities, and community-based initiatives.[134]

### Emerging Public Concerns

Public and professional reactions to perceived risks in the oral health care delivery system affect treatment modalities, service utilization, and ultimately oral health status. Well publicized reports of individuals contracting a number of conditions from fluoride, and amalgam restorations have prompted the dental research community to review the risks associated with the use of these fundamental components of

dental prevention and treatment.[135,136] Of even greater threat to the practice of dentistry and the recruitment of future dental personnel is the fear of contracting an HIV infection/AIDS in the dental office by both health-care providers and patients.[137,138] While dental public-health professionals have been at the forefront in ensuring access for patients infected with the AIDS virus, many dental practitioners are still reluctant to treat known AIDS patients. On the other hand, the revelation of the probable occupational transmission of the AIDS virus from a dentist to five of his patients has generated a high level of concern and anxiety about receiving dental care among the public.[138–140]

Dental public-health activities have been directed at preventing transmission of infectious diseases in the dental office by requiring dentists to comply with recommended ADA and CDC infection control guidelines and the Occupational Safety and Health Administration (OSHA) Bloodborne Pathogens Standard. However, implementation of these edicts is already dramatically changing the scope and cost of delivering oral health-care services in personal and public health-care settings.[141–143]

## Surgeon General's Report

In 1997, Donna Shalala, then Secretary of DHHS, commissioned the Office of the Surgeon General to create a report to, "Define, describe, and evaluate the interactions between oral health and general health and well-being (quality of life), through the life span, in the context of changes in society."[144] During the next three years, under the direction of the National Institute of Dental and Craniofacial Research, Project Director Dr. Caswell A. Evans supervised an impressive list of contributing authors and content experts. On May 25, 2000, at Shepherd Elementary School in Washington, D.C., Assistant Secretary for Health and Surgeon General, David Satcher, released *Oral Health in America: A Report of the Surgeon General,*[35] the first-ever Surgeon General's report exclusively dedicated to oral health issues. In his presentation to the Nation that day, Surgeon General Satcher summarized key themes of the report: 1) oral health means much more than healthy teeth, 2) oral health is integral to general health, 3) safe and effective disease prevention measures exist that everyone can adopt to improve oral health and prevent disease, and 4) general health-risk factors, such as tobacco use and poor dietary practices, also affect oral and craniofacial health.

The Surgeon General's Report was divided into five parts, each relating to a particular question. Part One asked *what is oral health,* Part Two asked *what is the status of oral health in America,* Part Three asked *what is the relation between oral health and general health and well-being,* Part Four asked *how is oral health promoted and maintained* and *how are oral diseases prevented,* and Part Five asked *what are the needs and opportunities to enhance oral health.* In answering these questions, the Surgeon General's Report listed several findings that reflected the four principal themes:

- Oral diseases and disorders, in and of themselves, affect health and well-being throughout life.
- Safe and effective measures exist to prevent the most common dental diseases—dental caries and periodontal diseases.
- Lifestyle behaviors that affect general health such as tobacco use, excessive alcohol use, and poor dietary choices affect oral and craniofacial health, as well.
- There are profound and consequential oral health disparities within the U.S. population.
- Additional information is needed to improve America's oral health and eliminate health disparities.
- The mouth reflects general health and well-being.

- Oral diseases and conditions are associated with other health problems.
- Scientific research is key to further reduction in the burden of diseases and disorders that affect the face, mouth, and teeth.

The Surgeon General's Report summarized dramatic changes in oral health issues during the last century, and it also brought to light some serious challenges for the future. It stated that, although oral health has improved in the United States, disparities in health still exist. Specific population groups, such as infants and young children, the poor, those residing in rural locations, the homeless, persons with disabilities, racial and ethnic minorities, the institutionalized, and the frail elderly, continue to experience a greater burden of oral and craniofacial diseases. The Surgeon General's Report also stated that there were great disparities in access to oral health care and utilization of preventive services, each crucial to the establishment and maintenance of optimal oral and general health. Finally, the report recognized that there were insufficient data to describe the population subgroups in greatest need for oral health-care services and dental public-health programs. The lack of data will make the development of relevant and effective dental public health programs a more difficult task.

By publishing the Surgeon General's Report, the Office of the Surgeon General has made available important and timely information to health-care practitioners, public-health professionals, policy makers, and the public. For access to the report, the Office of the Surgeon General provides an electronic version of the document and offers a free hardcopy of the report to all who request one.

## SUMMARY

The core functions of public health include assessment, policy development, and assurance. These functions are also essential components of dental public health, which is defined as the science and art of preventing and controlling dental diseases and promoting health through organized community efforts. It follows, then, that dental public-health programs are any organized efforts that strive to prevent and control oral and craniofacial diseases at the community level.

Dental disease has been a significant problem for Americans since the nation's early history. Arguably, one of the most successful dental public health programs ever created to address these problems has been community water fluoridation. As successful as fluoridation has been, however, new dental public-health programs need to be developed to meet the needs of population subgroups who have suffered from higher burdens of disease and have had poorer access to timely preventive and treatment services. The Surgeon General's Report on Oral Health in America highlighted some of these concerns and placed them in the context of existing programs and political realities. In addition, the federal government recognized that one way to address some of the oral health disparities that exist is to establish realistic national health objectives for 2010.

The initiation and implementation of any dental public-health program follows an established planning cycle, the first stage of which involves assessing the oral-health needs of the community. Once a problem is tentatively identified, it is addressed

through the use of six sequential steps of the public healthcare practitioner's method—survey, analysis, program planning, program operation, financing, and appraisal. ASTDD established a seven-step model for needs assessment which functions well during the first step.

When traditional dental public-health programs prove ineffective, they must be replaced by more cost-effective approaches. The combination of less disease, more effective use of personnel, and improved technology and preventive methods, particularly dental sealants, provides opportunities to create dental public-health programs for those who have been traditionally neglected. In order to fulfill these opportunities, however, a constituency of public and personal dental and non-dental advocacy groups is required.

Dental public-health programs play a critical role in the promotion and maintenance of oral health in America. The challenge for dental public-health practitioners is to devise programs that are effective, yet incorporate the principles of sound planning and implementation. The oral health of the public depends on it.

## ANSWERS AND EXPLANATIONS

1. B, D, and E—correct.

   A—incorrect. Children with the greatest treatment needs are usually at the bottom of the economic scale and have fewer resources available. Until access to care for these children is improved, they will continue to be in great need of oral-health treatment services.

   C—incorrect. In the United States, the incidence of oral clefts is three times higher among whites than it is among blacks.

2. A and D—correct.

   B—incorrect. The State Health Departments are under the administrative control of State government. There is often cooperation between the U.S. Department of Health and Human Services and State Health Departments, however, because many health programs are financed by the federal government.

   C—incorrect. The *examination* step of personal-health care is analogous to the *survey* step of public-health care.

   E—incorrect. The CPITN is a valid measure of treatment need. A valid measure of tissue destruction is an assessment of loss of periodontal attachment (LOA).

3. C and D—correct.

   A—incorrect. The American Dental Association is not under the auspices of the World Health Organization, however it is a member of the World Dental Federation (FDI).

   B—incorrect. The ten Regional Offices are of the U.S. Department of Health and Human Services, not the CDC.

   E—incorrect. The Surgeon General's Report on Oral Health in America was the first ever report of its kind.

## Self-Evaluation Questions

1. The core functions of public health include _____, _____, and _____.

2. By definition, dental public-health programs are _____.

3. According to 1998 estimates, approximately $_____ was spent on oral health-care services in the United States.

4. *DMFS* represents decayed, missing, and filled tooth surfaces, whereas, _____ represents a caries experience index for primary teeth.

5. By definition, a public-health problem is one that meets the following criteria: _____ and _____.

6. The following are comparative methods used in personal and public healthcare practice:

| Six steps of personal-health care | Six steps of public-health care |
|---|---|
| Examination | Survey |
| _____ | _____ |
| Treatment planning | Program planning |
| Treatment | _____ |
| Payment for services | Financing |
| _____ | Appraisal |

7. Two dental public-health program strategies for primary prevention of oral and pharyngeal cancer are: _____ and _____.

8. List three national oral health objectives for 2010: _____, _____, and _____.

9. List the four principle themes of the Surgeon General's Report on Oral Health: _____, _____, _____, and _____.

10. Health promotion consists of any: _____.

# REFERENCES

1. Harrell, J. A., & Baker, E. L. (2001). American Public Health Association Essential Services Workgroup. *The Essential Services of Public Health.* American Public Health Association web page [http://www.apha.org/ppp/science/10ES.htm#monitor]; accessed October 1, 2001.
2. Institute of Medicine (1988). *The Future of Public Health.* Washington, DC: National Academy Press.
3. American Dental Association Commission on Dental Accreditation (1988). Accreditation standards for advanced specialty education programs in dental public health. Typescript.
4. Cons, N. C. (1979). Using effective strategies to implement a program administrator's goal. *J Public Health Dent,* 39:279–85.

5. Graves, R. C. (1982). Aspects of the practical significance of current public health methods for the prevention of caries and periodontal disease. *J Public Health Dent*, 42:179–89.

6. Klein, H. (1941). The dental status and dental needs of young adult males, rejectable or acceptable for military service, according to selective service dental requirements. *Public Health Rep*, 56:1369–87.

7. Lewis, J. R. (1865). Exemptions from military service on account of loss of teeth. *Dent Cosmos*, 7:240–42.

8. Britton, R. H., & Perrott, G. J. (1941). Summary of physical findings on men drafted in World War I. *Public Health Rep*, 56:41–62.

9. Hollander, F., & Dunning, J. M. (1939). A study by age and sex of the incidence of dental caries in over 12,000 persons. *J Dent Res*, 18:43–60.

10. Fulton, J. T., Hughes, J. T., & Mercer, C. V. (1965). *The natural history of dental diseases*. Chapel Hill, NC: University of North Carolina School of Public Health, 80.

11. Moen, B. D. (1953). Survey of needs for dental care II: dental needs according to age and sex of patients. *J Am Dent Assoc*, 46:200–11.

12. Pelton, W. J., Pennell, E. H., & Druzina, A. (1954). Tooth morbidity experience of adults. *J Am Dent Assoc*, 49:439–45.

13. U.S. Department of Health, Education and Welfare (1979). National Center for Health Statistics. *Basic data on dental examination findings of persons 1–74 years: United States, 1971–1974*. DHEW Pub. No. (PHS) 79-1662, Series 11, No. 214. Washington, DC: U.S. Government Printing Office.

14. U.S. Department of Health, Education and Welfare (1979). National Center for Health Statistics. *Decayed, missing, and filled teeth among children, United States*. DHEW Pub. No. (HSM) 72-1003, Series 11, No. 106. Washington, DC: U.S. Government Printing Office.

15. U.S. Department of Health, Education and Welfare (1974). National Center for Health Statistics. *Decayed, missing, and filled teeth among youths 12–17 years, United States*. Pub. No. (HSM) 75-1626, Series 11, No. 144. Washington, DC: U.S. Government Printing Office.

16. Messner, C. T., Gafafer, W. M., Cady F. C., & Dean, H. T. (1936). Dental survey of school children, ages six to fourteen years, made in 1933–1934 in twenty-six states. *Public Health Bull*, 226.

17. Klein, H., Palmer, C. E., & Knutson, J. W. (1938). Studies on dental caries. I. Dental status and dental needs of elementary school children. *Public Health Rep*, 53:751–65.

18. Ast, D. B. (1983). Response to receiving the John W. Knutson distinguished service award in dental public health. *J Public Health Dent*, 43:101–5.

19. U.S. Department of Health and Human Services (1999). Centers for Disease Control and Prevention. National Center for Chronic Disease Prevention and Health Promotion. Division of Oral Health. Achievements in public health, 1900–1999: fluoridation of drinking water to prevent dental caries. *MMWR Morb Mortal Wkly Rep*, 48:933–40.

20. Russell, A. L. (1969). Epidemiology and the rational bases of dental public health and dental practice. In *The dentist, his practice and his community* (pp. 35–62). Philadelphia: Saunders.

21. Dean, H. T. (1938). Endemic fluorosis and its relation to dental caries. *Public Health Rep*, 53:1443–52.

22. McKay, F. S., & Black, G. V. (1916). An investigation of mottled teeth. *Dent Cosmos*, 58:477–84.

23. Churchill, H. V. (1932). The occurrence of fluorides in some waters of the United States. *J Dent Res*, 12:141–59.

24. Smith, H., & Smith, M. C. (July 1932). Mottled enamel in Arizona and its correlation with the concentrations of fluorides in water supplies. University of Arizona, College of Agriculture Experimental Station. *Tech Bull*, 43.

25. Dean, H. T., Arnold, F. A. Jr., & Elvove, E. (1942). Domestic water and dental caries. V. Additional studies of the relation of fluoride domestic waters to dental caries experience in 4,425 white children aged 12–14 years of 13 cities in 4 states. *Public Health Rep*, 57:1155–79.

26. Dean, H. T., Arnold, F. A. Jr., Jay, P., & Knutson, J. W. (1950). Studies on mass control of dental caries through fluoridation of the public water supply. *Public Health Rep*, 65:1403–8.

27. Ast, D. B., Finn, S. B., & McCaffrey, I. (1950). The Newburgh-Kingston caries-fluorine study. I. Dental findings after three years of water fluoridation. *Am J Public Health*, 40:716–24.

28. Blayney, J. R., & Tucker, W. H. (1948). The Evanston dental caries study. *J Dent Res*, 27:279–86.

29. Hutton, W. L., Linscott, B. W., & Williams, D. B. (1951). The Brantford fluorine experiment. Interim report after five years of water fluoridation. *Can J Public Health*, 42:81–87.

30. Centers for Disease Control and Prevention. (Feb. 2002). Populations receiving optimally fluorinated public drinking water—United States, 2000. *MMWR Morbidity and Mortality Weekly Report*, 51(07):144–47.

31. Easley, M. W. (1985). The new antifluoridationists: who are they and how do they operate. *J Public Health Dent*, 45:133–41.

32. Holt, R. D. (2001). Advances in dental public health. *Primary Dent Care*, 8:99–102.

33. Clarkson, J. J., & McLoughlin, J. (2000). Role of fluoride in oral health promotion. *Int Dent J*, 50:119–28.

34. Anonymous (2000). Position of the American Dietetic Association: the impact of fluoride on health. *J Am Dietetic Assoc*, 100:1208–13.

35. U.S. Department of Health and Human Services (2000). Oral Health in America: A Report of the Surgeon General. Bethesda, MD: U.S. Department of Health and Human Services, National Institute of Dental and Craniofacial Research.

36. Burt, B. A., & Eklund, S. A. (1999). The practice of dental public health. In Burt, B. A., & Eklund, S. A. *Dentistry, Dental Practice, and the Community* (5th ed.) Philadelphia: W.B. Saunders Co. pp. 34–42.

37. Kaste, L. M., Selwitz, R. H., Oldakowski, R. J., Brunelle, J. A., Winn, D. M., & Brown, L. J. (1996). Coronal caries in the primary and permanent dentition of children and adolescents 1–17 years of age: United States, 1988–1991. *J Dent Res*, 75(Spec Iss):631–41.

38. Ries, L. A. G., Eisner, M. P., Kosary, C. L., Hankey, B. F., Miller, B. A., Clegg, L., Edwards, B. K., Eds. (2002). *SEER Cancer Statistics Review, 1973–1999*. National Cancer Institute, Bethesda, MD. http://seer.cancer.gov/csr/1973-1999/.

39. Vargas, C. M., Crall, J. J., & Schneider, D. A. (1998). Sociodemographic distribution of dental caries: NHANES III: 1988–1994. *J Am Dent Assoc*, 129:1229–38.

40. Brown, L. J., Brunelle, J. A., & Kingman, A. (1996). Periodontal status in the United States, 1988–1991: prevalence extent, and demographic variation. *J Dent Res*, 75(Spec Iss):672–81.

41. Albandar, J. M., Brunelle, J. A., & Kingman, A. (1999). Destructive periodontal disease in adults 30 years of age or older in the United States, 1988–1994. *J Periodontol*, 70:13–29.

42. Ries, L. A., Kosary, C. L., Hankey, B. F., et al. (1999). *SEER cancer statistics review, 1973–1996*. Bethesda, MD: National Cancer Institute.

43. Schulman, J., Edmonds, L. D., McClearn, A. B., Jensvold, N., & Shaw, G. M. (1993). Surveillance for and comparison of birth defect prevalences in two geographic areas—United States, 1983–88. *MMWR CDC Survell Summ*. 42:1–7.

44. Burman, N. T. (1985). A case-control study of oro-facial clefts in Western Australia. *Aust Dent J*, 30:423–9.

45. Fraser, G. R., & Calnan, J. S. (1961). Cleft lip and palate: seasonal incidence, birth weight, sex, site, associated malformations and parental age. A statistical survey. *Arch Dis Childhood*, 36:420–3.

46. Habib, Z. (1978). Factors determining occurrence of cleft lip and palate. *Surg Gynecol Obstet*, 146:105–10.

47. Owens, J. R., Jones, J. W., & Harris, F. (1985). Epidemiology of facial clefting. *Arch Dis Child*, 60:521–4.

48. De Wet, F. A. (1981). The prevention of orofacial sports injuries in the adolescent. *Int Dent J*, 31:313–9.

49. Pinkham, J. R., & Kohn, D. W. (1991). Epidemiology and prediction of sports-related traumatic injuries. *Dent Clin North Am*, 35:609–26.

50. Sane, J. (1988). Comparison of maxillofacial and dental injuries in four contact team sports: American football, bandy, basketball, and handball. *Am J Sports Med*, 16:647–51.

51. McDonald, A. K. (1994). *The National Electronic Injury Surveillance System: A Tool for Researchers*. Washington, DC: U.S. Consumer Product Safety Commission.

52. U.S. Consumer Product Safety Commission (1987). *Tricycles. Reporting Hospitals and Estimates Reports, 1982–1986*. Washington, DC: National Electronic Surveillance System, U.S. Consumer Product Safety Commission.

53. Kaste, L. M., Gift, H. C., Bhat, M., et al. (1996). Prevalence of incisor trauma in persons 6 to 50 years of age: United States, 1988–1991. *J Dent Res*, 75(Spec Iss):696–705.

54. Gift, H. C., & Bhat, M. (1993). Dental visits for orofacial injury: defining the dentist's role. *J Am Dent Assoc*, 124:92–6,98.

55. Knutson, J. W. (1955). What is public health? In *Dentistry in public health* (2nd ed.) (pp. 20–29). Philadelphia: Saunders.

56. U.S. Department of Health and Human Services (1989). National Institutes of Health. National Institute of Dental Research. *Oral health of United States Children: The National Survey of Dental Caries in U.S. School Children, 1986-1987*. DHHS Pub. No. (NIH) 89-2247. Bethesda, MD: U.S. Government Printing Office.

57. Siegal, M. D., & Kuthy, R. A. (1995). *Assessing oral health needs. ASTDD Seven-step Model*. Jefferson City, MO: Association of State and Territorial Dental Directors.

58. Gruebbel, A. O. (1944). A measurement of dental caries prevalence and treatment service for deciduous teeth. *J Dent Res*, 23:163–68.

59. Löe, H., & Silness J. (1963). Periodontal disease in pregnancy. I. Prevalence and severity. *Acta Odont Scand*, 21:533–51.

60. Silness, J, & Löe H. (1964). Periodontal disease in pregnancy. II. Correlation between oral hygiene and periodontal condition. *Acta Odont Scand*, 22:112–35.

61. Greene, J. C., & Vermillion, J. R. (1964). The simplified oral hygiene index. *J Am Dent Assoc*, 68:25–31.

62. Russell, A. L. (1956). A system of classification and scoring for prevalence surveys of periodontal disease. *J Dent Res*, 35:350–59.

63. Ramfjord, S. P. (1959). Indexes for prevalence and incidence of periodontal disease. *J Periodont*, 30:51–59.

64. World Health Organization (1984). Community Periodontal Index of Treatment Needs, development, field testing, and statistical evaluation. Geneva, Switzerland: Oral Health Unit, World Health Organization.

65. Kuthy, R. A., & Odom, J. G. (1988). Local dental programs: a descriptive assessment of funding and activities. *J Public Health Dent*, 48:36–42.

66. Selwitz, R. H., Winn, D. M., Kingman, A., & Zion, G. R. (1996). The prevalence of dental sealants in the US population: findings from NHANES III, 1988–1994. *J Dent Res*, 75(Spec Iss):652–60.

67. Frazier, P. J., & Horowitz, A. M. (1995). Prevention: A public health perspective. In Cohen, L. K., & Gift, H. C., Eds. *Disease prevention and oral health promotion*. Copenhagen: Munksgaard. pp. 109–52.

68. Green, L. W., & Johnson, K. W. (1983). Health education and health promotion. In Mechanic, D., Ed. *Handbook of health, healthcare and the health professions*. New York: Wiley. pp. 744–65.

69. Kay, E. J., & Locker, D. (1996). Is dental health education effective? A systematic review of current evidence. *Community Dent Oral Epidemiol*, 24:231–5.

70. Faine, R. C., Collins, J. J., Daniel, J. (1981). Isman, B., Boriskin, J., Young, K. L., & Fitzgerald, C. M. The 1980 fluoridation campaigns: a discussion of results. *J Public Health Dent*, 41:138–42.

71. Bronstein, E. (1979). Letters to the editor: Fluoridation monitoring. *J Public Health Dent*, 39:248.

72. National Institute of Dental Research (1987). The oral health of United States adults: the national survey of oral health in U.S. employed adults and seniors, 1986–1986. U.S. Department of Health and Human Services, National Institutes of Health. DHHS Pub. No. (NIH) 87-2868. Bethesda, MD: U.S. Government Printing Office.

73. Kaste, L. M., Marianos, D., & Chang, R., et al. (1992). The assessment of nursing caries and its relationship to high caries in the permanent dentition. *J Public Health Dent*, 52:64–68.

74. American Dental Association (1982). Oral health status of Vermont nursing home residents. Council on Dental Health and Health Planning, Bureau of Economic and Behavioral Research. *J Am Dent Assoc*, 104:68–69.

75. Gift, H. C., Cherry-Peppers, G., & Oldakowski, R. J. (1997). Oral health status and related behaviours of U.S. nursing home residents, 1995. *Gerodontology*, 14(2):89–99.

76. Woolfolk, M., Hamard, M., & Bagramian, R. A. (1984). Oral health of children of migrant farm workers in northwest Michigan. *J Pub Health Dent*, 44:101–5.

77. Entwistle, B. A., & Swanson, T. M. (1989). Dental needs and perceptions of adult Hispanic migrant farmworkers in Colorado. *J Dent Hyg*, 63:286–89.

78. Little, J. W., & Falace, D. A., Miller, C. S., & Rhodus, N. L. (2002). *Dental management of the medically compromised patient*. St. Louis: CV Mosby.

79. Niessen, L., & Dunleavy, H. A. (1984). Meeting the oral health needs of the aging veteran. In Wetle, T., & Rowe, J. W., Eds. *Older veterans: Linking VA and community resources*. (pp. 369–407). Cambridge, MA: Harvard University Press.

80. U.S. Department of Health and Human Services (1980). *Special Report: Dental Care for Handicapped People*. DHHS Pub. No.(PHS) 81-50154. Washington, DC: U.S. Government Printing Office.

81. Gelberg, L., Linn, L. S., & Rosenberg, D. J. (1988). Dental health of homeless adults. *Spec Care Dent*, 8:167–72.

82. Gibson, G., Rosenheck, R., Tullner, J. B., Grimes, R. M., Seibyl, C. L., Rivera-Torres, A., Goodman, H. S., & Nunn, M. E. (2003). A national survey of the oral health status of homeless veterans. *J Public Health Dent*, 63(1):30–7.

83. Beck, J. D. (1988). Trends in oral disease and health. *Gerondontol*, 7:21–25.

84. Beck, J. D., & Hunt, R. J. (1985). Oral health status in the United States: problems of special patients. *J Dent Educ*, 49:407–25.

85. Klein, S. P., Bohannon, H. M., Bell, R. M., et al. (1985). The cost and effectiveness of school-based preventive dental care. *Am J Public Health*, 75:382–91.

86. U.S. Department of Health and Human Services (1986). National Institutes of Health. *Detection and Prevention of Periodontal Disease in Diabetes*. NIH Pub. No. 86-1148. Bethesda, MD: U.S. Government Printing Office.

87. Patton, L. L., Phelan, J. A., Ramos-Gomez, E. J., Nittayananta, W., Shiboski, C. H., & Mbuguye, T. L. (2002). Prevalence and classification of HIV-associated oral lesions. *Oral Dis*, 8 Suppl 2:98–109.

88. Kocaelli, H., Yaltirik, M., Yargic, L. I., & Ozbas, H. (2002). Alzheimer's disease and dental management. *Oral Surg Oral Med Oral Pathol Oral Radiol Endod*, 93(5):521–4.

89. Ship, J. A. (1992). Oral health of patients with Alzheimer's disease. *J Am Dent Assoc*, 123:53–58.11

90. Antczak, A. A., Branch, L. G. (1985). Perceived barriers to the use of dental services by the elderly. *Gerodontics*, 1:194–98.

91. Gilbert, G. H. (1989). "Ageism" in dental care delivery. *J Am Dent Assoc*, 118:545–48.

92. Cohen, L. A., & Grace, E. G. (1990). Infection control practices related to treatment of AIDS patients. *J Dent Pract Admin*, 7:108–15.

93. Strayer, M. S. (1995). Perceived barriers to oral health care among the homebound. *Spec Care Dentist*, 15(3):113–8.

94. Brunelle, J. A., & Carlos, J. P. (March 1989). Recent trends in dental caries in U.S. children and the effect of water fluoridation. International Fluoride Symposium, Pine Mountain, Georgia.

95. Bell, R. M., Klein, S. P., Bohannan, H. B., et al. (1984). *Treatment Effects in the National Preventive Dentistry Demonstration Program*. Santa Monica, CA: Rand; R-3072-RWJ.

96. Bohannnon, H. M., & Bader, J. D. (1984). Future impact of public health and preventive methods on the incidence of dental caries. *J Can Dent Assoc*, 50:229–33.

97. Brunelle, J. A., & Carlos, J. P. (1982). Changes in the prevalence of dental caries in U.S. schoolchildren: 1961–1980. *J Dent Res*, 61:1346–51.

98. Bryan, E. T., Collier, D. R., Howard, W. R., & Van Cleave, M. L. (1982). Dental health status of school children in Tennessee—a 25-year comparison. *J Tenn State Dent Assoc*, 62:31–33.

99. DePaola, P. F. (1983). The Massachusetts health survey. *J Mass Dent Soc*, 32(1):10–1, 23–5.

100. Glass, R. L. (1981). Secular changes in caries prevalence in two Massachusetts towns. *Caries Res*, 15:445–50.

101. Hughes, J. T., Rozier, R. G., & Ramsey, D. L. (1980). *The Natural History of Dental Disease in North Carolina, 1976–77*. Durham, NC: Academic Press.

102. Burt, B. A. (1985). The future of the caries decline. *J Public Health Dent*, 45:261–69.

103. Beazoglou, T., Brown, J., & Heffley, D. (1993). Dental care utilization over time. *Soc Sci Med*, 37:1461–72.

104. Friedman, J. W. (1977). A consumer advocate's view of community dentistry. *J Dent Educ*, 41:656–59.

105. Federation Dentaire Internationale (1988). Technical Report No. 31. Review of methods of identification of high caries risk groups and individuals. *Int Dent J*, 38:177–89.

106. Stamm, J. S., Disney, J. A., Graves, R. C., et al. (1988). The University of North Carolina caries risk assessment study. I. Rationale and content. *J Public Health Dent*, 48:225–32.

107. Galagan, D. J. (1976). Some comments on the future of dental public health. *J Public Health Dent*, 36:96–102.

108. Dunning, J. M. (1979). Guest editorial: the stone wall. *J Public Health Dent*, 39:175–76.

109. Institutes of Medicine (1988). The future of public health. Washington, DC: National Academy Press.

110. Milgrom, P., & Reisine, S. (2000). Oral health in the United States: the post-fluoride generation. *Ann Rev Public Health*, 21:403–36.

111. Glass, R. L. (1980). The use of fluoride dentifrices: a public health measure. *Community Dent Oral Epidemiol*, 8:278–82.

112. Health Care Financing Administration (2000). *National Health Expenditures 1998*. Washington, DC: Health Care Financing Administration.

113. Niessen, L. C. (1990). New directions-constituencies and responsibilities. *J Public Health Dent*, (Spec Iss);50:133–38.

114. Gaupp, P. G. (1990). New initiatives for advocacy in national maternal and child oral health. *J Public Health Dent*, (Spec Iss);50:396–401.

115. U.S. Department of Health and Human Services (1980). *Promoting Health/Preventing Disease: Objectives for the Nation*. Washington, DC: Public Health Service, 54.

116. U.S. Department of Health and Human Services (1991). *Healthy People 2000: National Health Promotion and Disease Prevention Objectives*, Washington, DC: U.S. Department of Health and Human Services.

117. American Public Health Association (1991). *Healthy Communities 2000: Model Standards*. Washington, DC: American Public Health Association.

118. U.S. Department of Health and Human Services (1992). *Healthy People 2000: Public Health Service Action*. Washington, DC: Government Printing Office.

119. U.S. Department of Health and Human Services. (1992). *Healthy People 2000: State Action*. Washington, DC: Government Printing Office.

120. U.S. Department of Health and Human Services. (1992). *Healthy People 2000: Consortium Action*. Washington, DC: Government Printing Office.

121. American Fund for Dental Health. (1992). *Proceeding of the National Consortium Meeting: Oral Health 2000*. Chicago, IL: American Fund for Dental Health.

122. U.S. Department of Health and Human Services. (2000). *Healthy People 2010* (2nd ed.) *With understanding and improving health and objectives for improving health*, 2 vols. Washington, DC: Government Printing Office.

123. U.S. Department of Health and Human Services. (2002). *A profile of older Americans: 2001*. Washington, DC: Administration on Aging.

124. Burt, B. A. (1982). New priorities in prevention of oral disease. *J Public Health Dent*. 42:170–79.

125. Hand, J. S., Hunt, R. J., & Beck, J. D. (1988). Incidence of coronal and root caries in an older adult population. *J Public Health Dent*, 48:14–19.

126. Stamm, J. W., Banting, D. W., lmrey, P. B. (1990). Adult root caries survey of two similar communities with contrasting natural water fluoride levels. *J Am Dent Assoc*, 120:143–49.

127. U.S. Department of Health and Human Services (1996). Office of Inspector General. *Children's Dental Services Under Medicaid. Access and Utilization*. Washington, DC: Office of Inspector General.

128. U.S. General Accounting Office. (2000). *Oral health: Dental disease is a chronic problem among low-income populations*. Washington, DC: U.S. Accounting Office.

129. Agency for Health Care Policy and Research (1992). National Medical Expenditure Survey: *Annual Expenses and Sources of Payment for Health Care Services*. Rockville, MD: Agency for Health Care Policy and Research.

130. Löe, H. & Drury, T. F. (1990). Future NIDR Initiatives in Risk Assessment. *In:* Bader J, Ed. *Proceedings of the Conference on Risk Assessment in Dentistry*, June 2–3 1989. Chapel Hill, NC: University of North Carolina Dental Ecology, 315–6.

131. U.S Department of Health and Human Services. (Sept 1992). Health Resources and Services Administration. *Health Personnel in the United States: Eighth Report to Congress, 1991*. DHHS Pub. No. HRS-P-OD-92-1.

132. Goodman, H. S., & Weyant, R. J. (1990). Dental health personnel planning: a review of the literature. *J Public Health Dent*, 50:48–63.

133. Interim Study Group on Dental Activities (1989). *Improving the Oral Health of the American People: Opportunity for Action*. Washington, DC: U.S. Department of Health and Human Services.

134. Machen, J. B. (1989). Education and dental environment: the future for dental schools. *J Am Coll Dent*, 56:33,42–44.

135. U.S. Department of Health and Human Services (1991). Review of fluoride benefits and risks. Public Health Service. Washington, DC: Department of Health and Human Services.

136. National Institutes of Health. (Aug 26–28, 1991). Technology assessment conference statement: effects and side effects of dental restorative materials. Department of Health and Human Services.

137. Cohen, L. A., Grace, E. G., & Ward, M. A. (1992). Maryland residents' attitudes towards AIDS and the use of dental services. *J Public Health Dent*, 52:81–85.

138. McCarthy, G. M., Koval, J. J., & MacDonald, J. K. (1999). Factors associated with refusal to treat HIV-infected patients: the results of a national survey of dentists in Canada. *Am J Public Health*, 89(4):541–5.

139. Ciesielski, C., Marianos, D., Ou, C-Y, Dumbaugh, R., Witte, J., Berkleman, R., Gooch, B., Myers, G., Luo, C. C., & Schochetman, G. (1992). Transmission of Human Immunodeficiency Virus in a dental practice. *Ann Int Med*, May 15;116:798–805.

140. Barnes, D. B., Gerbert, B., McMaster, J. R., & Greenblatt, R. M. (1996). Self-disclosure experience of people with HIV infection in dedicated and mainstreamed dental facilities. *J Public Health Dent*, 56(4):223–5.

141. American Dental Association (1992). Infection control recommendations for the dental office and the dental laboratory. Council on Dental Materials, Instruments, and Equipment; Council on Dental Therapeutics; Council on Dental Research; Council on Dental Practice. *J Am Dent Assoc* (Suppl);123:1–8.

142. Centers for Disease Control (1986). Recommended infection control practices for dentistry. *MMWR*, 35:237–42.

143. U.S. Department of Labor, Occupational Safety and Health Administration (1991). Occupational exposure to bloodborne pathogens, Title 29 CFR 1910.1030. *Fed Reg* Dec 6;56:64004–64182.

144. Evans, C. A., & Kleinman, D. V. (2000). The surgeon general's report on oral health in America: opportunities for the dental profession. *J Am Dent Assoc*, 131:1721–8.

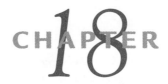

# CHAPTER 18

# Preventive Oral Health in Early Childhood

*Stephen J. Goepferd*
*Franklin García-Godoy*

## OBJECTIVES

*At the end of this chapter, it will be possible to*

1. Understand the rationale for professional preventive dental intervention for infants and toddlers.
2. Explain the type and process of early infant caries.
3. Provide appropriate recommendations for infant feeding that minimize the child's risks for developing *early-childhood caries* (formerly called "nursing caries").
4. Explain why it is so important that the mother and other members of the immediate family have a very high level of oral health, and especially a low *Streptococcus mutans* count from before birth until a mature, nonpathologic plaque is established in the infant.
5. Describe the six major areas to discuss with parents during the interview process.
6. Provide appropriate counseling on feeding/diet management, tooth cleaning, and fluoride management for parents of infants and toddlers.
7. Describe the timing, location, positioning, and steps for examining infants and toddlers.
8. Provide a rationale for determining the frequency of recall examinations.
9. Describe the process of anticipatory guidance and the age-specific information to be discussed during the dental visit.

# INTRODUCTION

*The dental profession possesses the knowledge and technology to assist parents in raising children free of dental disease.* Dentistry's goal is to help infants and toddlers avoid the pain and devastation that accompanies early childhood caries (formerly called "nursing caries"), provide them with a pleasant, nonthreatening introduction to dentistry, and to establish and reinforce the foundation of preventive dental habits. Although this potential exists, *the preventive process must begin early in infancy* (birth to 1 year of age),[1] to ensure a successful outcome.

As health professionals, it is necessary to identify the potential for the development of disease, and institute effective measures for preventing the initiation of the disease; it is then a sound and logical practice *to intervene prior* to the onset of the disease, rather than treat the effects of the disease. Examples exist in pediatric medicine with *"well-baby"* evaluations and immunization programs. Pediatricians recommend that the infant be evaluated five times during the first year, and three times during the second year of life. Although these visits are aimed at evaluating development, prevention, or early detection of disease, physicians are not trained to provide a thorough dental evaluation or proper preventive dental health counseling. *It is the dental profession that must be proactive and assume the responsibility.*

## Prenatal Considerations

In the short period after the diagnosis of pregnancy, an expectant mother is exposed to a barrage of information applicable to her health and that of her unborn child. Dentistry should be included in this routine. At the time of the dental counseling session, a knowledgeable dental professional should be the source of the essential information.

Dental counseling should come early, since the first trimester of pregnancy is a critical time. All organ systems are forming during this period. Tooth buds begin formation at the fourth to fifth week of gestation followed by the initial mineralization of bones and teeth from the ninth to twelfth week. Stress experienced by the unborn child at this time can produce dento-oral deformities. For example, a cleft lip or palate results when the maxillae fail to unite between the fourth to sixth weeks. These changes can result from a variety of etiologic factors affecting the mother such as genetics, stress of an injury, severe virus infection, alcohol toxicity, or smoking. An excessive stress to the fetus at any critical time in development can result in a temporary but often irreparable arrest in cellular growth.

Proper nutrition during pregnancy is essential. Although nutritional deficiencies in the mother usually must be severe to affect the unborn child, a daily balanced diet provides the necessary proteins, fats, carbohydrates, vitamins, and minerals. This requirement can usually be met by the adequate intake of the *four basic food groups*, although the obstetrician may desire to prescribe nutritional supplements. Bones of the maternal system form a large mineral reserve for use by the developing child.

*All* obstetric services should develop a positive referral system to assure that expectant mothers receive an early dental examination, preventive dentistry counseling for themselves and the future child, as well as necessary treatment. The referral may be to a private practice, a hospital dental service, or to a public-health facility.

If available, the mother-to-be should be encouraged to seek a flexible dental program where prevention, monitoring, and therapy is commensurate with the severity of the dental condition. Many women who become pregnant are already long overdue for treatment, and to postpone needed care for nine more months could cause severe oral problems. Dental radiographs for emergencies may be necessary, but *should be avoided whenever possible during the first trimester.* If radiographs *are necessary, careful gonadal and abdominal shielding* is required as with all dental patients. All dental treatment should be completed by the end of the second trimester, since the position of the baby by the third trimester affects the woman's posture, making long dental appointments quite uncomfortable.[2] Once the treatment is completed, the attending dentist should supply *feedback to the obstetrician,* indicating completion of the primary, secondary, and tertiary preventive dentistry treatment plans.

This emphasis on excellent maternal oral health is required for three reasons: (1) to reduce the possibility of onset and/or progression of caries and periodontal disease throughout the pregnancy; (2) because of the personal involvement of the mother with dental treatment, prevention, and counseling, there is a greater possibility of better care for the expected child; and (3) to *reduce the number of cariogenic organisms in the mother's mouth.*

## Dental Caries—An Infectious Disease

Evidence suggests that *dental caries is an infectious disease* process initiated via the transmission of S. *mutans* from parents to their infants.[3–5] The specific plaque hypothesis suggests microbial specificity in dental caries, and longitudinal evidence supports the role of S. *mutans* in caries initiation.[6,7] The following characteristics of S. *mutans* are important relative to dental caries in children.

- Permanent S. *mutans* colonization of the oral cavity in infants occurs only after the eruption of teeth.[8]
- S. *mutans* has difficulty colonizing in an oral cavity already colonized by mature oral flora.[9]
- Sucrose facilitates the adherence of S. *mutans* to the tooth surface.[10,11]
- The source of infection of the infant with S. *mutans* is from within the family, most likely the mother.[3–5,12–14]
- A minimum threshold level of maternal S. *mutans* is necessary for transmission of the microorganism to the infant.[12–14]

Transmission of S. *mutans* to the infant most likely occurs *during the first year of life, after the eruption of teeth.*[12–15] If the infant has a high sucrose diet in the presence of S. *mutans* the conditions are favorable for the initiation of caries. *The early establishment of oral hygiene measures and the adoption of a low cariogenic diet and low-risk feeding patterns should begin in infancy.*

With the above bulleted points as a backdrop, it is possible to develop the guidelines that minimize the possibility of transmittal of a cariogenic flora from the members of the family that will be most closely associated with the child. The most important goal is to reduce the bacterial challenge to the point that the *potential for transmission of S. mutans is minimal.* For the mother especially, this will require the continual maintenance of a high level of oral hy-

---

## Question 1

Which of the following statements, if any, are correct?

A. Dental counseling should be initiated in the first trimester of pregnancy.

B. Proper nutrition during pregnancy is not essential for the infant's oral health.

C. Mothers-to-be should seek a flexible dental program.

D. Dental radiographs should be avoided during the first trimester of pregnancy.

giene. Preferably, such a program should commence no later than the sixth month of pregnancy and continue throughout the time of the eruption of teeth and onward until a mature, stable, nonpathogenic plaque has been established (very low *S. mutans* count) on the child's erupted primary teeth.[15] Such a program includes appropriately spaced professional visits for prophylaxis, bacterial counts, and monitoring oral health. For the mother, the manual and chemical plaque control procedures may include, in addition to the toothbrush, irrigation devices and use of such antiplaque rinses as chlorhexidine, which can specifically target *S. mutans*. For the child, the most important procedure from time of birth would be a restriction of cariogenic foods, and oral hygiene attention, such as discussed later in this chapter.

## Question 2

Which of the following statements, if any, are correct?

A. Caries is an infectious disease transmitted to the infant mainly by the mother.

B. The most important bacteria associated with caries initiation is *Streptococcus mutans*.

C. *Streptococcus mutans* colonization occurs immediately after the child is born.

D. Sucrose facilitates the adherence of *Streptococcus mutans* to the tooth surface.

E. *Streptococcus mutans* can colonize any tooth with a mature plaque.

## The Mother-at-Risk

A pregnant woman is often at considerable risk of caries development. The mother's teeth do not lose calcium as postulated in a number of myths; instead, the risk of dental caries probably increases because of changes in eating habits. For example, the sucking of hard candy to reduce nausea, dietary cravings, and frequent between-meal snacks of refined carbohydrates can raise the caries potential of the dental plaque. In addition, the mother often *experiences* nausea or "morning sickness," causing vomiting with a regurgitation of stomach acid which may cause *erosion* and *demineralization* of the lingual surfaces of the teeth. Many times, only a toothbrush or a sudsy dentifrice is needed to trigger a gag reflex.

Avoidance of aberrant eating habits and snacking, and exercise of sugar discipline can greatly minimize the possibility of caries development. If the mother is living in a nonfluoridated area, fluoride supplements should be considered. There are few reports available that indicate a decrease in caries prevalence of children born to mothers taking fluoride.[16–18] Since the supplement brings the level of fluoride intake to one part per million—a level ingested daily by over 100 million other Americans—there is no danger of excessive intake by the mother. There is the *possibility* of some benefit to the child. In addition, the expectant mother should be provided with appropriate treatment and recall appointments during the period of pregnancy. Professionally applied topical fluorides and systemic fluoride supplementation can benefit from the additional daily home use of fluoride dentifrices and mouth rinses. These measures will both prevent demineralization of the teeth, as well as facilitate remineralization in the event of the development of an incipient lesion.

## Question 3

Which of the following statements, if any, are correct?

A. During pregnancy, the mother's teeth lose calcium.

B. If the pregnant woman lives in a nonfluoridated area, fluoride supplements should be considered.

C. The ideal amount of fluoride in water should range from 0.7 to 1 part per million.

D. Fluoride ingestion by the pregnant woman offers the possibility of some benefit to the child.

E. The use of fluorides both by mother and child prevents demineralization and facilitates remineralization of the teeth.

## Rationale for Early Preventive Intervention

### Early Childhood Caries

Dental caries can and does occur in infants and toddlers *well before 3 years of age*. Early infant caries has been observed in children as young as *12 months of age*.[19–21]

One of the first major hazards to the child's primary dentition is early childhood caries. This condition has also been referred to as "nursing caries," nursing bottle caries, *nursing bottle mouth, baby-bottle syndrome, baby-bottle tooth decay* (BBTD), and *bottle-mouth caries*. The caries pattern of this condition is highlighted by *rampant* dental caries *initially* involving the maxillary primary incisors,[6] and progressing to the first primary molars in later stages[22–25,27] (Figure 18–1). It is caused by continual, prolonged exposure of the primary teeth to milk, infant formula, fruit juices, soft drinks, or other sugar/carbohydrate-containing fluids placed in the nursing bottle.

Once teeth erupt, the practice of offering a child a bottle filled with cariogenic fluid as a pacifier or at naptime or bedtime should be discouraged. Once teeth erupt and plaque accumulates, the ingestion of sugar-containing fluids *during bedtime or naptime* places the child at considerable risk for dental caries since salivary

## normal

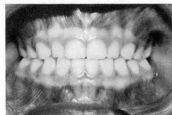

## very mild                    mild

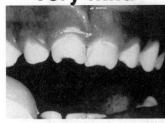
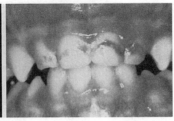

## moderate                    severe

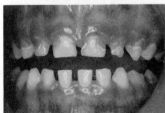
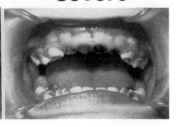

FIGURE 18–1   Different stages of early childhood caries according to García-Godoy, et al.[24,25]

flow decreases during sleep and the fluid pools around the teeth, creating a highly acidic environment. This permits the pooling of the oral fluids around the maxillary anterior teeth.[6] Not all primary teeth are equally attacked. During sucking of the nipple of either the bottle or the breast, the tongue overlies the lower incisors, which directs the sweetened liquid against the *maxillary incisors* and to the back of the palate. The mandibular incisors often are either completely intact or only slightly affected, while the maxillary incisors bear the brunt of the repeated acid attacks. The other primary teeth are involved to various degrees, depending on the suckling habits of the infant.

The caries attack begins with the appearance of white areas of demineralization around the gingival third of the teeth (see Figure 18–1). With time, these incipient lesions begin to turn brown as active caries progresses. Eventually, the carious lesions that ring the cervical areas of the teeth can result in entire crowns being lost, either by fracture of the undermined enamel or by the continuous action of the caries. In either event, only the exposed root is left in the alveolous (see Figure 18–1).

If a bottle is to be used as a pacifier, it should be filled with *water*.

Early childhood caries can also occur in some breast-fed children who are nursed every time the infant indicates a desire for feeding (demand feeding, with 10 or more nursing events over a 24-hour period).[26,27]

---

### Question 4

Which of the following statements, if any, are correct?

A. Dental caries may occur in infants and toddlers well before 3 years of age.

B. Early childhood caries is mainly due to continual, prolonged exposure of the primary teeth to milk, infant formula, fruit juices, soft drinks, or other sugar-containing fluids placed in the nursing bottle.

C. Once teeth erupt, the practice of offering a child a bottle filled with cariogenic fluid as a pacifier or at naptime or bedtime should be discouraged.

D. Early childhood caries does not occur in breast-fed children.

E. If a bottle is used as a pacifier, it should be filled with water.

---

The loss of teeth resulting from early childhood caries can have far-reaching effects on the child's eventual face growth.[18]

On occasion, there will be a pattern of multiple, severe caries in a toddler without a substantiated history of early nursing patterns that placed the infant at an increased risk. *The caries process is certainly multifactorial* and at times, a definite cause may not be identifiable. Nevertheless, sound primary preventive strategies early on will provide the appropriate environment for the prevention of dental caries.

### Disease Prevention—A Proactive Approach

As health professionals can identify the potential for the development of disease and have effective measures available for preventing the initiation of disease, it is a sound and logical practice to *intervene* prior to the onset of disease whenever possible rather than to wait and treat the effects of the disease. Examples of primary prevention exist in pediatric medicine with "well-baby" evaluations and immunization programs. Pediatricians recommend that the infant be evaluated five times during the first year and three times during the second year of life. Although these visits are aimed at evaluating development and prevention or early detection of disease, physicians are not adequately trained to provide a thorough dental evaluation or proper preventive dental health counseling. *The dental profession must be proactive and assume this responsibility.*

## Public and Professional Attitudes

Because of events such as early childhood caries, there is a *growing desire by parents* of infants and toddlers to receive an early dental evaluation and obtain information on the prevention of dental diseases in their children. According to parents, the major reasons for them seeking early dental evaluations are:

- Desire for information on preventing tooth decay for their child
- Desire to avoid unpleasant experiences that the parents had suffered
- Desire to learn what their role is in their child's oral health
- Recommended by their pediatrician or family physician.

The education process can probably best start with the obstetrician and pediatrician explaining to the expectant or new parents the cause and consequences of continued intake of sugar fluids. The physician can further aid in reducing the problem by prescribing those bottle formulae that contain the least sugar. For instance, there is a considerable range in the amount of sugar found in the various commercially available baby foods. Finally, the dental profession should emphasize the need for high school and community dental education programs to alert would-be parents of their responsibilities in dental care for their infant.

## Early Dental Care

The newborn should become accustomed to oral care early. After feeding, the ridges where the teeth will later appear and the palate should be gently wiped with gauze or a soft washcloth. This removes leftover food, and establishes a routine for the mother to clean inside the child's mouth. Children need directly supervised oral hygiene care throughout childhood. It was traditionally recommended that a child should visit the dental office no later than 2½ years of age. Ideally, the child's first dental visit should occur at 6 months of age and no later that at 1 year of age.[17] The purpose of this initial visit is to permit an evaluation of the mouth and jaws for proper formation and alignment of structures. A second objective of this visit is to allow the child to become familiar with the dental office and its personnel under pleasant circumstances and forestall future apprehension.

## Infant Oral-Health Education

According to the United Nations' Convention on "The Rights of the Child," articles 2 and 24, all children should have the same rights and have right to health and medical service.[28] Early childhood caries is a lifestyle disease with biologic, behavioral, and social determinants. An early screening of all children at around 1 year of age is an excellent opportunity for early detection of risk factors and risk indicators that may increase the possibilities for its prevention. The caries risk evaluation should form the base for appropriate recommendations of preventive measures.[28]

The American Academy of Pediatric Dentistry states: "*Infant dental care begins with dental health counseling for the newborn, which should include a dental office visit for preventive oral health counseling no later than 12 months of age.*[17] However, for those children who are delayed in erupting teeth, the first visit may be postponed, but should occur *within 6 months following the eruption of the first tooth.*"

The American Society of Dentistry for Children also recommends in *The Answer Book* that children should visit the dentist between 6 and 12 months of age.[18] Recently, a federal program called "Early and Periodic Screening, Diagnosis, and Treatment" (EPSDT), which *mandates* that medical and dental services be provided to children from low-income families, adopted the policy that children in the EPSDT program re-

ceive a dental screening by *12 months of age*. A recent survey among 54 dental schools pediatric dentistry programs showed that 86% teach students to see infants at 12 months of age or younger.[29]

One study evaluated an oral-health promotion program involving health visitors and mothers of 8-month-old babies in order to address some of the risk factors associated with nursing caries.[30] The oral-health promotion program significantly improved mothers recall of advice given by health visitors encouraging the use of a feeder cup, brushing their babies' teeth with fluoride toothpaste and restricting sugary foods and drinks. Significant improvements were also found in recall of advice regarding the use of sugar-free medicine and registering babies with a dentist. The program encouraged a higher proportion of the mothers to bring their children to clinics for a hearing check.[30]

The advantages of the infant oral-health approach are:

- Identifying and modifying detrimental feeding habits, reducing potential caries risk
- Assisting parents in establishing low caries-risk snacking and dietary patterns for their child
- Explaining and demonstrating tooth cleaning procedures for infants and toddlers
- Determining fluoride status and recommending an optimum fluoride program;
- Introducing dentistry to the child in a pleasant, nonthreatening manner
- Preparing parents for upcoming dental events for their child (anticipatory guidance).

### Question 5

Which of the following statements, if any, are correct?

A. Two major reasons for parents to seek early dental evaluations for their children are a desire for information on preventing tooth decay and a desire to learn what their role should be in their child's oral health.

B. After feeding the newborn child, the ridges where the teeth will later appear should be gently wiped with gauze or a soft washcloth.

C. The child's first dental visit should occur at 2½ years of age.

D. Some advantages of an infant oral-health approach are: identifying and modifying detrimental feeding habits and explaining and demonstrating to the parents tooth cleaning procedures for infants and toddlers.

E. The dental profession should emphasize the need for high school and community dental-education programs to alert would-be parents of their responsibilities in dental care for their infants.

## A Protocol for Early Preventive Intervention

### The Interview

The interview process and counseling session should be thorough and specific, yet concise. The attention span of the infant is limited and once the child becomes bored and seeks attention from the parent(s) their attentiveness to your discussion will be limited at best. Experience shows that the interview and preventive counseling are best accomplished *before* the examination of the infant for the following reasons:

- Specific parental concerns can be identified and addressed during the examination.
- Should the infant fuss during the examination (normal behavior) the parent(s) usually direct their attention toward the child during the ensuing discussion and not toward the dentist.

- The child can be kept busy with toys, etc., before the examination in a nonthreatening environment and the parent(s) will be better able to direct their attention toward the dentist.

The interview should begin with a discussion of the parents' reason for seeking care. Historical information gathered at the initial interview would assist the practitioner in developing the most appropriate and individualized preventive program for the family. Categories of helpful information are discussed in the following paragraphs.

1. GROWTH AND DEVELOPMENT. An abnormal pattern of development may be discovered or suspected, prompting a referral for further evaluation. Also, the date of the eruption of the first tooth will provide a baseline for determining dental development patterns and assist in answering future questions from parents regarding their child's dental development.

2. FEEDING HISTORY. Knowledge of the feeding patterns during infancy is critical to assist the dentist in assessing the child's risk for developing early childhood caries by discovering *potentially harmful feeding habits* and to help form a basis for recommendations regarding proper feeding practices that minimize the potential for dental disease.

3. MEDICAL HISTORY. A complete medical history is important. Knowledge of any systemic conditions that may adversely affect dental health will assist in developing appropriate preventive strategies. For example, long-term, frequent intake of sucrose-based medications may require additional recommendations for tooth cleaning to offset the increased caries risk from the sucrose intake.

4. PREVENTIVE ASSESSMENT. Information regarding dental development, dental health attitudes, and current oral hygiene practices will serve as a starting point for counseling

parents regarding an appropriate preventive program for their child. A history of tooth decay in the family ("soft teeth") will provide insight into the environmental influences as well as parental attitudes regarding dental health and serve to guide the dentist's discussion regarding preventive strategies.

5. FLUORIDE SUPPLEMENTATION. It is important to know if the child has access to fluoride in drinking water. It is not sufficient to establish that a family lives in a fluoridated community. On occasion, the family may drink bottled water, which contains an unknown quantity of fluoride. On the other hand, a family drinking well water may or may not be receiving systemic fluoride depending upon the concentration of fluoride in the water. Before any fluoride supplements are prescribed, the water should be tested for fluoride concentration and supplements prescribed accordingly. Some families live in rural settings with well water, but the child spends the majority of the day in a location with fluoridated water such as a day care facility or school. Therefore, an accurate assessment of all potential sources of fluoride intake should be explored before making any recommendations regarding fluoride supplementation.

If the daily intake of fluoride is insufficient, parents should be informed that small daily dosages are beneficial to a child's teeth. Appendix 18–1 will aid in determining the amount of fluoride supplementation needed. This can initially be best accomplished by the use of *fluoride drops*. Around the age of 3, the drops can be replaced by *fluoride tablets*, which are swallowed. Later, as the child gains skill in chewing the tablet, the fluoride-laden saliva can be swished around the mouth and then swallowed to provide a topical application as well as systemic benefits. The practice of using a tablet a day should continue until the child is at least 12 years old, although many believe that fluoride supplementation should be considered as long as the individual—child or adult—has a fluoride-deficient intake.

6. ORAL HYGIENE. An assessment of current tooth-cleaning activities is important to establish the parents' role in oral hygiene for their child. Many parents think that allowing an infant or toddler to brush their own teeth is adequate. If the infant's teeth are being brushed, it is important to **establish how, when, and by whom,** and inquire whether the parents experience any difficulties during the process.

In one study, almost half of the parents interviewed had started toothbrushing programs for their infants at 12 months and 75% had done so by 18 months. With such infant and toddler toothbrushing programs, only a small amount, approximately the size of a pea, of a fluoridated dentifrice should be used in order to avoid the possibility of the child ingesting an excess of fluoride. Around the age of 6, daily fluoride mouth rinses may be initiated as part of the total lifelong oral health program.

## Question 6

Which of the following statements, if any, are correct?

A. In a preventive oral-health program, the interview and preventive counseling are best accomplished before the examination of the infant.

B. The interview should begin with a discussion of the parents' reason for seeking dental care.

C. A complete medical history is not important in the initial visit.

D. A history of tooth decay is important to establish environmental issues as well as parental attitudes towards dental health.

E. It is important to know if the child has access to fluoride in the drinking water before prescribing any fluoride supplement.

## Counseling

Based upon the information gathered to this point, the practitioner is ready to provide recommendations on *how parents can play an active role* in preventing dental disease in their child by assuming the responsibility for the following procedures.

### Oral Hygiene

Parents should be educated regarding the following tooth-cleaning recommendations.

- A parent, other adult, or older sibling must assume total responsibility for tooth cleaning in infants and young children. Many children are unable to perform adequate plaque removal until 6 to 8 years of age.
- Tooth cleaning should be done in a comfortable location and pleasant environment. Positioning will be demonstrated during the examination.
- A dentifrice is not necessary for infants. In many cases, it may be a source for objection because of the taste and foaming action.
- If a dentifrice is used, only a pea-sized amount should be placed on the brush to avoid ingestion of excess fluoride.
- Tooth cleaning should be accomplished with a small, soft-bristled toothbrush.
- Tooth cleaning should be accomplished at least once daily.
- The evening tooth cleaning may be easier to accomplish following the infant's last feeding instead of waiting until just before bedtime since a tired infant can frequently be fussy during the procedure.

## Question 7

Which of the following statements, if any, are correct?

A. Tooth cleaning of infant's teeth should be done by a parent, other adult, or older sibling.

B. A dentifrice is not necessary in infants.

C. If a dentifrice is used, the entire length of the brush head should be filled.

D. In infants, tooth cleaning should be accomplished at least once a day.

E. A large toothbrush is adequate for cleaning infant's teeth.

*Diet Management*

Parents have control, for the most part, over their child's diet during the early years. The exceptions include time spent with babysitters and in day care settings. Parents can have some influence in those situations, however, if they make their wishes known. The following information should be shared with parents.

- Infants should be weaned from the bottle around 12 months of age.
- The bottle should not be used as a pacifier nor given during bedtime or naptime.
- Only formula or milk should be offered in the bottle.
- Frequent, prolonged episodes of breast-feeding could be a caries risk.
- Sleeping with the child and allowing nursing through the night should be avoided.
- Infants and young children generally will eat more frequently than three times daily.
- Between-meal snacks should consist of foods that have a low cariogenic potential.
- Total amount of cariogenic foods is not the issue, rather the frequency of ingestion and retentiveness of the food are the factors that contribute to the caries risk.

## Question 8

Which of the following statements, if any, are correct?

A. During the infant's oral health first visit, the parents should be informed that the infant should be weaned from the bottle around 12 months of age.

B. Only formula or milk should be offered in the bottle.

C. Between-meal snacks should consist of foods that have a low cariogenic potential.

D. Frequent, prolonged episodes of breast-feeding could be a caries-risk situation.

E. Total amount of cariogenic food consumption is more important than the frequency of cariogenic food consumption.

The Examination

Once the interview and counseling aspects of the visit are completed, the dentist is ready to proceed with the examination of the infant or toddler. The dental chair and overhead light are neither required nor very useful for examining children this young. Since one of the prime objectives is to provide a dental examination in a pleasant, nonthreatening manner, the procedure is best accomplished in the *knee-to-knee* position for children under 3 years of age (Figure 18–2). This position provides a stable, yet comfortable environment that incorporates the security of parental involvement, which may produce a calming effect on infants and toddlers who lack the cognitive ability to cooperate. Should the child offer resistance, the dentist can easily and gently stabilize the child's mouth and head cradled in the lap while the parent holds the child's hands and can stabilize the legs by cradling them with the elbows. Many of the infants and toddlers accept the examination procedures in this position without resistance. It is important in those instances where the children resist or cry that the parents be assured that the behavior is normal (and expected) for the child's age and should not be considered "bad" or "uncooperative."

The examination should begin with a soft touch, evaluating the extraoral head and neck

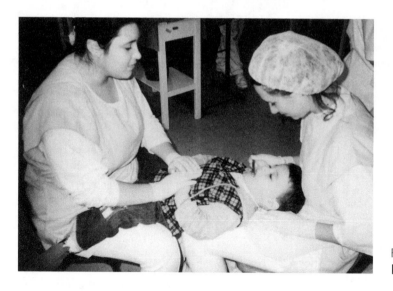

FIGURE 18–2    Knee-to-knee examination position.

conditions first, allowing the child to become accustomed to the dentist's actions. The examination of the oral cavity should begin by using the fingers to palpate the oral structures before introducing the dental instruments. Illumination can be provided with a penlight or flashlight held by the dental assistant. Access and stabilization of the mouth can be obtained by placing a finger on the gum pad distal to the most posterior tooth in a maxillary quadrant. Following inspection of the oral soft and hard tissues, a dental cleaning (plaque removal) is accomplished with a soft bristled, moist, child-sized toothbrush. Rarely will a rubber cup and polishing paste be required for stain removal. The tooth-cleaning process is discussed and demonstrated as you remove the plaque. At this point, it is very important that the child be repositioned with the head cradled in the parent's lap and the parent given the opportunity to practice the tooth-cleaning process with the dentist's supervision and guidance. This will help some parents get over their reluctance to clean their child's teeth, especially when the child resists. Occasionally, some infants and toddlers exhibit tight contacts between the an-

terior as well as the posterior teeth, which accumulate considerable plaque. The parent can be shown *how* to clean these areas using dental floss in a holder with relative ease. The parents are advised that they need to perform tooth cleaning for their child at least once per day, but preferably following each meal. The most critical time to clean the teeth is following the last meal or snack of the day. It is emphasized that toothpaste is not required and is usually objectionable to the infant. If it is used, only a minimal quantity should be placed on the brush.

It should also be emphasized early that when the child is becoming accustomed to the routine of having a parent brush the teeth, the tooth cleaning should not become an unpleasant struggle for those infants and toddlers who initially resist the procedure. On those occasions where the child struggles considerably, the procedure should not be abandoned. Rather, less attention can be placed on performing thorough plaque removal, while maintaining a consistent effort to establish a routine with the child. A more thorough tooth cleaning can be performed another day when the

child is more cooperative. Parents can be reminded of other routines that are accomplished in spite of the child's objections, such as washing the child's hair. If the tooth-cleaning routine is established during the first 12 months, strong objections and resistance to the procedure during the "terrible twos" can usually be avoided.

### Concluding the Appointment

The appointment is concluded by addressing the following areas.

- Provide the parents with a summary of your clinical findings.
- Make appropriate recommendations based upon the clinical findings.
- Solicit and answer any remaining questions that the parents may have.
- Reinforce the parents' role and responsibilities in their child's oral-health care.
- Establish an optimal fluoride program (pending any water analysis). (See Appendix 18–1.)
- Distribute educational pamphlets/brochures as desired.

- Provide anticipatory guidance information.
- Establish an appropriate recall schedule.

### Anticipatory Guidance

Anticipatory guidance is a process for preparing the parents for upcoming developmental changes and concerns that may arise before the next scheduled dental visit in order to minimize the negative effects that may arise. Wherever possible, *preventive oral health information* should be provided to expectant parents during prenatal education programs. Examples of such information are provided in Appendices 18–2 through 18–4.

### Establishing a Recall Schedule

The recall appointment may be scheduled for 3, 6, or 12 months depending upon the child's potential risk for developing dental disease based upon clinical findings, stage of dental development, and feeding or diet patterns. Examples for determining appropriate recall schedules are listed in Appendix 18–5.

## SUMMARY

The potential exists today for dental-health professionals to assist parents in raising caries-free children. The knowledge and technology are available and the request for this service is growing. The dental professional has the opportunity to accept this role with enthusiasm and continue to be a leader among the health professions in disease prevention. The dental profession must not ignore the oral health needs of infants and toddlers under 3 years of age. We must instead, take advantage of our knowledge and technology and begin our disease prevention efforts with children as infants and educate parents-to-be and new parents regarding their important role in the oral health of their children. By doing so, we can provide a pleasant and logical introduction to dentistry and promote the profession in a most positive way.

# ANSWERS AND EXPLANATIONS

1. A, C, and D—correct.

    B—incorrect. Although nutritional deficiencies in the mother must be severe to affect the unborn child, a daily balanced diet provides the necessary proteins, fats, carbohydrates, vitamins, and minerals.

2. A, B, and D—correct.

    C—incorrect. *Streptococcus mutans* colonization of the oral cavity in infants occurs only after the eruption of teeth.

    E—incorrect. *Streptococcus mutans* has difficulty colonizing in an oral cavity already colonized by a mature dental plaque.

3. B, C, D, and E—correct.

    A—incorrect. The mother's teeth do not lose calcium. Instead, the risk of dental caries occurrence probably increases because of changes in eating habits.

4. A, B, C, and E—correct.

    D—incorrect. Early childhood caries has been reported in several studies dealing with breast-fed children, although the prevalence is lower than in bottle-fed children.

5. A, B, D, and E—correct.

    C—incorrect. The child's first dental visit should be at 6 months of age and no later than 12 months of age to permit a complete examination of the child's mouth and jaws, to allow the child to become familiar with the dental office procedures under a pleasant situation, and to provide parents with early preventive advice.

6. A, B, D, and E—correct.

    C—incorrect. A complete medical history is important as some systemic conditions may adversely affect dental health.

7. A, B, and D—correct.

    C—incorrect. If a dentifrice is used, only a pea-sized or smaller amount should be placed on the brush to avoid ingestion of excess fluoride.

    E—incorrect. Although a large toothbrush may be carefully used to clean anterior teeth, a small soft-bristled toothbrush provides easier access to all areas of the teeth as well as more comfort to the infant's mouth.

8. A, B, C, and D—correct.

    E—incorrect. Total amount of cariogenic food is not the issue; rather, the frequency of ingestion and retentiveness of the food are the factors that contribute to the caries risk.


## Self-Evaluation Questions

1. Dental counseling to pregnant women should start _____.

2. Dental radiographs should be avoided during the _____ trimester of pregnancy.

3. The emphasis on excellent maternal oral health is required for three reasons: _____, _____, and _____.

4. Evidence suggests that dental caries is an _____ disease.

5. Dental caries is mainly produced by the bacteria _____.

6. The main source of transmission of *Streptococcus mutans* to the infant's mouth is mainly from _____.

7. Children of mothers taking fluoride at the time of the child's birth revealed less caries _____.

8. Three other terms that describe early childhood caries are _____, _____, and _____.

9. The caries process is _____ and at times a definite cause may not be identifiable.

10. Recently, it is recommended that a child should first visit the dental office at _____ of age.

# REFERENCES

1. García-Godoy, F. (1983). Oral health: Part of the socialization process. *J Pedodont*, 7:251–54.
2. Croll, T. P. (1994). A child's first dental visit: A protocol. *Quint Int*, 15:625–37.
3. Thorild, I., Lindau-Jonson, B., & Twetman, S. (2002). Prevalence of salivary *Streptococcus mutans* in mothers and in their preschool children. *Int J Paediatr Dent*, 12: 2–7.
4. Li, Y., Wang, W., & Caufield, P. W. (2000). The fidelity of mutans streptococci transmission and caries status correlate with breast-feeding experience among Chinese families. *Caries Res* 34:123–32.
5. Kozai, K., Nakayama, R., Tedjosasongko, U., Kuwahara, S., Suzuki, J., Okada, M., & Nagasaka, N. (1999). Intrafamilial distribution of mutans streptococci in Japanese families and possibility of father-to-child transmission. *Microbiol Immunol*, 43:99–106.
6. Ripa, L. W. (1988). *Baby bottle tooth decay (nursing caries): A comprehensive review.* Dental Health Section. Washington, DC: American Public Health Association, 1–13.
7. Tanzer, J. M., Livingston, J., & Thompson, A. M. (2001). The microbiology of primary dental caries in humans. *J Dent Educ*, 65:1028–37.
8. Berkowitz, R. J., Jordan, H. V., & White, G. (1975). The early establishment of *Streptococcus mutans* in the mouths of infants. *Arch Oral Biol*, 20:171–74.
9. Krasse, B., Edwardsson, S., Svensson, I., & Trell, L. (1967). Implantation of caries-inducing streptococci in the human oral cavity. *Arch Oral Biol*, 12:231–36.
10. Ooshima, T., Matsumura, M., Hoshino, T., Kawabata, S., Sobue, S., & Fujiwara, T. (2001). Contributions of three glycosyltransferases to sucrose-dependent adherence of *Streptococcus mutans*. *J Dent Res*, 80:1672–7.
11. Sheiham, A. (2001). Dietary effects on dental diseases. *Public Health Nutr*, 4:569–91.

12. Caufield, P. W., Dasanayake, A. P., Li, Y., Pan, Y., Hsu, J., & Hardin, J. M. (2000). Natural history of Streptococcus sanguinis in the oral cavity of infants: evidence for a discrete window of infectivity. *Infect Immun,* 68:4018–23.

13. Caufield, P. W., Cutter, G. R., Dasayanake, A. P. (1993). Initial acquisition of mutans streptococci by infants: Evidence of a discrete window of infectivity. *J Dent Res,* 72:37–45.

14. Li, Y., & Caufield, P. W. (1995). The fidelity of initial acquisition of mutans streptococci by infants from their mothers. *J Dent Res,* 74:681–5.

15. Brambilla, E., Felloni, A., Gagliani, M., Malerba, A., García-Godoy, F., & Strohmenger, L. (1998). Caries prevention during pregnancy. Results of a 30-month study. *J Am Dent Assoc,* 129:871–77.

16. Casamassimo, P. S. (2001). Maternal oral health. *Dent Clin North Am* 45:469–7.

17. Moss, S. J. (1988). The Year 2000 Health Objectives for the Nation. *Pediatr Dent,* 10:228–33.

18. Herbert, F. L., Lenchner, V., & Pinkham, J. R. (1994). In Starkey, P. A, Ed. *The Answer Book.* Chicago: American Society of Dentistry for Children.

19. Dimitrova, M. M., Kukleva, M. P., & Kondeva, V. K. (2000). A study of caries polarization in 1-, 2- and 3-year-old children. *Folia Med* (Plovdiv) 42:55–9.

20. Dimitrova, M. M., Kukleva, M. P., & Kondeva, V. K. (2000). Specificity of caries attack in early childhood. *Folia Med* (Plovdiv) 42:50–4.

21. Dimitrova, M. M., Kukleva, M. P., & Kondeva, V. K. (2000). Early childhood caries—incidence and need for treatment. *Folia Med* (Plovdiv), 42:46–9.

22. Behrendt, A., Sziegoleit, F., Muler-Lessmann, V., Ipek-Ozdemir, G., & Wetzel, W. E. (2001). Nursing-bottle syndrome caused by prolonged drinking from vessels with bill-shaped extensions. *ASDC J Dent Child,* 68:47–50.

23. Petti, S., Cairella, G., & Tarsitani, G. (2000). Rampant early childhood dental decay: An example from Italy. *J Public Health Dent,* 60:159–66.

24. Jones, D. L., Mobley, C. C., & García-Godoy, F. (1996). Validation of a clinical severity index of nursing caries in a preschool Hispanic population. *J Dent Res,* 75:14 (Abstr. 34).

25. García-Godoy, F., Mobley, C., & Jones, D. (Sept 1995). Caries and feeding practices in South Texas preschool children. *Report to the Centers for Disease Control and Prevention.*

26. Valaitis, R., Hesch, R., Passarelli, C., Sheehan, D., & Sinton, J. (2000). A systematic review of the relationship between breastfeeding and early childhood caries. *Can J Public Health,* 91:411–7.

27. Dini, E. L., Holt, R. D., & Bedi, R. (2000). Caries and its association with infant feeding and oral health-related behaviours in 3-4-year-old Brazilian children. *Community Dent Oral Epidemiol,* 28:241–8.

28. Twetman, S., Garcia-Godoy, F., & Goepferd, S. J. (2000). Infant oral health. *Dent Clin North Am* 44:487–505.

29. McWhorter, A. G., Seale, N. S., & King, S. A. (2001). Infant oral health education in U.S. dental school curricula. *Pediatr Dent,* 23:407–9.

30. Hamilton, F. A., Davis, K. E., & Blinkhorn, A. S. (1999). An oral health promotion programme for nursing caries. *Int J Paediatr Dent,* 9:195–200.

# APPENDICES

APPENDIX 18-1  Fluoride Supplementation Depends on the Fluoride Content
of the Drinking Water

| Age | < 0.3 ppm | 0.3–0.6 ppm | > 0.6 ppm |
|---|---|---|---|
| Birth–6 mos. | 0 | 0 | 0 |
| 6 mos.–3 yrs. | 0.25 | 0 | 0 |
| 3 yrs.–6 yrs. | 0.5 | 0.25 | 0 |
| 6 yrs.–16 yrs. | 1.0 | 0.5 | 0 |

## Anticipatory Guidance in Pediatric Dentistry

**APPENDIX 18-2  Prenatal Counseling (Developmental Age Range: Birth–12 Months)**

| Current Area | Dentist's Actions |
|---|---|
| **Oral Development** | |
| First primary tooth, molar eruption | Review of patterns of eruption |
| Formation of primary and permanent teeth | Review teething facts and myths |
| | Review oral anatomic landmarks |
| **Fluoride** | |
| Recommendation against fluoride use until 6 months of age | Discuss need to assess fluoride status |
| Systemic fluoride management after 6 months of age | Review dentifrice use |
| **Oral Hygiene/Health** | |
| Microflora acquisition in infants | Review of oral hygiene techniques for infants with parents emphasizing use of a soft brush and no dentifrice |
| Mouth cleaning techniques | |
| Periodicity for dental visits | |
| | Plan for baby's first dental care visit |
| **Habits** | |
| Pacifier use/thumbsucking | Review safe pacifier use and hygiene issues |
| | Review the mouth's exploratory role in infants |
| | Discuss effects of thumbsucking/pacifiers on oral structures |
| **Nutrition and Diet** | |
| Nursing caries patterns and causes | Discuss proper feeding practices |
| Role of sugars in the caries process | Encourage weaning by 12 months of age |
| | Discuss the role of "sugars" in dental caries initiation |
| **Injury Prevention** | |
| Oral trauma | Review appropriate response for parents if infant experiences oral trauma and provide emergency information/phone number |

## APPENDIX 18-3   First Dental Visit (Developmental Age Range: 12–24 Months)

| Content Area | Dentist's Actions |
| --- | --- |
| **Oral Development** | |
| Completion of primary dentition/concepts of occlusion | Discuss importance of space maintenance |
| Spacing/space maintenance | Discuss eruption patterns and concepts of spacing |
| Permanent tooth formation | Emphasize oral health to protect developing permanent teeth |
| **Fluoride** | |
| Dietary sources of fluoride | Assess fluoride status/need for fluoride supplementation |
| Fluoride sources outside the home | Review dentifrice use |
| Toxicity and safety (dentifrices, etc.) | Discuss procedures for accidental ingestion |
| **Oral Hygiene/Health** | |
| Type of brush, role and amount of dentifrice | Review of oral hygiene techniques |
| Parent and child's role in toothbrushing/flossing | Assist parents in overcoming oral hygiene difficulties |
| Frequency and location for oral hygiene | Plan for baby's next dental care based on risk assessment |
| **Habits** | |
| Pacifier use/thumbsucking | Review safe pacifier use and hygiene issues |
| | Discuss effects of thumbsucking/pacifiers on oral structures |
| **Nutrition and Diet** | |
| The role of plaque in the caries process | Emphasize weaning if not already accomplished |
| Role of sugars in the caries process | Review carbohydrates and sugar intake and frequency in the caries process |
| | Review diet patterns that occur outside the home |
| **Injury Prevention** | |
| Primary tooth trauma and sequelae | Discuss electric cord safety and childproofing the home |
| Electric cord injury/childproofing home | Discuss oral trauma management for preschool and other child care situations |

### APPENDIX 18-4  Second Dental Visit (Developmental Age Range: 2–6 Years)

| Content Area | Dentist's Actions |
| --- | --- |
| **Oral Development** | |
| Exfoliation of primary teeth | Discuss importance of space maintenance |
| Eruption of mandibular permanent incisors | Discuss eruption patterns and concepts of spacing |
| Eruption of permanent first molars | Emphasize oral health to protect developing permanent teeth |
| **Fluoride** | |
| Dietary sources of fluoride | Assess fluoride status/need for fluoride supplementation |
| Fluoride sources outside the home | Discuss procedures for accidental ingestion |
| Toxicity and safety (dentifrices, etc.) | Review dentifrice use in children |
| **Oral Hygiene/Health** | |
| Parent and child's role in toothbrushing/ flossing | Review of oral hygiene techniques and compliance |
| Frequency and location for oral hygiene | Child assumes more responsibility and parents supervise |
| Role of sealants in prevention of occlusal caries | Discuss sealants and radiographs
Frequency of dental visits based upon child's level of caries risk |
| **Habits** | |
| Pacifier use/thumbsucking | Discuss effects of thumbsucking/pacifier on oral structures
Discuss methods for terminating habits |
| **Nutrition and Diet** | |
| Snacking and sugar intake | Review carbohydrate and sugar intake and frequency in the caries process
Review diet patterns that occur outside the home |
| **Injury Prevention** | |
| Safety during sporting activities | Discuss use of safety equipment (helmets, etc.) and mouthguards |
| Permanent tooth injury | Review emergency trauma management |

### APPENDIX 18-5  Clinical Findings According to Child's Age and Expected Feeding or Diet Patterns and Dental Development Characteristics

| | Clinical Findings | Feeding or Diet Patterns | Dental Development |
| --- | --- | --- | --- |
| 3 months | Enamel decalcification
Considerable plaque build-up
Amelogenesis imperfecta
Dentinogenesis imperfecta | Bottle used at bedtime or naptime
Bottle used as a pacifier
Bottle used past 12 months of age
Frequent cariogenic diet or snacks | Stage of dental development has minimal influence on decision for a 3-month recall |
| 6 months | Posterior proximal contacts
No previous tooth cleaning
Primary dentition crowding
Moderate plaque build-up | Relatively cariogenic diet or frequent snacking on cariogenic foods | Second primary molar eruption is anticipated within 6 months |
| 12 months | Generalized spacing present
Good oral hygiene exhibited
Shallow occlusal anatomy | Good dietary habits exhibiting a low cariogenic potential | Second primary molar eruption anticipated within 12 months |

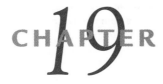

# CHAPTER 19

# Oral Health Promotion in Schools

*Alice M. Horowitz*
*Norman O. Harris*

## OBJECTIVES

*At the end of this chapter it will be possible to*

1. Explain why general and oral-health school programs are needed.
2. Discuss why many teachers are concerned about the prospect of teaching oral health and of conducting daily toothbrushing as a primary prevention measure.
3. Explain why school-based health clinics (SBHCs) offer the potential of providing access and funding for prevention and treatment programs.
4. Describe an effective primary preventive program that can be accomplished by *existing* school staff personnel.
5. Identify the reasons that school-based sealant and fluoride regimens should target "high-risk" students; explain how a dental hygienist can contribute to a preventive program; and finally, state the benefits that a dentist can add to the school health team.
6. Justify the need for a school tobacco intervention program to help prevent student use of smoking and smokeless tobacco products.
7. Describe the role of football helmets and intraoral mouthguards, as well as what to do if a player's tooth has been knocked out.
8. Explain how an expansion of a school's mission to include teaching about broad societal problems can be competitive with teaching a normal academic curriculum; suggest a solution to this dilemma.

We need to do a better job of weaving a safety net of understanding, appreciation and guidance in the family, in the community and school. We need to start thinking of health and education as interlocking spheres.

—C. Everett Koop, MD, Surgeon General

# INTRODUCTION

Today we have the ability to prevent or control most oral diseases or conditions of school-age children. Thousands of children and youths in the United States have benefited from the use of these preventive procedures. For example, dental caries has been reduced dramatically among U.S. children 5 through 17 years of age.[1-3] In fact, recent data show that nearly 55% of these children are caries-free in their permanent dentition, although the percentage *decreases dramatically* with age. In addition, an overall impression is that most students' mouths are cleaner with little noticeable exogenous stain and reasonably healthy gingiva. Unfortunately, preventive procedures have neither been available nor affordable by all children. This inequality likely explains why approximately 80% of caries lesions are found among one quarter of the U.S. child population.[1-3] Moreover, sharp disparities still persist in oral health status and use of dental services.[1] Poor children are more likely than non-poor children to have a *higher proportion of decay and are least likely to receive treatment.*[1-3]

Daily more than 6,000 U.S. youths 18 years of age and younger try their first cigarette.[4] It is well established that the use of *tobacco products*—smoking and smokeless tobacco—is the primary risk factor for oral and pharyngeal cancers.[5] Yet, the use of "spit" tobacco (chewing tobacco and snuff) among U.S. youths is on the rise and is not limited to lower socioeconomic groups. Purportedly, some youths believe that "spit" tobacco is a safe alternative to smoking. Moreover, when youths use spit or chew tobacco they are likely to switch to cigarettes. Equally or more disconcerting is that smoking cigarettes remains high and is increasing among the young.[6] One report showed that in 1998, 30% of high-school-senior girls reported that they had smoked in the past 30 days.[4] Also it is noteworthy that few health education texts include information that the use of tobacco and alcohol products are primary risk factors for oral cancers.[7]

The good news is that investing in comprehensive tobacco control programs, which includes schools, *does work.*[8,9] Two major contributing factors include: preventing the initiation of tobacco use among youth and promoting quitting among young people and adults.[8,9]

Equally important is the fact that large numbers of youth, especially minorities, do not complete high school.[10] And, many become parents at an early age. Thus, health literacy is especially important for youths who drop out of high school. It is important that they gain the knowledge and skills to attain and maintain good health, including oral health, for themselves and others who may depend on them. For these reasons, promoting oral health in schools is not only desirable but also a necessity.

Beyond the family, no other institution in our society can do more for child and adolescent health.[11] In today's fast-paced society in which children often live in single-

parent or dual-career families, the school may become the *only* bastion of constancy in a child's environment. But, oral health programs in schools *cannot be considered in isolation* from the maelstrom of conflicting needs and priorities of overall medical, dental, and social needs of children and youth.

## Definitions

For mutual understanding the following definitions are provided for use in this chapter.

*Diet* refers to the oral *intake of all foods and beverages*.

*Nutrition* is the study of metabolism that occurs *following the ingestion of foods and beverages*.

*Program* is an *organized* group of procedures designed to solve a defined problem.

*Health education* is any combination of *planned learning experiences* designed to facilitate voluntary actions conducive to health.[12] Health education must be an integral part of any school health program. Health education is used to inform, educate, and reinforce previous health messages. It is essential to educate a broad spectrum of individuals and groups to gain acceptance and use of health measures. Health education *alone* cannot function as a preventive method.[13,14] Still, accurate information and knowledge are important because they enable individuals, groups, and agencies or institutions to make *informed decisions* regarding oral health.[13,14]

*Health literacy* is the capacity of an individual to *obtain, interpret,* and *understand* basic health information and services and the competence to use, or not to use, such information and services in ways that are health enhancing.[2]

*Health promotion* is any *planned combination* of educational, political, regulatory, and organizational supports for actions and conditions conducive to the health of individuals, groups, or communities.[12] This definition differs from a more common use of promotion that is generally regarded as public relations or marketing activities. Although these kinds of activities frequently are a part of health promotion, this definition refers to actions intended to modify an individual's environment in a way that will improve health *regardless of individual actions* or to enable individuals to take advantage of preventive and treatment procedures by removing existing barriers. For example, one health promotion strategy to influence oral health might include providing a community-based fluoride regimen such as fluoride mouthrinse or tablets in schools that includes appropriate education for parents, students, and school personnel. Another example, using a regulatory support, might include the *prohibition* of any tobacco products on school property. This type of regulation along with appropriate education about the health effects of tobacco use as well as an increase in the *state's tobacco tax* would constitute a health promotion strategy.

*Comprehensive school health education* is a *planned*, systematic, and ongoing learning opportunity that enables *all students* (K–12) to be productive learners and to make well-considered health decisions throughout their lives.

*Comprehensive school health program* is an *organized* set of policies, procedures, and activities designed to protect and promote the health and well being of students and staff, which has traditionally included health services, a healthy school environment, and health education.

## Who is Responsible for Teaching Oral Health?

School age children, especially younger students, largely depend on parents and/or school-based programs for oral-health information or for inclusion in preventive dentistry or treatment programs. Many teachers believe that oral-health instruction should be the responsibility of parents and health educators—not teachers of academic subjects. This belief might be legitimate if, universally, parents were able to care for their children's oral health. To illustrate, Mandel has pointed out that there has been a profound drop in caries for 17-year-olds, with 50% being free of decay; at the same time he expressed concern for the 50% still experiencing caries.[15] In addition, the continued growth of numbers of children living in poverty, coupled with *cuts in public health programs,* may not bode well for the underserved population's access to dental services.[16,17] In fact, recent reports indicate that there is a huge disparity between low-income children and their higher-income counterparts.[1,2] A child reared in a home where the parents are subject to economic and educational disadvantages is often dentally neglected. In these homes, parental intercession in the oral-health care of a child frequently begins with seeking help to relieve pain, often a difficult task because access to dental care is not easy for them. Too many working mothers and single parents find it very difficult to take time off from work to tend to their children's health, especially when there are additional barriers to access. Others may be apathetic or so overwhelmed with how to feed their family that oral health simply is not a priority in their lives.

Even with highly motivated and educated adults, their knowledge about oral health is often minimal.[18–21] In addition, behavioral change may be more difficult to influence at home under parental guidance than under the tutelage of a teacher. In other words, many parents themselves do not know how to help their children help themselves and need the support of a school health program. Still, whenever possible, the parent must be included in a school-based, oral health program. Parents can provide strong positive reinforcement, either through role-modeling or verbal messages that support the attitudinal and behavioral changes promulgated in the school setting. Ideally, parent education should parallel child education; in this way, parents can learn to improve their own oral health as well as have the guidelines to assist their children. This educational process of parents is often necessary to help overcome the barriers raised by *their* past adverse experiences with dental treatment and its financial hardships.

The bottom line is that all children have *the right to a good education* to enable them to be knowledgeable, productive adults. A healthy child is better able to learn. Schools and health are inextricably linked; thus, school health programs are the underpinnings of promoting health and preventing diseases among our children.[22,23]

Typically school health programs have had three major components: health *education,* health *services,* and a healthful *environment.* More recently some have expanded this triad to an eight-component model that includes health education, physical education, health services, nutrition services, health promotion for school staff, counseling and psychological services, a healthy school environment, and parent and community involvement.[23] Those who advocate the eight-component model believe that it is more comprehensive to help solve complex problems now faced by communities. No individual model is best. Rather, school-based programs, like other health programs, should be comprehensive and *based on the needs of the population* they are designed to serve.

## Roles of Oral-Health-Care Providers

### Professional Volunteerism

In addition to parental support, *professional involvement* in school programs is desirable. The luxury of having salaried dentists or dental hygienists (or both) employed by school systems, however, is rare. Therefore, opportunities abound for dentists and dental hygienists to volunteer in school-based programs. Professional input is valuable for identifying teaching–learning resources, speaking to students, faculty, and parent groups, providing in-service training of faculty and administrators, and for assisting the schools on special occasions, such as career day and health fairs. The support of the professional community enhances a program's credibility, improves the image of dentistry and dental hygiene, and may be a *practice builder* for participating providers. A more consistent presence of the oral health professions throughout the academic year is needed to help strengthen school–community relationships.

Dentists, dental hygienists, and students of each provider group can and should play major roles in school health programs.[22] Their involvement may range from taking the lead in planning a comprehensive oral health program and implementing it, to participating by providing education to students, treatment or preventive services, or in-service training for members of the faculty. Or, they may simply play a role of being supportive of an appropriate procedure that is being recommended in a local school. Whatever the role one plays it requires that the provider be knowledgeable about the needs of students in the school(s), which necessitates conducting a needs assessment. And, it requires current scientific knowledge about how to prevent oral diseases and conditions identified among the children in the target school(s).[22]

Health care providers should support the use of valid procedures. That is, one should recommend, use, and provide accurate information about only those procedures known to be effective based on research.[22] For example in a school in which students have high-caries rates in chewing surfaces of posterior teeth, dental sealants should be recommended in addition to regular use of a regimen of fluoride (Figure 19–1).

Most important, oral-health-care providers must work with others who are involved in school-health programs. These groups include school nurses, health educators, physicians, nutritionists, school administrators, leaders of local religious organizations, members of the local and state health departments, parent–teacher associations, parents, students, and politicians. Ideally, oral-health-care providers should have solid community organization and communication skills.

## School-Health Programs Past and Present

School-health programs (SHP) originated around the beginning of the 20th century to help *cope with contagion, screening needs* for physical disabilities, *nutritional deficiencies*, and *first aid* ministrations. Since their inception, school-health programs have varied in quality and content by state and community. In the 1930s and 1940s, children were provided nutritional supplements, eye examinations, health education, smallpox vaccinations, and in some cases oral-health services. In the early 1950s, school-based fluoride regimens were introduced in the form of multiple applications of operator-applied, neutral sodium fluoride and school water fluoridation. In the 1960s, the outstanding success of rapid immunization of total school populations against polio-myelitis, and the almost universal establishment of nursing services within school systems to deal with day-to-day accidents and illnesses, is a legacy to the attainment of early school health objectives.

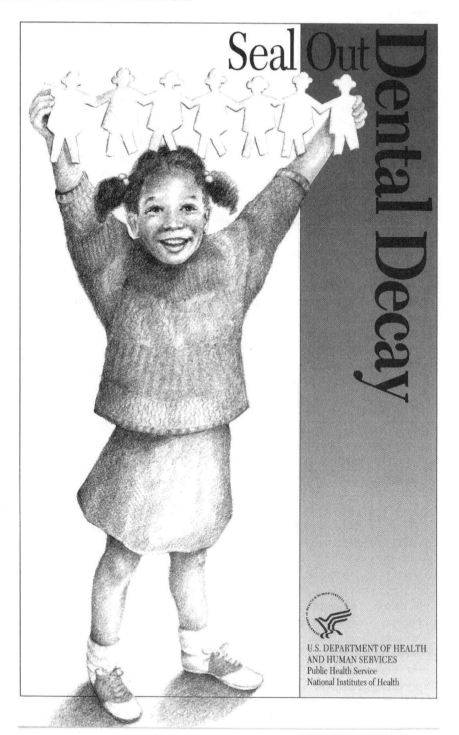

FIGURE 19–1    A leaflet explaining what sealants are and who needs them is available from the NIDCR (1 NOHIC Way, Bethesda, MD 208892-3500).

But, the concepts and requirements of school health programs have been greatly broadened over the last three decades. At the onset of the 21st century, *school-health services now include or attempt to address major societal health issues* that have invaded the schools. These include: alcohol, drugs, and tobacco use (smoking and "spit"); safe-sex, HIV, AIDS, other sexually transmitted diseases; gang violence and child abuse; and self-esteem, depression, homicide, suicide, and terrorism. In addition, health problems of dysfunctional families, migratory workers, and the poverty stricken are often addressed.[24-28] When these problems are mixed with those of ethnicity, race, religion, and politics, planning school-health programs becomes a complex and challenging exercise.[29] Further, while attempting to address more issues, most school systems have had a sharp reduction in health-related personnel. Today, it is a luxury for a school to have a full-time nurse or health educator on the premises. Although dental hygienists originally were trained to work in schools to improve children's oral health, relatively few schools today have access to this type of oral-health-care provider.

There is little doubt that schools, especially public schools, must become more involved in a wide range of health education and promotion to help cope with overwhelming societal health problems. This need is enunciated clearly in two documents, *Healthy People 2010 and Healthy Schools 2000*.[2,30] Appendix 19–1 shows the oral-health objectives related to schools contained *in Healthy People 2010*. Many states have their own health objectives that include oral health. Each state department of health has at least one person responsible for directing health education. Unfortunately, these *state-level health educators and the state dental directors rarely work together* to achieve oral health objectives. Some states even require health educators in attendance in elementary, junior, and senior high schools. Further, some states provide written guidance in the form of curriculum guidelines for health education.

Only a few states, however, elevate the status of health education to include *mandated testing*.[31]

In conflict with the expanding health role of the school system is the fact that *the primary mission of schools is education—not conserving health or preventing disease*. School administrators are sensitive to any change or expansion of their basic mission. There are limits to just how far schools can continue to assume greater teaching responsibilities.[32] Probably the most important factor is the *lack of time* in the curriculum for new teaching requirements. Unless school days or years are extended, any expanded health program becomes *competitive* with basic education needs. This competition is exacerbated by legislative mandates that require additions of specific school health workloads without allocating additional specific health funding.[33] It is little wonder that, at times, teachers consider themselves dedicated, beleaguered, and underpaid professionals who are being called on to discharge duties *which "society" itself cannot solve*.[34]

The needs of a community and its schools are intricately interwoven. To foster cooperation between the two, School Health Councils often are developed to help mobilize the health resources of a community. In schools, nurses, health educators, physical education teachers, guidance counselors, food-service directors, principals, students, and parents share responsibility, while the greater community taps the expertise of existing civic organizations, health agencies, and business and professional leaders.[35] A recent trend of School Health Councils has been to recommend implementation of *school-based health clinics (SBHC)* both within and outside of school hours.[24,28,29] These SBHC are now in 45 states and the District of Columbia. They have grown from 200 in 1990 to 1,380 in 2000.[36] These clinics are now operational primarily in high-risk urban and rural areas with higher levels of poverty where there is a lack of access and funding to conventional health care.[37] Some of the services provided include: athletic and pre-employment physicals, labora-

tory and diagnostic screenings, prescriptions on a limited basis, first aid, family planning, prenatal and postpartum care, drug and alcohol counseling, nutrition and obesity counseling, and *dental care* (Figure 19–2). Sponsorship of SBHCs may include community organizations, health departments, medical centers, hospitals, private not-for-profit organizations, and school systems.[38] Funding may be from private foundations, local funding, insurance, or government sources such as Medicaid. Should this trend continue, it is conceivable that schools of the future will need an assistant school superintendent for health affairs.

Members of Congress and many health providers including oral-health providers, are interested in this SBHC approach to health care for children and youth as it would make *Medicaid and other appropriated funds available for this use*. The Department of Education and the Department of Health and Human Services have funding mechanisms in place to promote research and development for these types of clinics. According to proponents, the development of this nontraditional component of a school health service will: (1) permit the school nurse to return to a more traditional purpose of the nursing service to support the classroom teacher as well as acting as a liaison with the SBHC; (2) return to teachers the responsibility for classroom teaching of subjects that match their academic training; and (3) *provide a method of access and funding* for all health care for school-age children and youth.

Today there is a national concern for achieving both excellence of education and for improved health for children. School-based programs appear to be a natural site for addressing both concerns. Students can stay in class, parents can continue at work, and cost-effective, comprehensive school health programs, *including those for oral health*, can be made available.[28,38] It is important to note that one of the oral health objectives in Healthy People 2010 is to increase the number of SBHC that include oral health (Appendix 19–1). A consensus exists that a student who is impaired by drugs or alcohol is as handicapped in learning as an individual who suffers from a sight or hearing deficiency. Thus, there is a need for schools to help shape social, psychological, and physical well being—*all in the name of school health*.

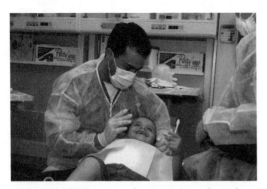

FIGURE 19–2   A student receives dental care in a school-based health clinic.

---

### Question 1

Which of the following statements, if any, are correct?

A. Oral health education, promotion, prevention, and treatment can be best provided within the framework of an overall school medical-health program.

B. Teachers are well prepared academically and through continuing education courses to act as facilitators in solving *societal* problems.

C. Teachers are well prepared academically and through continuing education programs to act as facilitators in teaching *oral-health education*.

D. School-based health clinics (SBHC) that include oral-health services, are *now* in operation.

E. Approximately 80% of caries lesions are found in approximately 25% of school-aged children.

# Creating Effective, School-Based Oral-Health Programs

To involve communities, families, or individuals in assuming responsibility for their own oral health, many ingredients are necessary. These include but are not limited to: knowledge, skills, motivation, access to preventive agents and treatment services, and a safe, healthy environment. Further, decision makers and teachers must be willing to include health education and health promotion in schools. Finally, *policy* is important. For example, smoke-free schools are a result of a policy that bans the use of tobacco products—by all—on school campuses. Such policies help deter students and faculty from using these products.

It is impossible for the approximate 152,000 active dentists[39] and over 100,000 dental hygienists[40] in the United States to assume the tremendous task of imparting essential oral health education to the public and encourage appropriate behaviors that are requisite to optimal oral health. Much of this education can be accomplished through *schools, mass media*, and *industry*.

## Planning—Key to Success

A successful school-based program does not just happen. An integrated plan of action for specified grades is essential, as is a clear delineation of program responsibilities and objectives.[20] It should be noted that, although including all grades—kindergarten through grade 12—is desirable and ideal, it rarely occurs regarding oral health. When oral health is addressed in a school setting, it is more often confined to kindergarten through grade 6.

Judicious planning ultimately will result in meaningful, target-specific programs that are integrated throughout the school years. Planning must include a community needs assessment, establishing priorities, developing a budget, and a strong component of evaluation. Developing a written plan of action is necessary for a variety of reasons. The plan can serve as an educational tool to inform individuals and groups, especially those that are needed to "buy in" as a partner in the endeavor. A written plan also can be used to solicit funds to help underwrite the proposed program. And, of course, the plan serves as a guide for all who are actively involved to help maintain focus on the objectives.[22]

A diverse and committed work group helps to ensure a greater variety of input, a representative audience, and a broad-based sense of ownership. It is essential that cooperative working relationships be established in the *initial* planning stages among parents, community leaders—both business and political—teachers, school administrators, and oral health professionals. A *dental representative should be a member of all state or local school advisory councils to ensure professional as well as political input*.[11]

## Educational Considerations

Traditionally, public schools have accepted the responsibility of teaching oral-health as a part of general health. Committed, knowledgeable teachers are the cornerstones of all effective, school-based oral-health education. However, the dental subject matter contained in many texts used in teachers' colleges relates mainly to the anatomy and physiology of the teeth, the supporting tissues, and salivary glands. Such a background enables schoolteachers to teach and promote basic information about the oral cavity. *Teachers cannot be expected to possess expertise* in a constantly changing pool of scientific knowledge relating to prevention and dental treatment options. As a result, they may be reluctant to teach what could be incorrect or obsolete information in these areas.

Periodic in-service training to upgrade teacher health knowledge, including oral health, would greatly help the faculty to develop greater competence and confidence.[41] To help attain this objective the state of Utah supplies

their teachers with a biannual update of advances in dentistry.[42]

Teachers and the dental profession alike have questioned the priority given to school oral health education programs. Sometimes the questions are asked by the educators because the time taken for dental education competes with the time needed for other subjects. Is oral health instruction more important than, for instance, mathematics or vocational training? Health professionals also question the time devoted to school programs that feature mainly information transmittal, rather than a *combination of education and preventive/treatment regimens*. Education, alone, rarely suffices. For example, it is pointless to provide plaque removal instruction if toothbrushes are not provided and the instruction is not practiced in the classroom. Individuals, who are not provided assistance in shaping health attitudes, beliefs, and habits early in life, are likely to suffer the consequences of reduced productivity in later years. Health-related knowledge and skills acquired in public school may become more meaningful in adult life when the importance of good health becomes more apparent.

The amount and quality of oral health taught in school is often too little to be assimilated by students, and not long-term enough to be amenable to good evaluation. A national school health evaluation conducted by the U.S. Public Health Service (USPHS), revealed that changes in health-related knowledge, practices and attitudes *increase* with the amount of instruction. The possibility of *securing that needed additional time is minimal* considering that in 1994, the annual average number of hours spent on health education, including oral health, was 13.8 hours![43]

## Educational Principles

Oral-health education involves the use of many communication and organizational skills and processes. These include conducting a needs as-sessment, listening, planning, facilitating group and individual participation, informing all relevant individuals and groups, leading, writing, speaking, providing feedback and reinforcement, and providing in-service training. These activities enlist the help of others and foster cooperation and the adoption and maintenance of effective health measures and programs by individuals, institutions, organizations, and communities. Educational principles necessary for oral-health education include:

- Health education must be an *integral part* of any preventive or restorative service or regulation or legislation relevant to a health program. This education functions to introduce and reinforce understanding and acceptance of, and participation in, whatever the health program consists of.

- Educational materials can be used effectively to gain attention on specific topics and to reinforce or clarify a procedure or regimen. But, *educational materials alone do not constitute an oral-health program*; they can be useful aids.

- Education materials should be *accurate* and *consistent* with current scientific knowledge.

- Educational materials must be appropriately designed for specific *ages, level of literacy, and cultural groups* for whom they are designed. One leaflet, for example, cannot be expected to be suitable for all racial-ethnic groups in a given community.

- Educational materials should be evaluated *prior to* their final production and use with the intended target group.

- Interactive teaching in which there is active *participation* and *involvement* on the part of learners is essential for all age groups and content areas.[22]

## Approaches for Health Education

Multiple channels of communication should be used to help ensure reaching as many of the tar-

get population as possible for purposes of informing and educating as well as for reinforcement. Oral health education should include *more than* one of the following approaches.

- *One-to-one communication* such as discussing the need for an oral-health program with a school superintendent.
- *Group presentations* of information and education, and demonstrations such as at parent–teacher meetings, in-service training for teachers, or organizational meetings.
- *Use of mass communication* such as newspapers, radio, television, web sites, and school newsletters to inform all groups about the need for an oral health program and plans to initiate a program, to solicit partners, and to provide feedback and reinforcement about the program's value and effectiveness.
- *Community organizational strategies,* such as coalitions, partnerships, councils, or committees to solve local health problems, gain commitment of resources, and conduct needs assessments.[22]

### Student Participation

*Philosophically, all children should be entitled to receive maximum information and primary preventive oral care.* Providing maximum oral health treatment for all children, however, is not feasible. Poor children have a higher percentage of untreated decayed teeth than nonpoor children.[1] Hence, a school-based program, other than classroom education, fluoride mouth rinses, or tablet program, should be selective *in targeting the children most at risk* as eligible for a higher level of care. Once criteria are established defining "high risk," all students meeting the high-risk criteria should be eligible for the same preventive and treatment benefits. For example, some states base eligibility for sealant programs on whether a child is eligible for free school lunches. The economic status of individual students, however, *should not* be the only

consideration because poor oral health occurs among the affluent as well as among the poor. Of importance in one study, it was found that following a few years of participation in an intensive caries prevention program, individuals were transformed *from high risk to low risk.*[44]

The extent of student involvement in program activities is an important issue. Personal involvement and participation tends to have a greater effect on behavior, attitudes, and beliefs. Active participation likely enhances interest in oral disease prevention measures and having a healthy mouth.

One opportunity for innovative student participatory learning comes during *Children's Dental Health Month held annually in February.* This activity, sponsored by the American Dental Association (ADA) and the American Dental Hygienists' Association (ADHA) was initiated in 1941 to provide an annual forum for oral health. Historically, both the dental and dental hygiene associations have participated in the program. Children's Dental Health Month has developed into the professions' *most widely supported and media-recognized oral-health event.* It is a time when schools, in cooperation with dental manufacturers, local dental and dental hygiene schools and associations, and other sponsors, organize oral health fairs for the public and for students. As a part of these health fairs, students engage in entertainment events, receive screening examinations, toothbrushes and toothpaste, watch demonstrations related to seat belt and air bag protection of the face and body, participate in discussions about the deadly effects of cigarette smoking and chewing tobacco or snuff, and learn about health-promoting behaviors (Figure 19–3).[45,46] During this time, students often develop group posters and exhibits, discuss nutritional information, and learn that dentistry is not a profession to be feared. The informality of these occasions may enhance student interest and fosters learning and development of desirable attitudes toward self-care and self-image.

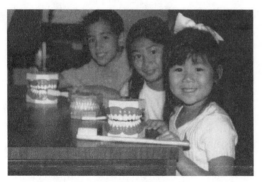

FIGURE 19–3 Students learn how to remove plaque during *Children's Dental Health Month.*

---

### Question 2

Which of the following statements, if any, are correct?

A. If the length of the present school year is maintained, any additional time commitments for teachers to adequately teach comprehensive health education and to address societal issues *must come from the teaching time used for other subjects.*

B. Teaching oral-health self-care is one of the most effective means for reducing oral disease.

C. Approximately *13.8 hours a year* is the average time devoted to *oral-health teaching.*

D. The annual Children's Dental Health Month is sponsored by the American Dental Association, and the American Dental Hygienists' Association.

E. Using multiple methods of communication is a better approach than using only one method in educating about oral health.

---

## What To Teach?

The needs of students in a particular school or district coupled with available resources—human, equipment, and financial—will dictate necessary preventive and treatment services, education, and policies. Appendix 19–2 provides a list of topics that students should be taught regarding prevention and early detection of oral diseases and conditions.

### Dental-Caries Prevention

*Fluorides and Dental Sealants*

Students need to learn that dental caries is an infectious disease with a multifactor etiology. And, they need to know that the disease can be *prevented, arrested and, reversed and how to do so.* Students should be taught that the appropriate use of fluorides and pit-and-fissure sealants are our best defense against this disease.[47] They also need to know about *systemic fluorides,* that is, fluoride intended for ingestion—community-water fluoridation, school-water fluoridation, and dietary-fluoride supplements—as well as *topical fluorides*—those fluoride products that are *not* intended to be ingested—toothpastes, mouthrinses, and operator-applied fluorides. Everyone needs to know that fluoride works both pre-eruptively and post-eruptively, but the primary ways that fluorides work are to *inhibit demineralization and to facilitate remineralization.*[48]

*Pit-and-Fissure Sealants*

Regarding dental sealants, students need to know how sealants protect occlusal surfaces of the teeth from decay; the ages at which teeth should be sealed and the need for possible reapplication of sealant material. Further, and very important, students and parents need to know that teeth that have been sealed should not need to be restored with a filling (see Chapter 10).

### Diet and Nutrition

The United States Department of Agriculture's food pyramid (see Chapter 15) makes it clear that sugars should be consumed only in moderation. Sweets not only are unhealthy for teeth but also are often in foods (cakes, pies, cookies,

etc.) that are laden with unhealthy fats. Basic information on diet and nutrition should be a part of all health education. Students need to understand that consumption of carbohydrates, especially sugar is a *key* component of the caries process and that sugar must be present for caries to occur. Ideally, when discussing diet in relation to oral health, information should be taught with a parallel emphasis on the preventive benefits of fluoride and how they remineralize incipient lesions, which prevent them from becoming overt, and on the use of pit-and-fissure sealants and oral hygiene measures. In the United States, especially in recent years, more emphasis has been placed on making the tooth more resistant to decay with the use of *fluorides and dental sealants*. Perhaps the best message about sweets is that *if you must consume sugars, do so at meals and in moderation*. It is important that in our efforts to encourage consumption of nonsweet snacks that we do *not* encourage the use of high fat and high sodium foods.

Often, after a teacher has taught that sugar is one factor that causes tooth decay and suggests that the child avoid excessive and frequent ingestion of refined carbohydrates, the child then goes to the cafeteria. There, the child is confronted with attractive, sugar-laden desserts. The question then is, "What message do students really get—the message they hear in the classroom or the message they see, smell, taste, and enjoy in the cafeteria?"

Schools should provide an *environment* that promotes avoidance of an excessive intake of sugar consumption. One important method of meeting this objective is for the *school dietitian* to reduce the number of days a week in which confections are available. Instead, desserts such as fresh fruits can be offered that are nutritionally sound and limit the amount of sucrose consumed.

A second strategy for reducing student sucrose intake is for the *school principal or superintendent* to remove all vending machines that dispense candy and junk foods and soft drinks.

Essentially, *the income from these machines uses the teeth of the children to subsidize nonbudgeted school expenses*.[49] Many schools have removed these kinds of machines or have substituted more nutritional snacks, including milk, fruit, and juices. Still, these machines remain a problem because selling sweets provides a major income for most schools in the United States. Recent evidence suggests that the consumption of fruits and vegetables may provide a protective effect against oral cancers (like several other cancers) and heart disease.[50] Further, several very successful 5-DAY programs have been initiated and evaluated.[50] These school-based programs are designed to increase student consumption of fruits and vegetables to at least five-a-day. Dietitians and school administrators can act as gatekeepers to better student health by exercising control of the menu and the items in the vending machines respectively.

## Preventing Gingivitis

### Classroom Toothbrushing

Thorough mechanical plaque removal on a routine basis will essentially *prevent and reverse gingivitis*. Thus, it is important for children and youth to know how to remove plaque using a toothbrush and dental floss without injuring their soft tissues. For some children daily toothbrushing in the classroom may be both needed and desirable; but, in most cases, *it is impractical*. Despite the need for emphasis on toothbrushing, some basic problems arise. Many teachers are willing to teach the mechanics of toothbrushing so long as they do not have to demonstrate the unfamiliar details of plaque control. In fact, the issue of toothbrushing is often played down since too-frequent repetition can be considered boring by students.[51]

Other than preschool teachers, very few teachers are willing to incorporate daily toothbrushing into their classroom schedule. The daily need for hygienic storage and continued replacement of worn-out and lost brushes also poses problems for a teacher. Unless replace-

ment toothbrushes are made available to the children without cost, dedicating classroom time for activities in which several students may not benefit due to economic or other factors is resisted. Finally, few classrooms have the water supply and the sinks necessary for conveniently scheduling daily brushing as a classroom activity.

Despite these problems, some classroom brushing programs have been a success. (See Appendix 19–3 for a suggested method of teaching toothbrushing.) Although little or no evidence supports toothbrushing *alone* as a means of preventing caries, *overwhelming evidence supports the fact that toothbrushing with a fluoride dentifrice is beneficial.* Thus, one objective of toothbrush instruction is to encourage children to use a fluoride dentifrice when brushing teeth and not simply to teach toothbrushing as an exercise.

Some volunteers go into schools to teach plaque removal without providing toothbrushes and toothpaste for the students to practice. This approach, while well intended, may send very poor messages, especially among lower socioeconomic children who cannot afford toothbrushes and toothpaste. That is, the importance of this procedure will be lost if the child does not own a toothbrush. If toothbrushing instructions are provided in a classroom, *it is critical not only to demonstrate proper procedure but also to provide brushes and toothpaste so that students can be observed practicing to help correct inappropriate methods.*

---

## Question 3

Which of the following questions, if any, are correct?

A. Topical fluorides can only be applied by a dentist or dental hygienist.

B. Sealants are most effective in preventing bicuspid and molar *occlusal* surface caries.

C. Sugar is the prime source of energy for cariogenic bacteria.

D. Daily toothbrushing in the classroom is *not* practical.

E. Toothbrushing alone does not significantly reduce the risk of caries; however, there is overwhelming evidence that brushing with a fluoride dentifrice does reduce caries incidence.

---

### Oral-Cancer Prevention and Early Detection

The use of tobacco products and alcohol can be found among U.S. students as young as 8 or 9 years of age.[52] Recently there has been an increase in use of cigarettes and "spit" tobacco products among youths. Both females and males tend to smoke while the use of smokeless tobacco products is used primarily by males. Young white females smoke more than young black females, often as a means of weight control.[53-55] Intervention programs, therefore, need to be implemented at *early grade levels* and supportive regulations must be in place throughout all schools. That is, *all schools should be smoke- and drug-free.* Use of tobacco products should not be allowed on school premises or at any school events. Further, state and local regulations regarding the sale of tobacco products or alcohol to minors should be strongly enforced by all communities.[9,54]

Students must be taught about the risk factors for and signs and symptoms of oral cancers (Table 19–1, 19–2). Also, they need to know that an oral cancer examination exists and that they should have the exam if they smoke or chew tobacco or consume alcohol. In addition, students should be taught how to look in their own mouths for abnormal lesions, especially if they are at high risk. *Any oral or facial lesion that does not heal within 2 weeks should be seen by a health professional.*[56]

#### Tobacco Avoidance and Cessation

Tobacco use interventions—avoidance, refusal skills, and cessation—must be included in the curriculum of any comprehensive school-based oral-health program. Experimentation with

**TABLE 19-1  Possible Signs and Symptoms of Oral and Pharyngeal Cancers**

- Red or white patch in the mouth
- A sore or lump
- Hoarseness or a feeling that something is caught in the throat
- Difficulty chewing or swallowing
- Difficulty moving the jaw or tongue
- Numbness of the tongue or other areas of the mouth

**TABLE 19-2  Risk Factors for Oral and Pharyngeal Cancers**

- All tobacco products
- Heavy Use of alcohol
- Certain viruses
- Low consumption of fruit and vegetables
- Marijuana
- Age
- Race/ethnicity
- Gender

smoking is occurring at earlier ages than ever; most users begin experimentation prior to adolescence.[6] Approximately 6,000 children and youth initiate smoking each day. Thirty thousand new cases of oral cancer are reported annually, with 8,000 people dying prematurely each year. People who use tobacco—smoke or smokeless—are at *several times greater risk* for oral cancers than are nonusers.[5,56]

*The Healthy People 2010* objectives, 27-2, 27-3, 27-4, 27-7, and 27-11 (Appendix 19–1) address *youth and tobacco*. To respond to these objectives, school-based programs in elementary, junior, and senior high schools must include smoking and smokeless tobacco use interventions and provide students with tobacco-free environments.

A recent Surgeon General's Report states that educational strategies, conducted in conjunction with community- and media-based activities, can postpone or prevent smoking onset in 20 to 40% of adolescents.[4] This information is particularly important given the current decreasing age of smoking initiation especially among young girls. By delaying the onset of smoking, school programs have the potential to (1) prevent some students from ever starting; (2) reduce the possibility that young students will become regular adult users; and (3) make it easier for those who do start tobacco use to stop. These same principles that apply to smoking *also can be applied to "spit" tobacco* intervention programs. The National Institute of Dental and Craniofacial Research and the National

Cancer Institute have produced a guide for quitting spit tobacco (Figure 19–4).

Curriculum content must receive significant attention. Ideally, the topics of smoking and use of "spit" tobacco should be introduced in *primary school* with continuing reinforcement through middle or junior high school with *major reinforcement sessions in senior high school*. Tobacco subject matter may be integrated into preexisting curriculum units on drug abuse prevention and/or incorporated into health or physical education classes. *Coaches can be very influential* in persuading school athletes to cease use of tobacco of any kind as part of their training program.

Another pivotal ingredient for success is inclusion of content on *refusal skills*. Children and youth must be taught how to resist peer and media pressure by developing decision-making and problem-solving skills that facilitate refusal of undesirable habits and influences.[57] Children and youths also must be taught to realize that tobacco use is *not the norm* and has both immediate and long-range adverse physical and aesthetic effects.

A strong supportive network among students, parents, and teachers promotes program success. Student involvement is paramount. Although a teacher, health educator, or school nurse should lead sessions, students can assist in program delivery. Student role-playing and modeling exercises enhance student participation. Parental support is another critical component; the parental values opposing tobacco

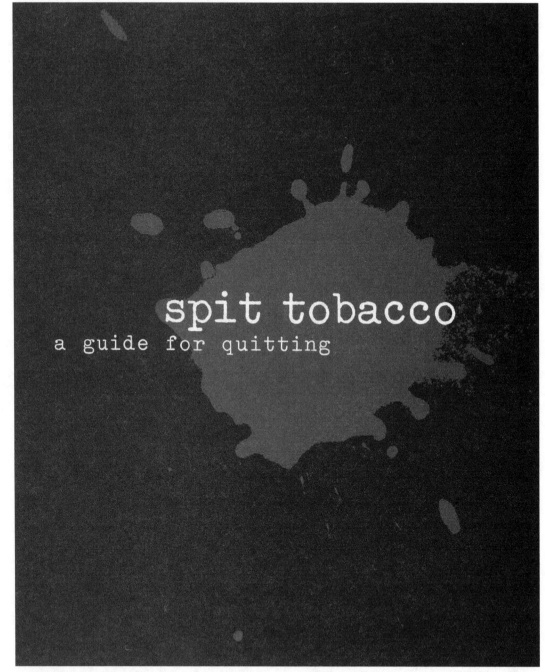

FIGURE 19-4    Spit tobacco a guide for quitting is available from the NIDCR (1NOHIC Way, Bethesda, MD 20892-3500).

use and favoring antiuse programs enhance program credibility.[58] Finally, teachers, health educators, or school nurses must be properly trained and committed to the program.

Examples of successful programs are mentioned briefly to provide guidance to future program planners.

Frequently smoking and "spit" tobacco use is related in a positive way to star athletes who often serve as role models to adolescent males.[59] Appropriately, in 1993, major league baseball's executive council, the governing body of the sport, announced an on-the-field ban of all tobacco products for every uniformed employee of minor league baseball. Under this policy, use of tobacco products of any kind is not permitted in any team area. Violators are subject to fines ranging from $100 to $300 and face game ejections.[59] Unfortunately, this ban does not extend to the major league level of the sport. The urgent need for establishing effective tobacco avoidance and cessation programs early is iterated by Glynn: *"Today, as in every other day of the year, more than 3,000 adolescents will smoke their first cigarette on the way to regular smoking. During their lifetime, it can be expected that of these 3,000 children, about 23 will be murdered, 30 will die in traffic accidents, and nearly 750 will be killed by smoking-related disease."*[60]

An outstanding article has been published that lends even greater *urgency* to achieving smoking avoidance and cessation by relating adverse changing in the body's immune system caused by smoking, to the onset, severity, and treatment of periodontitis (see also Chapter 13).[61]

## Preventive Dentistry in Sports

Sports are an important morale ingredient for both student athletes and the student body. During the 1989 to 1990 school year, in grades 9 through 11, the Ohio High School Athletic Association, which is the governing body for high school athletes in the state, listed 167,000 boys and 9,200 girls as competing in organized athletics with tournament play.[62] In many of the sports, the oral structures of these athletes are highly vulnerable to damage. The causative agents might be a hockey puck or a baseball speeding at 70 to 90 mph; a bone-crunching tackle or a thrown baseball bat; or an elbow following a spectacular basketball slam dunk. Yet, in a recent survey, results indicated that football was the only sport in which the majority of youth used mouthguards and headgear.[63]

In each session of competition, athletes face a 10% chance of orofacial injury, and a 33 to 56% possibility over a playing career. Protective equipment, rules, and regulations have been developed to reduce this toll. For instance, prototype leather football helmets with padding came into general use in the beginning of the 20th century, although were not required until 1939. By the 1950s, leather helmets had been replaced by a more protective hard plastic. Helmets protect the cranium and the ears, however, more than the lower face and mouth.

In 1960, the American Dental Association and the American Association of Physical Education issued a report that highlighted the fact that when high school players *did not* wear mouthguards *50% of all football injuries occurred in and around the mouth.*[64] The ADA House of Delegates soon passed a resolution urging that all athletes participating in contact sports wear intraoral mouthguards. This objective came to fruition in 1962, when several sports organizations mandated the use of mouthguards. It is estimated that as a result, from *100,000 to 200,000 oral injuries to football players are prevented annually.*[64]

Football is *not the only school sport* for which orofacial protection is needed. At the amateur level, sports that now mandate the use of mouthguards during practice sessions and in games are *boxing, football, ice hockey, lacrosse, and field hockey.* It is interesting that the Academy of Sports Dentistry has listed 40 different sports, including soccer, bicycling, skate boarding, and basketball in which cranial or orofacial protection should be considered.[64]

A mouthguard is constructed of soft plastic that is placed between the maxillary and

mandibular dentitions. These devices help to prevent violent contact between the lips, cheeks, and teeth, and between the upper and lower teeth. It reduces the possibility of fractured jaws as well as lessening the likelihood of neck injuries, concussion, cerebral hemorrhage, unconsciousness, serious central nerve damage, and death. Although 87% of Division I colleges have team dentists, it is the *team trainer* that usually selects the mouthguards.[65]

In football, for example, prior to a game, it is the responsibility of game officials to check with coaches to ensure that players are using required protective equipment.[65] When mouthguards and other protective equipment are not worn, penalties are levied, ranging from a reduction in the number of time outs to 5-yard penalties. It is the quarterbacks who are least compliant.[65] In the past decade, the thrust for protective equipment has been emphasized in an effort to reduce the possibility of *bleeding injuries*. In some states, any bleeding injuries are cause for officials to remove a player from the game due to the increased possibility of transmitting HIV.

When a mouthguard is not worn or fails, one of the most frequent orofacial injuries requiring emergency treatment by the dentist is the *avulsion of teeth*. Maxillary teeth are the most vulnerable. When avulsion occurs, a recovered tooth should be held by the crown to rinse and then *gently replaced at the site of origin*. If the tooth cannot be easily reinserted, it should not be allowed to dry. Milk is a good transport solution on the way for emergency treatment at a dental office. After replacement, a minimum 7- to 10-day splinting period is advised. All avulsed teeth with fully formed roots *eventually need endodontic treatment*.[66]

---

**Question 4**

Which of the following statements, if any, are correct?

A. The best grade level to introduce discussion of the health dangers of to-bacco smoking, cessation, and avoidance is in *senior high school*.

B. The on-the-diamond use of tobacco products (especially chewing tobacco) by *minor league* baseball players provides a role model for aspiring high school athletes.

C. More people die from tobacco-associated diseases in the United States than from violent crimes and traffic accidents.

D. Five organized amateur sports that mandate the use of helmets during practice and games are football, boxing, ice hockey, field hockey, and lacrosse.

E. Mouthguards are more important than helmets in preventing avulsion of teeth.

---

Equally or more important to prevent serious facial injuries is that the use of seat belts should be strongly advocated across all age groups but perhaps especially among youths who tend to believe they are not vulnerable. Car accidents involving youths frequently result in orofacial, head, and neck injuries, which could be *reduced with* the appropriate use of seat belts.

## Oral-Health-Programs for Preschool-Age Children

In 1965, Head Start, a national preschool program that provides early learning opportunities to poor and underprivileged children, was initiated under the Economic Opportunity Act of 1964. Health care and health education, including a dental component, have been a continual part of this program. The dental care component includes *annual examinations, preventive services, follow-up care, and classroom instruction*. Yet after four decades of existence, there is evidence that many Head Start centers *do not* comply uniformly with the U.S. Public Health Service Standards. As it now functions, Head Start is meeting the needs of *only a frac-*

*tion* of the eligible population.[67,68] However, some states have excellent Head Start oral health programs.

Today many other private and public preschool programs exist, with the number expected to increase dramatically if a national day care policy is established. The great majority of preschool programs will be under the auspices of private individuals or organizations with limited expertise in health education, specifically in oral health objectives and preventive practices.

Academically, preschool programs must include objectives, lesson plans, and the evaluation instruments needed to measure objective attainment. Even at preschool age, the important preventive dentistry related words, concepts, and skills can be introduced to young children to be reinforced later at higher grades. At preschool age, children are *especially eager to learn* and participate. Unlike most public schools, Head Start centers usually provide toothbrushes and toothpaste and the time to use both. Some Head Start programs that are located in communities without optimally fluoridated water also offer fluoride tablet programs.

Bright Futures is a health education innovation developed by the U.S. Department of Health and Human Services whose mission is to promote and improve the health, education, and well-being of children, families, and communities.[69] It offers expert guidance for providing health services to children and their families. This project includes an excellent section on oral health entitled, Bright Futures in Practice: Oral Health.[70]

## Helping Teachers Teach

In a school curriculum, teaching mathematics becomes more sophisticated as a child progresses from grade-to-grade. In first grade, the child is taught to add 1 and 1; yet at the high-school level the young adult is able to perform problems of calculus. In many courses, such as chemistry, the didactic information is reinforced by laboratory assignments; the combination of information and experience helps develop student understanding and motor skills. This same approach could be used to teach oral health. Oral-health programs should be planned so that each higher-grade level receives a greater diversity and complexity of subject matter and practical experience. For example, elementary schoolchildren have less dexterity than junior-high students. Flossing, therefore, is more easily taught and practiced in the upper grades.

At the high-school level, students should have an advanced lay knowledge of terminology, anatomy, and functions of the oral cavity and the etiology and consequences of oral diseases. They also should have the understanding to accept responsibility for (1) preventing and controlling oral diseases, (2) identifying the presence of their own oral diseases at an early stage, and (3) seeking treatment once oral disease is suspected or identified. In other words, *students should be taught to open their eyes when they open their mouths in front of a mirror.*

### The Tattletooth II Integrated Program

To construct an integrated curriculum for oral health that is applicable to a continuum of grade levels, it is first necessary to consider what information is relevant for each grade level. One example of a comprehensive grade-to-grade program developed for teaching dental health is exemplified by *Tattletooth II, A New Generation program, developed by the Texas Department of Health.*

This comprehensive oral health curriculum targets students from *preschool through grade 12.* In 1993, with funds appropriated by the state legislature, the Texas Bureau of Dental Health Services employed approximately 20 dental hygienists and dental assistants to promote the program statewide. Annually, thousands of children are served by this program with aid from the Texas Dental Hygienists' Association.

Each grade level has five core lessons and two enrichment lessons. Background informa-

tion *for the teacher* is provided as part of the lesson. Educational strategies are described for integrating oral health topics into discussions involving other subjects, such as languages, arts, mathematics, and science activities. To facilitate bilingual education, the program has been translated into Spanish.

In addition, the curriculum includes scope and sequence charts, a unit test, bulletin board suggestions, audiovisual lists, and suggested letters to be sent to parents. A videotape illustrating the appropriate techniques of brushing and flossing is available on loan to schools. The curriculum and training materials were designed, tested, evaluated, retested, reevaluated, and again revised. This program *matches subject matter with grade level*, provides teachers with guidance information, and is available in two languages to target major minority groups of the state. To obtain the program for their classroom, teachers must attend in-service training provided by a state regional dental hygienist who uses a multimedia approach in the training sessions. The program is copyrighted; however, *out-of-state educators may secure it gratis and reproduce it at their own expense*. Because the program has been in use for some time and still is, some of it will be replaced over the next few years with newer materials.

## Putting it all Together— Comprehensive Oral Health Programs

Treatment is not the answer to solving children's oral health problems; rather *primary prevention is the key*. From an economic viewpoint, there is little rationale for treating a disease at great expense, when the disease can be prevented at a much lesser cost. From a humane viewpoint, there is even less reason not to develop strong preventive programs supported with treatment programs when prevention fails. Research has shown that incipient dental caries can be largely controlled by techniques now available, such as *sealant placement and*

*remineralization therapy*—techniques that are little publicized and underused by the profession.[71] *Gingivitis also can be controlled by a combination of oral hygiene practices—prophylaxis, chemical, and manual plaque control.*

Many states and communities are focusing on how millions of underprivileged children can be provided with health care. As a keystone of this effort, care must be *acceptable, equitable, affordable, and accessible to all*. It is critical that the dental profession, health educators, and public health agencies take the steps necessary to ensure that oral health is represented in the planning and implementation of such national efforts. *State dental directors must play a major role in ensuring that dentistry's share of funds will be available*. Unfortunately, some states currently do not have state dental directors, and do not intend to fill these positions. At the same time some preventive activities have been curtailed or eliminated.[71]

There are several advantages to a comprehensive, school-based program: (1) students are available for preventive or treatment procedures; (2) school-based clinics may be less threatening than private offices; (3) school dental programs facilitate and increase the effectiveness of teaching oral health subjects; and (4) dental services supplement the school nursing services by providing total health care for schoolchildren.

A combined education, promotion, and preventive program in the school would greatly reduce the amount of classroom time lost in traveling to a treatment facility. Comprehensive school programs also would obviate the loss of study time due to pain and apprehension before and after treatment. This lost time can be considerable; for example, children missed more than 51 million hours of school in 1989 because of acute dental problems.[1] Combined school-based educational and preventive dentistry programs for all schools should be feasible and cost-effective in terms of staffing, money, and material. Most important, with comprehensive school programs the decayed, missing,

and filled teeth (DMFT) of students *should demonstrate a substantial and steady decrease over time*. A few of these kinds of programs have been established. Others could be established at different levels, depending on available funds as described below and shown in Appendix 19–4.

## Level 1

Level 1 should include the use of a comprehensive oral-health curriculum such as the *Tattletooth II program*. Providing such a curriculum minimizes the need for teachers or health educators to locate and organize lessons in an unfamiliar field. In addition, *the teacher with the help of a school nurse and or adult volunteer* can conduct weekly fluoride mouth rinses or administer daily fluoride tablet regimens. The nurse might be responsible for preparing the mouth rinses or making the tablets available on a schedule approved by the teachers. *Health educators*, if available, help coordinate and integrate all health education activities. They have extensive training in educational principles and health and are accustomed to working with school faculty. Fluoride mouth rinse or fluoride tablet regimens are easy to accomplish, economical, and effective. Table 19–3 compares the two school-based fluoride regimens. *Neither of these self-applied, school-based fluoride regimens should be used if community or school water fluoridation is available.*

### School Water Fluoridation

Fluoridating a school's water supply is similar to community water fluoridation in that *no direct action is needed by individuals to accrue its benefits* other than consuming the water or foods prepared with it. School water fluoridation is used only when the school has an independent water supply, usually in consolidated rural schools. Consolidated rural schools are ideal for this approach because all grades from kindergarten through 12 are housed in the same complex using one water source. In the past, this preventive measure was used in over 600 U.S. schools in many states. Today, the need for this preventive measure has diminished both because the water supplies of many rural schools have been incorporated into major community water systems that are optimally fluoridated and because there are numerous other sources of fluoride available including dentifrices and mouth rinses. The recommended concentration of fluoride for school water supplies is 4.5 ppm.[72] School water fluoridation was developed

---

TABLE 19-3 **Comparison of School-based Self-applied Fluoride Regimens**

| Fluoride Mouth Rinse | Fluoride Tablets[a] |
| --- | --- |
| Safe and effective | Safe and effective |
| Inexpensive | Inexpensive |
| Easy to learn and do | Easy to learn and do |
| Nondental personnel can supervise | Nondental personnel can supervise |
| Well accepted by participants | Well accepted by participants |
| Little time required—5 minutes weekly | Little time required—3 minutes daily |
| Provides topical benefits | Provides systemic and topical benefits |
| Waste materials need to be deposed | No waste materials |
|  | Suitable for preschool-age children |

[a]Provide to only those children whose drinking water is fluoride-deficient. (Modified from Horowitz AM. Community-oriented preventive dentistry programs that work. Health Values. 8(1):21–29.)

and tested in the United States in the 1950s and 1960s. Researchers found up to a 40 percent reduction in dental caries after 12 years. Installation costs are relatively expensive and workers must be trained to operate, monitor, and maintain the fluoridation unit.

### Dietary Fluoride Tablets

The use of fluoride tablets in schools is a method of administering systemic fluoride to children. This self-applied fluoride regimen is for use *only* in communities in which the water supply is fluoride-deficient and *has been used in the United States and abroad for over 40 years.*[47] All children who participate in self-applied fluoride programs must have parental consent. Usually, a classroom teacher who has been trained to supervise the procedure first dispenses the fluoride tablets to participating students. Students are then instructed to put the tablet in their mouth and to chew it for 30 seconds; the resultant solution is then vigorously swished between their teeth for another 30 seconds before the participants are told to swallow the solution. Using this approach, *both systemic and topical benefits* will accrue. The procedure is easy to perform, requires little time, and there are no waste products to dispose of. Studies conducted in the United States show that school-based fluoride tablet programs provide about a *20 to 30% reduction* in new caries lesions. A daily fluoride tablet appears to be *more effective* than a weekly mouth rinse, as well as being preferred by teachers.[73] The major drawback is that it is a daily procedure and some teachers object to it for this reason.

It is important to note that caries preventive effects of school fluoride regimens may not be permanent. After an 11-year follow-up study in Norway, it was concluded that the residual benefits of school-based fluoride programs decrease as the length of time between previous participation and follow-up increases.[74] It should be pointed out, that students should be educated to use a fluoride containing dentifrice during and following the school-based fluoride regimens. In contrast, Kobayashi and coworkers found good post treatment benefits after 11 years.[75]

### Fluoride Mouth Rinsing

Fluoride mouth-rinsing programs are *the most widely used* school-based fluoride regimen in the United States and usually are *supervised by classroom teachers* or other adult volunteers. Caries reductions range from *20 to 25%*, although few recent studies have been conducted.[76] Fluoride mouth rinse regimens as originally conceived consisted of mixing a preweighed packet of fluoride powder with a specified amount of water in a container with a plastic pump calibrated to dispense 5 or 10 mL of solution that would yield a 0.2 percent neutral sodium fluoride rinse. After mixing, the solution is dispensed into paper cups for use by the students. Today, most schools order premixed solutions that come in individual containers. This latter approach is somewhat more expensive but it simplifies the procedure for use in classrooms. Using premixed solutions *reduces the time required* of paid or volunteer staff to simply dispensing a container and napkin to each student and then supervising the rinse procedure. Students are requested to put the solution in their mouth and to rinse vigorously for 60 seconds (Figure 19–5). When instructed, students are asked to empty the contents of their mouth back into the cups and blot their lips with the napkin. The waste products are then put into a plastic bag for disposal. Fluoride mouth rinse used in schools is available in either a flavored or nonflavored and sweetened or nonsweetened varieties. Generally, this procedure is *not recommended for children before first grade* unless extensive training is conducted with the children to ensure that they do not swallow the contents of the cup. The weekly solution, if swallowed over time may contribute to fluorosis among children 6 years of age or younger because some of their permanent teeth are still developing. (See Appendix 19–5 for details on conducting a mouthrinse program.)

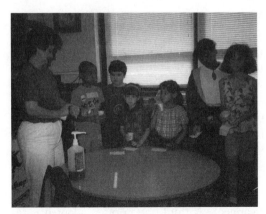

FIGURE 19-5    Students rinsing 60 seconds with fluoride under supervision of their teacher.

## Level 2

Level-2 programs *include level-1 activities plus the addition of a dental hygienist* to the school health staff. The inclusion of a dental hygienist in a comprehensive school health program is critical. A dental hygienist is educated to plan and participate in school programs that include oral prophylaxes, use of a variety of methods of fluoride application to foster remineralization, teaching oral hygiene procedures, counseling on diet, placement of pit-and-fissure sealants, and screening and referral for suspected oral pathology for definitive diagnosis and treatment. A dental hygienist also serves as a school-resource person.

Many school districts or public-health agencies have dental trailers that are *used to provide prophylaxis and screening programs* for students. Others use portable equipment that is set up in a room designated by school authorities. Older, *teenaged students are more likely to present with gingivitis and calculus.* A periodic prophylaxis by a dental hygienist during the school years may help avoid the onset of periodontitis later on. In addition, the personal contact with a dental hygienist can help motivate teenagers to develop satisfactory plaque removal techniques

and to understand the need to seek professional care when needed.

Dental trailers also may be used by hygienists *for placement of dental sealants.* Dental sealants are highly effective in protecting occlusal surfaces and lingual and buccal pits and fissures—sites where *up to 90% of all caries lesions occur.* In the 1988 to 1991 Third National Health and Examination Survey, phase 1 (NHANES III), *less than 19% of U.S. children and adolescents between 5 and 17 years of age had one or more sealants placed.*[76] In contrast, in Finland, so many of the occlusal surfaces are covered with sealant that these surfaces are often excluded in decayed, missing, and filled surfaces (DMFS) studies.[77]

The marked benefit of sealant placement in reducing caries incidence was reported by Sterritt and Frew in a study conducted in Guam.[78] Some 75,000 teeth of 15,000 children in grades 1 through 8 were sealed by *17 preventive dentistry technicians.* In a period of 2 years the average number of carious lesions per child *dropped from 5.35 to 2.92.* The first year retention rate for the self-curing sealant was 94% for first molars, 97% for premolars, and 75% for second molars. In one state program, it was demonstrated that, dental sealants reduced oral health disparities among school-aged children.[79] Sealant placement, when coupled with a *follow-up gel application of fluoride* helps provide protection to the *whole tooth.*[80] Ripa and colleagues have correctly pointed out that the combined use of sealants and exposure to a fluoride regimen in school *can result in a virtual elimination of dental decay in elementary school-children.*[81]

Cost per child for sealant placement varies depending on whether dentists, dental hygienists, or dental assistants are used. A 1989 estimated cost for sealants ranged from $13.07 to $28.37.[71] In contrast, the restoration of an occlusal lesion averages about $51.00.[82] Most important, it must be recognized that once a restoration is placed it will continue to need to be replaced which further weakens and com-

promises the tooth because the restoration becomes larger at each replacement.

A guide, "Seal America: The Prevention Invention," has been developed for purchase at a nominal fee. It was supported by the Maternal and Child Health Bureau of the Health Resources and Services Administration. The kit was designed for use in developing and implementing dental sealant programs in communities.

## Level 3

A level-3 program consists of all of levels 1 and 2 requirements plus the addition of a treatment delivery option. This level of a comprehensive school oral health program includes the ability to identify and refer all pathology for treatment as early as possible. To achieve this level, an annual screening is indicated for all children and a semiannual screening for children classified as high risk.

State practice acts permitting, *triage* with possible *referral* to a treatment facility can be accomplished by a dental hygienist.[83] During routine prophylaxis procedures and sealant placement, a dental hygienist can identify early pathology and refer the student for expeditious definitive diagnosis and treatment.

All too often, the present method of managing schoolchildren with oral problems is for the teacher or school nurse to send home a note indicating a need for treatment and recommending that a child be taken to a dentist. This approach *assumes* that the parent immediately seeks a private dentist or goes to a public-health clinic. In turn, it is *assumed* that when the dentist completes treatment, a postcard is returned to the school hygienist or nurse indicating that the referred pathology has been treated. Theoretically, this type of system has the advantage that it uses the professional delivery systems existing in the student's community. Unfortunately it does not always work. Not all parents respond positively because of lack of money or insurance, apathy, or lack of available time to take the child to a dentist. This formula of "no money, no priority, no dentist, equals no care" is an elementary equation repeated countless times each year in our schools.[84]

Another option for referral involves *contracting with local practitioners* to offer specific procedures for predetermined fees. In this case, the referral can be a direct transaction between the school system and dentist(s). The bill submitted by the dentist for completed work constitutes verification that the child received treatment. A third option often adopted is to *bus children to a public health clinic*. Or, in some communities dental societies have organized their dentists to volunteer to treat needy students.

The objective of whatever level of preventive care program is selected is that it be affordable, and accessible to all—*with a priority for high-risk students. Once the primary preventive dentistry procedures have reduced the incidence of oral disease to that of the annual treatment workload, the number of extractions for a school population should approach zero.*

## Foreign School-Based Programs

Sometimes we can learn other approaches to solving similar problems by looking at models in other countries. For example, the New Zealand School Dental Service reads like an exemplary level-3 program. It is *accessible* to all, being based in the schools, *equitable*, with all children being able to enroll, *affordable* because there is no charge for service, and *acceptable*, with 96% of the pupils being enrolled. The Service was formed in 1921 as a result of pressure on the government *by the dental profession* to help cope with the poor state of children's teeth. Originally, young women were trained to accomplish fillings and simple extractions. Today, both men and women are trained as dental therapists who can practice *only in state institutions*. They are not licensed for private practice. Supervision is

provided by public health service officers and senior dental nurses. The Service is based in clinics located in larger schools and takes care of all preschool, primary, and intermediate students between ages 5 and 13.

Children are examined annually, although those considered at *high risk are examined semi-annually*. The guidelines for high risk are:

1. Over 6 and under 9 years of age—Four or more deciduous teeth with full occlusal or compound fillings or new carious lesions other than buccal or lingual pits in permanent or deciduous teeth.

2. Over 9 years of age (permanent teeth only)—A full occlusal restoration or carious lesion on a first permanent molar, an interproximal cavity before age 9, or a new lesion in the previous 12 months other than a buccal or lingual pit.

The preventive program *focuses on high-risk children*. A 0.2 percent fluoride mouth rinse is used to prevent demineralization of "white spots," while fluoride varnish (Duraphat) is used for remineralization therapy of interproximal, enamel-limited lucencies. Finally, *fissure sealants are placed on all newly erupted vulnerable permanent molars to prevent occlusal caries*. This preventive emphasis and available treatment has resulted in a *drop* of DMFT of 10.7 in 1973 to 1.88 in 1992 (Figure 19–6), and a parallel drop in extractions from 18.20 per 100 in 1966, to 4.00 in 1992.[85]

Denmark also has an excellent and comprehensive school-based oral health care program.

There has been a long tradition of providing oral health care to Danish children, in fact the first school dental clinic was established in 1909. The Child Oral Health Care Act of 1971 is the basis upon which the current Danish child oral health care service was established. Essentially, this legislation mandated communities to provide free dental care for children 6 to 16 years of age. The process was an incremental one with emphasis on primary prevention and oral health education of all parties. Concomitantly, national epidemiologic data was established and maintained, which has provided the scientific evidence of the successful reduction of dental caries among Danish children between 1972 and 1992. In 1986, a new national law was introduced to replace the 1971 Act. The long-range goal of the revised national law was stated as: "The goal of the dental service is for the population to obtain healthy teeth, mouth and jaws, and to preserve them, in functional condition throughout life; this should be accomplished through a sufficient home dental care regimen, and a comprehensive preventive and curative dental health service." A major change in the 1972 Act was to include *all* children 16 years of age and younger. Again, the emphasis was on the use of fluorides, dental sealants, at least annual examinations and extensive educational interventions. Preventive regimens have been modified as new research has become available. The treatment of oral diseases and malocclusion also was included in the new legislation and by 1987 the system included all children. The law

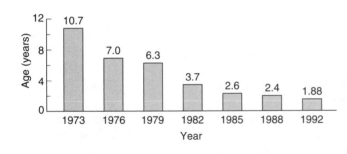

FIGURE 19–6    New Zealand Dental Service. Average DMF, ages 12-14 years, 1973-1991. Caries in permanent teeth has declined 78% in 18 years. (From internal data of the Department of Health, New Zealand, generated from annual returns prepared by principal dental officers.)

mandates oral health education for all children, parents and teachers. Education in schools is a part of the regular curriculum and, thus, is adjusted for age appropriateness and at the same time to maintain interest. Oral health instruction also is provided to gravid women and oral health instruction is included in home visits for newborn and young children. Older children are taught how to make dental appointments so that they can continue their oral health care as adults. The dental teams who provide these services include dentists, dental hygienists and dental assistants. Danish school children enjoy one of the lowest caries prevalence in the world.[86]

---

### Question 5

Which of the following statements, if any, are correct?

A. Preventive care for all Head Start children is authorized; as a result, preventive services are now provided to the *majority* of Head Start children.

B. Both incipient caries and gingivitis can usually be *prevented, arrested, or reversed.*

C. No fluoride tablet program should be conducted in a school serviced by a water system containing optimally fluoridated water.

D. Levels 1, 2, and 3 school oral-health programs provide highly effective dental care options ranging from education–prevention to education–prevention–treatment.

E. An abrupt drop in occlusal caries incidence can be detected *within a year* after the initiation of an occlusal sealant program.

---

### Research and Evaluation

There are approximately 48 million students in 110,000 elementary schools in the United States.[87] Many of these children currently benefit from preventive regimens previously described and supported by research. Many other children are not so fortunate, especially children from poor families. Research is needed to evaluate the success of currently used *programs* as well as the *feasibility* and *cost-effectiveness of future strategies* to promote oral health education, prevention, and treatment. Today, there is a need for research and evaluation on the best approaches to promoting oral health in schools with a focus on school-based clinics. The primary objective of such research programs must focus on the 3 M's—*manpower, money,* and *material,* plus the *amount of classroom* time it will take from conventional classroom education.

To improve cost-effectiveness and oral health for all, there is a need to develop *validated techniques to identify high-risk students* for both dental caries and gingivitis. To secure such information, research and evaluation is necessary. Finally, the use of *standardized methods of recording data including the use of computerized recording* is necessary to permit a comparison of data from studies to accelerate administrative decisions.

---

# SUMMARY

A large segment of our children and adolescents are at risk for dropping out of school before completing high school as a result of a wide range of health, economic, and behavioral problems. Moreover, a large proportion of our school-age children *do not have access to basic preventive and primary dental and medical care.* With the challenges posed by overwhelming need and limited resources, children deserve to receive information and

education that enables them to make informed choices about their health. Also, they deserve the opportunity to learn skills and develop attitudes that enable them to practice appropriate behaviors to enhance their oral and general health. Finally, they deserve to receive services that prevent and/or treat oral diseases. We have the ability to essentially eliminate most oral diseases among children. Less obvious are the *political and administrative means* needed to make these cost-efficient measures available to the children. School-based oral-health education and promotion programs give children and adolescents a chance to learn about their oral tissues in health and disease. Comprehensive, school-based oral-health prevention and treatment programs provide a means not only to learn about disease, but also to maintain the health of the oral tissues and structures. Dentists, dental hygienists, and students of each discipline have an opportunity and the responsibility to help make such comprehensive programs available.

The major successes of school-based oral-health programs have been achieved when education has been combined with active prevention and/or treatment programs.

Unfortunately, too few schools have routinely included active preventive dentistry regimens—fluoride mouth rinses and tablet programs, sealant applications, remineralization therapy, and a strong emphasis on the use of fluoride-containing dentifrices while brushing—*all of which can reduce the DMFS of a school population.* This reduction can be accomplished with only a minimal change in self-behavior or compliance required of the student. A few school systems have employed dental hygienists as resource personnel to aid in the teaching programs and/or to provide primary preventive services. The availability of a dental hygienist provides an effective and economic means for schools to plan and participate in higher-level preventive programs. Hygienists can function on the school staff as *oral-health educators, conduct preventive programs, accomplish triage, and arrange for referral and follow up to ensure completeness of treatment.*

The ubiquitous availability of sucrose-laden desserts and snacks can best be controlled by the school dietitian *reducing the availability and frequency of foods and desserts with high sugar content.* The school administrator also can aid in the objective by prohibiting the on-campus placement of vending machines to dispense high-sucrose snacks.

Protecting the oral health of future generations is a commitment that must be shared by parents, teachers, school administrators, and all health professionals. This shared responsibility is especially relevant now that national health objectives for total child health care are established. *Possibly the time is propitious to think in terms of a national school oral health policy*—one that endorses universal access to oral-health education, health promotion, preventive regimens, triage, and treatment referral capabilities for discerned pathology.

As a final note, if oral-health promotion is to be accomplished through the school systems, it must be integrated with the general medical health program. In order not to detract from the teaching of the classic academic curriculum, the school year must be lengthened proportionate to the increased time demands of promoting health, and the school system's budget must be increased in order to meet the requirements for additional facilities, manpower, and materials.

# ANSWERS AND EXPLANATIONS

1. A, D, and E—correct.

   B—incorrect. Teachers are certified by academic subject to be taught—English, mathematics, science, etc., but *definitely not* in in-depth comprehension of societal issues.

   C—incorrect. Same answer as B; teachers are not trained or certified to impart oral-health education.

2. A, D, and E—correct.

   B—incorrect. Substitute "least" for "most" and the answer becomes correct.

   C—incorrect. The 13.8 hours figure is for the *total* amount of health education; of this time, one cannot expect sufficient time will be allowed for oral health education and promotion.

3. B, C, D, and E—correct.

   A—incorrect. Every day, millions of people self-apply topical fluorides using fluoride dentifrices.

4. C, D, and E—correct.

   A—incorrect. The health dangers of tobacco should be started at the elementary school level in order to intercept the publicity and peer pressure to use cigarettes and smokeless tobacco at an early age

   B—incorrect. On-the-field minor-league baseball players and employees are not permitted to use tobacco products.

5. C, D, and E—correct.

   A—incorrect. The first part of the statement is *correct*; the second part, which is the most important, *is incorrect* and should be corrected. In other words, prevention is authorized but not implemented.

   B—incorrect. Since approximately 90% of the total lesions in the mouth occur on the occlusal surface, the reduction of caries incidence on this surface can be detected soon after the initiation of a sealant program.

## Self-Evaluation Questions

1. The expanded eight-compartment model for school health programs includes, in addition to health education, health services, and a healthy environment, at least two additional health attributes which are: _____ and _____.

2. Give five health tasks which *might* be assumed, or are assigned to a school-based health clinic: _____, _____, _____, _____, and _____.

3. It is estimated that 80% of carious lesions in a school population are found in only _____ % of the students.

4. Two nations with comprehensive school dental programs are _____ and _____.

5. The two most important explanations for the cariostatic properties of fluoride are that it inhibits _____, and equally (or more) important, facilitates _____.

6. The two most important school-system officials who are in a position to limit the ingestion of sugar-containing foods, desserts, and snacks during school hours are the _____ and the _____.

7. Give three reasons why daily classroom toothbrushing is impractical: _____, _____ , and _____.

8. Smokeless tobacco education includes: _____ techniques and _____ techniques.

9. One state school system that integrated an oral health teaching program that includes all 12 grades is the Texas _____ (name of program which may be obtained gratis by out-of-state health departments and major health providers).

10. Assuming that you are the coach, and an anterior tooth is avulsed by a hockey puck, describe how you would handle the situation _____.

11. One program that has been found to increase the number of fruits and vegetables consumed by school-aged children is the _____ program.

# REFERENCES

1. U.S. Department of Health and Human Services (2000). *Oral Health in America: A Report of the Surgeon General*. Rockville, MD: U.S. Department of Health and Human Services, National Institute of Dental and Craniofacial Research, National Institutes of Health.

2. U.S. Department of Health and Human Services (2000). *Healthy People 2010 (2nd ed.) With understanding and improving health and objectives for improving health*, 2 vols. Washington, DC:U.S. Government Printing Office.

3. Kaste, L. M., Selwitz, R. H., Oldakowski, R. J., Brunelle, J. A., Winn, D. M., & Brown, L. J. (1996). Coronal caries in the primary and permanent dentition of children and adolescents 1–17 years of age: United States, 1988–1991. *J Dent Res*, 75(Special Issue):631–41.

4. U.S. Department of Health and Human Services (2000). *Reducing tobacco use: A report of the Surgeon General*. Atlanta, Georgia: U.S. Department of Health and Human Services, Centers for Disease Control and Prevention, National Center for Chronic Disease Prevention and Health Promotion, Office on Smoking and Health.

5. Silverman, S. (1998). *Oral cancer* (4th ed). American Cancer Society. Hamilton, ON: B.C. Decker, Inc. 8–10.

6. Centers for Disease Control and Prevention (1996). Tobacco use and usual source of cigarettes among high school students—United States, 1995. *MMWR*, 45(20):413–18.

7. Gold, R. S., & Horowitz, A. M. (Oct 1993). Oral health information in textbooks. Presented at the 121st Scientific Session of the American Public Health Association. San Francisco, CA.

8. Centers for Disease Control and Prevention (2001). *Investment in tobacco control: State highlights—2001.* Atlanta, GA: U.S. Department of Health and Human Services, Centers for Disease Control and Prevention, National Center for Chronic Disease Prevention and Health Promotion. Office on Smoking and Health.

9. Centers for Disease Control and Prevention (Aug 1999). *Best practices for comprehensive tobacco control programs*—August 1999. Atlanta GA: U.S. Department of Health and Human Services, Centers for Disease Control and Prevention, National Center for Chronic Disease Prevention and Health Promotion, Office on Smoking and Health.

10. The Annie E. Casey Foundation (2001). *Kids Count Data Book*, 2001. Baltimore: The Annie E. Casey Foundation.

11. Kolbe, L. I. (1982). What can we expect from our school education? *J Sch Health*, 52:145–50.

12. Green, L. W., & Krueter, M. W. (1999). *Health promotion planning. An educational and ecological approach*, (3rd ed.) Mountain View, CA: Mayfield Publishing.

13. Frazier, P. J., & Horowitz, A. M. (1990). Oral health education and promotion in maternal and child health: A position paper. *J Public Health Dent*, 50:390–95.

14. Glanz, K., Lewis, F. M., & Rimer, B. K, Eds. (1990). *Health behavior and health education*. San Francisco: Jossey-Bass.

15. Mandel, I. D. (1996). Caries prevention: Current strategies, new directions. *J Am Dent Assoc*, 127:1477–88.

16. Lee, M. A., & Horan, S. A. (2001). Children's access to dental care in Connecticut's Medicaid managed care program. *Maternal Child Health J*, 5(1):43–51.

17. US General Accounting Office. (2000). *Oral health factors affecting the use of dental services*. GA01HEHS-00-149

18. Horowitz, A. M., & Nourjah, P. A. (1996). Factors associated with having oral cancer examinations among US adults 40 years of age or older. *J Public Health Dent*, 56:331–35.

19. Horowitz, A. M., Nourjah, P. & Gift, H. G. (1990). U.S. adult knowledge of risk factors for and signs of oral cancers: 1990. *J Am Dent Assoc*, 126:39–45.

20. Gift, H. C., Corbin, S. B., & Nowjack-Raymer, R. E. (1994). Public knowledge of prevention of dental disease. *Public Health Rep*, 109:397–404.

21. Horowitz, A. M., Moon, H. S., Goodman, H. S., & Yellowitz, J. A. (1998). Maryland adults' knowledge of oral cancer and having oral cancer examinations. *J Public Health Dent*, 58:281–87.

22. Horowitz, A. M., & Frazier, P. J. (1986). Effective oral health programs in school settings. In Clark, J., Ed. *Clinical Dentistry* (vol. 2). (pp. 1–17). Philadelphia: Harper and Row.

23. Institute of Medicine (1977). *School & Health: Our Nation's Investment*. Washington, DC: National Academy Press, 1997.

24. Feroli, K. L., Hobson, S. K., Miola, E. S., Scott, P. N., & Waterfield, G. D. (1992). School-based clinics: The Baltimore experience. *J Pediatric Health Care*, 6:127–31.

25. Stone, E. J., & Perry, C. L. (1990). United States: Perspectives in school health. *J School Health*, 60:363–69.

26. Good, M. E. (1992). The clinical nurse specialist in the school setting: Case management of migrant children with dental disease. *Clin Nurse Spec*, 6:72–76.

27. Dougherty, D., Eden, J., Kemp, K. B., et al. (1992). Adolescent health: A report to the U.S. Congress. *J School Health*, 62:167–74.

28. Morone, J. A., Kilbreth, E. H., & Langwell, K. M. (2001). Back to school: A health care strategy for youth. *Health Affairs*, 20(1):122–136.

29. Rienzo, B. A., & Button, J. W. (1993). The politics of school-based clinics: A community level analysis. *J School Health*, 63:266–72.

30. McGinnis, J. M., & De Graw, C. (1991). Healthy Schools 2000: Creating partnership for the decade. *J School Health*, 61:294–97.

31. Collins, J. L., Small, M. L., Kann, L., Pateman, B. C., Gold, R. S., Kolbe, L. J. (1995). School health education. *J School Health*, 65:302–03.

32. Burstrom, B., Haglund, B. J., Tillgren, P., Berg, L., Wallin, E., Ullen, H., Smith, C. (1995). Health promotion in schools: Policies and practices in Stockholm county, 1990. *Scand J Soc Med*, 23:39–49.

33. Auter, J. (1993). The comprehensive school health education workshop, background and future prospects. Closing session comment. *J School Health*, 63:38–39.

34. David, R. (1990). The fate of the soul and the fate of the social order: The waning spirit of American youth. *J School Health*, 60:205–7.

35. Killip, D. C., Lovick, S. R., Goldman, L., & Allensworth, D. D. (1987). Integrated school and community programs. [Review.] *J School Health*, 57:437–44.

36. http://www.healthinschools.org/

37. Dryfoos, J. G., & Klerman, L. V. (1988). School based clinics: Their roles in helping students meet the 1990 objectives. *Health Ed*, 154:71–80.

38. Palfrey, J. S., McGaughey, M. J., Cooperman, P. J., Fenton, T., McManus, M. A. (1991). Financing health services in school-based clinics. Do nontraditional programs tap traditional funding sources? *J Adolescent Health*, 1991; 12:233–39.

39. Personal communication (2001). American Dental Association, Chicago.

40. Personal communication (2001). American Dental Hygienist Association, Chicago.

41. Seffrin, J. R. (1990). The comprehensive school health curriculum: closing the gap between state-of-the-art and state-of-the-practice. *J School Health*, 60:151–56.

42. Bownian, P. A., & Zinner, K. L. (1994). Utah's parent, teacher, and physician sealant awareness surveys. *J Dent Hygiene*, 68:279–85.

43. Seffrin, J. R. (1994). *America's Interest in Comprehensive School Health Education*. A paper presented to the Second Annual School Health Leadership Conference, Atlanta. In National Health Education Standards, Achieving Health Literacy. Sponsored by American Cancer Society, 69.

44. Tonisson, C., Barenthin, T., & Sporre, D-M. (1992). Three-year follow-up study of teenagers with high risk for caries. *J Dent Res*, 71(Divisional Abstr.: 1093; Abstr. 57).

45. Horn, S. D., & Kaster, C. O. (1991). A model for a children's dental health carnival. *J Dent Child*, 58:320–27.

46. Harn, S. D., & Dunning, D. G. (1996). Using a children's dental health carnival as a primary vehicle to educate children about oral health. *ASDC J Dent Child*, 63:281–84.

47. Centers for Disease Control and Prevention (2001). Recommendations for using fluoride to prevent and control dental caries in the United States. *MMWR*, 50(No.RR-14):[inclusive page numbers].

48. Newbrun, E. (2001). Topical fluorides in caries prevention and management; A North American Perspective. *J Dent Edu*, 65:1083–88.

49. Meskin, L. H. (2001). Editorial outrageous II. *J Am Dent Assoc*, 132:10–11.

50. Potter, J. D., Finnegan, J. R., Guinard, J-X, et al. (2000). *5 A Day for Better Health Program Evaluation Report*. Bethesda, MD: National Institutes of Health, National Cancer Institute. November 2000; NIH Publication No. 01-4904.

51. Latho, M., Nyssonen, V., & Milan, A. (1983). Three methods of oral health education in secondary schools. *Scand J Dent Res*, 10:422–27.

52. O'Malley, P. M., Johnson, L. D., & Bachman, J. G. (1995). Adolescent substance use. Epidemiology and implications for public policy. *Ped Clinics N Am*, 42(2):241–60.

53. Faulkner, D. L., Escobedo, L. G., Zhu, B. P., et al. (1996). Race and incidence of cigarette smoking among adolescents in the United States. *J Natl Cancer Inst*, 88(16):1158–60.

54. Centers for Disease Control and Prevention (1994). Guidelines for school health programs to prevent tobacco use and addiction. *MMWR*, 43 (No. RR-21):1–17.

55. U.S. Department of Health and Human Services (2001). *Women and smoking: a report of the Surgeon General*. Rockville, MD: U.S. Dept. of Health and Human Services, PHS, Office of the Surgeon General; Washington, DC.

56. Ord, R. A., & Blanchaert, R. H. Eds. (1999). *Oral Cancer The dentist's role in diagnosis, management, rehabilitation, and prevention*. Chicago: Quintessence Publishing Co, Inc.

57. Simons-Morton, B., Haynie, D. L., Crump, A. D., Eitel, P., & Saylor, K. E. (2001). Peer and parent influences on smoking and drinking among early adolescents. *Health Ed Behavior, 28*(1):95–107.

58. Moss, A. J., Allan, K. F., Giovino, G. A., & Mills, S. L. (1992). *Recent Trends in Adolescent Smoking. Smoking Update/Correlates and Expectations about the Future*. Hyattsville, MD: U.S. Department of Health and Human Services, Public Health Service, National Center for Health Statistics.

59. O'Keefe, K. Baseball snuffs tobacco in minors. San Antonio, TX: *San Antonio Express-News*, June 14, 1993, 1B.

60. Glynn, T. J. (1990). School Programs to Prevent Smoking: *The National Cancer Institute Guide to Strategies that Succeed: Smoking Tobacco and Control Program*. Washington, DC: NCI, USD-HHS, NIH Pub. No. 90–500.

61. Barbour, S. E., Nakashimak Zhang, J. B. (1997). Tobacco and smoking: Environmental factors that modify the host response (immune system) and have an impact on periodontal health. *Crit Rev Oral Biol Med*, 8:437–60.

62. Ranalli, D. M. (1991). Prevention of craniofacial injuries in football. *Dent Clin North Am, 35*(4):627–45.

63. Nowjack-Raymer, R. E., & Gift, H. C. (1996). Use of mouthguards and headgear in organized sports by school-aged children. *Public Health Rep*, 111:82–86.

64. Johnsen, D. C., & Winters, J. E. (1991). Prevention of intra oral trauma in sports. *Dent Clin North Am, 35*(4):657–66.

65. Ranalli, D. M., & Lancaster, D. M. (1995) Attitudes of college football coaches regarding NCAA mouthguard regulations and compliance. *J Public Health Dent*, 55:139–42.

66. Camp, J. (1996). Special Report. Emergency. Dealing with sports-related dental trauma. *J Am Dent Assoc*, 127:812–15.

67. Nowjack-Raymer, R., & Gift, H. C. (1990). Contributing factors to maternal and child oral health. *J Public Health Dent*, 59(Special Issue):370–78.

68. Kupietzky, A. (1993). Teaching kindergarten and elementary school children dental health: A practical presentation. *J Clin Pediatric Dent*, 17:255–59.

69. Green, M., Ed. (1994). *Bright Futures: Guidelines for health supervision of infants, children and adolescents*. Arlington, VA: National Center for Education in Maternal and Child Health.

70. Casamassimo, P. (1996). *Bright futures in practice: Oral health*. Arlington, VA: National Center for Education in Maternal and Child Health.

71. Horowitz, A. M. (1995). The public's oral health: The gaps between what we know and what we practice. *Adv Dent Res*, 9:91–95.

72. U.S. Department of Health and Human Services, Public Health Service, Centers for Disease Control (May 1991). *Water fluoridation. A manual for engineers and technicians*. Atlanta: Centers for Disease Control, September 1986.

73. Driscoll, W. S., Nowjack-Raymer, R., Selwitz, R. H., Li, S., Heifetz, S. B. et al. (1992). A comparison of the caries-preventive effects of fluoride mouthrinsing, fluoride tablets, and both procedures combined: Final results after eight years. *J Public Health Dent*, 52:111–16.

74. Haugejorden, O., Lervik, T., Birkeland, J. M., Jorkjend, L. (1990). An eleven-year follow-up study of dental caries after discontinuation of school-based fluoride programs. *Acta Odontol Scand*, 48:257–263.

75. Kobayashi, S., Kishi, H., Yoshihara, A., Horiik, Tsutsui, A., Himeno, T., Horowitz, A. M. (1995). Treatment and postreatment effects of fluoride mouthrinsing after 17 years. *J Public Health Dent*, 55:229–33.

76. Selwitz, R. H., Winn, D. M., Kingman, A., et al. (1996). The prevalence of dental sealants in the US population: Findings from NHANES III. 1988-91. *J Dent Res*, 75 (Special Issue):652–60.

77. Sepp, A. I., Hausen, H., & Pollanen, L, et al. (1991). Effect of intensified caries prevention on approximal caries in adolescents with high caries risk. *Caries Res*, 25:392–95.

78. Sterritt, G. R., & Frew, R. A. (1988). Evaluation of a clinic-based sealant program. *J Public Health Dent*, 48:220–24.

79. Center for Disease Control and Prevention (2001). Impact of targeted, school-based dental sealant programs in reducing racial and economic disparities in sealant prevalence among schoolchildren—Ohio, 1998–1999. *MMWR*, 50:736–38.

80. Calderone, J. J., & Davis, J. M. (1987). The New Mexico sealant program: A progress report. *J Public Health Dent*, 48:220–24.

81. Ripa, L. W., Leske, B. S., & Sposata, A. (1989). The surface specific caries pattern of participants in a school-based fluoride mouth rinsing program with implications for the use of sealants. *J Public Health Dent*, 48:39–43.

82. Burt, B. (1989). Proceedings of the workshop: Cost-effectiveness of caries prevention in dental public health. *J Public Health Dent*, 49(Special Issue):250–344.

83. Wang, N. (1993). Substitution of dentists by dental hygienists in child dental care. *J Dent Res*, 72(Special Issue):172, Abstr.551.

84. Casamassimo, P. S. (1995). School oral health. [Editorial.] *Pediatric Dent*. 17:170.

85. Peterson, M. (1993). Personal communication. Dental Therapist. Community Health Services, Otago Area Health Board, Dunedin, New Zealand.

86. Friis-Hasche, E. (1994). Child oral health care in Denmark. Copenhagen University Press Copenhagen.

87. Kann, L., Collins, J. L., Pateman, B. C., et al. (1995). The school health policies and programs study (SHPPS): Rationale for a nationwide status report on school health programs. *J School Health*, 65:291–94.

# APPENDICES

## APPENDIX 19–1  Healthy People 2010 Oral Health Objectives Related to Oral Health in Schools

### Educational and Community-Based Programs

7-1    Increase high school completion

7-2    Increase the proportion of middle, junior high, and senior high schools that provide school health education to prevent health problems in the following areas: unintentional injury; violence, suicide; tobacco use and addition; alcohol and other drug use; unintended pregnancy, HIV/AIDS, and STD infection; unhealthy dietary patterns; inadequate physical activity; and environmental health.

### Health Communication

11-2    (Developmental) Improve the health literacy of persons with inadequate or marginal literacy skills.

### Injury and Violence Protection

15-19    Increase use of safety belts

15-23    (Developmental) Increase use of helmets by bicyclists

15-30    (Developmental) Increase the proportion of public and private schools that require use of appropriate head, face, eye, and mouth protection for students participating in school-sponsored physical activities

### Oral Health

21-12    Reduce the proportion of children and adolescents who have dental caries experience in their primary or permanent teeth

21-13    Reduce the proportion of children, adolescents, and adults with untreated dental decay

21-12    Reduce periodontal disease

21-12    Increase the proportion of children who have received dental sealants on their molar teeth

21-13    Increase the proportion of the U.S. population served by community water systems with optimally fluoridated water

21-14    Increase the proportion of children and adults who use the oral health care system each year

21-12    Increase the proportion of low-income children and adolescents who received any preventive dental service during the past year

21-13    (Developmental) Increase the proportion of school-based health centers with an oral health component

21-14    Increase the proportion of local health departments and community-based health centers, including community, migrant, and homeless health centers, that have an oral health component

### Tobacco Use

27-2    Reduce tobacco use by adolescents.

27-3    (Developmental) Reduce the initiation of tobacco use among children and adolescents.

27-4    Increase the average age of first use of tobacco products by adolescents and young adults.

27-7    Increase tobacco use cessation attempts by adolescent smokers.

27-11    Increase smoke-free and tobacco-free environments in schools, including all school facilities, property, vehicles, and school events.

**APPENDIX 19-2** **What to Teach About Preventing/Controlling Oral Diseases and Conditions**

## DENTAL CARIES

### Fluoride

What is fluoride

What is water fluoridation

How fluorides work to protect teeth from decay

Effectiveness of each procedure

Who needs fluoride

Recommended frequency of use and duration

### Pit-and-Fissure Sealants

What are dental sealants

How they work to protect teeth from decay

Who needs sealants and when reapplication of sealants

### Remineralization

Nature's way of repairing demineralized teeth

One of the most important functions of fluoride

Many times, it can be used instead of "fillings"

### Oral Cancer

Risk factors for oral cancers

Signs and symptoms of oral cancers

Components of a thorough clinical oral cancer examination and recommended frequency

Who needs oral cancer examinations; when
Protective factors against oral cancer

### Gingivitis

What is dental plaque

Role of dental plaque in oral diseases

How to remove plaque with toothbrush and floss

Frequency of plaque removal

Recommended types of toothbrushes

What may happen if gingivitis goes untreated

### Oral–Facial Injuries

Use mouthguards and headgear for sports

Use seat belts at all times, and air bags when possible

Wear helmets when riding bicycles and motorcycles

Use playground equipment safely

**APPENDIX 19-3 Small Group Toothbrushing Instruction**

| | |
|---|---|
| **Prerequisite** | Obtain permission from parents to participate |
| **Supplies Needed** | Toothbrush (individually wrapped) |
| | Disclosing tablets |
| | Paper cups |
| | Paper napkins |
| | Magnifying hand mirror |
| | Oversized dentoform model and large toothbrush |
| | Waste basket |
| | Dentifrice (for home use) |

**Routine**

1. Six to eight students sitting at a table can be taught as a manageable group.

2. Without removing the toothbrush from the cellophane wrapper, the students are asked to demonstrate how to remove some imaginary (and some not so imaginary) dirt from the cuticle of the thumbnail. (Place the brush at a 45° angle and use short vibratory strokes similar to those used in the mouth in performing the Bass technique.)

3. Reinforce the 45° concept on an oversized dentoform model, letting each child use the large toothbrush to demonstrate understanding and prowess.

4. Give each child a disclosing tablet to chew and swish around the teeth, expectorating excess saliva into the cup. Wipe the face with a napkin and force napkin into cup to avoid any spillage.

5. Encourage the children to look at the red-stained teeth of their neighbors. (They enjoy it.) Point out that all people have plaque.

6. Pass around the magnifying mirror to allow the students to look at their own teeth, explaining that where the red occurs bacteria live that cause decay and gum disease.

7. Begin dry toothbrushing (without dentifrice), emphasizing the need to brush the teeth in a definite sequence. (During the entire process, appropriate corrections and reinforcements should be made as soon as identified.)

8. Pass around magnifying mirror to demonstrate the success in removing the red plaque.

9. Place all cups and debris in wastebasket.

**APPENDIX 19-4** Comprehensive School-based Oral Health Programs

| | Education | Fluoride Rinse | Fluoride Tablets | School Water Fluoride | Prophylaxis | Sealants | Remineralization Therapy | Mouthguards | Oral Cancer | Referral | Treatment |
|---|---|---|---|---|---|---|---|---|---|---|---|
| **Level 1** | | | | | | | | | | | |
| Personnel | | | | | | | | | | | |
| Classroom Teacher | • | • | • | | | | | | • | | |
| Health Educator | • | • | • | | | | | | • | | |
| School Nurse | • | • | • | | | | | | • | | |
| Dietitian | • | | | | | | | | • | | |
| Coach | • | | | | | | | • | • | | |
| Administrator | | | | • | | | | | • | | |
| **Level 2** | | | | | | | | | | | |
| Personnel | | | | | | | | | | | |
| Classroom Teacher | • | • | • | | | | | | • | | |
| Health Educator | • | • | • | | | | | | • | | |
| School Nurse | • | • | • | | | | | | • | | |
| Dental Hygienist | • | • | • | | • | • | • | | • | • | |
| Dietitian | • | | | | | | | | • | | |
| Coach | • | | | | | | | • | • | | |
| Administrator | | | | • | | | | | • | | |
| **Level 3** | | | | | | | | | | | |
| Personnel | | | | | | | | | | | |
| Classroom Teacher | • | • | • | | | | | | • | | |
| Health Educator | • | • | • | | | | | | • | | |
| School Nurse | • | • | • | | | | | | • | | |
| Dental Hygienist | • | • | • | | • | • | • | | • | • | |
| Dietitian | • | | | | | | | | • | | |
| Dentist | • | | | | • | • | • | | • | • | • |
| Coach | • | | | | | | | • | • | | |
| Administrator | | | | • | | | | | • | | |
| **Recommended Grade** | | | | | | | | | | | |
| 1-12 | | | | | | | | | | | |

APPENDIX 19-5  **Conducting a Fluoride Mouthrinse Program**

| | |
|---|---|
| **Prerequisite** | Obtain written permission from parents for child to participate |
| **Supplies** | 1000-mL fluoride mouth rinse dispenser,[a] or Trays with individual 10 mL containers of fluoride mouth rinse. |
| | Paper cups |
| | Paper napkins |
| | Large plastic disposal bag |
| **Routine** | 1. Send a student to the school nurse's office to pick up supplies. |
| | 2. Teacher selects four children to pass out supplies: (1) a pump–pusher to dispense the fluoride; (2) a host or hostess to pass out the napkins; (3) a cup-passer to distribute the cups; and (4) a cleanup person to collect the cups at the end of the mouth rinsing. |
| | 3. a. All students pass the table supporting the fluoride solution dispenser and receive a 10-mLs of fluoride mouth rinse, or alternatively, |
| | b. All students receive a premeasured, sealed 10-mL container before returning to their seats to await instructions. |
| | 4. After cautioning against swallowing, the teacher tells the students to begin rinsing for 1 minute. |
| | 5. After the rinse is placed in the mouth the teacher keeps up a steady chatter—"the girls are doing better than the boys," "Monica is the best rinser in the class," etc. |
| | 6. At the end of the minute, the students are advised to carefully spit the rinse into the empty cup, and then wipe their mouths with the napkin before forcing it into the cup to absorb the liquid. |
| | 7. The cleanup person goes around the classroom to collect the cups and finally ties the plastic bag before placing it in the trash. |
| | 8. Students are instructed not to eat or drink for 30 minutes. |
| | 9. Return all excess supplies to the school nurse's office. |

[a]Medical Products Laboratories, Inc., 9990 Global Rd., Philadelphia, PA 19115

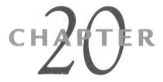

# CHAPTER 20

# Preventive Oral Health Care for Compromised Individuals

*Roseann Mulligan*
*Stephen Sobel*

*At the end of this chapter, it will be possible to:*

1. Explain why patients with the same handicaps can respond differently, based on communication and patient treatment techniques used by the dentist.
2. Discuss how visual, auditory, speech, and cognitive deficiencies can be identified and at least partially compensated for in preventive dentistry planning and implementation.
3. Illustrate how some functional deficiencies can be identified that require consideration in prescribing preventive dentistry techniques and devices.
4. Name and describe how new or modified devices or aids can be used to stabilize or aid patients with neurologic or physical disorders.
5. Cite at least three examples of how fluorides, pit-and-fissure sealants, and sugar discipline can be integrated into the preventive dental program for compromised individuals; also list possible exceptions.
6. Discuss the need to educate dental and dental-hygiene students, dentists, dental hygienists, and lay personnel to aid special patients in the home, in the office, and in institutional settings.

# INTRODUCTION

A compromised individual is a person who has one or more physical, medical, mental, or emotional problems that result in a limitation of the ability to function normally in fulfilling the activities of daily living (ADLs). More than 36 million individuals in the United States are compromised.[1]

When a patient presents for care, the clinician's judgment of the patient's capabilities may be biased. Unrealistic expectations of the ravages of a specific disease may have been formed in advance from reading the scientific literature or from firsthand treatment of another patient similarly afflicted. These experiences may produce unconscious and inaccurate generalizations about a person's capabilities. Such labeling can undermine a patient's preventive oral-hygiene program, because it does not consider the individual's actual capabilities.

This chapter presents information on how to assess the capabilities of a patient of any age within any disease category and offers suggestions on the development of individualized oral disease prevention programs. Oral-hygiene aids and techniques applicable to a preventive program for the compromised patient, as well as special management techniques, are included.

## Sensory Capabilities

Communication is compromised if the patient's hearing, vision, or speech is impaired. Communication is a critical factor in any attempt to engage the patient or caregiver in a behavioral change such as that required to improve the status of the patient's oral health.[2]

### Visual Deficits

A number of factors, from harmful prenatal and perinatal environments to the normal aging process, can alter visual acuity. These changes may range from correctable deficiencies to total blindness. Other common visual deficits include a loss of peripheral vision as occurs with glaucoma[3] or visual field cuts resulting from a cerebrovascular accident.[4]

A patient with a significant visual disability may be carrying a white-tipped cane or may arrive with an escort. If the individual requests, the nondental staff escort—whether human or guide dog—should be allowed to accompany the patient into the treatment room. The escort may then be permitted to stay if space is available in the treatment area and if the presence of the escort contributes to the patient's comfort. An escort who functions as an attendant may be involved in any oral hygiene instructions and demonstrations, and this person may be the crucial element necessary to a successful home care program.

Instructional materials to be used with patients who have decreased visual acuity could include commercial products that have been developed for pediatric dentistry programs, because such products have large pictures. Other commercially prepared pamphlets for self-instruction and information have limited value because the size of the print used in such pamphlets is too small for the visually impaired to see comfortably. Custom-made instructional sheets may be produced by the dental office using large black letters of at least 12-point type on off-white or white paper.[5] When appropriate, chairside instructions of tooth brushing

and flossing should be demonstrated on oversized models of the dentition with a giant-sized toothbrush (Figure 20–1). These large models allow the patient with limited visual acuity to see and to understand some of the more subtle aspects of tooth brushing, such as the correct angulation of the bristles into the gingival crevice. Red floss can help when demonstrating flossing to those with visual impairment who have difficulty seeing white floss. Green floss is also available and can be used, but red is easier for the aging eye to see.[6] Once the flossing technique is understood and visual acuity permits, the patient may switch to white floss for regular home use. This allows the patient to check the color of the floss for possible gingival bleeding.

To demonstrate brushing and flossing techniques in the office, an inexpensive magnifying mirror should be employed to assist the patient in observing his or her own performance. A similar mirror should be recommended for the patient's use at home. These mirrors, commercially available, are usually used for applying cosmetics. With attachments provided, they can be adapted to be hung around the neck, affixed to a wall, or placed on a countertop, thus allowing patients to keep their hands free for performing oral hygiene and still use the mag-

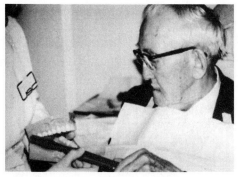

FIGURE 20–1    **Large dental models and a helping hand are needed to perfect toothbrushing habits in the visually impaired.**

nifying mirror to enhance vision. Many also feature a lighted mirror, another aid for enhancing vision. Some patients who have experienced a cerebrovascular accident lack the spatial–perceptual skills necessary to use a mirror. For these people, using a mirror causes confusion and therefore is contraindicated. If a patient has visual problems so significant that a mirror cannot be used, he or she must be sensitized instead to the "feeling" and "smell" of a clean mouth to attest to the success of oral hygiene measures.[7]

For individuals with visual field cuts or decreases in peripheral vision, be sure that demonstrations are within the patient's visual field. To check the limits of a patient's vision, perform a visual assessment by positioning your hand in various locations around the patient's face while holding up one or more fingers. For each position, ask the patient how many fingers can be seen, and note whether the patient moves the head rather than just the eyes to see your fingers.

Many patients with visual problems experience an increased sensitivity to light or glare. Indiscriminate positioning of the dental light so that it shines in the eyes of a patient can result in significant discomfort for such a patient. This can be avoided by carefully focusing and positioning the operatory light. Also, it is advisable to have sunglasses available; these can be disinfected after use.

With loss of orbital fat during aging, the eye becomes "sunken" with an increase in the upper lid fold and a decrease in peripheral vision. Extra-ocular muscle weakness by the age of 70 inhibits the ability to rotate the eye upward greater than 15° from the horizon.[8] Since arthritic changes in the cervical spine occur frequently among the elderly,[9] it may be difficult or impossible for some patients to tip the head back. Thus, to enhance communication with all patients, it is best to converse from a sitting position directly in front of the patient so that the clinician's eyes and the patient's eyes are at about the same level.

### Hearing Disabilities

Hearing problems can occur in all age groups. The sound of dental equipment in another room, background music, and street noises can hinder communication with the hearing-impaired, as these sounds often mask the sound of speech. The most common problem in communicating with the hearing disabled, however, occurs when the speaker is not directly in front of the patient, at the same eye level, face to face.[10]

Most patients with hearing disabilities do some speech reading (formerly termed lip reading), but even the best speech reader is able to decipher only about one fourth of a message conveyed entirely through this method.[11] The hearing-disabled patient also relies on the communicator's facial expression and body language.[10] Speaking distinctly and slightly slower, without exaggeration and in a well-modulated voice, facilitates communication.[12] The progressive loss of hearing of high-frequency tones that commonly occurs among the elderly may make a female voice more difficult to hear than a male voice. Avoid back lighting[13] that places the speaker's face in a shadow. Shouting at a hearing-disabled patient is not recommended, because loud sounds are actually more difficult for the impaired ear to comprehend.[10] When speaking to a patient, other than while doing a procedure, lower or remove your face mask.

Pantomime and demonstration may be necessary when working with the hearing disabled. When writing information, use a clipboard and a red felt-tipped pen. After providing oral-hygiene instructions, have the patient demonstrate the suggested oral-hygiene skills on models or in his or her own mouth to assess how well the message was comprehended.

Hearing aids are becoming more difficult to detect, as new technologies allow for decreasing size or positioning entirely within the ear canal. Long hair may mask their presence; therefore, a conscious effort should be made to look for such aids (Figure 20–2). If preventive

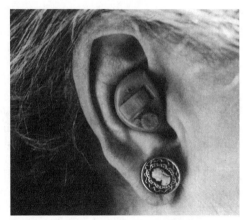

FIGURE 20–2    When longer hair is combed over the ear, this hearing device can be very inconspicuous—and vulnerable to handpiece noise.

instructions are to be given to a patient with a hearing aid, be sure the patient's aid is in place and turned on. Often patients turn off or remove their hearing aids in anticipation of dental treatment, because the proximity of the speaker's body to the aid may cause it to emit high-pitched squeals called "feedback." Providing dental care with the clinician seated in the 12 o'clock position places the operator's arm nearly in contact with the patient's ear, and the clinician's sleeve may accidentally dislodge an over-the-ear hearing aid. Handpieces can also cause many types of hearing aids to produce feedback. Suggest to the patient that the aid be removed or turned off prior to treatment and replaced or turned back on prior to receiving instructions.

Hearing aids are expensive devices, and individuals who wear them usually prefer to remove them themselves. Once removed, the aids should be placed in a secure spot, such as the patient's pocket or purse, rather than on the bracket table where they could be forgotten or gathered up and discarded. Individuals who have both hearing and visual deficiencies may have their hearing devices constructed as part of the frame of their glasses. In such cases it is

recommended that the glasses be left in place but with the hearing device turned off.

For patients with visual or hearing deficiencies, keep distractions to a minimum (it is advisable to have office background music turned off at this time). This includes any interruption of the clinician at chairside as well as the distraction created by auxiliary personnel entering and leaving the room.

## Speech and Language Disorders

Several conditions affect the motor or the cognitive components of speech or both. The patient with cerebral palsy may have speech impairment because of problems of the central nervous system affecting the muscular movements needed for speech.[14] With practice, a clinician who listens carefully and patiently to such speech can become adept at understanding much of it. This is the same sort of technique many dental providers have already achieved in learning to understand patients who attempt to speak with a rubber dam in place. Individuals, such as those who are mentally retarded, even though physiologically capable, may not use language because of their level of intellectual or emotional functioning. Those with neuromuscular diseases may have a weakness so severe that the muscles necessary to articulate sounds are unable to function. Deterioration of speech that once was normal may be due to progressive hearing loss. Individuals who are unable to hear the range of frequencies of the speech spectrum may develop a monotone voice. In addition, such a person often loses the ability to recognize how loudly he or she is speaking.

The patient who has suffered a stroke is particularly prone to language disorders. One type of disorder common to stroke patients is aphasia. In aphasia, the reception, integration, and expression of language are impaired. The aphasic patient, therefore, has difficulty finding the right words to communicate,[15] and this inability may be so pronounced that the patient may

become very frustrated. This is especially true for those individuals who are otherwise cognitively intact. When dealing with these individuals, frame questions so that they can be answered with "yes," "no," or just a shake or nod of the head.

The aphasic individual may also omit or substitute sounds for words. The words then may be meaningless by themselves but convey intent by the way in which they are expressed. The speech may consist only of nouns, verbs, or a few adjectives. An extreme example of an aphasic patient was a woman who suffered a stroke so severe that her verbal communication was reduced to two exclamatory words that were always said together. With the help of her facial expression, body language, and the force and intonation used in saying these words, dental appointments were completed to the satisfaction of the patient and the provider.

Dysarthria is a speech disorder resulting from a motor dysfunction of the speech-producing elements. This dysfunction may be caused by lesions in the central nervous system, the peripheral nervous system, or in the muscles themselves. The symbolic language is intact; however, the coordination necessary to produce speech is impaired. This type of disturbance occurs in patients with amyotrophic lateral sclerosis (ALS), Parkinson's disease, traumatic brain injury, myasthenia gravis, multiple sclerosis, and stroke.[16]

The substitution of written for verbal communication is a possible option for individuals in whom the recognition of language is still intact. Unfortunately, many of the causes of speech disorders result in slight or pronounced paralysis or tremors that prevent the patient from writing legibly. One solution is to provide the patient with a lapboard containing preprinted letters, common words, or pictures. Individuals with a knowledge of language but an inability to speak or to have their speech or writing understood can point to the letters or words or pictures to communicate. Another method is a sophisticated, small typewriter-like

device in which a keyboard is used to type out a tickertape message. Quadriplegic patients may be outfitted with a tongue control that permits very subtle movements of the tongue against a toggle switch. This action causes letters to be printed on a television monitor mounted to a wheelchair or bed.

Today's society places great importance on verbal communication; therefore, an individual with poor verbal skills is sometimes incorrectly perceived as having poor cognitive and intellectual abilities. This is not necessarily the case.

Although nonverbal communication, such as smiling, hand holding, and shoulder touching, plays a role in the clinician–patient interaction, it becomes extremely significant when there is no alternative. In such a case, the clinician needs to enlist either the patient's attendant or a family member who has become attuned to "reading" the patient's needs. Usually, these constant companions can help interpret the underlying message of such nonverbal actions as a rolling of the eyeballs or a fixed stare.

Most autistic patients are known to be unable to use language appropriately, and many present significant management challenges. Visual pedagogy was used for a group of autistic children in Sweden. Pictures of the location and the activities to be anticipated were shown to the autistic patient including the dental office, outside and inside, the dental chair, a wide-open mouth, a mouth mirror, and a toothbrush. The pictures were shown to the patient at home before the appointment and explanations were given thus familiarizing the patient with what was to come. The technique proved quite successful for clinical care and can be used for preventive activities as well.[17]

In summary, both verbal and nonverbal techniques play roles in the communication process between a dental-care provider and a compromised dental patient. Speaking directly to the patient from a sitting position in front of the patient in a well-modulated, well-articulated voice and reinforcing each step of the communication with nonverbal cues are all

techniques that should be used to produce a successful relationship with a patient who has impaired communication skills.

---

### Question 1

Which of the following statements, if any, are correct?

A. Many specialized preventive techniques applicable to one handicapping condition are applicable to other handicapping conditions.

B. During periods of patient–dentist communications, it is better that the dentist be able to clearly see the patient's face than vice versa.

C. An aphasic patient is one who has difficulty in articulating personal thoughts and observations.

D. When a patient is unable to form words because of a motor dysfunction problem, the condition is known as dysarthria.

---

## Cognitive Capacities

The functional capacity of a patient is of far greater importance than intelligence quotient (IQ) test results in determining the capability of benefiting from preventive dentistry instructions. For example, a patient who is mentally retarded is expected to have a low IQ, short attention span, and difficulty in understanding oral-hygiene instructions. Yet many of these patients, when properly taught and motivated, can successfully perform oral-hygiene procedures. To be successful, one must first determine the patient's level of cognitive ability and then direct all instruction to that level. Rather than attempting to analyze intelligence test scores, ask the patient a few simple questions to determine his or her functioning level. Questions of the type that might be asked of the patient, not the family member or attendant, could pertain to such everyday conversational topics as (1) What do you do in school (or at

work, or in retirement)? (2) What hobbies do you like? (3) Why do you like a favorite television show? or (4) What has been the most difficult task you performed lately? One mentally retarded patient who responded to a similar series of questions confided that he enjoyed his job as a file clerk in a sheltered workshop environment, but he was sometimes confused trying to remember the order of letters in the alphabet. He added that the most difficult job he faced was paying the rent at the first of each month. Even though he knew he had sufficient money, the responsibility of ensuring that the funds reached his landlord in time caused him a great deal of anxiety.

Such information from the patient offers insights into levels of responsibility, understanding, attention span, usual level of dexterity, and memory for details. These facts greatly assist the dental-care provider in selecting the appropriate vocabulary, level of complexity of instruction, and reward system for adherence to a customized preventive dentistry program.

If it is determined that the patient is intellectually or cognitively impaired, the traditional education program for oral-hygiene techniques must be modified. Brushing the teeth is a complex task that needs to be broken down into very simple, discrete steps. This allows the impaired patient to follow the instructions and to succeed at each step toward the final goal, thereby integrating the simple tasks into a final complex task.[11] At the first appointment it may be possible to address only the brushing of the occlusal surfaces of the teeth. This activity should be monitored and reinforced until a level of satisfactory compliance and incorporation into the patient's daily routine is achieved. Clinicians, in their quest to get the message across to the cognitively or intellectually impaired patient often tend to do and to say too much. It is important to keep instructional periods short with frequent repetition of the information. Using a level of language that is understood by the patient without being insulting is key. Written or tape-recorded reminders can be given for homework. At each appointment,

the patient should be asked to state or show what he or she has been doing since the last visit. This provides feedback about the effectiveness of the previous instructional period and the patient's memory and mastery of the technique.[11] Of course, one must use judgment and an understanding of the patient's cognitive functional level in assessing the validity of the patient's answers.

Demonstrations of appropriate behavior by any dental patient, especially those with decreased cognitive functioning, should always be followed by immediate and positive feedback.[19] Reinforcement throughout the learning period should be supplemented with both verbal and nonverbal rewards; for example, a smile or a gift of a new toothbrush is often motivating. Development of rapport aids in reducing stress, which can be detrimental to an individual's ability to learn. For this reason all learning should occur in an environment in which the dental staff can reflect warmth and friendliness.

Family members or guardians, teachers, or other caregivers must assume responsibility for oral health care programs of patients with little cognitive ability.[20] The selected individuals should be thoroughly instructed by the dental staff in the proper techniques for that patient's oral health.

## Functional Performance

Toothbrushing and flossing require the fine-motor skills or dexterity of the small muscles of the fingers and hands as well as the gross-motor skills of the larger muscle groups in the upper extremities.[21] The functioning of numerous muscles and nerves of the head, neck, and upper extremities are all involved, as is the range-of-motion capability of the joints, especially the shoulders and elbows. In many disabilities, one or more of these elements may be adversely affected or limited. Arthritis, for example, is a disease primarily of the joints and therefore often restricts the range of motion of the joint. Cerebral palsy is a central nervous system disorder. Because of aberrant neural sig-

nals transmitted to the muscle fibers, fine-motor skills are impaired. Muscle contractures also characteristically affect both the range and motion of the joints. A neuromuscular disease such as myasthenia gravis affects the nerve transmission process itself, resulting in a musculature so weak that dexterity, gross motor skills, and range of motion may all be affected.

An accurate assessment of a patient's ability to perform oral hygiene depends on the evaluation of each component of the task. Once a difficulty has been identified, either a device or a person is needed to compensate for the patient's inability. Gross motor skills such as grasping a toothbrush handle can often be improved by *orthotic*[a] appliances (Figure 20–3). Range-of-motion limitations may be altered by physical therapy, especially in the early stages of injury or disease, or in some cases by surgery. Dexterity necessary for the production of the small vibratory strokes recommended in tooth brushing usually cannot be enhanced through physical medicine, surgery or orthotic remedies. For certain patients, an electric toothbrush may provide effective compensation for this lack of ability.

### Assessment

Specific hand function tests employed by occupational therapists to evaluate a patient's ability to use his or her hands can help dental clinicians assess a patient's potential ability to accomplish oral-hygiene techniques. If the patient shakes your hand when first greeted, pay attention to the strength of the patient's handclasp. Individuals with a weak grasp should be asked to firmly grip the index finger of the clinician's hand. If the grip is weak, the patient should again be asked to grip the finger "as hard as you can." Repeating this procedure several times using two, three, and four fingers of the practitioner's hand in place of the one finger enables the practitioner to decide at what di-

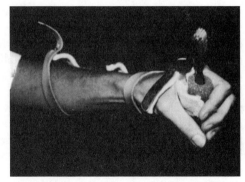

FIGURE 20–3    An orthotic device that permits a firmer grasp on a modified toothbrush.

ameter the patient has the strongest grip[22] (Figure 20–4). If it is determined that the patient would benefit from a manual toothbrush, the handle will need to be increased in diameter to match the number of fingers at which the patient had the strongest grasp.

The range of motion of the elbow and shoulder can be determined by having the patient extend and flex the lower arm, or rotate that arm about the shoulder. This information may be more quickly obtained by asking the patient, "Can you feed yourself?" Individuals who are able to do so, even if they use orthotic splints or other adaptive aids, are probably able to perform oral hygiene procedures. Patients who use

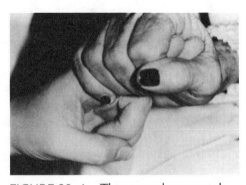

FIGURE 20–4    The muscular strength of a patient's hand can be assessed by handshake or by a grasp of the clinician's fingers.

[a]Orthotic appliances are devices, such as splints and braces, that are used to provide support to deformed or weakened limbs.

special devices to aid in self-feeding should bring these devices to the dental office so that toothbrushes and other oral hygiene aids can be modified to fit them. The best way to assess whether a patient has sufficient dexterity and cognition to perform adequate oral hygiene is to offer the patient a toothbrush and to directly observe his or her success in plaque removal. This accomplishes two objectives: 1) The clinician can assess the patient's current level of ability and understanding prior to any intervention. 2) The clinician can establish a baseline level of achievement against which future improvements or modifications can be measured.

Noticing the ease or difficulty with which each movement is accomplished (grasping the brush, angling, and moving it) and the care needed to synchronize these actions into purposeful motion gives the dental professional insight into the capabilities, training, and education of the patient to date. An understanding of the patient's current abilities allows the health care provider to determine the type and number of educational interventions to be introduced. Patients with compromised motor skills often compensate for their deficiencies in ingenious ways. Therefore, their ability to perform their own oral hygiene should not be prejudged, and they should be given opportunities to demonstrate their proficiencies. Many patients who appear unable to handle a toothbrush or floss, because of deformed fingers or decreased motor functions, can compensate and function reasonably well.

---

### Question 2

Which of the following statements, if any, are correct?

A. It is an inviolable rule that as the IQ decreases, so does the possibility of attaining cooperation from a mentally handicapped patient.

B. As an individual's disability increases, the need becomes greater for support from other individuals.

C. Explanations on primary preventive dentistry given to handicapped individuals should be detailed.

D. The hand strength and ability of a patient to use a toothbrush can often be determined by a handshake.

E. The best way to find out what a handicapped patient can do is to ask the person to accomplish a stated task.

---

## Attendant Care

To ensure dental care and compliance with home self-care preventive programs, complete cooperation must be established among the family or caregivers, the health provider, and, to the extent possible, the patient.[23, 24] Many compromised individuals are unable to handle their own hygiene due to sensory, cognitive, or physical deficits. For these individuals, an attendant or family member should be instructed in the proper oral-health care for the patient.[25] If long-term compliance with instructions is the goal, the comfort of both the caregiver and the patient in performing the oral hygiene program is paramount. For this reason, a number of positions have been recommended for the caregiver to assume when providing oral hygiene care to the patient. Facts to be considered include the patient's size and strength, the attendant's size and strength, and the amount of control that needs to be exerted over the intentional or unintentional movements of the patient. One position that has proven to be successful when the patient is an adult is for the attendant to stand behind the patient, who is seated in a straight-backed chair or a wheelchair. In this position, it is easy to stabilize the patient's head by resting it against the body of the attendant. Brushing then proceeds with the attendant using the same kind of arm and brush positioning as when cleaning his or her own teeth. Performing this operation in front of a mirror takes further advantage of the attendant's own brushing habits, although a mirror is not a necessity. Other recommended positions include having the patient lie on a sofa

or bed with the head in the caregiver's lap or sitting on the floor in front of a chair in which the caregiver is seated (Figure 20–5). As depicted in Figure 20-5B, note that the caregiver's legs are used as an additional restraint to the arms of the patient. Caregivers and patients should both be advised that the bathroom is not the only location in which to brush teeth. In fact, it is often the least convenient room in the house because of its space limitations and the need to share its use with other members of the family. Water is not always necessary for toothbrushing, as salivary flow is stimulated by brushing and thus provides moisture. If a patient has tender, friable gingival tissue that can easily become damaged by an initially dry toothbrush, the brush can be moistened beforehand to soften it. When no toothpaste is used, running water may not be needed. The elimination of the toothpaste increases visibility and decreases the possibility of gagging. In many cases, it has been found that when water and toothpaste were required, attendants or family members discontinued or decreased the number of toothbrushing sessions. Normally, a fluoride toothpaste is an important component of an oral-hygiene program in an uncompromised population. In compromised patients, however, if one must omit fluoride toothpaste from the routine, it can be compensated for by using fluorides in other forms.

Those patients who enjoy the taste or appreciate the aesthetic value of toothpaste can use a non-foaming, ingestible toothpaste[b] (originally developed for the astronauts). Because this toothpaste does not foam and can be swallowed, it is not necessary for the patient to be near a basin to expectorate.

If a patient likes to rinse with water or a mouthwash after brushing, a two-paper-cup technique can be used. One paper cup holds the rinse; the other is for the expectorate after the patient rinses. Because the cups are lightweight, patients can often hold both, bringing each of the cups up to their lips as needed. This two-cup technique provides a means of controlling drib-

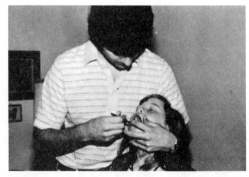

A

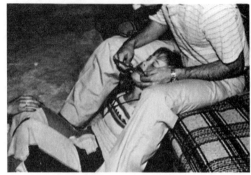

B

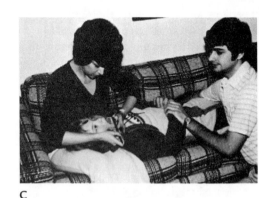

C

FIGURE 20-5    Three different positions for a caregiver to use in aiding toothbrushing. (Courtesy of Ionya Smith Ray and Gayla Hill Taylor.)

[b]NASAdent, Scherer Laboratories, Inc., Dallas, TX.

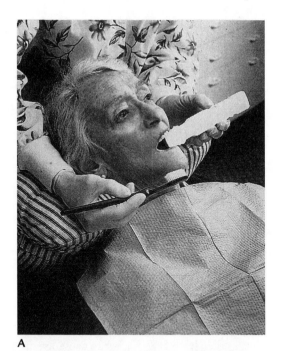

**A**

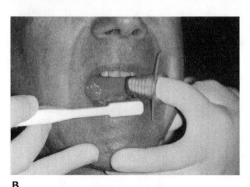

**B**

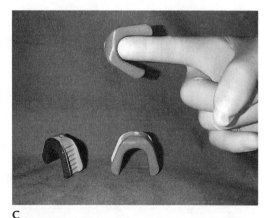

**C**

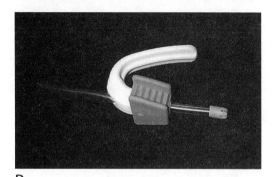

**D**

FIGURE 20-6    A. Open Wide® Disposable Mouth Prop.[c] B. Dental Shield.[d] C. C-shaped mouth prop with positioning concavity.[e] D. Open Wide® Wraparand Mouth Prop[f] with extraoral handle and opening to accommodate suction device.

bling or drooling, and it is valuable for an individual who is unable to lean over the basin, such as an arthritic patient, or for an individual who cannot purse the lips to expel the fluid, as is the case with muscular dystrophy patients.

## Specialized Equipment for Patient Management

### Mouth Props

Several types of mouth props can be used to assist in opening and holding open the patient's mouth for oral hygiene procedures (Figure 20–6). A simple, effective mouth prop can be easily fabricated with two or three tongue blades wrapped together, padded on one end with $2 \times 2$ gauze squares, and secured in place with adhesive tape.[26] This prop can be used with patients who are unable to understand or to cooperate due to decreased cognitive func-

[c]Specialized Care Co., Hampton, NH.
[d]Athena Nordic, Falun, Sweden.
[e]Logi Bloc, COMMONSENSE Dental Products, Nunica, MI.
[f]Specialized Care Co., Hampton, NH.

tioning, as seen in mental retardation, mental deficiency, senile dementia, or in patients exhibiting neuromuscular dysfunction, such as occurs in cerebral palsy or muscular dystrophy. This prop may be used initially to help open the patient's mouth. If necessary, it can then be replaced by a custom-made finger cover[27] or several different types of commercially manufactured props, which would then be placed on the opposite side of the arch from where the original gauze wrapped prop is initially placed and then removed once the more compact prop is in position. Not only is the gauze and tongue-blade mouth prop useful for initial examinations and screenings, it is economical and disposable as well.

Commercially available intra-oral mouth props are frequently available in different sizes to accommodate adult and pediatric patients, or as a one-size-fits-all unit designed to accommodate a range of mouth sizes. When using a prop of the former design, the correct size must be chosen and placed far enough back in the oral cavity to be held in place by the force of the jaws attempting to close. Otherwise, on closure, the prop slides forward along the occlusal surfaces of the teeth. It is not as likely that this will occur with the second type of prop because the serrations and graduated size over the length of the prop better resist slippage. When using either of these prop types, one should tie floss through the hole in the prop and allow the floss to extend from the patient's mouth. If inadvertent swallowing of the prop occurs, an occluded airway results. In such an event, the prop can be retrieved by means of the floss ligature.

The most critical aspect of placing a mouth prop is to protect the caregiver's fingers. Those props that require the fingers to cross the occlusal plane as part of the placement process pose the greatest jeopardy of being bitten. Therefore newer devices that have positioning concavities may be of help (Figure 20-6C). Another device is similar to a large thimble with flanges that fits over the thumb or one fin-

ger of the caregiver, freeing the other fingers and hand to stabilize the jaw during tooth brushing or a prophylaxis (Figure 20-6B). Because the patient's jaw might suddenly snap closed upon removal of a prop, use of the gauze-wrapped tongue blades during removal of any mouth prop should be considered.

An alternative to the gauze-wrapped tongue blade is a disposable, handheld, Styrofoam mouth prop with graduated notches (Figure 20-6A) that can be placed and controlled extra-orally. Another device controlled extra-orally is the Open Wide® Wraparound Mouth Prop with an extra-oral handle that can also be used with a suction device (Figure 20–6D). It is possible to hyperextend the mandibular muscles with an oversized mouth prop or the overzealous placement of one. This can cause a muscle spasm, resulting in considerable discomfort to the patient. Bite blocks must be used with caution, as they have been known to cause hypoxemia.[28] The smaller the patient with regard to height and weight, the greater the risk that oxygen desaturation will occur when bite blocks are used, particularly when the bite blocks are too large.

### Headrests

There are numerous ways of supporting and stabilizing the head and neck of compromised dental patients. For those individuals who remain in their conventional wheelchairs throughout treatment, a commercially available wheelchair headrest may be purchased and kept in the dental office. This headrest attaches to the hand grips of the wheelchair and adjusts to compensate for different chair widths and sitting heights of patients.[29] Other types of head stabilizers can be attached to the headrest of the dental chair with Velcro straps that extend around the back of the chair to secure the stabilizing device. Pillows designed for neck support are commercially available in retail stores. They can be used, with modifications if necessary, for patients with cervical spine defor-

mities. A cerebral palsy head support consists of a block of foam with a depression in the center to stabilize the patient's head.[30] Pillows sold to airplane travelers that contain buckwheat hulls as the filling material and are shaped as enlarged neck collars can also be used to stabilize the head and neck of a patient during preventive procedures.

## Soft Ties

Soft ties, which are cloth or soft leather straps, may be used to support and stabilize any part of the body, including the head.[31] Most commonly, soft ties are used to secure the upper and lower limbs to an appropriate leg or armrest. This prevents the limb from spasming, flailing, or hanging off the edge of the rest, a position that can compress nerves and lead to neural damage. Soft ties are not meant to be punitive or restraining devices. They are intended to provide positive support, stability, and security to the patient.

## Body Wraps and Other Limb Stabilizers

Full-body wraps, such as pedo-wraps and papoose boards, are often used to immobilize smaller adult patients during dental treatment.[31] A plastic elbow stabilizer, that begins as a flat sheet and is curled into a tube around the arm, keeps the patient from being able to bend the elbow to push away a caregiver (Figure 20–7). These devices have limited usefulness in preventive programs where purposeful attempts are being made to actively involve patients in their own oral hygiene. Body wraps and stabilizers should be considered when others give care, and the patient is unable to cooperate. For some compromised patients full body wraps are welcomed as a source of security and comfort.[32]

Some developmentally disabled patients exhibit self-injurious behavior causing significant peri-oral trauma. Management of this behavior is often difficult as restraining devices applied extra-orally are only appropriate during active treatment periods and may not prevent intra-

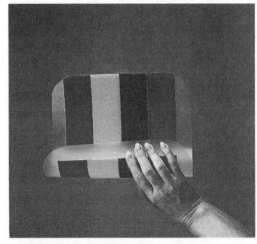

**A**

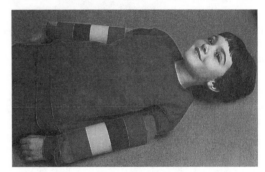

**B**

FIGURE 20-7    A. Rainbow™ Elbow & Knee Stabilizer[g] being rolled to fit around arm. B. Formed stabilizer in place.

oral chewing of the tongue and/or lips that may occur at any time of the day or night. In selected cases, oral appliances can be effective in preventing trauma by deflecting tissues from the occlusal plane.[33]

Mouth props, soft ties, wraps, and elbow stabilizers are all considered forms of restraint, and communities continue to struggle with the issue of the appropriateness of restraints.[34] The use of restraints is controversial, and each juris-

[g]Specialized Care Co., Hampton, NH.

diction may interpret what constitutes re-straints differently. Practitioners and caregivers should research their state and local guidelines before employing such restraints.[35] The intent to use any of these items should be included in the informed consent provided to the patient's guardian.

## Oral-Hygiene Devices

### Modifying Toothbrush Handles

In general, the principles and techniques of tooth brushing used for a compromised popula-tion are the same as for anyone else. In com-promised individuals, however, good oral hy-giene is much more difficult to achieve and maintain.[18] If it has been determined that the patient has adequate dexterity to produce the small strokes needed to brush properly, a man-ual toothbrush may produce satisfactory results. Toothbrush manufacturers are now providing a variety of different configurations[36] of brushes with increased handle dimensions, handles modifiable with hot water (Figure 20–8), an-gled brush heads, multiple brush heads, and curved bristles, all of which can be beneficial for special needs patients (Figure 20–9). One type of brush marketed for toddlers is designed with a large ovoid handle that prevents over insertion and potential intra-oral injury when a

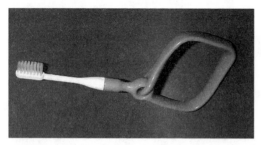

FIGURE 20-8    Commercially available toothbrush with handle that can be modi-fied by immersion in hot water.[h]

[h]Shape It™ Toothbrush, John O. Bulter Co., Chicago, IL.

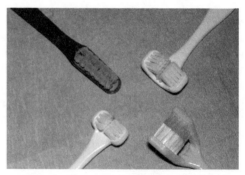

FIGURE 20-9    Commercially available toothbrushes designed for special needs patients. Clockwise from upper right: Curved bristle brush,[i] small triple brush head,[j] double brush head,[k] and large triple brush head.[l]

child is first learning to brush. Such a device may have application for an older compromised child (Figure 20–10). Even if the patient has a weakened hand grasp or uses orthotic splints or other adaptive appliances, a manual toothbrush can be modified to facilitate usage.[37,38] In a well-controlled study of children with cerebral palsy who received modified toothbrushes, plaque removal was increased by 28 to 35% over that achieved when conventional tooth-brushes were used.[39] Figure 20–11 illustrates different methods of quickly augmenting tooth-brush handles from commonly found materials. These include foam wrappings from packing materials, acrylic tray or bite registration mate-rial, the center foam piece from a hair curler, a bicycle grip with plaster anchoring the tooth-brush inside, or a juice can with a slotted ball inside to hold the toothbrush.[22] Inexpensive, cylindrical, closed-cell foam can be obtained from orthotic or medical supply stores. This foam cylinder has significant advantages over other types of foam materials because it is com-

[i]Collis–Curve™ toothbrush, Collis-Curve, Brownsville, TX.
[j]SUPER-BRUSH® Junior, Denta-Co., Bergen, Norway.
[k]action 2. Action Hygiene Products, Inc., Toronto.
[l]SUPER-BRUSH, Denta-Co., Bergen, Norway.

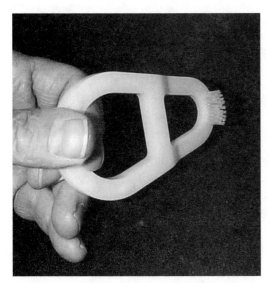

FIGURE 20-10    Tooth brush with large handle to prevent overinsertion.[m]

posed of closed plastic cells that shed water. This eliminates the increase in weight and the need to squeeze out absorbed water on completion of a hygiene procedure.

[m]INFANT-TODDLER SAFETY TOOTHBRUSH®, Preventive Dental Specialties, Inc., Rothschild, WI.

Handles augmented with foam can be used by a wide range of compromised individuals. They can be easily adapted to orthotic appliances such as splints. Handles modified with heavier materials, however, such as the bicycle grip or the juice can, should not be used with arthritics or those with neuromuscular weaknesses. These latter two types of modifications are more appropriately used with mentally retarded individuals, including those with Down syndrome, and with cerebral palsy patients who typically have strong grips and limb musculature (see Figure 20–11).

Patients who are unable to flex their elbows because of joint involvement can be given a toothbrush with an extended handle. This can be fabricated by inserting a bicycle or wheelchair spoke into, and parallel to, the original toothbrush handle and fabricating a new acrylic handle out of orthodontic resin or a similar material. The handle may be further modified if the patient has grasp difficulties. Other simple modifications include reshaping the plastic handle of the toothbrush by heating it in warm water and bending to the desired configuration or gluing the handle of a nailbrush to the toothbrush handle.

Several devices have been developed to assist individuals with limited function to

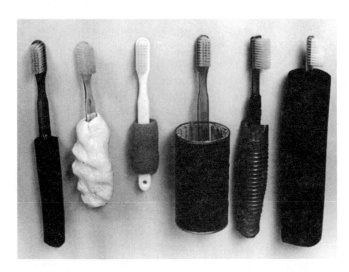

FIGURE 20–11    Readily available foam tubes, bicycle handles, cans, or dental tray material can be used to modify the size of toothbrush handles.

achieve independence. Often, products used to assist in feeding can be adapted for use in brushing the teeth, such as palmar cuffs or activities of daily living (ADL) cuffs.[n]

### Question 3

Which of the following statements, if any, are correct?

A. Dentifrices are essential to maintaining good oral-hygiene care among the handicapped.

B. Both mentally handicapped and individuals with neuromuscular dysfunction may need mouth props.

C. When it is necessary to constrain a neuromuscularly handicapped patient, it should be a nonpunitive action.

D. The appropriateness of using body wraps or pedo-wraps depends on the patient's size and stature.

E. A Bunsen burner flame is needed to modify a toothbrush handle.

### Electric Toothbrushes

Electric toothbrushes are valuable aids in assisting compromised patients.[40] They are especially useful when the patient has the strength to grasp the handle and place the brush in the mouth but does not have the manual dexterity needed to perform the fine movements necessary for the cleaning function. The length and diameter of the handle of an electric toothbrush approximates those of manual toothbrushes that have been modified for individuals with compromised hand function.

Recent models of electric toothbrushes display on/off buttons that are user-friendly. Unlike previous models, which had switches that were difficult to manipulate,[41] most now have pressure plates that activate the brush head and are easy to use. The weight of the electric toothbrush is still a problem for some individuals to manage, especially patients with poor upper extremity muscle control or strength. This can be compensated for by positioning the patient at a table and demonstrating brushing while the patient's elbows on the table are used to support the increased weight. If the patient is in a wheelchair, a countertop can be used to support the toothbrush handle while activating it (Figure 20–12).

For patients able to perform their own oral hygiene, the effectiveness of electric toothbrushes in plaque removal has been well established. Much less has been accomplished in attempting to establish the effectiveness of electric toothbrush use in compromised patients. However, one study did compare the Interplak® to manual toothbrushes in a population of persons with mental retardation/developmental disabilities (MR/DD). Those using the Interplak® showed significant improvement in the Gingival Index over the twelve months of the study.[42] The few other studies involve caregivers who are typically in the dental field delivering care to nursing home patients. In one of the studies, plaque and gingivitis levels were

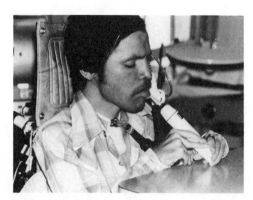

FIGURE 20–12 A pressure-activated toothbrush (Water-Pik) being used by a severely disabled individual.

[n]An ADL cuff is a generic term for any kind of appliance adapted to the upper extremity to which various implements can be added, as, for example, a toothbrush, so that the patient might perform his or her own daily living tasks without assistance.

compared after use of a manual and an electric toothbrush of a counter-rotational design with the care being delivered by a dental hygienist or dental assistant.[43] The results after the use of the powered toothbrush were significantly improved over the manual toothbrush. A second study compared plaque removal and gingival inflammation in a group of nursing home patients after using an electric rotary brush with a single tuft of brushes and a manual toothbrush. The care was delivered by dental students.[44] The electric toothbrush again effected a statistically significant improvement in the two parameters measured.

Even though electric toothbrushes seem to be indicated for use in a mentally handicapped population, Bratel and coworkers[45] were unable to demonstrate clearly the superiority of electric over conventional toothbrushes whether used independently or aided. It may be that electric toothbrushes are beneficial for this population, because patients and caregivers find them easier and more pleasant to use.[46]

It remains to be seen whether features such as smaller brush heads, sonic cleaning power, reciprocating brush heads, or a counter-rotational design may have unique effectiveness for this population (Figure 20–13).

In selecting which toothbrush is best for a particular patient, one should consider alignment of teeth in the arch, constriction of the arches, and whether an exaggerated gag reflex is present.

One additional note of caution should be considered before recommending an electric toothbrush for a compromised patient. An overzealously used electric toothbrush can cause considerable damage to the hard and soft tissues in a short time.

## Floss-Holding Devices

Dental flossing is not recommended for all compromised patients. Unless the task of toothbrushing can be learned, it is useless to superimpose the more complex task of flossing.

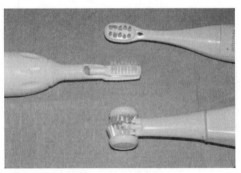

FIGURE 20–13    Electric toothbrushes. Top: multiple reciprocating brush head.[o] Center: sonic cleaning brush.[p] Bottom: counter-rotational design.[q]

To do so can be so discouraging that all attempts at oral hygiene are abandoned. This is true whether the patient or the attendant is performing the program. Flossing, therefore, should be introduced on a selective basis for those patients or attendants who have mastered toothbrushing and consistently show low plaque levels on tooth surfaces.

An adequate assessment of the patient's dexterity and ability to understand the technique must be determined before flossing is introduced.

For some compromised patients, flossing can be performed regularly if a floss-holding device is used. Eight such devices were evaluated by people with upper-extremity limitations.[21] This group rated one device significantly higher for its handle dimensions, ease of threading, and ability to keep the floss taut.[r] Although some compromised patients have learned adaptive techniques allowing them to thread floss-holders themselves, the majority of compromised patients have great difficulty in accomplishing

[o]INTERPLAK®, Bausch & Lomb Oral Care Division, Tucker, GA.
[p]Sonicare, Philips Oral Healthcare, Snoqualmic, WA.
[q]ORALGIENE™ USA, Inc., Culver City, CA.
[r]Floss-Aid Co., Santa Clara, CA.

this procedure. One patient with very limited use of his hands described how his wife kept five floss-holding devices threaded on the kitchen counter for use as he needed them. If one became unthreaded during a flossing routine, he simply obtained another. An alternative to multiple floss-holders is to create a plaster of Paris base for the floss-holding device, so that it can be stabilized by one compromised hand while the other completes the threading. The holder can then be used with or without the base, depending on the patient's strengths and desires. There are currently on the market several brands of floss holders claiming to be self-threading. There have been no comparative studies to determine if, in fact, they offer advantages to a compromised population. Therefore, manipulating the floss with or without a floss holder continues to be a barrier for this population.

### Interproximal Brushing

In older patients, gingival recession is a common experience. Often the recession is so pronounced that the use of regular dental floss is not effective in cleaning the long expanse of exposed root structure. In this situation some recommend Super Floss,[s] as it is considerably thicker at one end. If the gingival recession has occurred to the extent that the papilla no longer fills the interdental space, an interproximal brush may be beneficial.[47] Individuals who have never used floss or who have difficulty manipulating the dental floss or threading a floss holder seem to adapt more readily to the interproximal brush.

Interproximal brushing may be introduced near the beginning of the preventive program. Because handles of interproximal brushes are long and sturdy, they can easily be modified in the same manner as the toothbrush. Many interproximal brushes require the assembly of the proper brush head to the handle. This is an in-

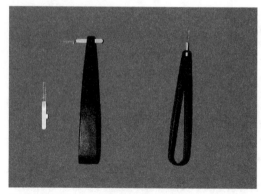

FIGURE 20–14    Interproximal brush handle that can accommodate brush at right (90°) or straight (180°) angle.[t]

tricate task and requires fine-motor skills. Additionally, some patients have severely constricted arches requiring unusual access and angulation of the brush head into the interproximal space. Therefore, the newer preassembled interproximal brushes, those with snap on brush heads and those where the angle of the brush to the handle can be changed from 90° to 180° are recommended for compromised patients (Figure 20–14). Demonstrations of assembly and use are definite requirements.

### Prosthesis Hygiene

Compromised patients who wear full or removable partial dentures may need assistance with maintaining proper hygiene of the appliances, which must be removed for thorough cleaning of the oral soft tissues and any remaining natural teeth. The appliances also must be cleaned appropriately and should be left out of the mouth for 6 to 8 hours per day. Modifications to denture-cleaning devices as well as modifications to the dentures may aid in helping compromised patients provide their own denture hygiene.[48] Oral hygiene care by nurses' aides in institutional settings should include removal of

[s]Oral-B Laboratories, Inc., Belmont, CA.

[t]Proxident holder. Athena Nordic, Fulan, Sweden.

all full or partial dentures and scrubbing and soaking of these appliances, as well as the care of the soft tissue and teeth. Dentures are often lost in institutions by the staff, as well as by the patients themselves. As a result, residents may experience digestive complaints, inadequate nutrition, and speech difficulties, all of which can contribute to a poor self-image. Therefore, it is important for the dental consultant to set up denture-identification programs to mark prostheses with the patient's name, Social Security number, or other means of identification. Then any misplaced appliances can be readily returned to their owner.

### Other Types of Oral Hygiene Aids

From time to time other oral hygiene aids are promoted for use with patients who are in some manner compromised (Figure 20–15). Frequently, these devices have not undergone any testing prior to their marketing, but are promoted on the basis of potential worth. When or if such testing is accomplished, claims are not always upheld. An example of such a product is the disposable "foam on a stick" device. In a study by Addems and colleagues,[49] able-bodied subjects showed marked increases in plaque and gingival index scores during the week when the foam sticks were used (compared with a week when conventional brushing was performed).

Another study[50] found some equality in removing plaque with the foam sticks in comparison to a regular toothbrush, but it was clear that the toothbrush was more effective in retarding plaque accumulation. Cotton swabs[x] are frequently used for oral hygiene in institutionalized settings. If swabs are used that contain citric acid, significant damage to the dentition can occur in the form of irreversible erosion of the enamel.[51]

In another study by Kambhu and Levy,[52] four devices were compared for efficacy when used on a simulated dependent care population by a nonprofessional caregiver. An unusual toothbrush with curved bristles,[y] as well as an electric toothbrush with ten different rotating tufts of bristles,[z] were more effective at removing plaque than a conventional toothbrush. A foam stick device came in a distant fourth in the study. The subjects rated the curved-bristle toothbrush as the most comfortable, and the caregiver rated it as the easiest to use.

Another device incorporates three different sets of brush tufts angled around an arc into one toothbrush head.[53] This allows the facial, occlusal, and lingual surfaces of each tooth to be brushed at the same time. Although no difference was found in plaque and bleeding indices when this brush was used in comparison to a regular manual toothbrush, it seemed to be easier to teach its use to mentally retarded individuals. However, this brush configuration does not work in cases of severe gingival recession.

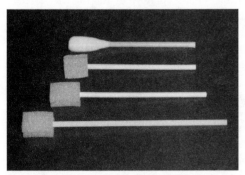

FIGURE 20–15  Oral hygiene aids. From top: swab on a stick,[u] foam on sticks of varying size (minifoam stick,[v] foam sticks with longer handles.[w])

[u]Moi-Stir®, Kingswood Laboratories, Inc., Carmel, IN.
[v]TOOTHETTE®, Halbrand, Inc., Willoughby, OH.
[w]MEDI-CLENZ®, Specialized Care Co., Hampton, NH.

[x]Moi-Stir®, Kingswood Laboratories, Inc., Carmel, IN.
[y]Collis-Curve™ Toothbrush, Collis-Curve, Brownsville, TX.
[z]INTERPLAK®, Bausch & Lomb Oral Care Division, Inc., Tucker, GA.

## Disclosing Techniques

Whatever the patient's age, disclosing products should be suggested to visualize plaque when a patient has difficulty in plaque removal. Disclosing solutions are readily available over-the-counter in multidose bottles. Recently, single-dose packaging of disclosing solution with its own cotton-swab applicator has become available and may prove practical for weekly plaque removal effectiveness checks in institutional settings (Figure 20–16). Should the price of disclosing solution serve as a deterrent the cost factor can be minimized by purchasing commercial food coloring, usually available in the bakery section of any grocery store. The food coloring can then be used in place of the disclosing solution to stain dental plaque. The color should be chosen on the basis of which is easiest to see in the mouth. For example, yellow is difficult to detect on teeth because the color is too close to that of natural tooth color. Blue and green, although suitable for teaching plaque control to children, are more difficult for the aging eye to see. Red food coloring is the easiest to visualize for all age groups. A popular color, it can be found packaged in a number of different containers, including individualized plastic bottles that are much easier

to use. Two drops of food coloring should be placed on the tongue and the patient advised to use the tongue to wipe the food coloring around all the surfaces of the teeth prior to brushing. An alternative technique when the patient is unable to follow these directions is to have the caregiver apply the food coloring to a cotton swab and gently dab it on the teeth. The plaque is well stained with either of these methods, and, as the volume of liquid used is minimal, little drooling or subsequent staining of the individual's clothes occurs.

## Preventive Therapies

### Dietary Considerations and Alternative Reward Systems

For many compromised patients, foods high in sugar are distributed throughout the day as a reward for having been compliant. Such a reward system encourages between-meal snacking and increases the consumption of highly cariogenic foods.[18] With patients who have decreased neuromuscular coordination or decreased salivary flow, it may be difficult to adequately clear the mouth.[20] Food may remain in the buccal vestibule and between the teeth until the next brushing. To reduce the cariogenic potential, it is necessary 1) to restrict between-meal snacking and 2) to limit the use of highly cariogenic foods.[20] If sweets are to be consumed at all, they should be presented at mealtime and the teeth brushed immediately after eating. Bedtime snacks should be discouraged.

An alternative to a reward system based on sugary treats[20] is to present tokens for later redemption for prizes, such as toys, noncarious food, or outings.

### Sealants and Fluorides

In spite of the normalization of handicapped individuals into the mainstream of society, it appears that the non-institutionalized handicapped do not have as high a level of oral health as the rest of the population. The F

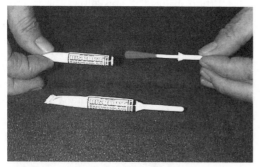

**FIGURE 20–16** Single dose disclosing solution with cotton swab applicator.[aa]

[aa]DISCLOSE® Beutlich Pharmaceuticals LP, Waukegan, IL.

(filled) value for the DMF (decayed, missing, or filled) scores is often lower in the compromised population, whereas the D and M values are higher than in the general population.[54, 55] Although becoming more common, preventive strategies that would really benefit this population group are often not available on a regular basis. The use of sealants and fluorides should be considered important preventive techniques to assist in caries control for compromised patients.[55]

Sealant application may be more difficult in compromised patients, because it may be more difficult to control moisture contamination. Salivary pooling is often seen in cerebral palsy and muscular dystrophy patients, because they have swallowing difficulties. For the short time needed to apply sealants, antisialogogue medications are usually not indicated. Instead, the sealant may be applied in the conventional manner using the techniques to control saliva flow indicated in Chapter 10. To aid in moisture control the patient should be seated upright rather than in a reclining position.

In a 30-month study of a preadolescent population with Down syndrome living in a hostel-like group setting, the application of dental sealants was 100% effective with a sealant retention rate of 97% in preventing caries over the term of the study.[56]

Regular topical fluoride applications by the dental staff are highly important for the compromised dental patient. A new fluoride-containing varnish developed for dentinal hypersensitivity is now available as a unit-dose application and can be used as a fluoride supplement. It is supplied in two doses: 25 mL for primary dentition and 40 mL for mixed dentition (Figure 20–17). The two may be combined to form a 65 mL dose for the permanent dentition. Fluoride varnish can be quickly painted on and is effective even in a moist field, a particularly important characteristic for some of the developmentally disabled and mentally retarded population who have a disordered swallowing mechanism and are therefore unable to

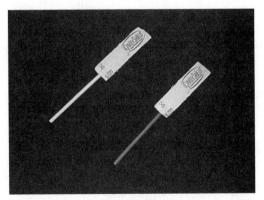

FIGURE 20–17     Unit-dose applicators of fluoride-containing varnish.[bb]

effectively clear their mouths of saliva. For the younger patient, water fluoridation or tablets are essential.[57] Equally important for this population is a home self-applied fluoride program. Several effective techniques are now available for home fluoride application, ranging from mouth rinses to fluoride gels applied with custom-made trays. Rinses are contraindicated for compromised patients who cannot effectively swish the solution around their mouths. Some individuals with muscular dystrophy and some post-stroke patients have an incompetent or hypotonic lip seal and cannot keep solutions in the mouth for the required period. Our experience with office-applied fluoride treatment delivered in a tray requiring the patient to keep the tray in place for a minimum of 4 minutes has demonstrated how difficult it is for many compromised patients to cooperate that long, particularly if there is an active gag reflex. A gel-filled tray also stimulates the flow of saliva, which is often difficult to confine. Neither the patient nor the caregiver likes the drooling that occurs. Therefore, home-fluoride treatments utilizing a tray-delivery method will probably not be successful. An alternative home-fluoride delivery method uses a foam applicator. In a

[bb]CavityShield™ OMNII Oral Pharmaceuticals, West Palm Beach, FL.

nursing home population, Saunders and colleagues[58] demonstrated that the level of fluoride in saliva was higher 3 hours following delivery by an intra-oral applicator when compared to the fluoride levels in saliva after residents rinsed with a fluoride mouthrinse. More independent populations may find brush-on fluoride gels easier to use, because their application takes advantage of an already learned toothbrushing behavior. Fluorides have been shown to reduce demineralization and enhance remineralization.[59] Therefore, brush-on gel fluorides should be considered for use by elderly compromised patients, particularly those with gingival recession. Fluorides should not, however, be indiscriminately given to patients for unsupervised use if some question exists as to the patient's ability to understand and follow instructions. Although Chan and O'Donnell[60] found little risk of toxicity when a fluoridated toothpaste was used independently by a population of mentally handicapped children, one must still exercise caution whenever recommending fluorides.

## Chemical Plaque Control

It has been recognized that treatments need to be developed to manage plaque control that are less dependent on the manual dexterity of the patient.[61] The efficacy of applying chlorhexidine (CHX) by swabbing for people with disabilities has been established. In one study[62] CHX was applied by a caregiver once daily, five times per week, for ten weeks using foam sticks.[cc] When compared with applying a placebo by swabbing, the CHX group showed consistent and significant improvement in lower plaque levels, gingivitis, and pocket depths. A subsequent study[63] demonstrated that CHX swabbing was effective at a reduced frequency (twice per week as opposed to five times per week) and was well tolerated with prolonged use (42 weeks).

Application of sustained-release varnishes of CHX and arginine also produced reductions in plaque, calculus, and pocket depths in a mentally retarded population.[64] The effectiveness of a very low concentration (0.06%) of CHX spray delivered by caregivers was evaluated in developmentally disabled patients,[65] and resulted in significant improvement in plaque scores. Thus, for severely disabled or mentally retarded patients, a caregiver can provide CHX applications by various means and improve the periodontal condition. However, it may not be possible for these patients independently to achieve these positive results as demonstrated in a study comparing CHX and an essential oil mouth rinse.[66]

## Implant Care for Compromised Patients

Patients who have become incapacitated subsequent to having dental implants placed are at significant risk for oral hygiene problems.[67] Once the patient or the family or the institutional staff has demonstrated the level of oral hygiene that is attainable, efforts should be made by the practitioner to modify the implant complex to ensure cleansibility. This should not be done until after a rehabilitation program, if warranted, is completed and it is clear that the level of ability has plateaued. During the interim period more dependence should be placed on chemotherapeutic efforts to maintain good oral health than would be appropriate to do over the patient's remaining life span.

Other compromised patients may be well served by implants if the implant design allows for easy cleaning. In a case report of a person with cerebral palsy, the use of magnetic keepers provided a highly cleansable surface.[68]

## Periodic Preventive Maintenance

Many compromised individuals have a higher incidence of caries and periodontal problems than noncompromised patients and, therefore, they should be seen more frequently.[69] The timing of preventive maintenance appointments

cc TOOTHETTE™, Halbrand, Inc., Willoughby, OH.

should be individualized and should reflect the patient's or caregiver's ability to perform oral hygiene procedures. Often, compromised patients are either on fixed incomes or have limited resources available to finance their dental care. Others who are enrolled in government or private insurance plans may have more flexibility in procuring dental care on a regular basis. Documentation by the dentist of the patient's disability and the subsequent oral problems often assists the patient in obtaining a more generous interpretation of the services covered by the third-party provider. This is particularly true for government plans. For some, the cost of dental care is assumed by the patient's family, who realize the importance of preventive oral care and are eager to see the patient benefit from such treatment. In general, the compromised patient has limited resources to expend on dental care. For these patients, the dental clinician may wish to consider some innovative financial arrangements to pay for preventive procedures. For example, it might be desirable if a contract could be established whereby the patient is brought in on a regular quarterly schedule for prophylaxis. Each appointment after the first one is performed for a reduced fee if the patient completes the entire series of scheduled visits. Concurrent treatment contracts should also be negotiated for restorative care.

### Provider Availability

Although compromised children are usually welcomed in most pediatric dentistry practices, it is often difficult for the similarly afflicted adult patient to find dental personnel with the training, empathy, and patience needed to deal with the patient's disabilities. In recognition of this problem, many dental schools are now providing training in special patient care to current students as well as to practicing dentists in continuing-education courses.[70] These actions should increase the number of dental clinicians with the expertise and willingness to render special care.

### Dental Care in an Institutional Setting

Many institutionalized persons have poor oral health.[71] It is often conjectured that this is because residents of institutions are likely to have more severe disabilities than those who are disabled but live in the community, or that the oral care of institutionalized populations is of poorer quality than those not institutionalized. A recent study examined the oral-hygiene habits, gingival bleeding, food diaries, and oral microorganisms of moderately or severely mentally retarded adults before and up to 21 months after relocating into the community from an institutional setting.[72] Of the oral-health parameters measured, none worsened and some improved, demonstrating that the institutional environment does place the compromised patient at greater risk for poor oral health.

The most common role for the dental provider in an institutional setting is that of consultant. In this capacity, the provider advises the administration about the dental needs of the residents and recommends the type and frequency of oral hygiene care to be delivered.[71, 73] The dental clinician should expect to provide in-service prevention-oriented educational training programs for the nursing staff. The administration and the staff must be kept aware of the importance of routine oral-health care.[74] The administrator of a facility may agree to a routine dental-care program, provided that the dentist or dental hygienist trains the staff. This requires an ongoing training program because of frequent turnover of nurses' aides in such facilities. Training aids may include videotape recordings of the important aspects of preventive care. The dentist should participate in staff meetings when needed. Periodic evaluation of the residents' oral hygiene using an established oral hygiene index helps determine if additional in-service training is needed. A more informed staff relative to the importance of oral hygiene has been shown to result in better oral health care for the residents.[74]

When appropriate, the residents of the various institutions should be encouraged to participate in their own oral hygiene efforts. Instruction in oral-hygiene methods, followed by staff supervision and encouragement, can result in improvements in various periodontal indices.[75]

Even the totally disabled or comatose patient who is no longer taking food by mouth but is being nourished via a gastric tube or intravenous line is subject to intra-oral plaque and calculus accumulation and should have daily oral-hygiene procedures performed. Ironically, it has been shown that, although plaque accumulates at about the same rate in tube-fed and normally fed patients, calculus accumulates faster in tube-fed patients.[76] The objectives for oral hygiene procedures for these patients are basically the same as for all patients except that more care must be taken, including such steps as lubricating the lips of the patient prior to the hygiene treatment. Petroleum jelly is an excellent, inexpensive lubricant that keeps desiccated lips from being injured by mouth props.

The teeth of comatose patients should be brushed in the conventional manner with a soft-bristled toothbrush. Edentulous areas should be wiped gently with gauze or a disposable foam sponge on a stick, both of which can be lightly moistened. If a mobile or central aspirating system is available, a toothbrush can be used that has been manufactured with an aspirating tube[dd] as a part of the brush head.[26] Such a device is an aid to controlling the salivary secretions in the debilitated or comatose patient.

---

### Question 4

Which of the following statements, if any, are correct?

A. Often, the intake of cariogenic foods can be better controlled by a guardian through judicious cooking than by a compromised patient.

B. Dry-field operation and patient cooperation are the two salient requirements for sealant placement.

C. Fluoride dentifrices should be utilized by all compromised patients.

D. Preventive care, even though more economic, usually has a lower priority than treatment.

E. The nurses' aides in institutions for compromised patients are usually well trained to take care of oral-health needs.

---

[dd]Plak-Vac, Trademark Medical, Fenton, MO.

---

## SUMMARY

Individuals with physical, medical, mental, or emotional problems often have a greater need for dental care than their healthy counterparts. This may be because the disability itself has oral manifestations, but more commonly it is because of (1) the limited capabilities of the individual or the family members to understand and to perform important oral hygiene tasks, (2) a lack of understanding of the importance of preventive dental care, and (3) an inability to finance dental care. When a compromised patient does present to a dental office, the clinician should develop a treatment plan that emphasizes prevention. Assessments should be made of the patient's sensory, cognitive, and functional abilities and be used to customize a preventive plan. When the patient

is unable to provide his or her own care, the family or an attendant needs to be taught the appropriate techniques.

Specialized equipment and easy-to-accomplish modifications of conventional oral hygiene devices may be employed to provide oral hygiene care. Strategies such as substituting a noncariogenic reward system to decrease caries incidence are often successful. Dental preventive procedures, such as sealants, fluorides, and chemical plaque control, should be considered for each patient as part of any treatment plan.

The rapport of the compromised patient and his or her family with the dental health provider and the entire office staff is critical to the comfort and compliance of the patient. All members of the office staff need to convey a warm, receptive attitude to these special patients.

Most institutionalized individuals have great oral health needs. The dentist can play a significant role in assessing those needs by communicating recommendations for a daily oral care program to the institutional administrator. Dentists and dental hygienists can offer training to the nurses' aides who provide that day-to-day care.

For many compromised individuals, the retention of teeth in a healthy mouth improves mastication and digestion, as well as helps maintain an adequate nutritional status. The pleasing aesthetics afforded by good oral health help people with disabilities to be more welcomed by others. Good preventive care enhances one's self-esteem. For some patients who are severely compromised, specially adapted appliances may be required to maintain oral health. Many individuals, because of neuromuscular problems, have difficulty functioning with any type of oral prosthesis. Because the natural dentition assumes such an important role in the total living environment of the compromised patient, it is of utmost importance that the patient, caregivers, and the dental team work together to achieve an effective preventive oral-hygiene program for such an individual.

## ANSWERS AND EXPLANATIONS

1. A, C, and D—correct.

    B—incorrect. The patient should be able to see the dentist's face to better understand and to note the dentist's body language.

2. B and E—correct.

    A—incorrect. Remember, do not generalize on what a patient might do because of a handicapping condition; there are always exceptions to the rule.

    C—incorrect. Directions given to the handicapped, especially mentally handicapped, should be as simple as possible to get the job done.

    D—incorrect. A handshake can determine hand strength but does not assess dexterity or cognition necessary to perform oral hygiene.

3. B, C, and D—correct.

    A—incorrect. It is the brush bristles that disturb the plaque—not the dentifrice.

    E—incorrect. Very hot water is sufficient to soften a toothbrush handle prior to modification.

4. A, B, and D—correct.

   C—incorrect. Fluoride dentifrices are desirable for those who have control of their oral musculature; otherwise, undesirable drooling or swallowing of the dentifrice occurs. Other methods of application of fluoride, however, should always be considered.

   E—incorrect. The high turnover of nurses' aides does not permit the development of a good teaching program.


## Self-evaluation Questions

1. A definition of a compromised individual is _____. Before initiating any preventive program, it is necessary to evaluate a range of functional, _____. intellectual, and _____ capabilities.

2. A patient may have a simple decrease in visual acuity, which can be noted when the patient begins to _____. If a human guide or guide dog accompanies the patient, they (should) (should not) be allowed in the treatment room. Other visual problems are _____ and _____.

3. Three precautions that should be taken to ensure that instructions are presented with maximum effectiveness to a person with loss of hearing are _____, _____, and _____. When a high-speed handpiece is turned on next to a hearing aid, it is uncomfortable for the patient because _____.

4. Patients with a history of previous _____ often have difficulty in speaking. In Parkinson's disease, multiple sclerosis, and ALS, there is often an impairment of speech, called _____. A severe impairment in the word sequence in speaking is termed _____. When speech impairment and body paralysis occur, communication can sometimes be accomplished by use of _____ (device).

5. The best way to determine the IQ of a patient is to _____. If a homebound patient cannot complete a task, the _____ (person) should be given the responsibility of helping.

6. A simple test to determine hand muscle strength is _____. To determine whether a patient has the cognitive and psychomotor ability to use a toothbrush, the easiest method is to _____.

7. One position that a caregiver might take in brushing the teeth of a compromised individual is _____. Two disadvantages of using toothpaste are _____ and _____.

8. Two mouth props are the _____ and the _____. Of these, the _____ needs to be secured with a piece of dental floss to prevent its being swallowed, while the second, the _____ prop, can cause an overopening of the mouth.

9. At least three modifications of a toothbrush are _____, _____, and _____. Electric toothbrushes can be used by severely weakened patients by

_____. One problem that might be experienced after compromised patients begin using an electric brush is _____. The _____ brush is often convenient for cleaning the interproximal embrasures.

10. A good substitute for commercially available disclosants is _____.

11. Patients with trouble in walking need either another person as an _____ to help or a wheelchair.

12. Reward systems should *not* include _____. In placing sealants, the two key factors to success are _____ and _____. In a nursing home, it is the _____ or the _____ who normally conducts in-service training for nurses' aides. To avoid the loss of dentures in a nursing home, it is desirable to _____ (action).

## REFERENCES

1. Meskin, L., & Berkey, D. (1989). The next step: A commitment to focus. *Special Care Dent*, 9(4):98–102.
2. Mowery, A. (1993). Communicating with the aphasic dental patient. *Special Care Dentistry*, 13(4):143–5.
3. Langston, R. H. S. (1996). The aging eye. In Jahnigen, D., & Schrier, R., Eds. *Geriatric medicine* (2nded.) (p. 375), Cambridge: Blackwell Science.
4. Evans, J. G. (1997). Stroke. In Wei, J. Y. & Sheehan, M. N. L., Eds. *Geriatric medicine: A case-based manual* (p. 44). Oxford: Oxford University Press.
5. Patients with physical and mental disabilities. (1991). *Oral health care guidelines*. American Dental Association, Chicago: 19.
6. Hooper, C. R. (1994). Sensory and sensory integrative development. In Bonder, B. R. & Wagner, M. B., Eds. *Functional performance in older adults* (p. 95). Philadelphia: F. A. Davis Company.
7. Morsey, S. (1980). Communicating with and treating the blind child. *Dent Hygiene*, 54(6):288–90.
8. Abrams, W., Beers, M., Berkow, R., & Fletcher A. (1995). *The Merck manual of geriatrics* (2nd ed). Whitehouse Station, NJ: Merck Research Laboratories, 215.
9. Collier, D. H., & Arend, W. P. (1996). Musculoskeletal diseases. In Jahnigen, D., & Schrier, R. *Geriatric medicine* (2nd ed.). Cambridge: Blackwell Science, 560.
10. Cherney, L. R. (1996). The effects of aging on communication. In Lewis, C. B., Ed. *AGING: The Health Care Challenge* (p. 103). Philadelphia: F. A. Davis Company.
11. Lange, B. M., Entwistle, B. M., & Lipson, L. F. (1983). *Dental management of the handicapped: Approaches for dental auxiliaries*. Philadelphia: Lee & Febiger.
12. Alpiner, J. G., & Roche, V. (1996). Hearing loss and tinnitus. In Jahnigen, D., & Schrier, R. *Geriatric medicine* (2nd ed.) (p. 365). Cambridge: Blackwell Science.
13. Mhoon, E. E. Otologic changes and disorders. In Cassel, C. K., Cohen, H. J., Larson, E. B., Meier, D. E., Resnick, N. M., Rubenstein, L. Z., & Sorensen, L. B., Eds. *Geriatric medicine* (3rd ed.) (p. 708). New York: Springer.
14. Sawczuk, A. (1990). Dental treatment of the patient with cerebral palsy. In Stiefel, D. J., Truelove, E. L., Eds. *A self instructional series in rehabilitation dentistry*. Seattle: Project DECOD, Module II(D).

15. Mulley, G. P. (1992). Stroke. In Brocklehurst, J. C., Tallis, R. C., & Fillit, H. M., Eds. *Textbook of geriatric medicine and gerontology.* (4th ed.) (p. 374). Edinburgh: Churchill Livingstone.

16. Cherney, L. R. (1996). The effects of aging on communication. In Lewis, C. B. *AGING: The Health care challenge* (p. 95). Philadelphia: F. A. Davis Company.

17. Bäckman, B., & Pilebro, C. (Sept–Oct 1999). Visual pedagogy in dentistry for children with autism. *J Dent for Children,* 325–31.

18. Entwistle, B. (1984). Private practice preventive dentistry for the special patient. *Special Care Dent,* 4(6):246–52.

19. Burkhart, N. (1984). Understanding and managing the autistic child in the dental office. *Dent Hygiene,* 58(2):60–63.

20. Nagel, J. A. (1987/88). Dental awareness for mentally handicapped children. *Dent Health,* 26(6):8–11.

21. Mulligan, R., & Wilson S. (1984). Design characteristics of floss-holding devices for persons with upper extremity disabilities. *Special Care Dent,* 4(4):168–72.

22. Ettinger, R., Lancial, L., & Peterson, L. (1980). Toothbrush modifications and the assessment of hand function in children with hand disabilities. *J Dent Handicapped,* 5(1):7–12.

23. Crespi, P. V., & Ferguson, F. S. (1987). Approaching dental care for the developmentally disabled: A guide for the dental practitioner. *NYS Dent J,* 53:29–32.

24. Dwyer, B. (1984). Professional tips for the nonhandicapped: Measuring expectations. *Dent Assist,* 53(1):21–23.

25. Udin, R., & Kuster, C. (1984). The influence of motivation on a plaque control program for handicapped children. *J Am Dent Assoc,* 109(10):591–93.

26. Napierski, G., & Danner, M. (1982). Oral hygiene for the dentulous total care patient. *Special Care Dent,* 2(6):257–59.

27. Geary, J. L., Kinirons, J., Boyd, D., & Gregg, T. A. (2000). Individualized mouth prop for dental professionals and carers. *Intl J Paediatric Dent,* 10: 71–74.

28. Ogasawara, T., Watanabe, T., Hosaka, K., & Kasahara, H. (1995). Hypoxemia due to inserting a bite block in severely handicapped patients. *Special Care Dent,* 15(2):70–73.

29. Napierski G. (1982). Positioning wheelchair patients for dental treatment. *Prosthet Dent,* 47(2):217–18.

30. Sinykin, S. (Jan–Feb 1984). The dental assistant and the special patient. *Dent Assist,* 24–26.

31. Hylin, D. (1984). Positioning of the cerebral palsy patient to facilitate dental treatment. *Texas Dent J,* 101:4–5.

32. Sklebinski, G. (Jan–Feb 1984). Different strokes. *Dent Assist,* 53:26–27.

33. Sæmundsson, S. R., & Roberts, M. W. (May–June 1997). Oral self-injurious behavior in the developmentally disabled: Review and a case. *J Dent for Children,* 64(3): 205–9.

34. Connick, C., Palat, M., & Pugliese, S. (2000). The appropriate use of physical restraint: Considerations. *J Dent for Children,* 67(4): 256–62.

35. Connick, C., & Barsley, R. (1999). Dental neglect: Definition and prevention in the Louisiana Developmental Centers for patients with MRDD. *Special Care Dentistry,* 19(3):123–27.

36. Mandel, I. D. (1993). The plaque fighters: Choosing a weapon. *J Am Dent Assoc,* 124:71–74.

37. Dickinson, C., & Millwood, J. (1999). Toothbrush handle adaptation using silicone impression putty. *Dent Update,* 26:288–89.

38. Arblaster, D. G., Rothwell, P. S., & White, G. E. (1985). A toothbrush for patients with impaired manual dexterity. *Br Dent J,* 159:219–20.

39. Soncini, J. A., & Tsamtsouris, A. (1989). Individually modified toothbrushes and improvement of oral hygiene and gingival health in cerebral palsy children. *J Pedodontics,* 13(4): 331–44.

40. Gratzer, P. (1982). Elektrische zahnpflege beim mehrfachbeninderten kind. *Rehabilitation,* 21:73–75.

41. Mulligan, R. (1980). Design characteristics of electric toothbrushes important to physically compromised patients. *J Dent Res*, 59:A731.
42. Carr, M., Sterling, E., & Bauchmoyer S. (1997). Comparison of the Interplak® and manual toothbrushes in a population with mental retardation/developmental disabilities (MR/DD). *Special Care Dent*, 17(5): 133–36.
43. Blahut, P. (1993). A clinical trial of the INTERPLAK® powered toothbrush in a geriatric population. *Comp Cont Ed Dent*, (Suppl. No 16):S606–S610.
44. Blahut, P., & Heisch, L. (1991). Clinical evaluation of an electric oral hygiene device in a geriatric population. *J Dent Res*, 70:366.
45. Bratel, J., Berggren, U., & Hirsch, J. M. (1988). Electric or manual toothbrush? A comparison of the effects on the oral health of mentally handicapped adults. *Clin Prev Dent*, 10(3): 23–26.
46. Bratel, J., & Berggren, U. (1991). Long-term oral effects of manual or electric toothbrushes used by mentally handicapped adults. *Clin Prev Dent*, 13(4):5–7.
47. Mulligan, R. (1984). Preventive care for the geriatric dental patient. *Calif Dent Assoc*, 12(1):21–32.
48. Kamen, S. (1997). Oral health care for the stroke survivor. *California Dental Assoc*, 25(4):297–303.
49. Addems, A., Epstein, J. B., Damji, S., & Spinelli, J. (1992). The lack of efficacy of a foam brush in maintaining gingival health: A controlled study. *Special Care Dent*, 12(3):103–6.
50. Lefkoff, M. H., Beck, F. M., & Horton, J. E. (1995). The effectiveness of a disposable tooth cleansing device on plaque. *J Periodontol*, 66:218–21.
51. Meurman, J. H., Sorvari, R., Pelttari, A., Rytomaa, I., Franssila, S., & Kroon, L. (1996). Hospital mouth-cleaning aids may cause dental erosion. *Special Care Dent*, 16(6):247–50.
52. Kambhu, P., & Levy, S. (1993). An evaluation of the effectiveness of four mechanical plaque-removal devices when used by a trained care-provider. *Special Care Dent*, 13(1):9–14.
53. Sauvetre, E., Rozow, A., deMeel, H., Richebe, A., Abi-Khalil, M., & Demeure, F. (1995). Comparison of the clinical effectiveness of a single and a triple-headed toothbrushes in a population of mentally retarded patients. *Bull Group Int Rech Sci Stomatol et Odontol*, 38(3–4):115–19.
54. Lizaire, A. L., Borkent, A., & Toor, V. (1986). Dental health status of nondependent children with handicapping conditions in Edmonton, Alberta. *Special Care Dent*, 6(2):74–79.
55. Nowak, A. J. (1984). Dental disease in handicapped persons. *Special Care Dent*, 4(2): 66–69.
56. Shapira, J., & Stabholz, A. (1996). A comprehensive 30-month preventive dental health program in a pre-adolescent population with Down's syndrome: A longitudinal study. *Special Care Dent*, 16(1):33–37.
57. Swallow, J., & Swallow, B. (1980). Dentistry for physically handicapped children in the International Year of the Child. *Int Dent J*, 30(1):1–15.
58. Saunders, R. H., Davilla, C. E., Hayes, A. L., Fu, J., & Zero, D. T. (1994). The effectiveness of sponge-type intraoral applicators for applying topical fluorides in institutionalized older adults. *Special Care Dent*, 14(6):224–28.
59. Shannon, I. L., & Edmunds, E. J. (1980). Reactions of tooth surfaces to three fluoride gels. *NY Dent J*, 46:426, 428–30.
60. Chan, J. C. Y., & O'Donnell, D. (1996). Ingestion of fluoride dentifrice by a group of mentally handicapped children during toothbrushing. *Quint Intl.*, 27(6):409–11.
61. Newman, H. N. (1998). The rationale for chemical adjuncts in plaque control. *Intl Dent J*, 48(3 Suppl 1):2989–304.
62. Stiefel, D. J., Truelove, E. L., Chin, M. M., & Mandel, L. S. (1992). Efficacy of chlorhexidine swabbing in oral health care for people with severe disabilities. *Special Care Dent*, 12(2):57–62.

63. Stiefel, D. J., Truelove, E. L., Chin, M. M., Zhu, X. C., & Leroux, B. G. (1995). Chlorhexidine swabbing applications under various conditions of use in preventive oral care for persons with disabilities. *Special Care Dent, 15*(4):159–65.

64. Shapira, J., Sgan-Cohen, H. D., Stabholz, A., Sela, M. N., Schurr, D., & Goultschin, J. (1994). Clinical and microbiological effects of chlorhexidine and arginine sustained-release varnishes in the mentally retarded. *Special Care Dent, 14*(4):158–63.

65. Steelman, R., Holmes, D., & Hamilton, M. (1996). Chlorhexidine spray effects on plaque accumulation in developmentally disabled patients. *J Clinical Pediatric Dent, 20*(4): 333–36.

66. McKenzie, W. T., Forgas, L., Vernino, A. R., Parker, D., & Limestall, J. D. (1992). Comparison of a 0.12% chlorhexidine mouthrinse and an essential oil mouthrinse on oral health in institutionalized, mentally handicapped adults: One year results. *J Periodontol,* 63:187–193.

67. English, C. E. (1995). Hygiene, maintenance, and prosthodontic concerns for the infirm implant patient: Clinical report and discussion. *Implant Dent,* 4:166–72.

68. Rogers, J. O. (1995). Implant-stabilized complete mandibular denture for a patient with cerebral palsy. *Dent Update,* 23–26.

69. Wathen, W. (1984). Geriatric Dentistry. *Tex Dent J, 101*(6):3.

70. Thorton, J. (1983). Dentistry and the handicapped child. *Ala J Med Sci, 20*(1):22–27.

71. Lange, B., Cook, C., Dunning, D., Froeschle & Kent, D. (2000). Improving the Oral Hygiene of Institutionalized Mentally Retarded Clients. *J Dent Hygiene, 74*(3): 205–9.

72. Gabre, P., Wikstrom, M., Martinsson, T., & Gahnberg, L. (2000). Move of adults with mental retardation from institutions to community-based living: changes in the oral microbiological flora. *J Dental Research, 80*(2):421–26.

73. Quinn, M. J. (1988). Establishing a preventive dentistry program in a long term health care institution. *Gerodontics,* 4:165–67.

74. Faulks, D., & Hennequin, M. (2000). Evaluation of a long-term oral health program by carers of children and adults with intellectual disabilities. *Special Care Dent, 20*(5): 199–208.

75. Shaw, M. J., & Shaw, L. (1991). The effectiveness of differing dental health education programmes in improving the oral health of adults with mental handicaps attending Birmingham adult training centers. *Community Dent Health, 8*(2):139–45.

76. Dicks, J. L., & Banning, J. S. (1991). Evaluation of calculus accumulation in tube-fed mentally handicapped patients: The effects of oral hygiene status. *Special Care Dent, 11*(3):104–6.

# Geriatric Dental Care

*Janet A. Yellowitz*
*Michael S. Strayer*

## OBJECTIVES

*At the end of this chapter, it will be possible to:*

1. Describe the demographic changes associated with the U.S. population 65 years and older since 1900, and how this segment of the population will appear in 2050.
2. Compare key age-related physiologic changes commonly found in older adults with disease related changes.
3. Identify the most prevalent chronic diseases found in the elderly population.
4. Describe the cognitive impairments generally associated with the older adult population.
5. Compare how patterns of oral-health status have changed since 1970, and how oral-health status will change among older adults by 2030.
6. Identify the three key oral disease processes commonly found in older adults.

## INTRODUCTION

During the latter half of the 20th century, the age composition of the population changed dramatically, with more people living to older ages and the older population getting older. This demographic change will have a major impact on the delivery of general and oral-health care, as well as on the providers of these services. Although some older adults have physical and/or psychological conditions that require special attention in the dental office setting, one should not assume that all older people share these

conditions. Yet, the greatest challenges in geriatric care focus on the oldest, sickest, frailest, as well as those with multiple medical and/or psychological problems.[1] In order to be best prepared for the future practice of dentistry, oral-health professionals need to be knowledgeable about the general and oral-health status of older adults, the physical changes associated with aging, and how best to optimally address these issues.

The "elderly" segment of the population is diverse and has been subdivided into the following categories:

1. People aged 65 to 74 years are the *new* or *young elderly* who tend to be relatively healthy and active;

2. People aged 75 to 84 years are the *old* or *mid-old,* who vary from those being healthy and active to those managing an array of chronic diseases;

3. People 85 years and older are the *oldest-old,* who tend to be physically more frail. This last group is the fastest-growing segment of the older adult population.

Although the elderly have traditionally been defined by as those over age 65 years, age 75 may be a more appropriate age to consider, allowing for some flexibility to account for the many variations found in this population.

## Demographic Trends

The 20th century has been experiencing an unprecedented "graying of America" (Table 21–1).[2,3] Today, 35+ million Americans or one in eight are age 65 or older, compared to only 3.1 million people at the turn of the century. Since 1990, the population 65+ years increased 10.6%, compared to an increase of 9.1% for the under-65 population.[2] The older population is also getting older. Compared to the population in 1900, in 1999 the 65 to 74 age group (18.2 million) was 8 times larger, the 75 to 84 group (12.1 million) was 16 times larger and the 85+ group (4.2 million) was 34 times larger, thus making the 85+ population the fastest-growing cohort of both older adults and the population as a whole.

By 2030, there will be about 70 million older persons, more than twice their number in 1999. Representing 13% of the population in 2000, the 65+ population is expected to grow to be 20% in 2030. In addition, the number of centenarians—people at least 100 years old—almost doubled in the past decade.

Although this growth pattern of the aging population slowed down during the 1990s, be-

TABLE 21–1 **Persons 65+ Years, 1900 to 2030 (in millions)**

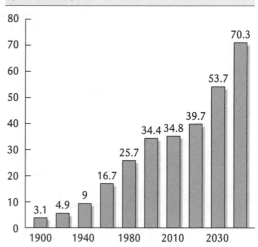

*Source:* U.S. Bureau of the Census.

Administration on Aging. U.S. Department of Health and Human Services. *Profile of Older Americans: 2000.* www.aoa.dhhs.gov/aoa/stats/profile. June, 2001.

cause of the decrease in the birth rate during the 1930s' Depression, a rapid increase is expected between the years 2010 and 2030, when

the "baby boomers" will reach age 65. By 2030, the 65+ population will rise to close to 20% of the population.[2]

Ethnic and minority populations are also projected to increase during this century, with the number of Hispanic-American and Asian-American populations to increase substantially by 2050. Minority populations are projected to represent 25.4% of the elderly population in 2030, an increase from 16.1% in 1999. Between 1999 and 2030, the white population is projected to increase by 81% compared to 219% for older minorities, including Hispanic-Americans (328%), African-Americans (131%), American Indians, Eskimos and Aleuts (147%), and Asians and Pacific Islanders (285%). These dramatic population changes will continue to alter the availability and delivery of general and/or oral health care.

## Life Span/Life Expectancy

Life span is generally defined as the maximal length of life potentially possible—the age beyond which no one can expect to live. Human beings have a life span of approximately 120 years. Life expectancy is the average number of years a group of individuals born during the same time period or cohort is expected to live. Between 1900 and 1997, life expectancy at birth increased from 46.3 years to 73.6 years for males, and from 48.3 to 79.4 for females.[4] (See Table 21–2.) Life expectancy also increased for the 65-year and older cohort, from 11.9 years in 1900 to 17.7 years in 1997 (Table 21–2).[4] These increases in life expectancy are primarily caused by advances in medical technology, and environmental and public-health measures. The increase in the population 75 and 85 years and older is of particular concern to health-care providers, since this age group tends to present with the highest frequency of physical and cognitive disorders.

As the population ages, the distribution of older adults varies greatly by gender. At age 55, there are approximately 100 females for every

**TABLE 21–2A  Life Expectancy, by Age Group and Gender, in Years, 1900–1997**

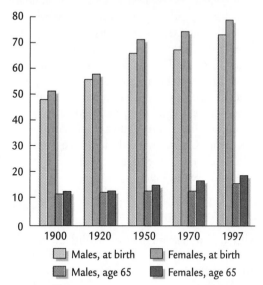

Males, at birth ◻     Females, at birth ◻
Males, age 65 ◻     Females, age 65 ■

*Source:* National Vital Statistics System.

**TABLE 21–2B  Life Expectancy, at Birth and at Age 65, by Gender, in Years, 1900–1997**

|  | 1900 | 1940 | 1960 | 1980 | 1997 |
|---|---|---|---|---|---|
| At birth, males | 47.9 | 61.6 | 65.5 | 70.1 | 73.6 |
| At birth, females | 50.7 | 65.9 | 66.8 | 70.1 | 73.6 |
| At age 65, males | 11.5 | 12.2 | 13.0 | 14.2 | 15.9 |
| At age 65, females | 12.2 | 13.6 | 15.8 | 18.4 | 15.9 |

Federal Interagency Forum on Aging-Related Statistics. *Older Americans 2000: Key Indicators of Well-Being.* Federal Interagency Forum on Aging-Related Statistics, Washington, D.C.: U.S. Government Printing Office. August 2000. Page 70.

100 males; at age 65 there are approximately 122 females for every 100 males; whereas at age 85, there are 259 females for every 100 males. Thus, as the size and proportion of elderly increases in the future, females will continue to outnumber males in the older age groups.

## Marital Status

Marital conditions and living arrangements of older persons vary tremendously by gender. Most men spend their later years married and in family settings, whereas most older women spend their later years as widows outside of family settings. This situation is primarily because most women marry older men, women have a longer life expectancy, and thus outlive their spouses. In addition, widowed or divorced men generally remarry rather than continue to live alone. Older widowed men have a remarriage rate that is over eight times higher than older widowed women.[5]

## Living Arrangements

Although approximately one-third of the elderly live alone, the majority of older non-institutionalized adults live in a family setting. However, these figures vary by gender and advancing years. Most men 75 years and older live with their spouses or other family member, compared to less than 50% of the women in this age group. Although only a small percentage (4.5%) of the 65+ population lived in a nursing home in 1997, the percentage increases dramatically with age, ranging from 1.1% for persons 65–74 years to 4.5% for persons 75–84 years and 19% for persons 85+ years of age.[6]

### Question 1

Which of the following statements, if any, are correct?

A. The new-elderly today are older than the new-elderly of yesteryear.

B. The oldest-old are dying off too fast to be a significant economic and health problem for the taxpayers.

C. The percentage increase in white population over the next thee decades will outnumber each of the following ethnic and cultural groups: Asian and Pacific

Islanders, African-American, Hispanic-American, African-American and American Indian, Eskimo, and Alaskan Aleut.

D. At age 85, there are more single men than single women.

E. The majority of individuals over 85 live in nursing homes.

## Education

The educational level of the older population is increasing. Between 1970 and 1999, the percentage of older adults having completed a high school education rose from 28% to 68%. This group varied considerably by race and ethnic origin, with 73% of whites, 68% of Asians and Pacific Islanders, 45% of African Americans and 32% of Hispanics.[2]

In summary, elderly of the future will be older, better educated, have better control of their finances, include more females, and have more minorities than ever before. With these changes, the elderly of the future will be significantly different than today's elderly population.

## Health Status

The study of aging includes not only diseases that cause morbidity and mortality but also the conditions that cause disability and decline in independent functioning. Table 21–3[7] lists the most common causes of death among elderly people in the United States, and Table 21–4[7] lists the most common chronic conditions effecting adults in different age groups.[7] The three leading causes of death in the elderly are: *diseases of the heart, malignant neoplasm* (cancer) and *cerebrovascular disease* (stroke). Eliminating deaths caused by heart disease would add an average of 5 years to life expectancy at age 65 and would lead to a marked increase in the proportion of older persons in the population.[8] Yet, if cancer as a cause of death were eliminated, the average life span would be extended by less than 2 years.

TABLE 21-3 **Population by Age and Type of Disability**

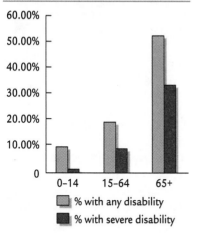

*Source:* Current Population Reports, "Americans with Disabilities, 1994-95, P70-61, August 1997.

Current Population Reports, U.S. Department of Commerce, Economics and Statistics Administration, Household Economic Studies, *Americans with Disabilities, 1994–1995:* Series p70–61. August 1997.

TABLE 21-4 **Persons 70+ Years with Select Chronic Conditions, by Gender, 1984 and 1955**

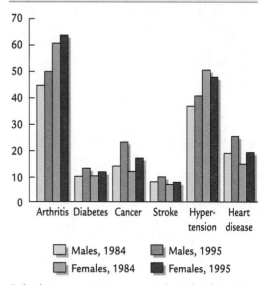

Federal Interagency Forum on Aging-Related Statistics. *Older Americans 2000: Key Indicators of Well-Being.* Federal Interagency Forum on Aging-Related Statistics, Washington, D.C.: U.S. Government Printing Office. August 2000, page 24.

The most common chronic conditions are arthritis, hearing impairment, hypertension and heart disease. The majority of health conditions and diseases are the result of the accumulation of ones' lifestyle, genetic factors and environmental conditions.

For many older Americans, chronic disease is a fact of life; however, most older adults perceive themselves in a positive manner. Approximately 80% of the elderly have at least one chronic medical condition. Yet, almost 71% of non-institutionalized older adults describe their general health to be excellent, very good or good, compared with others their age.[4]

### Physiologic Changes Associated with Aging

Physiologic changes have a cumulative effect as they relate to the continuum of biologic, psychologic, social, and environmental processes of aging. Many of the deficits traditionally thought to be associated with aging are actually signs of pathologic processes. Changes occur for all people, tissues, and organs, however these changes occur with differing rates and individual variability. Variations occur at every age and in every part of the body. Since many internal changes can mimic disease manifestations, and normal changes can mask signs of disease processes, it is very important for those who care for the aged to be knowledgeable about the changes that do occur with aging, rather than identifying changes either as pathologic or associated with the aging process.[9] The four characteristics of physiologic aging are: *universal, progressive, decremental,* and *intrinsic.*

The determinants of aging are complex, and include environmental exposures, genetics, lifestyle, and physiologic and psychological fac-

tors. Physiologic age-related changes are not mutually exclusive but rather synergistic and impact each other. In general, as the body advances in years, it tends to become less adaptive to stress. Physiologic changes associated with aging can modify every system in the body, and impact the style and manner in which dental care is delivered.

The major results of the aging process are: a) a reduced physiologic reserve of many body functions (i.e., heart, lungs, kidney); b) an impaired homeostasis mechanism by which bodily activities are kept adjusted (i.e., fluid balance, temperature control and blood pressure control); c) an impaired immunonologic system, as well as related increased incidence of neoplastic and age-related autoimmune conditions.[10]

The loss of elders' ability to function to capacity includes a decline in respiratory function and the inability to accommodate to temperature changes. It is important for the dental team to be aware of these changes; in particular when older adults are challenged by trauma, acute illness, or external temperature extremes. In each of the incidences, older adults tend to be less able to maintain a stable, internal physiologic state. As dental practitioners tend to maintain their office at a cool temperature, the decline in an older persons' baroreceptor function may cause the person to feel cold, which can impact their postural reflexes, causing the patient to be susceptible to orthostatic hypotension.[10] In addition, it is helpful to keep a blanket in the office to keep patients comfortable.

The cardiovascular system of older adults tends to be more likely to develop ischemia, arrthymias, and heart failure, especially when concurrent illness is present. With increased exercise and/or stress, there is an increase in cardiac output. For older adults, the work of the heart is increased as blood is pumped through a less compliant arterial system.

Slight increases in systolic blood pressure are not unusual for those in older age groups, however, one must ensure the pressure stays within acceptable values (<160/95 mm Hg) Systolic hypertension is a strong risk factor for stroke

and heart failure, and warrants treatment if it remains consistently elevated over 160 mm Hg, regardless of age. Diastolic blood pressure is not known to change with older age. Although both blood pressure lability and the prevalence of "white coat hypertension" are increased in the elderly, the clinical significance of these phenomena is controversial.[11, 12]

Nutrition deficiencies are common in the elderly patient. In community-dwelling elderly, anorexia and micronutrient deficiencies are common.[13] Anorexia is multifactorial, affected by changes in taste and smell, lifestyle, physiologic, and psychological changes. Multivitamin supplementation can often improve nutritional status and immune function in this population of older adults.[14]

Loss of subcutaneous fat and decrease in elastic tissue in the dermis render the skin of older adults more susceptible to tear-type injuries. In addition, wound healing is impaired in older adults.[15] Injuries from minor trauma, loss of the skin's effectiveness as a barrier, and a decrease in immune function renders the older person skin prone to infections.[16]

Age-related eye changes are common in older adults. The majority of older adults experience presbyopia, or age-related changes in the lens and iris of the eye. Persons with *presbyopia* have difficulty focusing on *near* objects, often requiring the use of reading glasses. In addition, those with presbyopia experience a greater loss of dynamic visual acuity (viewing objects in motion) than in static acuity. The ability to adapt to sudden changes of light and darkness also diminishes with age. An example of this change is experienced when moving from a brightly lit area to a darkened one, as when entering a movie theatre from the snack area. Yellowing of the lens and accumulation of insoluble protein in the center of the lens fibers eventually develop into *cataracts*, which not only reduce visual acuity, but also cause increases in light scattering, rendering the older adult with poor vision and a sensitivity to glare.[17]

Hearing impairment is common over the age of 60; with a prevalence of 25 to 30%

among community-dwelling elders and close to 70% in residents of long-term care facilities. *Presbycusis* is the most common type of hearing loss in older adults and is caused by both pathology and, in some cases, auditory processing.[18] Presbycusis causes gradual, progressive *bilateral hearing loss,* predominantly in the higher frequencies, as well as decline in speech discrimination. Both atherosclerosis and cumulative noise exposure may contribute to presbycusis. Communication with an individual affected by presbycusis is enhanced by slow, distinct vocalization at a low pitch. Shouting can actually be painful to the patient and does not improve the ability to understand what is being said.

## Question 2

Which of the following statements, if any, are correct?

A. The elimination of heart disease as a cause of death would result in a greater increase in life expectancy for the total population than if cancer were the first to be eliminated.

B. Each, and all of the following are major signs of the aging process: (a) reduced physiologic reserve of many body functions; (b) impaired homeostasis; (c) impaired immunologic system; (d) increased number of neoplastic conditions; (e) heart conditions, and (f) stroke.

C. Wound healing of the elderly following oral surgery would be expected to be slower than among the young.

D. Presbyopia and presbycusis are both common problems among elderly patients entering the dental office.

E. In counseling an older individual, it is advisable to evaluate if he/she can fully communicate and understand, as well as being able to consent and participate in a proposed treatment regimen.

Bone remains metabolically active throughout life. Age-related bone loss is extremely common, reflecting an imbalance between bone resorption by osteoclasts and bone formation by osteoblasts. *Osteoporosis,* a common problem in the elderly, is an age-related disorder characterized by a decrease in bone mass and by an increased susceptibility to fractures. Losses in bone mass with advancing age are multifactorial, including inactivity, estrogen deficiency, nutritional deficiencies and age-related changes. Clinically, advanced osteoporosis can present with chronic back pain, from mechanical strain caused by kyphosis or vertebral compression fractures. Recent studies indicate that changes in alveolar bone as a result of osteoporosis may contribute to the progression of periodontal disease.[19] Also, a significant decrease in bone mass of the mandible may lead to fragility and increased resorption, risk of fracture, and failure of osseointegration of implants. Prevention, rather than treatment, is the key to the management of osteoporosis. Exercise, vitamins, a balanced diet, dietary calcium, and estrogen play a role in the treatment and prevention of osteoporosis.

Despite extensive neuronal loss, cognitive function in the absence of pathology is well preserved for the most part. Certain neuropsychologic abilities do show decrement with age.[20] Difficulty with *word-finding* is a common complaint of healthy older adults, and a common symptom of cognitive disease. However, as most older adults do not experience cognitive diseases, with sufficient time older persons do find the desired word as successfully as those in younger age groups. *Processing speed* is also slower in older adults. Thus, complex tasks that require quick responses, especially in the context of distracting stimuli, can be hard for the elderly to perform. The central nervous system undergoes significant changes during the course of aging. Decreased response time is often seen in the elderly population, but there is a wide variation between individuals.

The immune system becomes less competent with age. However, the degree of defi-

ciency is not severe enough that opportunistic infections occur commonly in the elderly population.

It is the responsibility of the dental team to be aware and to address the commonly seen age-related changes of aging. Both modifications of office design and patient management techniques are best incorporated in the dental practice addressing the "graying of America."

Cognitive function in those ages 80 years and older is influenced by the high prevalence of dementing illnesses.[21] See section on Cognitive Function.

## Functional Status

Functional status is a critical indicator of health and well-being in the older person, and is one of the most challenging issues in health care of older adults. Functional status is often a better descriptor of an individual than the presence of specific diseases, as impairments in physical and cognitive functioning predict mortality, institutionalization, and the type and amount of health-care services needed. Identifying one's functional status requires a comprehensive *health assessment*, including an assessment of the individual's *functional abilities, health status, physical, psychological,* and *oral-health status*.

A functional assessment evaluates one's ability and limitations to complete basic tasks of daily life.[7] Functional status is defined in terms of Activities of Daily Living (*ADLs*) and Instrumental Activities of Daily Living (*IADLs*). Activities of Daily Living are those abilities that are *fundamental to independent living,* such as bathing, dressing, toileting, transferring from bed or chair, feeding and continence. Instrumental Activities of Daily Living (IADLs) are more complex *daily activities* such as using the *telephone, preparing meals* and *managing money*. The individual's ability to complete ADLs and IADLs will affect the person's ability to access and maintain their oral health care regimen.

Functional limitations serve as key indicators of an older person's ability to remain independent in the community, their quality of life and active life expectancy. Approximately 72% of the population aged 65+ years reported having no difficulty with ADLs and IADLs, while about 10% had difficulty with 3 or more ADLs.[22] As age increases, the percentage of the population having no difficulty with ADL's or IADLs decreases. The two most common IADLs identified by the elderly are *difficulty walking* and *getting outside*.[23] These common conditions may require dental-health professionals to modify the individuals' treatment plan, and to consider schedule times that are optimal for the patient.

## Cognitive Changes Associated with Aging

Inaccurate assumptions and false beliefs about mental health and the cognitive changes of aging have resulted in an overemphasis on decrements often associated with older adults. Recent studies of the aging brain show that major cognitive declines do not occur in the absence of disease, trauma, or stress. Developmental transitions, life events and environmental changes may interfere with older adults' ability to concentrate and to think clearly. Research has ascertained that one's intellect does not decline as an outcome of aging but rather, as a result of many conditions including poor nutrition, disease and hormonal changes.[24] An older person usually takes longer to learn the same information as a younger adult, but when given sufficient time, the end result is similar for both individuals. In general, more time is needed for an older person to encode, that is, to retrieve or to recall the information. In later life, mental health is measured by the capacity to cope effectively with relationships and environment and by the satisfaction experienced in doing so.

Because of the multiplicity of factors that relate to the treatment of the elderly, it is impor-

tant to evaluate the ability of the patient to communicate and to understand, consent to and participate in the treatment. The practitioner must determine, either through an interview or through professional services, the capacity of the individual to respond to treatment.

The *most common type of dementia* in the elderly is senile dementia of the *Alzheimer's type (SDAT)*, accounting for approximately 80% of all dementia's seen in the elderly. The second most common cause of dementia in the elderly is multi-infarct dementia or *vascular dementia,* accounting for 15 to 25% of cases.[25]

Alzheimer's disease is a progressive, degenerative, dementing illness that attacks the brain and leads to the loss of memory, intellectual capacity, thinking, and behavioral changes. SDAT is characterized by the accumulation of *neuro-fibrillary tangles* and *senile plaques* within the cerebral cortex.

Alzheimer's disease has an insidious onset that manifests as loss of recent memory, impairment of judgment and personality changes. Those with SDAT may experience confusion, personality and behavior changes, impaired judgment, difficulty finding words, finishing thoughts or following directions. When experiencing the early stages of the disease, the individual generally maintains good social skills and is often able to "disguise" the presence of the disease. In its early stage, the disease is often very difficult to assess, and is generally denied by family members.

The cause of SDAT is not known and currently there is no cure for it. Although SDAT has been found in younger age groups, it afflicts approximately 10% of those over the age of 65 and *47% of those over age 85.* The disease progresses from 2 to 20 years, and presents as a complex picture of overlapping symptoms, reflecting a continuous decline in memory, thinking, and behavior. Cognitive skills and competency in life skills decline. There is loss of memory, language, intellectual prowess, concentration, emotionality, and altered spatial

motor performance. Both verbal and nonverbal communication is affected.

There are numerous reversible causes of these symptoms in older adults including infection, dehydration and vitamin deficiencies. Attentive health-care professionals, in particular oral health-care professionals may be one of the first caregivers to detect some of the early, subtle changes associated with Alzheimer's. It is incumbent upon the health-care professional to assist the individual to obtain a comprehensive assessment to correct the reversible causes whenever possible and to assist the individual and family in the opportunity to address the care and management of the individual.

## Oral-Disease Patterns

During the past 50 years, one of the major changes in oral-disease patterns in the United States has been a steady *decrease in the rate of edentulism*. It is likely that for the first time in recorded history there are now more older adults with natural teeth than without teeth. In 1986, almost 30% of those 65 to 74 years were edentulous, whereas in 2024 it is predicted that only 10% of this group will be edentulous.[26] This decline in edentulism appears to be the result of water fluoridation, increased public awareness of preventive approaches, improved access to services, and a decrease in early tooth loss.[27]

Although the prevalence of edentulism increases in the non-institutionalized older age groups (10% of 45 to 54 years, 28.4% of 65 to 74, and 52.5% of 85+ years), these rates have steadily decreased over time.[26] This decline in tooth loss results in more natural teeth at risk for caries (coronal, recurrent, and root) and periodontal diseases. As these trends continue more restorative and preventive services will be needed in future dental practices.

Recent reports have found the prevalence of coronal caries is decreasing for children and young adults of middle to high socioeconomic status. Although dental caries has not traditionally been perceived as a problem for the el-

derly, decay rates have been found higher in some adult groups than in children. As long as teeth are present, individuals remain at risk of dental caries.[28] Unfortunately, many older adults do not place a priority on oral health care, and view seeing a dentist only to relieve pain and discomfort. For those not receiving routine dental care, and as a result of increased deposits of secondary dentin and a reduced sensory ability, many older adults tend to seek care only when their decay is in a late stage. A survey of Iowa's' population found 30% of dentate elderly had untreated coronal decay, with 77% having either a new coronal or root lesion in the last 3 years.[29]

Root caries is common and frequently occurs in this age group. Root caries has been found in 65% of the males and 53% of the females in the 1985–86 NIDR study.[30] With the use of new preventive approaches and restorative materials, the dilemma associated with restoring root-carious lesions is expected to diminish in the future.

Contrary to many long-held views, periodontal disease is *not* an age-related disease. Although the prevalence of periodontal disease appears to increase with age, this is likely due to the long-standing cumulative nature of the disease, with its onset earlier in adulthood. In addition, much of the available data reflects cross-sectional studies that do not present a generalizable view of the population. Longitudinal survey data is needed to document the progression of the disease. It is estimated that *90% of adults 65+ years* need periodontal treatment, with 15% needing complex treatment.[31] With the rate of periodontal disease progression partly related to the mass and composition of the oral microbiota and the host's ability to respond to this microbial population, research has focused on new diagnostic and treatment modalities, such as DNA diagnostic probes, enzymatic assays and bacterial analyses, the use of lasers, new pharmaceutical preparations and subtraction radiography. With new diagnostic methods complementing traditional clinical techniques, earlier identification of periodontal

disease and risk factors will be possible, as well as early treatment to help reduce disease progression and its subsequent loss of teeth.

---

### Question 3

Which of the following statements, if any, are correct?

A. Determining the ability of an individual to perform the Activities of Daily Living (ADL) and the Instrumental Activities of Daily Living (IADL) is a better means to evaluate a person's functional age than using age alone.

B. Periodontal disease is associated with the older individual; however, periodontal disease is not caused by aging—it is caused by oral neglect while aging.

C. The four general key admonitions to retaining teeth for a lifetime are: (1) have frequent recalls and dental examinations, and (2) have early diagnoses for disease and disease risk, followed by appropriate (3) early preventive and/or (4) restorative treatment.

D. Approximately 47% of individuals over 85 are afflicted with dementia of the Alzheimer's type.

E. Presbycusis, but not presbyopia, are physical problems of many seniors who will visit a dental office.

---

Like most cancers, oral cancer occurs primarily in the older age segments of the population, with the majority of cases diagnosed after age 65 and more than 95% occurring after age 40.[32] The key issue related to oral cancer problem is the need for *early and effective diagnosis*. Although the primary risk factors for the development of oral squamous cell carcinoma have traditionally included alcohol abuse and use of tobacco products, these risk factors do not have to be present for a lesion to develop. Thus, it is incumbent upon the oral health care professional to provide oral cancer examinations to

all patients on a regular (at least annual) basis. As the multifactorial etiology of oral cancer becomes evident, other factors including alterations in cellular oncogenes, as well as microbial and viral infections may be found to play a role in the pathogenesis of premalignant lesions and oral squamous cell carcinoma.[33] Given that early diagnosis of oral cancer greatly improves the prognosis of the disease, and that many factors influence the timing at which oral cancers are diagnosed, i.e., lack of access to care and patient delay in seeking treatment,[34] oral-health professionals must provide when appropriate, routine comprehensive intra- and extraoral examinations of their patient populations.

It is essential to recognize that no broad, generalized decremental changes in oral health occur simply with age. Healthy older people can expect to keep their teeth, throughout their lifetime. However, in the presence of one or more medical conditions and/or their treatments, oral functions may be altered which can then impact upon the patients' general and oral health status.

Through frequent recall visits and regular professional examinations, adults will be better able to maintain their dentition throughout their life. Prevention of oral disease is the critical component for oral-health maintenance. In addition to promoting and monitoring the basic oral-hygiene practices, the practitioner needs to be aware of the changing physical, psychologic, socioeconomic, and medication status of their older adult patients. In addition, the practitioner needs to be ready and willing to intervene and make necessary modifications to treatment as well as referrals to community resources. Older adults and their caregivers need to be educated and have their education reinforced so to enhance their knowledge of oral care protocols.

## Long-Term Care

Long-term care refers to health, social and residential services provided to chronically disabled persons over an extended time.[35] Longitudinal studies in the United States suggest that persons 65 years and older have a 40% chance of spending some time in a long-term care facility before they die. Of those who enter nursing homes, 55% will spend at least one year there, and over 20% will spend more than five years there. Two of the most common symptoms that lead to nursing home placement are incontinence and behavioral problems such as wandering or disruptive actions often associated with dementia and Alzheimer's disease.[36]

The majority of the 65+ population lives in the community, while only 4.5% are in nursing homes.[21] Of those institutionalized in 1990, 1% were 65 to 74 years, 6% were 75 to 84 years, 19% were 85 to 89 years, 33% were 90 to 94 years, and 47% were 95 and older. Given the growth of the 85+ population, a substantial increase in the future use of nursing homes appears inevitable.[37]

The delivery of oral-health care to residents in long-term care facilities or for those who are homebound presents special challenges for the professional. In addition to the mode of care delivery, this patient population tends to be frail, functionally dependent and often lacking any level of self-interest in their oral health. Cognitive declines, lack of motivation, physical impairment, and chronic medical problems all contribute to a decrease in self-care ability and increase risk of oral disease. This population has been characterized as having high levels of edentulism, coronal and root caries, poor oral hygiene, periodontal diseases and soft tissue lesions.[38, 39]

For the first time, the provision of oral-health care is mandated in long-term care institutions. The Omnibus Budget Reconciliation Act (OBRA) of 1987 (Public Law 100-203) requires all nursing facilities "must employ comprehensive assessments to determine specific health care needs of those residents who participate in Medicaid or Medicare Part B programs. The assessment must be conducted not later than 14 days after admission and can be amended up to 30 days after admission. Nursing facilities must review the resident's condition

for any changes in health status every 3 months and perform the comprehensive assessment annually. The assessments are conducted by a registered nurse, with input from a physician or other health care practitioner(s) as necessary." While these assessments are not required to be completed by a dental professional, dentists and/or dental hygienists need to be identified as part of the health-care team of the long-term care facility. Given a rapidly growing population of dentally aware older adults, future population growth patterns and technological advances in portable and mobile dental equipment, oral-health care programs in long-term care facilities will become feasible and common locations for providing dental care.

One major influence on dental utilization is having dental insurance. Since dental insurance is generally provided as an employee benefit, the elderly typically do not have this benefit. According to the 1989 NHIS[26], 50% of the 35 to 54 year, 37% of the 55 to 64 years and 15% of the 65+ population had private dental insurance. Dental benefits are not included in Medicare, and very few states provide dental service to adults through the Medicaid program. In 1990, nearly 75% of edentulous persons 35+ years did not have private dental insurance compared to about half of the dentate population.[40] Since edentulous persons are less likely to have visited a dentist for the past 5 years, routine examinations for and early treatment of oral soft-tissue diseases are precluded. Thus, the elderly edentulous population may be identified as one of the major underserved populations of this country.

> ### Question 4
>
> Which of the following statements, if any, are correct?
>
> A. The two most common causes of cancer are excessive consumption of alcohol and smoking; the two most important ways to insure recovery from cancer are early diagnosis and early effective treatment.
>
> B. Two out of every five (40%) of Americans over 65 will spend time in a nursing home before death.
>
> C. The majority of institutionalized individuals usually have private dental insurance.
>
> D. The two most common causes for nursing home attendance are incontinence and osteoporosis.
>
> E. Dental care is authorized for the elderly under Medicare.

## SUMMARY

With more older adults and more teeth per older adult, the composition of services rendered to this population will change dramatically in the next decade. The oral health professional of today and of the future will be called to treat an ever-increasing number of older adults. The future elderly will be different than the current cohort seen today. The future elderly will have more teeth, visit the dentist more often, have a higher level of education, better finances and a dramatically different perspective of needs. They are and will continue to be a heterogeneous mix of individuals with various levels of functional, socioeconomic and oral health status. Advances in materials and technology in combination with the changing patterns of oral diseases will continue to have dramatic effects on the practice of dentistry.

The role of the oral health-care professional will focus more on the diagnosis and treatment of oral diseases and disorders, using new aids and devices such as lasers, CAD/CAM, and molecular probes. As diseases of the hard tissues are resolved, more emphasis will be placed on the diagnosis and treatment of soft tissue lesions. With new and improved diagnostic skills, the older adult, the group identified as having the highest risk of oral cancer may no longer require the extensive and often disfiguring surgical remedies currently in place. Preventive oral-health approaches need to be maintained throughout the lifespan.

In order to provide optimal care to the aging population, one must remain current on oral medicine, pharmacotherapeutics and changing technologies. Oral health-care professionals must address how this aging population will manage in the dental facility, and, at a minimum, have accessible offices, large-sized type medical history forms available, as well as easy-to-read signs, health literature, and appointment cards.

## ANSWERS AND EXPLANATIONS

1. A—correct.

   B—incorrect. The elderly are living longer as a group, hence being the oldest, the sickest and the frailest, they constitute a major health (and political) challenge.

   C—incorrect. The truth is that between 1999 and 2030, the white population is projected to increase by a tremendous 81%; however this will be drawfed by the estimated 328% by Hispanic-Americans, 285% by Asian and Pacific Islanders, 147% by American Indians, Eskimos and Aleuts, and 131% by African-Americans.

   D—incorrect. There are more older widows because women marry earlier than men, hence often outlive their spouse.

   E—Incorrect. Majority means over 50%. The correct percentage of individuals over 80 living in nursing homes approximates 19%.

2. A, B, C, D, E—correct.

3. A, B, C, D—correct.

   E—Incorrect. BOTH presbycusis (hard of hearing) and presbyopia (far sightedness) are problems for the dental office; patient mobility and patient communication are jeopardized by these two impairments.

4. A, B—Correct.

   C—incorrect. The answer is that many nursing home residents do not have dental insurance. Part of this problem is due to the fact that many have dentures and do not believe they need insurance. Others do not have the money for insurance that buys access to professional care, nor do they have the motivation or physical ability to desire to maintain self-image.

   D—incorrect. Incontenence is one of the two major problems. Osteoporosis is not; (it can be coped with in home environments). The second major reason for institutionalizing individuals is the dementia characteristic of Alzheimer's disease.

   E—incorrect. Medicare does not subsidize routine dental care.

# REFERENCES

1. Hazzard, W. R. Bierman, E. L., Blass, J. P., Ettinger, W. H., & Halter, J. B. (1994). *Principles of geriatric medicine and gerontology.* New York: McGraw Hill.
2. The American Association of Retired Persons (2000). *A profile of older americans.* Washington, D.C.
3. U.S. Department of Health and Human Services. *Trends in the health of older Americans: United States, 1994.* DHHS, Vital and Health Statistics, Series 3, No. 30, 1995.
4. National Center for Health Statistics (1999). *Health: United States 1997.* Public Health Service.
5. U.S. Bureau of the Census (1991). *Marital status and living arrangements 1990.* U.S. Bureau of Census, Current Population Reports. P-20, No. 450.
6. Gabrel, C. S., & Jones, A. (2000). *The national nursing home survey: 1997 summary.* Vital & Health Statistics—Series 13: Data From the National Health Survey, (147): 1–121.
7. Adams, P. F., & Benson, V. (1990). *Current estimates from the National Health Interview Survey 1989.* Vital and Health Statistics, Series 10, National Center for Health Statistics.
8. U.S. Senate Special Committee on Aging (1991). *Aging in America: Trends and Projections.* U.S. Department of Health and Human Services.
9. Goldman, R. (1979). *Decline in organic function with age.* In Rosman, R. L., Ed. *Clinical Geriatrics* (2nd ed.) (pp. 113–116). Philadelphia: JB Lippincott.
10. Medalie, J. (1986). The practice of geriatrics. In Calkins, E., Davis, P. J., & A. B., Ford, Eds. *An approach to common problems in the elderly.* Philadelphia: WB Saunders.
11. Glen, S. K., Elliott, H. L., Curzio, J. L., Lees, K. R., & Reid, J. L. (1996). Whitecoat hypertension as a cause of cardiovascular dysfunction. *Lancet, 348:* 654–57.
12. Myers, M. G., Reeves, R. A., Oh, P. I., & Joyner, C. D. (1996). Overtreatment of hypertension in the community. *Am J Hyperten, 9:* 419–425.
13. Morley, J. E., Mooradian, A. D., Silver, A. J., Heber, D., & Alfin-Slater, R. B. (1988). Nutrition in the elderly. *Ann Intern Med, 109:* 890–904.
14. Chandra, R. K. (1992). Effect of vitamin and trace element supplementation on immune responses and infection in elderly subjects. *Lancet, 340:* 1124–27.
15. Chuttani, A., & G. B. A., Skin, in *Handbook of Physiology: Aging.* 1995, Oxford University Press: New York. p. 309.
16. Fenske, N. A., & Lober, C. W. (1990). *Skin changes of aging: Pathological implications, 45:* 27–35.
17. Liesengang, T. J. (1984). Cataracts and cataract operations. *Mayo Clin Proc, 59:* 556–67.
18. Jerger, J., Chmiel, R., Wilson, N., & Luchi, R. (1994). Hearing impairment in older adults. New Concepts. *J Am Geriatr Soc, 43:* 928–35.
19. Rose, L. F., Steinberg, B. J., & Minsk, L. (2000, October). The relationship between periodontal disease and systemic conditions. *Compendium Continuing Education in Dentistry, 21*(10A): 870–7.
20. Ciocon, J. O., & Potter, J. F. (1988). Age-related changes in human memory: Normal and abnormal. *Geriatrics, 43:* 43–48.
21. Fleming, K. C., Adams, A. C., & Peterson, R. C. (1995). Dementia Diagnosis and Evaluation. *Mayo Clin Prac, 70:*1093–107.
22. National Center for Health Statistics. (1993). *Health Data on Older Americans: United States.* Vital and Health Statistics, Series 3, No.27. Centers for Disease Control and Prevention.
23. Kart, C. S., Metress, E. K., & Metress, S. P. (1988). *Aging Health and Society.* Boston: Jones and Bartlett.

24. Jarvik, L. (1988). Aging of the brain. How can we prevent it? *Gerontol,* 28:739–47.
25. White, L., Cartwright, W. S., Cornoni-Huntley, J., & Brock, D. B. (1986). Geriatric epidemiology. *Ann Rev Gerontol Geriatr,* 6:215–311.
26. Weintraub, J. A., & Burt, B. A. (1985). Oral health status in the United States: Tooth loss in the United States. *J Dent Educ,* 49:368–78.
27. Bloom, B., Gift, H. C., & Jack, S. S., *Dental Services and Oral Health, 1989. Vital Health and Statistics, Series 10, National Health Interview Survey.* 1992.
28. Papas, A., Joshi, A., & Giunta, J. (1992). Prevalence and intraoral distribution of coronal and root caries in middle-aged and older adults. *Caries Research,* 26:459–65.
29. Hand, J. S., Hunt, R. J., & Beck, J. D. (1988). Coronal and root caries in older Iowans: 36-month incidence. *Gerodontics,* 4:136–39.
30. National Institute of Dental Research. (1987). Oral Health of United States Adults: National findings. *NIH Publ.* No. 87-2868.
31. Berg, R. L., & Cassells, J. S. (1990). *Oral Health Problems in the 'Second Fifty'.* In The Second Fifty Years: Promoting Health and Preventing Disability. Washington D.C.: National Academy Press.
32. Berkey, D. B., & Shay, K. (1992). *Geriatric dental care for the elderly.* In Baum, B. *Oral and Dental Problems in the Elderly, Clinics in Geriatric Medicine.* Philadelphia: WB Saunders.
33. Greer, R. O. (1993). *Recent clinical and molecular biological advances in diagnosis and treatment of oral cancer.* in *Scientific Frontiers in Clinical Dentistry, An Update.* National Institute of Dental Research, Washington, D.C.
34. Sadowsky, D. C., Kunzel, C., & Phelan, J. (1988). Dentists' knowledge, case-finding behavior and confirmed diagnosis or oral cancer. *J Cancer Ed.* 3:127–34.
35. Doty, P., Liu, K., & Weiner, J., (1985). Special Report: An overview of long-term care. *Health Care Financing Rev.* 6:69–78.
36. Ouslander, J. G., Osterweil, D., & Morley, J. E. (1997). *Medical Care in the Nursing Home,* 2nd ed. New York: McGraw-Hill.
37. Brody, J. A., Brody, D. A., & Williams, T. F. (1987). Trends in health of the elderly population. *Ann Rev Public Health.* 8:211–34.
38. Berkey, D. B., Berg, R. G., Ettinger, R. L., & Meskin, L. H. (1991). Research review of oral health status and service use among institutionalized older adults in the United States and Canada. *Special Care Dent,* 11:131–36.
39. Strayer, M. S. & Ibrahim, M. (1991). Dental treatment needs of homebound and nursing home patients. *Community Dent Oral Epidemiol,* 19:176–77.
40. Schou, L. (1995). Oral health, Oral health Care and Oral health promotion among older adults: Social and behavioral dimensions. In Cohen, L. K. & Gift, H. C. *Disease Prevention and Oral Health Promotio.* Copenhagen: Munskgaard.

# CHAPTER 22

# Preventive Dentistry in a Hospital Setting

*Norman O. Harris*
*Jeffery L. Hicks*

## OBJECTIVES

*At the end of this chapter it will be possible to*

1. Discuss the scope of dental services available at community, federal, and large metropolitan hospitals.
2. List at least eight categories of patients seen on a hospital service who benefit from a hospital dental service.
3. Name or describe the personal oral-hygiene items that, at a minimum, each hospitalized patient should possess at time of admittance, and that should also be stocked in the hospital store.
4. Cite several adverse side effects of chemotherapy and radiation therapy for cancer.
5. Outline the responsibilities of the oral surgeon, the speech therapist, the pediatrician and the pediatric dentist in the effort to make life as near-normal as possible for a cleft-palate individual.
6. Orient students about the administrative functions of a hospital and examples of a hospital dental and medical service in action.
7. Compare peritoneal dialysis with hemodialysis.
8. Explain why dentists favor pregnant women having folate during the first four months of pregnancy.
9. Tell another student what precautions you are going to take with this afternoon's high-risk cardiac patient.

# INTRODUCTION

The idea of providing for the delivery of dental services in a hospital setting is not new.[1] The first dentist to practice in an American hospital was Richard Courtland Skinner, who immigrated to Philadelphia in 1788.[2] Later, he was the first dentist to ask for and receive an official appointment to a medical institution. In the 1790s, Skinner created the first hospital dental clinic in the Dispensary of the City of New York to treat the indigent. It was not until the middle of the 19th century that Garretson and Hullihan laid the foundation for the practice of hospital dentistry.[3] Approximately 200 years after Skinner, in 1987, it was reported that about 40,000 dentists had hospital privileges.[4] In 1901, the Philadelphia General Hospital developed the first dental-intern training program. In spite of the fact that about 60% of all hospitals have dental programs, not all hospitals extend staff privileges to dentists. Presently, the *admission* of dentists to a hospital staff and the extent of dental *privileges* is a determination *made by each individual hospital* and is reflected in the hospital by-laws.

The following partial job description illustrates the typical daily tasks of a hospital dentist: "The hospital dentist focuses on serving those who cannot receive dental care through the traditional delivery systems. Patients who are medically and/or mentally compromised (e.g., with cancer, heart disease, HIV/AIDS, Alzheimer's Disease), often suffer from a debilitating anxiety towards dental treatment. In addition, the service provides care for victims of emergency and trauma to the head and neck regions, offers consultation services for other hospital services, and furnishes dental care to patients residing in the facility. Hospital dentistry renders the full range of surgical, restorative, consultative, maintenance and preventive outpatient procedures offered in private practice settings. The hospital practice also offers services for restorative and surgical procedures completed under general anesthesia."[5]

The majority of the dental care rendered in many hospitals is focused on the diagnostic and treatment care necessary to *support the recovery* of medically compromised patients or patients admitted for serious head and neck diseases, infection, or trauma. The U.S. health-care system recognizes that the training needed by dentists and dental hygienists for hospital practice can be incorporated into a teaching hospital's mission. To support this need for training dental personnel, teaching hospitals support training programs for *graduate students,* and rotate them through a dental department and other appropriate departments such as emergency medicine, internal medicine, and anesthesiology. Every year more than 1000 American dentists receive training in hospitals. At the same time, dental hygiene students and dental assistants have provided dental hygiene services for ambulatory and nonambulatory patients. The scope of the dental services within a hospital varies greatly, being dependent on such factors as bed capacity, economic support, level of specialty expertise, and proximity to medical and research centers.

As a result of the influence of these needs and limitations, dental services of hospitals can arbitrarily be placed in one of three categories:

1. Smaller nonfederal hospitals (private and community) that provide care to *only support recovery* of the patient's primary complaint from the time of admission. These

hospitals usually have only a *short-term* commitment to the patient for a period during which care is being rendered for a primary complaint. Accordingly, the dental service available is generally concerned with delivering maxillofacial care resulting from accidents. The oral surgeon may be on-call for cases arriving at the emergency room—or the problem may simply be handled by an attending surgeon. In these smaller hospitals, it is assumed that any patient requiring dental care, other than that pertaining to the primary complaint, will visit a private dentist following the period of hospitalization.

2.   Military and other federal hospitals that provide total oral-health needs for their active duty or eligible personnel. These services include diagnosis, treatment planning, preventive and treatment services, counseling and programmed recalls. Similarly, Veterans Administration and U.S. Public Health Service Hospitals provide complete care to eligible in-and-outpatients.

During war years, military hospitals are often at the forefront in innovative oral and general surgery.[6] The expertise gained in conflict is then brought back to the peacetime world. For instance, in World War I with its trench warfare, coupled with violent charges across battlefields blanketed with high explosives and a continual hail of high velocity small arms fire, produced devastating wounds of the face and body at a rate never known before.

It is of interest to know that in 1914, there was no general concept for reconstructing a destroyed mandible. It was between 1914 to 1918 that the transplantation of bone emerged as the best approach to restoring the lower jaw. Even then, there was a puzzle as to why one transplant would be a success and a failure in another. It was a Dr. Carl Partsch, a German Army Surgeon, who is credited for pointing out that the success of fracture healing and bone transplantation depended on the *tight contact* between undamaged surfaces, or between stumps and transplantation pieces.[7]

3.   Large metropolitan and university teaching hospitals have expanded their scope of dental services to include treatment for patients with serious systemic diseases associated with a *high risk for life-threatening emergencies*—such as heart disease. For these patients, when crises occur in the hospital, life-saving drugs and/or emergency teams are immediately available. Also, many patients are accepted who have a high risk for *transmitting of disease*, such as AIDS. Finally, to support advanced-degree programs, dental clinics are available to the public. Graduates from these degree programs often remain in hospital dentistry; others enter academia, while others go *well prepared* into private practice.

## Dental Needs of Hospitalized Patients

Dentists as well as other health professionals realize that oral health cannot be divorced from the general health of the hospitalized patient. Many oral conditions are intimately re-lated to systemic diseases. Optimally, total health care requires the *combined* efforts of the medical and dental professions.

Several reports indicated that long-term hospitalized or chronically ill patients had many significant dental needs. To verify these reports, the American Dental Association's

Council on Hospital Dental Services' surveyed 1,634 individuals. It was estimated that about 80% of all patients admitted to a hospital had some form of oral pathosis that *required* treatment. The majority of these patients was unaware of dental problems and typically did not have a family dentist. The six greatest dental treatment needs were the same dental needs as of the general population—dental caries, periodontal disease, plaque or calculus deposits, nonrestorable teeth, partial or complete edentulism. They also discovered that adequate, functional, fixed, and removable prosthetic devices were nearly nonexistent and that the level of dental care previously provided was very low. Poor oral hygiene, gingival inflammation, and papillary hyperplasia were the most prevalent periodontal problems. Almost all of the dentures examined were inadequate, with gross amounts of materia alba present on the denture and in the buccal vestibule. About 57% of patients with acute dental pain had not received palliative care.

There are several categories of hospital patients, each with special needs for dental services. Among others, such patients include: (1) head and neck cancer patients; (2) cleft-palate cases, (3) AIDS patients; (4) renal, liver, and heart-failure patients; (5) patients in need of prophylactic antibiotics; (6) comatose patients; (7) paraplegics, quadriplegics, and amputees; (8) postsurgical patients; (9) diabetic patients; (10) psychiatric patients; (11) obstetric patients; and (12) organ-transplant candidates and recipients. Each individual in each of these groups requires specialized care and counseling. No treatment plan fits all!

## Administrative Requirements

If a dentist or a dental hygienist is to be used in a hospital preventive dentistry program, the hospital administrator *must be receptive* to the idea. While dental hygienists may be employed by a hospital through normal employment channels, dentists must be *admitted* to the hospital staff and be *privileged to provide specific* services. Hospitals have well-defined regulations for the admitting and privileging processes. The existing medical staff and nurses must support any additional ward dental activity that has to be meshed with the other professional time requirements associated with patient care. Unfortunately, the subject of dental care is not emphasized in the formal training of the majority of nondental health professionals. Some medical professionals who have been trained in hospitals that sponsored post-doctoral dental-education programs may be more knowledgeable about hospital dental care. However, this education *usually* must come through continuing personal relationships between dental and medical staff personnel and through continuing education programs.

## The Hospital Dental Department

### Accreditation and Regulations

A hospital is administered by (1) a *governing body* entrusted with the responsibility for the overall organization and conduct of the institution. This body may be a Board of Directors, managers, or trustees and this body will establish policies that are in accordance with documents written by the Founders, the hospital administration and by the laws of the state and nation in which the hospital is located. Hospitals will appoint a (2) *chief operating officer* who has the day-to-day responsibility of maintaining administrative structure, decorum, quality of hospital care, planning and fiscal policies. The (3) *medical-dental staff* of a hospital is the third component of the hospital administrative structure and is composed of its appointed Chairpersons and elected representatives.

Hospitals, in order to be permitted by their respective states to deliver care and to receive reimbursement from federal payors, must participate in a formal accrediting process. Most, if not all hospitals in the United States are accredited by the Joint Commission on Accredi-

tation of Healthcare Organizations (JCAHO). The website of the JCAHO lists as its mission: "To continuously improve the *safety and quality* of care provided to the public through the provision of health care accreditation and related services that support *performance improvement* in health care organizations." In addition, teaching hospitals in the United States and Canada that sponsor postdoctoral dental education programs are *periodically assessed and accredited* by their respective *national dental associations*. In the United States, the accrediting agency is the Commission on Dental Accreditation of the *American Dental Association*. Goals and objectives for both U.S. and Canadian postdoctoral dental programs are similar. Postdoctoral teaching programs evaluate a variety of proficiencies—professional skills and practice management, restorative dentistry, prosthetics, endodontics, orthodontics and pediatric care, oral pathology, oral surgery, periodontics, pharmacology and hospital functioning. To add to this list may be emergency care, sedation anesthesia, and some aspects of public health.[8]

## Dental Department Administration and Sections

The Dental Department is the administrative and clinical hub for *all* dental operations in the hospital. The Department Chairperson is selected by the Hospital Board based on her/his demonstrated leadership and professional competence, and has equal status and responsibilities as the Chairs of other departments. Examples of these responsibilities include a requirement for interdepartmental cooperation and consultation, major and minor oral surgery, operation of a public clinic, clinical and basic research, Ward dental care of dental in-patients, recruitment of department manpower, and for budget preparation to meet expected department needs and for future institution expansion. To accomplish these tasks, many of the duties are delegated to the Section Chiefs—

surgery, prosthetics, periodontics, general practice, pediatric dentistry, and research.

The multichair dental clinic where the majority of routine dental care occurs, usually accepts an outpatient patient load as part of the postdoctoral training program. Many times, this patient load consists of the indigent, with or without government or insurance support. This general practice supervised teaching program is essentially a private-practice environment, and it is a splendid training background before entering practice. It also helps provide the dental manpower to meet the hospital's requirement for a fully functioning dental service.

The Dental Department's maxillofacial team is an essential component to a hospitals mission. In a large metropolitan hospital where emergency surgery is a daily routine, the operating room duties for major craniofacial surgery are usually shared by teams of *Board-Certified* medical and dental maxillofacial surgeons. Oral surgeons treat victims with major soft and hard tissue damage of the face and head. These injuries arise from many sources—automobile accidents, knife and gunshot wounds,[9] and societal and domestic violence.[10] The oral surgeons also provide orthopedic and plastic surgery to correct facial skeletal disharmonies and *developmental defects* such as cleft lip and palate.[11] Some oral surgeons specialize in more extensive *plastic* surgery, while oral *cancer surgery* is another major task for a well-trained oral surgeon.

The successful outcome of any minor or major surgery is determined by whether the patient feels as though he/she can socialize without impediment, whether there is acceptable speech, and whether dental appearance and oral function is satisfactory.[12]

The dental department's maxillofacial *prosthetic section* is an essential component of the maxillofacial team. The absence or loss of soft and/or hard tissue resulting from developmental defects, or following trauma or surgery, often is *too great for corrective surgery* alone.

With training beyond the usual prosthodontics graduate programs, some prosthodontists and laboratory technicians become proficient in sculpting customized dental or cosmetic prostheses.[13] Obturators are needed at times to bridge palatal clefts.[14] Some hospitals have established prosthetic centers specializing in the fabrication of eyes or facial parts lost by trauma or disease;[15] others have specialized in constructing ears lost because of trauma or congenital absence.[16]

In the past, these external and intra-oral prostheses usually *were* held in place with adhesives.[17] Now, whenever possible, they are magnetically connected to implants that are *integrated into bone* for more permanent fixation.[18] Once inserted, a *make-up artist* teaches the patient how to apply different shades of creams and powders to camouflage the prosthesis.

## Intra- and Extra-hospital Cooperation

Many times there is a need for cooperation between the physicians of other services and the personnel of the dental department. For example, there have been needs for endoscopic tooth extractions from the nasal cavity requiring the skills of a nose and throat professional.[19]

Physician intervention is often indicated to cope with seemingly routine tasks of a dental service that turn into emergencies. A few examples are: near-fatal bleeding following over self-medication with quinine,[20] treating of periodontal disease to help control diabetes mellitus (and possibly vice versa), reducing the possibility of a bacteremia of oral origin becoming a problem of cardiovascular pathology, or in receiving help in removing a denture that has lodged in a throat.[21] Some of these problems can be anticipated from a patient's history record, many cannot.

Daily there are requests for clinic consultations and examination of newly admitted patients. There are also many requests from the private sector for extractions under anesthesia, or for dental care of high-risk persons. Some are referred because of patient fear and anticipated difficult extractions, while still others are referred because of mental handicaps, moderate-to-severe behavioral problems or a history of seizures.[22]

Consultations between appropriate hospital services and private referring practitioners is encouraged, both as a form of courtesy to the referring professionals and to ensure that patient management is appropriate.

## Preventive Dentistry

In most smaller hospitals, there are no dental departments, hence no provisions for an active primary preventive program. In one study of short hospital stays, (at least one week) all 33 respondents to a questionnaire indicated they were unable to carry out their self-care as well as they could at home.[23] This finding would probably have been different if the hospital had had a policy of asking each self-sufficient patient admitted, to bring a small kit with a toothbrush and floss to carry out daily self-care procedures. In addition, the hospital store should stock high-demand dental products including fluoride dentifrices, floss threaders, disclosants, fluoride mouthwashes, and denture cleaners. The pharmacies should be in a position to dispense prescriptions for chlorhexidine.

In these hospitals, nurses or nurses' aides must provide essential post-operative dental procedures involving the oral structures.[24] An example might be the daily fluoride spray-cleaning of the mouths of mandibular fracture patients (where the interdental wiring makes mechanical plaque control difficult).

For military hospitals, the task is much easier. All essential dental items are stocked in the hospital exchange for patient purchase. A preventive dental officer is designated by the Chair to insure that the needs of Ward and clinic pa-

tients are served. Usually a visit to the clinic is scheduled for an examination as *soon as is appropriate* following admission. At this time, a dental examination is accomplished to determine preventive and treatment needs. Since, by policy, a military patient is held for recuperation before being returned to full-duty, there is often slack time for accomplishing needed dental services before being returned to his/her unit. During this time, counseling should be directed to the need and methods of self-care—mechanical plaque control (brush, floss, and irrigation), and chemical plaque control (use of fluoride mouth rinses for achieving limited reminerlization), and chlorhexidine (for temporary suppression of caries and gingivitis microbiota). Also, during this time, more intensive remineralization procedures can be instituted for interproximal radiographic lucencies that are without signs of overt cavitation. Since adults *do* develop occlusal caries, sealants should be placed in any deep pits and fissures.

For the clientele of the clinics of *large and university hospitals,* preventive dentistry takes on a more urgent and ominous tone. Many of these patients are high-risk patients who have serious chronic diseases that have been treated at the institution or elsewhere. For these patients, preventive dentistry means preventing the occurrence of life-threatening emergencies as well as protecting the oral structures from disease. The same procedures suggested in other chapters apply for these patients, except that (1) all the preventive actions and risk assessments are monitored at shorter intervals; and (2) all emergency precautions for each condition must be in place before treatment begins.

In total-care hospitals, a preventive dentistry cart should be available to the dental officer, dental hygienist or designated person making the ward rounds. Such a cart should be stocked with items such as disposable plastic mouth mirrors, a flashlight, a hand mirror for patient viewing, sterile tongue blades, cotton applicator sticks, mouth props, and seizure sticks (double tongue blades wrapped in gauze and taped securely). Additional aids can include a spray unit and high-volume, low-vacuum suction unit, aspirator tips, gauze squares, and disclosing tablets. Mouthrinses can be made up in quantity by the pharmacy for Ward use.

---

### Question 1

Which of the following statements, if any, are correct?

A. The first hospital dental service in America was established in New York only a few years after the Revolutionary War.

B. To become a professional member of a hospital staff, a candidate must be privileged.

C. A hospital dental service must be accredited by medical and dental rules and regulations established by the political and professional entities legally claiming jurisdiction.

D. The Chairman of the various departments of a hospital only vote on propositions pertaining to their respective services.

E. Pit-and-fissure sealants should be considered for adults with deep occlusal fissures.

---

To this point, hospital administration has been emphasized; this permits the business and professional aspects of a hospital to function harmoniously. From this point on, *examples* of the professional responsibilities and patient problems of a hospital population will be discussed. The diseases selected for brief discussion—cancer, cleft palate, HIV/AIDS, cardiovascular disease, renal disease, and diabetes mellitus are all pathologies that will be encountered by dentists and dental hygienists over a professional lifetime. These encounters will

occur regardless of whether the practice is a dental office, military facilities, academia, public health, or hospital clinic. The main focus should be in *recognizing* impending or actual emergencies and immediately *initiating a programmed and already rehearsed response*.

## Xerostomia

Many xerostomia ("dry mouth") cases that are seen in a hospital clinic are a combined physician-dentist concern. This hypo-secretion of saliva is seen in several medical and dental conditions—Sjogren's syndrome, intake of xerogenic drugs, dryness of psychogenic or idiopathic origin, diabetes, candidosis, and excessive alcohol consumption.[25]

Xerostomia is especially troublesome when it results from radiation therapy used in the treatment for cancer when the glandular tissue of the major and minor salivary glands are usually destroyed. A drastic *decrease* of saliva flow occurs, and an inverse *increase in salivary viscosity* soon follows. The xerostomia following radiation is generally *irreversible*, although some researchers have reported modest recoveries in some patients (Figure 22–1). Xerostomia diminishes the saliva's buffering capacity resulting in a *major increase of cariogenic organisms*

such as mutans streptococci and lactobacilli.[26–28] Cariogenic activity becomes rampant and accelerated under these "dry mouth" conditions. A radiation-induced caries, termed *radiation caries,* is especially destructive, displaying a cervical and incisal predilection on the teeth for, first plaque and then caries that can rapidly amputate the crown. (Figure 22–2). It should be emphasized that the caries is not caused by the radiation, but is a result of the xerostomia that allowed unrestricted growth of the cariogenic plaque bacteria.

Because the salivary changes following radiation are *permanent*, the threat of radiation caries exists for all teeth *throughout the reminder of the patient's life*. Preventive therapy involves meticulous attention to daily self-care consisting of oral hygiene, a low-carbohydrate diet, frequent dental checkups (at least every 3 months), topical fluoride gel, and chlorhexidine rinsing. Conversely, the xerostomia that occurs following the intake of xerogenic drugs and chemotherapy usually *regresses to normal* following discontinuance of the offending cause.

Salivary stimulants and saliva substitutes are options to provide some relief to the dry mouth. Generally, saliva substitutes consist of a wetting agent (carboxymethylcellulose or sor-

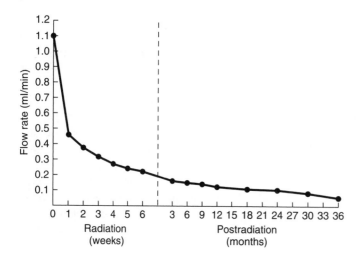

FIGURE 22–1   Mean flow rates of stimulated whole saliva in 42 patients with cancer before, during, and after radiotherapy. (From Dreizen S, Brown LR, Daly TE, et al. Prevention of xerostomia-related dental caries in irradiated cancer patients. *J Dent Res.* 1977; 56:99–104.)

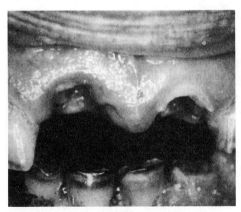

FIGURE 22-2    Severe radiation caries in the maxillary and mandibular anterior region of an adult treated for head and neck cancer. (Courtesy of the late Dr. Simon Katz, Indianapolis, IN.)

bital), electrolytes, fluoride, and flavoring. However, saliva substitutes are poorly accepted by patients because of their short duration of action (10 to 15 minutes). As such, the majority of xerostomic patients prefer frequent sips of water to the saliva substitutes.[29] Sugarless lemon drops and chewing gum, are recommended as methods for increasing salivary output.[26,30] A prescription for pilocarpine, a saliva stimulant, has also successfully increased salivary output in studies involving a variety of xerostomic populations.[31]

## Head and Neck Cancer

Cancer treatment is usually centered at major medical centers having both the facilities and personnel to continually seek new and better approaches to cancer therapy. Examples are the MD Anderson Hospital in Houston, Texas, and the Memorial Sloan-Kettering Cancer Center in New York City. For the year 2001 the American Cancer Society has estimated that there will be approximately 20,000 new cases of *oral cancer* in the United States. This same projection indicates that approximately 7,800 will die

of the disease.[32] Tobacco is the cause of an estimated 390,000 premature deaths in the United States annually. Despite the fact that the *incidence of cancer is increasing*, early diagnosis and significant advances in therapy have resulted in a *much longer and more productive life* for the cancer patient.[33]

Most head and neck cancers are *not* diagnosed early. In examining this problem with dentists in Maryland, where the mortality rate for oral and pharyngeal cancer is seventh-highest in the nation, focus groups found need for continuing education to correct: (1) inaccurate knowledge about oral cancer, (2) inconsistency in oral examinations, (3) lack of confidence in when and how to palpate for abnormalities, and (4) lack of time to routinely conduct oral cancer examination. Most cancers of the mouth are *easy* to see, while those of the floor of the mouth can be *easily* palpated.[34] The typical early intraoral lesion is usually an *indurated ulcer*. Any ulcer that persists for *3 weeks should be biopsied.*[34] The early detection, and early referral leading to a more favorable outcome of therapy, *is* a crucial responsibility of the *general dentist!*

### Cancer Prevention

A tragedy associated with many head and neck cancer deaths is that in *most cases* the disease *could have been prevented.* The great majority of head and neck cancers arise from *three* sources: (1) *smoking* and the use of smokeless tobacco, (2) exposure of the lips and face to the *sun,* and (3) excessive consumption of *alcohol.* Tobacco products account for *three-fourths* of all intraoral malignant (squamous cell) cancer cases (Figure 22–3) in the United States.[35] *Basal cell* carcinomas of the face are often caused by an excess exposure to the natural *sun* or to "*tanning devices.*" *Excess alcohol consumption* is also a major contributory factor to the development of oral and pharyngeal cancer[36,37] with alcohol appearing to synergize with tobacco as a risk factor for all the upper aerodigestive tract cancers.[38,39]

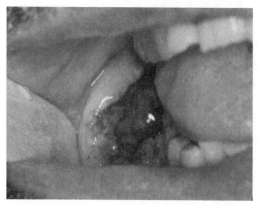

FIGURE 22–3    Intraoral squamous cell carcinoma. The patient was seen in a Hospital Dentistry Department for a complaint of oral pain. His social history reveled tobacco and excessive alcohol use for many years. A biopsy by the general dentist revealed squamous cell carcinoma. Despite appropriate referral for treatment, the patient died within 6 months. (Courtesy of Dr. Jeffery L. Hicks, University of Texas Dental School, San Antonio, TX.)

Even for those ignorant of, or who ignore the admonitions by the American Cancer Society concerning smoking, sun exposure and alcohol, there is frequently a second chance. Usually, there are early nonhealing, *precancerous* changes in the oral cavity or on the face that should alert an individual to immediately seek professional care. Cessation of the use of tobacco, avoiding excessive exposure to the sun, and consuming alcohol in moderation *will help* return the tissues to normal. Finally, if the cancer is diagnosed in the early stages, *immediate treatment* is usually followed by a "clinical cure," provided there is not a return to the original habits.

## The Profile of the Oral-Cancer Patient

The average oral cancer patient is over 40 years of age, with men afflicted more often than women. The most common intraoral cancer is a *squamous cell* cancer that might have been preceded by *leukoplakia*.[34] After a patient has been confronted with an often terrifying diagnosis of head or neck cancer, the scene becomes one of crisis. The patient will quickly undergo a series of examinations and tests by the various hospital services that will be involved in the treatment phase, including dentistry.[40] Following these examinations, the seriousness of the cancer is designated by a *TNM* classification system (staging) with scoring assigned in three areas of clinical assessment: (T)umor size, involvement of the lymph (N)odes draining the area and presence/extent of (M)etastasis. The greater the scoring numbers from 0 to 4 in each of the categories, the *more serious* the prognosis.

As a result of this whirl of activity, the patient is often left completely bewildered as to why teeth have suddenly become so important. Many of these individuals are in their fifth or sixth decade of life—some with a history of excellent oral hygiene, and some with a history of dental neglect. In addition to the impact of the diagnosis of cancer or the specter of possible facial mutilation and suffering from the cancer treatment, the patient is confronted with a possible full-mouth extraction. The result is additional stress to the patient's self-esteem and morale. Then, too, there is the fear of a family economic disaster as a result of medical expenses and loss of income, as well as fear of death. At this time, it is important to be cognizant of the *psychological and physical strain* placed on patients by their diagnosis and projected treatment. As such, patients may not be receptive to care and their pain reaction threshold may be depressed. Education, patience, and a compassionate demeanor will help establish rapport and facilitate care for most patients. However, in some cases the fear, economic, and social pressures are too great to cope with; in these cases pharmacosedation should be considered.[26,41,42]

## Treatment of Oral Cancer

Before treatment begins, all concerned departments comprising the Hospital Tumor Board convene to contribute of their expertise. Singh at the Eastman Dental Institute has pointed out that when the oncology team includes a dentist, the risk of development of serious complications, such as osteoradionecrosis (to be discussed later), are significantly reduced in the cancer patient. Other personnel such as family services workers and a chaplain may be included to contribute to issues that are not directly treatment oriented, yet important to a patient and family. In these meetings, the projected treatment details are discussed—chemotherapeutic agents to be used, the degree of anticipated immunosuppression, the total radiation dose, and the tissue fields (or ports) to be irradiated. Throughout the therapy, the progress of each patient will be evaluated—all with the object of achieving a better end result. Out of these meetings comes a consensus as to the best pretreatment, treatment and post-treatment regimens to be used for each patient.

The treatment for cancer of the oral cavity involves a choice of *surgery*, *radiation*, *chemotherapy*, or combinations thereof. Surgery is used to *excise* smaller cancerous lesions or to *debulk* large tumors (remove as much as possible of large volume cancers). As a co-therapeutic modality, *chemotherapy or radiotherapy* can be an option *following* surgery. The addition of radiotherapy adds two very disconcerting problems to the treatment regimen—*mucositis*[43] and *osteoradionecrosis* (*ORN*). Both are due to damage to the end arteries supplying the mucous membrane of the mouth or to the bone.

Chemotherapy and radiation produce their own complications; chemotherapy involves the use of plant alkaloids, and tumor antibiotics to *kill cells undergoing mitosis*, of which cancer cells are the most rapidly dividing. It is during mitosis that even a normal cell is most sensitive to chemotherapy.

The objective of using radiation has the same objective as chemotherapy—i.e., to *kill* rapidly growing cells. Unavoidably, in both cases other *normal* dividing host cells are also destroyed, such as *hemopoietic cells* (blood-forming cells) of the bone marrow, *epithelial* cells of the oral mucosa and gastrointestinal tract, and *endothelial* cells of terminal arteries are also killed. Host damage by radiation is usually *localized* to the field of irradiation, while the side effects of chemotherapy are *systemic*.

---

### Question 2

Which of the following statements, if any, are correct?

A. The xerostomia that often follows radiation therapy is permanent; that following the use of xerostomic drugs is usually confined to the period of drug use.

B. An ulcer that does not heal in two months should be carefully inspected and possibly biopsied by a professional.

C. The causes for most oral and orofacial cancers are self-inflicted—smoking, drinking, and tanning.

D. A large cancerous growth may be debulked by surgery prior to radiation therapy.

E. The damage from radiation therapy is local; the damage from chemotherapy is systemic.

---

## Mucositis

The mucositis resulting from damage to the mucous membrane is characterized by a mouth that has a raw, ulcerated, and painful mucous membrane that often makes eating and swallowing *very* painful.[44] There is often a reluctance of a patient to eat following the onset of mucositis. Patients will selectively eat cool, soft, high-carbohydrate foods that promote caries development. Patients must be encouraged to take vitamin supplements and eat balanced and creative diets that minimize mu-

cocitic pain, yet promote the desire to eat. Having the patient *consult a dietician* is salient to successfully manage this side effect.[45]

Since the effects of *chemotherapy* are systemic, there are several *systemic* complications. Aside from mucositis the complications include immune suppression (neutropenia—a low-neutrophil count), hemorrhage, and infection secondary to other foci of infection such as dental abscesses and periodontal infection. The use of chemotherapy, *does* suppress mitosis. However, it does *not* result in a marked *decrease in saliva* (xerostomia) production or in a prolonged mucositis such as seen following radiation therapy. Both the mucositis and any xerostomia tend to peak and to *regress within one or two weeks after treatment*.[46,47] Chemotherapy does *not* cause osteoradionecrosis (to be discussed later). However, chemotherapy is a significant source of morbidity and mortality. *Systemic infections resulting from the immunosuppression are responsible for 70% of deaths following chemotherapy.* Fortunately, mucositis occurs in only about 40% of the patients.

## Osteoradionecrosis (ORN)

Many serious complications result from radiation therapy. These include a permanent xerostomia with an accompanying accelerated caries and periodontal disease development, altered smell, dysphonia (speech), malnutrition, trismus, and osteoradionecrosis. But by far, the most serious complication is the potentially disfiguring occurrence and treatment of *osteoradionecrosis*.

Osteoradionecrosis is caused by a destruction of the end arteries *to the bone that were in the radiation beam*. There is a severe *reduction* or *cessation* of osteocyte and osteoclast activity.[48] A rough guideline defines ORN as "an area of exposed necrotic bone that has persisted *three months without signs of healing*" (Figure 22–4). A more optimistic viewpoint of osteoradionecrosis is that only 10% of all cases treated with radiation develop the condition; a more pessimistic outlook is that the risk of ORN is

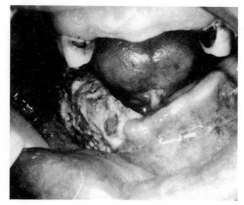

FIGURE 22–4    Massive mandibular osteoradionecrosis secondary to heavy x-ray irradiation for epidermoid carcinoma in the jaw. (Courtesy of Dr. Robert P. Johnson, San Antonio, TX.)

perpetual and continues to increase with the passage of time because the blood supply to the affected area *never* improves. As the total absorbed dose of radiation to bone *increases*, so does the likelihood of ORN developing. Any subsequent surgical trauma to the area, i.e., dental extractions, increases that risk. Because of the density and reduced blood supply to the mandible, one study found that the mandible was affected more than the maxilla by a 95 to 5% margin.[49]

Since the consequences of surgical treatment of osteoradionecrosis are so debilitating, *prevention is the crucial therapy*. The *conservative* treatment consists of analgesics, antibiotics, irrigation and debridement (removal of necrotic tissue) and occasionally, hyperbaric oxygen therapy.[50-52] Hyperbaric oxygen therapy (HBO) increases tissue oxygenation of the tissues by administering 100% oxygen to the patient while in a pressurized chamber (2.4 atmospheres). Under these conditions, tissue oxygenation is increased, which in turn promotes the healing process by encouraging the formation of a connective tissue matrix and *capillary budding*. Unfortunately, HBO is not effective as a singular therapy—and it is time-consuming and expensive.

When the necrotic bone of osteoradionecrosis is extensive, aggressive surgical *excision* of the necrotic areas often becomes necessary—a surgery that can be physically *disfiguring and disabling*.

The initial signs and symptoms of ORN include constant, throbbing pain, along with a soft tissue breakdown over the necrotic bone. Later signs and symptoms include suppuration, a fetid oral odor, possible pathologic fractures and orocutaneous fistulae. Attention to subtle oral changes is required for an early diagnosis.

### Dental Intervention, Cancer

If possible, all needed dental surgery for the newly diagnosed cancer patient should be accomplished *prior* to radiotherapy. All teeth with a questionable prognosis should be extracted, such as those with moderate-to-severe periodontal disease, extensive caries, impacted third molars and irreversible pulpitis. In making a decision to extract or retain teeth, consideration should be given to the past evidence of the patient having maintained a fastidious level of plaque control, overall prognosis, attitudes and expected compliance with written and verbal preventive dentistry instructions.

After exodontia there should be a 21-day waiting interval *before* radiation since the risk of developing ORN increases with a shorter interval elapsing between surgery and radiation therapy.

*Following* radiation, all dental care should be *conservative*, emphasizing endodontic and other tooth retention measures instead of extraction. Unfortunately, regardless of the adequacy of self-care of the preserved teeth, the risk of ORN is *perpetual*, even though the risk exists only for the osseous tissue that was within the field of radiation. Recognizing that patient compliance with oral care instructions following radiotherapy is reported to be less than 50%, frequent recalls are essential.[53] Research to date has clearly shown that routine self-care hygiene measures combined with use of fluoride therapy plus regular dental monitoring, significantly reduces the incidence of postradiation caries and the progression of periodontal disease.[54]

### Cleft Palate

Cleft palate is one of the most common of all birth defects, but very little is known of its cause.[55] Anatomically, it may involve either the right or left, or both the left and right sides of the embryonic incisal bone and lip, as well as the hard and soft palates. At the very minimum there might be evidence of only a slightly bifid uvula. Genetics has been believed to be an important factor in the development of cleft lip/cleft palate for the past 60 years, but no genes have been yet isolated.[56] Several environmental factors have been studied—cigarette smoking, alcohol consumption, organic solvents, and anticonvulsant drugs—with no conclusions.[57]

There is considerable interest that use of vitamin supplements during the first 4 months of pregnancy might have a protective effect.[58] Another study suggested that a folic acid deficiency may be responsible for different malformations through a common mechanism that interferes with embryonic development.[59]

In Europe, 1 out of *every 700 births* a cleft palate is present.[59] In the United States the Centers for Disease Control and Prevention have listed it as approximately 1 in 1,000 births with cleft palate alone, and 1 in 2,500 with cleft lip.[60] As soon as possible after the birth of the child with the cleft, the parents, the oral surgeon and a selected pediatrician must become involved in immediate decisions relating to the projected long series of primary, secondary and tertiary treatments that will be needed to provide the child with a life as near-normal as possible. Counseling should include a briefing with the parents about the future needs for surgery and rehabilitation procedures.

Surgical cleft-lip closure usually commences as early as age 3 *months*, and cleft palate repair at *1 year*. When speech begins, the advice and

corrective actions of a qualified speech therapist is essential to modify the hypernasal speech of a cleft palate individual as well as to insure the intelligibility of the child's speech. The next major surgery is at approximately 9 to 10 years of age, when bone grafting may be employed to restore the maxillary anterior alveolar ridge. After the healing of the anterior alveolar ridge surgery, there should be *orthodontic* corrections of the maligned teeth and jaws. *Prosthetic* appointments are needed to replace those teeth that are still missing, or to bridge the cleft for better eating, breathing, or speech. During this first decade of continual monitoring, it is the responsibility of the pediatrician to assure that the child remains well nourished and healthy. For example, ear infections are a persistent problem for the child with cleft palate. On the other hand, the pediatric dentist is similarly charged with continuously monitoring risk for oral diseases, and taking the necessary preventive actions to abort onset of the plaque diseases.[61]

The cost of care of a cleft palate case is considerable and requires outside help.[59] In Pisa, Italy, for the 800 children born with clefting, the cost is 80 million Euros (1 Euros = +/− 1 dollar), or $100,000 per child. This sum is not exhorbitant, when it is considered that the following members make up the lifetime Cleft Plate Team responsible for the care of each cleft palate birth:

- An audiologist (to assess hearing)
- A surgeon, usually a plastic surgeon, or an oral/maxillary surgeon, or a head-and-neck surgeon, or a craniofacial surgeon, or a neurosurgeon, (to perform corrective surgery)
- A pediatric or general dentist, (to prevent and treat dental problems)
- A dental hygienist, (to provide professional dental preventive care)
- A prosthodontist, (to provide specialized prostheses)
- An orthodontist (to align the remaining teeth prior to prosthetics)
- A geneticist, (to screen patients for craniofacial syndromes and consult parents about the risk of having additional children with clefts)
- An otolaryngologist, (to treat ear, nose, and throat problems)
- A pediatrician, (to monitor overall health and development)
- A psychologist or other mental health specialist, (to support the family and assess any adjustment problems)
- A speech-language pathologist (to assess and correct speech and breathing when swallowing)
- A school counselor (to aid in child's integration into school and educational programs.)
- A social services expert (to aid the family in securing financial help from government, services and fraternal/charitable organizations)

## Question 3

Which of the following statements, if any, are correct?

A. A child born with a cleft of the lip and palate should have both surgically corrected about 3 months after birth.

B. There are more clefts of the lip than of the hard palate.

C. Xerostomia is one of the symptoms of radiation damage to the salivary glands.

D. The identification of a pre- or early cancerous lesion is mainly the task for general practitioners.

E. Two major problem sequellae of radiation therapy are osteoradionecrosis and mucositis.

## AIDS

Acquired immune deficiency syndrome (AIDS) is a symptomatic infectious disease in which lymphocytes; specifically *T helper lymphocytes (CD4 cells)* are invaded and impaired by a retrovirus—the human immunodeficiency virus (HIV). The subsequent *gradual decline* in the number of protective CD4-lymphocyte cell population results in an *immunosuppression* (loss of effectiveness of the body immune defenses) that places the host at risk for *opportunistic infections and cancers*. Another commonly referred to lymphocyte is the *T-suppressor lymphocyte (CD8)*. The two lymphocyte cell populations *may* act in suppressing HIV infection *until they can no longer contain the virus.*

The AIDS virus is transmitted by blood and sexual contacts and the principal contributing behaviors are male-to-male sexual activity and parenteral drug abuse. Initially, the disease was confined mainly to those participating in these activities; however, the disease incidence is now increasing in the heterosexual population engaging in unprotected sex with females at greater risk of infection than males.[62] HIV/AIDS was projected to infect between 5 and 6 million persons worldwide by the year 2000.[62] Patients infected with the virus are termed HIV-positive (HIV+). Following initial infection, HIV patients may remain asymptomatic for years during viral dormancy. Nearly all patients *eventually* develop symptoms that classically consist of opportunistic infections such as pneumocystitis carinii pneumonia,[a] Candida esophagitis, toxoplasmosis, mycobacterial infections and cytomegalovirus.[63,64] Patients are considered to have progressed from HIV+ (Human Immunodeficiency Syndrome) to AIDS when the CD4 lymphocyte cell count

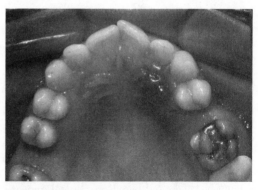

FIGURE 22–5   This HIV+ patient is exhibiting a Kaposi's Sarcoma on the hard palate. This lesion was treated with radiation to prevent its enlargement. (Courtesy of Dr. Jeffery L. Hicks, University of Texas Dental School, San Antonio, TX.)

drops below 500 cells per milliliter of blood.[b] Crossing this threshold results in patients being at increased risk of opportunistic infections.

AIDS patients are at risk for developing certain cancers and the development of these cancers signal a relatively *poor prognosis for survival.* The most common cancer-like disease developed by patients as a result of HIV infection is *Kaposi's sarcoma* (Figure 22–5).[64] Patient mortality attributable to AIDS is *nearly 100%* and is most often the result of an *opportunistic infection.*[63] Longevity has been increased by the use of *Highly Active Anti-Retroviral Therapy,* abbreviated HAART. HAART is a treatment where a combination of anti-HIV drugs—usually three—are administered even before the symptoms of AIDS develop.

Some of the opportunistic infections and cancers affecting AIDS patients are manifested orally, allowing *dental practitioners* to play a major role in diagnosis, patient monitoring, and management. The most common oral infection is *candidiasis—a yeast infection,* which

---

[a]There is no need to memorize the names of these diseases. That will come in Pathology. Just remember that an HIV patient becomes more susceptible to opportunistic diseases as the disease progresses from HIV to AIDS.

[b]The normal CD4 count ranges from about 600 to 1600.

afflicts 75% of all AIDS patients at least once in their disease course. The appearance of *hairy leukoplakia*, is another manifestation of AIDS. It is a corrugated, white, raised lesion located on the tongue.[65] The leukoplakia *cannot* be wiped off. The presence of this lesion appears to be an accurate *predictor* of progression from being HIV⁺ to AIDS. *Approximately 83% of patients who develop hairy leukoplakia are diagnosed with AIDS within 30 months*. This benign lesion does not require treatment and can usually be diagnosed based on clinical appearance without the need for biopsy.[65] *Aphthous ulcers* are also common in AIDS patients ranging from small, discrete lesions to large denuded areas. Kaposi's sarcoma appears as a flat or raised, purple to brown lesion and occurs orally in *50% of all AIDS patients*. The lesions are most commonly seen on the *hard palate* and when indicated, biopsy is suggested for definitive diagnosis. Treatment of these lesions is needed only when they interfere with patient function.[64] Oral Non-Hodgkin's Lymphoma (NHL) is another cancer which is increasingly seen in patients with AIDS. NHL occurs as a soft tissue mass, commonly on the palate or gingiva and may exhibit ulcerations. The occurrence of NHL signals a relatively *poor prognosis*. HIV⁺ dental patients who develop oral candidiasis, hairy leukoplakia, Kaposi's sarcoma, or NHL should be instructed to notify their physician. Development of these complications may indicate a need for a change of medical treatment.

*Acute periodontal infections* are common in AIDS patients. HIV gingivitis appears as an erythematous band of inflammation on the marginal gingiva that will *not* improve with oral-hygiene measures. HIV periodontitis is a rapidly progressive infection characterized by soft tissue ulceration and necrosis, and loss of periodontal attachment. Clinically, the disease mimics *acute necrotizing ulcerative gingivitis* (ANUG). Present treatment recommendations include aggressive scaling and root planing combined with chlorhexidine therapy and an-

tibiotics. *Early* treatment of the HIV gingivitis may prevent the development of HIV periodontitis.[66]

The immuno-compromised status of these patients requires the same aggressive *preventive* approach to caries and periodontal disease suggested for cancer patients. Potential sources of bacteremia should be definitively treated to prevent the development of an oral infection that threatens the patient's systemic health.[67] Xerostomia is a common finding in HIV⁺ patients. The decreased saliva production may be caused by HIV-associated gland disease or as a side effect of HIV medications.

## Perspectives, Responsibilities, Patient's and Dentist's Rights

The AIDS epidemic that came to the forefront in the 1980's has been a very serious disease characterized by a very high death rate. In the field of dentistry, all diagnostic or treatment procedures for HIV/AIDS individuals *is fraught with some degree of danger for the dental team*.[68]

The report of several years ago that a Florida dentist had transmitted the AIDS virus to six persons elevated the infection-control procedures of dentistry to public debate.[69,70] Much of the controversy was probably due to media reporting that favored sensation over rational discourse.[71] However, the debate brought to the forefront the *moral* and *legal* responsibilities of the *dentist to the patient*, and *vice versa*, the responsibilities of the HIV/AIDS patient to the dental team. Anti-discrimination laws restricted the ability of the practitioner to control admittance of new patients, while the Occupational Safety and Health Administration (OSHA) has forced an upgrade in the infection-control requirements of the dental office.[72]

There has been worldwide concern of the public that going to the dentist is beset with the possibility of transmission of the virus caused by incomplete sterilization of instruments. This concern has been exaggerated, but is not entirely baseless. In Hong Kong, teachers

and secondary-school students were polled to determine risk perceptions. Approximately one-half of each group was concerned about contracting HIV infection during dental visits, while 65% of the students and 57% of the teachers believed that a dentist did not have sufficient knowledge to identify AIDS patients.[73]

A mail questionnaire study was completed in Denmark to determine the time, steam and temperature settings used by Danish dentists to sterilize instruments. At the end of the study, it was concluded that 3.4% of the autoclaves had not operated properly.[74]

With the outbreak of a worldwide epidemic, dentists began to use additional disease barriers to protect themselves and their patients—operating uniforms, glasses, masks, and gloves. Yet there appears to be differences among the specialties in use of protective devices. For instance, general dentists outperform orthodontists in use of gloves (92 to 85%), masks (75 to 38%), eyewear (84 to 60%), gloves (92 to 85%) and heat sterilization of handpieces (84 to 57%). Additional precautions were increased in both groups when the patients were *known* to have HIV/AIDS.[75]

It is not known how many patients disclose their HIV status in the patient history form—one study set the figure at 70%. With this 30% uncertainty, dentists must provide maximum recommended barrier techniques and sterilization procedures on the assumption that any patient could be HIV infected.[76]

One of the omnipresent hazards of dentistry is living with the possibility of *needle-stick* and/or *cut* injuries. The actual injury pales in concern to the "terror factor," real or imagined, of contracting a potentially lethal injury.[77] This psychological effect is important considering that 60% of the dentists in a Denmark study reported having at least one needle-stick or cutting injury during the previous year.[74]

There is a *bias* by many dentists for caring for HIV/AIDS patients.[78] At times the bias has been caused by the concern of losing non-

HIV+ patients who discover that HIV/AIDS patients are being treated in a practice. At other times it is caused by sociocultural biases. In a study in Japan, 71% of the dentists surveyed felt as though they had a *moral responsibility* to treat HIV/AIDS patients, but only 16% were *willing* to treat HIV/AIDS patients.[79] In several studies it was believed that additional education is needed to improve knowledge and attitudes relative to the treatment of HIV/AIDS patients.[80] In a survey of dentists in Lothian, Ireland where care is mandated, the dentists considered that their professional background allowed them to cope with disease transmission problems in treating AIDS patients.[81]

As a final note for those worried about contracting the disease from dental professionals, it is worthwhile to quote from an abstract from a paper by Robinson and de Blienk: "The risk of acquiring human immunodeficiency virus (HIV) infection from a health-care worker is 2,000 times less than that of dying from a car accident. It is 700 times less probable than perishing from being struck by lightning or suffering a fatal fall. Despite the rarity of the risk of health-care-worker-to-patient, the transmission of the disease in the workplace has been the focus of investigation by congressional, federal, state, and local agencies. If all HIV transmission from health care workers to patients were prevented using current guidelines and legislation, the epidemic of AIDS would be reduced by 0.0006%."[82]

## The Patient with Cardiovascular Disease

Cardiovascular disease (CVD) is a term that embraces a *varied* array of cardiac pathoses. Generally, CVD patients can be subdivided into (1) ischemic heart disease (IHD—poor blood supply to heart muscle), (2) myocardial infarction (MI—scarred heart muscle from previous heart attack), (3) hypertension, (4) valvular and congenital heart disease, (5) dys-

rhythmias, (irregular and erratic pulse) and (6) congestive heart failure (CHF-failing heart muscle).

The following three sections on cardiovascular disease, renal disease, and diabetes mellitus is *not* meant to provide a detailed account of the drugs and detailed treatment modalities used in their treatment. Instead, it is another series of snapshots of what happens in different departments of a hospital—and are applicable for use in a private practice.

Each year, more than 350,000 adult Americans die each year of sudden cardiac arrest. The fatal event is unpredictable and can occur in patients with no history of cardiac disease or cardiac symptoms.[83] CVD is the *leading cause* of death in the United States and is responsible for twice as many deaths as cancer. Irrespective of the underlying cardiovascular problem, *all dental practices* should be prepared in case that a fatal events threatens or occurs in *your office, and to one of your patients*. Waters and others have laid out a path that should help prepare for such a catastrophe. The preliminary precautions begin on the initial contact with the patient. At this time an assessment is made of the *stress tolerance* of the patient. Such a tentative assessment is made following an interview that expands on the information contained in the patient's medical and dental history. Such details include the prospective patient's narration of health status, drugs being taken, any past heart attacks etc., followed by a possible consultation with the patient's cardiologist. For dental legal record purposes, an informed consent form should be completed outlining the expected treatment, and the expected compliance by the patient.[84]

## Preparing for an Office Emergency

The dentist should maintain a drug cabinet stocked with current fresh drugs. All office personnel should be included in an emergency plan—one that establishes who is to call EMS if necessary and who would secure the emergency drug(s). It is assumed that the dentist would accomplish the initial cardiopulmonary rescusitation, if necessary. A maneuver involving the office team should be rehersed at intervals to ensure an efficient operation if it is ever necessary to initiate an actual rescue plan.

## The Typical Appoinment

All appointments should be *short*—less than an hour if possible—and preferably in the morning.

The patient's chart is reviewed to refresh the memory about details of the patient's medical and dental background.

The treatment phase should be preceded with the taking of the patient's blood pressure. If it exceeds the systolic and diastolic limits suggested by the cardiologist, the appointment should be terminated until the blood pressure is within the established limits. If the treatment is of emergency nature (extraction), consultation with the cardiologist is recommended.

Effective stress management may include preoperative sedation with the decision being dependent upon the *expected stress tolerance* inherent in the proposed operation. *Stress tolerance is a gauge of the heart's ability to sustain additional stress*. Patients with poor stress tolerance (and high risk) include those with severe hypertension, uncontrolled cardiac heart failure, severe dysrhythmias (tachycardia, abnormally fast heart beat and bradycardia, abnormally slow heart beat), or hemodynamic instability (erratic blood pressure), unstable angina (new onset of chest pains, pain at rest, pain that is poorly controlled with medication, or pain that has recently changed character). Severe hypertension is characterized by a diastolic pressure greater than 115 mm of mercury, and a systolic blood pressure greater than 200 mm. There are an estimated 58 million cases of hypertension in the United States, with fewer than 5% having a curable cause. Many do not know they have high blood pressure, or its consequences, (usually heart attack or stroke) hence the term, *"the silent killer."*

At the end of the appointment, if the patient has been sedated, she/he should not be allowed to depart the office unless accompanied by a care giver who can help the patient in activities such as driving or crossing streets.

## On the Day of the Emergency

Everything is going along fine, until suddenly the patient complains of a chest pain. The dentist immediately and correctly ceases the dental treatment. It is now up to him/her to immediately assess the problem and react to the emergency. What is to be done? Not all chest pains are a serious heart attack.[85] Not all hyperventilation heralds a heart attack. The drugs in the emergency cabinet may be sufficient; however, if the dentist's diagnosis is that the pain is considered more serious, the EMS should be immediately contacted by the office personnel. This is a time that the dentist stands alone and must demonstrate decisive leadership as planned in past maneuvers. In a worst case scenario where the heart has stopped, (cardiac failure with unconsciousness) cardiopulmonary resuscitation (CPR) is absolutely necessary. It must be initiated immediately, with the stark reality that if the heart is not restarted in about 4 minutes, cerebral hypoxia jeopardizes life continuance.[86] Adding to the crisis is the fact that the chance of success towards getting the heart restarted is reduced by 10% for every minute that passes. There is not sufficient time to wait for the arrival of the EMS to apply advance resuscitation possibilities, such as the use of the automated external defibrillator. With its use, an electrical shock to the heart muscle offers a much better chance to restart heart action. Although dental offices do not usually have a need for a defibrillator over the lifetime of the practice, its early use instead of CPR, can mean the difference between life-or-death. Passenger planes carry defibrillators for passenger emergencies. They are usually available in large gathering areas such as sports arenas and industrial clinics.[83]

## Critique

There are several questions that can be asked. The most critical would question whether the dentist has the current level of training needed to correctly assess the severity of the case. A second question would be, "Should all dental offices stock defibrilators despite the fact that very few dentists experience a life-or-death situation during their entire professional careers." The third question would be, "If in the estimation of the cardiologist the victim is considered to be a very high risk patient, why was she/he not referred to a hospital with a dental clinic?" In such a facility, monitoring during the treatment is routine, all emergency drugs are available, and a crisis team is available within minutes of being summoned for any emergency.[87]

## Education Needs of the Dentist

In the United Kingdom, in 1999, senior officers in oral and maxillofacial surgery expressed dissatisfaction in their training in resuscitation.[88] These were professionals with graduate training, working with daily high risk operations. Yet, our above dentist was confronted with the same kind of critical decisions learned in a lecture hall some ten- or- fifteen years ago—or more— in dental school. He/she had the leadership, but not the academic background or experience to make the expeditious and informed decisions that were necessary. In view of the rarity of a life-or-death event in any dental office, there is a need for an intensive refresher course, much as given by the airlines to selected crew members to provide defibrillator resuscitation of airline passengers suffering a possible heart attack. Included in such a course should be a refresher session on CPR, mainly because "All healthcare professionals are expected to be competent in cardiopulmonary rescusitation."[88]

## A Final Topic—Antibiotic Prophylaxis

Once there is an invasive procedure involving blood and possible blood borne bacteria, there is the basis for a debate as to whether antibi-

otics should be administered to at risk patients (prophylactic antibiotic coverage). This category of patients includes immunocompromised patients and end-stage organ disease (kidney, liver), patients with certain cardiovascular manifestations (heart murmur, prosthetic valves) and patients with prosthetic joint replacements. The purpose of the antibiotic coverage is meritorious i.e., to get the antibiotic into the blood stream to eliminate the microorganisms before they reach the target organ; and secondly to get the antibotic into the target organ to eliminate any invading organisms. Acting on this common sense belief, antibiotics were used before all invasive procedures

to prevent infection. However, with the extensive use of antibiotics, it was soon noted that several strains of bacteria began to appear that were resistant to antibiotics. It was not long before the American Heart Association drew up some guidelines (Table 22–1 and 22–2) listing specific conditions for which antibiotics should definitely be used, with other conditions left to the judgement of the clinician. There are minor disagreements with these guidelines, but from a practical viewpoint (the medicolegal viewpoint) there appears to be a consensus to provide prophylaxic antibiotic coverage to at risk patients undergoing *oral surgery, periodontal treatment, and implant placement.*

---

TABLE 22–1  **Candidates for Antibiotic Prophylaxis According to the American Heart Association**

**Antibiotic Prophylaxis Is Recommended For:**

Prosthetic cardiac valves

Most congenital cardiac malformations

Surgically constructed systemic-pulmonary shunts

Rheumatic and other acquired valvular pathology

History of endocarditis

Mitral valve prolapse with insufficiency

Hypertrophic cardiomyopathy

**Antibiotic Prophylaxis Is Not Recommended For:**

Physiologic, functional, or innocent heart murmurs

Isolated secundum atrial septal defect

Surgical repair of congenital heart defects, without residua beyond 6 months

Previous coronary artery bypass graft surgery

Mitral valve prolapse without insufficiency

Previous Kawasaki disease without valvular dysfunction

Cardiac pacemakers and implanted defibrillators

Dental procedures not likely to induce gingival bleeding (i.e., adjustment of orthodontic appliances and supragingival restorations)

Intraoral local anesthetic injections except for intraligamentary injections

Shedding of primary teeth

---

(From: Prevention of bacterial endocarditis: Recommendations by the American Heart Association. JAMA, 1997; 277(22): 1794–1801.)

TABLE 22–2  **Recommended Antibiotic Prophylaxis Regimens According to the American Heart Association**

| Patient Type | Drug | Dosing Regimen |
|---|---|---|
| **Standard Regimen** | | |
| Nonpenicillin allergic | Amoxicillin | 2 g orally, 1 hr prior to procedure |
| Amoxicillin/penicillin allergic | Clindamycin | 600 mg orally, 1 hr prior to procedure |
| | or | |
| | Cephalexin | 2 g orally, 1 hr prior to procedure |
| | or | |
| | Cephadroxil | 2 g orally, 1 hr prior to procedure |
| | or | |
| | Azithromycin | 500 mg, 1 hr prior to procedure |
| | or | |
| | Clarithromycin | 500 mg, 1 hr prior to procedure |

For pediatric patients, the doses are amoxicillin 50 mg/kg, clindamycin 20 mg/kg, cephalexin 50 mg/kg, cefadroxil 50 mg/kg, azithromycin 15 mg/kg, and clarithromycin 15 mg/kg. The total pediatric dose should not exceed the adult dose.

| Patient Type | Drug | Dosing Regimen |
|---|---|---|
| **Alternate Regimens** | | |
| Cannot take oral meds | Ampicillin | 2 g, IV/IM, 30 min prior to procedure |
| Amoxicillin/penicillin/ampicillin allergic who cannot take oral meds | Clindamycin | 600 mg IV 30 min prior to procedure |
| | or | |
| | Cephazolin | 1 g, IM or IV, 30 min prior to procedure |

For pediatric patients, the doses are amicillin 50 mg/kg, clindamycin 20 mg/kg, and cefazolin 20 mg/kg. The total pediatric dose should not exceed the adult dose.

(From: Prevention of bacterial endocarditis: Recommendations by the American Heart Association. JAMA. 1997; 277(22): 1794–1801.)

## Question 4

Which of the following statements if any, are correct?

A. Patients are considered to have deteriorated from HIV to AIDS status when the laboratory count of the CD4 lymphocyte has decreased to less than 500 cells per milliliter.

B. As a safety precaution, barrier techniques (masks, glasses, rubber gloves, etc.) should be used while treating all patients on the common sense assumption that all patients are HIV/AIDS infected.

C. One of the best indicators of patient risk, is the patient's medical history.

D. Antibiotic prophylaxis is required for all cardiovascular patients.

E. A defibrillator is more effective than CPR in restarting the heart after heart failure.

## Renal Disease

Renal disease affects three percent of the United States population, of which 122,000 individuals require routine renal dialysis and approximately 40,000 have been recipients of kidney transplants. Renal disease is divided into *acute* (ARF) and *chronic renal failure* (CRF), the causes of which could include hypertension, drug reactions, renal obstruction and diabetes. Because ARF is an acute medical emergency, patients with this problem are *not* commonly encountered by dental practitioners and dental hygienists in a private practice setting. Chronic renal failure—also called *end-stage renal failure (ESRD)*, is usually the result of a progressive loss of renal function that *gradually* destroys the nephrons, (which accomplish the vital glomerular filtration) and eventually causes irreversible kidney damage. Few symptoms are manifest until up to 75 percent of glomerular filtration capability is lost. This loss of efficiency of blood filtration and increased build-up of waste in the vascular system affects *every organ* in the body.[89]

The two treatments for CRF are *dialysis* and *kidney transplantation.* One or the other is required or death ensues. The removal of wastes can be accomplished by *hemodialysis* and *periotoneal dialysis.* Dialysis is a palliative therapy that maintains life over a long and often demoralizing time as a patient waits till he/she reaches the top of a list to receive a donor kidney.

*Hemo*dialysis involves a requirement to surgically create a *shunt* which serves as a permanent access to the arterial and venous vascular systems. The usual sites of placement of the arterio/venous shunt is in the *forearm or upper arm.* By connecting the hemodialysis machine to this access, the patient's blood can be circulated through a dialyzer unit that acts as an artificial kidney and extracts the wastes from the patient's blood (Figure 22–6). *Nine to 12 hours* of hemodialysis is required *each week,* usually divided into three sessions on alternating days (M-W-F or T-Th-S).

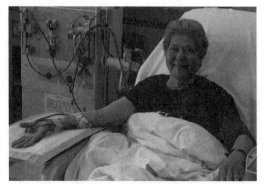

FIGURE 22-6   Patient and Hemodialysis Machine. An End Stage Renal Disease Patient is receiving dialysis treatment while connected to a dialysis machine. The patient is connected to the machine via tubing placed into a shunt in the patient's right arm. (Courtesy of Dr. Jeffery L. Hicks, University of Texas Dental School, San Antonio, TX.)

*Continuous ambulatory peritoneal dialysis* is a viable option for patients with poor vascular accesses for hemodialysis, or who prefer this method of dialysis. In continuous ambulatory peritoneal dialysis, dialysate is placed into the abdomen through a surgically placed permanent catheter and then drained after 4 to 6 hours. New dialysate is introduced after the old is drained, so that dialysis can be continued—if desired, throughout the day and night—hence the term *continuous.* It also permits the patient to be *ambulatory* during the dialysis period that can be accomplished at home with less risk of infection.[90] It is estimated that approximately one third of the Canadian chronic dialysis patients are on peritoneal dialysis.[91]

In contrast to dialysis, *kidney transplants* are the only means to normalize kidney function. They also provide a much better opportunity for survival than long term hemodialysis.[92] This

emphasizes the need for early transplantation once the diagnosis of ESRD is made.[93] The problem is that the number of individuals needing dialysis is growing by 10% to 15% per year—and there just are not enough donors.[94]

The donor source for renal transplants can be either from an immediately deceased corpse (cadaveric transplant), or from a living donor (allogenic transplant). Allogenic transplants are much more successful. Once a successful kidney transplant is in place, a *life-long* immunosuppression drug regimen is *required* to minimize the possibility of organ rejection.

## Salient Systemic Signs and Symptoms of ESRD Anemia

Dorland's medical dictionary defines anemia as "A reduction below normal in the number of erythrocytes per cubic mm., the quantity of hemoglobin, or the volumn of the packed cells per 100 ml. of blood." This definition sounds innocuous; however, one research group suggests a more ominous connotation applicable to the anemia of a dialysis patients, viz., "We suggest there is a triangular relationship, a vicious circle between chronic heart failure, chronic kidney insufficiency, and anemia where each of these three can both cause and be caused by the other."[95]

There are several important contributing factors to the development of an anemia of a hemodialysis patient: (1) Many *red cells are destroyed* by the hemodialysis unit; (2) there is a deficiency of *erythropoietin* (a protein that stimulates red cell production) and results in a *reduced output* of erythrocytes); and, (3) a lack of erythopoietin needed for normal formation of *hemoglobin*. A chronic or severe hemoglobin deficiency is highlighted by the results of a study of a group of hemodialysis patients, where "The relative risk of death and hospitalization are *inversely* associated with hemoglobin levels."[96]

The loss of erythrocytes is increased by *bleeding*. This is a platelet problem since they

are essential in the clotting process. Platelets can be destroyed during hemodialysis; their function to aggregate (clot) can be negated by the high blood urea content, or clotting can be prevented by the residual presence of heparin that is used during dialysis.

### Renal Osteodystrophy

Renal osteodystrophy[c] is a disorder of bone seen in the endstage of renal disease. Vitamin D is normally manufactured in the kidney, a source that is lacking in advanced kidney disease. In its absence there is a deficiency of calcium absorbed from the gut for essential body functions. To compensate, the parathyroid glands secrete a hormone that causes a withdrawal of calcium from bone. However, this secondry hyerparathyroidism results in any remodeled bone being dystrophic and often subject to spontaneous fracture. Renal osteodystrophy disease begins relatively early in the development of chronic renal failure.[97]

It is a challenge to the nephrologist to adjust the medications to simultaneously control the anemia, the deficient mineral metabolism of the ESRD patient, and other emergency medical needs as they arise. The *lack* of success is highlighted by the experienced mortality rates in patients with ESRD that are 10–100 times those without ESRD.[98]

### Hypertension

High blood pressure is considered a significant risk factor for the development of ESRD. Also, high blood pressure has been looked at as a possible predictor of mortality for hemodialysis patients.[99] Closely paralleling this risk factor is another of interest from a dental viewpoint, namely that uric acid might have a pathogenic role in the development of hypertension, vascular disease, and renal disease.[100] A few decades ago, American dentistry joined in the

---

[c]Dystrophy = not normal; osteodystropy = dystrophy of bone; renal osteodystrophy = bone dystrophy of renal origin.

campaign against high blood pressure by taking the blood pressure of all patients before providing dental care. Unfortunately, only an estimated 5% of those who are informed of their personal high blood pressure take active steps to reduce it as an *important* health hazard.[101]

### Infection

Infection is a constant companion of the ESRD patient. The shunt that is absolutely necessary for hemodialysis is vulnerable to infection from both within (blood borne bacteria) and from without (bacteria around the shunt). As much as 50% of hospitalization costs for ESRD is related to access problems.[102] The infections that occur are not a matter of just morbidity, but also of possible mortality. The solution is to use antibiotics to cope with blood borne pathogens, and exquisite cleanliness and hygiene around the shunt area. A clinician should make every effort to avoid traumatizing or infecting this vital arterio/venous access structure. For instance, the blood pressure sphygnomometer cuff should *never* be placed on this arm.

*Infection of dialysis patients with hepatitis B and C viruses* ranges from 20–30%. The probable source of the infection is probably from contaminated equipment and nosocomial transmission.[103] Because of the risk of transmission of the viruses, a consultation with the patient's primary care physician is recommended to determine the patient's infectious status before beginning dental care. However, *with appropriate vaccines and universal infection control measures, the risk to health care workers is minimal.*

### Antibiotic Prophylaxis

Antibiotic prophylaxis prior to any dental treatment for a hemodialysis patient that causes bleeding (calculus removal, scaling, and planing) *may be* recommended to avoid infection of the shunt by pathogenic blood borne bacteria. The decision concerning antibiotic prophylaxis should be *jointly made* between the dental prac-

titioner and the patient's nephrologist. However, antibiotic prophylaxis to prevent endocardidtis in the dialysis patient is no longer *specifically recommended* by the American Heart Association, thus leaving the decision up to the judgment of the practitioner and/or the nephrologist.

## Oral Manifestations of ESRD

There are several signs and symptoms of ESRD that are both of interest and important to the dentist and the dental hygienist. Most are due to the *high level of urea in the saliva*. (Under normal circumstances, the urea is filtered out in the urine by the healthy kidney). The changes in homeostasis that are attributable to urea are: (1) taste changes and breath malodor (halitosis) due to the urea in the saliva breaking down to ammonia; (2) a higher saliva pH and buffering capacity, also due to the high alkaline urea. Additional signs and symptoms of ESRD include: a lower flow of stimulated and unstimulated saliva, due to the excess loss of fluid through the diseased kidney; bone dystrophies seen in x-rays, such as a missing lamina dura around the roots of the teeth and abnormal trabeculae (the framework of bone) that can be traced to the secondary hyperparathyroidism; pallor of the oral mucous membrane, with ecchymosis and petechia[d] that are all caused by the anemia.

## Chronic Renal Failure and the Plaque Diseases

There is a consensus that there is a lower prevalence of caries in a ESRD population. Nunn et al found the prevalence of caries to be low in the ESRD patient.[104] It is believed that the lower caries prevalence that is characteristic of patients with ESRD, is due to the higher

---

[d]Ecchymosis = Area bleeding beneath the mucous membrane or skin; Petechia = Pinpoint bleeding beneath the mucous membrane or skin.

concentration of salivary (alkaline) urea nitrogen. Obry found the urea level in salivary analysis to be 513 +/− 210 mg/100ml *prior to* patient dialysis. *Following* dialysis, the saliva level dropped to 241 +/− 82 mg/100 ml. These figures are in contrast to 110 +/− 48 mg./100 ml. for the control group.[105]

It should be noted that in one study after the plaque was exposed to carbohydrate the configuration of the Stephan curve for both ESRD patients and the control group paralleled each other, but because the pH of the ESRD group being initially elevated, the drop did not as often reach the critical level required for demineralization.[106]

## Miscellaneous Factors Relating to the Care of ESRD Patient

Any routine dental appointment for a chronic renal failure patient should be scheduled for the day before, or the day after hemodialysis. This policy avoids the possibility of the patient coming to the dental office from one stressful appointment, to another equally or more stressful experience.

If *onset* of the renal failure begins *before* the development of the teeth is completed, there is the possibility of enamel *hypoplasia* and *intrinsic staining* caused by the high blood levels to urea and relative calcium deficiency.[104,107] These abnormalities probably date from the time of the onset of the ESRD.

The *intrinsic stain* of any teeth caused by uremia cannot be removed with scaling or prophylaxis (the same as for intrinsic stains of fluoride and tetracycline). This is because during the formation of the teeth, the stain completely permeates throughout the enamel.

If antibiotic coverage is *desired* in order to prevent infection of the shunt or cause further kidney damage, then the American Heart Association' recommendations (Table 22-1) should be followed. A simple way of achieving antibiotic coverage is to have the nephrologist administer intravenous vancomycin (an antibi-

otic) at the time of dialysis. For dialysis patients, the duration of coverage of vancomycin is approximately 5-to-7 days, giving the dental practitioner ample time to perform any needed dentistry.[108]

## Post Transplantation Dental Concerns

A successful transplant helps normalize daily activity. However, the patient is exchanging one problem for another. Infections are emerging as causes of morbidity and mortality because of the lifelong requirement for daily immunosuppressive drug therapy to prevent rejection of the kidney transplants.[109] Following the kidney transplant, *all* dental treatment expected to *cause bleeding* should be preceded by antibiotic prophylaxis (according to the American Heart Association guidelines).

Another problem generated by the immunosuppressant drugs is *hyperplasia* of the gingiva (Figure 22–7). There is a 30 percent incidence of gingival hypertrophy for patients taking the suppressive drug, cyclosporin A. This side effect can be minimized with scrupulous oral hygiene; however, if necessary, a gingivectomy or gingival flap is often needed.[110,111]

Of interest, in one study the data suggested that following a successful transplant, with the restoration of normal kidney function, there was again an increased risk of caries.[106]

There are very few studies that point out any specific periodontal problems in transplant patients not encountered by normal individuals. Once the diagnosis of ESRD is made, it should be the responsibility of the nephrologist to coordinate the patient's hemodialysis schedule and medical care. This schedule should also include provisions for an appropriate evidenced-based dental recall schedule to maintain as healthy periodontium as possible. (Chapter 23).

This need is well pointed out by Naugle et al. where 100% of ESRD patients on dialysis had some form of periodontal disease. Sixty four percent displayed a severe gingivitis (28%)

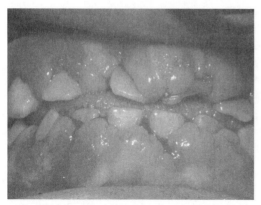

FIGURE 22–7    Several immunosuppressive drugs taken to prevent rejection of an organ transplant, and some taken to suppress seizures, produce the same gingival overgrowth. Surgery is indicted to remove the excess tissue, and patients must exercise excellent oral hygiene to prevent or delay regrowth. (Courtesy of Dr. Jeffery L. Hicks, University of Texas Dental School, San Antonio, TX.)

or early periodontitis (36%). Naugle also pointed out that these two periodontal conditions represent a bacterial foci that can contribute to a blood infection that can increase a patient's risk to morbidity or mortality.[112]

As a final note, not all successful transplants end happily. There are reports of transplants bringing with them problems that were part of the donor's legacy. This possibility is covered in a self-explanatory article entitled, "Risk for tumor and other disease transmission by transplantation: a population-based study of unrecognized malignancies and other diseases in organ donors."[113]

## Diabetes Mellitus

Diabetes mellitus (DM) is a *common endocrine* disorder. It is estimated that approximately *16 million* Americans are afflicted with the disease—a number that is projected to *double* by

2010. Twenty percent of U.S. citizens over 60 have DM.[114] An estimated 5.4 million of the 16 million do not realize they have the disease. This is unfortunate, since early and continued treatment helps prevent some of the disastrous consequences of DM. These consequences can range from blindness, to amputations of limbs, periodontal disease, renal failure, hypertension, neuropathy, cardiovascular disease and a *great* reduction in the quality of life. African Americans, Hispanics and American Indians are especially susceptible to diabetes.[115]

Diabetes mellitus is caused by an insufficient supply of insulin because of either a lack of production by the *islet cells of the pancreas*, a deficit of insulin receptors, or an error in insulin metabolism (insulin resistance). Insulin is the key that allows the blood glucose to *enter* the body cells to *provide for energy needs*. Without it, the body cells are literally starving for the energy-giving glucose, while just outside in the blood supply the needed glucose continues to build up to toxic levels in the blood and spill over into the urine.

There are two main sub classifications of DM, Type 1, and Type 2 (both with Arabic numerals, not Roman numerals). Type 1 is often the result of genetic omission, or as a result of an autoimmune destruction of the pancreatic beta cells *early in life*. By the time the disease is identified up to 80% of the beta cells have usually been destroyed. Approximately 5–10% of the cases of diabetes are in this category.

For glycemic control of Type 1, *exogenous insulin is absolutely necessary to maintain life*. This insulin is self-injected by the patient throughout life, or is automatically dispensed by a strapped-on insulin pump (Figure 22–8). The pump automatically senses a changing level of glucose in the blood, and adjusts the dose accordingly.

Type 2 usually develops *later in life* and is often associated with *overweight* and relatively *inactive individuals*. Approximately 90–95% of the cases fall into this category. Often Type 2 DM can be controlled by a combination of exercise, diet and/or oral hypoglycemic agents.[116] Both types can be recognized by the presence of

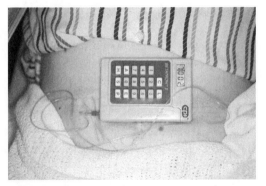

FIGURE 22–8    Insulin Pump. Worn beneath the clothes, this insulin pump is driven by an internal computer that can be programmed to inject specific amounts of insulin at specific times. More accurate glucose control is possible with the pump than with the typical 2 or 3 manual injections per day. (Courtesy of Dr. Jeffery L. Hicks, University of Texas Dental School, San Antonio, TX.)

three clinical signs: *polyuria* (frequent urination), *polydipsia* (frequent urge to drink), and *polyphagia* (frequent urge to eat). A positive diagnosis of DM usually follows a physician's clinical examination that is verified in routine blood tests as an excess of glucose, or in urine tests with the presence of glucose. Type 1 is increasing *slowly* in numbers. On the other hand, the number of Type 2 diabetics is escalating *rapidly* and is expected to *double* before 2010.[114] Many in the news media and public health call it an *epidemic*.

## The Relationship of Diabetes Mellitus to the CPITN

If there is a relationship between the level of blood serum glucose and periodontitis, then a high glucose level for an individual should have a significant parallel high CPITN score. There are two studies that verify this assumption.

A large-scale study involving 10,590 subjects in Israel charted abnormal blood glucose (levels over 120 ml/dl) with elevated CPITN scores of above 4.5.[117] In the second smaller study of 40 subjects—20 with diabetes, and 20 control subjects. It was found that there was a *steady increase* in blood serum glucose (142–173 mg/dl) that paralleled that of an increasing CPITN score (13.5–19.1).[118]

## Periodontal Disease and Diabetes Mellitus—Bi-Directional Diseases

In reviewing the literature, there is a consensus that periodontal disease has an adverse effect on the severity of DM, and vice versa that the severity of DM has an adverse effect on the severity of periodontal disease—a *bi-directional* relationship (Figure 22–9). The bi-directional etiology signals the need for cooperation between the medical and dental professions, as echoed in the following statements.[119]

**Statement:** *Poorly controlled diabetics* have a *greater incidence* of severe periodontal disease compared with those patients who are well controlled or have no diabetes mellitus.[120]

**Statement:** Periodontitis is a common problem in patients with diabetes. The relationsip between these 2 maladies appears bi-directional—insofar that the presence of one condition tends to promote the other, and that meticulous management of either may assists treatment of the other.[121]

**Statement:** New evidence suggests that advanced *periodontal disease may interfere with diabetes mellitus control* and the physician should be made aware of the patient's periodontal status.[122]

**Statement:** Not only does diabetes affect the periodontium, but periodontal infection can advesely impact glycemic control in diabetics.[123]

**Statement:** Equally important is the fact that there are *no* studies of acceptable design that refute this bi-directional relationship between periodontal disease and DM.[124]

In 1999 and again in 2000, the American Academy of Periodontology issued position papers about the relationship of diabetes and peri-

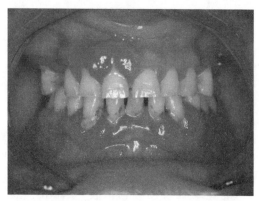

FIGURE 22-9 Periodontal disease as part of the Diabetes Mellitus problem. Examination and blood glucose testing of this patient with Diabetes Mellitus, Type 2, revealed severe periodontitis and hyperglycemia. The patient admitted to observing poor glucose control and to being chronically hyperglycemic. (Courtesy of Dr. Jeffery L. Hicks, University of Texas Dental School, San Antonio, TX.)

odontal diseases.[125,126] These two position papers point out that there *is* a relationship between the two diseases and that all patients should be informed of that relationship, especially where periodontal disease might increase the risk of DM complications and vice versa.

## Caries

Theoretically, there is a basis for *either* a decreased or increased caries prevalence for Type 1 diabetics. Normally, if there is a good self-care (with an effective mechanical and chemical plaque control regimen), there is a lower count of cariogenic organisms and a lower DMFS. If there is a diet with minimum carbohydrate there is a lower caries incidence. Another moderator is the flow of saliva, with an inverse relationship between flow rate and caries development. A look at several studies is necessary to determine what factor(s) are *most determinant* for the caries.

Twetman et al. after a three year study with adolescents of 8–15 years of age, concluded

that the *main most influencial determinants for high caries development over the period of the study were metabolic control*, poor oral hygiene, previous caries experience and high levels of lactobacilli. *Also there was a higher glucose in the resting saliva.*[127]

Other researchers have either confirmed or added to these findings. For instance:

**Statement:** *Poor control of diabetes* was found to be associated with caries.[128]

Moore et al. confined their studies to the flow of saliva, and reported that dry mouth (xerostomia) was more prevalent in diabetics than in the control subjects, with more complaints from diabetics with *poor metabolic control.*[129]

Xerostomia in diabetic patients is usually secondary to the dehydrational effects of the disease process itself. Greater amounts of fluids are eliminated via the urine (polyuria) and less is available for the saliva. Thus, the appropriate therapy for xerostomia of DM origin is to *restore insulin balance.*[130]

In another study, home care practices were similar, and all subjects had received similar regular dental treatment. In conclusion, *it was poor metabolic control of diabetes that was found to be associated with caries.*[131] Taking all previous statements into account, it is poor glycemic control that accounts for the excess prevalence and severity of the plaque diseases.

## First Appointment

Every dental office will treat diabetes patients.[122] Upon admittance, the patient will be asked to fill out a personal medical and dental history for the use of the dentist and the dental hygienist

The first appointment should have two major objectives. The first should be to establish rapport with the new patient, and the second is to learn more about the diabetic background of the patient. As the interview unfolds, any critical information should be added to the medical and dental history record.

This would include information on dosage, time schedules, method of administration, previous adverse experiences with insulin control, number of hospitalizations, and physician recommendations.

At this time, the dentist should carefully explain the relationship between DM and periodontal disease. According to an article by Sundberg, 83% of the DM patients were *not* aware of the linkage between the systemic and the oral disease. It is necessary that the patient should know in the beginning that there will be many visits to the dentist for prophylaxes, monitoring and possible periodontal treatment, that in turn will help maintain metabolic balance in the medical treatment.[132]

Another salient educational item is the subject of smoking. If the patient smokes or uses smokeless tobacco, cessation is required if periodontal health is to be maintained. In comparing the effects of smoking on diabetic and nondiabetic men, it was found that the parameters usually assessed for periodontal disease—plaque index, gingival index, bleeding score, probing depth, loss of attachment, and missing teeth were all greater for the diabetic men.[133] It is counterproductive and ridiculous for a periodontist to treat a disease, if at the same time the subject is practicing a habit that is *blocking* the effect of the treatment. (See Chapter 13 for a full discussion of the adverse effect smoking has on the periodontium.) Another reality is that if smoking continues, there is an increased risk for cardiovascular disease that is one of the serious consequences of diabetes mellitus. With the above education and counseling complete, routine treatment appointments can be made.

## Routine Appointments

When the known DM patient arrives for any appointments it is wise to determine whether she/he has had their prescribed insulin dosage and when the next dosage is due. Before treatment begins, the blood pressure needs to be recorded. If any surgery is contemplated, consultation with the patient's physician is desir-

able since the possibility of infection is omnipresent. There is always an *increased susceptibility to infection* of soft tissue as well as *a delayed healing of wound sites*. This increased hazard is probably due to the high content of glucose in the soft tissues that is ideal for bacterial growth. It is because of this increased risk of blood borne bacteria that all oral surgery (including periodontal treatment) should be accomplished with antibiotic prophylaxis.[122,134]

## The First DM Emergency—the Hypoglycemic Episode

The most common emergency is the *Hypoglycemic Episode*—an unexpected *decline* in the blood glucose level. This is manifest by the patient feeling weak, exhibiting mood changes, incoherence, sweating, and tachycardia. All operative procedures should cease, and the patient *immediately given a fast acting oral carbohydrate from the emergency cabinet*—glucose tablets or gel, candy, juice followed by a determination of the glucose level.[e] This can be determined easily with a relatively economic electronic glucose monitor, which is quite accurate. If there is no apparent progress after 10 minues, repeat ingestion of the fast acting carbohydrate. *If there is recovery*, the patient should eat a snack or a meal to prevent a rebound to the hypoglycemic state. If there is no apparent progress, the 911 phone call should be made, since with further delay, the symptoms begin to become ominous—unconsciousness, low blood pressure, hypothermia, seizures, coma and death.[135,136]

## A Day in the Life of a Diabetic

Like for any other disease diagnosis, compliance with an attending physician's advice can be expected to range from full to minimal cooperation. For the diabetic, glycemic control and his/her general health status directly de-

---

[e]Diabetic mellitus patients often carry a supply of fast acting carbohydrate agents of their choice. A soft drink (*not a dietetic* drink will often suffice.)

pend on this compliance. And what does this compliance entail????

Every morning, it will involve a *finger stick* to secure a drop of blood to determine the blood glucose level, using an electronic glucose monitor. If the blood glucose level is low, a decreased quantity of insulin is necessary. If breakfast is to include considerable more carbohydrate than normal, the amount of insulin must be increased. From 4 to 8 finger sticks a day is required to determine if glucose levels are remaining within pre established levels. A well controlled diabetic attempts to maintain a blood glucose level of 75–125 mg/dl. Additional finger sticks are necessary before events such as driving a car (safety) or before appointments (dental) to maintain a reasonably normal glucose blood level over the time to be involved. For some "brittle" diabetics where the insulin levels are erratic and unpredictable, night finger sticks may be necessary. Finger sticks and hypodermic self-administration of insulin become a monotonous way of life. However, they are *absolutely necessary day-in-and-day-out over the remaining years of life*. When the enormity of this daily task is fully realized, the unceasing support of a spouse, of the family, other diabetics, and the attendant medical community helps to *bridge the discouragement of the unending tasks necessary to preserve life*.

For those diabetics who have an insulin pump, the dosage is pre-programmed by the endocrinologist to inject insulin several times a day into the *abdominal cavity*. There is sufficient insulin in the pump reservoir for at least three days. The wearer must release additional insulin for any increased intake of carbohydrates or emergency. In addition, every third day, the patient must refill the pump reservoir, accomplish skin hygiene of the entry point, and replace the small catheter connecting the pump to the abdominal cavity.

For any diabetic, the holy grail is a cure that will eliminate the need for the repetitious finger sticks and self- or pump-adminis-

tered insulin. World-wide research programs to achieve such a cure abound. As reported in an excellent article in the New Yorker magazine, pancreatic cells have been implanted into humans that produce the needed insulin.[137] However, to offset this outstanding achievement, has been the fact that the availability of donor islet cells (from pancreases) is miniscule in relation to the tremendous need.[138-140] Yet, it is a very promising beginning, even though immunosuppressive drugs are still required.

The most promising preventive program that is immediately available as well as affordable for all ages is a personal crusade of *healthy eating, daily physical exercise,* and *maintaining a normal weight*.

---

**Question 5**

Which of the following statements, if any, are correct?

A. The saliva urea content of the average ESRD patient before hemodialysis is about twice as high as a ESRD patient undergoing hemodialysis; in turn, the saliva content of the patient undergoing hemodialysis is roughly twice as high as a non-diabetic control.

B. Dental foci of infection can damage either the shunt used for hemodialysis, or the transplant that replaces the need for hemodialysis.

C. Diabetes mellitus is charcterized by an insufficient amount of glucose within the cell membranes, and an excess of glucose in the blood supply outside the cell membranes.

D. Without a relatively continuous glycemic control in DM, an uncontrolled periodontitis can be anticipated.

E. The successful transplantation of islet cells still requires immunosuppressive drugs.

# SUMMARY

The first part of this chapter provided an overview of the objectives and the administration of a hospital. The second half related to some of the diseases that are being treated daily in a hospital. Most frustrating, in many cases prevention practiced before admission could have aborted the onset of the primary complaint. To cite a few examples: (1) in the case of facial cancer (basal cell) the etiology probably was excessive exposure to the sun in earlier days (and still continues with a generation that better understands the consequences). (2) For many, the more deadly intra oral cancer (squamous cell) could probably have been avoided by rejecting the earlier use of tobacco products (smoking and chewing tobacco). (3) Another failure in cancer prevention occurred when the individual failed to seek professional advice for that small mucosal ulcer that would not heal, but only enlarged in size; or, (4) the lesion could have been missed by the dentist in the last dental examination (if the person had access to a dentist). Another example of the need for close cooperation by Departments in the hospital is illustrated by the need for glycemic control by the diabetic patient. This control requires the combined effort by kidney specialists, endocrine experts, the periodontist. and other specialists to care for the complications, if and when they are diagnosed. The end result of this cooperation, is better health, and a better life for the diabetes mellitus patient. DM is truly an example of a bi-or-multi directional disease!

In dealing with diseased, traumatized, and mental and physically handicapped patients, there is always the concern for the unexpected. All hospital services have plans to react to most emergencies, ranging from use of emergency drugs to crisis teams that respond immediately when advanced resuscitation procedures are required. In all of these responses, someones life is often in balance. Even under the best of circumstances, the outcome is never guaranteed. In private practice, it is only a rare event such as the hypoglycemic episode that arises. Occasionally for some dentist in the United States a more serious emergency occurs. He/she is responsible for diagnosing and reacting to the emergency. The reaction must be immediate and correct. Like for the crisis team, it is an awesome responsibility, and the consequences can also be catastrophic, even though the response might have been correct.

For prevention of the plaque diseases in systemic disease, the guidelines outlined later in Chapter 23 apply. For self-care for most caries or periodontal patients, it is the usual need for mechanical plaque control with the "brush, floss, and flush" routine, coupled with chemical plaque control—fluoride mouthrinses and appropriate use of chlorhexidine (or other antimicrobial agents) to reduce the possibility of caries and gingivitis. It is not difficult to figure what is to be done, but instead, how to motivate individuals to do them. The main variable experienced in continuing care of chonically ill patients, is the time interval between recalls for prophylaxes and monitoring to avoid the need for secondary and tertiary prevention procedures. A second challenge is the question of how to best deliver preventive care to individuals who need help with self-care—such as the arm amputees, the unconscious, facial fractures, where the mandible and maxilla are wired together, and the mentally handicapped.

It is not long before a dentist in a hospital environment learns that dentistry does not end at the third molar. This chapter has pointed out how systemic disease can

modulate oral disease, and vice versa. In the case of renal disease, the accompanying uremia can even benefit caries control!

Hospital dental practice is now becoming an alternative dental career to the present options of private practice, academia, the military and public health. It is an exciting, challenging professional career of continual learning from colleagues and personal experiences. It is also a major contribution of the profession to insure better dental care for the disabled and diseased as well as for the healthy.

Finally, as a staff member of the hospital, there are four areas where there is a need for your participation in prevention: Your patient needs to be protected from body harm (Hippocratic Oath); you need to protect yourself and your co-workers from the transmission of diseases of patients; you need to protect yourself and your institution from malpractice suits; and if you are in a non-hospital environment (private practice) when an emergency occurs, you need to remember the numbers 911.

## ANSWERS AND EXPLANATIONS

1. A, B, C, E—correct.

    D—incorrect. The Department Chairpersons function as an Executive Board and act together for the good of the institution.

2. A, C, D, E—correct.

    B—incorrect. A non-healing ulcerous lesion should be carefully examined and possibly biopied after a period of about 3 weeks, not three months.

3. C, D, E—correct

    A—incorrect. At 3 months of age, only the surgical correction of the lip should be considered. The correction of the anterior alveolar ridge should await until the patient is about 10 years of age.

    B—incorrect. There are more clefts involving the hard palate than involving the lips and hard palate. During the embryonic period there is a cleft between the maxillary bones that fuses from the lip back towards the uvula. At times the fusion will proceed normally and for unknown reasons, leave a normal lip. This partial fusion accounts for the lips sometimes being spared and the palate being involved.

4. A, B, C and E—correct.

    D—incorrect. Since a cardiac emergency is probably the most serious occurrence that can happen in a dental office, probably the safest professional and safest legal position is to consult with the patient's cardiologist as well as review the current recommendations of the American Heart Association. If still in doubt, *empirical propylaxis* (prophylaxis coverage because the operator wants to be on the safe side) is a logical response.

5. A, B, C, D, and E—correct.

## Self-evaluation Questions

1. A dentist (and other hospital professional staff personnel) must be _____ to indicate competency to practice in a hospital dental service.

2. The accrediting agency for dental hospital services in the United States is the _____ (organization).

3. The prosthetic device used to bridge a palatal cleft is known as an _____.

4. The more scientific term for "dry mouth" is _____.

5. Bone necrosis that follows cancer radiation treatment is known as _____.

6. An HIV case becomes an AIDS case when the CD4 lymphocyte drops below _____ lymphocytes per milliliter of blood.

7. Relieving a patient's _____ is one of the best means to assure an uneventful appointment with a high risk cardiac patient.

8. A bi-directional disease is one where both can help influence the outcome or the severity of the other.

9. A systemic disease that reduces the incidence of caries is _____.

10. If you had a patient have a cardiac arrest in your office, would you have a better chance of resuscitation with (CPR) (a defibrillator). Circle your selection.

## REFERENCES

1. Salley, J. J., Van Ostenberg, P. R., & Gump, M. L. (1980). Dentistry and its future in the hospital environment. *JADA*, 101:236–39.
2. Asbell, M. B. (1969). Hospital dental service in the United States—A historical review. *J Hosp Dent Pract*, 3:9–11.
3. Cillo, J. E. (1996). The development of hospital dentistry in America—the first hundred years (1850–1950). *J Hist Dent*, 44:105–9.
4. Giangrego, E. (1987). Dentistry in hospitals: looking to the future. *JADA*, 115:545–55.
5. http://www.dent.unc.edu/careers/cid13.htm. Site visited in 2000–2001.
6. Godden, D. R., & Hall, I. S. (1996). Maxillofacial trauma at RAF War Hospital, Wroughton. *Brit Dent J.*, 23:180,231–3.
7. Brunner, P. P. (1996). Title not available. *Zur Medizingesch*, 264:1–125.
8. Epstein, J. B., Tejani, A., & Glassman, P. (2000). Assessment of objectives of post-doctoral general dentistry programs in Canada. *Spec Care Dentist*, 20: 191–4.
9. Gross, P. M., Peuten, M., Sequence, A., Schmidt, U., & Pollock, S. (2001). Mandibular fracture caused by absolute close-range gun shot with a blank cartridge fright weapon. *Arch Kriminol*, 208:88–95.

10. Le, B. T., Dierks, E. J., veek, B. A., Homer, L. D., & Pottery, B. F. (2001). Maxillofacial injuries associated with domestic violence. *J Oral Maxillofac Surg*, 59:1277–83.

11. Precious, D. S., Goodday, R. H., Morrison, A. D., & Davis, B. R. (2001). Cleft lip and palate; a review for dentists. *J Can Dent Assn*, 67:668–73.

12. Borlase, G. (2000). Use of obturator in rehabilitation of maxilloectomy defects. *Ann R Australian Coll Dent Surg*, 15:75–79.

13. Reisberg, D. J. (2000). Dental and prosthetic care for patients with cleft or craniofacial conditions. *Cleft Palate Craniofac J*, 37:534–37.

14. Markt, J. C. (2001). An endosseus, implant-retained obturator for the rehabilitation of a recurrent central giant cell granuloma: a clinical report. *J Prosth Dent*, 85:116–20.

15. Matthews, M. F., Smith, R. M., Sutton, A. J., & Hudson, R. (2000). The ocular impression: A review of the literture and presentation of an alternate technique. *J Prosthdont*, 9:210–16.

16. Taft, R. M., von Gonten A. S., & Wheeler, S. T. (2001). Assisted retention of hearing device in an implant—retained auricular prosthesis. *J Prosthetic Dent*, 86:386–9.

17. Shoen, P. J., Raghoebar, G. M., Van Oort, R. P., Reintsema, H., Vander Loan, Burlage, F. R., Roodenbur, J. L., & Vissink, A. (2001). Treatment outcome of bone-anchored craniofacial prosthesis after tumor surgery. *Cancer*, 92:3045–50.

18. Palmer, S., Brix, M., & Benateau H. (2001). The complex facial prosthesis. The value of bone-anchored maxillofacial prostheses in the treatment of extensive loss of facial tissue. *Rev Stomatol Chir Maxillofac*, 102:261–5.

19. Lee, F. P. (2001). Endoscopic extraction of intranasal teeth: a review of 13 cases. *Laryngology*, 111:1027–31.

20. Hawthorne, M., Sim, R., & Acton, C. H. (2000). Quinine induced coagulopathy—a near fatal experience. *Austr Dent J*, 45:282–84.

21. Stiles, B. M., Wilson, W. H., Bridges, M. A., Choudhury, A., Rivera-Arsas, J., Nguyen, D. B., & Edlich, R. F. (2000). Denture esophageal impaction refractory to endoscopic removal in a psychiatric patient. *J Emerg Med*, 18:323–6.

22. Hulland, S., Sigal, M. J. (2000). Hospital-based dental care for persons with disabilities: A study of patient selection criteria. *Spec Care Dentist*, 20:131–38.

23. Longhurst, R. H. (1999). An evaluation of the oral care given to patients when staying in a hospital. *Prim Dent Care*, 3:112–15.

24. Charteris, P., & Kinsella, T. (2001). The oral care link nurse: a facilitator and educator for maintaining oral health for patients at the Royal Hospital for neuron-disability. *Spec Care Dentist*, 21:6871.

25. Longman, L. P., Higham, S. M., Rai, K., Edgar, W. M., & Field, E. A. (1995). Salivary gland hypofunction in elderly patients attending a xerostomia clinic. *Gerodontology*, 12:67–72.

26. Redding, S. W. (1990). Hematologic and oncologic disease. In Redding, S. W., & Montgomery, M. T., Eds. *Dentistry in systemic disease*. (pp. 81–181). Portland, OR: JBK Publishing.

27. Liu, R. P., Fleming, T. J., Toth, B. B., & Keene, H. J. (1990). Salivary flow rates with head and neck cancer 0.5 to 25 years after radiotherapy. *Oral Surg Oral Med Oral Pathol*, 70:724–29.

28. Markitziu, A., Zafiropoulos, G., Tsalkikis, L., & Cohen, L. (1992). Gingival health and salivary function in head and neck irradiated patients. *Oral Surg Oral Med Oral Pathol*, 73:427–33.

29. Epstein, J. B., Stevenson-Moore, P. (1992). A clinical comparative trial of saliva substitutes in radiation-induced salivary gland hypofunction. *Spec Care Dent*, 2:21–23.

30. Aguirre-Zero, O., Zero, D. T., & Proskin, H. M. (1993). Effect of chewing xylitol chewing gum on salivary flow rate and the acidogenic potential of dental plaque. *Caries Res*, 27:55–59.

31. LeVeque, F. G., Montgomery, M. T., Potter, D., Zimmer, M. D., Rlieke, J. W., Steiger, B. W., Gallagher, J. G., & Muscoplat, C. C. (1993). A multicenter, randomized, double-blind, placebo-controlled, dose-titration study of oral pilocarpine for treatment of radiation-induced xerostomia in head and neck cancer patients. *J Clin Oncol*, 11:1124–31.

32. American Cancer Society (1990). *Cancer facts and figures*. New York: American Cancer Society, 1–7.
33. Fischman, S. L. (1983). The patient with cancer. *Dent Clin North Am*, 27:235–46.
34. Tan, I. B., Roodenburg, J. L., Copper, M. P., Coebergh, J. W., & van derwaal, J. (2001). Early diagnosis and prevention of malignant tumors in the head and neck region. *Ned Tijdschr Geneeskd*, 145:567–72.
35. Winn, D. M. (2001). Tobacco use and oral diseases. *J Dent Educ*, 65:306–12.
36. Hinddle, I., & Speight, P. M. (2000). The association between intra-oral cancer and surrogate markers of smoking and alcohol consumption. *Community Dent Health*, 17:107–13.
37. Gervasio, O. L., & Dutra, R. A., Tartaglia, S. M., Vasconcelbs, W. A., Barbosa, A. A., & Aquiar, M. C. (2001). Oral squamous cell carcinoma: a retrospective study of 740 cases in a Brazilian population. *Braz Dent J*, 12:57–61.
38. Waddell, W. J., & Levy, P. S. (2000). Interaction between tobacco and alcohol consumption and risk of cancer of the upper aero-digestive tract in Brazil. *Amer J Epidemeolo*, 52:193–4.
39. Johnson, N. (2001). Tobacco use and oral cancer: a global perspective. *J Dent Edu*, 65:328–35.
40. Singh, N., Scully, C., & Joyston-Bechal, S. (1996). Oral complications of cancer therapies: prevention and management. *Clin Oncol*, 8:15–24.
41. Allard, W. F, El-Akkad, S., & Chatmas, J. C. (1993). Obtaining pre-radiation therapy dental clearance. *JADA*, 124:88–91.
42. Wright, W. E., Haller, J. M., Harlow, S. A., & Pizzo, P. A. (1985). An oral disease prevention program for patients receiving radiation and chemotherapy. *JADA*, 110:43–47.
43. Feber, T. (1996). Management of mucositis in oral irradiation. *Clin. Onicol R Coll Radiol*, 8:106–11.
44. Hammelid, E., & Taft, C. (2001). Health-related quality of life in long-term head and neck survivors: a comparison with general population norms. *Br J Cancer*, 2001; 84:149–56.
45. Gavan, O., Sprinzel, G. M., Widner, B., et al. (2000). Value of a nutrition score in patients with advanced carcinomas in the area of the head and neck. *HNO*, 48:298–36.
46. Ohrn, K. E., Wahlin, Y. B., & Sjoden, P. O. (2001). Oral status during radiotherapy and chemotherapy: A descriptive study of patient experiences and the occurrence of oral complications. *Hogskolan Dalarna. Health and Caring Sciences*, 9:247–57.
47. The Joanna Briggs Institute. Prevention and Treatment of Oral Mucositis in Cancer Patients. http://www.joannabriggs.edu.au (site visited 2002).
48. Arcuri, M. R., Fridrich, K. L., Funk, G. F., Tabor, M. W., & LaVelk, W. E. (1997). Titanium osseointegrated implants combined with hyperbaric oxygen therapy in previously irradiated mandibles. *J Prosthet Dent*, 77:177–83.
49. Curi, M. M., & Dib, L. L. (1977). Osteoradionecrosis of the jaws: a restrospective study of the background factors and treatment in 104 cases. *J Oral Maxillofac Surg*, 55:540–41.
50. Shaha, A. R., Cordeiro, P. G., Hidalgo, D. S, Spiro, R. H., Strong, E. W., Zlotolow, I., & Huryn, J. (1997). Resection and immediate microvascular reconstruction in the management of osteoradionecrosis of the mandible. *Head Neck*, 19:406–11.
51. Ashamalla, H. L., Thom, S. R., & Goldwein, J. W. (1996). Hyperbaric oxygen therapy for the treatment of radiation-induced sequelae in children. The University of Pennsylvania experience. *Cancer*, 77:2407–12.
52. Lambert, P. M., Intriere, N., & Eichstedt, R. (1997). Clinical controversies in oral and maxillofacial surgery: Part one. Management of dental extractions in irradiated jaws: a protocol with hyperbaric oxygen therapy. *J Oral Maxillofacial Surg*, 10:1193–4.
53. Cachillo, D., Barker, G. J., & Barker, B. F. (1993). Late effects of head and neck radiation therapy, patient/dentist compliance and recommended dental care. *Spec Care Dent*, 13:159–62.
54. Axelsson, P., Lindhe, J., & Nystrom, B. (1991). On the prevention of caries and periodontal disease. Results of a 15-year longitudinal study in adults. *J Clin Periodontol*, 18:182–89.

55. Spritz, R. A. (2001). The genetics and epigenetics of orofacial clefts. *Curr Opin Pediatr*, 13:556–60.

56. Prescott, N. J., & Malcolm, S. (2002). Folate and the face: evaluating the evidence for the influence of folate genes on craniofacial development. *Cleft Palate Craniofac J*, 3:327–31.

57. Leite, I. C., Paumgarten, F. J., & Koifman, S. (2002). Chemical exposure during pregnancy and oral clefts of newborns. *Cad Saude Publica*, 18:17–31.

58. Loffredo, L. C., Souza, J. M., Freitas, J. A., & Mossey, P. A. (2001). Oral clefts and vitamin supplementation. *Cleft Palate Craniofac J*, 38:76–83.

59. Bianchi, F., Calzolari, E., Ciulli, L., Cordien, S., Gualand, F., Pierins, A., & Mossey, R. (2000). Environment and genetics in the etiology of cleft lip and cleft palate with reference to the of folic acid. *Epidemiol Prev*, 24:21–7.

60. Itikala, P. R., Watkins, M. L., Mulinare, J., Moore, C. A., & Liu, Y. (2001). Maternal multivitamin use and orofacial clefts in offspring. *Teratology*, 63:79–86.

61. Kauffman, F. L. (1991). Managing the cleft palate and lip patient. *Pediatr Clin North Am*, 38:1127–47.

62. Gicarra, G. (1992). Oral lesions of iatrogenic and undefined etiology and neurologic disorders associated with HIV infection. *Oral Surg Oral Med Oral Pathol*, 73:201–11.

63. Leggot, P. J. (1992). Oral manifestations of HIV infection in children. *Oral Surg Oral Med Oral Pathol*, 73:187–92.

64. Epstein, J. B., & Silverman, S. Jr. (1992). Head and neck malignancies associated with HIV infection. *Oral Surg Oral Med Oral Path*, 73:193–200.

65. Greenspan, D., & Greenspan, I. S. (1992). Significance of oral hairy leukoplakia. *Oral Surg Oral Med Oral Pathol*, 73:151–54.

66. Glick, M., Pliskin, M. E., & Weiss, R. C. (1990). The clinical and histologic appearance of HIV-associated gingivitis. *Oral Surg Oral Med Oral Pathol*, 69:395–98.

67. Scully, C., & McCarthy, G. (1992). Management and oral health in persons with HIV infection. *Oral Surg Oral Med Oral Pathol*, 73:215–25.

68. Spadair, F., Fazio, K., Lauritano, D., & Zambelini, A. M. (1997). Clinico-diagnostic and odontostomatologic therapeutic problems with HIV infection and AIDS. *Minerva Stomatol*, 46:307–28.

69. Comment (1996). *Ann Intern Med*, 124;255–6.

70. Barr, S. (1996). The 1990 Florida dental investigation: theory and fact. *Ann Inter Med*, 124:255–6.

71. Thomson, W. M., Stewart, J. F., Carter, M. D., & Spencer, A. J. (1997). Public perception of cross-infection in dentistry. *Austral Dent J*, 42:291–96.

72. Puplick, C. (1996). Washington's teeth: patient's rights and dentists' rights—where are we heading? *Ann R Austral Coll Dent Surg*, 13:221–36.

73. Chu, C. S., Chan, T. W., Hui, P. M., Samaranayake, C. R., Chan, J. C., & Wei, S. H. (1995). The knowledge and attitude of Hong Kong secondary school teachers and students towards HIV infection and dentistry. *Community Dent Health*, 12:110–14.

74. Scheutz, F., & Langeback, J. (1995). Dental care of infectious patients in Denmark. *Community Dent Oral Epidemiology*, 23:226–31.

75. McCarthy, G., Mamandras, A. H., & MacDonald, J. K. (1997). Infection control in the orthodontic office in Canada. *Am J Orthod Dentofacial Orthop*, 112:275–81.

76. Barnes, D. B., Garbert, B., McMaster, J. R., & Greenblatt, R. M. (1996). Self-disclosure experience of people with HIV infection of dedicated and mainstreamed. *J Publ Health Dent*, 56:223–5.

77. David, H. T., & David, Y. M. (1997). Living with needlestick injuries. *J Can Dent Assoc*, 63:283–6.

78. Greene V. A., Chu, S. Y., Diaz, T., & Schable, R. (1997). Oral health problems and use of dental services among HIV-infested adults. Supplement to HIV/AIDS Surveillance Project Group. *J Am Dent Assn*, 128: 1417–22.

79. Aizawa, F., Yonimizu, M., Aizawa, Y., Hanada, N., & Akada, H. (1996). A survey on infection control practices, knowledge and attitudes towards AIDS/HIV among dental practicioners. *Nippon Koshu Eisei Zasshi*, 43:364–73.

80. Kitaura, H., Adachi, N., Kobayashi, K., & Yamada T. (1997). Knowledge and attitudes of Japanese dental health care workers towards HIV-related disease. *J Dent*, 25:279–83.

81. Gibson, B. J., & Freeman, R. (1996). Comment. *Brit Dent J*, 180:53–56.

82. Robinson, E. N. Jr., & de Bliek, R. (1996). The college student, the dentist, and the North Carolina senator: risk analysis and risk management of HIV transmission from health care worker to patient. *Med Dec Making*, 16:86–91.

83. Alexander, R. E. (1999). The automated external cardiac defibrillator: lifesaving device for medical emergencies. *J Am Dent Assoc*, 130:837–45.

84. Waters, B. G. (1995). Providing dental treatment for patients with cardiovascular disease. *Ont Dent*, 72:24–6, 28–32.

85. Garfunkel, A., Galili, D., Findler, M., Zusman, S. P., Malamed, S., F., Elad, S., & Kaufman, E. (2002). Chest pains in the dental environment. *Refuat Hapeh Vahashinayim*, 19:51–59.

86. Kaeppler, G., Daubinder, M., Hinkelbein, R., & Lipp, M. (1998). Quality of cardiopulmonary resuscitation by dentists in dental emergency care. *Mund Kiefer Gesichtschir*, 2:71–77.

87. Woods, R. G. (2000). Improving safety of dental procedures with physiological monitoring. *Ann R Australas Coll Dent Surg*, 15:276–9.

88. Bassi, G. S., Cousin, G. C., Lawrence, C., Bali, N., & Lowry, J. C. (2002). Improved resuscitation training of senior house officers in oral maxillofacial surgery. *Brit J. Oral Maxillofac Surg*, 40:293–295.

89. Matthew, Cahill, Executive Director. (1997). 2nd Edition, *Diseases. Renal Urologic Disorders*. Springhouse, PA: Springhouse Corporation, pp. 1224.

90. Puttinger, H., & Vychytil, A. (2002). Hepatitis B and C in peritoneal dialysis patients. *Semin Nephrol*, 22:351–60.

91. Perez, R. A., Blake, P. G., Jindal, K. A., Badovinac, K., Trpeski, L., Fenton, S. S. (2003). Canadian Organ Replacement Register—EPREX Study Group. Changes in peritoneal dialysis practices in Canada 1996–1999. *Perit Dial Int*, 23:53–7.

92. Medin, C., Elinder, C. G., Hylander, B., Blom, B., & Wilczek, H. (2000). Survival of patients who have been on a waiting list for renal transplantation. *Nephrol Dial Transplant*, 15:701–4.

93. Meier-Kriesche, H. U., Port, F. K., Ojo, A. O., Rudich, S. M., Hanson, J. A., Cibrik Leichtman, A. B., & Kaplan, B. (2000). Effect of waiting time on renal transplant outcome. *Kidney Int*, 58:1311–7.

94. Klassen, J. T., & Krasco, B. M. (2002). The daily health status of dialysis patients. *J Can Dent Association*, 68:34–38.

95. Silverberg, D. S., Wexler, D., Blum, B., & Iaina, A. (2003). Anemia in chronic kidney disease and congestive heart failure. *Blood Purif*, 21:124–30.

96. Ofsthun, N., Labrecque, J., Lacson, E., Keen, M., & Lazarus, J. M. (2003). The effects of higher hemoglobin levels on mortality and hospitalization in hemodialysis patients. *Kidney Int*, 63:1908–14.

97. Ho, L. T., & Sprague, S. M. (2002). Renal osteodystrophy in chronic renal failure. *Semin Nephrol*, 26:488–93.

98. Block, G., & Port, F. K. (2003). Calcium phosphate metabolism and cardiovascular disease in patients with chronic kidney disease. *Semin Dial*, 16:140–7.

99. Luca, M. F., Quereda, C., Teruel, J. L., Orte, L., Marceen, R., & Ortuno, J. (2003). Effect of hypertension before beginning dialysis on survival of hemodialysis patients. (In Press) *Am J Kidney Dis*.

100. Johnson, R. J., Kang, D. H., Feig, D., Kivlighn, S., Kanellis, J., Watanabe, S., Tut, K. R., Rodriguez-Iturbe, B., Herrera-Acosta, J., & Mazzali, M. (2003). Is there a pathogenic role for uric acid in hypertension and cardiovascular and renal disease? *Hypertension*, 41:1183–90.

101. Little, J. W. (2003). The impact on dentistry of recent advances in the management of hypertension. *Oral Surg Oral Med Oral Pathol Oral Radiol Endod*, 90:591–9.

102. Anel, R. L., Yevzlin, A. S., & Ivanoich, P. (2003). Vascular access and patient outcomes in hemodialysis: questions answered in recent literature. *Artif Organs*, 27:237–41.

103. Zacks, S. L., & Fried, M. W. (2001). Hepatitis B and C and renal failure. *Infect Dis Clinic North Am*, 15:877–99.

104. Nunn, J. H. Sharp, J., Lambert, H. J., Plant, N. D., & Coulthard, M. G. (2000). Oral health in children with renal disease. *Pediatr Nephrol*, 14:997–1001.

105. Obry, F., Belcourt, A. B., Frank, R. M., Geisert, J., & Fischbach, M. (1987). Biochemical study of whole saliva from children with chronic renal failure. *ASDC J Dent Child*, 54:429–32.

106. Peterson, S., Woodhead, J., & Carall, J. (1985). Caries resistance in children with chronic renal failure: plaque salivary pH, and salivary composition. *Pediatr Res*, 19:796–9.

107. Wolff, A., Stark, H., Sarnat, H., Binderman, I., Eisenstein, B., & Drukker, A. (1985). The dental status of children with chronic renal failure. *Int J Pediatr*, 6;127–32.

108. Berns, J. S., & Tokars, J. I. (2002). Preventing bacterial infections and anti-microbial resistance in dialysis patients. *Am J Kidney Dis*, 40:886–98.

109. Oguz, Y., Bulucu, F., Oktenli, C., Doganci, L., & Vural, A. (2002). Infectious complications in 135 Turkish renal transplant patients. *Cent Eur J Public Health*, 10:153–6.

110. Thomason, J. M., Seymour, R. A., & Ellis, J. (1994). The periodontal problems and management of the renal transplant patient. *Ren Fail*, 16:731–45.

111. Pernu, H. E., Pernu, L. M., Knuuttila, M. I., & Huttunen, K. R. (1993). Gingival overgrowth among renal transport recipients and uraemic patients. *Nephrol Dial Transplant*, 8:1254–8.

112. Naugle, K., Darby, M. L., Bauman, D. B., Lineberger, L. T. & Powers, R. (1998). The oral health status of individuals on renal dialysis. *Ann Periodontol*, 3:197–205.

113. Birkeland, S. A., & Storm, H. H. (2002). Risk for tumor and other disease transmission by transplantation: a population-based study of unrecognized malignancies and other diseases in organ donors. *Transplantation*, 74:1409–13.

114. Varon, F., & Mack-Shipman, L. (2000). The role of the dental profession in diabetes. *J Contemp Dent Pract*, 1:1–27.

115. Lalla, R. V., & D' Ambrosio, J. A. (2001). Dental management considerations for the patient with diabetes mellitus. *J Am Dent Assoc*, 132:1425–32.

116. Matther, C., Executive Director. (1997). In *Diseases*, 2nd Ed. Springhouse, PA: Springhouse Corp., pp. 1224.

117. Katz, J., Chaushu, G., & Sgan-Cohen, H. D. (2000). Relationship of blood glucose level to community periodontal in the treatment needs and body mass index in a permanent Israeli military population. *J Periodontology*, 71:1521–7.

118. Almas, K., Al-Qahtani, M., Al-Yami, M., & Khan, N. (2001). The relationship between periodontal disese and blood glucose level among type II diabetic agents. *J Contem Dent Pract*, 2:18–25.

119. Bell, G. W., Large, D. M., & Barclay, S. C. (2000). Oral health care in diabetes mellitus. *SADJ*, 55:158–65, quiz 175.

120. Mattson, J. S., & Cerutis, D. R., (2001). Diabetus: a review of the literature and dental implications. *Comp Cont Educ Dent*, 22757–60, 762, 764.

121. Mealey, B. I. (2003). Clinical experience that many periodotists have had when treated as poorly controlled diabetic patients. *J Compend Continuing Educ*, 24:88.

122. Rees, T. D. (2000). Periodontal management of the patient with diabetes mellitus. *Periodontol*, 23:63–72.

123. Mealey, B. L. (2000). How does diabetes alter treatment in the dental office. *Compend Contin Educ Dent*, 21:943–6.

124. Taylor, G. W. (2001). Bidirectional interrelationships between diabetes and periodontal diseases: an epidemiologic perspective. *Ann Periodontol*, 6:99–112.

125. American Association of Periodontology. (1999). Diabetes and Periodontal Diseases. *J Periodontol*, 77:935–49.

126. American Academy of Periodontology. (2000). Parameters of periodontitis associated with systemic conditions. American Academy of Periodontology. *J Periodontology*, 7:876–9.

127. Twetman, S., Johansson, I., Birkhed, D. & Nederfors, T. (2002). Caries incidence in young type 1 diabetes mellitus patients in relation to metabolic control and caries risk factors. *Caries Res*, 36:31–35.

128. Karjalainen, K. M., & Knuuttila, Kaar, M. L. (1997). Relationship between caries and level of metabolic balance in children and adolescents with insulin-dependent diabetes mellitus. *Caries Res*, 31:13–18.

129. Moore, P. A., Guggenheimer, J., Etzel, K. R., Weyant, R. J., & Orchard, T. (2001). Type I diabetes mellitus, xerostomia, and salivary flow rates. *Oral Surg Oral Med Oral Pathol Oral Radiol End*, 92:281–91.

130. Greenspan D. (1996). *Xerostomia: diagnosis and management*. Oncology (Huntingt), 10:7–11.

131. Bjelland, S., Bry, P., Gupta, N., & Hirscht, R. (2002). Dentists, diabetes and periodontists. *Aust Dent J*, 47:202–7, quiz 272.

132. Sandberg, G. E., Sundberg, H. E., & Wikblad, K. F. (2001). A controlled study of oral self-care and self-perceived oral health in type 2 diabetic patients. *Acta Odontol*, 59:28–33.

133. Bridges R. B., Anderson, J. W., Saxxe, S. R., Gregory, K., & Bridges, S. R. (1996). Periodontal status of diabetic and non-diabetic men: effects of smoking, glycemic control, and socioeconomic factors. *IJ Periodontol*, 67:1185–92.

134. Mealey, B. I., & Rethman, M. P. (2003). Periodontal disease and diabetes mellitus. Bidirectional relationship. *Dent Today*, 22:107–13.

135. Bavitz, J. B. (1995). Emergency mangement of hypoglycemia and hyperglycemia. *Dent Clin North America*, 39:587–94.

136. Jowell, N. I., & Cabot, L. B. (1998). Diabetic hypoglycemia and the dental patient. *Brit Dent J*, 185:439–42.

137. Jerome Groopman. The Edmonton Protocol. *The New Yorker*, Feb. 10, 2003.

138. Ryan, E. A., Lakey, J. R., Rajotte, R. V., Korbutt, G. S., Kin, T., Imes, S., Rabinovit, A., Elliott, J. F., Bigam, D., Kneteman, M. N., Warnock, G. I., Larsen, I. & Shapiro, A. M. (2001). Clinical outcomes and insulin secretion after islet transplantation with the Edmonton protocol. *Diabetes*, 50:710–9.

139. Emerich, D. F. (2002). Islet transplantation for diabetes: current status and future prospects. *Expert Opin Biol Ther*, 2:793–803.

140. Robertson, R. P. (2002). Islet transplantation: travels up the learning curve. *Curr. Diab Rep*, 2:365–70.

# CHAPTER 23

# Rationale, Guidelines, and Procedures for Prevention of the Plaque Diseases

*Norman O. Harris*
*Marsha A. Cunningham-Ford*

## OBJECTIVES

*At the end of this chapter, it will be possible to*

1. Describe the two reversible stages that occur between histological normalcy and development of overt lesions for each of the plaque diseases, i.e., caries and periodontal disease.
2. Explain why the initial/annual dental examination is so important to the present and future dental health of a patient.
3. Name seven caries-activity indicators (CAIs), and four periodontal-activity indicators (PAIs) and explain why they should be included in the initial/annual examination.
4. Explain how the CAIs and PAIs that are included in the initial/annual dental examination can be used as an aid in preparing the patient's education, treatment, prevention, and maintenance plans.
5. Discuss two diagnostic scenarios in which the use (or misuse) of an explorer for caries diagnosis can result in the insertion of many unneeded occlusal and smooth surface restorations.
6. Propose a flexible recall schedule based on a patient's level of treatment urgency (risk), and explain how risk determination can be used to channel patients into a more closely monitored caries and/or periodontal maintenance program.
7. Critique the advantages and disadvantages for the development of national guidelines for preventive dental care.

8. State five (out of the six listed) clinical environments in which a zero-or-near-zero dental plaque disease prevention program can be fully implemented without major changes of present clinic facilities and manning personnel.
9. Contrast what you think *can be done to prevent the plaque diseases with what is being practiced.*

## INTRODUCTION

In the quest for a zero or near-zero incidence of the plaque diseases, i.e., caries, and periodontal disease(s), the critical requirement is that the signs and symptoms of impending disease be identified at a time when progression toward overt cavitation and/or periodontitis can be *prevented, arrested, or reversed.* Three salient factors make this preventive objective feasible: (1) both dental caries and periodontitis are the result of a prolonged presence of pathogenic plaques affecting the enamel, cementum, and/or contiguous gingiva; (2) in most cases, both diseases can be controlled by mechanical and chemical plaque control regimens; and, (3) both of the plaque diseases must go through a continuum of two *reversible* interim stages from histological normalcy to clinical pathology.

The earliest stage of the plaque diseases is *in situ* involvement. For caries, this stage is marked by the *microscopic demineralization* of the crystalline structure of the enamel rods.[1] For periodontal disease, it is the early *infiltration of inflammatory cells* beneath the sulcular epithelium.[2] Neither the early demineralization of caries nor the early cellular infiltration of gingivitis can be directly seen. However, these microscopic beginnings of impending plaque disease can be *suspected* on the basis of noninvasive caries and periodontal risk assessment tests and indices that are *now* available to dental and dental hygiene professionals.

An *in situ* involvement, unless arrested or reversed, merges into the next stage of progression of the caries process—*the incipient lesion.* For caries it is manifest by the clinical appearance of a *"white spot"* on the enamel that is due to a more extensive subsurface rod demineralization.[3] Incipient lesions can occur on any surface as a *precaries lesion.*[a] They may occur (1) interproximally, *apical* to the contact point, (2) as *cervical white spots,* (3) on the *walls* of the deep occlusal fissures, and (4) on *buccal* and *lingual surfaces*—wherever there is plaque stagnation. These precaries lesions can be easily seen on dry, well-lighted buccal, lingual, and gingival enamel surfaces.[4] They are more difficult to detect on the occlusal surface where "sticky" pits and fissures should always be highly suspect as having incipient or even early undetected carious lesions.[5] The presence of "white spots" on the smooth interproximal surfaces are usually first identified in radiographs.[6,7] In periodontal disease, the incipient lesion is an inflammation of the gingiva, i.e., *gingivitis* with gingival bleeding being one of the first noticeable manifesta-

---

[a]Precaries lesion; Since an incipient caries lesion can, in many cases, be remineralized, it should not be considered in the same category as an overt lesion where a restoration is usually indicated.

tions.[8] The incipient lesions of *both* caries and gingivitis can be reversed to histological normality—which by definition, represents a cure.

The third and final stage of the plaque diseases is the *overt* lesion. For caries, this stage is heralded by *cavitation* with bacterial infiltration. For periodontal disease, it is characterized by *nonreversible* changes in the periodontium such as an apical migration of the epithelial attachment and bone loss (periodontitis). At the overt lesion stage of the plaque diseases, treatment is usually indicated. There are two possible exceptions where noninvasive preventive regimens may possibly be used to reverse overt caries, namely the use of antibacterial agents and/or remineralization therapy to arrest root decay, and the use of sealants to arrest early pit-and-fissure caries.[9,10]

Not all *in situ* lesions progress to the incipient stage, nor do all the incipient lesions progress to the overt stage of caries and/or periodontitis.[11] However, it is extremely important to note that no overt plaque disease lesion occurs at any site without first beginning as an *in situ* manifestation, and then progressing to an incipient lesion before becoming overt. *Thus, any prevention program must focus on identifying and reversing the in situ and incipient stages of the plaque diseases with the same, or greater diligence than is now given to searching for and treating overt disease.* It is the purpose of this chapter to summarize how the dentist, the dental hygienist, and the other members of the office team can realistically accomplish this goal. Such an achievement will allow the profession to move from a traditional emphasis on secondary and tertiary preventive dentistry, *to a primary preventive focus and commitment.*

## The Initial and/or Annual Dental Examination

The *initial/annual dental examination* is a *most* important event in the entire oral health program of a patient. At this time, a person seeking dental care has the opportunity and *expectation* to have his or her current oral status carefully assessed by a professional, a treatment plan prepared, restorative care accomplished, and *a comprehensive preventive dentistry program initiated* that will help forestall future plaque disease. This baseline examination is one against which all future examinations should be compared to evaluate time–function deviations from baseline oral health.

The first phase of the initial/annual examination begins in the reception area of the dental office. Here the patient is asked to complete the usual paperwork that includes the patient's medical and dental histories. Included in these histories should be a carbohydrate-intake questionnaire and questions relating to systemic factors and behavior patterns that might affect past, present or future oral disease development. Before the clinical examination, the dentist and hygienist should carefully scrutinize the patient's history, both for evidence of transmittable disease, as well as for conditions indicating a relationship of systemic conditions to oral disease. For example, a patient taking antihypertensive medications, tranquilizers, or many other drugs, often has an accompanying xerostomia and an increased caries risk. The medical history also helps identify conditions such as Crohn's disease[12] or diabetes mellitus[13] that are background systemic factors that raise the risk for caries and periodontal disease, respectively.

The initial/annual examination should be divided into two stages: (1) a *clinical* and a *roentgenographic* phase to *locate, diagnose,* and to *record* sites of incipient and overt plaque disease; and, (2) *laboratory tests and indices* to help

identify the *risk* of in *situ* and/or incipient plaque disease. These are ultimately the responsibilities of the *dentist*[14,15] but the laboratory phases can be performed by the dental hygienist. The examination should include as a minimum:

- A visual examination of all the intraoral and craniofacial tissues for diseases, other than the plaque diseases (cancer for instance)
- A set of bitewing and periapical radiographs as part of the examination for interproximal enamel radiolucencies and loss of alveolar bone
- A *visual* and mouth mirror examination of all the teeth for incipient and overt coronal and root caries, and an explorer examination for suspected fractured restorations, and secondary (i.e., recurrent) caries
- A record made as to which occlusal surfaces need sealants
- A record made as to which "white spots," (interproximal radiolucencies *without* evidence of cavitation), and root surface caries that require remineralization therapy and,
- A periodontal probe examination of all gingival sulci

The *final phase of the initial/annual* examination can be accomplished by a dental hygienist as part of the first prophylaxis appointment. This phase should include: a plaque index, a calculus site recording, a saliva flow rate notation, and appropriate laboratory tests to establish caries risk. All can be easily accomplished in the dental office to furnish valuable baseline information on the background of the patient's plaque diseases. The indices also furnish valuable information needed to help establish the level of preventive treatment required.

A plaque index is both an indicator of caries *and/or* periodontal disease activity. However, it does not discriminate as to which plaque disease is involved. As the plaque score (Chapter 13) increases over 10% there is an increasing probability that the plaque bacteria are causing

damage to the teeth or to the periodontium. The plaque index also provides a means of evaluating, at sequential appointments, whether previously recommended plaque control measures have been implemented. The sites of calculus accumulation can be recorded at the same time, thus providing a further means of identifying areas of saliva stagnation where plaque control methods such as tooth brushing, flossing and irrigation have not been adequate.

Microbiologic caries activity tests provide a good assessment of caries risk, especially if the results are compared with previous baseline results. Dip-slide[b] kits are commercially available for evaluating the salivary levels of mutans streptococci and lactobacilli, respectively (Figure 23-1A and 1B). Any increase in the number of cariogenic bacteria between annual examinations should be viewed as indicating an increased risk for disease; therefore, it is prudent to take action to reduce the bacterial count. Microbiologic test scores when considered along with the carbohydrate intake score, serve as tools for assessing patient compliance with previous dietary and oral hygiene counseling intended to reduce the bacterial challenge.

Stimulated saliva should be collected in a calibrated tube in order to determine flow rate per minute. This latter datum—especially if the flow rate is below one milliliter per minute (xerostomia)—is often important in helping to identify the cause of an individual's caries. There is little difference between the data collected for treatment planning and the data needed for prevention programs. Perhaps the greatest contrast between the two is in the decision-making process of what to do with the data. The dentist making the initial/annual examination should have the knowledge and

---

[b]Dip-slide kits for office counts of mutans streptoccus and lactobacillus are available from Ivoclar Vicadent, Amherst, NY, 14228.

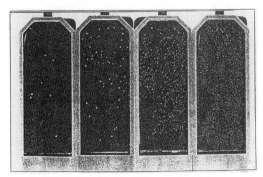

FIGURE 23–1A    After 48 hours, mutans streptococci become visible on test strip. The two left slides have less than 100,000 colony forming units (CFU) per milliliter of saliva and constitute a relatively low risk for caries. The two samples to the right indicate a high risk with more than 100,000 CFU/ml.

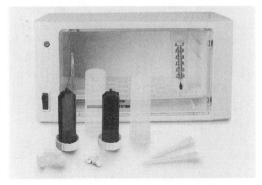

FIGURE 23–1B    A small convenient office incubator for processing Caries Risk Test slides. Both illustrations courtesy of Ivoclar Vivadent, Amherst, NY 14228.

experience to *identify* both incipient and overt lesions in the clinical and radiographic examinations, and the *wisdom* to differentiate between the two in selecting appropriate treatment options. A treatment-oriented decision of caries usually results in an invasive treatment procedure resulting in damage to the tooth, while a preventive-oriented decision usually leaves the tooth intact.[16]

A second major difference between the treatment and preventive aspects of the examination lies with office-time priorities. In the usual treatment plan, time commitments emphasize disease eradication. In an ideal preventive program, optimal time is allowed for *both* primary and secondary prevention. Another critical difference is that the treatment plan ends when the recorded pathology is successfully treated. In the preventive plan, the information gained in the initial/annual examination can be arrayed in a manner that permits the development of reasoned patient behavior modification and monitoring strategies that can be used to prevent future plaque disease development.

### The Computer Age

The percentage of dental practices using computers at the beginning of 1999 has been estimated at 89%.[17] Articles are beginning to appear in the literature on the advantages of hitech dental offices.[18–21] The initial use of computers was for administrative purposes— billing, recall appointments, electronic insurance claims, payroll and inventory control. However, with the passage of time, software became available that directly supported clinical needs. For instance, there are cosmetic imaging programs, interactive patient education CD-ROMs, self-administered patient histories, diet-analysis programs, software to determine the indications, contraindications, and incompatibilities of available drugs, on-line professional information and even remote consultations over the internet.[22] Even more benefits are coming.[23] However, three of the most current and promising areas for computer support of the dental clinical examination are: (1) *computerized charting*, (2) *the use of the intraoral videocamera (IVC)*, and (3) *(filmless) digitalized roentgenography (DXR)*.

Computerized charting programs are now commercially available for recording the pres-

ence of overt or incipient plaque disease lesions (Figure 23–2). Other parts of the computer software often permit *recording the presence and severity of selected caries and periodontal activity indicators* that are the basis of risk assessment *at the time of testing.* Commonly used evidence-based caries-activity indicators (CAIs) are the (1) plaque index, (2) quantification of cariogenic organisms, (3) saliva flow rate, (4) frequency of intake of refined carbohydrate (sugar). Equally important are the (5) number of "sticky" occlusal pits and fissures, (6) coronal and root caries, (7) incipient buccal and lingual smooth surface lesions, and the (8) number of interproximal lucencies (incipient lesions) *without cavitation.* For periodontal disease, the periodontal-activity indicators (PAIs) are the (1) plaque index, (2) calculus, and (3) gingival bleeding indices, and the (4) Periodontal Screening and Recording system (PSR) for

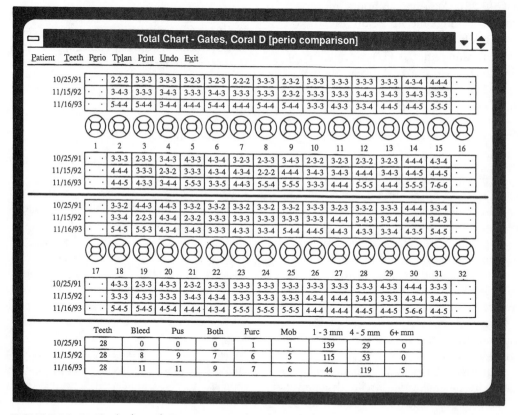

FIGURE 23–2  Periodontal Computer Assisted Record Form. A periodontal computer assisted record form that, along with other options available with the accompanying software, permits easy comparison with the details of previous periodontal examinations. When the probing is accomplished with the Florida Probe illustrated in Figure 13-6, entries can be automatically made on the record form. Color coding [not possible on this black and white photo] allows easy detection of differences in gingival sulci probing depths of 1-4 mm (black), greater than 5 mm (red). Note the other parameters that are part of a complete periodontal examination, such as PSR, plaque index, mobility, furcations, and recession. Courtesy of the Florida Probe Corporation, Gainesville, FL.

pocket depth.[24,25] These plaque disease indicators can be entered into the computer at chairside by use of a keyboard, mouse, touch screen, or voice activation. Note that the plaque index is useful as a risk indicator for *both* caries and periodontal involvement. Other indicators for either of the plaque diseases can be added or substituted in a computer format. For instance, the flow rate of gingival crevicular fluid might eventually serve as a PAI for dental offices having the necessary equipment.[26,27] However, the above four PAIs are now well known, easy to accomplish, and presently used by dentists and dental hygienists in caries and periodontal control programs.

---

### Question 1

Which of the following statements, if any, are correct?

A. Incipient "white spot" lesions are found only on the facial and lingual surfaces of teeth.

B. "White spots" in the enamel indicate that the carious process has passed the incipient stage.

C. The *in situ* stage of gingivitis is characterized by sulcular bleeding upon gentle probing.

D. The presence of dental plaque is an important evidence-based indicator for both caries and periodontal disease.

E. The CAIs and PAIs are more accurate in indicating *present vulnerability,* than of *predicting* future caries and/or inflammatory periodontal disease.

---

### The Intraoral Videocamera (IVC) and the Digitalized X-Ray (DXR)

The recent introduction of the intraoral videocamera (IVC) and the digitized dental x-ray (DXR) provide two powerful high-tech instruments, that when coupled with a computer, video recorder or color printer, facilitate a more accurate identification, charting, and understanding of the sites of both incipient and overt plaque disease.[28]

The IVC, which is a miniature camcorder, provides a uniform lighting at all sites being examined (Figure 23–3). It permits magnification of questionable areas to *improve* the possibility of locating incipient and overt lesions, as well as sites of plaque accumulation, calculus deposition, defective restorations, and periodontal problems. The IVC has the advantage of allowing an area to be freeze-framed to study a questionable site better, or if desired, to make high-quality color photographs by outputting the image to a high-resolution color printer. Cracked or fractured amalgams are easy to identify. A later replay of the examination tape on the high-resolution television screen is an outstanding means of educating and motivating patients.[29] Administratively, the modem of the computer can be used to transmit the necessary

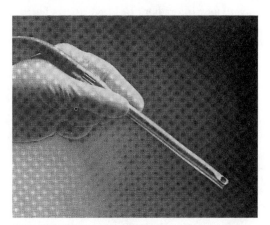

FIGURE 23–3   A high-tech merging of electronics and optics to make an intraoral video camera. Note the small camera lens at the end of the camera shaft. The images obtained are seen on the operatory monitor during the examination as well as being transmitted over the office hardwiring to the business center where it can be stored or printed, or if necessary sent out as an e-mail for insurance purposes.

images for immediate insurance verification of anticipated treatment and preventive costs, or to send treatment information to remote sites.

The digitalized x-ray (DXR) utilizes intraoral film-size *electronic sensors,* which are connected to the computer (Figure 23–4). The existing office x-ray unit provides the source of energy. No liquid processing is necessary as the image is processed electronically within the computer.[30] The digitalized image is more uniform in contrast than is now possible with film. By use of computer control, it is possible to zoom in on small details, and to use enhancement techniques to lighten or darken areas of the screen for better diagnosis.[31] An important advantage of DXR is that it only requires 50% *or less* ionizing radiation than is necessary in conventional dental radiography.[32] This improved safety factor results in a better balancing of the individualized need for more frequent radiographic monitoring against the ethical responsibility to minimize patient exposure to ionizing radiation.[33] Like the IVC, the

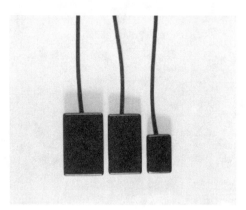

FIGURE 23–4  Three different intraoral film-size sensors—bitewing, anterior, and pediatric—used for DXR. Variations in energy received by the sensor are transmitted by the attached wire to the computer for electronic processing. The resulting image can be presented on a high resolution monitor, stored, printed or treated as e-mail if needed.

DXR images can be downloaded for patient education and study, insurance verification, or for use in treatment or preventive programs. There is no deterioration of the stored digitalized images with time. Finally, a most important point is that the diagnostic value of the image is considered equal to traditional bitewing radiography when downloaded to a *high-resolution* monitor or printer.[34]

## Caries and Primary Prevention

### Explorer Misdiagnosis and Misuse

The hi-tech advancements to dental diagnostic science discussed above, have arrived at a time when the traditional explorer is coming into question as often being an *accessory to iatrogenic dentistry.* With the millions of explorer diagnoses of caries-or-no caries being made every day in dental offices throughout the world, it is essential to look at any evidence that might indicate potential or actual patient harm, as well as possible solutions.

The use of the explorer to search for carious lesions is being questioned in Europe[35] and the United States.[36] This concern is generated by the fact that explorer examinations can possibly cause irreparable damage to the surface of immature enamel;[37-39] carry cariogenic bacteria from one infection site to other vulnerable deep pits and fissures;[40] and *most important, explorer catches have not proved to be valid indicators of the presence, or absence, of questionable occlusal caries.*[41,42] The diagnosis of pit-and-fissure caries with convoluted fissures is precarious by either visual or explorer techniques. The diagnostic value of an explorer examination of the occlusal surfaces *decreases* as the "stickiness" of the fissure increases—this at a time when *the need for validity increases.* For instance, the sensitivity of an explorer examination can decrease from 80% for wide fissures to 52% for those that are narrow.[42] Penning and coworkers employed an explorer to examine the occlusal surface of 100 extracted teeth that had *no visible cavitation,* and which were later x-rayed and

sectioned. Only 24% of the caries lesions that were eventually found were discovered by use of the explorer.[43] Lussi conducted a study involving 34 dentists who serially examined 61 extracted teeth. A histological study of the teeth was accomplished to provide the "correct" diagnoses. The results demonstrated that the dentists were more likely *not to treat decayed teeth than to "restore" sound teeth.* Forty two percent of the teeth were correctly diagnosed, only one tooth was correctly diagnosed by all, and two were never correctly diagnosed.[42] As a result of the lack of validity of the explorer-based examination of occlusal surfaces, *several clinical researchers have suggested that the explorer is no more effective for locating pit-and-fissure caries than is a visual examination coupled with professional judgment.*[44,45] This conclusion argues for the use of an *explorerless* mouth-mirror-only (or preferably the use of the IVC) in dental exami-

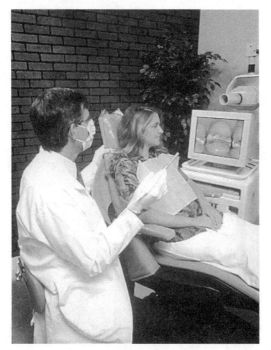

FIGURE 23–5   With a patient watching the monitor during the examination, much patient education can be accomplished.

nations, (Figure 23–5) but relegates the explorer to such tasks as locating calculus, checking the marginal integrity of newly placed restorations and sealants, and in searching for secondary caries. Even this latter use has been subject to question.[46]

An example of overtreatment caused by *misuse* of the explorer is the case of the incipient caries lesion. In a caries examination, "white spots" on the buccal and lingual surfaces can be easily seen; whereas, interproximal enamel lucencies ("white spots") are usually first detected by radiography. *Once incipient lesions are identified and recorded, there is no need to probe this precarious site.* To do so will often convert the incipient lesion into an overt lesion requiring a restoration. Lesions over 0.1 to 2.0 mm. can be created in extracted teeth by such misuse of the explorer.[37] Without the probing *penetration* of the surface zone that allows a subsequent bacterial invasion, remineralization therapy of the "white spots" can very often be successfully implemented with no eventual damage to the tooth.

As a general summarizing concept of *diagnostic errors*, Downer[47] and Bader[48] have both pointed out that in routine caries examinations, whether as a result of the x-ray diagnosis or from the use of an explorer, there is a high probability of *false-positive* and *false-negative* diagnoses. As that line of delineation between disease-and-no disease is approached, it becomes even more difficult, in fact impossible, to positively identify a tooth as carious-or-noncarious. In this gray area the toss of a coin can be as accurate as the explorer. These diagnostic errors are the result of perceptual and tactile variations between examiners, different criteria for treatment decisions, lack of precision of diagnostic technology, and differences in diligence to search for pathology and *impending* disease. This fallibility has been recognized for years, and several methods have been, or are being tested to provide more validity to caries diagnosis. Some of the more promising methods used are bite wing and digi-

talized roentgenography (the latter with its capability of image enhancement); fiber-optic transillumination (FOTI), visual examination especially when using a video intraoral camera, disclosing dyes, electrical conduction (or resistance) and high intensity focused light. In the latter cases, the reflectance from the tooth surfaces of the ultraviolet, fluorescent, laser, or infra red light are being measured by a light meter.[49] Until a better solution is developed, penetration of the surface zones of incipient lesions or false-positive diagnoses for caries can be as damaging to the teeth as is bacterial-induced cavitation, since in a clinical situation the end result is the insertion of unneeded restorations

Experience and studies also indicate that restorations are not-for-a-lifetime.[50–53] The high failure of amalgams from marginal defects, overhangs and recurrent caries has been noted for many years.[54,55] More contemporary studies show an improvement in longevity of restorations, but still the cycle of placement and replacement is strongly evident. Mjor et al., in a recent study of 6,761 restorations, found that the average longevity for an amalgam restoration placed in adults (> or = 19 years of age) was 11 years. Resin-based composites averaged 8 years, glass ionomers 4 years, and resin modified glass ionomer, 2 years.[56] Each successive replacement involves a greater loss of tooth structure and a greater danger of eventual tooth loss. Thus, preventing one new cavity results in a multiplier effect of preventing several recurrent lesions over a lifetime. For this reason, the present treatment of overt, and arrest, or reversal of incipient lesions, must be accorded an urgent priority of preventive care.

Probably the two most effective and economical dental-office preventive procedures available to rapidly reduce caries incidence, and often the least used, would be the early placement of sealants in all deep convoluted ("sticky") occlusal fissures, and the timely use of remineralization procedures for all noncavitated incipient smooth surface lesions. To epitomize the potential of the combined use of sealants and remineralization strategies, Ripa concluded that caries could practically be eliminated in U.S. schoolchildren by the combined use of sealants to protect the occlusal surfaces, and fluoride rinses to protect the smooth surfaces.[57]

> ## Question 2
>
> Which of the following statements, if any, are correct?
>
> A. The IVC camcorder documentation of the dental examination can be watched on a monitor screen by both the patient and the dentist.
>
> B. The main disadvantage of DXR is the fact that it requires more x-ray energy than bitewing films.
>
> C. Several clinical research studies have demonstrated that explorer catches are not valid indicators of the presence or absence of occlusal caries.
>
> D. According to several clinical researchers, an explorer examination of "sticky" occlusal surfaces results in many false-positive and false-negative diagnoses.
>
> E. A false-positive recording of caries status for a tooth usually results in the placement of a restoration in a non carious tooth.

## Sealants

The placement, replacement, and retention of a sealant in "sticky" caries-prone pits and fissures can prevent and/or arrest incipient occlusal lesions (Chapter 10).[58–62] Sealants provide a perfect solution to the dilemma of coping with the false-positive diagnoses of occlusal caries. Their placement in deep convoluted fissures of occlusal surfaces negates the possibility of wrongfully restoring the many teeth that would have received inadvertent false diagnoses for

caries. The sealing of a fissure also sequesters the cariogenic organisms to prevent the seeding of other areas in the mouth. Sealing of the fissures can be accomplished easily, quickly, painlessly and economically.

The sealant serves to interdict the nutrient supply to the fissure microorganisms, leading to their extinction, and the hardening of the underneath dentin.[63] The placement of an occlusal sealant is probably the most conservative solution to preventing or arresting the early caries process (if present), thereby avoiding the probability of future primary or recurrent lesions and their sequelae.[61] Sealant placement should be followed by a topical application of fluoride applied at the dental office, as well as a daily home exposure to a fluoride dentifrice and/or mouthrinse to help protect the whole tooth. Traditionally, the majority of sealants were placed on the occlusal surfaces of children's teeth. However, the *anatomy* of the occlusal fissure and the *risk assessment of the patient*, not the age of the individual should be the guide to any decision to place or not to place a sealant. *Lest we forget*, (1) *for every occlusal restoration seen at any age, a sealant was indicated previous to the development of the overt lesion and* (2) *for every smooth surface lesion seen at any age, remineralization was probably indicated previous to the development of cavitation!*

## Tooth, Heal Thyself— Remineralization

The microscopic loss (demineralization) and regaining of mineral (remineralization) on the *surface* of the teeth occurs *continuously* in a human environment.[64] Remineralization can be a *short-term* defense response to the daily microscopic loss of mineral from food abrasion and ingestion of acid foods and condiments such as oranges, pineapple, cola drinks and vinegar. Of equal importance is the body's ability, under *longer-term* favorable conditions, to repair radiographic lucencies that are seen in radiographs extending from the enamel surface

into as far as the outer 1/3 to 1/2 of the dentin. The rehardened subsurface lesions are usually microbiologically inactive with a hardness that approaches or exceeds that of the original enamel or dentin.[65]

The equilibrium between de- and remineralization can be greatly biased in favor of oral health by:

1. Reducing the population of cariogenic bacteria in the oral environment by mechanical and chemical plaque control measures. This is accomplished by frequent patient use of tooth brushing, flossing and irrigation ("brush, floss and flush"); it is also aided by the periodic use of therapeutic mouthrinses such as chlorhexidine and fluoride.

2. A drastic reduction of refined carbohydrate (sugar) intake.

3. Initiatiation of remineralization and protective strategies that enhance and supplement the crucial saliva-driven tooth remineralization.[66,67] Examples include multiple exposures to fluoride found in community-water supplies; of *professional* applications of fluoride varnish/gels, hygienist use of fluoride prophylactic pastes; and the *home use* of fluoride products such as fluoride dentifrices and mouthrinses.

4. Stimulating the flow of saliva with its mineralizing constituents. This can be accomplished by chewing non-sugar containing chewing gum, especially a gum flavored with xylitol, a non-acidogenic and non-cariogenic polyol[68] (Chapter 6.)

Remineralization of teeth is not a new concept. In 1884, one of Dr. J. D. White's "tips" in *Dental Cosmos* pointed out that "many teeth coming through the gums had an exceedingly defective look". For these teeth he suggested that the finger should be used to rub chalk on the teeth twice a day. As much of the chalk as possible should be allowed to remain.

Limewater was to be used to rinse the mouth instead of regular water.[69]

During the period of 1910 to 1920s, Head, a physician presented convincing experimental evidence that teeth could be hardened.[70] In one paper he wrote that he and several other dentists had seen *white spots* disappear, after which he asked, "If the spot disappears, would not this prove that the enamel is not a dead, inert substance that we are supposed to consider it?"[71]

By the 1920s, there was considerable agreement that recalcification (remineralization) could occur, but still considerable debate as to whether "calcification and recalcification" was physiological via the pulp, or a chemical phenomenon from addition of constituents from the saliva.[72,73]

It was not until the 1950s that there was more positive proof of caries arrestment. Muhler in his extensive research of a stannous fluoride dentifrice (Crest) found that the end-of-the-year examinations, many of the original charted lesions no longer existed. These he termed reversals.[74]

Following the initiation of water fluoridation, it was believed that the caries decrement that followed was caused by the formation of a more resistant fluorapatite crystal on the enamel surface, which to some extent was true. However, it was not till Silverstone described the carious lesion as comprised of a surface zone, the body of the lesion, and the dark and translucent zones, that it was demonstrated that with appropriate fluoride therapy, the subsurface carious lesion could be remineralized.[11] Today it is recognized that fluoride acts to *both* prevent demineralization and enhance remineralization. (Chapters 3 and 11.)

Remineralization therapy to arrest and reverse incipient smooth surface lesions is often mentioned in *research* journals, less mentioned in *practice-oriented* publications, and rarely employed *routinely* in clinical practice. Yet, the remineralization of incipient lesions with *no* evidence of cavitation is an essential *noninvasive*

preventive option to maintain a lifetime caries-free dentition. As early as 1970, von der Fehr and coworkers in a study involving multiple daily sugar mouthrinses, *visually* observed the development of "white spots" within 23 days. Remineralization of these "white spots" was successfully accomplished by use of dental hygiene and fluoride mouth rinses.[3] It was about 2 years later that a similar study was reported, only in this case, the students also used a 0.2% chlorhexidine mouthrinse twice-a-day to suppress the cariogenic organisms. There were no signs of early caries. *The chlorhexidine had made a difference.*

"White spots" are *not* rare occurrences. Mejare and colleagues visually inspected 598 surfaces of premolars extracted for orthodontic reasons as well as the adjacent surfaces of neighboring teeth and found that 51% had incipient lesions, of which only 5% demonstrated cavitation.[75] Mejare and Malmgren in another study found that at age 16, the mean number of incipient lesions per individual was 3.0[76] In a Scottish study, 2,917 incipient lesions were found visually on the buccal and lingual surfaces of the teeth of 2,854, 13-year-old school children. At the end of 2 years, approximately *three quarters* of the lesions had *remained static* or *regressed*. Furthermore, where incipient lesions were originally identified, there was a greater amount of plaque, as well as a greater possibility of locating other incipient lesions.[4] *The identification of one incipient lesion can be a warning sign of a more generalized caries status requiring attention.*

The *extreme importance* of considering all radiolucencies for remineralization is illustrated by a study in Denmark. The interproximal lucencies of 1,080 *preoperative* radiographs were examined *following* placement of restorations. Most lucencies found were those demonstrating demineralization but *not* cavitation. Only 10% demonstrated cavitations, meaning that 90% *should have been considered for remineralization in lieu of restoration.* As a result, it was concluded that the original diagnosing dentists needed to

better recognize lesions amenable to remineralization.[77] To further emphasize this problem of inappropriate over-treatment, Thylstrup and coworkers, in a roentgenographic study of interproximal caries, estimated the *only one out of four patients receiving restorations, needed restorations*.[78] Unfortunately, many believe that operative intervention is necessary to restore minimal interproximal lucencies despite a plethora of information that remineralization is a preferable *noninvasive* option for tooth longevity. For example, in a questionnaire study in Scotland, it was found that 44.2% of Scottish dentists would fill an approximal lesion confined to the enamel of a hypothetical 12-year-old *prior to* cavitation.[79]

Another factor to be considered when an interproximal surface of a tooth is prematurely restored is the *iatrogenic damage* caused to the proximal surface of the adjacent sound tooth. In one study, more than 50% of surfaces adjacent to approximal restorations were damaged, often presenting with radiographic changes.[80,81]

*Every* interproximal radiolucency *not showing cavitation*, should be considered for remineralization therapy and longitudinal monitoring; *only* when a lesion demonstrates cavitation should it be considered irreversible. Pitts and Rimmer, in examining 1,588 teeth, found that *100%* of the teeth with only "white spots" had sound enamel surfaces with no cavitation; even 89.5% of the enamel lucencies extending to the *dentinoenamel junction* had no cavitation. However, all lucencies extending into the proximity of the pulp *did have* cavitation.[82]

The New Zealand School Dental Service successfully uses fluoride varnish (Durophat) to enhance remineralization of the teeth of children having an interproximal lucency that is *not more than halfway through the enamel and no cavitation*.[83] Others use the dentinoenamel junction as the threshold.[84] For instance, Elderton believes that a radiolucency should extend *into* the dentin or *show cavitation* before operative intervention.[85] Dodds has suggested that even dentinal lucencies *without apparent cavitation* should be considered for possible remineralization therapy since further caries progression is often blocked by sclerosing or secondary dentin.[86]

Clinicians in Europe and globally are beginning to think conservatively.[87,88] The following 1999 paper from Scandinavia illustrates this trend. The study by Majare et al. is entitled "Caries assessment and restorative thresholds reported by Swedish dentists." The study included the responses of 651 (out of 923) dentists who indicated that for an adolescent with low caries activity and good oral hygiene, 90% would *not* automatically restore an approximal lucency if its radiographic appearance did not show obvious progression *to the outer* ⅓ *to* ½ *of the dentin*. Moreover, 67% would only consider immediate restorative treatment of an occlusal surface if *obvious cavitation* and/or if radiographic signs of dental caries could be observed. Other interesting findings were that the younger, more often than older dentists would postpone restorative treatment, and that dentists in private practice would restore approximal caries at an earlier stage of progression than dentists in the Public Health Dental Service.[89]

There are no U.S. reports available for comparison.

## The Remineralizable Root Caries Lesion

With an aging population retaining their teeth longer, there is an increasing prevalence of root caries.[90,91] Approximately 28% of the population seeking treatment who are under 60 years of age have root caries;[92] over 60 years of age, the estimate increases to approximately 40 to 63%.[93] Fifty-three percent of the root lesions are on the *facial* surface, followed in order by the distal, lingual and mesial surfaces.[94]

Like coronal caries, root surface caries occur in distinct and important stages—incipient, arrested, overt, and restored. The incipient stage that precedes frank (overt) cavitation is described as a "well-defined softened area, yellow-

ish or light brown in color, but *without* cavitation upon initial inspection, that is, undisturbed *before* probing.[95] There is no "white spot" or subsurface lesion as found in coronal caries. This softened mass can often be remineralized by daily plaque removal with a toothbrush and a fluoride dentifrice, plus appropriate spaced professional applications of fluoride.[96–98] As a part of surface rehardening, there is also a redistribution of mineral within the lesion.[99] Thus, like incipient coronal caries, the easily visible root caries site should *not* be subject to explorer manipulation if contemplating remineralization procedures. The influence of fluoride on root surface caries is the same as for coronal caries, i.e., reducing demineralization and enhancing remineralization.

Several chemotherapeutic approaches have been used to arrest root caries lesions. Billings and associates,[100] and Markitzui and colleagues used *topical fluorides.*[9] Nyvad and Fejerskove found that where root lesions were accessible (mainly *facial* surfaces) to brushing with a *fluoride dentifrice*, it was possible to convert 54% of the active root caries to an inactive status. Only 8% of the approximal lesions reverted to inactive status.[100,101] Schaecken et al. found that the use of chlorhexidine and fluoride caused a *hardening* of root caries as well as markedly suppressing the mutans streptococci over several months.[102]

Following a histopathology examination of extracted teeth with root caries, Schupack and associates concluded that remineralization depended on (1) the degree of active sclerosis of dentinal tubules underlying the lesion, (2) the degree of the bacterial infection of the dentin, (3) the degree of progression of the lesions, and (4) the location of the lesions at the various root surfaces[103]

The alternative to *preventing* active root surface caries is the insertion of restorations that soon become the sites of secondary caries. Fejerskov expressed this thought by stating, "The more fillings inserted, the more likely is the risk of developing more caries lesions."[104] Remineralization therapy of root caries, especially of the facial surface, appears to have an equal or better probability of success in restoring an incipient or early overt lesion to inactive status, than does the insertion of a restoration.

## Fluorides and Remineralization

Regimens to maximize the potential for remineralization as well as to minimize demineralization consist of the use of home and office chemical and mechanical plaque control techniques, multiple fluoride therapies, and a severely limited intake of sugar—exactly the same techniques as used to prevent the development of the incipient lesions in the first place. The multiple fluoride therapies include fluoride dentifrices and mouth rinses, office applications of topical fluoride liquids, gels, or use of a fluoride varnish or remineralizing paste at specific sites, and even the possible prescription of fluoride tablets in fluoride-deficient areas, regardless of age.[105] Once remineralization has been successfully accomplished in the presence of fluoride, the remineralized areas often are *more resistant to future acid attack than previous to demineralization.*

The two times when a tooth is especially vulnerable to demineralization and caries are (1) immediately after eruption and before maturation of the enamel, and (2) at any time during life following prolonged bacterial acid-induced demineralization. To meet the first of these two challenges, several *professionally applied fluoride* applications should be made from the time the first tip of the erupting cusp appears until the tooth is in occlusion. Even after full eruption is attained, fluoride should be applied several times professionally during the first year of intraoral maturation.

In the second instance, the many daily cycles of de- and remineralization at different periods throughout life are usually subclinical and are not possible to detect.[11] One of the best ways to ensure enamel protection from caries progression during such periodic negative min-

eral balances, is by the daily exposure of the teeth to fluoride, such as fluoridated water and by use of over-the-counter products such as fluoride dentifrices and fluoride rinses. (Figure 23–4).

## The Potential

The successful sealing of all deep pits and fissures and the remineralization of all incipient lesions would by definition, result in preventing all carious lesions (except for those caused by diagnostic error and explorer misuse) from progressing to the overt stage requiring restorations. Any concern of possible unnoticed caries progress during remineralization therapy or beneath a sealant can be allayed by shorter individualized recall schedules to permit longitudinal monitoring.[106,107] To further allay concern, the slow advance of the pre-caries front is seen in a report by Majare et al., where 50% of the lucencies at the dentinoenamel junction required an average of 3.1 years to progress into the dentin.[108] This provides ample opportunity to later substitute invasive operative treatment, if necessary.[109] To reinforce these previous facts, Pitts, in a 3-year study of regular adolescent attendees, found that 80% of the original radiolucencies apparently regressed or arrested spontaneously.[110] Thus, noninvasive approaches of sealant placement and remineralization therapy are viable and a preferred approach to maintaining intact teeth. *Dental caries is a preventable disease where even established precaries lesions can be arrested or reversed—with appropriate patient cooperation.*[111]

---

### Question 3

Which of the following statements, if any, are correct?

A. Sealants become more cost-effective as the fissures on the occlusal surface deepens and become more convoluted ("sticky").

B. Sealants should be placed over all "sticky" fissures where there is the possibility of a false positive or a false-negative diagnosis.

C. "White spots" result in a permanent change in color and surface topography of a tooth.

D. Usually, more "white spots" regress or remain static than those that progress to overt lesions.

E. Caries of both coronal and root surfaces can only occur when demineralization exceeds remineralization over time.

---

## Periodontal Disease and Primary Prevention

### A Rational Approach to Preventing Gingivitis

This short section will briefly review a few facts appropriate to this chapter that were learned from Chapters 4 and 13.

1. A high plaque-index score and/or the presence of calculus usually portends a gingivitis.

2. Gingivitis usually can be reversed by office-instituted and home self-care hygiene measures that remove or severely disturb the dental plaque. Since the periodontal tissues return to histological normalcy, this home and professional care represents a *cure*.

3. Once the gingivitis is successfully treated, the next recall interval should be based on the present treatment urgency, that is, the higher the apparent *risk*, the shorter the time interval should be before the next appointment.

Periodontal-activity indicators (PAIs) and guidelines for appropriate *therapy, counseling, and recall schedules* can be developed in the same way as previously discussed for caries-activity indica-

tors (CAIs). Again, the four evidence-developed indicators are the plaque index, calculus severity, number of bleeding sites on probing, and the Periodontal Screening and Recording system (PSR) for pocket depth (see Chapter 13). The PSR was introduced in 1993 by the American Dental Association and the American Academy of Periodontology as a method to screen all adult patients 18 years of age and older for evidence of periodontal disease.[24]

Only 5 minutes is needed to accomplish the PSR screening (probing). The zero-to-four coding system used for each of the sextants of the patient's mouth provides a numerical basis to suggest the periodontal treatment urgency as well as patient management guidelines commensurate with the patient's periodontal status. The PSR should be recorded at all initial/annual examinations, and at all recalls, especially where the previous periodontal treatment urgency was of concern. A color-coded, beaded probe tip is used to measure sulcus depth enabling the PSR to be quickly accomplished.

To increase the accuracy of determining the depth of the periodontal pockets, as well as to facilitate the ease of recording pocket depth, a computer-coupled periodontal probe was developed to automatically signal a computer to record the pocket depth of a tooth after encountering a given resistance at the base of the gingival sulcus.

Unlike the CAI laboratory tests in which caries risk is related mainly to mutans streptococci and lactobacilli levels, no parallel laboratory "*screening tests*" are available for periodontopathogens. A number of *diagnostic* laboratory tests for *Actinobacillus actinomycetemcomitans*, *Porphyromonos gingivalis*, and *Prevotelle intermedia* and other suspect periodontopathogens are used to aid in making treatment decisions, but their cost–benefit as routine microbiologic screening PAIs has not been adequately assessed. However, much research effort is now being devoted to finding some genetic marker for identifying present and future risk for periodontal disease.

## Plaque and Plaque Control

Dental plaque is *always* present at the interface between the saliva and the tooth surface. Any site with more than a minimal amount of plaque should be considered an *infected area* in need of constant and effective daily disruption or removal by use of a toothbrush, dental floss, and irrigation; and/or by the suppression of pathogenic bacteria with antimicrobial agents. Initially, a marginal gingivitis of local origin occurs as a result of bacterial metabolic end products in the supragingival plaque. This early periodontal involvement (gingivitis) is usually the first sign apparent to the patient in the form of "pink toothbrush" caused by blood on the toothbrush. Starting at an early age, it is essential that a person should learn to use plaque-control measures that remove or severely disturb plaque at least once a day. The tooth- brushing, flossing, and irrigation that are accomplished by the individual while the periodontium is healthy is intended to *prevent the onset* of gingivitis. Any eventual gingivitis may or may not progress to periodontitis. If it does, it was the supragingival plaque that probably served as the initial seeding loci of the microorganisms found in the subgingival plaque. If unsuccessful in maintaining gingival health, the preventive effort should immediately be directed to professional intervention to arrest the disease process before an entrenched subgingival plaque causes additional damage to the periodontium.

Periodontal maintenance care can reduce *both* the number of root caries and the number of pockets.[112]

## Chlorhexidine Gluconate

In August 1986, the U.S. Food and Drug Administration (FDA) approved the *prescription* sale of Procter & Gamble's Peridex, a 0.12% chlorhexidine gluconate solution as a mouthrinse. This action was soon followed by the American Dental Association (ADA) also approving the product as useful in the control of

gingivitis. Since that time, it has been found that chlorhexidine not only provides a potent adjunctive agent for the treatment of periodontal disease(s), but also is highly effective for suppressing cariogenic plaque bacteria.[112-116]

Chorhexidine is considered the "gold standard" for effectiveness as an oral antimicrobial agent. With the exception of fluoride, it is considered the most effective drug available in the war against mutans streptococci.[117] The effectiveness of chlorhexidine stems from its substantivity; that is, (1) it *adsorbs* to the infected tissue in the target area, (2) it is *released slowly*, and (3) it is *released in an active form*.

The dental uses of chlorhexidine are impressive.[118] For soft-tissue therapy it is used to treat gingivitis, periodontitis, stomatitis, herpes simplex, ulcers, and before and after oral surgery.[119] For caries control, it has been employed with success in mouthrinses, gels and varnishes. It has been combined with fluorides in varnishes to suppress Streptococcus mutans, and with fluoride to accelerate remineralization.[120,121] One three-year study of 12 to 14 year old high-risk students with >10$^6$ *Streptococcus mutans* that used 1% chlorhexidine gel experienced an 81% reduction in caries incidence.[122] There have been relatively few complaints, and these have have mainly targeted tooth stain (77% of the complaints), transient bitter taste (12%), excess calculus, and dry mouth (6%).[119] The small amount of tooth stain that occurs following continued use of chlorhexidine rinses can usually be easily removed at home by some of the rotary powered toothbrushes, or certainly by a prophylaxis. Some studies now being conducted indicate that when chlorhexidine is combined with peroxyborate, an antioxidant, the results are claimed to be superior to chlorhexidine alone, yet without the problems of taste and staining.[123]

In controlled mouthrinse programs, chlorhexidine has both *prevented* a buildup of plaque and *reduced* plaque accumulations, if used along with brushing.[124] Once gingivitis is diagnosed, chlorhexidine rinses plus other self-care oral hygiene measures are usually adequate to return the inflamed gingival to normal. Once the subgingival plaque becomes involved, subgingival irrigation with chlorhexidine becomes an option.[125] The irrigation instrument can be a powered pulsating jet stream, or as simple a device as a plastic canula attached to a plastic squeeze bottle.[83]

To briefly summarize its great utility in plaque disease control, chlorhexidine has been used with toddlers,[126] with high-risk schoolchildren,[127] with high-risk elders,[128] with the handicapped,[129] and with the mentally handicapped.[130] It has found use in orthodontics,[131] in periodontics,[132,133] in caries-control for overdenture patients,[134] and with post-radiation patients.[135]

### "Scorecards" and Guidelines

Professional *ethics* and the *law* mandate that health-care providers present patients with a disclosure of *full and accurate information* (informed consent)[136] about all contemplated invasive or noninvasive treatment procedures, as well as the likely costs and benefits of each.[137,138] Often *missing* from these discussions are science-based preventive regimens that offer options to both the patient and dental professional for the non invasive control of the plaque diseases.[139,140] In June 1995, *The Journal of the American Dental Association* supplement, entitled "Caries Diagnosis and Risk Assessment," aptly defined in *narrative style* the current needs for oral-preventive strategies and management.[141] Earlier, Anderson et al. concisely pointed out the same steps were required for a comprehensive preventive dentistry plan.[142] Needed is a way to bring all the narrative information into a workable paradigm at the time of the initial/annual examination.

Guidelines, or standards target specific diseases, help establish a patient's level of risk and suggest approaches to diagnosis, treatment and maintenance to meet that level of risk. The guidelines are intended to help in decision

making, as well as achieving a level of consistency of treatment throughout a population.[143] They should also increase the number of options to patient care, reduce patient costs, and improve the predictability of achieving desired outcomes.[144] *They should also leave room for professional judgment.* To accomplish these objectives, there are now efforts to develop nationwide professional guidelines of practice for both medical procedures[143–145] and for dentistry.[146–148]

As new research advances evolve for controlling or conquering the plaque diseases, any upgrading of standards should represent a consensus of the general practitioners, specialists, educators in dental and dental hygiene schools, research units, insurance servers and consumer groups. All guidelines should be subject to *continual review and change* as accomplished by the periodic updated recommendations by the American Heart Association,[149] the American Cancer Society and the American Academy of Periodontology.[150] As these guidelines continually evolve, parallel efforts are needed to educate the public and the profession about the new benefits resulting from use of new procedures and technologies.

## Putting it all Together—
## Examination, Treatment, Prevention

In the first edition of this text (1981), Harris introduced the concept of caries-activity indicators (CAIs) to develop a patient's oral-health profile ("scorecard") at the time of the initial/annual dental examination, and to link it with the treatment, prevention, patient education plans, and recall schedule.[151] This was followed in the second edition (1987) by Harris and Scheirton[152] suggesting that the same approach could be used for periodontal disease. These patient plaque disease profiles ("scorecards") can be used to match the severity of the evidence-based disease indicators with primary preventive dentistry responses commensurate with the severity of the plaque disease(s). This approach acknowledges that all individuals have different dental disease proclivities. Those at higher risk require more aggressive and closely monitored primary preventive therapies. Evidence-based indicators such as the plaque index, the bleeding index and semi quantitative microbiological testing should be employed to help establish whether a patient is at high, moderate, or low risk—and to adjust treatment and monitoring schedules accordingly.[153]

As an explanatory note, the CAIs and PAIs are *not being used as predictors* of impending plaque disease in terms of sensitivity and specificity;[154–156] instead they are being used *to estimate the patient's present vulnerability* and to take the necessary actions to return any indicator scores to as near zero as possible before the next appointment. A suggested approach to a guideline that uses the "scorecard" of the initial/annual examination to aid in selecting individualized treatment options is shown in Tables 23–1 and 23–2.

The first step following the entire examination is to secure a printout of the "scorecard" listing the oral health profile of the patient and the treatment urgency of each of the CAIs and PAIs. Tables 23–1 and 23–2 list the selected CAI or PAI clinical findings, laboratory tests, or indices considered important in the development of the plaque diseases and indicate the relative treatment urgency (risk) of the several indicators on a scale of 0 to 4. For example, if the finding for any of the caries indicators is negative, the zero in the appropriate column of the zero treatment urgency rows is circled—or entered into the computer. If, however, incipient or overt lesions are identified, circle the "1 or >1" listing found for each caries category in the Treatment Urgency 4 row. [Note: There is no intermediate possibility between Treatment Urgency 0 and 4—either a tooth is at risk due to incipient or actual lesions and should be given priority treatment, or it is at no risk]. In the example of Table 23–1, a Treatment Urgency of 4 is circled be-

cause of one incipient buccal lesion ("white spot") and two deep ("sticky") fissures—both without cavitation. The level-4 rating will be retained until the two fissures are covered with sealant, and remineralization therapy completed for the "white spot." If the two entries had been 0, the treatment urgency score would have been 3 because of the plaque index score. In these examples, the indicator values originally entered in the computer as part of the initial/annual dental examination are now highlighted (circled) in the appropriate columns and rows. The overall treatment urgency listing in the last column is based on the most urgent (highest number) entry in any of the columns, in this case, again 4 because of the incipient lesions and "sticky" fissures. With this Treatment Urgency of 4 established, a second printout is made that links the patient's "scorecard" to carefully considered individualized primary preventive dentistry suggestions (Tables 23–3 and 23–4). Thus, the CAI and PAI "scorecards" provide profiles of each patient's caries and periodontal health, respectively. As a summary listing of priority needs, they are understandable to the patient for discussing informed consent for treatment and economic options. For the practitioner, they are valuable in helping to provide guidelines suggesting the treatment for each of the levels of treatment urgency listed on the "scorecard." Thus, with the integrated caries and periodontal examination "scorecards", the dentist and the dental hygienist can use the original examination data as a patient-motivation instrument by highlighting *specific* patient oral health problems—and solutions.

Once "scorecards" and guidelines have been completed for the office records, a copy of each should be given to the patient as part of the informed consent, education-counseling process, and to emphasize the commitment the dental office has to prevention. Vice versa, it identifies the areas requiring patient cooperation. If desired, a printout can be supplied that lists the progress (or retrogression) of any/or all of the indicator scores recorded over the past several examinations.

### Question 4

Which of the following statements, if any, are correct?

A. The Periodontal Screening and Recording system (PSR) aids in diagnosis and suggests treatment options commensurate with the severity of the patients' periodontal status.

B. Chlorhexidine is used to suppress *both* cariogenic bacteria and periodontopathogens of the plaque.

C. Disease guidelines attempt to standardize disease diagnosis and to suggest treatment options based on disease severity, yet allow for professional judgment.

D. A nationally accepted guideline, i.e., one accepted by the American Dental Association, by state dental societies, by research authorities, dental school faculties, and by practitioners, would aid in improving uniformity of care and enhance the predictability of outcome of a disease process.

E. Computer storage of data contained in the initial/annual dental examination record permits convenient downloading of a patient's oral health profile ("scorecard") based on disease severity; with another keystroke, a guideline for suggested treatment, patient education, and preventive dentistry options can be displayed.

## The Recall Appointment

The recall appointment provides an opportunity for planned screenings and prophylaxes between annual examinations with the time interval being based on CAI and PAI findings at each successive recall. Philosophically, the re-

**TABLE 23-1  A Sample Patient's Caries Activity Indicator (CAI) "Scorecard"**

| Overt Caries | | | Incipient Caries | | | Laboratory | | Indices | | |
|---|---|---|---|---|---|---|---|---|---|---|
| Coronal | Root | Recurrent | Proximal | Bucco-Lingual | Caries Deep Fissures | Activity Tests[a] | Saliva Flow | Plaque Index[b] | CHO Index[c] | Treatment Urgency |
| (0) | (0) | (0) | 0 | (0) | 0 | (<100K) | >1.0/min | 10% | <4 | 0 |
|  |  |  |  |  |  |  | (1.0/min) |  |  | 1 |
|  |  |  |  |  |  |  |  | (15%) | (5–12) | 2 |
|  |  |  |  |  |  |  |  |  |  | 3 |
| 1 or >1 | 1 or >1 | 1 or >1 | (1 or >1) | 1 or >1 | (1 or >1) | >100K | <0.5/min | >25% | >12 | (4) |

Instructions: Circle the appropriate CAI notation in each *column*. The circled notation in the highest numbered *row* establishes the overall Treatment Urgency and suggested treatment and preventive dentistry options as seen in Table 23-3.

Key: Shaded areas allow for professional judgment as to whether the diagnosis should warrant a higher or lower Treatment Urgency.

[a]Using the Dentocult-SM dip-slide, under 100K is considered low risk, and over 100K is considered high risk.

[b]Plaque Index = Number of stained smooth surfaces/total number of smooth surfaces = %.

[c]CHO Index = Carbohydrate Intake Index. (See Appendix 23-2).


**TABLE 23-2  A Patient's Periodontal Disease Activity Indicator (PAI) "Scorecard"**

| PSRS | Pockets >3 mm | Bleeding Sites | Plaque Index[a] | Calculus Level[b] | Smoking Status | Treatment Urgency |
|---|---|---|---|---|---|---|
| 0 | 0 | 0 | <10% | 0 | Non Smoker[c] | 0 |
| 1 | 1 | 1 |  | 1 |  | 1 |
| (2) | (2) | 2 | (15%) | (2) |  | 2 |
| 3 | 3 | (3) |  | 3 |  | 3 |
| 4 | 4 or <4 | 4 or >4 | 25% | 4 | (Current smoker) | 4 |

Instructions: Circle the appropriate PAI notation in each *column*. The circled notation in the highest numbered *row* establishes the overall Treatment Urgency and suggested treatment and preventive options as seen in Table 23-4.

Key: Shaded areas indicate a need for professional judgment as to whether the diagnosis should warrant a lower or higher Treatment Urgency.

[a]Plaque Index = Number of stained smooth surfaces/total number of smooth surfaces = %. See Appendix 23-1.

[b]Calculus level: 0 = Insignificant; 1 = Slight; 2 = Moderate supragingival with isolated subgingival calculus; 3 = Moderate supragingival and moderate subgingival calculus; 4 = Heavy supra- and/or subgingival calculus.

[c]Since the original writing of this chapter, one outstanding article has been published that lends *urgency* to achieving smoking avoidance and cessation by relating adverse changes in the body's immune system to the onset, severity, and treatment of periodontitis (see Chap. 13). Barbour SE, Nakashima K, Zhang JB, et al. Tobacco and smoking: Environmental factors that modify the host response (immune system) and have an impact on periodontal health. *Crit Rev Oral Biol Med.* 1997; 8:437–450.

TABLE 23-3  Guide for Establishing a Primary Preventive Plan to Match the Severity of CAI Challenge

| Treatment Urgency | Restorations | Sealant Placement | Remineralization Therapy | Prophylaxis | Plaque Control Education | Nutrition Counseling | Chemical Control Office | Chemical Control Home | Recall Schedule (Months) |
|---|---|---|---|---|---|---|---|---|---|
| 0 | (0) | 0 | 0 | P | | | FA | FT, O | 6 |
| 1 | | | | P | E | E | FA | FT, O | 6 |
| 2 | | | | P | E | E | FA | FT, O | 3 |
| 3 | | | | | | | | | |
| (4) | R | (S) | (RT) | (P) | (C) | (C, M) | (FA, FV) | (FT, O, Rx) | (3 or <3) |

Instructions: Treatment Urgency level established in Table 23-1. Suggested treatment and preventive dentistry regimen(s) listed in circled Treatment Urgency *row*.

Key: Shaded areas allow for professional judgment as to whether the diagnosis should warrant a lower or higher Treatment Urgency.

R = Appropriate restorative treatment; S = Sealant placement; RT = Remineralization therapy; P = Prophylaxis; E = Education; C = Counseling session(s); M = Medical referral, if necessary; FA = Fluoride agent of choice; FV = Fluoride varnish; FT = Fluoride toothpaste; O = Over-the-counter antibacterial/antigingivitis rinses; Rx = Prescription mouth rinses (chlorhexidine).

TABLE 23-4  Sample Guide for Establishing a Primary Preventive Plan to Match the Severity of PAI Challenge

| Treatment Urgency | In-Office Preventive Treatment | Home Preventive Regimens | Flexible Prophylaxis Recall Schedule (Months) |
|---|---|---|---|
| 0 | P | B, F, O | 6 |
| 1 | P, E | B, F, O | 6 |
| 2 | P, E | B, F, O | 3 |
| 3 | | | 3 |
| 4 | T, P, S, R, C, SI, RP *Quit Smoking, Counseling* | B, F, SI, Rx *Quit Smoking* | 3 or <3 |

Instructions: Treatment Urgency level established in Table 23-2. Suggested preventive dentistry and/or maintenance regimens highlighted (circled) for treatment.

Key: Shaded areas indicate a need for professional judgment as to whether to place a patient in a higher or lower treatment level.

T = Appropriate periodontal treatment; RP = Referral to periodontist (if necessary); P = Prophylaxis; E = Education; C = Counseling; S = Scaling (if necessary); R = Root planing (if necessary); SI = Subgingival irrigation with antiplaque/antibacterial agent (chlorhexidine, stannous fluoride, listerine); B = Brushing; F = Flossing; O = Over-the-counter antibacterial, anticalculus, and fluoride-containing dentifrices and rinses; Rx = Prescription mouth rinses.

call period of high-risk patients should not exceed the time necessary for a pathogenic plaque to reform and to again allow its microbial population to damage the enamel, cementum, and/or gingiva. Once the pathogenic plaque is removed by prophylaxis, several studies have documented that it requires at least 3 months for the plaque to regain its disease-causing potential—even though there may be minimal compliance with home care plaque control programs.[157,158] Since *plaque and time* are the key factors in the development of both incipient caries lesions and gingivitis, each prophylaxis, by removing the pathogenic plaque, *essentially resets the time clock of plaque pathogenicity back to near zero*.

There is a need for a flexible recall interval, based *on the level of treatment need*, as suggested in Tables 23–3 and 23–4. Others have indicated that the same periodic oral hygiene procedures and monitoring are effective in reducing the incidence of *both* caries and periodontal disease.[116,159] If possible, the periodontitis and the caries maintenance visits should both be kept in synchrony on the same 3- to 6-month interval recall. In this way, a requirement for a 3-month recall for caries would aid in plaque prevention control for gingivitis, or vice versa, even though the *risk* of the other might be low. For example, fluoride applications for coronal caries would aid prevent root caries where the cementum is exposed. Chlorhexidine varnishes are effective in helping suppress *both the cariogenic and periopathodontic bacteria*.

Finally a high-plaque index can provide a warning sign for *either* caries or periodontitis. The index should ideally be 10% or less. When the plaque score increases markedly, it should cause professional concern. Additional education and counseling, laboratory tests and indices, such as bacterial quantification for caries, and/or the bleeding index for gingivitis is indicated. Thus, the accomplishment of a plaque index at each recall can alert the hygienist about the possible existence of *in situ* and incipient lesions for *either* or *both* of the plaque dis-

eases, while the accompanying prophylaxes can greatly aid in averting the initiation and progression of *in situ* and incipient lesions for *both* diseases. Recall programs can be easily handled by use of computer programs. With very little training, an office manager or dental assistant can enter changes in appointments and generate programmed recall notices that are automatically printed out for regular mailing or e-mailing appointment reminders. Such timesaving and improved administrative practices are essential, even in small dental practices.

### Carbohydrate Intake

The carbohydrate intake index provides an easy method to assess a patient's intake of refined sugars, especially if the intake is high. This sugar intake score is based on the patient filling out a carbohydrate intake short form administered by the dental office personnel. As the frequency of intake, and the retentivity of the different sugary foods increase, so does the carbohydrate intake score (Appendix 23–2).

### The Dental Hygienist— Primary-Prevention Specialist

As a primary dental prevention specialist in the dental office, the dental hygienist is salient in insuring emphasis on prevention. Academic dental-hygiene education provides a comprehensive curriculum that includes, among other requirements, clinical participation in applying pit-and-fissure sealant use, remineralization therapy, fluoride applications, patient education and oral-health promotion, dietary counseling, prophylaxis, root scaling, root planing and subgingival irrigation—all areas of expertise that are needed for an optimum plaque-disease prevention and control programs.

Under *a total immersion approach to prevention*, the "tooth-cleaning" appointments required for high-risk patients should *not* be perceived as prophylaxes performed mainly for aesthetic purposes, but rather as part of a caries

and/or periodontal disease prevention and maintenance program which will require longer appointment periods. Shallhorn and Snider[160] and Pfeifer and Pfeifer[161] found that it took approximately 53 and 57 minutes, respectively, to complete a recall appointment. The multiple appointments of individuals in these more intensive preventive programs will require additional hygienist time and responsibilities—*and compensation*. Additional hygienists will probably be required as well as an assistant due to the increased patient flow.[162] In turn, to administratively support the increased enrollment of patients in preventive programs, there should probably be one front desk individual who can act as an appointment coordinator to ensure that recall visits are scheduled, and followed up.

If patient compliance with home mechanical and chemical plaque control instructions for caries and periodontal involvement has been adequate between visits, the treatment urgency level for the average patient should drop and remain at a low score. This possibility will permit additional patients to enter the preventive program to maintain a full and expanding schedule for the office dental-hygiene sector.

## Patient Education

Traditionally, dentistry has been considered a treatment-oriented profession. The concept of going to the dentist to prevent disease is mainly associated with a twice-a-year prophylaxis and the use of fluorides. Probably the best way to start in the changeover from a treatment to prevention orientation is to conduct a separate appointment for *dental education and promotion devoted to the patient's own problems* as identified at the initial/annual examination (Appendix 23–3).[163] Like the annual medical examination and evaluation, this period should have a fee. It is essential to enlist the patient as a "co therapist" if a home prevention program is to be a success. For patients to assume this role, they need to know *what* is expected, *how* it is to be

accomplished, *why* it is necessary and *how much* it will cost. This is the same information as is required as part of informed consent

At the end of the session, the patient should fully realize that he or she is at risk, but that the plaque diseases can often be prevented or reversed as a result of recommended therapy. As a part of medicine's "one third rule," one third of all patients with chronic disease can be expected to comply with instructions, one third to comply erratically, and one third not to comply at all.[164] It is also necessary to inform the patient that all treatment eventually fails without a wholehearted and effective self-care commitment. Only the patient can decide whether he or she wants to pay to prevent disease—or to accept disease and pay for more expensive treatment. If the patient continually fails to comply with instructions, it is expedient to document a warning advisory in the dental record to counter any possible future legal repercussions.[165]

One individual from the dental office should be selected to carry out the main thrust of the education program. The person selected should be a dental hygienist or a health educator. The main attributes desired are that the person be mature, intelligent, and compassionate; has leadership ability; likes people; is persuasive; has the ability to improve on the daily presentations; and has the flexibility to adapt presentations to meet each patient's needs and attitudes. The entire education session can be facilitated by focusing on the "scorecard" listings for the CAIs and PAIs, especially when the Treatment Urgency level is above 2. At this time, the importance of plaque control can be introduced, using edited portions of the video camera tape to show the location and extent of plaque in the patient's mouth. The carbohydrate-consumption questionnaire previously filled out, becomes much more meaningful when discussed in context of the acid-producing capability of the bacteria in the patient's plaque. The need for laboratory tests to determine the number of acid-producing bacteria in

the patient's saliva becomes equally consequential when it is made clear that the risk of decayed teeth increases as the number of acidogenic bacteria increases. As stated by Krasse, "To run a caries preventive program without using microbiological methods is like running a weight control program without a scale."[166] Finally, the relationship of these CAIs to *in situ*, incipient or overt caries lesions can be related to the demineralization that occurs between the times of tooth health to tooth cavitation. This backdrop then provides the basis for introducing and discussing the "guidelines" for customized preventive strategies for the patient's own treatment urgency level.

At this point, probably the two most important subjects related to *caries* prevention and requiring discussion with a patient are: (1) the need and advantages of having *sealants* placed in all "sticky" fissures; and (2) the need to consider all incipient smooth surface lesions (without evidence of cavitation) for *remineralization therapy* and careful monitoring—not restorations. The advantage of these two exceedingly important prevention actions are not generally known and understood by the public, nor actively promoted by the profession.

Plaque-induced gingivitis is the most common form of periodontal disease.[123] All patients should be cognizant of the fact that "pink toothbrush" is an important warning sign of gingivitis that can be self-diagnosed. If not cleared up within a week by more vigorous self-care efforts at home, an immediate visit to the dental office is indicated. A combined professional and self-care program is usually all that is necessary to return the gingival to normal. On the other hand the neglect of this critical early stage of gingivitis creates an environment in the gingival sulcus that favors a more pathogenic flora. Intermittent episodes of gingivitis at a younger age *increase the risk* of a later periodontitis.[167]

The data acquired as part of the initial/annual dental examination as summarized in the "scorecards" and guidelines can form the basis for individualizing the educational presentation. The integration of all these subjects should make the educational phase for each patient much more motivational and longer lasting than an abstract discussion of preventive dentistry.

### Education of the Professionals

There is a need for the dental professionals to manage caries to the maximum extent possible by using non-invasive preventive measures. Both smooth-surface and pit-and-fissure lesions are preventable and reversible. Certainly, the restorative approach to caries control has not been successful, especially for those individuals without funds nor access to dental care—both in the United States and especially in nations without the resources of the United States.

In the past, few dental schools provided courses in *primary* prevention that rival those of secondary and tertiary preventive dentistry in terms of time, money, staff and commitment. In 1989, in an editorial in the *Journal of Dental Research*, Thylstrup identified two major reasons that the benefits of prevention are not universally available. First, dental schools do not yet inculcate in their students the importance of preventing disease. Second, and probably, most important, *no reward* is given for the prevention or reversal of ongoing plaque diseases which have been proved reversible.[78]

Anusavice has added another reason that appears as innocuous as it is important, viz., "*We do not examine for, or monitor incipient plaque disease.*"[88] Until the smooth surface and occlusal sites of incipient caries are identified and *recorded for priority care*, little non-invasive remedial action will occur for these pre-caries lesions. Until CAIs and PAIs as well as summarizing "scorecards" for caries and periodontal disease appear as part of the clinical record, there is no organized format to present each patient with individualized invasive and non-invasive preventive and treatment options.

Two other reasons might be cited. The first is the fact that many of the older dentists find it *difficult to accept the concept of remineralizing pre-caries lesions* seen as radiolucent areas—sites that in former dental school days were considered as diseased tissue that must be restored. Concurrent with this viewpoint is the fact that once a "white spot" develops, there is an *over-estimation* of the velocity of caries progression through the enamel and dentin.[168] Now it is realized that caries advances over a greatly varied time span that can range from months, years or to reversal.[108] Equally important is the fact that the advancing front of the incipient lesion can probably be remineralized until it has, according to Scandinavian studies, advanced to half way through the dentin, i.e., if cavitation has not occurred before reversal takes place.[108]

In evaluating Thylstrup's charge that the preventive care curriculum in dental schools is truncated, the ADA's Survey of Curriculum Clock Hours of Instruction is enlightening. In the 1997-98 school year, U.S. dental schools devoted a mean of 66 hours of curriculum time to prevention. Didactic instruction on *prevention* included mean of 93 hours out of a mean of 5228 hours in U.S. dental schools' curricula—or approximately 2% of the time.[169] In addition, the ADA's Accreditation Standards require that "graduates are competent in providing oral health care within the scope of general dentistry—including health promotion and disease prevention."[170]

In a 1999 questionnaire, Yorty et al. detailed some of the ongoing preventive initiatives being conducted in the dental schools. Forty-two of the fifty-five dental schools (76%) responded to the polling. Not all the queries were answered uniformly. Eighty-one percent reported having formal *risk training programs*, with 38% having criteria for low-, moderate-, and high-risk patients. Sixty-two percent had developed specific recall schedules based on that risk. Two-thirds of the respondents (17/25) consider the option of remineralizing or sealant placement for early primary (incipient) lesions. Thirty-seven of the schools indicated that the level of penetration of the caries front before restoration, was the outer one-third of the dentin.[171] Clearly, this study portends a trend towards a more conservative (preventive) approach to clinical dentistry.[171]

Economics can be a potent factor in changing health attitudes for both a patient and the professional. There is an acute need for *a reasonable reimbursement to dentists and dental hygienists practicing preventive dental care*, the same as is expected for dental treatment. The idea of purchase of good oral health is alien to Americans who have traditionally accepted restorations, extractions, and prosthetic devices as a means to cope with dental disease. The public *expectations* and *demand* for preventive dental care must change if the profession is to move into an era in which prevention replaces a need for restorations. In these opening years of this new millennium, the profession must prepare the *public* and *itself* for their new roles of dental prevention and full dentulism.

Clinical methods *now* exist to identify, arrest, or reverse the incipient plaque disease lesions that are precursors to overt lesions. It should be so easy to move the focus of dentistry to the practice of dentistry in this direction. The difference between prevention and treatment is simply an intact tooth, a restored tooth, or no tooth.

## Implementing Preventive Programs

There are six major treatment environments in which the aforementioned intensive preventive routines can be implemented immediately: (1) private practice environments, (2) military dental services, (3) public-health clinics, (4) public school dental programs, (5) industrial work sites and (6) dental-health maintenance organizations. In each instance, the strategies for reducing the incidence of both of the plaque diseases, involve few changes in clinical

physical facilities or in daily operating routine. Only a demonstration of leadership and a commitment to primary prevention is needed to identify and reverse the risk factors of impending plaque disease, rather than limiting the examination to a search for and treatment of pathology.

In the military, the economics of change from treatment to prevention should pose no major problem since appropriated funds are already available for dental care. In other dental settings, additional insurance and personal or public funds are initially required. However, a drastic reduction of later expenditures for the restoration of primary and secondary caries lesions, tooth fractures, periodontal treatment, endodontics, extractions, bridges, and dentures would soon compensate for the increased outlays from any of aforementioned sources. In private practices, it could lead to *contracts to prevent*, rather than treat dental disease

### The Immunity Factor

In 1960, Keyes[172] and Fitzgerald and Keys[173] demonstrated that S. *mutans* caused caries in rodents. Once it was established that caries was an infectious disease, it was realized that caries might be controlled by use of vaccines. Several institutions in the United States and England were already accomplishing vaccine research. There was the *prediction* that a vaccine would be available within 3 to 10 years.[174] In 1979 Cohen reported on a 9-year study where two *actively* immunized monkeys had zero and a small lesion respectively, whereas the three surviving control animals exhibited 56,69 and 73 decayed surfaces.[175]

The 3- to 10-year time-table was not realized for one major reason, viz., it was suggested that with active immunity, there might be a cross reaction with heart muscle.[176] With that possibility, (1) even if a vaccine was developed, there was no assurance it would be accepted by the Food and Drug Administration (FDA).

Even if approved by the FDA, potential manufacturers were wary of possible huge lawsuits.[177] Besides, caries was on the wane in developed countries and there appeared to be no urgency to risk major problems since caries was not a life-threatening disease. Much of the research stopped or slowed. Anticipation turned to disappointment. However, in Guys Hospital in England, the search was continued to develop a topically applied *passive vaccine* against *Streptococcus mutans*. This would by-pass the major problem of cross-reactions.

Every dentist should read the delightful easy-to-read article by JK-Ma.[178] It is a fascinating account citing some of the problems and successes that were encountered by the Guy's Hospital group over the past 20 years on the way to a prototype dental caries vaccine. The test vaccine has already successfully passed animal and a small-scale human tests. It is now in a Stage II test program with a larger number of subjects. The initial test answered two crucial questions, viz, (1) it is possible with the vaccine to *suppress Streptococcus mutans* (SM) and (2) to *prevent* caries. The vaccine is topically applied to the teeth, a process called *local passive immunization*, thus eliminating the possibility of involving the body's immune system. The antibody that has been developed by genetic engineering has targeted the *adhesins* responsible for the attachment of *Streptococcus mutans* (SM) to the tooth.

The development of the antibodies is a fascinating story in itself. In assembling the desired antibody by genetic engineering, it required four successive critical successes to develop the final antibody with the correct configuration to duplicate that of the human antibody. The amazing part of the genetic assembly process was the fact that each phase of the more-and-more complex antibody, was accomplished using the lowly tobacco plant that cannot ordinarily be induced to produce mammalian antibodies. Once developed, the continual harvesting of the plant *seeds* insured the

perpetuation of future crops of tobacco plants, with each generation duplicating the original created antibody configuration. This plant biotechnology supplied an economical and reliable source of antibodies needed for the study.

The preparation of the mouth for application of the vaccine was also ingenious. A two-week mouth rinse program using chlorhexidine was sufficient to clear the mouth of most *Streptococcus mutans*. If no further action was taken at this time, the mouth was quickly repopulated with SM. However, if the vaccine was applied to the acquired (salivary) pellicle of the teeth, this repopulation did not occur. It is estimated that this passive immunity would possibly last from three months to a year. To increase the universal value of these antibodies, studies are being conducted as to the feasibility of incorporating them into dentifrices and mouthrinses.[178,179]

A possible dental caries vaccine for the future? Remember, we are now in the beginning of the 21st Century.

### Question 5

Which of the following statements, if any, are correct?

A. The twice-a-year prophylaxis is adequate in helping to prevent, arrest, and reverse the progress of either of the plaque diseases.

B. The plaque is an etiologic factor for both caries and periodontal disease; therefore, a prophylaxis at appropriate intervals and recorded observations for PAIs and CAIs should greatly help to prevent, arrest, or reverse both plaque diseases.

C. Remineralization of overt carious lesions is a common practice in Scandinavia.

D. The cost of primary prevention to prevent one overt plaque-disease lesion can save a much greater cost of later successive secondary- and tertiary-prevention procedures.

E. Mammalian antibodies can be duplicated in plants.

# SUMMARY

By definition, if all incipient caries and all incipient periodontal lesions could be prevented, arrested or reversed in the incipient stages, there would be no overt lesions to treat. In order to approach this goal for all people, it will probably require an active public-health immunization program of the immensity and intensity that characterized smallpox elimination. We have not yet reached that point of dental disease suppression; however, the completion of the Human Genome Project does greatly enhance that possibility—not only for dental disease but for all infectious and genetic diseases. At the present time, the ravages of the dental plaque diseases can be greatly minimized for those individuals who have *access* to a dental facility, and the *commitment* to comply with a dental prevention and treatment programs established by a dentist. Guidelines would help establish a level of excellence and uniformity for both treatment and prevention intervention. When called upon, it is the responsibility of the dentist to examine, detect and perform—or delegate—the necessary primary and secondary procedures necessary to assure maximum patient dental health in the present and in the future. The initial/annual examination is a most important event in attaining these objectives. Here it is possible to simultaneously *identify and record treatment and preventive*

*needs, establish present risk level, specifically focus counseling and education addressing patients' specific needs, as well as making recommendations for home care.* Empirically, the home care involves daily oral-hygiene procedures—toothbrush (with fluoride toothpaste), dental floss, irrigation and supplemental mouthrinses recommended or prescribed by the dentist. The two most useful mouth rinses in the dentist's armamentarium are fluoride to increase tooth resistance and enhance remineralization, and chlorhexidine to suppress Streptococcus mutans, help *cure* gingivitis, and as an adjunct for treating periodontitis. If a short-time passive vaccine does becomes available, it will be a major step towards a lifetime of intact teeth for those *who have routine access* to dental care.

By the end of the initial treatment cycle, all overt lesions should be restored; all incipient smooth and root surface lesions should be undergoing remineralization therapy; all necessary sealants should be in place; and, all gingivitis should be under maintenance control. Also, by this time, the patient should have the knowledge and understanding to participate with the oral-health professionals in a team effort of self-care. The outcome of such a comprehensive, integrated, and personalized plaque disease prevention program involves the participation of the entire office team plus the compliance of the patient. As a result of such a controlled prevention and monitoring program, there should be an early dramatic reduction in the incidence of the plaque diseases and their sequelae. This is as it should be—the hallmark of the dental profession should be oral-health maintenance and enhancement, not just disease treatment.

## ANSWERS AND EXPLANATIONS

1. D, E—correct.

    A—incorrect. A "white spot" can occur on *any* surface; however, it cannot be visually observed on every surface. For instance, it cannot be seen at the bottom of pits and fissures. It is usually first observed as a radiolucency in x-rays of the interproximal surfaces.

    B—incorrect. The incipient stage begins as a "white spot" and continues until there is surface cavitation, which by definition is an irreversible overt carious lesion.

    C—incorrect. The *in situ* stage of gingivitis is characterized by an infiltration of body defense cells beneath the sulcular epithelium.

2. A, C, D, E—correct.

    B—incorrect. The opposite is true. Much less x-ray energy is required for the DXR images than with the intraoral film.

3. A, B, D, E—correct.

    C—incorrect. While "white spots" are a translucent white, once remineralized, they usually take on the hue of the enamel.

4. A, B, C, D, E—correct.

5. B, D, E—correct.

   A—incorrect. The twice-a-year prophylaxis is adequate for the majority of people; however, there are many who could benefit from a more frequent schedule. In other words, the interval between prophylaxes should be flexible and be based on risk.

   C—incorrect. Remineralization can only occur BEFORE the overt caries lesion stage.

## Self-evaluation Questions

1. The two stages of caries development, prior to the overt lesion development are _____ and _____; the two stages of periodontal disease prior to periodontitis are _____ and _____.

2. Three advantages of the intraoral videocamera are: _____, _____, and _____.

3. Three advantages of the digital X-ray are: _____, _____ and _____.

4. List five reasons for having the problem of false-negative or false-positive diagnoses for caries: _____, _____, _____, _____ and _____.

5. How does a sealant *prevent* caries on the occlusal surface? _____. How does a sealant *arrest* early caries on the occlusal surface? _____.

6. Define *substantivity*: _____. Give an example of the agent in a mouthrinse with this attribute: _____.

7. Give the reason why patients are not demanding remineralization therapy instead of restorations (YOUR evaluation).

8. Why do you believe, or not believe that a vaccine can be developed for periodontal disease?

## REFERENCES

1. Barakow, F., Imfeld, T., & Lutz, F. (1991). Enamel re-mineralization: How to explain it to the patients. *Quint Int.*, 22:141–7.
2. Brecx, M. C., Schlegel, K., Gehr, P., & Lang, N. P. (1987). Comparison between histological and clinic parameters during human experimental gingivitis. J *Periodontol Res.*, 22:52–7.
3. Von der Fehr, F. R., Löe, H., & Theilade, E. (1970). Experimental caries in man. *Caries Res.*, 4:131–148.
4. Nelson, A., Pitts, & N. B. (1991). The clinical behavior of free smooth surface carious lesions monitored over 2 years in a group of Scottish children. *Br Dent J.*, 171:313–8.

5. Konig, K. G. (1963). Dental morphology in relation to caries resistance with special reference to fissures in susceptible areas. *J Dent Res.*, 42:461–76.

6. Wenzel, A., Pitts, N., Verdonschot, E. H., & Kalsbeck, H. (1993). Developments in radiographic diagnosis. *J Dent Res.*, 21:131–40.

7. Espolid, I., & Tveit, A. B. (1984). Radiographic diagnosis of mineral loss in approximal enamel. *Car Res.*, 18:141–8.

8. Lang, N. P., Adler, A., Joss, A., & Nyman, S. (1990). Absence of bleeding on probing: An indicator of periodontal stability. *J Clin Periodontol.*, 7:714–21.

9. Markitziu, A., Rajstein, J., Deutsch, D., Rahdmim, E., & Gedalia, I. (1988). Arrest of incipient cervical caries by topical chemotherapy. *Gerodontics.*, 4:293–8.

10. Mertz-Fairhurst, E. J. (1992). Editorial: Pit-and-fissure sealants: A global lack of science transfer? *J Dent Res.*, 71:1543–4.

11. Silverstone, L. M. (1984). The significance of demineralization in caries prevention. *J Canad Dent Assoc.*, 50:157–67.

12. Benvenius, J. (1988). Caries risk for patients with Crohn's disease: A pilot study. *Oral Surg Oral Med Oral Pathol.*, 65:304–7.

13. Kneckt, M. C. (2000). Attributions of dental and diabetes health outcomes. *J Clin Periodontol.*, 27:205–11.

14. Edelstein, B. L. (1995). Case planning and management according to caries risk assessment. *Dent Clin North Am.*, 39:721–36.

15. Anusavice, K. J. (1995). Treatment regimens in preventive and restorative dentistry. *JADA*, 126:727–43.

16. Vehkalahti, M. (1997). To fill or not to fill: dentists decision on caries treatment. *J Dent Res.*, 76:88 (Abs. 596).

17. Martin, F., & Schnopf, K. (1999). Top 10 set the pace. *Dental Products Report.* December, 32,36,38.

18. Waiann, P. (1993). That is an electronic patient record. *Texas Dent J.*, 110:21–6.

19. Fair, C. (1996). The creation and integration of the high tech operatory. *J Can Dent Assoc.*, 62:20–2.

20. Manji, I. (1996). Beyond the bells and whistles: Hi-tech/high care dentistry. *J Can Dent Assoc.*, 62:658–61.

21. Heiert, C. L. (1997). Computer use by dentists and dental team members. *JADA*, 128:91–5.

22. Hirchinger, R. (2001). Digital dentistry; information technology for today's (and tomorrow's) dental practice. *J Calif Dent Assoc.*, 29:215–21.

23. Emmott, L. F. (2000). The future is coming and it will be amazing: computers in dentistry. *J Am Coll Dent.*, 67:33–6

24. Periodontal Screening and Recording (PSR) System. (1993). American Dental Association and the American Academy of Periodontology. Sponsored by Procter & Gamble, Chicago, IL.

25. Khocht, A., Zohn, H., Deasy, M., & Kuang-Ming, C. (1996). Screening for periodontal disease. *JADA*, 127:749–56.

26. Krasse, B. (1996). Discovery! Serendipity or luck: Stumbling on gingival crevicular fluid. *J Dent Res.*, 75:1627–30.

27. Page, R. C. (1992). Host response tests for diagnosing periodontal diseases. *J Periodontol.*, 71:1543–4.

28. Greenstein, G., & Lanster, I. (1995). Digitalized radiographs and computerized probes to facilitate more accurate measurement of disease progression. *J Periodontol.*, 66:659–66.

29. Willershausen, B., Schlosser, E., & Ernst, C. P. (1999). The intra-oral camera, dental health communication and oral hygiene. *Int Dent J.*, 49:95–100.

30. Don, C., & Daly, R. (1981). The first cassetteless x-ray department. *Electramedica*, 3:146–8.

31. Wenzel, A., Pitts, N., & Verdonshot, E. H. (1993). Computer-aided image manipulation of intra oral radiography to enhance diagnosis in dental practice: a review. *Intl Dent J.*, 43:99–108.

32. Homer, K., Shearer, A. C., Walker, A., & Wilson, N. H. (1990). Radiovisiography: An initial evaluation. *Br Dent J.*, 168:144–8.

33. American Dental Association. (1989). Council on Dental Materials, Instruments and Equipment. American Dental Association. Recommendations in radiographic practices. *JADA*, 118:115–7.

34. Wenzel, A., Hintze, H., Mikkelsen, L., & Mouyen, F. (1991). Radiographic detection of occlusal caries in noncavitated teeth. *Oral Surg Oral Medicine Oral Pathol*, 72:621–6.

35. Wenzer, A., & Fejerskov, O. (1992). Validity of diagnosis of questionable caries lesions of occlusal surfaces of extracted third molars. *Caries Res.*, 26:188–94.

36. Bader, J. D., & Brown, J. P. (1993). Dilemmas in caries diagnosis. *JADA*, 124:48–50.

37. Bergmann, G., & Linden, L. A. (1969). The action of the explorer on incipient caries. *Tandlak Tidsskr.*, 62:629–34.

38. Eckstrand, K., Qvist, V., & Thylstrup, A. (1987). Light microscope study of the effect of probing in occlusal surfaces. *Caries Res.*, 21:368–73.

39. Van Dorp, C. S. E., Exter kate, R. A. M., & ten Cate, J. M. (1988). The effect of dental probing on subsequent enamel demineralization. *ASDC J Child Dent*, 55:343–7.

40. Loesche, W. J., Svanberg, M. L., & Pape, H. R. (1979). Intraoral transmission of Streptococci mutans by a dental explorer. *J Dent Res*, 58:1765–70.

41. Brown, J. P. (1993). Introduction to the symposium ("Dilemmas in Caries Diagnosis"). *J Dent Res*, 57:407–8.

42. Lussi, A. (1991). Validity of diagnostic and treatment decisions of fissure caries. *Caries Res*, 25:296–303.

43. Penning, C. van Amerongen, J. P., Seef, R. E., & ten Cate, J. M. (1992). Validity of probing for fissure caries diagnosis. *Caries Res*, 26:445–9.

44. Kay, E. J., Watts, A., Patterson, R. C., & Blinkhorn, A. S. (1988). Preliminary investigation in the validity of dentist's decisions to restore occlusal surfaces of permanent teeth. *Community Dent Oral Epidemiol*, 16:91–4.

45. Mitropoulos, C. M., & Downer, M. C. (1987). Inter-examiner agreement in the diagnosis of dental caries among officers of the reference service. *Br Dent J*, 162:227.

46. Goldberg, A. J. (1990). Deterioration of restorative materials and the risk of secondary caries. *Adv Dent Res*, 4:14–8.

47. Downer, M. C. (1989). Validation of methods used in dental caries diagnosis. *Intl Dent J*, 39:241–6.

48. Bader, J. D., & Shugars, D. A. (1993). Need for change in standards of caries diagnosis—Epidemiology and health services research perspective. *J Dent Ed*, 57:415–21.

49. Stookey, G. K., Jackson, R. D., Zandona, A. G., & Analoui, M. (1999). Dental Caries Diagnosis. *Dent Clin North Am*, 43:666–77.

50. Qvist, J., Qvist, V., & Mjor, I. A. (1990). Placement and longevity of amalgam restoration in Denmark. *Acta Odont Scand*, 48:297–303.

51. Elderton, R. J. (1990). Clinical studies concerning restoration of teeth. *Adv Dent Res*, 4:4–9.

52. Allsopp, J. F., Matthews, J. B., Marquis, P. M., & Frame, J. W. (1996). Failure of amalgam restorations and their replacement in general practice. *J Dent Res*, 75:1134 (Abs. 35).

53. York, A. K., & Arthur, J. S. (1993). Reasons for placement and replacement of dental restorations in the United States Navy Dental Corps. *Oper Dent*, 18:203–8.

54. Cecil, J. C., Cohen, M., Schroeder, D. C., & Taylor, S. L. (1982). Longevity of amalgam restorations: A retrospective view. *J Dent Res*, 61:185 (Abs. 1956).

55. Allen, D. N. (1977). A longitudinal study of dental restorations. *Br Dent J*, 143:87.

56. Mjor, I. A., Dahl, J. E., & Moorhead, J. E. (2000). Age of restorations at time of replacement in permanent teeth in general dental practice. *Acta Odontol Scan*, 58:97–101.

57. Ripa, L. W., Leske, G. S., & Forte, F. (1987). The combined use of pit and fissure sealants and fluoride mouth rinsing in second and third grade children. Final clinical results after two years. *Pediatr Dent*, 9:118–20.

58. Weintraub, J. (1989). The effectiveness of pit and fissure sealants. *J Public Health Dent*, 49:317–30.

59. Meiers, J. C., & Jensen, M. E. (1984). Management of the questionable fissure. Invasive vs. noninvasive techniques. *JADA*, 108:64–8.

60. Swift, E. J. Jr. (1988). The effect of sealants on dental caries: A review. *JADA*, 116:700–4.

61. Mertz-Fairhurst, E. J., Shuster, G. S., & Fairhurst, C. W. (1986). Arresting caries by sealants. Results of a clinical study. *JADA*, 112:194–7.

62. Simonson, R. J. (1988). Editorial: Are we restoring what we should be preventing? *Quint Int*, 19:251–2.

63. Handlemann, S. I., & Jensen, O. F. (1980). The effect of an autopolymerizing sealant on the viability of the microflora in occlusal dental caries. *Scand J Dent Res*, 88:382–8.

64. Arends, J., & Ten Bosch, J. J. (1992). Demineralization and remineralization evaluation techniques. *J Dent Res*, 71: Supp (1) 924–8.

65. Anusavice, K. J. (1998). Chlorhexidine, fluoride varnish, and xylitol chewing gum: underutilized preventive therapies? *Gen Dent.*, 46:34–8.

66. Stephan, M. (1997). The role of diet, fluoride and saliva in caries prevention. *J Indian Soc Pedod Prev Dent*, 15:109–13.

67. Edgar, W. M., & Higham, S. M. (1995). Role of saliva in caries models. *Adv Dent Res*, 9:235–8.

68. Lamb, W. J., Corpron, R. E., More, F. G., Beltran, E. D., Strachan, D. S., & Kawalski, D. J. (1993). In situ remineralization of subsurface enamel lesion after the use of a fluoride chewing gum. *Caries Res*, 27:111–6.

69. White, J. D. (1865). Practical Hints. *Dental Cosmos*, 6;292.

70. Head, J. (1910). Enamel softening and rehardening as a factor in erosion. *Dent Cosmos*, 52:46–8.

71. Head, J. (1912). A study of saliva and its action on tooth enamel in reference to its hardening and softening. *JAMA*, 59:2118–22.

72. Wilson, L. A. (1928). Is the artificial calcification and recalcification of dental enamel possible? *Dent Digest*, 34:689–702.

73. Muhler, J. C. (1960). Stannous fluoride pigmentation-evidence of caries arrestment. ASDC *J Dent Child*, 28:157–61.

74. Löe, H., von der Fehr, F. R., & Schiott, C. R. (1972). Inhibition of experimental caries by plaque prevention. The affect of chlorhexidine mouth rinses. *J Dent Res*, 80:1–9.

75. Mejare, I., Grondhl, H. G., Carlstedt, K., Grever, A. C., & Ottosson, E. (1985). Accuracy at radiography and probing for the diagnosis of proximal caries. *Scan J Dent Res*, 93:178–84.

76. Mejare, I., & Malmgren, B. (1986). Clinical and radiographic appearance of proximal carious lesions at the time of operative treatment in young permanent teeth. *Scan J Dent Res*, 94:19–26.

77. Thylstrup, A., Bille, J., & Qvist, V. (1986). Radiographic and observed tissue changes in approximal caries lesions at the time of opertive treatment. *Caries Res*, 20:75–84

78. Thylstrup, A. (1989). Mechanical vs. disease-oriented treatment of dental caries: educational aspects. *J Dent Res*, 68:1135.

79. Nuttal, N. M., & Pitts, N. B. (1990). Restorative treatment thresholds reported to be used by dentistry in Scotland. *Br Dent J*, 169:119–26.

80. Medeiros, V. A. F., & Seddon, R. P. (1997). The prevalence of iatrogenic damage adjacent to restored approximal surfaces. *J Dent Res*, 76: 1070 (Abs. 414).

81. Qvist, V., Johanessen, L., & Brunn, M. (1992). Progression of proximal caries in relation to iatrogenic preparation damage. *J Den Res*, 173:210–2.
82. Pitts, N. B., & Rimmer, P. A. (1992). An *in vivo* comparison of radiographic and directly assessed clinical caries status of posterior approximal surfaces in primary and permanent teeth. *Caries Res*, 26:146–52.
83. MacKenzie, M., & Peterson, M. (1995). The New Zealand School Dental Service. In Harris, N. O., Christen, A. G., Eds. *Primary Preventive Dentistry*, 4th ed. Norwalk, CT: Appleton & Lange, 601.
84. Espelid, I. Tveit. A. B., & Skodje, F. (1997). Restorative treatment decisions on approximal and occlusal caries in Norway. *J Dent Res*, 76:1099 (Abs. 039).
85. Elderton, R. J. (1993). Overtreatment with restorative dentistry; when to intervene. *Int Dent J*, 43:20–4.
86. Dodds, M. W. J. (1993). Dilemmas in caries diagnosis—applications to current practice and need for research. *J Dent Educ*, 57:433–8.
87. Pitts, N. (1993). Current methods and criteria for caries diagnosis in Europe. *J Dent Edu*, 57:401–14.
88. Anusavice, K. J., Ed. (1988). Quality evaluation of dental restorations; criteria for placement and replacement. Chicago. *Quintessence*, 412–3.
89. Mejare, I., Sundberg, H., Espelid, I., & Tveit, B. (1999). Caries assessment and restorative treatment thresholds reported by Swedish dentists. *Acta Odontol Scand*, 57:149–54.
90. Shay, K. (1997). Root caries in the older patient: significance, prevention, and treatment. *Dent Clin North Am*, 41:763–93.
91. Jones, J. A. (1995). Root caries: prevention and chemotherapy. *Amer J Dent*, 8:352–7.
92. De Paola, P. F., Separkar, P. M., & Kent, R. L. Jr. (1989). Methodological issues relative to the quantitation of root caries. *Gerodontology*, 8:3–9.
93. Miller, A. J., Brunelle, J. A., Carlos, J. P., et al. (1987). Oral Health of United States Adults. NIH Publication No. 87-2868, 1–168.
94. Leske, G. S., & Ripa, L. W. (1989). Three year root caries increments: An analysis of teeth and surfaces at risk. *Gerontology*, 8:17–21.
95. Featherstone, J. D. (1994). Fluoride, remineralization and root caries. *Am J Dent.*, 7:271–4.
96. Emilson, C. G., & Berkhead, D. (1993). Effects of a 12-month prophylactic program on selected oral bacterial populations on root surfaces with active and inactive carious lesions. *Caries Res*, 27:195–200.
97. Wallace, M. C., Retief, D. H., & Bradley, F. L. (1993). The 48-month increment of root caries in urban population of older adults participating in a preventive dental program. *J Publ Hlth Dent*, 43:133–7.
98. Hoppenbrouwers, P. M., Groenendijk, N., Tawarie, N. R., & Driessens, F. C. (1988). Improvements of caries resistance of human dental roots by a two-step conversion of the root mineral into fluoridated hydroxylapatite. *J Dent Res*, 67:1254–6
99. Nyvad, B., ten Cate, J. M., & Fejerskov, O. (1997). Arrest of root caries in situ. *J Dent Res*, 76:1845–53.
100. Billings, R. J., Brown, L. R., & Kaster, A. G. (1985). Contemporary treatment strategies for root surface dental caries. *Gerodontics*, 1:20–7.
101. Nyved, B., & Fejerskov, A. (1986). Active root surface caries converted into inactive caries as a response to oral hygiene. *Scand J Dent Res*, 94:281–4.
102. Schaecken, M. J., Keljens, H. M., & van der Hoeven, J. S. (1991). Effects of fluoride and chlorhexidine on the microflora of dental root surfaces and progression of root surface caries. *J Dent Res*, 70:150–3.
103. Schupbach, P., Guggenhein, B., & Lutz, F. (1990). Histopathology of root surface caries. *J Dent Res*, 69:1195–204.

104. Fejerskov, A. (1994). Recent advancements in the treatment of root caries. [Review]. *Intl Dent J*, 44:139–44.

105. Horowitz, H. S. (1990). The future of water fluoridation and other systemic fluorides. *J Dent Res*, 69(Special Issue):760–7.

106. Pitts, N. B. (1991). The diagnosis of dental caries: diagnostic methods of assessing buccal, lingual and occlusal surfaces. *Dent Update*, 18:393–6.

107. Kidd, E. A. M. (1984). The diagnosis and management of "early" carious lesions in permanent teeth. *Dent Update*, 11:69–81.

108. Majare, I., Karlestral, C., & Stenlund, H. (1999). Incidence and progression of approximal caries from 11 to 22 years of age in Sweden: A prospective radiographic study. *Caries Res*, 33:93–100.

109. Ekanayake, L. S., & Sheiham, A. (1987). Reducing rates of progression of dental caries in British school children. A study using bitewing radiographs. *Br Dent J*, 63:265–9.

110. Pitts, N. B., & Deery, C. (1997). Radiographically monitored lesion behavior in Scottish adolescent regular attenders. *J Dent Res*, 76:260 (Abstr. 1976).

111. Elderton, R. J., & Osman, Y. I. (1991). Preventive versus restorative management of dental caries *J Dent Assn S Afr*, 46:217–21.

112. Alves, M. E. A. P., Allen, T., & Alves, M. C. (1997). Evaluation of long term periodontal maintenance therapy. *J Dent Res*, 76:54 (Abstr. 326).

113. Wallman, C., Krasse, B., & Birkhead, D. (1994). Effect of chlorhexidine treatment followed by stannous fluoride gel application on mutans streptococci in margins of restorations. *Car Res*, 28:435–40.

114. Lindquist, B., Edwards, S., Torrell, P., & Krasse, B. (1989). Effect of different carriers on preventive measures in children highly infected with mutans streptococci. *Scand J Dent Res*, 97:330–7.

115. Twetman, A. (1999). Interdental caries incidence and progression in relation to mutans streptocpcci suppression after chlorhexidine-thymol varnish treatment in schoolchildren. *Acta Odontol Scan*, 57:144–8.

116. Luoma, H., Murtomaa, H., Nuuga, T., Nyman, A., Nummikoski, P., Airamo, J., & Luoma, A. R. (1979). A simultaneous reduction of caries and gingivitis in a group of school children receiving chlorhexidine-fluoride applications. *Car Res*, 12:290–8.

117. Emilson, C. G. (1994). Potential efficiency of chlorhexidine against mutans streptococci and human dental caries. *J Dent Res*, 73:682–91.

118. Luoma, H. (1992). Chlorhexidine solutions, gels and varnishes in caries prevention. *Proc Finn Dent Soc*, 88:147–53.

119. Albandar, J. M., Gjermo, P., & Preus, H. R. (1994). Chlorhexidine use after two decades of over-the-counter availability. *J Periodontol*, 65:109–12.

120. Petersson, L. G., Magnusson, K., Anderson, H., Almquist, B., & Twetman, S. (2000). Effect of quarterly treatments with a chlorhexidine and a fluoride varnish on approximal caries in caries-susceptible teen agers: a 3-year clinical study. *Caries Res*, 34:140–3.

121. Twetman, S., & Petersson, L. G. (1999). Interdental caries incidence and progression in relation to mutans streptococci suppression after chlorhexidine-thymol varnish treatments in school children. *Acta Odontolog Scandinavica*, 57:144–8.

122. Zickert, I., Emilson, C. G., & Krasse, B. (1982). Effect of caries preventive measures in children highly infected with the bacterium Streptoccus mutans. *Arch Oral Biol*, 27:861–8.

123. Grundemann, L. J., Timmerman, M. F., Ijzerman, Y., van der Velden, V., & Weijden, G. A. (2000). Stain, plaque and gingivitis reduction by combining chlorhexidine and peroxyborate. *J Clin Periodontol*, 27:9–15.

124. Alves, M. E. A. P., Allen, T., & Alves, M. C. (1997). Evaluation of long time periodontal maintenance therapy. *J Dent Res*, 76:326(Abstr. 84)

125. Stein, M. (1993). A literature review: oral irrigation therapy. The adjunctive roles for home and professional use. *Probe*, 27:18–25.

126. Twetman, S., & Grindefjord, M. (1999). Mutan streptocci suppression by chlorhexidine gel in toddlers. *Amer J Dent*, 12:89–91.

127. Splieth, C., Steffen, H., Rosin, M., & Welk, A. (2000). Caries prevention with chlorhexidine-thymol varnish in high risk school children. *Community Dent Oral Epildemiol*, 28:419–27.

128. Clark, D. C., Morgan, J., & MacEntee, M. I. (1991). Effects of a 1% chlorhexidine gel on the cariogenic bacteria in high-risk elders: a pilot study. *Spec Care Dentist*, 11:101–3.

129. Martens, L., Marks, L., & Kint, J. (1999). The use of chlorhexidine as a preventive and therapeutic means of plaque control in the handicapped. Review of the literature and definitive advice for application. *Rev Belg Med Dent*, 52:27–37.

130. Burtner, A. P., Smith, R. G., Tiefenback, S., & Walker, C. (1996). Administration of chlorhexidine to persons with mental retardation residing in an institution: patient acceptance and staff compliance. *Spec Care Dentist*, 16:53–7.

131. Jenatschke, F., Elsenberger, E., Welte, H. D., & Schlagenkauf, U. (2001). Influence of repeated chlorhexidine varnish applications on mutans streptococci counts and caries increment in patients treated with fixed orthodontic appliances. *J. Orofac Orthop*, 62:36–45.

132. Corbet, E. F., Tam, J. O., Zee, K. Y., Wong, M. C., Lo, E. C., Mombelli, A. W., & Lang, N. P. (1999). Therapeutic Effects of supervised chlorhexidine mouthrinses on untreated gingivitis. *Oral Dis*, 3:9–18.

133. Piccolomini, R., Di Bonaventura, G., Catamo, G., Turmini, V., Di Placido, G., D'Ercole, S., Perfetti, G., & Paolantonio, M. (1999). Microbiologival and clinical effects of a 1% chlorhexidine-gel in untreated periodontal pockets from adult periodontitis patients. *New Microbiol*, 22:111–6.

134. Keltjens, H. M., Shaeken, M. J., van der Hoeven, J. S., & Hendriks, J. C. (1990). Caries control in overdenture patients: 18-month evaluation on fluoride and chlorhexidine therapies. *Car Res*, 24:371–5.

135. Epstein, J. B., McBride, B. C., Stevenson-Moore, P., Merilees, H., & Spinelli, J. (1991). The efficacy of chlorhexidine gel in reduction of Streptococcus mutans and Lactobacillus species in patients treated with radiation therapy. *Oral Surg Oral Med Oral Pathol*, 71:172–8.

136. Sfikas, P. M. (1998). Informed consent and the law. *JADA*, 129:1471–3.

137. Leake, J. L., Main, P. A., & Woodward, G. L. (1996). Report on the RCDS-CDHSRU workshop on developing clinical guidelines/standards of practice. *J Can Dent Assoc*, 62:570–7.

138. Surabian, S. R. (1996). Informed consent or refusal. *J Calif Dent Assoc*, 6:51–4.

139. Duckworth, R. M. (1993). The science behind caries prevention. [Review]. *Intl Dent J*, 43:(6 Suppl A); 529–39.

140. Horowitz, A. (1995). The public's oral health: The gap between what is known about preventing oral diseases is often extensive. *Adv Dent Res*, 9:91–265.

141. JADA Council of Access, Prevention and Interprofessional Relations. (June 1985). Caries diagnosis and risk assessment.

142. Anderson, M. H., Bales, D. J., & Omnell, K-A. (1993). Modern management of dental caries: The cutting edge is not the dental bur. *JADA*, 124:39–44.

143. Field, M. J., & Lohr, K. N. (1990). *Clinical Guidelines: Directions for a New Program*. Institute of Medicine. Washington DC: Academic Press.

144. Lohr, K. N., Eleazer, K., & Mauskopf, J. (1998). Health policy issues and applications for evidence-based medicine and clinical practice guide lines. *Health Policy*, 46:1–19.

145. Hayward, R. S. A., & Lawpacio, A. (1993). Initiating, conducting and maintaining guideline development programs. *CMA*, 148:507–12.

146. Anusavice, K. J. (1995). Treatment regimens in preventive and restorative dentistry. [Review]. *JADA*, 12:727–43.

147. Baker, J. D., & Shugars, D. A. (1995). Variation, treatment outcomes and practice guidelines in dental practice. *J Dent Edu*, 59:61–5.

148. Stephens, R. G., Kogon, S. L., & Bohay, R. N. (1996). Current trends in guideline development: A cause for concern. *J Can Dent Assoc*, 62:151–8.

149. Prevention of Bacterial Endocarditis. (1997). Recommendations by the American Heart Association. *Circulation*, 96:358–66.

150. Guidelines for Periodontal Therapy. (1998). The American Academy of Periodontology. *J Periodontol*, 69:405–8.

151. Harris, N. O. (1982). The clinical application of primary preventive dentistry procedures in the control of the plaque diseases. In *Primary Preventive Dentistry*, 1st ed. Reston, VA: Reston Publishing Company, Inc., 454–80

152. Harris, N. O., & Scheirton, L. S. (1987). In *Primary Prevention Dentistry*, 2nd ed. Norwalk, CT/Los Angeles, CA: Appleton & Lange, 533–73.

153. Frame, P. S., Sawai, R., Bowen, W. H., & Meyerowitz, C. (2000). Preventive dentistry practitioner's recommendations for low risk patients compared with scientific evidence and practice and guidelines. *Am J Prev Med*, 18:159–62.

154. Developing Clinical Teaching Methods for Caries Risk Assessment. (1995). Symposium Proceedings *J Dent Edu*, 59:7–15.

155. Bader, J. D., Ed. (1990). Risk Assessment in Dentistry. Chapel Hill, NC: University of North Carolina Dental Ecology.

156. Leverett, D. H., Proskin, H. M., Featherstone, J. D. B., Adair, S. M., Eisenberg, A. D., Mundorff-Shrestha, S. A., Shields, C. P., Shaffer, C. L., & Billings, R. J. (1993). Caries risk assessment in a longitudinal discrimination study. *J Dent Res*, 72:538–43.

157. Barrington, E. P., & Nevins, M. (1990). Diagnosing periodontal disease. *JADA*, 121:460–4.

158. Greenwell, H., Bissada, N. F., & Wittwer, J. W. (1990). Periodontics in general practice: Professional plaque control. *JADA*, 121:642–6.

159. Axelsson, P., & Lindhe, J. (1981). Effect of controlled oral hygiene procedures on caries and periodontal disease in adults. Results after six years. *J Clin Periodontol*, 8:239–48.

160. Shallhorn, R. G., & Snider, J. S. (1981). Preventive maintenance therapy. *JADA*, 103:227–161.

161. Pfeifer, M. R., & Pfeifer, J. (1988). Dental prevention: The oral prophylaxis. *Clin Prevent Dent*, 10:18–24.

162. Solomon, E. S. (1997). Results of the Texas Dental Association's Dental Hygiene Needs Survey. *Texas Dent J*, 114:17–22.

163. *Personal Communication* from RL Frazier, Austin, TX, 1981.

164. Levine, R. A., & Wilson, T. G. (1992). Compliance as a major risk factor in periodontal disease progression. *Comp Dent Edu*, 13:1072–9.

165. Wilson, T. J. Jr. (1998). How patient compliance to suggested oral hygiene and maintenance affect periodontal therapy. *Dent Clin North Amer*, 42:389–402.

166. Krasse, B. (1984). Can microbiological knowledge be applied in dental practice for the treatment and prevention of dental caries? *J Can Dent Assoc*, 50:221–23.

167. Robinson, P. J. (1995). Gingivitis: a prelude to periodontitis. *J Clin Dent*, 6: (Spec.) 41–45.

168. Lewis, D. W. (1996). Main, P. A. Ontario dentist's knowledge and beliefs about selected aspects of diagnosis, prevention and restorative dentistry. *J Canad Dent Assoc*, 62:337–44.

169. American Dental Association, Survey Center, 1997/98. (June 1999). *Survey of Predoctoral Dental Educational Institutions—Curriculum*, Volume 4.

170. Accreditation Standards for U.S. Dental Schools. (2000). *Commission on Dental Accreditation*, American Dental Association, Chicago.

171. Yorty, J. S., & Birgitti Brown K. (1999). Caries risk assessment/treatment programs in U.S. dental schools. *J Dent Edu*, 63:745–47.

172. Keys, P. H. (1960). The infectious and transmissible nature of experimental dental caries. Findings and implications. *Arch Oral Biol*, 1:304–20.

173. Fitzgerald, R. J., & Keyes, P. H. (1960). Demonstration of the etiologic role of streptococci in experimental caries in the hamster. *JADA*, 61:9–10.

174. Vaccine to prevent most tooth decay may be ready by 1990. *Wall Street Journal*, 14 July 1982.

175. Cohen, B., Colman, G., & Russell, R. R. B. (1979). Immunization against dental caries: further studies. *Brit Dent J*, 147:9–115.

176. Stinson, M. W., Nisingard, R. J., & Bergey, E. J. (1979). Binding of streptococcal cell components to muscle tissue. Meeting of the American Society of Microbiology. D80 (Abs).

177. Koshland, D. E. Jr. (1985). Benefits, risks, vaccines and the courts. *Science*, 227:1285.

178. Ma, JK-C. (1999). The caries vaccine: A growing prospect. 26:374–80.

179. Ma, J. K., Hikmat, B. Y., Wycoff, K., Vine, N. D., Chargelegue, D., Yu, L., Meim, M. B., & Lehner, T. (1998). Characteristics of a recombinant plant monoclonal secretory antibody and preventive immunotherapy in humans. *Nat Med*, 4:601–6.

Name:_____    Date: _____

Patient: Please check the column that best describes your consumption of the following foods.

Instructor: To derive score, multiply group number by column number.

   (*Example*: If check is in second column (2) × group 3, score = 6).

| | Group | 1<br>Seldom<br>(1 or 2 times<br>monthly) | 2<br>Not often<br>(1 or 2 times<br>weekly) | 3<br>Often<br>(1 or 2 times<br>daily) | Score |
|---|---|---|---|---|---|
| Group 1 | Tea or coffee with sugar | | | | |
| | Chocolate milk, or hot chocolate | | | | |
| | Soft drinks (regular, NOT diet) | | | | |
| | Milk shakes | | | | |
| | Dessert wines and cordials | | | | |
| | Fruit drinks | | | | |
| | Lemonade | | | | |
| Group 2 | Custards, puddings | | | | |
| | Whipped cream | | | | |
| | Ice cream, sherbert, popsicles | | | | |
| | Flavored yogurt | | | | |
| | Applesauce | | | | |
| | Canned fruit in syrup | | | | |
| Group 3 | Jams and jellies | | | | |
| | Whipped cream | | | | |
| | Cakes, coffee cakes | | | | |
| | Bananas | | | | |
| | Doughnuts | | | | |
| | Cookies | | | | |
| | Cereals, sugar-coated | | | | |
| | Pies | | | | |
| | Dried fruits | | | | |
| Group 4 | Candy bars | | | | |
| | Hard candy | | | | |
| | Chocolate candy | | | | |
| | Caramels | | | | |
| | Cough drops | | | | |

Group 1 = Liquids; Group 2 = Liquid to soft; Group 3 = Slowly dissolve;
Group 4 = Sticky

Total score:

(Courtesy of Dr. Carole A. Palmer, Tufts University School of Dental Medicine, Boston, MA.)

APPENDIX 23–3.  **Open Letter to New Patients**

Dear _____:

For myself and on behalf of my staff, I would like to extend a warm welcome to our dental practice. As we all readily admit, going to the dentist is not exactly our favorite pastime. Unfortunately many of us have had experiences in the past that have caused us to avoid dental visits. Although we cannot promise you that you will never have an uncomfortable moment while in our office, we can promise you to do all in our power to make your dental experience a pleasant one.

We believe that it is the right of every patient to know the cause of his or her dental disease and how he or she can prevent it. Ninety-five percent of dental disease is preventable, and it is our intention that the dental treatment we perform for you will last a lifetime. We believe that we should make every effort to preserve every natural tooth for life (with the possible exception of some wisdom teeth). We have organized a series of appointments with the express purpose of stopping your dental disease (tooth decay and gum disease). We believe that anyone with active dental disease should receive this counseling as the first phase of his or her treatment, after we relieve any emergency condition, of course. If we were to repair the damage of disease without stopping the disease, our treatment would eventually fail. If you accept and practice good home care, you should need little more than an annual checkup. This means low dental costs over the years. As you will find out, however, the only person who can truly stop dental disease is you, and we acknowledge that every person reserves the right to remain sick if they so choose.

I hope that you have more of an insight into how I practice and thus you can decide if I am the right dentist for you. I hope that this will mark the beginning of an enjoyable experience and continued good dental health.

(Courtesy of Dr. RL Frazier, Jr., Austin, TX.)

# GLOSSARY

Abrasive system: Abrasive agent + polishing agent = Abrasive system for toothpaste.

Abutment teeth: The teeth to which the two ends of a bridge are attached.

Adherence: The willingness of the patient to comply with the suggested plans of self-care proposed by dental-health professionals.

ADL: Activities of Daily Living. Toileting, preparing food, showering, getting into bed, etc. Instrumental Activities of Daily Living. (IADL). Using telephone, preparing meals, managing money.

Adhesin: The surface appendage of a bacterium that allows the microbe to attach to receptor sites on the tooth or on other bacteria in the plaque.

ADA: American Dental Association: The U.S. professional organization of dentists, with headquarters in Chicago, Illinois.

ADA Seal of Acceptance: An advisory to inform the profession and the public that a product meets the requirements of the ADA for safety and effectiveness. It does not have the force of law, as does an approval by the Food and Drug Administration. However, product manufacturers eagerly seek the Seal as an additional incentive for the public to buy.

ADA website: www.ada.org The ADA website is a source of information about dental subjects and dental products.

Aging: Young elderly—65–74 years of age.
Mid-elderly—75–84 years of age.
Oldest-old—over 85 years of age.

AIDS: Acquired Immunity Deficiency Syndrome. Usually contracted through sex and exchange of drug needles.

Aerobic bacteria: Bacteria that require oxygen for survival.

Anaerobic bacteria: Bacteria that survive only in the absence of oxygen.

Anorexia: No desire to eat.

Antiemetics: Emesis = vomiting. Antiemetics = Drugs to suppress vomiting.

Antismoking programs: Programs conducted to teach avoidance or cessation of use of tobacco products by nonusers, and to help existing smokers to break their addiction.

"Antibiotic prophylaxis": The administration of an antibiotic for patients where there is a possibility of causing a transient bacteremia.

Aphasia: A condition where reception (hearing), integration and expression (brain) of language is impaired. Difficulty in finding the right words to communicate.

Attached gingival: The mucous membrane extending from the muco-gingival fold to the marginal gingival on the facial side of the alveolar process.

Autistic: Self-centered in thought and behavior. Often difficult or unable to use language appropriately.

Avulsion: The traumatic removal of teeth. (accidents, sports)

Baby-bottle caries: Usually caused by an infant taking milk as nourishment when hungry, and then retaining the nipple and the milk in the mouth during "sleep time." Can also be caused by "demand" breast-feeding.

Behavior modification: A change in behavior due to motivation causing a shift in self-designated goals.

Biofilm: A layer of living organisms that can attach to a solid object, for instance moss or seaweed to rocks, or in a dental context, oral bacteria to the teeth.

Bis-GMA: The abbreviation of the chemical name of the plastic used for sealants. (Bisphenol A-glycidyl methylacrlate).

Biopsy: The excision (removal) and microscopic examination of tissue suspected of being cancerous.

Bleeding index: A record of the location of marginal bleeding following gentle probing of the free margin of the gingiva.

Body defense cells: Cells that identify the presence of antigens (foreign bodies), remove the

antigens, and/or repair the damage caused by the antigens.

**Body Mass Index:** BMI. A medical standard for defining obesity.

**Body wraps:** Blanket like wraps that fully enfold a young patient to restrain body parts or patient actions during a dental procedure.

**Buffering:** The ability to neutralize acidity (of the plaque) by use of alkaline substances.

**Bulimia:** Binge eating. Eating a meal, and then resorting to regurgitation to eliminate the stomach contents. Often accompanied by lingual erosion of teeth from stomach acid.

**Caloric sugar:** Containing calories. Natural sugars—Sucrose, glucose, fructose, lactose, etc.

**Cannula:** A small diameter tip of an irrigator syringe or device that allows a deeper irrigation of a periodontal pocket.

**Caregiver:** Members of the family, a friend, or hired personnel who assume responsibility of helping compromised persons to live as normal life as possible.

**Caries activity:** A level of caries risk as determined by use of laboratory methods, plaque index and other evidence-based evaluations.

**Caries-Activity Indictors (CAI):** Evidence-based predictors of the course and outcome of the dental caries process.

**Catheter:** A tube connecting a body cavity with the exterior for purposes of irrigation or drainage.

**Cavitated:** An incipient lesion in which the surface zone has collapsed over the body of the lesion, thus creating an overt cavity.

**Cemento-enamel junction:** The junction point between the coronal enamel and the cementum.

**Centers for Disease Control and Prevention (CDCP):** An arm of the United States Public Health Service located in Atlanta, GA. It is responsible for epidemiology studies to determine the presence, extent and recommended solutions to diseases in the United States and in collaboration with foreign governments.

**CFUs:** Colony-forming units (bacteria). The number of bacterial colonies that are found on a suitable agar after an appropriate period of incubation.

**Chemical plaque control:** The use of anti-microbial mouth rinses to aid in plaque control.

**Chemotaxis:** A response to a chemical signal that initiates the movement of body defense cells to an area of inflammation.

**Children's Dental Health Month—February:** A nationally sponsored month by the dental profession and dental hygienists' in which there is a coordinated effort by community leaders, industry, volunteer dentists, and students to demonstrate the advantages of dental care.

**Chlorination:** The addition of chlorine compounds to water supplies to kill pathogenic bacteria.

**Chlorhexidine:** An effective antimicrobial mouthrinse that is effective for suppressing cariogenic and periopathogenic organisms.

**Cleft palate:** An oral malformation in which there is a lack of union at the midline of the palate which may involve only a split uvula of the soft palate to a cleft of all structures of the palate and include the upper lip.

**Cognition:** Ability to concentrate and think logically.

**Colorado brown stain:** The early designation for severe fluorosis (with brown coloration of teeth) before its etiology was known.

**Collagen:** Collagen is the protein for the framework of soft and hard tissues of the body.

**Collagenase:** Is the enzyme that attacks collagen.

**Compliance:** A willingness of a patient to follow prescribed actions.

**Compromised individual:** A person with one or more physical, medical, mental or emotional problems that limit their ability to function normally.

**Concept:** After an individual has learned a sufficient number of facts relating to a subject, by reasoning these facts begin to form an overall belief called a concept.

**Coronal caries:** Caries located on the crown of the tooth.

**Cost-effective analysis:** A calculation of how much money is saved (or overspent) as a result of some action.

**CPITN: A Community Periodontal Index of Treatment Needs:** A world-wide standardized

periodontal index based on the severity (pocket depth) exhibited by a population.

**Crevicular fluid:** A tissue fluid that arises from the underlying connective tissue, flows slowly through the gingival crevice into the mouth; its two major functions are to (1) flush out catabolites, and (2) to act as a carrier for immune cells and antibodies that bathe (and protect) the four smooth surfaces on every tooth.

**Cytokine:** A proinflammatory blood borne agent of the body's immune system.

**Cure:** Occurs when a disease process terminates with a return to histologic normalcy of all tissues involved. The return to normal can be due to natural body defense mechanisms, or because of professional intercession.

**Debridement:** The mechanical or chemical removal of infectious or necrotic material from an inflamed, or potentially inflamed area.

**Demineralization:** The loss of mineral from the tooth because of bacterial acids, acid foods (soft drinks, acid juices, etc), or even toothbrushing abrasion.

**Demographic data:** Environment conditions relating to and having an effect on data found in a survey, such as population, socioeconomic status, race, age, unusual environmental conditions, etc.

**Dental caries:** A carbohydrate modified transmissible localized infection caused mainly by mutans streptococci and lactobacilli.

**Dental plaque:** A combination of bacteria, saliva and complex polysaccharides on the surface of the teeth.

**Dentate:** With teeth. The opposite is edentulous, i.e., not to have teeth.

**Dentifice:** A more scientific, but less used, term for toothpaste.

**Desquamate:** To shed skin cells.

**Dentacult SM and Denticult L:** Commercially available test kits that facilitate counting of mutans streptococci and lactobacilli, respectively.

**Dentino-enamel junction (DEJ):** The junction between the dentin and the enamel cap.

**Dextrose:** Common lay designation of glucose.

**Dietary Fluoride Supplement Schedule:** Recommended daily dosage of fluoride supplements.

(applicable to fluoride drops or tablets) to bring the daily intake to the equivalent of 1 ppm.

**Dietary Reference Intake (DRIs):** To address how foods can bridge the difference between healthy individuals and those with chronic and acute disease. This also will involve a study of different vitamins, minerals as they relate to health.

**Digitized x-ray:** Instead of a film that needs to be wet processed, an electronic sensor of similar size is used. The same office x-ray unit is used for energy. The resulting image is processed in the computer and can be shown on the monitor, recorded for storage on a tape or disk, or e-mailed for insurance claims.

**Disaccharide:** A combination of two simple sugars. Example—Glucose + fructose = sucrose.

**Disclosing tablet:** A red tablet that is chewed to mix with saliva and then swished around the mouth to disclose the presence and location of dental plaque on the teeth.

**Dysarthia:** A speech problem.

**Duraflor:** A commercial fluoride varnish for aiding remineralization and for reducing hypersensitivity of dentin. (Examples, Durophat and Fluor Protector).

**Early and Periodic Screening, Diagnosis and Treatment (EPDST):** A federal program that mandates that medical and dental services be provided to children from low income families to receive a dental screening within 12 months of birth.

**Edentulism:** Without teeth.

**Elderly:** Young elderly, from 65 to 74 years of age; mid-old, 75 to 84; and 85 > oldest old.

**Electrocardiogram:** A measurement of the electrical activity of the heart as a diagnostic measure.

**Electronic periodontal probes:** Electronic probes attached to a computer that automatically triggers a measurement of pocket depth when a given pressure on the bottom of the sulcus is encountered.

**Embrasure:** The inter-proximal space between two adjacent teeth. Classified as class 1 embrasures that occurs when a soft tissue papilla fills the entire space, type 3 when the papilla is missing, and type 2, intermediate.

Enamel maturation: A period of one or two years after eruption during which time the enamel becomes "fully" mineralized (matured).

Endodontics: The treatment of diseased root canals.

Endoscope: A small probe-like videocamera for examining areas that is not readily available, for visual examination—for example, intranasal examination, colonoscopy, intraoral dental examination, etc.

Endothelial cells: The cells lining blood vessels.

Epidemiological survey: A controlled study of the origin, presence, extent or consequences of a condition or disease.

Epithelial attachment: The junctional epithelial cells that attach the crevicular epithelium to the tooth.

Eruptive period, pre-: Before eruption. It is a period during which teeth are developing.

Eruptive period, post-: A short, indefinite period after eruption.

Ischemia: Lack of sufficient blood to a part.

Etchant: An acid (40 to 50%) phosphoric acid that is used to etch the tooth surface to provide more surface area that in turn enhances retention of sealants.

Etiology: The cause of a disease.

Evidence-based decisions: The basing of decisions on verified research evidence that certain signs or symptoms are predictive of certain outcomes. For instance, the finding of a greater number of mutans streptococci poses a greater risk for future caries development than does a low count.

Exodontics: The extraction of teeth.

Extrinsic stain: A stain that is on the outside of the tooth surface that can be removed.

Facultative aerobic and anaerobic bacteria: Bacteria that can survive in the presence, or absence of oxygen, respectively.

Fact: A positive or negative bit of information that a person consciously or unconsciously remembers temporarily or permanently.

Fimbria: Small microscopic projections from a bacterial cell wall.

Fistula: A tissue connection between a subsurface infected area and the surface of a mucosal membrane or skin.

Flap surgery (periodontal diseases): The removal of a sufficient circumferential portion of the marginal gingival to lessen pocket depth and open the subgingival area to self-care preventive procedures.

Fluoridated water, artificial: Water that is adjusted to 1 ppm of fluoride content (with annual temperature compensation).

Fluoridated water, natural: Ground water that is fluoridated by water flowing over rocks and soil containing fluoride.

Fluoridation, topical: The professional liquid or gel office application of fluoride to the surface of the teeth, or the home application of fluoride to the teeth by use of dentifrices and mouthrinses.

Fluoride diffusion effect: Also referred to as a "halo effect." It is the caries reduction experienced by individuals not living in a water fluoridated area, but getting its benefits by eating and drinking food processed in an area with optimum water fluoride content. Also, the term applies to those who commute between fluoridated and nonfluoridated communities.

Fluoride varnishes: Varnishes containing fluoride that is painted over tooth surfaces to provide a longer contact of fluoride with the enamel or cementum.

Frank lesion: Same as cavitated or overt caries lesion.

Fluorosis: Cosmetic deviation of enamel in development because of an excessive intake of fluoride during the development periods of the primary and the permanent teeth. Depending on amount of intake, the cosmetic effect ranges from mild veining to a severe brown coloration with a pitting of the enamel.

Food and Nutrition Board: A government Board established in 1941 by the National Research Council of the National Academy of Science to determine the food needs of the American people. It is a still functioning Board with a greatly enlarged mandate to study all aspects of food intake, as for instance, what are the detailed nutritional needs of pregnancy and lactation?

Foods Additive Amendment: Passed by Congress in 1958. A Bill that required all manufacturers to prove that a new food product was safe.

Furcation areas: The space between multi-rooted posterior teeth.

Gag reflex: A reflex to a tendency to vomit. Often encountered when patient irritate the posterior tongue or palatal area when cleaning the teeth. Also can occur with an obnoxious taste or with some cases of pregnancy.

Gingival crevicular fluid: Fluid that arises from the connective tissue beneath the gingival sulcus that slowly flows through the gingival crevice. Its purpose is to flush debris from the sulcus, and carry defense agents into the oral cavity.

Gingival sulcus: Around each tooth there is a collar of approximately 3 millimeters on depth of soft tissue. (A comparative soft-hard tissue junction might be the cuticle of the fingernail). Between that collar and the tooth there is a potential *sulcus* or *crevice*.

Glass ionomer: A hard plastic with fine incorporated glass powder to resist abrasion. Used for restorations and tried as a sealant substitute.

Glaucoma: An increased intraocular pressure that, unless treated, can lead to blindness.

Antibiotic environment or chamber: A sterile chamber that is used to give birth, feed, and accomplish studies of rodents or animals in a bacteria-free environment.

Goal orientation: An objective than an individual has decided to attain; it may be only a temporary short-term goal or a long-term goal; it may be a temporary short-term goal that is powerful only until attained.

Guideline: An established and agreed upon method for examining, treating, preventing and/or monitoring a disease.

Head Start: A national program that provides access to early learning for under privileged children.

Health promotion: Any planned combination of educational, political, regulatory and organizational efforts conducive to the health of a community or group of individuals in a definite geographical location.

HFCS: High fructose corn-sugar.

HIV: Human immunodeficiency virus. Usually a predecessor of AIDS.

Homeostasis: Occurs when the body is in normal metabolic balance. Reference to caries: a balance between demineralization and remineralization.

Hopewood House: An orphanage in Australia that demonstrated that children raised on a good diet, caries is minimal. It also proved that once the children left Hopewood House and its diet, caries again became a problem, proving that the acquired low caries status of the orphanage was not permanent.

Human Genome Project: Probably the greatest health research program of the 20th century. This has been a worldwide research effort to decipher "the molecule of life"—desoxynucleic acid.

Humeral body defenses: Genetic defense factors found in body fluids.

Hydroxyapatite: The basic building crystal in the formation of enamel rods. It is composed of mainly calcium, phosphate and hydroxyl, but also includes many other trace quantities of up to 30 or 40 elements.

Hyper-: Above normal.

Hypo-: Below normal.

Hypoglycemic shock: A decrease in the level of blood glucose (in diabetes mellitus) that can be accompanied by a variety of symptoms from confusion to coma and death.

Hypothesis, nonspecific: A belief that periodontal diseases arose from the conglomeration of bacteria making up the dental plaque. Now discounted.

Hypothesis, specific: A belief that the periodontal diseases arise from specific bacteria in the dental plaque.

Immune response: Any time a foreign substance penetrates the body's defenses, there is a cellular reaction (immune response) to seek out the antigen (foreign substance) and to neutralize or eliminate it.

Immunization: The injection, or ingestion of an antigen into the body to cause an enhancement of he body's capability to resist disease.

Incidence: The amount of disease that occurs *between* two surveys over an agreed upon time period.

Incipient caries lesion: A pre-caries lesion that exists before cavitation. Seen on the enamel as a "white spot." It can be remineralized.

Informed patient consent: Before any treatment is commenced, the patient is informed verbally, or in writing of all primary and treatment options, costs and expected results.

Implant: A metallic "root" (the implant) that is surgically inserted into the alveolus in the space of a missing tooth. Following healing, a crown is later constructed on the "root".

Incidence: A study of the rate of occurrence of a disease or condition over a given period of time.

Intense sweetener: Considered noncaloric because of their small bulk needed to deliver desired sweetness.

Interproximal: The area between the mesial and distal surfaces of two adjacent teeth.

Irrigator: A small device containing a reservoir for water that is pumped at relatively low velocity to cleanse the interproximal spaces or loosening plaque.

Intrinsic stain: A stain that was incorporated in the enamel during development, and which cannot be removed without damage to the enamel.

Kock's postulates: Kock, a German bacteriologist postulated that the etiology of an infectious disease could only be confirmed when the agent could be recovered from a patient, introduced into an experimental animal to produce the same disease with a re-recovery of the same original pathogen.

Lactobacilli: An acidogenic bacterial species that is an etiologic microorganism seen at the later stages of the incipient caries lesion.

Lucency: (As applied to dental x-rays), a darker area on the x-ray indicating demineralization (caries) or the enamel, dentin or cementum.

Leukoplakia: A white or reddish corrugated lesion found in the mouth that is often precancerous.

Level 1 school-preventive program: A fluoride mouth rinse program accomplished with the cooperation of the teachers, school nurse and volunteers from the Parent Teachers Association.

Level 2 school-preventive programs: All procedures of the Level 1 program, plus the addition of a dental hygienist to help in the teaching of dental subjects, plus the additional clinical duties of prophylaxes and sealant placement.

Level 3 school-preventive programs: All the procedures of Level I and II, plus the addition of a dentist to accomplish secondary and tertiary preventive requirements.

Life span: The maximum of life potentially possible—now considered 120 years-of-age.

Life stage groups: A logical division of a total population into various age groups according to their different nutritional needs. Also groups such as pregnancy and lactation.

Lysozyme: An antibacterial enzyme found in the saliva and other fluids of the body.

Malodor, oral: Halitosis

Mechanical plaque control: The use of toothbrushes, dental floss, and irrigators to aid in plaque removal.

Monomer: A liquid plastic that when mixed with a catalyst, polymerizes to a hard plastic (polymer); or a liquid plastic containing a catalyst that is activated with a light (light cured).

Monosaccharide: A simple sugar. Example—Fructose, and glucose.

Morbidity: A ratio of sick to a given number of persons per unit time. Example 12: 100,000/year.

Mortality: The number of deaths from a given cause in a population per unit time. Example: 1: 1000 per year.

Motivation: An inner drive of an individual to attain a self-designated goal.

Mucositis: An inflammation of a mucous membrane.

Multifactorial disease: A disease where several factors must coalesce in order to cause the disease.

mutans streptococci: A causative cariogenic organism linked to the early stages of an incipient caries lesion.

National Institute of Dental and Craniofacial Research (NIDCFR): Located in Washington, DC on the campus of the National Institutes of Health. It is responsible for planning, publiciz-

ing, accomplishing the government funding for research that is needed to improve dental and cranial-facial health.

National Labeling and Education Act of 1990. A Congressional Act that requires specified information being imprinted on the label indicating the nutritional content of the contained items of food.

New Zealand School Dental Program: For New Zealand students in New Zealand between the age 5 and 13, which includes most of the procedures embodied in Level 1, 2 and 3 performed by specially trained Dental Nurses trained for government service. 90% of the children in New Zealand are enrolled in the program.

Noninvasive care: Care that can be administered without damage to the body tissues.

Obturator: A specialized maxillary prosthesis constructed to facilitate speech and eating by a cleft palate individual, as well as to prevent food from entering the nasal cavity.

Occlusal surface: Each posterior tooth has five surfaces, mesial, distal, lingual, buccal and occlusal; the occlusal surface is the biting surface of the posterior teeth.

Omnibus Budget Reconciliation Act (OBRA) of 1987. [Public Law 203]. Requires comprehensive assessments to determine specific health care need by those residents of nursing homes participating in Medicate or Medicare Part B program. The assessment must be conducted not later than 14 days after admission.

OSHA: Occupational Safety and Health Administration. A Federal agency responsible for the enforcement of health and environmental safety laws passed by Congress.

Osteoporosis: A pathology of bone marked with fragility and porosity.

Octocalcium phosphate: The first mineral laid down for enamel formation before its conversion to hydroxyapatite.

Oral-health self-care: Any action taken by an individual to maintain optimum oral health, including carrying out daily mechanical and chemical plaque control regimens as well as complying with recommendations by the dentist or dental hygienist.

OTC drugs: Drugs sold over-the-counter without a prescription.

Overt caries lesion: A cavity where the undermined enamel has broken down into a cavity, a process called cavitation. Remineralization is not a possibility (at least at this point in time, 2002).

PAHO: Pan American Health Organization.

Papillae: 1. The triangular soft tissue that fills the inter-proximal embrasures. 2. The specialized projections from the surface of the tongue that allow reception of different taste sensations.

Passive smoking: Relates to the tobacco smoke inhaled by family members or bystanders who breathe second-hand smoke.

Pasteurization: The heating of a product (usually milk) to a given temperature (often 60° C) for a given time (30 minutes) in order to kill pathogenic bacteria, and extend the time before other bacteria become pathogenic.

Periodontal disease indicators: Signs and symptoms that usually precede the onset of periodontal disease. Also called "markers."

Periodontal pocket: An abnormal deepening of the gingival sulcus marked by an accompanying apical migration of the epithelial attachment.

Peri-implantitis: Following the placement of an implant, the same meticulous self-care is necessary as with natural teeth. When this care does not materialize, the same infection and apical migration occurs to the epithelial attachment as occurs with periodontitis.

Permiability (of teeth): The ability of fluids to pass from the surface to the pulp and vice versa.

Phagocytosis: The envelopment and destruction of an antigen by one of the body defense cells.

Plaque index: O'Leary's index charts the location of the location of plaque on the teeth. The index of Silness and Löe is much the same with the exception that the status of the adjoining index is also recorded.

Polyol (alcohol sugar): Sweeteners that have an alcohol grouping to each carbon atom of the polyol. Referred to as sugar alcohols. Examples: sorbitol, mannitol, and xylitol.

Polypharmacy: Excessive multiple useage of medications often seen with senior citizens.

Pontic: The artificial teeth that are a part of the bridge between the abutment teeth.

Prediction: A clinical decision as to the outcome of a disease process based on professional judgement and evidence-based information.

Predictive value, negative: Probability that the subject will not develop disease.

Predictive value, positive: Probability that the subject will develop disease.

Prevalence: The amount of disease that is found after an epidemiology survey of a population.

Presbycusis: Hearing deterioration.

Presbyopia: Far sighted. Opposite—myopia.

Prognosis: A synonym for "prediction."

Prophylaxis: A cleaning of the hard concretions, plaque and food particles (material alba) from the tooth surfaces. (It should involve a final polishing with fluoride paste.)

Prosthesis: An artificial replacement for a lost body part—bridges, dentures, artificial legs, etc.

PSR (Periodontal Screening and Recording System): Similar to the CPITN, with the exception that it offers suggested treatment to match each level of severity.

Quadriplegic: An individual who has lost the use of arms and legs due to spinal cord injuries.

Radiation caries: The rampant caries that often occurs because of the detruction of the oral salivary glands that have been in the x-ray beam as a part of cancer treatment.

Refractory disease: A disease that does not respond to accepted treatment therapies.

Remineralization: The replacement of tooth mineral (hydroxyapatite) that has been lost by demineralization. The minerals needed for the remineralization are derived from the saliva (or from man-made products).

Risk: The probability that a harmful or unwanted event will occur.

Risk assessment: A professional judgement on an individual's susceptibility or resistance to disease, based on evidence-based information.

Risk factor: An evidence-based sign, test, or circumstance reliably associated with the onset or progression of a disease process.

Root caries: Caries located on the root (cementum) of a tooth.

School-Based Health Clinics (SBHC) and School-Based Dental Health Clinics (SBDHC): Programs sponsored by the Robert Johnson Foundation and communities to set up SBHC and School-Based Dental Health Clinics to improve the total and dental health of school children. Funding is now beginning to come from the government.

School Health Council: A Council or committee made up of representatives from the community and from the school district to identify or to develop programs to improve the total health—including dental health—of school students.

"Scoreboard": A sumary profile of the key factors of a patient's oral health following a laboratory, x-ray and clinical dental examination.

Screening tests: A rapid examination to identify healthy from unhealthy individuals, and the characteristics that separate them.

Seal of Acceptance. The logo and overprint of the American Dental Association awarded to manufacturers who voluntarily submit products to the ADA for testing of safety and efficacy of a product or device used for preventing or treating oral diseases.

Sealant: A plastic that is flowed over the occlusal surfaces of posterior teeth, and lingual pits of upper incisors to form a barrier between caries risk sites and the hostile oral environment.

Sensitivity (of test): The proportion of diseased subjects who test positive is termed "sensitivity."

Snyder test: A colorometric test used to estimate the relative acidogenic potential of salivary lactobacilli.

Soft ties: Cloth or leather straps use to immobilize uncontrollable body parts resulting from imperfect neuromuscular control.

Specificity: The proportion of nondiseased subjects that test negative.

"Spit" tobacco: A contemptuous term for the habit associated with either chewing tobacco or use of snuff.

Stannous: Meaning, tin.

*Streptococci mutans*: A specific species of the mutans streptococci grouping.

Subgingival and supra-gingival plaque: The plaque that is located on the tooth below, and above the gingiva, respectively.

Suppuration: Pus. A puerulent discharge from an infected area.

Symbiosis (bacterial): Two or more species of bacteria that mutually support one another.

Tattletooth II. An integrated dental health teaching program conducted under the auspices of the Texas Department of Health. Teachers from K-12 are provided with prepared packets of dental information considered important for each grade level.

Tautness: The tension of dental floss that is maintained by the fingers, or by the prongs of the floss holder.

TNM: A method of evaluation of the treatability of cancer, based on the extent of the (T)umor, involvement of the lymph (N)odes and the extent of (M)etastases.

Tolerable Upper Intake (of food): A study to attempt to answer the question, "What food do you need to remain healthy, but not obese?"

"Topping": Flowing a sealant over a preventive dentistry restoration and the remaining fissure system of a posterior tooth.

Trismus: (As applied to dentistry). Difficulty in opening the mouth due to nerve involvement, pain and/or infection of the masticatory muscles.

USPHS: United States Public Health Service.

Vaccine: The introduction of beneficial agent into the body to enhance the capability of the immune system to challenge and/or eliminate and repair the damage caused by a foreign antigen.

Validity: The reproducible accuracy of a test as a predictive measure.

Value: A strongly held belief of an individual, based on an unknown number of positive or negative concepts, that in turn are based on an unknown number of positive or negative facts.

Vasculitis: Inflammation of blood vessels resulting in the leakage of fluid and the migration of defense cells through the capillary walls.

Vipeholm: A study conducted in a mental institution in Vipeholm, Sweden. The clients were fed cariogenic snacks at different frequencies, at mealtime, between meals, etc. to see which situation was the most cariogenic.

"White spots": A white translucent area on the enamel indicating that there is localized demineralization of the enamel and possibly extending as far as the underlying dentin.

WHO: World Health Organization

Xerostomia: Dry mouth. A lower than normal secretion of saliva (1 ml per minute). A symptom with Sjorgrens disease, also following exposure of the salivary glands to cancer radiation and after use of several psychogenic drugs, fear, etc.

Xylitol: A sugar alcohol that is used as a flavoring agent that is both non-cariogenic and anti-cariogenic.

# INDEX

abrasives. *See also* dentifrices
   dentures, use on, 170
   in dentifrices, 124–125, 263
   in whitening dentifrices, 131
   testing of, 125
abutment teeth, brushing, 111. *See also* tooth brushing
acesulfame-K, 410, 411–412
acid. *See also* demineralization; remineralization
   damage, reducing, 325
   demineralization role, 16, 63
   measuring, 433
   production, reducing, 324–325
acquired pellicle, 26–27, 28
actinomycetes, 324
Addis, William, 94
adhesins, role in plaque formation, 29
Administration for Children and Families, 481
adolescents, caries risk of, 429. *See also* children
Agency for Healthcare Research and Quality, 481
Agency for Toxic Substances and Disease Registry, 481
aging
   alveolar process, 438
   bone density, 438
   cognitive changes, 596–597
   demographics, 589–591
   edentulous rates, 2
   education, 592
   functional status, 596
   health status, 592–593
   life span/expectancy, 591
   living arrangements, 592
   long-term care, 599–600
   long-term care facilities, dental care problems in, 2
   loose teeth, 437
   marital status, 592
   nutrition status, 437–438
   oral and pharyngeal cancer rates, 2
   oral disease patterns, 597–599
   peridontal disease rates, 2
   physiologic changes associated with, 593–596
   smell, impaired, 437
   taste, impaired, 437
AIDS. *See* HIV/AIDS
ALS. *See* amyotrophic lateral sclerosis
alveolar bone, 76
Alzheimer's disease, 597
amalgams, 302–303
American Academy of Pediatric Dentistry, 507

American Academy of Periodontology, 381–382, 631–632
American Dental Association (ADA)
   Acceptance Program, 104–105
   Ad Hoc Committee on Dentinal Sensitivity, 131
   anticalculus formulas, lack of seal for, 130
   artificial sweeteners, position on use of, 410
   chemotherapeutic products, guidelines for acceptance, 123
   Children's Dental Health Month, 531
   Council on Dental Therapeutics, 263, 267, 302
   Council on Scientific Affairs, 121, 122, 131, 132
   dental public health definition, 468
   fluoridation, definition of, 183
   Journal of, 266
   periodontal screening, 381–382
   pit-and-fissure sealant requirements, 288–289
   Seal of Approval, 104, 122
   support for sealants, 306
   toothbrushes accepted by, 104–105
   toothbrushing frequency, recommendations for, 108
American Society of Dentistry for Children, 507–508
amyotrophic lateral sclerosis, 563
antibiotic prophylaxis, 623–624
antifluoridation groups. *See under* fluoridation
aphasia, 563
Aspartame, 400–401
aspartame, 410, 411
Association of State and Territorial Dental Directors, 473
attachment loss, determining, 379
attendant care, 567–569
autism, treating patients with, 564
automated interproximal cleaners, 163

B vitamins, 429. *See also* nutrition
baby bottle decay. *See* infants
bacteriocins, 27
bad breath. *See* halitosis
baking soda dentifrices, 127
basal cell carcinoma, 613. *See also* cancer
Bass toothbrushing technique, 106–107
behavior, human
   as interaction of multiple factors, 451
   change theories, 456–460
   client-provider relationship as method of influencing, 461
   consumerism, as method of influencing, 461
   default, as method of influencing, 461

behavior, human (*cont.*)
  motivation. *See* motivation
  mutuality, as method of influencing, 461
  paternalism, as method of influencing, 461
  value systems, 453, 454–456
Bis-GMA, 12, 288–290, 306, 308. *See also* pit-and-fissure
    sealants
Black, G. V., 46, 184, 469
bleeding gums. *See also* gingivitis
  dental consult for, 85
  prevalence, 470–471
  self-diagnosis of, 449–450
blind patients. *See* visually-impaired patients, dental care
    for
Bloom's taxonomy of educational objectives, 453
BMI. *See* Body Mass Index
Body Mass Index, 422, 423t
body wraps, 571–572
bone density, 438
bone loss, silent, 368
breast-fed babies, with caries. *See* infants
Bright Futures program, 539
bulimia, 436–437
Buonocore, 288

calcium bridging, 28
calcium fluoride, 63, 64
calcium fluorides. *See* fluorides
calcium, caries protection of, 432
calculus
  alkaline conditions, role of, 35
  as last stage in dental plaque maturation, 33–34
  attachment to teeth, 36
  dentifrices to control, 130
  inhibiting formation, 36
  supraginigival, 34, 35
  systemic conditions affecting, 34
calorie deficiency, 427
cancer
  dental intervention, 617
  head, 613
  mouth, link to mouthwash, 132
  mucositis, 615–616
  neck, 613
  nutritional status of patients, 438–439
  oral. *See* oral cancer
  osteoradionecrosis. *See* osteoradionecrosis
  pharyngeal. *See* pharyngeal cancer
  prevention, 613–614
  skin, 613–614
  smoking, relationship between, 2
  tanning devices, associated with, 613–614
  throat, link to mouthwash, 132
  tobacco use, associated with, 613. *See also* tobacco use
Candida albicans, 358
carbohydrates, dietary. *See also* sugar

caries development, role in, 15, 430–432
  dietary counteractions to, 430
  intake, 666
  liquid vs. solid and caries development, 432
cardiovascular disease
  appointments for patients with, 622–623
  emergencies, office, related to, 622, 623
  ESRD anemia, related to, 627–628
  in aged patients, 594
  overview, 621–622
  stress management of patients, 622
caries. *See also* plaque
  -activity indicators, 662, 664
  activity of, 341–342
  activity tests, 358–359
  activity tests, dental-office, 350–358
  ages of interest for risk assessment, 345
  as oral disease classification, 5
  as public health problem, 3
  as transmissable disease, 6
  background factors affecting development of, 348–349
  bacterial values, relationship between, 354–355
  clinical examination for evaluating, 349–350
  coronal dentin, 59–60, 325
  cost, to U.S., of treating, 6
  decline in prevalence, 485–486
  definition, 337
  etiology, complexity of, 344
  in pits and fissures, 8, 46
  individual approach to risk assessment, 346–347
  lesion. *See* carious lesion
  prediction, 341–342, 343
  prevention counseling, 429–430
  process of, 6–7
  public dental health. *See* public dental health
  risk, 341–342, 343–344
  root. *See* root caries
  secondary/recurrent, 46, 61–62
  smooth-surface, 46–47
  transmission, 338–341
caries-activity indicators, 662, 664
Cariogram, 346–347
carious lesion. *See also* caries
  appearance of, clinical, 646
  bacterial plaque, connection to, 52–53
  diagnosis, early, difficulty of, 50
  miscroscopic features of, 50–51
  physical features of, 50–51
  zones, 52
cataracts, 594
cavities, definition, 46
cementum, 76
Centers for Medicare and Medical Services, 481
cerebral palsy, dental care for patients with,
    565–566
chemiscoparasitic theory, 46

chemotherapy, diet advice during, 429. *See also* cancer

chewing gum. *See* gum, chewing

children. *See also* infants
  age at initiation of topical fluoride therapy, 260
  ages at highest risk for caries, 345
  anticipatory guidance, 513
  between-meal snacks, 431
  caries prevalence, 2
  Children's Dental Health Month, 531
  dental illnesses, impact on schooling, 2
  dentist visits, percent without prior to kindergarten, 2
  diet management, 511
  early childhood caries, 505–504
  examination, dental, 511–513
  fillings, rates of, 2
  flora of, as reflection of mother's flora, 12, 25, 338–339
  fluoride rinse programs in schools, 203, 267
  fluoride rinse use home, 267
  fluoride supplementation, 509
  Head Start oral health programs. *See* Head Start
  infection routes for caries-related bacteria, 338–339
  interview of parents, 508–510
  mutans streptococcus, prevalence related to age, 339
  oral care, 510
  parental brushing of teeth, 112
  prevention of caries, 506
  public attitudes toward dental care in, 507
  recall schedule, 513
  school-based dental health education. *See* school-based
    dental education
  screening for dental care, 507
  sugar intake reduction, 357
  toothpaste ingestion, 264, 272
  topical fluoride applications, 249–252, 254, 256. *See also*
    fluorides
  varnish use for very young, 259

Children's Dental Health Month, 531

chlorhexadine
  as primary preventive care for periodontitis, 371,
    660–661
  bacteria suppression, 10, 12
  plaque control, role in, 9, 133–134
  side effects, 133–134

Chong, Dennis, 207

Churchill, H. V., 184, 469

cleft lip/palate
  prevalence, 471, 617
  surgical closure, 617–618
  vitamin supplements, possible protective effects of, 617

cognitively impaired patients, dental care for, 564–565

Colgate MFP, 263

Colgate Total, 129–130

Committee on the Medical Aspects of Food Policy, 404

communication, between dental professional and client,
  461

Community Periodontal Index of Treatment Need, 475

Community Periodontal Index of Treatment Needs, 381

community risk assessment, caries, 343–344, 345

compromised patients. *See also* specific handicap or problem
  body wraps, 571–572
  chemical plaque control, 580
  dietary considerations, 578
  disclosing agents, 574–575
  elbow stabilizers, 571
  fluorides use, 578–580
  headrests for, 570–571
  implant care, 580
  institutionalized care, 581–582
  limb stabilizers, 571–572
  mouth props, 571
  mouth props for, 569–570
  preventive maintenance, 580–581
  provider availability, 581
  reward systems, 578
  sealant use, 578–580
  ties, soft, 571
  toothbrushes, powered, 574–575
  toothbrushing, 565–567

computers, use in dentistry, 649–651

Concise Sealant, 3, 299

consumerism, 461

corn syrup. *See* high-fructose corn syrup

coronal caries, 325

counseling, patient, 462–463

CPITN. *See* Community Periodontal Index of Treatment
  Needs

craniofacial disorders. *See also* cleft lip/palate
  as oral disease problem, 5–6
  prevalence, 471

Crest Extra Whitening, 131–132

Crest family of products, 263–264

Crohn's diseas e, 647

cyclamate, 412

deaf patients. *See* hearing-impaired patients, dental care for

Dean, H. Trendley, 185, 192

defluoridation, 198–199. *See also* fluoridation

demineralization. *See also* remineralization
  acid-induced, 16, 63
  caries, role in, 338, 340–341
  crystal size, 331
  fluoride, impact of, 329

Dental Department, of hospital. *See* hospital setting, preventive dentistry in

dental education. *See also* school-based dental health education
  importance of, 667–668
  of parents, regarding children's care, 510
  primary preventive dentistry, as component of,
    451

dental exam. *See* examination, dental

dental floss
  brand differences, 150
  dental tape, 149–150
  holder for, 154–155
  holder for, with compromised patients, 575–576
  knitting yarn used as, 162
  methods, 150–151, 153–154
  objectives of use, 149
  threaders, 155–156
  unwaxed, 149
  wax, 149
dental hygienist, role of, 451, 666–667
dental insurance
  lack of, impact on dental health, 3, 450
dental professionals, client behavior, influence on, 451
dental visits, 450. *See also* examination, dental
dentifrices
  abrasives, 124–125
  anticalculus, 130
  antisensitivity products, 131
  baking soda, 127
  definition, 123
  detergents, 126
  essential oil, 127
  FDA regulation of, 122
  flavoring agents, 126
  flourides in, 9–10, 188–190, 262–265
  high-fluoride, prescription-strength, 61
  humectants, 125–126
  ingredients, 124
  market, in dollars of sales, 123
  non-foaming, ingestible, 568
  packaging, 124
  soaps, 126
  sweetening agents, 127
  therapeutic, 127–128
  whiteners. *See* whiteners
dentist's rights, 620–621
dentures
  bacterial colonization, 169
  brushing, 111, 169
  cleaning, 169
  compromised patients, hygiene with, 576–577
  dietary guidance, 429
  fungal colonization, 169
  immersion cleaners, 169–170
  self-care instructions, 169–170
  soft tissue care, 169
  swallowing ability changes, 437
  taste changes, 437
Department of Health and Human Services, 480–482
diabetes mellitus
  appointment objectives, 632–633
  bi-directional etiology, 631–632
  caries in patients with, 632
  caries risk, 647

  CPITN score, 631
  cure, potentials for, 633–634
  emergencies related to, 633
  nutrition care plan, 438
  oral health, relationship between, 369
  oral infections, 438
  overview, 630
  Type 1, 630
  Type 2, 630–631
diet. *See also* Food Guide Pyramid; nutrition
  assessment by dental team, 421
  caries development, inhibition of, 432
  cariogenic, 429, 433
  children's/toddler's, considerations regarding, 511
  couseling by dental team, 421, 429–430
  definition, 523
  early studies of cariogenic effects of, 54
  eating disorders. *See* eating disorders
  education on, in schools, 532–533
  food labels. *See* food labels
  oral health, relationship between, 419–420
  retention of food on teeth, 432
  role in caries resistance, 11, 15
  sequence of foods eaten, 432
Dietary Guidelines for Americans, 421–422
Dietary Reference Intakes, 421
digitized X-ray, 651–652
disaccharides, 399
disclosing techniques, 578
disease, dental. *See also* gingivitis; periodontal disease; periodontitis; plaque disease
  as common reason for rejection of draftees in wartime, 468
  historical overview, 468–469
DNA analysis of periodontopathogens, 382
Down's syndrome, oral health, relationship between, 369
dry mouth. *See* xerostomia

eating disorders, 436–437
education, dental. *See* dental education
elbow stabilizers, 571
Elders, M. Jocelyn, 467
emergencies, office, 622, 623, 633
enamel. *See also* demineralization; remineralization
  composition, 47
  embryology, 47, 48–49
  histology, 47, 48–49
  inorganic phase, 325
  mineralization, 325
  spindles, 58
enameloplasty, 286
ESRD anemia, 627–630
Evans, Caswell A., 490
examination, dental
  computer support of, 649–651

digitized X-ray, 651–652
explorer misdiagnosis/misuse, 652–654
initial/annual, 647–649
intraoral video camera, 651–652
recall appointments, 665–666
extraction, as result of periodontitis, 85

FHA. *See* fluorhydroxyapatite
floss, dental. *See* dental floss
fluorhydroxyapatite, 63, 64, 245
fluoridation. *See also* fluorides
    antifluoridation groups, 192–193, 203, 207, 216–222
    as public health policy, 183, 203–205, 484–485
    as public health success, 469–470
    benefits, 188–190
    costs of, 193–194, 196
    definition, 182, 183
    defluoridation, 198–199
    demographics served by, 206–207
    dentists/hygienists, involvement in promoting, 215–216
    diffusion effect, 190
    discontinuation, 193
    educating public about, 208
    effectiveness, 188–190
    efficacy, 183
    engineering aspects of, 200–201
    Fluoridation Census, 186–187
    fluorosis. *See* fluorosis
    fundraising for, 208–209
    historical overview, 184–188
    levels, optimal, 196–197, 201–202
    mechanisms of action, 190–191
    media, role of in forming public opinion and policy,
        210–212
    monitoring, 201–202
    myths, 224–225
    of school water, 541–542
    prevalence in United States, 10
    public perception of, 209–210
    referenda, 205–206
    remineralization process, relationship between, 247
    risk communication, 222–226
    safety, 183, 197–200
    surveillance, 201–202
    technology transfer phase, 187–188
    voter turnout/apathy, 212–215
    Year 2010 Health Objectives for the Nation, 186, 206
fluorides. *See also* fluoridation
    acidulated phosphate, 249
    actions, key, 11
    advantages of topical applications, 260–261
    age at initiation of topical therapy, 260
    application period, 259
    application procedure for gels, 252–253
    application procedure for topical, 249–252
    bacterial metabolism, effect on, 247–248

calcium, 244
chronic exposure, 271–272
compromised patients, use in, 578–580
dietary supplements, 10
dietary tablets, 542
disadvantages of topical applications, 260–261
education on, in schools, 532
effectiveness, 188–190
efficacy of topical application, 255–257
emergency treatment following poisoning, 271–272
frequency of application of topical forms, 253–255
gels for home use, 268–269
home storage security of products containing, 272
in dental restorative materials, 269
in water. *See* fluoridation
ineffectiveness in occlusal surfaces, 286
ineffectiveness of single topical treatment, 259
ingestion, 270–271
Knutson technique of application, 254
mechanism of action of topical applications, 242–247
milk fluoridation, 203
mouthrinses, 134–135, 203, 266–268
multiple therapies, 265–266
overview of use, 9–10
plaque, effect on, 247–248
prophylactic pastes, 261
remineralization and, 658–659
rinses, 542
sealants, added to, 290
sodium, 248
stannous, 248–249, 330, 371
stannous salts, 129, 202, 244
supplementation, in children, 509
topical applications, 10
toxicity, 271
toxicology of, 269–271
varnishes. *See* varnishes
fluorosis, 191–193, 264
Food and Drug Administration, 481
    regulation of new products and foods, 403
    regulation of oral chemotherapeutic agents, 121–122
    Sugar Task Force, 404
Food Guide Pyramid, 422, 424
food labels, 425–426
Foods Additive Amendment, 403–404
FRAMES method of counseling, 462–463
fructose, 408
fructose intolerance, 406

gauze strip, used to clean proximal areas, 162–163
geriatric dental care. *See* aging
gingiva, healthy, 370
gingival crevicular fluid, 383–384
gingival disease, rates among adults, 2
Gingival Index, 475
Gingival Index of Loe and Silness, 376

gingival lesion, 80–82, 82
gingival recession, 25
  description, 380
  measurement, 380
gingival sulcus, 7, 77, 79–80, 81
gingivitis
  as precursor to periodontitis, 82
  curing, 370
  definition, 369
  fluoride, effect of, 248
  inflammation, and frequency of plaque removal, 148
  prevalence, 74, 370–371
  public dental health. *See* public dental health
  treatment guidelines, noninvasive, 371
glass-ionomer sealants, 303–304
glucosyl-transferase, 28, 56–57
gum, chewing
  beneficial effects, 135
  prolonged delivery of agent, 120, 135
  sodium bicarbonate-based, 135–136
  sorbital-based, 135
  xylitol-based, 12, 135
gums, bleeding. *See* bleeding gums

Haim-Munk, 369
halitosis
  causes, 132–133
  gum for, 136
  mouthrinses for, 133
  problems causes by, seriousness of, 133
  tongue, role of, 164–165
HAP. *See* hydroxyapatite
Head Start, 538–539
headrests, 570–571
Health Belief Model, 456, 457
health literacy, definition of, 523
Healthy People 2010, 450, 527, 535
Healthy People in Healthy Communities, 467–468
hearing-impaired patients, dental care for, 562–563, 594–595
high-fructose corn syrup, 400–401, 407–408
HIV/AIDS
  dentist's rights, 620–621
  false link to fluoridation, 218–219
  nutritional status of patients, 438–439
  oral condition arising from, 5
  oral infections associated with, 619–620
  overview of disease process, 619
  patient's rights, 620–621
  periodontal infections, acute, 620
Hopewood House, 405
hospital setting, preventive dentistry in
  accreditation, 608–609
  administrative requirements, 608
  cancer patients, 613–617
  Dental Department, 609–612

overview, 606–607
  patients, dental needs of, 607–608
  regulations, 608–609
  xerostomia, 612–613
human behavior. *See* behavior, human
Human Genome Project, 75–76, 382
hydroxyapatite, 63, 64
hypertension. *See* cardiovascular disease

immune system
  aging, changes associated with, 595–596
  compromised patients, nutritional health of, 438–439
  compromised patients, oral health of, 438–439
  defenses from plaque, 83–84
  preventive dental approaches, 620, 670–671
  role in caries development, 670–671
  vaccine for caries, future possibilities for, 382–383
implants
  bacterial flora and, 373
  brushing techniques with, 167
  care, periodontal, 373
  flossing with, 167
  maintenance, importance of, 166
  oral hygiene, poor, as contributor to, 166–167
  oral irrigators with, 167
infants. *See also* children
  advantages of early oral care, 508
  anticipatory guidance, 513
  baby bottle decay, 434, 505–506
  breast-fed, with caries, 506
  caries, severe, 434
  diet management, 511
  examination, dental, 511–513
  future caries risk, in infants with severe decay, 435
  interview of parents, 508–510
  mutans streptococcus, growth during teething, 57
  nursing caries, 505
  oral care, 507, 508, 510
  recall schedule, 513
  risk factors for caries, 434
  suckling habits, 506
  taste preferences at birth, 400
informed consent, 4
injuries, head/facial/teeth, 471–472
institutionalized settings, dental care in, 581–582
InterPlak powered toothbrush, 102
interproximal brushes, 159–161, 576
intraoral videocamera, 651–652
irrigation devices, 165–166

junctional epithelium, 77–78, 85

knitting yarn, used as floss, 162
Knutson technique of fluoride application, 254
Koop, C. Everett, 183

lactobacilli
    acid, role in, 324
    caries, role in development, 55, 56, 338
    counts, testing, 353–354, 357
    diet, relationship to, 350
    dip slide method of testing, 354
lactose, 408
Lee, Philip R., 467
Leonard's toothbrushing technique, 106
limb stabilizers, 571–572
lipids and food particle clearance, relationship between, 432
Listerine. *See also* mouthrinses
    as primary preventive care for periodontitis, 371
    plaque control, role in, 9

malnutrition, 426–427. *See also* nutrition
maltose, 408
mannitol, 409
manual toothbrushes. *See* toothbrushes, manual
materia alba, 28
maternal oral health, 502–503
McKay, Frederick, 184, 469
medications, xerostomia-causing. *See* xerostomia
Mentadent, 128
Metropolitan Life Insurance Company epidemiological studies, 468–469
milk fluoridation, 203
Miller, W. D., 46
minerals, dietary, 427–428
monosaccharides, 399
motivation
    Bloom's taxonomy of educational objectives. *See* Bloom's taxonomy of educational objectives
    complexity of, 452
    description/definition, 452
    interviewing. *See* motivational interviewing
    varying levels, on part of client, strategies for approaching, 460
motivational interviewing, 461–462
mouth props, 569–570, 571
mouthguards, 537–538
mouthrinses
    ADA approved, 120
    alcohol-containing, 132
    child-safety caps, 132
    essential oils, 134
    flouride, 9–10
    fluoride, 134–135, 203, 266–268, 542
    halitosis, combating. *See* halitosis
    market share, U.S., 132
    plaque control, role in, 9
    therapeutic, 133–135
muco-gingival junction, 79
mucositis, 615–616

multiple sclerosis, 563
mutans streptococcus
    adherence to saliva, 323
    adherence to tooth surface, 56–57
    as infectious disease, 503–504
    bacterial challenge test, 350
    caries, role in development, 55–56, 338, 407
    chlorhexadine, suppression by, 12
    count, lab test for, 15
    counts, 351–352
    growth, in teething babies, 57
    immune system, relationship between, 670–671
    mother-child transmission, 503–504
    prevalence, increase with age, 339
    saliva, presence in, 351–352
    Strip mutans technique for testing, 352–353

National Institute for Dental and Craniofacial Research, 482
National Institutes of Health, 481–482
Novello, Antonia, 183
NuPro, 295
NutraSweet, 12
nutrition. *See also* diet
    definition, 523
    eating disorders. *See* eating disorders
    education on, in schools, 532–533
    in aging patients. *See* aging
    in diabetic patients. *See* diabetes mellitus
    minerals, 427–428
    oral tissues, relationship between, 426–429
    periodontal disease, relationship between, 435–436
    vitamins, 428–429
Nutrition Facts panel, 425–426
Nuva-Cote, 290–291
Nuva-Seal, 290–291

O'Leary's Index, 374–375
octacalcium phosphate, 49
oral cancer. *See also* cancer
    as public health problem, 471
    chewing tobacco link, 2
    patient profile, 614
    rates among older adults, 2, 598–599
    school-based education on, 534
    smoking, relationship between, 384
    treatment, 615
oral health
    health overall, relationship to, 450
    national objectives, 487–489
    self-care, 147–148
    self-diagnosis, 449–450
    trends affecting, 489
Oral Hygiene Index, 375–376
oral hygiene aides, for compromised patients, 577
oral prophylaxis. *See* prophylaxis, oral

oral surgery, nutritional considerations following, 439
Oral-Hygiene Index-Simplified, 475
orthodontic appliances, brushing of, 111
orthotic appliances, 566
osteoradionecrosis, 616–617

Page, Roy, 76
Pan American Health Organization, 480
Papillon- Le Fevre, 369
Parkinson's disease, 563
paternalism, 461
patient education. *See* dental education
patient's rights, 620–621
peri-implantitis, 373
perikymata, 36
periodontal disease. *See also* gingivitis; periodontitis; plaque
    disease
    as oral disease classification, 5
    as transmissable disease, 5
    bleeding index, 374, 376
    cost, to U.S., of treating, 5
    indicators, 373–374
    microflora, 82
    predicting, impossibility of, 76
    prevalence, U.S., 75
    prevention, primary, 659–662
    public dental health. *See* public dental health
    rates among adults, 2
    risk factors, 369
    theories of, 368–369
Periodontal Index, 475
periodontal ligament, 76
periodontal pocket, 78. *See also* periodontal disease
    as sign of periodontal disease, 368
    depth, as determined by probes, 379
    plaque, in deepening, 82–83
    surgery needed, 86
periodontal probes
    caution during usage, 377
    electronic, 377–379
    purpose of usage, 379–380
    variations, 377
Periodontal Screening and Recording System, 381–382
periodontal surgery, 86, 372–373
periodontal-activity indicators, 659–660, 662, 664
periodontitis. *See also* periodontal disease
    biodirectional synergism with systemic diseases, 74
    control of, 74
    definition, 369–370
    dental treatment, focus of, 85–86
    gingivitis, role of, 82–83
    invasive treatments, 371–372
    irreversible nature of, 7
    preventive care, noninvasive, primary, 371
    refractory, 385

    smoking, relationship to, 385. *See also* smoking
    surgery for. *See* periodontal surgery
periodontium, 76–78
periodontopathogens, 9, 382
pH
    changes after eating, 62, 432
    fluorides, responses to, 243
    measurement tests, 358, 433
    saturation, relationship between, 62
    simple sugars, responses to, 62
pharyngeal cancer. *See also* cancer
    as public dental health issue, 471
    older adults, rates among, 2
    relationship to smoking, 2
phenytoin, dental consequences of taking, 82
phosphorus, caries protection of, 432
pilin, 29–30
pit-and-fissure sealants, 12–13
    adhesive potential, 294
    American Dental Association ADA standards,
        288–289
    application, 298
    carious areas, placing over, 300–302
    colored vs. clear, 300
    cost-benefit, 287, 543–544
    criteria for tooth selection for placement, 287–288
    dentist involvement, 307
    depth of, 295
    development background, 288
    dryness, importance of, 296–298
    economics of, 305–306
    education on, in schools, 532
    fluoride-releasing, 290
    glass-ionomer sealants, 303–304
    in compromised patients, 578–579
    introduction of, 286–287
    light source, high-intensity, 291, 294
    light-cured, 291
    manpower required, 305
    occlusal and interproximal discrepancies, 298
    overview of usage, 654–655
    polymerization, 290–291
    preventive package, as one part of, 305
    retention of, 299–300, 303
    retention of, requisites for, 294
    self-cured, 291
    surface area, increasing the, 294–295
    surface cleaning prior to applying, 295
    tooth preparation, 295–296
    vs. amalgams, 302–303
    Year 2010 Health Objectives for the Nation, 306–307
pits and fissures
    caries, 286, 300–302
    depth, 295
    options for protecting occlusal surfaces, 303–304, 308

plaque removal from, inadequacy of, 8
sealants. *See* pit-and-fissure sealants
plaque. *See also* caries; carious lesion; plaque disease
    acquired pellicle. *See* acquired pellicle
    as microbial biofilm, 25
    bacterial adhesion, 28–30
    bacterial colonization, 25–26
    calculus. *See* calculus
    colonizers, bacterial, 30–31
    compartment, 323–324
    disclosing agents, 578
    fluoride, effect of. *See* fluorides
    formation, 27–28
    forming rate, test for, 358
    Gingival Index of Loe and Silness, 376
    Index. *See* Plaque Index
    matrix, 31–32
    measurement, 374–376
    metabolism, 32–33
    O'Leary's Index, 374–375
    Oral Hygiene Index, 375–376
    pallisades, 31
    physical characteristics of, 324
    removal, 148–149
    Silness and Loe Index, 375
    water rinsing to loosen, 165
plaque disease. *See also* periodontal disease; plaque
    bacteria, 24
    chemical control, 9, 85, 128–129, 580
    controlling, 7
    mechanical control, 9, 85
    mineralizing ions, role of, 9
    reformation after removal, 8
    strategies for combating, 7
    subgingval, 7, 83, 370
    supragingval, 7, 83, 370
Plaque Index, 475, 648
plastic sticks, for tooth cleaning, 157
plastic tip, for interproximal cleaning, 161–162
polyols, 409
poverty
    disparities in dental care, poor vs. non-poor, 522, 524
    impact on dental care, 3
powered toothbrushes. *See* toothbrushes, powered
predentin, 58
prenatal dental considerations, 502–503, 504
preventive dentistry
    in hospital setting. *See* hospital setting, preventive dentistry in
    lack of, impact on public health, 3
    primary, 4, 5, 659–662
    primary, role of in preventing periodontal disease, 85–86
    secondary, 4
    tertiary, 4, 5

probes, periodontal. *See* periodontal probes
prophylaxis, oral, 8
props, mouth. *See* mouth props
prosthesis hygiene, in compromised patients, 576–577
protein
    caries protection, 432
    deficiency, 427
public dental health. *See also* public dental health education
    caries, 470
    changing practices of, 486–490
    concerns of public and professionals, emerging, 489–490
    diagnosis vs. analysis, 474–475, 478–479
    evaluation vs. appraisal, 477, 479–480
    examination vs. survey, 473–474, 478
    example program, 477–480
    for special population groups, 485, 489
    gingivitis, 470–471
    health education services, 484
    health promotion services, 483
    indexes, dental, 475–476
    injuries, 471–472
    levels of operation, 480–483
    oral cancer, 471
    oral health objectives, national, 487–489
    overview, 472
    overview of current situation, 470–472
    payment for services vs. financing, 476–477, 479
    periodontal diseases, 470–471
    pharyngeal cancer, 471
    Surgeon General's Report, 490–491
    treatment planning vs. program planning, 476, 479
    treatment vs. program operation, 476, 479
    trends affecting, 489
public dental health education. *See also* public dental health
    lack of, in schools. *See* school-based dental health education
    overview, 13–14
    population vs. number of dentists, 14
pyorrhea alvolaris, 368

radiation, diet advice during, 429
radiographs, assessment of remineralization, 656–657
range-of-motion assessment, 566–567
Recommended Dietary Allowances, 421, 426
remineralization. *See also* demineralization
    as short-term defense to food abrasion, 655
    crystal size, 331
    definition, 329
    depth of, 64
    equilibrum with demineralization, 329
    fluoride, impact of, 329
    fluorides and, 658–659
    from fluoride mechanism, 247

remineralization (*cont.*)
  ions, role of, 63
  of root caries lesion, 657–658
  overview, 16, 655–656
  radiograph evidence, 656–657
  repair process, 329–330
  saliva, role of. *See* saliva
renal disease, dental care for patients with,
    626–627
Riggs' disease, 368
rights, dentist's, 620–621
rights, patient's, 620–621
root caries, 46. *See also* caries
  prevalence, 60, 258
  prevention, 60–61, 258
  remineralization of, 657–658
  risk factors for development, 60
  topical fluoride applications to prevent, 258
  vs. coronal caries, 60
rubber tip, for interproximal cleaning, 161–162

S. mutans. *See* mutans streptococcus
saccharin, 410–411
saliva. *See also* xerostomia
  buffering capacity of, 356
  calculus formation, role in, 34
  derivation of, 320
  dip slide measurement of yeast, 358
  flow rate, 321–322, 355–356, 648
  flushing function, 321
  functions of, 321, 323
  glands, 320–321
  in malnourished persons, 427
  lubrication function, 321
  plaque compartment. *See* plaque
  re- and demineralization role, 321
  remineralization role, 11
  samples, collecting, 356–357
  sialorrhea, 322
  stimulants, 612–613
  stimulation of, 322
  Strip mutans technique for testing, 352–353
  substitutes, 612–613
  suppression of, 322
  tests, to determine caries risk, 351–352
  viscosity test, 358
  whole, 321
Satcher, David, 184, 490
school-based dental health education. *See also* dental edu-
    cation
  approaches to, 530–531
  classroom toothbrushing, 533–534
  clinics, school-based, 527–528, 540
  comprehensive programs, 540–544
  cost-effectiveness, 546
  definition, 523

  diet, teaching on, 532–533
  dietary fluoride tablets, 542
  disparities in, poor vs. non-poor, 522, 524
  during 1930s, 525
  during 1940s, 525
  during 1950s, 525
  during 1960s, 525
  early twentieth-century, 525
  fluorides, teaching on, 532
  in foreign countries, 544–546
  lack of, in majority of schools, 14
  Level 1 programs, 541–542
  Level 2 programs, 543–544
  Level 3 programs, 543–544
  New Zealand School Dental Service, 15
  nutrition, teaching on, 532–533
  oral cancer prevention training, 534
  planning, as key component, 529
  preschool programs, 538–539
  principles of education, 530
  research and evaluation, 546
  responsibility for teaching, 524
  sealants, teaching on, 532
  smoking, instruction on avoidance. *See* smoking
  sports, preventive dentistry in, 537–538
  student participation, 531
  Tattletooth II Integrated Program, 539–540
  teacher education/training, 539–540
  teacher knowledge, 529–530
  tobacco use, instruction on avoidance. *See* tobacco use
  twenty-first century initiatives, 527
  vending machine removal, 533
  volunteerism, among dental professionals, 525
  water fluoridation, school, 541–542
scurvy, 428–429
SDAT. *See* Alzheimer's disease
sealants, pit-and-fissure. *See* pit-and-fissure sealants
senile dementia of Alzheimer's type. *See* Alzheimer's dis-
    ease
Sensodyne F, 131
Seven-step Model for Assessing Oral Health Needs,
    473–474
Shalala, Donna, 490–491
Sharpey's fibers, 36
sialoliths, 322
sialorrhea. *See* saliva
silent bone loss. *See* bone loss, silent
Silness and Loe plaque index, 375
SLS. *See* sodium lauryl sulfate
smoking. *See also* cancer; tobacco use
  cessation and recovery, 385–386
  in youths, 522
  peridontal and other diseases, relation to, 2, 374,
    384–385
  refusal skills, for children, 535
  school-based education on, 534–535, 537

Snyder test, 358
Social Cognitive Theory, 456, 457–458
sodium lauryl sulfate, 126
soidum monoflurophosphate, 246
sorbitol, 409
speech and language disorders, patients with, 563–564
speech, teeth, role of, 3
Spelnda, 12
sports, preventive dentistry, 537–538
Stages of Change Model, 458–460
stannous salts. *See* fluorides
Stephan Curve, 62
Stillman's toothbrushing technique, 106
subsurface pellicle, 26
sucralose, 410, 412
sucrose
    caries formation, role in, 56–57, 351, 404–407, 430–431
    consumption rates, 402
    disadvantages in industrial use, 403
    health aspects, 403–404
    in between-meal snacks, 406
    prevalence of use, 402
    usage, 402–403
sugar. *See also* sucrose; sugar substitutes; sweeteners
    caries development, role in, 11–12, 430–431
    consistency of intake, 12
    frequency of intake, 12
    intake in industrialized countries, 431
sugar substitutes, 12. *See also* specific sugar substitutes
suprascrestal collagen fiber apparatus, 78–79
Surgeon General's Report on oral health, 490–491
Sweet 'n Low, 12
sweeteners. *See also* specific sweeteners; sucrose; sugar
    corn starch-based, 400
    corn syrup, 407–408
    historical overview of use, 400, 401
    intense, 410–412
    legislation governing use, 412–413
    nutritive vs. nonnutritive, 400
    overview of those in foods, 401t
    sweetness levels of various, 408–409

Tang dynasty, 94
taste, sensation of, 400
Tattletooth II Integrated Program, 539–540
teething, 57
Third National Health and Nutrition Examination Survey, 60
ties, soft, 571
tobacco use. *See also* cancer; oral cancer; smoking
    cancer source, as, 613
    chewing type and oral cancer link, 2
    peridontal and other diseases, relation to, 2, 374, 384–385
    school-based education on, 534–535, 537
    vs. non-tobacco users, in risk factors, 385

tongue
    black, hairy, 131, 384
    brushing, 110–111
    cleaners, 164
    halitosis, role in, 164–165
tooth compartment, 325–327
toothbrushes, manual. *See also* toothbrushes, powered; toothbrushing
    bristle, shapes, 96, 98, 100
    bristles, nylon vs. natural, 100–101
    handle designs, 100
    hardness/texture, 96, 100–101
    historical overview, 94–95
    modified handles, 572–574
    profiles, 96
    replacement pf brushes, 110
    sizes, 96
toothbrushes, powered. *See also* toothbrushes, manual; toothbrushing
    as aid for compromised patients, 574–575
    attachments for interproximal cleaning, 163
    bristle/design, 103
    brushing techniques with, 108
    efficiency, 104
    motivation for purchasing/using, 103–104
    overview, 102–103
    replacement pf brushes, 110
    safety, 104
    uses for, special, 112
toothbrushing. *See also* toothbrushes, manual; toothbrushes, powered
    anterior lingual surfaces, procedures for, 109
    Bass technique, 106–107
    clinical assessment of, 110
    for handicapped patients, 111–112
    for implants, 167
    frequency, 108–109
    in patients with functional disabilities, 565–567
    intructing patients in, 105
    Leonard's technique, 106
    modified techniques, 107–108
    natural methods, 106–107
    objectives, 105
    occlusal surfaces, procedures for, 109
    of abutment teeth, 111
    of tongue, 110–111
    or orthodontic appliances, 111
    powered toothbrushes, methods for, 108
    school-based training of children, 533–534
    sequence of brushing, 109–110
    Stillman's technique, 106
    time, 108–109
toothpicks
    historical use, 157–158
    holder for, 158–159
    usage, 158

Topex, 295
Toronto probe, 377–378
Total, Colgate, 129–130
Transtheoretical Model, 456, 458–460
Triclosan, 129–130

U.S. Department of Health and Human Services. *See* Department of Health and Human Services
U.S. Public Health Service survey of dental health, 469
uni-tufted brushes, 159–161
United States Pharmacopoeia Convention
    regulation of oral chemotherapeutic agents, 121

Vac-Ejector, 297–298
varnishes
    brands, 65
    effectiveness, 65
    efficacy, 259–260
    European usage, 64, 259
    fluoride-containing, 579
    usage, 64–65
veillonella, 324
Vipeholm study, 405–406, 432
visually-impaired patients, dental care for, 560–561, 594
vitamin A, 428
vitamin C, 428–429, 429
volunteerism, among dental professionals, 525

water fluoridation. *See* fluoridation

Water Pik Technologies, 105
White, J. D., 655–656
whiteners, 131
wood sticks, for tooth cleaning, 157
World Dental Federation, 480
wraps, body. *See* body wraps

X-ray, digitized, 651–652
xerostomia
    aging patients, 437
    causes, 322
    counseling for, 429
    diabetic patients, 632
    diagnosing, 322
    in eating-disordered patients, 437
    in hospitalized patients, 612–613
    medications causing, 647
    mouth rinses for, 133
xylitol
    composition of, 409
    gum, for minimization of mother-child transmission of dental flora, 12
    gum, plaque neutrality with, 135
    metabolic acid inhibition, 431
    noncariogenic properties, 409

yarn, knitting, used as floss, 162
yeast
    measurement of oral infection, 358
    overgrowth in HIV/AIDS patients, 619–620

# ENCYCLOPEDIA OF WORLD ART

## Vol. III
## CALDER – COSMOLOGY AND CARTOGRAPHY

# ENCICLOPEDIA
# UNIVERSALE
# DELL'ARTE

*Sotto gli auspici della Fondazione Giorgio Cini*

ISTITUTO PER LA COLLABORAZIONE CULTURALE
VENEZIA-ROMA

# ENCYCLOPEDIA
# OF
# WORLD ART

McGRAW-HILL BOOK COMPANY, INC.

NEW YORK, TORONTO, LONDON

ENCYCLOPEDIA OF WORLD ART

Paper for plates and text supplied by Cartiere Burgo, Turin — Engraving by Zincotipia Altimani, Milan — Black-and-white and color plates printed by Tipocolor, Florence — Text printed by "L'Impronta," Florence — Binding by Stabilimento Stianti, San Casciano Val di Pesa, Florence — Book cloth supplied by Kohorn Ltd., Egerton, near Bolton, England.

*Printed in Italy*

Library of Congress Catalog Card Number 59–13433
19456

# INTERNATIONAL COUNCIL OF SCHOLARS

Mario SALMI, University of Rome, President

Marcel AUBERT, Membre de l'Institut; Dean of Curators, Musées Nationaux, Paris, Vice President
Ernst KÜHNEL, Director, Islamic Section, Berlin Museum, Berlin-Dahlem, Vice President
Amedeo MAIURI, University of Naples; Sovrintendente alle Antichità della Campania, Vice President
Gisela M. A. RICHTER, Honorary Curator, Metropolitan Museum, New York, Vice President
Giuseppe TUCCI, University of Rome; President, Istituto Italiano per il Medio ed Estremo Oriente, Vice President

Alvar AALTO, Architect, Helsinki, Finland
Jean ALAZARD, University of Algiers
Andrew ALFÖLDI, University of Basel; Institute for Advanced Study, Princeton, N.J.
Carlo ANTI, University of Padua
Gilbert ARCHEY, Director, Auckland Institute and Museum, Auckland, New Zealand
A. S. ARDOJO, Jakarta, Indonesia
Bernard ASHMOLE, Oxford University
Jeannine AUBOYER, Curator, Musée Guimet, Paris
Ludwig BALDASS, formerly Director, Kunsthistorisches Museum, Vienna
Sir John D. BEAZLEY, formerly, Oxford University
† Bernard BERENSON
W. BLAWATSKY, University of Moscow
† Albert BOECKLER, late Staatsbibliothekar, Munich
Axel BOËTHIUS, formerly, University of Göteborg; Director, Swedish Institute, Rome
Helmut T. BOSSERT, University of Istanbul
Cesare BRANDI, Director, Istituto Centrale del Restauro, Rome
Henri BREUIL, Membre de l'Institut; Collège de France, Paris
Peter H. BRIEGER, University of Toronto
Joseph BURKE, University of Melbourne
A. W. BYVANCK, University of Leiden
Guido CALOGERO, University of Rome
Alfonso CASO, Escuela Nacional de Arqueología y Historia, Mexico City
Carlo CECCHELLI, University of Rome
Enrico CERULLI, Accademico dei Lincei, Rome
Jean CHARBONNEAUX, Curator in Chief, Musée du Louvre, Paris
Gino CHIERICI, formerly Superintendent of Monuments, Pavia
Fernando CHUECA Y GOITIA, Architect, Madrid
Sir Kenneth CLARK, Chairman, Arts Council of Great Britain, London
Giuseppe COCCHIARA, University of Palermo
George CŒDÈS, Honorary Director, Ecole Française d'Extrême-Orient, Paris
Paul COLLART, University of Geneva
W. G. CONSTABLE, formerly, Boston Museum of Fine Arts
Paolo D'ANCONA, University of Milan
† Sir Percival DAVID
Guglielmo DE ANGELIS D'OSSAT, Director General, Antichità e Belle Arti, Rome
Otto DEMUS, President, Bundesdenkmalamt, Vienna
Paul DESCHAMPS, Director, Musée des Monuments Français, Paris
R. DE VAUX, Director, Ecole Française, Jerusalem
Prince DHANINIVAT, President, Siam Society, Bangkok
Adrian DIGBY, Keeper of the Department of Ethnography, British Museum, London
Einar DYGGVE, Director, Ny Carlsberg Foundation, Copenhagen
Gustav ECKE, Curator of Chinese Art, Honolulu Academy of Arts; University of Hawaii
Vadime ELISSÉEFF, Curator, Musée Cernuschi, Paris
A. P. ELKIN, University of Sydney
Richard ETTINGHAUSEN, Freer Gallery of Art, Washington, D.C.
Bishr FARES, Institut d'Egypte, Cairo
† Paul FIERENS, late Curator in Chief, Musées Royaux des Beaux-Arts de Belgique, Brussels
Giuseppe FIOCCO, University of Padua; Director, Istituto di Storia dell'Arte, Venice
Pierre FRANCASTEL, Director, Ecole des Hautes Etudes, Paris
Giuseppe FURLANI, University of Rome
Albert GABRIEL, Director, Institut Français d'Archéologie, Istanbul
O. C. GANGOLY, Calcutta
Antonio GARCÍA Y BELLIDO, University of Madrid
Alberto GIUGANINO, Vice President, Istituto Italiano per il Medio ed Estremo Oriente, Rome
L. Carrington GOODRICH, Universities of Buenos Aires and Montevideo; Columbia University, New York

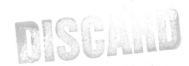

# ABBREVIATIONS

*Museums, Galleries, Libraries, and Other Institutions*

| | |
|---|---|
| Antikensamml. | — Antikensammlungen |
| Antiq. | — Antiquarium |
| Bib. Nat. | — Bibliothèque Nationale |
| Bib. Naz. | — Biblioteca Nazionale |
| Brera | — Pinacoteca di Brera |
| Br. Mus. | — British Museum |
| Cab. Méd. | — Cabinet des Médailles (Paris, Bibliothèque Nationale) |
| Cleve. Mus. | — Cleveland Museum |
| Coll. | — Collection, Collezione, etc. |
| Conserv. | — Palazzo dei Conservatori |
| Gal. | — Galerie |
| Gall. | — Gallery, Galleria |
| Gall. Arte Mod. | — Galleria di Arte Moderna |
| IsMEO | — Istituto Italiano per il Medio ed Estremo Oriente |
| Kunstgewerbemus. | — Kunstgewerbemuseum |
| Kunsthist. Mus. | — Kunsthistorisches Museum |
| Louvre | — Musée du Louvre |
| Medagl. | — Medagliere |
| Met. Mus. | — Metropolitan Museum |
| Mus. | — Museum, Museo, Musée, Museen, etc. |
| Mus. Ant. | — Museo di Antichità |
| Mus. Arch. | — Museo Archeologico |
| Mus. B. A. | — Musée des Beaux-Arts |
| Mus. Cap. | — Musei Capitolini |
| Mus. Civ. | — Museo Civico |
| Mus. Com. | — Museo Comunale |
| Mus. Etn. | — Museo Etnologico |
| Mus. Naz. | — Museo Nazionale |
| Mus. Vat. | — Musei Vaticani |
| Nat. Gall. | — National Gallery |
| Öst. Gal. | — Österreichische Galerie |
| Pin. | — Pinacoteca |
| Pin. Naz. | — Pinacoteca Nazionale |
| Pin. Vat. | — Pinacoteca Vaticana |
| Prado | — Museo del Prado |
| Rijksmus. | — Rijksmuseum |
| Samml. | — Sammlung |
| Staat. Mus. | — Staatliche Museen |
| Staatsbib. | — Staatsbibliothek |
| Städt. Mus. | — Städtisches Museum |
| Tate Gall. | — Tate Gallery |
| Uffizi | — Uffizi Gallery |
| Vict. and Alb. | — Victoria and Albert Museum |
| Villa Giulia | — Museo di Villa Giulia |

*Reviews and Miscellanies*

| | |
|---|---|
| AAE | — Archivio per la Antropologia e la Etnologia, Florence |
| AAnz | — Archäologischer Anzeiger, Berlin |
| AB | — Art Bulletin, New York |
| AbhAkMünchen | — Abhandlungen der Bayerischen Akademie der Wissenschaften, Munich |
| AbhBerlAk | — Abhandlungen der Berliner Akademie der Wissenschaften, Berlin |
| AbhPreussAk | — Abhandlungen der preussischen Akademie der Wissenschaften, Berlin |

| | |
|---|---|
| ABIA | — Annual Bibliography of Indian Archaeology, Leiden |
| AC | — Archeologia Classica, Rome |
| ActaA | — Acta Archaeologica, Copenhagen |
| ActaO | — Acta Orientalia, Leiden, The Hague |
| AD | — Antike Denkmäler, Deutsches Archäologisches Institut, Berlin, Leipzig |
| AEA | — Archivio Español de Arqueología, Madrid |
| AEArte | — Archivio Español de Arte, Madrid |
| AErt | — Archaeologiai Értesitö, Budapest |
| AfA | — Archiv für Anthropologie, Brunswick |
| AfO | — Archiv für Orientforschung, Berlin |
| AfrIt | — Africa Italiana, Bergamo |
| AJA | — American Journal of Archaeology, Baltimore |
| AM | — Mitteilungen des deutschen archäologischen Instituts, Athenische Abteilung, Athens, Stuttgart |
| AmA | — American Anthropologist, Menasha, Wis. |
| AmAnt | — American Antiquity, Menasha, Wis. |
| AN | — Art News, New York |
| AnnInst | — Annali dell'Instituto di Corrispondenza Archeologica, Rome |
| AnnSAntEg | — Annales du Service des Antiquités de l'Egypte, Cairo |
| AntC | — L'Antiquité Classique, Louvain |
| AntJ | — The Antiquaries Journal, London |
| AnzAlt | — Anzeiger für die Altertumswissenschaft, Innsbruck, Vienna |
| AnzÖAk | — Anzeiger der Österreichischen Akademie der Wissenschaften, Vienna |
| APAmM | — Anthropological Papers of the American Museum of Natural History, New York |
| AQ | — Art Quarterly, Detroit |
| ArndtBr | — P. Arndt, F. Bruckmann, Griechische und römische Porträts, Munich, 1891 ff. |
| ARSI | — Annual Report of the Smithsonian Institution, Bureau of Ethnology, Washington, D.C. |
| ArtiFig | — Arti Figurative, Rome |
| ASAtene | — Annuario della Scuola Archeologica Italiana di Atene, Bergamo |
| ASI | — Archivio Storico Italiano, Florence |
| ASWI | — Archaeological Survey of Western India, Hyderabad |
| AttiPontAcc | — Atti della Pontificia Accademia Romana di Archeologia, Rome |
| AZ | — Archäologische Zeitung, Berlin |
| BA | — Baessler Archiv, Leipzig, Berlin |
| BABsch | — Bulletin van de Vereeniging tot bevordering der kennis van de antieke Beschaving, The Hague |
| BAC | — Bulletin du Comité des Travaux Historiques et Scientifiques, Section d'Archéologie, Paris |
| BAcBelg | — Bulletin de l'Académie Royale de Belgique, Cl. des Lettres, Brussels |
| BACr | — Bollettino di Archeologia Cristiana, Rome |
| BAFr | — Bulletin de la Société Nationale des Antiquaires de France, Paris |
| BAmSOR | — Bulletin of the American Schools of Oriental Research, South Hadley, Mass. |
| BArte | — Bollettino d'Arte del Ministero della Pubblica Istruzione, Rome |

BByzI — The Bulletin of the Byzantine Institute, Paris

BCH — Bulletin de Correspondance Hellénique, Paris

BCom — Bollettino della Commissione Archeologica Comunale, Rome

Beazley, ABV — J. D. Beazley, Attic Black-figure Vase-painters, Oxford, 1956

Beazley, ARV — J. D. Beazley, Attic Red-figure Vase-painters, Oxford, 1942

Beazley, EVP — J. D. Beazley, Etruscan Vase-painting, Oxford, 1947

Beazley, VA — J. D. Beazley, Attic Red-figured Vases in American Museums, Cambridge, 1918

Beazley, VRS — J. D. Beazley, Attische Vasenmaler des rotfigurigen Stils, Tübingen, 1925

BEFEO — Bulletin de l'Ecole Française d'Extrême-Orient, Hanoi, Saigon, Paris

BerlNZ — Berliner Numismatische Zeitschrift, Berlin

Bernoulli, GI — J. J. Bernoulli, Griechische Ikonographie, Munich, 1901

Bernoulli, RI — J. J. Bernoulli, Römische Ikonographie, I, Stuttgart, 1882; II, 1, Berlin, Stuttgart, 1886; II, 2, Stuttgart, Berlin, Leipzig, 1891; II, 3, Stuttgart, Berlin, Leipzig, 1894

BHAcRoum — Bulletin Historique, Académie Roumaine, Bucharest

BIE — Bulletin de l'Institut de l'Egypte, Cairo

BIFAN — Bulletin de l'Institut Français d'Afrique Noire, Dakar

BIFAO — Bulletin de l'Institut Français d'Archéologie Orientale, Cairo

BInst — Bollettino dell'Instituto di Corrispondenza Archeologica, Rome

BJ — Bonner Jahrbücher, Bonn, Darmstadt

BM — Burlington Magazine, London

BMBeyrouth — Bulletin du Musée de Beyrouth, Beirut

BMC — British Museum, Catalogue of Greek Coins, London

BMCEmp — H. Mattingly, Coins of the Roman Empire in the British Museum, London

BMFA — Museum of Fine Arts, Bulletin, Boston

BMFEA — Museum of Far-Eastern Antiquities, Bulletin, Stockholm

BMImp — Bollettino del Museo dell'Impero, Rome

BMMA — Bulletin of the Metropolitan Museum of Art, New York

BMQ — The British Museum Quarterly, London

BPI — Bollettino di Paletnologia Italiana, Rome

BrBr — H. Brunn, F. Bruckmann, Denkmäler griechischer und römischer Skulptur, Munich

Brunn, GGK — H. Brunn, Geschichte der griechischen Künstler, 2d ed., Stuttgart, 1889

Brunn, GK — H. Brunn, Griechische Kunstgeschichte, Munich, I, 1893; II, 1897

BSA — Annual of the British School at Athens, London

BSEI — Bulletin de la Société des Etudes Indochinoises, Saigon

BSOAS — Bulletin of the School of Oriental and African Studies, London

BSPF — Bulletin de la Société Préhistorique Française, Paris

BSR — Papers of the British School at Rome, London

Cabrol-Leclercq — F. Cabrol, H. Leclercq, Dictionnaire d'archéologie chrétienne et de liturgie, Paris, 1907

CahA — Cahiers Archéologiques, Fin de l'Antiquité et Moyen-Age, Paris

CahArt — Cahiers d'art, Paris

CAJ — Central Asiatic Journal, Wiesbaden

CEFEO — Cahiers de l'Ecole Française d'Extrême-Orient, Paris

CIE — Corpus Inscriptionum Etruscarum, Lipsiae

CIG — Corpus Inscriptionum Graecarum, Berolini

CIL — Corpus Inscriptionum Latinarum, Berolini

CIS — Corpus Inscriptionum Semiticarum, Parisiis

Coh — H. Cohen, Description historique des Monnaies frappées sous l'Empire Romain, Paris

Collignon, SG — M. Collignon, Histoire de la sculpture grecque, Paris, I, 1892; II, 1897

Comm — Commentari, Florence, Rome

Cr — La Critica, Bari

CRAI — Comptes Rendus de l'Académie des Inscriptions et Belles-Lettres, Paris

CrArte — La Critica d'Arte Florence,

CVA — Corpus Vasorum Antiquorum

DA — N. Daremberg, N. Saglio, Dictionnaire des antiquités grecques et romaines, Paris, 1877–1912

Dehio, I-V — G. Dehio, Handbuch der deutschen Kunstdenkmäler, Berlin, I, Mitteldeutschland, 1927; II, Nordostdeutschland, 1926; III, Süddeutschland, 1933; IV, Südwestdeutschland, 1933; V, Nordwestdeutschland, 1928

Dehio, DtK — G. Dehio, Geschichte der deutschen Kunst, 4 vols., Berlin, 1930–34

Dehio-Von Bezold — G. Dehio, G. von Bezold, Die kirchliche Baukunst des Abendlandes, Stuttgart, 1892–1901

DissPontAcc — Dissertazioni della Pontificia Accademia Romana di Archeologia, Rome

EA — Photographische Einzelaufnahmen, Munich, 1893 ff.

EAA — Enciclopedia dell'Arte Antica, Rome, I, 1958; II, 1959

EArt — Eastern Art, London

EB — Encyclopaedia Britannica

EI — Enciclopedia Italiana, Rome, 1929 ff.

EphDR — Ephemeris Dacoromana, Rome

ESA — Eurasia Septentrionalis Antiqua, Helsinki

Espér — E. Espérandieu, R. Lantier, Recueil général des Bas-Reliefs de la Gaule Romaine, Paris

FA — Fasti Archaeologici, Florence

FD — Fouilles de Delphes, Paris

Friedländer — Max Friedländer, Altniederländische Malerei, Berlin, 1924–37

Furtwängler, AG — A. Furtwängler, Antiken Gemmen, Leipzig, Berlin, 1900

Furtwängler, BG — A. Furtwängler, Beschreibung der Glyptothek König Ludwig I zu München, Munich, 1900

Furtwängler, KlSchr — A. Furtwängler, Kleine Schriften, Munich, 1912

Furtwängler, MP — A. Furtwängler, Masterpieces of Greek Sculpture, London, 1895

Furtwängler, MW — A. Furtwängler, Meisterwerke der griechischen Plastik, Leipzig, Berlin, 1893

Furtwängler-Reichhold — A. Furtwängler, K. Reichhold, Griechische Vasenmalerei, Munich

GBA — Gazette des Beaux-Arts, Paris

GJ — The Geographical Journal, London

HA — Handbuch der Archäologie in Rahmen des Handbuchs der Altertumswissenschaft . . . herausgegeben von Walter Otto, Munich, 1939–53

HBr — P. Herrmann, F. Bruckmann, Denkmäler der Malerei des Altertums, Munich, 1907

Helbig-Amelung — W. Helbig, W. Amelung, E. Reisch, F. Weege, Führer durch die öffentlichen Sammlungen klassischer Altertümer in Rom, Leipzig, 1912–13

HJAS — Harvard Journal of Asiatic Studies, Cambridge, Mass.

Hoppin, Bf — J. C. Hoppin, A Handbook of Greek Black-figured Vases with a Chapter on the Red-figured Southern Italian Vases, Paris, 1924

Hoppin, Rf — J. C. Hoppin, A Handbook of Attic Red-figured Vases Signed by or Attributed to the Various Masters of the Sixth and Fifth Centuries b.c., Cambridge, 1919

HSAI — J. H. Steward, ed., Handbook of South American Indians, 6 vols., Bureau of American Ethnology, Bull. 143, Washington, D.C., 1946–50

IAE — Internationales Archiv für Ethnographie, Leiden

IBAI — Bulletin de l'Institut Archéologique Bulgare, Sofia

IG — Inscriptiones Graecae, Berolini

ILN — Illustrated London News, London

IPEK — Ipek, Jahrbuch für prähistorische und ethnographische Kunst, Berlin

| | | | |
|---|---|---|---|
| JA | — Journal Asiatique, Paris | NBACr | — Nuovo Bollettino di Archeologia Cristiana, Rome |
| JAF | — Journal of American Folklore, Lancaster, Pa. | NChr | — Numismatic Chronicle and Journal of the Royal Numismatic Society, London |
| JAOS | — Journal of the American Oriental Society, Baltimore | | |
| JAS | — Journal of the African Society, London | NIFAN | — Notes de l'Institut Français d'Afrique Noire, Dakar |
| JBORS | — Journal of the Bihar and Orissa Research Society, Patna, India | NR | — Numismatic Review, New York |
| JdI | — Jahrbuch des deutschen archäologischen Instituts, Berlin | NSc | — Notizie degli Scavi di Antichità, Rome |
| | | NZ | — Numismatische Zeitschrift, Vienna |
| JEA | — Journal of Egyptian Archaeology, London | OAZ | — Ostasiatische Zeitschrift, Vienna |
| JhbKhSammlWien | — Jahrbuch der kunsthistorischen Sammlungen in Wien, Vienna | ÖJh | — Jahreshefte des Österreichischen archäologischen Institut, Vienna |
| JhbPreussKSamml | — Jahrbuch der preussischen Kunstsammlungen, Berlin | ÖKT | — Österreichische Kunsttopographie, Vienna |
| | | OMLeiden | — Oudheidkundige Mededeelingen van het Rijksmuseum van Oudheten te Leiden, Leiden |
| JHS | — Journal of Hellenic Studies, London | | |
| JIAI | — Journal of Indian Art and Industry, London | | |
| JIAN | — Journal International d'Archéologie Numismatique, Athens | OpA | — Opuscola Archaeologica, Lund |
| | | Overbeck, SQ | — J. Overbeck, Die antiken Schriftquellen zur Geschichte der bildenden Künste bei den Griechen, Leipzig, 1869 |
| JISOA | — Journal of the India Society of Oriental Art, Calcutta | | |
| JNES | — Journal of Near Eastern Studies, Chicago | PEQ | — Palestine Exploration Quarterly, London |
| JPS | — Journal of the Polynesian Society, Wellington, New Zealand | Perrot-Chipiez | — G. Perrot, C. Chipiez, Histoire de l'art dans l'Antiquité, Paris, I, 1882; II, 1884; III, 1885; IV, 1887; V, 1890; VI, 1894; VII, 1898; VIII, 1903; IX, 1911 |
| JRAI | — Journal of the Royal Anthropological Institute of Great Britain and Ireland, London | | |
| | | Pfuhl | — E. Pfuhl, Malerei und Zeichnung der Griechen, Munich, 1923 |
| JRAS | — Journal of the Royal Asiatic Society, London | | |
| JRS | — Journal of Roman Studies, London | Picard | — C. Picard, Manuel d'Archéologie, La Sculpture, Paris, I, 1935; II, 1939; III, 1948; IV, 1, 1954 |
| JS | — Journal des Savants, Paris | | |
| JSA | — Journal de la Société des Africanistes, Paris | | |
| JSAm | — Journal de la Société des Americanistes, Paris | Porter | — A. Kingsley Porter, Romanesque Sculpture of the Pilgrimage Roads, Boston, 1923 |
| JSO | — Journal de la Société des Océanistes, Paris | | |
| Klein, GrK | — W. Klein, Geschichte der griechischen Kunst, Leipzig, 1904–07 | Post | — Charles Post, A History of Spanish Painting, 10 vols., Cambridge, Mass., 1930 ff. |
| KS | — Communications on the Reports and Field Research of the Institute of Material Culture, Moscow, Leningrad | ProcPrSoc | — Proceedings of the Prehistoric Society, Cambridge |
| | | PSI | — Pubblicazioni della Società Italiana per la ricerca dei papiri greci e latini in Egitto, Florence, 1912 ff. |
| Lippold, GP | — G. Lippold, Die griechische Plastik (W. Otto, Handbuch der Archäologie, III, 1), Munich, 1950 | | |
| | | QCr | — Quaderni della Critica, Bari |
| Löwy, IGB | — E. Löwy, Inschriften griechischer Bildhauer, Leipzig, 1885 | RA | — Revue Archéologique, Paris |
| | | RAA | — Revue des Arts Asiatiques, Paris |
| MAAccIt | — Monumenti Antichi dell'Accademia d'Italia, Milan | RACr | — Rivista di Archeologia Cristiana, Rome |
| | | RArte | — Rivista d'Arte, Florence |
| MAARome | — Memoirs of the American Academy in Rome, Rome, New York | RArts | — Revue des arts, Paris |
| | | RBib | — Revue Biblique, Paris |
| MAF | — Mémoires de la Société Nationale des Antiquaires de France, Paris | RDK | — Reallexicon zur deutschen Kunstgeschichte, Stuttgart, 1937 ff. |
| MAGWien | — Mitteilungen der anthropologischen Gesellschaft in Wien, Vienna | RE | — A. Pauly, G. Wissowa, Real-Enzyklopädie der klassischen Altertumswissenschaft, Stuttgart, 1894 ff. |
| Mâle, I | — E. Mâle, L'art religieux du XIIe siècle en France, Paris, 1928 | | |
| Mâle, II | — E. Mâle, L'art religieux du XIIIe siècle en France, Paris, 1925 | REA | — Revue des Etudes Anciennes, Bordeaux |
| | | REByz | — Revue des Etudes Byzantines, Paris |
| Mâle, III | — E. Mâle, L'art religieux de la fin du moyen-âge en France, Paris, 1925 | REG | — Revue des Etudes Grecques, Paris |
| | | Reinach, RP | — S. Reinach, Répertoire des Peintures Grecques et Romaines, Paris, 1922 |
| Mâle, IV | — E. Mâle, L'art religieux après le Concile de Trente, Paris, 1932 | | |
| | | Reinach, RR | — S. Reinach, Répertoire des Reliefs Grecs et Romains, Paris, I, 1909; II and III, 1912 |
| MALinc | — Monumenti Antichi dell'Accademia dei Lincei, Milan, Rome | | |
| Mattingly-Sydenham | — H. Mattingly, E. Sydenham, C. H. V. Sutherland, The Roman Imperial Coinage, London | Reinach, RS | — S. Reinach, Répertoire de la Statuaire Grecque et Romaine, Paris, I, 1897; II, 1, 1897; II, 2, 1898; III, 1904; IV, 1910 |
| | | Reinach, RV | — S. Reinach, Répertoire des Vases peints, grecs et étrusques, Paris, I, 1899; II, 1900 |
| MdI | — Mitteilungen des deutschen archäologischen Instituts, Munich | | |
| | | REL | — Revue des Etudes Latines, Paris |
| Mél | — Mélanges d'Archéologie et d'Histoire (Ecole Française de Rome), Paris | RendAccIt | — Rendiconti della R. Accademia d'Italia, Rome |
| | | RendLinc | — Rendiconti dell'Accademia dei Lincei, Rome |
| MemLinc | — Memorie dell'Accademia dei Lincei, Rome | RendNapoli | — Rendiconti dell'Accademia di Archeologia di Napoli, Naples |
| MGH | — Monumenta Germaniae Historica, Berlin | | |
| MIA | — Material and Research in Archaeology of the U.S.S.R., Moscow, Leningrad | RendPontAcc | — Rendiconti della Pontificia Accademia Romana di Archeologia, Rome |
| Michel | — A. Michel, Histoire de l'art depuis les premiers temps chrétiens jusqu'à nos jours, Paris, 1905–29 | RepfKw | — Repertorium für Kunstwissenschaft, Berlin, Stuttgart |
| | | REthn | — Revue d'Ethnographie, Paris |
| MInst | — Monumenti dell'Instituto di Corrispondenza Archeologica, Rome | RhMus | — Rheinisches Museum für Philologie, Frankfort on the Main |
| MLJ | — Modern Language Journal, St. Louis, Mo. | RIASA | — Rivista dell'Istituto d'Archeologia e Storia dell'Arte, Rome |
| MnbKw | — Monatsberichte über Kunstwissenschaft | | |
| MPA | — Monumenti della pittura antica scoperti in Italia, Rome | RIN | — Rivista Italiana di Numismatica, Rome |
| | | RLV | — M. Ebert, Real-Lexikon der Vorgeschichte, Berlin, 1924–32 |
| MPiot | — Fondation Eugène Piot, Monuments et Mémoires, Paris | | |
| | | RM | — Mitteilungen des deutschen archäologischen Instituts, Römische Abteilung, Berlin |
| MPontAcc | — Memorie della Pontificia Accademia Romana di Archeologia, Rome | | |
| | | RN | — Revue Numismatique, Paris |

| | |
|---|---|
| Robert, SR | — C. Robert, Die antiken Sarkophag-Reliefs, Berlin, 1890 ff. |
| Roscher | — W. H. Roscher, Ausführliches Lexikon der griechischen und römischen Mythologie, Leipzig, 1884–86; 1924–37 |
| RQ | — Römische Quartalschrift, Freiburg |
| RScPr | — Rivista di Scienze Preistoriche, Florence |
| RSLig | — Rivista di Studi Liguri, Bordighera, Italy |
| RSO | — Rivista degli Studi Orientali, Rome |
| Rumpf, MZ | — A. Rumpf, Malerei und Zeichnung (W. Otto, Handbuch der Archäologie, IV, 1), Munich, 1953 |
| SA | — Soviet Archaeology, Moscow, Leningrad |
| SbBerlin | — Sitzungsberichte der preussischen Akademie der Wissenschaften, Berlin |
| SbHeidelberg | — Sitzungsberichte der Akademie der Wissenschaften zu Heidelberg, Heidelberg |
| SbMünchen | — Sitzungsberichte der bayerischen Akademie der Wissenschaften zu München, Munich |
| SbWien | — Sitzungsberichte der Akademie der Wissenshaften in Wien, Vienna |
| Schlosser | — J. Schlosser, La letteratura artistica, Florence, 1956 |
| SEtr | — Studi Etruschi, Florence |
| SNR | — Sudan Notes and Records, Khartoum |
| SPA | — A Survey of Persian Art, ed. A. U. Pope and P. Ackerman, Oxford, 1938 |
| SymbOsl | — Symbolae Osloenses, Oslo |
| ThB | — U. Thieme, F. Becker, Künstler Lexikon, Leipzig, 1907–50 |
| TitAM | — Tituli Asiae Minoris, Vindobonae, 1901–44 |
| TNR | — Tanganyika Notes and Records, Dar-es-Salaam |
| Toesca, Md | — P. Toesca, Il Medioevo, 2 vols., Turin, 1927 |
| Toesca, Tr | — P. Toesca, Il Trecento, Turin, 1951 |
| TP | — T'oung Pao, Leiden |
| USMB | — United States National Museum, Bulletin, Washington, D.C. |
| Van Marle | — R. van Marle, The Development of the Italian Schools of Painting, The Hague, 1923–38 |
| Vasari | — G. Vasari, Vite, ed. Milanesi, Florence, 1878 ff. (Am. ed., trans. E. H. and E. W. Blashfield and A. A. Hopkins, 4 vols., New York, 1913) |
| Venturi | — A. Venturi, Storia dell'Arte Italiana, Milan, 1901 ff. |
| VFPA | — Viking Fund Publications in Anthropology, New York |
| Vollmer | — H. Vollmer, Allgemeines Lexikon der bildenden Künstler des XX. Jahrhunderts, Leipzig, 1953 |
| Warburg | — Journal of the Warburg and Courtauld Institutes, London |
| Wpr | — Winckelmannsprogramm, Berlin |
| WürzbJ | — Würzburger Jahrbücher für die Altertumswissenschaft, Würzburg |
| ZäS | — Zeitschrift für ägyptische Sprache und Altertumskunde, Berlin, Leipzig |
| ZfAssyr | — Zeitschrift für Assyriologie, Strasbourg |
| ZfBk | — Zeitschrift für bildende Kunst, Leipzig |
| ZfE | — Zeitschrift für Ethnologie, Berlin |
| ZfKg | — Zeitschrift für Kunstgeschichte, Munich |
| ZfKw | — Zeitschrift für Kunstwissenschaft, Munich |
| ZfN | — Zeitschrift für Numismatik, Berlin |
| ZfSAKg | — Zeitschrift für schweizerische Archäologie und Kunstgeschichte, Basel |
| ZMG | — Zeitschrift der morgenländischen Gesellschaft, Leipzig |

*Languages and Ethnological Descriptions*

| | |
|---|---|
| Alb. | — Albanian |
| Am. | — American |
| Ang. | — Anglice |
| Ar. | — Arabic |
| Arm. | — Armenian |
| Bab. | — Babylonian |
| Br. | — British |
| Bulg. | — Bulgarian |
| Chin. | — Chinese |
| D. | — Dutch |
| Dan. | — Danish |
| Eg. | — Egyptian |
| Eng. | — English |
| Finn. | — Finnish |
| Fr. | — French |
| Ger. | — German |
| Gr. | — Greek |
| Hung. | — Hungarian |
| It. | — Italian |
| Jap. | — Japanese |
| Jav. | — Javanese |
| Lat. | — Latin |
| Mod. Gr. | — Modern Greek |
| Nor. | — Norwegian |
| Per. | — Persian |
| Pol. | — Polish |
| Port. | — Portuguese |
| Rum. | — Rumanian |
| Rus. | — Russian |
| Skr. | — Sanskrit |
| Sp. | — Spanish |
| Swed. | — Swedish |
| Yugo. | — Yugoslav |

*Other Abbreviations (Standard abbreviations in common usage are omitted.)*

| | |
|---|---|
| Abh. | — Abhandlungen |
| Acad. | — Academy, Académie |
| Acc. | — Accademia |
| Adm. | — Administration |
| Ak. | — Akademie |
| Allg. | — Allgemein |
| Alm. | — Almanacco |
| Am. | — America, American, etc. |
| Amm. | — Amministrazione |
| Ann. | — Annals, Annali, Annuario, Annual, etc. |
| Ant. | — Antiquity, Antico, Antiquaire, etc. |
| Anthr. | — Anthropology, etc. |
| Antr. | — Antropologia, etc. |
| Anz. | — Anzeiger |
| Arch. | — Architecture, Architettura, Architettonico, etc.; Archives |
| Archaeol. | — Archaeology, etc. |
| attrib. | — attributed |
| Aufl. | — Auflage |
| Aufn. | — Aufnahme |
| B. | — Bulletin, Bollettino, etc. |
| b. | — born |
| Belg. | — Belgian, Belga, etc. |
| Berl. | — Berlin, Berliner |
| Bern. | — Berner |
| Bib. | — Bible, Biblical, Bibliothèque, etc. |
| Bibliog. | — Bibliography, etc. |
| Br. | — British |
| Bur. | — Bureau |
| Byz. | — Byzantine |
| C. | — Corpus |
| ca. | — circa |
| Cah. | — Cahiers |
| Cal. | — Calendar |
| Cap. | — Capital, Capitolium |
| Cat. | — Catalogue, Catalogo, etc. |
| Chr. | — Chronicle, Chronik |
| Civ. | — Civiltà, Civilization, etc. |
| cod. | — codex |
| col., cols. | — column, columns |
| Coll. | — Collection, Collana, Collationes, Collectanea, Collezione, etc. |
| Comm. | — Commentaries, Commentari, Communications, etc. |
| Cong. | — Congress, Congresso, etc. |
| Cr. | — Critica |
| Cron. | — Cronaca |
| Cuad. | — Cuadernos |
| Cult. | — Culture, Cultura, etc. |
| D. | — Deutsch |
| d. | — died |
| Diss. | — Dissertation, Dissertazione |
| Doc. | — Documents, etc. |
| E. | — Encyclopedia, etc. |
| Eccl. | — Ecclesiastic, Ecclesia, etc. |
| Eng. | — English, England |

| | |
|---|---|
| Ep. | — Epigraphy |
| Esp. | — España, Español |
| Est. | — Estudios |
| Et. | — Etudes |
| Ethn. | — Ethnology, Ethnography, Ethnographie, etc. |
| Etn. | — Etnico, Etnografia, etc. |
| Etnol. | — Etnologia |
| Eur. | — Europe, Europa, etc. |
| ext. | — extract |
| f. | — für |
| fasc. | — fascicle |
| Fil. | — Filologia |
| Filos. | — Filosofia, Filosofico |
| fol. | — folio |
| Forsch. | — Forschung, Forschungen |
| Fr. | — French, Francia, Français, etc. |
| Gal. | — Galerie |
| Gall. | — Gallery, Galleria |
| Geog. | — Geography, Geografia, Geographical, etc. |
| Ger. | — German, Germania, etc. |
| Giorn. | — Giornale |
| H. | — History, Histoire, etc. |
| hl. | — heilig, heilige |
| Holl. | — Hollandisch, etc. |
| Hum. | — Humanity, Humana, etc. |
| I. | — Istituto |
| Ill. | — Illustration, Illustrato, Illustrazione, etc. |
| Ind. | — Index, Indice, Indicatore, etc. |
| Inf. | — Information, Informazione, etc. |
| Inst. | — Institute, Institut, etc. |
| Int. | — International, etc. |
| Ist. | — Istituto |
| It. | — Italian, Italy, etc. |
| J. | — Journal |
| Jb. | — Jaarboek |
| Jhb. | — Jahrbuch |
| Jhrh. | — Jahreshefte |
| K. | — Kunst |
| Kat. | — Katalog |
| Kchr. | — Kunstchronik |
| Kg. | — Kunstgeschichte |
| Kunsthist. | — Kunsthistorische |
| Kw. | — Kunstwissenschaft |
| Lat. | — Latin |
| Lett. | — Letteratura, Lettere |
| Lib. | — Library |
| ling. | — linguistics, lingua, etc. |
| Lit. | — Literary, Literarische, Littéraire, etc. |
| Mag. | — Magazine |
| Med. | — Medieval, Medievale, etc. |
| Meded. | — Mededeelingen |
| Mél. | — Mélanges |
| Mém. | — Mémoire |
| Mem. | — Memorie, Memoirs |
| Min. | — Minerva |
| Misc. | — Miscellanea, etc. |
| Mit. | — Mitteilungen |
| Mnb. | — Monatsberichte |
| Mnbl. | — Monatsblaetter |
| Mnh. | — Monatshefte |
| Mod. | — Modern, Moderno, etc. |
| Mon. | — Monuments, Monumento |
| Münch. | — München, Münchner |
| Mus. | — Museum, Museo, etc. |
| N. | — New, Notizia, etc. |
| Nachr. | — Nachrichten |
| Nat. | — National, etc. |
| Naz. | — Nazionale |
| Notit. dign. | — Notitia Dignitatum |
| N. S. | — new series |
| O. | — Oriental, Orient, etc. |
| Ö. | — Österreichische |
| obv. | — obverse |
| öffentl. | — öffentlich |
| Op. | — Opuscolo |
| Pap. | — Papers |
| per. | — period |
| Per. | — Periodical, Periodico |
| Pin. | — Pinacoteca |
| Pr. | — Prehistory, Preistoria, Preystori, Préhistoire |
| Proc. | — Proceedings |
| Pub. | — Publication, Publicación |
| Pubbl. | — Pubblicazione |
| Q. | — Quarterly, Quaderno |
| Quel. | — Quellen |
| R. | — Rivista |
| r | — recto |
| Racc. | — Raccolta |
| Rass. | — Rassegna |
| Rec. | — Recueil |
| Recens. | — Recensione |
| Rech. | — Recherches |
| Rel. | — Relazione |
| Rend. | — Rendiconti |
| Rép. | — Répertoire |
| Rep. | — Report, Repertorio, Repertorium |
| Rev. | — Review, Revue, etc. |
| Rl. | — Reallexicon |
| Rom. | — Roman, Romano, Romanico, etc. |
| Rus. | — Russia, Russian, Russie, Russo, etc. |
| rv. | — reverse |
| S. | — San, Santo, Santa (saint) |
| S. | — Studi, Studies, etc. |
| Samml. | — Sammlung, Sammlungen |
| Sc. | — Science, Scienza, Scientific, etc. |
| Schr. | — Schriften |
| Schw. | — Schweitzer |
| Script. | — Scriptorium |
| Sitzb. | — Sitzungsberichte |
| s.l. | — in its place |
| Soc. | — Social, Society, Società, Sociale, etc. |
| Spec. | — Speculum |
| SS. | — Saints, Sante, Santi, Santissima |
| St. | — Saint |
| Sta | — Santa (holy) |
| Ste | — Sainte |
| Sto | — Santo (holy) |
| Sup. | — Supplement, Supplemento |
| s.v. | — under the word |
| Tech. | — Technical, Technology, etc. |
| Tecn. | — Tecnica, Tecnico |
| Tr. | — Transactions |
| trans. | — translator, translated, etc. |
| Trav. | — Travaux |
| u. | — und |
| Um. | — Umanesimo |
| Univ. | — University, Università, Université, etc. |
| Urb. | — Urban, Urbanistica |
| v | — verso |
| VAT | — Vorderasiatische Tafeln |
| Verh. | — Verhandlungen, Verhandelingen |
| Verz. | — Verzeichnis |
| Vf. | — Verfasser |
| Wien. | — Wiener |
| Yb. | — Yearbook |
| Z. | — Zeitschrift, Zeitung, etc. |

# CONTRIBUTORS TO VOLUME III

Hélène ADHÉMAR, Louvre, Paris
Rosario ASSUNTO, University of Urbino
Jean BABELON, Curator in Chief, Cabinet des Médailles, Bibliothèque Nationale, Paris
Virgil BARKER, University of Miami, Coral Gables, Fla.
Eleanor BARTON, Sweet Briar College, Sweet Briar, Va.
Giulio BATTELLI, Director, Scuola di Paleografia dell'Archivio Vaticano, Rome
Eugenio BATTISTI, Rome
Giovanni BECATTI, University of Florence
Jan BIALOSTOCKI, National Museum, Warsaw
Vera BIANCO, Rome
Sergio BOSTICCO, Florence
Stefano BOTTARI, University of Bologna
Giuseppe BOVINI, Catholic University of the Sacred Heart, Milan
Hermann J. BRAUNHOLTZ, Harpenden, England
Hermann BURSSENS, University of Ghent, Belgium
Mario BUSSAGLI, University of Rome
Antonio BUTTITTA, University of Palermo
Michelangelo CAGIANO DE AZEVEDO, Catholic University of the Sacred Heart, Milan
Maurizio CALVESI, Galleria d'Arte Moderna, Rome
Editta CASTALDI, Rome
Giancarlo CAVALLI, Bologna
Carlo CECCHELLI, University of Rome
Luigi CHIARINI, Rome
Renata CIPRIANI, Milan
George CŒDÈS, Honorary Director, Ecole Française d'Estrême-Orient, Paris
George COLLINS, Columbia University, New York
Enrico CRISPOLTI, Rome
Maria Laura CRISPOLTI, Rome
Fernanda DE' MAFFEI, Rome
Waldemar DEONNA, Geneva
Germaine DIETERLEN, Ecole des Hautes-Etudes, Sorbonne, Paris
David DIRINGER, Cambridge University
Victor H. ELBERN, Bonn
Andrea EMILIANI, Bologna
J. FILLIOZAT, Collège de France, Paris
Jan FONTEIN, Museum van Aziatische Kunst, Rijksmuseum, Amsterdam
Giovanni GARBINI, Istituto di Studi Orientali, University of Rome
H. Enno VAN GELDER, Koninklijk Kabinet, The Hague
Gabriel GIRALDO-JARAMILLO, Colombian Embassy, Caracas
Raniero GNOLI, University of Rome
Douglas H. GORDON, Hingham, Norfolk, England
Basil GRAY, Keeper of the Department of Oriental Antiquities, British Museum, London
Robert H. VAN GULIK, Minister for the Netherlands, Kuala Lumpur, Malaya
Louis HAMBIS, Institut des Hautes Etudes Chinoises, University of Paris
Werner HOFMANN, Curator, Museum of Modern Art, Vienna
James HOLDERBAUM, Princeton University, Princeton, N.J.
Henry R. HOPE, Indiana University, Bloomington, Ind.
Robert H. HUBBARD, Chief Curator, The National Gallery of Canada, Ottawa
Nicola IVANOFF, Fondazione Giorgio Cini, Venice
Willibald KIRFEL, University of Bonn
Ernst KÜHNEL, Director, Islamic Section, Berlin Museum, Berlin-Dahlem

Arthur LANE, Victoria and Albert Museum, London
Susanne LANG, London
Ernst LANGLOTZ, University of Bonn
Vittorio LANTERNARI, University of Rome
Raymond LANTIER, Membre de l'Institut; Curator in Chief, Musée des Antiquités Nationales, Saint-Germain-en-Laye, France
Oliver W. LARKIN, Smith College, Northampton, Mass.
Jean LAUDE, Attaché de Recherches au C.N.R.S., Boulogne sur Seine
Emilio LAVAGNINO, Soprintendente alle Gallerie e alle opere d'Arte medievali e moderne, Rome
Giuseppe LIVERANI, Director, Museo Internazionale delle Ceramiche, Faenza, Italy
Manuel LORENTE JUNQUERA, Curator, Museo del Prado, Madrid
Mariella LUCIDI, Rome
Valerio MARIANI, University of Naples
Guglielmo MATTHIAE, Soprintendente ai Monumenti e alle Gallerie degli Abruzzi, L'Aquila, Italy
A. Hyatt MAYOR, Metropolitan Museum of Art, New York
Arthur McCOMB, Boston, Mass.
John W. McCOUBREY, Yale University, New Haven, Conn.
Bernard S. MYERS, formerly The City College, New York
Franco PANVINI ROSATI, Museo Nazionale Romano, Rome
Senarat PARANAVITANA, University of Ceylon, Paradeniya, Ceylon
Renato PERONI, Rome
Terisio PIGNATTI, Musei Civici, Venice
Margaret C. PIRIE, University of Toronto
Mario PRAZ, University of Rome
John READ, British Broadcasting Corporation, London
Graham REYNOLDS, Deputy Keeper in charge of the Department of Paintings, Victoria and Albert Museum, London
Martin ROBERTSON, University of London
Robert ROSENBLUM, Princeton University, Princeton, N. J.
Benjamin ROWLAND, Harvard University, Cambridge, Mass.
Luigi SALERNO, Rome
Margaretta M. SALINGER, Metropolitan Museum of Art, New York
Roberto SALVINI, University of Trieste
Norman SCHLENOFF, The City College, New York
Marvin D. SCHWARTZ, Curator, American Decorative Art, Brooklyn Museum, Brooklyn, N.Y.
Tani SHINICHI, Bridgestone Art Gallery, Tokyo
William H. STAHL, Brooklyn College, Brooklyn, N. Y.
Wilhelm STAUDE, Houilles, Seine-et-Oise, France
Boleslav SZCZEŚNIAK, University of Notre Dame, South Bend, Ind.
Hans THÜMMLER, Landeskonservator von Westfalen-Lippe, Münster, Germany
Romolo TREBBI DEL TREVIGIANO, Catholic University of Valparaiso, Chile
Laszlò VAJDA, University of Munich
Lionello VENTURI, Professor Emeritus, University of Rome
W. Friedrich VOLBACH, Zentralmuseum, Mainz, Germany
Francis J. B. WATSON, Assistant Director of the Wallace Collection, Assistant Surveyor of the Queen's Works of Art, London
William WATSON, Department of Oriental Antiquities, British Museum, London
Harold E. WETHEY, University of Michigan, Ann Arbor, Mich.
Hellmut WILHELM, University of Washington, Seattle
Ernst ZINNER, Bamberg, Germany

# ACKNOWLEDGMENTS

The Institute for Cultural Collaboration and the publishers express their thanks to the collectors and to the directors of the museums and galleries listed below for permission to reproduce works in their collections and for photographs supplied.

AGRIGENTO, Sicily, Museo Civico Archeologico
AIX-EN-PROVENCE, France, Musée Granet
ALEXANDRIA, Egypt, Greco-Roman Museum
ALEXANDRIA, Egypt, Municipal Museum
AMSTERDAM, Allard Pierson Museum
AMSTERDAM, Museum van Aziatische Kunst
AMSTERDAM, Rijksmuseum
AMSTERDAM, Stedelijk Museum
ANCONA, Italy, Museo Nazionale
ANKARA, Archaeological Museum
ANTWERP, Ethnografisch Museum
ANTWERP, Musée Mayer van den Bergh
ARUNDEL CASTLE, Sussex, England, Coll. Duke of Norfolk
ATHENS, Acropolis, Museum
ATHENS, Benaki Museum
ATHENS, Byzantine Museum
ATHENS, Kerameikos Museum
ATHENS, Museum of the Agora
ATHENS, National Museum

BAMBERG, Germany, Staatliche Bibliothek
BARCELONA, Museos de Arte
BASEL, Switzerland, Kunstmuseum
BASEL, Switzerland, Museum für Völkerkunde
BELÉM, Brazil, Museu Paraense Emilio Goeldi
BERGAMO, Italy, Biblioteca Civica
BERLIN, Staatliche Museen
BIKANER, India, Coll. Maharaja of Bikaner
BODMIN, Cornwall, England, Coll. M. Cardew
BOLOGNA, Museo Civico
BOLOGNA, Pinacoteca Nazionale
BONN, Rheinisches Landesmuseum
BOSTON, Museum of Fine Arts
BRISTOL, England, City Art Gallery
BRUSSELS, Musées Royaux d'Art et d'Histoire
BRUSSELS, Coll. Stoclet
BUDAPEST, National Museum
BURSLEM, England, Wedgwood Institute

CAGLIARI, Sardinia, Museo Archeologico
CAIRO, Coptic Museum
CAIRO, Coll. J. O. Matossian
CALCUTTA, Indian Museum
CAMBRIDGE, England, Fitzwilliam Museum
CAMBRIDGE, Mass., Fogg Art Museum
CAMBRIDGE, Mass., R. Hobart Coll.
CANBERRA, Australia, National Library
CAPUA, Italy, Museo Provinciale Campano
CENTO, Italy, Pinacoteca Civica

CESENA, Italy, Biblioteca Malatestiana
CHAUMONT, France, Musée d'Art et d'Histoire
CHICAGO, Art Institute
CIRENCESTER, England, Ingram Coll.
CLEVELAND, Museum of Art
COLOGNE, Schnütgen-Museum
COLOMBO, Ceylon, National Museum
COPENHAGEN, Nationalmuseet
CORINTH, Greece, Archaeological Museum

DELPHI, Archaeological Museum
DENVER, Art Museum
DETROIT, Institute of Arts
DRESDEN, Gemäldegalerie
DUBLIN, National Gallery

EKOLSUND, Sweden, Coll. C. Kempe
EPERNAY, Marne, France, Bibliothèque Municipale
EPIDAURUS, Greece, Archaeological Museum

FAENZA, Italy, Museo Internazionale delle Ceramiche
FAYETTEVILLE, University of Arkansas Museum
FERRARA, Italy, Museo Archeologico di Spina
FLORENCE, Biblioteca Nazionale
FLORENCE, Gabinetto Nazionale dei Disegni e Stampe degli Uffizi
FLORENCE, Museo Archeologico
FLORENCE, Museo Nazionale
FLORENCE, Uffizi
FORLÌ, Italy, Pinacoteca e Musei Comunali

GENEVA, Musée d'Art et d'Histoire
GHENT, Belgium, Musée des Beaux-Arts
GODALMING, Surrey, England, J. C. Thomson Coll.
GÖTEBORG, Sweden, Ethnografiska Museet

THE HAGUE, Koninklijk Penningkabinet
THE HAGUE, Mauritshuis
HAMBURG, Museum für Kunst und Gewerbe
HAMBURG, Museum für Völkerkunde
HANOVER, Germany, Kestner-Museum
HANOVER, Germany, Landesmuseum
HERAKLION, Crete, Archaeological Museum
HONOLULU, Museum of the Academy of Arts

ISTANBUL, Archaeological Museum

JENA, Germany, Friedrich-Schiller-Universität, Hilprecht-Sammlung

KANAGAWA PREFECTURE, Japan, Kimpei Takeuchi Coll.
KANSAS CITY, Mo., Nelson Gallery of Art and Atkins Museum
KASSEL, Germany, Staatliche Kunstsammlungen

LAHORE, Pakistan, Central Museum
LA SERENA, Chile, Museo Arqueológico
LEIDEN, Netherlands, Rijksmuseum
LEIDEN, Netherlands, Rijksmuseum voor Volkenkunde
LENINGRAD, The Hermitage
LIÈGE, Belgium, Musée Curtius
LIPARI, Italy, Museo Eoliano
LONDON, British Museum
LONDON, D. Cohen Coll.
LONDON, Cunliffe Coll.
LONDON, Dulwich College Gallery
LONDON, D. Gure Coll.
LONDON, National Gallery
LONDON, V. Rothschild Coll.
LONDON, Coll. Mrs. Walter Sedgwick
LONDON, Seligman Coll.
LONDON, Tate Gallery
LONDON, University, Percival David Foundation of Chinese Art
LONDON, Victoria and Albert Museum
LONDON, Wallace Coll.
LUGANO, Switzerland, Coll. F. Vannotti
LUGANO, Switzerland, Von Thyssen Coll.
LYNGBY, Denmark, Museum
LYON, France, Musée Historique des Tissus

MADRID, Museo Arqueológico Nacional
MANRESA, Spain, Museo Municipal
MARBURG, Germany, Universitätsmuseum
MESSINA, Sicily, Museo Nazionale
MEXICO CITY, Museo Nacional de Antropología
MILAN, Biblioteca Ambrosiana
MILAN, Pinacoteca di Brera
MIYEGINO, Kanagawa, Japan, Hakone Art Museum
MUNICH, Bayerische Staatsbibliothek
MUNICH, Bayerische Staatsgemäldesammlungen
MUNICH, Residenzmuseum
MUNICH, Staatliche Antikensammlungen

NANCY, France, Musée Historique Lorrain
NAPLES, Museo di Capodimonte
NAPLES, Museo Duca di Martina alla Floridiana
NAPLES, Museo Nazionale
NEW DELHI, India, Museum of Central Asian Antiquities
NEW YORK, Brooklyn Museum
NEW YORK, F. Caro Coll.
NEW YORK, G. del Drago Coll.
NEW YORK, N. Heeramaneck Coll.
NEW YORK, Metropolitan Museum of Art
NEW YORK, Museum of Modern Art Film Library
NEW YORK, Mrs. Marius de Zayas Coll.
NÎMES, France, Musée Archéologique

OLYMPIA, Greece, Archaeological Museum
ORLEANS, France, Musée Historique de l'Orléanais
OTTERLO, Netherlands, Rijksmuseum Kröller-Müller
OXFORD, Ashmolean Museum
OXFORD, Museum of Eastern Art

PADUA, Italy, Museo Civico
PARIS, Bibliothèque Nationale
PARIS, Cabinet des Médailles
PARIS, Coll. Capitan
PARIS, Institut de France
PARIS, Louvre
PARIS, Musée Carnavalet
PARIS, Musée Cernuschi
PARIS, Musée de Cluny
PARIS, Musée Guimet
PARIS, Musée de l'Homme
PARIS, Coll. A. Patino
PARIS, Coll. Pellerin
PARIS, Musée du Petit-Palais
PARMA, Italy, Galleria Nazionale
PEKING, Ch'i Pai-shih Museum

PEKING, Jupéon Museum
PHILADELPHIA, Museum of Art
PHILADELPHIA, University Museum
PIRAEUS, Greece, Archaeological Museum
PISA, Museo Civico
POSSAGNO, Italy, Gipsoteca
PRAGUE, National Museum

RAVENNA, Italy, Museo Nazionale
REIMS, France, Bibliothèque Municipale
ROME, Biblioteca dell'Istituto di Archeologia e Storia dell'Arte
ROME, Capitoline Museum
ROME, Gabinetto Nazionale delle Stampe
ROME, Galleria Borghese
ROME, Galleria Colonna
ROME, Galleria Doria Pamphili
ROME, Galleria Nazionale d'Arte Moderna
ROME, Istituto Italiano di Numismatica
ROME, Lateran Museum
ROME, Museo d'Arte Orientale
ROME, Museo delle Arti e delle Tradizioni Popolari
ROME, Museo Nazionale Romano
ROME, Museo Pigorini
ROME, Museo di Villa Giulia
ROME, Museo della Zecca
ROME, Vatican Library
ROME, Vatican Museums

SAARBRÜCKEN, Germany, Saarlandmuseum
SAINT-GERMAIN-EN-LAYE, France, Musée des Antiquités Nationales
SANTA BARBARA, Calif., Museum of Art
SEATTLE, Wash., Art Museum
SÈVRES, France, Musée Nationale de Ceramique
SHANGHAI, Coll. Union of Chinese Artists
SINGAPORE, Raffles Museum, S. Y. Wong Coll.
STOCKHOLM, Museum of Far Eastern Antiquities
STRASBOURG, France, Musée des Arts Décoratifs
STUTTGART, Germany, Landesmuseum
SYRACUSE, Sicily, Museo Archeologico

TAICHUNG, Formosa, National Palace Museum
TAIPEH, Formosa, National Museum
TARANTO, Italy, Museo Nazionale
TARBES, France, Musée Massey
TEHERAN, Archaeological Museum
TEHERAN, Imperial Library of Gulistan
TERVUEREN, Belgium, Musée Royale du Congo Belge
TOKYO, Suzekō Idemitsu Coll.
TOKYO, Tatsuo Ishida Coll.
TOKYO, Japanese Palace Coll.
TOKYO, Baron Masuda Coll.
TOKYO, Takeo Nakazawa Coll.
TOKYO, National Museum
TOKYO, Nezu Art Museum
TOKYO, Kan Okabe Coll.
TOKYO, Kishichiro Ōkura Coll.
TOURANE, Vietnam, Museum
TRIER, Germany, Bischöfliches Museum
TRIER, Germany, Rheinisches Landesmuseum
TRIESTE, Italy, Museo Civico di Storia ed Arte
TRIPOLI, Libia, Archaeological Museum
TURIN, Italy, Biblioteca Reale
TURIN, Italy, Museo Egizio

UTRECHT, Netherlands, Universitätsbibliothek

VENICE, Accademia
VENICE, Biblioteca Marciana
VENICE, Museo Correr
VENICE, Scuola di S. Giorgio degli Schiavoni
VENICE, Seminario Patriarcale
VICENZA, Italy, Museo Civico
VIENNA, Albertina

VIENNA, Kunsthistorisches Museum
VIENNA, Naturhistorisches Museum
VIENNA, Nationalbibliothek

WASHINGTON, D.C., Dumbarton Oaks Coll.
WASHINGTON, D.C., Freer Gallery of Art, Smithsonian Institution

WASHINGTON, D.C., Phillips Coll.
WENDOVER, Bucks., England, Barlow Coll.

ZURICH, Coll. C. A. Drenowatz
ZURICH, Rietberg Museum, Coll. E. von der Heydt
ZURICH, Schweizerisches Landesmuseum

# PHOTOGRAPHIC CREDITS

The numbers refer to the plates. Those within parentheses indicate the sequence of subjects in composite plate pages. Italic numbers refer to photographs owned by the Institute for Cultural Collaboration.

A.C.L., Brussels: 130 (4, 5); 305 (4); 308 (2); 311 (2); 418 (1)
ALINARI, Florence: 12 (1–3); 13 (1,2); 19 (3); 29 (1); 43; 66 (1); 74; 102 (1); 105; 106 (1, 2); 135 (5); 137 (2); 138 (1, 2); 149 (2, 4); 299 (3); 301 (2); 303 (2–6); 304 (1, 2, 4); 305 (2); 306 (1, 3, 4); 307 (2, 4); 308 (1); 309 (1); 310 (3, 4); 311 (1, 3, 4); 312 (2); 313 (1, 3); 314 (3); 329 (1); 352 (2); 363 (2); 368 (4); 381; 386 (2); 388 (3, 4); 389 (4); 391 (3, 4); 392 (2); 411 (5, 6); 417 (2, 4); 418 (2); 465; 468 (1, 2); 469; 478 (1, 2); 479 (1); 483 (2); 487 (5); 490 (3)
ANDERSON, Rome: 12 (4); 34; 37; 70 (1, 3); 73; 76; 86; 107 (1, 2); 108; 135 (1); 207 (1, 2); 209 (3, 4); 210; 211 (2); 299 (5); 302 (1, 2); 305 (3); 306 (2); 309 (3); 310 (1, 2); 312 (3, 4); 313 (2); 314 (4); 324; 328; 350; 358; 359; 363 (1); 372 (2); 383; 390 (4); 391 (2); 392; (4, 5); 417 (1); 470; 471; 472; 477 (1, 2); 479 (2); 480; 483 (1); 487 (6); 488 (1)
ARCHAEOLOGICAL DEPARTMENT OF CEYLON, Colombo: 177; 178; 179 (1–4); 180 (1–3); 181 (1–4) 182 (1, 2); 183 (1, 2)
ARCHAEOLOGICAL SURVEY OF INDIA, Madras: 300 (2)
ARCHIVES PHOTOGRAPHIQUES, Paris: 49 (1); 50; 51 (1); 53 (1, 2); 54 (1); 59; 111 (3, 4); 152 (2, 4); 155 (2, 3); 211 (4); 361 (1); 388 (1); 490 (2)
ARTE E COLORE, Milan: 63 (1)
ARTS COUNCIL OF GREAT BRITAIN, London: 434 (1)
ATELIER ARTISTIQUE NELLYS, Athens: 367

BATTISTI, Rome: 173 (1); 486 (1)
BAYERISCHE VERWALTHUNG DER STAATLICHE SCHLOSSER, GÄRTEN UND SEEN MUSEUMSABTEILUNG, Munich: 160 (3)
BELZEAUX-ZODIAQUE, La Pierre-qui-vire, Yonne, France: 118
BESSEN, Amsterdam: 257; 288
BIBLIOTHÈQUE NATIONALE, Paris: 68 (3); 428 (1)
BILDARCHIV FOTO MARBURG, Marburg: 48 (1, 2); 49 (2); 57 (2); 60 (3); 65; 209 (2); 340 (2); 341 (2); 353 (3); 369 (3, 4); 390 (1); 484 (2)
BORCHI, Faenza, Italy: 173 (3)
BROGI, Florence: 320
BULLOZ, Paris: 185 (2)

CACCO, Venice: 30 (2)
CARRARO, Taranto, Italy: 376
CLEVELAND MUSEUM OF ART, Cleveland: 263 (1, 2); 264; 265; 270 (1); 283 (2); 291; 292
COURTAULD INSTITUTE OF ART, London: 208
CREA, Rome: 9 (2); 10 (1–4); 11 (1–3); 16 (1); 419 (1, 2); 420 (1); 428 (2, 3); 429 (2, 4, 5)

DA RE, Bergamo: 19 (1)
DE ANTONIS, Rome: 3 (2); 35; 36; 41; 42; 61; 81; 82; 87; 88; 99 (1, 2); 100; 21 (3); 122 (3); 124 (3); 131 (5); 132 (3); 136 (3); 139 (1, 2); 140 (1–3); 143; 147 (1, 2); 150 (1, 3); 154 (1–3); 157 (1–3); 158 (2); 228; 247; 298; 299 (2); 309 (2) 375; 378 (2); 463
DE LIBERALI, Tripoli: 387 (1)
DEPARTMENT OF ARCHAEOLOGY, GOVERNMENT OF INDIA: 121 (4); 211 (1); 485 (4)
DEUTSCHE PHOTOTHEK, Dresden: 467
DEUTSCHES ARCHÄOLOGISCHES INSTITUT, Athens: 342; 343; 344 (1); 368 (3); (3); 371 (2)
DEUTSCHES ARCHÄOLOGISCHES INSTITUT, Rome: 5 (1, 2); 347; 351; 353 (1); 354; 361 (2); 370; 382; 386 (3)
DEWSBURY: 174 (1, 2); 175 (1); 176 (1)
DIETERLEN, Paris: 486 (3)
DINGJAN, The Hague: 212 (4)
DRAYER, Zurich: 136 (4)

ECOLE FRANÇAISE D'EXTRÊME-ORIENT, Hanoi: 192 (1, 2); 193 (1, 2); 194 (1, 2); 195 (1, 2); 196

FALL, London: 229 (1)
FARINA, Monza, Italy: 68 (1, 2)
FERRANTE, Rome: 386 (1)
FERRUZZI, Venice: 24; 491; 495
FIORENTINI, Venice: 489 (1)
FLAMMARION, Paris: 111 (1); 112 (3)
FLEMING, London: 23; 441; 442
FORSTER: 330 (3)
FOTOTECA CENTRO SPERIMENTALE, Rome: 332 (1); 335 (1)
FOTOTECA FONDAZIONE CINI, Venice: 26 (1); 28 (1)
FOTOTECA UNIONE, Rome: 5 (3)
FOTOWERKEN F. CLAES, Antwerp: 416 (4)
FRANTZ, ALISON, Athens: 341 (1); 377 (2)

GABINETTO DI EPIGRAFIA, UNIVERSITÀ DI ROMA, Rome: 4 (4)
GABINETTO FOTOGRAFICO, GALLERIA NAZIONALE D'ARTE MODERNA, Rome: 184 (3)
GABINETTO FOTOGRAFICO, ISTITUTO CENTRALE DEL RESTAURO, Rome: 325; 326; 387 (2)
GABINETTO FOTOGRAFICO, SOPRINTENDENZA ALLE ANTICHITÀ, Agrigento and Caltanissetta, Sicily: 136 (1)
GABINETTO FOTOGRAFICO, SOPRINTENDENZA ALLE ANTICHITÀ, Ancona, Italy: 117 (4)
GABINETTO FOTOGRAFICO, SOPRINTENDENZA ALLE ANTICHITÀ, Rome: 416 (2)
GABINETTO FOTOGRAFICO, SOPRINTENDENZA ALLE ANTICHITÀ, Syracuse, Sicily, 122 (5)
GABINETTO FOTOGRAFICO, SOPRINTENDENZA ALLE ANTICHITÀ D'ETRURIA, Florence: 445 (2); 487 (1, 2)
GABINETTO FOTOGRAFICO, SOPRINTENDENZA ALLE GALLERIE, Florence: 201 (1–3); 323; 422 (1)
GABINETTO FOTOGRAFICO, SOPRINTENDENZA ALLE GALLERIE, Naples: 40 (2); 389 (1)
GABINETTO FOTOGRAFICO, SOPRINTENDENZA ALLE GALLERIE, Pisa: 327
GABINETTO FOTOGRAFICO, SOPRINTENDENZA ALLE GALLERIE, Trent: 57 (1, 3); 60 (1)
GABINETTO FOTOGRAFICO, SOPRINTENDENZA AI MONUMENTI, Venice: 30 (1)
GABINETTO FOTOGRAFICO NAZIONALE, Rome: 27; 38; 312; (1); 387 (3); 430 (4); 477 (3); 497
GILARDI, Rome: 164 (3)
GIRAUDON, Paris: 39; 63 (2); 75; 116 (1–4); 117 (1); 119; 120; 130 (1, 2); 131 (6); 133; 134; 137 (3); 139 (6); 144; 160 (1); 165 (1, 2, 4); 166 (1, 2, 4); 167 (1, 2); 168; 169 (3); 170 (1, 3); 172 (1); 187; 188; 189; 213; 214; 215; 216 (1, 2); 217; 218; 219 (2); 230 (2); 233; 246 (1); 248; 252; 258; 259 (2); 260 (1, 2); 261 (1, 2); 267; 268; 269; 274, (1, 3); 277; 278; 287; 297; 308 (3); 369 (2); 374 (2); 384 (4–9); 390 (3); 393 (1–23); 394 (1–4); 395 (1–16); 396 (1–18); 397 (1–7); 398 (1–12); 399 (1–12); 400 (1–10); 409 (1–8); 415 (6, 7); 430 (3); 449; 459 (1); 460; 461 (1); 462; 466

HEMAN, Basel: 18 (4)
HINZ, Basel: 355; 492
HIRMER, Munich: 3 (3); 52; 97 (3); 135 (3, 4); 301 (1); 329 (2); 337 (1, 2); 338; 339 (1, 2); 345; 346; 348; 349; 356; 357 (1, 2); 362 (1, 2); 364 (1, 2); 368 (1, 2); 369 (1); 377 (3); 378 (1); 379; 380; 391 (1); 392 (1)

KAUFMANN, Munich: 373
KONINKLIJK PENNINGKABINET, The Hague: 413 (1–13); 414 (1–13)

LABORATORIO RICERCHE SCIENTIFICHE, PINACOTECA DI BRERA, Milan: 21 (3)
LANDESDENKMALAMT WESTFALEN, Münster: 44 (1); 45
LAPEYRE, Tarbes, France: 111 (2)
LAROUSSE, Paris: 112 (4); 113
LAURATI, Florence: 496 (2)
LEHMANN, Paris: 485 (3)
LICHTBEELDEN-INSTITUT, Amsterdam: 135 (2)

MAGYAR NEMZETI MUSEUM, Budapest: 164 (1)
MAS, Barcelona: 7 (2); 46 (1, 2); 47; 51 (2); 117 (3); 137 (5); 145 (1, 2); 161 (1); 315; 316 (1–3); 317; 318; 319; 408 (9–11)
MAYER, Vienna: 476
McLEAN, Brussels: 365
MELETZIS, Athens: 340 (1)
METROPOLITAN MUSEUM OF ART, New York: 32; 33; 445 (1)
MOOSBRUGGER, Zurich: 232
MUSÉE GUIMET, Paris: 485 (2)

NATIONAL FILM ARCHIVE, London: 334 (1, 2)

OBERT, Santa Barbara, Calif: 246 (3)
OFFENTLICHE KUNSTSAMMLUNGEN, Basel: 307 (1)
ORLANDINI, Modena: 17 (1, 2); 18 (1, 2)
ÖSTERREICHISCHE NATIONALBIBLIOTHEK, Vienna: 422 (2)

PAPAFAVA, Padua: 158 (1)
PONTIFICIA COMMISSIONE D'ARTE SACRA, Vatican City: 90; 91 (1–3); 92; 95 (1, 2); 96; 97 (1, 2); 98 (1, 2); 101; 102 (2); 103 (1–4); 104 (1–4); 304 (3); 305 (1)

POZZI E BELLINI, Rome: 401 (1–10); 402 (1–12); 403 (1, 2); 404 (1–12); 405 (1–6).

RAMPAZZI, Turin: 450 (1, 2)
RHEINISCHES BILDARCHIV, Cologne: 67 (1, 2)
ROSENTHAL-PORZELLAN A. G. BILDERDIENST, Selb, Germany: 173 (2)

SAVIO, Oscar, Rome: 2; 49 (3); 93; 94; 121 (2); 123 (2, 3); 127 (1); 146 (1, 2); 204 (1–3); 205; 212 (2); 227; 231 (2); 344 (2); 360; 366; 371 (1); 385 (3); 406 (1–2); 407 (1–20); 410 (1–13); 412 (1–18); 415 (4, 5); 481; 482; 488 (3); 489 (1)
SCALA, Florence: 71; 72; 77; 78; 109; 110; 148; 321; 322; 411 (1–4); 473
SCHMIDT-GLASSNER, Helsa, Stuttgart: 388 (2)
SCUOLA ARCHEOLOGICA ITALIANA DI ATENE, Athens: 131 (4)
SIMONE DI SAN CLEMENTE, Florence: 300 (3, 4)
SIRÉN, Stockholm: 245 (1, 2); 255 (1, 2); 256 (1, 2); 273 (1–4); 279 (1, 2)
STEINKOPF, Berlin: 203; 392 (3)

TRAUTE LEHMANN, Bamberg: 389 (3)
TWEEDIE, M.W.F., London: 229 (2)

VAGHI, Parma: 474
VICTORIA AND ALBERT MUSEUM, London: 141 (2–4); 163 (3)
VILLANI, Bologna: 79; 80 (1, 2); 83 (1, 2); 84 (1, 20); 85; 89; 153; 421 (1)

WALLACE COLLECTION, London: 25
WARBURG INSTITUTE, London: 202 (1–4); 206 (1–6)
WELLS, Bergamo: 9 (1); 21 (2)

# CONTENTS - VOLUME III

| | Col. | Pls. |
|---|---|---|
| CALDER, Alexander | 1 | |
| CALLIGRAPHY AND EPIGRAPHY | 2 | 1–16 |
| CALLOT, Jacques | 25 | |
| CAMBODIA | 26 | |
| CAMEROONS | 35 | |
| CAMPIN, Robert | 38 | |
| CAMPIONESI | 39 | 17–21 |
| CANADA | 45 | |
| CANALETTO | 53 | 22–25 |
| CANO, Alonso | 56 | |
| CANOVA, Antonio | 57 | 26–30 |
| CARAVAGGIO | 62 | 31–43 |
| CAROLINGIAN PERIOD | 81 | 44–69 |
| CARPACCIO, Vittore | 128 | 70–78 |
| CARPEAUX, Jean-Baptiste | 133 | |
| CARRACCI, Ludovico, Annibale, Agostino, Antonio | 134 | 79–89 |
| CASSATT, Mary | 143 | |
| CATACOMBS | 144 | 90–104 |
| CAVALLINI, Pietro | 170 | 105–110 |
| CELLINI, Benvenuto | 174 | |
| CELTIC ART | 175 | 111–119 |
| CERAMICS | 186 | 120–173 |
| CEYLON | 325 | |
| CEYLONESE ART | 330 | 174–183 |
| CÉZANNE, Paul | 339 | 184–191 |
| CHAGALL, Marc | 356 | |
| CHAM, SCHOOL OF | 357 | 192–196 |
| CHAMPAIGNE, Philippe de | 363 | |
| CHAO MÊNG-FU | 363 | 197–200 |
| CHARACTERIZATION: PSYCHOLOGICAL, PHYSIOGNOMICAL, AND ETHNIC | 366 | 201–212 |

| | Col. | Pls. |
|---|---|---|
| CHARDIN, Jean-Baptiste-Siméon | 382 | 213–218 |
| CHARONTON, Enguerrand | 387 | |
| CHASSÉRIAU, Théodore | 388 | |
| CHILE | 388 | |
| CHINA | 393 | |
| CHINESE ART | 466 | 219–298 |
| CHIRICO, Giorgio de | 577 | |
| CHOREOGRAPHY: POSE, GESTURE, AND GROUPING | 578 | 299–302 |
| CHRISTIANITY | 587 | 303–314 |
| CHRISTUS, Petrus | 607 | |
| CHURRIGUERESQUE STYLE | 608 | 315–319 |
| CIMABUE | 614 | 320–328 |
| CIMA DA CONEGLIANO | 619 | |
| CINEMATOGRAPHY | 619 | 329–336 |
| CLASSIC ART | 632 | 337–384 |
| CLASSICISM | 673 | 385–392 |
| CLODION | 697 | |
| CLOUET, Jean and François | 698 | |
| COELLO, Claudio | 699 | |
| COINS AND MEDALS | 700 | 393–416 |
| COLE, Thomas | 748 | |
| COLOMBIA | 749 | |
| COMIC ART AND CARICATURE | 754 | 417–435 |
| CONFUCIANISM | 775 | 436–439 |
| CONGO | 782 | |
| CONSTABLE, John | 790 | 440–444 |
| COPLEY, John Singleton | 795 | |
| COPTIC ART | 796 | 445–458 |
| COROT, Jean-Baptiste-Camille | 810 | 459–464 |
| CORREGGIO | 818 | 465–476 |
| COSMATI | 829 | 477–483 |
| COSMOLOGY AND CARTOGRAPHY | 835 | 484–500 |

CALDER, ALEXANDER. Sculptor of the mobile, an American both by birth (Philadelphia, July 22, 1898) and by the characteristics of his art. Buoyant, exuberant, humorous, Calder's work is peculiarly an expression of the American vernacular of this century — the vernacular of science, engineering, and mechanics. The artist's grandfather and father were sculptors, the latter, A. Sterling Calder, a prominent academician; his mother was a painter. Calder was graduated from Stevens Institute of Technology in 1919 and entered the engineering profession. He began to draw at night school in New York, later studying painting at the Art Students League. As an illustrator for the *National Police Gazette*, he developed a simple linear style, seen in his animal and circus drawings. In 1926 Calder went to Paris, where he made a miniature circus of animated marionettes in wood and metal, which he manipulated for the amusement of his friends. His first sculptures in wire (*Josephine Baker*, 1926, ht., 28 in.; *Helen Wills*, priv. coll., 1928; *Portrait of Shepard Vogelgesang*, owned by S. Vogelgesang, Whitefield, N. H., 1930) resembled caricatures, but their wire execution gave them three-dimensionality.

In 1930 Calder began to meet some of the revolutionary figures in contemporary art, including Mondrian and Miró (qq. v.). His visit to Mondrian's studio marked a turning point: Calder soon abandoned the animated circus toys and humorous caricatures and turned to abstract art. Impressed by Mondrian's severe geometric planes and primary colors, he produced a series of abstract sculptures in wire and wood, painted in red and black. In 1931, he began to experiment with figures in motion, first with a simple swaying form on a fixed base, then with a motorized turning composition (*Dancing Torpedo Shape*, Berkshire Mus., Pittsfield, Mass., 1932). Finally he succeeded in making "two or more objects find actual relations in space" (*The Circle*, 1934). Marcel Duchamp (see DUCHAMP), whose earlier sculptures had perhaps shown the way, gave these new inventions the name "mobile." Later Calder developed the hanging mobile, making use of wind currents to set in motion the free forms which he balanced with rhythmic precision (*Hanging Mobile*, 1936). These are clearly related to the free curves and bright colors of Miró.

In 1933 Calder settled on a Connecticut farm, where he was able to develop a large standing *Steel Fish* (Richmond, Va., Mus. of Fine Arts, 1934; ht., 10 ft.). Its stately, graceful motion is repeated in the large hanging mobile, *Lobster and Fish Tail* (New York, Mus. of Mod. Art, 1939).

The mercury fountain at the Spanish Pavilion of the Paris Exposition of 1937, a mobile which splashed mercury into a basin, was perhaps Calder's most successful piece of large-scale sculpture. In the same year he constructed the *Whale* (New York, Mus. of Mod. Art; ht., 6 ft., 6 in.), a curvilinear abstract standing figure cut out of sheet steel; he called it a "stabile." Other large, nonmoving figures of abstract design were later combined with mobiles.

Since World War II, Calder has become an internationally celebrated artist. The suave curves of his wire rods, the flat metallic planes in red or black, whether shaped in geometric forms as in his early work (*The Circle*, 1934) or in organic shapes (*Red Petals*, Chicago, Arts Club, 1942), always have a crisp spirit both humorous and mechanistic. Perhaps the most significant characteristic of Calder's sculpture is its dynamic concept of space; rhythmically moving forms describe arcs which constantly shift yet make us aware of the area both within and without their orbits (I, PL. 132).

BIBLIOG. J. J. Sweeney, Alexander Calder, New York, 1951.

Henry R. HOPE

**CALLIGRAPHY AND EPIGRAPHY.** The term "calligraphy" means "beautiful writing" or "elegant penmanship" (from the Latin *calligraphia*; in turn derived from Greek καλλιγραφία, from κάλλος, "beauty," and γράφος, "writing" or "writer"). Today calligraphy generally refers to the art of beautiful writing as a profession or field of study, that is, of writing as dependent on esthetic considerations. Linguistic usage distinguishes between epigraphy (lapidary writing incised on durable materials with a chisel or similar instrument) and calligraphy proper (rendered on perishable materials with a brush or pen). The present article deals with the esthetic aspects of writing in all media.

Although writing serves a primarily utilitarian purpose, the styles of other art media have placed their imprint upon the development of its various forms, as in pictographic or iconographic script (Ancient Egypt, pre-Columbian America), ideographic or synthetic script (China and Japan), and alphabetic script (Kufic, Carolingian, Gothic, Renaissance, etc.). Writing in turn has always been of primary importance as a means of ornamental enhancement of painting, sculpture, and architecture. At its best, calligraphy may equal other forms of esthetic expression, and at certain times it has been regarded as an art not inferior to painting.

SUMMARY. Writing and art (col. 2). Primitive and ethnological pictographs (col. 4). Evolution of prealphabetic writing (col. 7): *Egypt; Cuneiform; Cretan-Mycenaean and Hittite scripts; China; Japan.* Major examples of alphabetic scripts (col. 11): *Greece and Rome; India and Farther India; Islam; Europe: the Middle Ages to the present.*

WRITING AND ART. A study of writing as art can, and to some extent must, proceed from the history of writing and the alphabet, with consideration of outstanding cases of creative originality and interrelationships with other art forms. In this sense writing may merge with painting (as in pictographs, especially in pre-Columbian America, or in Chinese and Japanese ideograms, as well as in some contemporary graphic art). It interpenetrates symbol and emblem (marks of ownership, trademarks, etc., which are perennial and ubiquitous) and monumental decoration (Roman and Humanist dedicatory epigraphs, sacred texts inscribed on the walls of Islamic mosques and, occasionally, of Protestant churches). Writing invades even the field of personal decoration; modern pins inscribed with initials reflect a long history of usage.

In all these cases an unquestioned esthetic intention exists along with both the mnemonic and phonetic functions of writing. The written form often acquires an importance beyond that of merely rendering meaning — almost as if the meaning could not be fully conveyed by the characters or ideographic symbols alone. This is especially clear in the calligraphic idiom

of religious, commemorative, and official texts, in which the writing is as a rule closely related to the best elements of the dominant artistic styles; this relationship is also evident in the development of the graphic arts (q.v.) after the invention of the printing press. Not infrequently the physical garment of a group of words is of more concern than textual meaning.

All civilizations have left some kind of record of the importance attributed to the esthetic aspect of writing. From the earliest times the Egyptians had the greatest veneration for books and writing; their esteem is suggested by the declaration of the wise Khety (Akhthoy) to his son Pepy, about 2000 B.C.: "I shall make thee love writing more than thine own mother; I shall make beauty enter before thy face." Similarly in Assyria the great king Ashurbanipal (669–626 B.C.) wrote in his inscriptions: "I, Ashurbanipal, learned the wisdom of Nabu, the entire art of clay tablets .... I received the revelation of the wise Adapa, the entire treasure of the art of writing ...." According to Philostratus (3d cent.), there were in the entourage of Apollonius of Tyana two scribes, one for daily needs and the other for purposes requiring ornate writing. During the Renaissance the creation of a library of perfectly transcribed codices was a matter of political importance. This preoccupation with the beauty of writing is amply confirmed by the exceptional quality of many of the written documents that have survived from ancient times. In China, Japan, India, and the Islamic countries, the profession of calligrapher was — and still is — held in high esteem; and in Europe and America the design of printing fonts that continue the stylistic evolution of calligraphy is the object of intense study.

A pictograph and a page of alphabetic script present different esthetic problems. Picture writings may be considered as art either individually (as imitations of nature and dependent on their power of evocation) or in stylized form (as a coordinated series which unfolds a consecutive discourse). Both in the primitive pictographic stage and in the synthetic or ideographic stage we find clear affinities with the prevailing art styles — often, in fact, a complete identity, as in Egypt and presumably in prehistoric times. The need for a comprehensible arrangement of the pictured tale — whether vertical or horizontal — accompanies a concern with order, balance, and clarity, which in turn look forward to problems of the ideographic or calligraphic page. Writing, however, remained in these cases a kind of monumental picture.

When the naturalistic image passes to a schematic, ideographic, or alphabetic symbol and mimetic or representational preoccupations disappear, the quality of the writing (as in modern nonobjective painting) depends on the independent structural values of harmony, fluency, elegance, and interrelation. This is true not only for Chinese and Japanese ideograms but also for all the alphabetic scripts (which today are thought to have derived from a single northwestern Semitic prototype; that is, from the region of Phoenicia and Palestine, ca. 1800–1700 B.C.). Both systems derived, undoubtedly, from the intentional stylization of natural forms, but they soon became divorced semantically from these forms through a process facilitated by a slow and continuous adaptation to the tools and materials used in writing. Lapidary writing, inscribed or incised with a chisel on stone, thus acquired a geometric quality, without curves or ligatures; in sharp contrast was the rapid writing permitted either by the reed pen (Gr., κάλαμος; Lat., calamus or canna) — a stick of common reed with its end frayed or split, for use on papyrus or parchment — or by the writing brush, made of elastic hair and used on silk. Thus two opposing principles developed: on the one hand, a monumental or official style (in the West, generally in classicizing terms) tending toward a rigidly formal organization, a symmetry and proportion of the individual signs and lines — indeed, of the whole written surface — with careful alignment and spacing; and on the other hand, a more pliant cursive style, eurythmic and intuitive, which often served to reveal the personality of the writer. (It was the observation of differences in calligraphy that gave birth to the concept of personal style in Renaissance artistic treatises.) By and large these two classes of writing — monumental and cursive — correspond to the two different fields of

epigraphy (the study of inscriptions on durable materials) and paleography (the study of writings on perishable materials). In practice, the two classes are often less distinct and give rise to continual interchange, as will be seen in the subsequent historical discussion.

The distinction between mimetic writing (pictograms) and totally schematic writing (alphabetical letters) seems to diminish in certain periods. There are noteworthy examples of illuminated schematic writing in which individual alphabetical letters are formed from pictorial representations, or the pictorial decoration of individual letters emphasizes the meaning of the written material; however, the intent of such alphabets is generally decorative rather than explanatory. In the process of formalization of writing, the abandonment of color as a determinant of meaning for the symbol is typical. But even when formalized and abstract, the written symbol or phrase does not lose its decorative function.

Illumination of manuscripts is the best-known example of embellishment, but other important cases of embellishment also exist. The Egyptian hieroglyphic script, when colored, was admirably suited to paintings on walls, tombstones, sarcophagi, etc., and was also common in architectural ornamentation, where it was engraved or embossed. We can cite the famous Chinese inscriptions of the Confucian classics on the stone drums and those on pottery vessels and jade; also the beautiful Mayan steles and altars with their elaborate cartouches containing several picture signs gathered into a single frame. The Arabic lapidary, or Kufic, style was employed mainly on walls of mosques and on coins. With the development of Arabic calligraphy, Kufic became more and more consistent in height, thickness, and form of the single characters. In fact, it became such an exceptionally beautiful script that it was often used in the Christian West for purely decorative purposes. The cartouches on medieval frescoes and panels are often also very effective, as are the legends which accompany the paintings, serving not merely as explanations but for the clearly decorative purpose of creating a pleasing frame.

The artist's signature constitutes a special case of insertion of writing into painting and sculpture. Its placement is often ingeniously calculated; sometimes the name is changed into a monogram. There also exist, especially in more recent works, exercises on the alphabetic theme that are fundamentally pictorial, as in surrealist and cubist paintings, where the introduction of letters serves as a symbolic suggestion or even as a structural fulcrum of the entire work (see CUBISM AND FUTURISM; SURREALISM). Certain of the works of Paul Klee (q.v.) illustrate this device. In the fields of graphic arts (q.v.) and cinematography the frequent use of a typically calligraphic arrangement of the lettering reflects the current tendency to a return to a unity of calligraphic style, probably stimulated by the achievements of nonobjective art (q.v.) and neoplasticism (see EUROPEAN MODERN MOVEMENTS).

* *

PRIMITIVE AND ETHNOLOGICAL PICTOGRAPHS. Pictography, or picture writing, is the most primitive stage of writing. A picture or sketch (pictogram) represents the thing shown; thus, a circle may represent the sun, a sketch of an animal may represent the animal shown, a sketch of a man may indicate a man. Straight narrative can thus be recorded in a sequence of pictures, drawings, or symbols that yield their meaning to later decipherers with a fair degree of clarity and can be expressed in speech in any language, as the symbols do not represent speech sounds. Curiously enough, the symbols employed assumed similar (though by no means identical) forms in picture writings of different lands and ages. For instance, the symbol of an eye shown with tear drops, to represent sorrow, is to be seen not only in a Californian rock painting but also in the more-developed Mayan and Aztec scripts, as well as in the early Egyptian hieroglyphic and Chinese scripts and even in modern primitive picture writings.

Picture writings are found everywhere. They are the work of ancient peoples in a primitive stage of culture, such as the prehistoric inhabitants of southern France, northern Spain,

Italy, Palestine, and Crete, or the work of modern tribes of North America, Australia, northeastern Siberia, and other areas. The bark of trees, wooden panels, skins of animals, bones, ivory, the surface of rocks, and the walls of caves were all, or are still, used for this purpose.

The first attempts to express ideas graphically, or rather pictorially, were undifferentiated from pictures, which, in primitive cultures, tend toward the abstract. These graphic representations probably had a magical character (see MAGIC; PAINTING). Very possibly we may include in the category of sympathetic magic the numerous river pebbles of the Azilian culture (Mesolithic period), which show dots and lines painted with peroxide of iron. The various geometric signs or conventional figures of men, painted or engraved on stones (known as petroglyphs) dating from the Paleolithic era down to modern times, can in some cases be considered as the crude beginnings of writing.

Mention may be made of distinguishing devices, which, generally speaking, belong to a more recent period. Examples are the *wusums*, cattle marks and brands of Arab tribes east of Damascus, and the *tamgas*, symbolical marks or seals of the early Turks and allied tribes. Ancient property marks have been found on pottery or masonry in Egypt, Palestine, Crete, Cyprus, and other Mediterranean countries.

Primitive picture writings are still being made in North and Central America, in Africa, among the Yukaghirs of northeastern Siberia, among the Eskimos, and by some other native tribes in various parts of the world.

David DIRINGER

The Eskimos have produced many graffiti, carvings on bone, horn, or ivory, which pictorially represent scenes of hunting and fishing, daily life, ritual dances, or shamanic activities (see ESKIMO CULTURES). Sticks also carry the pictographic record of several events, the individual scenes being separated, on a single surface, by vertical lines. While in Canada the Eskimos execute lively and naturalistic figures, in Alaska they content themselves with linear and stylized forms.

The "annual recital" of the northeast Siberian Yukaghirs is a pictographic account on manatee hide in which the various happenings are minutely recorded in a spiral, as in the winter counts of American Indians (see below).

In Cameroun, the Bamum alphabet, invented by Sultan Njoya about 1907, originally consisted of more than 300 naturalistic and clearly definable symbols; after 1918, the characters became more decidedly symbolic and were reduced to 70 in number. To the west, among the Vai (Vei) in Liberia, writing that is now diagrammatic still includes certain symbols that retain their realistic character. The tifinagh alphabet of the Tuaregs seems to have derived from an early Saharan alphabet of dots and lines.

The message sticks of Australia are well known. Used for both ritual and nonritual purposes, they are certainly a rudimentary form of writing. Round or flat short sticks are carved (or less often painted) with stylized figures; straight, crossed, or curved lines, bars and dots appear in numerous combinations which vary according to local cultures.

In the New Caledonia area, carvings on bamboo also constitute true pictographs, as has been indicated by the testimony of a chief of the island of Kunie (Île des Pins). The various scenes, depicted between the knots, represent traditional or colonial subjects (firearms, persons in uniform or European dress, etc.). Geometric decoration with probable symbolic value is frequent.

The 24 wooden tablets from Easter Island which have come down to us boast a type of writing which consists of linear symbols outlined in contour. They are generally boustrophedonic (that is, with lines running alternately left to right and right to left). Although it is not yet certain whether these characters form a symbolic script using ideograms for a rebus (pictures representing their homonyms), the approximately 500 characters may be either naturalistic or geometric; but even when they are naturalistic, a tendency to geometrization is evident. Predominating among the naturalistic characters are human figures with birds' heads, shown either in profile or

frontally, with rhomboidal ears projecting; the image of the god Make-Make, with human form; the head of a frigate bird, and the tail of a fish; and bizarre contorted anthropomorphous figures, always seen frontally. The various symbols seem to relate to a language of mimicry, as they indicate sleeping or sitting, bowing, working, etc. It is thought that the tablets contain genealogies, sacred hymns, records of feast days in honor of ancestors, chronologies, and lists of various kinds.

The picture writing of North American Indians (PL. I) is either of a public nature (calendrical records, historical documents, census lists, etc.) or used in ritual magic or for private purposes (records of events or deeds, biographies, messages, etc.); they are painted or carved on skin (buffalo, elk, deer), wood, or bark, and, more recently, on paper; sometimes they appear on shields (Crow), on teepees, and on the cloaks of warriors, medicine men, or members of secret societies. Styles vary from a vigorous realism, as in certain handsome Sioux battle scenes, to complete stylization and abstraction.

The most characteristic notations are the winter counts, or counts back, tribal annals that register the events of a long period of time; originally they may have been historical or biographical, but they came to be used as calendars of recorded events succeeding each other at regular intervals. These were disposed in a spiral, starting at the center; the date can be determined by counting either backward or forward from a known event. The Dakota Lone Dog's Winter Count records the events of 1800–71; the meanings of the designs, which are generally rendered only in outline, are almost always comprehensible at first sight. Sometimes, however, the designs are symbolic: a block for a horse, straight sticks for the fallen enemy, connecting lines between human figures to show relationship, etc.

The Navaho symbolic and narrative "sand paintings" are executed in the course of curing rituals and illustrate elements of traditional chants. Made with earth, sand, ashes, and mineral or vegetable colorings, they depict conventionalized figures of gods, animals, rain, lighting, plants of mythological import, etc. The scenes are frequently bordered on three sides by an anthropomorphous representation of the rainbow. The colors used are red, yellow, blue, black, and white, each symbolically significant. The pictures are destroyed at the conclusion of the ceremony and must be reproduced exactly from memory at each repetition of the ritual.

Some Peruvian figures may be picture writing; for instance, in the vase motif of runners holding sacks of beans, the beans represent messages borne by couriers, according to Inca custom. It is thought that the figures of deer, falcons, and hummingbirds with anthropomorphous characteristics may symbolize the messengers, and those of wolves and felines the interpreters and scribes. The beans and kidney-shaped tablets of the Mochica, covered as they are with engraved lines of various kinds (straight, curved, dashed, parallel) and often-repeated dots, circles, and crosses, must certainly have had conventional meanings. A similar graphic system is to be found also in weavings.

Editta CASTALDI

The great masterpieces of pictography are the magnificent pre-Columbian manuscripts, whose importance transcends calligraphy and which rightly belong to the history of painting (see MIDDLE AMERICAN PROTOHISTORY).

It is known that a large number of Mayan hieroglyphic manuscripts were in existence at the time of the Conquest, but only three, written on the bark of the wild fig tree, have survived; they are the beautiful Dresden Codex, the Madrid Codex, and the Paris Codex. Other Mayan written material has also survived: numerous steles — huge, vertical monolithic pillars — dating perhaps from the 4th to the 10th century of our era, carved all over in low relief with glyphs and figures; large oval stones or altars, similarly carved; some polychrome pottery painted with glyphs and figures; and carvings and engravings on metal and bone.

Mayan writing (PL. I) is almost entirely ideographic, although signs of a phonetic development are already in evidence. Five

stages can be distinguished, passing from the purely conventionalized glyph through increasingly naturalistic phases until the character of the writing becomes wholly realistic and pictorial.

The glyphs, or cartouches, are highly conventionalized groups of many picture signs gathered into a single frame; they have some external, but undoubtedly casual, resemblance to the Egyptian royal cartouches. The script is on the whole undeciphered, except for the calendar symbols and the notation signs.

Apart from a great number of manuscripts written under Spanish domination, there are less than a score of pre-Columbian Mexican manuscripts extant. The work of scribes, who belonged largely to the priestly class, these manuscripts (PL. 1) have been generally considered Aztec, but it would appear that the major part were more certainly Mixtecan and later (15th cent.) inspired the Aztec codices. Each of these manuscripts is painted on a long sheet of white-varnished coarse cloth made from the fiber of the *Agave americana* (century plant) or on *amatl* paper, folded in accordion style to form the leaves. A wide range of colors prevails — red, yellow, blue, green, purple, brown, orange, black, and white — some in more than one shade. The symbols are outlined in black. The coloring is precisely executed and laid on in flat planes without perspective but with a fine sense of design — at least in so far as the manuscripts attributed to the Mixtecs (ca. 650–900) are concerned. The sheet was fastened to what may be called the binding of the codex, which was of fine, thin wood covered with brilliant varnish. Each cover measured nearly the same as the leaves, and the binding had no back.

The script used by the Mixtecs and Aztecs is much better known than the Mayan and has been partly deciphered. The symbols of this highly pictographic script are crude pictures; there are numerous instances of pure ideographic writing, and sometimes the script is even more in the nature of mnemonic aid to be supplemented by oral description than of a true script. The migrations of the Aztecs, for example, were represented by footsteps from place to place; in the tribute lists objects such as shields, garments, mosaics, strings of beads, etc., were depicted, accompanied by pictographs of numbers.

In some respects, however, the Aztec script is more advanced; many conventional signs have phonetic value, either as word signs or as syllables. Historical events were ingeniously depicted by pictographs together with symbols which indicated the site and year of occurrence. Abstract ideas are represented by picture signs borrowed from homonyms.

EVOLUTION OF PREALPHABETIC WRITING. *Egypt*. Monumental hieroglyphic writing, derived from pictography, maintained representational characteristics during three millenniums (ca. 2900 B.C.–4th cent. of our era), even though some ideograms became phonograms; that is, they acquired a phonetic value independent of their graphic meaning.

The were about 500 picture signs in common use. These represented (in partial or complete stereotypes) men, women, gods, mammals, birds, amphibians, reptiles, invertebrates, plants, shrubs, buildings, boats, domestic and funerary objects, clothes, weapons, hunting and fishing equipment, farming implements, tools, cordage, baskets, stone and pottery vessels, writing tools, musical instruments, and various aspects of the sky, earth, and waters.

Relief hieroglyphics are either hollowed out or raised, while painted hieroglyphics are often in several colors. A monumental text may be made up of vertical or horizontal lines; the vertical is the earlier, as in the royal pyramids of the 5th dynasty (2480–2350 B.C.). The stonecutters did not leave spaces between the words, but concentrated on arranging the hieroglyphics within a given square area, a peculiarity which sometimes led to metathesis. The hieroglyphics generally go horizontally from right to left, which is indicated by the direction assumed by the hieroglyphics representing animate beings; they almost always turn toward the beginning of the writing. In texts accompanying painted or relief human figures, however, hieroglyphics face the same direction as the direction assumed by the personage to which the symbols refer.

Hieroglyphic writing was ubiquitous. It appears on the walls of temples and tombs, on steles, obelisks (PL. 2), statues, sarcophagi, domestic, funerary or farming implements, seals and scarabs, and even as ornamental motifs on gold and precious woods. The carved hieroglyphics of the Old Kingdom (2650–2200 B.C.) are of great perfection to the minutest detail.

The book hand had a development parallel to that of monumental inscriptions. The writing was done with a small, hollow reed pen and a solid black or red ink used with water, on the inner membrane of papyrus stalks (*Cyperus papyrus*). The introduction of papyrus also marked the emergence of the so-called "hieratic" script, which is merely a simplification of hieroglyphic writing.

In the oldest surviving hieratic papyri, dating to the 5th dynasty, the lines were written vertically, but during the 12th dynasty (1991–1778 B.C.) the tendency to horizontal lines appeared and became fixed. When a papyrus was of any considerable length, the text was divided into columns or pages. Inscriptions have been found also on ostraca — fragments of pottery and limestone — which date from the 6th century B.C. to the 4th century of our era.

In the course of time hieratic writing became increasingly divorced from its hieroglyphic prototypes: the ductus became more fluent and new ligatures appeared. Meanwhile differences according to content also appeared, resulting in three distinct types of hieratic scripts found in paleographic texts: a book hand, a script for official documents, and one for religious and funerary use, this last in the 21st dynasty (1085–932 B.C.) only. The funerary papyri of the 18th to the 20th dynasty (1570–1085 B.C.) were written instead in hieroglyphic characters.

From the 7th century B.C. onward hieratic script in everyday use was simplified to demotic writing, characterized by a reduction in the number of symbols, a greater number of ligatures, and greater cursiveness.

* *

*Cuneiform*. The earliest written documents extant are Mesopotamian clay tablets from the middle of the 4th millenium B.C. They are inscribed with a crude pictographic writing, many characters being purely pictorial and the picture symbols representing various animate or inanimate objects. The writing gradually developed from pictorial symbols, which were not very suitable for writing on moist and soft clay, into combinations of short strokes (straight, vertical, horizontal, or oblique, sometimes forming angles), having the shape of a wedge; each symbol represented a syllable. Hundreds of thousands of writings on clay tablets, stone, bronze, copper, and occasionally gold, silver, and ivory have transmitted a very rich literature of the Sumerians, Akkadians, Babylonians, Assyrians, Elamites, Kassites, Mitanni, Hurrians, Urartu, and ancient Persians for about 3,500 years, or nearly to the Christian era (PL. 3).

The two greatest periods of vigor in Assyro-Babylonian history — that of Hammurabi (18th cent. B.C.) in Babylonia and the 9th to the 7th century B.C. in Assyria — were marked by a corresponding flourishing of cuneiform writing. The rich libraries of the Assyrian kings contained many thousands of tablets of literature and scientific works. There are also complete records of royal campaigns and other activities, impressed on hollow cylinders or prisms, with six, seven, eight, or even ten faces, each covered with as much calligraphic, minute writing as it could possibly hold. The Assyrians simplified the whole cuneiform system and rendered the writing more square in appearance (PL. 3).

*Cretan-Mycenaean and Hittite scripts*. A rapid survey of other Mediterranean and Near Eastern civilizations, whose artistic and cultural capacities made for elaborate and pictorial scripts, should include the Minoan peoples (see CRETAN-MYCENAEAN ART), who had important systems of writing (PL. 3). Four such systems can be distinguished: pictographic class A, pictographic class B, linear class A, and linear class B. The last was deciphered by Michael Ventris and John Chadwick after World War II and proved to be an early form of the Greek language.

Mention should be made of the Phaestos disk (PL. 2), which can be assigned to about 1700 B.C. The disk contains pictorial sign groups impressed by means of separate stamps on both its faces. Hardly any of the numerous Cretan-Mycenaean tablets discovered have any outstanding esthetic merit.

The Hittites inhabited Asia Minor and northern Syria in the last two millenniums B.C.; their empire reached its height in the 14th and 13th centuries. They employed both cuneiform writing and an indigenous hieroglyphic script (PL. 3; known as Hittite hieroglyphic writing), which apparently evolved about the mid-2d millennium B.C. The majority of the inscriptions, coming mainly from northern Syria, belong to the 10th to 8th century B.C.; the latest is of about 600 B.C. Some of these inscriptions, particularly those carved in relief on stone, are truly calligraphic.

David DIRINGER

*China.* For more than 2,000 years the Chinese have considered calligraphy as the very essence of pictorial art (PLS. 14, 15). Until about the 5th century of our era painting was regarded as a mere skill and painters as artisans, while calligraphers were looked upon as the true artists. It took several centuries before painting could conquer a place of its own in cultural life, and till the present day it has not been able to oust calligraphy from the first place. Calligraphy is linked up with painting by the brush stroke; both the calligrapher and the painter use exactly the same brush, and its strokes constitute the common basis of the two sister arts. Chinese art critics have always considered the brush stroke as the main criterion in judging a painting. Moreover, the balanced composition of each individual calligraphic character and the spacing of a number of characters written together provided the basic principles that ruled the spacing and composition of Chinese paintings.

Authentic specimens of the calligraphy of the great old masters have always been rare, but copies are widely accessible in the form of rubbings. Since ancient times the Chinese have incised the works of famous calligraphers in stone or wood, with almost photographic accuracy; these engraved inscriptions are reproduced by placing a sheet of thin paper over the surface and then rubbing it with ink so that the writing shows in white on a black ground. Rubbings have always played a most important role in Chinese calligraphic and epigraphic studies; by placing the rarest works of the famous masters within everyone's reach, they have promoted and kept alive popular interest in this art (see ENGRAVINGS AND OTHER PRINT MEDIA).

The study of calligraphy and epigraphy starts with inscriptions on oracle bones and bronze vessels dating from about 1500 B.C., but it is only from about the 5th century B.C. (roughly the time of Confucius) that the epigraphical remains are sufficiently numerous and varied to give a general idea of the artistic qualities of the writing used at that time. Those archaic characters, called *chüan-shu,* commonly called "seal script," were written with a primitive brush and coarse ink or lacquer on bamboo or wooden tablets or silk. This script developed such a perfect balance and austere linear beauty that it has ever after remained in use for the legends of seals and calligraphic purposes. It is characterized by rounded curves and lines of uniform thickness ending in blunt tips.

During the last two centuries B.C. two other scripts came into general use: *li-shu* ("chancery script") and *ts'ao-shu* ("draft script" or "grass script"). The former is a simplified form of the seal script, but it has sharp corners and lines of varying thickness ending in broad sweeps and jagged ends. The draft script is a kind of shorthand in which even the most complicated characters are often reduced to a single scrawl; the strokes are of greatly varying thickness, and their tips show a great variety of shape. The modulation of the strokes is important.

In the first centuries of our era the technical perfection of the writing brush produced a new style of writing, a stylized form of the chancery script generally called *k'ai-shu* or *chêng-shu* ("regular script"); it has sharp, clear-cut corners, and straight strokes of varying thickness predominate. This regular script was also written in a more cursive way, a style called *hsing-shu* or "running hand."

All these five scripts have remained in use till the present day. The regular script is the model for printed type, first used in wood-block printing, and in modern times for movable type, while the running script is widely used for the practical needs of daily life. Seal, chancery, and draft script are still the favorite means of expression for calligraphers. Seal and chancery script have a static beauty that requires carefully adjusted proportions and expressive strokes, always within the limits of the rules for spacing evenly the characters composing a text; every character must be of approximately the same size. The draft script is dynamic; it is not bound by the rules for even spacing, and the characters need not be of the same size, thus giving the artist the fullest freedom for expression. It is, however, the most difficult of all and takes many years to master; its main beauty lies in what might be called the abstract line and the dynamic rhythm of the richly modulated strokes. It is not without reason that Chinese connoisseurs consider it as the highest expression of Chinese pictorial art. Masters in this style are reverently called *ts'ao-sheng* ("holy men of the draft script").

It was in the draft and the running scripts that the paragon of Chinese calligraphers of all times excelled, the celebrated Wang Hsi-chih (321–79). Even during his lifetime a few lines written by him were paid for in gold, and autographs ascribed to him are national treasures, still eagerly copied by everyone who aspires to become a calligrapher. The most famous specimen of his handwriting is the *Lan-ting-hsü* ("Essay on the Orchid Pavilion"). His son Wang Hsien-chih (344–88) shared his father's fame, and the pair are known as the "Two Wang."

Their work was especially popular during the T'ang dynasty (618–907), when under imperial patronage the art of calligraphy flourished as never before; the emperor Ming Huang (T'ang Hsüan-tsung; 713–55) himself was an excellent calligrapher. Of the great masters only a few can be mentioned here. All-round calligraphers were the scholar-officials Ou-yang Hsün (557–641), Chu Sui-liang (596–658), and Yü Shih-nan (558–638); they wrote in a great variety of styles, but favored especially the draft and the running hands. Also famous were the calligraphers Liu Kung–chüan (778–865), Yen Chêng-ch'ing (709–84), and Li Yang-ping (ca. 750), known for his seal script. The T'ang dynasty was the great age of the draft script; among its masters were Sun Kuo-t'ing, who wrote *Shu-pu,* a handbook on calligraphy; the priest Huai-su; and the drunkard artist Chang Hsü (ca. 700), who wrote in the very difficult *K'uang-ts'ao* or "inspired draft script."

Under the Sung dynasty (960–1279) there was published a collection of rubbings of selected specimens of calligraphy, *Ch'un-hua-ko-fa-t'ieh,* as well as a voluminous catalogue of calligraphic specimens of the imperial collection. The most famous calligraphers of the period were Su Shih (literary name Tung-p'o, 1036–1101), Huang T'ing-chien (Shan-ku, 1045–1105), Ts'ai Hsiang (1012–67), and Mi Fei (q.v.). Even during the Yüan period (1260–1368), when China was ruled by the alien Mongol dynasty, calligraphy was flourishing, the two most outstanding masters being Chao Mêng-fu (q.v.) and Hsien-yü Shu (1257–1302).

Under the Ming dynasty (1368–1644) there was a galaxy of artists who successfully followed the ancient masters. The six leading calligraphers were Tung Ch'i-ch'ang (q.v.), Chu Yünming (1460–1526), Wên Chêng-ming (q.v.), Chang Jui-t'u (ca. 1600), Wang To (1592–1652), and Hsing T'ung (ca. 1580). Also the emperors of the Ch'ing dynasty (1644–1912) were patrons of the art of calligraphy, and some were masters in this art; the emperor Ch'ien-lung published a collection of rubbings of ancient specimens of calligraphy (*San-hsi-t'ang-shih-chu-pao-chi-fa-t'ieh*). Some calligraphers created new styles: Chin Nung (Tung-hsin, 1687–1764), Chêng Hsieh (Pan-ch'iao, 1693–1765), Ho Shao-ch'i (1799–1873), Ch'ên Hung-shou (Man-kung, 1768–1822), and the statesman and reformer K'ang Yu-wei (1858–1916). Among the many calligraphers who specialized in the ancient styles were Chao Chih-ch'ien (1829–84), Têng Wan-po (1743–1805), and Wu Hsiang-chih (1797–1870). Excellent handbooks of calligraphy were compiled, such

as *I-chou-shuang-chi*, by Pao Shih-ch'eng (1775–1855), which was later supplemented by K'ang Yu-wei.

In the Chinese Republic, established in 1912, calligraphy retained its prominent position. Cheng Hsiao-hsü (d. 1938) became more famous as a great calligrapher than as the premier of the puppet state of Manchukuo. Wu Ch'ang-shih (1844–1927), Shen Yin-mo, the great master of Shanghai, and Yü Yu-jen, the aged calligrapher and statesman of Formosa, are other famous calligraphers of modern China.

*Japan.* The Japanese esteem calligraphy as highly as do the Chinese (PL. 15). Calligraphy started in Japan in the early 7th century with the copying out of the sacred Buddhist texts, in a special variety of the Chinese regular script, at that time favored by Chinese Buddhist monks. Prince Shōtoku (572–621) was an expert in this style. At a later period the Japanese monk Kūkai (Kōbōdaishi, 774–835) acquired during his stay in China great skill in all styles of Chinese calligraphy and introduced these into Japan. The Japanese emperor Saga (810–23) wrote an excellent running hand, and the emperor Daigo (898–930) wrote an impressive draft script.

After the invention of hiragana by Kūkai, the Japanese used this script, occasionally intermixed with Chinese characters (Kanji). Hiragana was a kind of syllabic writing which originated as abbreviated and conventionalized Chinese ideographs. The hiragana calligraphy of the great masters Ono Michikaze (Dōfu, 896–966) and Kino Tsurayuki (883–946) has the charm of graceful, light strokes. The early court novels (e.g., the *Genji-monogatari*) were written in this style.

Kublai Khan's (1216–94) attack on Japan severed relations of that country with China, and *wa-yō* (the Japanese style of writing) developed further at the expense of *kara-yō* (the Chinese style). With the renewal of the contacts with China, under the Tokugawa shogunate (1615–1867), there was a revival of interest in Chinese calligraphy, particularly among the warrior caste, poets and painters in Chinese style, and students of Confucianism; whereas students of Shinto (see SHINTOISM) and the poets and painters in the Japanese style continued to favor the *wa-yō*; of the latter calligraphers, we mention Kitamura Kigin (1618–1705), Kei-chū (1640–1701), and Kamo Mabuchi (1697–1769). Chinese calligraphy was cultivated by Konoe Nobutaka (1565–1614), Hon-ami Kō-etsu (1557–1637), Ishikawa Jōzan (1583–1672), and many others. Moreover, the Tokugawa shoguns, who patronized the study of Chinese for political reasons, founded a Confucianist academy in Edo (mod. Tokyo), where Chinese calligraphy was studied, and many Japanese calligraphers became masters in Chinese calligraphy: Hosoi Kōtaku (1658–1735), Ichikawa Bei-an (1779–1858), Nukina Kai-oku (1778–1863), and others.

Also in the last century, despite the Japanese interest in Western culture, calligraphy continued to flourish, and excellent work was done by Kusakabe Mei-kaku (1838–1922), Hidai Tenrai (1872–1939), Jamamoto Keizan (1863–1934), and Tashiro Shūkaku (1883–1946). Calligraphy is still immensely popular in Japan; the government organizes a yearly national calligraphic exhibition, just as it does for painting and sculpture.

Robert H. VAN GULIK

MAJOR EXAMPLES OF ALPHABETIC SCRIPTS. *Greece and Rome.* All the evidence appears to indicate that the Greek alphabet existed by about 1000 B.C. Serious scholars agree that it is of north Semitic origin. Occupying a unique place in the history of writing, it not only transformed the consonantal Semitic script into a modern alphabet (with appropriate consonants and vowels) but was also the progenitor of all the European and many non-European alphabets.

If we accept the principle that writing which is to rank as calligraphy should be formal, deliberate, and controlled, then numerous Greek inscriptions can be regarded as calligraphic (PL. 4). The writing of the many inscriptions discovered throughout the Hellenic world is, as a rule, monumental or lapidary. The earliest examples (from Athens, Thera, Boeotia, Corfu) belong to the late 9th or the 8th century B.C.

A craftsman who cut inscriptions was known as γλύφας. From late classical times the names of several such craftsmen are incised in the inscriptions, sometimes with the addition of ἔγραψα, "I have written"; in the Museo Nazionale in Palermo there is a tablet (CIL, X, 7296) in Greek and Latin advertising the trade of a certain stonecutter. Some of the men who cut inscriptions were artists in their craft; but from classical antiquity and the ancient Near East the name of only one professional calligrapher has come down to us, the lapidary scribe and miniaturist Furius Dionysius Filocalus, who composed in Rome the famous Chronographer, or Calendar of the Sons of Constantine (in Hellenistic style), about the middle of the 4th century.

As far back as the oldest preserved documents (4th cent. B.C.), we see side by side two classes of Greek cursive writing — the literary or book hand and the current or running hand, used for nonliterary writing (letters, accounts, receipts, etc.).

The two earliest Greek calligraphic book hands are known as capitals and uncials. Capitals, or large letters, were the older; in fact, they were adaptations from the monumental or lapidary style. They were formed chiefly by straight strokes meeting at angles and avoiding curves in so far as possible. The uncial forms developed from the capitals by being more rounded, curves becoming habitual, since they were more easily inscribed with the pen on soft material such as papyrus or parchment. The uncial style, probably the character best adapted for calligraphy, was the usual Greek book hand for several centuries; it was only after about A.D. 800 (when the minuscule style was adapted as a book hand) that the uncial went out of use for books.

Latin calligraphy and epigraphy go back to the Etruscans. Serious scholars now generally hold that the Etruscan alphabet was the link between the Greek and the Latin; it was also the progenitor of nearly all the Italic alphabets and perhaps also of several other scripts, such as the Germanic runes.

The main offshoot of the Etruscan alphabet — the Latin or Roman character — which has so much importance in the history of civilization, had itself a very poor history during the first five or six centuries of its existence; it showed little or no development, and calligraphically it had little significance. The oldest extant record of the Latin script dates from the 7th century B.C., but it is only from the 1st century B.C. onward that Latin inscriptions throughout the Mediterranean world become so numerous that they cannot be counted.

Roman literature, flourishing from the 3d century B.C. onward, was based on Greek models, and there seems little doubt that Latin calligraphy also followed Greek models.

There may well have been attempts at calligraphy in Rome before the 1st century B.C., but very little evidence of this has come down to us. There is no doubt, however, that in the 1st century B.C. the Latin alphabet was truly calligraphic; that is, regular, harmonious, well-proportioned, and elegant (PL. 5). This is particularly so in the monumental or lapidary style. This style, with insignificant changes, was constantly used not only in monumental writing and as the earliest book hand of the Roman period, but also for capital letters of the Latin alphabet during the Middle Ages; it continues to be used in printing even up to the present day. There are extant several Latin inscriptions up to 2,000 years old which are, or can be, employed nowadays as models for modern capital letters.

Although we have no direct evidence, we may assume that by the 1st century B.C. there existed calligraphic copies of literary works written in monumental style, known as square capitals. What little material in this style has come down to us is mostly late (4th or 5th cent.). As the manuscript fragments extant are mainly copies of Vergil, such as the Codex Vergilius Augusteus (Vat. lat. 3256) and Codex 1394 of the Stiftsbibliothek, St. Gall, Switzerland, it has rightly been suggested that the continuance of square capitals as a calligraphic book hand was a survival of a style first employed at an early period to do honor to the greatest Roman national poet.

Nearly all the earliest Latin manuscripts extant are written in rustic capitals derived from the square capitals. They are in a rather easier and somewhat negligent style, being light and quickly formed, but as a calligraphic book hand they were no

less carefully formed than square capitals. The strokes are more slender, cross strokes are short and more or less oblique, and there is a greater tendency to rise above the line. The best-known Vergil manuscripts written in rustic capitals are the Codex Vergilius (Vat. lat. 3225); the Codex Mediceus in the Laurentian Library at Florence; the Codex Vergilius Romanus (Vat. lat. 3867); and the Codex Palatinus (Vat. pal. lat. 1631). They belong to the 4th and 5th centuries. Other examples extant of manuscripts written in rustic capitals are copies of Cicero, Terence, and Prudentius.

By the end of the 5th century square capitals and rustic capitals appear to have fallen out of general use as book hands for entire texts, although they were not infrequently used in the Middle Ages for titles and initials (sometimes even for a few pages of text). On occasion they were used throughout the whole text, as in the finely executed 6th-century copy of Prudentius preserved in the Bibliothèque Nationale at Paris and the superb 9th-century Utrecht Psalter (Utrecht, Univ. Lib., Script. eccl. 484; PL. 58), which no doubt is a copy of an older codex.

From available evidence it seems that the Latin uncial script was already used in Roman documents of the 3d century of our era. In the 4th century it appears as a perfect book hand beside the square and the rustic capitals, and from the 5th century onward, for 500 years it was the main book hand of the Christian world, especially for de luxe codices. The Greek uncial character which was the script of the earliest Bible codices helped materially in the rapid diffusion of the Roman uncial writing.

The uncial style which, generally speaking, is a modification of the square-capital writing, was a mixed script. Although the majority of the letters were slightly modified capitals, some (*h, l, q*) were minuscules, that is, written according to the four-line scheme, and four letters (*a, d, e, m*) assumed the typical rounded shape, the main feature of the uncial hand (PL. 8). Uncial, then, is essentially a round hand, because in writing with the reed pen on a material more or less soft, especially parchment, the scribe tends to avoid angles by curving the "corners." The main vertical strokes generally rise above or fall below the line of writing.

Numerous Latin codices written in this beautiful book hand are extant. Particularly in those of the 5th and the 6th centuries the letters are generally formed with much beauty and precision of stroke; but from the 7th century onward this book hand becomes more artificial, forced, imitative, and badly formed.

Several Latin codices which have come down to us are written in a book hand known as "semiuncial" or "half uncial." This half-and-half style, easier than the uncials and more calligraphic than the formal cursive of minuscule writing, was also a mixed script, derived partly from capital letters and partly from the cursive. One of its earliest forms may be seen in a 3d-century papyrus fragment found in 1903 in Oxyrhynchus, Egypt (Oxyrhynchus Papyri, IV), and preserved in the British Museum; it contains an independent epitome of Livy's history for the years 150–137 B.C. The semiuncial is the book hand of many beautiful codices of the 5th to the 9th century.

David DIRINGER

*India and Farther India.* The Indian graphic system underwent innumerable changes during its course. With great vitality it spread widely over the central and eastern parts of Asia and Farther India and resulted in a number of diverse calligraphic types. The oldest securely dated writings are the inscriptions of King Aśoka (3d cent. B.C.), distributed from the territory of his ancient kingdom of Magadha (with its capital in modern Patna) in the east to modern Mysore in the south; they are carved with geometric simplicity on rocks and stone columns with two different hands, the Brahmi and the Kharoshthi. The former is lapidary in character, with absolutely rigid and vertical characters. When the latter appears on stone pillars, it is generally carelessly composed.

Kharoshthi script is a vulgarized cursive hand, without special attempt at calligraphy, but generally is fairly regular and uniform without the angularity of the Brahmi. In the manuscripts on parchment and wooden tablets of Central Asia the Kharoshthi is more calligraphic. This refinement is probably due to the use of ink and to an influx of the Iranian decorative taste so widespread in Central Asia.

In India true calligraphy was first attempted in the early centuries of our era and had a development parallel to the expansion and the differentiation of scripts which were to take different forms in the north and south of India.

In the north, writing was more refined. The vertical strokes became equalized and terminated more broadly in a curl, thus describing an upper line, called "matra," below which, as a result, each character was to be traced. Alignment was more regular and ligatures appeared. The early clearly distinguishable scripts are the Kṣatrapa and Kushan types.

Of the Kṣatrapa type ("of the satraps") of the north, the earliest inscription found is that of the satrap Śoḍāsa (perhaps A.D. 14). The Kushan type, named for the ruling dynasty of the Indo-Scythian empire and also recorded in Central Asia, displays the earliest ligatures and blunted angles; the upper appendages are developed in flamelike undulations. Inscriptions for this period are numerous in the west, though of an earlier type. Also in Ceylon archaizing forms similar to the Aśoka type subsisted, such as the Tonigala inscriptions of King Vaṭṭagāmanī Abhaya of the late 1st century.

In later centuries the different calligraphic schools became more clearly differentiated: the northern schools preferred linear and angular elements and sought after a harmonious regularity; the southern scripts, on the other hand, leaned toward rounded forms and curving lines, whose decorative effect was greater. This curvilinear quality was the result of the widespread practice of incising on palm leaves as a writing method. Although palm leaves lend themselves to the engraving of globular characters, they do not permit the tracing of the thick strokes with ornamental serifs favored by the use of ink in the north, so that southern calligraphers were forced to get their esthetic effects only from the inflection of line.

In the north in the Gupta period (4th–5th cent.) the various scripts underwent a final differentiation and expansion. In the numerous manuscripts found in Central Asia, Hoernle has identified two types of writing: the straight Gupta and the slanted Gupta. The Buddhist manuscripts in Sanskrit found at Bamian (Afghanistan) and Gilgit (Kashmir) show two more elaborated calligraphic types, with thick lines and very fine serifs. In type A the characters are rather low and wide and the matra above has become larger, but the balance is reestablished by an oblique weighting of the lower part of the characters. Type B has more slanted but straighter letters, with curves inclined slightly to the right and downward. Related scripts were in use in the basin of the Tarim River (Sinkiang) for Sanskrit and the local languages of the mid-7th century to the 10th century. Type B, widespread in the epigraphy of northern India with the name of Kutila, was transported to Japan, China, Korea, and Central Asia and was also used for magical formulas and for Sanskrit texts until after the 10th century. In Cambodia and in Kashmir (where it is called Sarada) it is in use to the present day. In Nepal scripts have followed the evolution of the Gupta alphabet since the 5th century. In Tibet from the 7th century on writing was formed after a post-Gupta model and had an erudite elaboration when used for Sanskrit.

From these ornamental types there developed a type known as the "boxhead type," in which the matras are transformed into small squares and the curves are replaced as often as possible by right angles. A variant with the lower dots turned toward the right is embellished with ornamental flowers.

After the 10th century the distinction between the common hands and the sophisticated hands became clearer. Many samples of the latter have been preserved in manuscripts, especially in western Bengal and Nepal.

The major type which is today more widespread is the Nagari (urban) or Devanagari alphabet, which was originally the local script of Benares. Because of the importance subsequently assumed by that city, Devanagari became increasingly widespread and was used to transcribe, besides the local language,

both Sanskrit and Hindi. In the early 19th century it was adopted for the printing of Sanskrit and Prakrit (Sanskrit vernacular) texts in Bengal and in Europe.

Nagari appears to be remotely derived from Brahmi, as it has the same system of transcription and the same direction from left to right. Its most original calligraphic element lies in the horizontal development of the matra so that when the characters are juxtaposed, they appear to have been written below a horizontal line. The effect of these linear elements is geometrizing; calligraphic embellishment and accentuated curves are absent.

The Jain Nagari, used in books on Jain doctrine and therefore most widely distributed in the West, differs somewhat from the ordinary Nagari. The Nepalese writings tended toward a form similar to the Nagari but were markedly calligraphic and varied. The two principal types are the Rañja ("elegant") and the Vartula ("round").

The Bengal scripts and those from near Mithila were similar in the Middle Ages to the Nepalese, but later they became more undulant, with bends and acute angles, curly bars, and slightly curved and straight matras which do not generally link one character with the other. In Orissa, north of the Bengal Gulf, Oriya script is characterized by rounded forms. Often the matra, developed in a convex curve, is larger than the rest of the character.

The Gurumukhi, used to transcribe the Punjabi tongue, is similar to the Nagari but is more cursive and rounded. The vernacular Gujarati alphabet is also cursive and simplified and is without matras. In the north and northwest various cursive hands exist.

In the south the two groups of inscriptions which have given birth to the two great groups of modern southern scripts, are those of the Pallava (6th–7th cent.) and Chalukya dynasties (7th–8th cent.). The inscriptions of the Pallava (who dominated the eastern coast, with Kanchipuram as their capital), from the lower basin of the Kistna River in the 4th to the 9th century, are ornamental by comparison with contemporary northern forms. Letters are slanted, strongly bent to the left and rising again toward the top of the foot, which becomes smaller and rounder. The Pallava forms for writing Sanskrit prepared the literary alphabet later called Grantha ("free"). Another hand for inscriptions developed into Tamil after the 7th century. This was the first Indian script to be printed (by the Portuguese mission in Malabar, 1577), although wood engravings of Sanskrit were being printed in Central Asia and China as early as the 10th century. The Tamil hand, at first in straight lines, became after the 19th century progressively more slanted. In the Tamil area the Grantha alphabet was also used for printing Sanskrit texts from the 19th century onward. Both Grantha and Tamil are elegant in themselves and are calligraphic in their regularity and the purity of their curves. They are accompanied by various cursives. The Tamil is also in use in northern Ceylon.

In Ceylon writing underwent its own evolution from the Aśoka types (see above). Editions de luxe of woven silk threaded with gold were executed with particular care; they are very beautiful. The calligraphic writing of Ceylon was in use not only for its own language (Singhalese) but also for Pali (the canonical language of Buddhism) and Sanskrit (the language of poetry and science).

The scripts of the Chalukya dynasty (both eastern and western), who ruled over the valleys of the Kistna and the Godavari, are less slanted than the Pallava script. They were to give rise to the Dravidian writings of the Telugu and Kannada regions in the north and west of the Tamil area.

The Telugu or Telinga script (east of Deccan) and the Kannada script (west of Deccan) are different, as to calligraphic qualities especially. Both are typified by letters formed of circles and arcs and topped by a matra forming a V-shaped flourish; but this assumes a quite different form in each of the two structures. Besides, in the earliest Kannada, forms tended to curls and curving verticals, which turned progressively upward where the curls first lengthened and then closed into circles. This ornamental hand inherited the calligraphic pecu-

liarities of the Hoysala inscriptions (12th cent.); it appeared in temple architecture with a particularly lively and complex ornamentation that suggests work in ivory. Kannada epigraphs have survived from the Katumba, Chalukya, Nastrakuta, and other reigns.

Thai (Tai) calligraphy is of great interest, as are Burmese and Cambodian. Like Singhalese, these are used for Pali texts. In the Thai script straight lines and right angles predominate over curves; the characters are well-spaced, their simple, self-contained forms creating a sense of regularity and order. Burmese script is completely different; its marked tendency toward rounded forms which enclose space displays points of resemblance with south Indian scripts. The characters, indeed, consist almost exclusively of curved lines forming circles and arcs which, uniformly repeated with little or no variation, give to the script a harmonious, if extremely simplified quality.

In Cambodia there are two types, Mul and Jrieng. In Mul ("fundamental"), used for Pali, the consonantal groups are formed by superposition; the characters, which lean slightly, are made up of generous lines rich in volutes and angles harmoniously interrelated in space and creating a particularly decorative effect. A slight variant of this type is Kham. Jrieng ("derived"), used principally for the Cambodian language, is more uniform and tends to be geometric, with right angles and straight lines predominating.

J. FILLIOZAT

*Islam.* As Islamic tradition tended to prohibit representational art, writing acquired a greatly enhanced artistic value (PL. 7). Calligraphers received honors elsewhere accorded to painters — even the names of minor calligraphers were well known — and their profession was esteemed above that of all other artisans. Leading princes became adepts at calligraphy.

Kufic script, which owes its name to the city of Kufa in Iraq, where it was invented (the names of its originators are not known), is the oldest of Arabic calligraphic styles. It appeared on the coins of the Ommiads and in the epigraphs on the earliest Palestinian mosques. It was successful in all fields: architecture, epitaphs, manuscripts, coins, textiles, and utensils. In the 8th century Qetba first established the relative sizes of the letters, and in the 9th century Ustād Ahwal of Seistan composed a calligraphic canon in Baghdad.

The irregular occurrence of the vertical strokes of the letters became rhythmical in time. After about 750 this omnipresent irregularity was obviated by an accentuation of the horizontals and of curves swinging below the line, and often by a leveling of the strokes, producing a style known as "gliding" Kufic. In monumental script the form of each symbol became more squat and compact, and after the early 9th century letters terminated in a wedge shape. From the 10th century on, on textiles, ceramics (especially Samanid wares), metalwork, epitaphs, and legends on coins, the vertical line became heightened, while the spacing was kept carefully even.

In response to a feeling for density of surface ornament, a "foliate" Kufic came into vogue in the late 10th century. The spaces between the strokes were filled with plant elements. At first springing organically from the characters themselves, this decoration was gradually enriched so as to become a decorative rinceau foil to the letters. The influence of the typically Islamic arabesque ornament is evident in this development. A more austere type of decoration was preferred for the Koran, but for inscriptions on stone, textiles, etc., graphic symbols were transformed (even at the expense of legibility) into burgeoning decorations. After about 1050 an "interlaced" Kufic became widespread, in which the strokes were developed into simple or complex interlacings that also helped decoratively to fill the voids. Another variant, the "speaking" Kufic, was mostly limited to Iran. In the 12th century it was used there primarily on bronzes, its strokes and curlicues terminating in heads of men, dragons, and birds.

In the 12th century the development of Kufic for the most part came to an end. In the manuscripts of the period it was no longer used, although it still served for decorative inscriptions and those on buildings, where it resulted in various "Ku-

ficizing" forms, such as the "geometric." Its ornamental appeal has had a certain influence on the West, where Kufic and pseudo-Kufic characters appear in decoration (see EXOTICISM).

Kufic was well-suited to calligraphy on parchment, the principal medium for copies of the Koran from the 8th to the 10th century. In the 10th century there developed from the cursive script a round, fluent hand known as Naskhi, which gave a new direction to calligraphy; in the 12th century it even penetrated monumental epigraphy. To the famous calligrapher vizier Ibn Muqla (d. 940) is attributed the introduction of Naskhi into the chancery of the caliphs of Baghdad: he prepared a round hand which was perfected and amplified by another vizier, Ibn al-Bawwāb (d. 1032). The beauty of this style was further enriched by the vizier Yaqūt al-Mustasimi (d. 1298), who introduced the pen with a tapering point to replace the reed pen with a straight slit; he had many disciples and imitators. From the 12th century on Naskhi was spread from Iraq to all the countries of Islam (with the partial exception of northern Africa and Spain).

In the decorative thuluth script, curves become rounder, while in the Rihāni they are open like the blade of a scimitar. In Riqa' all corners are blunted and the wavy lines accentuated; Tauqī', characterized by looped forms, was adopted for the chancery script for documents. Special forms were in use on ceramics, glass, metal, textiles, and faïence mosaics.

Baghdad, the old city of the caliphs on the Tigris, was the principal center of calligraphy and kept its position of leadership even after the conquest by the Mongols (1258). Certain fine copies of the Koran produced for the Mongol rulers, with solemn and majestic texts in black and gold, belong to the most splendid graphic works of the period. But soon Cairo preempted the first place. The Mameluke emirs (1250–1517) vied with each other in presenting precious, richly painted copies of the Koran to schools and mosques. Ibn al-'Afīf (d. 1335) and Ibn as-Sāigh (d. 1441) are the best-known of the calligraphers of the Cairo school. Many Iranian calligraphers were disciples of Mustasimi (see above) and were active at home and in Turkistan. Tabriz became an important center and was still a leader in the 16th century. At that time the fashion for *muraqqa'* became popular; these were bound volumes in which were brought together single pages of calligraphy and miniatures, often works signed by well-known masters. From the 15th century on Turkey also achieved a high place in Arabic calligraphy; many masters were called to Constantinople, the new capital: Sheikh Hamdullah (d. 1520), known as "Qiblet-ul-kuttāb" ("focus of writers"), also furnished models for the lapidary inscriptions of several mosques; Hāfiz 'Othmān (d. 1689) had various Ottoman sultans as disciples.

In the Islamic west in the region of Maghrib, from Tripoli to Morocco and Spain, a particular character was developed which was an intermediary form between the straight Kufic and the rounded Naskhi. It seems to have been flourishing at Kairouan about 1000. In the 12th century it was widespread in most of Maghrib, especially in Spain (where the principal centers were Seville and Valencia) and also in Sicily in Norman times. In the 14th and 15th centuries Granada was a center for the production of splendid, richly painted borders for copies of the Koran. But the Maghrib script did not penetrate the field of epigraphy, where various decorative forms of Kufic were still in use or Naskhi was introduced in a variant known as "Andalusian."

An early 13th- and 14th-century attempt at a national Iranian form through the use of the slant-cut reed is known as "taliq"; it is especially abundant on ceramics of the period. A book hand, the nastaliq, created by Mīr 'Alī of Tabriz (late 14th cent.), rapidly succeeded throughout Persia and thus became a national style. It recurs frequently in albums (*muraqqa'*). On the pages conceived as graphic models the verses, often in white on colored paper, are enclosed in clouds interspersed with vines and arabesque. Many of the 40 masters called by Prince Baisonqur (d. 1433) to the Academy of Artistic Book Production in Herat were disciples of Mīr 'Alī, whose style they spread far and wide. This was also propagated by

the sultan 'Alī of Meshed (d. 1513), who was also active at the court of Herat, together with the great poet Jami and the famous painter Bihzād (q.v.). Mahmūd of Nishapur (d. 1545) in Tabriz, Mīr 'Alī of Herat (d. 1558) in Bukhara, and, in the early 17th century, Mīr 'Imād (d. 1648) and 'Alī Rizā 'Abbāsī in Isfahan were masters of Naskhi as well.

From the 16th century on the nastaliq style spread to Turkey, where it was adopted as the norm for Turkish correspondence, and to India, where it enjoyed a great calligraphic success in the court of the Moghul emperors.

Toward the mid-17th century Shafī'a created in Herat the shikasta hand, a complicated, capricious, and difficult-to-read variation of the old taliq; another variant of the same, but (unlike the shikasta) ordered and measured, the Divānī replaced the old Tauqī' as the script for diplomas and other documents and was richly developed in calligraphy especially in the chancery of the Ottoman sultans. Of all these late styles only the nastaliq had an effect on epigraphy. After about 1500 it was common in Iranian, Turkish, and Indian inscriptions. Numerous other variants were of purely local importance. Here and there fanciful variations were in use, as the "trembling," "powdered," "curled," "peacock," "crescent-moon" etc. In other cases the fancy of the calligrapher produced animal figures, human heads, etc., which illustrated religious proverbs, thus placating the stern antirepresentational bias of Islam.

Ernst KÜHNEL

*Europe*: *the Middle Ages to the present.* With the disintegration of the Roman central authority in the West and the rise of separate states, a marked development took place in the Latin book hand. Although the Byzantine world maintained some unity of script and made use only of two types, majuscule and minuscule, for its book hand, several "national" hands assumed distinctive forms in western Europe. These were minuscules which developed from the Latin cursive script. The originality of the medieval period in calligraphy lies in its elevation of these scripts to the status of standard book hands. Introducing such features as punctuation, regular separation of words, and initials, these scripts form the basis for the so-called "roman" type in which almost all printed texts are composed today.

Until the invention of printing and the spread of the printed book, calligraphy was extensively practiced in monasteries, which supplied the large demand for beautifully executed liturgical texts and other religious books. Benedictine monks were the pioneers of medieval civilization in England, Germany, Poland, Bohemia, and Scandinavia. As other forms of monasticism arose, numerous monasteries became centers of literary and artistic activity. All the main monasteries seem to have produced books or at least in some way to have secured their production.

* *

The earliest of the new minuscules made its appearance in the 6th century in France. This was the Merovingian script, derived from the script used in decrees of the provincial Roman administration, continued and perfected in the diplomas of the chancery of the Frankish kings. Certain letters (*a, b, h, o, t*) and a kind of tangled complexity created a decorative effect, but the script was not well-suited to book use. Thus a whole series of adaptations and calligraphic variations resulted. The types elaborated in the 8th century in the monasteries of Laon, Luxeuil-les-Bains, and Corbie are most typical.

In Spain a book hand began to be evolved in the 7th century from the Latin cursive. This gradually became calligraphic and was perfected in the 11th century, when its general appearance, the product of slender lines and a slight effect of chiaroscuro, recalls certain elements of the Arabic script in use in Spain. The alphabet is all in lower case (the g excepted). The Arab fashion is more evident in the majuscule alphabet which often accompanies the text.

In central and northern Italy local expression was calligraphic only in a few cases (e.g., at the monastic center of No-

nantola), as such an evolution was interrupted by the spread of the Carolingian minuscule. But in the southern areas there was an independent evolution of writing known as Beneventan (after the Lombard duchy of Benevento; PL. 8), Lombardic or Lombardo-Cassinese (after the monastery at Monte Cassino, which was its most fruitful book-producing center). This script predominated in Italy south of Rome, spreading also to Dalmatia. A special effect of chiaroscuro, obtained with an obliquely cut pen, was typical, the alternation of thick and thin strokes being particularly effective. While the earliest examples date to the late 8th century, the peak of calligraphic stylization was reached in the 11th century. The codices of Monte Cassino of the time of the abbot Desiderius (1058–87) are among the most sumptuous examples in the history of book production. Beneventan continued in use until the 13th century, when it was supplanted by black letter.

In England and Ireland in the 7th to the 12th century, book hands derived from the script used for sacred texts brought from Italy to France had a development altogether different from those in continental Europe (except for a few rare cases of pure uncial). Both majuscule and minuscule scripts were in use, while a special, rather decorative majuscule alphabet occasionally served for titles. The finest examples of Insular majuscule script are the Gospels of Lindisfarne (London, Brit. Mus., Cotton Nero D. IV) and Kells (Dublin, Trinity College Lib., Ms. 58), the former written in England (late 7th cent.) and the latter in Ireland (ca. 800). The luxuriant decoration of these two manuscripts is of an exceptionally high quality (see ANGLO-SAXON AND IRISH ART).

Insular majuscule is rare for whole codices after the 8th century, although it was retained for titles. The minuscule, in common use until the mid-11th century, was used in general for less formal codices, but this fact did not lessen calligraphic quality. It also was accompanied by graceful initials. A fine example is the Cod. pal. lat. 577 in the Vatican Library. After the Norman Conquest in 1066, Insular was replaced in England by Carolingian script, although in Ireland it continued in use, especially in the Gaelic texts; even today the early minuscule is perpetuated in the Irish printing fonts. In the 8th and 9th centuries, Insular script was employed in the scriptoriums of monasteries founded by English or Irish monks at various sites in continental Europe, as at Corbie and Luxeuil-les-Bains (France), Mainz and Regensburg (Germany), St. Gall (Switzerland), Bobbio (Italy), etc.

Under Charlemagne, the *renovatio imperii* and the rebirth of ideas of universality (as opposed to the separatism responsible for the national hands and partly inspired by antique culture) brought forth a new script known as Carolingian minuscule (PL. 6). Ligatures were few, and the regular, well-proportioned letters maintained a constant form. An early example is the Godescalc Gospels (ca. 781–83; Paris, Bib. Nat., Nouv. acq. lat. 1203). The spread of Carolingian was rapid, as it met the need for a common direction for many schools; by about 800 it was in use in most of the Empire. In the 9th century it reached Catalonia, and in the 11th, England; in the 12th it reached the rest of Spain and began to penetrate southern Italy. See CAROLINGIAN PERIOD.

This return to classicism (q.v.), as against the barbaric taste for a crowded page incorporating zoomorphic motifs done in lively colors, is evident in the finest manuscripts of the period. Perfectly designed titles in capitals — either rustic or square — stand out clearly from the white of fine parchment, with ample space around each letter. One of the most important codices is the Alcuin Bible, executed about 800 in Tours (now Zurich, Zentralbib., C. I.): the text is in a beautiful Carolingian, but the titles embody at least four types of antique hands (square and rustic capitals, uncials, and semiuncials).

Carolingian deteriorated in the 10th and 11th centuries. With the rise of the universities in the late 12th century, writing tended toward a rigid stylization which was to transform its appearance. Gothic, or black letter (PLS. 8, 9), evolved directly out of Carolingian, although the two hands represent two different esthetic principles.

Decoration at the expense of clarity prevailed in black letter.

The letters are often tall and narrow, and always close together. The predominance of vertical lines gives the particular tone of this hand, the strokes being bent back at the ends. The notable contrast between the thick down- and the fine upstrokes produces a decorative effect. The page became a compact unit, and there was a tendency to fill even the spaces at the end of lines with small dashes or with words from the following line.

Black letter marked a return to uniformity of script in the Latin world, although regional styles existed as well as variations according to the nature of the text. Generally forms were more angular in France and England, heavier in Germany, rounder in Italy and in Spain. Books destined for study in the universities constituted a separate class with minute characters: their variants go by the names of Bologna, Paris, Oxford (littera Bononiensis, Parisiensis, Oxoniensis). Stylization reached its peak in liturgical books (especially in choir books), whose letters had to be written large for ease of reading. Black-letter capital letters which were used widely for monumental inscriptions, seals, and coins also served for titles. Deriving substantially from antique uncial, they were highly decorative. Besides the black-letter book hand, a black-letter cursive was commonly used in documents and letters; rapidly traced, this was sometimes very regular and beautiful even when there was no attempt at calligraphy as such.

A variant of cursive, traced with great care and embellished in the style of the royal chanceries (tall downstrokes, flourishes, decorative elements), was the lucid Italian chancery of Italian texts. The papal documents of the 13th century are particularly fine examples. Another variant in which a number of very beautiful texts were written in the 15th century in France is the *bâtarde* letter, such as in the handsome codices commissioned by the dukes of Burgundy (now mainly in Brussels, Bib. Royale). In Germany the high point was reached in Textura (i.e., for a text), written in bold, widely spaced characters.

Giulio BATTELLI

Because of their monumental character, epigraphic inscriptions remained faithful to the antique majuscules, so that before the 11th century it is not easy to establish the date of an inscription on the basis of the letters alone. There is, however, a certain parallel in the calligraphic level of inscriptions and the finest manuscripts, especially the title pages of the latter. From the 13th century on, black-letter majuscules were commonly used for monumental inscriptions, although the black-letter minuscule book hand was also widespread. The two forms also appeared in paintings and textiles, especially in France and Germany.

* *

In conformity with a general reaction against Gothic art in 15th-century Italy, the Florentine Humanists set in motion a comprehensive reform of lettering modeled on the calm and lucid forms of Carolingian minuscule. There were two types: a neat, rounded humanistic hand (now known as "antiqua"), and a cursive humanistic hand (*italica* or italics) deriving from black-letter cursive. The former served as a formal hand for literary productions. This *littera antiqua* was perfected in northern Italy, chiefly at Venice, where it was adopted in printing presses in the late 15th and early 16th centuries and became what is now known as the roman type.

The cursive humanistic hand for everyday purposes — letters, accounts, and so on — was adapted into a printing font by Francesco Griffi (Francesco da Bologna) for the great Venetian printer Aldus Manutius (1450–1515). Known as Aldine type, this font became the source of our modern italics. The italics are probably the most perfected and the most clearly legible form of printed letter which has yet been invented. The use of the roman type and of italics spread all over the world. They were brought into England from Italy in the 16th century. The black letter lingered on in England for some time; in Germany it is still used to some extent.

Movable printing type was invented about 1450, and in a quarter of a century printing presses were established through-

out western Europe. Johann Gutenberg (1400?–68?), probably the earliest European printer with movable types, copied the black letter; so did William Caxton (1422?–91), the first English printer; but in Italy the *littera antiqua* was used in Rome by Sweynheym and Pannartz, who had come from Germany, and by the Frenchman Nicolas Jenson (d. ca. 1480), the great printer who perfected it in Venice. With his superb sense of design, Jenson created a most legible and pleasing type, very accurate in alignment.

Thus by about 1500 the main letter forms of the West — Roman type, italics, and black letter — became definitely fixed.

The use of machines and the work of the type designers, such as William Caslon (1692–1766), John Baskerville (1706–75), and Giambattista Bodoni (1740–1813), did not cause any change in the essential forms of the letters, though it influenced their artistic appearance. In fact, the current private use of the typewriter has tended to establish printing types as the norm for the whole field of writing. Beautiful handwriting as an independent art did not completely disappear, however. Surprisingly enough — perhaps in reaction to the dominance of printing — it has become an important field of endeavor closely related to the new trends and problems of the other graphic arts (q.v.). Thus, while printing fonts at first attempted to reproduce the effects of manuscripts, they in turn — owing to innovations and widespread use — influenced calligraphy.

As a distinct branch of study, calligraphy may be said to have been born about 1463 with Felice Feliciano's book, the manuscript of which is preserved in the Vatican Library (Vat. lat. 6852). This deals with several aspects of the Roman alphabet. In the following century or so, when the printing press was firmly established throughout Europe, several more books appeared containing systematic studies of Latin and western European calligraphy.

In Italy the earliest printed treatise on calligraphy, by Damiano de Moyllis (Moile) of Parma, appeared about 1479. Of more importance is Fra Luca Pacioli's *De divina proportione*, Venice, 1509. Sigismondo Fanti of Ferrara, who in 1514 published a famous treatise on the forms and proportions of the main styles, may be regarded as the founder of calligraphic methodology. Also important are the treatises by Francesco Torniello, 1517; Giambattista Verini, 1526; Eustachio Cellebrion of Udine, 1525, and several others. Among the Italian calligraphers of the late 16th century we may mention Scalzini (1581), Curione (1588), and Orfei (1589).

In France the leading calligrapher was Geoffroy Tory (1480?–1533?), also a great type designer and bookbinder. In *Champfleury* (pub. 1529) he set forth the formula on which he believed antique capitals had been designed. It was in large part his influence that swung France from black letter to roman type. Other 16th-century French calligraphers were Jean le Moyne, Pierre Hamon, Estienne du Tronchet, J. de la Rue, Jean de Beauchesne, Jean Beaugrand, and Guillaume Legagneur. Later calligraphers were Materot (1604), Barbedor (1647), Pailasson (1787), and particularly Nicolas Jarry (1620–74). In Spain a beautiful *antigua* letter style was developed. The best-known calligrapher of the period is Juan de Ycíar (1547). Madariaga, Lucascon (and his pupils), Pedro Díaz Morante, Lorenzo Ortiz, Aznar de Polanco, Francisco Palomares and Torio de la Riva (1800) were also excellent calligraphers.

In Germany the great Albrecht Dürer (q.v.) wrote *Underweysung der Messung mit dem Zirkel und Richtsheyt in Linien, Ebenen und ganzen Corporen* (Nuremberg, 1525); he designed the prototype of the modern black letters. Christoph Stimmer, Johann Neudörffer the Elder, and Urbanus Wyss (PL. 9) also exercised some influence in the 16th century as calligraphers. In England the earliest professor of calligraphy was Jean de Beauchesne; with John Baildon he published in 1571 *A Booke Containing Divers Sortes of Hands*. That book is, in fact, the first writing master ever published in England. Fifty years earlier a papal scribe, Lodovico degli Arrighi, "il Vicentino," wrote the first Italian writing master, which was published in Rome in 1522 (PL. 10). It was followed by manuals published by Giovanni Antonio Tagliente (Venice, 1524), Giovan Battista Palatino da

Rossano (Rome, 1540), Vespasiano Amfiareo (Venice, 1544) (all, PL. 10), Ferdinando Ruano (1554), Gian Francesco Cresci (Rome, 1560), Giuliantonio Hercolani (Bologna, 1571), and several others. The Spaniard Juan de Ycíar, already referred to, published several really fine book hands.

In the course of time the writing master and manuals on calligraphy declined in importance, though there were still calligraphers in Italy, France, Germany, Spain, and England during the 17th, 18th, and 19th centuries. In the second half of the 19th century, the quill pen was outmoded, and calligraphy still further declined with the adoption of the steel pen; but the stage was set for a revolution in taste. Thanks to the work of Owen Jones (1809–74), a master in the black letter; William Morris (1834–96), a great master in the Renaissance hand; Edward Johnston (1872–1944); and William Graily Hewitt (1854–1952), calligraphy enjoyed a resurgence. These men were followed by Eric Gill, T. J. Cobden-Sanderson, Noel Rooke, Anna Simons, and others in England; Elbert Hubbard, Bruce Rogers, Daniel Berkeley Updike, Bertram G. Goodhue, Will Bradley, Fred Goudy, and others in the United States.

David DIRINGER

BIBLIOG. *General*: H. Wuttke, Geschichte der Schrift, Leipzig, 1875; K. Faulmann, Illustrierte Geschichte der Schrift, Vienna, Budapest, Leipzig, 1880; I. Taylor, The Alphabet, 2 vols., London, 1883, 2d ed., 1899; H. Bouchot, Le livre, Paris, 1886 (Eng. trans., London, 1890); F. Carta, C. Cipolla, and C. Frati, Monumenta palaeographica sacra, Atlante paleografico artistico compilato sui mss. esposti in Torino alla Mostra d'arte sacra, Turin, 1899; E. Clodd, The Story of the Alphabet, New York, 1900 (subsequent eds., 1907, 1912, 1938); L. Blau, Studien zum althebräischen Buchwesen, Strasbourg, 1902; Y. B. Schnitzer, Illustrated General History of Writing (in Russian), St. Petersburg, 1903; F. N. Skinner, Story of the Letters and Figures, Chicago, 1905; F. Ballhorn, Alphabete orientalischer und okzidentalischer Sprachen, Leipzig, 1906; C. Davenport, The Book: Its History and Development, London, 1907, New York, 1908; E. F. Strange, Alphabets, London, 1907; A. Cim, Le livre, 5 vols., Paris, 1908; F. Specht, Die Schrift und ihre Entwicklung, 3d ed., Berlin, 1909; A. W. Pollard, Fine Books, London, 1912; T. W. Danzel, Die Anfänge der Schrift, Leipzig, 1912, 2d ed., 1929; C. Biagi, Cinquanta tavole in fototipia da codici della R. Biblioteca Medicea-Laurenziana, Florence, 1914; K. Weule, Vom Kerbstock zum Alphabet, Stuttgart, 1915, 2d ed., 1921; E. Curtius, Wort und Schrift, Berlin, 1917; A. Hertz, Ein Beitrag zur Entwicklung der Schrift, Archiv für die Geschichte der Psychologie, 1917; W. Mieses, Die Gesetze der Schriftgeschichte, Vienna, Leipzig, 1919; W. A. Mason, A History of the Art of Writing, New York, 1920; M. Audin, Le livre, Lyons, 1921, 2d ed., Paris, 1927; M. Pardo, Storia delle scritture, Catania, 1922; Reichsdruckerei, Alphabete und Schriftzeichen, Berlin, 1924; H. Jensen, Geschichte der Schrift, Hanover, 1925; A. von Le Coq, Bilderatlas zur Kunst- und Kulturgeschichte Mittel-Asiens, Berlin, 1925; C. Fossey (ed.), Notices sur les caractères étrangers anciens et modernes rédigées par un groupe de savants, Paris, 1927, 2d ed., 1948; F. G. Kenyon, Ancient Books and Modern Discoveries, Chicago, 1927; H. Delitsch, Geschichte der abendländischen Schreibschriftformen, Leipzig, 1928; M. Heepe (ed.), Lautzeichen und ihre Anwendung, Berlin, 1928; A. von Le Coq, Buried Treasures of Chinese Turkestan, London, 1928; H. Degering, Die Schrift: Atlas der Schriftformen des Abendlandes, Berlin, 1929, 3d ed., 1952; A. Wodrze, Zum Problem der Schrift (dissertation), Breslau, 1930; B. Ducati, La scrittura, Padua, 1931; J. Evans, Pattern: A Study of Ornament in Western Europe from 1180 to 1900, 2 vols., Oxford, 1931; H. Tentor, Writing and the Origins of the Alphabet (in Croatian), Zagreb, 1931; The Dolphin, New York, 1933 ff.; J. Evans, Nature in Design, Oxford, 1933; R. N. D. Wilson, Books and Their History, New York, 1933; K. Löffler and J. Kirchner (eds.), Lexikon des gesamten Buchwesens, 3 vols., Leipzig, 1934–37; A. B. Allen, The Romance of the Alphabet, London, New York, 1937; D. Diringer, L'alfabeto nella storia della civiltà, Florence, 1937; E. Lesne, Les livres, "scriptoria," et bibliothèques, Lille, 1938; B. H. Newdigate, The Art of the Book, London, 1938; D. Fava, La Biblioteca Nazionale Centrale di Firenze e le sue insigni raccolte, Milan, 1939; J. Tschichold, Geschichte der Schrift in Bildern, Basel, Frankfort on the Main, 1941, new ed., 1946; E. Curtius, Schrift und Buchmetaphorik, Halle, 1942; A. Esdaile, The British Museum Library, London, 1946; C. Loukotka, The Development of Writing (in Czech), Prague, 1946; A. C. Moorhouse, Writing and the Alphabet, London, 1946; A. Carlier, Histoire de l'écriture, Cannes, 1947; J.-C. Février, Histoire de l'écriture, Paris, 1948; Société Asiatique, Ecritures et livres à travers les âges, Paris, 1948; D. Diringer, The Alphabet: A Key to the History of Mankind, London, New York, 1948, 4th ed., 1953; M. Cohen, L'évolution des langues et des écritures, Paris, 1949; O. Ogg, The 26 Letters, London, 1949; Bibliothèque Nationale, Trésors des bibliothèques d'Italie, IVᵉ–XVIᵉ siècle, Paris, 1950; J. Tschichold, Schriftkunde, Schreibübungen und Skizzieren, Berlin, 1951; A. Allen, Story of the Book, London, 1952; I. J. Gelb, A Study of Writing: The Foundations of Grammatology, London, Chicago, 1952; Hoffmanns Schriftatlas, Stuttgart, 1952; P. d'Angelo, Storia della scrittura, Rome, 1952; C. Bonacini, Bibliografia delle arti scrittorie e della calligrafia, Florence, 1953; M. Cohen, L'écriture, Paris, 1953; D. Diringer, Alphabet Exhibition, London, 1953; D. Diringer, The Hand-produced Book, London, New York, 1953; A. C. Moorhouse, A History of Writing, New York, 1953; J. Rambousek, Writing

and Its Use (in Czech), Prague, 1953; G. Cencetti, Lineamenti di storia della scrittura, Bologna, 1954; C. Higounet, L'écriture, Paris, 1955; E. I. Katsprzhak, History of Writing and of Books (in Russian), Moscow, 1955; R. Benz and U. Schleicher, Kleine Geschichte der Schrift, Heidelberg, 1956; S. A. Birnbaum, The Hebrew Scripts, London, 1957; M. Cohen, La grande invention de l'écriture et son évolution, 3 vols., Paris, 1958; D. Diringer, The Illuminated Book, London, New York, 1958; H. Jensen, Die Schrift in Vergangenheit und Gegenwart, 2d ed., Berlin, 1958; L. Ribeiro, História das letras e dos algarismos, Lisbon, 1959 (see also bibliogs. of GRAPHIC ARTS and MINIATURES AND ILLUMINATION). *Primitive and ethnological. a. Africa*: H. Baumann, R. Thurnwald, and D. Westermann, Völkerkunde von Afrika, Essen, 1940; O. F. Raum, The African Chapter in the History of Writing, African Studies, II, 4, 1943; R. Mauny, Gravures, peintures et inscriptions rupestres de l'ouest africain, Initiations Africaines, XI, 1954; H. Lhote, Les Touaregs du Hoggar, 2d ed., Paris, 1955. *b. Australia and Tasmania*: E. H. Giglioli, Tasmania, Milan, 1874; The Aborigines of Victoria, I, London, 1878; N. W. Thomas, Natives of Australia, London, 1906; B. Spencer, Native Tribes of the Northern Territory of Australia, London, 1914; F. D. McCarthy, Australia's Aborigines: Their Life and Culture, Melbourne, 1957; C. P. Mountford, The Tiwi: Their Art, Myth and Ceremony, London, 1958. *c. New Caledonia*: M. Leenhardt, Notes d'ethnologie néo-calédonienne, Travaux et mémoires de l'Institut d'Ethnologie, VII, 1930; M. Leenhardt, Documents néo-calédoniens, Travaux et mémoires de l'Institut d'Ethnologie, IX, 1932; M. and G. Lobsiger-Dellenbach, Traité d'agriculture néo-calédonienne gravé sur un bambou, Archives Suisses d'Anthropologie Générale, VIII, I, 1938; M. and G. Lobsiger-Dellenbach, Essai d'interprétation des gravures néo-calédoniennes incisées sur bambou, Archives Suisses d'Anthropologie Générale, VIII, 2, 1939; M. and G. Lobsiger-Dellenbach, Quelques aspects de l'existence des Néo-Calédoniens d'après leurs bambous gravés, Le Globe, LXXXI, 1942; M. and G. Lobsiger-Dellenbach, Trois bambous gravés de Nouvelle-Calédonie, Le Globe, XV, 2, 1950; M. and G. Lobsiger-Dellenbach, Trois bambous gravés de Nouvelle-Calédonie, Le Globe, XXII, 1, 1957; M. and G. Lobsiger-Dellenbach, Deux bambous gravés de Nouvelle-Calédonie, JSO, XIV, 1958. *d. Easter Island*: H. Balfour, Some Ethnological Suggestions in Regard to Easter Island or Rapanui, Folk-Lore, XXXVIII, 1918; A. Pietrowski, Deux tablettes avec les marques gravées de l'Ile de Pâques, REthn, VI, 1925; J. Imbelloni, Las tabletas parlantes de Pasqua, monumentos de un sistema gráfico indo-oceánico, Runa, IV, 1951; P. H. Buck, Les migrations des Polynésiens, Paris, 1952; R. Fijas, Nuevas indagaciones sobre Pasqua, Runa, VI, 1953–54; R. Heine-Geldern, La escritura de la Isla de Pasqua y sus relaciones con otras escrituras, Runa, VIII, 1956–57. *e. North America*: G. Mallery, On the Pictographs of the North American Indians, Bureau of American Ethnology, Annual Report for 1882–83, IV, 1886; W. Matthews, The Mountain Chant: A Navajo Ceremony, Bureau of American Ethnology, Annual Report for 1883–84, V, 1887; J. Stevenson, Mythical Sand Painting of the Navajo Indians, Bureau of American Ethnology Annual Report for 1886–87, VIII, 1891; G. Mallery, Picture Writing of the American Indians, Bureau of American Ethnology, Annual Report for 1888–89, X, 1893; H. Hale, Four Huron Wampum Records, JRAI, XVI, 1896–97; W. J. Hoffman, The Graphic Art of the Eskimos, Washington, 1897; F. G. Speck, The Functions of Wampum among the Eastern Algonkian, Memoirs of the American Anthroponomical Association, VI, 1, 1919; M. Covarrubias, The Eagle, the Jaguar and the Serpent, New York, 1954. *f. Mexico*: C. Thomas, Notes on Certain Maya and Mexican Manuscripts, Bureau of American Ethnology, Annual Report for 1881–82, III, 1884; J. M. A. Aubin, Mémoires sur la peinture didactique et l'écriture figurative des anciens Mexicains, Paris, 1885; G. V. Callegari, Introduzione allo studio delle antichità americane, Milan, 1930; G. V. Callegari, Dei sistemi grafici degli Aztechi, epoca pre-colombiana, B. dell'Accademia italiana di stenografia, 1934; J. E. Thompson, Maya Hieroglyphic Writing, Washington, 1950; P. Kelemen, Medieval American Art, 2d ed., New York, 1956. *g. Peru*: J. Imbelloni, La esfinge indiana, Buenos Aires, 1926; R. Larco Hoyle, A Culture Sequence for the North Coast of Peru, HSAI, II, 1946, pp. 149–75; G. Kutscher, Nordperuanische Keramik, Berlin, 1954; F. Boas, Primitive Art, New York, 1955; L. Boudin, La vie quotidienne au temps des derniers Incas, Paris, 1955. *Egypt*: G. Moeller, Hieratische Paläographie: Die ägyptische Buchschrift in ihrer Entwicklung von der fünften Dynastie bis zur römischen Kaiserzeit, 3 vols., Leipzig, 1909–12; A. Erman, Die Hieroglyphen, Berlin, Leipzig, 1912; P. Marestaing, Les écritures égyptiennes et l'antiquité classique, Paris, 1913; P. Lacau, Sur le système hiéroglyphique, Cairo, 1954; A. H. Gardiner, Egyptian Grammar, 3d ed., London, 1957. *Cuneiform*: G. A. Barton, The Origins and Development of Babylonian Writing, 2 vols., Leipzig, 1913; British Museum, Cuneiform Texts from Cappadocian Tablets in the British Museum, 4 vols., London, 1921–27; E. Chiera, They Wrote in Clay, Chicago, 1938; C. Clark, The Art of Early Writing, with Special Reference to the Cuneiform System, London, 1938; J. of Cuneiform Studies, 1947 ff. *Cretan and Mycenaean scripts*: A. Evans, Scripta Minoa, Oxford, 1909; Minos: Revista de Filología Egea, 1951 ff.; E. L. Bennett (ed.), The Pylos Tablets: Texts of the Inscriptions Found 1939–54, Princeton, 1955; M. Ventris, Documents in Mycenaean Greek, Cambridge, England, 1956; J. Chadwick, The Decipherment of Linear B, Cambridge, England, 1958. *Hittite script*: B. Hrozný, Les inscriptions hittites hiéroglyphiques, 3 vols., Prague, 1933–37; W. F. Albright, Hittite Scripts, Antiquity, VIII, 1934, pp. 453–55; B. Hrozný, Inscriptions "hittites"-hiéroglyphiques des rois de Tuvana-Tyana, Archiv Orientální, X, 1937, pp. 217–22; O. R. Gurney, The Hittites, Harmondsworth, 1952. *China*: L. Driscoll and K. Toda, Chinese Calligraphy, Chicago, 1935; Lin Yutang, The Aesthetics of Chinese Calligraphy, Tien Hsia Monthly, I, 1935, pp. 491–507; Sun Ta-yü (trans.), On the Fine Art of Chinese Calligraphy by Sun Kuo-t'ing of the T'ang Dynasty, Tien Hsia Monthly, I, 1935, pp. 192–207; Yang Yu-hsün, La calligraphie chinoise depuis les Han, Paris, 1937; Chiang Yee, Chinese Calligraphy, London, 1938 (with bibliog. of Chinese-language works); W. Willetts, Chinese Art, II, Harmondsworth, 1958, pp. 533–81. *Japan*: Juichi Iki, Nippon Shodō no Hensen (Development of Japanese Calligraphy), Tokyo, 1935; Heibon-sha Shodō Zenshū (Heibon-sha's Albums of Calligraphy), 25 vols., Tokyo, 1954–56. *Greece and Rome*: B. de Montfaucon, Palaeographia graeca, 6 vols. and appendix, Paris, 1708; T. Birt, Das antike Buchwesen, Berlin, 1882; E. Hübner, Exempla scripturae epigraphicae latinae, Berlin, 1885; P. Berger, Histoire de l'écriture dans l'antiquité, Paris, 1891, 2d ed., 1892; W. Wattenbach, Anleitung zur griechischen Paläographie, 3d ed., Leipzig, 1895; F. G. Kenyon, The Palaeography of Greek Papyri, Oxford, 1899; E. M. Thompson, Handbook of Greek and Latin Palaeography, 3d ed., London, 1906; T. Birt, Die Buchrolle in der Kunst, Leipzig, 1907; V. Gardthausen, Griechische Paläographie, 2 vols., Leipzig, 1911–13; L. Mitteis and V. Wilchen, Grundzüge und Chrestomathie der Papyruskunde, 2 vols., Leipzig, 1912; E. M. Thompson, An Introduction to Greek and Latin Palaeography, Oxford, 1912; W. Larfeld, Griechische Epigraphik, Handbuch der Altertumswissenschaft, I, 5, Munich, 1914; H. B. Van Hoesen, Roman Cursive Writing, Princeton, 1915; C. M. Kaufmann, Handbuch der altchristlichen Epigraphik, Freiburg im Breisgau, 1917; J. E. Sandys, Latin Epigraphy, Cambridge, England, 1919; A. Mentz, Geschichte der griechisch-römischen Schrift, Leipzig, 1920; L. Schiapparelli, La scrittura latina nell'età romana, Como, 1921 (with bibliog); T. Birt, Aus dem Leben der Antike, 4th ed., Leipzig, 1922; Palaeographia latina, II, 1923, pp. 74–93 (bibliog.); W. Schubart, Griechische Paläographie, Handbuch der Altertumswissenschaft, I, 4, Munich, 1925; P. Franchi de' Cavalieri and J. Lietzmann, Specimina codicum graecorum Vaticanorum, Berlin, 1929; R. H. Conway, The Ancient Alphabets of Italy, Cambridge Ancient History, IV, Cambridge, England, 1930, pp. 395–403; Jahresbericht für Altertumswissenschaft, 236, 1933, pp. 85–115 (bibliog.); R. H. Barrow, A Selection of Latin Inscriptions, Oxford, 1934; M. Norsa, La scrittura letteraria greca dal secolo IV a. C. all'VII d. C., Florence, 1940; P. Batlle Huguet, Epigrafía latina, Barcelona, 1946; H. L. Pinner, The World of Books in Classical Antiquity, Leiden, 1948; H. Foerster, Abriss der lateinischen Paläographie, Bern, 1949; G. Costamagna, Lineamenti estetici dello sviluppo della scrittura latina, Cogoleto, 1950; R. Bloch, Epigraphie latine, Paris, 1952; R. Devreesse, Introduction à l'étude des manuscrits grecs, Paris, 1954; C. H. Roberts, Greek Literary Hands, 350 B.C.–A.D. 400, Oxford, 1955; B. A. van Groningen, Short Manual of Greek Palaeography, 2d ed., Leiden, 1955; G. Klaffenbach, Griechische Epigraphik, Göttingen, 1957. *India and Farther India. a. General*: A. C. Burnell, Elements of South-Indian Palaeography, London, 1878; G. Bühler, Indische Paläographie, Strasbourg, 1896 (trans., J. F. Fleet, Indian Palaeography, appendix to The Indian Antiquary, XXXIII, 1904); G. H. Ojha, Bhara tiya Pracina Lipimala, The Palaeography of India, Ajmer, 1918; C. Śivaramamurti, Indian Epigraphy and South Indian Scripts, B. of the Madras Government Museum, N.S., general section, III, 4, Madras, 1952; L. Renou and J. Filliozat, L'Inde classique, Manuel des études indiennes, II, Paris, 1953, Paléographie, pp. 665–712; R. B. Pandey, Indian Palaeography, 2d ed., Benares, 1955. *b. Collections of material*: The Indian Antiquary, Bombay, 1872 ff.; Epigraphia Carnatica, Bangalore, 1886 ff.; South-Indian Inscriptions, Madras, 1890 ff.; Epigraphia Indica, Calcutta, 1892 ff. *c. Spread of Indian scripts*: K. F. Holle, Tabel van Oud- en Nieuw-Indische Alphabetten, Buitenzorg, 1877; A. Barth and A. Bergaigne, Inscriptions de Campâ et du Cambodge, Paris, 1885–93; Epigraphia Zeylanica, Oxford, Colombo, 1904 ff.; Epigraphia Birmanica, Rangoon, 1919 ff.; G. Cœdès, History of the Thai Writing, Bangkok, 1924; L. Finot and G. Cœdès, Inscriptions du Cambodge, 6 vols., Paris, plates, 1926–37, text (G. Cœdès), 1937–54; L. C. Damais, Les écritures d'origine indienne en Indonésie et dans le sud-est asiatique continental, BSEI, N.S. XXX, 4, Saigon, 1955, pp. 365–82. *Islam*: M. Amari, Le epigrafi arabiche di Sicilia, 2 vols., Palermo, 1875, 1879; J. Karabaček, Die Bedeutung der arabischen Schrift, Nuremberg, 1877; B. Moritz, Arabic Palaeography, Cairo, 1905; C. Huart, Les calligraphes et miniaturistes de l'orient musulman, Paris, 1908; B. Moritz, Arabische Schrift, Enzyklopädie des Islam, I, 1913; S. Flury, Islamische Schriftbänder, Basel, 1920; F. Babinger, Die grossherrliche Tughra, Jhb. der Asiatischen Kunst, II, 1925, pp. 188–98; V. Kratchkovskaya, Arabic Epitaphs of the Palaeographic Museum of the Soviet Academy of Sciences, Leningrad, 1929; J. David-Weill, Les bois à épigraphes jusqu'à l'époque mamlouke, Cat. du Musée Arabe, Cairo, 1931; E. Lévi-Provençal, Inscriptions arabes d'Espagne, Leiden, 1931; A. Musa, Zur Geschichte der islamischen Buchmalerei in Ägypten, Cairo, 1931; H. Hawary and H. Rached, Stèles funéraires, 1, Cat. du Musée Arabe, Cairo, 1932; L. A. Mayer, Saracenic Heraldry, Oxford, 1933; J. David-Weill, Les bois à épigraphes depuis l'époque mamlouke, Cat. du Musée Arabe, Cairo, 1936; G. Wiet, Stèles funéraires, 2, Cat. du Musée Arabe, Cairo, 1936, 4, 1936, 5, 1937; M. Minovi and P. Ackerman, Calligraphy: An Outline History, SPA, II, 1939, pp. 1707–42; S. Flury, Ornamental Kufic Inscriptions on Pottery, SPA, II, 1939, pp. 1743–69; V. Kratchkovskaya, Ornamental Inscriptions, SPA, II, 1939, pp. 1770–84; E. Kühnel, Islamische Schriftkunst, Berlin, 1942; A. Grohmann, From the World of Arabic Papyri, Cairo, 1952; E. Künel and L. Bellinger, Catalogue of Dated Tiraz Fabrics, Textile Museum, Washington, 1952; E. Kühnel, Die osmanische Tughra, Kunst des Orients, II, 1955, pp. 69–82. *Europe: Middle Ages to the present. a. Facsimiles*: Monumenta graphica Medii Aevi, 10 vols., Vienna, 1859–82; The Palaeographical Society, Facsimiles of Manuscripts and Inscriptions, 6 vols., London, 1873–1901; Archivio Paleografico Italiano, Rome, 1882 ff.; H. Omont, Fac-similés de manuscrits grecs des XV<sup>e</sup> et XVI<sup>e</sup> siècles . . . d'après les originaux de la Bibliothèque Nationale, Paris, 1887; H. Omont, Fac-similés des manuscrits grecs datés de la Bibliothèque Nationale, du IX<sup>e</sup> au XIV<sup>e</sup> siècle, 2 vols., Paris, 1890–91; H. Omont, Fac-similés des plus anciens manuscrits grecs, en onciale et en minuscule, de la Bibliothèque Nationale, du IV<sup>e</sup> au XII<sup>e</sup> siècle, Paris, 1892; A. Chroust, Monumenta palaeographica, series I–IV, Munich, 1902 ff.; The New Palaeographical Society, Facsimiles of Ancient Manuscripts, 5 vols., London, 1903–32; H. M. Bannister, Monumenti vaticani di paleografia musicale latina, 2 vols., Leipzig, Rome, Turin, 1913; F. Ehrle and P. Liebart, Specimina codicum latinorum Vaticanorum, 2d ed., Berlin, 1927; Exempla scripturarum, Vatican City, 1929 ff.; E. A. Lowe, Scriptura Beneventana, 2 vols., Oxford, 1929; F. Steffens, Lateinische Pa-

läographie, 2d ed., Trier, 1929; V. Federici, La scrittura delle cancellerie italiane dal sec. XII al XVII, Rome, 1934; K. and S. Lake, Dated Greek Minuscule Manuscripts to the Year 1200 A.D., 11 vols., Boston, 1934–45; E. A. Lowe, Codices latini antiquiores, Oxford, 1934 ff.; J. Mallon, R. Marichal, and C. Perrat, L'écriture de la capitale romaine à la minuscule, Paris, 1939; H. Foerster, Mittelalterliche Buch- und Urkundenschriften auf 50 Tafeln, Bern, 1946; A. Bruckner and R. Marichal, Chartae latinae antiquiores, Olten, Lausanne, 1954 ff.; J. de Ycíar, Arte Subtilissima, trans., E. Shuckburgh, Oxford, 1960. b. General: H. L. Bordier, Description des peintures et autres ornements contenus dans les manuscrits grecs de la Bibliothèque Nationale, Paris, 1883–85; J. W. Bradley, A Dictionary of Miniaturists, Illuminators, Calligraphers and Copyists, 3 vols., London, 1887–89; G. H. Putnam, Books and Their Makers during the Middle Ages, New York, London, 1896; W. Wattenbach, Das Schriftwesen im Mittelalter, 3d ed., Leipzig, 1896; S. Beissel, Geschichte der Evangelienbücher, Freiburg im Breisgau, 1906; W. Morris, The Ideal Book, London, 1908; E. M. Thompson, An Introduction to Greek and Latin Palaeography, Oxford, 1912; E. Cotarelo y Mori, Diccionario biográfico y bibliográfico de calígrafos españoles, 2 vols., Madrid, 1913–16; E. A. Lowe, The Beneventan Script, Oxford, 1914; C. Johnson and H. Jenkinson, English Court Hand, A.D. 1066 to 1500, 2 vols. Oxford, 1915; E. Bishop, Liturgica historica, Oxford, 1918; M. Gerlach, Das alte Buch und seine Ausstattung vom 15. bis zum 19. Jahrhundert, Vienna, 1918; A. Bauckner, Einführung in das mittelalterliche Schrifttum, Munich, 1923; H. J. Hermann, Die frühmittelalterlichen Handschriften des Abendlandes, Leipzig, 1923; M. Prou and A. de Boüard, Manuel de paléographie latine et française, 4th ed., Paris, 1924; B. Bretholz, Lateinische Paläographie, 3d ed., Leipzig, 1926; E. A. Lowe, Handwriting, in C. G. Crump and E. F. Jacob (ed.), The Legacy of the Middle Ages, Oxford, 1926, pp. 197–226; H. Jenkinson, The Later Court Hands in England from the Fifteenth to the Seventeenth Century, Cambridge, England, 1927; P. Lauer, Les Enluminures des manuscrits de la Bibliothèque Nationale, Paris, 1927; G. J. Sawyer and F. J. Harvey Darton, English Books 1575–1900, 2 vols., London, 1927; E. K. Rand, A Survey of the Manuscripts of Tours, 2 vols., Cambridge, Mass., 1929; A. Heal, The English Writing-masters and Their Copy-books, 1570–1800, Cambridge, England, 1931; A. Millares Carlo, Tratado de paleografía española, Madrid, 1932; S. de Ricci and W. J. Wilson, Census of Medieval and Renaissance Manuscripts in the U.S. and Canada, 3 vols., New York, 1935–40; O. Dobias-Rozhdestvenskaya, Istoriya pisma v srednie veka: Rukovodstvo k izucheniyu paleografii (History of Writing in the Middle Ages: Manual for the Study of Paleography), Moscow, Leningrad, 1936; L. W. Jones, The Script of Tours in the Tenth Century, Speculum, XIV, 1939, pp. 179–98; L. W. Jones, The Art of Writing at Tours from 1000 to 1200 A.D., Speculum, XV, 1940, pp. 286–98; W. H. Lange, Schriftbibel: Geschichte der abendländischen Schrift von den Anfängen bis zur Gegenwart, Stuttgart, 1941; J. Tchichold, Schatzkammer der Schreibkunst, Meisterwerke der Kalligraphie aus vier Jahrhunderten (1522–1940) auf Tafeln, Basel, 1945; H. Fichtenau, Mensch und Schrift im Mittelalter, Vienna, 1946; A. Floriano Cumbreno. Curso general de paleografía y diplomática, 2 vols., Oviedo, 1946; Scriptorium, 1946 ff.; Bodleian Library, Exhibition of Renaissance Manuscripts, Oxford, 1948; G. Battelli, Lezioni di paleografia, 3d ed., Vatican City, 1949; S. Morison, Notes on the Development of Latin Scripts from Early to Modern Times, Cambridge, England, 1949; A. F. Johnson, A Catalogue of Italian Writing-books of the Sixteenth Century, Signature, 1950, N.S. no. 10, pp. 22–48; J. Tchichold, Meisterbuch der Schrift, Ravensburg, 1952; W. Doehde, Bibliographie deutscher Schreibmeisterbücher von Neudörffer bis 1800, Hamburg, 1958; W. Fugger, Handwriting Manual, trans., F. Plaat, Oxford, 1960.

* *

Illustrations: PLS. 1–16.


**CALLOT, JACQUES.** French engraver and etcher (b. Nancy, ca. 1592, d. Nancy, 1635), son of the herald and master of ceremonies at the court of Lorraine. Callot was apprenticed to a Nancy silversmith and engraver in 1607, and a few years later was engraving in Rome. In 1612 he went to Florence, where he began to etch, covering the copper plate with a varnish of mastic and linseed oil then used by lutemakers. This new hard ground, unlike the old soft ground, could be scratched with very fine lines and did not flake off in the acid bath, thus ruining a plate with foul biting. With a dependable ground to work on, Callot became the first specialist virtuoso etcher.

In Florence he etched 50 small *Capricci di varie figure* — sprightly studies in which each figure appeared in outline and was repeated, fully shaded, to instruct artists in drawing. He also etched festivities of the Medici court and a remarkable large plate of the *Fair at Impruneta* (1620) which contained well over 1,300 figures. So many figures have rarely been combined in an orderly picture in any medium. On the death of Duke Cosimo II (Feb., 1621), Callot returned to Nancy.

To meet the French demand for his prints, he repeated various coppers such as the *Capricci* and the *Fair at Impruneta*, that he had left behind in Florence. He also used Italian sketches for the sets of etchings of *The Gypsies* (1621), the 20 *Hunchbacks* (or *Gobbi*, 1622), and the 24 *Italian Comedians* (or *Balli di Sfessania*). The *Balli* are the only pictures that suggest the ribald brilliance of the old improvised Italian *Commedia dell'arte*. He also recorded life at the court in Nancy in his etchings of *The Palace Garden* (1625), *The Tournament in the Place de la Carrière* (1627), and the *Combat à la Barrière* (1627).

In 1627 the regent of the Spanish Netherlands commissioned Callot to etch six large copper plates that join together to form a bird's-eye panorama of the Spanish capture of Breda by Spinola. Callot so vividly combined the accuracy of a map with the liveliness of news reporting that France's Louis XIII called him to Paris to make similar huge etchings of the *Siege of the Ile de Ré* (1631) and the *Siege of La Rochelle* (Louvre, 1631). In 1633 he etched six *Petites Misères de la Guerre* and 18 *Grandes Misères de la Guerre*, which are the first unromantic pictures of war, exposing its impersonal cruelty, casual violence, and senseless destruction. Two years later, Callot died at Nancy of a stomach ailment.

In his forty-odd years of life, Callot produced 1,428 etchings and engravings and over 2,000 drawings, but no paintings. Many of his copper plates still exist in the Musée Historique Lorrain at Nancy, where they were used to make prints until recent years. He taught all subsequent etchers how to combine lightly bitten and deeply bitten lines and established the basic professional procedure of etching. His technical brilliance and his zest for life influenced artists as diverse as Rembrandt and Watteau. The grandeur of the baroque opera stage was compressed by Callot into pictures no bigger than this page. His records of war — torture, rape, burning at the stake, the firing squad — are strikingly believable because he observed decorum, viewed events as dispassionately as only a Frenchman can, and made his figures move as delicately and precisely as deadly insects. Through his technical innovations and the excellence of his drawing he exerted an influence more profound than that of many greater artists. (See V, PL. 241.)

BIBLIOG. J. Lieure, Jacques Callot, Paris, 5 vols., 1927–29 (basic life, criticism, and completely illustrated catalogue); E. de T. Bechtel, Jacques Callot, New York, 1955 (brief and excellent account, in English).

A. Hyatt MAYOR


**CAMBODIA.** Kingdom in southeastern Asia situated between Vietnam, Laos, and Thailand, with its capital at Phnom Penh. Cambodia (Kambuja) lies within the sphere of Indian civilization. From the beginning of the Christian era it was subjected to the powerful influence of Indian culture, particularly in the realm of art. The art of ancient Cambodia is known as Khmer art (see KHMER). Important architectural remains date from the 7th to the 13th century and have been the subject of many studies. The best known of these remains are the world-famous ruins of Angkor.

SUMMARY. Historical survey (col. 26). Art centers (col. 28); *The Angkor group; The region northeast of Angkor; The region east of Angkor; The region southeast of Angkor: a. The Roluos group; b. The Sambor Prei Kuk group; The region northwest of Angkor.*

HISTORICAL SURVEY. The territory of present-day Cambodia was once occupied by a kingdom whose culture was of Indian origin and which is known chiefly through Chinese historians, who call it Funan. Its history began in the 2d century with the marriage of an Indian Brahman and the daughter of a native ruler. At the beginning of the 3d century, Funan extended its dominion to a large part of the center and south of the peninsula, and early in the 6th century it included among its possessions the principality of Kambuja, originally situated north of the Great Lake and later extended along the middle of the Mekong River, in the region of Bassac. In the second half of the 6th century the ruler of this principality, who was related to the royal family of Funan, became independent, conquered a portion of the ruling state, and moved its capital from the region of Ba Phnom to Angkor Borei. His successors completed the conquest, and on the ruins of ancient Funan the Kambujas founded the Khmer kingdom, which remained one of the principal Indianized states of the peninsula until its decline in the 13th century.

Its first historical period, prior to the establishment of the capital at Angkor, is called "pre-Angkorian." The capital was then at Iśā-

napura in the vicinity of Kompong Thom, to the east of the Great Lake. The succession of kings is well known until the 8th century, when a temporary schism occurred between "Cambodia of the Land" and "Cambodia of the Water," corresponding respectively to the basins of the middle and lower Mekong, which were in turn divided into numerous rival principalities.

At the beginning of the 9th century, Cambodia, a part of which had been forced to accept the sovereignty of the Kingdom of Java, regained its freedom. In 802 King Jayavarman II seized power and established his residence north of the Great Lake at Hariharālaya (ruins of Roluos), near the future site of Angkor. He proclaimed independence from Java from the summit of Mount Mahendraparvata (Phnom Kulên) during a religious ceremony, at the same time

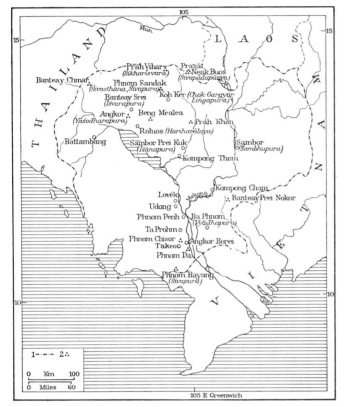

Cambodia: principal centers of artistic interest. *Key*: (1) Political boundaries; (2) ruins of monumental groups.

instituting the cult of the king-god, which identified the reigning sovereign with Śiva (Ang., Shiva), the guardian of the state. He then returned to Hariharālaya, where he died.

His two successors continued to reside there. Indravarman, in the year of his accession to power (877), ordered the excavation of a great artificial reservoir north of the capital. Two years later he dedicated the temple of Parameśvara (Prah Kô) to the funerary cult of his parents, and in 881 he inaugurated the first great stone monument, the Bakong, a stepped pyramid built for the royal lingam (Skr., *linga*), Indreśvara. In 893 his son and successor Yaśovarman (889–900) dedicated to him the funerary temple of Indravarmeśvara (Lolei) in the center of the artificial lake. He then established a new capital, Yaśodharapura, on the site of Angkor. On the hill of Phnom Bakheng, the center of the vast quadrangle which formed the limits of the palace precincts, he built a stone pyramid dedicated to the royal lingam Yaśodhareśvara. To the northeast of the city he undertook construction of a huge reservoir, the Yaśodharatāṭaka (East Baray).

Except for a brief period (921–41) during which Jayavarman IV, brother-in-law of Yaśovarman, moved the capital to Chok Gargyar (Koh Ker) in the north, Angkor, whose plan was altered many times, remained the capital until the 15th century. The return of King Rājendravarman (944–68) to Angkor coincided with the displacement of the center of the city toward the east, where he built the two major monuments of his reign, the Rajendreśvara and the Rajendrabhadreśvara (see below, *The Angkor group*).

His son, Jayavarman V (968–1001), undertook the construction of a new residence, Jayendranagarī, on the same site, the exact position of which is not certain. At the beginning of his reign his religious preceptor brought to completion the little temple of Iśvarapura (Banteay Srei) north of Angkor. The pyramid of Phimeanakas, in the

center of the Royal Palace, and Takeo, east of the city, were also built or at least begun during his reign.

In 1002 a new dynasty, founded by Sūryavarman I, extended the dominion of Cambodia westward. Except for the entrance gates of the Royal Palace at Angkor Thom, dating from the end of his reign, the constructions undertaken by this king are found mostly in the provinces: at Prah Vihar in the Dangrek (Donrek) Mountains, at Phnom Chisor in the south, and in the region of Battambang in the west.

His son and successor Udayādityavarman II (1050–66) built a great pyramid in the center of Angkor, the Baphuon, an imitation of the Mount Meru of Indian cosmology which rises at the center of the universe. He was also responsible for the construction of a vast reservoir (West Baray) with an island temple dedicated to Viṣṇu (Ang., Vishnu).

In the first half of the 12th century, following three reigns not associated with any important constructions, Sūryavarman II (1113–mid-12th century) built his mausoleum at Angkor Wat. After the disturbances and disasters following his death, particularly the capture of Angkor by the Chams in 1177, the country recovered through the efforts of the great Buddhist King Jayavarman VII (1181–1218). This king built the walls of Angkor Thom and many imposing monuments around the city: Banteay Kedei, Ta Prohm (1186), the funerary temple of the queen mother, Prah Khan (1191), the funerary temple of his father, and Neak Pean, in the middle of the artificial lake of Prah Khan. In each of the large cities of his realm a temple was erected to house a replica of the great statue of the royal Buddha in the center of the Bayon. He maintained 102 hospitals and built 121 roadhouses along the routes of his empire, which extended from Vieng Chan in the north to the valley of the Menam in the west, to the northern part of the Malay Peninsula in the south, and to the China Sea in the east.

From the 13th century on, many factors combined to effect the rapid decline of Cambodia: the decrease in relations with India, the adoption of Indian civilization by an ever-increasing number of natives, the appearance of Singhalese Buddhism, and above all, the gradual migration southward of two large ethnic groups, the Tais and the Vietnamese. The liberation of the Tais of the middle Menam and upper Mekong Rivers, who were still subjects of the Khmer empire in the 12th century, struck a fatal blow to Cambodia. By the 14th century it was surrounded by its former western and northern dependencies which had become sovereign states.

Very little remains from the medieval period that is worthy of mention, as stone was not used for construction. There are only traces of religious monuments in the successive capitals, as at Phnom Penh (15th cent. and after 1866), at Lovêk (16th cent.) and at Udong (mid-18th to mid-19th cent.).

ART CENTERS. There are a large number of monuments and architectural remains in Cambodia, of which more than 700 have been classified. The foregoing historical survey indicates the regions in which they are to be found. These are, first, in and around the ancient capitals of Funan (regions of Ba Phnom and Angkor Borei), in pre-Angkorian Cambodia (Sambor Prei Kuk, Sambor on the Mekong), then at Roluos, Phnom Kulên, Angkor, Koh Ker, and finally at Phnom Penh, Lovêk, and Udong. Next, there are the most venerated holy sites: in the north, at Wat Ph'u in Laos, at Prah Vihar on the cliffs of the Dangrek Mountains in Thailand, and in the region of Cheâm Khsan; in the south, at Phnom Chisor and Phnom Bayang; and the funerary monuments, Beng Mealea and Banteay Chmar. Finally, there are the areas of dense population — the regions to the northwest and southeast of Angkor and the region south of Kompong Cham. Khmer monuments also extend into the territories of Laos, Thailand, and Vietnam, recalling the period in which Cambodia dominated the Menam basin, the plateau of Korat, and the valley of the lower and middle Mekong.

The monuments described below include only those which are most important for their size or artistic interest and which are situated within Cambodia, beginning with Angkor and proceeding toward the four cardinal points.

*The Angkor group*. Angkor is not a single monument, but a complex of monuments, walls, embankments, bridges, and artificial lakes. It is the stone skeleton of an urban settlement from which all structures in perishable materials have disappeared. The terrain reveals the successive stages through which the city passed. Some of the major edifices are situated beyond the outer wall of Angkor Thom, the city of the late 12th century.

The plan of Angkor Thom, corresponding to the final stage of the city, is extremely simple. It consists of a square measuring about 2 miles on each side and surrounded by a wide moat. The surrounding wall, 26 ft. high, is interrupted at the center of each side by a monumental entrance surmounted by three towers decorated

with enormous human faces. Each entrance is preceded by a bridge with a balustrade in the form of a gigantic naga serpent, supported on one side by 27 figures of divinities and on the other by an equal number of demons.

Four roads lead from the four gates to the interior and meet at the geometric center of the city, which is marked by a temple, the Bayon. At first sight this temple appears to be a mountain of stone culminating in some thirty summits; in reality, these are towers adorned with huge human faces turned toward the four cardinal points (late 12th to late 13th cent.). From an architectural point of view, it is a pyramid of three steps, each of which consists of a complicated system of galleries. The lowest level is formed by a rectangular gallery measuring 492 ft. east to west × 328 ft. north to south. This gallery is open to the exterior, and its inner wall is covered with low reliefs inspired by the history and daily life of the Khmer people. The middle level contains another rectangular gallery, concentric to the first, with towers adorned with human faces surmounting the axial entrances and the corners. The inner wall of this gallery is also decorated with low reliefs representing religious and legendary subjects. The gallery in turn encloses an elevated earthfill, upon which rose the great central tower housing

some funerary function, is covered with low reliefs, subdivided into horizontal registers, representing the fabled beings who haunt the slopes of Mount Meru.

Still farther to the north is the great Buddhist monument of Prah Palilay (12th cent.), fronted by a terrace with two large standing and seated images of the Buddha.

Leaving Angkor Thom by the northern gate and proceeding northeast for 3/5 mile, one encounters the wall of Prah Khan (2,625 ft. from east to west × 2,297 ft. from north to south), the funerary temple of the father of Jayavarman VII, who is represented as Avalokiteśvara. Built in 1191 on the site of Jayaśrī, its plan includes a large number of galleries and chapels, and it is surrounded, like the city of Angkor Thom, by a moat traversed by four bridges analogous to those of the capital. East of the temple a basin was excavated measuring nearly 2 1/6 miles east to west and about 3/5 mile north to south. In the center, on the axis of Prah Khan, the Khmers built an island 1,148 ft. square, in turn containing a small basin 230 ft. square. In the center of this basin there is a circular island, set between the forms of two nagas, which supported a little temple dedicated to Avalokiteśvara. This complex, contemporary with Prah Khan and called Neak Pean (formerly Rājaśrī), was a pilgrimage

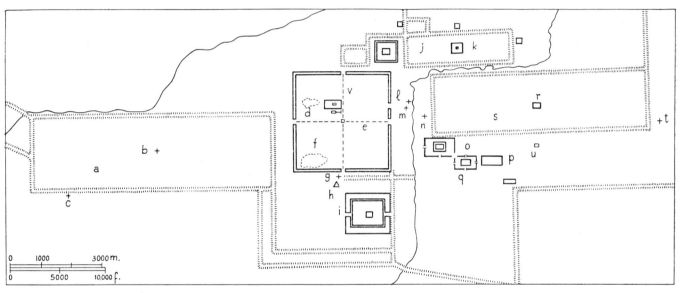

Monumental complex of Angkor, plan: (*a*) West Baray; (*b*) Mebon; (*c*) Ak Yom; (*d*) Baphuon; (*e*) Bayon; (*f*) Angkor Thom (Yaśodharapura); (*g*) Baksei Chamkrong; (*h*) Phnom Bakheng; (*i*) Angkor Wat (Yaśodharapura); (*j*) Prah Khan (Jayaśrī); (*k*) Neak Pean (Rājyaśrī); (*l*) Thommanon; (*m*) Chasuay Tevoda; (*n*) Takeo; (*o*) Ta Prohm (Rājavihāra); (*p*) Sra Srang; (*q*) Banteay Kedei; (*r*) East Mebon; (*s*) East Baray (Yaśodharatāṭaka); (*t*) Banteay Samrè; (*u*) Pré Rup (from a sketch of the terraces outlining the ancient artificial lakes).

the sanctuary of the Buddharāja, the image of Buddha that incarnated royalty.

To the north of the Bayon rise the principal monuments of Angkor Thom, built before the Bayon and the wall and later incorporated within the outlines of the new city.

The main monument is the Baphuon, an enormous pyramid of five levels, originally crowned by a tower faced with gilt metal sheets. The base of the pyramid measures 394 ft. east to west × 328 ft. north to south, and the top step is 79 ft. above the level of the surrounding terrain. The first, third, and fifth tiers have surrounding galleries. The gopuras of the middle gallery are covered with low reliefs, divided into small separate compartments, with scenes from the *Rāmāyana*, the *Mahābhārata*, and the legend of Krṣna (Ang., Krishna).

North of the Baphuon is the wall of the Royal Palace; the dwellings, constructed of light materials, no longer exist, but in the center there remains a pyramid of three levels, the Phimeanakas, surmounted by a vaulted gallery, perhaps the first built by the Khmers.

In front of the eastern façade of the Royal Palace there is a vast open area flanked on the east by 12 small towers and on the west, along the wall of the palace, by a long terrace, adorned with low reliefs representing the episodes of an elephant hunt (13th cent.). From the eastern entrance to the palace a fifth road leads eastward to a fifth gateway, the Victory Gate, identical with the others and located in the northern half of the eastern wall.

Slightly to the north and in prolongation of the Terrace of the Elephants is the Terrace of the Leper King, named after a mutilated statue covered with white lichens, representing Dharmarāja, the judge of the dead, whom the indigenous population identified with the legendary leper king. This construction, which probably served

site whose waters were believed to purify the soul and cure diseases. In its general aspect it symbolized Lake Anavatapta, which Indian cosmology placed in the region of the Himalayas.

Leaving Angkor Thom by the Victory Gate and proceeding eastward, one passes between two small temples of the 12th century, Thommanon and Chausay Tevoda, and reaches the pyramid of Takeo (end of 10th–beginning of 11th cent.) which has five levels and attains a height of 70 ft. It is crowned by five towers disposed in quincunx and left rough-hewn and undecorated.

Southeast of Takeo is Ta Prohm (1186), funerary temple of the queen mother, who was represented as Prajñāpāramitā. The outer wall measures about 3,100 × 1,900 ft., and the entrance ways, which are not preceded by bridges, are surmounted by towers adorned with human faces.

The southeast corner of the outer wall of Ta Prohm coincides with the northwest corner of Banteay Kedei, a contemporary temple of uncertain purpose. This monument is surrounded by a wall 2,298 × 1,640 ft. with entrances surmounted by towers with human faces. It comprises a system of two concentric galleries, connected to each other and crowned by towers. To the east of Banteay Kedei there is a magnificent lake, 2,298 × 984 ft., which is always filled with water; this is the Sra Srang, or Bath of the King, and dates from the late 12th century.

A great excavation, the East Baray, the ancient Yaśodharatāṭaka, dates from the reign of Yaśovarman (end of 9th cent.). It measures over 4 miles long east to west × about 1 1/4 miles wide, and extends to the east of Angkor Thom. Its western embankment can be seen from a certain distance to the east of the temple of Takeo. In its center, on a small island, rises the temple of East Mebon, a low pyramid surmounted by a quincunx of towers. It was built in 952

as the sanctuary of the royal lingam Rājendreśvara and is surrounded by the funerary images of the parents of King Rājendravarman.

Situated on the north-south axis of the East Mebon, but south of the southern embankment of the Baray, is the pyramid of Pré Rup. Its three steps are crowned by five towers in quincuncial arrangement, surrounded at their base by two concentric galleries which border long halls. This temple of the lingam Rājendrabhadreśvara was built in 961 by King Rājendravarman, who dedicated the four corner towers to various funerary images.

Beyond the southeast corner of the Baray is Banteay Samrè, a funerary temple of unknown purpose. Its main tower, analogous to those at Angkor Wat, is preceded by a vestibule and enclosed by two concentric galleries.

Leaving Angkor Thom by the southern gate, one passes to the small pyramid of Baksei Chamkrong (10th cent.). One then arrives at the base of Phnom Bakheng, a natural hill about 200 ft. high, which was chosen by King Yaśovarman, the founder of Yaśodharapura, to mark the center of the capital (889). On the summit rises the temple of Yaśodhareśvara, the lingam which personified royalty during the founder's reign. It is a stone pyramid of five levels, with five towers in quincunx at the top, 12 small towers on each level, and 44 towers around the base.

Southeast of Phnom Bakheng lies Angkor Wat, the major monumental complex in the Angkor group and perhaps the largest temple in the world. It covers an area of about 5,000 × 4,000 ft.; its surrounding moats are 623 ft. wide, and its inner wall measures 3,363 × 2,625 ft. A causeway paved with hard sandstone traverses the moat on the west side and leads to the central portico of the entrance building. This building itself is a veritable monument and is decorated with greater richness and elaboration than the central temple. A paved roadway 1,148 ft. long begins at the central portico and dominates the surrounding area; it runs between two small edifices, passes two large artificial lakes to right and left, and terminates at a small stairway of a dozen steps which commands the principal entrance to the temple proper. The temple has a very simple plan, consisting of three concentric galleries of over 4,500 ft. in total length, rising toward the center and separated by paved courts. In the center of the highest gallery, and joined to it by four colonnades disposed along the axes, is the large central tower, which stands 208 ft. above the level of the ground, and which, together with the four corner towers, forms the quincunx typical of the Khmer pyramids. The corners of the middle gallery are also surmounted by high towers, so that Angkor Wat presents the visitor with an array of nine towers harmoniously arranged in tiers. The unusual effect of this monument lies in the impression it gives, from a certain distance, of a three-stepped pyramid, while in reality it consists of concentric, progressively higher galleries. The lowest gallery (705 ft. east to west × 613 ft. north to south) opens toward the exterior, as at the Bayon, and its inner wall is decorated with large low reliefs of scenes from Indian myths and epics as well as a royal procession and scenes of the heavens and hells. On the western side this gallery is joined to the middle gallery by a sort of covered passage. This arrangement, with its imaginative transition from a lower to a higher level, is a triumph of the architect. Angkor Wat, with its entirely Vishnuite decoration, was constructed in the first half of the 12th century by King Sūryavarman II to house his mausoleum, with the posthumous name of Paramaviṣṇuloka.

To the west of Angkor Thom is the great West Baray excavated by Udayādityavarman II, which measures 5 miles in length east to west and over 1 1/4 miles in width. On an island in the center is the temple dedicated to Viṣṇu, who is represented by a large reclining bronze statue. Three-fifths of a mile from the southwestern corner, the southern embankment of this hollow partially covers the monument of Ak Yom, an unfinished pyramid which must date from about the 8th century.

*The region northeast of Angkor.* Banteay Srei. Thirteen miles northeast of Angkor Thom and formerly called Iśvarapura, this monument was built under Jayavarman V for the lingam Tribhuvanamaheśvara. It is one of the jewels of Khmer art, for its architectural proportions, for the perfection of the low reliefs which adorn the pediments, and for the profuse decoration of the walls. At the center of the inner wall there are three towers, aligned along the north–south axis and open toward the east, which rise from a single base; the central tower is preceded by a hall joined to the sanctuary by a vestibule. In the northeast and southeast corners of the court are two libraries opening toward the west. The entire complex, as well as the two gopuras at the east and west, is richly decorated. The second surrounding wall, concentric to the first, is encircled by a moat crossed by two elevated causeways on the east-west axis, and in turn is enclosed by another wall with two gopuras. Leading to the eastern gopura is a road lined with milestones, which continues on to the eastern gopura of the outermost wall.

Phnom Kulên. This sandstone plateau, some 25 miles long with a maximum elevation in the southeastern portion of 1,472 ft., is situated about 19 miles northeast of Angkor. Formerly an immense stairway, cut into the rock to permit the ascension of a cliff 640 ft. high, gave access to the southwestern part. This picturesque spot, the source from which the river of Angkor descends in small rapids and falls and the site of the sandstone quarries utilized by the builders of the monuments of Angkor, is rich in edifices dating largely from the beginning of the 9th century. The most important are, from west to east: Rup Arak, the original site of a beautiful statue of Viṣṇu; Prasat O Pong; Krus Prah Aram Rong Chen, an early pyramid perhaps related to the institution of the cult of divine kingship; Prasat Damrei Krap, possibly constructed by Cham architects (see CHAM, SCHOOL OF); Sra Damrei, with two large monolithic statues of animals; Prasat Neak Ta and Prasat Thma Dap, where three beautiful statues of Viṣṇu were found. The eastern cliff is dotted with caves where hermits left sculpture and inscriptions.

Koh Ker. Seventy-eight miles from Angkor, the former Chok Gargyar, also called Lingapura, was the temporary capital of King Jayavarman IV and his son from 921 to 944. It contains numerous edifices that constituted the religious core of the city and its surroundings. These unusually large monuments are oriented in relation to a great lake, the Rahal, north of which the city was located. The principal building is the temple of the king-god, an enormous five-level pyramid. Above it, at a height of 134 ft., rose the great tower which housed the lingam. The pyramid was enclosed by a wall, with a single gate on the eastern side that communicated with a group of buildings girded by a triple wall and consisting principally of 9 towers, aligned in two rows, on a terrace bordered by 12 small towers. The eastern gopura of the outer wall, of colossal dimensions, is proportionate in scale to the pyramid rather than to the aforesaid monuments; it housed a statue of the dancing Śiva. The gopura of the middle wall, of more modest size, contained six statues of Brahmanic divinities. It is connected to the eastern one by a terrace bordered by images of nagas driving off two standing Garuḍas. Besides this complex, the group of Koh Ker includes about thirty-five secondary monuments.

Prasat Khna Sen Keo. This monument, southeast of Koh Ker, consists of a tower, entered through a cruciform room and flanked by two libraries, all encircled by a wall with two gopuras of three passages to the east and west. It is particularly important for its low reliefs, identical in style to those of the Baphuon at Angkor Thom and certainly of the same period (second half of the 11th cent.).

Phnom Sandak. Situated northwest of Koh Ker, the hill of Phnom Sandak, about 128 ft. high, corresponds to ancient Śivasthāna or Śivapura. Within the inner wall, which opens to the west in a gopura of three passages, there are seven towers aligned in two rows. The group is completed by two subsidiary buildings and an outer wall with a large gopura on the eastern side. This temple, built in the 9th century, in its present state appears to date from the mid-10th.

Prasat Neak Buos. Northeast of the preceding group, 6 miles in the direction east-northeast from the town of Cheâm Khsan — at the center of a region rich in archaeological remains — is the monument of Prasat Neak Buos, situated against the lower southern slopes of the Dangrek Mountains. It is the ancient Śivapāda of the East, founded prior to the 8th century and venerated and visited through the ages. The central tower, of large dimensions and probably contemporary with the gigantic edifices of Koh Ker, is encircled by small sanctuaries, irregularly disposed. The complex is surrounded by a wall opening to the south in a gopura of three passages.

Prah Vihar. The ancient temple of Śikharīśvara (god of the summit) is built at an altitude of 2,392 ft. on a projection of the Dangrek chain that dominates the Cambodian plain; from the plain one approaches the temple by a stairway 3/5 mile long cut into the rock. From the north, that is, from the direction of Thailand, there is an access road 1/2 mile long. A stairway leads to an avenue flanked by nagas which ends at a cruciform portico constructed on a terrace. Then a broad roadway 1,148 ft. in length conducts one to a second cruciform portico, also on a terrace; a third roadway of 328 ft. opens on a third cruciform portico flanked by two rectangular buildings. Beyond an esplanade a short stairway leads to a gopura of three passages, whose eastern and western extremities adjoin two galleries. These open on the interior of a court containing two libraries and a hall which precedes the gopura of a second cloister. In the center of this cloister is the sanctuary of Śikharīśvara, giving access on the four cardinal points by means of vestibules. Most of these constructions date from the middle of the 11th century, but some parts may be older, and inscriptions attest to reconstructions in the 12th century.

*The region east of Angkor.* Beng Mealea. This monument, 43 miles east of Angkor, is slightly earlier than Angkor Wat. It has the same plan as the latter except that the concentric galleries remain at ground level and are not articulated in planes. Its ancient name is not known, nor is its purpose, which was perhaps funerary. The temple is surrounded by a 2½-mile moat (ca. ⁵/₆ mile east to west × ²/₃ mile north to south). Four roads lead to gates located at the center of each side of the outer wall and preceded by cruciform terraces. The monument comprises three systems of concentric galleries with four axial gopuras. The exterior gallery measures 594 ft. east to west × 499 ft. north to south, and has a tower both at the center of each side and at each of the four corners. The central and inner galleries are displaced toward the west to make room to the east, between the central and outer galleries, for two libraries and a cruciform court. The outer wall has four gopuras and four corner pavilions; the interior contained the central sanctuary, preceded by a long hall, that today is completely ruined.

Prah Khan. Thirty-nine miles east of Beng Mealea and 65 miles east of Angkor Thom, to which it is connected by a direct road, is the great complex of Prah Khan (Kompong Svay); the main part dates from the 12th century. Its site has been occupied since the reign of Sūryavarman I (first half of 11th cent.) and may have served as the residence of Jayavarman VII at the end of the 12th century during the construction of Angkor Thom. The outer wall, 3 miles on each side, is interrupted on the eastern face by an artificial lake 1 ⅓ miles east to west × ½ mile north to south, which was probably built by Jayavarman VII; the western half of this lake lies within the surrounding wall, while the eastern half lies outside of it. Beyond the southeast corner rises Prah Damrei, a stepped pyramid 23 ft. high. The center of the lake, located on the axis of the eastern wall, is marked by the cruciform sanctuary of Prah Thkol, which thus occupies the same position as the Mebon in the middle of the Angkor Thom lake. Centered in the west side of the reservoir is the Prah Stung with towers adorned with human faces analogous to those of the Bayon and the gates of Angkor Thom. The surrounding wall of the temple of Prah Khan, 1,640 ft. to the west of the Prah Stung, is preceded by a large moat traversed by a bridge, the lower part of which is decorated with *haṁsa* (swan or goose) caryatids while the parapets are formed by the bodies of two nagas. Further toward the interior, another concentric wall has axial gopuras; the eastern gopura, with five passages, is flanked on the inner side by four richly decorated buildings. A terrace extends from this gopura to a final innermost wall with four partially preserved monumental gopuras. This wall encloses the central sanctuary, which was merely begun and seems to have succumbed to systematic destruction.

*The region southeast of Angkor. a. The Roluos group.* This group of monuments, about 9 miles southeast of Angkor, corresponds to ancient Hariharālaya, the pre-Angkorian site at which Jayavarman II located his capital at the beginning of the 9th century and where his immediate successors reigned. Apart from some remnants of the pre-Angkorian period, the three most important complexes date from the reigns of Kings Indravarman (877–89) and Yaśovarman (889–900).

From north to south, the first of these monuments is Lolei (the Indravarmeśvara), in the center of the lake. Its four brick towers, consecrated by Yaśovarman in 893, are built on a quadrangular two-staged terrace, accessible by means of a stairway at the east. These identical towers, showing traces of stucco, are dedicated to the parents and maternal grandparents of the founder.

Prah Kô, south of Lolei, was built by Indravarman in 880 in the eastern part of a vast area contained by a surrounding wall. There are six brick towers with traces of stucco, aligned by threes in two rows and opened to the east onto a common terrace. The central tower of the eastern row is dedicated to Parameśvara, the posthumous name of Jayavarman II, and the others contain funerary statues of the parents and grandparents of the founding king.

Bakong, south of the preceding complex, was built in 881 by Indravarman for the royal lingam Indreśvara and was the first stone pyramid. It measures 217×210 ft. at the base and 66×58 ft. at the summit of the fifth story, which is about 50 ft. above ground level. Efforts at reconstruction (1936–43) have led to the restoration of a tower, datable not earlier than the 11th century, on this top level, as well as the restoration of 12 small stone towers to their original positions on the fourth story. The base of the pyramid, surrounded by eight brick towers and various secondary edifices, is enclosed within three walls; the outermost measures 2,953 ft. east to west × 2,296 ft. north to south, and the middle wall measures 1,312×984 ft.

*b. The Sambor Prei Kuk group.* About nineteen miles northeast of Kompong Thom is the former Iśanapura, the capital during the

first half of the 7th century, which is composed of three groups of buildings, mostly in brick, corresponding to the various religious centers of the city that was situated slightly to the west. Each of the three groups consists of a principal sanctuary and subsidiary buildings enclosed by a wall.

The central (or western) group, whose purpose is unknown, has a beautiful brick tower located at the center of a double wall. It is almost rectangular in plan, oriented toward the east, and is adorned with three false doors.

Immediately to the southeast, the southern group includes a sanctuary attributable to King Iśānavarman, located at the center of a double wall and preceded to the east by a rectangular edifice containing a mandapa (Skr., *maṇḍapa*) which housed an image of the bull Nandi. This sanctuary, open to the east and decorated with false doors, originally held the gold lingam of Prahasiteśvara, the "smiling god." The inner wall, which embraces five octagonal towers as well as this sanctuary, is decorated on the exterior with scenes in circular medallions placed between pilasters.

The northern group, located northeast of the central group, was dedicated to the god Gambhīreśvara, whose quadrangular sanctuary, built on a terrace, opens toward the four cardinal points by means of four axial bays; four small temples are located at the corners of the terrace. Four towers (the one at the southwest is octagonal) rise inside of the four corners of the surrounding wall, and three towers are located outside in the western part of the area contained by the outermost wall.

Sambor. Sambor on the Mekong, north of Kratié, is the former Śambhupura of the 8th century and was still known in the 17th century by the name of Sambabour. There exist eight groups of ruins, represented by elevations in the terrain, which have yielded sculpture and pre-Angkorian inscriptions.

Wat Nokor. This Buddhist monument of the age of Jayavarman VII (end of 12th cent.), situated 1 1/4 miles from Kompong Cham, consists of a cruciform sanctuary open toward the four cardinal points and preceded by a vestibule. Together with its two libraries to the southeast and northeast, it is enclosed within a double wall pierced by four gates.

Banteay Prei Nokor. This is an ancient city 25 miles southeast of Kompong Cham. In the center of a quadrangular wall with a perimeter of 5 1/2 or 6 miles, three quadrangular brick sanctuaries are aligned on the north-south axis. About 800 ft. east of these are three more towers open toward the north and aligned on the east-west axis. Banteay Prei Nokor may have been one of the capitals of pre-Angkorian Cambodia during the period of anarchy in the 8th century.

Lovêk. This city, 31 miles north of Phnom Penh, was the capital during a large part of the 16th century. Three sides of its surrounding wall are still visible for several miles. Two pagodas, Wat Traleng Keng and Wat Prah Ein Tep, date from an early period.

Udong. Twenty-eight miles north of Phnom Penh, the modern capital, is Udong, the ancient capital, of which very little remains. To the south, on the hill of Phnom Prah Reacheatrap, are the stupas that contained the ashes of the sovereigns who ruled at the end of the 18th and during the 19th century.

Phnom Penh. On the summit of the artificial hill that gives its name to the city, the present capital of Cambodia, stands the great bell-shaped stupa, which dates from the time when the court established itself there after abandoning Angkor.

Angkor Borei. About 60 miles south of Phnom Penh is the ancient city of Angkor Borei, the last capital of Funan in the second half of the 6th century. The oldest Buddhist statues of Cambodia originated here. South of the city, the hill of Phnom Da, dotted with caves made into sanctuaries, has yielded three magnificent Vishnuite statues representing the finest achievements of pre-Angkorian sculpture. A little farther west is the Asram Maharosei, the source of a Harihara of the same period. It is a quadrangular building with a compartment separated from the outer wall by means of a surrounding corridor from 24 to 32 in. wide. The two planes which constitute the elevation and reproduce the principal body on a reduced scale are crowned by a small onion-shaped finial. The gate opens to the north and is flanked by two windows; three windows illuminate each side of the inner corridor.

Ta Prohm of Bati. Situated 25 miles south of Phnom Penh, this monument from the period of Jayavarman II, with towers adorned with human faces, rises on an ancient site of the Funan

period. In it has been found one of the rare inscriptions, reused at a later date, which remain from this early kingdom.

Phnom Chisor. Thirty-five miles south of Phnom Penh, the two brick towers of Prasat Neang Khmau, constructed in the 7th century but rebuilt in the 9th, contain the few frescoes that we know of in Cambodia and mark the beginning of a road leading to the hill of Phnom Chisor. This is the former Sūryaparvata, whose summit, 328 ft. high, is crowned by a group of buildings datable to the reign of Sūryavarman I (first half of 11th cent.). A monumental stairway, 705 ft. long with 400 steps, ascends the eastern side and leads to a rectangular wall which encloses eight buildings: the central sanctuary, preceded by a vestibule and a nave with four columns; two libraries to the northeast and southeast; and two buildings of the same type aligned with the sanctuaries. The surrounding gallery is divided into 16 rooms not connected to one another; it is interrupted by gopuras of three passages at the center of the eastern and western sides.

Phnom Bayang. Situated about 78 miles south of Phnom Penh, the monument of Phnom Bayang, the former Śivapura, is one of the finest complexes of pre-Angkorian art. It is built at a height of 1,027 ft. on a narrow plateau. Entrance from the southeast is by a stairway of more than 1,300 steps which terminates at the summit in a straight, steep ramp enclosed between two walls with irregular indentations. The encircling wall, with a gopura in an almost total state of ruin, consists of a gallery around the central sanctuary, a vestibule (of later date), and seven small identical towers, one in each corner of the sanctuary and one at the extremity of each axis (except the eastern). The sanctuary, built of brick with the surrounds of the doors in sandstone, measures 33 ft. long × 26 ft. wide × 49 ft. high. It is composed of several elements: a ground floor including a sub-base, the principal body and a cornice, and three superimposed levels crowned by a barrel vault. These levels, which diminish in size and reproduce the main body, are false; the interior vault decreases gradually up to the apex. The façade of the ground floor is decorated with large replicas of buildings; these appear to each side of the entrance way, which opens to the southeast, and to each side of the false doors, framed by round colonnettes and lintels, on the other three sides. The interior of the sanctuary contains a mandapa of later date.

*The region northwest of Angkor.* In this area a considerable number of small ruins indicates a major concentration of population. Only the most important will be mentioned.

Banteay Chmar. A vast complex 38 miles from the city of Sisophon, Banteay Chmar has the aspect of a closed city: it is surrounded by a wall 5 1/2 miles in perimeter, with a Buddhist temple in the center built by King Jayavarman VII in memory of his son and companions in arms who fell in the course of the battles of the second half of the 12th century. The wall around the temple is 2,724 × 1,969 ft. Elevated causeways, bordered by gigantic figures as at Angkor Thom, lead to the four axial gopuras and continue into the interior to a sanctuary where, as at the Bayon, the crossings of the galleries are surmounted by towers adorned with human faces. The sanctuary is enclosed by a gallery open toward the exterior and measuring 804 × 262 ft.; its inner wall, like that of the Bayon, is covered with low reliefs of scenes of a historical and religious character.

BIBLIOG. Q. Aymonier, Le Cambodge, 3 vols., Paris, 1900–4; L. de Lajonquière, Inventaire descriptif des monuments du Cambodge, 3 vols., Paris, 1902–11 (Pubs. de l'Ecole Française d'Extrême-Orient, IV, VIII, IX); H. Parmentier, L'art Khmèr primitif, 2 vols. Paris, 1927 (Pubs. de l'Ecole Française d'Extrême-Orient, XXI, XXII); H. Parmentier, History of Khmèr Architecture, Eastern Art, III, 1931; H. Parmentier, L'art Khmèr classique; Monuments du quadrant Nord-Est, 2 vols., Paris, 1939 (Pubs. de l'Ecole Française d'Extrême-Orient, XXIX); M. Glaize, Les monuments du groupe d'Angkor, 2d ed., Saigon, 1948; L. P. Briggs, The Ancient Khmer Empire, Trans. Am. Phil. Soc., XLI, part 1, 1951 (with bibliog.).

George CŒDÈS

Illustrations: 2 figs. in text.

**CAMEROONS.** The Cameroons is a vast region of central west Africa that stretches from the basin of Lake Chad in the north as far as the eastern end of the Gulf of Guinea in the south. From 1884 to 1919 it was a German protectorate (Kamerun); after World War I about five sixths of it became a French mandate (Cameroun) and is now independent (capital Yaoundé);

the remaining sixth was placed under British trusteeship (capital Buea). It is bordered on the north by Nigeria; on the east, west, and south by French Equatorial Africa; and still farther south by Spanish Guinea. Archaeological exploration, limited to sporadic attempts, has not so far furnished material of particular interest; the production of the contemporary natives (about 4,500,000) is better known. There are no noteworthy contributions in the field of European-derived art.

Among the few excavation finds those of Djimoun should be noted. In 1948 a terra-cotta statue was brought to light there, buried in the laterite inside the perimeter of the first palace of the Bamum sultans and therefore datable about the 15th century. Old bronze ornaments were discovered in excavations at Makari.

There is a museum of indigenous art at Foumban, built by the sultan Njoya (first quarter of the 20th century) containing important

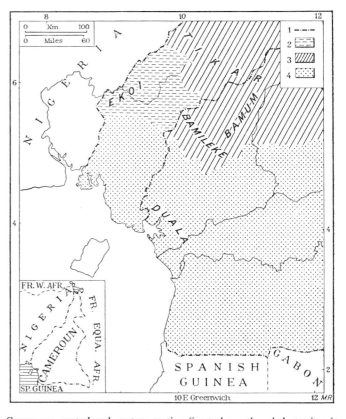

Cameroons, central and western section (inset shows the whole territory). Shading indicates the geographical division of art styles. Tribal names are in bold italic capitals. *Key:* (1) Political boundaries; (2) Cross River region; (3) grasslands region; (4) eastern forest region.

collections of Bamum art and of the art of neighboring grasslands groups. The sculptor Mose Yeyap, a rival of Njoya, created another museum at Foumban for his own works and those of other artists.

Cameroons sculpture can be localized in three distinct geographical zones: the Cross River region, the grasslands region, and the eastern forest region.

The Cross River region is inhabited by semi-Bantu groups with cultural elements common to the grasslands peoples as well as to the coastal Bantu; there are influences of the high Sudanese culture in the painted decoration on the outside of the houses (see GUINEAN CULTURES). The Ekoi, who constitute the largest group, are known for anthropomorphic wooden statues, heads in the round, and masks connected with the Egbo secret-society rites. Simple masks, originally covered with human skin, are covered today with antelope or monkey skin. Janus and androgynous masks are sometimes painted in two colors and surmounted by zoomorphic figures with a magical-symbolical significance. Analogous sculptures are found among the Boki. The Banyangi have masks in the shape of an antelope head; the Anyang make statuettes, sometimes covered with skin, of a seated figure with the head leaning on the right hand. In this area curved lines and floral motifs (decorative themes unusual for Negro Africa) are used in body embellishment, in tattooing, in decorating the exterior

walls of the houses, and in the secret-society symbols. The same inspiration appears in the *nsbidi* writing of the Ekoi and Efik. The former also make pottery of good quality.

The grasslands region (see BANTU CULTURES), occupying the central and northern parts of the territory, has supplied the most notable contributions, especially in the regions between the Bafum (properly Bum) and the Bangangte. Two style currents are distinguishable in the sculpture, one secular (doorframes and supporting posts, vases, bedposts, drums, stools with anthropomorphous and zoomorphic supporting figures), the other religious (ancestor masks and statuettes). Zoomorphic motifs with a precise symbolic significance predominate in the decoration: snakes, frogs, and lizards are fertility symbols, while among the Bamenda the spider and the chameleon are symbols of death.

In the Babassi zone a well-made pottery is produced. The Tikar, Bamum, and Bagam work in copper and bronze. The last are known for their fine pipe bowls cast in copper by the lost-wax process. Weaving also flourishes, and artificial colors are used. The Bamum have a method of dyeing similar to *plangi* (a form of resist dyeing). Beads of European import have supplied the material for an outstanding decorative art; the bead-covered throne of Njoya, now in the Museum für Völkerkunde in Berlin, is famous. In this area the Bamum and the Bamileke, both of the former French sector, exhibit an extremely fine artistic sense. Among the most outstanding works are the houses with sculptured doorframes and doorposts and with exterior walls covered with frescoes; the dance masks in wood, terra cotta, or bronze; the polychrome cloth embroidery in traditional geometric motifs; and the dressed skins, often decorated with reverse, or negative, designs. A typical Bamum decorative theme is the two-headed snake. The Kom group has features of its own and is noted for monumental sculpture (especially the royal thrones with life-size anthropomorphous back rests), decorative carving, and masks. An analogous type of monumental statuary is found among the Babanki, who produce fine covered jars supported by animal figures. The Wum, a small group situated between the Bum and the Kom, produce characteristic figurines of a seated person holding a large bowl. The Babenga and the Bamessing, two other minor groups of the grasslands zone, are known for their clay pipe bowls, generally cephalomorphic or in the form of a seated or crouched figure.

At Bafoussam the Bamileke have a school of sculpture and crafts where skilled teachers follow the traditional styles and techniques, but the quality of its productions is greatly inferior to the older works. Bamileke sculpture is generally of a court character: only chiefs' houses are decorated with sculpture, and their beds alone may be carved. The preferred subjects in the statues and the decoration of the drums are great political personages. The Bamileke also execute noteworthy ivory sculptures.

The contribution of the minor groups, Banen, Bafia, Balom, and Bali, is small. The last, of Sudanese origin, make fine clay pipe bowls, probably derived from the Bamileke and the Bamum but with original elaborations. The most common among the great variety of types is that of a seated anthropomorphous figure with a disproportionately large head — frequently a human body with the head of an animal. Also noteworthy are the stools supported by human, animal, or combined human and animal figures.

The eastern and southern forest zone is inhabited by little-known peoples of diverse origins. Among these the Duala should be noted. Their westward migration from the valley of the Sanaga River seems to have taken place two centuries ago. They have no statues of note but make fine cattle masks (*nyati*) painted in white, black, red, and blue. These masks belong to the Ekongolo society and are used at funerals; they also exist among the Bajong, the Bodiman, and the Wuri. The canoes of the Duala are remarkable for their carved prows, on which superimposed decorative motifs are surmounted by a bird holding a snake in its beak: behind the bird, on a lateral plane, is a man standing between two animals. The Kpe-Mboko, a small group of this area, produce elaborately sculptured biers and masks connected with the Nganya society.

European occupation has led to an urban type of building. Efforts are being made to adapt this to the local environment.

BIBLIOG. L. Frobenius, Der Kameruner Schiffschnabel und seine Motive, Halle, 1897; P. Germann, Das plastische-figürliche Kunstgewerbe im Grasland von Kamerun, 4 vols., Leipzig, 1910; L. W. G. Malcolm, Note on a Brass-Casting in Central Cameroon, Man, XXIII, 1923; E. von Sydow, Masque Janus du Cross-River, Documents, VI, 1930; E. Buisson, Quelques réalisations animales chez les Bamiléké, Togo-Cameroun, Paris, 1931; E. von Sydow, Die abstrakte Ornamentik der Gebrauchskunst im Grasland von Kamerun, BA, XV, 1932; S. Truitard and E. Buisson, Arts du Cameroun à l'exposition d'art colonial de Naples, Naples, 1934; Catalogue de la mission H. Labouret au Cameroun, Paris, 1935; Idrissou Mborou Njoya, Le sultanat du pays Bamoum et son origine, B. Soc. d'études camerounaises, VII, 1935; J. P. Lebeuf, Note sommaire sur l'habitation fali, JSA, XI, 1941; J. B. Jauze, Contribution à l'étude de l'archéologie du Cameroun, B. Soc. d'études camerounaises, VIII, 1944; M. D. W. Jeffreys, Le serpent à deux têtes bamoum, B. Soc. d'études camerounaises, IX, 1945; J. P. Lebeuf, Vêtements et parures du Cameroun français, Paris, 1946; J. B. Jauze, L'art inconnu d'une culture primitive africaine dans la région de Yaoundé, B. Soc. d'études camerounaises, XXIII–XXIV, 1948; J. P. Lebeuf and A. Masson-Detourbet, L'art ancien du Tchad, Afrique equatoriale et Cameroun, CahArt, 1951; R. Lecocq, Quelques aspects de l'arte bamoum, Présence africaine, X–XI, 1951; J. P. Beguin et al., L'Habitat au Cameroun, Paris, 1952; J. P. Lebeuf, Labrets et greniers des Fali (Nord-Cameroun), BIFAN, XV, 3, 1953; J. P. Lebeuf, Villes et palais du Nord-Cameroun, Rev. voyages, VIII, 1953; R. Lecocq, Les Bamiléké, Paris, 1953; M. McCulloch, M. Little-wood and I. Dugast, Peoples of the Central Cameroons, Ethnographic Survey of Africa, Western Africa, IX, London, 1954; E. Ardener, Coastal Bantu of the Cameroons, Ethnographic Survey of Africa, Western Africa, XI, London, 1956.

Jean LAUDE

Illustrations: 1 fig. in text.

**CAMPIN**, ROBERT. Flemish painter, probably to be associated with the Master of Flémalle (b. possibly Valenciennes, ca. 1378, d. Tournai, 1444). Campin was established in Tournai as a free master in 1406. In the course of that year and the next he executed a fresco, the *Annunciation*, for the Church of St.-Brice in Tournai, which was uncovered in 1940. In 1410 Campin acquired citizenship in Tournai; during the following decade he apparently became well known as a teacher, attracting apprentices to his workshop. He became dean of the painters' guild in 1423 and was a member of one of the governing councils of Tournai during the political upheaval that temporarily expelled the patricians from power. He was subsequently prosecuted for taking part in the revolt and, as a married man, was also condemned on moral charges involving his relations with a young woman named Leurence Polette. Documents record that Campin trained Jacques Daret in his workshop, as well as a painter named Roger de La Pasture, probably to be identified with the great Rogier van der Weyden (q.v.), who became the official painter of the city of Brussels in 1435. Except for the St.-Brice fresco, no signed or documented painting by Campin remains. There is good reason, however, to believe that Campin was the real name of the artist who has gone by the anonymous title of the Master of Flémalle, so-called from the three panels in the Städelsches Kunstinstitut in Frankfort on the Main that are supposed to have come originally from an abbey in Flémalle. If this identification is correct, Robert Campin was also the author of the triptych of the *Annunciation* (New York, The Cloisters) long known as the *Merode Triptych*, from the family name of former owners. This exquisite and startlingly realistic altarpiece has a representation on the central panel of the Annunciation, taking place in a fully furnished bourgeois interior; donors are depicted at the left, with St. Joseph at work in his carpenter shop on the right. The work is contemporary with, and may even be earlier than, the famous Ghent altarpiece of 1432 by the brothers Van Eyck (q.v.). Other paintings in the same style as The Cloisters *Annunciation*, and surely by the same artist, include the *Nativity* in Dijon (Beaux-Arts), the *Annunciation* and *Marriage of the Virgin* (V, PL. 279) in Madrid (Prado), the wings from the Werl altarpiece showing St. Barbara and the donor with St. John the Baptist in the same gallery (Prado; V, PL. 278), the *Madonna in Glory* in Aix-en-Provence (Musée Granet) the *Madonna by the Fireside* in Leningrad (Hermitage), and a number of portraits, especially that of Robert de Masmines, in Berlin (Staatliche Mus.). Emile Renders (followed by some other scholars) has declared that no such artistic personality as the Master of Flémalle ever existed, ascribing all the paintings usually so attributed to the early period of Rogier van der Weyden. The style of the entire group connected with the name of Flémalle does indeed show a clear relationship to that of Rogier van der Weyden in iconography, facial and bodily types, and nervous linear execution. There are, however, a robustness about the group and a quality of forthright vitality that distinguish them from Van der Weyden's paintings, which are without exception characterized by extreme sensitiveness and aristocratic elegance. Campin-Flémalle exerted a very strong influence on Netherlandish painting, not only as the teacher who shaped the early style of Rogier van der Weyden but also as the artist who, in his own right, formulated many

of the principles of composition and design that determined the character of Flemish painting for numerous succeeding generations. See also FLEMISH AND DUTCH ART.

BIBLIOG. M. J. Friedländer, Die altniederländische Malerei, II, Berlin, 1924; E. Renders, La Solution du problème Van der Weyden-Flémalle-Campin, Bruges, 1931; C. de Tolnay, Le Maître de Flémalle et les frères Van Eyck, Brussels, 1938; E. Panofsky, Early Netherlandish Painting, Cambridge, Mass., 1953; T. Rousseau, Jr., The Merode Altarpiece, and M. B. Freeman, The Iconography of the Merode Altarpiece, both BMMA, XVI, 1957, pp. 117–39.

Margaretta M. SALINGER

**CAMPIONESI.** Lombard sculptors, master builders, and stonecutters active from the end of the 12th through the 14th century; so called by 19th-century critics from their place of origin, Campione di Lugano, whose name was frequently added to their baptismal names. Unlike the Antelami (Bognetti), they do not constitute an officially recognized workshop, and only during the 12th and the first half of the 13th centuries do stylistic characteristics differentiate them from other north Italian currents in architecture and especially in sculpture. Thereafter their style becomes indistinguishable from that of artists from Arogno, Bissone, or even from the area between Lake Como and Lake Lugano. In spite of diverse influences and a particular ability to adapt themselves to local trends, the workshop as a whole consistently displays a compact solidity of form that indicates a common origin and common tradition.

SUMMARY. The Campionesi at Modena (col. 39). Activity in northern Italy to about 1250 (col. 39). Activity in Switzerland (col. 40). Lombard artists in Tuscany in the 13th century (col. 40). Masters from Arogno and the Cathedral of Trent (col. 41). The Campionesi and Antelami (col. 41). Activity from late 13th century to about 1330 (col. 41). Activity in Bergamo (col. 42). Tuscan influences (col. 43). The Campionesi and the Cathedral of Milan (col. 44). Criticism (col. 44).

THE CAMPIONESI AT MODENA. The first known document records that in 1244 a certain Enrico da Campione committed himself and his descendants to work for the Cathedral of Modena *in perpetuum* and that he was renewing previous contracts made by his father, Ottavio, and his grandfather, Anselmo. We may reasonably assume that during the second half of the preceding century Anselmo had supervised all work at the cathedral (which had been dedicated in 1184), for he immediately appears in the dual role of sculptor and architect. For example, the *pontile* (PLS. 17, 18) of the cathedral, which has been unanimously attributed to him, presents an architectural solution for the articulation of the nave and the chancel raised above the crypt. The further problems concerning the contributions of the Campionesi to the construction of the Modena Cathedral have not yet been examined by scholars. Those relating to the sculpture, however, have been fully resolved. The Provençal training of Anselmo and his workshop (Saint-Gilles, Arles, Beaucaire) has been demonstrated and their vigorous sculptural sense and pronounced tendency toward realism emphasized. A basic stylistic bond connects all the sculpture at Modena: the *pontile*, the reliefs of the campanile, the pulpit, the altar, the capitals of the crypt, the royal portal on the south side, and the rosette.

The royal portal (1209–31) was most probably built under the direction of Ottavio. Two of its columns are of special interest because they reappear in all buildings, both civic and religious, by later Campionesi. One is hexagonal and derives from Arles, the other is twisted and based on one in the Cathedral of Ferrara by the sculptor Nicolò. The last of the Campionesi active in Modena was the later Enrico under whom the campanile was completed in 1319 and who built the pulpit in 1322.

ACTIVITY IN NORTHERN ITALY TO ABOUT 1250. An important group of sculptures is associated with those by the Campionesi at Modena. First among them are the apostles, of red Verona marble (PL. 18), in the left aisle of the Cathedral of Milan. They date from about 1185–87 and come from the now-destroyed older cathedral, where they were probably part of a *pontile* of the same type as the one at Modena. Their close relation to the apostles of St. Trophime in Arles and the way of placing them between hexagonal columns once again reaffirms the Provençal training of the Campionesi. Other works belonging to this group are the capitals in San Vitale delle Carpinete, near Modena, and the seated figure of a man writing, possibly Vergil, in the Palazzo Ducale at Mantua; the red marble altar in the Cathedral of Parma; and the saint in the Museo S. Stefano in Bologna. Furthermore, the lion doors (1220) from the earlier cathedral of Bologna, which made such an impression on Vasari, may very well have been made by a branch of this workshop, at least judging from the extant fragments consisting of a telamon and two lions supporting columns (now in the Archbishop's Palace and the Cathedral, respectively). Characteristics pointing to a Veronese master of the early 14th century, however, exclude from this group the large figure of the "smiling" St. Zeno from the church of that name in Verona.

So far, scholars have failed to note the link between the sculpture of the Campionesi and that of the tripartite window set behind the Gothic gallery of the Cathedral of Ferrara. A capital of one of the pilasters and one of the paired columns of the window repeat the distinctive meander pattern of leaves with projecting animal heads in such a way that it seems to be the work of the same craftsman who was responsible for those on the royal portal in Modena.

ACTIVITY IN SWITZERLAND. During the closing years of the 12th century and the beginning of the 13th, the Campionesi extended their activities beyond the cities of the Po Valley into the region of the Alps. They worked on the Cathedral of Chur (ca. 1178), where sculptures from the old *pontile*, now dismembered, are still extant. The figures of the apostles (PL. 18) and the relief with scenes from the life of St. Lawrence in the Cathedral of Basel may also be assigned to the Campionesi; the iconography is characterized by elements clearly derived from Early Christian examples, as is that of the two figures of SS. Peter and Paul, today embedded in the wall of the cloister of S. Giuseppe fuori Porta Saragozza in Bologna.

LOMBARD ARTISTS IN TUSCANY IN THE 13TH CENTURY. The style of Guido Bigarelli da Arogno, known also as Guido da Como, which is completely independent of Benedetto Antelami, may be explained by the late-12th-century tradition with its double heritage of Provençal and Early Christian art. Together with a half-brother, Lanfranco, and other assistants, he was active in the mid-13th century in Tuscany, where he made the octagonal baptismal font in the Baptistery of Pisa (1248) and the well-known pulpit of S. Bartolomeo in Pantano in Pistoia (1250; PL. 19). As Salmi has pointed out, in the font he displays his ability to adapt himself to local taste by assuming the elaborate decorative formula of the carved ornaments of the cathedral. The figures of the pulpit in Pistoia indicate a familiarity with the work of the Campionesi in Modena as well as with sculptures similar to the apostles in Basel. He had, however, returned to the simple sculptural volumes used earlier, so that the rather squat figures stand out sharply against a background so smooth that it accentuates their solid projection. The calm and solid expanding and intersecting of planes and volumes typical of Guido's work, which also characterizes later Lombard sculpture, is perhaps due to the direct influence of Early Christian sarcophagi and to the fact that he himself was not actually trained in Provence.

Other works by Guido in Tuscany include the monumental Archangel Michael on the façade of the Church of S. Giuseppe in Pistoia and the lintel of the main entrance and the sculptures of the portico of the Cathedral of S. Martino in Lucca (Salmi). Still according to Salmi, the scenes from the life of St. Regulus in S. Martino in Lucca may be the work of Guido's half-brother, Lanfranco, and his assistants, and are certainly Lombard. Their author has found truly original solutions, as, for example, in the lunette with the martyrdom of the saint, where the composition displays great subtlety and elegance. The

figures in the other compartments, rigid as if they were hieratic apparitions, are vaguely reminiscent of the saint in the Museo S. Stefano in Bologna. Like those of Guido, the compartments are framed in strongly projecting rectangular moldings against which the halos are forced to curve out in the same manner as those of the apostles in Milan and of the figures on the *pontile* and the pulpit at Modena.

MASTERS FROM AROGNO AND THE CATHEDRAL OF TRENT. That Adamo d'Arogno, although much less gifted, belonged to the same artistic tradition as Guido is corroborated by the fact that they came from the same area, the village of Arogno being adjacent to Campione. For about a century Adamo and his descendants worked on the construction of the Cathedral of Trent, which, according to a tablet of 1295, still *in situ*, was begun in 1212. For it Adamo d'Arogno and his descendants built "circuitum chori... cum appendiciis intrinsece et extrinsece" ("the ambulatory with interior and exterior additions"). One need only compare the telamon supporting the pulpit at Pistoia with the badly weathered triple one in the porch near the small apse on the right in the Cathedral of Trent, which definitely dates from the time of Adamo. These, together with the insets of scenes of fighting on the bases, which are generally reminiscent of motifs favored by the Campionesi in many buildings in northern Italy, dispel any doubt of the close relation between the two workshops. At Trent the activities of the Lombard masters were much more architectural than sculptural; it is the extensive use of hexagonal columns throughout the building that most consistently characterizes their activity there.

THE CAMPIONESI AND ANTELAMI. Benedetto Antelami's strong personality was bound to leave a mark on most Lombard sculptors who, in turn, contributed to his formation. In all probability Campione stonecarvers worked under his direction, possibly at Borgo San Donnino (now Fidenza) and in the Church of S. Andrea at Vercelli. An important example in which these two currents meet is the plinth in the Museo Civico in Bologna. Moreover, an assimilation of elements derived from Antelami is evident in the Cathedral of Trent in the tympanum of the north portal with Christ in Glory surrounded by the symbols of the Evangelists, in the two carved bands in the two apses (today unfortunately almost completely hidden by the baroque altars), and in the statue of the "Madonna of the Annegati." It is also probable that this workshop was responsible for the porch of the Cathedral of Bolzano and the tympanum of the Franciscan church in Salzburg as well as the tympanum from the earlier portal (first half of the 12th cent., now in the Salzburg museum), to which the two supporting lions may also belong.

ACTIVITY FROM LATE 13TH CENTURY TO ABOUT 1330. During the course of the 13th century the Campione and Antelami styles gradually lost their distinctive qualities, so that, fusing into a common idiom, they became one, so to speak. The leadership of a strong personality, however, was lacking. Thus the Egidio di Campione who made the wheel of fortune in the Cathedral of Trent produced sentimental, doll-like figures, and Giambone di Bissone repeated shopworn forms in the lions of the porch of the Cathedral of Parma (1281). The various tombs from the first decades of the 14th century published by Baroni, as well as the baptismal font in the Cathedral of Varese, are the expression of a tradition handed down from father to son. In these works the only tie with the triumphs of the past is the deep undercutting of the moldings against which the saints' halos rest, for the figures themselves are heavy and lifeless. There is some originality in the tomb of Ottone Visconti in the Cathedral of Milan (1295), a solidly sculptural work in which the figure of the deceased lies on one side of the sloping lid, surrounded by the subtle repetition of the accordion-pleated drapery. The original structure of the tomb is unknown, but the general scheme was close to that of the tomb of Berardo Maggi (1308) in the old Cathedral of Brescia, probably by a Veronese master. Both schemes depend on the same prototype, the funerary monument of Robert, son of Richard, Duke of Normandy (beginning of the 12th cent.), formerly in the Church of St. Pierre in Chartres.

ACTIVITY IN BERGAMO. To find another group of works with distinctive characteristics one must turn to the Campionesi working in Bergamo. The earliest example there is the tomb of Guglielmo Longhi (PL. 19), which has been tentatively attributed to Ugo da Campione. While the 19th-century reconstruction responsible for the entire superstructure and one of the supporting lions appears to be wholly arbitrary, the tomb itself is original. It presents a new device in the four standing figures, two angels and two clerics, guarding the deceased, which have been substituted for the usual angels attached to the bier. An immediate stylistic precedent for the figures of the Longhi tomb may be seen in a Virgin and Child from the beginning of the 14th century (PL. 20) in the Art Institute, Chicago. This is the work of a capable sculptor, influenced by Arnolfo da Cambio, who, like other Campione masters of the period, blends disparate stylistic elements in one work. In the Longhi tomb this blending is evident in the telamons, especially the left one, which shows the influence of Nicolò, while the heads of the angels with their large flat curls distantly echo Antelami's manner. Though later and more developed, the tomb of a member of the Castelbarco family in Loppio (Trentino) is also derived from the tomb in Bergamo. Further additions to this rather provincial group of sculptures, listed by Baroni, are a Madonna on the front of a tomb in Loppio and the Madonna formerly on the high altar of the Cathedral of Como. These figures are linked with the nine statues of the Loggia degli Osii in Milan (1316–30), of which the St. Stephen (PL. 21), St. Dionysius, and one unidentified saint are by the workshop of the master of the Longhi monument. The rest of these figures, by another hand, awkwardly combine trans-Alpine Gothic elements and faint echoes of Giovanni Pisano with an all-pervasive and fundamental Romanesque. To this group should be added the statue on the portal of the Cathedral of Crema. It is by a cruder hand, perhaps the one that carved the relief, *St. George Slaying the Dragon*, in the Church of S. Giorgio in Palazzo, Milan (1308).

The most clearly defined personality active in Bergamo was Giovanni da Campione. In 1340 he signed the Baptistery and in 1351 one of the porches of S. Maria Maggiore, and in 1353 a statue of St. Alexander there. At Bellano he was listed as "magister de muro et de lignamine" ("master builder and wood carver"), and in the register of S. Maria Maggiore (1361–63) as head of the workmen employed in restoring the church. The porch, of which the uppermost loges are by Andreolo de' Bianchi, evinces his fine sensitivity. At times he returns to forms favored by Nicolò (Verona, Ferrara), but the twisted columns, perhaps derived from Giovanni di Balduccio (see below), lend the upper structure an unaccustomed animation. Giovanni da Campione's architectural ability, however, is most manifest in the Baptistery, which was virtually a separate structure within the Church of S. Maria Maggiore and, after various moves, was poorly reconstructed outside the church during the 19th century. A drawing of 1660, reproduced by D. Calvi, shows amid 17th-century ornamental baroque additions what must have been its original form. About halfway up the octagonal building, which is better proportioned in its present state, the blind arcade, so common to Lombard architecture, is repeated. Shallow niches, marking an easy transition at the corners, contain elongated figures (PL. 21) of a type traditionally placed on portals, representing the theological and cardinal virtues, to which the figure of Patience is added. Assistants may have collaborated on these statues, particularly the *Hope* and *Charity*, but there is no question of later recarving (A. Venturi). A fusion of diverse stylistic elements is evident, but the imprint of Giovanni di Balduccio's *Virtues* on the tomb of St. Peter Martyr (Milan, S. Eustorgio) emerges most clearly, while spontaneity and northern harshness are blended with assurance and coherence. The Baptistery's original internal structure is still unknown, but it certainly did not correspond to its present one. The six panels with scenes from the life

of Christ also remain a mystery. They may have been part of a baptismal font or been set into the walls above the cornice between the figures of the Virtues. These figures are by another hand, and though one is a 19th-century copy and the others were rubbed down and polished during the last century so that they have lost much of their original power, they are not made of plaster as has been alleged. The master who carved the reliefs of the life of Christ — and it was not Giovanni da Campione — had a good grasp of Gothic ivories, whose forms, in effect, he here enlarged.

Another signed and dated work by Giovanni da Campione in Bergamo is the monumental statue of St. Alexander (PL. 21) now in S. Maria Maggiore but, according to some critics, from the older church of that name. Quite obviously the equestrian statues of Oldrado da Tresseno in the Palazzo della Ragione, Milan, and of St. Martin with the beggar in the town hall of Treviglio are his antecedents. But the vital and witty statue of the Cangrande in Verona (1330) also impressed the Lombard artist, who, however, did not succeed in reproducing the self-confident smile in his St. Alexander. The latter keeps a rigid seat on a solid and well-nourished horse which has little in common with the nervous, almost prancing, thoroughbred of the Cangrande. Beside the St. Alexander are a statue of S. Proiettizzio, which is closely linked to the tomb of Guglielmo Longhi, and one of St. Barnabas, which, because of its richly Gothic drapery, seems to be not only by a different hand but also from another period.

The activity of this Campione family, who left an indelible mark on the city of Bergamo, came to an end with the death of Nicolino di Giovanni (1364).

TUSCAN INFLUENCES. The tomb of St. Peter Martyr in S. Eustorgio, Milan, carries the signature of Giovanni di Balduccio and the date 1339. When this artist was called to Milan by Azzone Visconti, he brought traditionally Tuscan methods and manners to Lombard sculpture, although local workshops undoubtedly assisted him in his sculptural enterprises as well as in the construction of the Church of S. Maria di Brera. Under his direction indigenous stonecutters strained to free themselves of the rigid and tightly bound forms of the Romanesque but succeeded only in softening their figures by giving them a more worldly and graceful appearance. The deep impression made by his marvelous caryatids and the gentle Madonna seated on the tabernacle above the tomb of St. Peter Martyr made possible sculptures such as those of the master of the Viboldone lunette (1348), while architectural elements such as twisted columns appear in various buildings. But Giovanni di Balduccio's influence is reflected most clearly in the so-called "tomb of St. Augustine" in the Church of S. Pietro in Cielo d'Oro in Pavia (1360), an overloaded structure of which only the individual pieces of sculpture have any true value.

By far the most eminent of the Campionesi of the second half of the 14th century was Bonino da Campione, whose artistic personality can be reconstructed by means of three dated works: the tomb of Folchino degli Schizzi (1357) in the Cathedral of Cremona; the tomb of Bernabò Visconti from S. Giovanni in Conca, now in the Castello Sforzesco, Milan, whose equestrian statue may have been executed in 1363 although the rest of the work was not completed until 1380–85; and the tomb of Cansignorio della Scala in Verona (ca. 1376; PL. 21). His œuvre has been considerably enlarged first by Bellone's studies and later by Baroni's and includes the tomb of Bishop Lambertino Balduino in the old Cathedral of Brescia and, in Milan, the tomb of Stefano and Valentina Visconti in S. Eustorgio (1352, badly reconstructed, see Baroni), that of Protaso Camaini in the same church, and most probably the one of Regina della Scala now in the Castello Sforzesco (1384), as well as the reliefs on the lintel of the portal of S. Marco. Bonino is close to Giovanni di Balduccio in some aspects of his style and is true to Campione traditions in the calm and symmetrical placing of his figures, which are rarely gathered into groups, and in his simple, traditional backgrounds. His masterpiece is the tomb of Bernabò Visconti, in spite of the fact that, for political reasons, it was never completed. The equestrian statue,

on a low plinth above a coffin decorated with reliefs, is a more forceful version of the St. Alexander in Bergamo. Bernabò sits, rigidly encased in his suit of armor decorated with heraldic serpents on the back and chest, the lance upright in his hand; he seems to be cut from the same block as the horse, who arches his neck, champs the bit, and turns his head slightly to the right.

In the tomb of Cansignorio in Verona, Bonino shows once again that adaptability to local forms so typical of the Lombard workshops. In order to conform to the Gothic structure of the other Scaligeri tombs, and particularly to that of Mastino II, which, like that of Cangrande, is the work of a Veronese master, Bonino complicated the tabernacle-like structure and made it heavier through the superabundant use of sculpture. Only the reclining figure of Cansignorio (PL. 21), the angels watching over him, and three reliefs on the side of the sarcophagus facing the church are by Bonino himself. The rest is by Veronese workmen or by his own workshop, as is the equestrian statue, an uninspired repetition of the one of Bernabò in Milan.

The Lombard current of the Campionesi ends with Matteo da Campione, who died in 1396. Like his predecessors he was architect and sculptor of the Cathedral works of Monza and was responsible for the façade of this church, the pulpit now used as choir gallery, and the no longer extant baptistery. Elements derived from Pisa and Orvieto infiltrate the façade and give it a trite decorativeness that dissolves the sculptural quality of traditional Lombard construction. The pulpit has a parapet of conchlike niches housing statues that is similar to the former frieze of the southern portal of S. Maria Maggiore in Bergamo (attributed to Andreolo de' Bianchi by Baroni). This motif had occurred in 1353 in the tomb of St. Agatha in the Cathedral of Verona, which must be attributed to a Campione master. The panel with the coronation of a king that forms the rear of this pulpit is much more interesting, but its greater fineness and singularly schematic linearism, reminiscent of the Master of S. Regolo in Lucca, suggests the presence of another hand (according to Baroni, Cino dei Sinibaldi). However that may be, Matteo was the most outstanding Lombard artist of the period, and in 1390 he was asked to direct the work on the Cathedral of Milan, though it is not known whether he assumed the post.

THE CAMPIONESI AND THE CATHEDRAL OF MILAN. During the years of construction the records of the Cathedral of Milan list a succession of Campionesi as builders and stonecutters, though they were gradually replaced by trans-Alpine masters. Among them was a certain Zeno whom some scholars consider the first architect of the Cathedral. None ever rose above the level of mere artisans, however, and the Giacomo who carved the relief above the north door of the sacristy (1390) is not a strong personality and seems to have absorbed German mannerisms. Thus that unity of taste and style which formed a close bond among Lombard workshops for two centuries was dissolved by the beginning of the 15th century.

CRITICISM. Aside from signed works and documents, the Campionesi are first mentioned in D. Calvi's *Effemeride* (1676–77) in reference to work executed in the city of Bergamo; then in S. Maffei (1732), who notes that he read Bonino da Campione's signature on the tomb of Cansignorio della Scala in Verona. Next follow Tassi (1793), G. L. Calvi (1859), and P. Locatelli (1869). The Campionesi, grouped together as a workshop, are mentioned in *Le glorie dell'arte lombarda* by Malvezzi (1882) and in Merzario (1893), who gives further general, though at times erroneous, information about them. The first scholarly discussion of their works was that of A. G. Meyer (1893), whom later criticism follows on the whole (A. Venturi, E. Bertaux, G. G. Vitzthum, and F. Volbach), although those of the Campionesi who contributed to the construction of the Cathedral of Milan were discussed at length by Boito (1889). More recently thorough studies of the sculptors of this school have been published by Baroni (1944) and Francovich (1952). But a complete or exhaustive discussion of Lombard-Campionesi art, including architecture, is still lacking. One need only consider what Bergamo owes to Giovanni da Campione in this respect, or Matteo's contribution to the Cathedral of Monza. The skill of the Campionesi was not only that of "magistri picantes lapides vivos" ("masters working in living

stone") but also of architects who were worthy successors of the masters of Como.

BIBLIOG. D. Calvi, Effemeride, III, Milan, 1676–77, p. 292; S. Maffei, Verona Illustrata, Verona, 1732, p. 79; F. M. Tassi, Vite dei pittori e architetti bergamaschi, Bergamo, 1793; G. L. Calvi, Notizie dei principali architetti, scultori e pittori che fiorirono a Milano durante il governo dei Visconti e degli Sforza, Milan, 1859; P. Locatelli, Illustri bergamaschi, Bergamo, 1869; L. Malvezzi, Le glorie dell'arte lombarda, Milan, 1882; C. Boito, Il Duomo di Milano, n.p., 1889; G. Merzario, I maestri comacini, I, Milan, 1893, pp. 235–54; A. G. Meyer, Lombardische Denkmäler des XIV. Jahrhunderts, Stuttgart, 1893; W. Vöge, Der provenzalische Einfluss in Italien und das Datum des Arles Porticus, Repfkw, XXV, 1902, pp. 409–29; E. Bertaux, La sculpture en Italie de 1070 à 1260, in Michel, I, 2, pp. 670–708; A. Venturi, Storia dell'arte italiana, IV, Milan, 1901 ff.; E. Gall, Die Apostelreliefs im Mailänder Dom, Ein Beitrag zur Geschichte der oberitalienischen Plastik im XII. Jahrhundert, MnbKw, XIV, 1921, pp. 1–13; G. Vitzthum and F. Volbach, Die Malerei und Plastik des Mittelalters in Italien, Handbuch der Kw., Potsdam, 1924; M. Salmi, Scultura Romanica in Toscana, Florence, 1928, pp. 109–13 (for Guido da Como); S. Vigezzi, La sculptura in Milano, Milan, 1934; G. Sinibaldi, La scultura italiana del trecento, Florence, 1934; G. P. Bognetti, I magistri Antelami e la Valle d'Intelvi, Periodico storico comense, II, 1938, pp. 17–72; L. Bellone, La scultura del '300 a Milano, Giovanni Balduccio da Pisa e Bonino da Campione, Arte, XXII, 1940, pp. 118–201; C. Baroni, Scultura gotica lombarda, Milan, 1944 (with extensive bibliog.); W. Arslan, Recensione a Scultura gotica lombarda di C. Baroni, Archivio storico lombardo, I, 1944, pp. 42–44; E. Jullian, L'éveil de la sculpture italienne, Paris, 1945; M. R. Rogers and O. Goetz, Handbook to the Lucy Maud Buckingham Medieval Collection, Chicago, 1945; M. L. Gengaro, Note a proposito della corrente pisana nella scultura lombarda del Trecento, Belle Arti, 1–2, 1946–48, pp. 49–50; W. R. Valentiner, Notes on G. di Balduccio and Trecento Sculpture in Northern Italy, AQ, X, 1947, pp. 57–60; Toesca, Md; G. de' Francovich, Benedetto Antelami, Florence, 1952, part 2, pp. 45–109 (with extensive bibliog.); F. de' Maffei, Le Arche Scaligere, Verona, 1954; W. Arslan, La scultura romanica milanese, Storia di Milano, III, Milan, 1954; C. Baroni, La scultura gotica, Storia di Milano, V, Milan, 1956; Catalogo della mostra lombarda "Dai Visconti agli Sforza," Milan, 1958.

Fernanda DE' MAFFEI

Illustrations: PLS. 17–21.

**CANADA.** Canada, a member state of the British Commonwealth, occupies a unique place among the nations of the world, being one of the largest in area (about four million square miles), yet one of the least populous (seventeen million). Canada is, nevertheless, one of the most prosperous and influential the "middle powers" today. Little is known of its prehistory, and little archaeological work was done prior to World War II. In the light of available information it is difficult to discuss the art of the native population before the coming of the white man (see AMERICAN CULTURES). Canadian art of the colonial and modern periods is a branch of Western art, but one that derives some distinctive features from its environment and history. It has been open to influences from France, England, and, principally, the United States (see AMERICAS: ART SINCE COLUMBUS); recently, international influences have become more widely felt.

SUMMARY. Primitive and contemporary native art developments (col. 45): *The Northwest Coast Indians; The Cordillera Indians; The Eskimos; The Woodland Hunters; The Woodland Farmers; The Plains Indians.* Colonial and modern periods (col. 50). Principal centers (col. 51).

PRIMITIVE AND CONTEMPORARY NATIVE ART DEVELOPMENTS. The native population may be grouped into six culture areas, which emerged because of diverse climatic and geographic conditions: the Northwest Coast Indians, the Cordillera (Rocky Mountain) Indians, the Eskimo, the Woodland Hunters, the Woodland Farmers, and the Plains Indians. None of these groups, including as they do tribes which are often of different linguistic stocks and which have migrated from different territories, can be called exclusively Canadian, since they were an integral part of the aboriginal life of the whole continent (see AMERICAN CULTURES). Some cultural areas extended southward into the United States, others westward into Alaska or eastward into Greenland. The wellsprings of most Canadian Indian cultures were to be found outside of Canada.

Since most tribes were nomadic, primitive art in Canada was usually small in scale. Only in the Northwest Coast area, where there was a surplus of material goods and the existence of fixed settlements was therefore possible, were monumental works of art produced. Canadian Indians never developed such complicated techniques as metal casting and welding, the true loom and the

weaving of tapestries, or the potter's wheel and the painting of pottery, possibly as a result of their nomadism and uneven cultural development, combined with their isolation from the centers of higher Indian culture to the south.

Only the art of quill embroidery was almost certainly originated and developed by Canadian Indians. In prehistoric times it was practiced in all culture areas of Canada, even though some tribes had to obtain the materials by trade. Designs consisting of geometric patterns in solid rather than outline form were made by wrapping, weaving, plaiting, or sewing colored bird and porcupine quills onto leather garments or small objects. Quillwork was largely abandoned in favor of beadwork when European trade beads became plentiful in the early 19th century.

Before their contact with Europeans, the men and women within the tribal or regional area had distinctively different art styles, according to their sex. Women were usually forbidden to create designs involving life forms. Ancient pottery, basketry, and embroidery designs were traditionally geometric and abstract, and it was not until after European contact that realistic flower and leaf motifs were adopted.

*The Northwest Coast Indians.* The Indians of the Northwest Coast (Tlingit, Haida, Tsimshian, Bellacoola, Kwakiutl, Coast Salish, Nootka) lived by the sea in the coniferous forests of British Columbia. Their economy, based on salmon fishing, provided an inexhaustible food supply, economic stability, and leisure time. The acquisition of wealth by the aristocracy was important, and clan or personal status could be enhanced by gift-giving feasts or potlatches. The Northwest Coast style of animal art is understandable only in terms of a life based on this prestige system, since the conventionalized animal symbols served as tribal, clan, or personal heraldic devices.

Exploration of this culture area was not completed until the mid-19th century, and its prehistory is still poorly known. Although most articles in early times were presumably made of wood — as they were in post-contact times — the only objects to survive are made of shell, bone, or stone: utilitarian or ceremonial mortars and pestles, charms and amulets, figures and heads, some of which were seemingly carved for esthetic reasons. The dates and makers of this stone sculpture are unknown, but all pieces were made in conformity with an art tradition which probably flourished between the 9th and 12th centuries. This ancient art was dramatic and descriptive, strong in expression, and large in scale, and with its vertically oriented or superposed figures, use of life forms, the eccentric curve, and black, red, or white pigment, foreshadowed modern totemic art in the Northwest Coast area.

There was little realistic art prior to contact with Europeans. Tlingit men did make a protective helmet-mask of wood to be worn with slat armor, which was a realistic portrait of a man afflicted with unilateral facial paralysis. The various heraldic and mythological animals, however, were usually portrayed symbolically. In the round they were portrayed by means of identifying "signatures" made by selecting some outstanding characteristic of the animal to represent the whole. In the two-dimensional arts, such as carving in low relief or painting, they were depicted by a method of dissection in which the animal was split up the front and laid flat, the various parts of the body were abstracted, symbolized, rearranged to form a pleasing design, and adapted to the surface to be decorated.

Found in this coastal area are pieces carved in bone, horn, antler, shell, wood, stone, and, after the introduction of European tools two hundred years ago, in native copper, black slate, and silver. They include spoons, ladles, bowls, boxes, and other household articles, as well as helmets, staffs, rattles, headdresses, masks, and other ceremonial and ornamental objects. Many wooden pieces were enhanced by abalone-shell inlays and other trimmings. The dimensions of these objects varied from miniature carvings 1 to 2 in. high up to mammoth totem poles 80 to 100 ft. high (see TOTEMISM), which illustrated the mythology of each clan and served as evidence of family wealth and pride. The significance, the order, and the color of the figures on the poles varied with each owner. Other large-scale objects, such as memorial poles, potlatch welcome figures, grave markers, canoes, clan houses, and interior and exterior house posts, also bore carved and painted heraldic and mythological figures. Painting was apparently the older art: in the precontact period, murals depicting clan myths were painted both inside and outside the large wooden houses, and clothing often bore painted clan crests. When carving became an important art, painting was combined with it to form a new art genre.

During the winter ceremonial season, religious and mythological ceremonies were dramatized by plays and dances held under clan or secret-society auspices which featured masked participants. Masks were worn to create startling and dramatic effects. Such materials as sea-lion bristles, otter fur, feathers, and human hair were added to the masks, and many of them had movable eyes and mouths which

could be manipulated by the wearer. Ingenious double or triple masks were made so that sections of the outer masks swung out to reveal a second or even a third face beneath. Northwest Coast masks were among the finest produced anywhere in the world.

Since women were forbidden to create designs involving life forms, they made use of geometric patterns. They produced excellent basketry, conical spruce-root hats, mats, cloaks and blankets from mountain-goat wool and shredded cedar bark. Only the Chilkat blanket, actually a fringed, oblong ceremonial dance cape of twine-woven wool-and-bark tapestry, bore patterns employing life forms, which the women copied from a pattern board created by the men and returned to them upon completion of the task.

severely limited in material resources, were skillful craftsmen who fashioned a tremendous variety of excellent tools by chipping flint and quartz, carving driftwood, reindeer antlers, bone, horn, ivory, and stone, and by pounding out nuggets of native iron and copper (see ESKIMO CULTURES). Their traditional art consists chiefly of objects for everyday use made by the men and artistically decorated with engraved or incised geometric designs, and in the postcontact period with naturalistic hunting scenes. In this primitive period, the men also carved ivory dolls and toys in the round for the children. In recent times the Eskimos have begun decorating objects with realistic forms in high relief as well as with the ancient engraving and incising. Since the climate has not changed perceptibly in the five

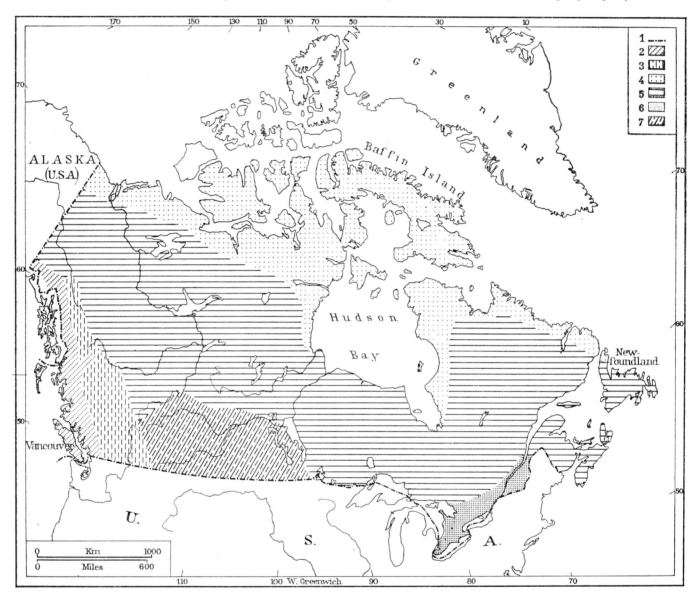

Canada: distribution of native cultures. *Key:* (1) Political boundaries. (2) Culture of the Northwest Coast Indians. (3) Culture of the Cordiller Indians. (4) Culture of the Eskimos. (5) Culture of the Woodland Hunters. (6) Culture of the Woodland Farmers. (7) Culture of the Plains Indians.

*The Cordillera Indians.* The Cordillera Indians (Tagish, Tahltan, Tsetsaut, Carrier, Chilkotin, Shushwap, Lillooet, Thompson, Okinagan, Lake Salish, Nicola, Kootenay) lived by hunting and gathering in the river valleys of the Rocky Mountains. They adopted many ideas from tribes in surrounding culture areas — the Plains Indians, the Woodland Hunters, and the Northwest Coast Indians — and, as a result, much of the art produced in this area was not distinctively different from that of surrounding tribes. Their finest development was a type of coiled basketry, produced by the women, which was round or rectangular and decorated by imbrication with traditional geometric or zoomorphic designs in black, pale yellow, or red, without symbolic or ceremonial significance.

*The Eskimos.* The Eskimo (Mackenzie, Caribou, Copper, Central, Labrador) hunters and fishers of the Arctic Coast, living in areas

thousand or so years the Eskimos have inhabited the Arctic Coast, there is no recognizable break between archaeology and ethnology. The ancient and modern cultures have blended imperceptibly.

*The Woodland Hunters.* The Woodland Hunters occupied the vast forest area stretching from Alaska to Newfoundland. Athapaskan-speaking tribes (Chippewayan, Beaver, Slave, Dogrib, Yellowknife, Hare, Kutchin, Sekani, Goat, Kaska) roamed the Yukon–Mackenzie basin where game was abundant, while the Algonquian-speaking tribes (Beothuk, Nascapee, Micmac, Malecite, Montagnais, Eastern Cree, Algonkin, Cree, Ojibwa) occupied the Hudson Bay–Atlantic basin, where game was scarce. In general, woodland hunting tribes had a simple culture, and their arts and crafts were rudimentary. The men used wood and bark for such objects as canoes, snowshoes, drums, lovers' flutes, dolls, grave markers, bows and arrows, tools

and household utensils, and, in precontact times, they also made mide rolls of birchbark which were used as mnemonic devices, containing charts and pictures utilizing over two hundred symbols in what was almost a true hieroglyphic system. The earlier tobacco pipes for ceremonial and everyday use were of wood and stone, the later ones are of brass, iron, pewter, copper, and metal-inlaid stone. The women made wicker, splint, and spruce-root baskets, which they often enhanced by weaving aromatic sweet grasses into the designs. Bags, sashes, straps, and mats were woven by basketry techniques, or by braiding, netting, looping, twining, or finger weaving and were decorated with geometric or conventionalized motifs. Birchbark utensils were decorated by engraving, scraping, painting, and the appliquéing of birchbark cutouts or by quill embroidery. Early designs were usually geometric hourglass, zigzag, or diagonal motifs, conventionalized floral forms or supernatural figures such as the thunderbird, the underground panther, butterfly, deer, and the like. Semirealistic and floral design units appeared soon after the arrival of the Europeans, and an elaborate scroll and double-curve motif appeared about 1860.

Tailored skin clothing was decorated with quill and moosehair embroidery until about 1800, when ribbon appliqué appeared; by 1860, beadwork was introduced and trade cloth such as velvet and broadcloth supplemented skins for clothing. Decoration of clothing in precontact times was limited mostly to continuous borders of geometric conventionalized flower and leaf patterns in varied colors; bead weaving, on the other hand, used isolated design units, usually adaptations of natural objects (the rose, leaf, claw, or feather) embroidered in up to three shades of the same color.

*The Woodland Farmers.* The Woodland Farmers were mainly Iroquoian-speaking peoples (Huron, Erie, Tobacco, Neutral, Seneca, Cayuga, Onondaga, Oneida, Mohawk) who lived by agriculture supplemented by hunting and fishing, following the pattern of life set by the higher centers in the southeastern United States and adapting it to life in the lowlands surrounding Lake Erie, Lake Ontario, and the upper St. Lawrence River.

Iroquoian men worked in antler, bone, stone, shell, clay, bark, wood, maize husks, maize cobs, and native copper and silver. Their antler and bone implements and jewelry were of fine quality, and their ancient use of stone for projectile points and pipes was excellent. Shell was made into gorgets and beads; the purple and white wampum strings and belts were of great ceremonial and political significance. Bark, wood, and maize products were made into all types of containers and implements, while native metals, handled by hammering and repoussé work, were made into ornaments, brooches, gorgets, etc. Copper was used until the 17th century, when, with the introduction of European tools, it was superseded by silver, which in turn was little used after 1865. The finest products of the Iroquois men were their zoomorphic or anthropomorphic clay pipes and their wooden masks. The masks, for symbolic reasons, were roughed out on the living tree, cut off, finished, painted red or black, and decorated with strands of basswood or elm as hair. These masks were intended to create fear and were used in the curing of disease by the Falseface Secret Society.

The Woodland Farmers were the only Canadian Indians who manufactured pottery. It appeared about the 14th century, reached its peak in the early 18th century, and gave way to European metal kettles late in that same century. The pottery, coil-made by the women, was varied in form and decoration, unglazed and unpainted. The women also did fine embroidery on skin clothing and ceremonial equipment, as well as making splint baskets, mats, dolls, and masks of maize-husk fibers, the latter being reserved for the Huskface Secret Society.

*The Plains Indians.* The Plains Indians (Assiniboin, Gros Ventre, Blackfoot, Plains Cree, Sarsi) acquired the horse in the late 17th century, abandoned agriculture and hunting on the edge of the plains, and became completely dependent on the wandering bison herds. This was the last cultural area to come into being in Canada; its people, nomadic, warlike, and individualistic, practiced four major crafts: skin preparation and sewing, quill embroidery, bead embroidery — all done by women — and skin painting, done by both sexes. Quillwork was the oldest decorative craft, and its designs were purely abstract and ornamental. The women also painted geometric designs on clothing and such rawhide articles as the parfleche.

Most skin painting was done by men. The motifs consisted of life forms and served as a pictorial record of history, biography, bison hunts, wars, as well as religious and winter counts of animals, and warlike decorations on clothing. The skin was identified by the pictographic signature of the owner. The men also decorated the skin tepee or lodge covers with religious symbols. These designs were oriented to the cardinal points and usually pictured constellations, the earth, and larger-than-life-size animals, all of which had

been disclosed to the owner in a vision. The lodge cover thus formed part of a complex of religious objects owned by an individual, and its decoration was considered the highest form of pictorial art of the Plains Indians. The men engaged in the minor crafts of pipe making in clay, gray slate, or stone, and the manufacture of fine feather bonnets.

Native Canadian arts, fallen in modern times to the level of production of curios for the souvenir trade, have nevertheless begun in recent years to enjoy a degree of revival, thanks to renewed interest on the part of the government and the public.

BIBLIOG. *a. General:* W. H. Holmes, Art in Shell of Ancient America, ARSI, II, 1880–81; G. Mallery, Picture Writing of the American Indian, ARSI, X, 1893; O. T. Mason, Aboriginal American Basketry, 1902, Ann. Rep. U. S. Nat. Mus., Washington, D.C., 1902; W. C. Orchard, Beads and Beadwork of the American Indians, Contributions, II, Mus. of the Am. Indian, Heye Foundation, New York, 1916; W. C. Orchard, The Technique of Porcupine Quill Decoration among the North American Indians, Contributions, IV, 1, Mus. of the Am. Indian, Heye Foundation, New York, 1916; H. I. Smith, An Album of Prehistoric Canadian Art, Ottawa, 1923; G. Weltfish, Prehistoric North American Basketry, Its Techniques and Modern Distributions, AmA, XXXII, 1930; The Denver Art Museum, Indian Leaflet Series, Denver, 1934; D. Jenness, The Indians of Canada, B. of the Nat. Mus. of Can., LXV, Ottawa, 1934; A. D. Harding and P. Bolling, Bibliography on North American Indian Art, Washington, D.C., 1938; G. C. Vaillant, Indian Arts in North America, New York, 1939. *b. The Northwest Coast Indians:* Publication of the Jesup North Pacific Expedition, Leiden, 1898–1930; G. T. Emmons, The Basketry of the Tlinkit, Mem. Am. Mus. of Nat. H., III, New York, 1903; G. T. Emmons, The Chilkat Blanket, Mem. Am. Mus. of Nat. H., III, 4, New York, 1907; L. Adam, Nordwest-Amerikanische Indianerkunst, Berlin, 1923; F. Boas, Primitive Art, Cambridge, Mass., 1927, New York, 1955; R. B. Inverarity, Movable Masks and Figures of the North Pacific Coast Indians, Bloomfield, Mich., 1941; A. Ravenhill, A Cornerstone of Canadian Culture, Occasional Papers, V, B. C. Provincial Mus., Victoria, B.C., 1944; R. T. Davis, Native Arts of the Pacific Northwest, Stanford, 1949; M. C. Barbeau, Totem Poles, Ottawa, 1950; R. B. Inverarity, Art of the Northwest Coast Indians, Berkeley, 1950; V. E. Garfield, The Tsimshian: Their Arts and Music, New York, 1951; P. S. Wingert, Prehistoric Stone Sculptures of the Pacific North West, Portland Art Mus., Portland, Oreg., 1952; People of the Potlatch, Vancouver Art Gall., Vancouver, 1956. *c. The Eskimos:* Reports of the Canadian Arctic Expedition, 1913–1918, Ottawa, 1918–28; D. A. Cadzow, Native Copper Objects of the Copper Eskimo, Heye Foundation, New York, 1920; Reports of the Fifth Thule Expedition under the Direction of Knud Rasmussen, 1921–24, 10 vols., Copenhagen, 1927. *d. The Woodland Hunters:* F. G. Speck, The Double-Curve Motif in Northeastern Algonkian Art, Mem. Nat. Mus. of Can., 42, 1914; Reports of the Canadian Arctic Expedition, 1913–1918, Ottawa, 1918–28; D. S. Davidson, Decorative Art of the Têtes de Boule of Quebec, Mus. of the Am. Indian, Heye Foundation, New York, 1928; F. G. Speck, Montagnais Art in Birchbark, A Circumpolar Trait, Indian Notes and Monographs, VII, 2, Mus. of the Am. Indian, Heye Foundation, New York, 1937; C. A. Lyford, The Crafts of the Ojibwa, Indian Handicrafts, 5, Ed. Div. ,U. S. Office of Indian Affairs, Phoenix, 1943. *e. The Woodland Farmers:* L. H. Morgan, The League of the Iroquois, New York, 1901–02; M. R. Harrington, Iroquois Silverwork, Am. Mus. of Nat. H., New York, 1908; "Wampum" Handbook of the American Indian, ARSI, XXX, 1912; W. N. Fenton, Masked Medicine Societies of the Iroquois, ARSI, 1940; M. Lismer, Seneca Splint Basketry, U. S. Office of Indian Affairs, Chilocco, Okla., 1941; C. A. Lyford, Iroquois Crafts, Ed. Div., U. S. Indian Service, Washington, D. C., 1945; R. S. MacNeish, Iroquois Pottery Types, B. Nat. Mus. of Can., 124, Ottawa, 1952. *f. The Plains Indians:* A. L. Kroeber, Ethnology of the Gros Ventre, Am. Mus. of Nat. H., New York, 1908; C. Wissler, Costumes of the Plains Indians, APAmM, XVII, 2, 1915; L. Spier, An Analysis of Plains Indian Parfleche Decoration, Univ. of Wash. Pub. in Anthr., I, 3, Seattle, Wash., 1925; L. Spier, Plains Indian Parfleche Designs, Univ. of Wash. Pub. in Anthr., IV, 3, Seattle, 1931; Denver Art Museum, Plains Beads and Beadwork Designs, Leaflet 73–74, Dept. of Indian Art, Denver, 1934; J. C. Ewers, Plains Indian Painting, London, 1939.

Margaret C. PIRIE

COLONIAL AND MODERN PERIODS. Canadian art (see I, cols. 331–34), which has been influenced mainly by England, France, and the United States, and in modern trends by the school of Paris, can be divided into five periods: (1) The French colonial period (1608–1760), during which the Church fostered a thriving activity among carvers of sacred images (among whom the Levasseur, Baillairgé, and Labrosse families are outstanding), silversmiths, and a few painters, as well as in other handicrafts, especially embroidery. In architecture, the most interesting developments were the rural cottages and churches, with steep roofs and uptilted eaves. (2) The English colonial period 1749–1867), during which the English Georgian and Regency styles were introduced into Canada in simple and charming forms. Landscape painting was introduced by English topographical artists, followed by such resident painters as Paul Kane and Cornelius Krieghoff. Portrait painting in Quebec was influenced by French classicism (Antoine-Sébastien Plamondon et al.). By 1850, there was a significant development of Gothic-revival architecture, already felt to a limited degree earlier in that century (Parliament House, Ottawa begun in 1859 by Thomas Fuller, and University College of Toronto,

begun in 1856 by Frederick W. Cumberland). (3) The Confederation period (1867–1900) saw the formation of national art organizations (Royal Canadian Academy, 1880) and the adoption of European academic standards in painting (Robert Harris et al.). (4) The early 20th century (1900–13), when the influence of the United States predominated, with pretentious styles in architecture (the Beaux-Arts and "château" styles) and sculpture of some elegance by Philippe Hébert. In painting, impressionism was introduced by Maurice Cullen, and postimpressionism by James Wilson Morrice. (5) The recent period (1913—), characterized by evolution toward contemporary taste, inaugurated by the Group of Seven (the landscapists Alexander Young Jackson, Lawren S. Harris, James E. H. MacDonald and others), to whom Emily Carr, who often used West Coast Indian motifs, is related in style. Unlike them was David Milne, an independent painter with a quiet, sensitive style. The Montreal school (Goodridge Roberts, Alfred Pellan, Stanley Cosgrove, Paul-Emile Borduas, et al.) used contemporary international modes. Younger painters in various regions show considerable variety of style: Jean-Paul Riopelle, Harold Town, William Ronald (nonfigurative); Bertram Charles Binning (decorative abstraction); Jack L. Shadbolt and Gordon Smith (nature-expressionism); Alexander

Quebec. Walled capital of Quebec, it is the only town of substantially European character in the French tradition. – Hôpital Général (1671). – Ursuline Convent (1686, with chapel wood carvings by Levasseur, 1732–34). – Seminary (1694). – Church of Notre-Dame (1744). – Hôtel-Dieu (chapel carvings by Baillairgé, ca. 1828). – Citadel (ca. 1830). – Parliament Building (1878). – Château Frontenac hotel ("château" style, 1889). In the region there are old churches, houses, especially on Ile d'Orléans. – Shipshaw, large dam (1941). – Palace called the Ecole des Beaux-Arts. *Museums*: Musée de la Province de Québec. – Musée de l'Université Laval (European painting).

Toronto. Metropolis rich in modern buildings. – Osgoode Hall (Palladian, 1829). – University College (Victorian Romanesque, 1856). – City Hall. – Parliament (Richardsonian Romanesque, 1888–91). *Museums*: Royal Ontario Museum (decorative arts; Chinese art; Canadiana). – Art Gallery of Toronto (European and Canadian painting, sculpture, graphic arts). The University has a Department of Art and Archaeology; Ontario College of Art has an art school.

Vancouver. Principal city of the West Coast, with many modern houses and buildings, including the Electrical Building of British

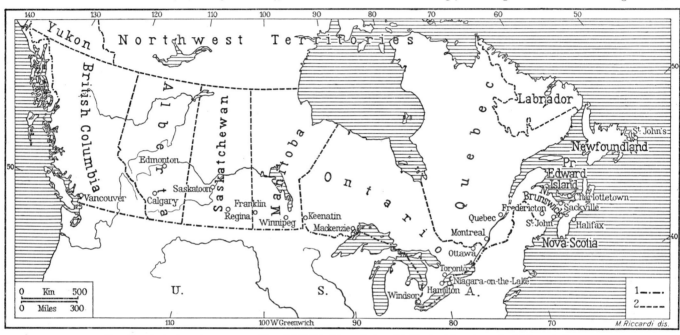

Canada: principal modern centers. *Key*: (1) Political boundaries. (2) Territorial and provincial boundaries.

Colville (magic realism); Jean Dallaire, Jean-Paul Lemieux (surrealism); and others. Significant sculptors (Louis Archambault, Anne Kahane) are emerging. In architecture, up to 1930 the chaos of styles inherited from the Victorian era persisted, but since then a great wave of building has caused the exploitation of Canadian materials and forms, especially in Vancouver.

PRINCIPAL CENTERS. Ottawa. Capital of Canada, it is the seat of the federal government and of official organizations encouraging the arts such as the National Gallery of Canada (1880) and the Canada Council (1957). – Parliament (three buildings, originally Gothic revival, from ca. 1859 and partly from 1916). – Modern buildings by the architects J. B. Page and Steele. *Museums*: National Gallery of Canada (collection of European painting, sculpture, graphic arts and large collection of Canadian art), which organizes programs of traveling exhibitions; its new building is under construction. – National Museum of Canada (Indian, Eskimo art). – Public Archives (early topographic painting, portraits).

Montreal. Largest Canadian city, bilingual and bicultural, is Montreal, metropolis of eastern Canada. *Art monuments*: Séminaire de St. Sulpice (begun 1680). – Church of Notre-Dame (early Gothic revival, begun 1824). – Christ Church Cathedral (Gothic revival, 1857). – Old houses, groups of modern buildings, with skyscrapers. *Museums*: Montreal Museum of Fine Arts (European and Canadian painting, sculpture, graphic arts). – McGill University museums. – Château de Ramezay (Canadian folk arts). *Art schools*: Montreal Museum school. – Ecole des Beaux-Arts. – Ecole des Arts Graphiques. In the region there are old houses and forts, especially in the Eastern Township and Carillon districts.

Columbia by the architects Sharp and Thompson, and the Civic Auditorium (1957; first prize to the architects Affleck, Michaud Desbarats, Sise, and Lebensold of Montreal). *Museums*: Vancouver Art Gallery (European and Canadian painting). – Vancouver City Museum and Art Gallery. – University of British Columbia Art Gallery. – Remarkable totem poles in Stanley Park and at the University of British Columbia's School of Art.

Victoria. Parliament (Victorian baroque, 1889). – Provincial Museum (Indian art objects). – Indian villages of Vancouver Island; totem poles and decorated houses.

Winnipeg. Capital of Manitoba, most important prairie city. – Parliament (Beaux-Arts style, ca. 1910). – Modern buildings, such as St. Paul College (University of Manitoba). *Museums*: Winnipeg Art Gallery (European and Canadian painting). – Gallery of the University of Manitoba, which has an art school. In the region: at Regina, capital of Saskatchewan: the Parliament (Beaux-Arts style, 1910); art school and Gallery of Regina College (decorative arts, European and Canadian painting). – Saskatoon, Saskatchewan: Arts Centre; University of Saskatchewan Department of Art. – Calgary, Alberta: Arts Centre. – Banff, Alberta: Summer School of Fine Arts. – Edmonton, capital of Alberta: Edmonton Art Gallery (Canadian art); University of Alberta Department of Art and Art Gallery.

Other centers. Halifax, Nova Scotia: St. Paul's Church (colonial Georgian, 1750); Government House (Regency, 1801); Province House (Palladian, 1811); and Nova Scotia Museum of Fine Arts. – St. John's, Newfoundland: Cathedral (by George Gilbert Scott, 1846). – St. John, New Brunswick: New Brunswick Museum (decor-

ative arts, Canadian painting). – Port Royal, Nova Scotia: Champlain's "habitation" (1606, reconstruction). – Annapolis Royal, Nova Scotia: Fort Anne (1797). – Fredericton, New Brunswick: Cathedral (Gothic revival, by F. Wills, 1845); Lord Beaverbrook Art Gallery. – Sackville, New Brunswick: Mount Allison University art school – Hamilton, Ontario: Dundurn Castle Museum (building of historic interest, 1826); Art Gallery of Hamilton (European, Canadian painting). – Niagara-on-the-Lake, Ontario: neoclassic houses, church, and fine modern hospital. – Kingston, Ontario: Fort and early 19th-century houses. – London, Ontario: McIntosh Memorial Art Gallery (Canadian painting). – Windsor, Ontario: Willistead Art Gallery (Canadian painting). – Stratford, Ontario: Shakespeare Memorial Theatre. – Kitimat, British Columbia: Industrial city (1950, city plan by C. S. Stein) and impressive dam.

BIBLIOG. G. Morisset, Coup d'oeil sur les arts en Nouvelle-France, Quebec, 1941; D. W. Buchanan, Canadian Painters, Oxford, London, 1945; H. Carver, Architecture in Canada, Studio, 129, 1945; W. Abell, The Arts of French Canada, Mag. of Art, 40, 1947; D. W. Buchanan, The Growth of Canadian Painting, London, 1950; J. Gréber, Le plan d'aménagement de la Capitale (Québec), Vie urbaine, 1950, p. 23; G. C. McInnes, Short History of Canadian Art, Toronto, 1950; P. Duval, Canadian Drawings and Prints, Toronto, 1952; P. Duval, Canadian Water Colour Painting, Toronto, New York, 1954; R. H. Hubbard, Canadian Gothic, Arch. Rev., 1956; R. H. Hubbard, Growth in Canadian Art, The Culture of Contemporary Canada, Ithaca, Toronto, 1957; The Arts in Canada (Canadian Citizenship Ser., Pamphlet No. 6), Dept. of Citizenship and Immigration, 1957. See also Canadian Art, 1924 ff.

Robert H. HUBBARD

Illustrations: 2 figs. in text.

**CANALETTO** (GIOVANNI ANTONIO CANAL, called CANALETTO). Italian painter (b. Venice, Oct. 18, 1697), son of a theatrical scene painter, Bernardo Canal, in whose studio he received his first training. In 1716 and the two years following, he is recorded as working with his father and brother at the Teatro S. Angelo and the Teatro S. Cassiano in Venice. During the carnival of 1719–20 all three were in Rome, where they painted the scenery for Scarlatti's operas *Tito Sempronio Gracco* and *Turno Aricino*. It must have been at this time that he renounced the theatre, as he himself told Antonio Mario Zanetti. Doubtless he found the rigid perspective system of contemporary stage scenery too restrictive of his natural bent for landscape painting, which had probably been stimulated by contact with the many Flemish landscape painters then working in Rome. Mariette's comment (possibly based on information from the artist himself) that Canaletto worked "dans la manière de Van Vytel" suggests that he may actually have studied under the Dutch painter of *vedute* ("views"), Gaspar van Wittel (Gaspare Vanvitelli). He probably returned to Venice in 1720, when his name first appears in the roster of Venetian painters; it was to continue to appear there until 1767. His early development was undoubtedly influenced by Luca Carlevaris, the leading view painter of Venice, although he does not seem to have been his pupil or his collaborator.

By March, 1722, Canaletto was already in contact with English patrons, who were to remain his chief support. He had recently completed his part in two curious allegorical paintings (belonging to the Earl of Plymouth and an English private collection), which commemorated Lord Somers and Archbishop Tillotson. Commissioned by the English operatic impresario, Owen McSwiney, the pictures were sold to the Duke of Richmond. Canaletto's contribution to these earliest documented works consisted only of the architecture, while the figures were painted by his collaborators G. B. Piazzetta, G. B. Pittoni, and G. B. Cimaroli.

He seems shortly thereafter to have begun painting those views of Venice which were to form almost his entire production. The earliest documented examples are a group of four (Montreal, Pillow Coll.), painted in 1725–26 for Stefano Conti of Lucca, for which the contracts survive. On the basis of topography, however, the four large Venetian views formerly in the Liechtenstein Collection would seem to date from about 1723. Of Canaletto's early works, the most important group is in the English Royal Collections at Windsor Castle. These are painted in an extremely broad, free style, with remarkable sensitivity for sunlight and shadow, cloud effects, and the texture of wall surfaces. Usually large in size, they are warm but somber in tone, and often dramatic in lighting. They have an almost preimpressionist character, and there is some evidence that Canaletto at this period actually practiced plein-air painting, a most unusual procedure. He seems to have continued to use this broad, early manner, with some modifications, until about 1730 or a little later.

Letters from Conti's agent at Venice confirm that by 1725 Canaletto's success already overshadowed that of Carlevaris; in 1727, McSwiney describes the artist as having "more work than he can do," and speaks of his whimsical temperament and unreasonable charges. This characterization is confirmed by that of the Swedish Count Tessin, in 1736, and by the Frenchman, Des Brosses, in 1739, who added, "the English have completely spoiled him by offering three times as much as he asks for his paintings."

The increasing pressure of commissions from his principal clients, the wealthy English visiting Venice on the grand tour, largely accounts for the development of Canaletto's style of rapid execution which could be readily taught to studio assistants. From about 1730 his broad, impressionist manner changed to a simpler, clearer, more linear style making use of semimechanical devices. In this his early training in perspective served him well, and his skillful use of the camera obscura for preliminary drawings (a common practice at the time) is well documented. There is a perceptible change between the two celebrated views now in the National Gallery, London: *The Stonemason's Yard* and the *Scuola di S. Rocco*, the former probably painted shortly before and the latter shortly after 1730. Marked signs of a change toward his later style with its cooler tones, lighter and brighter colors, lessening of atmospheric effect, and more precise drawing are to be found in a series of 12 small views of Venice (Windsor Castle), of which Antonio Visentini's engravings were completed by July, 1730, and issued by Joseph Smith in 1735. A letter from Zanetti to Gaburri dated July 24, 1728, and two paintings on copper of this date (London, Richmond Coll.), suggest that the change was already becoming noticeable. Possibly both styles were used concurrently at first.

Joseph Smith, an English merchant, publisher, art collector, and later British Consul at Venice, seems to have acted in some degree as Canaletto's agent, possibly under a contractual arrangement. To the 12 Visentini engravings issued in 1735, Smith added 26 plates in 1742. These 38 engraved views almost certainly provided a catalogue of subjects for Canaletto's clients; they were frequently repeated as paintings and also much used by imitators. Rich English clients often purchased Canaletto's Venetian views in large quantities: the fourth Earl of Carlisle bought some 15 about 1737–38, and the Duke of Bedford, 24, a little later. The Canalettos in Smith's own collection, when sold to King George III in 1763, were magnificent, numbering 54 paintings and 143 drawings. Among them was a series of large Roman views, several dated 1742 to 1743; 13 overdoors of fantastic architecture in the Palladian style, dated 1744; and other Venetian views, dated either 1743 or 1744 (PLS. 22, 23). The group of Roman subjects has led to a hypothesis that Canaletto may have returned to Rome about 1740–41, but no documentation has been found, and the views might equally well be based on drawings made during his early visit to Rome, or on engravings. In the paintings from 1740 to 1744, a new, darker tonality with heavy shadows and somewhat mannered drawing is apparent. By contrast, the group of etchings of the same period, many of a capricious landscape character and apparently executed for his own pleasure, are among the artist's most luminous creations.

The outbreak of the War of the Austrian Succession seriously interrupted Continental travel. In order to maintain contact with his English clientele, Canaletto went to England in May, 1745. He arrived in London with an introductory letter from McSwiney to the Duke of Richmond — both former patrons; his first commissions were for two views of London from Richmond House (London, Richmond Coll.).

Except for two short visits to Venice, Canaletto remained in England continuously until 1755. He seems to have en-

joyed considerable success both with his London views, especially those of the Thames, and with views of the town and country houses of the nobility, notably those of the Dukes of Northumberland and Beaufort. To combat some organized opposition from dealers in forged views of Venice, he publicly exhibited exceptionally large examples of his work in London in 1749 and 1751.

The majority of critics consider that Canaletto's sojourn in England had an adverse effect on his style. They ascribe its colder color and more mannered drawing in part to the northern atmosphere and in part to the influence of Dutch landscape painters working in England at the time. On the other hand, the characteristics of this period, observable even before his visit, may be attributed not only to excessive production but, to a certain degree, to a deliberate setting aside of the imagination. If at times this desire for objectivity seems merely prosaic, it nevertheless suggests a closer connection between the artist and nature.

After his return to Venice in 1755, Canaletto seems to have painted comparatively little, perhaps on account of increasing age and illness. His style became still harder and more mechanical, the figures especially being indicated by purely conventionalized blobs and twirled brush strokes. Much of his output at this period seems to have consisted of fanciful views (*vedute ideate*) and of *capricci* (PL. 25), such as the two executed in 1755 for Algarotti and based on Palladio's designs for a reconstructed Rialto Bridge (there are similar compositions in Parma, Pin.). He also composed many *capricci* for the engraver Giuseppe Wagner, for whom he had also worked just before his journey to England. His last important commission, undertaken for the publisher Furlanetto, was a series of drawings of the *Feste Dogali*, engraved by Giambattista Brustolon.

The fact that Canaletto, having twice failed to secure sufficient votes, was not elected to the Venetian Academy (founded 1755) until 1763 was probably due merely to the low esteem in which landscape painting was held, at this period, in the official hierarchy of the arts. His reception piece was a highly mannered scene of a palace courtyard, dated 1765 (Venice, Acc.; PL. 24). In this painting, as in all the others of these late years, such as the interior view of St. Mark's (Windsor, England, Royal Colls.) and the view of the Procuratie (London, Nat. Gall.), the quick spot method of painting suggests Francesco Guardi (q.v.), who may have been Canaletto's pupil.

Canaletto died in Venice on Apr. 20, 1768. The works he had executed in genres other than landscape are rare. There are records of a *Holy Family* at Mestre and a still life in an English private collection, both of which have disappeared. A self-portrait survives, however, apparently painted in London and perhaps intended for engraving.

He was a prolific draftsman, his drawings ranging from hasty preliminary notations made on the spot to highly finished views rich in detail, intended for sale or possibly for engraving. The principal assemblages of his drawing are at Windsor Castle and the Accademia in Venice.

Canaletto had a large number of assistants throughout his career. They certainly included his nephew, Bernardo Bellotto. Besides collaborating with Canaletto on at least two occasions, Cimaroli produced many pastiches of his views, as did also Visentini, Antonio Joli, and, to a lesser extent, Michele Marieschi. Documents suggest that Guardi may have worked in the studio for a short while about 1760; this has been disputed, but on insufficient grounds. Pastiches, copies, and forgeries of Canaletto's views, mostly anonymous, were made in great numbers in Italy and elsewhere in Europe, not only during his lifetime but throughout the 19th century.

Francis J. B. WATSON

The development of *veduta* painting is an aspect of the taste of English and German collectors in the 18th century. These "views," mostly of specific places, were wanted either by travelers as souvenirs or by landowners proud of the houses and estates they possessed. *Vedute* were considered a minor genre in the 18th century, particularly in Italy, and were valued mostly for their fidelity to the subject. Thus Canaletto's con-

temporary, Vertue, remarked of him that "his Excellence lyes in painting things which fall immediately under his eye." The judgment of Zanetti (1771) provides an exception. He discovers in Canaletto instances of "picturesque license," a wonderful clarity, and a tasteful facility in color and drawing, the effects of a serene mind and a happy temperament; he recalls the painter's use of the camera obscura, at the same time stating that the artist's talent transcended a reliance on purely mechanical aids.

The influence of Canaletto was widespread. In Italy, his nephew Bellotto continued his manner in a general way, and Guardi diverged to develop a kind of impressionism, while Marieschi transformed the master's "views" into the realm of fantasy. In England, particularly, Canaletto was a determining factor in the work of Samuel Scott, William Marlow, Thomas Girtin (q.v.), and, less directly, in that of the great landscapists of the turn of the century, Constable, Turner, and Bonington (qq.v.). He also exercised a clearly discernible influence on the general development of the picturesque (q.v.), and the closely allied system of "blot" painting — a technique he himself employed in typically "picturesque" paintings such as that of Alnwick Castle (London, Duke of Northumberland Coll.).

During the neoclassic period, Canaletto was decidedly preferred to Guardi; thus Lanzi (1789), while recognizing the *brio*, taste, and "fine effect" of the latter, ranked him after Canaletto with respect to "exactness of the proportions and the rational quality of his art."

Correspondingly, Canaletto was less esteemed during the esthetic reaction of the romantic period. Ruskin deplored in him "a miserable, heartless, virtueless mechanism" and granted him only "a dexterous imitation of commonplace light and shade" (*Modern Painters*, III, 216). On the other hand Turner, probably because of his interest in rendering perspective through color, thought highly of Canaletto, and a little later Whistler did not hesitate to regard him as comparable to Velázquez. With the rise of impressionism, however, Guardi began to be considered as a surprising forerunner of the new artists, and Canaletto suffered another eclipse. At the same time there was a decided preference for his earlier paintings with their lively contrast of light and shade, while his later English phase was regarded as a regression to academicism. A redress of this critical estimate is due to Maria Pittaluga (*L'Arte*, 1934), who recognized in the late works a new direction in the artist's style, rather than a falling off of his powers. Although he does not share this esteem for the late style, W. G. Constable (*Canaletto*, 1960) emphasizes the fanciful and imaginative elements in Canaletto's work, evident in the *capricci* and notably in the etchings, which transform the objectively seen facts into a personal vision. In recent years important historical contributions have been made by Detlev von Hadeln (1926, 1930) and K. T. Parker (1948) for the drawings; by Hilda Finberg (1923) for the English period; and by F. J. B. Watson (1949).

Nicola IVANOFF

BIBLIOG. E. Dayes, The Works of the Late Edward Dayes . . . , London, 1805; E. J. Dent, Alessandro Scarlatti, His Life and Works, London, 1905; W. H. Challenor, The Egertons in Italy and the Netherlands 1729–34, B. John Rylands Lib., XXXII, 2, 1950, pp. 157–70; Canaletto and English Draughtsmen, Exhibition Cat., Br. Mus., 1950; for other sources and bibliography see V. Moschini, Canaletto, Milan, 1954 (Eng. trans., London, 1956); F. Haskell, Stefano Conti, Patron of Canaletto and Others, BM, XCVIII, 1956, pp. 296–300; F. J. B. Watson, A Self-Portrait by Canaletto, BM, XCVIII, 1956, pp. 295–96; J. L. Howgego, A Recent Canaletto Rediscovery, Guildhall Misc., Aug. 7, 1956, pp. 21–9; W. G. Constable, Canaletto, London, 1960.

Illustrations : PLS. 22–25.

**CANO,** ALONSO. Spanish baroque master, who practiced all major branches of art (b. Granada, 1601; d. Granada, 1667). In 1616 Cano was apprenticed to the painter Francisco Pacheco in Seville. He moved to Madrid in 1638. Falsely accused of murdering his wife in 1644, Cano fled to Valencia, returning to Madrid in 1645. In 1652 he became prebendary of Gra-

nada Cathedral, but was expelled over a controversy with the canons in 1656. The years 1657–60 were spent at court in Madrid, after which the artist was reinstated at Granada (1660).

The paintings of Cano's Sevillian period (1624–38), in *tenebroso* style, were profoundly influenced by the young Velázquez (e.g., Cano's *St. Francis Borgia*, Seville, Mus. Provincial de Bellas Artes, 1624; *Portrait of an Ecclesiastic*, New York, Hispanic Society of America). Idealism and decorative qualities, notable also in his drawings, characterize *St. Agnes* (Berlin, destroyed in 1945) and *St. John's Vision of Jerusalem*, 1635–37 (London, Wallace Coll.). In Madrid, 1638–52, influenced by Venetian paintings of the royal collection, Cano's technique developed and his idealism increased. The principal paintings of this period were two altars in La Magdalena at Getafe, 1645 (partly workshop), *Immaculate Conception* (Vitoria, Mus. Provincial de Bellas Artes), *Miracle of the Well* (Madrid, Prado), *Madonna and Child* (Prado), *Christ Supported by an Angel* (Prado), *Noli me tangere* (Budapest, Nat. Mus.), and *Descent into Limbo* (Los Angeles County Mus.). In Granada, 1652–67, Cano developed a monumental style with increased baroque spatial organization, seen in seven large canvases illustrating the life of the Virgin, in the sanctuary of the Cathedral. Other major compositions of this period were *Immaculate Conception* (Granada, Cathedral oratory), *Holy Family* (Granada, Convento del Angel), *St. Bernardine of Siena and St. John Capistrano* (Granada, Mus. Provincial de Bellas Artes), and *Death of St. Francis* (Madrid, Mus. de la Academia de Bellas Artes de San Fernando). Later paintings include *St. Benedict* (Madrid, Prado), *Christ at the Pillar* (Avila, Carmelitas Descalzas), and his masterpiece, *Madonna of the Rosary* (Málaga Cathedral, 1665–66). As a painter, Cano ranks among the half dozen greatest figures of Spanish baroque art; he became founder of the Granadine school.

As a sculptor, Cano worked extensively with polychromed wood during his Sevillian period. In this city his fame was established by the high altar of S. María at Lebrija (1629–31), near Seville. Virtually abandoning sculpture in Madrid, Cano returned to it later (creating the Granadine school). Most famous are his statuettes of the *Immaculate Conception* and *Virgin of Bethlehem*, the busts *Adam, Eve*, and *St. Paul* (all in Granada Cathedral), and *St. Anthony of Padua* (Murcia, S. Nicolás). Three statues of Franciscan saints (Granada, Palace of Charles V), carved with the assistance of Pedro de Mena, have an introspective dramatic mood combined with a formal beauty.

In architecture, the Lebrija altar with its colossal Corinthian order, revolutionary for the era, and the altar of St. John the Evangelist (Seville, S. Paula, 1635–37) are the only survivals from the early Sevillian period. Cano's drawings provide the best evidence of his restrained architectural style and his richly inventive ornament. The destroyed church of the Convento del Angel, Granada (1653–61), copied in La Magdalena (Getafe, 1677–94), brought influential innovations in the design of capitals and column ornament. Attenuation of scale is noted here, as well as in the design for the façade (1667) of the Granada Cathedral, where the recessed plan was dictated by Renaissance foundations. See also BAROQUE ART; SPANISH AND PORTUGUESE ART.

BIBLIOG. A. L. Mayer, Der racionero Alonso Cano, JhbPreussKsamml, Beiheft, XXX, 1909, and XXXI, 1910; M. Gómez-Moreno, Alonso Cano, escultor, AEArte, II, 1926; H. E. Wethey, Alonso Cano, Painter, Sculptor and Architect, Princeton, 1955.

Harold E. WETHEY

**CANOVA**, ANTONIO. Italian sculptor, born in Possagno, near Venice, Nov. 1, 1757. Orphaned at an early age, he was brought up by his grandfather Pasino, a stonecutter and master builder. In 1768 he was apprenticed to Giuseppe Bernardi, called "Torretti," in Pagnano (Asolo). Torretti took Canova with him to Venice, where he studied the famed collection of plaster casts in the palace of Filippo Farsetti and frequented the Academy. In 1771–72 he carved two *Baskets of Fruit* (Venice, Mus. Correr) for Senator Giovanni Falier, who thereupon commissioned two statues, *Eurydice* (1773) and *Orpheus*

(1776) for the Villa Falier (Pradazzi d'Asolo), now in the Museo Correr in Venice.

After the death of Torretti, Canova set up his own studio (1774) and, having achieved a certain reputation for portraiture, carved a marble *Daedalus and Icarus* (1778; Venice, Mus. Correr) for the Procurator, Pietro Vittor Pisani. In the fall of 1779, after modeling an *Apollo* in terra cotta (Venice, Accademia), he left (Oct. 6) for Rome, where he was the guest of the Venetian Ambassador Girolamo Zulian, who provided him with a studio in the embassy palace. In the winter he visited Naples, Herculaneum, Pompeii, and Paestum, spent a short time in Venice, and early in 1781 returned to establish himself in Rome. June saw him at work on the model for *Theseus and the Minotaur* (London, Coll. Lord Londonderry), which was completed in marble in the following year. At the suggestion of Giovanni Volpato, Msgr. Carlo Giorgi commissioned in 1783 the monument to Clement XIV for the Church of SS. Apostoli in Rome (PL. 28), which was unveiled four years later. This was followed by the ambitious monument to Clement XIII in St. Peter's (1792). Simultaneously he was at work on *Cupid and Psyche* (Louvre), as well as on a model for *Adonis Crowned by Venus*, which was never to be translated into marble. In 1792 the Venetian senate commissioned the monument to Angelo Emo (Venice, Mus. Storico Navale), completed in 1795, as was *Venus and Adonis* (now in the Villa Fabre at Eaux-Vives, Geneva). In 1794 Canova made a few sketches for a projected monument to Titian (Possagno, Mus. Canoviano) for his friend Ambassador Zulian. In April, 1796, he had already finished the model for *Hercules and Lichas*, which was not, however, to be completed in marble (Rome, Gall. Naz. d'Arte Moderna) until 1815 (PL. 29). Also dated 1796 are the *Penitent Magdalen* (now in Cadenabbia) and the Berlin *Hebe* (Staat. Mus.). In May, 1798, after the French invasion of Rome, Canova took refuge in Possagno, but August found him in Vienna at work on the monument to Maria Christina for the Augustinerkirche. In November, 1799, he was back in Rome, where he completed *Perseus* (1801) and the *Pugilists* (1802), the only modern works in the Vatican's Belvedere. In September, 1802, he was summoned to Paris to do a portrait of Napoleon. The original plaster of *Napoleon as First Consul* is in Possagno. For Sta Croce in Florence the Countess of Albany, widow of the Young Pretender, commissioned a funerary monument for the poet Vittorio Alfieri, her lover, who had died the year before. In 1805 Pius VII named Canova Inspector General of Fine Arts and Antiquities for the Papal States. In the same year he began the portrait of Napoleon's sister, Pauline Borghese, as Venus Victrix (Rome, Borghese Gall.), which, according to Faldi, was probably not completed until 1807 (PL. 27). Between 1806 and 1810 he did the *Dancing Girl with Her Hands on Her Hips* (Leningrad, Hermitage), the *Terpsichore* for Count Sommariva's Paris palace (now in Cadenabbia, Villa Carlotta), the *Dancing Girl with her Finger on her Chin* (Rome, Gall. Naz. d'Arte Antica), and the *Dancing Girl with Cymbals* for Count Domenico Manzoni in Forlì.

In 1810 he was appointed director of the Accademia di S. Luca (Rome), for which he obtained from Napoleon important imperial concessions; four years later he was to be made its permanent director. Also in 1810 he went to Paris to do a bust of the empress Marie Louise. In 1812 he completed the *Venus Italica* (Florence, Pitti) and in 1813, the model for the *Three Graces* (completed 1816; Leningrad, Hermitage). In August, 1815, he was again in Paris, commissioned by Pius VII to recover the works of art looted by Napoleon's army. This difficult assignment successfully completed, Canova traveled in November to London to inspect the Elgin marbles recently transferred from the Parthenon. In 1816 he finished the statue of Marie Louise as Concordia (Parma, Gall. Naz.; PL. 28) and the plaster model for *Mars and Venus* commissioned by the Prince Regent of England (London, Buckingham Palace). In 1819 he completed *Theseus and the Centaur* (Vienna, Kunsthist. Mus.), unveiled the monument to the Stuarts in St. Peter's, laid the cornerstone of the Temple in Possagno, and finished the plaster model for *Endymion*, which was cut in marble (1821) for the Duke of Devonshire (Chatsworth), and the *Fainting*

*Magdalen* (1822) for the Duke of Liverpool (Possagno, Mus. Canoviano). In 1820 the equestrian statue of Charles III of Naples (Naples, Piazza del Plebiscito) was cast in bronze and the marble monument of George Washington in Roman dress was completed. (This was sent to the state capitol in Raleigh, N.C., where it was shortly afterward destroyed in a fire. A model survives at Possagno.) In 1821 Canova made a model of a *Deposition* (later translated into bronze by Bartolomeo Ferrari for the Temple in Possagno). He died on Oct. 13, 1822, in Venice.

Two periods can be distinguished in Canova's activities: (1) his youthful Venetian phase, during which he was linked to the sculptural tradition of the works he saw around him; and (2) a period that began with his decision to settle in Rome and his subsequent systematic study of classical sculpture. To the first period belong such works as the *Orpheus* and *Eurydice* and the portraits of the Doge Paolo Renier (1779; Padua, Mus. Civ.) and Gian Matteo Amadei (ca. 1776–79; Venice, Seminario; PL. 30). These works, like the portrait on canvas of Amedeo Svajer (Venice, Mus. Correr; PL. 30), display an acute psychological perception, but Canova's classicizing bent becomes ever more apparent — reflecting, of course, the prevailing European taste. Canova's conscious need for structural austerity is clearly expressed in *Daedalus and Icarus* and is, so to speak, the sculptural equivalent of the Venetian neo-Palladian fashion. However, the definite links between Canova's youthful oils and sculptures (even after 1780) and the works of the Cinquecento should not be overlooked.

With approaching maturity, in the decade between 1780 and 1790, Canova, fired by his direct contact with classical antiquities, to some extent set aside his Venetian legacy of naturalism. He was, however, able to handle in a highly personal manner the isolation and idealization demanded by the esthetic standards that had recently been established by Winckelmann; the *Genius of Death* seated next to the sarcophagus of Clement XIII in St. Peter's (Rome) breathes an exquisite Praxitelean wistfulness not too far removed from the popular Arcadian mood. This was a difficult moment in Canova's development as an artist; conflicting directions are clearly reflected in the Louvre *Cupid and Psyche* (the most important work of this period), the extremely lifelike figure of the *Penitent Magdalen* (1796) — which almost forecasts the naturalism of Bartolini — and the monumental model for *Hercules and Lichas*.

The following period, during which both classicism and naturalism had their day or were happily merged, saw Canova's success as a sculptor in the grand manner. His works were sought after: for example, *Perseus*, the *Pugilists*, the *Three Graces*, *Hebe* (PL. 29), and the *Dancers* were frequently repeated by his assistants. The period was also one of masterpieces: the portraits of Napoleon as First Consul and of Pauline Borghese, an image ideal yet quickened with life, wherein the elements of classicism, technical virtuosity, and a submerged sensuality are fused in a subtly evocative whole. After his trip to London, Canova's more successful works such as the *Sleeping Endymion* embody his vision of the Phidian marbles, which he had described with such excitement in letters to his old friend Quatremère de Quincy.

While the marble sculptures of Canova trace a subtle artistic evolution, his rapid sketches — most of them preserved in the Museo Canoviano in Possagno — retain the liveliness and spontaneity of original inspiration, together with those lasting values of mass, weight, and volume common to sculpture of all periods.

Canova also executed a certain number of paintings (PLS. 26, 30) that seem rather amateurish; among the best are the portrait of Svajer and the self-portrait in the Uffizi. His project for the solemn Temple in Possagno, to be placed in a lovely site in the Venetian countryside, was executed in collaboration with Pietro Bosio, Antonio Diedo, and the master builder Giovanni Zardo.

In the artistic circles of Rome, Canova — who had at first preferred the sculptures of Agostino Penna to those of Bartolomeo Cavaceppi, the famous restorer, copyist, and admirer of Winckelmann — soon found himself in the position of intermediary and conciliator between their different points of view. Something of his attitude may be gathered from his remarks on the Elgin marbles which he had seen in London in 1815. While they were still unappreciated by many art lovers, he found in them "no affectation, no hardness, nothing which could be called conventional or geometric . . . the works of Phidias are true flesh." He congratulated himself for "having steadfastly believed that the great masters have always worked in this manner and no other."

He wrote these words to Quatremère de Quincy (Nov. 9, 1815) at the height of his career and in a position of such authority that he succeeded through personal prestige in forcing the Congress of Paris to return the works of art seized by Napoleon in Italy. However, the younger artists were feeling restive under his artistic dominion. We find him complaining to his biographer Missirini: "There are many who, without knowing what they are talking about, speak of I don't know what geometric style . . . I think that the works of a frank and skilled hand are worth a great deal more than a scrupulous and timid diligence . . . ."

Clearly, the accusations that were embittering the aging sculptor stemmed from the circle of Thorwaldsen, even though Canova had had so high an opinion of Thorwaldsen as to get him appointed to the chair of sculpture in the Accademia di S. Luca in 1811. Canova himself had no students as such, although all the contemporary sculptors of Rome, and especially his numerous assistants, were more or less influenced by his work. Among these were Adamo Tadolini, Rinaldo Rinaldi, and Cincinnato Baruzzi. After the death of Canova, Baruzzi was to be entrusted by his heirs with the completion of his unfinished sculptures. These included the large Pietà intended for the Temple in Possagno, where a bronze cast now stands, the marble version (thanks to Antonio Sarti, the architect) having finally been placed in the Church of Il Salvatore in Terracina.

Emilio LAVAGNINO

Perhaps no artist has ever been more exalted in his own age than Canova — he was considered little less than divine and the supreme arbiter of taste — nor fallen so low in the esteem of more recent times. With rare exceptions (e.g., Karl Ludwig Fernow, who in his *Uber den Bildhauer Canova und dessen Werken*, Zurich, 1806, reflects the adverse opinion of his friend Jakob Asmus Carstens), the tone of those who spoke of him both during his lifetime (e.g., Ugo Foscolo and Pietro Giordani) and throughout most of the 19th century was eulogistic. In fact, P. Giordani's *Panegirico ad Antonio Canova*, written for the dedication of his bust in the Accademia di Belle Arti in Bologna (June 28, 1810) can speak for all: To Giordani, Canova was a "man without equal on the earth," "an angel of God." The artist's feminine type became proverbial as a paragon of ideal beauty in all the Western world. A contemporary of Edgar Allan Poe, speaking of Poe's young wife Virginia Clemm, wrote: "Her face would have challenged the genius of Canova to copy it." Flaubert, while visiting the Villa Carlotta, stood enchanted in front of the group of *Cupid and Psyche* (that same group which had scandalized Wordsworth, who, in exclaiming "Demons!" was implicitly confessing the profound emotion it produced in him). Flaubert wrote, "I didn't look at anything else in the gallery. I walked around it several times and the last time I kissed under the armpit the swooning woman who holds out her long marble arms toward Cupid. And the foot! And the head! The profile! May I be forgiven, this was the only sensual kiss that I have bestowed in a long time; it was something more than that, I was kissing Beauty itself. It was to genius that I was dedicating my burning enthusiasm."

Apart from these exponents of romanticism, however, romantic criticism was to follow another path, identifying neoclassicism with academic tyranny and exalting freedom of the imagination and the genuineness of all that is primitive. Once immediacy, a romantic fetish, had become the supreme criterion of judgment, neoclassicism was condemned as synonymous with frigidity. Among the works of the great neoclas-

sical artists were exempted only those rough drafts and spontaneous sketches still glowing with the divine fire that further elaboration was thought to extinguish. The romantic tenet had already been expressed in the Platonic theory of infancy of Wordsworth's "Ode on Intimations of Immortality from Recollections of Early Childhood." Here the child is the " best of the Philosophers," "the eye among the blind." This romantic prejudice considered as academic a work inspired by classical models in the Vatican but not that inspired by models in the Musée de l'Homme in Paris; i.e., it was academic to copy the *Apollo Belvedere* and the *Laocoön*, but it was pure and original art to borrow motifs and technique from those prehistoric drawings on stones known as "art mobilier"; he who copied from the Vatican Museums destroyed the marvelous leap into the unknown realms of fantasy, whereas he who copied from the caves of Altamira and Lascaux realized to the full the autonomy of art.

One can understand how such criticism condemned Canova's art, sparing, if anything, only his less typical productions — the quick sketches and drafts — even to the most careless indications of pose and movement, which were thought to reflect genuine inspiration not made artificial by academic discipline.

There are two schools of thought as to the work of Canova: (1) that he is an artist of the gracious, withdrawn from the turbulent political scene to dream of the Graces and the Muses; and (2) that his was an 18th-century artistic temperament congealed by a superimposed neoclassicism, that he was therefore a creator of works whose artificiality denies them the right to qualify as art. Both these positions find some support in the life of the artist: he did love to live quietly and at first even hesitated to go to Rome ("Nature can be found without going to Rome"); in his youth he was disinclined to listen to those who were urging him in the direction of classical imitation. The second opinion is temperately expressed by A. de Rinaldis, who sees no conflict between the declining spirit of the 18th century and the classical spirit in the most successful of Canova's works (the standing *Cupid and Psyche*, the *Dancing Girls*, *Endymion*). The same conciliatory tone is taken by E. Lavagnino, who seems to share the traditional views, combining them in the famous phrase of the French painter Suazy describing Canova as "a Venetian sculptor translated into Greek." C. L. Ragghianti attaches great importance to Canova's drawings, even while conceding their unevenness: he finds in them on the one hand "a highly cultivated refinement and an attenuated exquisiteness reminiscent of Prud'hon," on the other "a natural spontaneity and absence of style which can be related to the realistic sketches of David's *Revolution*." Ragghianti feels that this coexistence of artistic modes points up Canova's originality as an artist. Without wishing to negate the value of "all his more sophisticated works," he suggests, therefore, that the most vital works are those which reflect the spontaneous feelings of this "representative man," and that the more majestically monumental and "sublime" he became, the weaker was his production. This romantic concept would, in short, admit only the spontaneous work most expressive of the most fundamentally human qualities.

E. Bassi, in what is to date the best Italian monograph on Canova (1943), accepted the formula of the artist who, in order to put himself in unison with the spirit of his time, "had to suppress his youthful aspirations and almost always to deny his true self. Canova pleases us when he withdraws from his time, for example, in the portraits which continue a more frankly 18th-century tradition." C. Delogu in his anthology of Italian sculpture (1956), also spares the works in which Canova "sees the actual and is inspired by the human model, by human emotions," while noting that "frigidity, academicism, and mannerism are the visible constant of Canova's art." Less temperate, indeed deliberately damning, are the opinions of C. Brandi (1949): "To be cold and bombastic is Canova's secret.... Form, for Canova, becomes ritual. It is like a ritual gesture which has outlived its identity, its meaning, its relation to the action which it abridges and symbolizes.... It is almost worse when he threatens to become expressive. His miming is atrocious: he does not re-create, he imitates.... Canova's sculpture

turns marble into cement; it is opaque, never going beyond the surface.... In Canova occurs that fatal separation between the first vision of the image and its formulation which marks the end of the formal civilization of the Renaissance.... In Canova there is always a conflict between the initial impulse, which tends to arrange the image in a fluid contour, and the diabolical brake which overturns it." The same opinion is expressed by Kenneth Clark in *The Nude* (New York, 1956), and by Roberto Longhi, who writes (*Viatico per cinque secoli di pittura veneziana*, Florence, 1946): "Antonio Canova, the sculptor born dead, whose heart is in the Frari [Venice], whose hand is at the Academy, and the rest... is I don't know where."

However, M. Marangoni (*The Art of Seeing Art*, London, 1951) is more just. In comparing Canova with Bronzino, he speaks of "a manner — albeit full of dangers — of arriving at art by other paths."

There are signs of a trend toward a more balanced appraisal of Canova's work, forecast in 1932 by Osbert Sitwell (*Winters of Content*, London, 1932), who compared Canova with Ingres. This is especially true outside of Italy, where neoclassicism is being reevaluated (E. Kaufmann, *The Architecture of the Age of Reason*, Cambridge, Mass., 1955, and others). Just as in England since about 1930 there has been a reaction against the romantic criticism which, in the name of an art that is "all feeling," did not recognize Alexander Pope as a poet, it may be that David and Ingres will no longer be approved only for their sketches and that Canova will be appreciated for more than his sketches. Among the indications of a new view of Canova are R. Zeitler's favorable treatment (*Klassizismus und Utopia*, Stockholm, 1954); a commemorative exposition of Canova's work and that of his contemporaries held in the Museum of the R. I. School of Design on the occasion of the 200th anniversary of Canova's birth; and the appreciative evaluation by A. M. Clark in the catalogue of that exhibition (1956).

Mario Praz

Bibliog. M. Missirini, Della Vita di Antonio Canova, Prato, 1822; L. Cicognara, Biografia di Antonio Canova, Venice, 1823; A. D'Este, Memorie per servire alla vita di Antonio Canova, Venice, 1823; L. Cicognara, Storia della scultura dal suo risorgimento in Italia fino al secolo di Canova, Prato, 1829; P. E. Selvatico, Sulla architettura e sulla scultura in Venezia, Venice, 1847; A. Tadolini, Ricordi autobiografici di Adamo Tadolini, Rome, 1900; L. Coletti, La fortuna del Canova, B. del Regio Ist. di archeologia e storia dell'arte, I, 1927, pp. 21–96 (with bibliog.); E. Bassi, Canova, Bergamo, 1943; A. De Rinaldis, Arte e "mestiere" nel Canova, Arti Fig., I, 1945, p. 137 ff.; C. Brandi, Periplo della scultura moderna, Immagine, II, 1949, pp. 58–65; G. Fallani, Canova, Brescia, 1949; E. Lavagnino, Le invenzioni del Canova, Arte veneta, IV, 1950, pp. 86–94; P. Della Pergola, Paolina Borghese Bonaparte di Antonio Canova, Rome, 1953; I. Faldi, Galleria Borghese, Le sculture dal secolo XVI al XIX, Rome, 1954, pp. 45–7; R. Zeitler, Klassizismus und Utopia, Stockholm, 1954; E. Lavagnino, L'Arte Moderna dai neoclassici ai contemporanei, Turin, 1956; G. Delogu, Antologia della scultura italiana, Milan, 1956; Mostra Canoviana (cat.), ed. L. Coletti, Treviso, 1957; C. L. Ragghianti, Studi sul Canova, CrArte, XXII, 1957, p. 102; E. Bassi, La Gipsoteca di Possagno (with extensive bibliog.), Venice, 1957; A. Muñoz, Canova, Le opere, Rome, 1957; E. Lavagnino, A duecento anni dalla nascita di A. Canova, Ulisse, V, 1958, p. 1755 ff.; M. Praz, Gusto neoclassico, 2d ed., Naples, 1958.

Emilio Lavagnino

Illustrations: PLS. 26–30.

**CARAVAGGIO.** Michelangelo Merisi, called "Caravaggio," was born in Caravaggio (between Milan and Brescia) probably on Sept. 28, 1573, according to an epitaph composed by his friend Marzio Milesi (*Inscriptiones et Elogia*, a document known only in a late copy). The epitaph tells us that his father was Fermo Merisi, majordomo and architect of the Marquis of Caravaggio. Another document relates that on Apr. 6, 1584, the young man was placed by his elder brother Battista (we may assume his father had died) in the care of the painter Simone Peterzano, who was active in Milan between 1573 and 1596. The apprenticeship seems to have continued for five or six years, that is, up to the beginning of 1590. However, Milanese documents pertaining to Simone Peterzano are lacking between 1585 and 1590, and since they occur again between 1590 and 1596, it has been suggested that Peterzano was absent

from Milan during the years for which Caravaggio had been apprenticed (Calvesi, 1954).

Bellori mentions a visit that Caravaggio made to Venice prior to his arrival in Rome. Mancini, on the other hand, writes that, after having been in trouble in Milan and having had to leave the city, he arrived in Rome at about twenty years of age or, according to the birth date mentioned above, about 1593. For the time being this date can be accepted.

The apprenticeship to the mannerist Simone Peterzano was of some importance, but since the young artist soon surpassed his master, he could have learned little more from him than a technical skill. Peterzano, however, made available to him a sort of "anthology" of motifs, compositional schemes, and methods of drawing, whose influence, though not apparent in Caravaggio's early work, has been remarked by recent critics in his later work.

These reminiscences of Peterzano's work become evident in the art of Caravaggio when the painter is no longer confronted by problems of pictorial naturalism, but by those connected with the third dimension and especially of placing the human figure in a given space. It is reasonable to suppose that the years spent with Peterzano gave him some familiarity with the pictorial tendencies of the Lombard school and his master's compositional methods.

According to Baglione and a marginal note by Bellori to Baglione's *Vite*, Caravaggio became friendly in Rome with one Lorenzo from Sicily, presumably an art dealer and painter. Mancini records that he lived in the house of Pandolfo Pucci, who was a beneficiary at St. Peter's and majordomo of Camilla Peretti, the sister of Sixtus V. He executed several devotional paintings for Pucci, who took them to his home in Recanati. Pucci earned for himself a peculiar notoriety for having fed the artist so frequently with salad that Caravaggio ironically nicknamed him "Monsignor Insalata." From Bellori's marginal note to Baglione's *Vite* we learn that at this time Caravaggio took up with the painter Antiveduto Gramatica, whose few remaining paintings are in a Caravaggesque style. The sources agree that Caravaggio was for a while (according to some scholars between 1592 and 1593) an assistant to Giuseppe Cesari, known as the Cavalier d'Arpino, then the leading fresco painter.

Giulio Mancini gives us other information concerning the young artist's stay in Rome. He writes that, wounded by the kick of a horse, Caravaggio was admitted into the Hospital of the Consolation and that the Prior received some paintings from him which he later seems to have taken to Seville, his native town. In 1593 Camillo Contreras was Prior of the hospital, and to judge by his Spanish name, could be the Prior mentioned by Mancini. This is the first suggestion of an exportation of Caravaggio's works abroad, and it is interesting to note that the paintings taken to Spain were undoubtedly the early works and of a style, therefore, that could easily be apprehended by the Spanish artistic world. It seems that the period spent with the Cavalier d'Arpino (of eight months' duration, according to Mancini) terminated abruptly just at the time of Caravaggio's accident..

Among his early works sources cite a painting known only through copies, the *Boy Peeling Fruit*, and a group of paintings from the collection of the Cavalier d'Arpino, confiscated by the fiscal authorities on May 4, 1607, and given by Paul V to his nephew Cardinal Scipione Borghese, the art collector. This group included the *Boy with a Basket of Fruit* and the *Boy with Fruit* ("Bacchino Malato," PL. 35; supposedly a self-portrait of the young artist when he was ailing), both in the Borghese Gallery. It is likely that these works were executed while Caravaggio was still in the workshop of d'Arpino and that they remained there. According to Malvasia, a few years later d'Arpino was supposed to have asked Guido Reni to obtain for him paintings by Caravaggio, but this is a late and unreliable statement. Another painting cited by Mancini as a very early one is the *Boy Bitten by a Lizard*, known in two versions: one in the Roberto Longhi Collection, in Florence, and the other in the Vincent Korda Collection, in London. This painting must have been immediately successful, since

there are contemporary copies. Stylistically, it is related to the *St. Francis in Ecstasy* (Hartford, Conn., Wadsworth Atheneum), which was cited as early as 1597 as a work by the "very famous painter," Caravaggio, in the will of Don Ruggiero Tritonio, Abbot of Pinerolo, who had acquired it from Ottavio Costa, a contemporary connoisseur. According to Baglione, the first work executed by Caravaggio after he left the Cavalier d'Arpino was a *Bacchus*, now identified as the one in the Uffizi.

After he left the hospital Caravaggio found a patron in Monsignor Fantin Petrignani, a nobleman born in Amelia who had returned to Rome in 1595 after a long absence. Caravaggio went to live in his palace on Via dei Giubbonari, the present Monte di Pietà. But it was only when the art dealer Maestro Valentino, who lived near S. Luigi dei Francesi, introduced Caravaggio to Cardinal del Monte that he found an understanding patron who finally opened to him the doors of the Roman art world. Some canvases were painted for Del Monte in 1596 and 1597, and, from a document published by Bertolotti, we gather that in 1600 the artist was the Cardinal's guest in what is today known as Palazzo Madama. Among the paintings executed for the new patron are a *Medusa*, presented by Cardinal del Monte to the Archduke of Tuscany in 1608 (Florence, Uffizi), and a *Basket of Fruit*, that Del Monte gave to Cardinal Federico Borromeo in 1596, as we learn from a letter addressed to Borromeo in that same year. The painting, the bottom of which appears to have been repainted, is perhaps a fragment of a bigger work, possibly including figures (Milan, Pin. Ambrosiana). The care with which the young artist depicted these still lifes from nature is touching; but what is most surprising is the instinctive power of synthesis that he employed even in the smallest particular. From the veins of the leaves to the drops of dew, each detail is essential to him and lends exceptional meaning and worth to the most humble product of nature. The inner vitality that springs from this new pictorial approach is without equal in any painting of the kind.

The outstanding example of the new relationship between still life and figure is the *Bacchus* of the Uffizi, whose face is believed to resemble that of the painter Lionello Spada, who lived in Rome. The same model, perhaps, occurs again in *The Fortuneteller* (Louvre) and in some of the figures in the paintings in S. Luigi dei Francesi. Longhi dates the painting about 1589, but in the recent revision of Caravaggio's chronology, it has been suggested that the date be advanced about five years. Baglione mentions it as the first of the paintings executed by Caravaggio in Rome after leaving the Cavalier d'Arpino. He writes: "and the first was a Bacchus with some divers bunches of grapes, very diligently executed; but in a rather dry style." The biographer's observation evidently refers to the emphasis that the artist placed on the contours of objects and figures, which, as in the other early paintings in the Borghese Gallery, emerge from a uniform background not yet overladen with shadows. This permits the forms, which are carefully contained within their contours, to appear compact and taut, thus giving maximum realistic concreteness to the human figure. The apparent classicism of this Bacchus, which the artist purposely depicted in the antique pose of a reclining young man before a prepared table, is modified by the suppleness of the figure, painted with realistic color. The fruit and other objects resemble those in the *Boy with Basket*, in the Borghese Gallery, and the *Basket*, in the Ambrosiana. But in the beauty of the model, who seems barely to support the heavy crown of grapes, in the languor of eyes already torpid with wine, and in the unexpected novelty of the entire work, there is almost a synthesis of the early years of Caravaggio. The resulting vitality and sureness of hand justify a comparison with the artists of the golden age, from Raphael to Titian.

During the period when the artist worked for Cardinal del Monte he seems to have painted *The Musical Party* (PL. 31), referred to by Baglione as follows: "and he painted very expertly for the Cardinal a concert of youths drawn from nature." This is the beautiful canvas found in England and bought by the Metropolitan Museum of New York. In the lower left of the painting is a rather old inscription bearing the name of the painter in block letters. The four youthful figures are

carefully composed, their poses and gestures alternating harmoniously; the recurrent folds of their drapery form an ideal bond between the figures, and the boy in the center, tuning a lute, turns to the light his large, dark eyes and lips shaped in song. The musical instruments are related to those in the *Amor Victorious* (PL. 33), in Berlin; the boy at the far left is the same as the one in the *Boy Peeling Fruit*; and the young man with his back to the viewer is similar to the *Bacchus* in the Uffizi.

For the same Cardinal del Monte he also painted the *Lute Player* (Baglione), which has been at The Hermitage in Leningrad since 1815 and was formerly in the Giustiniani Collection, and the *St. Catherine*, which was owned by the Barberinis as early as 1627 and is now in Lugano (Von Thyssen Coll.). The *St. Catherine* is particularly praiseworthy. The clarity of the figure and loving attention to detail (especially the large wheel, an actual wheel of a carriage) and the care in differentiating textures place this painting among the most expressive. A long, pointed, bloodstained sword touches the martyr's palm (with obvious allusion) and provides a motif of foreshortened perspective that heralds the paintings in S. Maria del Popolo. Another group of works is considered to have been executed for Monsignor Fantin Petrignani and therefore dated a little earlier: a *Fortuneteller*, which Mancini seems to place among them, later part of the Collection of Alessandro Vittrice (Paris, Louvre) and known also through a copy in the Capitoline Gallery in Rome; the *Rest on the Flight to Egypt* (PL. 36); and the *Magdalen* (PL. 32), now in the Doria Gallery. Mancini is not very explicit, however, in giving the chronology of these early works and the names of their first owners.

The *Magdalen* in the Doria Gallery is mentioned by Bellori, and, although his discussion is intended to be merely descriptive, it is actually critical in tone: "He depicted a girl seated upon a chair, her hands in her lap, in the act of drying her hair; he painted her in a room and, by placing on the floor a small jar of ointment, trinkets and jewels, he pretended she was the Magdalen." The painting has in common with his other early works a genre character, but the isolation of the gentle figure in the shaft of light and the sweet melancholy that suffuses her face and body serves to transform her in a subtle way into the figure of the Magdalen, who is adequately identified by the modest objects lying on the floor. This figure, which bears an affinity to the Virgin in the *Rest on the Flight to Egypt* and was executed at the same time, is yet another proof of the artist's rigorous ideal, consistent since the very beginning in avoiding the clamorous representations of the prevailing style of painting by taking refuge in the intimacy of life itself.

The *Rest on the Flight to Egypt* (Rome, Doria Gall.) is a painting of great importance. It is among Caravaggio's earliest paintings and contains one of his rare examples of a landscape. The figures are grouped under a young oak whose branches are silhouetted against a heavy and sultry sky. On the right is an illusionistic group of trees with silvery trunks and in the foreground a few wild plants. The entire picture was executed with the same care already noted in the still lifes; but here the group appears enveloped and almost sealed in a pastoral lyricism. The splendid fall of the white garment around the young body of the angel constitutes the principal axis of the composition that still retains the charm of a Venetian *sacra conversazione* but is constructed with a realism that is entirely new. The angel and St. Joseph are bound together by a feeling of intimacy, and the unforgetable group of the Virgin with the Child on her lap seems enwrapped in the sweetness of a lullaby, in the silence and stillness of the hour. Again in the early *Conversion of St. Paul* (Rome, Coll. Odescalchi-Balbi) the landscape is a background to the agitated figures, illuminated by a light that is violent but not yet decisive and constructive. The atmosphere is stormy but, as in the *Flight*, the landscape is painted with firmness and subtle characterization, while manneristic motifs (the figure of the fallen saint) are accompanied by touches of realism (the old soldier), as one might expect in a great young talent that is brimming with new and conflicting ideas and not yet rid of reminiscences of the past.

A last example of an almost nocturnal landscape appears in the *St. Francis in Ecstasy*, another early work. Here, however, the light enters diagonally, throwing into relief the sharp folds of the garments and casting shadows over the figures, while the simple and convincing composition centers around the fall of the saint's body.

A painting not mentioned by the earliest sources but cited later by Scannelli (1657) and by Bellori (1672), the *Cardsharpers*, was executed for someone whose name is unknown. During the last century it was in the Sciarra Gallery but has since been lost; today it is known only through copies. The *Narcissus* (Rome, Gall. Naz.), presumably of the same time, is a typical interpretation of allegory in terms of realistic imagery and is very successful in its use of rich color.

The *Amor Victorious* (PL. 33), the *Portrait of a Young Woman*, and the first version of *St. Matthew* (see below) entered the collection of Vincenzo Giustiniani at the time when Caravaggio was busy in S. Luigi dei Francesi — about 1600. Later, in the 19th century, these works passed into the possession of the Berlin Museum. At the same time the artist seems to have executed several pictures for Ciriaco Mattei: a *St. John the Baptist*, mentioned by Bellori as in the Pio Collection, identified with the painting in the Doria Gallery and, recently, with the version in the Capitoline Museum; a *Christ at Emmaus* that some identify with the *Supper at Emmaus* in the National Gallery in London; and the *Incredulity of Thomas*, known through copies.

Caravaggio executed the portrait of Cardinal Maffeo Barberini, who became Pope Urban VIII in 1623. He also painted for the Cardinal a *Sacrifice of Isaac*, now in the Uffizi. Any attempt to establish a precise chronology of his works, however, even though hypothetical, would be rather arbitrary, since he was an artist who followed the inclination of the moment.

Caravaggio did not reject the contributions of artists of the 16th century when working out problems of composition or figure treatment. Proof of this is seen in his *Amor Victorious*, which is reminiscent of Michelangelo's *Victory* in the Palazzo Vecchio in Florence. The relationship has even greater value when we realize that Caravaggio borrowed the motif of Victory's raised, bent arm for his earlier *Boy with Fruit* ("Bacchino Malato") in the Borghese Gallery. Normally these comparisons are used to prove possible analogies in interpretation; in the case of Caravaggio, however, it is just the opposite. The theme is the same: a victorious adolescent. But in Michelangelo's work everything centers in the victory of the youth over the barbarian, prostrate under the boy's knee. In the *Amor Victorious* the youthful nude, painted with so much care and capability, is interpreted as though he were an unwilling model taken from the street and artfully arranged in a Michelangelesque pose. The musical instruments on the floor, the arms, and the sharply pleated garment are handled with the precision of the style of the early still lifes.

The same model appears in the *Sacrifice of Isaac*, in the Uffizi, where, notwithstanding the concentrated light, there is again a fragment of a landscape painted with breadth and flashing lights. A trace of the artist's early manner is still apparent in the clear glass vase, holding jasmine and carnations, on the desk in the *Portrait of Maffeo Barberini* (Florence, Coll. Corsini), a successful interpretation of the poet-cardinal.

In summary, the various tendencies that may have contributed to the formation of Caravaggio's art are predominantly Lombard, Bergamasque, and Venetian. Later came his peculiar license in the handling of Michelangelesque motifs, which he reinterpreted in a naturalistic manner, as if to show a distinct distaste for the "heroic" style of Michelangelo.

Lombard influences are evident in Caravaggio, while from his teacher Peterzano (who boasted of being a pupil of Titian) he may have derived his admiration for the Venetians and for Correggio. His nocturnal effects he derived from the Campis several years later. But the early works are not characteristic of the "tenebrosi," and the influence of Bergamasque painters has been correctly recognized by Longhi. Though Bellori claims that Caravaggio went to Venice, such a trip is not very likely before his arrival in Rome, especially since there is

nothing in his art to indicate the necessity of a direct contact with Venice. It was possible for him to assimilate Venetian characteristics of style through Savoldo and other Venetians of the 16th century in Lombardy.

The beginning of a more complex and mature style can be easily identified with the works of the Contarelli Chapel in S. Luigi dei Francesi. The French Cardinal Matteo Contarelli (Mathieu Cointrel), who died in 1585, had bought the chapel in 1565 and then had become a benefactor of that church. On Sept. 13, 1565, the Cardinal made arrangements with Girolamo Muziano for the painted decoration (Bertolotti), and it is interesting to note that, in general, the iconographic conception was then the same as that later formulated by the Cavalier d'Arpino and Caravaggio. It was very probably d'Arpino who accepted the commission (May 27, 1591) to complete the chapel within two years, but Virgilio Crescenzi (executor of Cardinal Contarelli's will) died in December, 1592, and the work was delayed. From other documents it appears that very little was done in the chapel from the death of Cardinal Contarelli (1585) to the end of 1596 and the beginning of 1597.

Finally, on Nov. 6, 1597, an agreement was signed for final payment to be made to the Cavalier d'Arpino after the completion of the decoration. At this time, though it was still d'Arpino who was commissioned to execute the paintings, he actually did no more than the frescoes on the vault. On the basis of this documentation Caravaggio's paintings can be dated about 1600, almost contemporary with his paintings in S. Maria del Popolo (Hess, 1951). On June 27, 1600, Caravaggio is mentioned for the first time in relation to the chapel. In December, 1600, October, 1602, and February, 1603, a carpenter was paid for paneling the areas in which the paintings were to be placed and for furnishing the stretchers.

We cannot believe that the Cavalier d'Arpino, of his own free will, left to Caravaggio the main decoration in the chapel, especially since the relationship between the two men had deteriorated into rivalry. According to Baglione, it was Cardinal del Monte who secured the commission for Caravaggio, while Bellori states that the artist was introduced to Virgilio Crescenzi by the Cavalier Marino. This notion, however, is unacceptable. Unlike Bellori, Baglione was an eyewitness, and we must remember that at this time Caravaggio was the guest of Cardinal del Monte in the Palazzo Madama, situated a few steps from S. Luigi dei Francesi.

It is quite likely that Caravaggio's earliest work for the Contarelli Chapel was the altar painting, the first version of *St. Matthew*, which was refused by the church authorities. In this first version the artist seems to have added to the results of past experience a vigorous naturalism. The protagonist is St. Matthew, depicted with a great book resting on his knee, patiently writing in large Hebrew characters. The youthful face of the angel has a patronizing look as he impatiently guides the rough hand of the saint. The conception shows a beautiful pattern of gestures, enhanced by a light precisely distributed over each figure and object. As in the *Amor Victorious*, the forms are firm and compact, and there is a clear desire to obtain a bold projection from the shadow, sustained by the position of the saint's legs, which are crossed in the foreground as though jutting from the canvas toward the viewer. The painting was conceived in relation to the actual daylight in the chapel, thus creating a unity between pictorial and physical light, a procedure which Caravaggio was to employ again.

The differences between the first, rejected painting and the second version, now on the altar, are not only in changed proportions. The first version was refused because the worshipers might have disliked the pose of the saint with his peasant's feet just at the edge of the altar, and consequently the artist painted the same subject from an entirely different point of view. The measure of Caravaggio's genius is apparent in the solution of this difficult problem. Compelled to reconsider a motif already executed, he was able, nevertheless, to deepen the emotional content of the first conception, even though he now had to face the problem (often to recur in his work) of making the angel appear from above. The figure of the angel, surrounded by the flowing drapery, was modeled by the light penetrating the shadow. St. Matthew, in a new and energetic pose, turns his fine, inspired face to the light. The general tone of the painting was profoundly modified, having lost a certain crudity of contours and presenting a better relation between figures and surroundings. The saint turns outward, his knee on a wooden stool which casts a shadow on the floor and barely seems to maintain its equilibrium, as if it were about to fall. The instability of the pose lends a new expressive intensity to the entire work.

The painting on the left wall of the chapel is the *Calling of St. Matthew* (PL. 41). In order to explain its composition we must take into consideration Caravaggio's determination not to abandon the technique of oil painting. He considered this technique more effective than fresco in rendering form realistically, more flexible in making unforeseen revisions, and above all, more intimately tied to the Venetian and Lombard traditions. It was normal to use fresco in decorating lateral walls of chapels, and Girolamo Muziano intended to decorate the Contarelli Chapel in this way. There was only one other example at that time of the use of oil painting for side walls, namely, the decorations by Cigoli and Santi di Tito in the chapel of S. Girolamo dei Fiorentini in 1599.

Caravaggio's use of light as a determining factor in the construction of figures assumes a definite importance for the first time in the *Calling of St. Matthew*. The scene occurs in a room into which light enters from the right and above, and this further emphasizes the clear profiles and the closed window in the background. The figures, as in the later *Death of the Virgin* (Paris, Louvre), are illuminated by the light penetrating the room almost without warning. Thus the impression is of an uncommon occurrence, instantaneous but without great activity. The famous gesture of Christ, who beckons Saint Matthew by slowly lifting his hand toward him, is very effective because of the cone of light that accompanies the gesture and moves in the direction of the saint. This is the core of the splendid painting that marks Caravaggio's victory over the difficulty of interpreting a religious scene "in the grand manner" and at the same time putting it in terms of contemporary realism (see the costumes of the ruffians and the saint). This revolutionary work, marking the beginning of a new era in painting, can be compared with works of the great innovators: Giotto's *Resurrection of Lazarus*, in Padua, Masaccio's *Tribute Money*, in the Brancacci Chapel, and Michelangelo's *Creation of Adam*, in the Sistine Chapel. The comparison, naturally, is limited to the portrayal of divine power exercised over human activity. It is significant that Caravaggio, usually considered indifferent to religious values, should surpass his earlier realistic manner and produce one of the most striking of religious paintings.

The crisis that Caravaggio experienced in these initial works of large dimensions is documented by the *Martyrdom of St. Matthew* (PL. 37), intended for the opposite wall. This painting, together with others in the same chapel, has been X-rayed, and two previous versions (mentioned by Bellori) were found under the present surface, thus revealing a development through various stages to the final composition (Venturi, 1952; Wagner, 1958). In the early versions there remains perhaps some reminiscence of the manner of Girolamo Muziano, but, while we find just one revision in the *Calling*, nothing of the previous versions is retained in the final composition of the *Martyrdom*. In the latter, despite its great pictorial quality, we feel an uncertainty and irresoluteness, as if Caravaggio had tried to combine contrasting elements. This, however, because it is disconcerting, increases the air of drama. In the *Calling* there is no trace of mannerism (q.v.), while in the *Martyrdom* the naked executioner in the center and the figures in the foreground stem from 16th-century models. They are much less meaningful than the beautiful group at the left, where the artist's interest in the everyday world is so evident. His bohemian companions participate in the drama, and he even portrays himself in the background, his face turned toward the scene of execution.

Almost contemporary with the Contarelli Chapel is the Cerasi Chapel in S. Maria del Popolo. The contract for the

execution of the two lateral paintings, the *Crucifixion of St. Peter* and the *Conversion of St. Paul*, is dated Sept. 23, 1600, and the final payment to the artist was made on Nov. 10, 1601. Again Caravaggio executed a first version of these paintings "which did not please the patron" (Baglione). Some scholars identify the first version of the *Conversion of St. Paul* with the one now in the Odelscalchi-Balbi Collection. This hypothesis, however, appears stylistically unsupportable. The Baldi painting is more immature than any of the works in S. Luigi dei Francesi and S. Maria del Popolo. Both the coloring and the composition seem to place the painting at the end of Caravaggio's first period, epitomizing but not yet surpassing his past achievements.

One factor, not sufficiently stressed by the critics, was Caravaggio's concern about effectively relating his paintings to the place they were to hang, even when the paintings were executed in his studio and not on the site. The two canvases in S. Maria del Popolo are the result of a careful study of the physical situation and lighting of the Cerasi Chapel, which is narrow, with barely enough space for the two paintings to be seen as a unit. Caravaggio obviously took advantage of foreshortening to make it possible to view his pictures also from outside the chapel. It is thus evident that the abrupt diagonal structure of the *Crucifixion of St. Peter* depends on its location. The figures are here compelled to move within the frame created by the inverted cross; and the result is of such a dynamic and plastic intensity as to recall some of the famous compositional solutions of the Renaissance. The same is true in the *Conversion of St. Paul* (PL. 34), but with a different expressive implication. In this scene the blinding light has prostrated the saint, who, lying on the ground, is on the verge of consciousness, while the gesture of his outstretched arms indicates very eloquently the new faith that begins to possess him. In contrast, the great horse, lifting his hoof to avoid striking his master, creates a zone of calm and realistic contemplation in this singular and tightly contained composition. The artist, who was not at his best in scenes of action, has here achieved a stillness paradoxically charged with movement. We imagine the previous rearing of the horse and the commotion created by an unusual event, so many traces of which are still apparent in the earlier painting in the Balbi Collection.

The *Deposition of Christ* (Vat. Mus.) was intended for the Vittrice Chapel in S. Maria in Vallicella and was executed between Jan. 9, 1602, and Sept. 6, 1604 (Lopresti, 1922), most probably in 1603. In this large canvas, always considered Caravaggio's strongest and most complete work, we have the most "classical" expression of three-dimensional space. The figures are held within an imaginary prism suggested by the stone that serves as their base. It is evident that the artist conceived the grandiose structure of the painting almost as if it were sculpture, carving into the block formed by the human figures and drawing each one gradually out of the shadows and into the light which focuses sharply on the figure of Christ held by the bearers. But a strong sense of humanity is contained in this geometric severity, thereby communicating a profound and lasting sentiment. The *Deposition* was always considered a great work because it has both the monumental qualities of "classic" painting and the realistic force of the new art. Rubens produced a free interpretation of the design (now, Ottawa, Nat. Gall.); and it is interesting to know of the existence of a water color by Cézanne inspired by a reproduction of this famous painting, for it clearly shows the volumetric aspect of Caravaggio's work.

From 1600 on, biographical information becomes fuller because of the many lawsuits in which Caravaggio was involved. On Oct. 25, 1600, the architect Onorio Longhi, a compatriot and friend of Caravaggio, declared in a lawsuit that the painter was convalescing (Bertolotti). On Aug. 23, 1603, a famous lawsuit initiated by Baglione charged Onorio Longhi, Orazio Gentileschi, Caravaggio, and Filippo Trisegni with circulating a defamatory pamphlet. The documents relating to it, and especially the well-known deposition by Caravaggio (published by Bertolotti and more recently by Samek Lodovici), reveal much about the Roman society of that time. Caravaggio was arrested on Sept. 11, 1603, but was released on the 25th of the same month through the intercession of the French Ambassador. In 1604 he was in the Marches, but he soon appeared again in Rome, where he was denounced by the servant of the tavern keeper Del Moro, in whose face Caravaggio had thrown a plate of artichokes.

Felice Cavalletti's bequest in favor of the first chapel on the left in the Church of S. Agostino (Sept. 4, 1603) determines the earliest date for the chapel's altar painting, the *Madonna di Loreto* (also known as the *Madonna of the Pilgrims*), while the latest date is Mar. 2, 1606, when the monks presented Cardinal Scipione Borghese with the painting that had adorned the chapel up to that time (Lopresti, 1922, p. 176). The Virgin and Child, bent toward the kneeling followers, can be compared to certain Hellenistic prototypes. However, this classical allusion was intended merely to give the figure of the Virgin a greater sculptural force. The main idea was to exploit the perspective foreshortening from below in order to make the worshipers appear more grandiose. Baglione speaks of this painting and the scandal it created. As with the first version of the *St. Matthew*, there was great objection to the dirty feet of one of the pilgrims. Baglione says, "He painted in a natural manner a Madonna di Loreto. There are two pilgrims, a man with muddy feet, a woman with a torn and dirty bonnet. The populace made a great clamor over the disparaging treatment of certain elements which should have been handled with more respect in such an important work." Distracted by such observations, Caravaggio's contemporaries did not notice the new dignity permeating the holy group and the great pictorial quality of the whole painting, especially in the young and vital figure of the Virgin.

A model called Lena (Hess, 1954), who seems to have been selected to pose as the Virgin, was the cause of another more serious fight, followed by a lawsuit. Caravaggio, motivated by jealousy, on July 20, 1605, in Piazza Navona, attacked and wounded his rival Mariano Pasqualone, assistant of the notary Spada, and was arrested. The story, which was told by Passeri almost seventy years later, is confirmed by the documents relating to the trial. Also documented is Caravaggio's flight from Rome and his arrival in Genoa before Aug. 6, though on the 24th of the same month the artist was once again in Rome.

The *Virgin and Child with St. Anne* (PL. 38), known also as the *Madonna dei Palafrenieri* or the *Madonna of the Serpent*, was painted for the altar that the Palafrenieri of the Vatican hoped in vain to obtain in St. Peter's (Hess, 1957). The painting was delivered at the beginning of 1606, and after having been placed for some time in St. Peter's, it entered the collection of Scipione Borghese. In the Madonna we can recognize the same model who posed for the S. Agostino painting (Hess, 1954). Notwithstanding some passages of vigorous realism, this is not one of Caravaggio's best paintings. The scene, which perhaps would have been more effective in smaller scale, is in complete contrast with the monumental intentions of the artist. It may well have been painted reluctantly, as the artist, because of religious symbolism, was obliged to represent mother and child simultaneously killing the serpent of heresy.

The great *Death of the Virgin* (Paris, Louvre, PL. 39), painted for the first altar on the left in S. Maria della Scala, was removed by the monks because it lacked decorum and because, as usual, there were traces of excessive realism. Nonetheless, the work is an undoubted masterpiece. The artist seems here to repeat the successful handling of the *Calling of St. Matthew* in giving a unity to the scene. Furthermore, the painting shows an increased stability and an exceptional dramatic power. Grief is almost audible, and the light unites the large figures in one great block from which emerge the sorrowful faces of the apostles. The figure of the Virgin lies on the modest bed in peaceful death, the beauty of the modeling enhanced by the treatment of the light. The painting is rich in details of profound significance. The lean, sensitive hand of the dead woman is placed gently against the shadow of the pillow, and the weeping Magdalen, crouched in the foreground with hidden face, presents a highly dramatic figure, but a still greater poetic effect is achieved by the heavy folds of a large red drapery

in the upper part of the painting. It is as though a curtain were about to be lowered on one of the most intense treatments of the subject ever produced in painting.

Toward the end of his stay in Rome Caravaggio painted for Cardinal Scipione Borghese the *David with the Head of Goliath* (Rome, Borghese Gall.). According to the catalogue of Manilli (I. Manilli, *Villa Borghese fuori Porta Pinciana*, Rome, 1650) we have a self-portrait of the artist in the severed head of the giant. The painting is based on a contrast between light and shadow and acquires an even stronger significance in the opposition of the classic beauty of the youthful figure to the bloody head of Goliath.

On May 29, 1606, Caravaggio fatally wounded one Ranuccio Tomassoni in a fight during a game of tennis at Muro Torto. The painter, also wounded, fled to avoid arrest and found refuge in one of the Colonna castles, probably Paliano, Zagarolo, or Palestrina. During this period, which could not have extended beyond the end of 1606, Caravaggio painted for his protector a *Fainting Magdalen* and a *Christ At Emmaus*, probably the one in the Brera. The *Madonna of the Rosary* (Vienna, Kunsthist. Mus.; PL. 40), which must have been completed in Naples, if we are to recognize in it the portrait of Don Marzio Colonna, Duke of Zagarolo, was also painted at this time. In April, 1607, the Duke of Mantua purchased the *Death of the Virgin*, following the suggestion of Rubens, and exhibited it to the public for a week in Rome.

Caravaggio's sojourn in Naples probably took place in 1607, an extremely active year; Baglione says that he did many things there. The artist may have considered his Neapolitan stay but a temporary pause in his travels and was perhaps already anticipating his trip to Malta and working for the Grand Master of the Order. Yet in Naples he was to find new stimuli in the city's way of life and its natural tendency toward a realism that discovered its greatest champion in Caravaggio.

Neapolitan painting received from Caravaggio a new impetus and a determination to overcome the mannerism that had taken hold of it. As in Rome, a group of painters were deeply impressed by his art. Although it is not possible to compile a complete list of the works executed by the artist in Naples, they include the *Flagellation of Christ* (Church of S. Domenico Maggiore), the *Seven Works of Mercy* (Church of Pio Monte della Misericordia), the *Madonna of the Rosary* (now in Vienna), a *Resurrection of Christ* (Church of S. Anna dei Lombardi, lost in the earthquake of 1805), the *Stigmatization of St. Francis* (lost), a *David* (now in Vienna, Kunsthist. Mus.), and a *Crucifixion of St. Andrew* (known through a copy in Toledo, Spain).

The very important painting of the *Madonna of the Rosary* (PL. 40), which was for sale in Naples in 1607, was evidently executed for an altar and, very probably, also refused. This canvas has the compositional clarity and the monumental structure of Caravaggio's main works; the group of the Madonna and Child contrasts sharply with the adoring multitude, to the characters of which, as always, the artist gave an assured individualization. Even the simple and essential gestures help to create that air of grandiose calm which, in Caravaggio, never results in immobility, but rather in a contained vigor.

In the composition of the *Flagellation* in S. Domenico Maggiore we seem to perceive once again a challenging attitude toward the painting by Sebastiano del Piombo in S. Pietro in Montorio in Rome. The Michelangelo influence evident in this celebrated painting had its effect on Caravaggio's well-composed grouping of contrapuntal figures, but his own imagination comes forth in the pose of the nude figure of Christ, carved with sculptural vigor from the shadows, the proud and sorrowful face turned downward. The figures of the three ruffians are, by comparison, rough and almost peasantlike as if bent by manual labor.

The composition of the *Seven Works of Mercy* (PL. 40) was far more complex and difficult, for the artist had to group in one painting the seven episodes pertaining to the religious theme and, furthermore, to represent the Virgin and Child among the angels above. All these figures were organized by Caravaggio into a unified synthesis of intertwining gestures and drapery. Some of the groups (such as the one at the left representing the elegant young man cutting his cape and giving half of it to the beggar) are quite beautiful; others seem handled more summarily and are made to stand out by the flashing light. A surprising manneristic intrusion is created in the upper group by the angel in violent foreshortening, reminiscent of Michelangelo's Christ in the *Conversion of St. Paul* in the Paolina Chapel. The group of the Virgin and Child, looking sadly upon the sorrows of the world, is extremely tender.

The works executed in Naples show an increase of movement in the figures and a breaking up of light into reflections and sharp accents. Typical of this is the *David* in Vienna, especially if we compare it to the stillness of the one in the Borghese Gallery. The rectangular shape of the canvas seems to have been chosen by Caravaggio in order to develop more freely the concept of movement; the figure seems to proceed briskly toward the right, holding the severed head of Goliath as a trophy.

His trip to Malta, which took place at this time, might have been the "great adventure" of his feverish and unstable artistic career, if we are to judge from the reception that was extended to him and the bestowal of the cross of *cavaliere di grazia*, on July 14, 1608. He could have become, had his exceptional temperament permitted it, something similar to what Mattia Preti later became, the "official" painter of the Order, heaped with work and with glory. Instead, his stay there was, as usual, quite brief, from 1607 to Oct. 6, 1608, the day he climbed down the wall of the jail in which he had been imprisoned for a slight inflicted on a knight, and fled by ship to Syracuse, so rapidly, as Bellori puts it, that "he could not be overtaken."

While in Malta he seems to have executed five paintings: *St. Jerome Writing* and *The Beheading of John the Baptist* for the Cathedral of S. Giovanni at La Valletta, *Portrait of Alof de Wignacourt*, standing (Paris, Louvre), and another portrait of the same person seated (now lost), and the *Sleeping Cupid* (Florence, Pitti). Some scholars doubt the authenticity of the handsome portrait of the standing Grand Master, with the page next to him holding his cloak and his headpiece; but the qualities of the painting, though somewhat less finished in the lower part, remind us of Caravaggio's manner. The chronological objections to this portrait do not seem to constitute a serious difficulty in identifying it as by Caravaggio. The importance of the figure is reminiscent of the 16th-century Venetian and Bergamasque traditions, but with a novel approach. Encased in his gleaming armor, the Grand Master holds with both hands the staff of command, like an early-17th-century Pippo Spano (I, PL. 245) at the same time foreshadowing, in the innate pride and humanity of the figure, the great portrait style of Diego Velázquez.

On the right-hand border of the *St. Jerome* we see the coat of arms of Father Ippolito Malaspina, a friend of Alof de Wignacourt, who evidently commissioned this painting for the Italian Chapel in the Cathedral of S. Giovanni. This is not only one of the most successful interpretations of a theme already treated by Caravaggio several times, but also a painting of extraordinary vigor and realism.

On the back of the *Sleeping Cupid* in the Pitti Palace we read, in contemporary writing, "Opera di Michelangelo Maresi da Caravaggio i(n) Malta 1608." Even though the painting is considerably yellowed by age, there are noticeable those characteristics of color, almost silky in the light and warm in the shadows, which are to be found later in the Sicilian works. The singular effects of the radiant light in this realistic painting are in strong contrast to the classical theme. The hypothesis that it was painted under artificial lighting might explain the livid hue of the flesh and the rough and sharp shadows. In an attempt to determine its origin more precisely, we could presume that it was related to an allegorical theme, and since it represents Cupid asleep after having unstrung his bow, the artist might have been commissioned by one of the Knights of Malta, who were under vows of chastity.

Bellori gives interesting details in describing the great canvas (11 ft., $10^{1}/_{8}$ in. × 17 ft., $^{3}/_{4}$ in.) of the *Beheading of John*

*the Baptist* (PL. 42), painted by Caravaggio for the Cathedral of S. Giovanni in Malta, and it is worthwhile to quote his words. He says that the Grand Master Alof de Wignacourt, having awarded the painter the Cross of Malta, had him paint "for the Church of S. Giovanni the *Beheading of St. John* who has fallen to the ground while the executioner, as though he had not quite killed him with his sword, takes his knife from his side and grasps the saint by the hair to cut his head from the body . . . . In this work Caravaggio used every power of his brush, having worked at it so feverishly that he let the canvas show through in the halftones." Recent painstaking restorations have confirmed the high quality of this exceptional painting, which had been reduced to a seeming monochrome by time and previous unskillful restorations. The artist's signature was clearly revealed, drawn at the bottom of the painting, on the ground, in the same maroon color as that of the puddle of blood gushing from the neck of the saint. The canvas was ordered by the Grand Master for the Oratory annexed to the Cathedral of S. Giovanni at La Valletta, and the artist himself decided on its position at the far end of the bare room, rather high above the altar, so that it could be seen by anyone entering the Oratory. A splendid carved and gilded frame, bearing the coat of arms of Wignacourt, still frames it today and helps isolate the dramatic action of the painting from the space of the room itself. The Oratory, of severe 16th-century style, was later redecorated in the baroque manner; canvases by Mattia Preti were added to it and elaborate pieces of goldsmith work, designed by Bernini, were placed on the altar.

The *Beheading* marks the beginning of a more complete synthesis in Caravaggio's method of composition. The few figures, grouped at the left around the agonized body of the Baptist, are arranged in a semicircular scheme which is repeated in the background by the rusticated archway. At the right, behind a grate, two prisoners are looking on at the execution with foreboding. A rough rope, almost a symbol of torture, hangs from above and slides through a large ring attached to the wall. All has become essential: the gestures stem from an irresistible logic, and only the presence of the young woman, who rushes forward on her gruesome errand (her white arm bare, and the reflection of the rich basin mirrored on her shadowed face), adds an accent of pathos to the sinister atmosphere of the painting.

After landing in Syracuse, the fugitive artist painted, during the last months of 1608, the vast composition of the *Burial of St. Lucy*, for the Church of S. Lucia. There are evident traces of the Malta *Beheading* in the emphasis given the bare rear wall and in the gigantic figures of the gravediggers in the foreground. In Messina he painted a *Nativity* for the Church of the Capuchins, now in the Museo Nazionale there, one of the most harmonious and charming canvases of Caravaggio's late period. The artist painted it on a dark ground, modeling the faces of the shepherds with simplicity and barely defining the ox and the ass in the back of the barn. But the group of the Virgin and Child is permeated with an intimate spirituality.

The *Raising of Lazarus* (Messina, Mus. Naz.; PL. 43), another large work executed by the artist in his Sicilian refuge (where agents of the insulted Knight of Malta could not have been very far away), was painted between 1608 and 1609. According to a document published by Saccà (1906), the painting was executed between Dec. 6, 1608, and June 10 of the following year and commissioned for the Church of the Crociferi by the Genoese merchant Giovan Battista de' Lazzari, whose home was in Messina. The name of the patron accounts for the theme of the painting, which is one of the most dramatic of Caravaggio's works, even though here and there we see traces of a certain haste in those large areas which are barely covered by paint. The theme of divine intervention, represented with absolute realism, as in the famous *Calling of St. Matthew*, acquires here a three-dimensionality approaching high relief. The radiant light, which throws the figures into sharp relief against the bare background, emphasizes the faces and the folds of the garments. The costumes are now composed of grand sweeps of drapery and no longer reflect contemporary taste. The action, though gravely solemn, is made more dramatic by the gesture of Christ and the immediate response of Lazarus, whose body is almost crucified in space by the impaling force of the light and whose rigid gesture of response is appropriate to one who has only partly come back to life.

The last important painting of Caravaggio known to us is the *Adoration with St. Francis and St. Lawrence*, executed for the Oratorio di S. Lorenzo in Palermo. Smaller than the other paintings of the same period, this canvas concentrates the light upon the gentle figure of the Virgin adoring the Child. This young Caravaggesque Madonna is perhaps the last homage paid by the artist to his personal feminine ideal. Seated on the ground, without trinkets or rhetorical flourishes, she is a humble plebeian flower in the midst of his violent and hectic life. At the right there is a beautiful realistic passage in the shepherd with the wide hat, one of the most vivid examples of Caravaggio's genius as a precursor of artists from Velázquez to Courbet.

Caravaggio's art and life were to be concluded in a dramatic finale, as though his destiny had led him fatally to a premature death. Caravaggio had gone from Palermo to Naples by Oct. 24, 1609, at which time there is a report that he was once again involved in an armed fight. Evidently under surveillance, since his arrival in Sicily, by men engaged by the knight with whom he had had difficulties at La Valletta, he was recognized at the entrance of the tavern of Cerriglio, attacked, and wounded so seriously that, as Baglione said, "because of the blows received he was almost unrecognizable." Though close to death, he nevertheless recovered, and some months later, about the end of June, 1610, sailed to Port'Ercole, then occupied by Spain. While there it was rumored that, through the intercession of Cardinal Gonzaga, he had been granted an amnesty to return to Rome. But the tragic destiny that had accompanied him all his life still persecuted him, for, after landing in Port'Ercole, he was arrested by mistake and imprisoned for a few days. When he regained his freedom, he could not find his belongings or the boat he had rented. After wandering aimlessly on the beach, desperate, without help, and plagued by violent fevers, he died on July 18, 1610. On July 28 of the same year the *Avvisi* of Rome announced his death: "Word has been received of the death of Michel Angelo Caravaggio, the famous painter, renowned in the handling of color and painting from life, following an illness in Port'Ercole."

Caravaggio's biography reveals the tragedy of a personality in rebellion against the contemporary world and has always influenced any evaluation of Caravaggio's art.

Van Mander (*Schilderboek*, Alkmaar, 1604) bears out the legend of the peculiar and quarrelsome temperament of Caravaggio when he writes about his art: "For he is one of those who pay little attention to the work of others, and yet will not even praise his own work . . . . Consequently he does not execute a single brushstroke without close study from life, which he copies and paints . . . ." That the tale of a revolutionary painter, individualistic, defiant of study and tradition, and interested only in the direct imitation of nature, should have originated so early can be explained by presuming that Caravaggio himself openly advocated this policy in words and behavior. Biographers attribute to him polemic statements, and his patron Vincenzo Giustiniani (letter to Teodoro Amideno, ca. 1620–1625, published in *Raccolta di Lettere*, ed. G. Bottari, VI, Milan, 1822, p. 121 ff.) recalls a statement of principle expressed by Caravaggio in a very concise manner: "And Caravaggio said that it took as much care and skill to produce a good painting of flowers as it did of figures." This principle was contrary to the whole theoretical system of mannerism: to the hierarchy of themes he opposed the thesis that everything is worth painting, thus the subject becomes almost a pretext for painting and the value of art is transferred from subject to style.

To understand Caravaggio's statement more fully, we must realize that the artist meant to dignify still life to the same degree as figure painting. He insisted, indeed, on the "good" painting of flowers, which thus acquire the same dignity as the human figure. All this was contrary to the deep-seated conviction that the painting of figures was more "difficult" and required more application than other types of painting.

The peremptory, expressive, and rebellious vigor of Caravaggio's work created immediate interest; and since he worked in Rome, the artistic capital of Europe, his impact was very great. However, his contemporaries did not, in general, value Caravaggio's work much more highly than that of the Cavalier d'Arpino, or even of Cristoforo Roncalli. Rubens himself, who showed so much interest in him, considered one of his paintings inferior to one of Roncalli's, a judgment we find very surprising today. The true critics and partisans of the artist were a number of painters who were impressed by the novelty and the high quality of his style and so began to imitate him, while to some merchants goes the credit for having discovered the artist while he was still young. As for the great collectors who bought his paintings, they often preferred works by the Carraccis and their followers. In other words, none of them, though adding to their collections paintings by the innovator, consciously accepted his essential quality. Centuries passed and Courbet and impressionism appeared before Caravaggio's contribution was understood and accepted as an illuminating factor in art.

The hostility of the Cavalier d'Arpino and Federico Zuccari — the fashionable artists of the time and the exponents of conceptual painting or mannerism — against the young Lombard artist was completely implacable. Baglione writes that, as soon as the Chapel in S. Luigi dei Francesi was unveiled, "Federico Zuccari came to look at it and said in my presence: 'What is all the fuss about?' and as he carefully examined the entire work, he added, 'I don't see anything here but the thought (*pensiero*) of Giorgione in the picture of the saint called to the Apostolate by Christ.' Smiling and marveling at all this excitement, he shrugged his shoulders and then turned his back and left." This was probably meant to be an open accusation of plagiarism, denying the idea of absolute imitation of life maintained by the artist, who claimed he had no other teacher but nature. Zuccari's comment was meant to show that Caravaggio did, in fact, have teachers and that he even resorted to old and outdated Giorgionesque models.

However, we must stress the fact that this reference to Giorgione is actually to the "thought," which at that time meant "manner" and "custom," while nothing is said of the great innovation in the use of light. Pure "mimesis" (or imitation) was, in fact, condemned by theoreticians. A few years later Giovan Battista Agucci wrote (1606–1615): "Bassano can be compared to Peraikos in that he depicted the worst in nature, and many of the modern painters have done the same. Among these, Caravaggio, most excellent in color, can be compared to Demetrius, since he abandoned the idea of beauty and was interested in depicting reality." In these words we already find the distinction between "manner of painting" and "content," so prejudicial to the correct appreciation of Caravaggio's art by his contemporaries.

Another current theory that Caravaggio undermined was that of "decorum," meaning not a sense of moral propriety, but rather, according to the classicistic theory, fidelity to the historical image. And since religious literature, encouraged by the hierarchy, exalted the beauty and nobility of the Virgin and saints in accordance with an idealized official art, Caravaggio was criticized for his choice of gross models, and therefore many of his paintings were removed from altars. This was the case with the *Death of the Virgin*, originally in S. Maria della Scala, in which he is said to have used the body of a young woman who had drowned to represent the Virgin.

His attitude opposing "decorum" was, in fact, the result of a different religious sentiment, and accusations could be uttered only by passive followers of the prevailing Counter Reformation point of view. Courageous collectors, such as Sannesio, Del Monte, Giustiniani, Scipione Borghese, and the Duke of Mantua, were happy to secure the paintings that were rejected as altarpieces. They did not particularly care that Caravaggio's works were unorthodox, since they admired above all the quality of his art. On the other hand, these works did not enter their collections as altarpieces. It was only later that the accusation of lack of decorum and of vulgarity became widespread. It is to the credit of art lovers and (what is more important) of high prelates that they developed a collector's appreciation of his art.

The well-known lawsuit of 1603 (Bertolotti; Samek Ludovici) reveals the relationship between Caravaggio and the Roman artistic world. "In my use of the word," he declares in one of his depositions, "a good artist means a man who knows how to paint well and to imitate natural things well." In this deposition he includes among the good artists Annibale Carracci, whose painting in S. Caterina dei Funari he admired, Prospero Orsi, Antonio Tempesta, and Sigismondo Laer, painters with a style different from his own, while, besides d'Arpino, he is antagonistic to the very painters who imitated him most: Orazio Gentileschi, Baglione, Tommaso Salini.

His refusal to have collaborators and his contempt for his followers were other aspects of Caravaggio's independence. He was opposed to schools of art and the imitation of the masters, and understandably did not want to assume the role of master himself. This exclusiveness is due also to the high opinion he had of himself and to the innate conviction that his artistic credo was inimitable, since everyone must rediscover for himself the values of concrete reality.

The antithesis between Caravaggio and Annibale Carracci was not yet deeply felt when they were still both alive, as is demonstrated by the consideration they had for one another. A further confirmation of this lies in the fact that Vincenzo Giustiniani places them on the same level, both opposed to mannerism: "The twelfth category is the most perfect," he writes in the aforementioned letter to Amideno, "because it is more difficult in that it joins the tenth and the eleventh categories, that is, painting in a manneristic style but deriving the model from nature. Many of the great masters painted in this way ... and in our age Caravaggio, Carracci, Guido Reni, and others. Some of these inclined more to 'manner,' others to 'nature,' though without ever departing too much from either way, emphasizing good design and true coloring, and proper and true lighting...." Giustiniani did not consider Caravaggio's art imitation, but rather detected in it a certain "idealism" or "manner," in which there was an affirmation of the value of "style" which differentiated it from realism. Giulio Mancini, who wrote about 1620, was the first to define the cleavage between Caravaggio and the Carracci, describing the style of the former with particular insight: "It is peculiar to this school [the Caravaggesque] to use a unified light coming from above and without reflections, as would occur in a room with one window and with the walls painted black. The result is that the light areas would be very light and the dark areas very dark, giving relief to the painting, though in an unnatural manner never conceived by previous masters." This indicates that Mancini recognized the originality of the Caravaggesque style in terms of its contrasts of light and shade but, in the last analysis, considered it to be antinaturalistic in light and color, in spite of the fact that the painter worked directly from a model. Elsewhere, Mancini declares that Caravaggio's portraits do not achieve likeness, while he credits Annibale Carracci with this particular ability. Caravaggio's realism is, a priori, an abstraction from the reality of life, which consists of movement and action and is determined by an occurrence in time. Caravaggio, because of his attachment to the model, as Mancini notes, lacks movement and action. He implicitly acknowledges Caravaggio's intention of using "as much care and skill" in a still life as in a painting of figures, but he rebukes him for painting figures as if they were still life. Mancini also introduced the accusation of lack of "decorum" into the evaluation of Caravaggio's work. Thus we find in him the first expression of the theories that culminated in Bellori's criticism.

Mancini's opinion is that the point of contact between Caravaggio and Carracci is in their opposition to mannerism (q.v.) as a result of the return to a study of nature, but that their individual interpretations of what constitutes "nature" are antithetical. Annibale Carracci exalts and idealizes nature. He selects and synthesizes natural detail and the "idea" of beauty; from the particular he proceeds to the universal through the experience of history; he combines imitation and invention,

nature and idea, truth and probability. Caravaggio, on the other hand, halts at the natural event, eliminating any narrative, historical, or dynamic development. The moment portrayed by Annibale is continuous and includes at the same time what preceded and what will follow, thus making his painting "speak." The immobility of Caravaggio's figures, on the other hand, is revealed by the ray of light which defines them. In substance, Mancini points out not so much Caravaggio's lack of classical idealization as the limitation of his art, which, in rejecting movement and action, rejects also the narrative and decorative possibilities of painting.

After 1620, about the time Mancini was writing his biography, Caravaggio's popularity began to decline. Most of the artists who in the second decade of the 17th century had followed his example left Rome, while the fame of Guido Reni, Domenichino, and Albani, followers of the Carraccis and the strongest rivals of Caravaggio, was increasing. Malvasia records the hostile statements made by Albani in regard to Caravaggio (*Felsina Pittrice*, Bologna, 1678), and later writers (such as Scannelli, *Microcosmo della Pittura*, Cesena, 1657) bear traces of this anti-Caravaggio attitude, yet they maintain their admiration for him and regard him as the founder of naturalism, an artistic current that continued to live in every Italian movement.

Baglione devotes three and one-half pages to the life of Caravaggio, and his attitude is influenced by the dissension between them. Of this there is ample documentation in the archives of the lawsuit in which Giovanni Baglione had sued the artist, together with Onorio Longhi, Orazio Gentileschi, and Filippo Trisegni for libel. This happened in 1603, yet Baglione, 40 years later, even though he could not deny the originality and the great quali y of the painter, was unable to remain entirely unbiased. In his biography he praises Caravaggio's ability to paint objects and figures with great realism. Typical is his accurate description of the *Lute Player*, painted by the artist in his early Roman years: "In it is a carafe of flowers filled with water in which one can easily distinguish the reflections of a window and other objects in the room. On the flowers is fresh dew which is rendered with exquisite accuracy." We seem to perceive a certain satisfaction in the manner in which the biographer, a former friend and imitator of the artist, carefully lists paintings rejected because of "lack of decorum" or because they caused a scandal. On the other hand, Baglione is compelled to close his short biography (useful especially for its information on Caravaggio's works) with a positive judgment that defines quite well his critical position. He writes, "If Michelangelo Amerigi had not died so soon, he would have done a great deal for art through his great ability to paint from nature, even though he lacked judgment in choosing the good and omitting the bad." In these words there is an echo of the esthetic classicistic tradition favored by official academicism and largely subscribed to by the Carraccis themselves.

Giovanni Pietro Bellori made marginal notes in Baglione's *Vite*, where he maintained that they had not really been written by Baglione but by Tronsarelli, who knew nothing of painting.

It is interesting to examine Bellori's marginal notes in the edition at the Accademia Nazionale dei Lincei in order to understand Caravaggio's influence on art in Rome. In one of these notes we read that "Michelangelo painted all his figures in a medium light, and he placed them all in one plane, without grading them." When Baglione asserted that the success obtained by the paintings in S. Luigi dei Francesi was due to people envious of the fame enjoyed by the Cavalier d'Arpino, Bellori brusquely wrote, "Baglione, idiot!" and added, "Caravaggio deserves great praise, as he was the only one who attempted to imitate nature, as opposed to the general trend in which painters imitated other painters." In this important statement Bellori, though mainly stressing Caravaggio's realism, anticipated that description of Caravaggio as a painter "without teachers" which became so popular with later critics.

We owe the first systematic criticism of Caravaggio to Bellori who, by influencing Félibien, Dufresnoy, and other outstanding writers of the late 17th century, established the antithesis between Caravaggio and the Carraccis in those rigorous terms that have been maintained to the present. Bellori condemns the mannerism of d'Arpino and of Zuccari, and the mere fact that he selected Caravaggio from among the most important artists of his century and wrote his biography is proof of his substantial appreciation of the artist and his historical importance.

Though the antimanneristic revolt of Caravaggio is praised by Bellori, his art is found lacking in "idea" and in "decorum." "Idea" originates in nature, yet supersedes it and becomes unique in art, but Caravaggio works without "idea" and achieves art through mere technique. While the Bamboccianti (q.v.) imitated the baser aspects of nature, their choice of a theme in nature could be justified as genre; Caravaggio's art, on the other hand, is without choice, lacks imagination, and is antinaturalistic, inasmuch as impressionable nature is not perfect nature, a condition achieved only through "idea."

Bellori criticizes his "excessive relief" (just as earlier Mancini had criticized the lighting which gives relief, but is not natural). That is, he disapproves of Caravaggio's representation of figures as divorced from an intelligible spatial perspective organization. The literary translation of the painting, which Bellori makes so effectively, attests to his ability to understand the stylistic value of Caravaggio's art, even if he criticizes it on a theoretical basis. Some of his very perceptive notes on the varied technique used by Caravaggio are quite useful, and his insight has often been confirmed by direct examination of Caravaggio's painting in more recent times, after cleaning has brought the paintings back to their original state.

Classicism later offered criticism of much the same tenor: lack of design, anatomical errors, inability to compose, lack of decorum and of nobility. The situation grew worse when Caravaggio's style began to be confused with the luministic and naturalistic trend. For example, Passeri (*Vite de' pittori, scultori ed architetti*, ed. Hess, Vienna, 1934), about 1673, claimed that Guercino was a follower of Caravaggio, a statement that, at least in this form, appears inexact. In the 18th century Francesco Algarotti (*Saggio sopra la pittura*, Bologna, 1762) spoke of a particular "manner" common to Caravaggio, Velázquez, Ribera, Rembrandt, Piazzetta, and Tiepolo — the "naturalistic" and "luministic" style. With the low ebb of interest in Caravaggio's work during the 18th and 19th centuries, it became common to attribute to him any painting representing vulgar figures in a somber style — peasantlike saints, soldiers, or cardplayers.

Neoclassicism, with Winckelmann and Mengs, attacked both the Carraccis and Caravaggio as representing two opposed types of excess: the former because they were considered eclectic, the latter because he lacked discipline and was indifferent to antiquity and to Raphael, that is, to beauty in the classicist sense.

Romanticism inherited these traditional preconceived ideas and accentuated the mythical qualities of Caravaggio's personality. Franz Kugler (*Handbuch der Geschichte der Malerei seit Constantin dem Grossen*, Stuttgart, 1837) speaks of the "opposition of the naturalists (Caravaggio and followers) to the eclecticists (Carracci and followers); an opposition that was manifested not only with the brush, but even with dagger and poison." In Kugler's opinion, there is an almost tragic pathos in Caravaggio's paintings which contrasts with the wild passions that characterized his life, and in order to define this tragic and anticlassical beauty, he compares him with Michelangelo Buonarroti. With the exception of these rare demonstrations of intuition, the 19th century until the appearance of the *Cicerone* by Burckhardt (1st ed., Leipzig, 1858) universally condemned the vulgar or criminal aspect of his personality.

A reevaluation was initiated in 1906 by Wolfgang Kallab and was continued by Lionello Venturi in his study of 1910, and most notably by the numerous essays of Roberto Longhi. The latter extended his research into the vast group of Caravaggio's followers, thus laying the foundations for distinguishing the authentic works and evaluating the Caravaggesque phenomenon. While the first documents were being published (Orbaan, Lopresti, De Rinaldis, Venturi, Longhi, Pevsner, etc.), the reputation of the painter was undergoing a radical change.

In 1922, the exhibition of 17th- and 18th-century art at the Pitti Palace focused attention on Caravaggio and his realism. Paintings thus far neglected were being rediscovered (such as the *Bacchus* in the Uffizi), and it became apparent that Caravaggio was aiming at a purity of style that went beyond realism and achieved results equivalent to those of classicism and of the Renaissance. Caravaggio was coupled with artists such as Bronzino and Ingres and was finally described as the last of the classical Renaissance artists. In this we discern a leaning of taste and criticism toward the study of form, as opposed to that of content, which had so preoccupied the 19th century. Indeed, in 1922 Marangoni denied the artist's extreme realism, pointing out that this was often limited to the subject and not to the style.

Roberto Longhi energetically refuted the popular academic interpretation of mere naturalism, as well as the more recent view of the artist as the last Renaissance master. He established Caravaggio as of antibaroque orientation and an original phenomenon of the 17th century. As early as 1911 he placed the artist's formative phase in Lombard art of the 16th century, and cited as his predecessors, in addition to Peterzano, the Campis, Romanino, Moretto, and Savoldo, an opinion that is universally accepted today.

Longhi was perhaps not entirely free of the romantic "myth." He referred to Caravaggio's "indescribable precocity" and consequently established a chronology for the "child prodigy" that proved, in the light of more recent studies, to be not quite so exceptional. Longhi's numerous contributions to the study of Caravaggio and of his school culminated in the large exhibition of 1951 in Milan. His introduction to the catalogue of this exhibition — along with the biographical chronology that precedes the individual discussions of paintings — is a concise, comprehensive profile of the master and is especially important for its searching discussion of the artist's use of light, the result of which is to create form through a play of shadows that carves out the figures. Longhi's brief introduction is interesting also in that it defines the influence of Caravaggio's art. His early works introduce that "emotional atmosphere" that "was to permeate the neat exteriors and interiors of the great Dutch masters of the 17th century." In his approach to objects are seen the beginnings of the art of Velázquez and Franz Hals, and, in the incidence of the beam of light, a prelude to the "nocturnal magic" of Rembrandt.

The exhibition of 1951 was an important milestone in the history of Caravaggio studies and a starting point for new discoveries, new documents, and authentication of works (see especially the series of personal contributions by R. Longhi, D. Mahon, J. Hess). It also produced numerous monographs on Caravaggio that have examined critical problems thus far neglected, such as those by R. Longhi, L. Venturi, B. Berenson, W. Friedländer, R. Hinks, F. Baumgart, J. Bialostocki, and H. Wagner.

In the light of the most recent criticism (Friedländer, Wagner), the myth of Caravaggio as the anticlassical painter who acknowledged no teachers and scorned the study of other masters is greatly weakened. Caravaggio himself originated the myth; but though he professed to have no teacher but nature, he certainly used his eyes and his memory, so that many years later he could recall the works of Correggio, Raphael, Michelangelo, and Lorenzo Lotto. He also looked at the contemporary works of Annibale Carracci and at ancient sculpture. Careful analysis has revealed Caravaggio's dependence on his cultural environment. This revelation denies the tale of his being uneducated, primitive, or romantic.

Yet his cultural environment was employed by the artist in an extremely personal manner. He not only selected the motifs of his compositions with instinctive vigor, but often appropriated them with a critical intent, avoiding the meaning they might have had in the works of other masters. This is evident from his frequent use of motifs from Michelangelo to which, however, he gave entirely opposite meanings. The absence of original drawings by the artist, though signifying that he did not attach too much importance to them, does not prove that he did not possess sketchbooks (very popular among artists) in which he annotated, in addition to "first ideas," rapid notes of the work of others. This would explain the reminders of movement of figures and compositional attitudes, rather than of precise pictorial details.

The transition from genre to monumental painting, which occurred in 1600 with the Contarelli Chapel in S. Luigi dei Francesi, is typical of the growth of the artist. Caravaggio develops from genre to a kind of secular "conversazione," and, finally, to the great religious compositions, almost as though he wanted to maintain his prestige before the "grand manner" of Annibale Carracci and the Cavalier d'Arpino. But he never gave up his conviction of the power of realism, which he continued to employ with deepening effect.

Friedländer studied the religious ideology and the social conscience of Caravaggio. To deal with the supernatural as though it were sensible reality was in agreement with the religious basis of the spiritual exercises of St. Ignatius Loyola, which teach spiritual comprehension through the use of the senses. These spiritual exercises were very popular and were practiced by St. Charles Borromeo, Archbishop of Milan (the city in which Caravaggio was an apprentice) and by St. Philip Neri. Caravaggio painted for the Augustinians, the Carmelites, the Dominicans, and the Oratorians. He was very close to such people as the Vittrice, the Crescenzi, and Pomarancio, all of them associated with the Oratorians.

Caravaggio, therefore, worked within a particular religious current that preached humility, simplicity, and loyalty to the Holy Scriptures and demanded that the Virgin not be represented as a beauty of courtly elegance. This inner religious feeling is undeniably present in his art and becomes more dramatic in his later works, where the thought of death and martyrdom becomes almost an obsession. Caravaggio's saints, unlike those of Guido Reni, do not gaze heavenward, and their visions seem to originate from within. It is a surprising observation that the characters he uses in "worldly" themes lend themselves equally effectively to compositions of religious allegory: modern clothes indicate the everyday world, while classical vestments indicate eternity.

The contrast with the religious painting of his time is constant in Caravaggio, and not just because of the attractive simplicity of his compositions; it is manifest also in his obvious uneasiness in dealing with supernatural phenomena. Celestial apparitions, the intervention of angels on the scene, all those motifs that the newborn baroque had inherited from mannerism, found this artist unresponsive and sometimes clumsy.

Though he could not translate everything into human terms, he was definitely oriented toward a realistic and concrete interpretation even of religious events. When he had to portray them, therefore, Caravaggio made his apparitions substantial and "true," introducing them with sudden flashes in the dark background of the canvas, as though the shadows were bursting open to sustain his young angels leaning, from the platform of clouds or drapery, toward mankind on earth.

SOURCES. G. Mancini, Considerazioni sulla pittura, ed. A. Marucchio and L. Salerno, 2 vols., Rome, 1956–57; G. Baglione, Le vite de' pittori, scultori ed architetti, Rome, 1642 (fac. ed., Rome, 1935); G. P. Bellori, Le vite de' pittori, scultori ed architetti moderni, Rome, 1672 (repr., Rome, 1931); A. Bertolotti, Artisti lombardi a Roma nei secoli XV, XVI e XVII, Milan, 1881; S. Samek Ludovici, Vita del Caravaggio dalle testimonianze del suo tempo, Milan, 1956.

BIBLIOG. For the bibliography prior to 1951 consult the Catalogo della mostra del Caravaggio e dei caravaggeschi (Milan, 1951), Florence, 1951. In addition: H. Voss, Die Caravaggio-Ausstellung in Mailand, Kunstchronik, IV, 1951, pp. 165–9; H. Voss, Caravaggios europaische Bedeutung, Kunstchronik, IV, 1951, pp. 258, 287–94; D. Mahon, Caravaggio's Death: A New Document, BM, XCIII, 1951, pp. 202–4; W. Arslan, Appunti su Caravaggio, Aut-Aut, V, 1951, pp. 444–51; J. Hess, The Chronology of the Contarelli Chapel, BM, XCIII, 1951, pp. 186–201; D. Mahon, Egregius in Urbe pictor: Caravaggio Revised, BM, XCIII, 1951, pp. 223–34; D. Mahon, Caravaggio's Chronology Again, BM, XCIII, 1951, pp. 286–92; R. Longhi, Il Caravaggio e la sua cerchia a Milano, Paragone, 15, 1951, pp. 3–17; R. Longhi, Alcuni pezzi rari nell'antologia della critica caravaggesca, Paragone, 17, 1951, pp. 44–62; R. Longhi, Il Caravaggio e i suoi dipinti a San Luigi dei Francesi, Paragone, 17, 1951, pp. 3–13; R. Longhi, La Giuditta nel percorso del Caravaggio, Paragone, 19, 1951, pp. 10–18; R. Longhi, Sui margini caravaggeschi, Paragone, 21, 1951, pp. 20–34; R. Longhi, Volti della Roma caravaggesca, Paragone, 21, 1951, pp. 35–39; R. Longhi, An-

tologia della critica caravaggesca, Paragone, 21, 1951, pp. 43–56; R. Longhi, Antologia della critica caravaggesca, Paragone, 23, 1951, pp. 28–53; L. Venturi, Il Caravaggio, Novara, 1951; R. Longhi, Il Caravaggio, Milan, 1952; F. Baumgart, Die Anfänge Caravaggios, ZfKw, VI, 1952, pp. 85–106; R. Hinks, Michelangelo Merisi da Caravaggio, His Life, His Legend, His Works, London, 1952; D. Mahon, Addenda to Caravaggio, BM, 94, 1952, pp. 3–23; D. Mahon, An Addition to Caravaggio's Early Period, Paragone, 25, 1952, pp. 20–31; C. Baroni, Tutta la pittura di Caravaggio, Milan, 1952; B. Berenson, Caravaggio, His Incongruity and His Fame, London, 1953; D. Mahon, Contrasts in Art Historical Method: Two Recent Approaches to Caravaggio, BM, 95, 1953, pp. 212–20; D. Mahon, Die Dokumente über die Contarelli Kapelle und ihr Verhältnis zur Chronologie Caravaggios, ZfKw, VII, 1953, pp. 183–208; L. Venturi and G. Urbani, Studi Radiografici sul Caravaggio, Rome, 1953; J. Bousquet, Documents inédits sur Caravage, La date des tableaux de la Chapelle Saint-Mathieu a Saint-Louis-des-Français, RArts, 1953, pp. 103–5; F. Klauner, Eine Notiz zur Arbeitsweise Caravaggios, JhbKhSammlWien, N. S., XIV, 1953, pp. 137–40; M. Calvesi, Simone Peterzano, maestro del Caravaggio, BArte, 39, 1954, pp. 114–33; J. Hess, Modelle e modelli del Caravaggio, Comm, 5, 1954, pp. 271–89; R. Longhi, L'"Ecce Homo" del Caravaggio a Genova, Paragone, 51, 1954, pp. 3–13; R. Longhi, Ambrogio Figino e due citazioni del Caravaggio, Paragone, 55, 1954, pp. 36–8; R. Longhi, Il Caravaggio e la "patria" del Priore della Consolazione, Paragone, 57, 1954, pp. 54–5; R. Longhi, Una citazione tizianesca nel Caravaggio, Arte veneta, VIII, 1954, pp. 211–12; A. Czobor, Autoritratti del giovane Caravaggio, Acta H. Artium Acad. Sc. Hung, II, 1955, pp. 201–13; F. Baumgart, Caravaggio, Kunst und Wirklichkeit, Berlin, 1955; W. Friedländer, Caravaggio Studies, Princeton, N.J., 1955; E. Battisti, Alcuni documenti su opere del Caravaggio, Comm, 6, 1955, pp. 173–85; J. Bialostocki, Caravaggio, Warsaw, 1955; R. Jullian, Caravage à Naples, RArts, 1955, pp. 79–90; C. Maltese, Noterelle di critica figurata sul Caravaggio, Comm, 6, 1955, pp. 111–16; L. Salerno, Caravaggio e il priore della Consolazione, Comm, 6, 1955, pp. 258–60; J. Hess, Caravaggio, d'Arpino und Guido Reni, ZfKw, X, 1956, pp. 57–72; R. Jullian, "Lombardisme" et "venetianisme" chez Caravage, Arte lombarda, II, 1956, pp. 112–21; D. Mahon, A Late Caravaggio Rediscovered, BM, 98, 1956, pp. 225–28 (and Paragone, 77, 1956, pp. 25–34); G. C. Argan, Il "realismo" nella poetica del Caravaggio, Scritti di storia dell'arte in onore di Lionello Venturi, II, Rome, 1956; R. Longhi, Il Caravaggio, Milan, 1957; H. Wagner, Michelangelo da Caravaggio, Bern, 1958; R. Longhi, Un anticipo a "20 postille caravaggesche," Paragone, 105, 1958, pp. 75–6; P. Della Pergola, La Galleria Borghese, I dipinti, II, Rome, 1959; R. Longhi, Un'opera estrema del Caravaggio, Paragone, 111, 1959, pp. 21–32.

Valerio MARIANI

Illustrations: PLS. 31–43.

## CARICATURE. See COMIC ART AND CARICATURE.

## CAROLINGIAN PERIOD.

The artistic revival that western Europe witnessed between the middle of the 8th and the end of the 10th century is properly described as the "Carolingian renaissance," as its main inspiration came from Charlemagne and his court, and later from Charles the Bald. It was an art dependent on the ruling classes, and it flourished in the major political and religious centers of the empire. It was also characterized by a renewal and strengthening of connections with the Mediterranean world as a result of the consolidation of disciplinary and liturgical links between the Frankish and the Roman churches about the middle of the 8th century. Elements surviving from previous as well as contemporary north European cultures (see ANGLO-SAXON AND IRISH ART; EUROPE, BARBARIAN; SCANDINAVIAN ART) converged and developed in the new ambient. But innovation was so prevalent that — except for some sporadic survivals (see PRE-ROMANESQUE MEDIEVAL ART) — a clear break must be noted, a break that had a decisive influence on the development of European art (see ROMANESQUE ART).

SUMMARY. Introduction (col. 82). Architecture (col. 82): *Hall churches; The basilicas of Saint-Denis, Lorsch, and Regensburg; Churches with westwork; Churches with facing chancels; Churches with Latin-cross plans; Crypts; Vaulted buildings; The Palatine Chapel in Aachen*. Monumental painting (col. 104): *Western Frankish region; Eastern Frankish region; Alpine regions and northern Italy; Spain; Mosaics*. Sculpture (col. 107): *Western Frankish region; Eastern Frankish region; Alpine regions and northern Italy; Bronzes*. Illumination (col. 110): *The Court School of Charlemagne (Ada Group); The "New Palace School"; Reims; Tours; The style of Charles the Bald; Franco-Saxon style; Minor western Frankish scriptoriums; Eastern Frankish region; Salzburg; St. Gall*. Ivories (col. 116): *Ada Group; Liuthard Group; Metz Group; Minor schools*. Gold- and silverwork (col. 118): *Early Carolingian works; The golden altar of Milan; Western Frankish region; Spain; Eastern Frankish region; Alpine regions and northern Italy; Rome*. Engraved rock crystal (col. 123).

INTRODUCTION. Carolingian art should be regarded as a product not so much of artistic and esthetic movements as of political and religious forces. Its development can be explained only by reference to the grand imperial idea of Charlemagne, who would never have been able to achieve his educational aim without the help of Church and clergy. The construction of cathedrals and abbey churches was therefore an important political matter, though the immediate occasion was often provided by the translation of a saint's relics. The imperial family and the great nobles were in many cases related to the principal ecclesiastics and often acted as founders. Many religious foundations were built between the Seine and the Weser, a territory of which Aachen was the focal point; considered as a group, they display a common character which they owe to the fact that neither Charlemagne nor his successors ever had a fixed residence; the court moved from one center to another.

Cathedrals and monasteries sheltered artists' workshops in their schools. These schools were subsidized and encouraged by Charlemagne in every way. As the Frankish people lacked a cultural background, he thought that representations of historical and religious events, with their emphasis on the human figure, would provide a means for conveying to the Franks some notion of the empire he was trying to revive. Models were drawn variously from Early Christian, Byzantine, and Greco-Italian sources; in this very diversity, due to the convergence of elements of the most disparate origins, the Carolingian workshops display an underlying unity. The influence of their art, and of course of Carolingian architecture, reached the Spanish March (the region bordering the Pyrenees), the Asturias, Britain, and — with lesser force — Italy.

Hans THÜMMLER and Victor H. ELBERN

ARCHITECTURE. Only a few Carolingian buildings have survived, and of those none can be considered free of alterations with any certainty. Old illustrations and written accounts tell of the existence of other buildings, but they rarely provide a substantial picture of their structure. Excavations carried out in the foundations of churches destroyed in World War II have, however, made a great contribution to our knowledge and have led to many discoveries. These have caused a reformulation of previous conceptions of this period, so that church buildings can be classified in fairly coherent groups and even local styles may be distinguished.

*Hall churches.* The largest of these groups is that of small and simple hall churches (FIG. 87). This type reproduced the earliest form of Christian religious buildings; it was widely diffused; and since it was used in rural areas without appreciable development until the 12th century, the date of individual buildings is hard to establish in the absence of external evidence. The origin of this plan may be appreciated in the remarkable series of early church buildings, dating from the 4th to the 8th century, which have been traced through the excavations carried out under the Church of St. Viktor at Xanten. The remains of other churches were found after World War II under Ste-Gertrude at Nivelles (ca. mid-7th cent.), St. Willibrord at Echternach (ca. 700; rebuilt early 9th cent.), and St. Maria in Mittelzell on the island of Reichenau (before 750); under the Abdinghofkirche at Paderborn the earlier foundations (ca. 777) of the Salvatorkirche, rebuilt after 799, were discovered. The Chapel of St. Sylvester at Goldbach on Lake Constance (9th-10th cent.), which is still standing, gives a clear idea of this type of church. There are also some similar buildings in Italy; the oldest church at Garbagnate near Milan (dated by Arslan in the 6th or 7th cent.) is one of the few extant examples.

Hall churches of the 8th-9th century have so far not been found in France, though it may be presumed that they existed, since this very type of church, with an additional polygonal choir, appears at St.-Bertrand-de-Comminges in southwestern France as early as the 5th century and reappears frequently in the 10th. Before World War II it was generally held that hall churches were introduced on the Continent by the Irish-Scots missionaries, since similar buildings existed in Northumbria

(Monkwearmouth, ca. 675; Escomb, ca. 700). In the church at Escomb, which has hardly been altered, the nave and choir are emphatically separated; this feature was to become the rule in Irish hall churches of the 10th century. Such a division is found also in Continental examples: Mittelzell on Reichenau (before 750); Müdehorst (ca. 800), the forerunner of the Herford convent church, which is modeled on it; and Minden

S. Maria in Cosmedin in Rome, again of the 6th century, was of this type also.

Hall churches soon acquired extensions in the form of small lateral chapels which, in plan, practically assumed the character of transepts. The chapels were lower than the nave, however, and were often connected to it only through a narrow aperture; occasionally they were provided with an eastward apse.

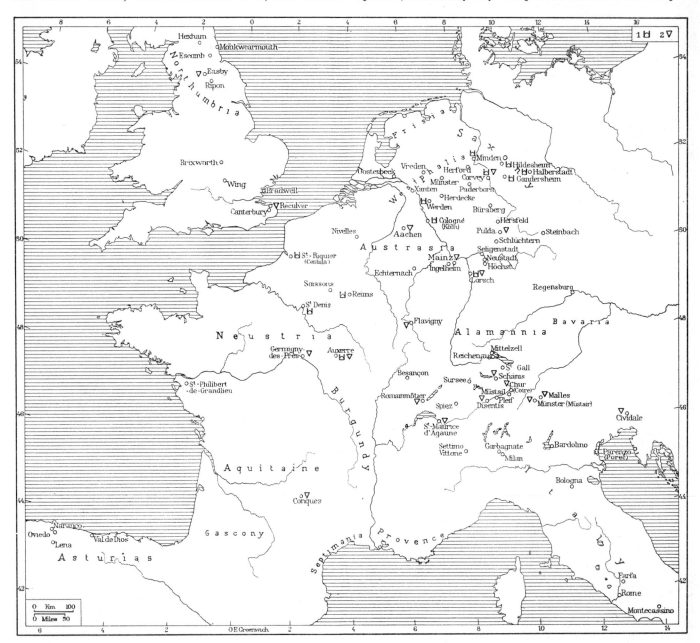

Main centers of the development and diffusion of Carolingian architecture and sculpture. *Key*: (1) Churches with westwork; (2) sculpture.

Cathedral (ca. 800; FIG. 87). But there are also early examples of buildings (FIG. 87) in which a square chancel opens into the nave along its whole width: the chapel at Büraberg near Fritzlar, raised in 742 to cathedral status by St. Boniface (Winfrid), and the first monastery church "auf der Kreuzwiese," at Lorsch. The hypothesis of a British influence on the relation of nave and choir must therefore be revised.

Unsubdivided hall churches with semicircular apses, on the other hand, are rare in the Carolingian period. The earliest and best-known German example is the small monastery church at Hersfeld, founded in 775. The rebuilt 6th-century chapel of S. Benedetto at Montecassino is thought to show an important stage in the development of the plan that derives from the apsidal halls of pagan antiquity. The original Church of

This type of church is rather common in Switzerland; excavations have revealed the existence of early examples at Romainmôtier (first building consecrated about 630, the second in 753), at Spiez (after 765), and at Sursee (mid-9th cent.). In the south of England it occurs even earlier and has the same features; for instance, the Church of St. Pancras (first half of 7th cent.) in Canterbury, Reculver (founded in 669), and Bradwell (after 653; see I, FIG. 460). The source for this type should certainly be sought in Early Christian architecture, and such common origin provides sufficient explanation for the resemblances between buildings as widely separated as the original church under S. Abbondio in Como and the 5th-century building at Silchester in Hampshire.

A separate group among the early hall churches is formed

by many churches in the canton of Graubünden (Grisons). They are characterized by a choir consisting of three contiguous apses, of which the central one with the main altar is only slightly larger (FIG. 87). The two churches of St. Maria and St. Martin at Disentis (first half of 8th cent.) provide the most ancient instances; the only one still intact is the Church of St. Peter at Müstail, built in the second half of the 8th century.

of the Carolingian empire: at Werden on the Ruhr (St. Clement, consecrated in 957) and at Oosterbeek in Holland, where the three apses terminate in a straight east wall.

*The basilicas of St.-Denis, Lorsch, and Regensburg.* The important Carolingian innovations must be sought not in small hall structures but in such buildings as the abbey church of

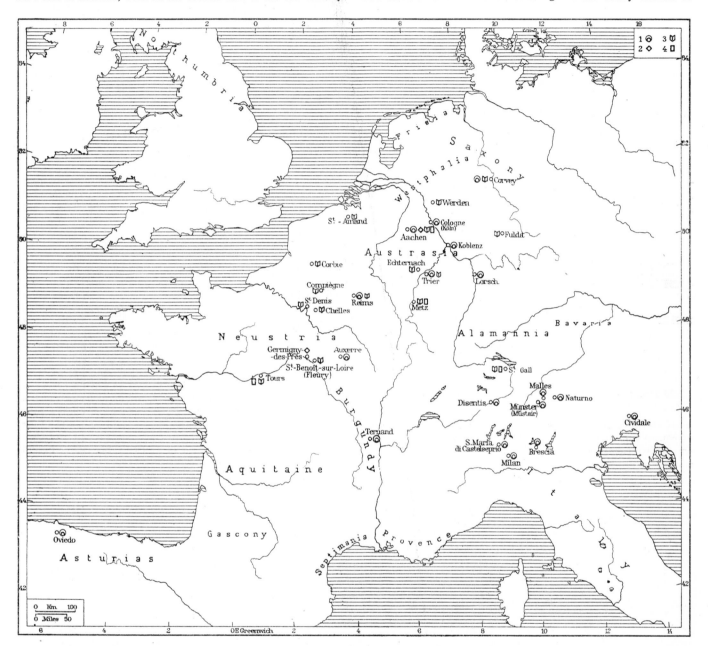

Main centers of the development and diffusion of Carolingian painting and minor arts. *Key*: (1) Painting; (2) mosaics; (3) illumination; (4) ivory carving.

The churches of St. Martin and St. Lucius in Chur (Coire), probably built about 800, also had three-apsed choirs. Other examples of the early 9th century are the abbey church of St. Johann at Münster (Müstair), S. Benedetto at Malles Venosta (Mals), and St. Vincenz at Pleif. The Eastern origin of this plan is generally accepted. One of the earliest instances of it is the *consignatorium*, or confirmation chapel, of the cemetery basilica at Abū Mīnā in Egypt, of the 5th century. There are examples of the transitional stage of this plan among the churches of Istria, such as the 6th-century pre-Euphrasian Cathedral of Parenzo (Poreč), as well as among Lombard buildings, such as the choir of the early-8th-century Church of S. Maria di Aurona in Milan, where the lateral chapels are rectangular. Later evolutions of this plan appear in the northern territories

St.-Denis (FIG. 87), which might well be described as the first Carolingian state church. It was begun by Abbot Fulrad after 754, while Pepin was still alive, and solemnly consecrated in 775 in the presence of Charlemagne and all his court. The plan of this church — which was replaced by a new Gothic building in the 12th century — was revealed by the excavations of Viollet-le-Duc in 1869 and those of Sumner Crosby in the period 1938–48. It was a three-aisled basilica, with a sharply projecting transept. The apse, which stood over an annular crypt, opened directly onto the transept. The western approach with two towers — as reconstructed by Crosby in 1942–44 — was expressly mentioned in the records when the old church was destroyed to make way for Abbot Suger's new construction. In all probability this was part of a larger west structure, and

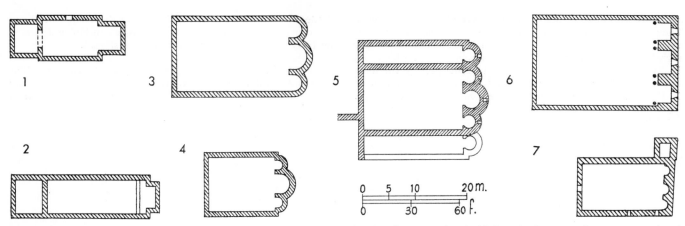

Plans of hall churches from the 8th to the 10th cent. (1) Büraberg near Fritzlar, Germany, chapel; (2) Lorsch, Germany, first monastery church "auf der Kreuzwiese" (*both after Lehmann, 1938*); (3) Disentis, Switzerland, St. Martin; (4) Müstail, Switzerland, St. Peter; (5) Münster, Switzerland, St. Johann; (6) Malles, Italy, S. Benedetto; (7) Disentis, St. Agathe (*last five after RDK, IV, p. 398*).

the twin towers were simply stair towers preceding or flanking a larger central tower containing a gallery. The remains of some solid foundations at this end of the church have not yet been

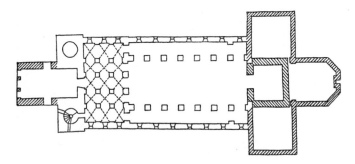

Minden, reconstructed plan of cathedral (*after Thümmler, 1957*).

satisfactorily explained; but whatever the final interpretation may turn out to be, there is little doubt that we are dealing with a "westwork" (*Westwerk*; see below). The whole building assumes a programmatic importance, inspired as it was by the

spatial scheme of the great Constantinian basilicas, with their ample, undivided transept and continuous apse. This kind of transept is in fact known as "Roman." The conscious return to the architectural schemes of the first Christian emperors is paralleled by Charlemagne's championing of the Roman rite against the Oriental liturgy that had so far dominated the Frankish state church.

The excavations of F. Behn have shown that the Church of St. Nazarius in the imperial abbey of Lorsch (FIG. 89), built between 768 and 774, was also a basilica with three aisles, though without transept; it was basically the old type of hall church — of which another example in Lorsch is the monastery church "auf der Kreuzwiese" (FIG. 87) — enlarged, however, by the addition of aisles, while the chancel retained the plain rectangular form. The extensive and highly articulated west end may constitute an innovation; since its walls are extremely thick, we can only interpret it as having served as support for a grand tower complex, subdivided by piers at ground level and containing a gallery above. Probably three towers rose above the basilica — in all likelihood, one of the first instances of the westwork, so characteristic of Carolingian architecture. The west façade of Fulrad's St.-Denis basilica must have been a very similar structure (FIG. 87).

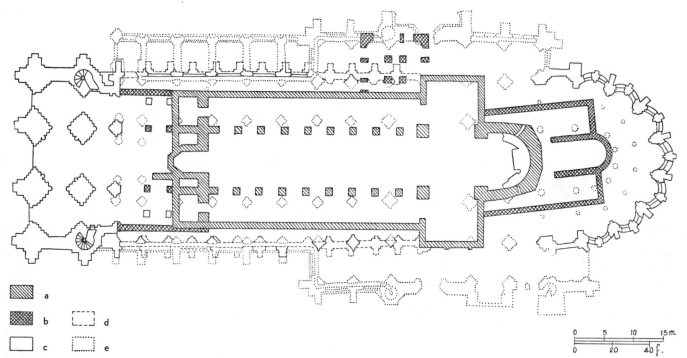

St.-Denis, plan of the abbey church. (*a*) 8th-cent. walls (in part hypothetical); (*b*) 9th-, 11th-, and 12th-cent. additions; (*c*) walls of the Gothic period; (*d*) planned but unexecuted Gothic walls; (*e*) additions made since the 13th cent. (*after Crosby, 1953*).

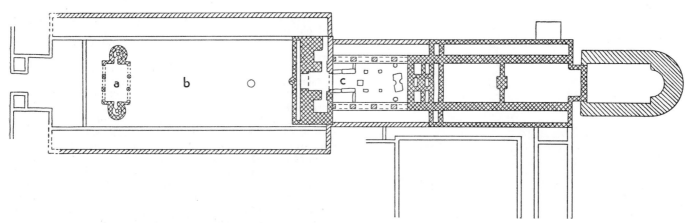

Lorsch, Germany, plan of the abbey church of St. Nazarius. (*a*) Gateway (*Torhalle*); (*b*) 10th-cent. atrium; (*c*) 8th-cent. structure. Hatching shows the different phases of construction (*after RDK, I, p. 1202*).

Bishop Liutpert (consecrated in 768) ordered, with the support of Charlemagne, the rebuilding of the old abbey church of St. Emmeram in Regensburg. It was a three-aisled basilica terminating to the east in three parallel apses. Around the main apse ran an annular crypt which, to the east, opened into a rectangular chapel. The chapel was already in existence when the relics of St. Emmeram were transferred to it in 740 and had belonged to the original building, probably a hall church.

The three basilicas, St.-Denis, Lorsch, and Regensburg, were all built about the same time. Charlemagne showed a great interest in these foundations, and all three display the main programmatic features of Carolingian architecture. First of all the basilican plan was taken over, particularly the Early Christian Latin-cross variant. Then the chancel was opened out into three apses instead of one, and many-chambered crypts were built underneath. The triapsidal chancel — the earliest example of which is to be found in the basilica at Emmaus in Palestine — was frequent in Syrian buildings and soon appeared in the West, where it occurred about 550 in Parenzo Cathedral and at the end of the 6th century at St.-Martin in Autun. Its appearance in Regensburg is therefore hardly an innovation; it only indicates that the type, which had in any case already been used in churches in the Alps in the early 8th century, was becoming more widely diffused. Neither was the annular crypt a Carolingian invention; it harks back to Early Christian practice in Rome. The annular crypt under St. Peter's goes back to the 5th or 6th century, and the one at S. Pancrazio is attributed to Pope Honorius I (625–38). However, it was only under Adrian I (772–95) that annular crypts became at all common, whether in Rome or beyond the Alps. Their development is connected with the growth of the cult of relics in the 8th and 9th centuries; annular crypts provided an ideal place for exhibition and veneration of the remains of martyrs, which had formerly been placed behind the high altar.

*Churches with westwork.* The westwork (*Westwerk*) was a new feature of church plans. This complex consisted of two stair towers, one on each side of the west entrance of the church; the stair towers gave access to a raised gallery, or tribune, inside the church, from which the emperor and his entourage could follow the services. West towers incorporated in the façade had existed in Syrian buildings as early as the 6th century (Termânîn, Kalb-Lauzeh, Ruweha) and not much later in Frankish architecture, at St.-Martin in Autun, but they were not important features of the building, nor did they rise above the height of the nave. In Carolingian churches the towers are not the principal element of the west façade, but rather extensions in height of the whole many-storied tall west structure, whose flanks they are. The increasing use of bells, recorded in many documents, is often advanced as an explanation for the system of façades with belfries, but it does not account for either the fortress character of westworks or their complex internal structure. To understand the underlying conception of a westwork, the towers must be seen as symbols of power

and justice. On coins and in manuscript illuminations Rome and Jerusalem, the two most important cities of the medieval world, were represented by a gate flanked by two defending towers. Symbolically within the tower-fortress of the Frankish church stood the emperor, the new protector of the Roman Church, for whom the spacious gallery between the stair towers was intended. In the Palatine Chapel at Aachen this three-towered structure rises to the west of the central-plan church and forms, as it were, a monumental canopy over the imperial throne in the gallery.

The imperial throne in the gallery was the true *raison d'être* of Carolingian westworks; it determined the corresponding spatial articulation of the gallery level, subdivided into principal chambers for the emperor and secondary ones for his entourage, so that they could either take part in the divine service at a private altar or follow the monastic choral liturgy. This is why the arcades of the galleries opened over the nave of the church. By placing the emperor's throne on a higher level, it was possible to leave free the main west entrance of the church while a convenient access to the galleries could be gained by the ample staircases in the twin towers. A third tower was erected over the principal chamber, and the lateral chambers surrounded it on three sides. This arrangement determined the exterior three-tower configuration of the westwork, which documents of the time already designated as *triturrium* ("triple tower") or *tres turres* ("three towers").

One instance of a westwork that has survived almost intact is that of the Benedictine abbey church at Corvey on the Weser (consecrated in 884; PL. 44; FIG. 92). The upper sanctuary, the so-called "Johanneschor," extends over an entrance hall at ground level which is treated as a three-aisled colonnaded and vaulted crypt. Also vaulted are, or rather were, the lateral chambers, above which another flat-ceilinged gallery extends. The central chamber, however, rises through the two floors and is covered by a timbered roof. The side galleries open onto the main chamber through three double arcades. The great arch of the main chamber extends to the floor of the gallery and has no parapet; the imperial throne probably stood just

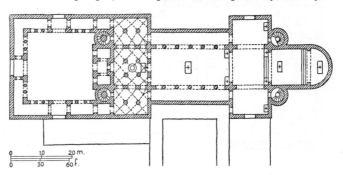

St.-Riquier (Centula), France. Effmann's reconstruction of the church plan (*after Gall, 1930*).

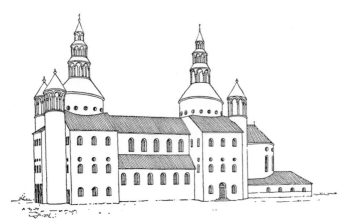

St.-Riquier (Centula), France. Effmann's reconstruction of the church (*after Gall, 1930*).

within it (PL. 45). The two orders of the gallery arcades look down upon a narrow bay inserted between the Johanneschor and the nave; the bay had the character of a transept and stressed the central-plan aspect of the westwork because, thanks to it, the emperor's chamber was surrounded on all sides by subsidiary spaces. Such a bay, however, east of the galleries, appears only at Corvey.

The westwork at Corvey was added to the church between 873 and 885, but the abbey church of St.-Riquier (Centula), built between 790 and 799 under the special protection of Charlemagne's privy councilor Angilbert, already had a westwork (PL. 44; FIG. 91). Although nothing remains of it, a detailed description and an old view of the building enabled Effmann (1912) to make a reconstruction. The most ancient westworks of which traces remain are those of Lorsch, consecrated in the presence of Charlemagne in 774, and of St.-Denis, which was finished in the following year. The western foundations of Lorsch were brought to light by Behn, but he interpreted them wrongly; today they are generally recognized as the substructure of an entrance hall in the form of a three-aisled crypt under a westwork with flanking stair towers. The fragments that Crosby discovered beyond the twin-towered west façade of St.-Denis are not sufficient to allow such an easy interpretation; given the special position this building occupied in the imperial Frankish Church and in the imperial family, it could not have lacked a large west gallery, and most probably the stair towers would have been set back as at Lorsch.

The parallel development of westworks in the western and eastern parts of the Frankish empire is borne out by their even distribution. The foundations discovered by Deneux and the records of the demolition of 976 facilitate the reconstruction of a large westwork in Reims Cathedral, founded by Archbishop Ebbo of Reims (816–35) and consecrated by his successor Hincmar in 862. The upper part of this building was also supported by an entrance hall in the form of a three-

aisled crypt. Similar schemes existed — according to the sources and old illustrations — both in the abbey church of St.-Germain at Auxerre, consecrated in 865, and in the cathedral there (westwork built 879–87).

After World War II foundations for westworks were found in Germany: in the cathedrals of Halberstadt (consecrated in 859), Hildesheim (consecrated in 872), and Minden (westwork and rebuilt nave consecrated in 952) and in the Church of St. Pantaleon in Cologne (second half of 10th cent.), the plan of which has definite affinities with the scheme of Corvey (FIG. 91). In Minden Cathedral (FIG. 87) the fragments of Carolingian walls, embedded in the structure of the surviving later westwork, suggest a reconstruction on the lines of Corvey.

It is strange that no westworks have as yet been discovered in any French or German regions besides those already named; and it is also remarkable that this type of structure was most frequent in the second half of the 9th century.

In Italy there is an isolated example of a westwork. Between 830 and 840 Abbot Sichartus added to the existing church (S. Maria) of the Benedictine abbey at Farfa an oratory dedicated to the Saviour; it was joined to the west flank of the church and had twin stair towers. The south tower survives, but only its lower floors belong to the Carolingian period; of the north tower nothing but the foundations remains. The

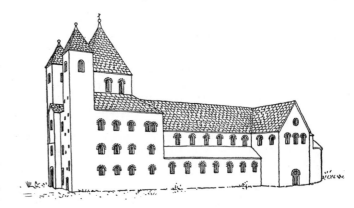

Corvey, Germany. Effmann's reconstruction of the abbey church (*after Gall, 1930*).

stair towers suggest a western portion with several stories, which one may conceive as a westwork, especially since the monastery was raised to the rank of imperial abbey in Carolingian times.

The westwork is one of the most original features of Carolingian architecture, even if it owes something to central-plan Byzantine buildings and to the twin-towered façades of Syrian churches. It seems to set forth the double mission of the Frankish empire as protector of both state and Church (*regnum* and *sacerdotium*). Monumental stone construction was practically limited to religious buildings in the Carolingian period.

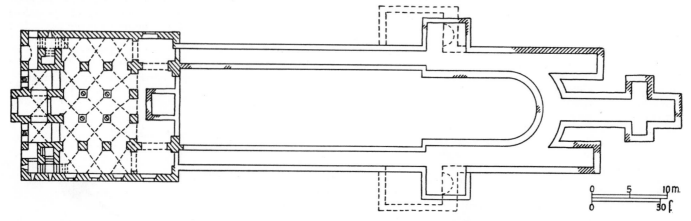

Corvey, Germany, abbey church, plan at crypt level (*after Claussen, 1957*).

Therefore the ceremonies of homage to the emperor, the investitures, and the administering of the law must have taken place mostly in churches and specifically in the westworks, which were large enough for such occasions and separated to a certain extent from the rest of the church. Westworks remained important until the middle of the 10th century. Then, as the power of the empire decayed and that of the Church increased, westworks diminished in size and importance. The westwork of Reims Cathedral was demolished in 976; that of Halberstadt Cathedral was replaced, after its collapse in 965, by a west chancel and that of Hildesheim Cathedral by a shallow western construction (1022–38). In the early 11th century the entrance hall of St. Pantaleon in Cologne was no longer handled as a crypt, and the floor of the new westwork was raised to the same level as the adjoining nave, as had already been done in the westwork (consecrated in 943) of the abbey church of Werden on the Ruhr.

*Churches with facing chancels.* An important group of Carolingian churches have facing chancels (FIG. 93). This type cannot be considered a Carolingian innovation like the west-

in the western part of the church, furnished the occasion for adding the monumental west choir to the ancient basilica. It is quite possible that Early Christian examples of this type of plan in North Africa were the result of a similar cult of a saint or martyr. It is not known, however, why west choirs were built at Paderborn or Cologne; and the ideal plan of the St. Gall parchment does not make clear the liturgical function of the west chancel, which had its own altar. At Fulda the west chancel opens onto a vast transept and gives the appearance of being the principal sanctuary. In fact the western portion of the building is elaborate and carefully developed, and when cathedrals were rebuilt in Ottonian times, this arrangement became standard.

*Churches with Latin-cross plans.* Among the pressing programmatic requirements of the time, however, was the return to the Latin-cross basilican plan (FIG. 95). One of the most remarkable instances is the abbey church of St.-Denis, already mentioned, but it must be considered in conjunction with the monastery church at Seligenstadt, the palatine chapel at Ingelheim (Hesse), and Reims Cathedral. Although this

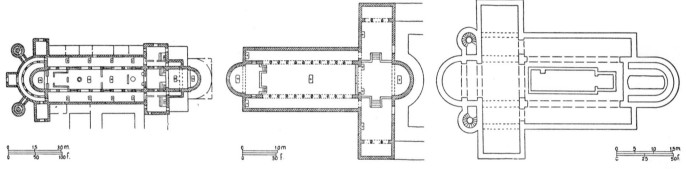

Plans of churches with facing chancels. *Left*: St. Gall, Switzerland, abbey church as projected in plan of early-9th-cent. parchment; *center*: Fulda, Germany, abbey church; *right*: Paderborn, Germany, Salvatorkirche according to Ortmann's reconstruction (*after RDK, I, p. 864*).

work, since basilicas with two apses — one at either end of the nave — existed in early Christian times. However, a deliberate return to such models did not occur until the time of Charlemagne, when they were developed as Latin-cross basilicas with two facing apses, one at each end of the nave. The facing-chancel arrangement was to last until the end of the Romanesque period. The ideal plan of the abbey church of St. Gall, preserved in the famous parchment drawing of about 820 (St. Gall, Stiftsbib.), is the best-known Carolingian example of the type. Given the programmatic nature of the drawing, there is every reason to suppose that this scheme was widely diffused during the period. For a long time, however, few actual examples of churches with facing chancels were known; excavations have revealed that the basilica of St.-Maurice d'Agaune is perhaps the oldest example (end of 8th cent.). Then follow — in chronological order — the abbey church in Fulda (PL. 44), consecrated in 819; the Salvatorkirche in Paderborn (after 799); the abbey church of St. Willibrord in Echternach, the cathedral traditionally ascribed to Archbishop Hildebold (785–819) at Cologne, and Besançon Cathedral (all three early 9th cent.); the abbey church of St.-Remi at Reims, consecrated in 852; Auxerre Cathedral (857–73); and the monastery church at Oberzell on Reichenau (ca. 890). That these west apses were not just secondary or subsidiary chancels is shown by the fact that in some cases — as at Fulda, Paderborn, and in the rebuilt Cathedral of Cologne (consecrated in 870) — the west chancel also opened into a second transept. At Fulda the transept was so large that it resembled — as may be seen from the plan and from surviving views (FIG. 93) — the great Constantinian basilicas, which are, in fact, the only possible models for churches with elaborate apsidal developments to the west. In the life of Abbot Eigil the plan at Fulda is described as arranged *Romano more* ("in the Roman manner"); from the same source we learn that the growing veneration of the tomb of St. Boniface, which lay

type of plan developed most readily in the north, it was taken up in Rome as well; and in the 8th century the Constantinian system of basilicas with continuous transepts was resumed, as may be seen in S. Anastasia and S. Stefano degli Abissini, built under Leo III (795–816), and S. Prassede, built under Paschal I (817–24). While the first two examples show included transepts, in S. Prassede the transept projects beyond the aisles.

In Britain there is an exceptional instance of the Roman basilican scheme at Hexham Priory in Northumberland, which may be reconstructed from ecclesiastical documents and excavated foundations; this building also had a generous transept. It was built during the tenure of Bishop Wilfrid of York (ca. 675–80), soon after the Synod of Whitby, which secured the triumph of the Roman over the Irish party of the Church. During this period many churches were erected in Britain.

Even in northeastern Spain, under the Asturian kings, when a singularly independent Visigothic architecture was flourishing, some churches were built that display affinities with Latin-cross Roman basilicas; for instance, S. Julián de los Prados (Santullano) in Oviedo (812–42; PL. 46; FIG. 95), the largest pre-Romanesque church still extant in Spain. The architectural idiom of the Carolingian empire, whose overwhelming political power had spread to the Spanish March, a region incorporated into the empire in 812, is reflected in the huge "Roman" transept, segregated from the nave by a triumphal arch, and in the use of a round instead of a horseshoe arch (which had been common practice until then) in the nave arcades resting on piers. The choice of a simple basilica with three-aisled nave divided by piers instead of the more frequent central plan of Eastern origin would be unaccountable were it not for the impact of Carolingian influence. St. Peter near Fulda (PL. 48) and the basilican abbey church of Schlüchtern are beyond a doubt the prototypes of S. Salvador at Val de Dios (dedicated in 893; PLS. 46, 47), where the basilican

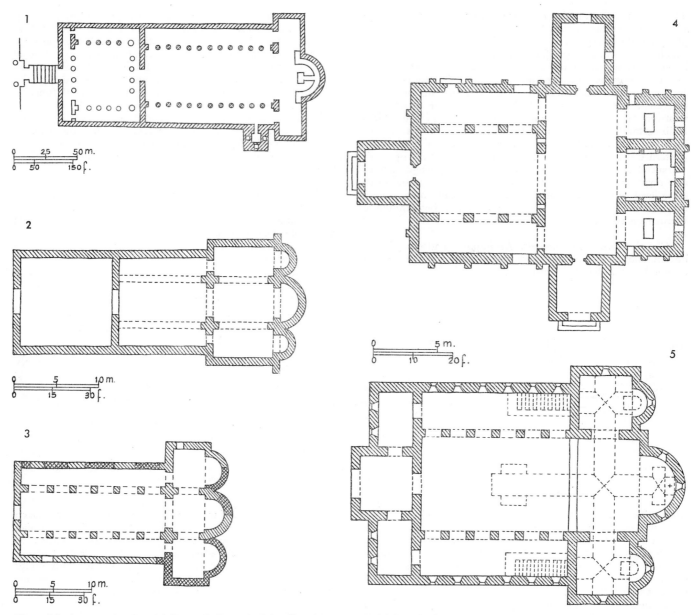

Plans of Latin-cross churches. (1) Rome, S. Prassede (*after Krautheimer, 1942*); (2) Lorsch, Germany, church on the Seehof; (3) Höchst, Germany. monastery church (*after Gall, 1930*); (4) Oviedo, Spain, S. Julián de los Prados (*after Ars Hispaniae, 1947*); (5) Steinbach, Germany, basilica (*after Müller, n.d.*).

scheme is combined with a tripartite chancel terminating in straight walls.

The basilica with transept soon developed a step further in the central territories of the Carolingian empire. Even while the plain and unarticulated Roman transept, into which the apse opens directly, was still being built, there appeared a type in which the transept was separated from the apse by a chancel bay, as at Neustadt on the Main, St. Gall, Vreden, Cologne Cathedral (first building), St.-Riquier, and Mittelzell on Reichenau. The extension of the main apse into a separate spatial unit was motivated by the desire to isolate and stress the importance of the high altar, at which all the choral services were held, and to provide more space for the officiating clergy.

Sometimes there are two transepts, one east, the other west, as in the rebuilt Cathedral of Cologne (consecrated in 870) and in the 9th-century Cathedral of Besançon. That St.-Riquier also had two transepts is proved by a 17th-century engraving; the difference between this example and the others is that here the second transept was incorporated in the westwork and contained galleries. The arms of the east transept may also have contained galleries, as the disposition of windows on several levels, exactly reflecting the fenestration of the west

transept, would otherwise be difficult to account for. St.-Riquier anticipates formal principles that were not to be realized until the Ottonian period and are best reflected in St. Michael in Hildesheim (consecrated in 1033).

The fact that the true Latin-cross basilica had not become common in Carolingian times is shown by a group of churches in which the transept is an important external feature but does not correspond to the effect inside the building. This may be seen in churches in which the exterior apse walls are straight, as in the basilica at Schlüchtern or of St. Peter near Fulda (PL. 48), or else terminate in a semicircular projection, as at Herdecke on the Ruhr, Höchst, and Steinbach in the Odenwald. In spite of its ruined condition, the Steinbach basilica (FIG. 95) can be reconstructed without great difficulty, from the description of Einhard, Charlemagne's biographer and confidant, who built the church between 821 and 827. The basilica had a nave divided into three aisles by piers. The transept was lower than the nave and had a double-pitched roof; its arms joined the nave in such a way that from the outside, and particularly from the east end, the building appeared to have the Latin-cross form; this impression was confirmed by the triapsidal chancel, with an enlarged and dominant central apse. It is therefore surprising that in the interior the rhythm of the

narrowly spaced piers is not emphatically interrupted at the chancel. The nave arcading, however, is so narrow that the aisles are hardly visible from the nave, and the nave therefore gives the impression of a single hall. At the point where the regular movement of the arcade should open into the transept, the piers are heavier, but the transition into the transept occurs through a round arch less than twice the span of the nave arcade; and the transept itself is completely walled off from the aisles. Hence what appear to be the arms of the transept are in fact two segregated chapels, modeled not on the Roman transept, but on Early Christian pastophoria.

Before Charlemagne the Western church was strongly influenced by the Eastern, whose dominance found expression both in liturgy and in art; but Charlemagne established a link with the Early Christian heritage of Rome. Therefore the pastophoria of Steinbach may seem in the interior like small chapels opening from the nave, but from the exterior they take on the form of a true transept. During the restoration of the old church of the convent at Herdecke, carried out between 1930 and 1940, the original form of the church was revealed as it had been first built in the early 9th century. It repeated quite literally the scheme of Steinbach. St. Alban in Mainz, too, as has been proved, had a similar structure; however, in the monastery church at Höchst (FIG. 95) — most of it still standing — the transept, obtained by fusing of the lateral chapels, is also clearly recognizable from within.

When only the foundations of a Carolingian church remain, it is often very difficult to tell whether the transept formed an integral part of the space or was segregated by walls and subdivided into several chambers. In Cologne Cathedral and the Salvatorkirche in Paderborn the four foundation walls of the three-aisled nave are carried through the transept area, so that a narrow opening into the transept, similar to that at Steinbach, must be postulated. In the early single-nave Latin-cross churches the arms of the transept were isolated as a rule and built only as side chapels, lower than the body of the building; at a later period the nave was intersected by a transept as wide and high as itself, and an identifiable square crossing was formed. But the origin of such developments may be traced to Carolingian buildings, such as the monastery church at Neustadt on the Main and St. Maria at Mittelzell on Reichenau (rebuilt by Abbot Heito); in both cases the crossing forms a square, and the arches on all four sides are sprung from the same height.

*Crypts.* The increased size of the chancel is closely connected with the development of the crypt. How this took place is not clear; yet many examples (FIG. 99) show that crypts had become an established element of episcopal and monastery churches as early as Carolingian times.

At first the most prevalent type was the annular crypt, which consisted of a semicircular barrel-vaulted passage underneath the apses. It surrounded the tomb of the martyr, which was generally connected with the high altar above it through an aperture.

Annular crypts existed as early as the 5th and 6th centuries in Rome in Old St. Peter's and in S. Pancrazio (attributed to Honorius I, 625–38). By the 8th and 9th centuries crypts had become an integral part of Roman churches, as is shown by many surviving in whole or in part: at S. Crisogono (built under Gregory III, 731–41), at S. Marco (built under Adrian I, 772–95), at S. Stefano degli Abissini (built under Leo III, 795–816), at S. Cecilia and at S. Prassede (built under Paschal I, 817–24), at SS. Quattro Coronati (built under Leo IV, 847–55), at S. Martino ai Monti (built under Sergius II, 844–47), at S. Nicola ai Cesarini (9th cent.). Contemporary with these are the annular crypts in S. Apollinare Nuovo (856) and S. Apollinare in Classe (9th cent.), both in Ravenna.

With the spread of the cult of relics exhumed from the catacombs, the annular crypt was adopted in the north, in both the eastern and western parts of the Carolingian empire. The most remarkable instances are the crypt of St. Emmeram in Regensburg (ca. 740), St. Lucius in Chur (mid-8th cent.), St.-Denis (consecrated in 775), St.-Maurice d'Agaune (end

of 8th cent.), Seligenstadt (828–40), and the abbey church of Werden (consecrated in 875); only the first two and the last of these survive. In St. Emmeram the crypt was built under a preexisting apse, so that the underground annular passage is actually outside the limits of the building. The annular crypt was in use also in England, as in Canterbury Cathedral and in the churches of Brixworth and Wing (all of 9th–10th cent.), where enough of the original foundations remain to allow reconstruction.

Contemporary with the annular crypt is another form, known as the "tunnel crypt." It consists of several parallel, barrel-vaulted aisles in the form of narrow rectangles cut through by a connecting passage. Examples of this form are the crypt of St. Peter near Fulda (FIG. 99) and of the abbey church of Schlüchtern — both built about 800 and still extant. Another example was found in the course of excavations under the church at St.-Quentin (835). In some of these crypts the aisles are placed both to the east and to the west of the connecting passage, as in the Church of St. Willibrord at Echternach and in St.-Médard at Soissons (817–41), where there are no fewer than 10 intercommunicating galleries (PL. 49).

This form of crypt derives its arrangement from the burial chambers in the Roman catacombs, which at that time were the objects of much reverence because they were an inexhaustible source of martyrs' relics. The crypts of two Northumbrian churches — Hexham and Ripon, both founded by Wilfrid in the last quarter of the 7th century — are transitional structures, for they do not tie in organically with the churches above them and lack the strict symmetrical organization of the tunnel-crypt system. In the basilica of Steinbach the passages are so disposed under the presumed location of the transept as to form three successive crosses. One section of the central aisle extends under half the length of the church nave; the other is shorter, but both terminate in cruciform chambers (FIG. 95). Altars stood at the east ends of the three longitudinal aisles, the northernmost of which dates back to the founding of the church. In these altars were kept the precious relics that Einhard's emissaries had abstracted secretly from a martyr's grave in the Roman catacombs. But Einhard relates that three months after their installation in Steinbach the sacred bones revealed to him in a dream that they wanted to be translated to Seligenstadt, the other church he had founded.

Besides the annular and the tunnel crypts there came into use, though somewhat later, a third type — the hall crypt. The most ancient of these as yet discovered is the small three-aisled crypt under the Church of S. Maria in Cosmedin in Rome (PL. 49). Built under Adrian I (772–95) at the same time as the church was reconstructed, its plan is that of an apsidal basilica with included transept. The nave columns do not support arches but a straight architrave on which rests a flat ceiling made of great stone slabs. The specific function of this small structure — that of an exhibition hall for a collection of relics — is obvious from the many horizontally shelved niches, built into the wall like cupboards, which provided space for 32 reliquaries. There is a similar hall crypt under the Church of St.-Germain at Auxerre, where it constitutes the core of a vast crypt development (see below). Here, too, the aisle columns support a straight entablature, which, however, bears not a flat ceiling as in S. Maria in Cosmedin, but a barrel vault. The two crypts under the east and west choirs of the abbey church at Fulda — if the evidence of the excavations is to be trusted — also had nave and aisles. The various forms taken by the development of crypts must be related to multiple variations in the cult of relics, but, as far as we know, the annular crypt was the only form of construction exclusively reserved for this purpose.

Crypts became so complex because they were enlarged by the constant addition of subsidiary chapels, which extended underground beyond the actual church and were dug out of the earth at the same level as the core of the crypt. This development is characteristically Carolingian and a result of the desire, for which there is much documentary evidence, to be buried close to a protecting saint. The chapels, at first simple rectangular chambers, assume all sorts of complex forms through

the combination of annular, tunnel, and hall crypts. A rectangular chapel built before 830 for the tombs of St. Liutger's family was later connected with the annular crypt of the abbey church at Werden (FIG. 99).

The crypt of Hildesheim Cathedral (consecrated in 872) terminated in a chamber flanked by two small projecting apses which opened into the semicircular passage (FIG. 99). The exterior crypt of the abbey church at Corvey (consecrated in 844) had lateral passages which extended so far beyond the annular

The multiplication of altar spaces may be observed also in the development of the simple tunnel crypt. In St.-Médard at Soissons (817–41) there were no fewer than 10 spatial units (FIG. 99). For the same purpose little projecting chapels were added at the west end of the two lateral galleries of the crypt at Corvey; later two regular transept arms were hollowed out into these chapels (FIG. 91). There are similar lateral chapels in the annular crypt of the abbey church at Vreden (FIG. 99), consecrated in 839; small semicircular niches were

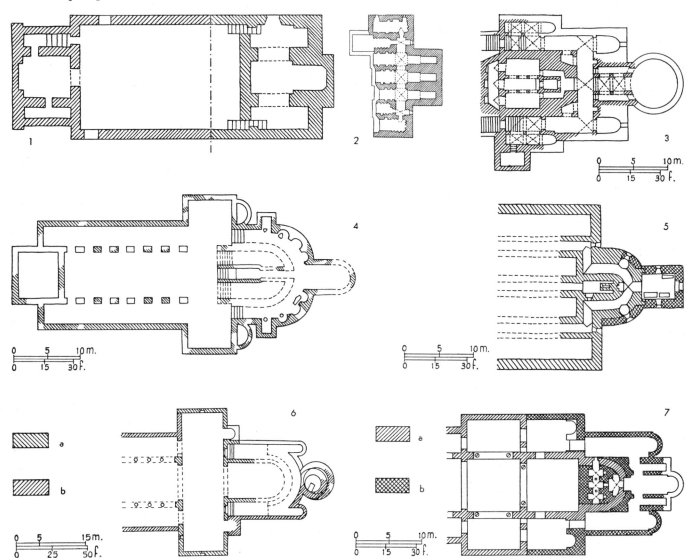

Plans of 9th-cent. crypts. (1) Fulda, Germany, abbey church of St. Peter on the Petersberg, near Fulda (*after Lehmann, 1938*); (2) Soissons, France, St.-Médard (*after Lefèvre-Pontalis, 1894–96*); (3) Auxerre, France, St.-Germain (*after Louis, 1952*); (4) Vreden, Germany, abbey church (*after Winckelmann and Claussen, 1953*); (5) Werden, Germany, abbey church (*Effmann's reconstruction; after Claussen, 1957*); (6) Hildesheim, Germany, Cathedral (*after Bohland, 1953*): (a) remains incorporated in the later superstructure; (b) plotted after excavation; (7) St.-Philibert-de-Grandlieu, France, church: (a) 9th cent.; (b) later building (*De Lasteyrie's reconstruction; after Claussen, 1957*).

crypt as to enclose a Latin-cross chapel. Excavations have revealed a similar ground plan for the exterior crypt of Halberstadt Cathedral (consecrated in 859).

The exterior crypt spread from the north to Italy, where a good example is provided by the crypt foundations, believed to be somewhat earlier than 887, that were brought to light in 1914 in the immediate vicinity of the Church of S. Stefano in Bologna. Like the crypts of Corvey and Halberstadt, it consisted of two lateral aisles terminating in straight walls and of a central chapel in the form of a Latin cross which differed from the two northern examples only in that the eastern arm of the cross ended in a semicircular rather than a square apse. Inserted between the chapel and the aisles were two small apses in the shape of horseshoes. Thus the chambers which could receive altars were, in this case, increased to seven.

cut into the walls of the annular gallery which opened into an apsed hall toward the east. In France other partially preserved examples of the exterior crypt are to be found at St.-Denis, St.-Philibert-de-Grandlieu, and St.-Germain at Auxerre (PL. 49). The crypt at St.-Denis, three-aisled and with an apse projecting from the nave, was added about 832 to the choir of the abbey church, which already had an annular crypt. The crypt built under the church at St.-Philibert-de-Grandlieu after 847 (FIG. 99) consists of a group of very small cruciform cells flanking the burial chamber of St. Philibert, installed under the old apsidal choir of the church. The exterior crypt proper, of five chapels en échelon, is disposed around the chancel. There was probably an upper story over the three middle chapels, to which access was gained by two narrow staircases in the small galleries flanking the central chapel. Even more compli-

cated is the crypt of St.-Germain at Auxerre (841–54; FIG. 99). Originally, as at St.-Philibert, the five exterior chapels *en échelon* were connected by a many-cornered passage. The whole complex culminated in a rotunda which, like the present one, rebuilt in the Gothic period, must have been two-storied. What is remarkable about the whole complex is that in the side chapels the groined vaults rest on arches, as though presaging the classic type of hall crypt. In fact there is a crypt of just this shape under the choir of the church, though the architrave is still straight and the vault is a barrel vault. The resulting architectural character of the whole is rather confused and recalls a Roman catacomb. That these underground churches came into being almost independently of the upper churches suggests that the cult of relics had by then a considerable importance.

It is remarkable that this cult was most popular in the regions in which the westwork also developed. From the evidence now available it would appear that Italy, Spain, and Britain had no part in its development.

*Vaulted buildings.* Crypts and westworks were both important preliminaries to the revival of monumental vaulted buildings. In annular crypts, as well as in tunnel crypts, the barrel vaults of antiquity persisted; in the atriums of westworks — similar in form to large hall crypts and often referred to as "cryptae" in documents — the classic cross vault (or groin-vault) system developed with the intersection of two barrel vaults of equal diameter and height. The entrance hall of the westwork at Corvey is an impressive instance of this, while more advanced examples are the cross vaults of the crypt at St.-Germain at Auxerre, where the bays are separated from one another by bands, which in turn determine the articulation of the supporting piers.

In the Carolingian period the vaulting of entire churches was at first limited to the central-plan type or to small churches related to this type by virtue of a more or less marked cruciform structure. There are several examples in Italy, such as S. Zeno at Bardolino (873–81) and S. Lorenzo at Settimo Vittone near Turin (850–900; FIG. 102), both Latin-cross hall churches with a prolonged nave; the barrel vault of the four arms meets over the square crossing to form a groined vault. This type of building belongs to a probably uninterrupted tradition which, through Spanish examples such as S. Comba at Bande (ca. 670), goes back to the Mausoleum of Galla Placidia in Ravenna (mid-5th cent.). The high springing of the barrel vault of the nave and the way it rests on pilastered arcades backed by a wall are unthinkable without immediate Spanish precedents.

A remarkable flowering of ecclesiastical architecture took place in Spain, more precisely in the kingdom of the Asturias — the only part of the country that did not submit to Islam — in the reign of Ramiro I (842–50). The single-nave churches of S. María at Naranco (PL. 51) and S. Cristina at Lena, for instance, and others still nearly intact, show a more highly developed vaulted construction than anything produced by Carolingian builders. The balance between structural elements and spatial relationships makes S. María a masterpiece without contemporary equal. Its form is so close to the Early Christian churches of Armenia that it actually seems directly inspired by the castle chapel at Ani (consecrated before 622), where the blind arcades and engaged columns support the barrel vault articulated by bands.

Another element common to Spanish and Armenian architecture is the arcade with horseshoe arches. The first entirely vaulted basilica in Spain is S. Salvador at Val de Dios in the Asturias (PL. 47), with three-aisled nave and horseshoe arches resting on piers. It has no transept; its three contiguous chancels are closed by a straight wall; much lower than the rest of the building, they are divided into two stories. The church, dated by an inscription in the year 893, is barrel-vaulted throughout. S. Julián de los Prados at Oviedo (812–42) also has three aisles, but the barrel-vaulted chancel is the usual single-level kind. As early as 661 three rectangular barrel-vaulted chancels are to be found in S. Juan Bautista at Baños de Cerrato, though originally they were not contiguous as they are now: the two lateral ones projected in the manner of pastophoria. The scheme

of the little Lombard Church of S. Maria in Valle (762–76) at Cividale — the "tempietto longobardo" — is probably also derived from Visigothic prototypes; although it is a hall church, it has a tripartite barrel-vaulted chancel supported by two rows of columns with straight architraves. The western section of the building is taller and is roofed by a groined vault.

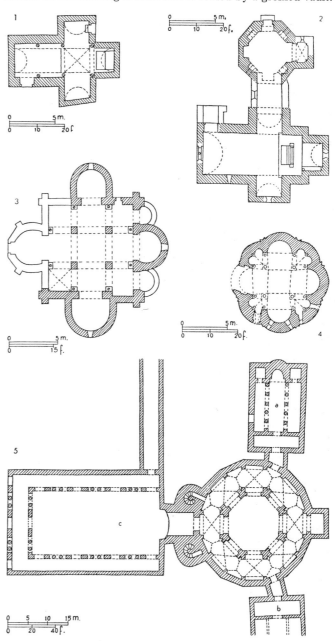

Plans of vaulted buildings. (1) Bardolino, Italy, S. Zeno; (2) Settimo Vittone, Italy, S. Lorenzo (*both after Verzone, 1942*); (3) Germigny-des-Prés, France, oratory (*after Conant, 1959*); (4) Milan, S. Maria presso S. Satiro, Cappella della Pietà; (5) Aachen, Germany, Palatine Chapel and adjoining structures at ground level: (*a, b*) buildings contemporary with the chapel but of uncertain function; (*c*) atrium.

S. Maria in Valle is one of the earliest medieval vaulted structures in Italy, and therefore of primary importance.

In France the little funerary chapel of St.-Laurent in Grenoble (ca. 800), originally freestanding, is similar in structure to the Italian and Spanish barrel-vaulted hall churches with blind arcades. Its vaulting is dependent on the central-plan system, for the ground plan is cruciform with four terminal apses, of which the west one projects somewhat more than the rest.

How closely linked Carolingian architecture was with the East, through Spain, is shown by the oratory at Germigny-des-Prés near Orléans (PLS. 50, 51). This church is interesting

not only because of its place in the history of architectural development, but also because it is the only surviving Carolingian church in France. It was founded in 806 by Theodulf, abbot of the neighboring monastery, St.-Benoît-sur-Loire (or Fleury), and bishop of Orléans. Theodulf was a Visigoth by birth and had estates in the district. Unfortunately the building was badly restored and extended westward in 1869. Originally it was a central-plan church (FIG. 102); four piers at the crossing marked off the four arms of the cross, each barrel-vaulted and ending in an apse. The four compartments in the angles of the cross were a little smaller than the squares contained within it and were roofed with groined vaults much lower than the barrel vaults of the arms. The towerlike crossing was covered by a dome on a drum and pendentives. The stepwise increase in height from the outward portions of the church to the elevated crossing produces a Byzantine effect; the horseshoe arches of the arcade and of the three apses were probably motivated by the Visigothic tastes of the builder. The closest parallels to Germigny-des-Prés are in Armenia: the Cathedral of Echmiadzin (see ARMENIAN ART) is so similar in both plan and section that the little French oratory could almost be described as an Armenian outpost in the Carolingian realm.

The influence of Armenian architecture is not limited to a single instance; it is also manifest in the Cappella della Pietà (ca. 876; formerly S. Satiro) adjacent to the Church of S. Maria presso S. Satiro in Milan (FIG. 102). Despite Bramante's alterations about 1480 during his work on the main church, much of the original building remains. The four internal supports in this case are columns, not piers. The arms are barrel-vaulted; three terminate in apses, and the fourth, on the west, contains the entrance. The small square corner sections are covered by groined vaults. Bramante's lantern over the crossing must once have been a tower, roofed in the interior by a groined vault. The chapel differs from Germigny-des-Prés in that, in the interior, it has less the character of a hall church and is more emphatically centralized. The apses are drawn closer to the crossing, and the small corner bays are hollowed out into niches, so that the cross-in-square plan expands rhythmically into an octagon emphasized on the exterior perimeter by niches on either side of the apses. This scheme is comparable to that of the Cathedral of Bagaran in Armenia (624–36; see ARMENIAN ART), which may have been its prototype. More rigorously centralized than the Cathedral of Echmiadzin, it is spatially dominated by its square crossing, while the angle bays are reduced to mere passages behind the piers. According to a detailed description of 1127, the chapel of the Great Palace of the Emperors in Constantinople had a similar plan, though on a larger scale; it was dedicated in 881 by Basil I, the founder of the Macedonian dynasty. The chapel in Milan, begun about the same time, may have been directly influenced by it. Its original dimensions were somewhat modified when the floor and the four columns were raised about 26 inches.

*The Palatine Chapel in Aachen.* The most important centralized building of the Carolingian period is without doubt the Palatine Chapel in Aachen (PL. 52; FIG. 102), consecrated in 805. Closely connected with the personality of Charlemagne, it was the court chapel of his favorite residence, and he chose it as his final resting place. Complex and daring in structure, it is the best-preserved of all Carolingian buildings; it was not altered materially until fairly late in its history.

It is a vaulted octagon, surrounded by an ambulatory with galleries above. The original chancel, destroyed by the Gothic additions, was a small square bay which contrasted sharply with the grand three-towered westwork: the latter contained a porch at ground level, and above, between the access towers, a portion of the gallery. The grandeur of this scheme is significant; it made possible the expansion of the west bay of the gallery, where the famous imperial throne was installed. The opposite bay of the gallery, above the chancel, was also enlarged to accommodate a special altar; thus the octagon appeared to be set between two projecting bodies.

There were also two lateral buildings, contemporary with the octagon, in the form of three-aisled chapels with apses; their two-storied porches were connected with the octagon by galleries and round-arched doors, still visible though walled up. We do not know to what use these side buildings were put.

The ambulatory was conceived as a support divided into compartments with vaults resting on heavy piers; the structural system seems to anticipate much Romanesque construction. The complex vaulting of the upper story or gallery level is intended to support the dome that covers the octagon and to relieve the pressure it exerts on the corners of the piers, a system masterfully employed by Justinian's architects.

Unlike Byzantine architecture, however — so compact and undifferentiated in its membering — the Palatine Chapel is subtly and clearly articulated and forecasts the Romanesque styles. In this it differs from S. Vitale at Ravenna, often considered its prototype. The relation between the two buildings is spiritual rather than formal. In the Carolingian period Ravenna still retained some of its glamor as the last capital of the Roman emperors in the West, and S. Vitale was considered the imperial palace chapel. This is why Charlemagne, confirming his authority through the symbols of tradition, chose it as a model for his chapel at Aachen and caused marble columns and pavement slabs to be brought from Ravenna, as well as the equestrian statue of Theodoric. Seen in this light, the Palatine Chapel of Aachen is the link between the twilight of the ancient world and the dawn of the Middle Ages.

Hans THÜMMLER

MONUMENTAL PAINTING. The prominence given to Carolingian wall painting in contemporary texts is amply justified by the important remains of fresco cycles discovered in the 20th century. Such decoration continued a practice common in ancient times, and the antique world was surely an ever-present source of inspiration. Our knowledge of Carolingian wall painting is further enlarged by the known tituli, texts of inscriptions intended to be placed below the paintings, which indicate the subjects depicted and give a general idea of their diffusion and iconographic schemes. Through these accompanying inscriptions, the cycles, of which they were an integral part, became painted sermons in the truest sense.

One aspect typical of the symbolic character of representations based on sacred texts (see BIBLICAL SUBJECTS) may be deduced from the writings of Deacon Florus of Lyons (d. ca. 860; Carmen XX). He describes the Heavenly Jerusalem with Christ in Majesty surrounded by the symbols of the four Evangelists, above figures of martyrs and with Paradise represented by the Lamb of God and the four rivers.

That extensive cycles of the life of Christ and of many saints also existed is indicated by the frescoes discovered in Münster (in Graubünden). The typological schemes of many of these cycles, known from documents, favor a Roman, or at least Italian, origin.

Almost no secular mural painting remains, but the written sources give a general idea of their scope. Charlemagne had scenes of his war in Spain painted in his palace in Aachen. Representations of the seven liberal arts and of the seasons occurred in Aachen and in the residence of Theodulf, bishop of Orléans (799–818). Louis the Pious (814–40) had the imperial palace at Ingelheim (Hesse) decorated with a series of heroes, all historical figures, beginning with Alexander the Great and ending with Charlemagne. There seems to be an intentional parallelism between them and the cycle of the life of Christ in the Palatine Chapel in Aachen.

The sources also bear witness to the existence of panel painting (Servatius Lupus), while stained glass, though of little importance, is known to have existed at Werden and Zurich.

From both the technical and the artistic viewpoints a catalogue of colors in a letter of about 827 (*Monumenta Germaniae historica*, Epistola V, p. 292 f.) is of great interest. Its author requests "ut nobis mittas ad decorandas parietes colores diversos, qui ad manum habentur, videlicet auri pigmentum, folium indicum, minium, lazur atque prusium et de vivo argento iuxta facultatem" ("that you should send us various colors

that you have at hand for the decoration of walls, to wit: gold pigment, Indian leaf, minium, azure, emerald, and as much quicksilver as possible").

*Western Frankish region.* Fragments from two distinct fresco cycles uncovered in the crypt of St.-Germain in Auxerre in 1927 are the only ones remaining in this region. The first consists of three scenes from a cycle of the story of St. Stephen (PL. 54), which are framed by painted columns and plant motifs, the other of two frescoes with two bishops each. Forceful gestures and lively movements animate the scenes from the life of St. Stephen, and their expressiveness is heightened by the small number of figures in each. The artist's awareness of the interrelation between architectural setting and decoration is indicated by the type of framing elements employed and by the position of the frescoes within the lunettes. These frescoes are generally dated in the period between the construction of the crypt in 841 and the translation of the relics of St. Germain and other bishops of Auxerre (859–61); such a dating finds confirmation in the late Carolingian character of the rich foliate ornament. The static figures of the bishops are perhaps slightly later.

Major stylistic differences separate the frescoes of Auxerre from those of Ternand (Rhône), which some French scholars attribute to the Carolingian period.

*Eastern Frankish region.* Remnants of Carolingian frescoes have been found in many localities of the eastern Frankish empire; excavations have brought them to light, for example, in St. Florin at Koblenz, at Lorsch, beneath the present Cathedral of Cologne, and in the westwork of Corvey. But the frescoes from the crypt of St. Maximin in Trier (transferred to the Trier Landesmus.; PL. 54), discovered in 1917 and restored 1936–39, best reflect what the wall paintings of this region must have been like. The crypt was a reused late-antique tomb chamber. The rest of the church was destroyed during the Norse raid of 882 and probably rebuilt during the first half of the 10th century. According to some scholars the frescoes were painted before this attack (Eichler, 1952); according to others they were executed shortly thereafter (Grabar, 1957). The frescoes were in the eastern part of the crypt. On each side of the monolithic altar there is a procession of four martyrs, and in the lunette above a large Crucifixion (ca. 6½ × 11 ft.) with the Virgin, SS. John, Longinus, and Stephaton, as well as the rarely shown feature of the nails at the foot of the cross. Unfortunately the upper portion of the scene was destroyed during later construction. In the vault there appear the Evangelists, prophets, and inscriptions naming the virtues, all framed by wide ornamental bands and painted architectural elements. Notwithstanding common stylistic elements, the iconographic sources of the cycle in St. Maximin are to be found not in miniatures but in Italian fresco cycles. A date toward the end of the 9th century is supported by the pronounced linearism, which emphasizes the expressive quality and slight plasticity of the frescoes.

The remains of monumental painting in the "solarium" of the gateway (*Torhalle*) at the abbey of Lorsch (FIG. 89) are of particular importance because of their secular character. A dado simulating multicolored marble slabs is surmounted by delicate columns, widely spaced, which support a richly profiled architrave, thus giving the illusion of an opening into space. Evidently antique models inspired this architectural rendering.

*Alpine regions and northern Italy.* By far the most important examples of Carolingian painting have been preserved in remote Alpine valleys. The imposing spectacle of such a decorative scheme can still be seen, partially intact, in the Church of St. Johann at Münster (PL. 57), founded at the end of the 8th century and first mentioned in a document of 805. The east wall was occupied by an *Ascension* (detached; now in Zurich, Schweizerisches Landesmus.); in the central apse Christ in Majesty appears above scenes from the life of St. John the Baptist; in the south apse is a jeweled cross with medallions

and, below, scenes from the life of St. Stephen; and in the north apse are the Traditio Legis, or Christ investing SS. Peter and Paul with the New Law, and, below, scenes from the lives of the apostles. Facing these, on the west wall, is the oldest extant monumental representation of the Last Judgment. No less important than the two great complementary scenes of the Majesty and the Judgment are the three cycles unfolding in 82 framed scenes, displayed in five registers, on the walls of the nave. The uppermost zone consists of 20 scenes from the story of David and Absalom. The 48 scenes from the life of Christ in the three following zones constitute the most extensive early medieval cycle of this type. The poor state of preservation of the lowest zone makes identification of the theme uncertain, and the whole south wall has been damaged beyond recognition by the elements. The original color scheme has suffered seriously, but the overpowering impact of the brick red must have been balanced by other colors and contrasting highlights. In place of a linear presentation of outlines and internal divisions, volume is rendered in large areas of color. Details were handled in a manner sometimes called "impressionistic," and white hatching was used extensively, though it has all but disappeared. The stocky, rather uniform figures, unclear in their volumetric forms, differ considerably from the Ottonian frescoes of Oberzell on Reichenau and S. Vincenzo in Galliano (Lombardy). Though the isolated abbey of Münster was open to influences from the great monastic centers of Reichenau and St. Gall, their close affinity to Italian, particularly Roman, works suggests an Italian source beneath the provincial manner.

Not far from Münster, in one of its dependencies, the tiny chapel of S. Benedetto at Malles (PL. 57), there are frescoes which were probably painted before 881 according to Garber (1928). The east wall is decorated with stuccowork which frames the apses. In the main one Christ is depicted surrounded by saints and angels, and on the narrow wall between the apses there are portraits of the founders. The scenes from the life of St. Paul on the north wall are in a poor state of preservation.

Compared to the frescoes of Münster and Malles those in S. Procolo at Naturno (PL. 57) seem strangely exotic. The lower portion of the south wall of the nave is decorated with scenes from the story of St. Paul, the triumphal arch with cherubs and elders. The figures, which seem composed of variously colored bands and appear as multicolored silhouettes against the light background, bring to mind Irish work on the Continent (St. Gall, Salzburg), but their similarity to Lombard and Merovingian works, illustrated respectively by the frescoes at Cividale and the Sacramentary of Gellone (Paris, Bib. Nat., Lat. 12048), has also been recognized. A parallel may also be seen in traces of Merovingian art as reflected in Spanish illumination of the 10th century. Hence the frescoes at Naturno, though their 9th-century date is uncertain, may furnish a clue to what central European painting of the 8th and 9th centuries might have been like had there been no revival of the antique.

Few remains of monumental painting have survived in northern Italy aside from the works in Malles and Naturno, just mentioned, which, however, belong stylistically and historically to the Alpine group. The fragments in S. Salvatore in Brescia may be as early as the dedication of the church in 760, although Cecchelli (1954) relates them to Malles. Some historians also date parts of the fragments in S. Maria in Valle (the "tempietto") at Cividale to this period. The fragmentary figures of saints in niches in the Cappella della Pietà in S. Maria presso S. Satiro in Milan, built by Archbishop Ansperto about 876, are from the end of the 9th or the beginning of the 10th century, but even they do not have the same sense of volume as the frescoes in Malles, although they have been compared to them.

*Spain.* In Asturias, Spain's only Christian kingdom, monumental painting of the 9th century reverted to Early Christian traditions in a manner comparable, in its general direction though not in its specific formal aspects, to the developments within the confines of the Carolingian empire. The frescoes in the Church of S. Julián de los Prados (San-

tullano) in Oviedo are the best-preserved example. Though they are badly faded, their general scheme has been reconstructed by De Selgas (1916) and by Schlunk (1957). Their character is essentially decorative. The lowest register imitates a revetment of colored marble slabs sunk into the wall to form geometric patterns. Above it rise several bands of architectural motifs with niches and aediculae similar to the mosaics in the dome of the Baptistery of the Orthodox in Ravenna and in St. George in Salonika. The vault of the apse is decorated with floral and geometric motifs in panels reminiscent of coffering. These frescoes are close to Early Christian works not only in subject matter and composition but also in their choice of colors: once-luminous ochers, carmine reds, blues, and whites stand out against a blue-gray background. The frescoes were executed most probably soon after the church was built, during the last years of the reign of Alfonso II the Chaste (d. 842). Aside from their general dependence on late-antique and Early Christian prototypes, nothing certain is known about the sources of this type of decoration, least of all to what extent it was based on now obscure local traditions. This style is apparent in various places in Spain up to the end of the 10th century, and it is only during the Romanesque period that the representation of the human figure becomes usual in Spanish painting. In fact the decoration of S. Miguel at Lillo, though mainly ornamental, is exceptional in its figures of the 9th century.

*Mosaics.* By far the most important mosaics of the period must have been those in the dome of the Palatine Chapel in Aachen. It has been possible to reconstruct their original composition with the help of a drawing by Ciampini (1699) and the underdrawings brought to light during the restoration of 1879–81. Early Christian iconography is followed: Christ appears in a *mandorla* surrounded by the symbols of the Evangelists, while the elders of the Apocalypse hold gold crowns.

The only Carolingian mosaic to retain some original elements is the one in the apse of the oratory at Germigny-des-Prés (PL. 53). Built by Theodulf, bishop of Orléans, one of Charlemagne's advisers in the revival of learning, it must have been constructed after the Palatine Chapel was completed. The background is partly gold, partly deep blue with golden stars; the ark of the covenant is represented in the center with the hand of God above and angels at the side. Most of the adjacent ornamental areas, lost during the restoration of 1869, contained scrollwork and palmettes under arches which, according to Grabar (1954), show Ommiad influence, while the impetuous movement of the angels is close to the style of the Ada Group of illuminations.

SCULPTURE. Less is known of sculpture than of any other phase of Carolingian art, and almost nothing has survived (apart from works in small dimensions usually considered in the category of minor arts). It was Charlemagne's intention to enrich the churches and palaces of his domain with sculpture, and to this end he had models brought from Italy, among them the marble capitals in the Palatine Chapel in Aachen and the bronze equestian statue of Theodoric. Further, it is known that there were "images" of him in the cloister of the monastery at Lorsch and on the gilded arch above his tomb in Aachen; it is certain that the latter was a relief. Though it is debatable whether the small equestrian bronze in the Louvre represents Charlemagne (see ANTIQUE REVIVAL; I, PL. 303), there can be no doubt that the much-admired antique equestrian statues exercised a considerable influence on Carolingian sculpture. Sparse remains scattered throughout the empire indicate that an ornamental sculpture closely linked to Merovingian traditions was predominant. Much of the architectural sculpture, mainly limited to capitals and moldings, revived antique forms which had fallen into disuse. In the decoration of ambos and closure slabs the Merovingian low relief and incised interlacings gave way to a deeper and more decisive carving without, however, changing its fundamental character.

Marble was almost never used; its place was taken by other stone, though stucco was also popular because it could be worked with great ease. "Imagines in gypso vel testa formatae" ("images

made of stucco or terra cotta") are specifically mentioned in the *Libri carolini*. Almost everywhere stucco was the most important material in the decoration of churches — a technique that derived from Merovingian usage. It is known that the three main altars at St.-Riquier were encased in gold, while the side altars had stucco reliefs with painted frames incrusted with stones; evidently they were imitations of gold altars (see below) and could be produced quickly and cheaply.

The mention of not only stucco reliefs but also stucco statues raises the problem of sculpture in the round. Although no extant remains date earlier than the end of the 10th century, sources attest to their use much earlier. Furthermore Charlemagne is said to have donated to the basilica of St. Peter's in Rome the cross of which a copy still exists in the sacristy. Undoubtedly Italy was an important source for Carolingian sculpture in the round (Keller, 1951), even if the majority of the many *imagines* mentioned in the *Liber pontificalis* ("Book of the Popes") were reliefs.

*Western Frankish region.* Although it is particularly difficult to assess the sculpture of the western Frankish region, the little that remains permits one to trace a development in architectural sculpture from the capitals of St.-Denis and Germigny-des-Prés (ca. 806) to those of St.-Germain in Auxerre. The best works are also the earliest, and in their structure they evince an undisputed preference for antique forms. In contrast, the Merovingian tradition dominated in such works as the square pillar decorated with rinceaux and rosettes in St.-Pierre at Flavigny and also continues to be utilized in church decoration in other parts of the empire.

Since certain works in Reims and Autun, called Carolingian by Porter (1927), have been reassigned to a later period, our knowledge of the lost sculpture of France is based exclusively on the few reliefs found in England that reflect its style. Thus the figure that may be identified as Christ on a fragment of the Reculver cross in the crypt of Canterbury Cathedral is typically western Frankish and probably dates from the middle of the 9th century. Fragments of the Easby cross (London, Vict. and Alb.), probably of the 9th century, are badly weathered, but a Christ in Majesty, busts of the apostles, and vine scrolls with birds and animals are still visible (I, PL. 291).

Aside from the modest fragments of scrolls, palmettes, rosettes, and interlace at Germigny-des-Prés nothing remains, in the western Frankish lands, of the considerable wealth in stucco decoration mentioned in contemporary documents. Monumental crucifixes, already in use during the Merovingian period, must have been common, as well as figures of Christ in Majesty and figures of saints similar to the one of Ste-Foy in Conques, which dates well into the 10th century and testifies to the high quality of western Frankish sculpture in the early Middle Ages.

*Eastern Frankish region.* Little sculpture has survived in the basins of the Meuse and the Moselle and to the east of the Rhine. Besides the capitals of Lorsch, Fulda (PL. 60), and Corvey, some of which display exceptional workmanship, sandstone fragments have been excavated at Lorsch; they were probably carved there, since this kind of stone is quarried nearby. Unfortunately the poor state of preservation of the head found there makes an attribution more precise than early Carolingian impossible, and an identification with the Ada Group has to be rejected (Boeckler, 1954). The most important finds of the period are the so-called "window of Hatto" and the "priest's stone" (*Priesterstein*) from the Church of St. Alban in Mainz (Dom- und Diözesanmus.). The window's scrolls and small panels with scenes are close to the ivories of the Ada Group. The "priest's stone" is worked on four sides. On the front, within an arched niche, appears a figure in priestly vestments, carrying a crozier. In his left hand he holds a book bearing the inscription *venite benedicti* ("come ye blessed"). This figure may be identified as Christ, particularly as the cross on the rear of the stone is inscribed *sca crux salva nos* ("holy cross, save us"). Both the fine acanthus decoration and the epigraphy suggest a date shortly after 800.

*Alpine regions and northern Italy.* Important work in stucco, some with figures, has been preserved in the monasteries of these regions. Excavations of the Church of St. Martin at Disentis (Graubünden) have brought to light numerous fragments of heads, drapery, hands, etc., some of them with traces of polychromy. Originally these large figures must have decorated the walls of the apse while purely decorative motifs enriched the church's moldings.

Enough of the 9th-century stuccowork in S. Benedetto in Malles remains to permit a reconstruction of the entire east wall of the small church. Here the frescoes were framed by columns and arches or moldings. A particularly well-preserved fragment of a head carved in low, flat relief is reminiscent of the frieze in S. Maria in Valle in Cividale (of controversial date) and the sandstone head from Lorsch. Indeed, the same flat modeling is typical of all stuccowork of the early Carolingian phase.

In the territories of the Roman empire, in the countries south of the Danube, in Switzerland, Italy, France, and even Spain — most markedly in northern Italy and Rome — much sculptural decoration in stone and stucco has been found which was once considered Lombard but which should be dated in the Carolingian period. These works were meant to decorate pulpits, chancel barriers, ciboriums, and altars, and the motifs employed were limited to consistently repeated interlaces, volutes, rosettes, and other rather abstract plant elements, particularly various forms of leaves, all carved in a low, flat relief. Some of the finest surviving examples are the slabs from chancel barriers in Chur, the abbey churches of Münster and Schänis (PL. 60), and S. Benedetto in Malles, as well as the ambos in the churches of St.-Maurice d'Agaune and Romainmôtier. All this material, not yet fully classified, should be assigned to the 9th century. Furthermore the origins of this style must be sought in the late-antique period and may have been spread by Italian craftsmen.

In Italy proper no Carolingian figure sculpture has been preserved, for the Byzantinizing stucco figures in S. Maria in Valle at Cividale, previously assigned to this period, should probably be dated in the 10th or 11th century.

*Bronzes.* Bronzes provide a much clearer idea of the artistic importance and technical accomplishment of Carolingian sculpture than do works in stone. Much of what is extant can be connected with the foundry in Aachen, which was discovered during excavations. It was responsible for the four doors of the Palatine Chapel in Aachen (PL. 65). Despite their size each door was cast in a single piece. The extraordinary esthetic impact is due to the careful balance of the square and rectangular fields, to the moldings — finely profiled and decorated with ornamental motifs derived from the antique — and to the powerful projection of the lions' heads. Both the technical perfection and the faithful imitation of antique ornament suggest foreign artisans.

The famous bronze railings around the octagonal gallery of the Palatine Chapel in Aachen were also made in this workshop. The way some of the rectangles are subdivided into squares with diagonal divisions is typically antique; many of them are enriched with a delicate plant ornament related to the ivories of the Ada Group, especially the Deventer chalice. The *pigna* (pine cone) of the Palatine Chapel in Aachen, which copied the one in the atrium of Old St. Peter's in Rome, is perhaps also by this workshop. The difficulty of dating it has been increased by the loss of the decorative elements on the corners.

The so-called "throne of Dagobert" in the Louvre (PL. 68) also seems to be a Carolingian work and probably from the same workshop. Its transfer to St.-Denis seems quite plausible because of the close relations between the two foundations at this time. It is a folding chair (*sella plicatilis*) with some traces of gilt. That the curved legs terminate in panthers' heads above and in animal claws below is additional proof that the chair was intended as a royal throne (compare the one in the Psalter of Lothair, London, Br. Mus., Add. 37768). The restorations undertaken by Abbot Suger of St.-Denis, according to documents, cannot have altered it very much, and a

date in the beginning of the 9th century seems probable. A much simpler folding stool, with original Carolingian ornamental inlay in gold and silver, was discovered at Pavia during excavations for a new bridge over the Ticino in 1950. It probably dates after Charlemagne's conquest of Lombardy in 774.

If one adds to the works that have survived those mentioned in documents, such as the bronze figures crowning the chancel barriers of the church of St.-Riquier, a fuller picture of Carolingian bronzes emerges. The only bronze representation of the human figure that has survived from this period is the previously mentioned small equestrian statue of a Carolingian emperor with crown, sword, and imperial globe in the Louvre. Although it is most frequently identified as Charles the Bald (843–77), Deér (1953) demonstrated its similarity to the work of the Ada Group and identified it as a portrait of Charlemagne. In either case the little statue, with its close ties to antiquity, is a significant expression of the spirit and forms of Carolingian art (I, PL. 303).

ILLUMINATION. Because of their quantity and variety, the illuminated manuscripts are by far the most important form of Carolingian art. The rapid development in manuscript production was concomitant with the general revival of learning which stressed both sacred and secular texts. The greater concern with accurate sacred texts was connected with the reforms in script, encouraged by Alcuin of York, that led to the creation of the Carolingian minuscule (see CALLIGRAPHY AND EPIGRAPHY). Not only Charlemagne but also his successors, particularly Charles the Bald, were so interested in books that book production changed from an anonymous craft to an art linked to the names of leading scribes and their powerful patrons.

At first the main centers of illumination were in the old eastern Frankish regions, but later they shifted to the north of France, particularly Reims and Tours. For a long time the eastern Frankish regions retained insular (i.e., Anglo-Irish) and Merovingian traditions; this local style should not be overlooked, although it was overshadowed by the aristocratic current emanating from Salzburg, St. Gall, Echternach, and other centers that exercised a decisive influence during the first period of Carolingian book illumination.

The conscious revival of the antique, apparent in all phases of artistic endeavor during the 8th and 9th centuries, is fundamental to the development of miniature painting. Hence it is one of the primary tasks of scholarship to trace the process of assimilating and transforming diverse earlier prototypes in the different schools. This process is of wider concern also, inasmuch as the models used for miniatures had a considerable influence on the other arts as well, so that the conclusions in this field are also valid for other forms of expression.

The Italian and Byzantine manuscripts that served as prototypes for Carolingian illumination have been lost, but it is known that such manuscripts came into Frankish hands by many routes. Furthermore there is ample indication that foreign artists were working in the Frankish empire. But the awareness that Carolingian manuscripts reflect their models in varying degrees should not obscure the recognition of original and creative elements contained in them. The models copied most faithfully were nonreligious works whose content and form were to be "as far as possible accurately mastered" (Goldschmidt, 1928). Secular texts used in an educational system controlled by the Church are, however, relatively rarer than sacred texts. Among the latter the most common during the early Carolingian period were Gospel books. Their miniatures were determined by the texts, but their subject matter was considerably more limited than during other periods, being reduced on the whole to presentations of Christ in Majesty and portraits of the Evangelists. Though no New Testament cycles have come down to us, completely illustrated Gospels did most probably exist (Koehler, 1952). The heritage of illustrative material of the Old and New Testaments and of secular themes is revealed in all its wealth in the Psalter in Stuttgart (Landesbib., Bibl. fol. 23) and to an even greater extent in the one in Utrecht (Univ. Lib., Script. eccl. 484; PL. 58); the latter can readily be considered an inventory of illustrative resources of the time.

Carolingian illuminators showed much originality in the selection and interpretation of decorative elements, which they took from many sources, the most important being the Insular school. The full-page initial stems from Insular manuscripts, as do some of the ornamental elements around the arcades of the Eusebian canon tables (concordances of the four Gospels arranged in tabular form).

Different techniques were used. Tempera, occasionally with some gold illumination, was preferred by the schools associated with the imperial court; ink drawings, sometimes on a colored ground, were favored in St. Gall, in the areas around Lake Constance, and, in the 10th century, by the Westphalian and Saxon group; the two methods were combined by the Reims school and, in the 10th century, by the English schools. These variations are probably to be explained, in large part, by the differences in the models; for example, the antique texts used for instruction were often filled with many simple pen-and-ink drawings.

*The Court School of Charlemagne (Ada Group).* The earliest group of Carolingian manuscripts was first isolated by Janitschek (1889), who named it after a Gospel book (Trier, Stadtbib., Cod. 22) commissioned by Ada, the supposed half sister of Charlemagne. One of the earliest manuscripts of the group, the Godescalc Gospels (Paris, Bib. Nat., nouv. acq. lat. 1203), was probably made between 781 and 783 to commemorate the baptism of the Emperor's son Pepin. Besides the portraits of the Evangelists and Christ in Majesty, there is a full-page representation of the Fountain of Life (PL. 55) that probably alludes to Pepin's baptism; the rich gold uncials on parchment dyed a regal purple are appropriate to the importance of the event. The insular manner in the decoration of the initials points to the connections established between the British Isles and the palatine scriptorium through Alcuin of York, who directed the scriptorium until 796, when he became abbot of Tours.

In rapid succession the palatine scriptorium produced the other masterpieces of the Ada Group: the Gospels in London (Br. Mus., Harley 2788), the Gospels of St. Médard of Soissons (Paris, Bib. Nat., Lat. 8850), the Codex Aureus from Lorsch (in two parts, one in Alba Julia, Romania, Cathedral Lib., and the other, together with the cover, Rome, Vat., Pal. lat. 50), as well as others, including the so-called small "Psalter of Dagulf" (Vienna, Nationalbib., Cod. 1861) presented to Pope Adrian I by Charlemagne. The last two still have the ivory plaques of their original bindings. All these manuscripts are artistically superior to the Godescalc Gospels and comprise the first classicizing phase of Carolingian illumination. The figures of the Evangelists, monumentally enthroned, achieve organic coherence chiefly through the linear presentation aided by some modeling of the volumes. The golden highlights and angular breaks of the drapery folds are as surely derived from Byzantine models as the backgrounds imitating antique theatrical scenery. But the Byzantinizing Italian style is responsible for the habit of setting figures into arcades, as may be seen from a comparison with English manuscripts influenced by Italian prototypes, such as the Codex Aureus of Canterbury (Stockholm, Royal Lib., A. 135). The diversity of sources the palatine scriptorium drew on is further emphasized by the fundamental role played by Insular influences in the development of ornament and by the use of Syriac models for the iconography of certain of the full-page miniatures.

That the pictorial range of the Court School was much more extensive than the few extant full-page illustrations would indicate is known from marginal illustrations with lively little figures in narrative scenes in the Soissons Gospels. Another important contribution to our knowledge of early Carolingian illumination is the cycle of New Testament episodes reconstructed by Koehler (1952).

Although today only some ten codices, chiefly Gospels, make up the main body of the Ada Group, its influence on the Continent, particularly at Fulda, was considerable and extended even to Ireland, as may be seen in the Book of Kells (Dublin, Trinity Coll. Lib., Ms. 58).

*The "New Palace School."* Tradition has it that Otto III found the Coronation Book (Vienna, Schatzkammer) in Charlemagne's tomb. Hence it would seem that even before the Emperor's death a style very different from that of the Ada Group had come to dominate the palatine scriptorium, one closely related to late-antique illusionistic painting. A Greek name, "Demetrius Presbyter," on folio 118 of the Coronation Book supports the thesis that foreign artists participated in the new movement. The new style is variously associated by scholars with Charlemagne's coronation, rich in consequences for the artistic world, with his recognition in 812 by the Byzantine emperor, and with the succession of his son Louis the Pious (814).

The Gospels of the Cathedral Treasury in Aachen and the Xanten Gospels (Brussels, Bib. Royale, Ms. 18723) belong to the same group as the Coronation Book. All three are sumptuous works with few but exceedingly fine decorations. Full-page illustrations are limited to the Evangelists; in the Aachen Gospels they are placed against a blue-gray background hinting at a landscape, while the Brussels Gospels reflect a late-antique composition similar to the portrait of Galen in the Vienna Dioscorides (Nationalbib., Med. gr. 1), probably made shortly before A.D. 512. A portrait of an Evangelist (fol. 17) stitched into the Brussels manuscript and placed against a purple background is perhaps by the same hand as the Coronation Book. This page, which is related to Hellenistic art, is one of the most beautiful works of this school.

The sources and genesis of the new style remain a mystery, but it undoubtedly flourished and developed most fully at Reims. Although frequently considered a work of the "New Palace School," the Gospels of Cleve (Berlin, Staatsbib., Theol. lat. fol. 260) may possibly form a transition to the Reims school, as indicated by its close stylistic relation to the Gospel book of Ebbo (Epernay, Bib. Municipale, Ms. 1) and the Psalter of Lothair in London (Br. Mus., Add. 37768). The complex interrelations between the "New Palace School" and the Reims workshop largely reflect the personality of Archbishop Ebbo of Reims, who was active in the palatine scriptorium in Aachen before his investiture in Reims (816–35).

*Reims.* Stylistic affinities with the Palace School are still considerable in the Epernay Gospels made for Archbishop Ebbo in the monastery of Hautvillers near Reims (PL. 59). Here too the portraits of the Evangelists are the most important decoration, although numerous lively little figures, animals, and scenes have been added to the canon tables. A characteristic trait of the Reims school is the expressive and animated manner of painting the Evangelists. Already in this manuscript the rapid, pliant brush strokes are only superficially related to the opaque coloring of late-antique illusionistic illumination.

In the second masterpiece of the school, the Utrecht Psalter (Utrecht, Univ. Lib., Script. eccl. 484; PL. 58), pen-and-ink drawings replace painted illustrations. This manuscript is not only of scholarly interest as a repertory of the late-antique heritage of religious and secular iconography but is also one of the greatest artistic achievements of the period. The drawings, which seem to have been executed freehand, adhere closely to the phrases and words that inspired them. The close interdependence of illustrations and text has made it possible to ascertain that the prototype must have been an example of the so-called *Psalterium duplex* or *triplex*, in which different versions appeared in parallel columns. On the other hand, the illustration of text passages added to the Psalms in the Carolingian period has allowed Wormald (1953) to demonstrate important original contributions by Carolingian artists — contributions inconceivable, to be sure, without these artists' reference to ancient sources. Similarities to the illustrations of the Stuttgart Psalter (Landesbib., Bibl. fol. 23), which is most probably based on a 6th-century prototype of which there is unfortunately no precise knowledge, indicate a model at least as old for the Utrecht Psalter. This Psalter is by far the most important single work of the period by virtue of its influence on the later development of Carolingian art, particularly ivories and metalwork, and on manuscript illustration in England, where the manuscript was taken at an early date.

Another series of Reims-school manuscripts, both secular and religious, combine the style of the Ebbo Gospels with the more classical tendencies of the "New Palace School." They include the Troyes Psalter (Cathedral Lib.), the Gospels of Blois (Paris, Bib. Nat., Lat. 265), and the Bern Physiologus (Stadtbib., Cod. 318) as well as others.

The diversities of style evident within the Reims school as early as the 9th century suggest the existence of a number of subsidiary scriptoriums in northern France, particularly in Lorraine, but the only one that can be clearly identified is the one in Metz. Its most outstanding work is a sacramentary (Paris, Bib. Nat., Lat. 9428; PL. 56) made for Archbishop Drogo (826–55). The numerous small scenes follow the style and iconography of Reims, but the ornamental element is given new prominence, and the initials, with their rich decoration of golden acanthus leaves, are modest forerunners of late Carolingian ornament.

*Tours.* Although the abbey that grew up near the tomb of St. Martin at Tours had an old and powerful tradition, strengthened under the direction of Alcuin of York (796–804), its scriptorium developed a style of its own only under Abbot Fridugisus (807–34). The Tours manuscripts are characterized by a script based on antique models and by a well-defined ornament structurally contained in a framework. At first the illustrations were small and the figures seemed silhouetted, as in the Bamberg Bible (Staatliche Bib., Bibl. 1; PL. 329) and the Gospels of St. Gauzelin in Nancy (Cathedral Treasury; PL. 63).

However, larger illustrations became usual later, as in the Stuttgart manuscript (Landesbib., Bibl. II. 40), in which the manner of Reims was united with a vigorous linear articulation and a marked emphasis on volume.

Artistically the Tours school may be regarded as intermediary between the Ada and Reims groups. Its greatest achievements are the Bible of Moutier-Grandval of about 840 (London, Br. Mus., Add. 10546) and a cycle of illustrations of the Old Testament in the Vivian Bible of 846 (Paris, Bib. Nat., Lat. 1). Through the series of illustrations of Genesis its model can be identified as a sumptuous Bible, now lost but known to have been made in Rome for Leo the Great (440–61; Koehler, 1930–33). An important addition to the iconographic repertory was the late-antique emperor portrait. In the Vivian Bible it appears in the dedicatory miniature, in which the monastery's lay abbot, Count Vivian, is shown presenting the Bible to the emperor Charles the Bald (PL. 64); in the somewhat later Gospels of Lothair (Paris, Bib. Nat., Lat. 266) it is a monumental throned figure flanked by two attendants.

One of the artists working on the Vivian Bible was also responsible for the portraits of the Evangelists in the Prüm Gospels (Berlin, Staatsbib., Theol. lat. fol. 733), but thereafter the level of artistic achievement in Tours declined rapidly and was brought to an abrupt end by the Norse raid of 853.

*The style of Charles the Bald.* A group of manuscripts of the second half of the 9th century particularly rich in ornamental and illustrative decoration — a group previously linked to Corbie (near Amiens, Somme) by Janitschek (1889) and to St.-Denis by Friend (1923) — is now generally associated with Charles the Bald, who ruled from 843 to 877. Important manuscripts made for him include the Psalter now in Paris (Bib. Nat., Lat. 1152; PL. 62), the Book of Hours (Munich, Residenzmus.), the Coronation Sacramentary (Paris, Bib. Nat., Lat. 1141; only partially preserved), and the Codex Aureus of St. Emmeram in Regensburg (Munich, Bayerische Staatsbib., Clm. 14000), still bound in its original sumptuous cover. But by far the most outstanding work of this group is the Bible of S. Paolo fuori le Mura (PL. 61); the arguments advanced by Kantorowicz (1955) that it was made for Charles the Bald himself are convincing. The basic stylistic traits of Reims and Tours come together in this Bible, but the iconography of the Old Testament scenes of its Tours-school model has been extended considerably. This lavish work represents one of the peaks in Carolingian book illumination.

Even before he became lay abbot of St.-Denis in 867,

Charles the Bald possessed a large and outstanding collection of manuscripts, among them the Vivian Bible. The close connections between St.-Denis, Reims, and other northern Frankish monasteries explains the stylistic diversity of these manuscripts; they can be attached to any of the imperial foundations. Nordenfalk (1957) has proposed Compiègne as the focal center. In these manuscripts the almost baroque magnificence of the acanthus ornament and the scenes resplendent with figures show the full range of Carolingian illumination. As shown by three of its most important manuscripts, this phase of illumination covered a relatively short span of time, one that falls within a period when the influence of the Tours school was still felt and that of Reims was at its height. There is internal evidence for dating the Codex Aureus in Munich and the Bible of S. Paolo fuori le Mura about 870, and the same scribe, one Liuthard, who was responsible for the Codex Aureus, also did the Psalter of Charles the Bald.

*Franco-Saxon style.* Boutémy (1949) has advanced reasons for considering St.-Amand, near Tournai, the center for the Franco-Saxon group of manuscripts, sometimes also called "Franco-Insular" or "Anglo-Frankish," after the dual heritage of its style. This school produced large numbers of Gospels and sacramentaries, most of which show no close connection with the production of contemporary scriptoriums, but exercised a major influence in the 10th century. The only important manuscript in the group which can be related to the school of Reims is that of the so-called "Gospels of Francis II" (Paris, Bib. Nat., Lat. 257). In the earliest works portrait medallions are frequently placed at the summit of the arches of the canon tables as in Insular texts; in general, ornamentation is predominantly of the insular type but, unlike this type, is contained within heavy frames characteristic of the Carolingian style. A particularly good example is the Second Bible of Charles the Bald (Paris, Bib. Nat., Lat. 2; PL. 56), presented by the Emperor to the abbey of St.-Denis.

*Minor western Frankish scriptoriums.* A vast network of local workshops, most of which can no longer be isolated, grew up alongside the major centers; they produced some outstanding works, particularly during the early Carolingian period. Several Bibles made at the beginning of the 9th century in the monastery of St.-Benoît-sur-Loire (or Fleury), the residence of Theodulf of Orléans, are noteworthy, and a number of later manuscripts with lively decoration, but devoid of scenes or figures, are to be attributed to Corbie, once regarded as the seat of the palatine scriptorium of Charles the Bald (Homburger, 1957).

*Eastern Frankish region.* The influence of the schools associated with the imperial court was confined largely to the western half of the empire. Even such centers as Cologne lacked important scriptoriums. Hildebold, who was archbishop of Cologne (785–819) as well as Charlemagne's personal chaplain, familiarly known as "Aaron" at court, had to import manuscripts for his own library. This probably explains the heterogeneous character shown by the remnants of the Carolingian library of Cologne. Three early Carolingian manuscripts (Cathedral Treasury, Mss. 63, 65, 67) have been attributed to the convent at Chelles, near Paris (Bischoff, 1957); the *Collectio canonum* (Ms. 213) has Insular decorations and script; the rather primitive Gospels of Hiltfredus (Ms. 13) are of western Frankish origins; the large and lavish Codex 14 is the product of a secondary Franco-Saxon workshop; and the illustrations of Codex 56 are provincial versions of the style of Reims.

The ancient bishopric of Trier was at first influenced by the Insular style, transmitted by way of Echternach (Trier, Cathedral Treasury, Cod. 63) and later mingled with Byzantinizing Italian elements. Furthermore the early Franco-Saxon manner is exemplified in works such as the lectionary in the Trier Stadtbibliothek (Cod. 23).

The most important scriptorium east of the Rhine was in the monastery of Fulda. At first it employed Insular models, but later followed the Court School closely, though always retaining some original elements in the ornamentation and

especially in the choice of colors, which, however, never achieved the subtlety of those of the Ada Group.

That scriptoriums also existed in the various newly founded monasteries of Westphalia and Saxony is a mere hypothesis, but the close ties between these monasteries and their mother houses in the older imperial lands, for example, between Corvey (Westphalia) and Corbie (near Amiens, Somme), are documented by numerous translations of reliquaries to the new monasteries and the frequent activities of insular or Frankish bishops there. Their presence accounts for many manuscripts brought to these monasteries, for example the Terence manuscript (now Rome, Vat., Lat. 3868), which had been at Corvey. The traditions of Reims in particular remain evident in the early Ottonian manuscripts produced in the monasteries on the Weser. In the abbey of Werden on the Ruhr the Frisian abbot Liutger formed a library which housed the early-6th-century Codex Argenteus (now Uppsala, Univ. Lib.). The late-9th-century Epistles of St. Paul, possibly from Essen, in Düsseldorf (Landes- und Stadtbib., A. 14) has two pen-and-ink author portraits in which late-antique prototypes are imperfectly assimilated. The early Carolingian Gospels of the abbey at Essen however, still follow the indigenous Merovingian style of decoration.

Very little has come down to us of the manuscripts from Mainz, Lorsch, and Wissembourg (Alsace), though the Gospels of Otfrid of Wissembourg (Vienna, Nationalbib., Cod. 2687) should be mentioned.

*Salzburg.* Long the ecclesiastical center of the area comprising modern Bavaria and parts of Austria, Salzburg was the site of an important and well-defined school of illumination. The earliest manuscripts, such as the Cutbercht Gospels (Vienna, Nationalbib., Cod. 1224), show strong Insular influences, while the Psalter in Montpellier (Bib. de l'Ecole de Médecine, H. 409), dating from the time of Charlemagne, is stylistically related to the Tassilo Chalice (see ANGLO-SAXON AND IRISH ART; I, PL. 287). That the scriptorium of Salzburg had absorbed the forms of Carolingian imperial art by the beginning of the 9th century may be seen in the full-length author portrait in the Homilies of St. John Chrysostom (Vienna, Nationalbib., Cod. 1007); the influence is even more pronounced in the representations of the months in a collection of astronomical treatises (Vienna, Nationalbib., Cod. 387; II, PL. 24). In considering the transmission of this style to Salzburg, one should bear in mind that Arno (d. 821) was abbot of St.-Amand before he became archbishop of Salzburg in 798.

*St. Gall.* The only eastern Frankish scriptorium to produce manuscripts significant to the development of book illumination was St. Gall. The dominance of the insular manner during the 8th century was followed, up to the middle of the 9th century, by the Merovingian fish-and-bird ornament; but under Abbot Grimald (841–72) a new style came to the fore. Its rich and impressive ornamentation of heavy interlaced bands terminating in large, flat leaves and flowers and punctuated by delicate animal heads may be seen in the Psalter of Folchard (St. Gall, Stiftsbib., Cod. 23). As Boeckler (1951) has shown, large initials with this kind of decoration attained a classical monumentality which changed to a more "baroque" manner in the Psalterium Aureum (St. Gall, Stiftsbib., Cod. 22) and the Evangelium Longum (Cod. 53), both written under Abbot Salomon's time (890–920). The extensive use of figures and the color range employed in the Psalterium Aureum indicate a familiarity with the major movements of Carolingian illumination. The influences of the school of Reims and the style of Charles the Bald are fruitfully employed.

In conclusion, a trait peculiar to the St. Gall scriptorium must be noted. In numerous manuscripts besides the Psalterium Aureum — a codex containing various texts (Zurich, Zentralbib., Ms. 59247), a compendium of astronomical texts (St. Gall, Stiftsbib., Cod. 250), and the Homilies in Basel (Universitäts Bib., Ms. IV 26) — painted prototypes are translated into pen-and-ink drawings. The many drawings in Prudentius' *Psychomachia* (Bern, Stadtbib., Cod. 264) exemplify the full development of its style, the final stage of which is embodied in the overanimated scenes of the Book of the Maccabees in Leiden (Univ. Lib., Cod. Perizoni 17).

In the 10th century the Reichenau school, to which no Carolingian manuscript can be attributed with certainty, took up the ornamental initials of St. Gall, which were of profound importance to the development of Ottonian miniatures.

IVORIES. The renewed predilection for ivories is another indication of the conscious revival of antiquity. Carolingian ivories were limited to religious use, however, and therefore never achieved the variety of their ancient prototypes. In addition late-antique ivories, which might be completely recut or left almost unchanged, were used in a new context, perhaps partly owing to a shortage of the raw material. The relatively large number of surviving ivories compensates, at least to some extent, for the lack of monumental sculpture. It also permits extensive study, though the lack of information on the provenance and original intent of most of the pieces has made definitive attributions difficult. As a result the classification of ivories must depend on comparative stylistic analyses based partly on the classification of schools established for miniatures. Additional help is derived from iconographic comparisons which furthermore not only contribute to our knowledge of the Carolingian thematic repertory and to its sources but may also indicate the type of book for which the ivory originally served as cover. Christ in Majesty, the Virgin, the Crucifixion, and the Evangelists were used for Gospels; King David or illustrations of individual Psalms on Psalters; the Crucifixion, St. Gregory, or liturgical scenes on sacramentaries.

*Ada Group.* Some forty ivories have been related to the Court School of miniatures and share fundamental characteristics with it. Single figures or scenes with few figures predominate. Like the simple diptychs or diptych leaves composed of five panels of late-antique times, the Carolingian ones are usually narrow and high; they are also classicizing in the modeling of the figures. The perfection of the workmanship can be explained only by the high quality of their late-antique models, and such models would have been available only at the imperial court. The subjects, echoing those of the miniatures and as limited in range, are Christ, either standing or enthroned, the Virgin and Child, monumental figures of angels or apostles, and Evangelists, as well as rather abbreviated scenes from the New Testament (diptych in the Aachen Cathedral Treasury). There are also a few isolated pieces with purely ornamental decoration, such as the ivory chalice of Lebuinus in Deventer (Netherlands). By far the most outstanding ivory of the Ada Group is the diptych that once was the cover of the Codex Aureus of Lorsch; the front cover, composed of five panels, is in the Vatican (PL. 66), and the back one is in the Victoria and Albert Museum, London. The cover in the Vatican shows on the central panel Christ trampling a lion and a dragon; an angel appears on each side panel. The London cover shows the Virgin enthroned between SS. John and Zacharias, an allusion to the Incarnation of Christ. Though based on different stylistic sources, the compositions of both panels reflect the decorations of Early Christian church apses. The one in the Vatican, using a model from the Theodosian period, stresses sculptural qualities in the figures and relates the modeling to the linear presentation of the drapery with great delicacy. In the leaf in London, which follows Eastern models of about A. D. 500, volume is less important and linear values are emphasized instead. Out of these two opposing tendencies the medieval style was to develop (Schnitzler, 1950).

The diptych from Genoels-Elderen (Brussels, Musées Royaux d'Art et d'Histoire; PL. 305), reminiscent of the Godescalc Gospels and still under strong insular influence, must be dated earlier than the Lorsch panels. A decisive development in Carolingian ivory carving falls between this piece and the covers of the so-called "Psalter of Dagulf" (Paris, Louvre; the manuscript it originally covered is in Vienna, Nationalbib., Cod. 1861; the book was among the objects Charlemagne presented to Pope Adrian I). These two panels, adorned with

scenes of the writing and translation of the Psalms, reflect the artistic atmosphere of the imperial court. The combination of powerful modeling, particularly in the heads, with the flat quality of the whole — a quality emphasized by the iconographically related medallions in the corners — links these panels both with the late-antique tradition and, by virtue of the new pictorial conception expressed in them, with the early Middle Ages. Another work in this group, the splendid panel in Florence (Mus. Naz.), has two scenes, each with a victorious warrior who has been interpreted as a symbolic portrait of Charlemagne (Deér, 1953). What we know of this group of ivories points to a place of origin in the Rhine-Meuse region.

The ivories of the Ada Group do not present a stylistic unity, and the divergencies become more pronounced in the later pieces, dating in the 10th century. Thus the fragment with the Ascension (Darmstadt, Landesmus.) is in very flat relief and has expressive accents foreign to the school. Quite a different impression is created by the Christ in Majesty in Berlin (PL. 66), in which a vigorous treatment of volumes is fused with a supple and nervous handling of drapery in a manner recalling Reims. Like the miniatures of this school, the ivories played a considerable part in forming the Ottonian style.

*Liuthard Group.* A new painterly trend characterized by a lively narrative manner, which contrasts sharply with that of the Ada Group, arose about the 9th century. Many new subjects, probably taken over from paintings, were introduced. Diptychs lost importance. The panels, evidently planned as book covers, were varied in format in accordance with subject matter and the size of manuscripts.

This new group of ivories is named, rather inappropriately, after Liuthard, the scribe of the Psalter of Charles the Bald (Paris, Bib. Nat., Lat. 1152; PL. 62); it was made between 860 and 870. Its covers, treated in the new painterly style, show dramatic scenes, full of life, illustrating Psalms 51 and 57. These covers, as well as two small panels (Zurich, Schweizerisches Landesmus.; Zurich, priv. coll.) that possibly once belonged to the cover of the Book of Hours of Charles the Bald (Munich, Residenzmus.), undoubtedly used the Utrecht Psalter as model. Furthermore the Crucifixion on the cover of the Pericope of Henry II (Munich, Bayerische Staatsbib., Clm. 4452; II, PL. 284) is by the same hand as the ivories of the Book of Hours.

Goldschmidt (1914) included in the Liuthard Group a number of works which are stylistically similar though often less effective. The rapid and expressive movement, the painterly interplay of light and dark, frequently achieved through abrupt undercutting around the figures, and the framing ornament, characteristic of these pieces, indicate a northern French origin. Alongside these somewhat mannered reliefs are secondary groups which developed in more remote areas. Those stemming from the monasteries of Saxony (Goldschmidt, I, 1914, pls. 52 ff.) have the strong modeling of the Ada Group. Outstanding among them are the casket reliquary in Quedlinburg (Stiftskirche, Treasury) and the related fragments in Munich (Bayerisches Nationalmus.), both dating as late as the 10th century.

*Metz Group.* Among the manuscripts that in 1802 came to the Bibliothèque Nationale in Paris from the Cathedral of Metz are two large books (Lat. 9388 and Lat. 9393) with sumptuous bindings decorated with ivories carved in openwork. Each has three scenes from the New Testament, one above the other, enclosed within a wide band of finely carved foliage tracery. Scenes dealing with the early life of Christ appear on Ms. 9393, Passion scenes on Ms. 9388. Despite important divergencies these pieces belong to the same development as the ivories of the Liuthard Group. This is also true of the stylistically related cover of a manuscript in Frankfurt (Stadtbib., Barth. typ. 2), with the Temptation of Christ surrounded by marginal scenes, which probably drew on the same iconographic sources. These ivories are closely related to the small illuminations in the Drogo Sacramentary (Paris, Bib. Nat., Lat. 9428; PL. 62), though the liturgical scenes on its ivory cover are less delicately carved.

Most probably the production of the Metz Group was initiated under Archbishop Drogo of Metz (826–55). The precise stylistic relations between these early Metz ivories and the Liuthard Group, as well as the date and provenance of both, remain highly problematic. The assumption that a previous school of ivories was located in Metz is all the more justified as the masterpiece of the Liuthard Group, the Psalter of Charles the Bald, came to Paris from Metz in 1674 together with other manuscripts.

In the later Metz ivories there is considerable variation in style and quality, though the range in subjects diminishes. The Crucifixion, presented with a wealth of symbolic detail, is the main theme. Its prototype seems to be the above-mentioned ivory of the Liuthard Group in Munich (Bayerische Staatsbib., Clm. 4452).

By the end of the 9th century ivories found a more widespread application. They were used not only as book covers but as reliquaries and other objects such as the comb of St. Heribert in Cologne (Schnütgen Mus.; PL. 67), which on the front has a sober and impressive Crucifixion, on the back a vigorously designed acanthus scroll.

*Minor schools.* The majority of Carolingian ivories may be classed with either of two main tendencies, that represented by the sculptural Ada Group or that represented by the painterly Reims and Metz groups. The numerous ivories that defy precise classification are usually dominated by the painterly point of view, perhaps because some of the minor workshops were located in what is now northern France and Belgium. The handle of the flabellum of Tournus (Florence, Mus. Naz.), with scenes from Vergil's *Eclogues*, is from this area. Another small group stems from Tournai; the diptych of Nicasius in the Cathedral Treasury there (Goldschmidt, I, 1914, nos. 159–62) is a recut late-antique piece and has much in common with the late Metz Group both in its figures and in its ornament, while the acanthus and scrollwork are closer to the style of Charles the Bald. Although Tours had a leading scriptorium, no important ivories can be assigned to it.

The ivories from St. Gall, many of them exclusively ornamental in character, can be identified with precision. The most important work is the diptych (now cover of Cod. 53, St. Gall. Stiftsbib.) made shortly before 900 by a monk named Tuotilo. One panel has Christ in Majesty; the other, the Assumption of the Virgin and scenes from the legend of St. Gall. The crowding, the emphasis on decorative elements, and the use of parallel lines in the drapery all point to a provincial, Alpine interpretation of the late Carolingian style. An interesting phenomenon is the striking similarity, especially in the drapery forms and the predilection for diptychs, in the St. Gall and Tournai ivories, since they originate from two widely separated provinces of the empire. Nor should relations between St. Gall and northern Italy be overlooked. The simple, almost classical frames are a common characteristic. There are also affinities with the cover of the Sacramentary of Berengar and the diptych with King David and St. Gregory, probably a recarved, late-antique consular diptych, both in Monza, Italy (Cathedral Treasury).

GOLD- AND SILVERWORK. Though in comparison to miniatures the number of works in precious metals still extant is rather small, such works have an important place among the minor arts of the period. Gold was prized particularly among the Germanic peoples, not alone for its material value: the belief in its magical powers led to the Christian viewpoint that it was the most fitting offering to God.

Carolingian cathedrals and monasteries were extremely rich in furnishings of gold and silver: chalices, patens, aquaemanalia, basins, censers, crowns, ciboriums, candlesticks, reliquaries, and most especially crosses, as well as many other objects. Also notable were the altar frontals, or antependiums, of chased gold, documented throughout the Carolingian empire by contemporary sources and sometimes by later accounts (e.g., Hincmar's antependium in Reims).

The different uses to which gold was put go hand in hand

with a variety of techniques: chasing, engraving, niello, and filigree; it was incrusted with precious stones and pearls and enhanced with enamel work, both cloisonné and champlevé. Many of these works were decorated with scenes from the life of Christ or with individual figures of saints or the Virgin. The tombs of the more venerated saints were richly furnished with an altar, ciborium, coffin, and innumerable decorated objects (Tours, Fulda, St.-Denis, S. Ambrogio in Milan, St.-Riquier). As in the ancient Germanic world, goldsmiths were held in high regard in the Carolingian period. They are often mentioned in the contemporary literature, and they portrayed themselves on important works, such as the golden altar of Milan.

The extraordinary flowering of the "sumptuous" arts was the result of the reformation of the Frankish Church, the founding of innumerable monasteries, and the increased contact with Mediterranean culture, especially with Rome. Indeed, an intentional imitation of the great Roman basilicas and the tombs of the apostles is documented for Auxerre. Thanks to the capture of the Avar treasure, the supply of gold increased considerably, permitting Charlemagne to present the Pope with massive barbaric pieces worked in gold. The will of Eberhard, Margrave of Friuli, who died in 837, indicates what a wealth of precious metals minor feudal lords possessed.

Because of the importance of gold as a possession of stable value, most early pieces made of gold were later melted down, and the remaining works are too few to permit more than a partial reconstruction of the development of this aspect of Carolingian art. Its main outlines, however, can be traced, and a gradually developing preference for figures and scenes over purely coloristic and abstract ornament is clear.

*Early Carolingian works.* The Tassilo Chalice (I, PL. 287) in the abbey of Kremsmünster can be dated before 788 on the basis of its inscription. For this reason it is the focal piece of a group of objects decorated in the Insular style introduced into large areas of the Germanic territories by missionaries. Contrary to earlier opinion, it can thus be localized within the sphere of Insular influence around Salzburg. Significant links between the chalice and the early Salzburg miniatures support such a provenance (G. Haseloff, 1951). Moreover, only Continental origins would explain the shape of the chalice and some of its ornamentation, or the oval medallions formed of bands of interlace containing figures — Christ in Majesty and the symbols of the Evangelists on the bowl, and busts of four saints on the foot.

Among the various works that can be related to the Tassilo Chalice either by their style or by their ornamental motifs, the most important is the slightly earlier lower cover of the Lindau Gospels (New York, Pierpont Morgan Lib., Ms. 1; I, PL. 287) also probably made on the Continent. Against a background completely covered with zoomorphic interlace is placed a cross with arms that flare slightly at the ends. Into these arms interlaces and medallions of champlevé enamel are set in a pattern that outlines another cross. The center was most probably occupied by a large cabochon signifying the "image" of Christ, as the slightly later inscription and the busts of Christ around it indicate. There are tiny enamel animals set into the arms of the cross, and decorative enamel plaques set into the angles formed by the cross make up much of the outer frame. Bosses with convoluted animals have also been set into the four fields. The allover decoration of the background, contrasting sharply with the solid structure of the cross, indicates an 8th-century date.

The same stylistic tendencies are apparent in the reliquary of Enger (Berlin, Staat. Mus.), which legend identifies as Charlemagne's present to Wittekind, Duke of Saxony, to commemorate the latter's baptism (785). The rear and sides with their crude chased figures are secondary to the front, which gains prominence through the rich, colorful decoration of zoomorphic interlace, studded with cabochons and ancient engraved gems. Around a central cabochon 12 stones are set to form two crosses. This motif is common on pre-Carolingian works, for example, in the fibula from Mölsheim (Darmstadt, Landesmus.). Here, too, the center is accentuated by means of a raised central

gem, an antique agate carved with the head of Medusa, no doubt then considered to represent Christ.

Among works connected with these pieces are the small reliquaries of Andenne and Maeseyck and a larger one in the Cathedral Treasury at Chur, the front of which is reminiscent of the Enger reliquary and has interlace ornament that possibly reveals Italian influences. Like the Enger reliquary, the one in Ennabeuren (Württemberg) has guardian lions attached to the upper fastenings. Finally, among the early Carolingian works influenced by the Insular style is the portable altar from the monastery of Adelhausen (Freiburg im Breisgau, Augustinermus.). The porphyry altar slab is flanked by two silver plaques with interlacings into each of which is set an enamel cross made up of circular motifs. Technically the work is close to the Tassilo Chalice, with which it is probably contemporary. The oft-mentioned analogies to Milanese enamels can be regarded as no more than a generalized Mediterranean influence. Large quantities of enamels were produced in various centers north of the Alps during the early Carolingian period. Among these are a precious little enamel cross in Munich (Bayerisches Nationalmus.) and the Frankish medallion from the Guelph Treasure (Cleveland, Mus. of Art).

The evident love of precious materials, used with truly barbaric sumptuousness in these earlier works, later manifested itself in the goldsmith work of Charlemagne's court. The only work that can be associated with the court workshops with certainty is the setting, with fine acanthus scrolls, of the Sassanian enamels on the ewer of St.-Maurice d'Agaune (ca. 800). Stylistic similarities are evident in the reliquary of Charlemagne known from drawings. This style is the basis of the western Frankish manner of decoration discussed below.

*The golden altar of Milan.* A decisive change occurred in the development of Carolingian metalwork with the introduction of figures. The reliquary of Einhard, known only from drawings, which was made either at the end of the reign of Charlemagne or at the beginning of that of Louis the Pious, may be one of the earliest examples with figures. Einhard gave this reliquary, in the form of a late-antique triumphal arch less than 16 in. high, to his monastery of St. Servatius in Maastricht. In its form as well as in its three zones of scenes, culminating in a representation of Christ enthroned, it is a perfect expression of Carolingian attitudes, and its style suggests the Court School. This work supplied the needed transition to the most significant goldsmith work of the period, the golden altar of S. Ambrogio in Milan (PL. 63). It is in the form of a large casket, about 7 ft. long, 3 ft. high, and 4 ft. deep. The surfaces of the four sides are divided into framed compartments. In a medallion occupying the central compartment in front appears Christ, enthroned among the apostles and holding a bejeweled cross and book. The two compartments flanking the central one are filled with scenes from the life of Christ. On the back are scenes from the life of St. Ambrose. The *fenestella confessionis*, an opening through which the relics of the saint might be viewed, indicates that the altar, which is structurally derived from sarcophagi, was regarded as the tomb of a martyr. Inscriptions in the dedicatory medallions tell us that Archbishop Angilbertus II (824–59) was the donor and one "Wolvinius magister phaber," the chief artist. Its historical position, size, and artistic quality assure the altar's preeminent position. However, because it is a unique piece in which a variety of stylistic currents come together, its provenance is still debated. Bascapé and other scholars have isolated several hands; two basic styles can be detected: on the front the painterly-illusionistic manner, on the back linear simplification of strong volumes. The heavy geometric construction of the altar is lightened by delicate colorful decorations of enamels, precious and semiprecious stones, and filigree work on all four sides. The altar presents a unified whole, from the point of view of both style and iconography, for the discrepancies are merely different phases of a single style in much the same manner as in the two ivory covers of the Lorsch manuscript.

Where did the artists who made the golden altar come from? Wolvinius, whose name suggests eastern Frankish origins,

undoubtedly received his training in the most important art centers of his time. He must have been the master in charge and most probably designed the project. He may also have been responsible for the front, although his portrait appears in a medallion on the back that is stylistically consistent with the rest of the panel. The altar cannot be assigned to any one school, neither Reims, to which earlier scholars assigned it, nor Tours, as suggested in the 1950s, although connections with both are undeniable. An attribution to a single school ignores the magnitude of the undertaking and the evidence, internal and external, for Milan as its place of origin. It must be remembered that even foreign artists working there could not have escaped local influences altogether.

*Western Frankish region.* Contemporaneously with book illumination and ivory carving, metalwork flourished in northwestern France toward the middle of the 9th century. Most of the important pieces were probably made for that great patron of the arts, Charles the Bald. The precise location of the workshop is not known; it may have been at Reims or at St.-Denis, where some of the most important pieces were preserved until the French Revolution. The two stylistic tendencies noted in the altar of Milan — one depending wholly on the color and design of the precious stones and the gold settings, the other adding small repoussé figures to the rich ornamentation — achieve their full development in these pieces. To the figured group belongs the reliquary of St. Stephen in Vienna (Schatzkammer). On the front of the reliquary a large quantity of pearls, precious stones in flat settings, and gold claws are placed according to a symbolic system, in a pattern vaguely suggesting a cross. An approximate date is suggested by the figures in medallions on the sides, which imitate the style of the Utrecht Psalter.

The cover of the Psalter of Charles the Bald (Paris, Bib. Nat., Lat. 1152), dated between 860 and 870, is close to this reliquary. While the heavy frame around the upper panel gives the impression of a decorative band composed of stones, that of the much simpler lower panel consists of large-grained filigree surrounding a cross made up of a few stones. The processional cross from the Ardennes (Nuremberg, Germanisches National-Mus.) is closest to this cover.

The leading work of this group was doubtless the "screen" of Charlemagne, destroyed, except for the crowning medallion (Paris, Cabinet des Médailles), during the French Revolution. According to an 18th-century drawing, it consisted of an upper structure of three arcades made up of bands of pearls and precious stones mounted on the actual reliquary. As a whole and in its details, as well as in its use of sumptuous materials, this work belongs with the antependium of Charles the Bald for the high altar of Saint-Denis. This work, known only from a 15th-century painting (Master of St. Giles, *Mass of St. Giles*, London, Nat. Gall.; V, PL. 386), was a large repoussé gold panel with arcades containing figures. In the center was a figure of Christ enthroned, holding a book and cross, with smaller figures of the apostles on either side and above them angels holding jeweled crowns. The antependium furthermore supplies the transition to a number of later works probably produced by the same northwestern French workshop.

The cover of the Codex Aureus from St. Emmeram in Regensburg (Munich, Bayerische Staatsbib., Clm. 14000), probably contemporary with its manuscript, dated 870, is linked to the school of Reims by its vigorous acanthus scroll and by certain technical peculiarities that follow the so-called "cup of Ptolemy" (Paris, Louvre). An articulation by means of color and relief is more pronounced than in the Psalter of Charles the Bald. The raised settings of the framing stones give greater prominence to the figure of Christ in Majesty in the center, and the other fields, created by the outlines of the cross, are also surrounded by bands of heavy stones in ornate settings. The figures continue the painterly style of the Utrecht Psalter, but in a manneristic-decorative vein that corresponds to the style of Charles the Bald. This trend is even more pronounced in the upper cover of the Lindau Gospels (New York, Pierpont Morgan Lib., Ms. 1). On the strength of the close

similarities between the figures of the Munich and New York covers, Boeckler, perhaps erroneously, has attributed the two book covers to the same hand, and H. Swarzenski (1955) has added to the group another piece, the cross known only from a reproduction within a larger crucifix of Henry II. Presumably the last work in this series is the unique ciborium and portable altar (Munich, Residenzmus.; PL. 68), executed with great skill for Arnulf of Carinthia and donated by him to St. Emmeram in Regensburg together with the Codex Aureus.

Among the few extant pieces made for secular use during the 9th century is the ceremonial gold fibula of the Hon find (Oslo, Univ., Coll. of Antiquities), whose decorative ornament shows affinities to the later cover of the Lindau Gospels. Here we have evidence for a parallel development of profane and religious objects; further support is supplied by the finely made Carolingian rings and perhaps by a late Carolingian silver cup in the British Museum, with heavy plant ornament, whose original use is not certain.

*Spain.* The last echoes of goldsmith work in northwestern France are found in the Asturian capital of Oviedo. Legend has it that the "angel cross" in the Cámara Santa, according to an inscription donated by Alfonso II in 808, was made by angels; most likely it is the work of traveling craftsmen. In form close to the cross of Desiderius in Brescia, it has carefully disposed precious stones and is covered by floral patterns in filigree. Toward the end of the century Alfonso III had an exact replica of it, now lost, made for the church of Santiago de Compostela.

Alfonso III also had a ceremonial cross made in 908, La Cruz de la Victoria (Oviedo, Cámara Santa), which measures 36 × 28 in. The relations between the King and western Frankish workshops, for which there is documentary evidence, suggest that it was the work of French artisans. Moreover the sculptural make-up and specific thematic and technical details link it to works in the style of Charles the Bald as well as to the Berengar cross in Monza (PL. 68). The gold disks at the intersection of the arms, though clumsily designed, show great technical ability.

During the 10th century Asturian smiths, possibly in the footsteps of western Frankish artists, produced works of considerable artistic merit. The silver casket reliquary in Astorga was another gift of Alfonso III. The Caja de las Agatas, a casket reliquary given to the Cathedral of Oviedo in 910 by Fruela II (d. 925), is made up of colorful plaques of agate set among repoussé ornament. Its somewhat earlier cover with cloisonné enamels similar to those of the Enger reliquary and the earlier, lower cover of the Lindau Gospels is most probably a Frankish import.

*Eastern Frankish region.* Compared to the works from northeastern France the eastern Frankish region offers little of significance from the middle period of the Carolingian era, although minor centers, such as the old monastery of Fulda, were still active.

*Alpine regions and northern Italy.* Various minor works from the Alpine regions have survived. The masterpiece of the St. Gall workshop is the frame around the Tuotilo ivories (ca. 900), in which the influence of northern Italy, perhaps Milan, is evident. Of the several reliquaries worth mentioning the least ornate is that of the Treasury of St.-Maurice d'Agaune. On the front it has a number of heavy stones and on the back, large but awkward scrolls. The ornaments of the small reliquary of Muotathal (Schwyz) may be given a Eucharistic interpretation. The Altheus reliquary (Sion, in Valais), antedating 799, has outstanding figured enamels which have been attributed to the school of Milan (Hackenbroch, 1938) but are most likely later additions. How problematic the Milan school of enamels is becomes clear when one considers that the enamels of the reliquary of Pepin at Conques, as well as the later ones of the Victory cross at Oviedo, would for technical reasons have to be attributed to this school.

The "iron crown" of Monza, as well as two similar pieces

known only from documents and reproductions — diadems found near Kazan (U.S.S.R.) — were probably made in northern Italy, most likely toward the end of the 9th century. Originally to be worn by a woman (Elze, 1955), the Monza crown is decorated with gilded enamel flowers alternating with repoussé ones and rows of precious stones. Its artistic appeal derives from the contrast of gold and colorful stones and enamels. A similar effect is even more pronounced in the reliquary in Monza (PL. 68); both technically and formally it is the finest piece of late Carolingian goldsmith work in northern Italy. Against a gold background of delicate interlace the pattern of the precious stones is developed in a contrapuntal color scheme. In the center is a raised central stone, the *lapis nimirum pretiosus* ("marvelously precious stone"), which represents Christ. The crucifix on the back is closest to one in a manuscript by Otfrid of Wissembourg (Vienna, Nationalbib., Cod. 2687). Its provenance is not known, but it was part of the treasure of Berengar I (888–924) in Monza, to which the magnificent pectoral cross with three rows of precious stones in raised settings also belonged (PL. 68). The acanthus ornament of the settings is most reminiscent of such western Frankish work as the covers of the Codex Aureus.

*Rome.* A clear distinction can be drawn between north Italian and Roman works of about 800. The character of the latter is exemplified by several objects made under Pope Paschal I (817–24). One of the most sumptuous is the cross in the Vatican with enamels depicting scenes from the youth of Christ. They are similar to those of the Beresford-Hope cross (London, Vict. and Alb.), in which the Byzantine influences current in Rome during the 8th and the beginning of the 9th century are evident. In contrast, the influence of 9th-century Roman mosaics is apparent in the crude Christological representations in flat repoussé on the two silver crosses in the chapel of the Sancta Sanctorum near the Lateran.

The wealth of decorations and furnishings in the Roman churches, known from references in the *Liber pontificalis*, and the sumptuous works produced for the Byzantine court must have served as manifold inspiration to north European artists.

ENGRAVED ROCK CRYSTAL. The engraving of vessels cut out of rock crystal not only was a further expression of the love of precious materials and fine workmanship but was an art form almost unique to the Carolingian period. Rock crystal was used for seals engraved either on the lower surface of a flat disk or on the flat surface of the cabochon. These pieces can be classified according to their function. The most beautiful of the three remaining seals on the cross of Lothair in Aachen has given it its name, for the inscription on it probably refers to Lothair II of Lorraine (855–69). Most objects of engraved rock crystal were meant for liturgical use, and the most common subject is the Crucified (Chicago, Art Inst.; Paris, Cabinet des Médailles; Esztergom, Hungary, Cathedral; London, Vict. and Alb.; Freiburg im Breisgau, Münstermus.). The Baptism of Christ also occurs (Freiburg im Breisgau, Münstermus.; Rouen, Cathedral), while an angel appears on the Rogerus cross from Herford (Berlin, Staat. Mus.).

Sources tell of other altar furnishings of rock crystal, now lost, but the most important extant piece is the crystal of Lothair in London (Br. Mus.; PL. 69). It is a flat disk, 4 7/16 in. in diameter, on which eight scenes from the story of Susanna are engraved; the judge on his seat appears in the center. The precision of execution and the lively figures not only assure its artistic position but make it the heir of the Reims school, whose masterpiece, the Utrecht Psalter, must have served as its model. However — no doubt justifiably — it has not been assigned to Reims but has been described more generally as "Lotharingian." That there was a relation between Lotharingian centers, such as Metz, and Reims in the middle of the 9th century is undeniable.

Victor H. ELBERN

BIBLIOG. *Architecture.* E. Lefèvre-Pontalis, L'architecture religieuse en France dans l'ancien diocèse de Soissons au XIᵉ et XIIᵉ siècle, 2 vols., Paris, 1894–96; W. Effmann, Die karolingisch-ottonischen Bauten zu Werden, I, Strasbourg, 1899, II, Berlin, 1922; W. Effmann, Centula-St. Riquier, Forschungen und Funde, II, Münster, 1912; J. Strzygowski, Die Baukunst der Armenier und Europa, Vienna, 1918; J. Vonderau, Die Ausgrabungen am Dom zu Fulda in den Jahren 1919–1924, 17. Veröffentlichung des Fuldaer Geschichtsvereins, Fulda, 1924; Die Kunstdenkmäler der Rheinprovinz, X, 3: Die profanen Denkmäler und die Sammlungen der Stadt Aachen, Düsseldorf, 1924; G. B. Giovenale, La basilica S. Maria in Cosmedin, Rome, 1927; J. Hecht, Der romanische Kirchenbau des Bodenseegebietes, I, Basel, 1928; W. Effmann, Die Kirche der Abtei Corvey, Paderborn, 1929; A. W. Clapham, English Romanesque Architecture before the Conquest, Oxford, 1930; E. Gall, Karolingische und ottonische Kirchen, Burg bei Magdeburg, 1930; J. Hubert, Germigny-des-Prés, Congrès Archéologique, XCIII, 1930, pp. 534–68; V. Lampérez y Romea, Historia de la arquitectura cristiana en la Edad Media, I, 2d ed., Madrid, Barcelona, 1930; C. Rauch, Die Königspfalz Karls des Grossen zu Ingelheim am Rhein, Neue deutsche Ausgrabungen, 23–24. Heft: Das Deutschtum in Ausland, Münster, 1930, pp. 266–77; E. I. R. Schmidt, Kirchliche Bauten des fröhen Mittelalters in Südwestdeutschland, Katalog des Römisch-Germanischen Zentralmuseums, Mainz, 1932 (corrects the dating of the most ancient buildings); F. Behn, Die karolingische Klosterkirche von Lorsch an der Bergstrasse nach den Ausgrabungen von 1927–28, 1932 und 1933, Berlin, Leipzig, 1934; H. Buscow, Studien über die Entwicklung der Krypta im deutschen Sprachgebiet, Würzburg, 1934; J. Vonderau, Die Ausgrabungen am Büraberg bei Fritzlar 1926–1931, Fulda, 1934; O. Müller, Die Einhards-Basilika zu Seligenstadt a. M. und ihre Instandsetzung, Deutsche Kunst und Denkmalpflege, 1936, pp. 254–59; E. Lehmann, Der frühe deutsche Kirchenbau, Berlin, 1938; S. Steinmann-Brodbeck, Herkunft und Verbreitung des Dreiapsidenchores, ZfSAKg, I, 1939, pp. 65–95; G. Croquison, La basilica carolingia dell'abbazia imperiale di Farfa, Atti del V Congresso nazionale di studi romani, 1940; T. Meyer, Das deutsche Königtum und sein Wirkungsbereich: Das Reich und Europa, 1941; R. Krautheimer, The Carolingian Revival of Early Christian Architecture, AB, XXIV, 1942, pp. 1–38; P. Petermeise, Die Stiftskirche zu Herdecke und die Verwandten der steinbacher Baugruppe, 10. Sonderheft der Z. Westfalen, Münster, 1942; P. Verzone, L'architettura religiosa dell'alto Medioevo nell'Italia settentrionale, Milan, 1942; S. M. Crosby, The Abbey of St. Denis, New Haven, 1942; S. M. Crosby, AJA, XLVIII, 1944, p. 220 ff.; H. Schlunk, Arte visigodo, arte asturiano, Ars Hispaniae, II, Madrid, 1947; L. Blondel, Les anciennes basiliques d'Aguane, Vallesia, III, 1948, p. 28 ff.; W. Bader, Der Dom zu Xanten, Kevelaer, 1949; H. Beumann and D. Grossmann, Das Bonifatiusgrab und die Klosterkirche zu Fulda, Marburger Jhb. für Kunstwissenschaft, XIV, 1949, pp. 17–56; H. Claussen, Heiligengräber im Frankenreich, dissertation (typescript), Marburg, 1950; J. Hubert, La "crypte" de Saint-Laurent de Grenoble et l'art du sud-est de la Gaule au début de l'époque carolingienne, Atti del II Convegno per lo studio dell'arte dell'alto Medio Evo tenuto presso l'Università di Pavia nel settembre 1950, pp. 327–34; A. Verbeek, Die Aussenkrypta: Werden einer Bauform des frühen Mittelalters, Z. für Kunstgeschichte, XIII, 1950, pp. 7–24; J. Hubert, L'architecture religieuse du haut Moyen-Age en France, Paris, 1952; R. Louis, Les églises d'Auxerre des origines au XIᵉ siècle, Paris, 1952, pp. 41–42; H. Reinhardt, Der St. Galler Klosterplan, St. Gall, 1952; R. M. Staud and J. Reuter, Die kirchlichen Kunstdenkmäler der Stadt Echternach, Luxembourg, 1952; W. Zimmermann, Das Münster zu Essen, Essen, 1952; J. Bohland, Der Altfrid-Dom zu Hildesheim, dissertation (typescript), Göttingen, 1953; S. M. Crosby, L'abbaye royale de Saint-Denis, Paris, 1953; F. J. Esterhues, Zur frühen Baugeschichte der Corveyer Abteikirche, Westfalen, XXXI, 1953, pp. 320–35; E. Gall, L'abbaye carolingienne de Lorsch, Mémorial d'un voyage d'études de la Société nationale des antiquaires de France en Rhénanie, Paris, 1953; W. Winckelmann and H. Claussen, Archäologische Untersuchungen unter der Pfarrkirche zu Vreden, Westfalen, XXXI, 1953, pp. 304–19; E. Arslan, L'architettura dal mille, Storia di Milano, II, Milan, 1954; W. Böckelmann, Die abgeschnürte Vierung, Forschungen zur Kunstgeschichte und frühmittelalterlichen Archäologie, Baden-Baden, I, 2, 1954, pp. 101–11; O. Doppelfeld, Stand der Grabungen und Forschungen am alten Dom von Köln, Forschungen zur Kunstgeschichte und christlichen Archäologie, Baden-Baden, I, 2, 1954, pp. 69–100; A. Khatchatrian, Notes sur l'architecture de l'église de Germigny-des-Prés, CahA, VII, 1954, pp. 161–69; A. Mottart, La collégiale Sainte-Gertrude de Nivelles, Nivelles, 1954; W. Sulser, Die St. Luciuskirche in Chur, Frühmittelalterliche Kunst in den Alpenländern (Akten zum III. Internationalen Kongress für Frühmittelalterforschung), Olten, 1954, pp. 150–66; R. Tournier, Les églises comtoises, Paris, 1954; E. Kubach and F. Bellmann, Übersicht über die wichtigsten Ausgrabungen in Deutschland, Kunstchronik, VIII, 1955, pp. 117–24; G. Bandmann, Über Pastophorien und verwandte Nebenräume im mittelalterlichen Kirchenbau, Kunstgeschichtliche Studien für Hans Kauffmann, Berlin, 1956, p. 44 ff.; W. Böckelmann, Grundformen im frühkarolingischen Kirchenbau des östlichen Frankenreiches, Wallraf-Richartz-Jhb., XVIII, 1956, pp. 27–69; H. Christ, Die sechs Münster der Abtei Reichenau, Reichenau, 1956; E. Lehmann, Vom neuen Bild frühmittelalterlichen Kirchenbaus, Wissenschaftliche Z. der Martin-Luther-Universität, Halle, Wittenberg, VI, 1956–57, pp. 213–20; H. Claussen, Spätkarolingische Umgangskrypten im sächsischen Gebiet, Karolingische und ottonische Kunst (Forschungen zur Kunstgeschichte und christlichen Archäologie, III), Wiesbaden, 1957, pp. 118–40; D. Grossmann, Zum Stand der Westwerkforschung, Wallraf-Richartz-Jhb., XIX, 1957, pp. 253–64; B. Ortmann, Baugeschichte der Salvator- und Abdinghofkirche zu Paderborn nach den Ausgrabungen, 1944–56, Westfälische Z., 1957, pp. 255–364; H. Thümmler, Die karolingische Baukunst in Westfalen, Karolingische und ottonische Kunst (Forschungen zur Kunstgeschichte und christlichen Archäologie, III), Wiesbaden, 1957, pp. 84–108; H. Borger, Die Ausgrabungen im Bereich des Xantener Domes, Neue Ausgrabungen in Deutschland, Berlin, 1958, pp. 380–90; F. Kreusch, Über Pfalzkapelle und Atrium zur Zeit Karls des Grossen, Aachener Beiträge zur Baugeschichte, IV, 1958; K. J. Conant, Carolingian

and Romanesque Architecture, Harmondsworth, 1959; O. Müller, Die Einharts-Basilika zu Steinbach bei Michelstadt im Odenwald, Seligenstadt, n.d.; P. Glazema, Ausgrabungen in der durch den Krieg zerstörten mittelalterlichen Kirche von Oosterbeek, Amersfoort, n.d.; H. Deneux, Dix ans de fouilles dans la cathédrale de Reims (1919–1930), Conférence donnée à la Société des amis du vieux Reims le Ier Juin 1944, Reims, n.d.; L. Blondel, Les édifices antérieurs à la cathédrale actuelle, Les monuments d'art et d'histoire de la Suisse, n.d., pp. 27–59.

Hans Thümmler

*Representational and minor arts.* J. von Schlosser, Schriftquellen zur Geschichte der karolingischen Kunst, Vienna, 1892; Michel, I, 1, p. 321; J. Baum, Die Malerei und Plastik des Mittelalters, II, Handbuch der Kunstwissenschaft, Wildpark, Potsdam, 1930; A. Boeckler, Abendländische Miniaturen, Berlin, 1930; R. Hinks, Carolingian Art, London, 1935; J. Hubert, L'art préroman, Paris, 1938; C. R. Morey, Medieval Art, New York, 1942; H. Fichtenau, Das karolingische Imperium, Zurich, 1949; W. v. d. Steinen, Karolingische Kulturfragen, Welt als Geschichte, X, 1950, p. 156 ff.; P. Lehmann, Das Problem der karolingischen Renaissance, I problemi della civiltà carolingia, Spoleto, 1954, p. 309 ff.; E. Kitzinger, Early Medieval Art in the British Museum, 2d ed., London, 1955, p. 36 ff.; W. Otto, Die karolingische Bilderwelt, Munich, 1957. *a. Monumental painting.* E. Steinmann, Die Tituli und die kirchlichen Wandmalerei im Abendlande vom 5. zum 11. Jahrhundert, Leipzig, 1892; F. F. Leitschuh, Geschichte der karolingischen Malerei: Ihr Bilderkreis und seine Quellen, Berlin, 1894; P. Clemen, Die romanische Monumentalmalerei in den Rheinlanden, Düsseldorf, 1916; E. W. Anthony, Romanesque Frescoes, Princeton, 1951; A. Grabar and C. Nordenfalk, Early Medieval Painting, Geneva, New York, 1957. (1) *Western Frankish region.* E. S. King, The Carolingian Frescoes of the Abbey of St.-Germain d'Auxerre, AB, XI, 1929, p. 359 ff.; P. Deschamps, Peintures murales de l'époque carolingienne en France, Arte del I millennio, Pavia, 1950 p. 335 ff.; P. Deschamps and M. Thibout, La peinture murale en France: Le haut Moyen-Age et l'époque romane, Paris, 1951. (2) *Eastern Frankish region.* O. Doppelfeld, Die Domgrabung, Kölner Domblatt, 1950, p. 141 ff.; H. Eichler, Die karolingische Krypta von St. Maximin und ihre Wandgemälde, Rheinischer Verein für Denkmalpflege und Heimatschutz, 1952, p. 65 ff. (3) *Alpine regions and northern Italy.* J. Zemp and R. Durrer, Das Kloster St. Johann zu Münster in Graubünden, Mit. der Schw. Gesellschaft für Erhaltung historischer Kunstdenkmäler, N.S., V–VII, 1906–11; G. Gerola, Gli affreschi di Naturno, Dedalo, VI, 1925–26, p. 415 ff.; J. Garber, Die romanischen Wandgemälde Tirols, Vienna, 1928; H. Torp, Note sugli affreschi più antichi dell'Oratorio di S. Maria in Valle a Cividale, Atti del II Congresso internazionale di studi sull'alto Medioevo, Spoleto, 1953; E. Arslan, La pittura della conquista longobarda al mille, Storia di Milano, II, Milan, 1954, p. 623 ff.; L. Birchler, Zur karolingischen Architektur und Malerei in Münster (Müstair), Frühmittelalterliche Kunst in den Alpenländern (Akten zum III. Internationalen Kongress für Frühmittelalterforschung), Olten, 1954, p. 167 ff.; C. Cecchelli, Pittura e scultura carolingie in Italia, I problemi della civiltà carolingia, Spoleto, 1954, p. 199 ff.; G. de' Francovich, Il ciclo pittorico della chiesa di S. Giovanni a Münster (Müstair) nei Grigioni, Arte Lombarda, II, 1956, p. 28 ff.; M. Girard, Studien zu den karolingischen Wandmalereien von Müstair, unpublished dissertation, Basel. (4) *Spain.* F. de Selgas, La basilica de S. Julián de los Prados, Boletín de la Sociedad Española de Excursiones, XXIV, 1916, pp. 97–139; H. Schlunk, Arte asturiano, Ars Hispaniae, II, 1947; H. Schlunk and M. Berenguer, La pintura mural asturiana, Madrid, 1957. (5) *Mosaics.* M. van Berchem and E. Clouzot, Mosaïques chrétiennes, Geneva, 1924; J. Hubert, La mosaïque disparue de la chapelle du Palais de Charlemagne, BAFr, 1936, p. 132 ff.; A. Grabar, Les mosaïques de Germigny-des-Prés, CahA, 1954, p. 171 ff.; J. Deér, Die Vorrechte des Kaisers in Rom, Schw. Beiträge zur allgemeinen Geschichte, XV, 1957, p. 23 ff. *b. Sculpture.* P. Clemen, Merowingische und karolingische Plastik, Jhb. des Vereins von Altertumsfreunden im Rheinland, XCII, Bonn, 1892; L. Coutil, L'art mérovingien et carolingien, Paris, 1930; H. Keller, Zur Entstehung der sakralen Vollskulptur in der ottonischen Zeit, Festschrift für Hans Jantzen, Berlin, 1951, p. 71 ff. (1) *Western Frankish region.* A. K. Porter, The Tomb of Hincmar and Carolingian Sculpture in France, BM, XL, 1927, p. 75 ff.; L. Bréhier, L'art en France des invasions barbares à l'époque romane, Paris, 1930; L. Stone, Sculpture in Britain, The Middle Ages, Harmondsworth, 1955, p. 19 ff. (2) *Eastern Frankish region.* K. Schumacher, Frühmittelalterliche Steinskulpturen aus den Rheinlanden, Die Altertümer unserer heidnischen Frühzeit, V, 1911, p. 269 ff.; A. Boeckler, Malerei und Plastik im ostfränkischen Reich, I problemi della civiltà carolingia, Spoleto, 1954. p. 173 ff. (3) *Alpine regions and northern Italy.* R. Kautzsch, Die römische Schmuckkunst in Stein vom 6. bis zum 10. Jahrhundert, Römisches Jhb. für Kunstgeschichte, III, 1939; K. Ginhart, Die karolingischen Flechtwerksteine in Kärnten, Carinthia, I, 1942, p. 132 ff.; G. de' Francovich, Arte carolingia ed ottoniana in Lombardia, Römisches Jhb. für Kunstgeschichte, VI, 1942–44, p. 116 ff.; J. Baum, Frühmittelalterliche Denkmäler der Schweiz und ihrer Nachbarländer, Bern, 1943, p. 29; I. Müller and O. Steinmann, Zur Disentiser Frühgeschichte, Frühmittelalterliche Kunst in den Alpenländern (Akten zum III. Internationalen Kongress für Frühmittelalterforschung), Olten, 1954, p. 133 ff.; P. Deschamps, A propos des pierres à décor, d'entrelacs et des stucs de St.-Jean de Mustair, Frühmittelalterliche Kunst in den Alpenländern (Akten zum III. Internationalen Kongress für Frühmittelalterforschung), Olten, 1954, p. 253 ff.; G. de' Francovich, Problemi della pittura e della scultura provinciale, Settimana di studio del Centro italiano di studi sull'alto Medioevo, II, I problemi comuni dell'Europa post-carolingia, Spoleto, 1955, p. 370 ff.; G. de' Francovich, La decorazione pittorica e in stucco del tempietto di S. Maria in Valle a Cividale, Venezia e l'Europa (Atti del XVIII Congresso internazionale di storia dell'arte, 1955), Venice, 1956, p. 139 ff.; T. von Bogyay, Zum Problem der Flechtwerksteine, Karolingische und ottonische Kunst (Forschungen zur Kunstgeschichte und christlichen Archäologie, III), Wiesbaden, 1957, p. 262 ff. (4) *Bronzes.* P. E. Schramm, Das Herrscherbild in der Kunst des frühen Mittelalters, Vorträge der Bibliothek Warburg, II, 1922–23, p. 156 ff.; A. Goldschmidt, Die deutschen Bronzetüren des frühen Mittelalters, Marburg, 1926; W. Meyer-Barkhause, Ein karolingisches Bronzegitter als Schmuckmotiv des Elfenbeinkelches von Deventer, ZfBK, I, 1930, p. 244; J. Hubert, Le fauteuil du roi Dagobert, Demareteion, I, 1935, p. 17 ff.; N. Degrassi, La sella plicatilis di Pavia, Arte del I millennio, Pavia, 1950, p. 56 ff.; J. Deér, Ein Doppelbildnis Karls des Grossen, Wandlungen christlicher Kunst im Mittelalter (Forschungen zur Kunstgeschichte und christlichen Archäologie, II), Wiesbaden, 1953, p. 139 ff.; P. E. Schramm, Die Throne und Bischofsstühle des frühen Mittelalters, Herrschaftszeichen und Staatssymbolik, I, Stuttgart, 1954, p. 326 ff. *c. Illumination.* S. Beissel, Geschichte der Evangelienbücher in der I. Hälfte des Mittelalters, Freiburg im Breisgau, 1906; A. Boinet, La miniature carolingienne, Paris, 1913 (plates only); A. Goldschmidt, German Illumination, I, Florence, Paris, 1928; E. Lesne, Histoire de la propriété ecclésiastique en France, IV, Les livres, scriptoria et bibliothèques du commencement du 8e à la fin du 11e siècle, Lille, 1938; P. Buberl and A. Boeckler, RDK, II, s. v. Buchmalerei; A. Boeckler, Buchmalerei, Handbuch der Bibliothekswissenschaft, Wiesbaden, 1952, p. 275 ff.; C. Nordenfalk, Book Illumination, in Early Medieval Painting, Geneva, New York, 1957, p. 89 ff. (1) *The Court School of Charlemagne (Ada Group).* K. Menzel, P. Corssen, H. Janitschek, and others, Die Trierer Ada-Handschrift, Leipzig, 1889; W. Koehler, An Illustrated Evangelistary of the Ada-school, Warburg, XV, 1952, p. 48 ff.; A. Boeckler, Die Evangelistenbilder der Adagruppe, Münchener Jhb. für bildende Kunst, III–IV, 1952–53, p. 144 ff.; A. Boeckler, Die Kanonbögen der Adagruppe und ihre Vorlagen, Münchener Jhb. für bildende Kunst, 1954, p. 7 ff.; A. Boeckler, Formgeschichtliche Studien zur Adagruppe, Bayerische Akademie der Wissenschaften, Philosophisch-historische Klasse, Abhandlungen, N.S., XLII, 1956; E. Rosenbaum, The Evangelist Portraits of the Ada School, AB, XXXVIII, 1956, p. 81 ff.; W. Koehler, Karolingische Miniaturen, II, Die Hofschule Karls des Grossen, Berlin, 1958. (2) *The "New Palace School."* H. Swarzenski, The Xanten Purple Leaf and the Carolingian Renaissance, AB, XXII, 1940, p. 7 ff.; A. Boutémy, Quelques manuscrits contemporains de Lothaire Ier, B. de l'Académie des Inscriptions et Belles Letters, 1954, p. 27 ff. (3) *Reims.* G. Swarzenski, Die karolingische Malerei und Plastik in Reims, JhbPreussKSamml, XXIII, 1902, p. 81 ff.; L. Weber, Einbanddecken, Elfenbeintafeln, Miniaturen, Schriftproben aus Metzer liturgischen Handschriften, I, Jetzige Pariser Handschriften, Metz, Frankfort, 1912; E. T. Dewald, The Stuttgart Psalter, Princeton, 1930; H. Woodruff, The Physiologus of Bern, AB, XII, 1930, p. 266 ff.; G. R. Benson and D. Tselos, New Light on the Origin of the Utrecht Psalter, AB, XIII, 1931, p. 13 ff.; E. T. Dewald, The Illustrations of the Utrecht-Psalter, Princeton, 1933; D. Panofsky, The Textual Basis of the Utrecht Psalter, AB, XXVII, 1945, p. 50 ff.; F. Wormald, The Utrecht Psalter, Utrecht, 1953; H. Swarzenski, Monuments of Romanesque Art, London, 1954; D. Tselos, The Influence of the Utrecht Psalter in Carolingian Art, AB, XXXIX, 1957, p. 87 ff. (4) *Tours.* E. K. Rand, a Survey of the Manuscripts of Tours, Cambridge, Mass., 1929; W. Kochler, Die karolingischen Miniaturen, I, Die Schule von Tours, Berlin, 1930–33; E. K. Rand and L. W. Jones, The Earliest Books of Tours, Cambridge, Mass., 1934; C. Nordenfalk, Beiträge zur Geschichte der touronischen Buchmalerei, ActaA, VII, 1936, p. 281 ff.; P. Lauer, Iconographie carolingienne, Vivien et Charlemagne, Mél. F. Martroye, Paris, 1941, p. 191 ff.; J. Croquison, Une vision eschatologique carolingienne, CahA, IV, 1949, p. 105 ff. (5) *The style of Charles the Bald.* G. Leidinger, Der Codex Aureus der Bayerischen Staatsbibliothek in München, 1921–25; A. M. Friend, Carolingian Art in the Abbey of St. Denis, Art Studies, I, 1923, p. 67 ff.; A. M. Friend, Two Manuscripts of the School of St. Denis, Speculum, I, 1926, p. 59 ff.; H. Schrade, Untersuchungen zu der karolingischen Bilderbibel von St. Paul vor den Mauern, Munich, 1954 (unpublished thesis); E. H. Kantorowicz, The Carolingian King in the Bible of S. Paolo, Late Classical and Medieval Studies in Honor of A. M. Friend, Princeton, 1955, p. 287 ff. (6) *Franco-Saxon style.* C. Nordenfalk, Ein karolingisches Sakramentar aus Echternach und seine Vorläufer, ActaA, II, 1931, p. 232 ff.; G. L. Micheli, L'enluminure du haut Moyen-Age et les influences irlandaises, Brussels, 1939; C. Niver, A Study of Certain of the More Important Manuscripts of the Franco-Saxon School, Cambridge, Mass., 1941; A. Boutémy, Le style franco-saxon de St.-Amand; Sources inutilisées, Scriptorium, III, 1949, p. 260 ff. (7) *Minor western Frankish scriptoriums.* J. Porcher, Les manuscrits à peintures en France du VIIe au XIe siècle, Paris, Bib. Nat. (exhibition cat.), 1954, no. 81 ff.; O. Homburger, Eine spätkarolingische Schule von Corbie, Karolingische und ottonische Kunst (Forschungen zur Kunstgeschichte und christlichen Archäologie, III), Wiesbaden, 1957, p. 412 ff. (8) *Eastern Frankish region.* P. Jaffé and W. Wattenbach, Ecclesiae metropolitanae coloniensis codices manuscripti, Berlin, 1874; E. H. Zimmermann, Die Fuldaer Buchmalerei in karolingischer und ottonischer Zeit, Halle, 1910; L. W. Jones, The Script of Cologne from Hildebald to Hermann, Cambridge, Mass., 1932; R. Drögereit, Werden und der Heliand, Beiträge zur Geschichte von Stadt und Stift Essen, no. 66, Essen, 1950; E. Jammers, Die Essener Neumenhandschriften der Landes- und Stadtbibliothek Düsseldorf, Düsseldorf, 1952; B. Bischoff, Die Kölner Nonnenhandschriften und das Skriptorium von Chelles, Karolingische und ottonische Kunst (Forschungen zur Kunstgeschichte und christlichen Archäologie, III), Wiesbaden, 1957, p. 395 ff.; R. Drögereit, Zur Einheit des Werden-Essener Kulturraumes in karolingischer und ottonischer Zeit, Karolingische und ottonische Kunst (Forschungen zur Kunstgeschichte und christlichen Archäologie, III), Wiesbaden, 1957, p. 60 ff. (9) *Salzburg.* G. Swarzenski, Die Salzburger Malerei von den ersten Anfängen bis zur Blütezeit des romanischen Stiles, II, Leipzig, 1913; H. J. Hermann, Die frühmittelalterlichen Handschriften des Abendlandes, VIII, Beschreibendes Verzeichnis der illuminierten Handschriften in Österreich, N.S., I, Nationalbibliothek, Vienna, 1923; P. Lauer, Le psautier carolingien du président Bouhier (Montpellier Univ. H. 409), Mél. d'Histoire du Moyen-

Age offerts à M. F. Lot, Paris, 1905, p. 359 ff.; K. Holter, Die Schreibschulen von Mondsee und Kremsmünster, Dreiländertagung für frühmittelalterliche Forschung, Linz, 1950, p. 61 ff. (10) *St. Gall.* R. Rahn, Das Psalterium Aureum von St. Gallen, Saint Gall, 1878; F. Landsberger, Der St. Galler Folchardpsalter: Eine Initialstudie, Saint Gall, 1912; A. Merton, Die Buchmalerei in St. Gallen vom 9. bis zum 11. Jahrhundert, 2d ed., Leipzig, 1923; A. Bruckner, Scriptoria Medii Aevi Helvetica, Schreibschulen der Diözese Konstanz, St. Gallen I und II, Geneva, 1936–38; K. Löffler, Die St. Galler Schreibschule in der 1. Hälfte des 9. Jahrhunderts, Neue Heidelberg Jhb., N.S., 1937, p. 28 ff.; A. Boeckler, Zwei St. Galler Fragmente, Festschrift für Hans Jantzen, Berlin, 1951, p. 37 ff. *d. Ivories.* A. Goldschmidt, Die Elfenbeinskulpturen aus der Zeit der karolingischen und sächsischen Kaiser, I, Berlin, 1914; L. Eitner, The Flabellum of Tournus, New York, 1944; W. F. Volbach, Elfenbeinarbeiten der Spätantike und des frühen Mittelalters, 2d ed., Mainz, 1952; Mostra degli avori dell'alto Medio Evo, Ravenna, 1956 (cat. ed. by G. Bovini and L. B. Ottolenghi. (1) *Ada Group.* H. Schnitzler, Die Komposition der Lorscher Elfenbeintafeln, Münch. Jhb. der Bildenden Kunst, I, 1950, p. 21 ff.; Deér, Ein Doppelbildnis Karls des Grossen, Wandlungen christlicher Kunst im Mittelalter (Forschungen zur Kunstgeschichte und christlichen Archäologie, II), Wiesbaden, 1953, p. 102 ff.; A. Boeckler, Malerei und Plastik im ostfränkischen Reich, I problemi della civiltà carolingia, Spoleto, 1954, p. 169 ff. (2) *Liuthard Group.* A. A. Friend, Carolingian Art in the Abbey of St. Denis, Art Studies, I, 1923, p. 67 ff.; D. Tselos, The Influence of the Utrecht-psalter in Carolingian Art, AB, XXXIX, 1957, p. 93 ff. (3) *Metz Group.* H. Swarzenski, Monuments of Romanesque Art, London, 1954, p. 18 ff. *e. Gold- and silverwork.* E. Molinier, Evolution des arts mineurs, Michel, I, 2, p. 836 ff.; O. von Falke and G. Lehnert, Illustrierte Geschichte des Kunstgewerbes, I, Berlin, 1908–09; M. Rosenberg, Geschichte der Goldschmiedekunst auf technischer Grundlage, I–IV, Frankfurt, 1908–21; J. Braun, Meisterwerke der deutschen Goldschmiedekunst, I, Munich, 1922; J. Seligmann, L'orfèvrerie carolingienne: Son évolution, Trav. d. Et. du Groupe d'Histoire de l'Art de la Faculté des Lettres de Paris, Paris, 1928 p. 137 ff.; P. Metz, Das Kunstgewerbe von der Karolingerzeit bis zum Beginn der Gotik, Geschichte des Kunstgewerbes, ed. H. T. Bossert, V, Berlin, 1932, p. 197 ff. (1) *Early Carolingian works.* E. Molinier, Le trésor de la cathédrale de Coire, Paris, 1895; M. Rosenberg, Erster Zellenschmelz nördlich der Alpen, Jhb-PreussKSamml, XXXIX, 1918, p. 90 ff.; G. L. Micheli, Reliure de l'Evangéliaire de Lindau, RA, VIII, 1936, p. 70 ff.; F. Rademacher, Fränkische Goldscheibenfibeln, Munich, 1940; A. Alföldi, Die Goldkanne von St.-Maurice d'Aguane, ZfSAKg, X, 1948–49, p. 7 ff.; G. Haseloff, Der Tassilokelch, Münch. Beiträge zur Vor- und Frühgeschichte, I, Munich, 1951; V. H. Elbern, Der Adelhauser Tragaltar, Nachr. des deutschen Inst. für merowingische und karolingische Kunstforschung, nos. 6–8, Erlangen, 1954; V. H. Elbern, Werdendes Abendland an Rhein und Ruhr (exhibition cat.), 4th ed., Essen, 1956. (2) *The golden altar of Milan.* J. Brassinne, Monuments d'art mosan disparus, B. de la Société d'Art et d'Histoire du Diocèse de Liège, XXIX, 1938, p. 155 ff.; G. de' Francovich, Arte carolingia e ottoniana in Lombardia, Römisches Jhb. für Kunstgeschichte, VI, 1942–44, p. 115 ff.; B. de Montesquiou-Fézensac, L'Arc de Triomphe d'Einhardus, CahA, IV, 1949, p. 79 ff.; V. H. Elbern, Der karolingische Goldaltar von Mailand, Bonn, 1952; V. H. Elbern, Der Ambrosiuszyklus am Goldaltar von Mailand, Mit. des Kunsthistorischen Inst. in Florenz, VII, 1, 1953; G. Rosa, Le arti minori dalla conquista longobarda al mille, Storia di Milano, II, Milan, 1954, p. 678 ff.; C. Bascapé, L'altare d'oro di S. Ambrogio a Milano, Ragguagli della basilica di S. Ambrogio, III, 6–8, 1955 (résumé of an unpublished thesis); B. de Montesquiou-Fézensac, L'Arc de Triomphe d'Eginard, Karolingische und ottonische Kunst (Forschungen zur Kunstgeschichte und christlichen Archäologie, III), Wiesbaden, 1957, p. 43 ff.; W. Otto, Die karolingische Bilderwelt, Munich, 1957, pp. 44 ff., 74 ff. (3) *Western Frankish region.* W. M. Schmid, Zur Geschichte der karolingischen Plastik, Repertorium für Kunstwissenschaft, XXIII, 1900, p. 1 ff.; G. Swarzenski, Die karolingische Malerei und Plastik im Reims, Jhb. für Kunstwissenschaft, 1902, p. 92 ff.; M. Conway, The Abbey of St. Denis and Its Ancient Treasures, Archaeologia, 1914–15, p. 103 ff.; M. Conway, Some Treasures of the Time of Charles the Bald, BM, XXVI, 1915; M. Rosenberg, Das Stephansreliquiar im Lichte des Utrecht-Psalters, JhbPreuss-KSamml, 1922, p. 169 ff.; H. Arbman, Schweden und das karolingische Reich, Stockholm, 1937; J. Hubert, L'escrain dit de Charlemagne, CahA, IV, 1949, p. 71 ff.; R. Otto, Zur stilgeschichtlichen Stellung des Arnulf-Ciboriums und des Codex Aureus aus St. Emmeram in Regensburg, ZfKG, XV, 1952, p. 1 ff.; J. de Borchgrave d'Altena, Reliefs carolingiens et ottoniens, Revue Belge d'Archéologie et d'Histoire de l'Art, XXIII, 1954, p. 21 ff.; H. Swarzenski, The Dowry Cross of Henry II, Late Classical and Medieval Studies in Honor of A. M. Friend, Princeton, 1955, p. 301 ff. (4) *Spain.* H. Schlunk, Ars Hispaniae, II, Madrid, 1947, p. 406 ff.; H. Schlunk, The Crosses of Oviedo, AB, XXXII, 1950, p. 91 ff. (5) *Alpine regions and northern Italy.* Y. Hackenbroch, Italienisches Email des frühen Mittelalters, Ars Docta, II, Basel, Leipzig, 1938; O. Homburger, Früh- und hochmittelalterliche Stücke im Schatz des Augustinerchorherrenstiftes von St. Maurice und in der Kathedrale zu Sitten, Frühmittelalterliche Kunst in den Alpenländern (Akten zum III. Internationalen Kongress für Frühmittelalterforschung), Olten, 1954, p. 339 ff.; G. Rosa, Le arti minori dalla conquista longobarda al mille, Storia di Milano, II, 1954, p. 678 ff.; R. Elze, Die eiserne Krone von Monza, in P. E. Schramm, Herrschaftszeichen und Staatssymbolik, II, Stuttgart, 1955, p. 450 ff. (6) *Rome.* H. Grisar, Die römische Kapelle Sancta Sanctorum und ihr Schatz, Freiburg im Breisgau, 1908, p. 58 ff.; J. Colin, La plastique "gréco-romaine" dans l'Empire carolingien, CahA, II, Paris, 1947, p. 87 ff.; C. Cecchelli, La vita di Roma nel Medio Evo, I, Le arti minori e il costume, Rome, 1951–52. *f. Engraved rock crystal.* E. Babelon, Histoire de la gravure sur gemmes en France depuis les origines jusqu'à l'époque contemporaine, Paris, 1902; O. Dalton, The Crystal of Lothair, Archaeologia, IX, 1904, p. 25 ff.; J. Sauer, Ein unbekannter Kristallschnitt des 9. Jahrhunderts, Festschrift für Paul Clemen, Bonn, 1926, p. 241 ff.; H. Wentzel, RDK, II, s.v. Bergkristall; J. Baum,

Karolingische geschnittene Bergkristalle, Frühmittelalterliche Kunst in den Alpenländern (Akten zum III. Internationalen Kongress für Frühmittelalterforschung), Olten, 1954, p. 111 ff.

Victor H. ELBERN

Illustrations: PLS. 44–69; 14 figs. in text.

**CARPACCIO,** VITTORE. Italian painter, son of Pietro, a fur merchant, born in Venice about 1465. He was descended from an old family of sailors and shipbuilders who resided along the estuary of the river Po. All the family documents use the Venetian dialect form Scarpaza for the surname, which the artist was to change to the Latinized Carpathius and the Italian Carpaccio. The theory that the artist was born at Capodistria is unfounded, though he may perhaps have died there (see P. Stancovich, *Biografia degli uomini distinti dell'Istria*, Trieste, 1928–29).

In 1486 Carpaccio paid rent for rooms in the Procuratie Vecchie in his father's name, according to a document which gives the impression that he was under age at this time (Ludwig and Molmenti, 1906, p. 57). In 1488, documents from the Scuola di S. Orsola, preserved in the Venice State Archives, record the decision to commission paintings depicting the history of this saint; it is safe to refer this entry to Carpaccio's canvases. Possibly Carpaccio traveled, in his early years, to Dalmatia (where at the turn of the century he was to paint a polyptych for the Cathedral of Zara) and to the Near East (see C. Vecellio, *Degli Habiti antichi e moderni di tutto il mondo*, Venice, 1590).

In the St. Ursula cycle *The Arrival of St. Ursula at Cologne* (PL. 73) bears the inscription "Op. Victoris Charpatio Veneti MCCCLXXXX m. Septembris." The other paintings in the cycle follow in this order: *The Meeting of St. Ursula and the Pope in Rome* (PL. 78), *Martyrdom of St. Ursula* (1493), *Departure of the Betrothed* (1495), the three compositions with the *Arrival*, *Dismissal*, and *Return of the Ambassadors*, the *Dream of St. Ursula*, the *Altarpiece of St. Ursula*. Although the *Altarpiece* is dated 1491, it is most likely of a later period because it is painted in the style of the second decade of the 16th century. We know that the altar was renovated in 1504, and it may well be that on this occasion Carpaccio's original canvas, probably dated 1491, was set aside. When it was replaced by the present *Altarpiece*, the old date might have been inscribed upon the new one for commemorative reasons (Berenson, 1952, pp. 11–12). However, on this point compare also Fiocco (1932, p. 64), who insists upon an early date for the extant painting.

Much has been written about the precise location in Venice of the Scuola di S. Orsola and the arrangement of the paintings within the building. Attempts have been made to identify the oratory of the school with the now-demolished small chapel with a side porch, somewhat in the rear of the Church of SS. Giovanni e Paolo (Pignatti, 1956, p. 180). The oratory appears in De' Barbari's plan of Venice in 1500. Carpaccio's paintings might have been placed around the walls of the chapel by starting on the right, facing the altar, with the lower portion of the *Arrival of the Ambassadors* partially cut by the single entrance door. Such an arrangement takes into consideration the documents, the logical unfolding of the legend, and the fall of shadows within the pictures — as does the present reconstruction in the Venice Accademia (see Moschini, 1948).

In 1496, for the Church of S. Pietro Martire in Udine, Carpaccio painted *The Blood of the Redeemer*, now in the Museo Civico of that city. About this time he worked with Gentile Bellini (q.v.) on the cycle of the legend of the True Cross for the Scuola di S. Giovanni Evangelista in Venice. Carpaccio's canvas showing the episode of *The Healing of the Madman* (PL. 72) might be dated between 1494 — on the basis of a canvas by Mansueti for the same cycle (see F. Zanotto, *Pinacoteca della I. R. Accademia di Venezia*, Venice, 1834, fasc. 34) — and 1496, which is the date of Gentile's *Procession in St. Mark's Square*. However, the most exact point of reference for Carpaccio's dated work is *The Departure of the Betrothed* of 1495.

In 1501–02 he executed a painting for the Sala dei Pregadi in the Doges' Palace (destroyed in the fire of 1577) and was

paid 50 ducats for it (Ludwig and Molmenti, p. 58). In 1502 he worked in the Scuola di S. Giorgio degli Schiavoni, dating two of his paintings, *The Calling of St. Matthew* and *The Funeral of St. Jerome*. The later paintings in the series, according to the sources, were probably finished in 1507, the date of the *Miracle of St. Triphonius* (Zanetti, p. 37). The *Annunciation* (1504) in the Ca' d'Oro, Venice, is one of six episodes from the life of the Virgin for the Scuola degli Albanesi near the Church of S. Maurizio. A document of the school in 1500, however, alludes to paintings and frames in the hall of its hostel (Ludwig and Molmenti, p. 199), where we later find Carpaccio's works. Therefore it is not certain that the *Annunciation* was the first to be painted — particularly since it is chronologically the fourth episode of the cycle. Edwards in 1808 remarked that the *Birth of the Virgin* seems to date from about the end of the 15th century (Ludwig and Molmenti, p. 208). We can conclude, then, that the series on the life of the Virgin in the Scuola degli Albanesi may antedate — at least in part — the paintings in S. Giorgio degli Schiavoni; but the problem is of limited interest because of excessive workshop participation.

A contract by which Carpaccio and Giovanni Bellini were to execute a canvas each for the Sala del Maggior Consiglio in the Doges' Palace is dated 1507. These paintings, which perished in the fire of 1577, represented *Pope Alexander III in St. Mark's* and *The Meeting of the Pope with the Doge in Ancona* (Ludwig and Molmenti, p. 58). A record of the latter is to be found in two drawings in the British Museum and in the Crocker Art Gallery in Sacramento, Calif. (H. and E. Tietze, nos. 615 and 635). The *Altarpiece of St. Thomas* in the Staatsgalerie, Stuttgart, is dated 1507 and was commissioned by Tomaso Licinio for the Church of S. Pietro Martire in Murano. The *Adoration* in the Gulbenkian Collection, now on loan to the National Gallery, Washington, belongs to the same year. In 1508 Carpaccio competed unsuccessfully for the commission to paint a processional banner for the Scuola della Carità, losing to Benedetto Diana. Also in 1508 he served on a committee with Lazzaro Bastiani and Vittore Belliniano to appraise Giorgione's frescoes on the Fondaco dei Tedeschi (Ludwig and Molmenti, p. 58). The *Death of the Virgin* in the Pinacoteca, Ferrara, once in S. Maria in Vado, also belongs to 1508. The large *Presentation of Christ in the Temple* (PLS. 76, 77) for the Sanudo altar in S. Giobbe, Venice, now in the Accademia in Venice, is dated 1510. In 1511 he wrote Francesco Gonzaga suggesting that the Duke acquire *A View of Jerusalem* and reminding him that they had met while Carpaccio was painting *The History of Ancona* for the Sala del Maggior Consiglio in the Doges' Palace (Ludwig and Molmenti, p. 58). Also in 1511, the artist began painting a series of episodes in the life of St. Stephen for the guildhall of the Scuola di S. Stefano, inscribing the date 1511 on the *Communion of the Seven Deacons*, now in the Staatliche Museen, Berlin. He continued to work intermittently for S. Stefano, with Bissolo as his principal assistant, producing in 1514 *St. Stephen Disputing with the Doctors* (now in the Brera, Milan) and probably the *St. Stephen Preaching* (Louvre; PL. 75). *The Stoning of St. Stephen* in the Staatsgalerie, Stuttgart, is from the year 1520.

In 1514 Carpaccio completed the polyptych of S. Fosca, dating the *St. Sebastian*, which, with the *St. Peter Martyr* of the same altarpiece, is now in the Museo Correr, Venice; the *St. Roch* is in the Galleria dell'Accademia Carrara, Bergamo. For the parish priest of S. Vitale in Venice he painted a large canvas of the saint on horseback, which is still preserved in the church. Dated 1515 are *The Meeting of Joachim and Anna* (Accademia, Venice; formerly in S. Francesco, Treviso) and *The Martyrdom of the Ten Thousand*, once part of the altarpiece of the Ottoboni family in the Church of S. Antonio di Castello in Venice and now in the Accademia there. Dated 1516 are the *St. George* in S. Giorgio Maggiore in Venice and the *Lion of St. Mark* in the Doges' Palace. In this year Carpaccio moved to Capodistria, where he painted a *Madonna and Saints* for the Cathedral. *The Entry of Captain Contarini* is dated 1517 and is in the Museo Civico in Capodistria. To the year 1518 belong the *Madonna and Saints* for the Church of S. Francesco at Pirano and the altarpiece in the Church of S. Tommaso at Pozzale di

Cadore. The *St. Paul* in S. Domenico, Chioggia, is dated 1520. In 1522 Carpaccio was paid for an altarpiece and other paintings, now lost, for S. Pietro di Castello (Ludwig and Molmenti, p. 59). Several documents of the same year bear his name. He returned to Capodistria and painted for the Cathedral a *Massacre of the Innocents* and a *Presentation in the Temple*, perhaps for the organ shutters; the *Two Prophets* for the organ railing are in the Pola (Pulj), Yugoslavia, Museum. Carpaccio was still alive in October, 1525 (Ludwig and Molmenti, p. 59); but in a document dated June 26, 1526, the artist's son Pietro alludes to his father's death.

Carpaccio's first dated work is *The Arrival of St. Ursula at Cologne* (PL. 73), in the series which he began in 1490 for the Scuola di S. Orsola in Venice. This is probably an early work that was preceded by a formative period to which may be attributed paintings which, as *juvenilia*, remain undocumented.

The earliest painting before the St. Ursula series is probably the *Christ* in the Contini Bonacossi Collection, Florence. This work should be connected with the similar *Head of Christ* (ca. 1485) in the Accademia in Venice or with the *Arrival at Cologne*. The Contini *Christ* conforms closely to the manner of Antonello (q.v.) as passed on by Alvise Vivarini (q.v.). Other paintings of the late 15th century which display affinities with Antonello but have been attributed to Carpaccio are the *Venetian Lady* (Amsterdam, Rijksmus.) and a *Madonna and Saints* (Vicenza, Mus. Civ.), once ascribed to Montagna but probably painted by Carpaccio, since it closely resembles a drawing in the Albertina in Vienna which is his beyond question.

Following these early paintings there was a productive period in the artist's development during which the incisive geometry of Antonello was gradually translated into forms of greater amplitude and more intense color. At this point Carpaccio seems to have come in contact with the school of Ferrara, either directly or, less probably, through Ercole de' Roberti (q.v.), who was in Venice about 1480. Evidence for this hypothesis is the presence of the Este eagle in the *Tournaments* (London, Nat. Gall.), attributed to Carpaccio, a painting which is intimately connected with the *Cavalcade* in the frescoes of Francesco del Cossa (q.v.) in the Palazzo Schifanoia in Ferrara. Further evidence is the Ferrarese vigor and forthrightness in the *Portrait of a Man with a Red Cap* in the Museo Correr. Most important, however, is the spatial definition of the school of Ferrara in the St. Ursula cycle. Iconographically the various episodes of the legend also contain surprising analogies with the copies of the lost frescoes of Ercole de' Roberti for the Garganelli Chapel in S. Petronio, Bologna, while the ambassador incidents in the cycle recall the trains of noblemen in the Schifanoia frescoes of Francesco del Cossa.

The St. Ursula cycle develops independently of the traditional story in Jacobus de Varagine's *Golden Legend*, which had been republished in an Italian translation in Venice some years before. In the *Arrival at Cologne* Carpaccio lays out his perspective of castles and canals with nearly Flemish pedantry and barely enlivens his subdued browns and off-greens with the brilliant, rapidly sketched soldiers in the background. A step forward in the atmospheric treatment of color may be seen in the *Martyrdom of St. Ursula*, especially in the luminous green meadow under the castle. The axis of the composition is carefully calculated according to a perspective arrangement that proceeds from the wings in the foreground back to the more distant planes. An increasing interest in color already appears in the third canvas, *The Meeting of St. Ursula and the Pope in Rome* (PL. 78), with the splendid array of the bishops' white mitres under the reddish flags and the brilliant procession that unfolds on the green field. In *The Departure of the Betrothed*, of 1495, we have a peaceful seascape punctuated by towers in perspective, each architectural detail precisely recorded and enlivened by intent onlookers whose garments sparkle with rich touches of color. The true light of the Venetian atmosphere comes to life within the composition.

Carpaccio rises to an even higher level in the three ensuing canvases of the *Arrival, Dismissal,* and *Return of the Ambassadors* and in *The Dream of St. Ursula*, where the warm, dense air of the interiors foreshadows his work in S. Giorgio degli Schia-

5. III.F.W.A.

voni. *The Healing of the Madman* (Venice, Accademia; PL. 72) follows immediately after these and is even more refined.

With these works Carpaccio's youthful period comes to a close, and for a while he seems curiously uncertain, as if torn between the wish to pursue his experiments with color and the need to keep abreast of the changing taste of the times. The group of works beginning with the *Blood of the Redeemer* (1496; Udine, Mus. Civ.), the *Madonna* in the Staedel Institute in Frankfurt, the *Pietà* in the Serristori Collection in Florence, the *Meditation on the Passion* in the Metropolitan Museum in New York, up to and including the *St. Martin* polyptych in the Cathedral of Zara give proof of the artist's embarrassment when confronted with Venetian painting in the grand manner as practiced by Giovanni Bellini.

However, color triumphed again in the new cycle for the Scuola di S. Giorgio degli Schiavoni (1502–07). The first dated canvas, *The Calling of St. Matthew* (1502), harks back to the climate of the later St. Ursula compositions. Issuing from the tax-collector's office, Matthew joins Christ and His followers; the passage from the warm, subdued shadow to the brilliant sunlight establishes a rhythm and endows the colors with an intensity that seems to pulsate in the light. In the succeeding pictures of *St. Jerome in His Study* (PL. 71), *St. Jerome and the Lion*, and *Funeral of St. Jerome*, color plays a dominant role, obliterating the evidence of calculated perspective planning. Whereas color had the character of inlay in the St. Ursula cycle, in the St. Jerome series it envelops all things in luminous space. The legendary, exotic subject of the latter and the gentle, dreamy unfolding of events evocative of past myths make Carpaccio famous as an enchanting storyteller; but his distinction here is in the handling of color as enhancement: The golden atmosphere of St. Jerome's study and the lacquer-red seal that seems suspended in the air, cassocks in a rhythm of lively blues counterpointed by the green-gold of a monastery yard (*St. Jerome and the Lion*), the violet mantle of an old monk in the *Funeral* — these are lyrical motifs that exist independently of subject matter. In the ambassador episodes of the St. Ursula legend, light was treated naturalistically; sky and water spread out with unforgettable breadth. But in the Schiavoni cycle, forms live for themselves alone, in the integrity of their color. Memorable also in the Schiavoni series are certain details of *St. George and the Dragon* (PL. 70), *Triumph of St. George*, *Baptism of the King*, and *Miracle of St. Triphonius*.

In these later paintings, however, quality falls off and continues at a lower level, as in the series on the life of the Virgin for the Scuola degli Albanesi, approximately of the same period and now dispersed among Venice, Bergamo, and Milan (PL. 74). Such a sudden desiccation of the creative instinct in a relatively young artist is difficult to understand; and there is no evidence of the excessive use of helpers or pupils. When we consider the best works of this decade, such as the *Knight in a Landscape* (Lugano, Von Thyssen Coll.; PL. 70), the *Adoration* (Lisbon, Gulbenkian Coll., on loan to Nat. Gall., Washington; 1507), the *Madonna* in Caen (Mus. B.-A.), the *St. Thomas* (Stuttgart, Gemäldegalerie, 1507), or the *Death of the Virgin* (Ferrara, Pin. Civ., 1508), we cannot fail to realize that Carpaccio's lyrical phase practically came to a close with the Schiavoni series. In the Von Thyssen *Knight* some passages are reminiscent of the fairy-tale mood of the St. Ursula legend, and in the Caen *Madonna* we find Oriental elements that recall the Schiavoni canvases. A new interest in portraiture makes its appearance in the Gulbenkian *Adoration*. Despite the apparent loss of lyricism in the Stuttgart and Ferrara works, however, these two squared, pedantically composed paintings have an enamel-like quality, brilliance of surface, and an incisive style of drawing that is close to Cima da Conegliano.

About 1510 Carpaccio came under the classicizing influence of the Venetian architecture and sculpture of the Lombardo family. Certain works of the succeeding decade hark back, however, to a more direct lyrical feeling: the large *Presentation of Christ in the Temple* (1510; PLS. 76, 77) seems to recapture in its cool and changeable colors, recently revealed by restoration, a sense of space intimately handled, as well as a placid narrative rhythm; and the famous *Courtesans* (PL. 70) of the Museo Correr has a chromatic density that surpasses the late works of Giovanni Bellini and those of Giorgione's followers.

Carpaccio's relentless activity and his professional specialization caused him, in his later years, to accept the commission for the decoration of the Scuola di S. Stefano (1511–20). This work, extending through nearly a decade, showed a gradual deterioration. The *St. Stephen Preaching* (PL. 75) is still organically designed and rich in fine amber tones, but not so the *Stoning of St. Stephen* (Stuttgart, Staatsgalerie), which brings the series to an end. A *St. Peter Martyr* and *St. Sebastian* in the Venice Museo Correr, which belonged to a polyptych for the Church of S. Fosca in Venice (1514), give the impression that Carpaccio can no longer make his figures live harmoniously in a pastoral setting. This was the crisis; his later production, listlessly executed with the aid of his two sons, Benedetto and Pietro, in the provincial churches of Istria and the Venetian mainland, was negligible. In the 16th century, Venetian naturalism and the religious acceptance of all things accessible to the senses, predicated by the works of Giorgione and Titian, came into conflict with the timidly humanistic vision of Carpaccio. The vital impulse of the new Venetian climate overpowered and submerged him.

Terisio PIGNATTI

HISTORY OF CARPACCIO CRITICISM. Vasari considered that Carpaccio was the first of the Venetian painters to make "works of real importance," and he called him a "very diligent and practical master." The word "diligent" was customarily applied to artists of the 15th century who could not go beyond a simple imitation of nature. From Vasari onward, the early historians judged Carpaccio accordingly. Thus he was praised by Ridolfi for a "a diligence that departs from the absolute inflexibility of the ancients" and for having "sweetened" his style. The considered opinion of Charles Nicolas Cochin, who saw some merit in Carpaccio, reflected the taste of the 18th century: His manner, according to Cochin, was "dry and without comprehension of light and shadow." For the rest, he continued, there was vigor in the color and in "things rendered with ingenuousness and precision of a lowly nature and without taste, but true" (*Voyage d'Italie*, III, Paris, 1758). During the neoclassic period the artists of the Quattrocento were first regarded with a certain sympathy for their "purity," although they were reevaluated only in the light of the then-current reaction against the baroque. One of the first admirers of Carpaccio was A. M. Zanetti, who in 1771 commented on the St. Ursula cycle: "Truth, imitated or painted only with reason, even without the help of art, exerts great power upon the senses of the spectator . . . . It is not that I suggest that one should paint like Carpaccio but that one should attempt to report on canvas, vividly, the simple truth just as Carpaccio did." In the romantic period Pietro Selvatico praised his religious inspiration; later, H. A. Taine admired his narrative vein and saw him as an illustrator and chronicler of his times. One of the few sensible appraisals was that of Théophile Gauthier, who admired in Carpaccio the "purity," the "graceful seductiveness" of the painter of Urbino in his earliest manner, combined with the admirable Venetian coloration that no other school could attain.

The true rediscoverer of Carpaccio was John Ruskin, whose criticism is however, excessively focused on content and its possible allegorical interpretation. Nor did Roger Fry display any greater visual sensibility when he singled out Carpaccio as the inventor of genre painting, thereby connecting him with the Flemish. While the early writers based their appraisal on the more impersonal altarpieces in which the artist was attempting to achieve the monumental aspects of Antonello and Giovanni Bellini, later critics shifted their interest to Carpaccio's imaginative use of fable and legend and his skill as a painter of scenes. The first monograph on Carpaccio is by Ludwig and Molmenti (1906). A truly critical investigation was undertaken by Fiocco, who was the first to establish certain basic connections between Carpaccio and Gentile Bellini and correctly to reduce to the role of mere disciple the modest personality of Lazzaro Bastiani. Fiocco was also the first to study Carpaccio's drawings, observing the varied and lively hatching. Longhi, while exploring the spread of Piero della Francesca's art in the Venetian region, mentioned Antonello's influence on Carpaccio, reflected in the search for structure, "harmony of proportions," and "colored forms within a clearly defined space." Later, as we have seen, some interesting connections with the school of Ferrara came to light (Pignatti, 1955); and finally, Coletti perceived in Carpaccio's lyrical inspiration a prelude to the suspended animation of Giorgione's subjects. The variety of present

critical opinion, while reflecting the contrasts of modern taste, serves to confirm the hitherto unsuspected complexity of Carpaccio's paintings.

Nicola IVANOFF

BIBLIOG. Vasari, III (Am. ed., trans. E. H. and E. W. Blashfield and A. A. Hopkins, 4 vols., New York, 1913); M. Boschini, Carta del navegar pitoresco, Venice, 1660; C. Ridolfi, Le meraviglie dell'arte, Venice, 1668; A. M. Zanetti, Della pittura veneziana, Venice, 1771; L. Lanzi, Storia pittorica . . . , Bassano, 1795–96; P. Selvatico, Sulla architettura e scultura di Venezia, Venice, 1847; H. A. Taine, Lectures on Art, New York, 1875; J. Ruskin, St. Mark's Rest, Keston (Kent), 1877; J. Ruskin, Fors clavigera, London, 1896–99; S. Colvin, Ueber einige Zeichnungen des Carpaccio, JhbPreussKSamml, 1897, p. 183; G. Ludwig and P. Molmenti, Vittore Carpaccio, Milan, 1906; V. Goloubeff, Due disegni del Carpaccio, Rass. d'Arte, 1907, p. 140; H. A. Taine, Voyage en Italie, Paris, 1907; L. Venturi, Le origini della pittura veneziana, Venice, 1907; R. E. Fry, A Genre Painter . . . , Q. Rev., Apr., 1908; A. Venturi, Storia dell'arte italiana, VII, Milan, 1911–15; J. A. Crowe and G. B. Cavalcaselle, A History of Painting . . . , London, 1912; T. Gauthier, Voyage en Italie, Paris, 1912; D. von Hadeln, ThB, s.v.; R. E. Fry, Vision and Design, London, 1920; D. von Hadeln, Venetianische Zeichnungen des Quattrocento, Berlin, 1925; Van Marle, VIII, 1927; G. Fiocco, Vittore Carpaccio, Rome, 1932, 2d ed., Rome, 1942; G. Fiocco, Nuovi documenti intorno a V. Carpaccio, BArte, Sept., 1932, p. 115; G. Fogolari, Pre' Sebastiano Bastiani, suo padre Lazzaro e il Carpaccio, R. di Venezia, 1932, p. 279; R. Longhi, Per un catalogo delle opere di V. Carpaccio, Vita Artistica, 1932, p. 115; G. Fiocco, A proposito dei pittori L. Bastiani e V. Carpaccio, R. di Venezia, 1933, p. 31; C. L. Ragghianti, Due disegni del Carpaccio, CrArte, 1936, p. 277; F. Hartt, Carpaccio's Meditation on the Passion, BMMA, Mar., 1940; H. and E. Tietze, The Drawings of the Venetian Painters . . . , New York, 1944; R. Longhi, Viatico per cinque secoli di pittura veneziana, Florence, 1946; R. Longhi, Calepino Veneziano, Arte Veneta, 1947, p. 188; V. Moschini, La leggenda di S. Orsola, Milan, 1948; B. Berenson, The Italian Painters of the Renaissance, 2d ed., rev., London, 1952; T. Pignatti, Carpaccio, Geneva, 1955; M. Muraro, Vittore Carpaccio, alla Scuola degli Schiavoni, Milan, 1956; T. Pignatti, Proposte per la data di nascita di Vittore Carpaccio e per la identificazione della Scuola di S. Orsola, Atti dell'VIII Congr. di Storia dell'Arte, Venice, 1956; B. Berenson, Italian Pictures of the Renaissance, Venetian School, London, 1958.

Terisio PIGNATTI

Illustrations: PLS. 70–78.

**CARPEAUX, JEAN-BAPTISTE.** French sculptor, etcher, and painter of the Second Empire (b. Valenciennes, May 11, 1827; d. Courbevoie, Oct. 12, 1875). He trained in his native Valenciennes and in Paris from 1842, where he studied under François Rude, a leading romantic sculptor. In 1854 Carpeaux won the Prix de Rome with *Hector* (Paris, Mus. de l'Ecole Nat. des Beaux-Arts). In Italy he modeled his famous *Neapolitan Fisherboy* (versions in Louvre; Washington, Nat. Gall; etc.; 1858), a lively urchin surpassing Rude's prototype but endowed with the formal graces and slender elegance of the rococo (q.v.), recalling Falconet (q.v.). The tragic sculpture *Ugolino and His Starving Sons* (Paris, Louvre, 1857–61), conceived under the gloomy spell of Michelangelo's *Last Judgment* and Dante's *Inferno* and thus very unlike Carpeaux's usually joyful works, is a culminant masterpiece of romanticism, with its passion for medieval themes and emotional excesses. Carpeaux always conceived in terms of clay modeling rather than stonecutting. Though he has compressed his allusions to Michelangelo into a dense cluster of anguished bodies in the *Ugolino*, the mass is broken by undulating currents of space. Always Carpeaux's vivid reality bespeaks the age of the photograph.

In spite of conservative opposition, he received enviable commissions — first, for the Pavillon de Flore (Paris, Tuileries, 1863–66), for which he executed the pediment sculptures and a splendid, unprecedentedly deep relief of *Flora with Dancing Cupids*; again, rococo images as ebullient and sensuous as Clodion's are enriched by Michelangelesque *contrapposto*, yet at the same time conserve the fleshy particularity of the model with unabashed voluptuousness. Carpeaux's masterpiece, the nine-figure group, *The Dance* (1865–69), for the architect Garnier's opera house, created a scandal because this pagan romp was wholly emancipated from the academic chill which conservative opinion then identified with art. Today *The Dance* seems a brilliant reconciliation of movement and abandon with an easy formal symmetry that makes it magnificent architectural decoration, perfectly attuned to the exuberant luxury of Garnier's building.

Many fine likenesses of the imperial family and other leading contemporaries demonstrate that Carpeaux was also the best portraitist of the time, as can be seen in the charming statue *The Imperial Prince with His Dog Nero* (Paris, Louvre, 1865). Later works include the figures personifying the Four Continents on the fountain in the Luxembourg Gardens (1872), the marble *Daphnis and Chloë* (1873), and the memorial to his fellow townsman Watteau in their native Valenciennes (1869; completed posthumously).

BIBLIOG. O. Grautoff, ThB, s.v.; L. Clément-Carpeaux, La Vérité sur . . . Carpeaux, Paris, 1934–35; Catalogue de l'Exposition J.-B. Carpeaux, Petit-Palais, Paris, 1955–56.

James HOLDERBAUM

**CARPETS.** See TAPESTRY AND CARPETS.

**CARRACCI,** LODOVICO, ANNIBALE, AGOSTINO, ANTONIO. A family of Bolognese painters, among the most important of the Italian Seicento.

SUMMARY. Lodovico (col. 134). Annibale (col. 136). Agostino (col. 139). Antonio (col. 141). The Carraccis in the artistic milieu of the Seicento (col. 142).

LODOVICO. He was baptized on Apr. 21, 1555, in the Cathedral of Bologna and died in Bologna on Nov. 13, 1619. Neither Lodovico's principal biographer, Canon Malvasia (1678), nor the most recent research furnishes sound documentation concerning the artist's youth. Lodovico first studied with Prospero Fontana between about 1570 and 1580. Since this alone did not satisfactorily explain his development, Malvasia assumed that the artist traveled to Florence, Parma, Mantua, and Venice and served an apprenticeship with Passignano. It is very likely that Lodovico also studied with Camillo Procaccini, as stated by Bellori. Although the exact chronology of his early years remains uncertain, Arcangeli's (1956) admirable study has somewhat clarified the problem. In 1578 Lodovico became a member of the Compagnia dei Pittori (Malvasia), but we have no authenticated works prior to the frieze with the story of Jason in the Palazzo Fava, Bologna (1583–84). Lodovico's participation in this enterprise is actually much smaller than Malvasia would have us believe. The frieze in the second room of the Palazzo Fava, representing the story of Aeneas, is also problematical. Here some parts — the Trojans and the Harpies, for example, as well as some of the decorative figures — seem to suggest a date contemporary with that of the Jason room, in contrast to other sections which are obviously much later. Such a dating would partially explain why Lodovico contributed so little to the planning and execution of the Jason frieze. Arcangeli recently indicated the following as contemporary with the Jason frieze: *St. Francis* and *Portrait of a Youth* (Rome, Mus. Cap.), *Mystical Marriage of a Saint* (Bologna, Beretta Coll.), and the *Baptism of Christ* (Munich, Bayerische Staatgemäldesamml.), which is slightly later and somewhat closer to the *Annunciation* (PL. 80) in the Pinacoteca Nazionale, Bologna, from the now destroyed Church of S. Giorgio. With this *Annunciation* we presumably reach the year 1585. The first definite documentary reference is dated 1587 and concerns the *Conversion of St. Paul* (Bologna, Pin. Naz.), doubtless executed before the final payment in 1589. The year 1588 is inscribed on the Bargellini *Madonna* (Bologna, Pin. Naz.; PL. 79).

*The History of Rome* in the Palazzo Magnani (now Salem) in Bologna was probably begun about 1588. The date 1592, inscribed on the fireplace in the room where the fresco appears, probably refers to the completion of the work. Lodovico contributed the splendid *She-wolf* (PL. 80), *The Rape of the Sabines*, and *The Sabines Intervening in the Battle*.

Subsequent works are *Supper in the House of Simon*, *Martyrdom of St. Ursula*, and *Preaching of the Baptist* (Bologna, Pin. Naz.) of 1592. About 1593–94 Lodovico collaborated with Annibale and Agostino in the decoration of several rooms of the Casa Sampieri (now Talon) in Bologna. Also to be dated 1592–93 are the *Flora* and the *Opis* that, together with two

other ovals by Annibale and Agostino, were executed for the Palazzo dei Diamanti in Ferrara and are today at the Estense in Modena. It is not improbable that, on Annibale's departure for Rome (1595), Lodovico put the finishing touches on the large painting, *St. Roch Giving Alms* (Dresden, Gemälde gal.).

The decoration of the second room of the Palazzo Fava (the story of Aeneas) dates from about this time or slightly earlier; it was begun about 1583–84 and subsequently interrupted. At the onset of the new century, Lodovico undertook the second version of the *Martyrdom of St Ursula* (Imola, Church of SS. Nicola e Domenico, 1600) and, the following year, the *Assumption* (Bologna, Church of Corpus Domini). Lodovico's trip to Rome, documented with extreme precision (May 31–June 13, 1602), marked a new phase: to the already mature immobility of his deliberately "provincial" style was added a Romanism altogether alien to such a restrained and naturalistic painter. A suggestion of this Romanism was already apparent in the three paintings dedicated to three women of the New Testament, executed by the Carraccis about 1595 for the Sampieri family (Milan, Brera). At the beginning of this classicistic crisis, which made the first decade of the 17th century the most disconcerting period of Lodovico's life, we may place the aforementioned *Assumption* (1601) in the Church of Corpus Domini in Bologna, the *Divine Providence* (Rome, Mus. Cap., ca. 1604–05), and *Christ Healing a Blind Man* (Rome, Gall. Pallavicini).

The main undertaking of Lodovico and his workshop in Bologna was the fresco decoration of the cloister of the Convento di S. Michele in Bosco, which reveals great personal and dramatic vigor. The final payments for this series on the life of St. Benedict were made Apr. 9, 1605, and included compensation for Lodovico, who painted 7 of the 37 frescoes and numerous caryatids, and for his assistants — Reni, Massari, Garbieri, Cavedone, Tiarini, etc. In November, 1606, work was begun for the Cathedral of Piacenza and was definitely completed Aug. 24, 1609. It consisted of frescoes in the choir and vault (some of them today in the Episcopal Palace) in addition to two enormous paintings — the *Funeral of the Virgin* and the *Apostles at the Tomb of the Virgin* (Parma, Gall. Naz.). After Annibale's death, Lodovico, now alone, continued working in his native city. Of this period are the *Virgin in Glory* and the *SS. Orso and Eusebio* (Cathedral of Fano, 1613), *The Crucifixion* (Ferrara, Church of S. Francesca Romana, 1614; PL. 82), the *Martyrdom of St. Margaret* (Mantua, Church of S. Maurizio, 1616), and the *Adoration of the Magi* (Milan, Brera, 1616). In 1619 he signed and dated the *S. Bernardino Saving the City of Carpi*, in 1939 recovered in Notre-Dame in Paris. Finally, between 1618 and the beginning of 1619 he painted the large fresco of the *Annunciation* on the triumphal arch of the Cathedral of S. Pietro in Bologna.

OTHER IMPORTANT WORKS (in approximately chronological order). *Vision of St. Anthony* (Amsterdam, Rijksmus., ca. 1585; copy in Bologna, Pin. Naz., ca. 1586). – *Assumption* (Raleigh, N. C., Mus. of Art). – *Sacrifice of Isaac* (Rome, Mus. Vat., ca. 1586–87). – *The Tacconi Family* (Genoa, private coll., ca. 1589–90). – *The Holy Family with St. Francis and Donors* (Cento, Pin. Civ., 1591; PL. 81). – *Adoration of the Magi* and *Circumcision* (now destroyed; formerly Bologna, in S. Bartolomeo, ca. 1591–92). – *Madonna of the Scalzi* (Bologna, Pin. Naz., ca. 1592). – *Alexander and Thais* (Bologna, private coll., ca. 1592). – *Trinity* and *Dead Christ* (Rome, Mus. Vat., ca. 1592). – *Charity* and *St. Francis* (Bologna, Church of S. Domenico, ca. 1592). – *St. Jerome* (Florence, Coll. M. Salmi, 1593). – *Virgin with S. Giacinto* (Paris, Louvre, 1594). – *Crowning with Thorns* and *Flagellation* (Bologna, Pin. Naz., ca. 1595). – *Christ and the Canaanite Woman* (Milan, Brera, ca. 1595). – *Christ at the Pool of Bethesda* (Bologna, Pin. Naz., ca. 1596). – *Martyrdom of S. Angelo* (Bologna, Pin. Naz., ca. 1596–98). – *St. Jerome* (Bologna, S. Martino, ca. 1596–98). – *Transfiguration* (Bologna, Pin. Naz., ca. 1595–97). – *Ascension of Christ* (Bologna, S. Cristina, ca. 1597). – *Flight into Egypt* (Bologna, private coll., ca. 1598). – *St. Roch* (Bologna, S. Giacomo Maggiore, ca. 1600). – *St. Sebastian* (Rome, Gall. Doria Pamphili, ca. 1602). – *Mystic Marriage of St. Catherine* (Berlin, formerly in Bieber Coll., ca. 1602–04). – *Birth of St. John the Baptist* (Bologna, Pin. Naz., ca. 1602–04). – *Annunciation* (Genoa, Palazzo Rosso, ca. 1603). – *Calling of St. Matthew* (Bologna, Pin. Naz., ca. 1603–05). – *Assumption* (Modena, Gall. Estense, ca. 1605–06). – *St. Catherine in Prison* (Bologna, Coll. Co-

munali d'Arte, ca. 1605–06. – *Fall of Simon Magus* (Naples, Mus. Naz., 1605–07). – *Annunciation* and *Nativity of the Virgin* (Piacenza, Episcopal Palace, ca. 1606–09). – *Apostles at the Tomb of the Virgin* and *Funeral of the Virgin* (Parma, Convento di S. Domenico, ca. 1612). – *Visitation* and *Flagellation* (Bologna, S. Domenico, ca. 1612). – *S. Carlo Praying* (Bologna, S. Bartolomeo, ca. 1612–14). – *S. Carlo and the Child* (Forlì, Pin., ca. 1614–16). – *Paradise* (Bologna, S. Paolo, ca. 1616). – *St. Peter Repenting* (Bologna, S. Pietro, Sacristy, 1617).

Andrea EMILIANI

ANNIBALE. Painter and engraver, Agostino's younger brother and Lodovico's cousin, he was born in Bologna on Nov. 3, 1560, and died in Rome on July 15, 1609. Nothing is known about Annibale's early training except that he was introduced to painting by Lodovico. However, the earlier works of Annibale and Lodovico, which fall between 1582 and 1585, show altogether different artistic orientations, though an equally high level. Annibale, who was engaged in engraving paintings by Sabbatini and Barocci, indicated a preference for the local late mannerism, as is confirmed by his earliest known public works, *The Crucifix* (Bologna, Church of S. Nicolò, 1583), *The Butcher's Shop* (Oxford, Christ Church; PL. 83), and *The Bean Eater* (Rome, Gall. Colonna). In the last mentioned, Annibale openly yields to the realism of Bartolomeo Passerotti, thus paralleling the work of the Campis, a family of painters from Cremona with whom Annibale was certainly familiar. *The Baptism of Christ* of 1585 (Bologna, S. Gregorio; PL. 84) also contains late-manneristic elements; here Annibale combines the suffused tenderness of Barocci with the poetic sensuality of Correggio (q.v.). To the same phase belong the *Allegory* (London, Hampton Court) and the frieze with the story of Jason in the Palazzo Fava in Bologna, done in collaboration with Lodovico and Agostino. Annibale seems to recall here the intricately entwined compositions of Nicolò dell'Abate, but with Tuscan drawing and color. Even more Correggesque than the *Baptism* is the *Deposition* (Parma, Pin.), also of 1585. This phase, which was dominated by the influence of Correggio, finally culminated in the altarpiece of the *Assumption* of 1587 (Dresden, Gemäldegalerie). The other altarpiece in Dresden, *The Virgin and Child with SS. Matthew, Francis, and John the Baptist* (PL. 84), of 1588, marks Annibale's first turning to the great masters of the Venetian Cinquecento and to the painterly approach to color and light popular in northern Italy. The work that earned for the Carraccis their true recognition was the frieze containing the story of Romulus and the legendary history of Rome, 14 sections, executed in the Palazzo Magnani in Bologna in fresco between 1588 and 1590. Here mutual artistic exchange and the neo-Venetian influence can best be observed in an almost gradual development. While the scenes are still separated by heavy borders and caryatids supporting the architrave, painted in grisaille to imitate marble statues, a new trend is initiated by the illusionism of framing a series of canvases in moldings of architectural sculpture. This is a precociously baroque idea that was fully realized a decade later in the Galleria Farnese in Rome. In the Palazzo Magnani, as in the Palazzo Fava, the Carraccis worked in such close cooperation that critics of the mid-17th century found it difficult to distinguish the various parts. Malvasia has the painters themselves utter the famous phrase: "It [the work] is by the Carraccis; we all have done it." To Annibale is attributed: *Remus Punishes the Brigands*, *Remus before Amulius*, *Romulus Sets Out the Boundaries of Rome*, *The Plague* (?). To Lodovico is attributed: *The She-wolf*, *The Slaying of Amulius*, *The Sabines Intervening in the Battle*, *The Slaying of Titus Tatius*, *The Pride of Romulus*. To Agostino is attributed: *The Refuge on the Capitol*, *Romulus with the Remains of Acron*, *Battle of the Romans and Sabines*, *Defiance of the Captain of Veii*, *Romulus Appears to Proclus*, *Lupercalian Sacrifices*.

A little later, Annibale's neo-Venetianism focuses on Veronese and Tintoretto, as in the *Assumption* (Bologna, Pin. Naz.) and *Madonna with SS. Luke and Catherine* (Paris, Louvre, 1592). A second phase in Annibale's study of the great masters of the Cinquecento had begun, in which the various artistic references were resolved into a personal style. His neo-Venetianism is expressed in many diverse works which may be either sacred

or profane, a direct impression or an elaborate conception, an exaggerated, bizarre realism or an allegorical, disciplined, composition. Among these works are the *Madonna of S. Ludovico* (Bologna, Pin. Naz.), *Venus and Adonis* (Vienna, Kunsthist. Mus.), *Baccante* (Florence, Uffizi), *Portrait of a Musician* (Dresden, Gemäldegalerie), *Portrait of a Man* in Munich (Alte Pinakothek), *Self-portrait* in the Uffizi, *Venus and Cupid* (Modena, Gall. Estense), *Assumption of the Virgin*, dated 1592 (Bologna, Pin. Naz.), and the *Resurrection* in the Louvre (1593). Already germinating in Annibale's mind, however, was the idea of a compositional harmony springing from a determination to reinstate the forms of nature through the study of tradition. Exemplifying this are the *Samaritan at the Well* (Milan, Brera) and the frescoes on the ground floor of Casa Sampieri in Bologna (1593–94), of which we can attribute to Annibale the ceiling with *Hercules Instructed by Virtue* and the fireplace with *Hercules and Anteus*. Annibale's last work in Bologna is *St. Roch Giving Alms* (Dresden, Gemäldegalerie), which he had been commissioned to do in 1587–88 by the Confraternità di S. Rocco of Reggio Emilia and at which he worked, with interruptions, until his departure for Rome in 1595.

There is documented evidence that Annibale was in Rome on Nov. 8, 1595, in the service of Cardinal Odoardo Farnese, who commissioned him to decorate the ceiling of the Camerino in the Palazzo Farnese. This work lasted two years and is of marked interest because it can be considered the introduction to a new attitude of Annibale, based on the study and revival of classical forms. In the center of the ceiling is the painting of *Hercules at the Crossroads* (Naples, Capodimonte; PL. 85); at the sides, two ovals with *Hercules Supporting the World* and *Hercules Resting*; and in the two main lunettes, *Ulysses and the Sirens* and *Ulysses Receiving the Chalice from Circe*. The entire decoration of the Camerino is Annibale's work as demonstrated by the preparatory drawings (Paris, Louvre; Windsor, Royal Colls.; Besançon, Mus.; Montpellier, Mus. Fabre; Turin, Mus. Civ. d'Arte Antica).

The works in the vault of the Galleria, begun toward the end of 1597, were probably finished by the end of 1599, when Agostino left Rome after completing two of the principal scenes, the *Galatea*, and *Aurora and Cephalus*; in the cornice below the *Galatea* we read the date 1600, presumably referring to the completion of the vault. The work on the walls, however, continued beyond 1602, the year Domenichino arrived in Rome. Annibale probably assigned to him the execution of the large *Liberation of Andromeda* on the end wall. Intended to celebrate the deeds of Alessandro Farnese, who died in Flanders in 1592, the theme underwent a profound but slow development in allegorical content, deriving inspiration from Alexandrian mythology. The development occurred in successive stages according to Annibale's "method," as is proved by a very large series of drawings (Paris, Louvre; Windsor, Royal Colls.; Leicester, Coll. Lord Ellesmere; Vienna, Albertina; Besançon, Mus.; Florence, Uffizi; etc.). Notwithstanding the consciously literary approach imparted to the new theme by Monsignor Giovanni Battista Agucchi, the literary friend of Annibale and chamberlain of Cardinal Pietro Aldobrandini (Bellori), the imaginative inspiration of the painter was not hampered. We see, then, that the revival and evolution of the Bolognese frieze of the Cinquecento tradition, after the intermediate developments in the Fava and Magnani palaces, find their highest and freest expression in the Galleria Farnese (PL. 86; see Louvre drawings, nos. 7422 and 8048). The decorations have the significance and illusionistic function of a homogeneous complex in which architecture, sculpture, and painting are integrated. In the opening of the vault, with light and sky visible through the false wall structure, the sense of space becomes real. This is the first indication of the free spatiality that later dominates the baroque period (q.v.) and is the most authoritative precedent for Pietro da Cortona and Luca Giordano. Annibale's general idea was to produce the illusion of a series of gold-framed paintings hung under the vault, at the center and sides, thus creating a highly original pictorial-architectural structure. At the center of the vault, between the two smaller paintings of *Mercury and Paris* and *Pan and Selene*, is the large rectangular composi-

tion with the *Triumph of Bacchus*. The theme was partially inspired by an analogous subject by Giulio Romano in the Palazzo del Tè in Mantua, and the figures by Raphael's composition of *Psyche Received in Olympus* in the Farnesina. Against the two end lunettes, supported by nude figures, lean the paintings of *Polyphemus and Galatea* on one side and *Polyphemus Killing Acis* on the other. The same scenic device is repeated on the frieze. It is undeniable that a study of the remains of Greco-Roman art and, more importantly, of Raphael in his evocations of antiquity enriched Annibale's developing poetic style in 1595. This is proved by the numerous extant drawings that are actually fragmentary studies — for the most part notations, analyses, detailed research. Together they comprise a passionate, persistent work, with nature as the model. To the drawings Annibale applied classical quotations derived from direct archaeological study and from the large body of figure drawings and paintings of the Renaissance, particularly Raphaelesque; further inspiration were the prints of Marcantonio and Caraglio. In this atmosphere Annibale created masterpieces such as the small engraving of the *Temptation of St. Anthony* (London, Nat. Gall.) and two splendid small works, *Bacchus and Silenus* and *Silenus Gathering Grapes* (London, Nat. Gall.).

Annibale had a lively interest in landscape as a separate subject, and initiated the modern approach to landscape — a colloquy between man and nature — which is in different aspects both heroic and romantic. In the friezes of the Fava and Magnani palaces, between 1583 and 1590, Annibale already seemed to echo Nicolò dell'Abate's Ariostesque fable in terms of a naturalistic pictoricism oscillating between Bassano (q.v.) and Dosso (see DOSSI). This is the origin of the "meteorological" character of certain very youthful landscapes, such as the two examples of *Hunting and Fishing* (Paris, Louvre), the *Vision of St. Eustace* (Naples, Capodimonte), *Festa Campestre* (Marseilles, Mus.), and the *Landscape* in Berlin (Staat. Mus.; PL. 83). Among the newest and most poetic landscapes in the first years of the Seicento we must include the engraving of the *Sacrifice of Isaac* (Paris, Louvre) and the *Preaching of the Baptist* (Grenoble, Mus.). Annibale went beyond the Flemish perspicacity in subtle observation of light or the Nordic taste for the picturesque; altogether new was the spiritual breadth of his image of nature, poetically observed and permeated with a melancholy yet intimate feeling of life. Illustrating this is one of the greatest masterpieces in 17th-century Italian landscape painting — the famous *Flight into Egypt* (Rome, Gall. Doria Pamphili; PL. 89), one of six lunettes on canvas painted for the chapel of the Palazzo Aldobrandini by Annibale and his pupils about 1603–04. The problem of collaboration has not yet been entirely clarified. Certainly *The Deposition*, in this group, should be attributed to Annibale; but the *Flight* indeed deserves the fame of leading in the development of heroic classic landscape. From the serene and resigned melancholy of Annibale's classicism, from his "feeling of time," was to derive, a little later, Poussin's more lucid classicism (see POUSSIN) and the more romantic classicism of Claude Lorrain (q.v.). The decoration of the Aldobrandini Chapel corresponds with the climax of Annibale's classicistic revival in Rome, in which two periods can be distinguished. The first begins with the *Coronation of the Virgin* (London, Mahon Coll.) and the Farnese Camerino and includes the finishing of the vault in the Galleria Farnese up to the cornice (1595–96 to 1600). The second period, which opened the brief final phase of Annibale's activity, begins with the *Assumption* in S. Maria del Popolo in Rome (1600–01) and includes the remainder of the Galleria, which Annibale did not execute but only directed. Authentic masterpieces of this second phase are, besides *The Flight into Egypt* (PL. 89) in the Galleria Doria Pamphili, the *Domine, Quo Vadis?* (London, Nat. Gall.), *The Samaritan at the Well* (Vienna, Kunsthist. Mus.), the *Pietà* in Vienna (Kunsthist. Mus., ca. 1603; PL. 87), the dramatic scene of the *Three Marys at the Tomb* (London, Nat. Gall.), and the *Martyrdom of St. Sebastian* (Paris, Louvre), datable about 1604. From 1600 on, Annibale's work is marked by a unity of touch, a loftiness of content as if the canvas were a fresco, and a sculptural approach that exalts design. This

rigorous, formal equilibrium needs but a touch of hedonism and a slight suggestion of Correggesque softness, as in the *Pietà* in Vienna, to be transformed into that other baroque naturalism that resulted in Bernini's blissful sensuality. Unavoidably, however, Annibale's poetic tendency gave way to gesticulation and rhetoric, as can be seen in the late *Pietà* in the Louvre (ca. 1607).

At the beginning of 1605, struck by the first attack of his disease "with apparent danger of apoplexy" (Mancini), Annibale left the service of Cardinal Farnese. By this time his work was limited to the slow preparation of the drawings for works to be executed mainly by his assistants — Albani, Domenichino, Lanfranco, Antonio Carracci, Sisto Badolocchio, and Innocenzo Tacconi. A typical product of this period is the decorative complex of the Herrera Chapel in S. Giacomo degli Spagnuoli in Rome, with the *Stories of the Life of S. Diego* (1602–07). Executed almost entirely by Albani, this work was dismantled during the 19th century and is now divided between the Prado and the Museo de Bellas Artes in Barcelona. Probably the last composition completed by Annibale was the Louvre *Pietà*. On July 14, 1608, he agreed with his assistants to spend two hours a day in the workshop; a year later, on July 15, 1609, after another attack of illness, Annibale died. He was barely forty-nine years of age.

OTHER IMPORTANT WORKS. *St. Francis Adoring the Crucifix* (Rome, Mus. Cap., ca. 1584). – *Portrait of G. F. Turrini* (Oxford, Christ Church, 1585). – *St. Francis Adoring the Crucifix* (Venice, Accademia, ca. 1585–86). – *Marriage of St. Catherine* (Naples, Palazzo Reale, ca. 1586). – *Christ Crowned with Thorns* (Dresden, Gemäldegalerie, 1586–87). – *Portrait of C. Merulo* (Naples, Capodimonte, 1587). – *Annunciation* (Bologna, Pin. Naz., 1586–87). – *Self-portrait with Father* (Milan, Brera, 1587–88). – *Bacchus* (Naples, Capodimonte, 1590–92). – *Self-portrait* (Florence, Uffizi, 1590–92). – *The Genius of Glory* (Dresden, Gemäldegalerie, 1590–92). – *Madonna of the Swallow* (Dresden, Gemäldegalerie, 1590–92). – *Madonna with SS. Luke and Catherine* (Paris, Louvre, 1592). – *Self-portrait* (Parma, Gall. Naz., 1593). – *Samson Imprisoned* (Rome, Gall. Borghese, 1593–94). – *River God* (Naples, Capodimonte, 1593–94). – *Crucifixion* (Berlin, Staat. Mus. 1594). – *Madonna in Glory above the City of Bologna* (Oxford, Christ Church, 1593–95). – *St. John the Baptist in the Desert* (London, Denis Mahon Coll., 1594–95). – *St. Margaret* (Rome, S. Caterina de' Funari, 1595–96, perhaps in collaboration with Massari). – *Vision of St. Francis* (London, John Pope-Hennessy Coll., 1595–96). – *Christ Mocked* (Bologna, Pin. Naz., 1596–98). – *Birth of the Virgin* (Paris, Louvre, 1598–1600). – *Madonna of the Silence* (London, Hampton Court, 1598–1600). – *St. John in the Desert* (London, Nat. Gall., 1598–1601). – *Sleeping Venus* (Chantilly, Mus. Condé, probably in collaboration, ca. 1604).

Giancarlo CAVALLI

AGOSTINO. Annibale's older brother and Lodovico's cousin, he was baptized in the Cathedral of Bologna Aug. 16, 1557. According to Malvasia he first became an engraver with a goldsmith; later he studied painting with Prospero Fontana and then, in a brief apprenticeship, with Passerotti. After that he was again in the workshop of an engraver, Domenico Tibaldi, brother of Pellegrino. His artistic evolution can be traced through his engravings; the earliest ones, up to 1579, are influenced by the major representatives of local mannerism, especially Samacchini and Sabatini. Later Agostino concentrated on older artists, particularly Michelangelo. It is not unlikely that this direction resulted from a visit to Rome about 1580. Each of a series of small pictures of saints, signed and dated 1581, bears the word "Rome," although Malvasia believes this was added later. Between 1580 and 1582 he engraved works by Francia, Raffaellino da Reggio, and Cort; the only contemporary Bolognese artist whose works he engraved was Calvaert. This might indicate an inclination of taste, as is later confirmed in painting by the small *Communion of St. Francis* (London, Dulwich College Picture Gall.), dated about 1582–83. For the *Communion* Agostino borrowed a composition by Calvaert (Turin, Gall. dell'Accademia Albertina) and adhered to his style; but he introduced a more accomplished naturalism. The closeness to the reserved approach of Calvaert was motivated by Agostino's progressive rejection of the more involved forms of the late Cinquecento — a rejection that ap-

peared more decisive after a trip to Venice (1582). There he engraved numerous plates, especially from Veronese, in which he tried to combine in a clear spatial volume a quality of color and atmosphere with a definite and patient "truth" of design. In 1583–84 he collaborated with Annibale and Lodovico in the decoration of the Palazzo Fava. The general conception of the complex was probably by Agostino, who was recognized as the most cultivated of the three Carraccis. We can undoubtedly attribute to him the scenes in which Venetian influences are most obvious, since they are stylistically similar to a series of engravings of apostles after his own designs (1583). Thus in the room of Europa, at least two of the four episodes represented are his, and probably others as well, such as the *Golden Fleece Being Given to King Pelias*, and *Jason Killing the Sleeping Dragon*, in the room of Jason.

As early as the time the works in the Palazzo Fava were done, a Parmese influence was added to the Venetian, first through engravings of Parmigianino (q.v.) and, especially, Caraglio. A precise reference to engravings of Caraglio is documented by the fresco of *Bacchus and Ariadne* (Bologna, Pin. Naz.), which should probably be placed between 1584 and 1585. The culmination of these influences was a trip to Parma, which Agostino probably made with Annibale about 1586; while there, Agostino engraved two paintings by Correggio. His *Virgin with Child and Saints* (Parma, Gall. Naz., 1586) illustrates, in its archaic and programmatic composition, the confluence of Veronese and Parmese elements. Another trip to Venice occurred in 1588–89, during which he engraved a large print of the *Crucifixion* by Tintoretto, earning the master's praise. Probably to this period should also be attributed the famous *lascivie*, a series of amatory scenes taken from classical mythology. Between 1588 and about 1591 he collaborated with Annibale and Lodovico on the large frieze in the Palazzo Magnani, henceforth devoting himself wholeheartedly to painting. The *Pluto* of the Galleria Estense in Modena, dated 1592, is a tribute to the gigantic style of Titian. Between 1591 and 1593 can be placed the celebrated *Communion of St. Jerome* and the *Assumption of the Virgin* (both in Bologna, Pin. Naz.). In these works Agostino was concerned with naturalism and design. He combined the atmosphere and pictorial breadth of Veronese with the compositional and spatial organization of Raphael. To the softness of Correggio he added a rich, elaborate, and precious impasto. At this time Agostino also became more attentive to Tuscan-Roman plastic constructivism, probably through the study of Pellegrino Tibaldi, the engravings by Marcantonio, the frescoes in the Casa Sampieri (ca. 1593–94), and the Prado painting representing the *Last Supper* (ca. 1594). In *Christ and the Adulteress* (Milan, Brera; PL. 88) we notice a direct though somewhat sketchy influence of the Roman school, particularly of the Stanze of Raphael in the Vatican. This could be the result of Agostino's and Annibale's brief sojourn in Rome in 1594. In 1596 or 1597 Agostino probably joined Annibale in Rome for the work at the Palazzo Farnese. The two large paintings in the Galleria — the *Galatea* and the *Aurora and Cephalus* — are by Agostino (cartoons in London, Nat. Gall.); here the heavy rounded modeling of *Christ and the Adulteress* emerges as a massive plasticity, with which Agostino attempts to give a more animated naturalism to ancient statuary. Agostino's participation in the over-all scheme of the Galleria vault must have been considerable, especially in the choice of iconographic material (also related to the graphic repertory of Marcantonio and his school). Not much later than *Christ and the Adulteress*, perhaps when he was already in Rome, Agostino painted *Composition with Figures and Animals* (Naples, Capodimonte). This work was formerly attributed to Annibale and somewhat arbitrarily interpreted, probably in the 19th century, as a satire against Caravaggio. The *Portrait of Giovanna Parolini-Guicciardini* (Berlin, Staat. Mus.) is dated 1598. It was probably in 1599 that Agostino returned to Bologna, his departure hastened by disagreements between the two brothers (Malvasia) during their association in Rome. In the same year Agostino completed one of his best engravings, *Pan Overpowered by Cupid*. In this work the forms, suggesting a soft Raphaelesque quality, are suffused by a gentle melancholy,

as in the contemporary *Holy Family with St. Margaret* (Naples, Capodimonte).

In July, 1600, Agostino was summoned to Parma by Duke Ranuccio to decorate a small room in the Palazzo del Giardino. The vault of the Camerino was divided into five sections, four of which were frescoed by Agostino with mythological scenes; in the fifth a tablet was placed, commemorating the artist's death, which occurred on Feb. 23, 1602. The style of these frescoes, as in the *Holy Family* in Naples, results from a pleasing fusion of Roman idealism with Bolognese sensuality in an elegant and dreamlike classicism. Though the quality of Agostino's work was inferior to that of Annibale and Lodovico, his importance in the Academy established by the Carraccis in Bologna is not to be underestimated; his extensive traveling and the documentation of his engravings must have performed an eminent cultural function. Since Agostino's principal role was probably that of theoretician of the school, as tradition holds, it is perhaps through his personality that the concept of "eclecticism" can be historically reevaluated. The concept stands, in any case, not as a closed and rigidly codified formula but rather as a stylistic search, through progress and integration, that continues in various cultural directions (see ECLECTICISM).

OTHER IMPORTANT WORKS. *Marriage of St. Catherine* (Milan, private coll., attrib. Arcangeli). – *Adoration of the Shepherds* (Bologna, S. Bartolomeo). – *Marriage of St. Catherine* (Göteborg, Art Gall., attrib. Arcangeli). – Four canvases with erotic subjects (Vienna, Kunsthist. Mus., attrib. Kurz; according to Longhi, Pallucchini, and Fiocco, by Paolo Fiammingo). – *Susanna and the Elders* (signed; Sarasota, Ringling Mus.). – *Venus and Cupid* (Vienna, Kunsthist. Mus., usually attrib. to Lodovico). – *Double Portrait* (London, Stonor Coll.). – *Last Supper* (Ferrara, S. Cristoforo alla Certosa). – *Diana and Acteon* (Brussels, Mus. Royaux des B.-A.). – *St. Jerome* (Naples, Capodimonte). – *Holy Family* (Montecassino, Abbey, attrib. Salerno). – *Pentecost* (Bologna, S. Domenico, attrib. Volpe).

ANTONIO. Agostino's illegitimate son, he was born in Venice in about 1583 (Baglione) or about 1589 (Bellori). After the death of Agostino, Antonio left Emilia for Rome, where, according to both biographers, he entered the workshop of his uncle Annibale. When Annibale died, Antonio went to Bologna for a year to join Lodovico. In 1610 we find him again in Rome, assisting Guido Reni (q.v.) in the decoration of the Pauline Chapel in the Quirinal Palace; his style is recognizable in two lunettes (the *Presentation of Mary in the Temple* and the *Annunciation of the Angel to Joachim*) and in two figures (Adam and a saint). From 1614 to 1616 Antonio's name appeared in the archives of the Accademia di S. Luca. On Feb. 25, 1615, he married Rosa Leoni of Cyprus. After a short stay in Siena, he died in Rome on Apr. 8, 1618.

If the frescoes in the presbytery of the Church of the Madonna del Piano in Capranica were actually done by Antonio (as attributed by Salerno), their date of completion was probably earlier than 1611–12, at least for the two lateral frescoes of *The Birth of Mary* and *The Death of Mary*; the manneristic features of the Mary frescoes, clearly reminiscent of Cesi, had not yet been substantially modified by Reni and Albani, whose influence is apparent in Antonio's works at the Quirinal. Two ceilings of the Palazzo Mattei — *Jacob and Rachel at the Well* and *Isaac Blessing Jacob* — formerly attributed to Domenichino, were later attributed to Antonio and dated about 1612 (Salerno). Accordingly the date of the frescoes in the Capranica vault, which are stylistically linked with the frescoes at the Galleria Farnese, must be about 1614. Very likely the cycle of frescoes at S. Bartolomeo dell'Isola in Rome was also done in 1614; it is undoubtedly a product of Antonio's full maturity. The work on which the artist's fame rests is *The Deluge*, executed about 1615–16 in the frieze of one of the rooms in the Quirinal Palace and then duplicated in a painting in the Louvre. The fresco displays an elegance reminiscent of certain compositions by Agostino, but it goes beyond it in neoclassical anticipations.

OTHER WORKS. *The Lord and Saints* (Rome, S. Sebastiano). – *Madonna and Child with St. Francis* and *The Annunciation* (Naples, Capodimonte, attrib. Cavalli). – *Madonna and Child with St. Francis*

(Rome, Mus. Cap., attrib. Salerno). – *Jupiter and Juno* (Rome, Gall. Borghese, attrib. Salerno). – *Burial of Christ* (Rome, Gall. Borghese, attrib. Longhi; assigned by Mahon to Sisto Badalocchio). – *Coronation of St. Cecilia* (Montpellier, Mus. Fabre, attrib. formerly, now rejected, by Longhi; reattrib. Salerno).

Maurizio CALVESI

THE CARRACCIS IN THE ARTISTIC MILIEU OF THE SEICENTO. The Carraccis exercised an enormous influence upon art and the literature of art. At first a recognition of the naturalistic element in their work caused them to be grouped with Caravaggio (q.v.) in an antimanneristic reaction. This view, however, was soon superseded by another which was later to become traditional: the superiority of the Carraccis in idealizing nature through a systematic program of eclecticism. As early as 1602, the writer Lucio Faberio, in his oration on the occasion of Agostino's death, praised the Carraccis for their ability to amalgamate the best qualities of the great masters of the past — a eulogistic convention which became a critical cliché. Giulio Mancini, in about 1620, wrote that Annibale joined "the manner of Raphael with that of Lombardy"; and in the same period Monsignor Agucchi commended Annibale's late style, in which color and drawing were skillfully blended. Giuseppe Bellori expanded this concept, praising the Carraccis for their classical idealism uniting the study of nature, "idea," and the diverse qualities of the great masters of the Renaissance. Malvasia, notwithstanding his anticlassicism, strengthened the cliché by publishing a sonnet written by Agostino that constituted a declaration of eclecticism. Agostino's statement became the backbone of the critical tradition and prevented an unbiased examination of the art of the Carraccis: as long as eclecticism had a favorable connotation, they were praised; but when the term acquired negative implications — during the decline of classicistic theory and the rise of romantic esthetics — the Carraccis were condemned as critical and theoretical artists and therefore uncreative. It was not until Lanzi and the manuals of the first half of the 19th century that some objectivity was possible. A number of modern scholars, especially Friedländer, have emphasized the antimanneristic and naturalistic character of the Carraccis; others have doubted the authenticity of Agostino's famous theoretical sonnet; in various studies, Denis Mahon has disputed the traditional eclectic and classicistic interpretation. In addition, careful examination of the marginal notes in Vasari made by Agostino or Annibale reveals an instinctive preference for Venetian naturalistic color. It has also been demonstrated that the Academy "degli Incamminati" did not have the characteristics that later became typical of such institutions. And finally, just as Caravaggio's intellectual and cultivated approach is now better understood, so also is the pictorial and imaginative instinct of the Carraccis. Only Annibale and Agostino adhered to a precise classicistic discipline; Agostino, less gifted, was perhaps more susceptible to theory. Annibale, in contrast to the mannerists, realized that it was a question not of imitating the "manner" of the great masters or the results they achieved but rather of repeating their creative process — turning to nature and idealizing it. To seek the "idea" in art yielded a mode of painting invigorated by nature, yet historical and believable as well as decorative and elegant — a mode of painting that could express the classic or Renaissance ideals of beauty and decorum. We cannot, therefore, deny the impact of theory on the development of Annibale. In his view, theoretical and literary premises remain in the sphere of content — "ut pictura poesis" — and are allegorically expressed; thus they constitute the chief presupposition in Bellori's concept of a work of art. But it is precisely the contrast between Annibale's northern, naturalistic education and the new content which determines his evolution toward the late sculptural style that seems to be the negation of his early work. This development can be traced year by year, and its variety explains how contrasting personalities — from Brill and Elsheimer to Domenichino and Claude Lorrain — could be influenced by it. Annibale was master to such diverse artists as Poussin and Rubens (q.v.), and from his work two opposite trends developed — one toward classical idealism (Domeni-

chino, Reni, Albani, Poussin, Claude Lorrain), and another toward decorative eloquence (Lanfranco, Pietro da Cortona).

BIBLIOG. G. Mancini, Considerazioni sulla pittura, ed. A. Marucchi and L. Salerno, 2 vols., Rome, 1956–57; G. P. Bellori, Le vite de' pittori . . . , Rome, 1672; C. C. Malvasia, Felsina pittrice, Bologna, 1678; A. Foratti, I Carracci nella teoria e nella pratica, Città di Castello, 1913; H. Voss, Die Malerei des Barock in Rom, Berlin [1924]; C. L. Ragghianti, I Carracci e la critica d'arte nell'età barocca, Cr, XXXI, 1933, pp. 66, 74, 223, 233, 382, 394; R. Longhi, Momenti della pittura bolognese, L'Archiginnasio, XXX, 1935, p. 111 ff.; H. Bodmer, Ludovico Carracci, Burg, 1939; D. Mahon, Studies in Seicento Art and Theory, London, 1947; F. Arcangeli, Sugli inizi dei Carracci, Paragone, VII, 79, 1956, p. 17 ff.; G. C. Argan, I Carracci, Comunità, 1956; F. Bologna, Lo sposalizio di S. Caterina di Annibale Carracci, Paragone, VII, 83, 1956, p. 3 ff.; M. Calvesi, Note ai Carracci, Comm., 4, 1956, p. 263 ff.; M. Calvesi, Pinacoteca di Bologna . . . , stampe di Agostino Carracci, Bologna, 1956; Catalogo critico della mostra dei Carracci, Bologna, 1956 (with complete earlier bibliog.); G. Fiocco, Per Paolo Fiammingo, Arte Veneta, X, 1956, p. 187 ff.; J. Jaffé, Some Drawings by Annibale and by Agostino Carracci, Paragone, VII, 93, 1956, p. 12 ff.; C. L. Ragghianti, Una mostra della prosa nell'arte figurativa, Sele-arte, 26, 1956, p. 21 ff.; L. Salerno, L'opera di Antonio Carracci, BArte, XLI, 1956, p. 30 ff.; L. Dunand, Les estampes composant le lascivie du graveur Agostino Carracci, Lyons, 1957; W. Friedländer, Mannerism and Anti-mannerism in Italian Painting, New York, 1957; M. Gregori, Una segnalazione per Annibale Carracci, Paragone, VIII, 85, 1957, p. 48 ff.; R. Longhi, Annibale 1584?, Paragone, VIII, 89, 1957, p. 33 ff.; D. Mahon, Afterthoughts on the Carracci Exhibition, GBA, 49, 1957, pp. 193–207, 267–98.

Luigi SALERNO

Illustrations: PLS. 79–89.

**CARTHAGE.** See AFRICA, NORTH; PHOENICIAN-PUNIC ART.

**CARTOGRAPHY.** See COSMOLOGY AND CARTOGRAPHY.

**CARTOONS.** See COMIC ART AND CARICATURE; DRAWING.

**CASSATT,** MARY. American painter, pastelist, and print maker (b. Allegheny City, Pa., May, 1845; d. Paris, June, 1926). From 1861 to 1865 she studied at the Pennsylvania Academy of Fine Arts in Philadelphia, and in 1866 settled in France. Rarely returning home during her lifetime, she nevertheless thought of herself as an American (Sweet), although according to some (Adhémar, 1949) she considered herself French because of her ancestry.

In 1872 Miss Cassatt studied with Raimondi in Parma, and in 1874 with the fashionable French painter Charles Chaplin. Her paintings appearing at the Paris Salons of those years inspired Degas to remark: "This is someone who feels as I do." In 1877 he asked her to join the impressionists. *The Cup of Tea* (New York, Met. Mus., 1879), her first work exhibited with them, reflects the taste of other women members of the group, such as Berthe Morisot. Mary's sister Lydia was the model for *The Cup of Tea*. The next year Lydia and their mother appear in a painting with the same title (Boston, Mus. of Fine Arts); the emphasis here is not on the depersonalized sitters but rather on the asymmetry and a boldly diagonal quality in the work. *Lady at the Tea Table* (a portrait of Mrs. Biddle; New York, Met. Mus., 1885), which Degas felt was "distinction itself," is characterized by a sedate horizontal movement. *The Bath* (Art Inst. of Chicago, 1892; I, PL. 110) is another oil, showing the influence of Japanese art, which she and Degas rediscovered in an 1890 exhibition. In 1893 Mrs. Potter Palmer commissioned *Modern Woman* for the Chicago exhibition of that year. Pastel was a congenial medium for Mary Cassatt's style: *In the Garden* (Baltimore Mus. of Art, 1893) captures the decorative and patterned quality she admired in Japanese and Persian art. "Mary Cassatt has charm," Gauguin remarked of her work, "but she also has force."

Although Degas praised her competence as a print maker, for some critics Mary Cassatt's prints are "poorly drawn, but have much charm" (Adhémar); for others they are "mature graphic works of first quality" (Breeskin). Colored prints influenced by the Japanese Utamaro and Toyokuni are much admired. In 1891 *The Fitting, Women Bathing,* and *The Letter*

showed simply delineated flat surfaces contrasted with audacious Oriental floral patterns; these prints no doubt influenced Matisse, whose work Miss Cassatt denigrated. Her colors in this medium are usually muted, and, as in her paintings, blacks are absent.

The theme which ran through most of Miss Cassatt's work was the *douceur de vivre*, which she rendered with detached gentleness. A friend of the impressionists and hostess to many distinguished people in her Château de Beaufresne at Mesnil-Théribus (near Beauvais), wealthy Mary Cassatt preferred portraying the people she knew — her friends, her family, and their children. She never sold her portraits. As a friend of the Havemeyers she helped form their collection. Mary Cassatt remained unmarried during her 81 years and was blind during the last decade of her life.

BIBLIOG. A. Segard, Mary Cassatt, un peintre des enfants et des mères, Paris, 1913; F. Watson, Mary Cassatt, New York, 1932; L. Venturi. Les archives de l'impressionisme, Paris, New York, 1939 (the artist's letters); A. D. Breeskin, The Graphic Work of Mary Cassatt, New York, 1948; J. Adhémar, Inventaire du fonds français, Paris, 1949. Catalogues of Cassatt Exhibitions: A. D. Breeskin, Baltimore Mus. of Art, 1941; A. D. Breeskin, Wildenstein Gall., New York, 1949; F. Sweet (Sargent, Whistler, and Cassatt), Art Inst. of Chicago, 1954; F. Sweet, Met. Mus., New York, 1954; F. Sweet, Centre Culturel Américain, Paris, 1959–60.

Norman SCHLENOFF

**CASTAGNO,** ANDREA DEL. See ANDREA DEL CASTAGNO.

**CATACOMBS.** The beginnings of Christian art are documented primarily in the subterranean cemeteries, commonly known as "catacombs," which lie outside Rome and other ancient cities. A knowledge of these monumental complexes has therefore a special value for the student of both the official (see ROMAN IMPERIAL ART) and the popular trend (see ITALO-ROMAN FOLK ART) in the art, especially painting, of late imperial Rome. The study of the catacombs is also of particular importance for the light it sheds on contemporary or later manifestations of the new Christian content in the art of late antiquity (see LATE-ANTIQUE PERIOD) and of the early Middle Ages. The art of the catacombs can thus be considered as a legitimate chapter in the development of Western art and almost as an introduction to medieval art.

SUMMARY. General characteristics of the catacombs (col. 144): *Name, origins, development; The exploration of the Roman catacombs; Topography and structure.* Painting (col. 149): *Artistic problems. Iconography.* Architecture, sculpture, and minor arts (col. 154); List of the catacombs (col. 157): *Orthodox Christian catacombs of Rome and its environs; Catacombs in other parts of Italy; Principal catacombs outside Italy; Heretical catacombs; Syncretistic catacombs; Jewish catacombs.*

GENERAL CHARACTERISTICS OF THE CATACOMBS. *Name, origins, development.* The name "catacomb" appears in the 9th century and derives from the Greek κατὰ κύμβας ("by the hollows"), a term that refers to the site of the sepulchers in the declivity along that part of the Via Appia extending from the 2d to the 3d milestone outside Rome, where the Church of S. Sebastiano now stands — and where also the Basilica Apostolorum, referred to as "in catacumbas," formerly stood. The name soon came to include all those burial sites which in ancient times were known as κοιμετήρια, that is, places of rest (from κοιμέω, "I sleep"). In the earliest days the Christians had their burial places in pagan necropolises, as can be seen from the tombs of SS. Peter and Paul; but very soon, even as early as the 2d century, they had their own burial grounds, both because from the very beginning they adopted the practice of inhumation rather than cremation, which the pagans practiced, and because some pagan cemeteries were sacred to pagan divinities.

In accordance with the general practice throughout the ancient world — in Rome sanctified by law — the Christian cemeteries were outside the pomerium (the free space within and without the city walls protected from building by decree,

in the interests of defense) and almost always beside the consular roads, within a radius of 3 miles from the walls. Those which were more distant belonged to the pagi, that is, to the outlying rural districts.

Contrary to popular belief, the catacombs were never a place of refuge during the persecutions, and their origin was not in sand quarries (arenariae) dug by the pagans. They were exclusively burial places and as such enjoyed the protection of Roman law. Furthermore, although subterranean cemeteries were very extensive in Rome, they were not limited to that city. In fact, there are many in other regions of Italy and elsewhere, as far afield as Malta and North Africa. Moreover, we know that the custom of excavating tombs in the subsoil was not a Christian invention, not even in the strictly limited sense of catacombs, since there has been found at Anzio a pagan cemetery made up of several galleries into whose walls loculi, or graves, have been dug, one above the other (L. Morpurgo, *RendPontAcc*, XXII, 1946–47, pp. 155–66).

It is not entirely improbable that even in the late 1st century some Roman nobles and wealthy Christians, among them the Flavii and the Acilii, had placed their burial grounds at the disposal of the faithful. Thus, with the protection of Roman property and funerary laws, the Christians were able quite early to have burial grounds virtually for their exclusive use (F. De Visscher, *Analecta Bollandiana*, LXIX, 1951, pp. 39–54). In the 2d century others of the faithful, for example Praetextatus, must have opened their lots to their fellow Christians, and, in the 3d century, Maximus, Thraso, Basilla, Pontianus, etc., whose names have remained to indicate the cemeteries which were originally their property. We know that St. Agnes was buried on the Via Nomentana "in agello suo," and of St. Eugenia we learn that she was buried on the Via Latina "in praedio suo"; that is, both were buried "in their own ground." At the same time, however, we note in the Christian community the establishment of a cemeterial property strictly its own: we are thus informed that Church property had been substituted for private property. A passage in the *Philosophumena* (XI, 12) informs us that Pope Zephyrinus (ca. 199–ca. 217) placed in charge of the cemetery on the Via Appia the deacon Callixtus, whose name, in fact, became attached to this cemetery. From the testimony of the *Philosophumena* it is clear that this necropolis was the first to be administered in the name of the Church, under the direct auspices of the bishop of Rome, and for this reason was known simply as "the cemetery." Here Callixtus designated the site for papal interment, and here, indeed, many 3d-century popes were buried. During the course of the 3d century the Church gained strength and converts, so that the various communities came to need additional cemeteries; these sites the Church itself probably acquired. It is perhaps for this reason that cemeteries appeared which — probably because they were no longer private property — were not designated by the name of an owner but by a topographical term such as "in catacumbas," "ad septem palumbas'" ("by the seven doves"), "ad duas lauros" ("by the two laurels"), etc. This new institution must have been established about 260, after Gallienus revoked Valerian's edict of persecution and, as Eusebius tells us (*Historia ecclesiastica*, VII, 13), restored to the bishops (ἐπίσκοποι) the places dedicated to religious worship and the "so-called cemeteries" (καλούμενα κοιμητήρια).

But other communities as well, the Jewish, for example, and several syncretistic sects, buried their dead in catacombs, either because this type of cemetery was traditional, as with the first, or because it was borrowed from the Christians, as with the second.

*The exploration of the Roman catacombs.* After Pope Damasus, in the 4th century, had revived the veneration of the early martyrs, the Christians sought out their graves and relics in the various cemeteries. The remains of these martyrs were for the most part transferred to the urban churches during the 8th and 9th centuries. The catacombs were abandoned; during the Middle Ages even the approaches to them were lost sight of, except for those cemeteries which extended under the principal extramural basilicas. Not until the 15th century

were occasional devoted searchers able to enter some of the cemeteries. But the real spur to a revival of interest in the catacombs was the chance discovery on May 31, 1578, on the Via Salaria Nuova, of the Catacomb of the Jordani, which was at the time erroneously thought to be the Catacomb of Priscilla. After this fortuitous find, Antonio Bosio undertook, in 1593, a systematic search for ancient subterranean Roman cemeteries. He found about thirty. Toward the middle of the 19th century, Father Marchi, a Jesuit, brought the study of the catacombs to a new peak. But it was G. B. De Rossi who really systematized, under rigorously scientific controls, the search and exploration of the ancient catacombs. He divined that the discovery of the crypts which had contained the graves of the martyrs was of vital importance and would facilitate the retracing of the history of cemeterial topography. He did find them, and it was thus that almost every subterranean cemetery regained its true name and its true boundaries and many false names were corrected.

*Topography and structure.* There is a strict relationship between the geological structure of the subsoil and the way in which the ancient cemeteries were excavated. The great variety in the structure and hardness of the various strata must be considered the principal reason why the fossores, or gravediggers, did not always align the galleries perfectly [G. De Angelis d'Ossat, *B. dell'Ufficio Geologico d'Italia*, LXX, no. 3, 1945–46 (1947), pp. 1–33, pl. 1]. As to the degree of cohesion, the rock strata can be divided into the following categories: cohesive, semicohesive, and noncohesive. The noncohesive volcanic rock (pozzuolana) lent itself poorly to excavation because of its tendency to cave in. The only cemeteries cut in this type of rock are that of Pontianus near the Via Portuense and the one known as "ad duas lauros" on the Via Labicana, and these were possible only because the rock hardened immediately upon being dug, a very unusual occurrence. The cohesive tufa, on the other hand, was not much exploited because, although structurally absolutely stable, its hardness made it difficult to work. An exceptional example of its use is the Catacomb of St. Valentine on the Via Flaminia. Only the semicohesive tufa, the *tufa granolare*, gave good results. This stratum of terreous rock, widely dispersed beneath the surface humus of the Campagna, was honeycombed with subterranean cemeteries. It was both easy to work and resistant enough to ensure durability. Most important, it permitted the excavation of lofty galleries.

The complex development of the Roman cemeterial networks, according to recent calculations (Kirschbaum, 1949, p. 27), would appear to have a range of 60 to 90 miles, with the number of tombs, excavated in the course of two and a half centuries (ca. 150–400), somewhere between a half and three-quarters of a million. In many cemeteries the galleries are developed in several tiers (*catabatica*). The Catacomb of Thraso has five such tiers.

If the ground was level at the entrance, access to the subterranean cemetery was achieved by hollowing out a stairway which descended to a mean depth of 23–26 ft. from the ground level. A gallery proceeded horizontally from the stairs, sometimes for more than 650 ft., while several other galleries opened laterally from this one and ran parallel to it. If, on the other hand, the ground had a steep enough inclination, the first gallery, either level or inclined, was cut directly into the side of the hill.

The galleries (PL. 90), usually 30–35 in. wide and about 8 ft. high, are today designated as *ambulacra*, or "ambulatories," although they had previously been termed *cryptae* by the gravediggers, as can be seen in an inscription scratched on the tomb of one Gregory on the second level of the Catacomb of Priscilla: "undecima cripta, secunda pila, [locus] Glegori" [*sic*] ("11th crypt, 2d *pila*, loculus of Gregory"). It is thought from this epigraph that the word *pila* was meant to designate the vertical section of wall containing a series of superimposed graves — the loci, or, in today's language, loculi (PL. 90). These consisted of rectangular cavities, an average of 5 3/4 ft. long, 12 in. high, and 18 in. deep, or much

deeper, depending on whether they housed one or more bodies, on whether they were *monosomi, bisomi, trisomi,* or *quadrisomi.* When a tomb contained a larger number it was designated by the Greek word *polyandrion.*

All four edges of the opening of the loculus were recessed, to facilitate the insertion of marble slabs or tegulae (flat tiles), which were then cemented in the aperture. Sometimes there was a layer of mortar (this varied in thickness) over the slab,

glasses, small bronzes and ivories, statuettes, tiny balls, little dolls, etc. (PL. 104).

Opening off the sides of the galleries (PL. 91) at intervals were cubicula, or sepulchral chambers, generally square or rectangular in plan; the occasional round or octagonal ones indicate derivation from the mausoleums *sub divo* (under the open sky). Each of these crypts, housing several graves, formed the private tomb of some wealthy family or of members

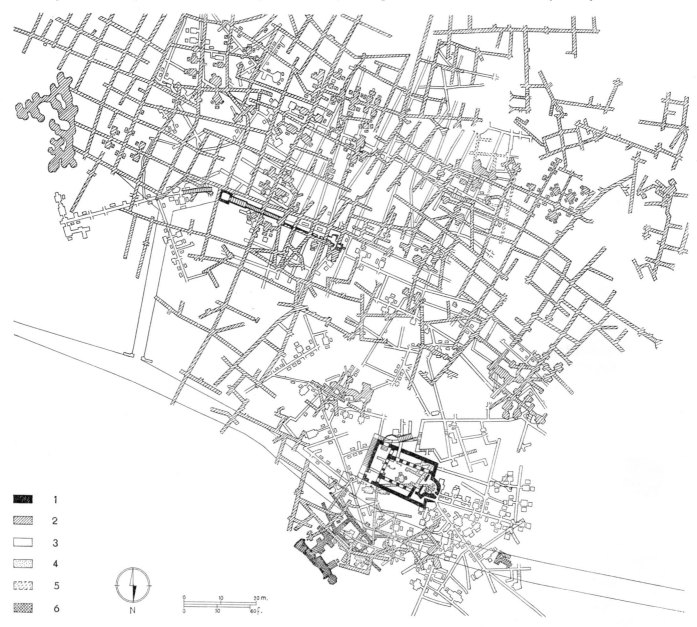

Rome, Catacomb of Domitilla or of SS. Nereus and Achilleus on the Via Ardeatina: general ground plan including the basilica erected over the tomb of the martyrs at the end of the 4th cent. *Key*: (1) Construction in masonry; (2) first or uppermost level; (3) second level; (4) third level; (5) fourth level; (6) pagan hypogeum and Hypogeum of the Flavii (*from Commissione di Archeologia Sacra, Pianta del cimitero di Domitilla, Rome, 1914*).

with a brief inscription incised or painted, in red or black. More rarely, a mosaic might be applied, or perhaps a layer of stucco worked to look like the front of a sarcophagus, as in the loculus cut into one of the lateral chambers opening on the gallery that leads into the Hypogeum of the Flavii in the Catacomb of Domitilla. Frequently the slabs and the tegulae were not entirely coated with mortar; instead it was applied only to the edges to ensure a hermetic seal. Often, on these narrow borders of mortar, brief inscriptions (graffiti) were incised or modest mnemonic symbols were inserted in order to make identification of the grave possible. Among the objects used were coins, paste gems, phials for perfume, lamps, gold

of some organization, as inscriptions indicate. At the center of the apse in some of the crypts in the cemeteries in Malta, funerary triclinia (couches) have been found, cut into the rock in the form of a sigma; these served for the fraternal agape, or mystical love feast (C. Zammit, *RACr*, XVII, 1940, pp. 293–97).

Fairly common in these cubicula, as well as along the walls of some of the ambulatories, are the arcosolia. Since these are tombs of major distinction, they consist of a *solium* (a sarcophagus sealed with marble or brick slabs), over which an arch is cut into the rock or constructed of masonry. Their form derives from that of several ancient pagan mausoleums,

in which the sarcophagi were placed below large niches or alcoves. The lunette (*parieticulum*), the vault, and in some cases even the extrados of the arch were decorated with frescoes or mosaics, as can be seen in the Roman catacombs of St. Hermes and St. Hippolytus and, more frequently, in the catacombs in Naples. An occasional grave, called a *forma*, was even cut into the floor of the galleries or the cubicula, primarily to satisfy the desire of those faithful who wished to be buried near the venerated remains of a martyr ("ad sanctos").

An unusual kind of grave of the so-called "baldachin" type consists of one or more *formae*, raised a little above the level of the floor. Four colonnettes are cut into the tufa at the corners, reaching the ceiling in such a way that the tombs are arched over; the effect is of a canopied shrine. *Puticoli*, or graves dug in a kind of well, are rare. Sometimes urns for bones, true ossuaries, were used.

A more clearly defined architectural form in frequent use was the *basilicula*, or miniature basilica, in which the relics of martyrs were often placed.

The hexagonal chamber on the axis of the second-level gallery of the catacomb discovered in 1955 on the Via Latina (FIG. 151) has a purely architectural function as a focal point of traffic: here the architecture is admirably related to the decoration, as the six painted segments of the semicircular vault supported by six corner columns are joined above by a circular panel which also serves as the vault key (cf. A. Ferrua, *Civiltà Cattolica*, Q. 2540, 1956, p. 124).

For the location of catacombs see map (FIG. 159); for a typical plan, FIG. 147; and for characteristic forms, FIG. 153.

PAINTING. *Artistic problems*. The catacombs of Rome, Naples, and Syracuse are particularly rich in frescoes, especially in comparison with those elsewhere. The frescoes date from the 1st century of the Christian era until about the 10th century. This dating includes those in the subterranean cemeteries of Naples; although these were reused during the late Middle Ages for victims of the plague, they belong largely to the same period.

The Christian artists of the catacombs naturally borrowed the contemporary stylistic idiom. In the earliest time they worked predominantly in two distinct styles, one linear, the other, often called *compendiario*, rapid and sketchy in the illusionistic manner. In several cases, an approach employing elements characteristic of both styles was developed. A clearly naturalistic tendency is basic to the linear style. All the elements are compositionally balanced and stand in proper spatial relation to one another. Frescoes done in the sketchy manner, on the other hand, are executed in rapid and summary strokes without rigid organic forms, so that the pictorial vision is realized through a shifting play of light and shade produced by patches of color.

The chronology of cemeterial frescoes is still a matter of controversy, especially in regard to the earliest examples. While some scholars feel that the frescoes go back as early as the 1st century, others maintain only that they definitely antedate the beginning of the 3d century. Of course the dating of the frescoes hinges on the dating of the regions of the cemeteries in which they are found. Some of these regions are datable, if not with absolute certainty, at least very closely.

Perhaps the most ancient paintings in Rome's subterranean cemeteries are those which adorn the Cubiculum of Ampliatus in the Catacomb of Domitilla (Wilpert, 1903, pls. 30–31). The walls, above a dado of marbleized plaster, are divided by slender columns whose fragility does not preclude a sense of architectural function. This decorative system, unique in the catacombs, reproduces the décor of a house, and recalls the so-called "Style IV" of Pompeii, which continued in use even into the 2d century, as is shown by certain frescoes in a villa under S. Sebastiano on the Via Appia (Wirth, 1934, pl. 19) and others in a house in Ostia on the Via delle Corporazioni (Wirth, 1934, p. 104, fig. 47), which Wirth has assigned respectively to A.D. 140–60 and 160–70. It is on the basis of this comparison that the paintings in the Cubiculum of Ampliatus, previously attributed by De Rossi to the 1st century and by Styger to the 3d, can be placed a little later

than A.D. 150. The frescoes on the vault of the gallery of the Hypogeum of the Flavii, also in the Catacomb of Domitilla, can be assigned to a period about a decade later, as can those on the vaults of some large niches lateral to them. Here, delicate geometric dividers are drawn on a clear ground. Set into them are flowers, birds, or small winged genii realized with great swiftness of touch (Wilpert, 1903, pls. 2–7). On a section of the wide ambulatory that opens into the hypogeum is painted a kind of wide bower intertwined with vines (Wilpert, 1903, pl. 1), which recalls a similar motif in a stucco relief on a tomb found under the Basilica of S. Sebastiano (Wirth, 1934, pl. 286) assigned by Wirth to about 200.

In none of these frescoes do we meet specifically Christian motifs. Such are to be found in the cubiculum known as Urania's and as the "Cubiculum of the Passion," in the Catacomb of Praetextatus. There the symbolic image of the Good Shepherd appears on the ceiling, framed by the slender geometric dividers which in later works were to become much thicker (P. Markthaler, *RQ*, XXXV, 1927, pp. 53–111). The walls are also decorated with scenes taken from the New Testament (Wilpert, 1903, pls. 7–20). The figures appearing there, especially that in the so-called "Crowning with Thorns," are rendered in graduated tones, over which are laid rapid touches of whites and yellows. With these paintings we are perhaps at the beginning of the 3d century, when the decoration of Lucina's Crypt in the Catacomb of Callixtus was completed (Wilpert, 1903, pls. 24; 25; 26, no. 1; 27, no. 1; 28; 29, no. 1), as well as the paintings in the so-called "Cubicula of the Sacraments" (Wilpert, 1903, pls. 38, 39, 41), in the same catacomb. All the ceilings of these rooms are provided with linear dividers in geometric designs, but the Christian iconographic elements are more developed. Besides the image of the Good Shepherd, there are orants, representations of Daniel in the lions' den, and, along the walls, scenes from the story of Jonah and others alluding to baptism and the Eucharist (Wirth, 1934, pls. 45, 41b). On the ceiling of Lucina's Crypt there appear also a few heads of women, symbolic of the seasons, which, as Calza has observed (*La necropoli del porto di Roma nell'Isola Sacra*, Rome, 1940, p. 141, fig. 67), recall stylistically those on a tomb in the Isola Sacra assigned to the early 3d century. Heads of putti emerging from clusters of leaves, painted in this same technique, adorn the so-called "Greek Chapel" (Wilpert, 1903, pl. 13; De Wit, 1938, pl. 8, no. 1) in the Catacomb of Priscilla. Here appear also — on a reddish background — scenes of Noah in the ark, of Daniel in the lions' den, and the famous *Fractio panis* ("Breaking of Bread"; Wilpert, 1903, pls. 15, no. 1; 16; PL. 93). Other subjects, for example the episodes from the Susanna story by another hand (Wilpert, 1903, pl. 14), are set off against a light yellowish background. Scholars are not in agreement as to the date of these pictures: Byvanck thinks about 140, De Wit 220 and a little later, while Wirth puts them at 320–30; most likely they are from the end of the 2d or the beginning of the 3d century.

To the first decades of the 3d century most probably can also be attributed the almost completely ruined fresco of the Virgin and Child on the vault of a gallery in the region in the Catacomb of Priscilla known as the "arenaria" (Wilpert, 1903, pl. 22). This is the oldest image of the Virgin as yet discovered. The paintings that adorn the Hypogeum of the Aurelii, near the Viale Manzoni, are of fairly high quality. They are in the linear style, which is manifest chiefly in the soft modeling of the austere figures of the apostles (Wirth, 1934, pl. 47), rather than in the more narrative scenes of other sections in this hypogeum (Wirth, 1934, pls. 48, 50). These paintings are almost universally ascribed to the period 220–40. To the same period belong the fresco of the healing of the woman with the issue of blood on the lunette of an arcosolium in the Catacomb of SS. Peter and Marcellinus (De Wit, 1938, pl. 10), and, perhaps, the frescoes of the so-called "Cubiculum of the Veiled One" in the Catacomb of Priscilla (Wilpert, 1903, pls. 79–81; PL. 94). It must be noted, however, that although in this last-named fresco the beautiful veiled figure of the orant has been expressed with a sense of chiaroscuro — so that the colors are extraordinarily fused and mellow — the other groups display touches

in the sketchier manner. This style becomes much more frequent toward the middle of the 3d century, as in some of the paintings in the Catacomb of SS. Peter and Marcellinus; for example, in the heads of the personified seasons or in that of Moses (De Wit, 1938, pls. 11–12, 18; PL. 96). Here details of feature and form are resolved in patches of light and shade rather than in clearly defined outlines.

Countering this dissolution of organic form, in the age of Gallienus (260–68) a trend toward a more "classical" vein developed. This brought with it a note of idealism, as in the luminously transparent fresco of the orant in the Catacomb of Callixtus (Wilpert, 1903, pl. 88). The figure here wears the helmetlike hairdress affected by Salonina, wife of Gallienus.

given such explicit characterization as to evoke the term "expressionistic" (PL. 97).

Toward the mid-4th century, such striking effects were no longer in vogue, and painters turned to a more naturalistic vision; we are in the period which, precisely because of this "classicistic" direction, has been called that of the *stilo bello*, or grand style. Its finest expression is in the frescoes of the catacomb on the Via Latina discovered in 1955; for example, the fresco showing the crossing of the Red Sea and one probably representing a lesson in anatomy (A. Ferrua, *Civiltà Cattolica*, Q. 2540, 1956). In this same artistic current is the painting in the arcosolium of Veneranda (Wilpert, 1903, pl. 213) in the Catacomb of Domitilla (PL. 98), assignable to the time of Pope

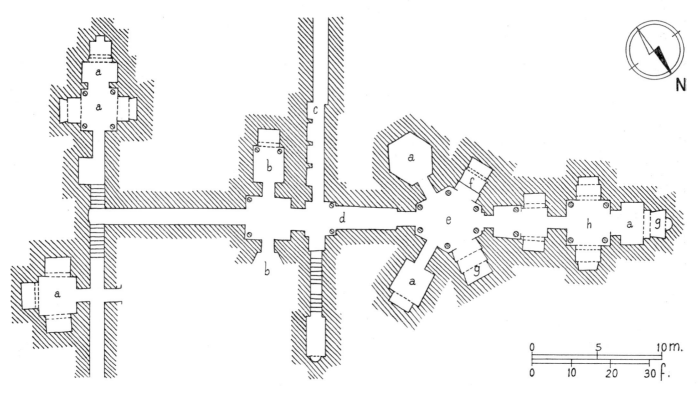

Rome, hypogeum on the Via Latina discovered in 1955: ground plan. Typical architectural forms: (*a*) cubicula; (*b*) crypts; (*c*) gallery with loculi; (*d*) cryptoporticus; (*e*) hexagonal chamber; (*f*) niches; (*g*) arcosolia; (*h*) chamber with arcosolia (*from A. Ferrua, Civiltà Cattolica, 1956*).

Late-3d-century funerary frescoes show an effort to consolidate further the organic structure of the figure, largely by means of drawing lines to define the color masses and to give more coherence to the forms. Thus there originated a new type of painting which might best be termed "plastic-constructive"; examples are the figures of Dionysia, Nemesian, Procopius, Heliodorus, and Zoë in the so-called "Cubiculum of the Five Saints" in the Catacomb of Callixtus (Wilpert, 1903, pls. 110–11). Incidentally, this period (after the division of the empire by Diocletian in 286) gave rise also to the type of painting known, because of its fresh and lively narrative style and subject matter, as "popularizing"; the type is exemplified by the frescoes of the so-called "Cubiculum of the Coopers" in the Catacomb of Priscilla (Wilpert, 1903, pl. 202; PL. 97) and those in the Hypogeum of Trebius Justus; the latter include scenes of gardening and of the building of a country house (O. Marucchi, *NBACr*, XVII, 1911, pls. 10–15). Solid composition also characterizes the fresco of Christ among the apostles in the Catacomb of the Jordani. In this fresco, the faces of the apostles are illuminated by a fixed and penetrating look (De Wit, 1938, pl. 34). This style, with its synthetic linear values and firmness of composition, continued until about 340; it found its most characteristic expression in the fine, richly dressed figures of orants in the Catacomb of Thraso (Wilpert, 1903, pls. 174–76) and in the Coemeterium Majus (Wilpert, 1903, pls. 207–08). The faces of these figures are

Damasus (366–84). Great structural solidity is here achieved by means of clearly delineated contours. Even in the Theodosian era (379–95), these same "classicizing" touches appear, albeit in company with a few rapid brush strokes and patches of color, especially in the figures of Moses unlacing his sandals and Moses striking the rock in the so-called "Crypt of the Little Sinners" in the Catacomb of Callixtus (Wilpert, 1903, pls. 237–38).

Several examples of catacomb painting from this era reflect the decorative idiom of the cult buildings; this is clear in the figure of Christ at the center of the college of the apostles in one of the semicircular niches in the crypt named for the *pistores*, or millers, in the Catacomb of Domitilla (Wilpert, 1903, pl. 193) and in the Crypt of the *Traditio legis* (Delivery of the New Law) in the catacomb "ad decimum," at the 10th milestone, on the Via Latina near Grottaferrata (J. Wilpert, *Die römischen Mosaiken und Malereien der kirchlichen Bauten vom IV. bis XIII. Jahrhundert*, Freiburg, 1916, pl. 132). To the late 4th or early 5th century belongs the somewhat disjointed fresco in the Catacomb of SS. Peter and Marcellinus which shows Christ enthroned between apostles and, above, the mystic Lamb among four of the martyrs venerated in the cemetery (Wilpert, 1903, pls. 252–54).

The development of funerary painting throughout the 5th century can be more easily traced in the frescoes of the Neapolitan catacombs (PLS. 99, 100). To the early 5th century can be attrib-

uted the fresco on the arcosolium of a high civil functionary in the Catacomb of St. Januarius (S. Gennaro dei Poveri) (Achelis, 1936, pl. 34). The deceased appears with SS. Peter and Paul and two other saints on a transparent bluish-green ground. Nearly contemporary is the painting in the Catacomb of St. Gaudiosus that represents, against an undefined background, the deceased Pascentius between SS. Peter and Paul (Achelis, 1936, pl. 39). In this fresco we note that plastic form has given way to a kind of academic calligraphy. In yet another fresco, in the tomb of Vitalia in the Catacomb of St. Januarius (Achelis, 1936, pl. 28), we find a strongly balanced composition. Here the deceased appears among the open books of the four Evangelists. A certain rigidity can be noted, more in the out-

complete figures or heads, amoretti, landscapes, vases, floral candlesticks, garlands, and scrolls (PL. 95). The last often contained an obvious symbolic reference to the words of Jesus: "I am the vine, ye are the branches." It was common practice to allude symbolically to Christ, to the faithful, to the soul of the deceased, to the hope for peace in the afterlife, etc. Symbols in most frequent use were the fish (the letters of the Greek word ΙΧΘΥΣ, "fish," form the acrostic, 'Ιησοῦς Χριστὸς Θεοῦ Υἱὸσ Σωτήρ, "Jesus Christ, Son of God, the Saviour"), the Lamb (Agnus Dei), the A and Ω ("I am Alpha and Omega, the beginning and the end"), the Good Shepherd ("I am the good shepherd"), the orant, the anchor, the palm, the peacock (PL. 92), the phoenix, etc. But soon there appeared also scenes

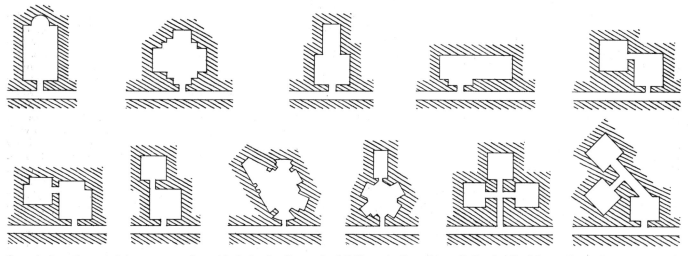

Ground plans of some of the more complex cubicula in the Catacomb of Callixtus in Rome (*from G. De Angelis d'Ossat, Catacombe romane, 1939*).

line of the hands than in the face. Vitalia's hairdress is strikingly like that of Maria, wife of Honorius (395–423), on the well-known cameo in the Rothschild Collection in Paris; thus the probability is great that this fresco is correctly assigned to the first quarter of the 5th century.

About a decade later is the fresco in another arcosolium in the same catacomb, which represents St. Januarius between two candelabra and the orant figures of Nicatiola and Cominia (Achelis, 1936, pl. 38). We can ascribe to mid-5th century the painting on the tomb of a certain Eleusinus, who is shown within the hollow of a shield at the center of radiating vine sprays with his face turned ecstatically heavenward (Achelis, 1936, pl. 26). His face recalls that of the consul Asturius (who was invested in 449) delineated on a panel of an ivory diptych now in the Landesmuseum in Darmstadt. A greater stiffness of feature is apparent in the bust of the young Proculus, which is roughly cut between two tall candelabra in the center of a lunette of yet another arcosolium, also in the Catacomb of St. Januarius (Achelis, 1936, pl. 27). The scarlet *lacerna*, or overcloak, in which he is clothed is furrowed by striated and angular folds. These, together with the impassive, yet penetrating, expression of his face, announce the formation of a new artistic temper.

*Iconography.* The most striking feature in the content of catacomb painting is the perfect harmony of the representations with the symbolic-eschatological concepts of the earliest Christians, as Kirsch has so well explained (*RACr*, IV, 1927, pp. 259–87) — in contradiction to the theory of Styger (*Die altchristliche Grabeskunst*, Munich, 1927, *passim*), who saw in the frescoed subjects only historical meanings, devoid of reference to or expression of Christian faith.

The earliest paintings in the catacombs were limited to ornamental and symbolic motifs, which though drawn from contemporary pagan art were nevertheless open to symbolic interpretation by the Christians: the story of Cupid and Psyche, Orpheus calming the wild beasts, the seasons personified in

from the Old and New Testaments. Favored were those which bore witness to the Messianic idea so closely allied to the hope for salvation (II, PL. 281): scenes of Noah in the ark, Daniel in the lions' den, the three Hebrew children in the fiery furnace, Susanna, Job, Jonah, David, etc., not to mention the raising of Lazarus and the healing of the paralytic, of the woman with the issue of blood, of the blind man, of the leper, etc. Nor were other narrative and historical subjects lacking — representations of the Fall (PL. 97), of Moses unlacing his sandals before the burning bush, of Jesus foretelling Peter's triple denial, etc., as well as representations referring to the advent of Christ on earth to redeem mankind and having eschatological import, such as the Virgin and the prophet Balaam (or Isaiah), the Annunciation, the birth of Jesus, the Adoration of the Magi (PL. 95), the baptism of Christ, the miracle of the transformation of water into wine at the marriage of Cana, the multiplication of the loaves and fishes, etc. (see also BIBLICAL SUBJECTS; CHRISTIANITY).

The scenes taken from real life have a unique character, as do those which reflect the painting in the basilicas, such as illustrations of the Traditio legis or the Traditio clavium (Delivery of the Keys) or Christ the Teacher (PL. 305) among the college of the apostles.

ARCHITECTURE, SCULPTURE, AND MINOR ARTS. The structural character of the catacombs is closely related to the method of excavation, which was almost always conducted with common ditch-digging techniques, according to the exigencies of the terrain. Nevertheless, occasional galleries or cubicula, as well as various crypts or miniature basilicas, display true architectural qualities (FIGS. 151, 153). Thus, for example, the high, ample, rather long gallery on the second level of the Catacomb of Priscilla — with other corridors leading from both its sides at right angles — cannot fail to impress the observer. A sense of grandeur is achieved by the long, flat surfaces, interrupted at fairly regular intervals by lateral ambulatories and by the continuous repetition of the horizontal lines of the several tiers of loculi.

The plan of the cubicula — which are for the most part of fairly small dimensions — is the same as is found in some of the interiors of secular buildings designed for the most varied uses: thus we find cubicula that are square, rectangular, round, pentagonal, hexagonal (PL. 91), and octagonal; cubicula with more or less distinct and individualized additions, whose format varies from the simple to the complex; cubicula that are doubled, and not infrequently those formed of three or four communicating enclosures. These have either flat ceilings or domical vaults, often with columns at the corners. The columns, like their capitals, may be cut out of the tufa or constructed of bricks. However, a sense of spatial vastness is rarely achieved, occurring in only a few of the largest rooms. We may cite St. Januarius' Crypt in the Catacomb of Praetextatus, where the ceiling is opened by a large skylight; also a few interiors of the previously mentioned catacomb on the Via Latina discovered in 1955.

A more defined architectural character is displayed by those crypts which, with the passage of time, were transformed into veritable little basilicas because they housed the bones of martyrs and became as a result centers for worship, to which the faithful flocked in numbers.

The enlarging of these primitive interiors brought with it the adoption of masonry structures not only along the walls but also on the vault. There thus evolved small basilicas (basilicula) which were either entirely subterranean — the "Greek Chapel" in the Catacomb of Priscilla, the Papal Crypt in the Catacomb of Callixtus (FIG. 153), the small basilica of St. Hermes in the cemetery of the same name, etc. — or semisubterranean, in that their surrounding walls jutted partly above ground. (Sometimes these walls were very extensive, as in the case of the Basilica of SS. Nereo e Achilleo on the Via Ardeatina.)

Various sculptures and objects with direct bearing on the history of Early Christian art have been found in the most widely scattered catacombs, especially in Rome. The sculptures are certainly the most important. As a rule they are affixed to the fronts and the ends of sarcophagi as well as to the funerary slabs covering the loculi. Frequently there are funerary steles in the cemeteries above ground.

Sarcophagi have been found in the cubicula and under the arcosolia within the ambulatories. They belong almost exclusively to the 3d and 4th centuries, and their style is, naturally, that of contemporary pagan sculpture.

The oldest sarcophagi are sculptured with scenes alluding to the spiritual life of the deceased or showing them in the garden of Paradise, in company with either the Good Shepherd or the symbolic Fisherman. There is an occasional episode from the Jonah cycle. A well-defined narrative sense is lacking in these early sarcophagi. The figures, emerging distinctly from their plain background, are without any close relation, but they are executed with just proportions and lively modeling.

Contemporaneously with this type of sarcophagus, however, was produced another, adopted from pagan usage — the columnar sarcophagus. In such sarcophagi the fronts are divided into three or, more frequently, five fields. The panels with figures usually occupy either the middle or the outer area — occasionally both. In the center panel an orant or the Good Shepherd often appears; at the sides, especially toward the middle of the 3d century, are either protomas or the complete figures of two lions, often devouring their prey. The outer ends of the front are often decorated with small pilasters, colonnettes, or small figures symbolizing death or dressed as philosophers. A medallion is rather frequently carved on the central section, sometimes in the form of a sea shell, with the bust or busts of the deceased, generally husband and wife (PL. 102). The presence of these images, especially when there is an attempt at portraiture, is of great value in establishing dates for the sarcophagi, as they are mostly devoid of consular inscriptions and therefore not epigraphically datable.

Sarcophagi whose fronts are carved with pastoral and rural scenes are characteristic of the second half of the 3d century. A new type of sarcophagus appeared late in the century, after Diocletian's division of the empire, namely the frieze sarcophagus, so termed because the whole space is filled with an uninterrupted series of scenes, taken generally from the Old or the New Testament. The figures are decidedly vertical and are crowded considerably in the effort to introduce as many Biblical scenes as possible (PL. 102). The use of this type of sarcophagus was very widespread during the age of Constantine; in the second quarter of the 4th century the front frequently assumed a new form with two registers, one above the other. By comparison with the earlier style, that of the late 3d century and the age of Constantine is less rounded and much less plastic. The forms are more square and rigid, and illusionism has given way to violent contrasts of light and shade. These contrasts are produced by long drilled grooves serving to indicate the folds of the garments. This "negative" manner of working the marble achieves effects that are no longer tactile; they are purely optical.

It should be noted that contemporaneously, albeit unobtrusively, another style developed, which tended to bring back the naturalistic vision, by means of a return to plasticity and to a modified pictorialism. Here the drill was not in use.

A reaction against the distortion of organic form is more evident in the sarcophagi of the mid-4th century, especially those with two registers, which, like the "Tomb of Lot" discovered in the Catacomb of St. Sebastian, date a little after 350 (PL. 102). The reconquest of volume is very apparent. The figures are again animated with a sober movement that endows them with a sense of grace. No longer crowded, they are knowingly dispersed so that there is a free circulation of space about them. Even the high polishing of the marble has been brought back.

To this same period belong the sarcophagi whose fronts are divided by columns so as to form niches. The rhythmic division into niches, usually numbering five or seven, slows the continuity of the narrative, so that the individual scenes — often referring to the Passion of Christ — tend to be completely isolated. Occasionally the rhythmic division is obtained by means of the trunks of trees, whose leaves form arches, rather than by means of columns. The central panel in these sarcophagi often represents the Anastasis (Resurrection), the Victoria Christi, or even the Maiestas Domini or the Traditio legis.

The sarcophagi that belong to the late 4th century frequently present the crossing of the Red Sea (also to be found in the preceding century) or the apostles in attitudes of deference (acclamante) or carrying crowns, often against a background of city walls.

Stucco decoration in the catacombs is infrequent, a fact due to the lack of durability of the material itself, made as it is of lime and marble powder (PL. 91). Among the ornamental motifs of greatest interest are those in the vault of a cubiculum in the Catacomb of Apronianus, which is divided into four trapezoidal sections whose upper edges form a central medallion in which is represented the Good Shepherd. At the corners of the four segments of the vault are amorini which support a spiraling vine, lush with bunches of grapes and foliage (cf. G. Bottari, Sculture e pitture sacre estratte dai cimiteri di Roma, 3 vols., Rome, 1737–54, pl. 93). A similar decoration is recorded by Bosio (1632, p. 488) in the Catacomb of Thraso. Very unusual is a kind of small aedicula of a sculptural character found in the Catacomb of Cyriaca on the Via Tiburtina and now in the Lateran Museum. It is an arch supported by two columns, with a medallion containing a cross centered below.

Among the objects found in the catacombs the most numerous are small terra-cotta funerary lamps (PL. 104) — those of bronze are rare — and gold glasses.

The earliest lamps are of a fairly fine clay, so that the sides are thin; hence they are light in weight. For the most part the form is round and the handle is a ring; the designs are rather elaborate. In a second type, dating chiefly from the 4th century and later, the clay is cruder and thicker, so that the lamps are somewhat heavy. The form is prevailingly oval; the handle is no longer a ring, but solid; the neck is more or less elongated and is devoid of ornament. These lamps, almost always found with blackened spouts, were used mainly for illumination; we cannot discount entirely, however, the possibility of their use as tokens of funerary piety. On the flat surface of the lamps

images often appear: the Good Shepherd is represented on the oldest examples, as are several surviving pagan divinities, which of course no longer had any idolatrous significance.

Symbolic animals are fairly common: fish, lambs, doves (sometimes with olive branch in bill or claws), stags, cocks, lions, leopards, horses, phoenixes. The palm tree often figures in the vegetation. Christian emblems recurring most frequently are the cross and various forms of the monogram of Christ. Biblical scenes are less common; fairly popular among them is the Three Hebrew children in the fiery furnace. Some of the lamps are entirely without ornamentation. In the Jewish catacombs are lamps with representations of the seven-branched candlestick.

Gold glasses are also very numerous (PL. 104). These can be considered as having originated in the catacombs. Usually small medallions but sometimes the bottoms of cups or plates, they are glass disks polished with emery, to which has been applied, with a very fine layer of resin, a thin gold leaf incised with the contours of figures. An important collection is in the Museo Sacro of the Vatican Library. The scenes which appear on these gold glasses refer to both the Old and the New Testament (Adam and Eve, the sacrifice of Abraham, Daniel in the lions' den, the Hebrew children in the fiery furnace, the Jonah cycle, Moses striking the rock, etc.; the miracle at Cana, the raising of Lazarus, the healing of the paralytic, the three Magi, etc.); other subjects are the Good Shepherd, the orant, SS. Peter and Paul, saints in attitudes of adoration, busts of various personages, the *dextrarum junctio* (marriage), etc. Often to be found is the exclamation "Pie zezes in deo" ("Drink and good luck to you").

Bone and ivory objects are rare in subterranean Christian cemeteries; many that are said to come from there are forgeries. Among the authentic objects in this category, the most unusual — indeed it is the only example — is a hexagonal medallion made of vitreous paste and layers of colored bone which was inserted into the left end of a slab for a loculus in the Catacomb of St. Agnes. It is inscribed with the name of a certain Ulpia Siricia. Within the hexagon is a square in which is drawn a bust of the deceased (M. Armellini, *Il cimitero di Sant'Agnese*, Rome, 1880, pl. 8).

Other small bone or ivory objects were inserted in the mortar right on the loculi or in their immediate vicinity, primarily to facilitate recognition of the tomb; these include small dolls, rings, tesserae, pins terminating in small busts, and lamins (thin plates of metal or ivory that served as charms; PL. 104).

Coins, medals, and bronzes have been found affixed, for this same purpose, to various loculi, especially in the catacombs of Praetextatus, Callixtus, and Domitilla. Boldetti asserts that the medallion with the busts of SS. Peter and Paul facing each other, now in the Museo Sacro in the Vatican Library, is from the Catacomb of Domitilla, but its authenticity is seriously questioned by Romagnoli, who is supported by Cesano.

Small glass phials have frequently been found near the loculi. Since a number of these showed reddish traces, it was believed in preceding centuries that they had contained the blood of martyrs; they were therefore held to be almost certain signs of martyrdom. This belief was shown to be completely without foundation by G. B. De Rossi, in a note ("Sulla questione del vaso di sangue") that remained unpublished until 1945, when it was issued in its entirety by A. Ferrua. De Rossi was of the opinion that these small phials held balsam or aromatic oils.

LIST OF THE CATACOMBS. *Orthodox Christian catacombs of Rome and its environs.* The following list takes into account the topographical arrangement followed by those guidebooks which (like the Salzburg one) enumerate the sanctuaries of the martyrs interred in the catacombs by proceeding clockwise from the Via Cornelia, where St. Peter rested, to include the areas bordering the great highways that radiated from Rome. On the Via Cornelia itself, however, there is no subterranean cemetery.

Via Flaminia. Catacomb of St. Valentine. It shows a notable regularity of excavation and is on three levels; the lowest, with an entrance in the slope of the hill, is the oldest. On this level the original crypt was excavated; on its walls were found traces of rather late paintings, which suggests that devotions here continued over a long period of time. Notable among the frescoes is a 7th-century image of Christ crucified. The upper levels are characterized by low, narrow galleries, reached by a stair. Toward the middle of the 4th century, Julius I constructed a basilica above this cemetery, which was restored in the 7th century by Popes Honorius and Theodore. The body of St. Valentine, who suffered martyrdom under Claudius Gothicus (268–70), reposed in the crypt beneath the church until the 16th century, when it was transferred to S. Prassede (O. Marucchi, *Il cimitero e la Basilica di San Valentino*, Rome, 1900, p. 140).

Via Salaria Vecchia. (1) Catacomb of Pamphilus. It has three levels. Again, the lowest is the oldest: it reaches the noteworthy depth of 62½ ft. Here are the graves of Pamphilus, Candidus, and Quirinus, "cum multis martyribus." An original crypt was found near the entrance stairway (G. P. Kirsch, *RQ*, XXXIV, 1926, pp. 1–12). The ambulatories of the lower level were filled with earth during an early period, so that they have been found completely intact (E. Josi, *NBACr*, XXVI, 1920, pp. 60–64; *RACr*, I, 1924, pp. 11–119, III, 1926, pp. 51–211). The deepest galleries go back to the 3d century. Here the loculi are sealed with tegulae smoothed over with mortar, on which were incised or painted epigraphs. Most of these were fairly simple, being limited to the name of the deceased. Often a symbol, such as an anchor, a fish, or an equilateral cross, was added. Loculi devoid of inscriptions are not rare; they usually have set into them instead some mnemonic sign: coins, glasses, or small objects of bone, ivory, or metal. One cubiculum has an arcosolium flanked by two cathedras cut into the tufa. (2) Catacomb of Basilla or of St. Hermes. This is best known for its underground masonry basilica (R. Krautheimer, *Corpus basilicarum Christianarum Romae*, Vatican City, 1937, pp. 195–208). Constructed in the 4th century for veneration of St. Hermes, to whom Pope Damasus (366–84) dedicated an epigraph, it was restored by Pope Adrian I (772–95). Another historic center in this hypogeum is the cubiculum of the brother saints, Protus and Hyacinth, who were martyred under Valerian (253–60). The tomb of Hyacinth was found still intact by G. Marchi, because the loculus enclosing the remains of this martyr — found carbonized among the remains of a garment of cloth interwoven with a few gold threads — had remained since antiquity under a pavement, the level of which was raised in later times (E. Josi, *RQ*, XXXII, 1924, pp. 10–32). The cemetery was partially excavated in 1894–95 (see G. B. De Rossi, *BACr*, 1894, pp. 14–31, 70–75; G. Bonavenia, *BACr*, 1896, pp. 99–114, 1898, pp. 73–93). In 1939 Carletti found in a niche, at a height of 44 ft. above the level of the basilica, a block altar and a fresco showing the bust of Christ between two angels. Below them is the Virgin with the Holy Child flanked by two archangels and SS. Hermes, John the Evangelist, and Benedict. Josi assigns this painting to the 8th century (*RACr*, XVII, 1940, pp. 195–208).

Via Salaria Nuova. (1) Catacomb of St. Felicitas or of Maximus. It takes one of its names from the celebrated St. Felicitas, who very probably was martyred in Rome under Marcus Aurelius (161–80), along with seven other martyrs whom legend has made her sons; she was buried there with the youngest, Sylvanus. It was also named after the owner of the ground, Maximus. The catacomb's two levels are cut into old, earthy (and therefore not very consistent) tufa, and it reaches a depth of 36 ft. The guidebooks indicate that St. Felicitas was buried "in ecclesia sursum," that is, in the small basilica above, which was excavated in the 4th century as an enlargement of the cubiculum that originally held the grave of the martyr, while Sylvanus was buried "sub terra deorsum," that is, in the catacomb itself. The relics of these two martyrs were transferred by Pope Leo III (795–816) to the Church of S. Susanna. The entrance to the cemetery was recognized by De Rossi (*BACr*, 1863, pp. 21, 41–46), who then explored the original crypt (*BACr*, 1884–85, pp. 149–81), which was found to contain a fresco of Christ bestowing the symbolic crown of martyrdom on St. Felicitas, while the seven sons, lined up on either side of her, show that they have already received theirs. It is thought that Boniface I (d. 422) is buried in the little subterranean basilica. (2) Catacomb of Thraso or of St. Saturninus. The dual name derives from the owner of the property in which this cemetery developed and from the most famous of the martyrs buried there, the Carthaginian St. Saturninus, who was condemned to work in the stone quarry for the construction of the Baths of Diocletian. The cemetery, which is about 49 ft. deep, spreads out on five levels, which do not adhere rigorously to the usual horizontality. A part of this hypogeum is also occupied by a fairly extensive arenaria (sand quarry) whose galleries are devoid of loculi; it is thought that here, during the persecution by Valerian (253–60), were buried SS. Chrysanthus and Daria (G. B. De Rossi, *BACr*, 1873, pp. 5–21, 43–76). There are various paintings preserved in the hypogeum: most important are those with two large portraits of women buried there, depicted as orants and dressed in richly ornamented garments

(Wilpert, 1903, pl. 163, 2). (3) Catacomb of the Jordani. This is a small cemetery, but it is rich in cubicula and arcosolia; its network of galleries (46 ft. deep) develops in a rather irregular fashion. It is known that three (Martialis, Vitalis, and Alexander) of the presumed seven children of St. Felicitas were buried here, but their graves have not yet been located. When the hypogeum came to light in 1578, it was thought to be the Catacomb of Priscilla. It was De Rossi (*BACr*, 1873, p. 12) who identified it as belonging to the Jordani, although he was unable to penetrate it, as all traces of it had been lost since its previous discovery. It fell to Josi to rediscover it in 1921 (*RACr*, V, 1928, pp. 167–227, VIII, 1931, pp. 183–284). (4) Catacomb of Priscilla. This is one of the most ancient and illustrious of the Roman catacombs. It takes its name from its founder, who belonged to the noble family of the Acilii Glabriones, whose Christian branch had a hypogeum there. In this large catacomb,

the apsidal basin showing the agape, or mystical banquet (J. Wilpert, *Fractio panis*, Freiburg, 1895, p. 140). A representation of a phoenix near the entrance is a later find. Various independent stairways communicated with the second level, among them one, discovered by Bonavenia (*NBACr*, IX, 1903, pp. 135–43), which led to the first as well. The second level has a very regular plan. Of interest here is a fairly long gallery, interrupted almost at its center by a large skylight. About twenty lateral galleries emerge at right angles from the main gallery. These were not yet fully explored by 1960. Because of its size and extent, this area is one of the most impressive in all of *Roma sotterranea*. Here, also, many of the loculi were sealed with tegulae on which the names of the deceased were painted in red. Several reservoirs of water have also been found in the Catacomb of Priscilla, which led Marucchi to surmise that the cemetery was the one called "ad nymphas," where, according to tradition,

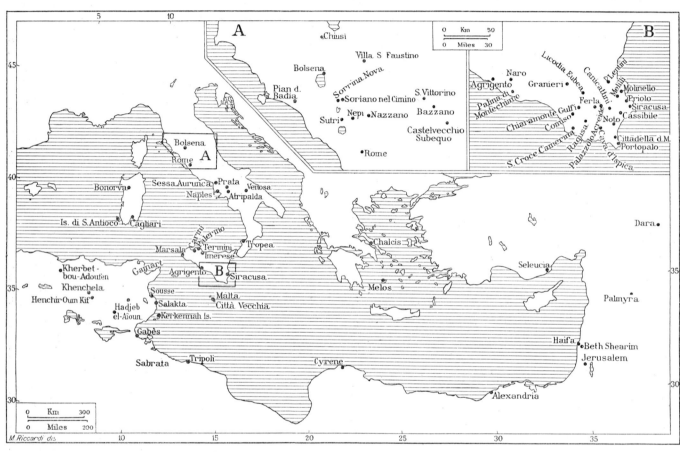

Distribution of catacombs along the central and eastern Mediterranean.

whose two levels reach the impressive depth of 75 ft., were buried the martyr Crescentius and Pope Marcellinus (296–304) as well as two of the presumed sons of St. Felicitas, Felix and Philippus, and other popes: Marcellus, Sylvester, Siricius, Celestine, and Vigilius; these last were buried beneath the floor of the basilica erected by Pope Sylvester (314–35) (O. Marucchi, *NBACr*, XIV, 1908, pp. 5–125). Originally the cemetery was made up of various distinct hypogeums, one of the oldest of which is that of the Acilii (G. B. De Rossi, *BACr*, 1888–89, pp. 15–66, 103–33). This is formed by a wide gallery in the shape of a gamma along whose walls were recessed niches and arcosolia. Not far away was discovered the cubiculum in which St. Crescentius was buried. A nearby stairway communicated with the Basilica of S. Silvestro above. Another section with a distinct character of its own is the arenaria, where the loculi were usually closed with tegulae. These often had seals on them, with the name of the deceased directly painted on in red. One of the galleries contains a fresco with the oldest known image of the Virgin and Child, next to a prophet who is thought now to be Balaam rather than Isaiah (E. Kirschbaum, *RQ*, XLIX, 1954, pp. 157–64). Next to this section is the so-called "cryptoporticus" which houses the "Greek Chapel," thus named by fossores and later even by scholars because on one of its walls were found two painted Greek inscriptions. The interior, divided in two by an arch and decorated with stuccoes and paintings, must have served as a gathering place for worship. Among the frescoes should be mentioned particularly the one above

St. Peter conferred baptism. Marucchi believed he had recognized a baptistery in one of these reservoirs (*NBACr*, VII, 1901, pp. 71–118).

Via Nomentana. (1) Catacomb of St. Nicomedes. According to De Rossi, this cemetery, which owes its name to a martyr who was executed under Domitian (81–96), is probably the one that Bosio had previously seen (*BACr*, 1864, p. 95). It has two levels of limited extent; in the first is a catacomb which, as it was dug in pozzuolana, or soft volcanic rock, required frequent fortification with masonry. In the second, which is 44 1/2 ft. deep, is a spacious gallery almost 164 ft. long that terminates in a water reservoir. It was perhaps the presence of this vein which prevented the further excavation of this large ambulatory. According to Josi and Marucchi, this would appear to be a hypogeum of uncertain denomination, perhaps having belonged to the gens Catia. They hold that the actual cemetery of St. Nicomedes was made up of about thirty galleries which were found during the excavation for the foundations of the Ministry of Communications (E. Josi, *NBACr*, XXVI, 1920, pp. 44–45). (2) Catacomb of St. Agnes. It extends partially under the Basilica of S. Agnese, which was erected over the tomb of the celebrated martyr by Constantina, the daughter of Constantine, and was reconstructed in the 7th century by Pope Honorius. Several sections of this cemetery are certainly of earlier date than the deposition of St. Agnes, who was buried "in praedio suo" or "in agello suo," that is, on her family's property (M. Armellini, *Il cimitero di Sant'Agnese*, Rome, 1880,

p. 424). This catacomb has no important paintings. It was apparently built on two levels; below are cavities which De Angelis d'Ossat thinks were probably hydraulic tunnels. (3) Coemeterium Majus or Catacomba Maggiore. The "Greater Cemetery" was probably so called because of the vast size of its network of ambulatories, but the name may also derive from comparison with the fairly small Catacomb of St. Agnes, which is contiguous to it. De Rossi thought he could identify this catacomb, called "St. Agnes" by the earliest explorers, with the Ostrianum Cemetery and with the site of the veneration of the *sedes Sancti Petri* ('chair of St. Peter'). But this hypothesis was vigorously opposed by Marucchi, who identified the Ostrianum Cemetery as that of Priscilla. Within are cathedras hewn out of the tufa, which G. Marchi thought to be seats intended for the confessional; De Rossi saw here a reproduction of the apostolic throne and therefore associated them with St. Peter. On the other hand, Josi (*RACr*, I, 1924, p. 104) thinks they were provided for comfort, while Cecchelli (*La Chiesa delle Catacombe*, Rome 1943, p. 66) sees them as a symbol of the heavenly throne prepared by the Saviour for the elect. Also characteristic of this cemetery, which has only two levels, are the occasional crypts decorated with architectural motifs; for example, cornices with small corbels cut directly from the tufa. One of these crypts has been recognized as that of St. Emerentiana (M. Armellini, *Scoperta della Cripta di Santa Emerenziana*, Rome, 1877, p. 118). The graves of the other martyrs in the cemetery, Victor, Felix, Papia, and Alexander, have not been located. The catacomb is rich in paintings, among which should be noted the head of an orant with her baby before her, flanked by two Constantinian monograms (the image probably represents the Virgin and Child). Another, a *prostratio* (E. Josi, *RACr*, X, 1933, pp. 11-12), is unique among funerary paintings: a man and a woman (perhaps a couple who were invoking the aid of St. Emerentiana) are kneeling on either side of an orant.

**Via Tiburtina.** (1) Catacomb of Cyriaca or of St. Lawrence. The galleries of this cemetery — which owes its fame to the fact that St. Lawrence was buried "in Cyriacae viduae praedio in agro Verano" ("on the estate of the widow Cyriaca in the Verano field") (P. Guidi, *RACr*, XXVI, 1950, pp. 147-80) — radiate to the southeast and northeast of the basilica (S. Lorenzo) erected by Constantine on the highly venerated tomb of the martyr. The hypogeum has four levels, of which only three are accessible by the many entrances. The oldest region is to the northeast of the church. Its galleries are narrow; they are devoid of cubicula and paintings, which are, in contrast, very numerous in the southeastern region. A painted cubiculum, on whose walls were various graffiti, was seen by Stevenson (*NBACr*, I, 1895, pp. 74-105) but was later destroyed. Some of the paintings show rare subjects, notably the one depicting the miracle of the manna and the one inspired by the Parable of the Wise Virgins. In this catacomb were the graves of the martyrs Justinus, Crescentius, Romanus, etc., which have, however, not been rediscovered. (2) Catacomb of St. Hippolytus. When Bosio visited this catacomb, he read an inscription that commemorated St. Hippolytus, but he held that this hypogeum was a part of that of Cyriaca. The explorations of Armellini and Marucchi led to the finding of a small 4th-century undergound basilica which enlarged the site of the tomb of the saint from whom the cemetery received its name (G. B. De Rossi, *BACr*, 1883, p. 60 ff.). Near the entrance was a graffito with the inscription: "Ippolite in mente [habeas] Pet[rum] [p]ec[cat]or[em]" ("Hippolytus, recall the sinner Peter"). In the *basilicula*, Pope Damasus (366-84) placed an inscription (G. B. De Rossi, *BACr*, 1881, pp. 26-55) which was certainly read by Prudentius (see *Peri stephanon*, XI). The original crypt, which was damaged during the Gothic invasion, was restored by "praesbiter Andreas" about 538, during the pontificate of Vigilius (538?-555). The Hippolytus interred in this cemetery was a celebrated 3d-century author, as is confirmed by the recovery of the statue, now in the Lateran Museum, which represents him seated *in cathedra*, on the sides of which is a list of his works (G. Bovini, *BCom*, LXVIII, 1940, pp. 109-28). Together with Hippolytus were buried SS. Tryphonia and Cyrilla and the martyr Genesius, but their tombs have not been rediscovered.

**Via Labicana.** (1) Catacomb of St. Castulus. This is a small hypogeum "juxta aquaeductum," that is, next to the Claudian aqueduct. Fabretti found there an epigraph concerning several persons buried on the second level on a stairway near the tomb of the martyr: "catabatico secundo ad martyrem domnum Castulum in scala" (G. B. De Rossi, *BACr*, 1865, pp. 9-10; A. Bartoli, *NBACr*, XIV, 1908, pp. 129-30; O. Jozzi, *Il cimitero di San Castulo*, Rome, 1904). (2) Catacomb "ad duas lauros" or of SS. Peter and Marcellinus. The two names of this cemetery derive respectively from its location ("by the two laurels"), near the Mausoleum of Helena — the area is also known as "in comitatu" — and from the two best-known martyrs of the persecution under Diocletian, who were buried there with SS. Tiburtius, Gorgonius, the four crowned martyrs, and many others. When the cemetery was rediscovered, it was explored by De Rossi (*BACr*, 1882, pp. 111-30) and later by Stevenson, who was able to bring to light the apsidal crypt, which, as can be seen from the presence of graffiti invoking SS. Peter and Marcellinus, actually contained the tomb of these two martyrs (O. Marucchi, *NBACr*, IV, 1898, pp. 137-93). This crypt was much restored by Popes Damasus and Vigilius. Later, Pope Adrian I (772-95) opened a stairway for the convenience of pilgrims. It is probable that St. Gregory was buried in the cubiculum whose vault is frescoed with images of Christ flanked by SS. Peter and Paul and of SS. Gregory, Peter, Marcellinus, and Tiburtius, who stand on either side of the Lamb of God. The crypt of St. Clement, who was one of the martyrs buried "in comitatu," that is, with many others, was identified by a graffito on one of the walls (O. Marucchi, *NBACr*, XXI, 1915, pp. 4-11). The catacomb is extraordinarily rich in cubicula and paintings (J. Wilpert, *Ein Cyclus christologischer Gemälde aus der Katakombe der hl. Petrus und Marcellinus*, Freiburg, 1891, p. 58). Represented are orants, fossores, and personages holding books. Various scenes must allude to the celestial banquet, as the servants are identified by the symbolic names of Irene (Peace) and Agape (Love). Somewhat rare subjects, Job on the dung heap (J. Wilpert, *NBACr*, IV, 1898, pp. 118-21) and the healing of the crippled woman (E. Josi, *NBACr*, XXVI, 1920, pp. 78-87), are encountered in a series of similar cubicula frescoed with Old and New Testament scenes (J. P. Kirsch, *RACr*, VII, 1930, pp. 31-46, 203-34, IX, 1932, pp. 17-36).

**Via Prenestina.** Anonymous catacomb, fairly small, near the Villa of the Gordiani (A. Ferrua, *BCom*, LXXV, 1953-55, pp. 167-71).

**Via Latina.** (1) Catacomb of SS. Gordianus and Epimachus. Josi (*RACr*, XVII, 1940, p. 31) thinks that to the cemetery of these two saints belong the galleries explored in 1933 at the level of the Vicolo dell'Acqua Mariana as well as those seen previously by Boldetti in the Vigna Moiraga and all the archaeological material found in the Vigna Aquari (E. Josi, *RACr*, XVI, 1939, pp. 197-240, XX, 1943, pp. 9-45). (2) Catacomb of St. Eugenia or of Apronianus. This cemetery, according to Josi (*RACr*, XVII, 1940, pp. 7-39), can probably be identified with the wide net of galleries stretching out on three levels which was explored in 1937-38 at the high point where the Via Latina crosses the Via Cesare Correnti. Of interest are two clay slabs found here together with numerous inscriptions. A layer of stucco was applied to the slabs (now in the Lateran Museum) which sealed a loculus. Mosaic tesserae depicting three scenes from the Jonah cycle were set into this. Josi is of the opinion that the Hypogeum of Trebius Justus can perhaps be assigned to this same area, as well as the galleries which were found in 1910 by Schneider-Graziosi on the Tinagli property on the Vicolo dello Scorpione.

**Via Appia Antica.** (1) Catacomb of Callixtus. This is one of the best-known cemeteries of subterranean Rome. Originally made up of various independent areas, it was already church property in the year 200. During the papacy of Zephyrinus (ca. 199-ca. 217) it was administered by the deacon Callixtus, who himself later became pope. The cemetery took its name from Callixtus, although he was not buried here. In identifying the cemetery, De Rossi made use of the Latin epitaph of Pope Cornelius, who was known to have been buried in the Catacomb of Callixtus. The region in which Pope Cornelius is buried, known as that of Lucina, is one of the oldest (P. Styger, *RendPontAcc*, III, 1924-25, pp. 269-87; G. Belvederi, *RACr*, XXI, 1944, pp. 121-64). The best known of the paintings which it contains are those of the baptism of Christ and of two fish, placed symmetrically and supporting on their backs a basket containing bread, with a small jug of wine behind — clearly Eucharistic symbols. Another fairly important area is that known as the "Region of the Popes and of St. Cecilia" (P. Styger, *Zeitschrift für katholische Theologie*, 1932, pp. 67-81). Here De Rossi found a crypt in which several 3d-century popes were buried and, nearby, another cubiculum whose frescoes show St. Cecilia as an orant (S. Scaglia, *NBACr*, XX, 1914, 2, pp. 23-27). In the Papal Crypt (J. Wilpert, *Die Papstgräber und die Cäciliengruft in der Katakombe des hl. Kallistus*, Freiburg, 1909, p. 109) were found the epitaphs of Popes Anterus, Pontianus, Fabian, and Lucius. Near these is the epitaph of Eutychianus. The tomb of Sixtus II, to whom Damasus dedicated an inscription, must have occupied the back wall. On either side of the entrance to the crypt, the walls were covered with graffiti, some of which invoke Sixtus and Pontianus. Fairly close to the Papal Crypt is a gallery (P. Styger, *Rend Pont Acc*, IV, 1925-26, pp. 91-153) which has six cubicula on one side, some of these quite early. They have been wrongly called "Cubicula of the Sacraments" because five of them contain paintings which can be interpreted as alluding to baptism and the Eucharist (J. Wilpert, *Die Malereien in den*

*Sakramentskapellen der Katakombe des hl. Callistus*, Freiburg, 1897). Not far off is what De Rossi called the "Region of Pope Miltiades" because he thought he recognized the site of that pope's grave in one of the cubicula opening into it; but there is no certain proof of this (G. Schneider-Graziosi, *NBACr*, XX, 1914, pp. 51–93). The martyrs Calocaerus and Parthenius were buried here in a single cubiculum, while Popes Gaius (283–96) and Eusebius (309 or 310) rest in two separate cubicula, one in front of the other, in an area where the deacon Severus obtained permission from Pope Marcellinus (296–304) to excavate a "cubiculum duplex cum arcosoliis et luminare" ("a double cubiculum with arcosolia and light shaft"). Opposite is the "Cubiculum of the Five Saints," so called because five orants, two men and three women, are pictured on the back wall in a garden symbolizing Paradise. Also part of the Catacomb of Callixtus is the area which extends a little to the north and which was designated as the "Liberian Region" by De Rossi because it was found to contain several graffiti from the time of Pope Liberius (352–66). The adjacent region, once said to belong to St. Soter — whose sanctuary has not yet been identified — is very characteristic, as it contains several round, domed crypts (E. Josi, *Il cimitero di Callisto*, Rome, 1933, p. 108). (2) Catacomb of Praetextatus. This large cemetery, on two levels only, must be considered one of the oldest in Rome. The name derives from that of the owner of the ground in which it was excavated. Perhaps its earliest nucleus was in the area found by De Rossi (*BACr*, 1872, pp. 63–80), in which one of the galleries was deepened to make room for the setting of new graves into the walls. Here is Urania's Cubiculum, known also as the "Cubiculum of the Passion" and as the "Cubiculum of the *Coronatio*" — after one of its paintings identified variously by scholars as the crowning with thorns and as the testimony of John the Baptist before the baptism of Christ (J. Wilpert, *RQ*, XII, 1908, pp. 165–72; O. Marucchi, *NBACr*, XIV, 1908, pp. 131–42, XV, 1909, pp. 157–85; A. De Waal, *RQ*, XXV, 1911, pp. 3–18; A. Baumstark, *RQ*, XXV, 1911, pp. 112–21). The region containing the large gallery known as the "Spelunca Magna" ("Great Cave") is also fairly early. Its walls contain recessed cubicula, of which the entrances are surmounted with brick pediments. In one of these cubicula, whose floor and walls have marble revetments, is a large skylight decorated with graceful allegorical scenes of the seasons. In this cemetery were buried St. Januarius (E. Josi, *RACr*, IV, 1927, pp. 218–55), the martyrs Urban, Tiburtius, Valerian, Maximus, and perhaps SS. Agapetus and Felicissimus (R. Kanzler, *NBACr*, I, 1895, pp. 172–80; M. Armellini, *Scoperta di un graffito storico nel Cimitero di Pretestato*, Rome, 1874). (3) Catacomb of St. Sebastian or Cemetery "ad catacumbas." The name of the locality near the Via Appia in which this cemetery extends — called, in fact, "ad catacumbas" because of the notable depressions characteristic of the terrain — was given to this small hypogeum as early as the 4th century and came several centuries later to be applied to any subterranean Christian cemetery. The great fame of this catacomb derives primarily from the fact that it extended near the devotional center created in the area in 258 when the remains of SS. Peter and Paul were temporarily transferred there. On this apostolic memorial, naturally an object of great veneration, as its graffiti testify (O. Marucchi, *NSc*, 1923, pp. 80–103), Constantine erected the basilica dedicated to the apostles, which after the 8th century was called S. Sebastiano. In the catacomb were laid St. Sebastian and, in one of the adjacent mausoleums, the bishop St. Quirinus of Siscia, whose remains were transferred in the 5th century from Pannonia. Among the paintings in this cemetery should be noted that of the manger, the only example of this scene among funerary paintings.

Via Ardeatina. Catacomb of Domitilla or of SS. Nereus and Achilleus (FIG. 147). Domitilla was the name of the wife of the consul Flavius Clemens, who was condemned to death by Domitian for "atheism" and "foreign" religious practices. In early sources this catacomb is also named after SS. Nereus and Achilleus because these soldier saints were buried there — as was St. Petronilla. The cemetery is one of the largest in Rome. Bosio began his famous excavations here; he was, however, under the misapprehension that this was the Catacomb of Callixtus. It was De Rossi who identified the catacomb as Domitilla's (*BACr*, 1865, pp. 17–24). Originally it was made up of several independent hypogeums; one of the oldest is named for the Flavii. Its entrance, faced with masonry, is cut into the side of the hill (G. B. De Rossi, *BACr*, 1865, pp. 33–46; A. M. Schneider, *RM*, XLIII, 1928, pp. 1–12) and leads to a vestibule with a bench around the sides. From a wide gallery descends, its vault decorated with a long vine and graceful cupids which are found also in the lateral galleries. The region named for Ampliatus is also very old. It has a regular stairway and decorative paintings (P. Testini, *RACr*, XXVIII, 1952, pp. 77–117). Between these two early nuclei there developed a large area which was once independent. The large basilica, complete with nave and side aisles, was erected

late in the 4th century over the tomb of the martyrs (G. B. De Rossi, *BACr*, 1874, pp. 5–34). Behind the apse is a cubiculum containing a fresco of St. Petronilla leading the deceased, Veneranda, to heaven (G. B. De Rossi, *BACr*, 1875, pp. 5–37). A section of the cemetery was probably reserved for employees of the annona (the imperial distribution of free grain), since in one crypt which is made up of two semicircular niches, various paintings depict the loading of grain. Above these are images of the Good Shepherd and Christ among the apostles; the composition of the latter is clearly derived from apsidal paintings in basilicas. This crypt is also known as that of the *pistores*, or millers. There is a painting on a partition between two loculi in a gallery not far from here showing the Adoration of the Magi — whose number, for symmetry, has here increased to four (O. Marucchi, *Monumenti del cimitero di Domitilla*, Rome, 1909–14, p. 259; P. Styger, *RendPontAcc*, V, 1926–27, pp. 89–147).

Via Ostiense. (1) Catacomb of Commodilla. In this cemetery were buried SS. Felix and Adauctus, martyred during the persecutions of Diocletian (303), and SS. Nemeseus and Emerita. The original crypt (G. Bonavenia, *NBACr*, XXVI, 1920, pp. 277–89; O. Marucchi, *NBACr*, X, 1904, pp. 11–160, XI, 1905, pp. 5–66) has an arcosolium at the far end and two lateral apses; furnished by Pope Damasus (366–84) with an inscription, it was restored soon after by Pope Siricius (384–98) (G. Bonavenia, *NBACr*, X, 1904, pp. 171–84). On one wall is a 6th-century fresco of the Virgin and Child enthroned between SS. Felix and Adauctus. The latter is presenting a woman by the name of Tortora, who is also buried there. Another painting, from the second half of the 7th century, depicts St. Luke as a doctor (J. Wilpert, *NBACr*, X, 1904, pp. 161–70; A. Muñoz, *L'Arte*, VIII, 1905, pp. 55–59). Near this sanctuary is a gallery which was sealed off in early times, after being filled with sepulchers, and was therefore discovered intact. For increased capacity, several unusual rather deep square pits were dug along the margins of some of the galleries in the central area. There are rows of loculi in all four sides of these pits (B. Bagatti, *Il cimitero di Commodilla*, Vatican City, 1936). (2) Catacomb of St. Thecla. This is a fairly small hypogeum. The crypt, which must have housed St. Thecla's grave, is here in the guise of a cubiculum with pilasters (*RQ*, III, 1889, pp. 343–53, IV, 1890, pp. 259–73).

Via Portuense. Catacomb of Pontianus. The name of this catacomb, which was in the region known as "ad ursum pileatum" ("by the hooded bear"), derives from a rich landowner in the district. SS. Pollio, Pigmenius, and Milix were buried there. Their cubicula have no door, only a tiny window (*fenestella confessionis*), through which the remains could be viewed. Also buried here were SS. Vincent, Candida, and the famous Persian martyrs Abdon and Sennen, to whom above-ground oratories were dedicated. The original centers in this cemetery, which is located in a clay ground ill adapted to excavation, were ornamented with frescoes in a Byzantine style. Armellini found here a cubiculum with traces of mosaic in the vault. A monument unique in Roman cemeteries was excavated in another cubiculum, probably of the 6th century. This is a baptistery decorated with a fresco of the baptism of Christ and a large jeweled and flowered cross. It was probably connected with the cemeterial church and may have been used by the local population. In another cubiculum is a scene painted from daily life, in which a boat with a shipment of amphoras is depicted (O. Marucchi, *NBACr*, XXIII, 1917, pp. 111–15; B. Manna, *BCom*, LI, 1923, pp. 163–224).

Via Aurelia Antica. (1) Catacomb of St. Pancras or of Octavilla. It underlies the property of a certain Octavilla. During the time of the Diocletian persecution (303), the martyr St. Pancras was buried in one of its galleries (J. P. Kirsch, *Miscellanea Ehrle*, Rome, 1924, II, pp. 65–71). Above ground, Pope Symmachus (498–514) erected a church which was rebuilt and enlarged by Honorius I (625–38). The whitewashed loculi are characteristic of this cemetery, as are the several graves cut into shelves of tufa which jut from the walls. One cubiculum is decorated with cupids and marine animals. Here SS. Dionysius, Artemius, and Paulina were also venerated, as well as the matron Sophia and her daughters Agape, Elpis, and Pistis (E. Fusciardi, *Catacomba, basilica e convento di San Pancrazio*, Rome, 1929). (2) Catacomb of SS. Processus and Martinian. The cemetery in which these two saints — thought to be the jailers of St. Peter mentioned in the Acts of the Apostles — were buried may be identified as the cluster of galleries which extend beneath the Villa Doria-Pamphili. (3) Catacomb of the Two Felixes. This cemetery, which legend affirms contained the remains of the "pontifices et martyres Felices duo," probably corresponds to a small network of galleries found under the Pellegrini vineyard (J. P. Kirsch, *Miscellanea Ehrle*, Rome, 1924, II, pp. 76–81; J. P. Kirsch, *RQ*, XXXIII, 1925, pp. 1–20). (4) Catacomb of Calepodius. Not far from the Catacomb of the Two Felixes. Here Pope Callixtus was buried in 222.

On his tomb Julius I (337–52) erected a basilica whose apse was discovered by Stevenson (*BACr*, 1881, p. 105; Kirsch, *Miscellanea Ehrle*, II, pp. 82–86).

Catacombs in the suburban areas, that is, about three miles beyond the Aurelian wall, occupy for the most part the territories of the episcopal seats of suburban Rome (see Armellini, 1893).

Via Flaminia. (1) Catacomb "ad rubras" at the 9th milestone (Boldetti, 1720, p. 577). (2) Anonymous catacomb at the 20th milestone, between Morlupo and Leprignano, not far from Capena (O. Marucchi, *NBACr*, XVII, 1911, pp. 239–40; XVIII, 1912, pp. 183–84). (3) Catacomb of Theodora at the 26th milestone, near Rignano (G. B. De Rossi, *BACr*, 1883, pp. 134–59). (4) Catacomb of SS. Hyacinth, Alexander, and Tiburtius at the 25th milestone, near Monteleone (Armellini, 1893, p. 543).

Via Salaria. Catacomb of St. Anthimus at the 23d milestone, near Montelibretti (Boldetti, 1720, p. 575).

Via Nomentana. (1) Catacomb of SS. Alexander, Theodulus, and Eventius at the 7th milestone (O. Marucchi, *Il cimitero e la basilica di Sant'Alessandro*, Rome, 1922, p. 36; G. Belvederi, *RACr*, XIV, 1937, pp. 7–40, 199–224, XV, 1938, pp. 19–34, 225–46). (2) Catacomb of SS. Primus and Felician at the 14th milestone, in a district called in ancient times "ad arcus nomentanos" (Bosio, 1632, p. 416). (3) Catacomb of St. Restitutus at the 16th milestone, no longer accessible (Bosio, 1632, p. 416).

Via Tiburtina. Anonymous catacomb at Acquoria (G. De Angelis d'Ossat, *RACr*, XXV, 1949, pp. 125–27).

Via Labicana. (1) Catacomb of St. Primitivus, near ancient Gabii (G. B. De Rossi, *BACr*, 1873, p. 115; Armellini, 1893, pp. 561–63). (2) Catacomb of Zoticus at the 10th milestone (E. Stevenson, *Il cimitero di Zotico*, Modena, 1876; G. De Angelis d'Ossat, *B. della Regia Deputazione di Storia Patria, Sez. Veliterna*, IX, 1941, pp. 5–16).

Via Prenestina. (1) Catacomb of St. Agapetus near Palestrina (O. Marucchi, *Guida archeologica della città di Palestrina*, Rome, 1912). (2) Catacomb of St. Hilary "ad bivium" ("at the crossroads") at the 30th milestone, not far from Valmontone (Boldetti, 1720, p. 566). (3) Anonymous catacomb at the 36th milestone at Colle San Quirico near Paliano (O. Marucchi, *NBACr*, XX, 1914, pp. 131–136; G. De Angelis d'Ossat, *RACr*, XXII, 1946, pp. 89–99).

Via Latina. (1) Anonymous catacomb near Tavolato (R. Kanzler, *NBACr*, IX, 1903, pp. 173–86; O. Marucchi, *NBACr*, IX, 1903, pp. 282–84). (2) Anonymous catacomb at the 10th milestone (S. Scaglia, *Le catacombe tusculane "ad decimum" della via Latina*, Grottaferrata, 1903; O. Marucchi, *NBACr*, XIX, 1913, pp. 230–37; A. De Waal, *RQ*, XXVII, 1913, pp. 151–61; F. Grossi-Gondi, *Catacombe tusculane, scoperta di un'importante iscrizione greca*, Grottaferrata, 1914; F. Grossi-Gondi, *NBACr*, XXIV–XXV, 1918–19, pp. 87–94; G. De Angelis d'Ossat, *B. della Regia Deputazione di Storia Patria, Sez. Veliterna*, 1942, pp. 3–10).

Via Appia Antica. (1) Anonymous catacomb at Boville, described in 1712 by Boldetti (1720, p. 558) but not since found (G. B. De Rossi, *BACr*, 1869, p. 79). (2) Catacomb of St. Senator at the 14th milestone near the Church of S. Maria della Stella in Albano (G. B. De Rossi, *BACr*, 1869, pp. 65–78; O. Marucchi, *BACr*, 1892, pp. 89–111; G. De Angelis d'Ossat, *B. della Regia Deputazione di Storia Patria, Sez. Veliterna*, 1942, pp. 11–19). (3) Anonymous catacomb near Velletri (G. Schneider-Graziosi, *BCom*, XLI, 1913, pp. 225–55).

Via Ardeatina. Anonymous catacomb at the 10th milestone, near the church called "La Nunziatella" (G. B. De Rossi, *BACr*, 1877, pp. 136–41; O. Marucchi, *BACr*, 1882, pp. 168–70).

Via Ostiense. Catacomb of St. Cyriacus at the 7th milestone (Bosio, 1632, p. 233).

Via Portuense. Catacomb of Generosa "ad sextum Philippi," at the 6th milestone, near Magliana (De Rossi, 1864–77, III, pp. 647–697; G. B. De Rossi, *BACr*, 1869, pp. 1–16; C. Huelsen, *NBACr*, VI, 1900, pp. 121–26; E. Josi, *RACr*, XVI, 1939, pp. 323–26).

Via Aurelia. (1) Anonymous catacomb at the 4th milestone, near Monte Mario, not far from Via Trionfale (G. B. De Rossi, *BACr*, 1894, pp. 133–46). (2) Catacomb of Basilides at the 12th milestone, near the ancient Lorium (Boldetti, 1720, p. 538; E. Stevenson, in Kraus, *Real-Encyklopädie der christlichen Alterthümer*, II, 1886, 128;

G. De Angelis d'Ossat, *La geologia e le catacombe romane*, II, Rome; 1933–35, pp. 45–49).

Via Cornelia. Catacomb of SS. Marius and Martha and Their Children, "ad nymphas Catabassi," at the 13th milestone (Boldetti, 1720, p. 538).

*Catacombs in other parts of Italy*. To the Roman catacombs listed above can be added those in the following localities (names within parentheses are modern provinces):

Sessa Aurunca (Napoli). (O. Marucchi, *BACr*, 1879, p. 140.)

Naples. (For the various catacombs of this city, see A. Bellucci, *Atti del III Cong. Int. di Archeol. Cristiana* [1932], Rome, 1934, pp. 327–70; Achelis, 1936, p. 101, pl. 60; D. Mallardo, *Ricerche di storia e di topografia degli antichi cimiteri cristiani di Napoli*, Naples, 1936.) (1) Catacomb of St. Januarius (S. Gennaro dei Poveri) (R. Garrucci, "Il cimitero cristiano di Napoli detto la catacomba di San Gennaro," extract from *Civiltà Cattolica*, series VIII, vol. V, 1872, pp. 551–59; V. Schultze, *Die Katakomben von S. Gennaro dei Poveri*, Jena, 1877; G. A. Galante, *Atti della Regia Acc. di Napoli*, XXV, 1908, p. 115 ff.). (2) Catacomb of St. Gaudiosus or "della Sanità" (Bellucci, *Atti...*, pp. 358–70; A. Bellucci, *RACr*, XI, 1934, pp. 73–105). (3) Catacomb of St. Euphebius or of Severus (Bellucci, *Atti...*, pp. 327–58; A. Bellucci, *BACr*, XI, 1934, pp. 105–18).

Atripalda (Avellino). Hypogeum of St. Hypolistus (G. A. Galante, *Il cemitero di S. Ipolisto*, n.p., 1891).

Prata (Avellino). (G. Taglialatela, *Basilica e catacomba di Prata*, Naples, 1878.)

Tropea (Catanzaro). (P. Toraldo, *RACr*, XII, 1935, pp. 329–37, XIII, 1936, pp. 155–60.)

Castelvecchio Subequo (Aquila). Anonymous catacomb (A. Ferrua, *RACr*, XXVI, 1950, pp. 53–83; G. De Angelis d'Ossat, *RACr*, XXVI, 1950, pp. 89–92).

San Vittorino (Aquila). (A. Bevignani, *NBACr*, IX, 1903, p. 190.)

Bazzano (Aquila). (A. Bevignani, *NBACr*, IX, 1903, pp. 187–90; G. De Angelis d'Ossat, *RACr*, XXVI, 1950, pp. 98–100.)

Villa S. Faustino near Massa Martana (Perugia). (G. Sordini, *Atti del II Cong. int. di Archeol. Cristiana* [1900], Rome, 1902, pp. 109–21.)

Viterbo. Catacomb of S. Salvatore di Rovello, located in the "Grotta di Riello" (F. Orioli, *Viterbo e il suo territorio*, 1848, p. 291; Armellini, 1893, p. 653).

Nepi (Viterbo). (Boldetti, 1720, pp. 579–81; G. B. De Rossi, *BACr*, 1874, p. 113; A. Baumstark, *RQ*, XVI, 1902, p. 245.)

Sutri (Viterbo). Catacomb of St. Juvenal (Boldetti, 1720, p. 581).

Sorrina Nova. Ancient city 2 1/2 miles from Viterbo (Armellini, 1893, p. 663).

Soriano nel Cimino (Viterbo). Catacomb of St. Euticius (Germano da S. Stanislao, *Memorie archeologiche e critiche sopra gli atti e il cimitero di Sant'Eutizio a Ferento*, Rome, 1886).

Bolsena (Viterbo). (1) Catacomb of St. Christina (G. B. De Rossi, *BACr*, 1880, pp. 71–72, 109–43; E. Stevenson, *NSc*, 1880, pp. 3–23; E. Stevenson, *RQ*, II, 1888, pp. 327–50). (2) Anonymous catacomb near "Le Grotte" (Armellini, 1893, p. 663).

Pian della Badia, ancient Vulci (Viterbo). (O. Kellermann, *BInst*, 1835, pp. 177–80; G. B. De Rossi, *BACr*, 1877, p. 107.)

Nazzano (Roma). (Armellini, 1893, p. 625.)

Chiusi (Siena). (1) Catacomb of St. Mustiola (B. Pasquini, *Ragguaglio d'un antico cimitero di cristiani in vicinanza di Chiusi*, Siena, 1831; B. Pasquini, *Relazione di un antico cimitero...*, Montepulciano, 1833). (2) Catacomb of St. Catherine (A. Bartolini, *DissPontAcc*, 1853, pp. 1–58; C. Cavedoni, *Ragguaglio storico-archeologico di due antichi cimiteri della città di Chiusi*, Siena, 1872, p. 348).

Sicily. Many sites on the island where Christian catacombs have been found have been completely explored and described by

two German scholars (J. Führer and V. Schultze, *Die altchristlichen Grabstätten Siziliens*, Berlin, 1907). They include Canicattini, Carini, Cassibile, Cava d'Ispica, Chiaramonte Gulfi, Cittadella dei Maccari, Ferla, Granieri, Lentini, Licodia Eubea, Marsala, Melilli, Palermo, Palazzolo Acreide, Priolo, the Sant'Elia district of Palazzolo Acreide, Santa Croce Camerina, Termine Imerese.

Other catacombs in Sicily: Agrigento (C. Mercurelli, *RACr*, XXI, 1944-45, pp. 5-50; C. Mercurelli, *MPontAcc*, VIII, 1948, pp. 1-105; P. Griffo, *Atti del I Cong. Naz. di Archeol. Cristiana* [1950], Rome, 1952, pp. 191-99). – Comiso and the area of Camarina (C. Mercurelli, *RACr*, XXI, 1944-45, pp. 59-104). – Molinello (J. Führer, *RQ*, XVI, 1902, pp. 205-31; P. Orsi, *NSc*, 1902, pp. 411-434). – Naro (C. Mercurelli, *RACr*, XXI, 1944-45, pp. 50-59). – The well-known Noto neighborhood (G. Agnello, *RACr*, XXX, 1954, pp. 169-80, XXXI, 1955, pp. 201-22). – Palma di Montechiaro (G. Caputo, *NSc*, 1931, pp. 405-08). – Portopalo (S. L. Agnello, *RACr*, XXIX, 1953, pp. 167-83). – Ragusa (altipiano) (G. Agnello, *RACr*, XXIX, 1953, pp. 67-87). – Marina di Ragusa near the "Grotta della Taddarita" (L. Bernabò-Brea, *NSc*, 1947, p. 255). – Syracuse. The various catacombs of the city have been studied by Führer ("Forschungen zur Sicilia sotterranea," *AbhAkMünchen*, XX, 1897, p. 671 ff.), Barreca (*Le catacombe di Siracusa alla luce degli ultimi scavi e recenti scoperte*, 3d ed., Rome, 1934), and S. L. Agnello (*Problemi di datazione delle catacombe di Siracusa: Scritti in onore di G. Libertini*, Florence, 1958, pp. 65-82). Various minor hypogeums have been studied by Orsi (*RQ*, XI 1897, pp. 475-95, XIV, 1900, pp. 187-290; *NSc*, 1915, pp. 205-08), by S. L. Agnello ("Scavi recenti nella catacomba di Vigna Cassia Siracusa," *RACr*, XXXII, 1956, p. 7 ff.), by Bernabò-Brea (*NSc*, 1947, pp. 172-90), and by Puma (*Atti del I Cong. Naz. di Archeol. Cristiana* [1950], Rome, 1952, pp. 251-57). (1) Bonaiuto Catacomb (L. Bonomo, *Atti del I Cong. Naz. di Archeol. Cristiana* [1950], Rome, 1952, pp. 93-100). (2) Führer Catacomb on the estate of Adorno Avolio (P. Orsi, *RQ*, IX, 1895, pp. 463-88). (3) Catacomb of St. Lucy (P. Orsi, *NSc*, 1918, pp. 270-85; S. L. Agnello, *RACr*, XXX, 1954, pp. 7-60). (4) Catacomb of St. John (P. Orsi, *NSc*, 1893, pp. 276-99, 1895, pp. 477-521; C. Barreca, *Le catacombe di San Giovanni in Siracusa*, Syracuse, 1906). (5) Catacomb of Vigna Cassia (P. Orsi and J. Führer, *AbhAkMünchen*, XXII, 1902-05, p. 107 ff.).

Sardinia. Cagliari: catacomb of the Collina di Bonaria (F. Vivanet, *NSc*, 1892, pp. 183-89; G. Pinza, *NBACr*, VII, 1901, pp. 61-66). – Bonorva (G. Pinza, *NBACr*, VII, 1901, pp. 66-69).

*Principal catacombs outside Italy.* Malta. Catacombs of Abbatia, of St. Agatha, of St. Catald, of S. Maria delle Virtù, of St. Paul, of St. Venera (A. Caruana, *Ancient Pagan Tombs and Christian Cemeteries in the Island of Malta*, Malta, 1898; A. Mayr, *RQ*, XV, 1901, pp. 216-43, 252-384; E. Becker, 1913, p. 203; A. Ferrua, *Civiltà Cattolica*, III, 1949, pp. 505-15).

Greece. Chalcis in Euboea (G. Lampakis, *Neue kirchliche Z.*, III, 1892, p. 903 ff.; P. Strzygowski, *RQ*, IV, 1890, p. 2). – Melos: catacomb near Tripiti (*BCH*, II, 1878, pp. 347-59; R. Schultze, *Die Katakomben*, Leipzig, 1882, pp. 275-79).

Mesopotamia. Dara (ancient Anastasiopolis).

Cilicia. Seleucia (*BCH*, IV, 1880, p. 195 ff., VII, 1883, p. 230 ff.).

Palestine. Haifa (*Z. des deutschen Palästina Vereins*, 1890, p. 175 ff.).

Egypt. Alexandria (Néroutzos-Bey, *L'ancienne Alexandrie*, Paris, 1888, pp. 38-54): catacombs of Karmuz, with frescoes (C. Wescher, *BACr*, 1865, pp. 57-61; G. B. De Rossi, *BACr*, 1865, pp. 61-64, 73-77); of the Rufini, of Mustafa, and of Abu-al-Ashen (G. Botti, *B. de la Soc. Archéologique d'Alexandrie*, I, 1898, pp. 5-24); of Gabbari (G. Botti, *B. de la Soc. Archéologique d'Alexandrie*, I, 1898, pp. 37-56); and of Agnew (H. C. Agnew, *Archaeologia*, XXVIII, 1840, pp.150-70).

Cyrenaica. Cyrene (J. R. Pacho, *Relation d'un voyage dans... la Cyrénaïque...*, Paris, 1827-28; H. Weld-Blundell, *BSA*, II, 1895-96, p. 132 ff.; Schultze, 1882, pp. 286-90).

Tripolitania. Sabrata (G. Caputo, *Schema di fonti e monumenti del primo cristianesimo in Tripolitania*, Tripoli, 1947, pp. 25-26). – Tripoli (Caputo, *op. cit.*, p. 26; Jewish or Christian cemetery?).

Tunisia. Catacombs in various localities: Hajeb el Aioun, Kerkennah, Gabès (anc. Tacape), Salakta (anc. Sullectum; Leynaud, 1936); Sousse (anc. Hadrumetum): (1) the catacomb called the Good Shepherd's and (2) the catacomb called that of Severus (Leynaud,

1936, pp. 19-332, 357-446). Also in Sousse was discovered a pagan catacomb, named Agrippa's (Leynaud, 1936, pp. 335-53).

Algeria. Catacombs at Oum Kif (anc. Cediae; see Leynaud, 1936, pp. 451-59), at Kherbet-bou-Adoufen, in the region of Sétif (S. Gsell, *Monuments antiques de l'Algérie*, II, Paris, 1901, pp. 183-84), at Khenchela (anc. Mascula; C. Vars, *Rec. de la Soc. Archéologique de la Province de Constantine*, XLIII, 1898, pp. 362-70).

*Heretical catacombs.* Just as there was a clear separation between pagan and Christian cemeteries immediately after the earliest Christian period, so it was with the orthodox Christian and the heterodox burial grounds. It must immediately be noted, however, as Cecchelli has made clear (*Monumenti cristiano-eretici di Roma*, Rome, 1943), that the distinction is often very difficult to make, as the presence of an occasional fresco outside the usual iconographic cycle, together with an inscription whose content is open to question, is not enough to establish as heretical a cemetery in which such a painting and an epigraph have been found. Nor can the sole fact of a cemetery's being limited in extent and isolated from the large ecclesiastical hypogeums be adduced as conclusive indication of heterodoxy. In fact, if we take into account that, especially in the early period, there were groups of hypogeums entirely distinct from one another and that very large necropolises (as in the post-Constantinian period) did not exist, it becomes clear that such a separation need not be construed as necessarily the result of a religious schism. See HERETICAL SUBJECTS.

The following subterranean cemeteries of Rome are generally held to be heretical: (1) Anonymous catacomb in the Viale Regina Margherita near the beginning of the Via Tiburtina (F. Fornari, *RACr*, VI, 1929, pp. 179-239; E. Josi, *RACr*, X, 1933, pp. 187-233). An epigraph found here — "Novatiano beatissimo martyri Gaudentius diac[onus] fec[it]" ("The deacon Gaudentius made it for the blessed martyr Novatianus" — seems to refer to Novatianus, a noted schismatic of the 3d century. Also discovered were two epigraphs of consular date painted on the plaster that covers the tiles sealing the loculi. One, in Latin, is dated 266; the other, in Greek, is dated 270. These are the oldest dated inscriptions still preserved *in situ* in all subterranean Rome. (2) Small hypogeum in the Via Ardeatina, between the catacombs of Domitilla and Callixtus (G. Marangoni, *Delle cose gentilesche o profane*, Rome, 1744, pp. 461-62), thought to be Sabellian. In an arcosolium is a mosaic which represents Christ on a sphere between the seated figures of SS. Peter and Paul. At the bottom is the inscription: "qui et filius diceris et pater inveniris" ("You who are called the Son and are found to be the Father also") (see Cod. Vat. Lat. 9071), which Schultze (*Z. für Kirchengeschichte*, XLV, 1926, pp. 513-16) has thought to be a typically Sabellian statement, on account of its identification of the Son with the Father. Cecchelli, however, tends to regard it as a Montanist expression. (3) Hypogeum between the 2d and 3d milestones of the Via Prenestina, not far from the Villa of the Gordiani. Although all traces of this cemetery have been lost, transcriptions of epitaphs were made in the 17th century by Suarez, bishop of Vaison (Cod. Vat. Lat. 9140). All of these refer to members of the same family, originally from Cyprus, a few of whom held ecclesiastical posts (see G. Schneider-Graziosi, *Bessarione*, 1915, p. 107 ff.). (4) Hypogeum of the Aurelii, near the Viale Manzoni, within the Aurelian walls (G. Bendinelli, *NSc*, 1920, pp. 123-41). It contains some very fine frescoes from the second quarter of the 3d century that represent various Christian themes, as well as mystic ceremonies in which women are participating (G. Bendinelli, *MALinc*, XXVIII, 1922, cols. 290-510; J. Wilpert, *AttiPontAcc*, XVIII, 1924, pp. 1-42). Mingazzini has questioned the hypothesis that these are heterodox themes (*Rend PontAcc*, XIX, 1942-43, pp. 355-69), but Cecchelli has recently countered his argument (*Monumenti cristiano-eretici di Roma*, Rome, 1943, pp. 235-44).

It is far from certain that the following hypogeums belong to the heretical category into which they are so often thrust. (1) At Cava Rossa near the 1st milestone of the Via Latina (R. Kanzler, *NBACr*, IX, 1903, pp. 173-86). The paintings, often showing chalices (one of them very large) with handles, have been linked by Marucchi (*NBACr*, IX, 1903, pp. 301-14) to the superstitions of the Valentinian heretic Marcus. (2) Near the Via della Caffarella (G. Schneider-Graziosi, *NBACr*, XXVII, 1921, pp. 177-80). (3) Near the tomb of the Scipios between the Via Appia and the Via Latina. This cemetery came to light a little before 1850 but has not been rediscovered. It was decorated with Christian paintings. Among the inscriptions referring to people from Asia and the Orient was that of Veratius Nicatora, now in the Lateran Museum (A. Ferrua, *Epigraphica*, I, 1940, pp. 7-20); in his reading of it Schneider-Graziosi saw an allusion to the heretics (*BCom*, XLI, 1913, pp. 61-66).

*Syncretistic catacombs.* These belonged to pagans who attempted a synthesis of precepts from various religions or to Christians still

imbued with pagan thought. Among their subterranean cemeteries can probably be numbered the following: (1) The Hypogeum of Trebius Justus on the Via Latina (R. Kanzler, *NBACr*, XVII, 1911, pp. 201–07), in which, besides a graffito invoking divine vengeance, were discovered paintings of the first half of the 4th century showing scenes of mystic content and of gardening, the building of a villa, etc. (O. Marucchi, *NBACr*, XVII, 1911, pp. 209–35, XVIII, 1912, pp. 83–99; sup. *RQ*, 1913, pp. 297–314; J. Wilpert, sup. *RQ*, 1913, pp. 276–96). According to Josi (*RACr*, XVII, 1940, p. 39), the possibility should not be excluded that this was a part of the nearby Catacomb of St. Eugenia or of Apronianus. (2) The Sabazian and Christian hypogeum on the Via Appia not far from the Catacomb of Praetextatus, with interesting paintings of mystic subjects and a pagan banquet executed by Vibia and Vincentius, devotees of Bacchus Sabazius (R. Garrucci, *Tre sepolcri con pitture e iscrizioni appartenenti alle superstizioni pagane del Bacco Sabazio e del persidico Mitra*, Naples, 1852). (3) The so-called "Hypogeum of the Hunters" on the Via Appia, near the Sabazian cemetery (R. Kanzler, *NBACr*, XXII, 1916, p. 102). It contains various paintings of hunting scenes from the first half of the 4th century (K. Wurmbrand-Stuppach, "Die Jägerkatakombe an der Via Appia," *Belvedere*, VI, 1927, pp. 289–94). The possibility of its being orthodox cannot be excluded. (4) The hypogeum on the Via Latina (A. Ferrua, *Civiltà Cattolica*, Apr., 1956, pp. 118–31; W. Artlet, "Der verkannte Katakombenfund: Ezekiel-Vision, Aufweckung oder 'Anatomie-Szene'?" *Rheinischer Merkur*, June, 1957). It contains an extensive cycle of paintings, among the most beautiful in the Roman catacombs, with scenes from the myths of Alcestis and Hercules as well as from the Old and the New Testament, many of them entirely new.

*Jewish catacombs*. The Jews generally had their cemeteries separate from those of the Christians, although their appearance was quite similar. Greek inscriptions predominate; Latin are few, and Hebrew really rare. A few of these last record notables of the synagogues. The loculi, arranged in rows, are usually sealed with tegulae, which are covered over with a layer of white lime in Oriental fashion. It is this practice to which Jesus alluded in the expression "whited sepulchers." Occasionally one encounters a sepulcher *a forno* (in the shape of an oven), into which the corpse is introduced endways. The painted decor is largely ornamental and, like the sculpture and the graffiti, symbolic; included, for example, are the seven-branched candlestick which burns in the temple, the horn of unction, the palm tree recalling the land of Palestine, the fruit of the citron tree and the *lulav*, or sheaf of aromatic grasses, used in the Feast of Tabernacles, the *aron*, or aedicula, containing the tablets of the Law.

The following Jewish cemeteries have been found in Rome: (1) Between the Via Appia Pignatelli and the Church of S. Sebastiano (R. Garrucci, *Il cimitero degli antichi ebrei recentemente scoperto in Vigna Rondanini*, Rome 1862); (2) on the Via Appia Pignatelli (*RM*, II, 1886, pp. 49–56); (3) near S. Sebastiano under the Cimarra vineyard (G. B. De Rossi, *BACr*, 1867, p. 16); (4) at the 2d kilometer marker of the Via Labicana (O. Marucchi, *AttiPontAcc*, II, 1884, pp. 499–532), a cemetery in which there was also an occasional tomb with a niched arcosolium, called an *absis*; (5) on the Via Portuense at Monteverde, almost entirely destroyed except for the inscriptions, which are preserved in the Lateran Museum (N. Müller, *Die jüdische Katakombe am Monteverde zu Rom*, Leipzig, 1912; *AttiPontAcc*, XII, 1915, pp. 205–318; G. Schneider-Graziosi, *NBACr*, XXI, 1915, pp. 13–56; R. Paribeni, *NSc*, 1919, pp. 60–70; N. Müller and N. A. Bees, *Die Inschriften der jüdischen Katakomben am Monteverde zu Rom*, Leipzig, 1919); (6) at the 1st milestone on the Via Nomentana under the Villa Torlonia (R. Paribeni, *NSc*, 1920, pp. 143–155; O. Marucchi, *NBACr*, XXVI, 1920, pp. 55–57; B. Manna, *BCom*, LX, 1922, pp. 205–23; H. W. Beyer and H. Lietzmann, *Die jüdische Katakombe der Villa Torlonia in Rom*, Berlin, 1930; K. H. Rengstorf, *Z. für neutestamentische Wissenschaft*, XXXI, 1932, pp. 33–60). In a cubiculum in this catacomb, in the four lateral semicircles of the vault, were painted four dolphins twined around tridents; Frey (*RACr*, VIII, 1931, pp. 301–14) has pointed out that this motif, unique in Jewish art, is no more than a purely decorative element borrowed directly from classical art.

The main Jewish catacombs outside Rome are the following: (1) That of Venosa (R. Carrucci, "Cimitero ebraico di Venosa in Puglia," *Civiltà Cattolica*, series XIII, vol. I, 1882, pp. 707–20; C. Lenormant, *Revue des Etudes Juives*, VI, 1883, pp. 200–07); (2) those at the Capuchin monastery in Syracuse (P. Orsi, *RQ*, XI, 1897, pp. 475–495; XIV, 1900, pp. 187–209); (3) that on of Sant'Antioco near Sardinia (P. Orsi, *NSc*, 1908, pp. 150–52); (4) those in Malta (Becker, 1913); (5) the small catacombs southeast of Palmyra, made up of a cluster of small cubicula with paintings, among which are the well-known Victories bearing shields (J. Strzygowski, *Orient oder Rom*, Leipzig, 1901, pp. 11–39); (6) a small hypogeum in Jerusalem (L. H. Vincent, *RBibl*, 1909, pp. 297–304); (7) the catacomb of Beth Shearim [N. Avigad, "The Beth She'harim Nekropolis," *Antiquity and Survival*, II, 2–3, 1957, p. 244 ff.; B. Mazar (Maisler), *Beth She'arim: Report on the Excavations during 1936–40*, I, *The Catacombs*, Jerusalem, 1957 (Hebrew text with English summary)]; (8) the burial chambers in the hill of Gamart north of Carthage (A. L. Delattre, *Gamart ou la nécropole juive de Carthage*, Lyons, 1905).

BIBLIOG. *a. General*: A. Bosio, Roma sotterranea, Rome, 1632; M. A. Boldetti, Osservazioni sopra i cimiteri de' SS. Martiri ed antichi cristiani di Roma, Rome, 1720; L. Perret, Les catacombes de Rome, Paris, 1852; G. B. De Rossi, La Roma sotterranea cristiana, Rome, 1864–77; F. X. Kraus, Roma sotterranea: Die römischen Katakomben, Freiburg, 1873; F. Becker, Rom's alchristliche Coemeterien, Düsseldorf, 1874; J. S. Northcote and W. E. Brownlow, Roma sotterranea, or An Account of the Roman Catacombs, London, 1879; T. Roller, Les catacombes de Rome, Paris, 1881; V. Schultze, Die Katakomben: Die altchristlichen Grabstätten, Leipzig, 1882; G. Marchi, Monumenti delle arti cristiane primitive nella metropoli del Cristianesimo, I, Architettura della Roma sotterranea, Rome, 1884; M. Armellini, Gli antichi cimiteri cristiani di Roma e d'Italia, Rome, 1893; J. Führer and V. Schultze, Forschungen zur Sicilia sotterranea, Munich, 1897; E. Becker, Malta sotterranea, Strasbourg, 1913; G. P. Kirsch, Le catacombe romane, Rome, 1933; O. Marucchi, Le catacombe romane, Rome, 1933; P. Styger, Die römischen Katakomben, Berlin, 1933; P. Styger, Römische Martyrergrüfte, Berlin, 1935; H. Achelis, Die Katakomben von Neapel, Berlin, 1936; A. F. Leynaud, Les catacombes africaines: Sousse-Hadrumète, 3d ed., Algiers, 1936; C. Cecchelli, Monumenti cristiano-eretici di Roma, Rome, 1943; C. Cecchelli, La Chiesa delle Catacombe, Rome, 1943; J. F. Aerts, De Catacomben van Rome, Louvain, 1949; E. Kirschbaum, Le catacombe romane e i loro martiri, Rome, 1949; G. Bovini, Rassegna degli studi sulle catacombe e sui cimiteri "sub divo," Vatican City, 1952; E. Kirschbaum, E. Junient, and J. Vives, La tumba de San Pedro y las catacumbas romanas, Madrid, 1954; A. Amore, Note di toponomastica cimiteriale romana, RACr, XXII, 1956, p. 59 ff.; A. Ferrua, Lavori e scoperte nelle catacombe, Triplice omaggio a S.S. Pio XII, II, Vatican City, 1958, pp. 49–60, 18 pls.; P. Testini, Archeologia cristiana, Rome, Paris, Tournai, New York, 1958. *b. Geology*: M. S. De Rossi, Analisi geologica ed architettonica (della Roma sotterranea cristiana), in G. B. De Rossi, La Roma sotterranea cristiana, I, Rome, 1864–97 (appendix); M. S. De Rossi, Analisi geologica ed architettonica (del cimitero di Callisto), in G. B. De Rossi, op. cit., II (appendix); G. De Angelis d'Ossat, La geologia e le catacombe romane, Memorie della Pontificia Accademia delle Scienze, Nuovi Lincei, series II, XIV–XVI, 1930–32, I (catacombs of the Via Tiburtina, Nomentana, Salaria Vecchia, Salaria Nuova, Flaminia), pp. 125–65, 267–310, 529–73, 629–65, 873–911, XVII, 1933–34, II (catacombs of the Via Cornelia and the Via Aurelia), pp. 43–74, 1–49; G. De Angelis d'Ossat, La geologia delle catacombe romane, in Roma sotterranea cristiana, III, Vatican City, 1938, fasc. I (Via Portuense and Via Ostiense), fasc. II (Via Ardeatina and Via Appia), fasc. III (Via Latina and Via Labicana). *c. Painting*: L. Lefort, Chronologie des peintures des catacombes de Naples, Mél., 1883, pp. 67 ff., 183 ff.; J. Wilpert, Le pitture delle catacombe romane, Rome, 1903; J. P. Kirsch, Sull'origine dei motivi iconografici nella pittura cimiteriale di Roma, RACr, IV, 1927, pp. 259–87; P. Markthaler, Die dekorativen Konstruktionen der Katacombendecken Roms, RQ, XXXV, 1927, pp. 53–111; M. Dvořak, Katakombenmalereien: Die Anfänge der christlichen Kunst, Kunstgeschichte als Geistesgeschichte, Studien zur abendländischen Kunstentwicklung, Munich, 1928, pp. 3–40; R. Kömsted, Vormittelalterliche Malerei, Augsburg, 1929; A. Schuchert, Die römische Katakomben-Malerei in Wandel der Kunstkritik, RQ, XXXIX, 1931, pp. 7–22; A. W. Bijwanck, De Dateering der Schilderingen in de Romeinsche Katakomben, Mededeelingen van het Nederlandsch Historisch Instituut te Rome, 1932, pp. 45–78; F. Wirth, Römische Wandmalerei vom Untergang Pompejis bis ans Ende des dritten Jahrhunderts, Berlin, 1934; H. Achelis, Die Katakomben von Neapel, Berlin, 1936; J. De Wit, Spätrömische Bildnismalerei, Stilkritische Untersuchungen zur Wandmalerei der Katakomben und verwanter Monumenten, Berlin, 1938; G. Agnello, La pittura paleocristiana della Sicilia, Vatican City, 1952; G. Bovini, Momenti tipici del linguaggio figurativo della pittura cimiteriale d'età paleocristiana, Corsi di cultura sull'arte ravennate e bizantina, Ravenna, 1957, fasc. I, pp. 9–30. *d. Sculpture*: J. Wilpert, I sarcofagi cristiani antichi, Rome, I–V, 1929–36; F. Gerke, Die christlichen Sarcofage der vorkonstantinischen Zeit, Berlin, 1940. *e. Lamps*: G. P. Bellori, Le antiche lucerne sepolcrali figurate raccolte dalle cave sotterranee e grotte di Roma, Rome, 1691; H. L. Schurzfleisch, De lucernis veterum christianorum sepulcribus, Wittenberg, 1810. *f. Gold glasses*: R. Garrucci, Vetri ornati di figure in oro trovati nei cimiteri cristiani primitivi di Roma, 2d ed., Rome, 1864; H. Vopel, Die altchristlichen Goldgläser, Freiburg, 1899; W. Fröhner, Verres chrétiens à figures d'or, Paris, n.d.; O. Dalton, The Golden Glasses of the Catacombs, Archaeological Journal, 1901, p. 227 ff.; Complete catalogue of C. R. Morey in process of preparation (1960) at the Poliglotta Vaticana under the direction of G. Ferrari.

Giuseppe BOVINI

Illustrations: PLS. 90–104; 4 figs. in text.

**CAVALLINI**, PIETRO. Painter, born in Rome, probably about 1240. He was a member of the noble family of the Cerroni, who owned estates in the city. The name Cavallini, by which we know him today, is derived from the nickname Caballinus, or Cavallinus, bestowed by his contemporaries.

There are three extant documents which refer to Cavallini. The earliest of these is preserved in the archives of S. Maria

Maggiore. It relates how, on Oct. 2, 1273, "Petrus dictus Cavallinus de Cerronibus" and "Bartholomaeus Johannis Cerronis" witnessed and acted as guarantors in a sales contract drawn up by Giovanni di Jacopo di Meta, "Sanctae Romanae Ecclesiae criniarius." The second is a contract written in Naples and dated Dec. 15, 1308, which refers to another contract of June 16 of the same year. In the December contract Robert d'Anjou confirms a promise made by his father to "Magistro Petro Cavallino de Roma pictore" that the treasurer of the Court of Naples pay the latter a certain sum of money annually "usque ad beneplacitum regium" ("as long as the king wishes").

The third document is a note written by Pietro's son, Giovanni, in the margin of a codex (now in the Vatican Library) containing the writings of Valerius Maximus. The note says: "Huic commemoro Petrum de Cerronibus, qui centum annorum vitam egit, qui nullo unquam frigore caput vestimento cooperuit qui fuit et pater meus idest mei Joannis Caballini domini papae scriptoris." ("Here I commemorate Peter of the Cerroni family, who lived one hundred years, who never covered his head in the cold, and who was also my father — that is, the father of Giovanni Cavallini, scribe of our master, the Pope.") We do not know the exact year in which Giovanni Cavallini wrote this solemn and unique memorial to his father, stating that like the ancients he always went bareheaded, but it is believed that all Giovanni's explanatory notes in the Vatican codex were written between 1330 and 1360. Therefore Pietro, whose activity may be dated roughly from 1270 to 1330, was dead by 1360 at the latest.

Some of the works generally accepted as Cavallini's can be dated quite accurately. Between 1270 and 1279, Cavallini began the paintings which decorated the whole interior of S. Paolo fuori le Mura, returning to the task in later years. In 1291 he signed the band of mosaics under the conch of the apse in S. Maria in Trastevere. It is also known that about 1293 he painted the interior of S. Cecilia in Trastevere, and that between 1316 and 1320 he frescoed the Church of S. Maria Donnaregina in Naples. Ghiberti and Vasari tell us that during the pontificate of Pope John XXII (1316–34) Cavallini also composed the façade mosaics of the old basilica of S. Paolo fuori le Mura. But the mosaics were totally disfigured when an attempt was made to transfer them to the interior of the church after the fire of 1823.

The first biography of Cavallini was written by Lorenzo Ghiberti. To the artist he ascribed, in addition to the Roman works mentioned above, paintings in Old St. Peter's and the churches of S. Crisogono and S. Francesco. The Anonimo Magliabechiano chronicle repeated Ghiberti's attributions. Vasari expanded the list, crediting Cavallini with works in the transept of the Church of S. Maria d'Aracoeli and some frescoes in S. Maria in Trastevere as well as various mosaics on its façade; he also named him collaborator with Giotto in the mosaic of the navicella in Old St. Peter's. Vasari further attributed to Cavallini certain paintings in Florence and Orvieto which are definitely not his. In addition, Vasari recorded that "it is likewise said by some that Pietro made some pieces of sculpture . . . and that the crucifix in the great church of S. Paolo fuori le Mura — the very one that spoke to St. Bridget in 1370 — is by his hand."

Pietro Cavallini, like Cimabue and Duccio, belonged to the generation preceding Giotto's. Certainly Cavallini must have known, as did other artists of the mid-13th century dependent upon the papal court, the work of Eastern masters of the various Byzantine schools and periods. Fine examples of these were to be found even in the city of Rome. Austere and meditative in temperament, Cavallini searched deeply into traditional attitudes in order to express through them his own experience. He thus came to understand some of the values of classical art so well that he could use them to represent new concepts. His interest in the antique, however, did not cut him off from the more typical developments of his own times, which gradually led him completely beyond the conventions of the Romanesque idiom until he was able to express in his later works the spirit of the changing times.

Of the paintings which, according to Ghiberti and Vasari,

decorated S. Paolo fuori le Mura, nothing remains but a vague reflection in early representations of the basilica interior and some drawings by Antonio Ecclissi in a Vatican Library codex. The oldest work of the master which has come down to us is, therefore, the band of mosaics below the conch of the apse in S. Maria in Trastevere. These mosaics, divided into seven panels, were commissioned by Giotto's protector, Bertoldo di Pietro Stefaneschi. Until the middle of the 17th century it was possible to read an inscription on a border of the central panel bearing the artist's name. The panel shows the kneeling donor on the right being presented to the Virgin and Child by St. Peter. To the left stands St. Paul, and immediately below the Virgin is an invocation with Cardinal Stefaneschi's name and coat of arms. The other scenes show, from left to right, *The Birth of the Virgin, The Annunciation* (PL. 110), *The Nativity* (PL. 106), *The Adoration of the Magi* (PL. 105), *The Presentation in the Temple,* and *The Death of the Virgin.*

The iconographic schemes of these compositions largely correspond to those of other contemporary representations of the same subjects, which were painted so frequently in the areas of Byzantine and Byzantine-influenced culture. Yet as Coletti has observed, some of the panels (*The Annunciation,* for example) reveal an effort to provide convincing backgrounds for the figures, even though the scenes are always iconic rather than episodic. Also conventional are the figures, though Cavallini frequently seems to want to depart from the traditional rendering of certain specific images in an attempt to recreate the classical spirit of his models. The figures have a firmness and delicacy derived not only from their three-dimensional appearance, emphasized by the drapery folds often based on antique types, but also from the gradual modulation of brilliantly colored highlights into deep shadows often verging on black. This method of making mosaics strongly resembles that of painting (PLS. 105, 106).

The pictorial decorations in S. Cecilia once covered all the walls of the church. On the side walls only a few traces of the frescoes remain. They showed scenes of the Old and New Testaments, a large image of St. Michael, and figures of saints in Gothicized niches. On the wall of the nuns' choir at the back of the church was painted a *Last Judgment,* of which there remains only the central portion showing Christ as Judge, the Virgin, St. John the Baptist, the Twelve Apostles, the symbols of the Passion, and trumpeting angels who announce the Judgment (PLS. 107, 109; I, 304). The monumental figures appear to represent a heroic race of beings revealed here for the first time. They belong to a different world from that of the Byzantine-influenced Italian painters, who were affected to a greater or lesser extent by Neo-Hellenism. Above all, they reveal the presence of a profound personality who was fully capable of revealing his vision in appropriate visual terms.

Although the figures in these frescoes, like those in the mosaics of S. Maria in Trastevere, recall traditional types, Cavallini has taken liberties with every iconographic element in an attempt to individualize the figures and express his own sentiments. The compassion of Christ as Judge expresses not only His lofty spirit but also the artist's inner peace. Another obvious innovation, compared with the mosaics of S. Maria in Trastevere, appears in the modeling of the heavy woolen drapery which falls in deep, broad folds and recalls classical painting and sculpture. Antique painting is further suggested by the use of nearly black hues for the background, by the repeated combination of reds and greens with black, by the application of greenish shadows over vivid flesh tones, and by the use of beautiful violets and infinite gradations of rose and gray, which in their transitions from light to dark impart a plasticity to the figures. Cavallini's technique was to create the contours of his forms in heavy color, modulating from dark to lighter areas with delicate tones, until the correct values of the forms were achieved (PL. 109). The highlights were then accented by touches of pure white lead.

By 1308, more than twenty years after the execution of these paintings, which from a technical point of view have many characteristics in common with ancient encaustic paint-

ings, Pietro Cavallini collaborated on the decorations for the Church of S. Maria Donnaregina in Naples. Most of the paintings in the great choir of the nuns must be ascribed to various Roman, Neapolitan, and perhaps Sienese assistants. They are responsible for *The Last Judgment, The Ascension, The Pentecost*, the scenes from the Passion, and the lives of SS. Agnes, Catherine, Ladislaus, Stephen, and Elizabeth. To what extent Cavallini directly influenced these frescoes with their lively sense of narrative and realism — either through drawings, projects, or advice — is difficult to determine. Only the pairs of apostles and prophets represented standing, one on either side of a palm tree, in vertical rows of panels near the presbytery, can be considered his (PL. 108). They are related to the figures of the apostles in S. Cecilia. Although the stylistic traits of the Donnaregina frescoes are not identical with those of the master's earlier works, they derive from the latter and suggest Cavallini's developing powers of design and naturalistic expression. The best of these figures in Naples no longer express medieval sentiments. Their faces, glances, and poses convey with intensity new ideas and affirm moral values which are of more interest to the painter than the myth or symbolism expressed by the figures. The new moral emphasis is almost always conveyed in a style entirely free from traditional stylization. Clearly, Cavallini's work did not evolve stylistically along the same lines as Giotto's, even though in the 20-year interval between the frescoes of S. Cecilia in Rome and those of S. Maria Donnaregina in Naples, Giotto's innovations were the most influential factor in determining the future course of painting. Surely these innovations were known to Cavallini.

Cavallini's new expressive manner results from the gradual synthesis of antique conventions as he gained insight into their original function. At the same time, he reveals a spontaneous and more human spirit, a poignancy of Christian origin. It is very probable that this development of Cavallini's art influenced not only Giotto but Arnolfo di Cambio (q.v.) as well.

Arnolfo spent the last three decades of the 13th century in Rome. His ability to transform even classical elements into a language full of modern allusions brought him recognition as the most important living master. The younger architects and sculptors were drawn to him as to a magnet. To what extent the structural clarity and plasticity of Arnolfo's style may have influenced Cavallini, or Cavallini's paintings may have affected Arnolfo, it is difficult to gauge with any accuracy. Certainly the two masters, of almost the same age, were the most important figures in the restricted artistic world of Rome, whose population numbered a scant few thousand. For 30 years they lived side by side, and occasionally were even commissioned to work in the same church at the same time, as in S. Paolo fuori le Mura and S. Cecilia. The two men surely knew one another's work thoroughly and thereby influenced one another, even though the differences of medium and temperament limited this influence to an orientation of taste. A precise comparison between the two masters reveals Cavallini's more profound understanding of anatomy at S. Maria Donnaregina, a freer drapery style, and, as has been said, a developing tendency toward less rigorous stylization, through which his figures achieve a powerful individuality.

Among the first attributions to Cavallini, which Vasari also accepts, is the carved wooden crucifix, now preserved in the Chapel of the Sacrament in S. Paolo fuori le Mura. Although it is a beautiful work, much influenced by Arnolfo di Cambio, it contains a number of unfused stylistic elements: a Hellenistic influence, a renewed admiration for antiquity, and a vitality derived from popular art. It is not absolutely certain that the crucifix is by Cavallini, but many factors favor such an attribution.

None of the other works often ascribed to Cavallini display the high quality of those already discussed. For the most part they belong to his followers, the best of whom executed the lunette above the tomb of Cardinal Matteo of Acquasparta in the Church of S. Maria d'Aracoeli. Recently discovered fragments of older paintings in this church suggest that Vasari was correct about Cavallini's extensive activity here. A *Tree of Jesse* in the Cathedral of Naples is by one of the most ac-

complished of Cavallini's large Neapolitan following. This same painter may also have worked in S. Maria Donnaregina. Traces of Cavallini's influence have been found among painters in Umbria and in the minor centers of Lazio and Campania. His influence is certainly at the base of the so-called "school of Rimini." These minor artists signal the diffusion and dissolution of the great Roman master's art in numerous separate directions; for in his own city, torn by factions and political struggles throughout the 14th century, there was no worthy successor to his position.

BIBLIOG. L. Ghiberti, I Commentari, ed. J. von Schlosser, Berlin, 1912, I, p. 39, II, pp. 134–7; Anonimo Magliabechiano, ed. K. Frey, Berlin, 1892, pp. 56–7; Vasari (Am. ed., trans. E. H. and E. W. Blashfield and A. A. Hopkins, 4 vols., New York, 1913); E. Bertaux, Santa Maria Donnaregina e l'arte senese a Napoli, Naples, 1899; G. B. de Rossi, Musaici Cristiani, Rome, 1899; F. Hermanin, Gli affreschi di Pietro Cavallini in S. Cecilia in Trastevere, Le Gallerie Nazionali Italiane, V, Rome, 1902, p. 61 ff.; F. Hermanin, ThB, VI, p. 224; G. Ferri, Un documento su Pietro Cavallini, volume per le nozze Hermanin-Hausmann, Perugia, 1904; A. Venturi, Pietro Cavallini a Napoli, L'Arte, IX, 1906, p. 120; A. Venturi, Storia dell'arte italiana, V, Milan, pp. 153–68; C. R. Morey, Lost Mosaics and Frescoes of Rome, Princeton, 1915; S. Lothrop, Pietro Cavallini, Memoirs of the American Academy of Rome, II, Bergamo, 1918, pp. 17–24; P. Fedele, Per la biografia di Pietro Cavallini, Arch. della Soc. Rom. di Storia Patria, V, 43, 1920, pp. 157–9; Van Marle, I, p. 505 ff.; F. Hermanin, Due pitture inedite di Pietro Cavallini, R. Roma, I, 1923, pp. 403–6; A. Busuioceanu, Pietro Cavallini e la pittura romana del Duecento e del Trecento, EphDR, 1925, pp. 259–406; E. Lavagnino, Pietro Cavallini, R. Roma, III, 1925, pp. 305–13, 338–48, 385–93; A. Muñoz, Il restauro della Basilica di S. Giorgio in Velabro in Roma, Rome, 1926; L. Coletti, Esordi di Giotto, CrArte, June, 1937, pp. 104–7; L. Coletti, I primitivi, I, Novara, 1941, p. 37 ff.; E. Lavagnino, Il Crocefisso della Basilica di S. Paolo, RIASA, VII, 1941, pp. 217–27; P. Toesca, Giotto, Turin, 1941, p. 124 ff.; O. Morisani, Pittura del Trecento in Napoli, Naples, 1947, p. 26 ff.; R. Longhi, Giudizio sul Duecento, Proporzioni, II, 1948, pp. 5–55; E. B. Garrison, Italian Romanesque Painting, Florence, 1949; P. Toesca, Md, pp. 981–8; P. Toesca, Tr, p. 448; A. Prandi, Pietro Cavallini a S. Maria in Trastevere, RIASA, I, 1952, pp. 282–97; E. Lavagnino, Pietro Cavallini, Rome, 1953; P. Cellini, Di fra Guglielmo e di Arnolfo, BArte, III, 1955, pp. 215–29; J. White, Cavallini and the Lost Frescoes in S. Paolo, Warburg, 19, 1956, pp. 84–95.

Emilio LAVAGNINO

Illustrations: PLS. 105–110.

## CAVE PAINTING. See ARCHAEOLOGY; PREHISTORY.

**CELLINI,** BENVENUTO. Florentine goldsmith, sculptor, and writer (b. Florence, 1500; d. Florence, 1571). The son of an architect and musician, Cellini was apprenticed as a goldsmith and ultimately received commissions from princely and papal patrons for sculpture both small and monumental in scale. Cellini's spirited account of his stormy and colorful life has made him one of the most widely known figures of the Renaissance; his *Autobiography*, left unfinished in 1558 and finally published in 1728, enchanted Goethe, who made the first of countless translations. The autobiography also served as the basis for an opera, *Benvenuto Cellini*, by Berlioz (1837).

The restless pattern of Cellini's life was formed early in his career when at sixteen he was forced to flee his native city and spend several months in nearby Siena for participating in violent strife. He had already achieved great technical facility in his craft. From this time on he maintained an intense pride and absorption in his work, developed strong rivalries with other artists, engaged in endless quarrels, and pursued a life of constant travel. Among the most sympathetic traits in his curiously mixed character were devotion to his family and loyalty to the city of Florence. The latter remained strong despite his years of activity elsewhere, including short stays in Pisa, Bologna, and Venice and longer sojourns in Rome (1532–40) and Paris (1540–45).

In Rome, Cellini served Pope Clement VII and Pope Paul III, working chiefly on various minor objects, portrait medallions, coins, and jewels. An increasingly tense relationship with Pope Paul III and a series of violent incidents led to Cellini's imprisonment in Castel S. Angelo, a dramatic escape, and finally the journey to France. There Cellini served Francis I in different capacities — sculptor, decorator, and even designer of some architectural projects for Fontainebleau. He completed

for Francis I the famous and elaborate saltcellar (1543; Vienna, Kunsthist. Mus.) from a model prepared earlier (1539) for the cardinal of Ferrara. This, together with the bas-relief of the *Nymph of Fontainebleau* (1545; Paris, Louvre), is one of the relatively few surviving works by Cellini. His return to Florence, probably hastened by rivalry with Primaticcio, was followed by an extremely active decade executing for Duke Cosimo de' Medici a bronze portrait (Florence, Museo Nazionale), some figures of classical themes (wax and bronze studies, 1545–54, Florence, Museo Nazionale), and the bronze *Perseus* (Florence, Loggia della Signoria). These years saw a continuation of the pattern of Cellini's difficulties — a gradual intensification of problems with his patron and bitter conflicts with other artists, especially Bandinelli and Ammanati.

Cellini's autobiography breaks off in 1558, a year when he took preliminary religious vows which were never carried further, perhaps because of the complication of his domestic affairs. In his later years Cellini's productivity as a sculptor diminished; but he completed and published treatises on sculpture and the goldsmith's art (1568), married, and left two legitimate children.

The years during which Cellini lived were years of tension and crisis in every sphere — religious, political, social, and military. Cellini himself fought against the imperial troops in Charles V's sack of Rome (1527) and in the defense of Florence and Paris. This background of strife colors his writing and, at least indirectly, his sculptural style in its complexity and tension. His subjects were complicated by a wealth of allegorical allusions, and his style retained the qualities of the goldsmith's craft, with intricately wrought surfaces contrasted with highly polished smooth areas bounded by carefully chiseled edges and lines. The precious and elegant effect resulting from such contrasts was enhanced by his use of graceful, elongated figures. In his portrait of Duke Cosimo, a greater force is apparent in the tense pose and the biting characterization.

In his pride in technical ability and worldly success, in both his skepticism and superstition, his egoism and religious faith, Cellini seems to have been a typical figure of his day. He seems at the same time to be a virtual prototype of the romantic conception of an artist — a fiercely independent person living, according to his own code of behavior, a violent and intensely dramatic life. See also GOLD- AND SILVERWORK.

WRITINGS. Trattati dell'Oreficeria e della Scultura, Florence, 1568; La vita di Benvenuto Cellini, Naples, 1728; I discorsi e i ricordi . . . , Florence, 1857.

BIBLIOG. E. Plon, Benvenuto Cellini, Paris, 1883; H. Foçillon, Benvenuto Cellini, Paris, 1911.

Eleanor BARTON

**CELTIC ART.** Celtic art constitutes the most mature and original chapter in the evolution of art forms by the indigenous peoples of ancient west-central Europe. These forms were developed through a blending of local prehistoric traditions, Eurasian elements transmitted from the Orient over Continental routes, and preclassical and classical Mediterranean influences (see EUROPEAN PROTOHISTORY). The art of the Celts has definite stylistic characteristics, above all in the field of decoration, and occasionally in the handling of figures as well; these are revealed with considerable coherence through the entire area of expansion of the Celtic peoples and were handed down with singular tenacity throughout their history. In fact the Celtic artistic patrimony is sustained through the protohistoric period into the Roman era (see especially GALLO-ROMAN ART), and it continues through antiquity into the early medieval period, especially where the Celts had the opportunity for an autonomous existence and a cultural revival, as in the British Isles (see ANGLO-SAXON AND IRISH ART).

SUMMARY. Historical foundations (col. 175). Architecture (col. 179). Sculpture (col. 179). Decorative art (col. 180).

HISTORICAL FOUNDATIONS. One of the major achievements of archaeology and the history of ancient art in the 20th century

has been the discovery of the art forms of the "barbarian" cultures of Europe: those of the Italic, Celtic, and Iberian peoples. To students of ancient civilizations a new chapter has been opened, covering the attempts made by European peoples to fix their native imagery within the framework offered by Mediterranean classicism. Although the critical process of defining and evaluating these phenomena is still in process, we are in a position to discern with some clarity the fundamental character and development of Celtic art.

Its foundations lie in that great transformation of metallurgy which took place in Continental Europe during the 1st millennium B.C., when iron was substituted for bronze in the production of weapons, tools, and ornaments. This revolution made possible the establishment of a relatively homogeneous European culture that lasted for centuries, beginning with the so-called "Hallstatt" phase and continuing, from the 5th century B.C., with the La Tène phase, in which the main creators and carriers were the Celts.

The Hallstatt culture shows contacts, established across the Balkans and the Alps, with the Near East, with the Aegean, and with Italy (see MEDITERRANEAN PROTOHISTORY); across southern Russia and the Caspian steppes it reaches the centers of metalwork in the Caucasus and in central Asia, advancing as far as China (see ASIATIC PROTOHISTORY). On the other hand, about 500 B.C. a direct Oriental influence penetrated into central Europe with the Scythian nomads, whose presence has been clearly established by archaeological evidence; they were experts in metalwork. Although the Celts soon pushed them back beyond the Dnieper, Scythian influence on the formation of Celtic art was undoubtedly strong, especially with regard to animal motifs and the fantastic decorative vocabulary of curves, countercurves, spirals, and interlaces ultimately traceable to inner Asia (see also STEPPES CULTURES). The Eurasian impact on the development of Celtic art explains better than any esthetic theory its fundamental difference from the art of the Mediterranean.

But the importance of Mediterranean influences on Continental Europe, particularly from the start of Greek colonization and the vigorous thrust of Greek and Italic trade toward the North, should not be overlooked — notwithstanding the fact that too often there is a tendency to confuse trade connections with cultural ones. We have ample evidence of import from the Mediterranean world of pottery and metal vessels, of certain types of weapons and ornament, of coral and glass pastes, etc., and of building methods and techniques as well. The wealth of funerary objects found in the princely tombs of Vix in Côte-d'Or (Châtillon-sur-Seine, Côte-d'Or, Mus. Archéologique) and Reinheim in the Saarland (PL. 114) testifies to the taste of the tribal chieftains for imported works of art. These imports must have profoundly inspired Celtic bronzeworkers by suggesting new ways of giving expression to living forms.

However, we are not dealing only with indirect contacts. The Celts' restless and adventurous spirit of conquest and expansion determined the fundamental cycle of events in their history; it was the decisive element in the direct encounter between the Mediterranean and the European world. The Gauls, having spread from western Europe to the Danube, invaded Italy in the 5th century B.C.; in the 4th they entered Greece and established themselves in Asia Minor; their mercenaries were found in almost all Hellenistic armies (and it would be a grave error to minimize the function of these mercenaries in the development of Celtic art).

These manifestations of ethnic and political vitality have their counterpart in an indubitable artistic originality. As the heirs of ancient traditions of craftsmanship going back to the Neolithic and Bronze Ages, and enriched by Eurasian and Mediterranean influences, the Celts, if they took up themes and models, were capable of adapting and transforming them in accordance with their talent. In this connection the rather vague term "national genius" is not inexpressive. In the second phase of the Iron Age the modes of thought and life and the forms of art shared by the Celts within a wide territory had reached that high state of development and differentiation usually subsumed under the term "nation." The processes of reception, adaptation, and transformation produced new

forms that underwent a full development. The result was an art so well defined as to be readily identifiable both geographically and chronologically.

To interpret the art of the Celts as a conscious reaction of Continental European primitivism to Mediterranean classicism is only partially correct. The opposition between north and south goes back to prehistoric times and is without doubt a basic factor affecting all aspects of culture; it cannot be under-

Avoiding the balance of forces characteristic of classical Mediterranean art, this inorganic art covers the surfaces of stone or metal with a kind of embroidery of ornament, abstract in character or at least foreign to the real world, and reduces the forms of men, animals, or plants to an aggregate of spirals — and if, by chance, reasons of cult demand the representation of a living being, it refuses to make the image too similar to reality. However, this world of forms so far removed from life

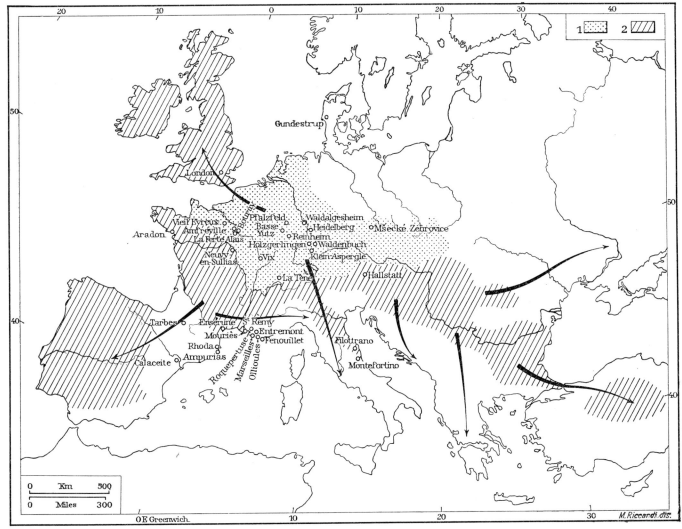

Spread of the Celts and places of archaeological and artistic interest. *Key*: 1) Original home of the Celts; (2) area of expansion (*adapted from Moreau*).

stood simply as an artistic dichotomy. The contrast persists even after the end of the ancient world, so much so that the hypothesis that certain forms of culture always correspond to certain spiritual predispositions is a tempting explanation. What we are dealing with is a fundamental divergence in mythological conception of the universe. The Celt lived in a world in which gods and heroes were always present, and he never knew whether he was dealing with men or with spirits. Man was subject to reincarnation, and it was possible for him to recall his former states of being. The world of the dead dominated the realms of ideas and of art. Like their later literature, full of mystery and hidden meaning, the art of the Celts translates the eternal process of exchange between our world and that of the dead. The Olympus of the Celts is different from that of the Greeks; there is an indeterminate boundary between the divine and the human — between gods and heroes conceived as superhuman but not supernatural beings who live and die but are limited in afterlife to haunting the earth. Like the Celtic epic, Celtic sculpture tried through the image of the hero to eternalize and magnify the cult of individual valor, personal strength, and spiritual energy.

is not one of pure imagination or of mere decoration. On the contrary, sculpture and ornament are full of significance, immersed in an atmosphere of myth and magic; the spirit that animates them rests on an individual and original conception of the world. Celtic art is based on the concept of the gods as warriors, healers, donors of goods, but also as artisans and teachers. It is not without significance that Manawyddan, Gobniu, and Pryderi are imagined, in the course of their travels, as goldsmiths, saddlers, and metalworkers, as owners or makers of miraculous tools. In the world of the Celts it seems difficult to separate the exercise of art from that of mechanical skills and of handicraft; this leads us to surmise that artists and artisans, grouped in corporations like those of the Middle Ages, worked under the protection of the great mythical artisans.

However, the Celtic society reflected in these manifestations had not yet passed the mental stage of the Greek and Italic peoples of the Geometric period. Hence an archaic, somewhat *retardataire* character — indeed, the character of a folk art in that religious themes are employed in which deities appear under zoomorphic forms or symbols.

It might seem illogical to speak of a national art in a society

represented neither by a definite ethnic type nor by a true and genuine nation in the political sense of the word, nor by a well-defined civilization of its own, if it were not that religion and art gave it unity within the geographical limits of the tribal territory.

Among the territories occupied and inhabited by Gallic tribes, one appears to have been especially fortunate in its contacts with the great routes of civilization in the ancient world: this was the area of Provence and Languedoc, bounded on the south by the Mediterranean and crossed by the "Road of Hercules." The latter, across southern Gaul, connected Italy with Spain; from south to north in the valley of the Rhone goods and influences were carried by water deep into the interior of the country. The crossing of these two routes determined the distinct character of this zone in contrast to the Continental Celtic regions farther north. The impact of Greek colonization of the Ligurian and Iberian coasts (starting with the founding of Marseilles by colonists from Phocis in Greece about 600 B.C.), the contact with currents of Etrusco-Italic culture, and the artistic developments among the local Ligurian and Iberian population reflecting Mediterranean art (see MEDITERRANEAN, ANCIENT WESTERN) were also elements that determined the particular character of the art produced by the Celts who had come into this territory. In some cases these elements were carried even farther afield.

ARCHITECTURE. Until the beginning of the Roman conquest Celtic life, at least on the Continent, was essentially rural, with urban development still rudimentary. The Celtic settlement was primarily a fortified village, the *oppidum*. In a sense the Celts were innovators in defensive construction; in choosing a site they looked for a natural projection such as the spur of a ridge which could be easily defended by a moat reinforced with earthworks and wooden palisades. The stability of the elements of the "Gallic wall" was assured by an interior structure of wooden posts (thus one might speak of competent carpentry rather than of true architecture). The urban and rural houses, developed from rectangular or circular huts, were also essentially connected with the technique of wooden construction. Exceptions such as the stone constructions of the British Isles must be attributed to regional geographic variations or surviving local prehistoric traditions. Typical of the Celtic dwelling in colder regions was the semisubterranean construction, reflected later in the cellars of Gallo-Roman houses.

In the south the building practices of the Mediterranean peoples, especially Greek techniques, had been known from early times; these systems tended to spread to the interior, toward the Celtic regions of the Rhine and the Danube. Greek techniques were used in stone fortifications — thus confirming the statement of Justin (a Roman writer of the 3d cent.) that the Celts had learned their military architecture from the Greeks — and in private houses, particularly in the Hellenistic period. The southern territories give evidence, in the plans of sacred buildings and also in cult images in sculpture, of the oldest and most intense activity in the field of religious architecture. Cult sites have been found at Mouriès, Roquepertuse, Entremont, Saint-Rémy, Nages (all Bouches-du-Rhône), and Ollioules (Var); they may be placed chronologically in the period from the beginning of the Hallstatt to the end of the middle La Tène phase. The plans of these sanctuaries do not show great differences. They are essentially *heroa*, tombs of heroes, sometimes on a monumental scale. The ornamental and symbolic elements are mainly of Mediterranean inspiration. The influence of this type of building was to spread widely over the Celtic world, even to the Danube area; it was still a characteristic element of local religious architecture in Roman times, especially in temple schemes consisting of a temenos, or enclosed sanctuary, preceded by a portico (see DANUBIAN-ROMAN ART; GALLO-ROMAN ART).

SCULPTURE. The sculpture that developed in southern France after the arrival of the Celts was strongly influenced by local Mediterranean as well as Etruscan and Greco-Oriental traditions of the representation of the human figure. The main type is that of the dead hero, conceived with hieratic immobility, following conventions inherited from archaic traditions, but with all the realistic detail of battle dress (PL. 111). Characteristic of the figure structure is a slender body with broad shoulders; correspondingly, the face is given a broad forehead. Both torso and face taper toward the bottom. Other common stylistic features are large mouths with straight, thin lips, pronounced cheekbones, deep eye sockets with bulging oval eyes and heavy eyelids, and hair shaped in domical fashion with decoratively stylized curls. Originating in the south, these stylistic formulas were broadly diffused in northern and eastern Europe, so that they became hallmarks of Celtic art as a whole.

The Celtic conception of the figure, altogether at variance with classical canons of proportion, bears the imprint of the individual personality of the hero. The main human type contrasts with that employed in the theme of "severed heads" (*têtes coupées*), which have the stiff and conventional appearance of masks (PL. 111). This theme was inspired by Greco-Italic concepts and iconography, but because of its essentially funerary significance became an important motif in Celtic art.

The sculpture of the Mediterranean Celts was not limited to the human figure; in addition there are fantastic and monstrous animals of ultimate eastern Mediterranean origin. These are found in Iberian and Celtic-Ligurian sculpture but became a favorite motif in Celtic art as well, possibly reinforced by the stimulus of late manifestations of the age-old animal art of Eurasia. Finally, the diffusion of representations of horses, due to Veneto-Alpine influence, should be mentioned.

The sculpture of the Mediterranean Celts is marked by a nobility and a grandeur that differentiate it from the rougher and more pronouncedly archaic work found in other parts of the Celtic world. Metalwork and stone sculpture of the Gallic sanctuaries of the Pyrenees, of the regions beyond the Loire, of the Rhineland, and of the eastern Celts in Czechoslovakia can seldom be dated accurately, especially since certain forms continue to appear up to the time of the height of the Gallo-Roman period. The repoussé metal masks of Tarbes (Hautes-Pyrénées; PL. 111) and of Vieil-Evreux, Eure (Evreux, Mus. Municipal) have moon-shaped faces, with broad cheeks, almost flat elongated triangular noses, and extremely oblique eye sockets which were probably filled with enamel or glass paste; hair and beard are stylized in double spirals, undulating lines, and scallops. The bronze statuette of a god from Bouray (Seine-et-Oise), patterned closely after the statues of heroes of southern Gaul, represents the last phase in the development of Celtic figure sculpture; the date is close to the Roman conquest, if not after it (PL. 113). The seated body is in repoussé, with the anatomy following an ornamental pattern; the head, cast in two separate pieces, front and back, is fastened to the body at the base of the hollow neck.

The freestanding stone sculpture of the northern Celts, for example the xoana, or pillar figures, of Greuten in Württemberg (Stuttgart, Landesmus.) and of Euffigneix (Haute-Marne; PL. 112), shows the inability of the artist to detach the members of the body or the religious attributes from the columnar core. This is still more clearly seen in works found between the Rhine and the Neckar — in the pillar from Pfalzfeld (PL. 112), in the statue from Holzgerlingen (Stuttgart, Landesmus.), and the head from Heidelberg (Karlsruhe, Landesmus.) — with their schematic faces flanked by heavy ornaments in the form of inflated bladders, a distant echo of the hairdress of the Egyptian goddess Hathor. The head of a Celtic chieftain from the *oppidum* of Mšecké-Žehrovice (Bohemia) dating from the end of the 1st century B.C. or the beginning of the 1st century of our era seems to be a translation into a block of limestone of a mask that decorated a bronze fibula (PL. 112). Its flat face and lack of volume recall the masks of Tarbes and Vieil-Evreux; noteworthy are the treatment of the eyebrows and mustache as curvilinear elements terminating in spirals and the geometric division of the ear into two volutes.

DECORATIVE ART. In the world of the Celts, attracted as they were to abstraction and geometric stylization, the most authentic expression, even in the treatment of figures, is to be

seen in that exuberance of decoration which covers the surfaces of a work with a fantastic vesture of entangled ornament. As the conception of art is predominantly two-dimensional, the animated form is sacrificed, transformed, schematized, dissolved by the irresistible pull to abstraction and geometry. This is expressed in an infinitely varied ornamental repertory — dogtooth, checkerboard, and zigzag patterns, circles, waves, and volutes. With these traditional Continental motifs surprising effects are achieved. The treatment of certain motifs tends toward a "flamboyant" style, in which curves oppose counter-curves, creating an extraordinarily variegated and complex mixture of teardrops, flame shapes, double spirals, curvilinear pinwheels, and chains. These designs may be deeply incised

Tène phase, and inserts of coral were used for enrichment. The use of coral, however, stopped suddenly in the 4th century; it was replaced by enamel, the scintillating polychromy of which does even more to enhance the effect of metalwork. Enamel-work abounds in the entire territory of the Celts, in Gaul, Celtic Spain, and Britain, where flourishing workshops produced shield bosses, personal ornaments, parts of weapons, and finials in champlevé technique. From these regions the technique passed to Ireland, giving birth to the splendid local production of the Christian centuries (see ANGLO-SAXON AND IRISH ART). Irish art was the heir of the techniques and the esthetic of the Continental Celts. The artist is closely linked with the aristocracy because his work is intended for the chieftains and for

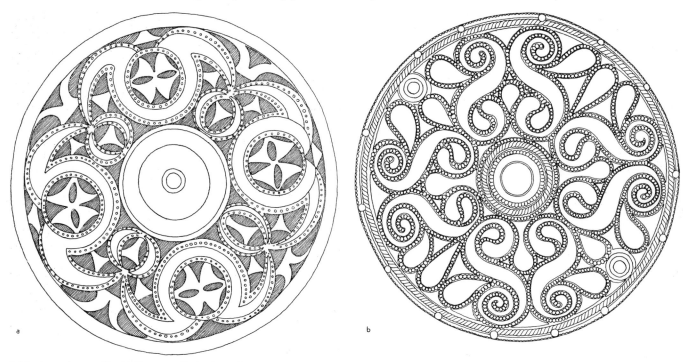

Celtic decorative motifs. (a) Bronze roll-rim from Somme-Bionne (Marne), 5th–4th cent. B.C. (*original, London, British Museum*); (b) gold appliqué disk from Auvers (Seine-et-Oise), 5th–4th cent. B.C. (*original, Paris, Cabinet des Médailles*).

into the surface of objects or delicately engraved, hollowed out or raised.

The decoration of objects, of swords, jewelry, cups, coins, shows the influence of the naturalistic ornament of the Mediterranean. The objects themselves may take on animate form, or organic motifs may be applied to them. The borrowed classical forms undergo changes as they meet northern motifs. The Greek palmette, for example, may become a curved pinwheel or a series of lozenges; classical foliate motifs may be juxtaposed with geometric patterns.

The decoration of the La Tène period continues to use the motifs of the Hallstatt stage but with an emphasis on greater harmony. Sometimes the ornament is austere, as in the relief bosses of the bracelets from Aradon (Morbihan); sometimes it reaches a baroque synthesis in combinations of triangular masks with dots, circles, and horns. Such combinations of the anthropomorphous and the geometric are found on twisted torques whose screwlike projections are tipped with floral motifs (Fenouillet, Haute-Garonne, and Lasgraïsses, Tarn; Toulouse, Mus. St. Raymond) and on fibulas, harnesses, chariots, and sword hilts. In some of this work polished coral pieces heighten the glitter of metal, for example in the vessels from Basse-Yutz (Moselle), produced during the 4th century B.C. by workshops in eastern Gaul. The animal motifs of their handles, reminiscent of Scythian, Altai, Siberian, and Chinese forms (see ASIATIC PROTOHISTORY), are mixed with abstract geometricizing ornament (PL. 115).

The ancient technique of pierced metalwork, already employed in the Hallstatt period, was taken up again in the La

the churches; he carries his age-old repertory of motifs and figures directly into the realm of Christian subject matter. For in the ancient ornamental patrimony the artist discovers a symbolism which makes it possible for him to progress smoothly from the pagan to the Christian world.

The Celts' rejection of naturalism in favor of stylization and symbolism is seen in a most extraordinary form in their coins (PL. 116). At first these were copies of the drachmas of Marseilles found in the valley of the Rhone and, from the 3d century B.C., in Languedoc, Roussillon, and the colonies of Marseilles in the Garonne basin. Toward the middle of the 2d century B.C. the stater of Philip II of Macedon, an international monetary unit in the Mediterranean world, penetrated the western Celtic area and became a highly prized coin. The currency used in the eastern Mediterranean area to pay the Celtic mercenaries in Hellenistic armies furnished models for widespread imitation in the Danube region.

The philippus — with the head of Apollo crowned with laurel on the obverse and a galloping horse-drawn chariot with driver on the reverse — was originally, like all the other coins, copied faithfully; but by a process of formal dissolution of the image it very soon lost its naturalistic aspect altogether and ended as an abstract schematization (FIG. 183). This process is the same everywhere: the various elements of the face are treated separately, isolated, rearranged, and grouped in balanced combinations of circles, palmettes, S motifs, pinwheel forms, and rinceaux. A strange effect of unreality is generated by this mélange, which might be taken as the expression of a disordered imagination were it not that it seems to translate into a now

obscure symbolism beliefs of which certain themes (severed heads, ships, horses' heads forming swastikas, overlapping pinwheels, rosette spirals) give us an occasional glimpse. There is a certain progression in the development of this deformation. In the territory of the Belgae the decoration of the coins of Tarentum (mod. Taranto) and the philippi are first transformed into a rich over-all surface treatment in which one element pre-

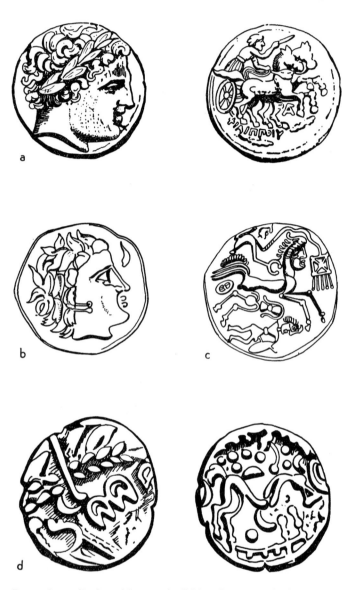

Progressive stylization of imagery in Celtic coins: type imitating the gold stater of Philip II of Macedon (obverse, head crowned with laurels; reverse, chariot). (a) Arverni, 2d cent. B.C. (obverse and reverse); (b) Aulerci Cenomani, 2d cent. B.C. (obverse); (c) Armoricani, 2d cent. B.C. (reverse); (d) Atrebates, 1st cent. B.C. (obverse and reverse).

dominates. For example, in a coin of the Bellovaci the hairdress spreads over almost the entire surface, while the area of the face is reduced to a minimum (PL. 116); later this decoration is split up into a series of rigid and static elements — a crown of laurels is transformed into a series of chevrons; the mass of hair forms an epsilon (ε). At the end of the period of Celtic independence these are the only clearly visible motifs on a round, formless mass, the last vestige of the face (FIG. 185). In the gold and copper coins of Brittany facial profiles are concave, like crescent moons, and the accentuated details of chin, eyes, eyebrows, and hair form curvilinear patterns. In the Rhineland the head is reduced to a single oversize eye.

The same development takes place in the case of the obverse of coins. The chariot of the philippus is combined with other themes; a Victory is transformed into a floating mass of hair;

one horse and one wheel stand for a chariot, the wheel becoming a rosette placed under the horse. In Brittany the horse has a human head and is set above figures with raised arms, reclining genii, wheels, and lyres, all possibly symbolic. The rider of such a horse carries a branch of mistletoe or a vexillum (banner of a Roman legion) as attribute. In the coins of the Elusates from Ampurias (Spain) the horse is nothing but a series of disks and lines. In the coins of Rhoda (mod. Rosas, Spain) a dolphin becomes a curved line and a rose a cross with various elements between the arms. The disintegration in the coins of Brittany is almost incredible: the body of the horse is attenuated, its legs are disengaged; the driver, the Victory, and the chariot are dissolved into a mesh of curved lines and dots, forming fan patterns or triangles above the back of the horse.

The realistic side of Celtic taste reappears in certain bronze coins found along the great commercial route linking Gaul, Switzerland, and Bohemia. The decoration of these coins is closely connected with the more naturalistic style of folk art. Human figures and animals are represented with an emphasis on movement rather than careful modeling. There are men sitting cross-legged, men carrying lances or wearing torques and walking with slow steps, goats standing upright, all caught in characteristic poses.

All these variations fall into stylistic groups that parallel the geographic divisions of the Celtic world. The central regions remain faithful to an archaizing stylization of classical types; elsewhere the trend is toward a freer interpretation that retains little connection with the models and may even transform them into ideograms. The individual regional styles interact with one another. Belgian coins were imitated in the British Isles, although the British Celts were more nearly related to the tribes of Brittany. The coinage of Brittany is close to Irish stone carving and foreshadows later Irish bronzework and manuscript illumination.

Related to the decoration of coins is the zoomorphic, astrological, and anthropomorphous ornament of the swords of the La Tène site; these traditional motifs are frequently combined with Greco-Oriental themes, such as the affronted goats on a sword signed by Korisios in the Historisches Museum in Bern.

In the 4th century B.C. numerous centers situated along the Rhine, in Switzerland and in Gaul, developed the so-called "style of Waldalgesheim," which spread across central and eastern Europe to the Balkans (cf. PL. 119). After this phase, which marked a high point, there was a turn away from geometric stylization and Eurasian influence toward closer contact with the classical civilizations of the Mediterranean. The result was the formation of a new decorative style, which was to lead to the "Hungarian arabesque style" and the development of monumental figure sculpture in southern Gaul. It seems as if during the last vital period of Celtic art the centers of production were displaced toward the east and south, while the old centers of the Rhine and of Gaul became arid.

Due consideration should be given to the diffusion of Celtic decorative art in Italy, especially in the region of Picenum, where the Celtic taste met and struggled with Greco-Italian models and formulations, producing a pronounced eclecticism. This trend is predominant in some objects of high quality, such as the goldsmith work from the tombs of Montefortino (Ancona, Mus Naz.); it is less manifest in the weapons that show the influence of the victorious Gauls (see ETRUSCO-ITALIC ART). A more compact and more purely Celtic development is found in the Spanish Meseta (PL. 117).

Celtic art made one of the most important contributions to the formation of European art. It was not only in Ireland that it survived. The artistic homogeneity imposed on the provinces conquered by Rome was only apparent; the old Celtic forms still remained a source of inspiration, especially in the geographically more isolated regions. In fact it is sometimes difficult to decide whether a work was executed during the last period of independence or under Roman rule. Particularly in the representation of divinities intended for popular devotion, the exterior aspects, attributes, and symbols of the ancient cults were retained, though the dress became Roman. In stone sculpture the artists harked back to the old mixed

wood-and-metal techniques; in bas-reliefs there still appeared squares and lozenges reminiscent of enamel decoration; in figures there was no visible relation between the drapery and the underlying anatomy. These popular tendencies were still more pronounced in the field of applied arts, especially in ceramics and metalwork. In the 3d century a group of goldsmith works marks a kind of Celtic renaissance in England, in Gaul, and in the Rhineland. The most outstanding example of the

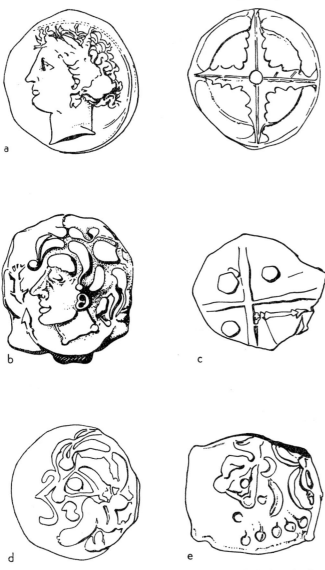

Progressive stylization of imagery in Celtic coins: type imitating the Syracusan silver stater, signed by Euainetos (obverse, female head; reverse, the rose of Rhodes). (a) Rhoda (mod. Rosas), Spain, 5th–4th cent. B.C. (obverse and reverse); (b-e) Volcae Tectosages, 2d–1st cent. B.C.

survival of Celtic taste is the Gundestrup cauldron, made in the territory of the Scordisci (middle Danube region) and found in Denmark; it displays all the variety of Celtic iconography, Celtic motifs, and Celtic stylization (PL. 118).

While it is correct to speak of a direct continuation, indeed of the last chapter, of Celtic art in the British Isles, especially in Ireland (see ANGLO-SAXON AND IRISH ART), it is no less true that the great decorative production of many European peoples during the Migration period was to be inspired, in varying degree, by techniques and motifs inherited from the decorative world of the Celts (see EUROPE, BARBARIAN).

BIBLIOG. S. Reinach, Les Gaulois dans l'art antique, Ra, XII, 1888, p. 273 ff., XIII, 1889, p. 11 ff.; Espér; J. Romilly Allen, Celtic Art in Pagan and Christian Times, 2d ed., London, 1912; J. Déchelette, Manuel d'archéologie préhistorique, celtique et gallo-romaine, III, Paris, 1913; S. Reinach, Catalogue illustré du Musée des antiquités nationales, Paris, 1921; RLV; British Museum, The Anglo-Saxon Antiquities, Guide to the Early Iron Age, London, 1925; M. Hoernes, Urgeschichte der bildenden Kunst, 3d ed., Vienna, 1927; P. Bieńkowski, Les Celtes dans les arts mineurs gréco-romains avec des recherches iconographiques sur quelques autres peuples barbares, Crakow, 1928; A. Schober, Zur Entstehung der Bedeutung der provinzialrömischen Kunst, ÖJh, XXVI, 1930, p. 9 ff.; A. Mahr, Christian Art in Ancient Ireland, Dublin, 2 vols., 1932–41; F. Henry, Emailleurs d'occident, Préhistoire, II, 1933, p. 65 ff.; P. Jacobsthal and J. Neuffer, Gallia Graeca, Recherches sur la hellénisation de la Provence, Préhistoire, II, 1933, p. 6 ff.; E. T. Leeds, Celtic Ornament in the British Isles Down to A.D. 700, Oxford, 1933; K. Bittel, Die Kelten in Württemberg, Stuttgart, 1934; W. von Jenny, Keltische Metallarbeiter aus heidnischer und christlicher Zeit, Berlin, 1935; A. Grenier, Sanctuaires celtiques et tombe du héros, CRAI, 1943, p. 360, 1944, p. 222; P. Jacobsthal, Early Celtic Art, London, 1944; R. Lantier and H. Hubert, Les origines de l'art français, Paris, 1947; F. Henry, Irish Art in the Early Christian Period, 2d ed., London, 1949; H. Hubert, Les Celtes depuis l'époque La Tène et la civilisation celtique, 2d ed., Paris, 1950; O. Klindt-Jensen, Foreign Influences in Denmark's Early Iron Age, Copenhagen, 1950; H. Vetters, Zur Frage der keltischen Oppida, Carinthia, I, CXLI, 1951, pp. 677–716; R. Lantier, Guide illustré du Musée des antiquités nationales, 2d ed., Paris, 1952; A. Malraux, Les voix du silence, Paris, 1952, pp. 129–42 (Eng. trans., The Voices of Silence, New York, 1953, pp. 131–44); O. Klindt-Jensen, Bronzekedelen fra Brå (The Bronze Cauldron from Brå), Aarhus, 1953; R. Joffroy, Le trésor de Vix (Côte-d'Or), Paris, 1954; L. Lengyel, L'art gaulois dans les médailles, Paris, 1954; W. Drack, Ein mittel-La Tène Schwert mit drei Goldmarken von Böttstein, ZfSAKg, XV, 1954–55, p. 193 ff.; F. Benoit, L'art primitif méditerranéen de la vallée du Rhône (Publications des Annales de la Faculté des Lettres d'Aix-en-Provence, N.S., IX), 2d ed., 1955; Musée pédagogique, Pérennité de l'art gaulois, Catalogue de l'exposition (Feb.–Mar., 1955), Paris, 1955; Musée des Augustins, De l'art des Gaulois à l'art français, Toulouse, 1956; R. Bianchi Bandinelli, Organicità e astrazione, Milan, 1956; A. Varagnac and G. Fabre, L'art gaulois, La Pierre-qui-vire, 1956; R. Wyss, The Sword of Korisios, Antiquity, XXX, 1956, pp. 27–28; Catalogue of the exhibition Kunst und Kultur der Kelten, Schaffhausen, Switzerland, 1957; O. Klindt-Jensen, Denmark before the Vikings, London, 1957; J. Moreau, Die Welt der Kleten, Stuttgart, 1958; T. G. E. Powell, The Celts, London, 1958; P. M. Duval, Celtica arte, EAA, II, 1959, pp. 457–67; O. Klindt-Jensen, The Gundestrup Bowl: A Reassessment, Antiquity, XXXIII, 1959, pp. 161–69.

Raymond LANTIER

Illustrations: PLS. 111–119; 5 figs. in the text.

**CERAMICS.** The term "ceramics," from κέραμος ("clay," "earthenware"), is generally used to designate objects modeled of clay and hardened by fire. These comprise a large number of types in all parts of the world, as the availability of clay and the ease of manufacture have made them a frequent and varied medium of expression. For this reason they are important to the study of the history both of civilization and of art.

Clay is used principally for containers and other useful objects made primarily for practical purposes, whose esthetic quality, as in other classes of functional objects, is a product of traditional taste and the adherence to established forms. For these objects the term "ceramics" has been adopted by students of ancient and primitive civilizations. But in its wider sense "ceramics" also embraces small terra-cotta objects (figurines, groups, reliefs, etc.) whose specific techniques often coincide with those of contemporary earthenware, especially in Western postclassical times and in the civilization of the Far East. In this case the purpose is esthetic and clearly related to the more general objectives of sculpture (q.v.). Further, we shall include terra cotta which has been modeled, painted, and glazed for the embellishment of architecture, at least within certain civilizations and within certain technical limits.

To this typological definition and classification, which is based on the *purpose* of manufacture, must be added a definition based on *technique* (terra cotta, faïence, porcelain, modern earthenware, etc.). Techniques are often highly specialized and elaborated within the individual classes and are an excellent instrument for the expression of current taste.

SUMMARY. General problems (col. 187): *Techniques and ceramic types: a. Terra cotta and its development, especially in ancient times; b. Glazed wares, faïence, majolica; c. Stoneware; d. Porcelain; e. Modern earthenware; Ceramic art: relation to sculpture, painting, and architecture.* Protohistoric "ceramic cultures" and cultures with protohistoric traditions (col. 196): *Origins of ceramics; Characteristics and development in Europe and Asia: a. Impressed ware; b. Incised ware; c. Painted ware; d. Monochrome ware; e. Protohistoric European pottery; Primitive cultures: a. Africa; b. Southeastern Asia and Oceania; c. The Americas: 1. North America; 2. Mexico and Central America; 3. South America.* The ancient world (col. 221): *Civilizations of*

the ancient Near East: a. Egypt; b. Mesopotamia; c. Syria and Palestine;¦ d. Anatolia; e. Cyprus; The Aegean and Greece: a. Bronze Age; b. Iron Age: proto-Geometric and Geometric styles; c. Archaic period; d. Attic red-figure and its origins; Pre-Roman Italy and the western Mediterranean; Hellenistic, Roman, and provincial pottery; Iran. Late antiquity and the Middle Ages (col. 245): Early Christian, barbarian, and Byzantine ware; Sassanian Iran; Islam: a. Origins; b. Period I: 9th–12th century; c. Period II: 12th–13th century; d. Period III: 14th century; e. Period IV: 15th–18th century; f. Hispano-Moresque ware; g. Tilework. Western ceramics in modern times (col. 259): The 15th and 16th centuries; The 17th and 18th centuries; Porcelain in the 17th and 18th centuries; The 19th century; The 20th century; Developments in the United States and European derivations. Folk art (col. 289). Asia (col. 292): India and southeastern Asia: a. Protohistoric period; b. Early historic and medieval period; c. Islamic period; d. Modern times; China: a. Neolithic and Shang-Yin period (1523–1028 B.C.); b. Chou period (1027–256 B.C.); c. The Han period and that of the Six Dynasties (206 B.C.–A.D. 221 and 221–589); d. Sui period (581–618); e. T'ang period (618–906); f. Sung period (960–1279); g. Yüan period (1260–1368); h. Ming period (1368–1644); i. Ch'ing period (1644–1912); Japan: a. Jōmon period; b. Yayoi culture; c. Tumulus period; d. Nara and Heian periods; e. Seto group; f. Karatsu ceramics; g. Porcelain.

GENERAL PROBLEMS. *Techniques and ceramic types.* The term "ceramic art" (or more properly "ceramic production") now designates the complex of operations necessary to the production of objects made of solid, nonmetallic, inorganic materials fashioned while cold and hardened by firing. Mechanical manufacturing methods since the industrial revolution in art have maintained these basic techniques but have greatly increased the range of substances usable as raw materials. Besides organic products, the definition of ceramics excludes cements and glasses (see GLASS) — cements because they lack the requisite consolidation by heat, glasses because they are formed while hot — and objects obtained with metallic powders, although they are formed while cold and consolidated by heat.

Clearly a classification based on the technique of manufacture covers a very large span of products all of which, however, can be assigned to a few main types. Some of these types or subtypes are of only practical or technological interest, e.g., refractories (useful for their properties of enduring high temperatures without softening) and artificial abrasives. In a broad sense these can be included among terra cottas, but as they are of no esthetic interest, they will not be considered here.

Ceramics have a white or colored body and are porous or compact in structure. They may also have one or more partial or total coatings (slip, varnish, glaze, enamel, luster). Various basic families can be distinguished for both body and coating: (1) terra cotta, with porous, colored body, with or without coating; (2) faïence (including majolica), with porous colored body and a coating of transparent or opaque glaze (especially glaze containing metallic oxides); (3) stoneware, with compact, vitrified colored body; (4) porcelain, with compact white body; (5) modern earthenware, with porous white body. Obviously such classifications are of use only for identification of techniques. In this sense specialists have adopted traditional terminology and terms used at specific times and in specific places (and therefore often of shifting meaning). Well-suited to modern production, they become inadequate if applied too rigidly to the products of the ancient world. Still, some of these types do correspond to certain historical traditions, as will be seen in the sections that follow.

*a. Terra cotta and its development, especially in ancient times.* The oldest and simplest product of the large ceramic family is terra cotta. The raw material, clay, is to be found almost anywhere. It has been used in differing degrees of purity — according to time and place — from the coarse primitive fabrics, which contained natural minerals and particles of carbon, to the finest clay fabrics (sometimes blackened by fumigation superficially or *in toto*, e.g., ancient Etruscan and American *bucchero* wares).

The primitive pot is fashioned either freehand or by applying the clay to a rudimentary mold (a basket, which after removal or desiccation leaves its imprint on the clay), or from a patty or "bat" (i.e., pressed or rolled out like a piecrust), or by the strip method. This last consists of systematically placing one above the other cylindrical strips of clay of varying thickness according to the dimensions desired and then joining them by manual pressure. Hardened in the sun, burnished when leather-hard with a stick of wood or bone or a stone to reduce the porosity, the object is placed directly into the coals for a rudimentary firing, which, by giving it a definitive consistency, changes its color. The resulting oxidation of metals in the paste (especially iron, the most common impurity in clay) creates occasional patches of lighter reddish spots.

The adoption of the wheel effected a revolution in the making of pottery, for by rotating his lump of clay, the potter was able to fashion symmetrical vases in round sections with finer walls of uniform thickness. This discovery, made in the ancient Near East, soon spread throughout the Old World.

Primitive potting equipment was later improved with the construction of the kiln with a grate, i.e., with a cooking chamber separated from the flames. More uniformly distributed, the heat completely penetrated the pot walls. The superficial spots disappeared, as did the bands of red and black formerly distributed from the most to the least fired (from the most to the least oxidized) according to the thickness of the clay. Firing in an atmosphere lacking oxygen made possible the perfecting of fumigation. Kiln firing also favored the development of painted ornamentation and the application of outer coatings whose waterproofing properties provided a good substitute for primitive burnishing.

In the ancient world these coatings generally had as base a blend of iron and manganese and tended toward the two tones red and black. Particularly important for metallic luster and fineness of application are the black "glaze" on Attic vases, whose imitation was vainly attempted outside Athens, and the red "glaze" on Arretine vases of the early Roman Empire, whose molded reliefs were copied after embossed metalwork. These last were largely diffused throughout Roman Europe (terra sigillata).

For decoration in relief the potter also used the barbotine technique, whereby slip clay was laid with a brush or a holder of some kind onto the surface of the vessel as soon as it was shaped. The custom, not unknown to pre-Hellenic potters, took hold in Hellenistic and late Roman times and gave rise to a polychrome barbotine decoration of white slip on a reddish ground or vice versa, which continued in use in the peasant pottery of many regions of Europe through the Middle Ages and even beyond the late Renaissance.

*b. Glazed wares, faïence, majolica.* In its broadest sense faïence can include all glazed wares, but in practice it applies primarily to glazed wares with a porous body.

From the earliest days of the civilized Near East, Iranian, Minoan, Mesopotamian, and Egyptian wares made of sand held together with a kind of cement were covered over with an alkaline glaze of quartz mixed with a flux of sodium and potassium. Later an admixture of metallic oxides, such as lead, produced a characteristic true lustrous polychrome glaze (especially green and white). The enameling applied to goldwork and metalwork (see ENAMELS) is an allied technique sometimes used in ceramics; channels or sockets impressed in the clay are thickly filled with varicolored vitreous enamels.

Glazed products, which were widespread in the ancient Orient, are generally of considerable esthetic merit. This is true not only of earthenware and small figurines but also of architectural decoration (e.g., the Neo-Babylonian reliefs on the Gate of Ishtar in Babylon, 6th cent. B.C.; the Achaemenian friezes in Susa, 7th–4th cent. B.C.). These represent the point of departure for a ceramic technique that was to have an imposing development in both Asia and Europe, not only in antiquity but especially in the Middle Ages and in modern times.

Outside the classical tradition which was to remain faithful to its clay pastes, the spread of this technique is already to be noted in late antiquity and the Byzantine world, which made free use of vitreous glazes, sometimes applied on intermediate layers of white slip. The imitation of precious metal pro-

totypes can be seen in the vases with molded decoration under a glaze of green or in a warm scale from ivory to ocher. Also imitative of metal prototypes are fabrics with fine decorations incised on the slip (sgraffito) so as to uncover the red color of the body, or with larger designs obtained with a spatula, or those with a depressed background, i.e., with the surface cut away, as in champlevé enamel, so as to display a light relief against the colored background. The resulting contrasts of ivory and white are sometimes heightened by the addition of dots of slip in another color beneath a clear glaze or more often under ocher or green glazes.

Stone models (agate, onyx, lapis lazuli) were imitated in marbled wares obtained by allowing a second, red slip with drops of ferrous, copper, or cobalt oxides to fall on the still-liquid white slip and then rotating the object. Mosaics also helped to encourage color development in Byzantine ceramics. Indeed, in some places on the edges of the empire — in Bulgaria and Asia Minor — there have been found tiny plaques and bits of molding of whitish clay painted in juxtaposed colors: brown, yellow, green-blue, rose, evidently in an economical attempt at the effects of the much more costly mosaic art. Painted polychrome decoration can also be found abundantly on earthenware, often with a characteristic blue color which reappears in later Italian majolica.

The use of glazes reached from the Near East as far as China in the Han dynasty (206 B.C.–A.D. 221), where pots and funerary terra-cotta figurines were glazed in a uniform color, green or brown, then in two colors, and finally, especially during the T'ang dynasty (618–906), with spots and speckles and the frequent addition of a grayish blue. The technical evolution of glazes seems to have followed the same rhythm in the West as in the Far East.

Excavations at Samarra indicate that Chinese porcelains, introduced at least as early as the 9th century, gradually brought back into fashion the white siliceous fabrics of Iran, Mesopotamia, Syria, Egypt, and later Asia Minor. With the old siliceous fabric the Islamic potters aspired to achieve the effects of porcelain. Suggestive of Sung models (960–1279) are designs incised or in very low relief that are brought out by the varying thickness — greater in the depressions, lesser on the surfaces or protruding parts — of the green, yellow, purple, or blue glazes. On the other hand, painted decoration in black, polychrome, or blue slip on a clear or more often green, turquoise, or blue glaze excited pictorial ambitions in the potters of the Far East, especially with the intensification of contacts under the Yüan dynasty (1260–1368), which contributed certainly to the spread and appreciation in China of Iranian precious minerals — particularly cobalt, which made possible a blue of intensity and purity not previously known.

The Near Eastern alkaline fluxes also contributed to a knowledge of glazes and enamels with a copper base of a turquoise color, used especially in wall facings. The opaquing of the glazes, thus transformed into enamels, furnished the basis for the use of colored pastes with a high percentage of clay as well as siliceous pastes. Decoration on top of an opaque enamel background — white or less frequently ivory, lapis-lazuli blue, and turquoise — was developed; in Iran it became the characteristic polychrome decoration of the *minai* and *lajvardina* types, obviously inspired by miniatures. Painting with metallic lusters over clear or opaque glaze was widespread in all Islamic countries. Luster pigments containing copper or silver especially (but other metals as well) are laid in a very fine film onto the glazed and protectively fired pot and refired in an atmosphere that is poor in oxygen and therefore absorbs the oxygen of the coloring oxides. The pigments, reduced to a metallic state, produce an iridescent surface wherever they have been applied.

Metallic lusters over glazed earthenware apparently prevailed in the products of the Abbassides (750–1258) at Samarra in Mesopotamia and of the Tulunid dynasty (868–905) at Fostat (Old Cairo) in Egypt (in contrast to the later fabrics of the Fatimid dynasty (909–1171) in Egypt and Syria and the Iranian wares, in which glazed siliceous fabrics obtained). They spread by way of North Africa to Moorish Spain, where they appeared in the 10th century as lustered earthenwares whose greenish tone was in the same tradition as those found in Samarra. These were perhaps imported.

"Hispano-Moresque" luster, which ranged from honey color to golden brown, had its own subsequent development. Pots covered with a cream-colored slip were fired sometimes with a blue pigment, in the *grand feu* — that is at the same temperature as the glaze, in which the pigment became inextricably incorporated — while the luster, like all the colors fired onto the glaze at a lower temperature in the *petit feu*, was only superficial. These methods obtained in the purely Moorish workshops of Málaga and Granada as well as in those of the 15th century and later, at Manises, near Valencia, and Barcelona, which came more and more under the influence of Western culture. Exportation to many European countries — to France, Flanders, and England and to Italy by way of Pisa, Genoa, Naples, and Venice — was considerable; it is assumed that these wares were given the name "majolica" after the nearest port of origin, the island of Majorca.

Oriental contributions became an increasingly important factor, especially where palette was concerned, in the evolution of medieval ceramics, which at least until the year 1000 remained faithful to late-antique and Byzantine traditions. The old and new processes are recorded in treatises: e.g., *Praeciosa Margarita Novella* by the Ferrarese doctor Pietro Bono Lombardo, who noted the proceedings of the potter in obtaining a glass by calcination of lead and tin (ca. 1330); and especially by the *Tre trattatelli dell'arte del vetro e del musaico* attributed to the Florentine Benedetto di Baldassare Ubriachi (b. 1337), who recorded and minutely described in Chapter 46 the method of preparing stanniferous glaze and in Chapter 40 that of preparing the nacreous luster of *maiolica*.

The technique of preparing the glaze and colors described by Ubriachi is also a springboard for numerous succeeding specialized treatises on the question, from Cennino Cennini (ca. 1370–ca. 1440) to Jerome Cardan (1501–76), Julius Caesar Scaliger (1484–1558), Vanoccio Biringuccio (1480–1539), and the theorist Cipriano Piccolpasso (1524–79) of Castel Durante, who dictated about 1550 his *Tre libri dell'arte del vasaio*.

The combustion of wine lees or the tartar from wine casks produces alkalis (carbonates of soda and potassium) which, mixed with siliceous sand and table salt (sodium chloride) and then fused together in a sagger (container) in the furnace, produce a "frit" or *marzacotto*. This frit is mixed with calcined lead, or galena (*cofollo* in Italy, *alcohol* in Moorish Spain, *alquifoux* in France), then newly fused and ground. When it is applied to the terra-cotta pot ("biscuit") and fired, it forms a transparent glass or crystal film on the surface. An opaque white glass or enamel can be obtained by the addition of tin to the mixture. Piccolpasso termed the joint oxidation of lead and tin, which in old workshops was achieved in a calcining furnace, *accordo* or *piombo accordato*. The process of coating the biscuit with the enamel which has been dissolved in water and applied while wet is called "glazing"; the ware thus enameled is "glazed" (see Cennini and Piccolpasso). The biscuit or *bistugio* covered with a white slip was said by Piccolpasso to be *sbiancheggiato*, or whitened — a term still used in Italian workshops.

The combination of metallic oxides (e.g., copper, iron, and antimony) with the frit and the use of minerals in their natural state (e.g., zaffer and manganese) produce the colors; they are sometimes mixed or superposed in order to widen the range of intermediary tones. The colors, distempered in water, are spread with a brush over the dry powdered glaze and are absorbed and incorporated into it during firing. A layer of clear glaze is often sprinkled over all as a final coat and fired at 900–20°C for a uniform brilliance. The immission of oxides of cobalt, copper, or antimony into the glaze colors it more or less intensely. Cobalt produces a grayish or pearly blue known as *berettino* in Romagna, *latesino* in Venetia.

The white glaze is prepared in different opacities and tonalities according to the use to which it is put (for the interior or exterior of the pot, as a background for decoration, or only as a waterproofing agent), to the period, and even to the workshop. In the earliest period, for example, the impure materials used and the scarcity of tin produced glazes which

barely covered and often leaned strongly toward a pinkish hue. In the deeper shapes (vases and jugs) the white glaze was applied only to those outer surfaces which were to receive the decoration, while the foot and the interior were made waterproof with clear glaze. In the flatter shapes (bowls and cups) it was reserved for the interior, which was the decorated area. After its perfection in the 15th century, white glaze was generally applied both inside and out and had, especially in the 16th century, a stable and glassy appearance in the potteries of Romagna and generally around the Adriatic; in Tuscany, Umbria, and Latium it was thinner and more fragile, with a tendency to chip. In Umbria, because of the requirements of luster — greenish brass-colored at Deruta and gold, silver, or ruby red at Gubbio — the glazes on pieces of the period were heavily plumbeous and were often laid on a slip background in order to facilitate the incorporation of the pigment during the third firing. In the potteries of the Marches (Castel Durante, Urbino) the tin glaze acted as binder for the colors and tints of *istoriato* ("narrative") decoration and was itself of a neutral tone, not very white or covering. The raised white tin-glaze backgrounds of Raphaelesque decoration were carefully brushed onto the uncolored parts only. Toward 1550 the composition and application of the glaze in the Faenza potteries was revolutionized. The changing of the ornamental style from polychrome *istoriato* to the sober *compendiario* style (a rapid, sketchy, impressionistic style) gave wide scope to the expression of form modeled and defined by a glaze left for the most part without overpainting. These potteries achieved an intensely opaque and milky whiteness with an enrichment of lead in the calcine and a thickness of application at least double that of previous glazes. It was the beginning of the *bianchi di Faenza* (Faenza whiteware), whose invention Piccolpasso appears to have attributed to the Duke of Ferrara, Alfonso II (1559–97). The volume of exportation of Faventine wares in the 16th century made the name of Faenza famous beyond the Alps. They were copied in France, then became known and adopted in other countries as "faïence," a substitute for the prior term of *lavori di preda* or *de vedrame*. The name *faenza* was also adopted in southern Italy, where the makers of glazed pottery are still called *faenzari*. After 1550 also in certain parts of middle and northern Italy the name *maiolica* lost its meaning of metallic luster derived from the Spanish origin of these wares and became synonymous with glazed faïence. In Spain, however, *pisa* was used for unlustered faïence painted in several colors, first imported from Italy and then produced locally.

It must also be noted that the term *porcellana* ("porcelain") was used in the 16th-century inventories to designate wares which were probably majolica. The confusion is the result of the influence exercised in the late 15th century by Oriental porcelain, which was prized as rare and exotic and which stimulated imitations in the majolica potteries that could easily be confused with true porcelain. In Holland throughout the 17th and 18th centuries the majolica from Delft, inspired by models imported in large quantities from the China of the Ch'ing dynasty in the ships of the Dutch East India Company, was called "Delft porcelain." Dutch commerce contributed to the introduction into England of the majolica wares of Delft and then to their production, so that in England majolica was called "delftware."

The introduction of porcelain into Europe made known the use of enamel colors on top of a tin glaze which had already been fired. These adhered only superficially, as they were fired at a lower temperature, about 600°C, known as *petit feu*; they were used by Dutch, French, Italian, and German potters in an effort to give the appearance of porcelain to majolica.

*c. Stoneware.* Stoneware, a ceramic product with a compact, opaque body that is almost without exception colored, is obtained with both simple natural clay and artificial pastes. The natural products are classified by some as vitrified terra cottas. To this group belong also the "clinkers" (bricks) and commercial stonewares made from a mixed paste and used in architecture, the latter often being colored artificially. Also

artificially colored are various types of 18th-century stoneware made by the factory of Josiah Wedgwood in England: e.g., the "black basalt" or "Egyptian ware" and "jasper ware," with an unglazed blue, lilac, or green body as a background for applied white relief decoration. Stoneware is an extension of terra cotta: the peculiar nature of a few clays or the addition of fluxes as correctives causes the paste to lose its porosity when fired at 1200–1300°C. The process was discovered spontaneously and independently in both the Orient and the West. In the Orient stoneware led to porcelain; in the West, much later, to modern earthenware.

That stoneware was known in Europe after the late Middle Ages is attested by examples preserved in the Altertumsmuseum at Mainz; in the Rhineland between Coblenz and Cologne, in France in the region around Beauvais, and in the Low Countries both south and north it was used for utility wares.

Molded wares were added to the wheel-thrown or hand-modeled wares late in the 16th century; casting was added more recently. Decoration in relief (impressed on the moist clay of the newly thrown pot or molded separately and then applied) and incised decoration are characteristic of Europe. Because the paste is so fine-grained and the vitreous shell of the glaze is so thin, the relief decoration retains all its immediacy. The glaze on stoneware is the result of the introduction of table salt to the kiln during the firing: the temperature decomposes the salt, and the sodium combines with the silica in the paste to form a vitrified surface. The use of a slip as well as firing in a reducing or oxidizing atmosphere turns the pot a characteristic gray or rusty color. Near-white fabrics are also produced.

Stoneware is sometimes provided with thicker alkaline lead glazes. Here the decoration results from the effects of devitrification, crystallization, etc. (similar to the frost on window glass), which occur during cooling in the kiln. Another deliberate art is *flambé* glazing: it consists of the reduction of copper oxide present in the glaze in the atmosphere of the kiln, thus conferring on the subject a brilliant blood-red color with a tendency toward violet.

Stoneware decoration has also been varied with polychrome glazing or enameling and the application of cobalt or manganese glazes to certain details; e.g., in the 17th and subsequent centuries on German beer tankards, especially at Kreussen (Bavaria). In the Orient stoneware is often also painted brown, black, or white.

*d. Porcelain.* Porcelain has a white, translucent, extremely fine-grained body whose qualities lend themselves to certain types of plastic and pictorial expression. The invention of Chinese potters, this refined product was discovered gradually from the compact stoneware bodies made up of petuntse (*pai tun-tzŭ*) and kaolin (*kao-ling*), or white china clay. The long period of transition from one to the other makes it difficult to distinguish the structure of stoneware from the more complex product we define as "porcelain." In the past the distinction was based only on the whiteness, translucence, and nonporosity of the latter.

The oldest surviving examples of Oriental porcelain are preserved in Japanese temples. The oldest-known in the West are the previously mentioned examples found at Samarra in Mesopotamia. The first person to have spoken of it in Europe and to have given it the name *porcellana*, which was to be universally adopted (alongside "china," widely in use in the modern English-speaking world), seems to have been Marco Polo (1254?–1324). Detailed information as to the techniques of Chinese porcelain reached Europe only in the 18th century, in the *Lettres édifiantes et curieuses* (1712–24) of the Jesuit Père d'Entrecolles.

In the prosperous late T'ang period (618–906) and under the Sung (960–1279) porcelain was given plastic or incised decoration under a monochrome white or colored glaze which, accumulating in little pools in the low parts, created a delicate motif of overcolor. The commonest glaze was a ferrous envelope of varying shades of jade green, known in Europe as "celadon," which also covered large crude stoneware vases from Martaban. Also, the "hare's fur" and *œil de perdrix* ("partridge-eye")

glazes have a ferrous coloring base: the first are mottled with brown and black; the second, on bowls known by the Japanese as *temmoku*, are dotted with black and white. But copper was at the base of the *flambé* glazes of various shades of vivid red splotched with lighter areas of blue or vice versa. To this family belong the reds known as *sang de bœuf* ("oxblood") or "pig's liver." The Chinese obtained a special tonal effect (a large or small network of crackle) by mixing a certain kind of stone in the glaze and thus artificially differentiating the coefficient of dilation of body and glaze.

Painted decoration under glaze in cobalt blue or ferrous red appears under the Mongolian invaders who established themselves as the Yüan dynasty (1280–1368); they facilitated contacts with Middle Eastern and Islamic countries and made their rich cobalt known in China. Decoration in blue was much developed under the following local Ming dynasty (1368–1644), and the style and technical development of porcelain were influenced by the manufacture founded in Ching-tê-chên by Hung-wu, first Ming emperor, to service the court at Nanking, later at Peking. Polychrome Oriental modes were added to monochromy; decoration in enamel or glaze was traced onto the biscuit, while designs were outlined in relief (much like cloisonné) or painted under the glaze; in the latter case colors were mixed with organic adhesives for immediate adhesion as well as with fluxing agents for permanent adhesion to the glaze after firing.

The Ch'ing dynasty (1644–1912) continued the traditional fabrics and developed polychrome overglaze decoration: the five-color group known as the *famille verte*; the *famille noire* (*famille verte* on a black ground); and the *famille rose*. Ch'ing potters also developed a technique for achieving a close-grained powder-blue ground, known in Europe as "blue *soufflé*," which was blown onto the body through a tube. This often was given an overdecoration of gilt, yellow, or green arabesques.

In 15th- and 16th-century Europe descriptions and the few pieces which arrived from the Orient by caravan generated attempts at imitation. The only one of these to have been developed subsequently was made at Florence about 1575 by Francesco Maria I de' Medici, grand duke of Tuscany (1574–87), in collaboration with potters from Faenza and Urbino. His recipe for "Medici porcelain" included a frit of white sand, rock crystal, and salt, fused together and then mixed with a white clay, and a coating of plumbeous glaze made from a similar frit. This was an artificial soft porcelain which late in the 17th century and early in the 18th was to appear in France and bring fame to French production in this medium. To this tradition also belonged the phosphatic English porcelain, or "bone china" (with calcined bones used as flux, and a lead glaze), as well as the soft-paste porcelain containing magnesia, characteristic of the Officina Reale in Vinovo (near Turin), established about 1770 by Giovanni Vittorio Brodel and then entrusted to Vittorio Amadeo Gioannotti (1729–1815).

Hard porcelain similar to the Chinese prototypes was the fruit of the research conducted at Meissen, near Dresden, for Augustus the Strong (elector of Saxony and king of Poland) by the alchemist Johann Friedrich Böttger (1682–1719) in collaboration with the celebrated physicist Ehrenfried Walther von Tschirnhausen (1651–1708). The first laboratory pieces, which followed preliminary works in red stoneware, appeared in 1708; Böttger then made up a "mother-of-pearl" luster glaze (pale purple in color) and studied and constructed kilns, but at his death he had not succeeded in discovering the composition of either the *grand* or *petit feu* colors which his successors, among them Johann Gregor Heroldt (or Höroldt, 1696–1765), adapted. The hard porcelain of Meissen and other European potteries can be distinguished from Oriental wares primarily by an esthetic appraisal of form and decoration, but it, of course, displays a constant attention to exotic models.

Another type of porcelain is "biscuit," unglazed porcelain that enjoyed a great vogue in the late 18th century, its dense white surface suggesting the characteristics of marble.

*e. Modern earthenware.* This type, with a porous white paste, was the last to appear in order of time. Perfected in England during the 18th century, it developed from earlier efforts of John Dwight of Oxford (1637?–1703), at Fulham in Staffordshire. The fine-grained white paste which, when thin, was translucent, was made with light-colored plastic clay and calcined ground "flints," after the methods of German stoneware production.

The original product, indeed, was from Staffordshire, a white-paste stoneware with a salt glaze added during the firing. From the same paste, fired at a lower temperature and therefore not vitrified, comes a lead-glazed earthenware whose persistent ferrous impurities give a yellow-ivory tone that earns it the name of "creamware." It was cast in bronze, alabaster, or terra-cotta molds in which the decoration was already incised. After 1750 the body was often diluted to slip, poured into a plaster-mold, and cast. Salt-glazed ware was decorated with molded or incised reliefs or painted with enamel colors which were fixed in the *petit feu*. The incised decoration was sometimes heightened with blue paste (known as "scratch blue") so as to appear in relief on the finished pot. Decoration of lead-glazed ware, other than relief and pierced work, was a polychrome marbleizing — either exterior ("tortoise shell") or in the paste itself ("agateware") — or a black ("black ware") or green glaze.

A factory on an industrial plan for the production of utilitarian ware was established by Josiah Wedgwood (1730–95) at Burslem in 1759; the protection granted by Queen Charlotte resulted in the name "queen's ware" for creamware. This was generally undecorated, but later the collaboration of John Sadler (1720–89) and Guy Green (b. ca. 1749) of Liverpool resulted in the introduction of transfer printing. The system of distributing among various shops the different phases of manufacture — shaping and firing, decoration — was instituted and made famous by Wedgwood, who maintained it even when in 1769, together with Thomas Bentley, he established a new factory, "Etruria," for the production of ornamental objects.

Giuseppe LIVERANI

*Ceramic art: relation to sculpture, painting, and architecture.* In objects and in parts of monuments made of terra cotta, glazed or unglazed, a practical end does not necessarily exclude esthetic value. Even within the limits imposed by function there is a certain freedom in the selection of forms; and a variety of developments, traditions, and innovations is therefore possible. Such freedom, such a variety of development, is obviously absent in the production of parts and objects used in construction, such as bricks — which, if they relate to art, do so for other reasons (see STRUCTURAL TYPES AND METHODS) — or in the metallurgical, chemical, and electrical industries. Even thus limited, the field of ceramics covers a wide range of objects, but the term is generally applied to the production of receptacles, these being the oldest and most widespread of all utilitarian objects.

Probably from earliest times pottery was assigned functions beyond the immediate practical ones. Objects were made to be offered to divinities, to be deposited in tombs, to be given to important personages, or to satisfy standards of taste or a demand for luxury. Such aims, as well as the artist's inventiveness and considerations of cost, contributed to the continual refinement of techniques, to the creation of ever more harmonious forms, and, of course, to the use of decoration.

It would be impossible — indeed, it would be an error — to separate the history of ceremonial ceramics from that of contemporaneous domestic wares or to apply the name of "art" to the former only. Especially in the ancient world and less-developed cultures the two are closely interlinked and usually indistinguishable; customary forms are constantly observed to affect the shapes of costlier products, while the technical and decorative innovations of the ateliers attached to temples, courts, and the nobility are reflected in the general production. One can only recognize that in certain cultures ordinary pottery tends to reproduce more archaic types and embody coarser techniques ("coarse ware"), and that in others ceramic products are created for a consciously esthetic purpose, in specialized

shops and factories and even by masters who feel the personal value of their work and underline it with a signature, first in ancient Greece, then from the Renaissance to the present day. A modern factor is the industrial standardization of domestic wares, often after good designs and under the seals of traditional manufacture.

Broadly considered, ceramic wares represent current taste in both form and decoration and are therefore an integral part of the history of culture and the history of art. Vase forms, either modeled by hand or wheel-thrown, reflect the plastic sense of craftsmen and, indeed, constitute one of its most basic expressions. Within the special conditions imposed by function, essential forms, pleasing and often of great elegance, are sought and found. But often a more knowledgeable and complex use of plastic methods enriches the basic forms of body, handles, and mouth and contributes to their embellishment with figured or abstract ornament. The decoration is sometimes in relief or molded (often in imitation of *repoussé* metalwork, as in the fine Hellenistic-Roman pottery with a coralline glaze known as "terra sigillata"); occasionally it is in the round; or it may be an admixture of complex forms, ornamental articulation, and applied relief, at times pompous, overdecorated, and devoid of positive esthetic values. Of particular interest are pots partially or totally shaped in imitation of other forms: inanimate (wooden boxes, casks, baskets, etc.) or animate (flowers, animals), sometimes human. Even in remote times a symbolic parallelism has existed between the individual parts of a pot (still called "foot," "body" or "belly," "neck," "mouth," "lip," etc.) and the corresponding members of a person. Hence, no doubt, the appearance of anthropomorphous vases in civilized areas quite independent of one another, such as Trojan vases (3d millennium B.C.), Egyptian and Greek balsam containers, Etruscan funerary urns of ancient Clusium (known as "canopic"), or pre-Columbian pottery in Peru. In modern Western wares the vessel's form is not bound to traditional types but depends entirely on the fancy of the artist. The same holds true for fictile statuary.

Besides the essentially plastic qualities of pottery, the modifications of surface through design and color are also of esthetic interest. Color plays a role even before the application (or deliberate omission) of extrinsic decoration, as it results from the quality of the paste and the procedures of firing, of burnishing, and finally and primarily of glazing. Some monochrome products equal and, indeed, surpass many-colored pots in elegance and purity of chromatic effect — so much so that in some cultures they were knowledgeably preferred. This is true of protohistoric pottery, Greek black-glazed vases, faïence and porcelain with monochrome glazes, etc.

Surface decoration can be achieved by impressing, punching, incising, molding, etc., with eventual addition of white or colored pastes; by brushing designs directly onto the burnished or slipped opaque paste; by leaving figures in the original color of the ground when painting with slip or glaze, or finally by the application of polychrome glazes. The possibilities for thematic development of incised design are naturally more limited, geometric rectilinear motifs being preferred, while painting allows every kind of ornament and figure drawing.

Whatever their sources of inspiration or their development, ceramic painting and design are generally conditioned by the form of the object and the space to be decorated. In the simplest and oldest productions, but also to a greater or lesser degree in all others, decoration accompanies and underlines the plastic elements of a pot, delimits them, and points up their contours. Typical, constant motifs are created for the individual ornamental sections (mouth, rim, feet, etc.) and are often repeated across the centuries through major cycles of ceramic civilizations or transmitted from one to the next. Bands, rays, meanders, palmettes, ivy leaves, interlace, grape clusters, etc. (see also ORNAMENTATION) are recurrent motifs. The decorative scheme, whether geometric, floral, or representational, generally is closely related to the shape of the object. Compositions with figures are adapted to the available fields — for example, to the round centers of cups and plates. The surface of large vases, however, are sometimes subdivided into

sections, each containing a separate composition. More rarely minute ornament, seemingly inspired by the decoration of materials and rugs, is spread over the entire surface of the object, without regard for structure. It is difficult to say at what point these paintings, monochrome or polychrome, reflect models from "high art." In some cases derivation is demonstrable; in others one is reminded of original works or at least of filterings through the invention of ceramic painters endowed with a truly personal style, as in ancient Attic vase painting or in modern ceramics. But as a whole, "ceramic painting" belongs to the field of painting (q.v.) as a special rather than as a "minor" category. It is clear that ceramic wares, so far as function, forms, and certain aspects of decoration are concerned, are closely interrelated with vessels of other materials — e.g., stone (which appears to have preceded clay pots somewhat in time), wood, metal (see METALWORK), glass (q.v.), and, more recently, artificial compositions — not to mention natural containers (e.g., gourds) and baskets (see BASKETRY). A continuous process of imitation occurs among these different types. Save for the initial inspirations given by natural containers and baskets to the earliest pottery (see below), this imitation is generally exercised as the influence of more costly material on the less costly, principally of metal on pottery. Fictile statuary, unhampered by such structural requirements as that imposed by the hollow form of a pot, allows full freedom of expression. Generally, although not necessarily, produced in the same technique as pots and plates, it is included with "ceramics" primarily because of the identity of methods of manufacture and therefore of fabric, especially in China and the modern West. On the other hand, the common, simple, unglazed figurines (usually painted in polychrome colors) of the classical world are not generally designated as ceramics. Terra-cotta statuary, major or minor, enters rather — even though with its own technical and stylistic qualifications and special functions — into the field of sculpture (q.v.). Similar considerations hold true for reliefs.

Architecture has largely availed itself of ornamental clay products for wall facings and pavements. Architectural terra cottas, both archaic and classical (sometimes made by the same methods as pots), belong to this category, even though, like figurines, they are not generally included among ceramic works. The glazed tiles of Mesopotamia, Egypt, and Iran, on the other hand, are included here; their techniques and traditions were highly developed in the Islamic world, as is evident in the superb glazed tiles (*azulejos* and *regolas*) of Spain. Modern Europe has made full use of this technique in pavements and glazed wall tiles.

\* \*

PROTOHISTORIC "CERAMIC CULTURES" AND CULTURES WITH PROTOHISTORIC TRADITIONS. *Origins of ceramics.* Pottery making first made its appearance with the stabilization of food-gathering communities and among agricultural peoples in the Orient, Europe, and around the Mediterranean during the shift from mesolithic to neolithic cultural stages.

Some authors believe that the shape of certain primitive pottery was dictated by that of receptacles made of animal skins or vegetable materials (especially gourds). Further, the shape of the round-bottomed pots of the earliest neolithic periods in Europe, Africa, and Asia, as well as their usually impressed decoration, suggests that baskets of woven vegetable fibers (e.g., in the excavations of predynastic sites in the Fayum), daubed on the inside with clay, gave rise to the form and decoration of the oldest pottery, after the removal of the basket itself.

More concrete than the problem of how pottery came to be made are the questions of where and why. Recent radiocarbon analyses would assign the prepottery Neolithic era (with or without the presence of stone vessels) to the late 7th and early 6th millenniums B.C., in both the Near East (Jericho) and the Middle East (caves of Hotu and Belt in northern Iran), and the oldest pottery-making cultures, at least in Iran, to the second half of the 6th millennium. In Jericho the moment of passage from one phase to the other is more clearly discernible: after the neolithic strata which contain vessels

made only of stone, there follow levels containing first soft, sun-dried pottery of pure clay, later of crudely fired clay mixed with chopped grass, and finally of clay mixed with siliceous materials; but from the first all have painted decoration in bands of red or brown. Also of coarse body and imperfectly fired are the large pots in the deepest levels at Hassuna, probably one of the oldest inhabited areas of northern Mesopotamia. A body of clay mixed with chopped grass is to be found at Jarmo on the Kurdistan plateau at the site of successive neolithic prepottery settlements, but here radiocarbon dating shows a much later passage from one state to the other.

At any rate it is probable that these fabrics originated in western Asia, and from there they must have spread both east and west to most inhabited areas.

*ramikum* — R. Pittioni), the full development of the cultures predominantly characterized by their pottery extends also to the age of metals or at least to stages in which metalwork is already present (as much in western Asia and the Mediterranean as in eastern Asia and the Americas). A unified study of these cultures as far as it concerns pottery, however, is justified by the wide diffusion of "classes" with substantially uniform and continuous appearance in certain areas and different times.

*a. Impressed ware.* One of the earliest efforts at ornamentation of pottery is the rough application of minute impressions to the outer surface of a vase ("impressed ware"; FIG. 197). In the area of its primary diffusion (southern Anatolia, Syria, northern Mesopotamia) this class seems at least as old as the

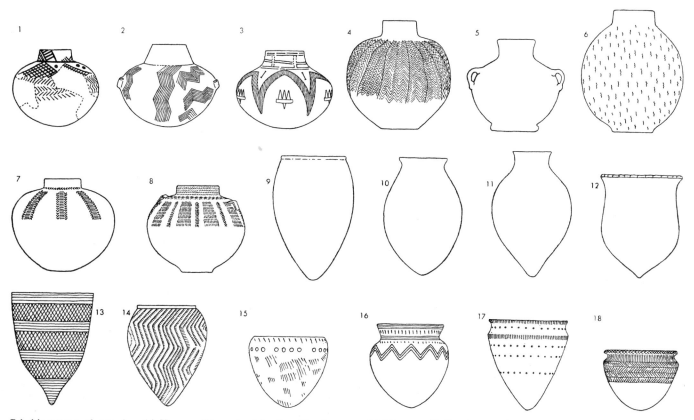

Primitive stages of ceramics. (1) Hassuna (Mesopotamia), 5th millennium B.C.; (2) Matrensa (Sicilian impressed ware), late 4th millennium; (3) Frankfort on the Main (*Bandkeramik* culture), 4th millennium; (4) Hassuna, 5th millennium; (5) "cardial" ware, Iberia, 4th millennium; (6) Terlizzi (impressed Apulian ware), 4th millennium; (7) Novosvobodnaya (Pontus I), 3d millennium; (8) Złota culture (Poland), late 3d millennium; (9) El Amrah culture (Egypt), 4th millennium; (10) Maadi culture (Egypt), late 5th millennium; (11) El Garcel (Spain), late 4th millennium; (12) Ertebølle (Denmark), 5th millennium (?); (13) early Jōmon (Japan), early 3d millennium (?); (14) Afanasievo culture (north-central Asia), 3d millennium; (15) central Russia, 4th–3d millennium; (16) Yatskovice, Kiev (Pontus culture, middle phase), late 3d or early 2d millennium; (17) *Kammkeramik* culture (Baltic), 4th–3d millennium; (18) Peterborough culture (England), early 2d millennium.

*Characteristics and development in Europe and Asia.* Earthenware was of relatively greater importance to the ancient world than to our civilization, whose technological structure has made for an extreme variety and complexity of instruments needed to satisfy the most elementary requirements of life. In more advanced civilizations of the ancient world pottery assumed the character of a specialized production. On the other hand, early historical cultures and the Neolithic Age that immediately preceded them seem to have been predominantly dependent on pottery and its many uses, granted, of course, that all wooden objects and textiles that may have been wrought in these remote periods have perished. Pottery therefore serves to distinguish these early cultures — in fact, sometimes to provide a qualifying name for them, so that one speaks of a "Banded-Pottery culture" (*Bandkeramikkultur*) or a "Geometric" one. Pottery constitutes the surest guide to the classification of stages of development, local variants, etc. Although to some authors it has seemed possible to define the "Neolithic Age" or "neolithic cultural level" by the term "Ceramic" (*Ke-*

earliest painted wares (Jericho, Hassuna), with which, indeed, some of its shapes offer interesting comparisons. Of a generally dark body, from blackish to reddish, this ware is often burnished and sometimes decorated with very simple geometric motifs, incised before firing (and then sometimes filled with white substance) or scratched after firing. Polishing is also fairly frequent. But the impressed technique assumes particular importance in the regions around the Mediterranean (North Africa, Iberia, southern France, Liguria, Apulia) and in the islands (Sicily, Malta). In the Aegean (Crete), in continental Greece (Sesklo), in the Balkans (Starčevo, Vinča), and in the region of the Danube (Körös) impressed ware is found at the deepest levels of neolithic settlements. Especially near the coast and on the islands the decoration of this type shows the imprint of the largely food-gathering economy of the community, as their makers used the lips of spiral shells to make their designs (especially the Cardium or cockle shell, whence the name "cardial" for a whole class of pottery). But wherever impressed ware survives until the influx of painted-pottery

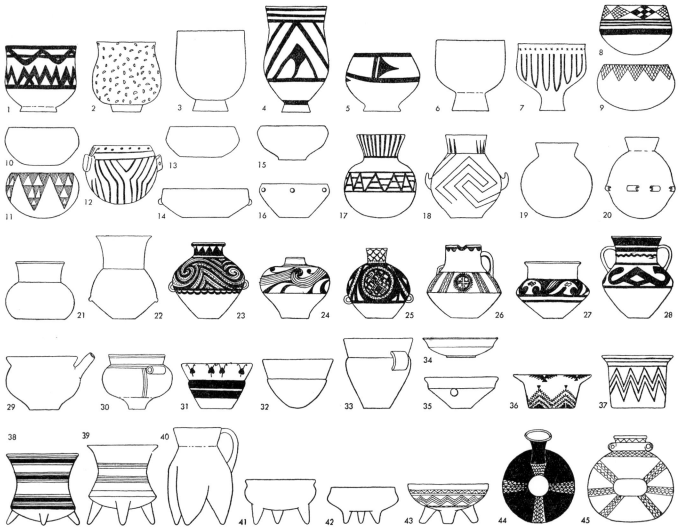

Protohistoric painted wares and related types. (1) al-'Ubaid (Mesopotamia), 4th millennium B.C.; (2) Körös culture (Hungary), 4th millennium; (3) Ripoli (Abruzzi, Italy), late 4th or early 3d millennium; (4) Periano (India), late 3d millennium; (5) al-'Ubaid, 4th millennium; (6) Körös culture, 4th millennium; (7) Bubanj (Yugoslavia), late 4th millennium (?); (8) Tepe Gawra (Mesopotamia), 4th millennium; (9) Chassey culture (France), 3d millennium; (10) Samarra (Mesopotamia), early 4th millennium; (11) Matera (Apulian-Materan scratched ware), 3d millennium; (12) *Bandkeramik* culture (Austria), 4th millennium; (13) Samarra, early 4th millennium; (14) Upper Austria (Painted Ware culture), 3d millennium; (15) Tell Halaf (Mesopotamia), early 4th millennium; (16) Upper Austria (Painted Ware culture), 3d millennium; (17) Samarra, early 4th millennium; (18) *Bandkeramik* culture (Austria), 4th millennium; (19) Tell Halaf, early 4th millennium; (20) Michelsberg culture (Germany), 3d millennium; (21) Tell Halaf, early 4th millennium; (22) Strelice (Moravia), 3d millennium; (23) Yang-shao culture (China), late 3d millennium; (24) Tripolje culture (Ukraine), 3d millennium; (25) Ma-ch'ang culture (China), first half of 2d millennium; (26) Ljubljana culture (Yugoslavia), late 3d millennium; (27) Cucuteni culture (Romania), 3d millennium; (28) Yang-shao culture, late 3d and early 2d millennium; (29) Tell Halaf, early 4th millennium; (30) Serra d'Alto (Apulian-Materan painted ware), 3d millennium; (31) Tell Halaf, early 4th millennium; (32) Windmill Hill culture (England), late 3d millennium; (33) Setteponti (Apulian-Materan ware), 3d millennium; (34) Samarra, early 4th millennium; (35) Upper Austria (Painted Ware culture), 3d millennium; (36) Sesklo (Thessaly), 4th millennium; (37) Jutland (Danish Individual Tomb culture), late 3d millennium; (38) Tepe Jamshidi (Iran), late 3d or early 2d millennium; (39) *chia (kia)* tripod (China), early 2d millennium; (40) *li* tripod (China), early 2d millennium; (41) Tepe Giyan (Persia), late 3d or early 2d millennium; (42) *ting* tripod (China), early 2d millennium; (43) Sardinia, 3d or early 2d millennium; (44) Tepe Gawra, 4th millennium; (45) Vučedol (Yugoslavia), late 3d millennium.

cultures, it arrives at more complex decoration, as in the stations in Sicily (Stentinello, Matrensa), Spain (Montserrat, Cueva de la Sarsa), and North Africa (cave of Acchakar near Tangier).

Aside from the primary centers in the Near East and the regions around the Mediterranean, impressed ware is also widespread in Asia, where its territorial or chronological limits are not yet well-defined. We can cite the ware with basketry impressions from the Quetta valley culture (Pakistan), the ware with impressions from weavings from the Celebes, and that from certain localities in China. The early earthenware of Hong Kong is distinct, as the influence of Chinese bronzes is already evident.

Substantially akin to impressed ware, but territorially distinct and perhaps of different genesis, is another great class of pottery, produced along the whole northern strip of Europe, especially among the populations of food-gatherers bound by mesolithic traditions. Notable are the large vases

with pointed base from the Danish culture of Ertebølle, which recall similar forms in early neolithic Iberia and North Africa; the conical long-necked pots, also with pointed base, of the *Kammkeramik* culture distributed from the Baltic to the forests of northern Russia, with "combed" decoration or small circular "dimples"; the round- or flat-bottomed globular jugs decorated with broken lines reminiscent of certain motifs on impressed wares of the Mediterranean or of agricultural groups in south-central Russia (Pontus, Ural, Fatyanovo). Many of these forms and decorative techniques are to be found in the territories of north-central Asia (from the Aral Sea to Lake Baikal to the Pacific shores of Siberia). The most easterly groups exhibit other techniques which link them to the "mat-marked" ware of southeastern Asia (impressions from weavings or braided fibers), or to the Japanese neolithic (Jōmon) decoration which, from its inception (proto-Jōmon), was the product of a confluence of Siberian and southeast Asian cultures (see ASIATIC PROTO-HISTORY, II, FIGS. 9, 21, PL. 16). In the islands of Japan,

where there was no painted ware, ornamentation consisted first of applied rope decoration and later (final Jōmon) of rough, uneven bands projecting from a smooth background. The shapes were jugs, spouted vases, and tall-stemmed chalices.

*b. Incised ware.* Unlike impressed ware, incised ware is far from constituting a single, uniformly distributed type. In many centers of the Near East impressed ware is accompanied from the first by the incision of unfired ware or geometric decoration (zigzags, triangles) scratched on after firing. While the motifs of the incised Hassuna ware (best known also as one of the earliest painted wares) recall impressed or related classes, it was actually the product of a later stage of development. Even in the deepest levels at Byblos or in the early neolithic levels at Knossos, the technique of incision, while appearing first, already reveals — in bands or triangles filled with dots,

Sialk I) with its repertory of rectilinear geometric elements (triangles, squares, rhombuses, zigzags, horizontal and vertical parallel lines, etc.) became progressively more complicated by the repeated interjection of representational motifs and their later stylization to the point of absolute abstraction; there arose a whole catalogue of complex motifs such as the Maltese cross and the swastika (styles of Samarra, Tell Halaf, al-ʿUbaid, in Mesopotamia, all apparently with affinities to Iranian styles: Tepe Sialk, Tepe Hissar, Tepe Giyan, Tell-i-Bakun, Susa). There were also important technical innovations, such as polychromy and the use of the wheel. In later phases pot shapes were more varied and better articulated, while wavy lines and spirals derived from stylized animal horns were added to the rectilinear geometric repertory (PL. 122).

Even before the end of the 4th millennium, in the earliest painted pottery which spread westward (Sesklo culture in

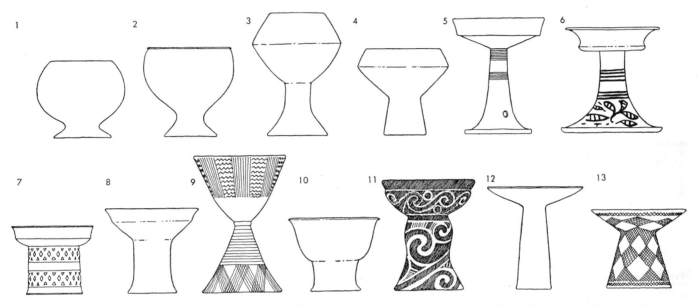

Shapes of chalices in Europe and Asia. (1) El Argar culture (Spain), mid-2d millennium B.C.; (2) Tepe Hissar (Iran), first half of 3d millennium; (3) Vinča (Yugoslavia), 3d millennium; (4) Lengyel culture (Hungary), 3d millennium; (5) Japan, Yayoi period 1st millennium; (6) Harappa civilization (Pakistan), late 3d millennium; (7) Samarra (Mesopotamia), early 4th millennium; (8) Strelice (Moravia), 3d millennium; (9) Pyrgos (Cretan sub-neolithic), 3d millennium; (10) Yang-shao culture (China), late 3d millennium; (11) Ariuşd (Erösd) culture (Transylvania), 3d millennium; (12) Lengyel culture, 3d millennium; (13) Nordic Megalithic culture, corridor-grave phase, 3d millennium.

incisions filled with white or red matter, or zones of decoration enclosed in a framework — a taste for color and a dependence on a decorative syntax akin to that of painted pottery. Elsewhere incised wares (even though they have something of the same genesis) tend to make use only of the simplest geometric elements, without curved lines or animal figures. This difference is apparent in a comparison of the triangles, lozenges, and checkerboards of Apulian-Materan incised pottery with the spiral meanders of generally contemporary painted ware from the same region; or, similarly, in a comparison of the carved or incised meanders and triangles on the glazed Lung-shan ware with the curvilinear motifs on the polychrome earthenware of the aëneolithic Chinese culture of Yang-shao. One of the few exceptions to the reigning geometric style is the oldest incised ware of continental Europe (*Linearbandkeramik*), whose spirals and slanted meanders are freely distributed over the surface of the vase (FIG. 199). But this free decoration generally accompanies a repertory of fairly primitive shapes: bowls, either hemispherical or with narrower mouths, and round-bottomed globular bottles with pierced lugs.

*c. Painted ware.* Vase painting on the outskirts of the Eurasian world had a fairly late flowering (late 4th–3d and even 2d millenniums B.C.). Spreading generally from centers where the Near and Middle East met, its development was long and complex, sometimes extending over a thousand years. The simple style of primitive painted-ware cultures of Mesopotamia (Hassuna) and of the Iranian Plateau (Tepe

Thessaly, earliest Apulian-Materan painted ware, Ripoli culture), the geometric ornamentation, though still rectilinear, was of some complexity.

The first diffusion of painted geometric ware (also 4th millennium) to the north and to the east of the Iranian Plateau is a similar case: To the east, in the lower valley of the Indus River (Amri culture) appeared, perhaps through the influence of southern Iranians, a buff ware with geometric decoration in black and reddish brown. To the north in Turkistan the oldest ware of Anau I culture, with north Iranian links, was decorated with rectilinear motifs in red and black on yellow or ocher ground; polychromy was not yet practiced.

But the second great wave of painted ware in Europe and Asia (3d millennium) went far beyond these rather narrow geographic confines (FIG. 199). To the west, from the Ukraine to the Carpathians and the upper valley of the Danube in the heart of central Europe, and to the south as far as Thessaly the neolithic centers producing painted ware were numerous: Tripolj, Cucuteni, Ariuşd (Erösd), Lengyel, Gumelniţa, Dimini (PL. 122). The wares display a fundamental unity of decorative concepts based particularly on the meander and the spiral (which are, however, often combined with the older rectilinear elements) and a growing tendency to free over-all decoration, at first primarily spiral and later arranged on the structural areas of the vase (neck, shoulders, body). White-on-red or red-on-light slip replaced the polychrome motifs, often outlined in black or, conversely, in white (e.g., at Tripolje, Ariuşd, Cucuteni, Dimini). The more westerly groups, however, to

whom these methods were not known, contented themselves with contrasting different-colored surfaces (yellow, red, brown, white, and black).

In southern Italy (latest phases of Apulian-Materan painted ware) two phases evolved, distinct both as to time and space: red or brown bands outlined in black, or an exuberantly inventive spiral-meander repertory.

Accompanying the painted ware in these areas were other decorative techniques more or less influenced by it, such as deep incisions filled with colored paste and ribbon motifs filled with dots (Tibisco, Butmir; PL. 123).

Tubular supports, carinate bowls, truncated cone bowls with vertical lip, tall-stemmed cups, biconical jugs, vases with modeled *décor* (anthropomorphous and zoomorphic), and one-piece jars (i.e., with a body consisting of continuous curves) with separate neck and elegant shape are the most common forms in the regions of the Balkans and the Danube. The individual groups also boast their own peculiar forms; e.g., the small Tripolje twin ("binocular") vases, tripod or polypod bowls, or vases with tubular spout.

In the Orient the Anau culture (Turkistan) and the cultures of Kot Diji, Quetta and those related to it, Harappa, and Mohenjo-daro (all in the Indus River valley) introduced new shapes (bowls, dishes, chalices), the use of the wheel, and

and of history. In Mesopotamia during the Uruk phase, which straddled the 4th and 3d millenniums, vase painting disappeared in favor of a slipped ware, red or gray or even polished black, whose uniform coloration was obtained by particular methods of firing. To this ware belong long open spouts depending from the lip, small tubular spouts added to the shoulder, tall handles extending above the rim and apparently inspired by metalwork, zoomorphic sculptured vases, and vases with several openings. Also in Iranian territory (e.g., Tepe Sialk) red monochrome ware supplanted the local painted ware whose traditions continued instead in the vast region of the plateau.

A class with polished gray-blackish surface and long spout and tripod took hold in Iranian centers after the middle of the 2d millennium. At about the same time, China's first historical dynasty, Shang-Yin (ca. 1500–1000 B.C.), produced a smooth gray ware. Only much later, in the last centuries B.C., did the flourishing chalcolithic civilization (Yayoi) of the Japanese archipelago produce a monochrome ware, with light-red surface, wheel-thrown, and sparsely decorated, perhaps the invention of Korean potters.

The spread of the new stylistic tendencies toward the west across Anatolia was more precocious. From the first half of the 3d millennium the Thermi and Trojan (Troy I, II) cultures produced a monochrome ware of black to brick color enhanced

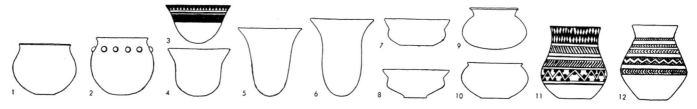

Monochrome wares and persistent early forms. (1) Samarra (Mesopotamia), early 4th millennium B.C.; (2) Cortaillod culture (Switzerland), 3d millennium; (3) Tepe Gawra (Mesopotamia), 4th millennium; (4) Michelsberg culture (Belgium), 3d millennium; (5) al-'Ubaid (Mesopotamia), 4th millennium; (6) Michelsberg culture (Germany), 3d millennium; (7) Tell Halaf (Mesopotamia), early 4th millennium; (8) Lipari (Italy, culture of Diana), late 3d millennium; (9) Tell Halaf, early 4th millennium; (10) Lipari (culture of Diana), late 3d millennium; (11) Samarra, early 4th millennium; (12) bell beaker from Garlasco (Lombardy), first half of 2d millennium.

polychromy with plant and animal motifs (PL. 121). In the steppes, from the Aral to the Altai, the influence of these centers was added to that of Tripolje and gave rise to various classes of painted ware, among which that of Afanasievo was characterized by triangles and stairs in red and white.

Vase painting in Mongolia in cultures bordering on China was practiced in the 3d millennium B.C. It is probably through these cultures that the influence of the late Tripolje civilization, straddling the 3d and 2d millenniums, penetrated as far as China. The pottery of the Yang-shao civilization in Honan and in eastern Kansu, decorated in red and black on a light ground, shows, in fact, a marked preference for curvilinear motifs, spirals, and triangles with concave sides, very like the Tripolje ornamental schemes; while the variations on the swastika and the stylized animal motifs, such as horns and claws, go back to the distant traditions of Mesopotamia and the Iranian Plateau. The same variety of influences is to be seen in the shapes: the one-piece jugs with short neck and those with body tending to a biconical or cylindrical neck echo the shapes of Tripolje and Cucuteni; and among the widespread tripod pots, besides a hollow-footed variety with breasts (*li*) which recall, perhaps, types from the cultures around Lake Baikal, some that are undecorated, with small, solid feet (*ting, chia*), show connections with Iranian forms (Tepe Giyan, etc.) from the Middle Bronze Age (2100–1700 B.C.).

*d. Monochrome ware.* After primitive impressed and incised pottery and the later great flowering of vase painting came monochrome ware, whose vogue extended through most of Europe and Asia. We cannot, of course, speak of three distinct and successive stages except occasionally, as in some regions in Europe where they correspond roughly to early, middle, and late neolithic (FIG. 203). Again, the primary center is in the Near East, now at the threshold of urban civilization

only by surface smoothing and occasionally by simple rectilinear designs in depressions or incisions. Shapes included jugs with oblique spout, pyxides with cylindrical lid, and vases with tripod or human feet. Handles were developed. While the wheel was in use, the period of Troy II also authored characteristic anthropoidal vases, tall two-handled goblets, zoomorphic askoi, and multiple vases.

The same tendencies were present in Greece, in the Rachmani culture and, a little later, in the early Helladic period. Tall ribbon-shaped handles (more than any of the other elements familiar to the Near East) were here adapted to globular or biconical pots with slanted neck (amphoras and two-handled cups, biconical jugs, askoi, and jugs with neck cut obliquely). Monochrome ware prevailed: unadorned, dark, black, gray, or reddish brown with burnished surfaces. A later stage of the early Helladic introduced a dark, brilliant glaze (*Urfirnis*) that reproduced the effects of burnished ware. Helladic influence penetrated deep into the regions of the Balkans and the Danube, where in the late Neolithic and Aëneolithic periods (Bubanj, Bodrogkeresztur, Jordansmühl, and Baden cultures) there flourished one- and two-handled cups, amphoras and decanters with spheroid bodies and separate neck, vases with multiple openings, globular pyxides with cylindrical lid. These were undecorated, incised, or impressed.

During the early Aëneolithic period Tyrrhenian Italy produced a dark undecorated ware, often glossy black (Rinaldone, Gaudo), featuring flasks, askoi, cylindrical lids, twin vessels. The aëneolithic cultures of the Early Bronze Age in Sicily (Serraferlicchio, Castelluccio), however, descended from the main stream of painted ware surviving in the Aegean world.

While remaining essentially outside the Orientalizing current, about this time the agricultural peoples of western Europe elaborated a monochrome ware of their own. This ware, neolithic in its traditions, was generally undecorated. South-

eastern Spain (Almería), southern France (Chassey), north-western Italy (Lagozza), the region northwest of the Alps extending to Belgian territory (Cortaillod, Michelsberg), and the British Isles (Windmill Hill) shared elementary and little-articulated forms of a predominantly archaic nature, such as the round bottom. Typical are hemispherical or carinate bowls, one-piece pots and narrow-necked bottles, cylindrical supports for vases (Chassey), and tulip-shaped vases (Michelsberg). In the best ware the walls are often very thin; the surfaces (black, gray, brown, sometimes red) are highly polished. Handles were replaced by projections pierced with one or more holes ("panpipe handles" of Lagozza and Chassey). Chassey developed a quiet but individual decoration, rare in the civilization of Lagozza, with bands of right angles, triangles, zigzags, or checkerboards finely engraved on the polished slip. The vogue for smooth wares was still current in the Bronze Age: e.g., El Argar (Spain), where, however, the esthetic interest was concentrated on the elegance of the well-articulated profile (stemmed cups, biconical vases; FIG. 201).

*e. Protohistoric European pottery.* The "bell beaker" is the independent creation of western Europe. Its sinusoidal profile is unmistakable, as are the deeply incised and molded motifs disposed in horizontal bands on the body and a sometimes radial foot. Of probably Iberian origin, this type was widespread in Europe during the Aëneolithic period — on the Mediterranean (Sardinia, Sicily) and the Continent (from France north to the British Isles and east to northern Italy, Bohemia-Moravia, and Hungary). In the northern regions (Germany and Low Countries) it appeared together with corded ware (*Schnurkeramik*) proper to some cultures of Scandinavia and numerous groups of eastern Europe from Poland to the Kuban River (FIG. 203).

In the full Bronze Age, about 1500 B.C. and thereafter, there was no longer any stimulus from the Aegean and the East (where the tradition of painted ware persisted, though gradually becoming commercialized), and European pottery lost much of its impetus. It reelaborated various local traditions and occasionally achieved a large repertory of shapes and designs of neolithic origin. In the Balkan-Danube area especially, the development of a glossy black ware, with an accompanying decorative technique of depressions traditional to those regions (with its high point in the Baden culture), made possible a fine plastic decoration applied with a stick (channels, facets, bosses, breasts, etc.) so as to catch and reflect the light. This class was fully matured by about 1500 B.C. in the middle Danube (Tószeg civilization) and was the cornerstone of terra-mara ware (Po valley, Lausitz area, and Germany and the upper Danube, where the *Urnenfelder* — urn-field — culture flourished). In the Iron Age the terramara culture was to overtake much of the Italian peninsula as well as other regions (PL. 124). Its shapes were well articulated: pyriform, biconical, or one-piece bodies with cylindrical or truncated-cone necks. The profiled shapes, with sudden marked transitions, enhanced the metallic aspect of the surface and the effects of modeled ornamentation. Vase painting had completely disappeared. Incised techniques now tended also to give way to the new influence of metalwork.

Early Bronze Age ornamentation was a monotonous repetition of a few geometric and rectilinear motifs of aëneolithic heredity. Only two European groups were excepted. The first, in a restricted area of the Danube, with closer links to the Aegean world, produced a repertory of baroque spirals, lattices, etc., disposed in centralized arrangement; the style sought effects of color reminiscent of white-paste filling (Pannonian ware). Less original is the decorative style of the Apennine civilization common to the Italian peninsula, often reminiscent of the taste of Butmir and late *Bandkeramik*; its wealth of rectilinear and curvilinear motifs (among them especially the meander and spiral) appeared in linear and ribbon versions. The latter especially were inspired by the dots and lines of the color techniques which included deep incision, intaglio, filling with white paste, etc. Other groups, also, with a more simple decorative repertory, made use of intaglio; e.g., the central

European civilization of the "Tumulus Builders" (*Hügelgräberkultur*).

The early Iron Age saw the rise of a new decorative vogue in pottery and the creation of various local geometric styles (Hallstatt, Villanovan) contemporaneously with the development of Greek Geometric. But they made no innovations, though the meander and the swastika emerged with greater importance in the Iron Age cultures of Villanova and southern Italy. In Hallstatt, too, there appeared a rudimentary form of vase painting with designs incised on the surface. Among Villanovan and Hallstatt wares the favorite shape, subject to innumerable variations, was the biconical urn, the joint inheritance of the urn fields of Europe. The application of modeled elements (figures of people and animals) on the surface was, of course, new, but Hallstatt fabrics began to show the effect of the great new Mediterranean civilizations (Greece, Etruria) only in their final phase, and then only in a few Orientalizing motifs. The introduction of the wheel in Iron Age II (La Tène, 5th–1st cent. B.C.) made for the first great renewal of production in central Europe since neolithic times.

Renato PERONI

*Primitive cultures.* In all the principal extra-European regions with which we are concerned — Africa, America, and parts of Asia and Oceania — pottery is a craft of considerable antiquity. Known almost universally to agricultural peoples, it is generally absent among hunters (Eskimo, Australians, and South African Bushmen); it is uncommon among nomadic herdsmen, for whom the transport of heavy and fragile objects is both burdensome and uneconomic. In one continent only, Australia, was pottery completely unknown, while its complete absence among Polynesians can be explained by the lack of suitable clay in the coral islands which they inhabited and which they must have passed in their migrations.

Few precise dates have been established; there are indications that in Africa south of the Sahara and in America pottery appeared much later than in Europe. In Mexico it was known during the "archaic" or early "formative" period by about 2500 B.C.; in Africa (Nigeria, the Sudan, and Kenya) the earliest examples seem to date from about 1000 B.C. The evidence does not enable us to say whether pottery was invented in Negro Africa or in America independently of the Old World. The emergence of pottery among the Pueblo peoples (Anasazi) as a direct sequel to the clay-lined baskets and unbaked clay vessels of the "Basket-Maker" cultures certainly suggests the possibility of independent discovery in this region, although it appears much later (ca. A.D. 400) here than in Mexico.

Primitive ceramics, best defined by the absence of the potter's wheel and of the closed kiln, without which accurate control is impossible, have the same general characteristics as prehistoric pottery. The clay used is coarse, oxidation during firing is incomplete, and the ware is porous and almost never vitrified. The only known examples of true glaze in primitive pottery occurred locally among some American Pueblo and in the so-called "plumbate" ware of Middle America (ca. A.D. 1100). Gum or resin was often applied to the surface of a vessel while hot from the fire to give it a bright varnish, but this coating must not be confused with a genuine glaze, as it would be destroyed in the heat of a fire.

Most pottery made by primitive peoples is utilitarian in purpose. Although its principal functions are for cooking and containing liquids, it is also used for dishes, corn bins, tobacco pipes, musical intruments, toys, etc. Many peoples also make pottery vessels for ritual and mortuary purposes, for offerings to spirits in shrines and graves. These are usually more elaborate than domestic wares and often assume human or animal shapes. Among them one may recognize a special class in the terra-cotta figurines, statuettes, heads, and other representations of life forms, which are used in religious ceremonies to promote fertility or to invoke other kinds of supernatural aid (PL. 126). The question of esthetic values among primitive peoples has been little studied, but there can be no doubt that much of the decoration of pottery is intended to please

the eye of the beholder and to satisfy the artistic impulse of the maker; and while the general form of these objects is inspired by other than esthetic considerations, their decoration, whether graphic, plastic, or both, is explicitly esthetic in intention.

Plastic decoration is the more ancient and widespread. It is produced by incising, punching, combing, stamping, or impressing dots, lines, or other patterns on the soft surface of the clay, usually, though not invariably, before it is dried and fired. Ornamental details in relief such as bosses, lugs, and flanges may also be applied to the pot after shaping. Among the "tools" used for plastic decoration are pointed sticks, shells, the fingernails, pieces of string, textiles, combs, and patterned beaters or spatulas.

Certain kinds of plastic decoration are the automatic result of the process of manufacture; others may be functional as well as ornamental. When a pot is made on a basket or textile fabric, its surface receives an impression of the texture ("mat-marked" ware), which may be retained for the sake of its decorative effect. Again, the impressions made by rolling a piece of cord or a patterned wooden cylinder, known as a "roulette," over the soft clay not only are ornamental but enable the pot to be grasped more firmly (FIG. 207). Rouletting has a further function in making the clay more compact, and by increasing the

and varnishing all serve a useful purpose, while being decorative as well, by rendering a vessel watertight and easier to clean, a fact which may have given rise to the process.

*a. Africa.* Africa south of the Sahara can be divided broadly into two main regions of artistic production, east and west, separated by the Ruwenzori mountain range and Lake Tanganyika. The entire eastern zone from the Sudan and Somaliland to Mozambique and South Africa is almost destitute of representational art and greatly inferior to West Africa in variety and decoration of earthenware. With rare exceptions representational art in pottery (as in other materials) is confined to the western zone (West Africa, French and Belgian Congo, northern Angola) where an astonishing wealth of ritual pottery bears witness to the inventiveness of its creators (FIG. 207).

Many of the characteristic features of modern East African pottery were already present in the earliest-known wares from the Sudan, Kenya, and Tanganyika, where they are exclusively abstract or geometric. Bowls and jars from Jebel Moya and Abu Geili, southeast of Khartoum, from the Napatean period (ca. 750 B.C.) are typically decorated with incised bands of crosshatching, fine dotted lines, and string impressions arranged in zigzags, chevrons, and triangular patterns. Some of these patterns were produced by means of pottery stamps or "rockers."

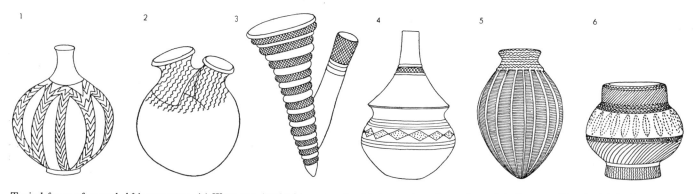

Typical forms of central African pottery. (1) Water pot, inspired by a gourd, with impression of a roulette, Acholi group, Uganda; (2) double-mouthed pot with impressions from a roulette; Jopadhola-Luo group, Uganda; (3) pointed-base pipe with black polish, Batutsi group, Ruanda; (4) bottle from the maritime region of the Congo; (5) pot with decoration inspired by basketry, from the Aruwimi river region (Congo); (6) pot with incised decoration, from the Aruwimi River region.

surface area exposed to evaporation, it reduces the danger of cracking in the fire. The decoration is often so modified and restricted as to become purely ornamental.

Another example of plastic decoration resulting from a technical process is the "corrugated" ware of the ancient Pueblo cliff dwellers (see below), where the "ripple" effect of the overlapping coils used in their manufacture are deliberately retained, and even emphasized, in the finished vessels. Some wares (Belgian Congo, ancient Colombia) have sharp angular patterns cut deeply into the surface in obvious imitations of wood carving.

The simplest kind of graphic ornament consists in burnishing parts of the surface or coating it with a slip, that is, a creamy wash of clay, powdered lime, mica, graphite, etc. Over this slip designs may be painted in one or more colors, generally red, black, or orange, but this technique is rare outside America. Paint or varnish may also be applied directly without a previous coating of slip, while a transparent varnish may be superimposed on painted decoration to protect it or give it luster (e.g., on the upper Amazon).

Designs may be naturalistic (generally zoomorphic), stylized, abstract, or geometric, and their purpose may be symbolic, magical, or purely ornamental. A special technical style, much used in ancient America, is known as "negative" or "lost-color" painting, achieved, after the manner of batik cloth, by first painting the design in a resistant material such as wax, then covering the whole pot surface with paint, and finally melting off the wax. The design emerges in the original color of the pot or of the slip with which it was coated. Burnishing, painting,

The lower part of the body is often marked with mat-work impressions. Lugs or small handles and indented fillets in relief are decoratively applied, and some of the finer waves are painted with thin red lines on an orange ground. Similar features are observable in early Nubian pottery (ca. 700 B.C.). Potsherds of approximately the same antiquity excavated in Kenya at Njoro and Elmenteita reveal similar styles of incised and dotted-line ornament, decorative lugs and bosses, and occasional looped curvilinear patterns on globular jars with pointed base and on wide shallow bowls. Analogous shapes and forms of decoration recur in the prehistoric cultures of Tanganyika at Mumba Cave and somewhat later in Sandawe, where red and black burnished ware recalls some of the early Sudanese styles. The Mumba Cave culture is exceptional in the prevalence of beakers with straight or slightly curving sides. All these early wares appear to be strictly utilitarian, but the remains found at some Sudanese sites also include spindle whorls with stamped patterns; ornaments in the form of rings and disks; and figurines of oxen, camels, and stylized human beings, probably children's toys, or perhaps votive offerings. It is interesting that similar small clay figures of cattle are still modeled by children among many of the pastoral peoples of East and South Africa.

A unique utilitarian ware of a later Iron Age period (bowls with beveled rims, globular jars, beakers with constricted sides) occurs in certain valleys north of Kavirondo Gulf, Kenya; it is known as "dimple-based" pottery from the shallow depressions made in the center of the rounded bases. The decoration is incised, combed, or pricked, in parallel straight or

wavy lines, scrolls, circles, zigzags and triangles, thus apparently continuing the horizontal style of the earlier Stone Age wares of East Africa (see AZANIAN ART, II, FIG. 198).

There have been few esthetic innovations in modern wares. Ethiopia produces a large variety of jars, jugs, and bowls in black ware with bands of incised ornament and small lugs pierced for suspension. The shapes are often rather angular and suggest the influence of Oriental metalwork. Pottery fumigators and incense burners here and in Somaliland resemble those of the Hadramaut. In the Nuba Mountains to the west of Ethiopia burnished black bowls are sometimes incised with a graceful reticulate "giraffe" pattern. Here and elsewhere in the eastern and western Sudan the clay is often pounded in a depression in the ground over which a mat has been laid, thus producing a style known as "mat-marked," of apparently direct descent from prehistoric times.

South of these regions earthenware production of the eastern and southern Bantu is limited to useful vessels, with some variety in decoration (dots in parallel or wavy lines, impressions from cylinders, etc.).

The Kamba in Kenya make only the simplest cooking pots, decorated with the maker's incised "trade-mark." Kikuyu pots with small pierced lugs bear shallow grooves and dimples. In the Rift Valley pottery is made by coiling, while the prevalent decoration around Lake Victoria is impressed with string, braided fiber, or small carved wooden cylinders. Some Uganda tribes combine incised work with rouletting. Banyoro (Kitara) milk bottles are painted with a graphite slip which takes a high polish. Their globular body and funnel-shaped neck are perhaps derived from vessels from ancient Meroë. The delicately incised and painted tobacco pipes were doubtless due to royal patronage, which certain professional male potters enjoyed. As for Uganda and Ruanda, ritual two-mouthed beer pots, vessels studded with sharp bosses, and small narrow-necked, flat-based bottles of polished red and black ware predominate. Representational art is absent in these regions except for a few ancient and crude statuettes excavated at Luzira and the figurines made secretly in Tanganyika and by the Ndau (Vandau) in Mozambique. Figures also appear on a small scale in the anthropomorphous pipes of the Wasambara (Shambala) and cleverly modeled animals (especially hippopotamuses) from Northern Rhodesia, but the esthetic merit of these figures is disputed. (See BANTU CULTURES).

West Africa, on the other hand, is extremely rich in ceramic art. In certain regions not strongly influenced by Islam, ritual pottery attains a high degree of elaboration, while at several culture centers, both ancient and modern, outcrops of representational art of striking beauty and originality occur. Ceramic decoration is mainly plastic, and painting is limited to a few tribes and localities. Even in prehistoric times there were relatively advanced cultures, e.g., in northern Nigeria (Plateau and Benue provinces), where a series of remarkable quasi-naturalistic terra-cotta heads and human and animal figures have been excavated in geological deposits dating from about 900 B.C. – A.D. 200 Very different was the succeeding Sao (Sau, Sô, Sù) culture in the Lake Chad region (ca. 9th or 10th cent.). Large quantities of pottery artifacts and ritual art have been excavated here: human and animal heads (horse, giraffe, sheep, etc.) and vigorously impressionistic or grotesque statuettes in great variety (PL. 126), some of which suggest Oriental influence; funerary urns with lids, double-mouthed vases, bowls, beakers, plates; whistles, bells, pipes, spindle whorls, counters believed to be "money," toys, ornaments, etc. Vase decoration is plastic and painting is absent.

The excavation of a number of tumuli, cemeteries, and village sites in the French Sudan has revealed the ceramic relics of "protohistoric" Iron Age cultures comprising both domestic wares and ritual objects, again with largely plastic decoration: jars and bowls and a number of crude statuettes and heads and an equestrian figure. But archaeological work is not sufficiently advanced to establish the chronology of these civilizations (see SUDANESE CULTURES).

The sculptural achievement of Ife, the old Yoruba religious center in southwestern Nigeria, stands forth as a unique phenomenon (10th–15th cent.) and marks the culmination of naturalistic art in Africa. The celebrated terra-cotta heads are modeled with an excellence and restraint which have little in common with the traditional stylizations of most African sculpture. Later (15th–17th cent.) and inferior are the surviving works of art from Benin City in southern Nigeria. The portraiture is less naturalistic than that of Ife, though probably inspired by it. Other, stylized, heads have been excavated in ancient sites of southern and central Ghana, together with a good many potsherds. The heads were intended for funerary rites which continued into the 19th century. The pottery was very diversified (see GUINEAN CULTURES).

Modern West African pottery (the best of it in Nigeria and the Cameroons) is so diverse, especially in its ritual aspects, that only a few of the more characteristic examples can here be mentioned. In the arid region bordering on the Sahara, water jars have a special importance. Some of the ritual vases made by the Nupe (PL. 125) and Yoruba are superb examples of the adaptation of ornament to ceramic shape. In the region of Kano in northern Nigeria use of a local micaceous clay imparts a fine golden luster to the surface. In Sokoto a pedestal water jar has a broad band of polychrome painted decoration around the rim. Fantastically elaborate vases ("pagodas," stylized elephants, etc., on globular bases) were placed on men's graves by the Dakakari. Whole Ashanti villages (Ghana) specialize in smoke-blackened wares with varied plastic treatment. Representational art, rare in the north, is to be seen in the sensitively modeled female statuettes for the fertility rites of the Ankwe of the Muri region (Nigeria) and the flattened clay heads of the Ewe. Vase painting is uncommon.

The pottery of the Cameroons, as in Nigeria, is exceptionally fine and varied, especially in ritual items. Large tripod vases, twin cups, etc., as well as realistic painted figures of unbaked clay, are made by the Ekoi, Ibo, and other tribes. Decoration is plastic and painted. Bamenda votive bowls and oil lamps are richly embossed with designs in relief, sometimes zoomorphic; these have odd lobed handles. Bowls like chalices have openwork pedestals with several legs or conical stands decorated with reticulate patterns in relief and colored red, black, or yellow. A characteristic pipe bowl of the Bamum, Bali, and Bamileke is exceptionally large and richly ornamented with reticulate patterns in high relief or modeled in stylized human or animal form. The Kapsiki make tripod bowls for cooking, crudely anthropomorphous funerary urns, and ritual beer pots marked with sex symbols. Representational art is mainly in applied decoration with symbolic significance.

The Congo region, so prolific in wood sculpture, is much poorer than West Africa in ritual pottery but has a great wealth and variety of domestic jars and bowls (PL. 126), many of which show a classical perfection of form. Decoration both painted and incised is as varied as the forms. Representational art is rare (see CONGO).

*b. Southeastern Asia and Oceania.* Although the potter's wheel is in general use in the higher cultures of India, some of the more primitive hill tribes still make their jars and cooking pots by hand. Simple globular bodies with constricted necks are the rule, and little decoration except burnishing is applied. The Toda of the Nilgiri Hills make hemispherical bowls for batter, and the Bhumij of Chota Nagpur use a special kind of bowl with a concave lid containing a small oil lamp at wedding ceremonies. Pottery drums are also found in India, e.g., among the Gonds of the Central Provinces. In northern Ceylon a bowl for washing rice has its interior heavily grooved with radiating scroll patterns. The simplest pottery is made by the Veddas; it is roughly spherical in shape and crudely decorated with wavy lines incised around the neck. In the Andaman Islands only rough undecorated conical pots are made for domestic use. In the Nicobar Islands the manufacture of pottery is limited to a single island, which supplies the whole group. A peculiar method of decoration is practiced there by pressing strips of coconut fiber about 1 2/3 in. wide on the vessel while hot from the fire, so as to mark it with black stripes. Simple geometric patterns in the form of rectangles, arrows,

or crosses are incised on the rims or body surface and serve as owners' marks.

In some parts of Malaya (e.g., Perak) bottles are commonly made in the shape of gourds, with vertical constricted necks and small mouths. Some have their bodies ornamented with series of longitudinal ridges, resembling an open basketry framework or string carrier. The upper part of such bottles is sometimes actually made of a piece of gourd attached to a pottery body. Spherical water jars are ornamented with delicate incised work and indented rims; large jars with wide flattened bodies, well-defined shoulders, and widely everted rims have bands of small incised or impressed triangles, chevrons, etc. Some of the older Iron Age pottery excavated in Perak and Selangor appears to have been coated with a gum or bituminous varnish.

In Borneo handmade pottery was formerly widespread. The excavation of old deposits in caves and on the Sarawak River delta indicates a more elaborate and varied decoration, although some patterns impressed with carved wooden beaters have survived to the present day. Pottery is now to be found only among the Dayak (Dyak), Murut, Kelabit, Dusun, Bajau, and a few other inland tribes, as along the coasts and rivers it has been displaced by imported brass and iron vessels, while fresh green bamboos are commonly used for cooking. Pottery jars and bowls for cooking rice and vegetables are globular or ovate with necks; the Dayak cover them with shallow chevron, check, or plaited patterns impressed with a carved wooden beater. Cord patterns, impressed with a roulette or a beater wrapped in string, are also present, e.g., among the Kenyah of Sarawak. All tribes except the Murut regard decoration as essential, either for traditional and esthetic reasons or as a magical protection against evil spirits. Patterned surfaces are also useful in resisting thermal shock, facilitating a firm grip, and offering a suitable surface for varnishing.

The simple pots of the Murut of the upper Trusan River, adjoining Indonesian Borneo, have either a rounded base or a flat-ring pedestal; they are made by inserting sticks and smooth, long stones into the center of a clay cylinder, while a flat wooden trowel with incised surface is used to beat the surface into shape. The mouth is added by freehand modeling. A coating of yellow varnish is applied by rubbing dammar gum all over the pot while it is still hot from the firing. The Bajau of Tempasuk (North Borneo) make both domestic and commercial pottery. It is reddish brown and rather roughly finished with small bits of embedded mica. Decoration, if present, is in roughly incised or impressed lines, or indented fillets applied longitudinally at widely spread intervals. The Bajau also use a gum varnish. Some of their cooking bowls and water jars have lids or covers with a central knob around which radial lines are incised. A special goglet or water cooler made here, with a small spout and flanged stopper, is similar to a Malayan type.

In the coastal area of North Borneo covered bowls and wide-lipped cooking pots are often elaborately painted after firing. The designs vary: white zigzags enclosing large red and white spots on a terra-cotta or yellow ground; or complex scrolls in red and black on white ground covering the whole body. The paddle and anvil shaping process (probably deriving from the mainland of southeastern Asia) is much used in Borneo.

Farther east, pottery is plentiful in New Guinea and is made at a number of other islands throughout Melanesia as far east as Fiji. But it tends to be localized in widely separated villages whose inhabitants enjoy a monopoly of the trade and export their wares in large quantities to the surrounding districts. Usually made by the coiling method, the finished products vary greatly in quality, shape, and decoration from one region to another. Decorative patterns are often the private property of certain families and enjoy a kind of "copyright."

Prehistoric pottery of uncertain age has been excavated at a number of sites in Melanesia and New Guinea. Superior in construction and ornament to the modern wares, vessels are large and well-fired and furnished with ornate lips and flanges. The designs are modeled. Several features suggest a relationship with early Japan. In New Caledonia early pottery fragments have been excavated from a number of middens and cave sites where no pottery is made today. Provisionally dated by the carbon 14 process at periods between 840 B.C. and the 16th century, it is associated with polished stone and shell artifacts beneath deposits containing European trade objects.

Modern production, where it is still practiced, is generally debased (see MELANESIAN CULTURES). Pottery villages are dotted along the northern coast of mandated New Guinea, but the most striking ware is made in the middle region of the Sepik River (PL. 127): cooking pots with small ears, large urns 2 ½ ft. tall for storing sago, shallow conical covers. Appliquéd designs in high relief are composed of "eyes," stylized human faces, or pigs' heads sometimes emphasized in color. The more ornate pots were placed in the "ghost houses" apparently for ritual use. Similar, more delicate, ovate bowls from the Shortland Islands (Solomons), large numbers of globular cooking pots from the Port Moresby region (Papua), exceptionally thin-walled open bowls from Tube Tube (New Guinea), sand-tempered cooking ware made by the women of the northwestern Solomon Islands, and the fanciful, varied vases of the Fiji Islands, decorated and coated over with a glossy kauri gum varnish varying from green to gold, represent the not very ample range of Melanesian pottery.

*c. The Americas.* Most American Indian pottery is prehistoric or pre-Columbian. Only the Pueblos in the southwestern states of North America and the Indians in some of the remoter parts of South America have continued to make traditional pottery unaffected or only slightly modified by colonial influence. America illustrates the principle that ceramics accompany a settled agricultural mode of life: The Eskimo and the Indian tribes of the Northwest Coast and the Great Plains, who lived by hunting, fishing, and food gathering, had no pottery; nor did the seminomadic inhabitants of Patagonia and Tierra del Fuego. Throughout the rest of the American continent, from the Great Lakes in the north to the Pampas region of Argentina, pottery was known in almost every place where suitable clay was available. In southeastern and southwestern North America and in the high civilizations of Mexico, Central America, and Peru the ceramic arts were practiced with intensity and originality, attaining high standards of craftsmanship and creative artistry (FIG. 213). The wares embrace almost every conceivable shape and decorative style, and their inclusion in the category of "primitive ceramics" is justified only by the fact that the makers were ignorant of the potter's wheel and of the refinements of the modern firing kiln. In spite of these limitations an incipient form of vitreous glaze was achieved in the so-called "plumbate" ware of Central America in the 11th century, and glaze paints appeared as a decorative feature at several periods in Pueblo pottery.

In a broad sense American Indian pottery falls into three stylistic groups: (1) utility wares of simple shapes with plastic decoration made by incising, impressing, or modeling in relief; (2) wares with zoomorphic shapes or attachments and other fanciful shapes, used chiefly for mortuary purposes; and (3) wares distinguished by their painted decoration.

Utility vessels include cooking bowls, food bowls, plates or dishes, roasting griddles, jars, bottles, cups, mugs, and ladles. A great variety of other objects also were made for ritual purposes, especially in the higher cultures. Particularly characteristic of Middle America are the abundant votive or fertility figurines (ca. 1500 B.C. in Mexico) and the musical instruments, comprising whistles and ocarinas (often in the form of effigies), flutes, panpipes, trumpets, drums, and rattles. Incense burners were much used in religious worship, and terra-cotta statuettes were made to represent deities and priests. Among the minor ceramic products are tobacco pipes (almost universal in North America) and flat or cylindrical stamps (*pintaderas*) for imprinting patterns on textiles or the human body; also spindle whorls (often decorated), potter's tools, toys, dolls, game disks, and personal ornaments such as earplugs and labrets. Characteristic of Middle America is the tripod vase. The use of negative painting is peculiarly American.

*1. North America.* In the more remote regions, around the Great Lakes and the Middle Atlantic area of North America and in the Pampas of southern Argentina, the ceramic arts remained at a rather crude and archaic level. Iroquois and Algonquian pottery was restricted to domestic wares and tobacco pipes. Shapes are simple, and the paste is coarse in texture. Painting and burnishing are absent. As with archaic ceramics generally, decoration is limited to simple geometric patterns, incised or impressed, and occasional fillets or bosses in relief. In Virginia vessels often have the entire surface marked with coarse textile impressions. A jar made by the Iroquois and on the Atlantic seaboard is an obvious imitation of birchbark receptacles; the rim projects in the form of a heavy squarish collar incised with straight lines resembling porcupine-quill embroidery on birchbark. Some tribes produced punctate patterns by rolling a notched spindle to and fro over the surface. The best products of the Iroquois were their

known in their earliest phase as Basket Makers for their sun-dried clay vessels and baskets lined with clay for receptacles. Pottery did not appear till later (ca. A.D. 500), perhaps as an independent discovery through the accidental burning of clay-lined baskets. Alternatively, it may have been introduced from the south, where it existed much earlier. Pueblo culture has been divided into three main periods (500–1700), of which the Great Pueblo phase corresponds with that of the cliff dwellers (ca. 1050–1300). Unlike most of their pottery, their cooking vessels were never painted. A special kind of gray "corrugated" ware was in use until the end of the Great Pueblo period, during which the overlapping coils of clay used in building up the body were retained and emphasized in the finished pot. The ornamental effect of these corrugations, covering part or all of the vessel, was often enhanced by means of finger indentations, frequently so distributed as to resemble basketry patterns. Bowls and jars, with or without handles,

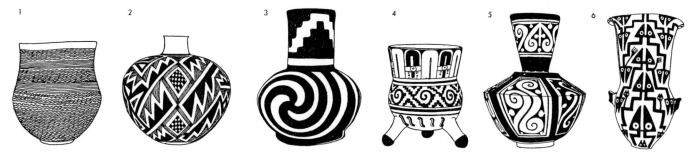

Typical forms of pre-Columbian American pottery. (1) Apache pot with wavy-line motif, Arizona; (2) pot in black-on-white style from Socorro (central New Mexico), ca. 13th cent.; (3) painted water bottle, Arkansas; (4) tripod in Mixtec-Zapotec style, from Mitla (Oaxaca, Mexico); (5) water bottle from Coclé (Panama); (6) funerary urn, S. María type, Chile.

tobacco pipes, whose bowls are the open mouths of well-modeled human or animal heads. In the south Appalachian region (Georgia and Alabama) there is a greater variety of shape and plastic ornament. The types include large caldrons and burial urns with covers, crude figurines, and effigy tobacco pipes. Carved wood spatulas were used to imprint elaborate patterns of lacelike texture, composed of curvilinear swastikas or "lover's knots." Ceramics were much more highly developed in the Mississippi and Ohio valleys, the region of the ancient Mound Builders and the Hopewell culture. The potters here excelled in modeling rather than painting and surpassed the Pueblos in variety and refinement of shapes. Especially characteristic of Arkansas and Missouri are the effigy bowls, designed to represent birds, animals, fish, and reptiles, whose heads and tails project from the rims of the vessels and whose bodies constitute the bowl itself. Typical well-shaped bottles or decanters with long necks and globular or gadrooned bodies are generally gray or black (less commonly red), with a highly polished surface and decorated with skillfully incised scrolls. Relief ornament was also applied in thin fillets. Scalloped rims, tripods, and various erratic forms occur, including boat-shaped vases with stirrup spouts reminiscent of Peru and realistic human death's-heads, with closed eyes and curiously striated cheeks. On the middle and lower Mississippi and in Florida slips and geometric painted decoration in red, white, and black scrolls, meanders, guilloches, zigzags, checkers, etc., are also common on jar surfaces and bowl interiors. Some of the designs are probably symbolic; step frets symbolize clouds and rain, while circular and stellate figures seem to have astronomical significance.

The ancient pottery of the Pueblo region in the southwestern states has been thoroughly studied and classified with the help of tree-ring dating (dendrochronology) and carbon 14. Its chief interest lies in its painted decoration rather than in fictile form. For both the beauty and originality of its designs and the skill in sheer draftsmanship, it ranks high among the ceramics of both the Old and the New Worlds.

The ancestors of the modern Pueblo Indians (e.g., Hopi and Zuñi) were the Anasazi of Arizona and New Mexico,

were made in this style, which became so refined that some examples contain as many as 12 corrugations to the inch.

Slip-painted pottery (which has persisted down to modern times) appeared early in the Pueblo period, perhaps under Mexican influence. The principal types comprise shouldered jars (*ollas*) for storing water (a vital necessity in this arid climate), globular seed jars, open food bowls, mugs with handles, and ladles or dippers. Shapes are simple but well-proportioned. For decoration the surface was first coated with a smooth slip, and over this designs were painted with a brush of chewed twig or leaf. In the early and "great" periods the patterns were chiefly in black on white and were entirely geometric; but black on red, produced by firing in an oxidizing atmosphere, and polychrome combinations of white and black on red, or red and black on orange were used locally. The designs were composed of such simple geometric elements as zigzags, triangles, checkers, frets, steps, spirals, etc.; and from the first one finds the "step and hook" device (*klimankistron*), which in various forms is one of the most distinctive and widely distributed traits of American decorative art. A number of the patterns used were undoubtedly symbolic in origin, such as steps or terraces symbolizing rain clouds and scrolls for whirlwinds, but later the meaning of the symbols seems to have been forgotten, and they were altered and elaborated from purely esthetic considerations. The exteriors of jars were generally covered with angular or scroll meanders of endless varieties arranged in broad bands; but the interior of the open bowl offered an even more suitable field for graphic virtuosity. To the south of the Anasazi, in the Gila and Salt valleys of Arizona, distinctive styles in red on buff were developed by the Hohokam. Early designs included small figures of birds and animals; later, from 900 to 1200, a geometric style was evolved in which the interspaces of the framework, which resembled plaiting, were filled out with elaborate scrolls. Some of the most beautiful painting was done by the Mogollon of the Mimbres valley in southern New Mexico. The interiors of open bowls are adorned with quasi-naturalistic figures of animals, birds, or insects (PL. 128). Sometimes a single figure appears in a central medallion on a white ground; in other cases a succession of figures

enclosed in oval cartouches forms a marginal border, the center being left blank. The radial composition, with all the figures facing in one direction, produces a dynamic effect of rotation, e.g., scenes of men fighting animals. These bowls were made for burial and were generally "killed" ritually by having a hole knocked in the bottom, thus releasing their spirit, a custom widespread among the American Indians.

The old pottery of the Hopi at Sikyatki and Shumopovi (Arizona) was beautifully decorated in black and red on a finely burnished yellow ground. Geometric and scroll patterns are combined with stylized figures of animals and birds, and detached zoomorphic elements (feathers, wings) are treated freely in the composition of heraldic designs. On the Rio Grande and at two periods in the Zuñi area of New Mexico lead or copper glazes (not intended to make vases watertight) were combined with mat painting for decorative purposes. In recent times, under Western influence, floral elements have been introduced into painted designs, and animal effigy vases have become common. Modern Zuñi *ollas* bear alternating figures of deer and floral rosettes (PL. 128). Elements of Chihuahua painted pottery in northern Mexico (15th cent.) recall the Mimbres style; geometric patterns are combined with stylized life forms in black and red on a buff ground. Some vases also depict human faces in a combination of modeling and painting.

*2. Mexico and Central America.* In Mexico pottery which appeared contemporaneously with agriculture (ca. 1500 B.C.) changed and developed considerably during the 3,000 years preceding the Spanish conquest. During the first 1,500 years known as the "archaic" or "formative" period, it remained at a relatively simple utilitarian level. Geometric patterns by incising, and painting with slip appeared early and were followed by such characteristically American features as effigy and tripod vases, spout handles, and negative painting. The growth of religious cults is evidenced by the terra-cotta figurines, among the most characteristic artistic products of Mexico and Central America. The modeling of the torso and limbs is elementary; the facial features and details of hairdress and costume are rendered by incising, punching, or the application of pellets of clay in relief. Many of these figurines (generally female) are vigorous and individual and possess a kind of naïve charm. The emphasis on sex suggests their use in fertility rites. In all subsequent phases of Mexican culture figurines continued to play an important role and were made in enormous quantities. In the "classic" period of Teotihuacán (200–900) the heads of these figurines were often modeled with the delicacy of true portraiture, but later mass production with molds made for a loss of individuality. In the Toltec and Aztec periods they are largely iconographical.

Among the Tarascan peoples of western Mexico something of the naïveté and charm of the early figurines survived in figures modeled on a larger scale for mortuary use. Although impressionistic, and showing little regard for anatomical accuracy, the figures are often expressive in feature and pose, and some appear to be deliberate caricatures. Among the best-known types are figures of squatting women and standing armored warriors (Nayarit); long-faced female deities (Guadalajara); and the hairless fat-bellied dog (Colima), more realistic than the human figures. They are generally red and highly polished with details added in white paint.

With the rise of the higher cultures of the Valley of Mexico at Teotihuacán (followed by the Toltec and Aztec), of the Zapotec and Mixtec in the south, and of the Olmec, Totonac, and Huaxtec (Huastec) along the Gulf of Mexico, the ceramic arts developed a bewildering diversity of forms and decorative styles. Their production, like that of the other arts, was stimulated by the religious needs of the great ceremonial centers. Designs are therefore often derived from religious concepts and should be studied in context (see MIDDLE AMERICAN PROTO-HISTORY). The classic period of Teotihuacán produced several new and distinctive types of vases, among them the small globular *florero* with high flaring neck and the massive cylindrical tripod jar with a conical cover. New decorative techniques included scraping away parts of the slip-painted surface, en-

graving after firing, and a kind of cloisonné or champlevé style, whose effect resembles that of medieval enamels. This was achieved by coating the surface with a thick plaster or stucco, from which the design was cut out and the cavities filled in with color in pastel shades of blue, green, and pink. Vases of this type were traded as far south as Kaminaljuyú in Guatemala. Effigy vases representing deities, especially the long-toothed face of the rain god, Tlaloc, were common, along with vases with one or two vertical spout handles attached to the neck. The early Zapotec culture of Oaxaca also produced these several-handled vases and distinctive flamboyant funerary vases, gray or red, whose cylindrical body is entirely obscured by seated or standing figures of deities or priests modeled in high relief. The rain god, bat god, and jaguar god are most commonly represented in elaborate costumes, animal helmet masks, and handsome feather headdresses. Nude lay figures such as the so-called "scribe of Cuilapán" are modeled with a high degree of realism.

Perhaps the most sensitive modeling of the human form was achieved by the Totonac of the Gulf region, masters of plastic technique. A well-known type depicts a laughing face. Totonac pottery vessels (PL. 128) include tripod and pedestal beakers, tripod bowls, plates, and bottles ornamented with gadroons. The fine-quality orange or buff paste is decorated with step, scroll, or zoomorphic patterns painted in a thick white, brown, or black slip. In the Huaxtec region a type of spouted vase resembling a kettle or teapot was characteristic.

The finest painting was done by the Mixtec. The beautiful polychrome designs on tripods and ewers contain many symbolic and iconographic motifs similar to those in their codices. A wax polish gave brilliance to the colors. The famous wares of Cholula show an exceptionally wide range of brilliant color and a strong sense of balance in formal compositions.

Aztec pottery was thin and well-fired. At first, patterns in thin, calligraphic black lines were painted on the mat orange surface. Later animal and floral patterns and ritual motifs such as skulls and crossbones were treated decoratively. Among their distinctive forms were oval tripod dishes with a depression at one end and bowls with roughened floors for grating cereals. Biconical drinking cups ornamented with black lines on a polished red surface had thicker walls. Huge braziers were made for temple use. Life-size human figures, built up in sections, showed technical ability but were stiff and lifeless.

The wares of the classic period of the Maya (ca. 300–900) show great virtuosity in color and freedom of decorative style, often inspired by religious themes. Calendrical hieroglyphs served as decorative borders, while processional and other religious scenes are depicted encircling the body of the vase. The drawings are precisely outlined in black and embellished mainly in red or orange tints on a buff or cream ground. A brilliant turquoise blue was also employed in some localities. But this painting, though highly decorative and skillfully adjusted to the available space, is really a pictorial art and would be better seen on a flat surface, as it has little relevance to ceramic form. Similar pictorial scenes were executed either in intaglio or in bold relief by carving out the background after firing. Among wares thus painted are large shallow dishes, with flanged or tripod bases, and massive cylindrical jars or beakers; tripods may be in the form of grotesque animals or shells containing pebbles to make rattles. The Maya also excelled in modeling terra-cotta statuettes and incense burners with details elaborated in appliqué relief. Among large numbers of molded whistle figurines at some sites (e.g. Lubaantun in British Honduras) some depict ball-game players in costume or secular subjects, such as hunting and grinding corn. The postclassic period (ca. 1100–1200) produced two distinctive kinds of wares known respectively as "fine orange" and "plumbate." The former is unusual for its fine texture and the absence of any tempering material in the paste and is known for its lustrous vitrified surface, produced by firing a special kind of clay in a reducing atmosphere at a temperature of about 950°C. The term "plumbate" is a misnomer, since there is no lead in the composition of the glaze; but the predominant color is a leaden gray, often mottled with patches

of orange or olive green resulting from imperfectly controlled firing conditions. It was a trade ware, which seems to have originated in the Guatemala highlands or Salvador, but was carried as far as nothwestern Mexico and Nicaragua. Apart from its iridescent luster, it is not particularly attractive. Globular and tapering jars, often tripods with gadrooned bodies, are prevalent forms, commonly adorned with incised loops and scrolls. Some of the many animal and human effigy vases show considerable realism, but modeling tends to be rough and carelessly finished.

The pottery of the Isthmian region of Central America (Nicaragua, Costa Rica, Panama) reveals a mixture of influences emanating partly from the higher cultures of Mexico and partly from those of South America. But several centers developed distinctive styles of high quality during the last few centuries before Columbus. The characteristic "Luna ware" of Nicaragua is decorated with delicately drawn, spacious, linear patterns on a white slip. Other Nicaraguan wares are monochrome reds and browns, bearing incised ornament often filled in with white pigment; large burial urns are in globular or shoe forms. In Costa Rica wares from at least three centers can be distinguished. The most beautifully decorated is the polychrome ware of Nicoya, made by the Chorotega of the western coast. Its typical forms are ovoid and pyriform jars with ring bases or tripod legs and flaring tripod bowls with zoomorphic legs. Some jars and bowls are in the form of jaguars, armadillos, turkeys, etc. The boldly modeled heads project laterally from the vase body, while the limbs are shown in low relief; or one pair of limbs together with the tail may furnish a tripod support. Jars may take the form of human heads, with facial features applied in relief. Nicoya ceramics are, however, most notable for the richness of their painted decoration, which is founded on geometrically stylized animal figures. Rendered in red or orange outlined in black on a cream or yellowish ground (originally coated with a lustrous varnish), the designs show clear stylistic affinities with Maya symbolism, especially in the figures of plumed serpents and monkeys; but many other animals — jaguars, turkeys, alligators, crabs, scorpions, and two-headed dragons — are depicted, and occasionally scenes of combat between men and jaguars. Decorative borders were composed of interlocking step and scroll patterns.

The pottery of the Guetar (Guetare) in the highlands resembles that of Nicoya, but is generally inferior artistically. Vase bodies are often of pointed oval shape with long zoomorphic tripods, and the decoration consists mainly of appliqué details in relief. Farther south on the eastern coast of Costa Rica and Panama, Chiriquí or Talamancan wares reveal several distinctive styles. One of these is called "biscuit" or "armadillo" ware, from the frequent use of motives derived from that animal and applied as relief decoration; the armadillo may also be represented as a complete figure. Tripod bowls and jars, which may have handles or twin mouths, show exceptionally fine craftsmanship and refinement of shape; the unpainted mat surface is of a uniform buff color, resembling the "biscuit" stage of European pottery before it is glazed. The tripod feet are usually hollow and contain rattles. Another style, "alligator ware," is rather thick and has a cream slip ornamented with red and black designs, all derived from the anatomy of the alligator in more or less conventional form. Some details, e.g., scutes, are isolated, simplified, and recombined into purely abstract patterns. Lost-color ware, in which geometric, textile, reptilian, and octopus patterns are rendered in negative painting, is also typical of the Chiriquí. A number of other styles have been defined as "scarified," "chocolate-incised," "black-incised," "maroon," "red and white line," etc.; Chiriquí pottery musical intruments are numerous: cylindrical drums, gourd-shaped rattles, and a variety of whistles commonly in the form of birds, animal, or human beings.

For sheer beauty and richness of decorative design the polychrome wares excavated from graves at Coclé in Panama (ca. 1300–1500) are unsurpassed in America. The varied shapes include rectangular trays and bowls, plates, carafes, bottles, spouted jars, and effigy vases. The bodies of the carafes are often sharply angled, with a flattened shoulder and a tall flaring neck, the whole shape being suggestive of metalwork. The spouted jars have globular bodies, and the spout which springs vertically from the shoulder is joined to a widely flanged mouth. Vases often occur in pairs identical in shape and decoration. Square shapes, which are found elsewhere only rarely (e.g., Mexico and southeastern United States) are common here, as in the Chimu culture of Peru. On a whitish slip, designs are outlined in black or brown and the spaces filled in with red, brown, and purple shades. Among the geometric designs, which include zigzags and concentric rings, a strong preference is shown for broad scrolls, subject to infinite variation. Executed with precision and artistry, they are either enclosed in well-spaced bands and panels or treated as continuous meanders encircling jars or the interiors of bowls; they are often associated with crocodile figures. The most original designs are composed of stylized monsters or dragons, in which the features of crocodiles, snakes, monkeys, crabs, turtles, and birds are variously combined and often displayed in heraldic fashion. They appear to greatest advantage on shallow bowls, either singly or repeated in a bisected or a quartered field, or again as a bordering meander. Even in the most elaborate and flamboyant examples, the basic composition is always controlled by a strong sense of balance and symmetry; luxuriance never degenerates into meaningless confusion. In the later period effigy jars in animal, fish, or, more rarely, human form become more frequent; the heads and limbs are only partly modeled in relief, some of the features being completed in polychrome painting. Some jars have covers representing human heads.

*3. South America.* South American ceramics present a very uneven picture. The best were produced by the series of high cultures which developed in Peru between 1000 B.C. and the Spanish conquest. Not until the rise of the Inca Empire in the 14th century did Peruvian influence seriously affect the surrounding regions, chiefly in Bolivia, Argentina, and Chile, and to a lesser extent in the highlands of Ecuador. The pottery of large areas of the continent from Patagonia to Brazil remained at a simple utilitarian level with little pretense at artistic expression, although large burial urns were widely distributed. The Arawak peoples constitute an exception. Their burial pottery, recovered from mounds in the Amazonian region of Brazil, was varied and beautiful; and many tribes of the middle and upper Amazon were still making finely painted wares until recent times.

The pottery of Colombia and Ecuador (I, PLS. 173, 174), esthetically inferior to that of the Isthmian region, offers variety of modeling rather than painted decoration. The Chibcha of northern Colombia made many small erect or seated idols with flat, rectangular heads whose facial features are crudely indicated by incised slits or modeling, while bodies and limbs are rudimentary, legs being often bulbous. Commonest are globular jars, often with faces modeled on the neck, and pedestal bowls (*compoteras*). They are cream- or buff-colored, and decorated by incising, stamping, or red paint. The Quimbaya wares of southern Colombia are superior, especially in geometric, negative painting. The over-all decoration of narrow elongated jars with flattened shoulders and lugs in red, black, and white is made up of long narrow triangles marked with white spots. Other distinctive Quimbaya styles are "brown-incised" and "chip carving," with geometric patterns in a kind of champlevé relief, the background being carved out as in woodwork. Double-spouted and double-figure vases after the Peruvian manner were also made.

The pottery of Ecuador differs markedly in the highlands and coastal regions, and until the Inca period it shows closer general affinities with Colombia and Central America than with Peru. Standard and tripod bowls are common in the highlands, with incised or appliqué decoration (stylized monkeys, reptiles, birds). Shapes, often complex, include both animal and poorly modeled human effigies, sometimes supine. Linear patterns were painted in red on buff. In the north a trichrome negative-painted style (Tuncahuán) on pyriform jars and flaring

bowls closely resembles the Quimbaya style. In the southern highlands thick white designs were painted on a chocolate slip.

The fine pottery of the coastal regions of Esmeraldas and Manabí includes well-burnished standard bowls and cups, sometimes painted in black, brown, yellow, and blue. Modeled heads and figurines are outstanding. Of gray paste, they are either impressed in molds or modeled hollow for whistles or ocarinas. Of the two cultures, Guangala and Manteño, distinguishable on the southern coast of the Santa Elena peninsula, the former recalls the Nicoya polychrome style of Costa Rica. A unique type of shallow bowl has five or six pointed feet. Manteño wares are mostly gray; decoration is engraved, appliqué, or produced by selective burnishing on a mat surface. A striking type of effigy jar has a bulbous neck with an appliqué modeled face and the limbs indicated by burnishing. Other ceramic products of Ecuador include stamps and molds (*pintaderas*), spindle whorls finely engraved with monkey and bird figures, braziers, conch-shaped trumpets, and graters set with stones.

The art of ancient Peru reached its peak in ceramics. Distinguished vases were produced in each of the major cultural periods, both in the Andean highlands and on the coast. The earliest pottery, dating from about 1200 B.C., was utilitarian. By about 800 B.C. in the gray vases of Cupisnique on the northern coast the peculiarly Peruvian stirrup spout was already in use. This form of spout, which persisted on the coast down to the Spanish conquest (I, PL. 175), served also as a handle and was contrived to counteract evaporation in an arid climate. The highest artistic level, both in modeling and painting, was reached in the Mochica culture, about 200 B.C. to A.D. 800. Many of the wonderfully realistic portrait heads must rank as true sculptural masterpieces. In the clearly delineated types there is often a touch of humor or caricature. More than a hundred species of animals, birds, and crustaceans are faithfully represented in a pictorial style rendered by admirably controlled drawing in red on buff or cream, as well as every kind of religious and secular activity, though the figures are slightly conventionalized. Purely geometric patterns, such as scrolls, as well as weapons and trophies are also used. Plastic and graphic techniques are often combined, and figures are modeled in "pressed" (i.e., low) relief. The double vase is characteristic: one of the bodies represents a human or an animal or bird, often holding a small whistle in the mouth. Although the Mochica plastic style reappeared later in the Chimu period (ca. 1200–1500), the wares were gray or black, and mass production and the use of molds had deprived them of much of their spontaneity (I, PLS. 200–202).

At Nazca on the southern coast of Peru the emphasis was on rich polychrome painting on bowls, beakers, and bottles, the latter usually with two small spouts connected by a bridge. The designs in as many as eight colors are outlined in black to represent demons, mythological figures, birds, and animals, and they vary from quasi-realism to complete stylization, often showing that strong textile influence (I, PLS. 190–192, 197, 198) which dominated later Ica style of the same region.

The vase paintings of Tiahuanaco in the highlands (ca. A.D. 1000) made much use of stylized pumas and condors, either complete or with their elements broken down into geometric patterns (I, PLS. 196, 199, 203, 205). Recuay in the north is known as the earliest site of negative painting. Inca wares (15th–16th cent.) are limited to a few standard types, of which the aryballus, or water jar with pointed base and small handles (I, PL. 208), is the most common. The well-fired vases have a certain classical dignity and restraint of shape and proportion. Decoration, painted in three or four colors, is mainly geometric, but a stylized plant motif and bees, butterflies, and other insects occur. Plate handles in the form of bird heads are the only Inca examples of modeling from life.

Before the arrival of Inca influence, as revealed in modified versions of the aryballus type, a number of indigenous styles had developed in Chile and Argentina, among them those of the Diaguita (PL. 129). The exteriors of bowls with vertical sides, characteristic of Chile, are painted in red, white, and gray with zigzags, step frets, and other geometric patterns, sometimes combined with stylized faces some of whose features

are modeled in low relief. Polychrome or plain brown oval "duckpot" jars with handles are also found, as are thinner bowls with flaring sides, on whose interiors appear small animal figures in black on white. In northwestern Argentina the best Diaguita wares are large infant burial urns from the Calchaquí valley. Of two main types the first, from Santa María, has a tall ovoid body, a flaring neck, and a pair of strap handles low down; it is painted all over with complex designs in black and red on white; the neck usually has a stylized face, often with "weeping" eyes, and the body has figures of snakes or birds intermingled with checkers and step frets. The other, from Belén and Tinogasta, has a squatter body and is more simply decorated with frogs, double-headed curling snakes, and fret patterns. From Los Barreales another type of bowl is adorned with geometric animals, engraved and inlaid with white lime on a black or gray surface.

In the great central plains of the Gran Chaco and Mato Grosso pottery tends to be purely utilitarian, though large burial urns occur throughout this region from the Río de la Plata to the Orinoco. In the south decoration is predominantly incised, impressed, or punctate, while "fingernail" impressions are characteristic of the Guaraní. Human forms are absent. In the Paraná River region vase handles often have the form of bird heads. In the state of Paraná in southern Brazil both cooking and storage pots are marked with fingernail impressions or horizontal grooves resembling the Pueblo "corrugated" style. The Paraná delta features cord impressions filled with white pigment and interspaced with red and black designs. Painted decoration, generally in red and black on a white slip, becomes increasingly common northward through the Mato Grosso till it prevails in tropical Amazonia.

Among modern wares unaffected by colonial influence the painted pottery of the Chiriguano in the Bolivian foothills of the Andes is especially attractive. Small bowls and globular jars show ancient Andean influence in their designs: scrolls and solid triangles surmounted by scrolls variously combined with angular meanders and zigzags. Colors are black and several shades of ocher.

At both the upper and lower ends of the Amazon valley, Brazilian pottery is distinguished by persistent features, comprehensively designated (Kroeber) as the "Amazonian ceramic style." The finest and most elaborately decorated of these wares, probably of Arawak origin, come from ancient burial mounds in Marajó Island and neighboring sites of the Amazon delta. They comprise funerary urns, bowls, seats, and women's triangular pubic coverings (*tanga*), richly decorated by incising, modeling, painting, and a kind of champlevé carving, where the relief portions may be painted white or red to contrast with the natural orange color of the carved background. Several of these methods may be combined in a single vessel. While over-all patterns are mainly composed of intricately interlocking frets and angular spirals, stylized faces often appear in low relief on the necks or bodies of large globular urns (sometimes over 3 ft. high). A peculiar feature of the painted designs is the duplication of heavy lines with thinner and paler "shadow" lines, in a kind of integrating framework, in which curved and angular elements are effectively combined. There occur zoomorphic urns, urns with reptilian appliqué moldings, seated figurines, mostly female, with the legs parted, and engraved discoid stamps (*pintaderas*).

At Counany (Cunani) on the coast of Brazilian Guiana similar wares have been excavated from subterranean galleries. Here effigy urns have faces modeled in low relief on a broad rim and attenuated limbs straddling across the body. Rectangular flat-bottomed dishes and oval boat-shaped vessels are finely painted with spirals and frets and a unique pattern of interlocking "commas." At Maracá on the northern bank of the lower Amazon a distinct type of funerary urn represents the human figure, with tubular trunk and limbs, seated on a low bench, the head forming a detachable cover.

In their fantastically modeled shapes and profusion of zoomorphic ornament the extraordinary wares of the Santarém region, at the junction of the Tapajoz and Amazon rivers, differ radically from all other ancient Amazonian wares. Not

burial urns, and with only slight traces of painting, they comprise multilobed jars, bowls supported by caryatid figures, and effigy vases in seated attitudes; also a characteristic bottle with a six-lobed body, a high flanged neck, and a pair of lateral branches in the form of bird or reptile heads encrusted with various small animals modeled in the round. The modeling suggests Caribbean wares and shows vivid imagination and technical virtuosity but also an overabundance of detail (PL. 129).

Several of the typical features of the Marajó style, e.g., interlocking fret patterns and thick and thin parallel lines, have survived in the modern pottery of the Montaña tribes (Conibo, Panobo, Chama, etc.) of the upper Amazon and Ucayali rivers. These wares are usually painted in black and red on a white slip and are competely covered after firing with a lustrous resinous varnish. The manufacture of enormous ceremonial vessels (sometimes over 3 ft. in diameter) for fermented drinks, decorated in the same style, represents a considerable technical feat.

Pottery of various styles has been found at a number of ancient sites in Venezuela, principally on the shores of Lake Valencia, at Los Barrancos on the Orinoco delta, and at Ronquín on the middle Orinoco. Valencia types include double-spouted jars, small bottles with bulbous effigy necks, and roasting griddles, plain gray or ornamented with red slip and broad incisions or punctations. Crudely stylized standing or seated female figurines with laterally projecting oblong heads and long slit eyes are characteristic of the later Valencian phase. Bowls, plates, and griddles from Los Barrancos are painted with black, red, and orange slips, and in both these regions the modeled animal and bird heads (adornos) are often attached to the rims. Somewhat similar adornos, serving as handles, are also common on jars, bowls, and plates in the Antilles (q.v.). In Jamaica they often represent human and parrot heads; grotesque heads are typical for Puerto Rico, and dash-and-dot incised patterns for Cuba and Santo Domingo. Slip decoration is confined to the Lesser Antilles, where the wares are superior both technically and artistically, and the zoomorphic adornos show a more refined finish. In Trinidad frog-shaped bowls occur, and reptilian heads are used as adornos, the eyes frequently emphasized by surrounding spiral incisions. On St. Kitts a finely polished red ware is ornamented with incised patterns filled with white pigment.

H. J. BRAUNHOLTZ

THE ANCIENT WORLD. *Civilizations of the ancient Near East.* The oldest painted wares appeared in the heart of the agricultural communities of the Near East. Local traditions, which especially characterized the most ancient stages of civilization, developed in Egypt, Mesopotamia, Syria, Palestine, Anatolia, and Cyprus.

*a. Egypt.* The oldest examples of Egyptian pottery were found in the neolithic stations of Fayum, Merimdeh in the western Delta, and Deir Tasa in middle Egypt. Recurring Fayum types are spherical and globular cups, rectangular plates, and large kettles. The color is red, the body coarse and modeled by hand, and the firing uneven. The red or black Merimdeh wares are slightly more developed: there appear the first handles, holes pierced for suspension, and certain incised linear motifs. Peculiar to Deir Tasa are brown or black calyx vases decorated with lines over which triangular elements are incised and filled with white paste. Ceramic fabrics underwent their greatest development in the Aëneolithic Age, while products of the north became differentiated from the better-documented wares of the south. The oldest civilization of this period was the Badarian. Here decoration was more interesting than the shapes themselves: parallel striations diagonal to the base were obtained with a comb of six or eight teeth. Firing having improved, red and brown pots with black rim were added to the monochrome wares. Carinate pots are characteristic, but handles are not usual. The late Aëneolithic Age in both areas coincided with the predynastic period and is commonly designated as the "Naqada period." The Naqada pottery types are diver-

sified. A finely polished red class includes the first narrow-necked bottle types; barrel-shaped pots; and black-rimmed pots with pointed base and several cups with a foot. An important class with wavy handles ranges from a wide one-piece jar (without indentation in the line of the body) to a small cylindrical vase with a little cord about the neck. Red decorated pots comprise two distinct categories: the earlier with white decoration, the other with a rich repertory of geometric, floral, and animal motifs in pale violet. Representations of boats are very frequent. Other forms are pots with plastic decoration (fertility goddess or "Dea Mater"), twin pots, zoomorphic pots (birds, fish), and spouted pots. But during the period of the Thinite dynasties (ca. 2850–2650 B.C.) pottery began to decline in the face of the manufacture of stone vessels. Decoration, handles, and feet disappeared; production became monotonous; the brown or red color was enlivened only by tinting with a hematite base. To this period belong the earliest examples of opaque-glazed pots and small vases.

During the Old Kingdom (2980–2475) techniques were improved by the gradual adoption of the handwheel. Pointed-base amphoras made of a soft, brown homogeneous material are characteristic of the 4th and 5th Dynasties (ca. 2600–2350). The pottery of the 12th Dynasty (1991–1786) displays a predilection for brown globular and pyriform pots. During the period of the New Kingdom (ca. 1580–950) a revival of quality brought with it bulbous forms with high necks and two handles, bottles, and lenticular flasks with small papyriform columns. The decorative repertory, in pleasant colors, was inspired by stylized floral motifs, and occasionally there are lively representations of animals; sometimes the decoration imitates the spots and veinings on stone pots. A few jugs of this period show figures and figurines in high relief emerging from the body; some pots are zoomorphic or in the shape of a bunch of flowers. Multiple vases in various arrangements also occur, as well as some canopic urns of painted terra cotta. Also during the New Kingdom the glazed ware often called "faïence" played an important role. In this category (with a blue or green glaze predominating) is a slender lotiform calyx with a circular, lobed, or squared mouth (PL. 130). The petals and veins are raised or painted in brown or violet. Glazed cups are decorated with a great variety of motifs: the more common are groups of nymphs sporting in a pool; while among more complex designs there are figures of dancers and musicians, boating scenes, and caricature motifs, among which the most widespread is that of a monkey musician.

From the Middle Kingdom (2400–1580 B.C.) on, small glazed figures were also produced in great number. They were funerary models whose purpose was generally protective or designed to avert evil (apotropaic). The bulk consisted of female figures known as "concubines," often nude and with prominent sexual features, and the mummiform figures called "ushabtiu" which were to substitute for the deceased in the manual labors of the nether world. The production of these last became standardized, with green or blue glaze, and continued from Saite to Roman times (4th cent.–30 B.C.). Also numerous were animal figurines, among them remarkably natural hippopotamuses, monkeys, and dogs. Many glazed amulets and pectoral plaques for mummies were made, and there was a contemporary mass production of figures of gods and sacred animals. Particular mention, finally, should be made of polychrome enameled tiles (PL. 130), the most significant examples of which are those in the Palace of Ramses III at Medinet Habu.

Sergio BOSTICCO

*b. Mesopotamia.* In Mesopotamia the oldest decorated pots appeared toward the end of the Neolithic period in the 5th millennium B.C.: they are large vessels with a fabric of clay mixed with grass, carinate, and with painted and incised geometric designs. To this ware, whose Oriental origin is demonstrated by its contemporary presence in Iran in the lowest levels of Tepe Sialk and Tell-i-Bakun (near Persepolis), the name of Tell Hassuna has been given from the locality (near Kirkuk) in which it was found. From the 4th millennium

another north Mesopotamian ware has been identified, also of Iranian origin (Tepe Sialk, Anau, Tepe Giyan) and named for its discovery in Samarra. Besides the dominant geometric decoration, naturalistic elements were also introduced: fish, birds, and other animals as well as highly schematized human figures (dancers), stags, and birds. Through successive stages these motifs evolved into very elegant pure abstract forms, the most common being the swastika, which evolved from the form of four dancing women with their hair blowing in the wind. Tell Halaf pottery, not much later than Samarra ware, had a largely contemporaneous development. The most flourishing center of its production seems to have been Tell Arpachiya. Although affinities with Iranian pottery (Tepe Sialk, Tepe Hissar, Tepe Giyan, Tell-i-Bakun) are present, development was largely autonomous. Especially toward the end of the Halafian period, geometric decoration became very elegant and shapes very delicate, their carinate profile suggesting metalwork models (FIG. 203). The oldest Halafian pots were profusely decorated with lively naturalism: human figures, birds, quadrupeds, leopards, cobras, plants. While northern Mesopotamia developed its civilization under the influence of cultural currents from Iran (which sometimes borrowed from Mesopotamia in return), the southern part of the country also began to be peopled and to depend culturally on its northern and eastern neighbors. The sites of Hajj Mohammed and the ancient city of Eridu especially have given us a brilliantly varnished handmade monochrome ware (the color varies from pot to pot), decorated with geometric motifs; while maintaining a certain originality, the ware shows the influence of the styles of Samarra and Tell Halaf.

Probably as the result of an immigration of peoples from the southeast, southern Mesopotamia underwent a cultural development which was progressively imposed on the north as well (Tepe Gawra, Tell Arpachiya). The pottery of this period, still partly contemporary with Tell Halaf and called "al-'Ubaid," shows a rich variety of pot forms: plates, cups, long-necked vases, jugs, incense burners; all handmade and with monochrome decoration over a slip background. This included at first the usual geometric motifs, but especially in the northern regions it evolved a somewhat naturalistic repertory with stags (which bring us back to the Iranian Plateau) and birds predominating. The al-'Ubaid culture extended as far as the Mediterranean, with a special development in the Iranian Plateau (Susa I).

The Uruk phase (corresponding to the levels IV–VI of the city of that name; late 4th–early 3d millennium) in southern Mesopotamia represented a sudden break in ceramic production: Monochrome handmade pots with red or grayish slip, or black-burnished, took the place of painted wares. A coarser ware, without slip or decoration, was even more widespread. It was both wheel-thrown and handmade and often characterized by long spouts or handles. This change also made itself felt to some degree in the north: In Nineveh and Tepe Gawra a similar coarse undecorated ware superseded the al-'Ubaid pots. The Uruk pottery marks a break in the evolution of Iranian wares as well. But Mesopotamian pottery did evolve beyond Uruk wares, and pots of the next "Jemdet Nasr," or "predynastic," period often bear a monochrome painted or incised decoration much as at al-'Ubaid, even while repeating the shapes of the preceding period.

The rise of Sumerian civilization coincided in Mesopotamia with the nearly total disappearance of painted pottery, which was generally replaced by a monochrome material devoid of all artistic merit. Even temple wares gave way to stone pots richly carved in relief. But about 1500 B.C., in northern Mesopotamia, painted wares reappeared — with a glaze. This pottery, known by various names (Mitannian, Tell Atchana, Tell Billa), was distributed in the East as well (Syria) and was characterized by an elegant Mediterranean-inspired decoration with stylized, geometric plant motifs. The glazes which appeared on Mitannian ceramics, were not limited elsewhere to vase production. Among other glazed objects, a figure of a lion was found at Nuzu.

In the Neo-Assyrian period (early 1st millennium B.C.) painted pottery made a late reappearance in Assyria: polychrome jugs and cups decorated with geometric motifs, in which curved lines predominate, or with scenes, generally a pair of goats rampant on either side of a tree or climbing down opposite sides of a hill. The presence of elements typically Iranian, at least in their origin, strengthens the hypothesis that this vase painting represents the last phase of a style which emerged under the influence of Iran in the latter half of the 2d millennium.

Mesopotamian ceramics are not limited to pots. Besides the fairly numerous large terra cottas of historical times (see SCULPTURE), little pottery figures were produced during the whole course of Mesopotamian civilization. Their iconography in prehistoric times was limited almost entirely to the representation of the nude goddess and of animals, but with the passage of time and the perfecting of technique the repertory was enlarged. The best examples of small terra cottas are those found by American excavators in the Diyala River district (late 3d millennium). Their iconography is still incomprehensible (e.g., a hero kills a monster whose head is a sun with a single eye), as no literary work has produced the mythological key. The workmanship is very fine. Many little terra-cotta models, perhaps domestic, for sanctuaries have been found at various sites, as well as the small terra cottas used in divination which show coiled intestines or the face of the demon Humbaba (Huwawa), who was thought to assist the reading of entrails (PL. 131). Finally we shall mention the fragments from Chagar Bazar, representing chariots and bridled horses, with painted details.

Terra cotta also had its architectural uses in Mesopotamia. Even in prehistoric Uruk ceramic nails with polychrome heads decorated massive brick columns. During the Kassite rule in Babylonia (1746–1171 B.C.) terra cotta was widely used to face sacred buildings and palaces. Later simple sculptured terra cotta gave way to enameled brickwork, sometimes put together to make up large reliefs.

*c. Syria and Palestine.* The Syro-Palestinian region did not have a truly autonomous and original production of painted pottery in antiquity. Foreign pottery was imported or imitated, especially from the Aegean. The oldest decorated pots have straight or wavy, brown or red lines in a prevailingly vertical direction over the whole surface of the pot. In a second phase (Early Bronze II; 2900–2600 B.C.) high stump pots with burnished red slip were produced; as in the preceding phase, Palestinian wares rather faithfully mirrored Egyptian models, while the northern region remained under the prevailing Mesopotamian influence (e.g., pottery from Tell esh Sheikh, late 4th millennium, which substantially reproduced Tell Halaf motifs). The most important phase of Syro-Palestinian culture of the Early Bronze Age was the third (2600–2300). The pottery of this period, known as Khirbet Kerak (from the modern name of ancient Beth-yerah, where it was first found), was handmade, in black or red and sometimes both. Forms are elegant; decoration is geometric with the spiral occurring frequently. Northern influence continued to play a role for some time: in the Middle Bronze I period (2100–1900) the calyx form of Caucasian-Anatolian origin (Alaca Hüyük) reached as far as Syria (Hama) and Palestine. But Palestine was to be more influenced by Egyptian models. In the Middle Bronze II period (1900–1600) wheel-thrown pots continued the traditional imitation of metalwork, the illusion being heightened with the application of red or cream-colored slip. Handmade pots were now limited to the coarser kitchen wares. Palestine passed under the direct political control of Egypt in the Late Bronze Age (ca. 1500 B.C.), a period which saw also the introduction of Aegean wares into the area. Vase decoration now included painted bands of alternating geometric and naturalistic motifs (fish, birds, goats) arranged in metopes. So-called "Philistine" pottery was added to this production in the last two centuries of the 2d millennium, this being an autonomous development of the regions of Palestine, rather than the production of immigrants from Egypt. A strong Mycenaean influence is here mingled with some Iranian-Mesopotamian motifs.

Productions of forms other than vases was very ancient in Palestine. A mask, or rather a very flattened sculpture from Jericho, dates to the Neolithic period; it bears traces of overpainting and the eyes are shells. The use of terra cotta was widespread in a later period (2d millennium): anthropoid sarcophagi, temple furnishings (especially incense containers and burners), domestic altars, models of sanctuaries. Examples have also been found in Phoenician cities (e.g., a cart with two people, from Ugarit). Anthropomorphous vases (common to Mitannian ware from northern Mesopotamia) were widespread throughout the region about 1500 B.C.

*d. Anatolia.* The oldest pottery of Anatolia is the neolithic ware from Mersin in Cilicia (the only one of its regions where the Neolithic Age has been documented). During the 5th and 4th millenniums this pottery faithfully reflected the evolution taking place contemporaneously in Mesopotamia, displaying the successive styles of Tell Hassuna, Samarra, and Tell Halaf. An original Anatolian ware did not make its appearance until the late 3d millennium in the so-called "Cappadocian" ware; handmade, its largely geometric polychrome designs are in black, red, and white. Zoomorphic rhyta are abundant. This type, which continued for several centuries, became ever more elegant in form, thanks partly to the use of the wheel, and acquired a red slip. It was in use during the Hittite period (2d millennium). Excavations conducted at Alishar Hüyük (the most important Anatolian region for the study of pottery) have revealed the duration of pot shapes after such metal prototypes as those of distant Caucasian provenance from nearby Alaca Hüyük. Iranian motifs also figured in the decoration. The evolution of Alishar pottery until the destruction of the Hittite empire (12th cent. B.C.) is of some interest; vases became bigger (especially at the base) and two-handled, while naturalistic motifs of clearly Aegean inspiration were added to the geometric meanders, especially birds (I, PL. 527). This evolution, which seems to owe its existence to new arrivals on Anatolian soil, was to culminate in the lively pottery of the Phrygians (first half of 1st millennium; (see ASIA MINOR, WESTERN).

Giovanni GARBINI

*e. Cyprus.* From the Early Bronze Age in Cyprus (roughly the second half of the 3d millennium B.C.) is a red polished ware, with incised (sometimes filled) designs or geometric and stylized animal motifs in relief (IV, PL. 91). It has four chronological phases. The principal shapes are bowl, jar, and jug in imitation of gourds and later of leather (askos), wood (bowl), and basketwork (lidded pyxis), as well as animal-shaped vases. It was later joined by a closely related black polished ware as well as red-slip and black-slip wares. The more important white painted ware first produced at the end of the Early Bronze Age became the most typical Bronze Age Cypriote pottery, going through five chronological phases. The earliest specimens, though closely related to the red polished ware, also show influence from Asia Minor and Syria. The pots are covered with a slip, on which simple geometric ornaments are applied in red or buff paint. Also found are double and ring vases and a gradually developing variety of bowls, jugs, bottles, and amphoras with concave necks and vertical handles. The white-slip ware is distinct and consists largely of hemispherical bowls and jugs, decorated with variously treated bands in black, which seem to imitate the seams on leather vessels. Also important is the base-ring ware, of brown or gray clay with a lustrous brownish black slip: bowls, flasks, and jugs, and other shapes showing Mycenaean influence — pyxides, three-handled jars, and bull vases (in the form of a bull's head). Imitation of metal is apparent in some forms and also in relief bosses, handle rings, etc.; occasional relief or a little decoration in white paint appears. All these wares are handmade.

Small clay sculptures were produced (both single and grouped votive figures) as well as such objects as the *Temenos* of the Cyprus Museum in Nicosia (see CYPRIOTE ART, ANCIENT; IV, PL. 91), a complex religious scene.

During the early Iron Age there developed from a fusion of native with sub-Mycenaean traditions (IV, PL. 92) a Cypriote geometric style principally manifested in the white painted and bichrome wares (IV, PL. 93), which run parallel, during seven chronological periods, from the end of the 2d millennium B.C. to the Hellenistic age. Common shapes are plate, bowl, cup, footed goblet, crater and krateriskos, and several forms of large amphora, whose geometric ornament is disposed in zones or panels or so as to leave much of the vase plain. Concentric circles are popular in the third phase, and in the fourth there is a distinction between vases with rectilinear decoration, mainly from the southern and eastern parts of the island, and those with circle decoration, favored in the north and west. The lotus pattern introduces Eastern influence which becomes pronounced in the fifth phase. Figure work, showing influence from Greek vase painting (first Ionian and later Attic black-and red-figure), is sometimes found on vases of the last three phases. Black-on-red and red bichrome wares are also important. The small, mostly votive, figurines are poor in quality.

*The Aegean and Greece. a. Bronze Age.* Evans's classification of Cretan Bronze Age pottery into Early, Middle, and Late Minoan, each divided into I, II, and III with some further subdivision, was based primarily on his excavations at Knossos. Early Minoan (or EM), which forms a transition from the Neolithic to the Bronze Age, he dated from about 3000 B.C. Work at Phaestos, however, suggests that this period was much shorter than has been supposed. Neolithic and EM pottery was handmade: gray polished ware with incised decoration, light ware with dark painted decoration, and later (EM III, conventionally ca. 2500–2200) dark-slipped ware with decoration first in white and then also in red paint. Patterns were abstract: rectilinear and curvilinear, or, in the "light-on-dark," occasionally stylized animal forms. The principal shapes were various forms of jug, sometimes beaked, cup, and bowl, sometimes spouted. Rare examples of anthropomorphous jugs exist, for example, the Koumasa jug (Heraklion, Archaeological Mus., inv. no. 4137), apparently the oldest of this type; they are related to the production of votive figures found at Palaikastro and Hagia Triada and perhaps derived from marble prototypes from the Cyclades (J. D. S. Pendlebury, *The Archaeology of Crete*, London, 1939, pp. 72, 86).

In MM I (end of 3d millennium) the introduction of the slow wheel made possible a great refinement of fabric and shapes (under metal influence). The light-on-dark decoration (elaborate florals, occasional animal and human figures), was also refined, with its peak in the Kamares ware of MM II (ca. 1900–1750, a period which also saw the introduction of the fast wheel). Delicate cups and jars, sometimes spouted, and large pithoi of coarser make were favorite shapes (PL. 131). Dark-on-light decoration also occurs, sometimes combined with relief (barbotine), especially on pithoi. Enormous hand-built storage jars with simple relief decoration and tiers of handles are also found.

Figurines, mainly votive, such as a warrior with a dagger or a wide-skirted orant with a high headdress are common. Also of the period is a glazed, or "faïence," ware, including vases and figurines, the best known of which are fish, bulls, and dancers with snakes (see CRETAN-MYCENAEAN ART).

During MM III and LM I (ca. 1750–1450), dark-on-light decoration supplanted light-on-dark, with a prevalence of naturalistic motifs, at first chiefly floral, later marine, under the influence of wall painting. Narrow-necked jugs, stirrup vases, funnel vases, and alabastra were favored, as well as tall three-handled jars, the principal vehicles of the "palace style" (LM II, ca. 1450–1400; PL. 131). This form appeared also on the Greek mainland, which had begun importing Cretan vases in quantity in LM I, and was probably produced there as well. The fine technique and great elegance of form and drawing of "palace-style" vases was soon accompanied by increasing stylization of natural motifs. This tendency grew in LM III (ca. 1400 into 12th cent. B.C.) when Cretan pottery was incorporated into the Mycenaean "koine."

Neolithic handmade polished wares in red and black, with decoration incised and sometimes filled, resembling those of

Crete and Asia Minor, are found in the Cyclades. Jars, pyxides, beaked jugs, and ring vases were favorite shapes. There was also an Early Bronze Cycladic ware: generally painted, dark-on-light, with rectilinear and curvilinear motifs and occasional stylized animals. Pithoi, beaked jugs, and various forms of cup are found, as well as remarkable kernoi (multiple vases presumably of ritual use). The Middle Bronze Age saw an increasing interest in natural forms, especially elaborately stylized birds. During the Late Bronze Age the local island tradition died out or was absorbed in the Mycenaean koine.

At the end of the Neolithic age distribution of wares from Thessaly to the Peloponnese was fairly uniform: polished pots, sometimes incised; painted pots with linear designs in black or red (sometimes both) on a white or buff ground. A special class was covered with white paint, then with red, which was scraped away while still wet to leave geometric patterns in the white. In the Early Bronze Age a polished ware continued, sometimes incised with linear patterns or stamped with concentric circles. More characteristic was a light ware on which a dark glaze paint was laid in linear patterns or in a plain wash over all or part of the vase, linear patterns in white being sometimes added on top. Shallow bowls, tankards, askoi, and "sauceboats" are the commonest shapes of these wares, but cups, jars, and jugs, all handmade, are also found. Wheel-made pottery was introduced in the Middle Helladic period, corresponding approximately to the Middle Minoan in Crete. Most important was the gray Minyan, perhaps introduced by the Achaeans late in the 3d millennium: polished vases with wide flat rims and angular profiles suggesting metal models, stemmed goblets, deep bowls, jugs, jars, and cups. Yellow Minyan was a development of this ware, while a red-slip ware and coarser imitations were also related. Concurrent were painted wares, some large coarse vases, others smaller and finer with a fabric related to yellow Minyan, decorated with geometric patterns and occasional natural motifs in mat paint, black, brown, or red. The coarse ware includes pithoi, jugs, basins, and jars; the fine ware, stemmed goblets, cups, jugs — sometimes beaked — bowls, and jars. There are also some with two-color decoration. Toward the end of the Middle Helladic period (perhaps ca. 1700 B.C.), luster-painted imitations of Cretan fabrics began, both dark-on-light and light-on-dark, the latter continuing during LH I, and in LH II becoming the norm.

During LH III (from the 14th cent. B.C. onward) a common style with its center at Mycenae was established throughout the Aegean area. This Mycenaean pottery was produced not only in the Peloponnese and Crete, but in Attica, Rhodes, and Cyprus. It was traded to Asia Minor, Syria, and Egypt in the East, Sicily and the Aeolian (Lipari) Islands in the West. Besides shapes of Cretan origin (stirrup vase, alabastron, jug, three-handled jar), new favorites in this period were the tall-stemmed goblet, perhaps modeled after earlier mainland types, craters (especially the amphoroid crater) and, in the late 13th century B.C. the deep bowl. Decoration became increasingly stylized. A special late-13th-century class are the "pictorial vases," mainly craters, decorated with human figures, from Mycenae and especially Cyprus. From Mycenae the most famous example is the *Warrior Vase*. Others, mostly fragmentary, have been found also on the mainland. But the largest distinctive group is rarely found outside Cyprus and was probably made there by Achaean settlers. Craters and other vessels were decorated with bulls, birds, chariot groups, etc. During the decline of the Achaean civilization (12th–11th cent. B.C.) forms became more stylized and the fabric coarser and weaker. Some deep bowls were decorated in a "close style" of massed abstract patterns which anticipated those of the next period.

Small fictile art, still ritual or votive, appeared in reliefs or figurines.

*b. Iron Age: proto-Geometric and Geometric styles.* The Achaean civilization gave way before the rise of the city-states of historical Greece, and the Aegean Sea became a Greek lake. Well before 1000 B.C. Mycenaean styles were supplanted by a new Athenian style which, though widely imitated, showed more and more marked local deviations. This characteristically varied proto-Geometric ware departed from sub-Mycenaean in shapes, decorative schemes, and motifs, but it was clearly a renaissance within Attic workshops and not the importation of a foreign style. Traditional shapes and others quite new — the neck-handled amphora, the globular pyxis, and a tall conical foot for cups and craters — show a precision foreign to Mycenaean, but the originally naturalistic motifs were ousted by abstract forms both old and new. With an increasing tendency to pack patterns close, whole areas of the vase were covered with paint; and in late proto-Geometric all the vase was thus covered, except the zones of pattern, so that the general effect was very dark, influenced, perhaps, by the quality of the black color perfected by Attic potters. Vases in the form of animals also appear.

Many centers evolved true Geometric styles out of proto-Geometric ones, but by far the richest and fullest was Attic (II, PL. 32). The Geometric style (q.v.) is defined by changes of shape, but more especially by selectivity in the abstract patterns used and much greater elaboration and subtlety in their disposition. The wide areas of black shrank, while the principle of covering the surface was maintained by the use of delicately graded bands of pattern circling the whole height of the vase. The hallmark of the period was the meander, but other patterns were also in use: the hatched swastika especially on the central zone, often divided into panels; concentric circles with a cross in the center; and the *mandorla*, a leaf or flower motif unique in the Geometric repertory. Shapes were amphoras with belly or neck handles and tall wide necks, round-mouthed jugs with similar necks, trefoil-mouthed jugs with narrow and often tall necks, high-footed craters, several variations of low cup, and low pyxides with flat lids.

The one exception to proto-Geometric abstraction was the appearance on late vases of little silhouette horses, sometimes tucked away under handles, drawn in a few simple straight and curved lines. However, bands of birds or grazing beasts as well as rigidly geometric funerary figures increased in frequency, the earliest probably on enormous amphoras and craters about 5 ft. high. From the grave jar the practice spread to smaller vessels, especially amphoras and oinochoai, funerals and battles by land and sea being the most popular scenes. Indeed, geometric ornament weakened during the 8th century B.C., and vases were covered with little more than thin stripes diversified with bands of zigzag, while the picture, when there was one, was given greater prominence in relation to the whole.

Geometric pottery was produced in many centers. Most of it, e.g., Attic, was for home consumption, but Cycladic and Corinthian were increasingly exported during the 8th century to the east and west Mediterranean. Rhodes had an impoverished style strongly reminiscent of the proto-Geometric, especially in a taste for wide black areas and crosshatched triangles. The false spiral often appeared on the sparsely decorated Cycladic ware. Birds were the only figures; they were also prominent in the Geometric of Crete, where motifs from the Bronze Age also survived. There was a lively production of clay figures (as at Karphi), of masks (as at Vrokastro), of anthropomorphous vases, e.g., the lady with the "Lybian wig"), and also of pinakes — clay tablets decorated in relief. One of the oldest manufactures of clay figures from this period has been identified at the Temple of Hera in Samos, where large, unsophisticated female figures were produced. Boeotian was simply a provincial imitation of Attic, and much the same can be said of production of the Argolid. Geometric earthenware votive idols, both plaques and bell shapes, were of some importance and tended to translate into sculpture the motifs on the pottery of the period (II, PL. 43).

Corinthian wares, the finest produced outside Athens, are simpler, but their clay and glaze are exceptionally fine. Early vases are largely black with a single panel of simple geometric design. Later ware, and finally the "sub-Geometric" of the succeeding period, is covered with even, fine, and close-set lines, while shapes show individuality and refinement. The forms of craters — with or without tall foot — jugs, and occasional amphoras and hydrias are closely related to those of other wares, though they are more elegant. From the ordinary Geo-

metric cup, low and wide with offset rim, comes a neater type, very fine-walled and with no modulation of contour at the lip: the kotyle or skyphos, which with the aryballos (and at a later date the column crater) was Corinth's chief contribution to the Greek pottery repertory. The aryballos, a small round scent bottle, perhaps derived from a Cypriote shape; it seems in any case to be connected with the Eastern trade which was reawakening in the 8th century B.C. Many of these and other Corinthian vases are found in the Western colonial sites that were settled from the mid-8th century on. Good imitations were made at Cumae and perhaps in other colonies; rougher ones in Italy and Sicily. Laconian pottery is a provincial ware, which also looks to Corinth. In the pottery of Ithaca, a sub-Mycenaean strain remains, even with the development of a local Geometric style under Cycladic and Corinthian influence that lasted into the Orientalizing period.

Crude clay figures and fine plaques in low relief were produced in all these centers, as well as in Corinth and Argos, Magna Graecia, Ephesos and Rhodes, and especially Asia Minor; also figures hollowed out by cylindrical stamps, with heads worked with a stick.

The Geometric style was disintegrating when works in a more sophisticated convention, imported from the East, opened Greek eyes to new possibilities. The new style was gradually absorbed into vase painting. Swinging curves were substituted for rectlinear precision, with corresponding modification of vase shapes. The repertory of figures was enriched: Eastern plant motifs, beasts, and monsters were combined with human figures, generally in mythological scenes. The thin silhouettes of Geometric ware were expanded into more lifelike shapes drawn in outline; details were incised on the black, white, red, and occasionally yellow ground. "Orientalizing" vases were made in most of the centers that had produced Geometric wares, but the Corinthian and Athenian were unrivaled (PL. 132; II, PL. 35).

The tradition of large vases continued in Athens; some were modified from the old forms: stemmed craters, neck amphoras, and tall slender hydrias based on the neck amphora; others were new: stemless craters, large lidded vessels (pyxides and lekanai), and a variety of small jugs and cups. Vessels were divided into graded zones, with the pattern bands reduced to forms of zigzag and sown over the background, making a shimmering surface on which the figures stand out. This form of decoration was to continue in use for centuries. Often one picture occupies most of the vase. On most archaic vases the foot is rayed with a conventional flower pattern. A simple pattern of loops is a feature on the back of many large Attic and Cycladic vases of this period, suggesting that they were made for ornament rather than use. Some were certainly grave vases in the Geometric tradition. The heads of some of the figures — people or animals — are in contour, the bodies in silhouette, with details added in white.

Some vases were sculptured, notably the jug from the Kerameikos (II, PL. 34). In the mid-7th century B.C. many Attic vase painters used almost as much white as black, and both white and black figures appeared together on the same vase. The "black-figure" technique, with figures in black silhouette and details incised or in color, appeared in most fabrics from the early Orientalizing period; after its early development into a consistent style by the potters of Corinth, it eventually became the norm for archaic vase painting, triumphing in Athens before the end of the century (see ARCHAIC ART; ATTIC AND BOEOTIAN ART).

As the Corinthian Geometric style had no important tradition of figure drawing, development there was different from that in Athens. The vases are comparatively small: aryballoi (first globular, soon ovoid, from the mid-7th century pyriform, from the last quarter round); alabastra from the mid-7th century: kotylai; small pyxides and oinochoai, including two Corinthian specialties — a conical form and, from the mid-7th century, olpai. There was less experiment in technique of drawing. Black-figure, developed with technical virtuosity and exceptional feeling for calligraphy, soon became the rule, its perfection being Corinth's most important contribution to Greek ceramic

development. Mid-century Corinthian potters also produced polychrome vases with figure scenes whose complex groupings clearly derived from free painting. These were mostly tiny aryballoi, but slightly larger works were made later. The decline of Corinthian ware, which began late in the 7th century, was almost complete by the second half of the 6th. Vases with friezes of animals and occasional human figures against a thick sowing of rosettes were more and more mass-produced. It is true that more careful figure work is found on the large column-craters (a Corinthian invention of the later 7th century) and on cups, plates, oinochoai, neck amphoras, and one-piece amphoras (see below), but the best of these, though competent, are dull next to the best contemporary Attic ware. Later Corinthian potters (ca. 550 B.C.) were to imitate Attic ones by washing their pale clay with orange, but their polychromy was typically bright and their compositions complex. Some very fine small perfume pots in the form of animals or occasionally human beings are a feature from before 650 B.C. into the 6th century. After the 8th century, Corinthian had displaced almost all other wares in the West, but it was rivaled and eventually driven out by Attic ware early in the 6th century.

Painted Orientalizing vases from Boeotia were largely imitated from Attic. More individual are big pithoi with designs in relief (patterns, animals, figure scenes). Similar relief pithoi were produced in Crete and Rhodes, and other relief vases in Corinth. The Argolid produced a few impressive pieces, but there is no evidence of Argolid painted pottery after 650 B.C. Laconian Orientalizing wares developed out of local Geometrical ones under Corinthian influence; apart from certain local shapes, especially the lekane, they had little individuality.

Distinctive Orientalizing vases in black-figure and mixed techniques have been found at Knossos, Afrati, and other parts of Crete. Ovoid pithoi of Geometric derivation from Knossos were sometimes white-slipped and painted in red and blue. Production of painted pottery on the island seems to have died out by about 650 B.C.

Cycladic black-figure is rare, (see GREEK ART, AEGEAN), but the big amphoras known as "Melian" were made in the mid-7th century, with large floral motifs and figure work in outline and added color. There were also smaller vases, including large aryballoi, Corinthian in shape and decorated in the eastern Greek "wild-goat style." Cycladic pottery seems to have died out by the 6th century. Some Orientalizing vases, showing Cycladic, Attic, and Corinthian influence, were produced at Eretria in Euboea.

From all the eastern islands and the Asia Minor coast come vases in the "Rhodian" or "wild-goat style." The oinochoe is commonest, with a band of lotus and bud at the foot, one or more bands of running goats or spotted deer, and on the shoulder animals and monsters sometimes flanking an elaborate floral design (see GREEK ART, AEGEAN). These designs are in both silhouette and outline with color added, but without incision. Stemmed dishes, squat oinochoai, and toward the end of the century olpai, plates, and dinoi were probably produced in this style in Rhodes, Samos, Ephesos, Miletos; a provincial version has been found at Larisa in Aeolis, and related wares in Lydia and Phrygia. Late in the 7th century black-figure decoration showing Corinthian influence was introduced, especially in the shoulder-friezes of oinochoai and dinoi. The style did not continue after 575 B.C. The vases are of a dark reddish clay covered with white slip. Concurrent was a "sub-Geometric" series in pale brownish clay without slip, mainly small, shallow, low-footed cups decorated with birds or rosettes.

The ware of Chios ("Naucratite" — previously thought to have been made at Naucratis) is remarkable for the fineness of its white slip and its drawing, the popularity of the distinctive "chalice" shape, and the introduction of polychrome human figures. Later Chios adopted the familiar black-figure technique, but quality degenerated.

Molded perfume pots are also a feature of eastern Greek ware, particularly in the form of human or animal heads.

*c. Archaic period.* Attic grave vases gave way to other forms of funerary monument in the late 7th century B.C.; the last

were in pure black-figure technique and style. Certain pinakes, made for votive and perhaps funerary purposes, were either all painted or partly in relief and partly painted, a fact suggesting their manufacture by professional potters. Small earthenware votive figures were the work of a special group of craftsmen, whose style showed slight regional variations. Sculptures, also produced in the pottery workshops, were generally of standing women or of animals but were characterized by their decoration in glaze paint: red or black, clear or opaque. When they became an art in their own right and no longer the work of vase makers, they lost all sign of painted decoration.

Solon's reforms and the commercial rivalry of Athens and Corinth may have contributed to diminishing production in the next generation. At any rate Attic ware shows intensified Corinthian influences by the second quarter of the 6th century B.C. especially in cups of a form widespread in Athens as well as in Corinth and eastern Greece. At the same time some workshops perfected the fine orange clay and bright black glaze, and achieved a wonderful refinement in potting and drawing, typified by the *François Vase* in the Museo Archeologico in Florence (signed by the potter Ergotimos and the painter Kleitias, who were among the earliest masters). This vase is a new shape, the volute crater, perhaps originating in Laconian metalwork; the decoration is on a miniature scale, arranged in zones, as on Geometric vases (I, PL. 348; II, PL. 36). Small figures also appear on the so-called "little master" (or "miniaturist" style) cups, in which the signatures of the potter or painter are part of the decoration (PL. 135). Other painters worked in a larger style, especially on the one-piece amphora, probably a Attic invention of about 500 B.C. (e.g., the one by Exekias; I, PL. 349). Here parts are not sharply offset, but merging curves unite the whole vase, checked only by the moldings of mouth and foot. A new decorative scheme fits the new shape: the vase is painted black, a panel reserved on each side for the picture, often a pair of horsemen.

Outstanding in the more monumental tradition were the painter Lydos (mid-6th cent.), the potter Amasis (second half of 6th cent.), and the potter-painter Exekias (q.v.), whose combination of the grand and exquisite makes him the greatest of vase painters. One of his favorite shapes was the neck amphora, which he remodeled from its tall slender form to a squat one (Amasis also made a variant) with short neck and elaborate floral motifs at the handles occupying as much of the surface as the picture at back and front. Perhaps the inventor of a new shape, the calyx-crater (later immensely popular), he elaborated the theme of the one-piece amphora. Both he and Amasis tried new cup forms with less demarcation than in the "little master" cups and more picture space, a scheme developed by their successors. Exekias and Lydos also painted pinakes for the adornment of tombs. Their pupils invented the revolutionary red-figure technique, but Attic black-figure continued important until the end of the 6th century and in some connections far beyond; in the 7th century it was still made largely for home use. Its exportation, begun in the early 6th century, was appreciable after 550 B.C., soon winning the Italian market and being sold throughout the Mediterranean region.

Imitations of Attic black-figure were produced in Eretria and Boeotia. As for Corinthian ware, besides that under Oriental influence noted above, there was an enormous production of painted pinakes.

Laconian vase painters of the 6th century specialized in stemmed cups (deriving from the Attic "little master" cups), white-slipped and decorated outside with a network of pattern and inside with mythological or everyday scenes in rather crude black-figure. They were also exported to Italy and to Cyrene, where they were once thought to have been made.

In eastern Greece the "wild-goat style" was succeeded (second quarter of 6th cent.) by the "Fikellura," produced in workshops in both Rhodes and Samos. On the favorite broad neck amphoras, as well as on oinochoai and slender amphoriskoi, a pale slip is used with a pseudo black-figure silhouette without incision. Make and drawing are rough; it is a peasant ware compared with the related but sophisticated products of Athens. The ware continued at least until after 525 B.C. Some very

fine eastern Greek "little master" ware in black-figure, perhaps made in Samos, is also related.

Various eastern Greek black-figure fabrics of about 575–525 B.C., some probably from Klazomenai (Clazomenae), are called "Clazomenian" (see GREEK ART, EASTERN). Of brownish clay, they comprise mainly two types of neck amphora, slim and broad, the body often circled by women in procession or dance or by mythological scenes. On either side of the neck is a single motif, often a palmette or a sphinx. This ware differs from Attic in the use of white for some male figures and white lines and dots for details, as do other loosely related vases. The "Northampton group," which closely imitates mid-century Attic and was perhaps made by a Greek settled in Etruria, is the finest. Also at Klazomenai are clay sarcophagi similar to the vases in decoration but sometimes copying early Attic red-figure. Others, of the early 5th century, are at Rhodes, with subsidiary decoration in the "wild-goat style" of a century earlier, the link being perhaps through textiles.

Fragments of many large vases of a tall cylindrical form, known as "situlae," decorated in black-figure in varied styles, were found at Tell Defenneh in Egypt and probably made there, though earlier examples of this shape come from Rhodes, where an occasional black-figure vase seems to have been made.

The best eastern Greek black-figure is on a group of hydrias, most if not all found at Caere (mod. Cerveteri) in Etruria (I, PL. 362). Round pots in orange clay, they are decorated by one or two painters in a style of eastern Greek origin with amusing mythological scenes, animal groups, and florals. In pure Greek style of the second half of the century (one has Greek inscriptions), their provenance and some likeness to Etruscan vase and tomb painting suggests that their creators may have worked in Italy.

The most important class of black-figure pottery produced outside Athens and Corinth presents a similar problem. Its name, "Chalcidian," is from the alphabet used by its first painter, but the many pieces of known provenance were all found in the West and it was probably made in a Greek colony or by Greeks settled in Etruria. The work of two generations, it appeared before 550 B.C. Clay, technique, and general character emulate Attic, but there are also affinities with late Corinthian and eastern Greek. Shapes are the favorite early ovoid neck amphora, often with a picture all around, sometimes black with panel decoration; the one-piece amphora; and a double-walled cooling vessel, a variety of amphora-psykter or neck amphora-psykter (found also occasionally in Attic) with a spout on the shoulder. Also common are column craters and hydrias and, in the later phase, oinochoai and especially a new form of cup, a lipless wide shallow bowl on a big foot with almost no stem. Though similar to a popular contemporary Attic form, it differs in detail, especially the foot. Like its Attic counterpart the outside always has a great pair of eyes on each side, but also a nose and ears, rare in Attic; the face is sometimes spoiled by the addition of figures, such as the satyr mask or gorgoneion common on Attic and earlier Corinthian cups. Round the inside of the lip runs a broad frieze with mythological and Dionysiac scenes, a favorite subject for Greek vase painting after 700 B.C.

*d. Attic red-figure and its origins.* Red-figure was invented about 530 B.C., probably by an anonymous painter who worked with the potter Andokides (the "Andokides Painter"; he was perhaps that same black-figure pupil of Exekias known as the "Lysippides Painter"; II, PL. 37). In red-figure, which is the reverse of black-figure, the background is filled in with shiny black, and the figures are silhouetted in the orange of the clay. It first gained a hold on the one-piece amphora, which was already largely covered with black. Early unsuccessful attempts to apply it to the light-colored neck amphora led to a remodeling of the shape.

Innovations of form, an early feature of the new technique, were not at first accompanied by a new style. Figures were still disposed as in black-figure and covered with the same fine decorative detail, but they were drawn with a brush instead of a graver, and with less red and white. Some vases were in

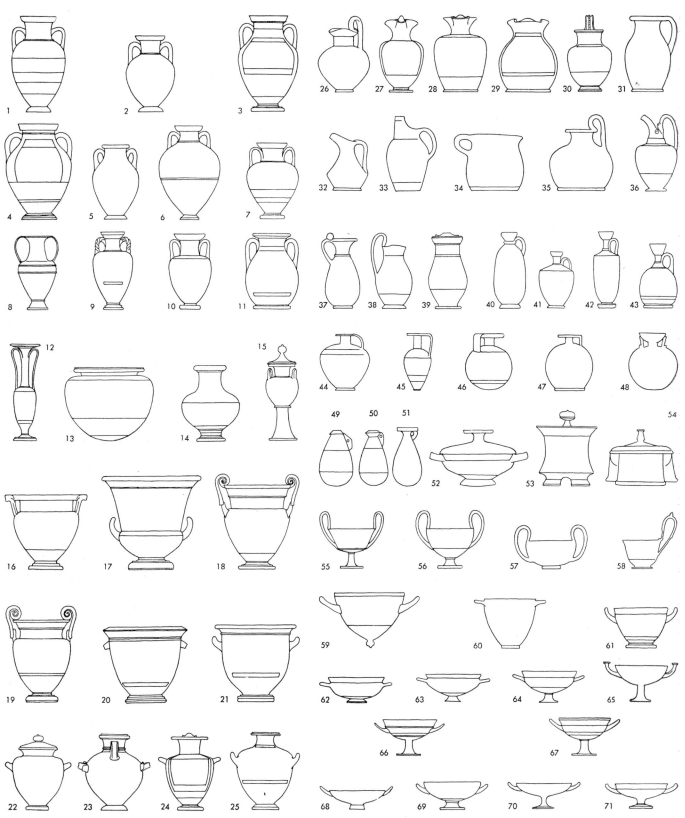

Greek pottery types (not in scale except within a single group). (1–10): Amphora: (1) Tyrrhenian (580–550 B.C.); (2) ovoid (600–540); (3–5) with panels (570–450); (6) Panathenaic (570–350); (7) neck amphora (550–500); (8) from the workshop of Nikosthenes (530–510); (9) with corded handles (500–420); (10) from Nola (490–400). (11) Pelike (520–400). (12) Loutrophoros. (13) Deinos (600–400). (14) Psykter. (15) Lebes gamikos. (16–21) Craters: (16) column crater (570–440); (17) calyx-crater (540–450); (18) volute crater (black-figure) (550–500); (19) volute crater (red-figure) (510–400); (20) stepped bell crater (480–450); (21) normal bell crater (450–400). (22) Stamnos. (23, 24) Hydria: (23) Corinthian and Attic (580–550); (24) normal (550–470). (25) Kalpis (510–400). (26–36) Oinochoe: (26) Corinthian; (27–36) Attic shapes. (37–39) Olpe: (37) Corinthian; (38) archaic (580–560); (39) normal (530–480). (40–43) Lekythos: (40) archaic, Corinthian, and Attic (620–580); (41) black-figure (560–530); (42) red-figure (510–420); (43) aryballoid (450–400). (44–48) Aryballos; (44) early proto-Corinthian (8th cent.); (45) middle and late proto-Corinthian (7th cent.); (46, 47) globular Corinthian (650–550); (48) Attic (520–480). (49–51) Alabastron: (49) proto-Corinthian (680–650); (50) Corinthian (680–630) (51) Corinthian (630–550). (52) Lekane. (53) Pyxis (480–440). (54) Tripod or Coton tripod pyxis (600–580). (55–57) Kantharos. (58) Kyathos. (59) Mastos. (60, 61) Skyphos: (60) Corinthian; (61) Attic. (62–71) Lekythos: (62) Corinthian (650–550); (63) komast (600–570); (64) Siana (570–550); (65) with button handles (570–550); (66) lip cup (550–540); (67) hand cup (550–530); (68) Chalcidian (540–520); (69–71) with eyes: type A (540–500); (70) type B (510–400); (71) type C (500–400) (selected by Enrico Paribeni).

both techniques. But the freer flow of the brush led to more lifelike drawing and to a decorative effect of contour rather than of surface pattern, while draftsmen soon learned to vary the sharp "relief line," perhaps drawn with a pen, with a thin brown or gold line. By the end of the 6th century the invasion of the picture background by the black had produced a new compositional ideal: figures enlarged and contrasted against the bright black ground, with less reliance on subordinate ornament. To the generation which first evolved a red-figure style belongs Epiktetos, mainly a painter of cups and plates, and one of the most attractive. The new style was popular and much poor work was mass-produced, especially cups, mugs, and column craters. In the late 6th century a new group, the "pioneers," created that pinnacle of Greek vase painting, the late archaic red-figure style; among these painters were Euphronios and Euthymides, working with lesser companions. Related artists, the Leagros group, still produced black-figure in the "pioneer" spirit, much of it excellent in a big free style; but the old technique was less suited to the spirit of the time than the new, and theirs was the last great black-figure ware. Both groups preferred big pots: the amphora, neck amphora, calyx-crater, volute crater, and hydria, as well as new shapes, the stamnos, pelike, and psykter (FIG. 233), a cooler designed to fit into the calyx-crater. Older forms of hydria had given place in the mid-century to one with a sharp angle at the shoulder, which bears a small picture separate from the main one on the body. A new red-figure form was round-bodied, its picture on the shoulder or later sometimes spreading onto the body.

Most early red-figure and contemporary black-figure cups are of "type A": a deep bowl set off from the stout stem by a fillet, often with eye decoration. This type was adopted, by Nikosthenes, among others, whose workshop produced an amphora of characteristic shape (PL. 135). "Type B," a wide shallow bowl with a continuous double curve and a slender stem, is often decorated on the outside with many-figured scenes. The vase painters of the early 5th century are divided into two groups: pot painters and cup painters who, about 500 B.C., began to sign their works and who worked in both black- and red-figure into the Hellenistic age. Painting was largely in red-figure after 500 (e.g., on the characteristic prize vase for the Panathenaic games, an egg-shaped oil jar with narrow neck, which had previously always been decorated in black-figure), but until the mid-century there were still workshops specializing in black-figure (I, PL. 299). They made only hastily produced vases, however, mainly lekythoi (oil bottles), cups, and skyphoi. It was red-figure pot painters who produced the Panathenaic amphoras and lekythoi; the amphora was the Berlin Painter's favorite shape, and the lekythos was made famous by his pupil, the Achilles Painter.

Red-figure, like black-figure, with its emphasis on surface decoration through sharp silhouette, was essentially suited to an archaic style. By clinging to it classical vase painters cut themselves off from contemporary developments, and it is not surprising to find the finest painter of the generation, the Pan Painter, looking backward for his inspiration. Other painters worked with limited success in various styles, the best of them directly influenced by the contemporary revolution in wall painting, whose most important formal feature was the abandonment of the single base line for the picture, so that figures are set on different levels in an attempt to create some illusion of depth. But as the silhouette technique of vase painting contradicts the idea of depth, few painters used the new style.

In Attic potteries, from late archaic to classical times, many pinakes were produced in the same techniques as vases; also terra-cotta reliefs (known as "Melii" from the site of their first discovery) and figurines.

A white slip in use in eastern Greece and elsewhere after 600 B.C. became popular in Athens among certain black-figure artists, especially on oinochoai, lekythoi, skyphoi, and cups. Some late archaic red-figure painters, abandoning silhouette and drawing in outline, made use of this white slip, mainly on cup interiors but also on exteriors or on oinochai and alabastra. The drawing, at first in relief line, was supplanted about 480 B.C. by a softer outline in dilute golden glaze with washes of the same and of a dark violet-red, whose effect must approximate contemporary easel painting. The white-ground ware, however, never rivaled red-figure in quantity, partly perhaps because the surface is more perishable, partly because of the deep-seated love of silhouette, and it all but died out about the mid-5th century, except in grave lekythoi fashionable about 450–375. These were not exported; they are found exclusively in Attica or in Athenian settlements such as Eretria (PL. 365; II, PL. 48). Originally domestic, subjects soon came to show the tomb or offerings for it, Charon and his boat, or Sleep and Death carrying off a soldier's body. At first a clumsy "second white" was added for women's flesh, but it was soon abandoned. Later there was another technical change: the outline was no longer drawn in thinned glaze but in mat paint, black or red, susceptible of a sketchier handling. Some painters worked in all three styles. Two other shapes for private Athenian occasions — weddings or the funerals of those who died unmarried — were the lebes gamikos, a round jar on a tall stand, and the loutrophoros, a very tall, thin amphora or hydria derived perhaps from an early Orientalizing type. These were decorated in black- or red-figure with appropriate scenes (see ESCHATOLOGY).

Although the finest late-5th-century vase painting was in this white-slip technique, red-figure remained dominant. Early in the century a rather conventional picture was painted on one side of a vessel — a draped youth or youths — but the quality of drawing was not distinguished. The backs, indeed, soon degenerated, particularly on the cheap, popular bell craters which tended by 400 B.C. to replace red-figure column craters as mixing bowls. These red-figure bell craters first appeared in the work of the Berlin Painter. Their form, originally simple, perhaps adapted from wood, with lugs for handles and at first no foot, was finally stabilized with loop handles and disk foot with narrow stem. The psykter, always rare, and the large one-piece amphora died out, but the stamnos and the slender-neck amphora remained popular throughout the 5th century, and the pelike to the end of red-figure. The mass-produced, cheap small vases in red-figure increased in number after the demise of black-figure during the second half of the century, especially in various forms of squat lekythos and oinochoe, but they also became vehicles for the highly elaborate late-5th-century style associated with the name of Meidias, one of a whole group of good artists. The delicate elaboration and sweetness of their style, however, tended to fussiness in the second generation, when it became the dominant manner in Attic vase painting. Workshops also featured miniature versions of some of the large shapes. Particularly charming are small, fat oinochoai of a special shape (chous) used by children at the Anthesteria and decorated with scenes of child life. Decorated cups, both the stemmed and the stemless kylix, introduced before 450, were popular far into the 4th century. The best cup painters of the later 5th century are the Eretria and the Kodros Painters; of the 4th, the Jena Painter. As an antidote to the fussiness of Attic vase painting some workshops of the second quarter of the 5th century revived a simple, if rather empty, style known as "Kerch" from the rich find spot (anc. Panticapaeum) in southern Russia (II, PL. 54), which was perfected in the third quarter. Also from southern Russia is a late-5th–early-4th-century production of painted and gilded clay figures which were used in petitioning. These and similar products from Tarentine workshops are closely related to the "Melian" reliefs mentioned above.

By the end of the 4th century Attic pottery had not only lost the Western markets but died out in Athens itself, except for the black-figure Panathenaic prize amphoras which remained as a wretched travesty of an old fashion even into the 2d century B.C.

Plain black ware was plentiful at Athens after the later 6th century. Most common in this class were small traditional vases or miniature versions of large shapes. The insides of many stemless cups and pointed amphoriskoi of a century later were decorated with impressed palmettes and other patterns, while the outsides still bore red-figure designs. Later still, in the 4th century, large black vases were ribbed and some-

times decorated with wreaths in gilded relief. Red-figure indeed was supplanted almost entirely by plain black ware, which probably flourished to about 100 B.C. — e.g., the ware found on the Acropolis known as "west slope," deriving from the 4th-century wreathed vases whose decoration combined thinned clay, white mat, and incision. Wreaths gradually yielded to panels of geometric ornament, perhaps in imitation of proto-Geometric and Geometric pottery found in graves around the Acropolis.

At Athens the production of earthenware figures, both votive and secular, was such in the late 4th century B.C. that the city is now considered to have been the center of production of the prototypes for the famous Tanagra figurines. Elsewhere they were produced from molds, but in Athens they were produced freehand, or at least freely retouched. In the early 3d century these figures were of very high quality (PL. 138).

After Athens had gained the monopoly of fine vases, undecorated or slightly decorated wares continued to issue from the potteries of Corinth, eastern Greece, and Boeotia. The Corinthian production is unimportant, as is the Boeotian except for the black-figure "Kabeiric skyphoi" (II, PL. 54) with burlesqued heroic scenes, the Homeric cups (a Megarian ceramic type with epic subjects), and figurines of the Tanagra type. But soon after 450 B.C. the workshops of southern Italy became serious rivals to those of Athens and some outlasted her in the production of figured pottery. The work is so close to Attic as to be certainly the production of emigrant potters and painters, perhaps colonists of Thurii in 443 B.C. Of the two main early classes the works of the Amykos group (possibly made at Heraklion) are found largely to the west of the Gulf of Taranto and in Lucania. Although the best work of the early-4th-century Dolon Painter has a bigness and wit that make it superior to contemporary Attic, by 350 the style had declined into a crudely provincial Lucanian. Attic shapes were preferred (bell crater commonest, calyx-craters for better work) along with the local nestoris. Another group (the Sisyphos Painter with his followers, the Sarpedon and the Dionysiac Painters) almost certainly worked in Tarentum (PL. 376).

The bell crater was their favorite form also, though their best work is on volute craters, from which stemmed the central line of south Italian vase painting, Apulian, which flourished through the middle and late 4th century. This was a vast mass production of bell craters, pelikai, skyphoi, plates, lekanai, etc., decorated mainly with women and Erotes, with much added white and yellow; and enormous volute craters with many-tiered scenes, of great accomplishment and no esthetic worth. In a pretty technique known as "Gnathia," their necks, and complete smaller vases, sported women's heads among flowers or other motifs, in color added over the black and incision. The style, which appears in other south Italian fabrics, outlasted red-figure. During the early 4th century red-figure began to be produced in Campania, at Cumae, Avellae, and Paestum. Only the last is important. Two painters have left us their names, Assteas and his pupil Python, on calyx-craters and bell craters with scenes from comedy, and "Phlyax" vases, often partly or wholly in Gnathia technique (PL. 417). These "Phlyax" vases also figured in Apulian and Lucanian wares. On late-4th-century Sicilian red-figure ware, mostly lekanai and characteristic pyxides, color was added in steadily increasing amounts until there resulted a polychrome rather than a red-figure style. This type led to a class of vases made at Centuripe in the late 3d and 2d centuries B.C., covered with a white slip and bearing multicolored painting in a purely pictorial style (PL. 138). Large white-slipped askoi with much plastic decoration were made during the same period. At Canosa in southern Italy contemporary large white-slipped askoi bore much plastic decoration as well as some polychrome decoration in a far less pictorial spirit.

*Pre-Roman Italy and the western Mediterranean.* Rough handmade pottery, plain or with simple decoration, was produced in many forms but in a fairly regular tradition throughout the Italian peninsula and the western Mediterranean during the Neolithic and Bronze Ages — notably at Terramara

in the Po valley — until the colonizations by the Greeks and Phoenicians in early historical times. The earlier diffusion of Orientalizing techniques and motifs did make for some individual developments, as on the aëneolithic fabrics of southern Italy and Sicily. Mycenaean influences have been detected in the later bronze culture of the Apulian coast, in Sicily, and in the Lipari Islands (second half of 2d millennium). A characteristic "plumed" ware of the 8th century B.C. has been found in Sicily, especially at Cassibile. It should be noted that while these southern fabrics, with their "proto-Geometric" and "Geometric" decoration, reflect the direct influence of Greece, the northern Iron Age fabrics in geometric style with incised decoration depend largely on continental traditions.

While Punic influence was very limited, Greek production in all its phases was fundamental to the formation and development of the various fabrics of the western Mediterranean from the beginning of historical times to the Roman era. This is primarily true for Italy.

In those areas which were subject to direct colonization, Greek products as well as Greek artisans and techniques were imported and gave rise to well-defined local developments. Other areas, however, were characterized by an independent production of local archaic painted wares (which have been studied and classified at Megara Hyblaea in Sicily) and especially of archaic ceramic sculpture, common in both southern Italy and Sicily. Local imitation of Attic wares was to give rise to the Italiote and Siciliote productions at the begining of the 5th century B.C. (see above).

Still more interesting is the constant influence of Greece on Etruscan, Italic, and Apulian Iron Age pottery, in which the "impasto," or coarse reddish fabric, of protohistoric tradition originally dominated. It is characteristically used in the funerary urn, especially the biconical "Villanovan" urn (9th–7th cent. B.C.) of Etruria and Emilia, on whose lustrous black surface geometric decorations were incised. Inventiveness in forms is notable in smaller vases on which sculptured figures were often added in a naturalistic or schematic style similar to that of contemporary bronze vases. Some of these Etruscan vases are already imitations of Greek shapes (e.g., kantharoi, kyathoi, etc.), expecially the Etruscan wheel-made ware known as *bucchero*, whose characteristic highly polished body was obtained by fumigation (PL. 136). The finest *bucchero sottile*, with its ultimately rich repertory of forms, appeared as early as the 7th century and continued into the 6th. The mold-made *bucchero pesante*, with its animals and figure decorations in reliefs, lasted into the 5th century, especially within Etruria (see ETRUSCO-ITALIC ART).

Few Etruscan vases were exported. The 8th-century wheelmade and painted imitations of Greek pottery introduced the Geometric style. The "Italo-Corinthian" aryballoi, oinochoai, and olpai followed in the 7th and early 6th centuries. These were decorated with Geometric and Orientalizing ornaments, animal friezes, and some human figures, often in incision or painted on black in a technique then current in Corinth and eastern Greece and later in Attica. With the "Pontic" neck amphoras and oinochoai, imitations of Attic and eastern Greek black-figure were added in the mid-6th, and soon the large Micali group and its outliers boasted neck amphoras, hydrias, and kyathoi whose black-figure décor was varied, though centaurs and sirens predominated. After 500 B.C. came red-figure imitations, though at first they were mostly in a pseudo red-figure: the figures painted in light color over black. Its most important examples are the Praxias group (early 5th cent.): amphoras, neck amphoras, stamnoi, column craters, hydrias, oinochoai, etc.; and the Sokra group (4th cent.): largely cups. Although both groups bear occasional Greek inscriptions, they were certainly made in Etruria. The later Hesse group of kantharoi, apparently from southern Etruria or Latium, is indistinguishable from good Greek Gnathia. Bowls inscribed *pocolom* and the related plate with a war elephant are of the same provenance.

While some true red-figure was made in Etruria in the 5th century (the better pieces used relief line), only in the late 5th and early 4th centuries did groups crystallize; most of the best work was on cups and stamnoi. The first distinguishable

local fabric, Faliscan (PL. 137), introduced about 400 B.C. perhaps by immigrants from Athens, also favored cups and stamnoi, though their repertory included other familiar shapes. A contemporary group from Clusium consists mainly of cups but also of fine skyphoi, askoi in the form of ducks, etc., which fostered a class of column craters (at least part of which must have been made at Volaterrae) that continued into the 3d century. Lesser products, among them skyphoi and other large vases (mostly decorated with profiles of maenads and satyrs), goose-shaped askoi, etc., were widespread. In the 4th century a class of pottery known as "north Adriatic" developed a tendency to cursive design — even to the complete dissolution of outline. The painted Faliscan and Etruscan fabrics are so similar to their southern counterparts (Apulian, Lucanian, Campanian, Sicilian) that a single "facies," independent of national origin, may be said to have existed.

No other groups in these areas were notable for originality or continuity of development except the Apulian wheel-made painted vases, perhaps of Greek proto-Geometric and Geometric extraction, which flourished into the Hellenistic age. Its three groups, Daunian, Peucetian, and Messapian (on the Salentine peninsula), developed both monochrome and polychrome geometric designs, as well as many local shapes, notably plates of exceptional fineness and hardness. Campania in the 5th century produced barbarous imitations of red-figure unconnected with her 4th-century Greek styles. At Canosa during the Hellenistic age a ware was produced in which the basic geometric patterns were derived from Greek decorative elements; at the same time, the application of entire figures and even of groups came into use.

Martin ROBERTSON

In the western Mediterranean — except in isolated areas such as Sardinia, with modest local fabrics in the protohistoric tradition — colonization by Greece and the Near East resulted in the spread of an "Orientalizing" civilization. The simpler Phoenician pottery — mainly amphoras, jugs, and plates without added color or painted-in bands — is to be found on the African coast, western Sicily, Sardinia, Iviza in the Balearics, and as far west as southern Spain. Greek fabrics, however, are in the forefront: 8th-century Greek Geometric vases have been found at Carthage, and other familiar fabrics along the coasts of southern France and Spain. Phocaeans, after 600 B.C., are thought to have introduced their monochrome vases of Asiatic origin: a fine gray body with bands of incised wavy lines, from which was to issue the "Ampuritanian" gray ware (from Ampurias, the modern name of Emporion in Catalonia).

Iberian pottery, which developed from the painted sub-Geometric Ionic fabrics, was (like Apulian in Italy) to remain faithful to Geometric traditions until the beginning of the Roman era. Only in a few particularly favorable locations and fairly late was Iberian painted ware to be enriched with figures and plant motifs in exuberant curvilinear stylizations (Elche-Archena group, whose chronology is a matter of dispute among students of Spanish history; PL. 137), or with complex battle, hunt, and dance scenes (San Miguel de Liria style), or with rug motifs of Celtic influence (Azaila in Aragon, 2d–1st cent. B.C.). Iberian fabrics spread from Andalusia to Ensérune in southern France and were also exported to Italy in Hellenistic times. The techniques are modest: generally a red coloring on the pinkish clay, a few shapes, the most usual being the cylindrical kalathos without handles.

In midwestern Europe Celtic Iron Age pottery of the La Tène culture (500 B.C. to the 1st cent. of our era) started with traditional Hallstatt forms, especially biconical vases, but was transformed by the wheel into a varied formal repertory. Its typical body, graphite mixed with clay, is gray, sometimes partly lustrous. Painting had no vogue until the late La Tène era: the polychrome decorations (red, orange, white, black) are largely arranged in panels and horizontal bands, often with geometric designs (especially wavy lines) between the bands. The most common form of this class of painted ware is the elongated egg-shaped vase with short, narrow cylindrical neck.

\* \*

*Hellenistic, Roman, and provincial pottery.* Painted ceramics as well as decorative products continued to be produced throughout the Hellenistic world. Painted ware from Hatra is typical; also black "Megarian" bowls with floral and figure motifs in relief on the outside. These perhaps originated in 3d-century Athens but were certainly made also in Alexandria, Syria ("Pergamene" pre-Augustan ware), and southern Russia. They were widespread in Greece, especially in Boeotia (e.g., the Homeric cups). The glaze on both these classes is black, often poor but sometimes with a perhaps deliberate metallic sheen. Similar black relief ware began to be produced in the 1st century B.C. at Arezzo, where from about 30 B.C. to about A.D. 30 a beautiful red-glazed ware with very fine molded decoration was also made. Far superior to its Hellenistic predecessors, it set the fashion for Roman imperial pottery (bowls, several forms of craters, cups, and jugs; PL. 138). It was exported as far as India (R. E. M. Wheeler, D. Gosh, and K. Deva, "Arikamedu," *Ancient India*, II, 1946, pp. 32 ff.), as well as to the rest of Europe. Rougher imitations were soon made throughout Italy and the Roman Empire, especially in Gaul, which became chief producer of this so-called "Samian" ware. The type is to be found in Asia Minor ("Çandarli" ware). Also in Asia Minor, in Myrina, Tanagra-style figurines were produced in imperial times.

The production of the so-called "Campana reliefs," similar in style to the Arretine ware, and architectural in function, was popular in imperial Rome. Under Tiberius an Arretine type of industry was established in southern Gaul (La Graufesanque is the largest factory so far uncovered); under Claudius it spread to central Gaul (Lezoux and other places), where by the 2d century it achieved some importance (PL. 138; see GALLO-ROMAN ART). The decoration of the earlier Gaulish bowls and pots was almost exclusively floral, but later animals and human figures, especially in hunting scenes, became common. There was a tendency to formalization and ultimately a decline, still more marked in the more provincial wares of Britain, Germany, Spain, and Pannonia. Other classes of pottery were produced in the northern and western provinces, especially a dark-slipped ware with light barbotine decoration, such as the footed cups from the British factory at Castor. Bowls with a marbled surface were made in Italy and Gaul during the 1st century of our era. Of true glazes both a lead glaze and a glazed quartz frit were known to Roman potters. The latter is a technique anciently practiced in Egypt and used there in Roman times for the production of brilliant blue vessels. Yellow and green lead-glazed pottery began to be made in the Near East in the 1st century B.C. and continued under the Empire, the principal center being always Asia Minor. More properly known as "Parthian," or in Rome as "murrhine," it was everywhere imitated, even in Italy and Gaul. Made in molds, the favorite shape was a two-handled cup, often with floral, occasionally with figure decoration. It also included the luxury vessels for the Roman table. Innumerable classes of rough undecorated ware were, of course, produced under the Roman Empire, including the long pointed amphoras used for transport and storage of wine. Aside from vessels, some lamps and sarcophagi were glazed, the latter sometimes in imitation of mummies. Other Roman amphoras have representational decoration.

Martin ROBERTSON

TERRA-SIGILLATA POTTERIES. *a. Arezzo*: The potteries were either in the town itself (especially the oldest ones, near the present Church of S. Francesco) or in its immediate vicinity (Cincelli, Ponte Buriano). As to their chronology, after an initial phase (Rasinius, C. Memmius, Publius, etc.) contemporary with the earliest production of the pottery of M. Perennius, there followed a second group, contemporary with the middle and late products of the Perennii (C. and L. Annius, C. Tellius, P. Cornelius, etc.); M. Perennius, at Arezzo, lasted throughout the period of production. A branch at Cincelli was important. – Rasinius, at Arezzo, oldest phase. C. Memmius, at Arezzo, partly contemporaneous, in part successor to Rasinius. Publius, at Arezzo, latest phase. C. and L. Annius, at Arezzo, perhaps two distinct potteries, respectively middle and late Augustan. C. Tellius, at Ponte Buriano, late Augustan. L. Pomponius Pisanus, not located, intermediary period. L. Titius Thyrsus, not located, prob-

ably early phase (the L. Titius mentioned by Gamurrini may be another one). C. Volusenus at Arezzo, intermediary phase. L. Avilius Sura, not located, perhaps intermediary phase. P. Cornelius, at Cincelli, late Augustan and Tiberian. C. Cispius, at Cincelli, Augustan. C. Gavius, at Cincelli, probably more recent phase. Cn. Atenius, at Arezzo, late Augustan. C. Amurius, not located, date uncertain. *b. Other potteries in Italy*: According to Pliny, the centers of ceramic production (the so-called "Late Italic sigillata") were at Hasta, Pollentia, and Mutina (Modena). We have no archaeological data about the first two, but at Modena a good deal of terra sigillata has been found in which the name of L. Gellius recurs frequently. Paduan terra sigillata originated in the Augustan age or even before and flowered under Tiberius and Claudius; at Aquileia, for example, the potters' stamps carry prevailingly northern names. These products were also exported to Germany and to Noricum and Pannonia even under Vespasian. A separate class is the production of C. Aco. He must also have been very active, with a numerous group of slaves; in the Po valley; some products of this pottery, found at Oberaden (Germany), date before 8 B.C. A group with applied relief decoration continued in the Paduan valley until the early 2d century. Another center for Italic terra sigillata, probably founded by Arretine potters (L. Rasinius Pisanus, Sex. Murrius Pisanus), apparently flourished at Pisa. But the best-known group of fabrics of Italic terra sigillata, comtemporary with late Arretine wares, is from Pozzuoli: from the potteries of Numerius Naevius Hilarus, of Q. Pompeius Serenus, and of L. Valerius Titus. *c. Eastern Gaul and Germany west of the Rhine*: The area of distribution is limited almost exclusively to the more northerly regions of the Empire (the Danube, Rhineland, Belgian Gaul, Germany, and Britain). Very little is to be found in central and southern Gaul. Exportation into Britain began in the late 1st and early 2d centuries and continued throughout the 2d and into the 3d. Characteristic of Rheinzabern are pots with barbotine decoration; of Trier, a dark-yellow paste containing a good deal of quartz and coated with a dark-red glaze. – Luxeuil, according to Oswald-Pryce: A.D. 80–200; Comfort: 80–120. Heiligenberg, according to Forrer: 85–165; Oswald-Pryce: 95–160; Comfort: 100–30. La Madeleine, according to Oswald-Pryce: 95–135; Comfort: 100–30. Aachen (Aquisgranum)-Schönforst, 100 (of short duration). Baden in Aargau, 100–20. Windisch (Vindonissa), 100–20. Chemery-Falquemont (pots by Satto and Saturninus), according to Oswald-Pryce: 90–140; Comfort: 105–35. Blickweiler, 105–40. Trier (Augusta Treviorum), according to Oswald-Pryce: 120–260; Comfort: 110–240. Ittenweiler, according to Oswald-Pryce: 100–30; Comfort: 110–30. Mandeure, 110–30. Lavoye, according to Oswald-Pryce: principally 120–40; Comfort: 120–200. Avocourt I, according to Oswald-Pryce: 120–80; Comfort: 120–200. Acovourt II, according to Comfort: 270–400. Rheinzabern (Tabernae Rhenanae), according to Oswald-Pryce: 120–260; Comfort: 130–200. Eschweilerhof, according to Oswald-Pryce: 140–80; Comfort: 130–60. Les Allieux, according to Oswald-Pryce: 120–80; Comfort: 130–200. Pont-des-Rèmes, 130–200. *d. Southern Gaul*: Southern Gallic or Ruthenian terra sigillata; distribution: primarily southwestern France, England, and Germany. The products of La Graufesanque have been found throughout France, including the north, in Italy, Switzerland, Austria, Germany, the Netherlands, England, Scotland, and Africa. Characteristics of La Graufesanque is a yellow glaze veined with red in imitation of marble; of Banassac, pots with ornamental inscriptions. – Montans, according to Oswald-Pryce: A.D. 15–100; Comfort: 15–90 or even later. La Graufesanque (Condatomagus), according to Hermet: 14–117; Oswald-Pryce: 15–100; Comfort: 25–30 to the Trajan era. Banassac, according to Oswald-Pryce: 40–110; Hermet, Comfort: 30–100. Rozier, according to Hermet, Comfort: 60–80–85. *e. Central Gaul*: Arvernian terra sigillata; distribution: central and northern France, territories of the Rhine, England, etc. Characteristics: at Saint-Rémy-en-Rollat and Vichy, light-colored paste tending to white, gray, or yellow, with a yellowish glaze; at Lezoux, in the late products, an appliqué technique prevails. – Saint-Rémy-en-Rollat, post-Augustan, A.D. 69–96. Vichy (Aquae Calidae), 80–130. Lezoux (Ledosus), according to Dechelette, Oswald-Pryce: 40–260; Comfort: 40–170. Saint-Bonnet, 110–20. Martres-de-Veyre, 120–60. Lubie-La Palisse, 120–60. Pulon-sur-Allier, 130–60. Nouatre (and Le Mourgon)? Altenstadt, 140–50. Schiltigheim-Strasbourg, 150–60. Jebsheim, 160–70. Sinzig, 180–200. Pont-des-Quatre-Enfants, 270–400. *f. Regions beyond the Rhine and Pannonia*: Lehen, A.D. 90–100. Bregenz (Brigantium), according to Oswald-Pryce: 90–114; Comfort: 100–20. Heddernheim, 120–30. Beinstein, 130–40. Kraherwald, according to Oswald-Pryce: 140–80; Comfort: 140–200. Westerndorf, 160–200. Ptuj (Poetovium), Antonine age. Sisak (Siscia), first half of 2d century. Budapest (Aquincum), third quarter of 2d century. *g. Spain and Portugal*: Pliny, Juvenal, and Martial record the fabrics of Saguntum, but there have been no archaeological finds. – Tricio (Tritium), late 1st century. Abella, second (or perhaps first) half of 1st century. Solsona, second half of 1st century (or perhaps

before). Portugal, Flavian age. *h. Britain*: Colchester (Camulodunum), second half of 2d century. Castor (Durobrivae), from the 2d century on. *i. Africa*: Decorated terra sigillata was produced at El Auja and especially at El Djem (Thysdrus) in the early 3d century. Characteristic of this production is the technique, unique in terra sigillata, of making a pot in sections and then mounting them. As to distribution, several examples have been found at Cyprus and one in Germany. *j. Oriental fabrics*: According to Comfort's classification: (A) The so-called "Pergamene" ware of the pre-Augustan (Hellenistic) age. It appears about the middle of the 3d or in the 2d century B.C. Distribution: Athens, Antioch, Samaria, etc. The name is conventional: the fabric may have been produced elsewhere as well (e.g., at Samos or Antioch). Potters' stamps are not known. (B) In a broad sense, all Pergamene fabrics, from the early imperial Roman period. Most notable: (B1) "Romano-Pergamene." The influence of Italic terra sigillata is in evidence in the shapes. This fabric has been identified at Pompeii, and a piece from Corinth dates to the late 1st or 2d century. (B2) "Olbio-Pergamene"; similar to the Çandarli wares. (B3) From Olbia; similar to Samian ware; mostly Tiberian. (B4) Continuation of B3; lasted until the 4th century; nonepigraphic stamps often used as decorative motifs. (B5) "Nabataeo-Pergamene." Much of the copious production of Pergamene fabrics must have been at Nabataean places, from the early 1st century to the late 2d century (all forms published to date, however, belong to the 1st century). (C) Group including the other Oriental fabrics of early imperial Rome: (C1) Nabataean terra sigillata; of the same period and with the same distribution as "Nabataeo-Pergamene." (C2) "Tralles ware." Its existence seems to have been demonstrated by inscriptions on pieces found at Notium. (C3) "Çandarli ware." This is the only Eastern fabric located with certainty: near the mouth of the Caicus (Sakir Çayi) (at Pitane?). There are two phases: the first (Tiberian) shows Arretine influences; the second, however (ca. 50–100), shows similarities with Gallic terra sigillata. At Olbia, Corinth, and Athens this fabric has been documented from the late 1st to the early 2d century. (C4) "Samian ware." It is often mentioned in Latin sources. There are technical similarities to Arretine, but the characteristic paste contains many brilliant particles. The chronology is uncertain; the ware may be pre-Augustan (Pliny, *Historia naturalis* XXXV, 160; according to Zahn: late 2d–1st cent. B.C.; but no find is certainly pre-Augustan, and the closest analogies are with early-1st-century Arretine. (C5) Continuation of C4. According to Knipowitsch (class D), it is primarily Tiberian, but is to be found throughout the 1st century (Pompeii, Herculaneum). The latest piece, from Corinth, is from the late 2d century. Maximum distribution in the eastern Mediterranean and the Black Sea. (C6) Red ware from Alishar; a fairly late derivation of Samian ware. (D) Eastern terra-sigillata fabrics from the middle imperial period. These represent a departure from true terra sigillata: (D1) To be found at Olbia, but not at Soli; derives from "Samian" and "Olbio-Pergamene"; about A.D. 50–300. (D2) To be found at Soli, but not at Olbia (Westholm's "mat red ware"); dates from 50 B.C. or later to the early 4th century. (E) Late Roman Eastern ware. Waage has subdivided it into four classes: A, B, and C were largely imported into Athens from Egypt and were distributed throughout the Mediterranean. D is an imitation of the first three; it was made at Athens, but has no distinctive characteristics. Class A flourished during the 3d century of our era; B from the 3d (according to Westholm, from the early 4th) to the 7th century; C, which often employs Christian symbols, from the late 4th–5th to the 7th century.

Vera BIANCO

*Iran.* One of the earliest flowerings of painted pottery probably took place in the central Iranian Plateau, where the principal finds by archaeologists have been at Tepe Sialk. Indeed, the south Iranian wares from both Susa and Tell-i-Bakun (near Persepolis) and the northern wares of Tepe Giyan, Tepe Hissar, and Anau (Turkistan) appear to have felt the influence of this oldest known center in Iran. Abstract designs were to become continuously more frequent and defined from the 5th millennium onward: from stylized organic forms they passed through deformations and modifications to an ever more decorative and exclusively geometric repertory. This process of simplification and stylization culminated in the production of Sialk II and III (4th millennium) as well as of other Iranian centers.

Thus a few motifs of Sialk vase painting, bands of triangles, herringbones, checkers, etc., recur also in the pottery of Giyan, Hissar, and Anau (II, PLS. I, 3); and the presence of the "bird-arrow" motif links Hissar (level I) and Giyan (level V B of the ninth station) even more closely to Sialk. All these sites,

however, are apparently later than Sialk II–III, except Tell-i-Bakun in the south, which is earlier and which developed a more individual character during this period.

With the appearance of the human figure on vessels from Sialk (III S) as well as Hissar (I B), Susa, and Persepolis (thus suggesting contacts and contemporaneity between these cultures), purely geometric stylization was abandoned in favor of a return to simplified natural forms. It was the apogee of all Iranian pottery: each center boasted its own variety of shapes and decorative motifs. The chalice was preferred by the potters of Sialk, Hissar, and Giyan; the truncated cone by the craftsmen of Persepolis; Susan potters favored a large, thin-walled bowl or a jar. Painted decoration is enriched and varied, even in the color of the paste, which varies from gray to red, from red to green, as a consequence of the perfection of firing techniques. In this phase the motifs with their origin in the human figure display a dynamism (from the attitudes of running or motion) that distinguishes them from those of the preceding phases. Silhouettes replace more linear forms. Animals, for instance, are indicated rather than drawn (PL. 121).

While a cup from Susa (A, style I) directly recalls a motif from Sialk, the esthetic sensibility in the south is essentially different. Here color serves primarily to heighten stylization. Susa's decorative repertory is also enriched with other motifs: the "combed" motif and the Maltese cross, which was common also at Persepolis.

Elam in Susiana, Iran's first state organization, gradually incorporated all these varied and flourishing local cultures into its sphere of influence, both peacefully and otherwise: the violent end of the Sialk III culture was probably the result of an Elamite military conquest. In the later station (Sialk IV) painted pottery was suddenly interrupted and supplanted by a red monochrome fabric similar to style II at Susa. Dependence on the new Elamite culture in the contemporary ceramic industry of Giyan IV appears less close (II, PL. 9), as Giyan is still represented by a painted ware very similar to that of Susa I in lively silhouetted geometric forms and a few characteristic motifs. But this phase marks the end of that great flowering of Iranian painted pottery which had been so important in the formation of contemporary Mesopotamian styles, notably in the invention and elaboration of numerous motifs, especially zoomorphic. From this time forward different external influences were brought to bear. In Giyan III a new pot form, the tripod, appeared alongside the traditional pots. The introduction of this form, not only in the region of Giyan, but in all the area occupied by the Kassites (mid-18th cent. B.C.) and in the most recent strata at Sialk, may have coincided with the advance of the Indo-Europeans. The tripod was a form diffused especially in the district of the Zagros Mountains and remained in Luristan, where many examples have been found in certain tombs which contain bronzes dating from the 1st millennium. But the data at our disposal on the development of Iranian Bronze Age pottery are scarce and poorly coordinated. There is a very long hiatus at Sialk lasting through the 3d millennium and past the middle of the 2d, and the levels known as Sialk V or Necropolis A and Sialk VI or Necropolis B are at the threshold of the Iron Age.

The pottery of these two cultures has notable affinities with that of the latest levels at Giyan and Hissar III (PL. 121), indicating that links with the centers on the plateau had been reestablished. The culture at Sialk V was apparently brought by a wave of invaders. Their presence would explain the appearance of a new type of pottery: a gray-black burnished ware, thrown on the wheel, and incised before firing and often filled with a white substance. A second wave, recognizable in the culture of Sialk VI and identical with that of the "Luristan type" tombs at Giyan, seems to have been responsible for a class of unburnished tripods. Also characteristic was a painted ware with a porous body, whose geometric decoration recalls the oldest tradition of lozenges, checkers, and crosses, including the Maltese cross. The household pots of Sialk V are completely different from those of the following period, Sialk VI, in which gray ware reappeared along with a painted ware with stylized natural motifs in red or a fine

shiny black. There is also a return to motion, to the contrast of blank and filled spaces, and to the representation of people and animals, the horse now being often preferred to the goat.

The shape which most differentiates this late production is a particular type of funerary vase with elongated spout. This form of spout is to be found also at Giyan and other centers on the Iranian Plateau, in Luristan, Solduz, and even in Afghanistan at Nad-i-Ali, on the banks of the Helmand River and on the outskirts of the desert of Seistan.

It has been thought that the horse, which distinguishes the work of the population that emigrated to Sialk, and also the solar symbol, which recurs with similar importance and frequency, have historical connections with a migration of peoples from the steppes. It should not be forgotten, however, that even in historical times the sun and the horse were attributes of the Iranian concept of royalty.

During and after the period illustrated by this station (perhaps 9th cent. B.C.), in some Iranian areas such as Azerbaijan, Kurdistan, Gilan, Mazanderan, and Tabaristan, a gray fabric was produced contemporaneously with another type with a red ground sometimes decorated. This last has been documented by the series of finds at several sites dating from about 1500 to about the 8th century B.C., or immediately before the Achaemenian period. At Hasanlu also a type of red ware is associated with a gray ware (perhaps in wider use) represented by tripod vases or long-spouted vases. One of these last, without a handle, bears on its sides two stylized figures of goats in relief. Spouted vases from Amlash have a red background painted in ocher with geometric motifs. The gray ware from Lahijan and Khurvin, which is scarce, includes a stylized terra-cotta bird.

The necropolis of Kalar Dasht has preserved terra-cotta objects showing largely Hittite foreign influences, but also a clearly Iranian local taste. Comparison with the pottery of the region of the Talysh Mountains in Iran suggests a date about 11th–10th century B.C. and indicates the existence of an Iranian art in the regions of the northwest. Zoomorphic terra cottas and long-spouted vases (II, PLS. 3, 4) have also been found at Garmabak (near Kalar Dasht). In the terra cottas from Zawiyeh (Ziwiye) and thereabouts (9th–7th cent. B.C.) geometric decoration — of Assyrian inspiration — is widespread and often accompanied by animal motifs. A spouted vase in the shape of a goose head has an incised geometric decoration and on the neck raised designs and circles imitating the reinforcements and neck decoration of metal vases.

Little is known about Achaemenian pottery because of the meager archaeological data at our disposal and also because it was peripheral to production in metal. Pottery received new suggestions and influxes but also preserved elements from the old traditions of Iran. These developments are best documented in three levels of the Achaemenian village of Susa (7th through 5th cent. B.C.). Decoration, rare in this group, is exclusively incised. From a series of fragments red ware has been identified as well as a scarce, perfectly fired ware with a fine café-au-lait body and decoration in a *lie de vin* color, generally geometric, in horizontal bands running over the entire body of the vase or in checkers and triangles reminiscent of prehistoric fictile traditions. A handsome horse-shaped rhyton belonging to this group, with a saddle blanket finely decorated with geometric and stylized animal motifs, was found in stratum I (7th–6th cent.). It closely recalls another horse-shaped rhyton from Maku (Azerbaijan), but its particular type of decoration links it primarily to the funerary pottery of Sialk VI (Necropolis B), showing the persistence of certain funerary customs. A gray-black ware of little distinction is also recorded.

Parthian pottery is known especially in examples from Dura-Europos, Assur, Samarra, Seleucia, Ctesiphon, and Babylon — all Mesopotamian centers — more than by Iranian examples: indeed, the wares of Susa, Rhages (Rayy), Kuh-i-Khwaja (Seistan) are less numerous. It is possible to identify various tendencies: Hellenistic and Syro-Roman, those of the new Persian overlords, and elements from preceding periods.

Handmade, wheel-thrown, and molded wares now existed side by side: some types, such as lamps and the so-called "pilgrim flasks," were made in sections put together with

plaster, the bottles being decorated with rosettes with a star at the center or with ribbons and bands. Lamps, sarcophagi, and amphoras have a generally floral molded decoration, sometimes with figures beneath an arch with Ionic columns. Animals are missing from the motifs, a notable omission considering the place they had in vase painting of preceding periods.

Molded wares were widely distributed in Babylon, where the technique was introduced under the Achaemenians, and at Dura-Europos. The usually round molds are of stars, hooked crosses, crosses with points between the arms, and more or less rudimentary leaves. A red ware was also common; some vases found at Nineveh have a painted decoration limited to a band below the rim; numerous shards display a preference for geometric designs, among them slanted spirals. Glaze was now common, though the range of colors was limited: cream, manganese yellow, brown, blue, green; polychrome combinations were practically unknown. The glazes varied considerably in chemical composition and technique of application. Sometimes bright and silvery and sometimes opaque, surfaces were porous, polished, or crackled. Amphoras were generally glazed.

The amphora, more than other types, betrays Hellenistic influence and coincides with Roman examples found at various sites in Syria. The decoration is simple and sparse: ribbons, lines, and zigzags and little disks and nodules applied on the neck. The jar was a closely related shape, but the most characteristic product of this period was the rhyton. A whole series of vases and bowls which repeat traditional types has a glazed decoration (some from Rhages). The classical influence diminished slowly: Hellenistic schemes were abandoned for simpler and traditional forms that bear witness to the rebirth of an archaizing and "national" taste in an evolution yet more recognizable in Sassanian products (see SASSANIAN ART).

Mariella LUCIDI

LATE ANTIQUITY AND THE MIDDLE AGES. *Early Christian, barbarian, and Byzantine ware.* Pottery lost much of its importance in late antiquity, especially in Early Christian art. Luxury items such as those produced by the terra-sigillata potteries of Arezzo, southern Gaul, and Argonne decreased steadily, and potters both in these places and in other parts of the Empire returned to the various traditions of local craftmanship. Plastic decoration was replaced in the 4th century by geometric motifs, as in the terra-sigillata vases with wheel patterns. Merovingian ware illustrates the next stage of this development; relief work, though still practiced, lost its plasticity and became flat and isolated, as in several plates given by emperors or by other functionaries on such occasions as circus games. These plates, which evidently took the place of the ancient silver dishes, are round: e.g., a plate in Vienna from Ephesus or one in Madrid showing the *Venatio* (artificially staged hunt). Christian scenes in relief are rare on dishes. An example with Christ surrounded by the apostles belongs to the Barberini Collection in Rome, and a fragment bearing the figure of a saint beside the Constantinian cross is in the Cairo Museum. Plates deriving from terra sigillata with incised or relief decoration of Christian themes have been found especially in North Africa (Carthage, Tipasa, Egypt). Ceramic lamps of the 4th-5th century made in North Africa are notable for their introduction of this same technique and decoration into the Christian world. Examples in the Museo Nazionale in Rome and in Berlin are easily datable, as they are impressed with a Theodosian coin (408-50). These lamps bear many nonreligious scenes, especially of beasts, as well as subjects from the Old and New Testaments (Christ standing on the basilisk, the return from the Promised Land, figures of saints) or symbolical figures (chalice, peacock, etc.).

Christian motifs began to appear on Italian lamps probably in the 3d century, but some — such as that of the Good Shepherd — which can be interpreted in a Christian sense, go back perhaps to pagan fabrics of prior date. There are no technical differences between Christian and pagan lamps. The stamps on the bottom of many are of Italian names such as Florent[inus] or Anni[us] Ser[apidorus]; on these also represen-

tations of animals frequently have a Christian meaning (e.g., the fish). The influence of African imports effected a change in the decoration on Italian lamps; scenes from the Old and New Testament appeared, or the monogram of the emperor Constantine (306-37).

By the 4th century lamps of Coptic (African Christian) origin had a radical influence on the predominantly Hellenistic shapes as well. A great variety resulted: the usual round disk assumed an ovoid form, others (especially in finds from Asia Minor) the form of a shoe, while still other 7th-8th-century lamps are closer to the Moslem type. Of major iconographical importance are the small flasks carried in the West by pilgrims to sacred sites such as Palestine, Ephesus, and the Basilica of St. Menas near Alexandria. A saint (St. Menas, the apostles, etc.; PL. 139) usually figured on these flasks. The most-prized (perhaps prototypes) were of silver, but terra-cotta examples are preserved in the treasures of Bobbio (in Piacenza) and Monza. A considerable number of poor votive terra-cotta statuettes have been found in the holy places of the Early Christian world, especially the city of St. Menas. Domestic ware, pots, plates, or amphoras for containing liquids (e.g., from the Church of SS. Giovanni e Paolo in Rome) do not speak well for Italian production; in Egypt, on the other hand, Coptic centers produced a great quantity of pots and plates painted, in few colors, with human and animal figures (PL. 139). Examples from the excavations at Bawit are now in Cairo, Berlin, Paris, and London. The technique continued until the Moslem period (7th cent.).

Merovingian pottery from the 5th to the 8th century and Carolingian times was fairly simple in form and little decorated. Normally linked to Roman provincial prototypes, it also resumed old indigenous motifs of the local La Tène style. Each profile is a typical form and falls into a particular group: Saxon, Frankish, Alamannian, Lombard, or Visigothic. Painted wares appear to have come from the Rhineland, but they are not earlier than Carolingian. Designs were very simple; the pots are white with red (*Pingsdorfer Ware*). Production was scanty in Italy also; typical examples found in the Roman Forum probably dating to the 8th-9th century are vases and jugs in the ancient tradition with rough surfaces covered with buttons. Glazed wares of the period, on the other hand, reflect a Byzantine influence ever more pronounced in later centuries. It is not at present possible to establish to what potter the few remaining Italian wares belong (Rome, Brescia, or Padua).

Oriental influence, especially from Iran, played a greater role in Byzantine potteries. Indeed, Parthian (ca. 250 B.C.-A.D. 226) wares cannot always be easily distinguished from Sassanian (A.D. 226-641), which immediately followed. Nor do examples found in excavations in Mesopotamia, Dura-Europos, Samarra, Ctesiphon, or Seleucia give many clues as to their date. Both Parthian and Sassanian potters produced green-glazed amphoras. Notable examples of vases with relief decoration (with or without glaze) in animal motifs or rosettes (5th-6th cent.) have been found at Kish, Ctesiphon, and Qasr-i-Abu-Nasr. The pottery from Susa is of better quality, a type with black glaze, lasting until Moslem times. From this group is the so-called *Chalice of S. Girolamo* (now in the Vatican, Mus. Sacro), with white glaze and a relief decoration of birds perching in vines; it is quite similar to Samarran types. Many examples of Byzantine pottery from excavations on the frontiers of the Empire at Istanbul, Cyprus, and Sparta are preserved in the Archaeological Museum of Istanbul, in Berlin, and elsewhere. Its close links with Moslem ceramics, though sometimes simplifying the problems of dating, make classification difficult. There was, in fact, a great importation of Moslem wares into the Byzantine Empire. The existence of various local potteries, e.g., at Sparta (active 1100-1250) or at Pergamum (before 1325), helps solve chronological problems. An important group without slip between body and glaze has relief and molded decoration. Excavations in the atrium of St. Sofia at Istanbul permit a dating of this type to the early Byzantine age, perhaps prior to Justinian (527-65). The dependence on Sassanian pottery in technique and decoration is clear, especially on the fabrics of nearby Mesopotamia and Samarra (griffins, winged

creatures, eagles, stags; all datable to the 4th–6th cent.). Constantinople was evidently the center of this production, and the pieces with relief decoration found in the Crimea must be considered local fabrics. A large vase from Constantinople with reliefs of Christ, the emperor, the Archangel Michael and the apostles (Berlin) does not belong to this group, however, as its style indicates an attribution to the 11th–12th century.

The very numerous remains found in the countries bordering on the Mediterranean, the Pontus, and the upper Adriatic are for the most part covered with glazes of various colors and have sgraffito designs cut through to reveal the background color. Another group includes plates and painted vases. Relations with Iranian wares are in evidence, especially on the sgraffito wares. A red class with simple designs apparently belong to a later period, among them a fragment, now in Berlin, bearing the monogram of the Palaeologi. Such late dating is confirmed by comparisons with the production of Fostat (Old Cairo).

A group of painted tiles from various excavations (Istanbul, Bulgaria, Patleina, Preslav), decorated with motifs of Oriental origin as well as Christian subjects — e.g., the Louvre tile showing the Virgin and Child — served mainly as wall decoration. The colors in greatest use were cobalt blue and copper green. The most probable dating is 10th–11th century, the last phase being represented by the tin-enameled pavement at Ozaani (Georgia). The technique reappeared in Italy especially in the tiles of Orvieto and in the green ware of Tuscany. Even earlier, tin-enameled tiles decorated the bell towers of Italian churches (Rome, Pomposa, Pavia, Pisa, etc.). Design and color show a number of the tiles to be of Oriental origin. In the 14th century began the most flourishing period of Italian majolica, an art that was to reach its peak during the Renaissance.

Wilhelm Friedrich VOLBACH

*Sassanian Iran.* Ceramics, like all the art of the Sassanian period (A.D. 226–641), followed in the path of former Iranian art, but with renewed vitality.

Centers where clearly Sassanian wares have been found are largely Mesopotamian: Nineveh, Ctesiphon, Barghutiyat, and Kish; in Iran proper at Susa, Rhages (Rayy), Damghan, Qasr-i-Abu-Nasr; and in Seistan and Makran. Fine pottery has been discovered at Susa, but the archaeological finds have been few. Most examples, unfortunately, were recovered by untrained excavators or antique dealers who, without offering archaeological documentation, have made their attributions on the basis of style alone. Three groups are generally distinguished: (1) similar to Parthian (and perhaps from that period); (2) clearly Sassanian, but more probably proto-Islamic, since it has been confirmed that Sassanian traditions continued in Islamic art; (3) represented by terra cottas in the form of carafes, certainly of Parthian derivation, with technically more developed decoration. The motifs are incised, modeled, in applied barbotine, or molded; decoration on glazed pots is more detailed and complex than on Parthian wares. This period also saw the production of vessels that were pierced in various patterns and then filled with glaze, as in the fine pierced, spouted vase with a green glaze in the collection of Kirker Minassian.

The range of glaze colors is generally the same as in the Parthian period: green of all shades predominates. Glazed three-handled jars from Kish are poor; far better examples come from Susa. Those made at Kish are probably datable to the 5th and 6th centuries, as they were found with a coin of Justinian I (527–65) and hence are late Sassanian.

A small unglazed pot from Susa (Louvre), its neck unfortunately missing, belongs to group 2 and is truly Sassanian in style: its floral decoration in high relief is similar to contemporary work in stucco.

In the late Sassanian period a squat round carafe appears. Examples, unglazed and with a single handle and a crude neck, were found at Quasr-i-Abu-Nasr. The sprinkler was an innovation of the period and was to become very common in both glass and faïence.

Another innovation was the magic bowl. Although the cups or bowls for magical uses (which were unglazed) have no artistic merit, they are of special historical and literary interest. They are often conical, sometimes representing the face of a demon, especially Lilith, or bearing a knot in the center, and are covered with black inscriptions. Texts are generally of magical apotropaic formulas. These bowls have frequently been found at Kish and belong therefore to the 5th and 6th centuries. But many, found in Mesopotamia in the region between Nippur and Assur, may be later and closer to the Islamic period, when many tendencies and styles of Sassanian art continued to have an influence.

Mariella LUCIDI

*Islam. a. Origins.* Islamic potters had inherited few technical resources from their immediate predecessors. Colored glazes had been used in Mesopotamia under the ancient Assyrian and Achaemenian empires, especially for large-scale wall decoration; but in the Parthian (ca. 250 B.C–A.D. 226) and Sassanian (226–641) periods only blue-green alkaline glaze survived on rather rough pottery vessels. In Egypt too, at the time of the Islamic conquest (A.D. 641), a long tradition of colored alkaline glazes on ornamental pottery was almost extinct. One class of fine pottery does appear to have had an unbroken if obscure history in Egypt from about the 1st century B.C. until its further development by Egyptian and Mesopotamian potters of the 9th century of our era: small vessels, with relief ornament imitating metalwork, and colored lead glazes. Islamic potters at first developed their art principally in their various lead glazes to meet an unsatisfied demand for the fine porcelain and stoneware from China which, according to an Arab historian, first reached Baghdad about 800. Fragments of Chinese vessels and contemporary Mesopotamian wares in a great variety of experimental techniques have been found in excavations at Samarra near Baghdad, built and occupied by the Abbasside caliphs between 836 and 883.

Chinese wares, imported overland or by the sea route, periodically influenced the Islamic potters to reform their own technique, especially in the 9th, 12th, and 15th centuries. But the lack of hard-firing china clay (kaolin) prevented the making of true porcelain of Chinese type in the Near East, though attempts to imitate it long anticipated similar European efforts during the Renaissance and later. The white tin glaze of 9th-century Mesopotamia passed by lineal descent, probably through Moorish Spain, to the makers of Italian majolica; the 12th-century composition of ground quartz and white clay is essentially similar to the soft-paste (*pâte tendre*) French porcelain of the 18th century.

Islamic pottery was intended for practical use, and it was not customary, as in China, to bury intact vessels with the dead. The pieces recovered by excavation on medieval sites are therefore largely broken and only a few pieces have survived. Exceptionally well-preserved pieces were found in 1942 at Gurgan in Iran, southeast of the Caspian Sea; they had been buried in large jars by the pottery merchants before the Mongol invaders destroyed the city in 1220. Vessels of the 16th century and later that have survived above ground are well represented in the museums of London, Paris, and Berlin. Good examples of the very important glazed tilework used for architectural decoration survive *in situ* in mosques in Turkey and Iran.

Unglazed water vessels of soft buff or whitish clay have at all times been a basic type throughout the Islamic territories. Commonly formed in molds with elaborate relief ornament appropriate to their period, their porous walls keep the contents cool through surface evaporation. Until the 12th century even the finest wares were made of ordinary low-fired buff or reddish potter's clay, with glazes fluxed by oxide of lead. The transparent lead glaze, which became very fluid in the kiln, was not immediately adaptable for use with painted decoration. Polychrome lead glazes were applied over molded reliefs on small vessels made in Egypt (8th–9th cent.); and related 9th-century Mesopotamian wares show the earliest application of "gold luster" as an even coat over the glaze, imitating precious

metal. On a ubiquitous type the lead glaze was laid over sgraffito decoration incised through white slip: subvarieties had green, yellow-brown, and purple mottling in the glaze, after a Chinese prototype (9th–10th cent.); others, less conspicuously polychrome, borrowed their more elaborate ornament from contemporary engraved metalwork (Iran, 10th–12th cent.; Mameluke Egypt, 1260–1517). In a second main type variously colored clay slips were boldly laid on in a thick paste that was not dissolved by the overlying glaze (eastern Iran, 9th–11th cent.).

A modified lead glaze, made white and opaque by particles of suspended tin oxide, was introduced in Mesopotamia (9th cent.) as an imitation of white Chinese porcelain. Laid over the buff clay body, it proved to be sufficiently stable in firing to retain simple patterns painted on its raw surface in cobalt blue, copper green, manganese purple, and antimony yellow. Even more revolutionary was the application to the fired tin glaze of designs painted in metallic gold luster (PL. 141). This pigment, apparently discovered in Egypt, consisted of sulfur in various forms combined with silver oxide (which acted as a yellow stain) and copper oxide (which contributed the lustrous element). After painting, vessels were fired a second time at a lower temperature in a kiln specially controlled to exclude oxygen. By this reducing process the metals were precipitated onto the surface of the glaze in a glittering film which resembled solid gold or copper or gave iridescent "mother-of-pearl" reflections where the film was thin. Luster painting passed from Mesopotamia to Egypt, Syria, Iran, and Moorish Spain, whence it reached the Italian potters of Deruta and Gubbio at the close of the 15th century.

Ancient Egyptian and Mesopotamian glazes had been fluxed with an alkali (plant ash or soda) and would adhere only to a body containing similar alkaline glassy matter. After an apparent lapse into obscurity during the early centuries of Islam, they were rediscovered and greatly improved about the middle of the 12th century in Iran and Egypt. For the glaze, finely powdered quartz was melted into glass with an approximately equal proportion of potash. The same materials, with a stiffening of white plastic clay, gave a white translucent body that united perfectly with the glaze. This technique, used henceforth for all fine pottery made in the Near East, was originally adopted with the intention of imitating the Chinese porcelain and celadon wares of the Sung period. Following the Chinese method, the decoration was at first incised, carved, or molded in low relief before the thick transparent glazes were applied. Copper oxide yielded a wonderful turquoise blue, sometimes made opaque with tin oxide; and the exceptionally pure cobalt from Qansar near Kashan produced a rich azure.

In the second half of the 12th century various techniques of painting were successfully attempted with the new alkaline glaze. Gold luster and a new range of overglaze enamel colors that included leaf gilding (so-called *minai* colors) required a second firing; but cheaper wares were painted directly on the body under the transparent glaze in black and blue (PL. 142). After 1300 the more complicated gold luster and enamel colors were gradually abandoned. Attention was concentrated on underglaze painting, the range of colors being greatly expanded in the 16th century, especially in Turkey.

From the 9th to the 12th century the principal motifs common to Islamic pot painters and craftsmen working in other materials were ornamental inscriptions in the angular Kufic script; stylized human and animal figures, shown against a background of coiling foliage derived from the Greco-Roman vine; and bold palmettes, half-palmettes, and rosettes from the more strongly surviving Sassanian tradition. The palmette motifs were often carried on interwoven dotted bands, which later developed into the typical arabesque complex. Motifs were drawn rather large, with little sense of movement.

The second half of the 12th century, especially in Iran, witnessed a great change of spirit: inscriptions now mainly in the cursive Neskhi scripts, a plant ornament freed from rigid convention, and lively figures were reduced in scale and crowded onto the available space so as to achieve an effect like that of miniature paintings in illuminated manuscripts.

From the beginning Chinese wares influenced the technique and, to a lesser degree, the shapes. But Chinese motifs were little imitated till about 1300, when China and Iran were both under Mongol rule. The dragon, phoenix, lotus, and cloud scroll then began to appear alongside the traditional Islamic motifs. A more assiduous and literal imitation of Chinese ornament and color schemes set in after "blue-and-white" porcelain became a standard import in the second half of the 14th century. As a notable exception to this prevailing fashion, the 16th-century Turkish wares of Iznik (Nicaea) reflected the vitality of the Ottoman Empire in their vivid palette and highly naturalistic plant designs (PL. 142).

Though simple glazed and unglazed wares were made almost everywhere, manufacture of the finer types was concentrated in relatively few centers, from which they were exported far and wide. The locations were chosen as much for their marketing facilities as for a local source of raw materials; and though there is little evidence of direct official protection, the chief schools of fine pottery correspond closely with the major dynasties which from time to time ruled over different parts of the Islamic world. Among fragments found in excavations at Fostat (Old Cairo) were many pieces from Syria, Mesopotamia, and Iran; this diffusion ensured a general resemblance in contemporary styles in different areas, while techniques were in many cases transmitted through mass migration of potters at a time of political or economic disaster.

*b. Period I: 9th–12th century.* The Ommiad (Umayyad) dynasty of caliphs (661–750), with its capital at Damascus was superseded by the Abbassides (700–1258), who moved their court eastward to Baghdad. This probably became the main ceramic center; but its wares are best known through the well-conducted archaeological excavations at Samarra, built and occupied by the court between 836 and 883. The finds included imported Chinese and native Mesopotamian wares in a great variety of techniques, some clearly experimental (I, PLS. 4, 8–10). Lead-glazed sgraffito ware, mottled in green, yellow-brown, and purple, imitated a Chinese type. An experimental class of small vessels with delicate relief molding has an even coat of gold luster over lead glaze, imitating the effect of metalwork. Some of the important white tin-glazed pieces were unpainted and of the same lobed shape as Chinese porcelain bowls; some were painted with wreaths, palmettes, and interlacements in blue, green, purple, and yellow; yet others were painted with patterns in overglaze gold luster. The luster, at first combined with other polychrome colors in somewhat incoherent patterns, became standardized before the end of the 9th century as a greenish-yellow monochrome, with palmettes, inscriptions, and highly stylized figures of men and animals in silhouette on a dotted ground. Polychrome lustered wall tiles survive in the great mosque at Kairouan in Tunisia, some imported from Mesopotamia and some made on the spot by a Baghdad potter in 862. Mesopotamian luster ware exported during the 9th and 10th centuries has been found in Iran, Egypt, and Spain (at Medina Azzahra near Córdoba, founded 937). Its manufacture died out late in the 10th century, when the potters, who kept their technique secret, apparently migrated to Egypt.

The seeds of some of the techniques that flowered in Mesopotamia were probably introduced by craftsmen from Egypt, where luster painting appeared on glass vessels (but not on pottery) in the 7th or 8th century. After Egypt gained political independence from Baghdad under the Tulunid (868–905) and the brilliant Fatimid (909–1171) dynasties, a very fine series of native luster-painted wares was introduced in the late 10th century, probably by immigrant Mesopotamian potters, who continued and developed the Mesopotamian style. The bold designs became much more elaborate, the figures, palmettes, coiling foliage, and inscriptions being often reserved in a ground of solid luster. Some pieces were signed by the potters Muslim, Sa'd, and others. About 1150 came a sketchier style of drawing, and the new transparent glaze laid on a white composite body of ground quartz partially superseded the old tin glaze laid on buff or red clay. The new materials were used also in a

class of wares with very lively designs carved or incised in the paste before application of the transparent glazes, which were often stained in bright monochrome colors. The carved wares continued into the 13th century, but luster painting apparently ceased altogether when the Fatimid dynasty fell in 1171. The potters probably migrated elsewhere with their technical secrets. Innumerable fragments found at Fostat give a comprehensive picture of medieval Egyptian pottery, though complete items are rare.

In Iran the powerful Samanid dynasty (874–999) widely extended its rule from Transoxiana (western Turkistan) with capitals at Samarkand and Bukhara. Its characteristic pottery, with a fine pink clay body, differs completely in technique and spirit from the contemporary Mesopotamian tin-glazed wares, being very boldly painted in clay slip of various colors under a thin transparent lead glaze. Kiln wasters were found at Afrasiyab near Samarkand, but there have been other centers; at Nishapur especially fine pieces were found in the American excavations (unpublished). Among the earliest pieces are dishes and straight-sided bowls with superb Kufic inscriptions in purple-black on an ivory-white ground. An olive-green slip was used to imitate the effect of Mesopotamian gold-luster

turquoise, deep blue, purple, green, or brown; relief tended to supersede the freehand intaglio designs. On one rare experimental early class (so-called *lakabi* ware) glazes of different colors were applied to various parts of the carved design. Technical comparison with the more easily identified painted wares suggests that those with monochrome glazes were at first made in the two principal centers of Rhages (Rayy), near Teheran, and Kashan about 120 miles to the south.

Among the techniques of painting rapidly developed between about 1150 and the first Mongol invasions of 1219–20 was gold luster, whose almost simultaneous introduction at Rakka in northern Mesopotamia and Rhages and Kashan in Iran may have been due to potters who left Egypt when the Fatimid dynasty collapsed in 1171. A Rhages bottle in the British Museum dated A.H. 575 (A.D. 1179) shows certain stylistic similarities with the late Fatimid Egyptian style. The recognizably Iranian figures, animals, and foliage are drawn in a vigorous but rather sketchy manner, for the most part reserved in a dark ground. The white alkaline glaze (which contains some tin oxide) is often supplemented by areas in transparent blue glaze. The manufacture of luster ware apparently ceased at Rhages after the city was sacked by the Mongols in 1224.

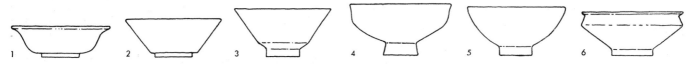

Typical shapes of Islamic bowls, 9th–15th cent. (1) Mesopotamian, 10th cent.; (2) Nishapur, 9th–10th cent.; (3, 4) Kashan, 12th–13th cent.; (5) Sultanabad district, 14th cent.; (6) Sultanabad, 15th cent.

ware, fragments of which have been found at Samarkand; other colors of design or background were a fine tomato red, reddish purple, and shades of brown. Inscriptions, interlaced dotted bands, palmette motifs, and highly stylized birds were common; there were few animals and no human figures. Manufacture apparently continued, with deterioration of quality, into the 11th century or even later. A class of coarse quality, made at Nishapur, often shows human and animal figures with incoherent background ornament of small birds, rosettes, and inscriptions (PLS. 141, 143); a strong yellow is conspicuous.

Several distinct types of 9th–12th-century sgraffito ware from west Iranian rustic potteries not precisely located suggest the influence of engraved metalwork. Those from the Garrus region have considerable areas of the white-slip ground cut away around the bold but clumsy human figures, birds, and animals. In a class attributed to Aghkand the incised animals and foliage are colored in green, yellow-brown, and purple. Sketchier designs, partly incised, partly painted in green and brown, are found on a relatively late group thought to have been made at Amul (PL. 140).

*c. Period II: 12th–13th century.* In this period Islamic pottery reached its highest accomplishment, especially in western Iran, which had hitherto produced nothing more sophisticated than sgraffito ware. Civilization here and in Mesopotamia had revived under the firm rule of the Seljuk Turks (1055–1157). The "Seljuk style," at once lively and refined, developed later in pottery than in the other arts (perhaps owing to the technical difficulties). It was from the first associated with the new white composite material of ground quartz with an alkaline glaze which was adopted in Egypt before the fall of the Fatimid dynasty and soon became widespread in the Near East.

The earliest Iranian pieces suggest a desire to imitate contemporary Chinese white porcelain and celadon ware, not only in material, but also in their shadowy ornament lightly carved in the surface under the thick transparent glaze. The actual designs, however, were with few exceptions Islamic — animals, coiling foliage, and inscriptions. To emphasize the translucency of the material, patterns were sometimes pierced through the walls of the vessel and filled with "windows" of molten glaze. The normally colorless glaze was often stained

At Kashan painting in gold luster probably began somewhat later than at Rhages, the earliest of many dated pieces being of A.H. 598 (A.D. 1202). The shapes, the glaze (made very white with tin oxide), and the painting reach a higher degree of refinement. On some splendid early dishes and bowls groups of large moon-faced figures, with elaborately patterned dresses, stand against a background relieved by tiny white spirals scratched through the luster. Quatrains of Persian verses are inscribed in an elegant cursive hand round the borders. A specialty of Kashan was lustered tilework with interlocking star- and cross-shaped pieces and a cornice of larger rectangular tiles at the top, to form a dado around the lower part of the walls. Of special magnificence were the ubiquitous prayer niches (mihrabs), which with their flanking pilasters and molded cornices form a quasi-architectural composition up to 13 ft. high. The largest of the many Koranic inscriptions in high relief, picked out in blue, contained signatures of Kashan potters and dates ranging between 1203 and 1339. The poorer draftsmanship of later examples shows the Chinese dragon, phoenix, and lotus among the designs. There is no evidence to support a suggestion that similar luster-painted tiles and vessels were made at factories in the Sultanabad region.

The so-called *minai* wares, whose effects closely approach those of contemporary miniature painting, are shown by dated examples to have been made from 1186 onward, but it is not possible to distinguish with certainty between the styles of Kashan, Rhages, and perhaps other centers. The painting, laid on an opaque white or turquoise glaze in numerous stains, enamel pigments, and leaf gilding, required two or more separate firings. After the Mongol invasions came a progressive simplification of this *haft paikar* ("seven-color," i.e., polychrome) technique, as it is called in the ceramic treatise written by Abulqasim in 1301. The *lajvardina* wares of Kashan which he described as contemporary can readily be identified. They are painted only in red, white, black, and cut gold leaf applied over turquoise or dark blue glazes; the designs are simple and monotonous, and the shapes rather clumsy. Their manufacture, which included tiles, apparently ceased before the middle of the 14th century.

Painting under the transparent alkaline glaze began at Rhages in the second half of the 12th century (PL. 141). The very strong designs of simple human and animal figures, floral

complexes, and inscriptions were laid on the white body in thick black slip, details of the silhouette being picked out with a pointed tool, a technique which imposed considerable stylization. On many pieces the transparent glaze was stained turquoise. A very much more fluent and sensitive style was practiced at Kashan between 1203 and 1220, on the evidence of dated pieces; the brush painting is in a thin black, with certain areas stained in deep blue, and, as at Rhages, the glaze is often stained turquoise. The human and animal figures are simplified versions of those on the Kashan luster wares, which were probably made in the same factories, but certain calligraphic motifs are local. Unlike the Kashan luster ware, this attractive type appears not to have been made after the Mongol attack on the city in 1220; but there is a later 13th-century class with rather slight and uninteresting painting in black under clear turquoise glaze.

The Ayyubid dynasty (1169-1250), which overthrew the Fatimids, had austere tastes. The luxurious luster-painted ware was no longer produced in Egypt, and its makers apparently departed to Iran and elsewhere. Rakka, an important caravan city on the northern border of Syria and Mesopotamia, had a thriving ceramic industry until the city was destroyed by the Mongols in 1259. The local ground-quartz material was softer and coarser than that made in Iran, and the thick transparent glaze had a green tinge. As no tin was used to whiten it, it gave a comparatively dingy appearance to the vessels painted in a characteristic chocolate-brown luster. The designs resembling those on the Rhages luster ware were more carelessly drawn. Rakka had its own monochrome-glazed wares, with decoration carved or molded in relief (PL. 140), and also a very characteristic series of wares painted under the glaze in black and blue with touches of opaque brownish red. The rather large designs of human and animal figures, arabesques, and a flower resembling the ancient Egyptian lotus are carelessly drawn, but have a jagged vitality that contrasts with the smoother rhythms of contemporary Persian drawing.

*d. Period III: 14th century.* The invasions begun by Genghis Khan led to the establishment of related Mongol dynasties, the Il-khans in Iran (1260-1335) and the Yüan in China (1280-1368). Efficient policing of the roads made contact between the Far and Near East closer than ever before. But in Iran, where the first devastating raids started in 1219, cultural life was virtually paralyzed until Ghazan Khan (1295-1304) embraced Islam and sponsored a great revival of art and architecture in his capital, Tabriz. Isolated Chinese motifs began to appear on the Kashan luster ware, an obsolescent survivor of the Seljuk tradition. A more specifically Mongol taste developed in miniature painting, textiles, and pottery after the beginning of the 14th century. The pottery is now conventionally named after the modern town of Sultanabad. The shapes are clumsy, the material coarse and not very white. In one main class figures in Mongol dress, running animals, and flying birds appear among dense foliage. The whole design tends to be broken up into medallions and panels of various sizes. In an unfamiliar effect suggesting textiles, outlines, dots on animals and draperies, and hatching in the interstices of the background are painted in a soft black which gives a predominantly grayish color scheme relieved by touches of dark blue, pale blue slip, and turquoise. Another class, probably made in the same unknown factories, had a ground color of brownish-gray slip, over which the designs are painted in thick white slip with black outlines and occasional touches of blue. In a third class, probably made at Kashan, more of the white ground is allowed to show. Inscriptions and dotted or hatched diapers in thick black and broader blue lines alternate in radiating panel design on dishes and bowls.

When the Mongols destroyed Rakka in 1259, some potters may have escaped to Damascus, where painting in brassy yellow luster on a deep blue ground continued through the 14th century. Intact examples of Damascus jars and albarellos, in which dried fruit and spices were sent to Europe, were found in Sicily and gave rise to the erroneous belief that they were made there. Much Syrian and Egyptian 14th-century pottery was painted in black and blue with paneled designs (PL. 142) like those on the Sultanabad ware. Signatures of Ghaibi and other potters are common on smaller and more delicately painted pieces made in Egypt.

*e. Period IV: 15th-18th century.* In the 14th century, probably under influence from the Near East, China adopted underglaze blue-and-white painting for the porcelain made in new factories at Ching-tê-chên. This rapidly became a standard export ware, and many 14th-century examples have survived in the great collections of the Topkapi Serayı, Istanbul, and the shrine of Sheik Safi at Ardebil (now removed to the Archaeological Museum of Teheran). They in turn set a new fashion in the Near East, and the transition to the new style can be well observed in surviving vessels and tilework made at Damascus. Excavation in Iran has yielded very little native blue-and-white of the 15th and 16th centuries, though it is frequently represented in miniature paintings of the period. Kerman and Meshed were main centers of manufacture.

Asia Minor was first conquered for Islam by a branch of the Seljuk Turks after 1071. Though tilework had developed earlier, no important pottery vessels were made till kilns were set up at İznik (Nicaea) late in the 15th century. The first İznik type (ca. 1490-1525) borrowed the Chinese blue-and-white coloring, but the crowded and carefully drawn arabesques were suggested by illuminated manuscripts. Between 1525 and 1550 a new range of polychrome colors included blue, turquoise, olive green, purple, and black. The tulip was conspicuous among the bold seminaturalistic floral designs of this class; also a pattern of slight spiral stems with florets. After 1550 a radical change of colors, with a superb scarlet (so-called "Armenian bole"), deep blue-green, blue, and black outlines, was specially suited to the painted tilework made in great quantities between 1550 and 1620 (see below, *Tilework*).

A series of dishes and bowls from an unidentified manufacture of northern Iran survived as house decorations at Kubachi, a remote town in the Caucasus. Early pieces (1473-95) were painted in black under turquoise glaze; others in Chinese blue-and-white style. A polychrome group, made about 1580-1630, had very freely drawn bust portraits of men and women among arching foliage recalling miniature painting of the time of Shah Abbas I the Great. The Kubachi ware is soft and the crackled glaze defective. Less interesting polychrome wares made in the 17th century at Kerman show slight arabesques, running animals, and growing flowers, painted in red and celadon green and often enclosed in shaped panels among blue-and-white ornament. A class of unknown origin (late 17th and early 18th cent.) revived gold luster with a brown tone; it was sometimes applied over a deep blue glaze. The vessels were small: bottles, spittoons, and bowls. Minor polychrome wares included tiles with relief-molded figures in 16th-century dress; they were made after 1850 at Teheran.

Close imitations of the gray-green Chinese celadon ware were made from the 14th century onward. In the 17th century fluted dishes of similar shape were glazed in other colors, especially turquoise and a very fine warm blue. At Kerman they were sometimes painted over the glaze in white, red, and blue slip with patterns found also on the Kerman polychrome ware. A distinct class of bottles and flasks, perhaps made at Isfahan about 1580-1630, has hard green or yellow-brown glazes laid over elaborate relief decoration of human figures, animals, and landscape in the style of the Shah Abbas I miniature paintings. The so-called "Gombroon ware" of the 18th century is of very fine white material, resembling white glass rather than porcelain. Simple designs were incised in the paste or pierced through the sides, the glaze filling in the perforations.

*f. Hispano-Moresque ware.* Imperfect evidence suggests that early medieval Spanish pottery fell short of the technical and artistic standards set in the Near East. Fragments of luster-painted ware imported from Mesopotamia have been found in the palace of the Cordovan caliphs at Medina Azzahra (built 937). A contemporary lead-glazed Spanish ware had slightly

painted animals and inscriptions in green and purple on a white-slip ground. Unglazed vessels of all dates, some very large, had stamped or relief-molded ornament; others were painted with simple patterns in mat black or in vitreous colors.

There is an obscure reference by Al-Idrisi (ca. 1150) to "gilded pottery vessels" made at Calatayud in Aragon; and Ibn Said of Granada said that about 1240 "glazed and gilded pottery" was made at Murcia, Almería, and Málaga. The Málaga luster-painted wares, made and exported between 1240 (or earlier) and 1420 (or later), became internationally famous as "opus de Melica." A derivation from the Egyptian Fatimid vases is suggested by the technique (tin glaze on red clay) as well as by the style of the earliest presumed Málaga pieces — some bowls preserved as architectural ornament at Saint-Antonin (Tarn-et-Garonne), Ravenna (S. Apollinare Nuovo), and Rome (SS. Giovanni e Paolo). An intact 14th-century bowl in Berlin, painted with arabesques and inscribed "Malaga," helps to identify the mainly unpublished fragments found at Fostat and at Málaga itself. Of the late 13th and 14th centuries are the huge wing-handled ornamental vases, 4 ft. and more in height, which take their name from the late and somewhat decadent example still preserved in the Alhambra at Granada. Earlier vases in Leningrad and Palermo have large Kufic inscriptions and strong, well-arranged arabesques. Manufacture probably ceased well before the capture of Granada by Ferdinand and Isabella (1492), the potters having moved north to settle in Christian territory near Valencia.

Tin-glazed wares made throughout the 14th century at Paterna, near Valencia, were sketchily painted in green and purple with figures and animals mainly of Gothic inspiration, though many of the potters were Moors (PL. 145). Luster painting was introduced from the south, probably about the end of the 14th century, and practiced especially at Manises. Early pieces are almost indistinguishable from those of Málaga, having heavy arabesque ornament partly in blue. A new repertory of elegant Gothic foliage and superb heraldic animals was soon added, and many pieces were painted to order with the arms of Spanish and Italian families. While an Islamic suppleness remained in the well-spaced, rhythmic drawing throughout the 15th century, a steady decline set in thereafter. Simple blue-and-white wares from Manises were exported along with the luster ware to Italy, where they strongly influenced the early majolica.

*g. Tilework.* Some of the glazed tilework so important from the 13th century onward can be considered along with vessels made and painted in the same workshops (*e.g.*, Kashan luster ware, 13th cent.; Turkish İznik ware, 16th cent.). Other techniques were purely architectural in application.

Glazed tilework, used as wall decoration, has a natural affinity with the baked or sun-dried brick that has been a basic building material in the Near East from very ancient times. Bricks painted with patterns or figures in colored glazes and glazed bricks molded to form large figures in relief adorned the palace at Susa of the Achaemenid Persian king Artaxerxes II (404–359 B.C.). This tradition died out after the Eastern conquests of Alexander the Great (356–323 B.C.). Under the Sassanian kings it became customary in Iran to decorate inner walls with panels of richly carved or molded stucco, a practice adopted widely by the Islamic conquerors after the 7th century. The later glazed tilework was often used in association with carved stucco, which it tended to supersede.

Painted tiles were made in the same factories and by the same technique as painted pottery vessels. At Samarra near Baghdad, a temporary capital of the Abbasside caliphs between 836 and 883, excavations have revealed a limited use of rectangular earthenware tiles with "marbling" and patterns painted in gold luster over a white tin glaze. Similar tiles, imported from Baghdad about 862, survive in the Great Mosque at Kairouan in Tunisia. Between 1200 and about 1340 the potters of Kashan specialized in painting delicate designs in gold luster on tiles exported throughout Iran (*kashi* is still the generic Persian name for a tile). Thirteenth-century Seljuk buildings at Konya have remarkable tile mosaics, and under the

Ottomans (ca. 1299–1922) fine tilework in various techniques was applied to early-15th-century buildings at Bursa and Edirne.

In the 15th century Syrian potters at Damascus painted hexagonal wall tiles with underglaze blue-and-white patterns derived from Chinese porcelain vessels. After 1550 the İznik factories greatly increased their production of tiles for interior decoration of the new stone-built mosques in Istanbul and elsewhere. Large bold designs of arabesques and seminatural-istic growing plants now spread over whole panels of adjacent rectangular tiles (PL. 144). Technique is irreproachable: the body, of ground quartz and white clay, forms a pure white ground for the brilliant underglaze colors, used also in vessels, a deep blue-green, turquoise, and the vivid Armenian bole, that stands up from the surface in relief. In the 17th century the industry at İznik declined, to be briefly revived in the Tekfur Seray quarter of Istanbul after 1724. Tiles made at Damascus from about 1560 onward resemble those of İznik in design but are technically inferior, being painted in blue, green, and purple (without the red).

In the 18th century tiles were made by Armenian potters at Kütahya (Asia Minor), sometimes with Christian themes and Armenian inscriptions. These tiles were exported and used in decorating churches along the whole eastern Mediterranean. (The same potters also produced delicate coffee services with popular designs in gay colors.) After 1850 Teheran produced polychrome tiles with decoration in relief.

Tile mosaic was quite different in principle and origin from painted tilework. It had no connection with the manufacture of pottery vessels, but derived from the brickwork on medieval Persian buildings, which was often disposed to form geometric patterns or Kufic inscriptions. The Mongol invasions after 1219 checked architectural construction in Iran, and true tile mosaic first appeared in the Ala-ad-Din Mosque (1220) and other 13th-century buildings of the Seljuk Turks at Konya in Asia Minor. Here the designs were chiefly geometric inter-lacing bands, Kufic inscriptions, and friezes of strongly styl-ized plant forms in austere purple-black, pale turquoise, blue, white, and yellow-brown. Somewhat similar mosaics were applied to the tomb-mosque of Uljeitu at Sultaniya (1304–16) in Iran, where development continued through the 14th century. In such famous examples as the Mausoleum of Tamerlane at Samarkand (1404) and the Blue Mosque at Tabriz (1465) curvilinear arabesques combine with lotus patterns of Chinese derivation, and the color scheme is warmer and richer, dominated by a deep blue. Isfahan has a notable series of tile mosaics ranging from the 14th to the early 17th century, often covering the whole façade of a building. Persians from Tabriz reintroduced tile mosaic into Turkey (the Green Mosque and Green Tomb at Bursa, ca. 1424; Çinili Köşk at Istanbul, 1472).

Since tile mosaic was a laborious and costly technique, it was imitated in Iran, from the late 14th century onward, by painting similar designs on clay slabs in glaze colors. The colors were prevented from mingling by outlines painted in a greasy manganese that burned to a mat black (called in Spain *cuerda seca*, "dry cord"). Early examples are found at Samarkand and in the above-mentioned Green Mosque and Tomb in Bursa. In Isfahan (e.g., the Great Mosque of Shah Abbas I, 1616) glaze-painted tilework was also used, in a way unknown elsewhere, for "tile pictures" with large-scale human figures festively grouped in a garden setting. The colors included bright opaque yellow, blue, and green.

The carved and molded stucco wall decoration so fashion-able among the Islamic peoples was hardly weatherproof enough for outdoor use, but its effect was reproduced in a class of carved and glazed tilework made in the district of Samarkand from about 1369 onward. Similar work is found also at Bukhara. Inscriptions on a background of coiling foliage, interlac-ing geometric figures, and geometrically coffered panels are carried on thick slabs of coarse sandy clay. The background is deeply cut away, the angle of cutting being steeper on the underside so that the patterns appear from below to stand out in sharp relief against the shadow. Green or turquoise glaze was applied over most of the surface, and inscriptions or other motifs were picked out in white, purple, or blue. In the late

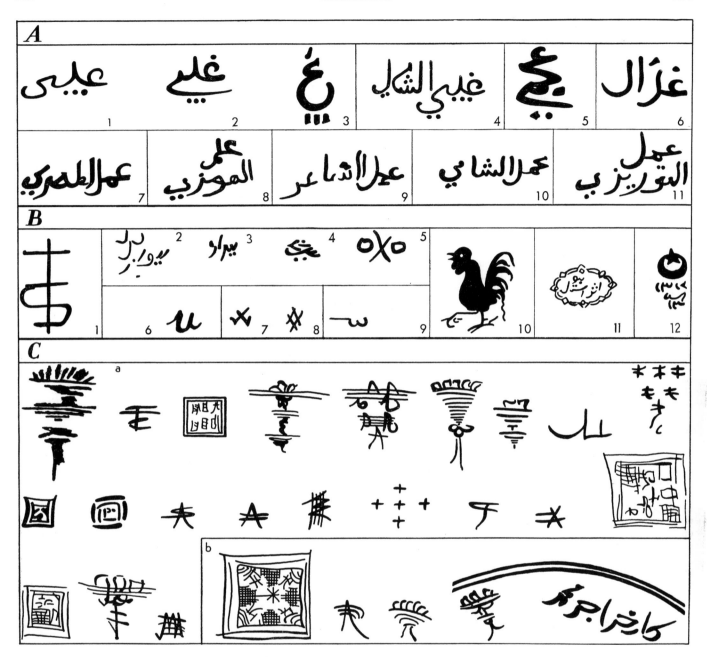

Marks on Islamic pottery. (*A*) Egypt: marks with potters' signatures, 10th–16th cent. (1–3) Chaïbī, on black-and-blue and blue-and-white ware; (4) Chaïbī al-Shāmī, on blue-and-white ware; (5) 'Ajamī; (6) Jazāl; (7) aml ("work of") al-Misrī; (8) aml al-Hormūzī; (9) aml al-Shāmī; (10) aml al-Shā'ir; (11) aml al-Tawrīzī. (*B*) Turkey (16th–20th cent.), marks: (1) on wares dating ca. 1570–80; (2–6) on wares from Kütahya, 18th cent.; (7, 8) on coffee cups from Kütahya, imitating a Meissen mark; (9) from the Samson works in Paris on imitations of wares from Kütahya and other Near Eastern wares (this mark is usually omitted); (10) of the Cantagalli factory in Florence, on imitations of Īznik wares; (11) on wares from Istanbul, second half of 19th cent.; (12) of the factory of Yildiz Koşk, 19th–20th cent. (*C*) Iran, marks: (*a*) on wares from Kerman, 16th–17th cent. in imitation of an imperial Chinese mark of the Ming dynasty; (*b*) on 17th–cent. wares perhaps from the factory at Yezd.

14th and early 15th century whole buildings might be covered with panels of this kind.

Islamic art in medieval Spain and North Africa followed the same basic trends as farther east, with a strong regional accent. Andalusia fostered a school of brick-built architecture with its concomitant wall decoration of carved stucco and glazed tilework. In the Aragonese kingdom of Valencia and Catalonia, following general European practice, decorated tiles were mainly laid on the floor.

The 14th century brought tile mosaic to full development in southern Spain, where in the Alhambra of the Moorish kings at Granada we find it forming a dado (*alicatado*) about 6½ ft. high around the inner walls. The individual pieces of tile (*aliceres*) are mostly cut into straight-sided geometric forms and arranged in radiating star-shaped patterns with a cornice of stepped battlements, along the top. Colors are soft: green,

light blue, purple, yellow-brown, and white. In the 15th century the star patterns were further complicated by adding narrow white strips as outlines to the colored *aliceres*.

As in the Near East, tile mosaic in Spain was superseded by glaze-painted rectangular tiles with similar patterns and coloring. The technique was adopted at Seville toward the end of the 15th century and sometimes used for figure subjects of late Gothic character.

Early in the 16th century the even more economical *cuenca* (hollow) technique was introduced at Seville and Toledo. Patterns, characteristically in the Renaissance vein, were molded on the square tiles whose raised outlines kept the colored glazes in their appropriate areas.

Early in the 13th century the Near Eastern technique of painting pottery in gold luster on a tin-glazed ground had been transmitted to Málaga. It was at first little used for tile-

work, though 14th-century wall tiles are found in the Alhambra and the Cuarto Real de S. Domingo at Granada, and there are a few very large luster-painted wall plaques inscribed with the titles of the Nasrid king Yusuf III (1408–17). About the end of the 14th century the center of the luster-painting industry shifted north to the Christian kingdom of Valencia. Their luster pigment being too vulnerable for use on the floor tiles in demand here, the potters produced through the 15th century a series of tiles painted in blue-and-white alone, designs being an admixture of surviving Islamic and adapted European Gothic motifs. Similar in style were the much coarser unglazed Valencian *socarrats*, long rectangular tiles made for insertion between the rafters of a ceiling. After the beginning of the 16th century immigrant Italian potters diffused from Seville a fashion for wall tiles painted with Renaissance designs in the bright colors of contemporary Italian majolica.

Arthur LANE

WESTERN CERAMICS IN MODERN TIMES. *The 15th and 16th centuries.* The transition from the Middle Ages to the Renaissance was marked by a ceramic evolution which culminated in late-14th-century majolica in both Spain and Italy. To overcome the color limitations imposed by uniform glazing and create a white ground on which to lay colors and to draw the decoration, potters first learned to clothe the body with a layer of slip clay that fired white, after which the decoration could be painted or incised. The whole was then covered with a thin coat of glaze which at the same time fixed the decoration and eliminated porosity. This slipped and glazed ware is known as *bianchetto*, or more often as *mezza maiolica*.

Later the invention of tin-enamel glaze almost completely supplanted the *bianchetto* technique. This glaze, in fact, thanks to the introduction into the former plumbeous mixture of a certain percentage of tin oxide, combined the properties of slip (white color) and of lead glaze (impermeability). The adoption of this single white, shiny coating into which the painted decoration becomes incorporated during firing signaled the birth of true majolica, but the name did not attain its present meaning until the second half of the 16th century, as previously it had been used only for metallic luster. (The name is thought to derive from the island of Majorca.)

In the 14th century Paterna in Spain and Orvieto, Siena, and Faenza in Italy were the most important centers of a production known as "archaic," from the stage of its technical development (PLS. 146, 147). In the 15th century the application of tin glaze became usual; new colors were added to the manganese and copper green, notably zaffer blue (*damaschino*).

As a whole the production of Spain in the 15th century was superior to that of Italy, although it was less varied and less open to development. Metallic luster, probably the discovery of Islamic potters (ca. 800), appeared in Málaga by the 13th century. Its many colors ranged from bronze to greenish, from light gold to reddish. It was not applied on any scale until the 15th century, when it became characteristic of a copious production known as "Hispano-Moresque," centered around Valencia and its suburb Manises (which was noted especially for its *azulejos*, or glazed tilework). Luster, alternating with dark blue, wove a shimmering web of reflections about the close-meshed decoration: geometric motifs, flourishes often borrowed from Kufic script, stylized leaves joined by the slenderest of stems (PL. 142). At the center of specially fine, large plates were heraldic figures or the eagle of St. John, which was especially venerated at Valencia. The most frequent shape was the albarello, a cylindrical wide-mouthed dry-drug jar generally without lid, which perhaps originated in Syria. Heavy nd slightly waisted to prevent slipping in the hand, in Spain it often had two massive handles.

Hispano-Moresque albarellos and those produced in the East invaded Italy, influencing the local fabrics (FIG. 261). The distribution of the albarello cannot be considered separately from the revival of pharmacies. An outgrowth of the monasteries, pharmacies in the 14th century became regular bazaars where valuable objects of various kinds were sold alongside drugs and spices. Pots were lined up on large shelves; the albarello was already conceived as belonging to a series, so that the search for a "type" was reflected on all ceramic fabrics. With the form, decoration was also radically changed and combinations after Hispano-Moresque and Oriental schemes were infused with a new meaning. Since the form of the jar gave no clue to the content — whether drug or spice — the decoration served to describe its properties. Thus the soberly colored designs of archaic wares were fractured by pictorial effects; light touches of blues, yellows, greens crackled on the pasty white glaze, the effects of luster being imitated by touches of yellow-green or lime yellow over the blue.

Besides the albarello there is a type of squat two-handled jug, often decorated in relief in a good blue color, or with an oak-leaf pattern derived from Oriental types. The brilliant deep blue oak-leaf motifs, connected by slender branches indicated in manganese, sometimes frame armorial bearings or animal figures (PL. 154). The highest achievements of 15th-century Italian ceramics, especially from Florence, belong to this group.

*Famille verte* decoration was produced after 1425, appearing on great flat dishes with an animal figure or man's bust. The large figures were placed with an eye to the form of the plate. The palette was temperate, manganese violet for the outline and green for the figures; the quality of the glaze was poor, not yet bright or free of impurities.

After 1460 and until about 1490 a motif consisting of long, stylized leaves, late Gothic in taste, was particularly developed. The motif appeared either alone or often in company with other motifs which became fashionable in the latter half of the century: peacock-feather eyes and the Persian palmette. The Gothic leaf seems to have made its first appearance at Faenza, where blue (zaffer) relief decoration was limited to the center of the vase.

In Florence it made a very early appearance on a few plates before 1460, where it was used to frame animal motifs and heads of men and women (PL. 149). These plates are very fine; the blue tone was used very discreetly, and the whites, yellows, greens, and violets are of exceptional delicacy. Although certain heads, in their Gothic cast and incisive lines, suggest the remote influence of an Alesso Baldovinetti or a Domenico Veneziano, it is more likely that the derivation is from niello work or early Florentine engravings.

Luca della Robbia (q.v.) did not invent tin glazing, as Vasari claimed, but he understood its potential application to sculpture: indeed, not only did he find an economical substitute for costly marble, but his lush, soft sculptural style was particularly adapted to envelopment in the thick brilliance of enamel glaze. While framing his compositions, especially roundels and lunettes, with rich festoons of flowers and fruit in tones of yellow, green, and violet, Luca normally made use of a combination of the two colors white and blue, the image being clearly isolated in its unnatural simplicity on a blue ground which represents the sky, but which in its uniformity has the quality of abstraction.

The Della Robbia formula was successful, but the increasing demand resulted in a decline in quality. Already in the work of Luca's nephew, Andrea della Robbia, the master's chromatic balance tended to become mannered; color was employed for a realistic effect, a use widely exploited by Andrea's sons — of whom Giovanni was the most active — as well as by his followers, Benedetto Buglioni, Santi Viviani, Filippo Paladino. The Della Robbia production was impressive: altar frontals, baptismal fonts, tabernacles, and lavabos; architectural applications were extended to the more complex forms: friezes over doors and on candelabra, ceiling coffers, pavements, and wall plaques.

The work of Luca della Robbia raised pottery to a higher esthetic plane, and for this reason ordinary pottery had no contact with it. Only when the glazed terra cottas of Luca's and Andrea's followers became popular were some bonds established. At Faenza especially the Della Robbia influence resulted, after about 1475, in the rise of a new type of sculpture (small groups, reliefs, and shields or panels), which continued into the first decade of the 16th century.

But the differences in types of production remained considerable, even for the same classes of objects, e.g., pavements and wall plaques. While the Della Robbia type imitated costlier materials, independent creations were elaborated, especially at Faenza, as potters availed themselves of the repertory of Quattrocento terra cotta (pavements of the Vaselli Chapel in S. Petronio at Bologna, dated 1487 and signed "Pietro Andrea da Faenza"; of the Lando Chapel in S. Sebastiano in Venice, dated 1510; of the Caracciolo Chapel in S. Giovanni a Carbonara, in Naples, maker unknown).

Faenza, at the center of a great rebirth in the late 15th and the early 16th centuries, saw a qualitative and a quantitative increase in production (PLS. 148-151), as well as a conquest of new markets. Documentary evidence permits us to follow the increasing consumption of raw materials in relation to increasing production. The most significant index is the consumption of lead, for which information exists for several potteries, although the data are not conclusive: 661 lbs. of lead were acquired in 1461 (potter: Pederzano di Checco), 2,813 lbs. in 1481 (potter:

is also probable that the increased competition with goldwork, along with the greater availability and reduced cost of silver and other precious materials, induced the makers of majolica to seek a new style. It is certain that the birth of engraving as a stylistic derivation of niello work was instrumental in the invention of *istoriato*: a phase in the imitation of niello is clearly apparent in some late Quattrocento pottery, especially sgraffito.

The first sign of the influence of engravings and woodcuts was the rise of a new exclusively decorative type, the painted shield. Not only did the object no longer serve a useful function, but the subject matter generally changed from secular to sacred. At the same time a new specialist emerged: the potter-painter, who selected motifs and elaborated and painted them in a personal style that no longer relied on a preestablished repertory. Production had to some extent been "industrialized," and he therefore limited himself to painting objects already fashioned and prepared.

The most important painter of this first phase of Faventine *istoriato*, the Master of the Resurrection, is known to have

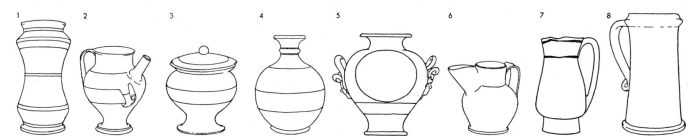

Typical shapes of European pottery in the 14th–18th cent. (1–5) Pharmaceutical pots: (1) Albarello, Faenza, 1470–80; (2) Castel Durante, ca. 1550; (3) Genoa, late 16th cent.; (4, 5) Faenza, early 17th. cent. (6) Umbrian panata, 14th cent.; (7) Faventine jug, 14th cent.; (8) majolica jug, Germany, 1742.

Lorenzo di Bartolo), 5,512 lbs. in 1517 (by three associated potters), 13,415 lbs. in the same year (by two potters), and finally, in 1518, the same quantity (by a single potter, Giuliano Manara). Without our entirely accepting the conclusion (Grigioni) that production between 1460 and 1500 increased tenfold, it is clear that the productive rhythm was continuously accelerated. The data relative to Francesco Mezzarisa (or Mezzarixa), head of one of the most flourishing Faventine potteries, suffice: in 1545 he engaged himself to produce 3,500 pieces of majolica, and the following year 7,025, half of which were to be delivered after 72 days (an average of nearly 50 pieces a day) and the other half after 133 days.

The wider distribution of Italian pottery was stimulated by the novelty of the *istoriato* ("narrative") style, credit for which must be given Faenza, even if early dishes of the Florentine Gothic-leaf group (ca. 1460) had accorded some importance to the human figure. The slightly later developments of slipped and sgraffito work also played a part. About the turn of the 15th century this particular technique flourished especially in northern Italy — Piedmont, Lombardy, Venetia (at Legnano and Padua), and Emilia (at Modena, Bologna, Ferrara, and Ravenna) — though it was seldom attempted at the two major centers of Florence and Faenza. With a decorative repertory all its own, it is clearly linked to such techniques as niello and enameling. The figure is given new prominence, though its elegant stylization and its decorative relation to the plant motifs that frame it preserve a late Gothic quality. But it was the change of the figure from the purely decorative or heraldic to the "historical," in the spirit of Humanism, that was to encourage the rise of *istoriato* decoration and the consequently greater cultural importance of majolica. Beginning with this change, Faventine majolica proceeded through phases also to be found in sgraffito work. Noteworthy is a portrait dish (*coppa amatoria*; Bologna, Mus. Civ.), dated 1499, in which the robust figure of a woman continuously outlined, as in plates from Legnano or Ferrara, fills the whole bowl (PL. 151).

The invention of the *istoriato* style helped extend the market to the wealthy and to introduce pottery into the noble houses side by side with the products of the goldsmith's craft. But it

been at work in Faenza and Forlì about 1510–23. Especially in his best-known work, in the Victoria and Albert Museum in London — the tile with the Resurrection, after which he was named — one perceives an evident wish to imitate on a crowded and vibrant stage the refined sensibility of German and Flemish engravings: especially of Dürer or Lucas van Leyden. It is primarily in great refinement of color that he displayed his mastery: blue, the dominant and characteristic color of Faventine potters, became lilac and violet and mingled with a range of oranges, pale greens, intense and soft yellows. The technique is outstanding in rapid touches that introduce spots of light and in glazes that flux and graduate the colors. His other works include the shield with the Martyrdom of St. Sebastian (Florence, Mus. Naz.; PL. 148); the panel with St. Jerome in the Desert, and the panel picturing the Original Sin (London, Vict. and Alb.).

But the panel with sacred and profane subjects soon fell into disuse, and *istoriato* was applied more commonly to plates and bowls, which were actually more closely associated with this art, especially because of their traditionally functional purpose. A group of *istoriato* dishes can be attributed to the Master of the Death of the Virgin, so called after his best-known work (London, Br. Mus.; ca. 1510), which is taken from an engraving by Martin Schongauer. Another group belongs with the Perseus and Andromeda plate at the Victoria and Albert Museum, which derives from a woodcut of the 1493 Venetian edition of Ovid.

The production of Faenza had a great impact on other Italian potteries. The most important center was at Cafaggiolo, near Florence. Active throughout the first half of the 16th century, it served the Medicis and other noble families, whose blazons almost always appear on the fabrics. The production, of a high order, consisted predominantly of dishes, generally pieces for show rather than use. The palette is very similar to the Faventine: deep blue background laid on in broad horizontal brush strokes, some brighter blues, some purple or a deep red, whose viscosity distinguishes it from the dark red of Faenza. But here, because of the nearness of Florence, works by Donatello, Botticelli, and Filippino Lippi served as models.

The best Cafaggiolo majolica pieces are largely the work of one man, Jacopo Fattorini.

Sienese pottery flourished until about 1520. Characteristic colors are yellows, deep oranges, and a fine black uncommon in majolica painting. There is evidence of the immigration of potters from the Faenza area into Siena; for instance, that Master Benedetto who signed the famous plate with the figure of a warrior saint at the center — blue with highlights of mat white (PL. 150) — is the son of one Giorgio da Faenza. While at Cafaggiolo the human figure was largely painted in the style of the miniaturists, Siena produced very little work in true *istoriato* style. The graceful figures, walking in a characteristically Umbrian landscape, are inscribed among concentric rings of arabesques and grotesques which recall the ornamental repertory of Bernardino Pinturicchio.

As in Siena, but with different results, *istoriato* decoration was taken up in a limited way in Deruta, which had been a pottery center since the Middle Ages; indeed, pottery was its principal industry. The 16th-century production of Deruta has links with the Trecento and Quattrocento in the surfaces emulating precious materials and in the unusual effects of light and color. The first Italian metallic lusters, after Hispano-Moresque models, were apparently introduced at Deruta, where shining iridescent tones of gold and mother-of-pearl were achieved during a third firing. Lustered decoration is often devoid of figures, the nearest thing being a few geometric compositions using stars. As in Hispano-Moresque wares, the geometric decoration is used to heighten the illusion of a covering of some precious material, such as gold leaf or mother-of-pearl. Its geometrization and incisive outlines persist in representational decoration as well. At Faenza the *istoriato* formula was the result of an increase of narration at the expense of purely decorative motifs, but at Deruta the stylization of outlines of single figures resulted in their standardization and reduction to a decorative motif. Thus, while recent engravings were copied at Faenza, at Deruta there was recourse rather to the earlier Umbrian traditions of Perugino or Signorelli.

A production of household ware flourished at Faenza especially, where the *istoriato* style had achieved a character of its own. This commercial class was primary in the principal Faenza pottery, Casa Pirota (which had its own stamp). A relation to the traditional Faventine décor — already well-defined in 14th- and 15th-century jugs — is seen in some plates with putti or coats of arms in the center and a wide ornate rim; a relation of blue to white was basic to the color scheme. *Berettini*, pieces with a characteristic slate-blue glaze and decoration in opaque white, constitute a special type. Rackham has suggested that the recurrence of formulas in these non-representational dishes indicates an industrial production. Various ornaments from the Renaissance repertory appear on the base color. Grotesques are in the forefront; indeed they are at this moment the finest and most complex of the various motifs. Cipriano Piccolpasso (1524–79), the author of *Li tre libri dell'arte del vasaio*, which he wrote about 1556, when grotesques had fallen into disuse, records that they brought a higher price than any other type of decoration, including even the *paesi* (landscapes), but excluding the *candelieri* (candelabrum designs), which, of course, belonged to a related type. (Piccolpasso does not mention the prices commanded by *istoriato*.) Apparently grotesques were also prized at Faenza in the early Cinquecento. It is also probable that, unlike the simpler and more formalized designs, they were often entrusted to masters who specialized in *istoriato*. Zoan Maria Vasaro was primarily a painter of grotesques, and Niccolò Pellipario did not consider himself above practicing this art. The grotesque theme was introduced into Faenza after 1487 (pavement in S. Petronio at Bologna). It became increasingly popular not only for borders but also for the whole surface of the plate. Among the best-known examples are two dishes dated 1508. In the first, polychrome grotesques are disposed in a candelabrum arrangement on a lead-blue ground and recall the engravings of Pellegrino Cesena (Liverani); and in the center of the plate two of the many figures are taken from the Dürer engraving *The Satyr's Family*. The design of the second (Modena, Gall.

Estense) is more clearly mechanical. Comparison with the David and Goliath plate (1507) in Florence (Mus. Naz.) shows a similar compositional scheme: a central axis precisely established, bunches of grapes in the upper section, two superposed curvilinear motifs that frame the composition of the bottom section, and the themes distributed laterally. This arrangement demonstrates how the process of "redecoration" of an illustration, so characteristic of the *istoriato* style, is often as fixed and schematic as in purely ornamental compositions. The plate with grotesques described above shows the same tendencies and represents the transition to *istoriato*; but here the design is broken up by the variety and liveliness of pictorial effect. Cafaggiolo grotesques have similar qualities. During the second decade of the 16th century, the grotesques on *berettini* became progressively standardized, while the *istoriato* painters, especially Francesco Xanto Avelli di Rovigo, gradually liberated themselves from the decorative formulas in order to concentrate on the interpretation of literary themes.

*Istoriato* decoration was to find its most extensive development in potteries established along the Metauro River, where prized clay was abundant. The most important of these centers was Castel Durante (now Urbania), whose name appears for the first time on a plate decorated with putti and grotesques, with the arms of Pope Julius II (1503–13) in the center. It is dated 1508 and signed by Zoan Maria Vasaro, to whom other pieces are also attributed and who may have worked at Faenza too. He usually painted grotesques and trophies among putti and monsters dancing a weird saraband about the center of the dish, which depicts the torments of Love (PL. 150). His lively representations break up the old symmetrical decorative scheme, and even extend out toward the rim. Zoan Maria's imagination was nourished by German engravings and woodcuts, especially Dürer's, but his principal source (hitherto unrecognized) is in the magnificent engravings of Francesco Colonna's *Hypnerotomachia Poliphili*, published by Aldus in 1499. His energetic idiom is coupled with a lively sense of color; the use of a gray blue tending to black and a luminous yellow amber in place of the usual orange is characteristic. Indeed, his work marks a break in the balanced Faventine canon and the adoption of a brighter palette, in which yellows predominate, by the potteries on the Metauro.

*Istoriato* had in Niccolò Pellipario an artist of unusual skill. Born not later than 1480, probably at Castel Durante, where he worked for many years, in 1527 he was at Fabriano and in the next year at Urbino, where he remained until his death between 1540 and 1547. Before 1521 he produced a service (now distributed among the Vict. and Alb., London; the Louvre; the Mus. Civ. of Bologna; and private collections) for Isabella d'Este; the supposed Ridolfi service (17 plates of which are in Venice, Mus. Correr); and other pieces belonging to unidentified services. Subject matter is drawn largely from the classics, especially Ovid and Lucian. His palette at the time was soft and harmonious, a mellower fusion of tones replacing the crowded thin brush strokes of the Master of the Resurrection; the concept of landscape is completely transformed. This master is eclectic; besides painting, his most important stylistic and iconographical source among engravings was the *Hypnerotomachia Poliphili* (I, PL. 308). The hypothesis (A. Venturi) that the dishes in the Ridolfi service were designed by Timoteo Viti has no stylistic foundation; nor is Pellipario's style a derivation (Wallis) from the works of Giorgione and Venetian painting; it is related, rather, to the Roman idiom of the Villa Farnesina in Rome and especially the friezes of Baldassare Peruzzi. After 1521 his plates show a classicizing trend and impoverishment of style; the happiest exceptions are the portrait plates of "beautiful women" (*belle donne*), e.g., the plate inscribed "Silvia Bella" (London, Vict. and Alb.; PL. 151). His subjects came more and more to be taken from Raphaelesque engravings, especially those of Marcantonio Raimondi, (e.g., a plate dated 1527 showing the Madonna of the Stairs). A vivid yellow, which was to remain typical of the Urbino school, appears for the first time in the famous plate (1528) taken from another Marcantonio engraving, *The Martyrdom of St. Cecilia*, and executed at Urbino in the workshop of Pellipario's son. In the

later works the approach is summary, with barely suggested backgrounds and few figures.

The back of a Pellipario plate at the Museo Civico in Bologna showing the Presentation in the Temple bears the inscription "M. G. finj de maiolica." This is a reference to Master Giorgio Andreoli (1465/70–1533?), born at Intra and established at Gubbio after 1498 with his brother. The inscription further testifies that he completed the work of Pellipario by adding metallic lusters in a third firing (PL. 153). The first Italian lusters (which were golden or nacreous) were achieved in Deruta. Master Giorgio lent his name to a ruby-red luster. The importation of the art of luster from Deruta to Gubbio seems confirmed by the properties of the Gubbio product. It is not known whether Master Giorgio limited himself to lustering pieces painted by others or whether, as is likely, he painted them himself. It is almost certain that pieces destined for luster were produced at Gubbio and that many potters sent their products to that city for this supplementary process. Lusters, which the less exuberant Deruta potters limited to undecorated pieces, were here applied on *istoriato* designs. A certain unity of style was achieved when the luster, instead of being applied merely as an embellishment of surface, was used as an integral part of the design, as in certain storm-struck landscapes with streaks of luster in gold and ruby red. It is thought that some of these works can be attributed to other artists working at Gubbio side by side with Master Giorgio, for example, the "Master of the Three Graces," so named after a famous plate (1525) now in the Victoria and Albert Museum (PL. 150).

During these years *istoriato*, which had been revived by Pellipario at Castel Durante, was to inspire many other painters, all under his influence. A fairly uniform group of plates datable to 1520–30 was assembled by Rackham and ascribed by him to an anonymous Durantine artist known as "Pseudo-Pellipario," from certain family resemblances of technique rather than of style. This master is the only one to have inherited Pellipario's lyricism — though in a more subtle vein — and the airiness and depth of his scenes, of which he tempered the luminosity by a uniform transparency, and to which he gave an archaizing clarity and unity of composition. His palette is low-keyed, with light greenish hues, pale blues, and grays.

At Urbino, where Niccolò Pellipario moved in 1528 and took the name of Fontana, his son Guido Fontana worked and lived from 1520 until 1576 and after. He established the Urbino potteries, which owed their prosperity to the patronage of the dukes of Rovere: Francesco Maria (1490–1538) and Guidobaldo II (1514–74). Guido's personal idiom is not easy to distinguish, as many pieces from his pottery bear the name of his father or his son Orazio (PL. 150).

The most interesting work from Urbino is that of Francesco Xanto Avelli di Rovigo. Born early in the 1500s, he was signing works after 1530 (his seal F.X.A.R., combinations of those letters, or even just a simple X). Recently a group of works signed F.R. or sometimes F.L.R., executed for the most part at Faenza, have been identified as his youthful work. Avelli took his cue from Pellipario, but very quickly his palette developed density and weight and his construction became solidly based on isolated elements. These, especially the figures, are often taken from engravings. They became largely imaginary portraits which, with certain greater or lesser changes, could be made to represent different personages. But where Pellipario's creative fancy had been abundant, Avelli's tended to be mechanical and to pay little attention to the form of the plate, whose blank areas he merely filled with figures taken from engravings. The new *istoriato* formula, which Avelli perfected, was also especially influenced by the late publications of Marcantonio, such as the *Phrygian Plague* or especially the *Quos ego*, in which the engraving tends to change from mere illustration to actual narration. There is always an inscription on the front or the back of Avelli's plates, often a rhyme, which the painted "story" illustrates — mostly incidents from literature, but also current events, politics, or history.

Pellipario's heirs, the Fontanas, also worked at Urbino and specialized in sumptuous services inspired by the more complex forms of contemporary silver, such as the celebrated ducal service now for the most part in the Museo Nazionale in Florence. The Fontana works are in warm colors skillfully handled, with yellows predominating. Designs were reproduced in series through considerable use of pricked drawings. The generally Raphaelesque decoration tends increasingly toward miniature, with intense chiaroscuro effects. Among the late potteries at Urbino that of the Pantanazzis should also be mentioned; their style pushed pictorial elaboration to an extreme and included networks of arabesques, etc. Forms were capricious and varied: fruit bowls, inkwells, candelabra, sculptured groups, garden fountains, vases, and cups, whose form and relief decoration were inspired by plant forms.

In Venice the influence of Urbino was dominant after 1520. Wares were decorated with flowers and fruits; *istoriato* became lively and pictorial, with outlines rapid and impressionistic. The most important potteries were directed by Master Domenico and Master Ludovico.

In Faenza the new *fiorito* ("floral") style became emancipated in the so-called *compendiario* ("shorthand") style. Shortly after 1550 Francesco Mezzarisa and especially Virgiliotto Calamelli and such masters as "Don Pino" and Giovan Battista dalle Palle introduced into the "story" a sketchy, shorthand decoration, almost monochrome, with thick lines of watered blue, yellow, and green spread over the excellent thick white enamel, which earned the name of *bianchi* (white ware) for this type of majolica. The *bianchi* spread rapidly in Italy and elsewhere; the name "faïence" came to be applied to all majolica fabrics. The masters of the *compendiario* style were much sought after and went to Turin, Genoa, Verona, Padua, Deruta, Castelli in Apulia, France, Holland, England. Other potters, expelled from Faenza for their allegiance to the Reformation, spread the same style to Germany, Hungary, and Switzerland.

The imitation of Italian majolica accounts for a good part of European 16th-century production, especially in France. The floor of the abbey at Brou (ca. 1530) is similar to the floor of S. Sebastiano in Venice (1510) and is the work of Italian potters. At Nîmes Antoine Syjalon (1548–90) executed plates and albarellos with decoration in the Faventine style. At Montpellier Pierre Estève (d. 1596) produced drug jars in a style similar to that of Syjalon. At Rouen the potter Masseot Abaquesne (fl. ca. 1526–60) specialized in drug jars and tiles in the Faventine style, at the same time introducing motifs borrowed from the Fontainebleau school and the grotesque ornaments of Cornelis II Floris. Lyons, where wares in the style of Urbino were produced, welcomed Italian majolica artists.

The works of the French pottery of Saint-Porchaire (1525–60) were more original. They are light, fragile pieces, with a fine hard body, often with filled-in decoration in a technique reminiscent of engraving. The interlaced geometric design is very quiet and subtle. At first the models were Oriental porcelains and contemporary goldwork; later, through the influence of Urbino, architecturally elaborated designs in relief predominated (PL. 152).

The greatest exponent of French 16th-century majolica was the sculptor, naturalist, and physicist Bernard Palissy (b. Agen, ca. 1510; d. 1589/90). In 1539 he established himself at Saintes and about 1554 invented a new type of majolica with plastic decoration known as *rustiques figurines*. These are plates and vases bearing leaves, shell fossils, flowers, fish, lizards and salamanders, frogs, snakes, eels, molded in high relief (PL. 152). The type may have been inspired by certain passages in the *Hypnerotomachia Poliphili* and has a counterpart in the contemporary work of the Nuremberg silversmith Wenzel Jamnitzer. Palissy's work, though often confused with that of his school, is outstanding for the ability with which the colored glazes are applied and superposed on the body. Their esthetic value is the result of a splendid harmony of colors — blue, purple, pale yellow, grayish white — as shown in the decoration of the Tuileries grotto commissioned by Catherine de Médicis and destroyed about 1590 (fragments at Sèvres, in the Louvre, and the Mus. Carnavalet in Paris). While Italian potters relied upon the illustrative impact of their subject matter and the pleasing composition and web of colors, the French potters pointed more directly to the beauty of material. In 1576 Palissy

moved to Paris. The production attributed to him and his school is enormous. Besides majolicas in the *style rustique*, there are the important *terres jaspées*, whose decorative hollows heighten the beauty of the glazes that cover them; this fabric is a refinement of a green-glaze ware, of medieval derivation, once produced at La Chapelle-des-Pots and in Saintonge. Also to be noted are plates and cups decorated in relief and allegorical compositions such as Water, Fertility, etc.

The Netherlands were also under Italian influence. The presence of Guido Savino of Castel Durante is recorded at Antwerp in 1512. In that city, about 1540, an original type of scroll decoration (*ferronnerie*) developed as a result of the influence of the engraving school of Cornelis II Floris. This genre also inspired certain majolicas from Seville and Talavera. In Spain, where majolicas of the Italian type went by the name of *pisa*, the Pisan potter Francisco Niculoso was active between 1503 and 1526. At Seville, Tentudia, and Flores de Ávila there are panels by his hand in the manner of Faenza with sacred subjects framed by grotesques.

The Italian fashion also throve in Switzerland, in the Tirol, in Moravia, probably in England, and in Germany, where Nuremberg underwent Venetian influence. But in England, Holland, and especially Germany the production between 1450 and the first decades of the 16th century is typified by pottery with decoration in relief and with glazes having a base of galena (lead sulfide) or lead oxide: a ware of direct medieval descent, not very different from the type produced in France by Palissy's circle. In Germany, Austria, and Switzerland a particular flowering of these lead glazes used in conjunction with tin enamel was due to stovemakers, whose green glaze was of a high technical order. Occasional applications of two or more colors appeared a little before 1500. The most original work, however, was done by a family of potters named Preuning, active at Nuremberg about 1550, who invented a robust, ample type of relief decoration; by the stovemaker Hans Kraut (1532–92) of Villingen in the Black Forest; and by an anonymous potter of Silesia who soon developed a similar style of great vigor.

Rhenish stoneware (*Steinzeug*), the most typical and most valued ceramic production of the German 16th century, is of medieval origin and achieved artistic dignity only in the second quarter of the 16th century, when it developed on an industrial scale at Cologne, Siegburg, and Raeren almost simultaneously. Finely executed reliefs are cut into the almost pure white or warm gray-brown surface; the forms are of a severity and solidity becoming to the very hard quality of the material. The first attempts at plastic decoration were made at Cologne. But the most highly prized type was a large spherical vase with molded relief of oak leaves or roses with long ornate stems in a Gothic style suggestive of the Italian *famille verte* designs of a century earlier. The jugs and wine bottles made at Cologne enjoyed a great success and were much sought after even in England. Rhenish stoneware reached its highest point in the work of Jan Emens Mennicken and Baldem Mennicken of Raeren. Jan Emens began working in the manner of Cologne in the 1560s, then elaborated an effective style of fine intaglio, as in the vase showing the history of Joseph (1587; Cologne, Mus.), which seems to stem from an imaginary metal model. Baldem, less versed as an engraver, was equally skilled in the invention and energetic detailing of measured forms that move freely in space. A notable group of potters, whose seals were F. T. (F. Trac), L. W., and H. A., worked at Siegburg; here also Anno and Christian Knütgen worked more in a Renaissance vein; their elegantly proportioned stoneware with fine reliefs was suggestive of ivory. In the 17th century, the school continued at Westerwald, Höhr, Grenzau, and Grenzhausen, where potters repeated motifs introduced by Jan Emens. New shapes and decorative forms were developed in Saxony and in Bavaria (at Kreussen) by the Vest family.

*The 17th and 18th centuries.* Although majolica was now at the end of its historical development and was gradually being supplanted by porcelain, it continued to flourish in the 17th and 18th centuries. The term "majolica," here used in a broad sense for the sake of clarity in discussions of techniques, is usually confined by students of ceramics to the tin-enameled wares of Renaissance Italy or their direct descendants, and the term "faïence" (its technical equivalent) is generally used instead for Dutch majolica of the 17th and 18th centuries and, generally, for all late majolica made in imitation of Oriental porcelain, as well as the more or less original production of tin-enameled wares of France, Germany, and other centers.

Baroque production in Germany was more varied and personal. Here craft tradition of enameling and metalwork were also in the ascendant, especially at Nuremberg and Augsburg. In the 1660s at Nuremberg Johann Schaper approached the *Schwarzlot* technique (black-enamel painting) for his exquisite landscapes, while in the late 17th century the style of Abraham Helmhack, Wolfgang Rössler, Johann Wilhelm Heel, and, at Augsburg, Bartolomäus Seuter showed similarities with contemporary engravings. Also after engravings were the leaves and strapwork (*Laub- und Bandelwerk*) which correspond exactly to the Bérain style in France and which were widely used during the first half of the 18th century after their introduction on early silvered or gilded Meissen porcelains (PLS. 157, 160).

In Holland the town of Delft very soon assumed primary importance. Majolica was produced there after 1500, and by 1700 the number of manufactures increased to nearly 30. A century later Dutch production underwent a crisis over the importation of English wares and European porcelain. Light and elegant, Delft majolicas compared at least in appearance with oriental porcelains. Their distribution was considerable, especially in England, where the name "delft" was applied to majolicas from everywhere. The use of an overglaze which was both compact and transparent, applied on the raw glaze (and similar to the Italian *marzacotto* described above), gave these majolicas a particular brightness and chromatic vigor (PL. 156). The first phase of Delft production (until ca. 1650) is typified by a rather heavy decoration outlined in deep purple and filled in with blue. Subjects include kermesses, battles, and other historical events, crowded with figures. The middle phase (ca. 1650–1710) is concerned with the imitation of Oriental porcelains. In the general mediocrity we can distinguish the blue majolica of Aelbregt de Keiser, the blue, red, and gold of Adriaen Pynacker (d. 1707), the black, blue, and purple of Samuel van Eenhoorn (1655–before 1687) (PL. 155): these are majolicas with polychrome decoration on a black-glaze background and also landscapes, rural scenes, and historical subjects painted in monochrome blue, as well as portraits on panels. In the late period there was a highly commercial production of every kind of object, even bird cages and musical instruments. The clay used was very fine and light. Oriental porcelains as well as those of Saxony were imitated, and although from the 16th century on polychrome decoration began to give way in the Netherlands to imitations of Chinese porcelain, nevertheless the large production of wall tiles at Rotterdam and other Dutch centers continued its traditions in the 17th century. At Delft itself there also flourished an independent production which, though it showed the influence of Chinese wares, had a more distinctly European flavor in its baroque decoration: e.g., some works by Rochus Hoppesteyn (V, PL. 198) or those attributed to Frederik van Frijtom (elected to the Guild in 1658), which echo Dutch painting. Certain fine 17th-century English delftware is also in the majolica tradition, as is also the work of the stove factories at Winterthur and Steckborn in Switzerland.

In Italy the *bianchi* (white ware) of Faenza continued to be distributed widely. The most complex baroque forms and the strangest objects (cages, obelisks, pyramidal or open-hand flower holders, shoes, hammers, violins) were made of white majolica. In the first half of the 17th century Montelupo regained prominence with its round jugs decorated in a popular vein, executed in a technique inspired by the *compendiario* style, but with a lively sense of construction and robust colors (PL. 154). In Naples and in Campania, polychrome majolica was used a good deal in architecture — panels with flowers, leaves, and baroque scrolls. One of the finest examples is in the cloister of S. Chiara in Naples (1742), where walls, pillars, and benches are faced with majolica panels in a rustic vein, with landscapes, rural and mythological scenes, masques and carnival processions.

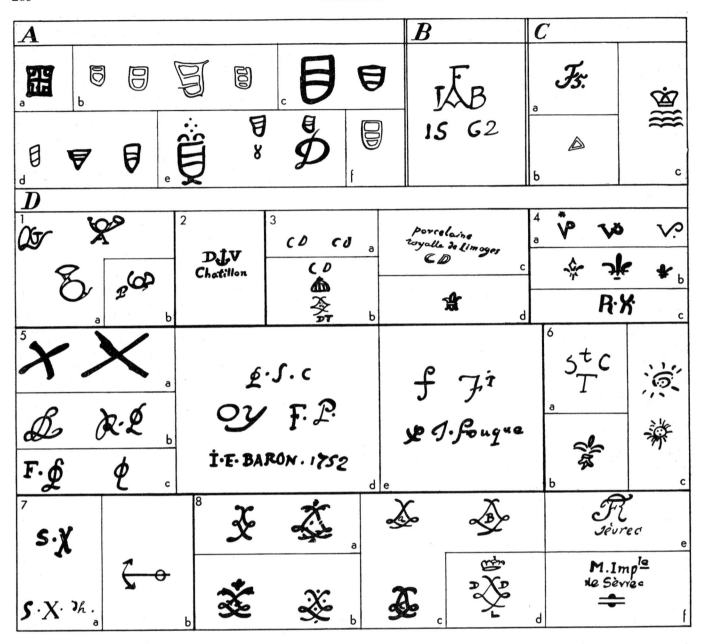

European marks. (*A*) Austria. Vienna: (*a*) 1718–1864; (*b*) impressed marks, 1744–49; (*c*) 1749–70, 1770–1810; (*d*) 1810–20, 1820–29, 1749–1827, and 1850–64; (*e*) before 1784; (*f*) impressed mark, 1827–50. (*B*) Belgium. Antwerp (16th–17th cent.), majolica: Probably the mark of Jan Boghaert (1552–71). (*C*) Denmark. Copenhagen: (*a*) Østerbro, soft-paste porcelain, mark of L. Fournier (1759–65), in blue enamel, referring to Frederick V of Denmark; (*b*) Royal Factory (act. from 1779), hard porcelain, impressed mark of F. H. Müller (in use from 1771); (*c*) Royal Factory, 1905. (*D*) France. (1) Chantilly (ca. 1725–1800), soft-paste porcelain: (*a*) Mark in red or sometimes black enamel for the initial period, blue under luster and sometimes crimson for the later period; (*b*) late 18th cent. and early 19th, gold mark on white ware. (2) Chantillon (from ca. 1775), hard porcelain, mark in red. (3) Limoges (from 1736), majolica: (*a*) Monogram of the Comte d'Artois, protector of the factory (1761–84), incised or painted, generally in red; (*b–d*) marks used from 1784 on white wares to be decorated at Sèvres: (*b*) incised and in blue enamel; (*c*) incised and inscribed initials in red; (*d*) impressed or incised. (4) Marseilles: (*a*) Veuve Perrin works (ca. 1740–95), marks of C. Perrin; (*b*) Savy works, act. from ca. 1770; (*c*) Robert works, ca. 1750–95. (5) Moustiers, from 1679 to 19th cent.: (*a*) 1710–40; (*b*) marks of J. Olerys and J. B. Laugier, ca. 1738–90; (*c, d*) seals attributed to J. Olerys and J. B. Laugier; (*e*) marks of J. Fouque, in use from 1749. (6) St.-Cloud, from ca. 1760: (*a*) On majolica, mark in blue; (*b*) incised mark on soft-paste porcelain, ca. 1678–1766; (*c*) mark in the shape of the sun, in blue. (7) Sceaux, ca. 1748–94: (*a*) Incised marks on porcelain; (*b*) mark painted on majolica. (8) Sèvres (from 1738), soft and hard porcelain: (*a*) In blue enamel, before 1753; (*b*) in blue under luster and in blue enamel, before 1753; (*c*) in blue enamel, from 1753; (*d*) in blue and red enamel, from 1781; (*e*) mark of the First Republic, in blue; (*f*) mark of the First Empire, in red.

Sicilian 17th-century production is also of a high order (Palermo and Trapani). The Ligurian production of Genoa, Savona, and Albisola is related; besides a richly decorative type inspired by models of the local school or directly practiced by such painters as the Guidobonos, another also existed which precociously reflected the influence of late Ming and Ch'ing models in their calligraphic rendition of bunches of long leaves on plates, trays, albarellos, drug jars, and little parallelipiped flasks. In Abruzzo, Castelli production in the 17th and 18th centuries was outstanding and elaborated an original *compendiario* style. The Grue family took up an *istoriato* style of the Urbino type. Its founder,

Francesco Antonio (1618–73), also executed shields and altar frontals. His son Carlantonio (1655–1723) took his inspiration from the baroque style of the Carraccis, Pietro da Cortona, and the Neapolitans and brought *istoriato* to a new level of splendor, treating it with softness and a refined, warm, quiet palette often enriched with gold. His successor was Carmine Gentile (1678–1763).

In France majolica was highly developed in the 17th and 18th centuries. Potteries multiplied at Nevers from 1630 to the first half of the 18th century. Between 1630 and 1660 decoration of a Persian cast was in vogue, with flowers and

birds in white and yellow on a handsome blue ground. After 1660 decoration inspired by Chinese models of the transitional period appeared. Another type of plate was decorated with scenes taken from Simon Vouet, Michel Dorigny, and Jacques Stella. In the 18th century the wares of Rouen and Moustiers were copied. Rouen indeed produced a ware of unusual quality and abundance. Among the many potteries which were established after 1650 and in the 18th century we can distinguish the pottery founded by Edme Poterat (d. 1687) and his son Louis (d. 1696). The invention of lambrequins (with scallops and lacelike decoration) in the *style rayonnant*, which dominated the production of Rouen, is probably attributable to Louis Poterat; this type of majolica has a body that fires from red to gray; the glaze was first limited to blue on white, but was then varied with a fine red, yellow ochre, and green. Objects of all kinds were produced in the *style rayonnant*, which went through phases of Chinese, then Persian, then rococo inspiration: round and oval plates, cruet stands, bidets, closestools, soapdishes, etc. At Moustiers, in the 17th and early 18th centuries, the Clérissys had some prominence in a production of vessels and devotional and other objects. Their *plats de chasse* (showing hunting scenes) were especially well known; within *rayonnant* borders appeared compositions after prints of Antonio Tempesta, Jean Leclerc, Frans I Floris, Jacques Callot, etc. The influence of Nevers as well as of Rouen was in evidence. Refined blue-and-white ornamental motifs, whose prototypes were the designs of Jean Bérain, became widespread in the early 18th century. It was probably Joseph Olerys (d. 1749) who first applied them to majolica and later brought them to Alcora (in Valencia). Similar derivations occur in various centers of southern France and in Italy, at Turin and Lodi, in the work of Giorgio Giacinto Rossetti and his family. At Saint-Jean-du-Désert (near Marseilles) the production of the 17th and 18th centuries was first under the influence of Savona and Nevers, then of Moustiers. At Strasbourg, after the arrival from Holland of Charles-François Hannong in 1709, a majolica with magnificent white glaze and lambrequins was produced first in blue, then, about 1740, in polychrome, by his son Paul-Antoine Hannong.

After 1750 high-fired majolica decoration was abandoned in France for the new technique of enamel colors applied in the *petit feu*, a technique already explored after 1747 in Germany, at Höchst, and thence imported to Strasbourg by the German painter Adam Friedrich von Löwenfinck. These tin-glazed wares, enameled like porcelain, included *faïence-porcelaine*, which copied porcelain and was first applied in the *fleurs des Indes* designs, which then evolved into the more lighthearted "flowers of Strasbourg." A similar transformation took place in Holland in the *Delft dorée*. The *petit feu* colors of Strasbourg were imitated in the majolica of Niderviller (where figurines and vessels were treated with a more subtle palette), at Marseilles, Rouen, Moustiers, and Sceaux, where Jacques Chapelle (1721–73) produced services and statuettes in the style of Strasbourg and Marseilles (PLS. 159, 160).

Alcora saw a flowering of the Bérain style after its introduction by Joseph Olerys. But Miguel Soliva, Francisco Grangel, and others soon offered a new form of freely inspired panel painting that was particularly successful in color and design.

A lush rococo style was adapted to majolica at Kiel and Eckernförde in Schleswig-Holstein ("Baltic rococo"), especially by Johann Buchwald and Abraham Leihamer, and in Scandinavia (Marieberg, Herrebøe).

*Porcelain in the 17th and 18th centuries.* The most sought-after ceramics in the 17th and 18th centuries were porcelains. The decoration and colors first of Oriental and then of European porcelain had therefore a great influence on majolica. Indeed, the adoption of majolica services at princely tables in the 17th century was in part due to the new prestige that Chinese porcelain had conferred on ceramics in general. The first news of the existence of Chinese porcelain was brought to Venice in 1295 by Marco Polo. In the 14th and 15th centuries porcelain was considered one of the most exquisite expressions of Oriental civilization; it was costly and jealously guarded.

The first attempts at imitation were made at Venice in the early Cinquecento, then at Ferrara, Urbino, and elsewhere. Between 1565 and 1620 the Medicis placed the Florentine kilns of the "Fonderia" in the Palazzo Pitti at the disposal of chemists and ceramists. The resulting "Medici porcelain" was only an approximation and did not achieve the cold crystal beauty of porcelain. But it was of a high esthetic order, and the rare and precious qualities of the Oriental models were transmuted into a delicate elegance of form and decorative effect.

Attempts at imitation of Chinese porcelain multiplied in the 17th century after the rise of Dutch commerce made possible its regular importation. Particularly important to its new vogue was its perfect adaptability to the new beverages: tea, coffee, and cocoa. After 1610 Dutch potters turned to the imitation of porcelain. What was then improperly called *Hollandsch porselein* was, as pointed out earlier, really majolica with decoration in a warm blue instead of in several colors. Toward 1650 the potteries of Delft gave a new impetus to these imitations, under the inspiration of the porcelain of the late Ming dynasty and also of the transitional period before K'ang-hsi. Besides the direct copying of Chinese models, there was from the sixties onward an output of *chinoiseries* fancifully interpreted motifs from the Orient. Originating in Delft, these *chinoiseries* soon spread throughout Europe (PL. 156).

Between the fall of the Ming dynasty in 1644 and the advent of the Manchu K'ang-hsi in 1662, imports from China were probably interrupted. Toward 1700 commerce was renewed by English and French trading companies and new types of Chinese porcelains as well as the hitherto unknown Japanese wares became plentiful in Europe. This new wave produced a new imitative phase (ca. 1700–30), originally characterized by the use of sumptuous reds, which began about 1720 to influence Chinese products in their turn. Thereafter new European styles developed truly independent forms.

Porcelain was a luxury throughout Europe and one of the principal objects of exchange when at last the chemical secret of its composition was discovered. The credit goes to the German alchemist Johann Friedrich Böttger (1682-1719), a jeweler in the service of Augustus the Strong who made use of the Saxon kaolin of Kolditz (ca. 1709) and thence moved to Meissen, where in 1710, in the Albrechtsburg, Augustus established the first European manufacture of hard porcelain.

The establishment of the factory at Meissen gave the signal for an intense rivalry among the reigning powers and nobility of Europe. According to Charles Eugene Duke of Württemberg (1758), the establishment of its manufacture was now an indispensable requisite of princely dignity. The vogue for porcelain constituted in fact one of the most typical aspects of 18th-century society. All kinds of objects were translated into porcelain: from sumptuous table ornaments to the equipment of entire rooms; statues and vases of all kinds, furniture, mirror frames, chandeliers, wall panels, all were made of porcelain. Chinese blue-and-white porcelain and Japanese Imari ware were used for the earlier furnishings (Charlottenburg Palace in Berlin; the "Japanese Palace" of Augustus the Strong in Dresden). For the later rooms (e.g., in the Palace of Capodimonte on the outskirts of Naples and the Buen Retiro Palace outside Madrid) porcelain was supplied by the local manufactures (PL. 158).

The factory of Meissen was of fundamental importance, especially in the products of its early decades. The painter Johann Gregor Heroldt (Höroldt, 1696–1765), who began work in 1720, gave the major impetus to the new style, resolving technical and chemical problems of color and achieving a happy union of material, decoration, and function. From about 1725 his *chinoiseries* displayed his rich invention and feeling for his medium: the ingenious figures, in a style akin to that of the miniaturists, reach their finest expression in the vases marked "A.R." (Augustus Rex). In the 1730s landscapes and marines were produced, still in a miniature style, with dominant tones of gold and red and luminous backgrounds like those of Sèvres; they were made by Carl Friedrich Heroldt, Johann Christian Heintze, and Adam Friedrich von Löwenfinck. Porcelain statuary was also important at Meissen, where it was first copied after Chinese porcelains and ivories and then was developed

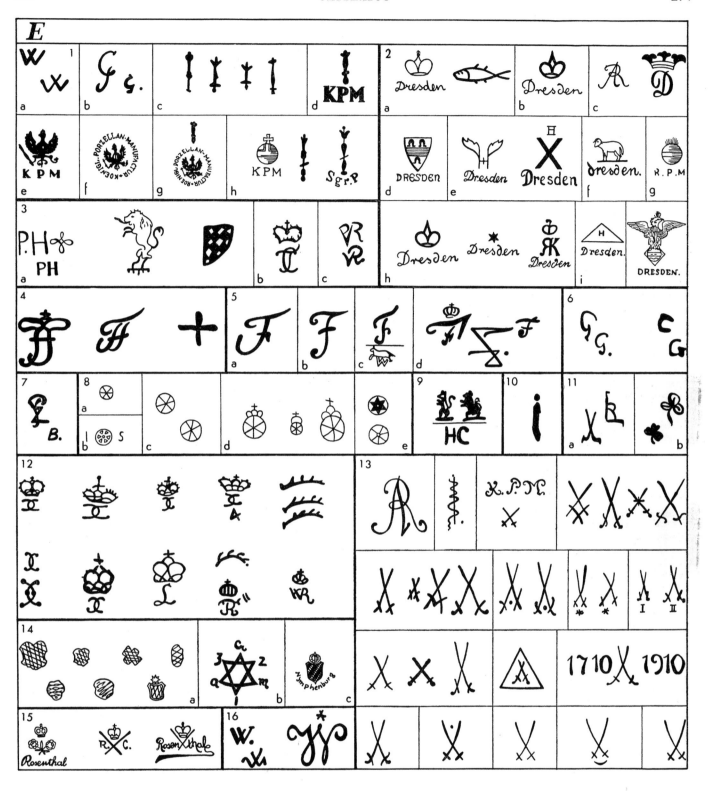

European marks. (E) Germany. (1) Berlin: (a) Wegely works, 1751–57; (b) Gotzkowsky works, 1761–63; (c-h) Königliche Porzellan Manufaktur: (c) KPM, 1763–1837; (d) KPM, 1837–44; (e) KPM, 1844–47; (f) KPM, 1847–49; (g) KPM, 1849–70; (h) KPM, left to right: from 1832, from 1870, from 1882. (2) Dresden, painters' marks: (a) A. Hamann; (b) Donath & Co.; (c) H. Wolfsohn; (d) F. Junkersdorf; (e) F. Hirsch; (f) A. Lamm; (g) H. Richter; (h) K. R. Klemm; (i) Heufel & Co.; also unidentified mark. (3) Frankenthal (1775–99), hard porcelain: (a) Marks of the Hannong brothers, 1755–56, 1756–62, ca. 1756 respectively; (b) reign of Charles Theodore, 1762–95; (c) marks of the Van Recums, 1795–99. (4) Fulda, 1764–90. (5) Fürstenberg, from 1747: (a) 1755–75; (b) ca. 1800; (c) impressed mark; (d) modern marks. (6) Gera, from 1779. (7) Gutenbrunn, 1767–75. (8) Höchst, 1746–96: (a) Mark in red and gold, 1750–62; (b) impressed mark, 1760–65; (c) 1762–96; (d) ca. 1765–74; (e) rare marks. (9) Kassel, 1766–88: mark used 1770–88. (10) Ilmenau, from 1777. (11) Limbach, from 1772: (a) Mark in purple or red, 1772–87; (b) in black, from 1787. (12) Ludwigsburg, 1758–1824, from left to right and from top to bottom: 1759–60, ca. 1765,1765–70,1770–75,1770–80, ca. 1790, 1793–95, 1800–10, 1806–16, 1816–24. (13) Meissen (from 1710), from left to right and from top to bottom: Augustus Rex, until 1733; ca. 1715–25; ca. 1723; ca. 1724–30; ca. 1730–63; era of the point, 1763–74; era of Marcolini, 1774–1813; ca. 1815 and 1830; 1815–60; mark impressed on biscuit, 1774–1815; mark of the bicentennial of the founding of the factory, 1910; 1860–1924; 1924–34; 1934–45; 1945–46; from 1946. (14) Nymphenburg (from 1747), impressed or incised marks: (a) From left to right and from top to bottom: 1755–65, 1766–80, 1780–90, 1780–90, ca. 1800, 1810–50, 1850–62; (b) 1763–65; (c) modern mark. (15) Selb, Rosenthal & Co. (19th and 20th cent.). (16) Wallendorf (from 1764), 1764–88 and after.

autonomously, especially by the sculptor Johann Joachim Kaendler (1706–75). After having been one of the principal executors of Augustus the Strong's project for the adornment of an entire palace with colossal porcelain figures of people and animals and fantastic vases, Kaendler devoted himself in the thirties to modeling small figures with lively play of light and color — mordant impressions of contemporary life — and imposing "architectonic" table services.

The rococo style did not particularly interest French ceramists, although it was prominent in German production. After a trip to Paris in 1747, Kaendler abandoned baroque grandeur in favor of a capricious lightness of form. Arcadian scenes after Boucher and Watteau were substituted for the landscapes and marines with small figures, and a softer red for the intense reds. *Deutsche Blumen* ("German flowers") in the new rococo vein also replaced the Oriental floral motifs.

Notwithstanding the efforts of Meissen to preserve the secret of porcelain, it soon leaked out, and Vienna was able to open a factory in 1718. In the latter half of the 18th century, Meissen production diminished during the Seven Years' War (1756-63), and the final publication of the recipes of the Viennese Joseph Jakob Ringler (1730–1804) encouraged a number of other manufactures throughout Germany. Nymphenburg in Bavaria enjoyed a golden age between 1761 and 1767. Its fame was linked to Franz Anton Bustelli (1723–63) from Switzerland, who usurped Kaendler's role in guiding contemporary taste. At first under the influence of the sculptor Ignaz Günther, then in an elegant and spirited style of his own, he modeled figures and groups inspired by religious and gallant themes or by Italian comedy.

In 1746 the manufacture of Höchst was established by Adam Friedrich von Löwenfinck. In three years it was producing porcelain. The best work, of 1753–58, consists of groups and figurines; the best artists were Simon Feilner, the anonymous "Chinesenmeister," and Johann Peter Melchior. In 1747 Charles I, duke of Brunswick, established a factory at Fürstenberg, whose best work was of 1770–1814. Ludwigsburg, established in 1758 by Charles Eugene of Württemberg, produced its best work during 1760–75, especially in the porcelains of the delicate modeler Wilhelm Beyer (1725–1806). Frankenthal in the Palatinate, one of the most important factories in Germany, was established in 1755 by Paul-Antoine Hannong (d. 1760) and acquired in 1762 by the Elector Charles Theodore. In the latter half of the century it was producing the work of Konrad Linck. After 1770 the most important German fabric was from the royal factory in Berlin, established in 1763, where rococo flourished in a palette of unrivaled intensity and purity until after the death of Frederick the Great. While the Berlin table services remained among the most interesting creations of German rococo, the figurines copied after Meissen were mediocre. From 1764 to 1790 the manufacture at Fulda, founded by Prince Heinrich von Bibra, produced groups of children and other small figures.

After Meissen, Vienna was the first to establish a manufacture of hard porcelain (1718) under the direction of the Dutchman Claudius Innocentius du Paquier. Two fugitives from Meissen, Christopher Konrad Hunger and Samuel Stölzel, as well Joseph Philipp Danhofer were employed there after the first year. The period of Du Paquier's directorship is characterized by a decoration of leaves and tangled ribbons similar to the Nuremberg *Laub- und Bandelwerk*. After its sale to the state in 1744, the factory was especially productive, thanks to the discovery of the important beds of kaolin in Hungary.

About 1720 Francesco Vezzi established a manufacture in Venice with the help of Hunger, who also persuaded Stölzel to come to that city. The factory remained active for 20 years. Its production was dependent on Meissen and Vienna but was distinguished by a clear trasnslucent glaze. Besides various *chinoiseries* and satirical and burlesque subjects, the best products were direct imitations of Oriental models. After the failure of Vezzi's factory, the Senate was able to insure Venetian production of porcelain. Nathaniel Friedrich Hewelcke and a companion, who left Meissen after the crisis of 1757 provoked by the Seven Years' War, found refuge in Udine, where they were at work between 1758 and 1761, and thereafter for two years in Venice, after which they returned to Meissen. Few of their works, which are of poor quality, are known to have survived. In 1763 the Venetian Senate licensed Pasquale Antonibon to manufacture porcelain in Nove near Bassano. This factory first produced majolica as well, added earthenware of the English kind after 1784, and continued active until 1825. The Nove body is almost indistinguishable from the porcelain made in the factory of Geminiano Cozzi in Venice, with which it also has many colors in common, especially red-brown, violet, and green. Original shades were subsequently added: a transparent rose, a soft gray-green, and very fine gilding. Characteristic are sugar bowls and teapots decorated in relief; cups and plates with slight landscapes and figures of peasants and animals; sculpture groups and figures portraying popular or mythological subjects. In 1764, taking advantage of the transfer of workmen from Nove, Geminiano Cozzi (who had already worked at the Hewelcke factory) opened a porcelain manufacture in Venice, which continued active until 1812; in 1769 he added the manufacture of majolica and in 1781 that of earthenware of the English type. The Cozzi factory produced cups, sugar bowls, coffeepots, grotesque figurines and various *chinoiseries*, tobacco boxes, and cane handles, all in German-style porcelain. The rococo forms are often eccentric, with much application of a plant decoration which was, however, rigid and less pliant than the German models. Color contrasts were lively: blue with fine gilding in the enamels, violet-red, emerald green. The influence of Sèvres was added to that of Germany rather later. After about 1790 neoclassicism was dominant. At Este, near Ferrara, craftsmen from Nove produced porcelain from 1765 to 1781. Between 1795 and 1840 a porcelain similar to the Cozzi fabric was produced at Treviso.

The factory of Doccia near Florence, established in 1735 by the Marquis Carlo Lorenzo Ginori (1702–57), was of major importance. Two years later Ginori was able to recruit the painter Wandelein, who had been working in Vienna in the Du Paquier factory. After several years of experimentation Ginori succeeded in producing a porcelain from a gray-blue hybrid paste known as *masso bastardo*, which was in use for half a century. The earliest work of any esthetic interest stems from the modeler Gaspare Bruschi, who designed table ornaments, groups and figures, basins decorated with floral motifs, and masks in high relief. Plastic production was much developed in grandiose baroque compositions and reproductions of classical originals on a bold scale. Lorenzo I (1734–91) succeeded his father Carlo Ginori on the latter's death, and under his direction porcelain was used in ingenious and bizarre forms: for brackets, frames, ornamental applications, entablatures, capitals, masks, putti, chimeras. Table services were executed in Chinese, Japanese, floral, and landscape styles. After the death of Lorenzo I, earthenware in the English manner was produced. In 1819 the ingenious kiln with four stories, invented by Leopoldo Carlo Ginori (1788–1837), gave a new impetus to Doccia production, as it permitted the simultaneous firing of pots at different temperatures. The neoclassical style appeared in soup bowls in the form of tripods, sugar bowls shaped like pyxides, vases inspired by Greco-Roman antiquities, with meanders and laurel or oak crowns framing mythological figures.

The manufacture of Capodimonte, near Naples, was established by Charles III of Bourbon in 1743; after his accession to the throne of Spain it was virtually transferred to Madrid to the Buen Retiro Palace; it closed down in 1808. It is often very difficult to distinguish between the fabrics of Capodimonte and those of Buen Retiro because the management, the workers, and even the materials were the same and the mark is the same. L. O. Schepers and especially his son Gaetano supervised the composition of the paste, which was soft, translucent, and almost pure white. Giuseppe Gricci was the chief modeler; Giovanni Ceselli was in charge of the pictorial aspect and was succeeded at his death (1752) by the Saxon J. S. Fisher. The initial production was inspired principally by the Meissen shapes, the preferred subjects for decoration being battle scenes, marines, landscapes, mythological scenes, garden parties in contemporary dress; fruit decoration is common. After 1755 a more spirited

rococo invaded the late baroque German forms. Gricci's group sculptures are particularly important; masques and subjects from the Italian stage, sacred and mythological scenes, peasants, tradesmen, fishermen, and animals were modeled with a fine sense of folklore and a vivid palette with soft luminous touches. The furnishings for a room once in the Villa Reale in Portici (now, Palace in Capodimonte) is a Ginori masterpiece and an especially fine example of European rococo. After the transfer of the factory to Madrid, Charles Ferdinand IV opened the Manifattura Reale for porcelain in Naples (1771), which flourished until 1806, its style borrowed from Capodimonte and Buen Retiro.

Hard-porcelain factories multiplied throughout Europe: in St. Petersburg, Copenhagen, Marieberg (Sweden), Zurich and Nyon (Switzerland), Weesp near Amsterdam, Loosdrecht and the Hague (Holland), Brussels and Schaerbeek (Belgium), Lisbon and Vista Alegre near Oporto (Portugal).

Hard porcelain arrived relatively late in France, where soft

The earliest work of the Vincennes-Sèvres factory was influenced by Saint-Cloud and Chantilly. The paste was originally a poor white, but it improved steadily. In an effort to emulate the success of Meissen works, which soon served as models for floral decorations and minute landscapes with figures, the manufacture was progressively emancipated from German influence until it arrived at a formula that was perhaps the best expression of contemporary French culture. Seeking a pleasing, joyous effect, one of feminine grace (not for nothing did Madame de Pompadour exert her influence on the development of style), Sèvres porcelains soon displaced Meissen in the European market. It became for the latter half of the 18th century what Meissen had been for the first: the richness and variety of its production fixed the style of European porcelain. The colors first were refinements of the *gros bleu* and the gold of Vincennes. Soft airy profiles of birds were contrasted against the pure white glaze; Arcadian figures after Boucher were painted in purple and blue, and finally elegant landscapes and

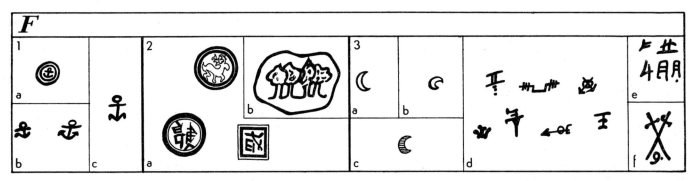

European marks. (*F*) England. (1) Chelsea, ca. 1749–52: (*a*) Mark in applied relief; (*b*) in red, in blue under luster, in red or purple enamel, 1752–56; (*c*) in gold, ca. 1758–69. (2) Staffordshire: (*a*) Bradwell Wood (17th–18th cent.), impressed marks; (*b*) Burslem, mark of Ralph Wood, ca. 1770. (3) Worcester, from 1751. (*a–d*) 1755–90: (*a*) in blue under luster; (*b*) in red; (*c*) impressed in blue; (*d*) craftsmen's marks, all blue under luster; (*e*) in blue under luster in imitation of Japanese marks, ca. 1760–75; (*f*) in blue under luster in imitation of a Meissen mark.

porcelain, fragile and difficult to work, was in vogue for a long time. Its invention preceded the discovery of hard porcelain in Europe by more than 30 years, if, as seems probable, it was the invention of Edme Poterat, who in the name of his son Louis procured the royal privilege for manufacturing porcelain in Rouen (1673). A single piece is securely attributable to the Poterat works: it is in the *style rayonnant*, which was to die with Louis in 1696. At Saint-Cloud, from the early 18th century on, the first important manufacture of soft porcelain worked in the Rouen style: lambrequins, Bérain designs, Chinese flowers; then, under inspiration of the Far East, *blancs de Chine* and polychrome pieces with flowers, birds, figures, and landscapes *à la haie* were produced. The influence of Saint-Cloud predominated in the soft porcelain from Lille (manufacture established in 1711). At Chantilly (1725–1801) soft porcelain was first covered with an opaque white tin-enamel glaze which set off to advantage the polychrome decoration in red, soft blue, light green, yellow, and black. Ornament was inspired by the Japanese Kakiemon style. Subsequently it underwent the influence of Sèvres. Soft porcelain was also produced at Mennecy from 1740 to the end of the century (coffee and toilette services as well as statuettes and ornamental pieces with floral decoration) and at Sceaux, Orléans, Crépy, Etoilles, Arras, and Saint-Amand-les-Eaux.

Because of the poor ductility of *pâte tendre* (soft-paste porcelain), but also because of a concept of refinement to which excesses and bizarreness were unsuited, rococo did not have so unbridled an application in France as in Germany. A more graceful measure prevailed with reliance on harmony of line and exquisite combinations of color. The most important French factory was the Manufacture Royale, established in 1738 by private citizens at Vincennes, removed in 1756 to Sèvres, and nationalized in 1760 by Louis XV. Only after 1768, the year in which kaolin was discovered at Saint-Yrieix, was hard porcelain produced. But soft porcelain, now a national tradition, continued to be made until 1804.

bouquets by Jean-Jacques Bachelier (1724–1806) were rendered in delicate, warm colors which were studiously original and were made possible by the soft glaze into which they sank deeply: ultramarine blue, the turquoise of Jean Hellot, Persian green, violet, *jaune jonquil* (an intense yellow), *bleu de roi*, *bleu céleste*, *rose Pompadour*, etc. The royal goldsmith and sculptor Claude-Thomas Duplessis furnished models in a subdued rococo; his forms recall silverwork.

In small sculptures, on the other hand, color soon was replaced by the white of the biscuit, first in the creations of Bachelier, later especially in the very delicate and affected groups after models by Etienne-Maurice Falconet (1716–91), who, inspired by Boucher, produced pastoral and gallant subjects. This statuary is more delicate than the German, but the effect of marble sought through the elimination of both glaze and color tended to considerable coldness. The groups were the work of the best-known French sculptors: Falconet, Louis-Simon Boizot, Clodion, Jean Le Riche. Boizot, Falconet's successor, arrived at Sèvres in 1774. Here he showed a preference for a hard-paste biscuit porcelain which suited his chill neoclassical taste. The advent of neoclassicism, which had already been heralded in the stiff and sumptuous forms of the vases produced in the seventies, brought an end to the dominant influence of Sèvres on European porcelain.

English porcelain is distinguished by a subtle color range and a wealth of imagination (PLS. 162, 163). Even the early experiments have a special fascination which lies in the very imperfections of technique. The best-known fabric was an especially fine soft porcelain made at Chelsea (1747–83). English figurines, often copied after Meissen models, are among the most highly prized of European productions; at first only modestly colored, these were soon painted in a profusion of colors. Vases and services were still inspired by Meissen wares in their unrestrained rococo flowers and figures, or they richly interpreted Sèvres motifs and colors, such as *gros bleu* and *rose Pompadour*. Some of the most original soft-paste porcelains were from the

factory of Bow (active 1745–75). After 1775 the factory at Derby (1749–1848), under the influence of both Meissen and Chelsea, repeated Bow models. Toward the turn of the century, able artists such as J. J. Spengler and William J. Coffee treated biscuit figures in a neoclassical style. Worcester (1751–83; 1783–1852), after Chelsea probably the most important English soft-porcelain center, combined motifs from Meissen, Sèvres, Chelsea, and the Orient. Mention should also be made of the factories at Longton Hall (1749–60) and Liverpool (1756–1841). Hard-paste porcelain was produced only in a factory established in 1768 by William Cookworthy (b. 1705) at Plymouth. Cookworthy then went to Bristol (1770) and subsequently to New Hall (1781–1830). The predominant influence was from Sèvres. Bristol figurines have a nervous and original flair and often carry the mark of a certain Mr. Tebo.

The first original independent English porcelain drew on rustic medieval traditions for inspiration; originating in Staffordshire, it was of prime importance in the progress toward a more modern style. During the 17th and nearly 18th centuries, a "slip ware" (i.e., painted with slip) was produced in forms that were simple, well-proportioned, and appropriately decorated with stylized designs in warm, pleasing reddish browns and yellows. Toward the end of the 17th century, John Philip Elers and his brother David, from Holland, introduced the production of a red ware subtly fashioned in the manner of the Chinese, and brought to the attention of Staffordshire potters the refinements of porcelain and the problems of invading the European market. New research into technique was undertaken, resulting after 1720 in the first salt-glazed stonewares and earthenwares. The glaze, a thin hard shell produced on a special clay with the addition of sodium cloride (ordinary table salt) during firing, provided a cheap substitute for tin-enamel glazes. Some fabrics continued the old traditions, while the new "Astbury ware" (linked to the name of Thomas Whieldon) was distinguished for its warm oat and red tones, relief decoration, and gray, green, and black glazes. Ralph Wood and John Voyez excelled in figurines and groups executed in a vigorous and popular style, a production which, although influenced by porcelain models, achieved a marked stylistic independence in the beauty of its colors and the spirited effects of its stylized modeling. The development in ceramics was one of the most interesting manifestations of the early British industrial period. The increased use of tea and coffee after the 17th century, as well as a growing scarcity of tin and lead, made for a gradual substitution of ceramic wares for metal. While porcelain graced the tables of the well-to-do, the needs of the poorer class were met by an intelligent use of the new economical earthenwares. New manufacturing skills and new systems of decoration were developed to meet the accelerated rhythm of production.

Josiah Wedgwood (1730–95), born into a family of Staffordshire potters, was to have an enormous impact on this type of production, thanks to his combination of practical, commercial, and technical skills. While confronting new problems of style and insisting on artistic quality, Wedgwood understood that the widest margin of profit was in the manufacture of useful earthenware on an industrial scale. Although he used steam to turn his wheels and grind his materials, the greatest part of the work was still done by hand, and it was in the subdivision of labor that he achieved a reduction of costs which was to gain for his wares the markets of England, Europe, and America. With Thomas Whieldon, Wedgwood perfected between 1754 and 1759 hardness and resistance to fire in earthenware and produced services in various forms: cabbages, cauliflowers, or pineapples, in "agate" (i.e., marbled) wares, which consisted of two or more mingled clays, and in so-called "tortoise shell" ware, with colored glazes on a creamware body. In 1759 at Ivy House he began to produce the earthenware known as "creamware," using copper plates for the impressed decoration. In 1769 he established between Hanley and Newcastle-under-Lyme the Etruria factory, which introduced neoclassical taste to English pottery. It was his new associate, Thomas Bentley (1730–80), a connoisseur of classical and Renaissance art, who interested him in antiquity. Reacting against rococo forms, Wedgwood reduced his wares to simple rational lines, often to the form of a classical urn, and so perfected his ivory color that he was able to eliminate painted decoration entirely. Wedgwood's creamware had many imitators, and at Leeds its production was of a very high order. Another of Wedgwood's ambitions was to produce pottery in the Greek manner. By perfecting a black ware already produced at Staffordshire, he created his "black basalt" (PL. 163), in which he copied Greek vases and classical cameos, employing John Flaxman, William Hackwood, and other sculptors to design the reliefs which he applied to the surface of a vase. Flaxman worked for Wedgwood from 1775 to 1787 and also modeled figures, such as the famous chessmen. In 1774 Wedgwood achieved a stained stoneware body which he called "jasper," in white, blue, lavender, green, or black. With reliefs in white paste applied on blue-black jasper, he completed in 1790 a copy of the celebrated *Barberini* (later *Portland*) *Vase* which G. Hamilton had sold to the Duke of Portland for 1,029 pounds sterling. The extreme agility of line, the quiet elegance, and the submerged romanticism in which the classical form is reborn completely redeem the imitative impulse that gave birth to such creations and make them a valid expression of the taste of the period: the ease with which they blend into an Adamesque interior is remarkable. At first the imitation of these products was limited to the English potters John Turner and William Adams, but it spread to Sèvres and Meissen, to Fürstenberg, Höchst, Nymphenburg, Kassel, Königsberg, and Copenhagen.

Late neoclassicism was characterized by the arrival of the Empire style in France and by a new popularity of Egyptian motifs resulting from the Napoleonic conquest. Its tumultuous forms, so unrelated to medium, announced the end of the historic cycle of porcelain. Spode in England, nevertheless, enjoyed a great success (1796–1847), and in Russia porcelain production was outstanding under Alexander I (1801–25).

*The 19th century.* After the neoclassical phase production was disorganized and eclectic throughout Europe. The wide application of mechanical methods and the manufacture of porcelain by industry brought to an end a long tradition of craftsmanship. But the work of an isolated artist and experimenter frequently opposed itself to the organized production of the great factories.

Rococo was revived between 1820 and 1850, especially in France under Louis Philippe. Its best exponent was Jacob Petit, who between 1830 and 1862 directed, first at Fontainebleau and thereafter in Paris, a factory which produced vases, chandeliers, pendulum clocks, and figurines with decorations in the style of Capodimonte, in an exquisite range of colors from pale rose to a soft green and black and gold. Before 1850 the study and imitation of ancient and Renaissance pottery became widespread. As early as 1835 Aimé Chenavard (1798–1838) revealed this new interest in antiquity in his *Album de l'ornemaniste*, while in 1838 J. C. Ziegler (after studying the manufacture of glass and porcelain in Germany) established a stoneware factory at Voisinlieu (France) which was dedicated to the imitation of products of the German Renaissance. Among his works, which were decorated in relief, was the famous large *Vase of the Apostles* (1842). Palissy's rustic style, after 1840, was imitated by C. I. Avisseau at Beaumontles-Autels.

In Italy D. Zoppi, G. Baldassini, and B. Becheroni initiated at Doccia, about 1830, a decorative vocabulary of mythological and historical subjects, portraits, idyls after the Swiss poet-painter Salomon Gessner, landscapes, bunches of flowers done in miniature as if on ivory. Between 1830 and 1850, in Milan, Pietro Bagatti-Valsecchi made porcelain in miniatures in the style of the painter Andrea Appiani. After 1850 there were imitations at Doccia of the century-old Capodimonte style, and the chemist Lorenzini and the painter Giusti reproduced metallic lusters (as did others throughout Italy) in the manner of Renaissance majolica. In Naples (1820–50) Biagio Giustiniani and his sons reproduced antique vases and sculpture groups in Egyptian, Etruscan, and other styles, while unglazed French porcelains were imported and then decorated by local painters, among them Raffaele Giovine of the school of Posillipo. After 1850 some Italian ateliers revived Renaissance

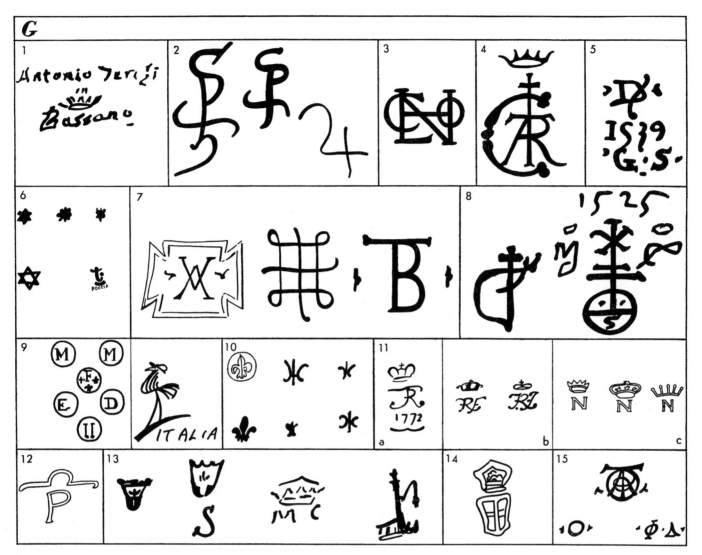

European marks. (*G*) Italy. (1) Bassano (18th cent.), majolica: mark of A. Terchi. (2) Cafaggiolo (early 16th cent. onward), majolica, *left and center*: SPR (Semper); *right*: 1514. (3) Castel Durante (16th cent.), mark of N. Pellipario, painter, 1528. (4) Castelli (17th–18th cent.), majolica: mark of the Carthusian order, 1697–1727. (5) Deruta (from ca. 1490), majolica. (6) Doccia (from 1735), *above*: in blue, red, and gold, late 18th cent. and early 19th; *below left*: in red, 18th cent.; *right*: one of the Richard-Ginori marks. (7) Faenza (14th cent. onward), majolica, *left*: ca. 1490; *center*: 1510–15; *right*: one of the Casa Pirota marks, sometimes used by Faenza painters who had emigrated to other manufactures. (8) Gubbio (from 1495), majolica: two of the many marks of Master Giorgio's manufacture, 1514–41. (9) Florence (ca. 1575–ca. 1587), soft-paste porcelain, *left*: FMMDEII [Franciscus Maria (or Medici) Magnus Dux Etruriae II]; *right*: Cantagalli, modern mark. (10) Naples (environs), Capodimonte (1743–59), *above left*: impressed mark; *below*: in gold, ca. 1745; other marks generally used on domestic wares, also at Buen Retiro. (11) Naples: (*a*) Mark of the Fabbrica Reale at Portici, before 1775; (*b*) monograms of the Fabbrica Reale Ferdinandea (1773–87), in red or in blue; (*c*) impressed mark, late 18th cent. (12) Pesaro (from ca. 1486), mark of early 16th cent. (13) Savona (16th–18th cent.): four typical marks (the last on the right is for the Levantino family at Albisola). (14) Turin (16th cent. onward), majolica: coat of arms of Savoy, probably the mark of the Parco works, act. from 1646. (15) Urbino (from ca. 1520 to 18th cent.), majolica: marks of O. Fontana, mid-16th cent.

majolica: Devers in Turin, Cantagalli in Florence, Minghetti in Bologna, Marabini and Farini in Faenza, etc.

In England, however, Staffordshire traditions were still in force, especially in the figures of ordinary people and portraits of historical personages, which remained popular throughout the century.

Toward 1840 the archaeological vogue was to find expression in the new Parian body (an imitation of the early biscuit) at Copeland, Garret, and Minton, where elegant classical figurines were drawn from models by sculptors of the period. After 1850 elaborate decorative pieces in a Renaissance manner were modeled by noted foreign artists, such as A. E. Carrier-Belleuse, Hugues Protat, V. E. Symian, and Emile Jeannest.

The study of Persian and Turkish styles followed the enthusiasm for the Renaissance; after 1860 the fashion was Japanese wares; later Chinese wares. Théodore Deck, established in Paris in 1856, drew from his studies of Persian wares the blue-green with which his name has been associated. In 1878 he decorated an entire façade with majolica; about 1880 he produced a Chinese type of porcelain as well as plates in

the style of Gubbio and Castel Durante; from 1887 to 1891 he was director of the factory at Sèvres. Late in the century certain students, through a development of technique and a study of Arabic majolica and of Chinese porcelain and stoneware, attempted to free themselves of the stylistic formulas that had characterized previous production. Productive cycles on a new scientific basis and new chemical research were also initiated, and with them a progressive specialization. Ernest Chaplet, who had been trained at Sèvres, established a factory at Choisy-le-Roi. Here, following a method revived by Devers, he produced a majolica whose decoration was painted on the raw glaze and fired in the *grand feu*. Japanese styles received a personal interpretation by Albert Dammouse in France, who created a stoneware decorated in *grand feu* glazes with plant motifs, and by Jean-Charles Cazin in England, whose quiet and elegant shapes met with considerable success. Also in France, the sculptor Jean Carriès used stoneware effectively to model grotesque masks and forms inspired by plants. August Delaherche, early under the influence of Jules Claude Ziegler, took over Chaplet's factory at Choisy-le-Roi; he sub-

ordinated decoration to the problems of form and medium. Delaherche's dark red stonewares with stylized ornament were very successful; his glazes were often lively, the forms simple and rounded, the surfaces rough and enriched by polychrome drops crystallized from metallic oxides. Edmond Lachenal achieved golden majolicas and collaborated with Rodin and Louis Dejean in the production of glazed sculpture. Emile Massou studied Far Eastern, Hispano-Moresque, and Persian wares, which he interpreted in a personal manner.

*The 20th century.* In England, the only ceramist in the group of craftsmen who founded the Arts and Crafts Exhibition Society was a friend of William Morris, William de Morgan (active at Fulham). His chief interest lay in perfecting color and glaze techniques, and he succeeded in the faithful reproduction of Persian and Middle Eastern models. While in most cases his works were deliberate pastiches, his finished and polished creations preserved the flavor of English 19th-century fabrics and have some resemblance to Morris's weavings. De Morgan had no successor. In the latter half of the 19th century and the first decade of the 20th, the four brothers Martin (Robert, Walter, Edwin, Charles) revived the technique of English stoneware at Southall; their original fabrics in the shape of fantastic birds and grotesque heads, or with decorations derived from plants and shells, made imaginative use of the plastic resources and inherent colors (principally gray and brown) of clay. Though the Martins had no direct successors either, their plastic concepts and craftsman's approach were fundamental in the revival of English pottery between 1920 and 1940, which drew its inspiration from the precious and jadelike qualities of Chinese stoneware. In the forefront of these developments were William State Murray, who worked at Bray and taught at the Royal College of Art in London, and Bernard Leach, who headed the modern school of the British Studio Potters. After a trip to Japan, Leach established about 1920 a manufacture at St. Ives, England, where for the first three years he collaborated with the Japanese potters Hamada and Matsubayashi, making experiments in a Japanese type of majolica called "raku," which is fired at rather low temperatures; in hard porcelain; in English medieval pottery; and especially in high-fired Oriental stoneware. Leach hoped to show the beauty of fabric in relation to both medium and function and thus applied to pottery the ideals of workmanship and good design that had already pervaded other areas of British industrial craftsmanship. In 1933 he went to teach at the Darlington School, where he found a friend and collaborator in the American painter Mark Tobey. His principal coworkers were his son David, Kenneth Quick, and Bill Marshall. Almost all modern British pottery has felt Leach's influence. The first to break with his precepts was probably Thomas Samuel Haile, who attempted long, irregular forms, subtly decorated with sgraffito designs and patches of color. After studying in Vienna, Lucy Rie opened a pottery (1939) where she collaborated after 1949 with Hans Coper, producing stoneware and porcelain vases and household ware; the rather precise forms are executed with an excellent feeling for medium and are decorated with sgraffito designs and bands of color. Also of note is the work of Norah Braden, one of Leach's first students, and Reginald Marlow, Heber Matthews, James Tower, Stephen Sykes, Kenneth Clark, Eleanor Whittall; on a high level also are dishes and zoomorphic wares by Nicholas Vergette, Margaret Hine, William Newland, all vaguely suggestive of Picasso. Since 1921 a modern English household ware, very precise in its execution, has been produced on an industrial scale at Poole, with the participation of top designers (John Adams, Truda Carter, Harold Stabler). The Derby Pottery (near Derby) and the Briglin Pottery, London, should also be noted.

In France the movements of the turn of the century, already described, were followed by a great revival, due especially to the collaboration of outstanding painters; the type of ware produced was ornamental rather than utilitarian. An important attempt at a break with decorative traditionalism was made in about 1903 at Asnières by the potter André Metthey (1871–1920), to whom Ambroise Vollard sent his painter friends:

Renoir, Odilon Redon, Maurice Denis, Matisse, Pierre Bonnard, Edouard Vuillard, Rouault, Maurice de Vlaminck, André Derain, Henri Rousseau. This collaboration lasted five years, during which majolica dishes, cups, and vases, animated by a lively pictorial sense and decorated with great freedom and lightness of color, were produced and exhibited at the Salon d'Automne and the Salon des Indépendants. Among the most active participants, also between 1903 and 1907, was Othon Friesz (1879–1949): at Sainte-Adresse he and Metthey decorated a whole building, facing balconies with large ceramic panels decorated with flowers and fish. Joseph Llorenz Artigas (b. 1892) produced an interesting undecorated stoneware between 1922 and 1932. He also collaborated actively with Raoul Dufy and in 1932–33 with Albert Marquet, and in 1949 he produced an important series with Georges Braque. Stoneware was also successfully translated into useful objects with a solid rustic feeling by Paul Beyer (1873–1945). Emile Decoeur (b. 1876) used stoneware and porcelain in undecorated, pure classicizing forms. Also to be mentioned are Emile Lenoble (1875–1939), who continued the work of Chaplet and produced a glazed rustic ware with strong, full colors from well-incorporated metallic oxides; Jean Mayodon (b. at Sèvres, 1893), who made monumental ceramic sculptures, pools, and garden fountains. From 1932 Marc Chagall (PL. 158) and Maurice Savin (painter, engraver, medalist, and specialist in tapestry) also devoted themselves to ceramics; the latter produced small porcelains, stoneware, and majolica sculptures. Fernand Léger occupies a special place; in New York (1945) and after his return to Paris (1947) he produced large polychrome wall sculptures. Also well known are the ceramics of Pablo Picasso, which he began producing in 1947 after his transfer to Vallauris (PL. 173). Besides numerous single pieces, he has issued works in series; the *éditions céramiques*, produced at the Madoura Studio (Suzanne and Georges Ramié), are faithful reproductions from an original or examples made from a single matrix. A similar experiment was attempted by Metthey in 1903 and was repeated 50 years later by the ceramist Henry Plisson, who gathered about him some of the representatives of the new French school (Aizpiri, Roger Bezombes, Lagrange, Lucien Coutaud). Plisson's group also work through the national factory at Sèvres. Independents at work are Edouard Pignon at Vallauris and the Italian Manfredo Borsi at Saint-Paul-de-Vence, known for his fine pictorial panels. The last ceramics of Henri Matisse are in the chapel at Saint-Paul-de-Vence. Alfred Manessier, Maurice Estève, Léon Gischia, Singer, Hans Hartung, and Bernard Buffet also devote themselves to ceramics. The Porcelaine de Paris, which was established in 1773, throughout the 19th century and the first half of the 20th confined itself to eclectic imitations and reproductions of the most successful traditional models (Sèvres, Lowestoft, Chantilly, Capodimonte); since 1950 it has experimented with transfer printing on wares which, while still traditionally decorated, are simpler in form.

In Spain the generous application of polychrome ceramics to buildings, an invention of Antonio Gaudí's (1852–1926), occupies a unique position in the history of architecture no less than of modern ceramics. The balustrade in the Güell Park (I, PL. 466) is one of the happiest of Gaudí's creations, in which the varied and contrasted motifs of ceramic tiling already forecast the later movements of cubism and abstract art. Of Spanish birth, but active in France, were a number of important innovators in modern ceramics — from Artigas, who also collaborated with Joan Miró, to Picasso. In current Spanish production the vases and bottles of Antonio Cumella Serret (b. 1913) are distinguished for their unusually imaginative and sensitively modeled forms.

In Italy as in France the first efforts at revival were connected with the work of painters and sculptors, especially Arturo Martini, who in the twenties produced at the Albisola kilns ceramic sculptures and vases: animated forms bursting with energy or large still lifes such as the *Cornucopia* and numerous small works. Also at Albisola about 1925 worked a futurist group, the *aereoceramisti*, including Tullio Mazzotti, Enrico Prampolini, Alf Gaudenzi, Fillia, Munari, who produced in collaboration with Giuseppe Mazzotti vivacious and geo-

metrically stylized ceramics and plastic complexes (*complessi plastici*). Albisola saw the successive work of Lucio Fontana (b. 1899), one of the most authentic masters of contemporary Italian ceramics, Agenore Fabbri, Aligi Sassu, Luigi Broggini, De Salvo, Rambaldi, Trucco, and others. The example of Albisola was soon followed at Faenza by Pietro Melandri, Anselmo Bucci, Rambelli, Angelo Biancini, Melotti; and in other centers by Guido Gambone and Andrea Parini. One of Italy's most promising young ceramists, Salvatore Fancello, produced at Albisola, before his untimely death at the age of twenty-three, a work marked by imaginativeness, technical ability, and a vigorous, elegant style. After World War II, in the same center, worked such sculptors as Giacomo Manzù, Garelli, Cherchi, and also such foreign artists as the Swedish-born

forms. Wagenfeld and Löffelhardt (who succeeded Gretsch in 1950 at Arzberg) attempted an overthrow of the purely utilitarian and functional approach in favor of quiet and concrete plastic form. At Nymphenburg a tired line of figurines by Hubert Gerhard, Dominikus Auliczek, Joseph Wackerle, Resl Lechner, tracing its descent from Franz Anton Bustelli (1723–63), gave way to the elegant porcelains of Wolfgang von Wersin.

In Sweden the Society of Manual Arts had brought about (1916) a new collaboration between artists and industry in the production of tablewares. Ceramics, though backward in other areas, had something of a flowering in this field. After 1917 the factory at Gustavberg, active since about 1850, was given a new impetus by Wilhelm Käge, whose works from 1930 on were characterized by robust constructivism and delicate tech-

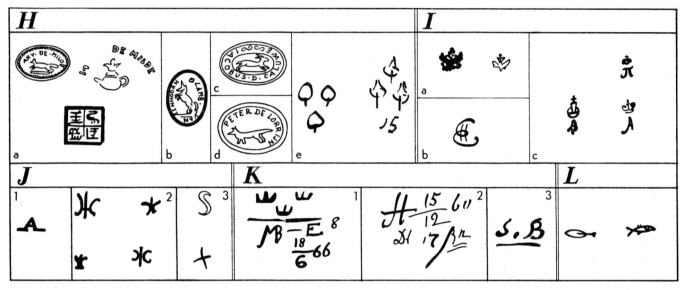

European marks. (*H*) Holland. Delft: (*a*) Marks of A. de Milde, 1680–1708; (*b*) mark of L. van Eenhoorn, 1680–ca. 1721; (*c*) mark of J. Caluwe (d. 1730); (*d*) P. de Lorrijn; (*e*) "De 3 Klokken," 1671. (*I*) Russia. St. Petersburg (from 1744), hard porcelain: (*a*) Imperial Russian porcelain works, impressed marks from the reign of Elizabeth Petrovna, 1741–62; (*b*) mark in blue of Catherine II, 1762–96; (*c*) *above:* mark of Paul I, 1796–1801; *below:* marks of Alexander I, 1801–25. (*J*) Spain. (1) Alcora, from 1726. (2) Madrid (environs), Buen Retiro (1760–1808), soft-paste porcelain (1760–1804), hard porcelain (1804–08), marks in blue; (3) Sargadelos, 1804–29. (*K*) Sweden. (1) Marieberg (from 1758), marks of J. E. L. Ehrenreich, 1760–66. (2) Rörstrand, from 1725. (3) Sölversborg, 1773–93. (*L*) Switzerland. Nyon (from ca. 1780 to 19th cent.), in blue under luster.

Hans Hedberg and the members of the "Cobra": Jorn, Karel Appel, Sebastiano Antonio Matta, and Corneille. Among independent ceramic artists is the sculptor Leoncillo Leonardi, a resident of Rome, who began in the forties to work out a successful personal idiom (*barocchetto*) related to Roman expressionism. After a bout with neocubist constructivism, he became interested in nonobjective experiments in which choice of materials, made with thorough technical knowledge, plays an essential part; as a result, his work belongs to the most modern artistic trends (PL. 173). As to household ware, besides the work of Giuseppe Pagano, there is that of Gio Ponti for the Richard-Ginori factory and of Guido Andlovitz and Antonia Campi at Laveno. The "Ernestine" factory at Salerno, established after World War II, is distinguished for its production on modern lines.

In Germany Max Laeuger (1864–1952) had a great personal impact; his panels and sculptures regained for ceramics a soft, yet vibrant pictorialism. As to household wares, the work of Philip Rosenthal, who at the beginning of the century obtained results of unusual brightness, should be recorded. The positive influence of the Werkbünde and the Bauhaus was reflected after 1930 in the work of a group of innovators who introduced functional forms into porcelain; the more important among them are Herman Gretsch at the factory of Arzberg, W. Wagenfeld at Fürstenberg, Trude Petri at Berlin. After World War II the factories at Arzberg, Schönwald, and Berlin maintained a rigidly modern line along with an increasing number of copies of older wares. The Rosenthal works retained the American industrial designer Raymond Loewy and the Finn Tapio Wirrkala to design new models that are also influenced by Japanese

nical innovations, such as the "Argenta" glaze (green, decorated with silver). Along with Käge, Stig Lindberg (after 1941) and Berndt Friberg (after 1934) achieved highly elegant results. The younger artists include Anders Liljefors, Karin Biörkvist, and the Bregers. Louise Adelborgè and Gunnar Nylund worked after 1930 at the old Rörstrand porcelain factory (founded in Stockholm, 1726; reestablished at Lidköping); Nylund produced robustly functional vessels as well as sculptures in variously glazed stoneware. From 1940 on, Carl-Harry Stålhane's sharply stylized forms have been produced at the same factory. An important and varied output at the Ekeby factory in Uppsala was due to Arthur Percy, Iven Erik Skawonius, Hjördis Oldfors, Ingrid Atterberg. Also to be mentioned are Eva Björk and Ewald Dahlskog at the Boberg majolica factory; the little pottery of the Trillers at Tobo specializing in stoneware; Edgard Böckmann, active in Stockholm and Höganas.

In Finland the revival of ceramics was due to the activities after 1900 of an Englishman, A. W. Finch, at the Iris factory in the town of Borgä. His influence spread not only in the field of ceramics but also in many other areas of Finnish industrial production. He was responsible for the introduction of the *Jugendstil* (Art Nouveau) in decoration. Finch's teachings were particularly beneficial to a group of younger artists at the Arabia porcelain factory in Helsinki (established 1874 and from 1947 a part of the great complex of Wärtsilä); among them were Tyra Lundgreen, Rut Bryk, Toini Muona, Kyllikki Salmehaara, Kay Franck, Birger Kaipiainen, Michael Schilkin, Gunnel Nyman, Saara Hopea, Friedl Kjeleberg, Marita Lybeck, Anne Siimes, Raija Tuumi, Kaarina Aho, Raija Uosikkinen.

Denmark's first artistic stirrings were expressed by a group

of potters — among them Thorvald Bindesbøl — who copied old Italian majolica (ca. 1880). The royal factory at Copenhagen, under the direction of the architect Arnold Krog, produced porcelain with landscape decoration. After 1878 Danish production centered on stoneware. Toward the end of the century the Dane J. F. Willumsen, in Paris, learned to treat stoneware in a manner influenced by Paul Gauguin; on his return to Denmark, he founded a school. The national manufacture launched stoneware in 1904; in 1911–12 Bing and Grøndahl became established; and in 1930 the potter Nathalie Krebs founded her atelier, Saxbo, where — often in collaboration with Eva Staehr Nielsen — she achieved conspicuous results: round, sure forms, in which decoration is provided by the surface play of light. Axel Salto's wares, by contrast, are distinguished by the polychrome play of glazes, by incised and relief decoration, in burgeoning forms of a naturalist spirit. Stoneware was widely used for sculpture by Mogens Bøggild, Knud Kyhen, Jais Nielsen, Jean Gauguin, Helge Christoffersen, and Johannes Hedegaard. The younger potters include Christian Poulsen, Ebbe Sadolin, the delicate and nimble decorator Bjørn Wiinblad, Per Linnemann-Schmidt with his atelier Palshus, Gudrun Meedom, Gertrud Vasegaard, Gerd Bøgelund, Thorkied Olsen, Lisbeth Munch Petersen, Axel Brüel, and Richard Kjaergaard.

Maurizio CALVESI

*Developments in the United States and European derivations.* Pottery was made by Europeans in America from the time of the first settlements. At Jamestown, Va., and sites in Massachusetts and New York there is evidence of the activity of potters before 1700. Fragments of simple red-ware forms covered with brownish glazes and occasionally decorated with slip, found at the sites of early settlements, have been attributed to local makers. A more ambitious pottery was organized by Dr. Daniel Coxe of London and opened in 1688 in Burlington, N.J.: "For ye promoting setting up ye Trade or Art of making white & painted Earthenware & Pottery vessells within the Province of West New Jersey in America." The ware made was probably very much like English delft, but no examples remain to substantiate the hypothesis. There is little physical evidence of any of the activity in ceramics before 1750, but the records suggest that pottery was produced throughout the American colonies and that the outstanding ware was a glazed red ware decorated with slip or scratch decoration.

An early distinctive ware was made in Pennsylvania by the German settlers, commonly called the Pennsylvania Dutch. They made decorative pottery out of red ware, glazed in any of a number of earth colors, with scratch or slip designs. The patterns they used are related to the folk-pottery tradition of northern Europe. The tulip, a motif derived from the tree-of-life design which permeated northern Europe as an Eastern influence, is frequently encountered, but bird and fish motifs occur as well; often a Biblical quotation or homely saying in the Pennsylvania German dialect frames the plate. Such plates, their edges crimped to serve as pie plates, most often were presentation pieces meant for display.

A fine white earthenware in imitation of porcelain was produced by the Philadelphia firm of Bonin and Morris in 1771 and 1772. Their designs were inspired by English blue-and-white wares such as those made at Worcester and Bow.

Shortly before the Revolution a higher-fire utilitarian ware was introduced. It was a salt-glazed earthenware used mainly for storage jars in which wine, spirits, and pickles might be kept. Classical shapes were favored for these jars and dark blue swag ornamentation was popular. This salt-glazed ware was produced in potteries all along the coast.

Probably the first successful manufacture of porcelain was that undertaken by Dr. Henry Mead of New York in 1816. The one known example is an Empire-style soft-paste porcelain vase with caryatid handles. Other attempts followed in short order. In 1824 Abraham Miller of Philadelphia showed a specimen of porcelain at the exhibition of the Franklin Institute. In 1826 the Jersey City Porcelain & Earthenware Company made its first porcelain, but by 1828 the property had been

taken over by David Henderson and was known as the American Pottery Manufacturing Company. One of the more famous early porcelain factories was started by William Ellis Tucker in about 1827 and was productive until 1838. It produced simple Empire-style wares, at first without decoration, then with sepia or gold decoration, and finally with elaborate polychrome floral designs. In 1830 Smith, Fife & Co. were competitors, making wares in Grecian designs in a different body.

Molded wares achieved great popularity in the second quarter of the 19th century. These were generally made of earthenware and produced in the larger-scale potteries that made utilitarian wares. One of the earliest manufacturers was David Henderson, mentioned above. Tea sets molded in naturalistic leaf patterns, Rockingham pitchers with various kinds of decoration, and plates with blue transfer-print decoration were among the output of the firm, which was largely under British influence. In Bennington, Vt., there was another center of large-scale production. In about 1850 the United States Pottery Company produced decorative wares in bodies that included Parian ware, a white unglazed porcelain, and the same type of porcelain with a pitted blue background. In Greenpoint, Brooklyn, a soft-paste porcelain factory headed by Charles Cartlidge opened in 1847 with Josiah Jones as the chief modeler. Its best-known product was a squat white, porcelain pitcher in an over-all relief oak-leaf pattern. Busts, tablewares, buttons, and door furniture were made there as well. The factory closed in 1856 and was succeeded the next year by William Boch and Brothers, who produced similar wares until 1861, when Thomas C. Smith took over the firm and changed the name to the Union Porcelain Works, which had a long and successful history. They produced ornamental wares and tablewares; in the seventies they had the services of Karl Müller as modeler. Rococo designs were a main source of inspiration, with realism as a factor in rendering detail.

A protective tariff introduced in 1861 proved its worth after the Civil War, when the ceramics industry flourished and was able to develop finer bodies. Trenton, N.J., and East Liverpool, Ohio, emerged as two of the most active centers of the industry, and in both places a new thin porcelain body based on the Irish Belleek was developed for the production of the new forms in the exotic taste. Near Eastern designs were an important influence on ceramic forms of the eighties.

A development that evolved by the time of the Philadelphia Centennial in 1876 was art pottery, wares made by artist potters who followed the teachings and philosophy of William Morris. One result of the new approach was the rather large and very successful Rookwood Pottery of Cincinnati, Ohio. It was formed by a group of ladies who had taken up china painting as a cultural pursuit and had gradually become interested in the production of the forms as well as the decoration of the surfaces. What began as a club became a business within a few years and won a long series of awards for excellent techniques and designs. A number of individual artist-potters developed small studios producing experimental wares; Oriental and Near Eastern influences were most important in these studios. The artist-potter has continued to play an important role on the American scene with certain changes of interest. After a long period of work on functional forms that were inspired by folk pottery, particularly the work of the primitive Japanese periods, potters have begun experimenting with forms that are sculptural and not functional, with decorative quality as the all-important objective. Rough-textured asymmetrical abstract forms with splashes of color in calligraphic designs are typical of contemporary output.

In the manufacture of tablewares a certain traditionalism was dominant in the choice of forms until fairly recently. Experimentation in decoration brought out few new developments in the shapes chosen, and even when novelties were sought, relief or painted ornament was applied to known and tried forms. One of the few to experiment with basic shapes was Russell Wright, whose innovations in design were on the market in the thirties.

Marvin D. SCHWARTZ

By and large, studio ceramics produced in the United States after World War II are characterized by an emphasis on textural enlivenment of surfaces, often achieved through the exploitation of new technical processes. Even in utilitarian vessels there is a tendency toward asymmetrical balance and sculptural variation of shape. In the work of a number of potters the influence of Chinese and Japanese historical styles is evident in shape and surface decoration. Contemporary potters of distinction include Carlton Ball, Fong Chow, Thomas Ferreira, Maija Grotell, Gertrud and Otto Natzler, Henry Varnum Poor, Antonio Prieto, Peter Voulkos, David Weinrib and his wife Karen Karnes, and Marguerite Wildenhain. For other aspects of modern American ceramic production see INDUSTRIAL DESIGN.

\* \*

FOLK ART. Pottery thus classified, either because of its distribution among particular classes or regions (usually far from the great cultural centers) or because of the esthetic concepts it expresses, originates in large part from the same factories that have long produced "works of art" and reflects the same history, the same changes in taste and tendencies, as other productions, even though it shows a lag in acceptance of new styles and themes. This fact would seem at first sight to support the thesis (Scerbakivskyj) of nonoriginality in popular artistic expressions, especially in the field of ceramics: a thesis according to which folk craftsmen merely appropriate and democratize and popularize the styles of the higher arts. This is only partly true, however. Actually the ceramic factories serve as one of the meeting grounds between sophisticated trends and popular styles, so that their products reflect the often perfect confluence of two cultural streams (PL. 164).

The simultaneous presence of "cultured" and "popular" motifs in pottery sometimes makes it impossible to classify them rigidly. It must also be remembered that there is often a considerable delay in popular acceptance of more sophisticated styles, so that the "work of art" of a certain epoch may reappear as a "popular expression" at a later date. The socioesthetic classification of ceramic products is less difficult if one keeps in mind that, besides a decorative purpose, popular wares always have a functional one. Indeed, in folk pottery usefulness and beauty are inseparable: though decoration is always concordant with function, the impression of usefulness, and hence the value, of a piece is heightened by its esthetic qualities.

The anthropomorphous lamps of Sicily are among the most remarkable products in which artistic quality and function are one. The Museo Etnografico in Palermo houses a rich collection of these lamps from the traditional Sicilian pottery centers of Caltagirone and Collesano. Mostly made in the 19th century, they display a perfect plastic and pictorial harmony and often gently satirize the worlds of town and country. Ladies of fashion and women of the people, cavaliers and shepherds, *carabinieri* and brigands file past, portrayed in their most characteristic attributes. At times, however, the usual themes are abandoned for representations that are unexpected, though of noble iconographic lineage: nude ladies on horseback, deer, peacocks. But whether they represent types and figures from daily life or fantastic subjects, these Sicilian anthropomorphous lamps are always of impressive artistry.

Italy is very rich in centers for the production of folk pottery: in Apulia, Grottaglie, Fasano, San Pietro in Lama, Laterza, and Taranto; in Abruzzo, Campli, Teramo, Altri, Penne, Pescara, Chieti, Orsogna, and Guardiagrele.

Fine folk pottery has been produced in Spain, where the manufactures have been numerous for several centuries. In Catalonia, about the 18th century, excellent glazed tiles were made; for the most part (like certain popular prints), they illustrated types and professions with grace and simple realism. A good collection is in the Archivo Histórico of Barcelona; it includes cavaliers, ladies, itinerant peddlers, shopkeepers, craftsmen, all with typical attributes and activities. Each piece is an esthetic statement in itself. Well-known Spanish centers are still operating in Valencia, Palencia, and Toledo and its province. The folk pottery of Valencia, the earliest examples

of which date from the 17th century, are distinguished by their many lively colors and varied decoration. Most in favor were yellow, green, blue, and sometimes red, always on a white glaze; decorative motifs included flowers, trees, stylized suns, birds, fountains, and houses. The jugs and dishes made for weddings are especially interesting. In the province of Toledo, besides the well-known manufacture of Talavera de la Reina, there were others producing excellent fabrics: especially the factory in Menasalbas, opened by the Duke of Frías after the destruction of the famous old factory at Buen Retiro by the English and French. Menasalbas wares owe their typical character to harmonious alternations of geometric decorations: zigzags, saw-tooth patterns, broken lines, and zoomorphic motifs (domestic animals, but also, and especially, butterflies).

The popular fabrics of France, England, Scandinavia, Germany, Austria, and Switzerland have been and still are of poor quality and scanty in number in spite of the plentiful supply of good clays. Though important centers have always existed in Bavaria, production in that region has generally showed an artistic rather than a popular tendency.

Folk pottery once flourished in France, each region having a distinct decorative style and palette. Wares from the Ile-de-France usually had a single coat of undecorated white glaze; those from Saint-Omer in Artois had, besides the white glaze, decorations in blue; those from La Chapelle-aux-Pots in Beauvais were glazed in brown and had relief decoration; those from Oberbetschdorf were gray with blue decoration; those from Alsace had dark red glaze with a green dotted decoration; those from the famous La Borne factory in Berry were usually an undecorated gray. Of some esthetic quality are the so-called "patronymic plates," a particular type of plate for hanging on the wall, on which newlyweds are portrayed with the signs of their calling. A fine example at the museum of Angers, of Nevers pottery, is marked "Pierre Gerraud et Françoise Ménard, 1774" and represents a pair of young swineherds.

Folk pottery is very abundantly produced in eastern Europe. Production in Czechoslovakia is of especially good quality. It was introduced into that country by 16th-century Swiss and Italian Anabaptist refugees from the southern Tirol, who set up many manufactures. Quality was so high that until the mid-19th century Slovak and Moravian wares were exported to Bohemia, Austria, Hungary, and Silesia. Though religious restrictions limited the Anabaptist craftsmen to the use of purely floral and geometric motifs, no two vases are alike — such was the inspiration and ingenuity with which the few ornamental motifs were mixed together and complicated in a thousand diverse ways. These patterns did not remain static throughout the centuries but were, of course, subject to the fluctuations of fashion. Indeed, Italianizing Anabaptist motifs were fused and harmonized with ornamental elements from the Empire style, as can be seen in the pottery produced in the first half of the 19th century at Vyskov. Unlike the Anabaptists, Catholic potters preferred representations of religious subjects. There is a large number of jugs from Stupava and Moravia, as well as from Vyskov, bearing pictures of the Virgin, the Crucifixion, and saints, in which predilection for linear design and bright colors is displayed to the full. Also of great interest — both for their documentation of popular plastic concepts and for the comparisons they suggest — are the anthropomorphous vases, largely religious, that were produced in Slovakia until the early 20th century.

In Hungary various potteries making household wares existed even in the Middle Ages, but a true pottery art cannot be said to have existed until the 16th century, when the Tirolian Anabaptists established potteries there, just as in Czechoslovakia. The common origins of Hungarian and Czechoslovak pottery have not, however, resulted in identical characteristics. Hungary, in fact, also underwent the Asiatic influence of Turkish invaders in the 16th and 17th centuries. Only toward the end of the 18th century did painted and decorated wares penetrate the homes of peasants. The most important centers for Hungarian folk pottery, which developed from that time forward, are on the Great Hungarian Plain. Very fine examples, decorated with flowers on a yellowish ground, are produced in the city

of Mezötúr. The potters of Mezöcsát are famous for their anthropomorphous jugs (*miska*). These, along with brandy bottles in the shape of a bird with a blossoming branch held in the beak (made both at Mezöcsát and Tiszafüred), are the finest productions of Hungarian folk pottery. The decorative technique is barbotine, while to the north of the Great Plain, at Gyöngyös and at Pásztó, the gay designs are brushed on in blue, green, and red on a white ground. In southern Hungary one of the most famous pottery centers is at Sárköz, where the craftsmen paint tulips, daisies, roses, and birds on a dark ground.

In Romania, pottery is one of the most important of the local folk arts. Decorative techniques vary: painting, incision, or relief decoration are used alone or together with reliefs and incised designs covered over with glaze. The commonest is painting. An interesting variant, employed in Hungary as well, is a black unglazed ware, ornamented only with incised designs, which comes from around Suceava and Iași. Zoomorphic and anthropomorphous wares from Oboga, Pisc, and Pucheni are on a high level. The decorative vocabulary of Romanian potters is ample, the more common motifs being geometric: spirals, circles, broken lines. Floral motifs, dominant in Transylvania, are also employed, while representational decoration is scattered throughout the country. Since the 18th century a ware colored brown, red, and green, with relief decoration, has been produced at Horezu in Oltenia and at Curtea-de-Argeș in Muntenia.

German and Hungarian minorities in Romania also produce fine pottery. The German potters in Transylvania have a predilection for cobalt, both as a background for incised designs painted in white and as decoration on a white ground. The most common motifs are in a stylized floral vein similar to that on the wares produced by the Hungarian minority, which, however, are decorated in green or yellow with dark outlines.

In the Ukraine, especially in the villages of Opochnia and Dybyntsi, folk pottery has ancient and illustrious traditions. A particular method of coloring and decoration, in which colors are dribbled onto a pot that is being rotated on the wheel, results in a series of yellow or green spirals on the reddish ground of the biscuit. Over the spirals, at a short distance and perpendicular to them, brief lines are added in green or some other dark color. After firing, the pots are given a clear glaze to ensure impermeability and to add brightness. After a second firing this glaze makes the pots both more functional and decoratively more interesting.

The peasant potters of Kiev use a different technique. By making a few lines across the freshly painted spirals and thus slightly distorting the colors, they produce a series of small, graceful transverse streaks. This process is encountered also beyond the Carpathians up to the Don basin or wherever there have been immigrations of Ukrainian potters.

Although perhaps not one of the aspects of Greek folk art most in evidence, Hellenic pottery is of considerable interest. An index of the dynamic quality of the popular culture is its dissimilarity to classical pottery. (Commercial wares for the tourist trade still employ classical formulas, but these are not true folk productions.) Hellenic pottery also documents the interesting results of a meeting of two disparate artistic cultures, in this case the Greek West and the Turkish East. At Rhodes, one of the best-known centers for Greek folk pottery, productions clearly display this merging of the Turkish geometric and floral patterns with the more representational repertory of the West.

A similar phenomenon is even more apparent in Latin American pottery, whose forms, colors, and decorations of clearly Iberian descent are shot through with Inca elements as well as motifs from the artistic repertory of various pre-Inca peoples of South America. In the well-known folk pottery of Quinchamali (Chile), for instance, Iberian, Inca, and Araucanian elements have been identified.

South American pottery shapes, besides vases of largely European types, include sculpture as well. Pottery birds known as *jarrospatos* ("duck vases") in Chile are widely distributed along the Pacific as well as in Argentina. Ceramic decoration in South America is painted, incised, or in relief, while the ornamental repertory is almost exclusively floral.

Antonio BUTTITTA

ASIA. *India and southeastern Asia. a. Protohistoric period.* The earliest recorded Indian pottery (ca. 3100–2850 B.C.) is that of Baluchistan: handmade coiled wares, occasionally coated with a slip. Painted decoration of plain bands or simple geometric patterns is rare, the most common mode being that of mat marking.

During the period about 2950–2800 B.C. neolithic peasant farmers from the Iranian Plateau introduced wheel-thrown painted pottery to Baluchistan and Sind, as indicated by the allied wares of Kechi Beg near Quetta, Loralai in the Zhob, and Amri in Sind. This is a bichrome ware of black and bright red decoration on a red slip (see above: *Protohistoric "ceramic cultures" and cultures with protohistoric traditions*).

Next are the pottery industries named after type sites in Baluchistan, of which that of Togau, a red-slipped ware decorated with animals, horn fringes, and geometric patterns in black, is preeminent as a link with the approximately fixed chronology of the Harappa culture (see INDUS VALLEY ART). Comparative stratigraphy has shown that Togau is contemporaneous with the contacts of early Nal-Nundara and of Amri with southern Baluchistan and Makran; the late phase of Kechi Beg corresponds to middle Amri and early Nal in Sind; and since early Nal (at the site of Pandi Wahi in Sind) just overlaps earliest Harappa, but Togau probably does not, these contacts can be fixed at appproximately 2600 B.C.

The bichrome ware of Kechi Beg, Amri, and Loralai consists mainly of bowls, globular pots, and straight-sided beakers. These are decorated with geometric designs of a style common in the repertory of ancient Iran (see above). Loralai pots have zones of animals derived from an earlier, enigmatic, short-lived industry which introduced bull and antelope motifs, painted in brown on a buff slip.

The ceramics of the type sites of Kulli and Mehi and of Nal and Nundara are the chief remains of two cultural traditions dominating southern Baluchistan, contemporary with the rise and fall of the Harappa culture (ca. 2600–1550 B.C.). Kulli culture pottery shapes include canister jars, pedestal dishes, and narrow vases of Harappan type. Ornament combines bulls and pipal trees of the Indus valley with ibex, sigmas, and fringes of Iran, painted in black on pale red and whitish slips. Contacts are widespread and there are strong Kulli influences at Bampur in Iranian Makran and at Ghazi Shah in Sind.

The pottery named after the Sohr Damb of Nal has for the most part been derived from a cemetery on that site. In its early stages, as seen at Nundara, there are clear contacts with Amri. Fish, birds, antelope, and lions appear as decoration in polychrome on buff-slipped bowls, beakers, and canisters. The production of red-slipped bowls and beakers spread from Periano Ghundai in the Zhob south to Nal, where their makers settled. These settlements of painted-pottery makers were all swept away by Aryan invaders about 1800–1700 B.C.

The Indus civilization turned out thousands of mass-produced, well-fired pink pots in a limited range of shapes, of which pedestal dishes, pointed-base beakers, and narrow vases are the most characteristic. Handsome pots with black decoration on a polished red slip and rare polychrome vases are the less common painted wares. The earlier examples of painted ware are characterized by naturalistic pipal trees growing from a small mound, like the trees on Kulli sherds. Later examples have close geometric patterns, notably of intersecting circles.

The period of invasions which witnessed the appearance of Aryan or Aryan-led peoples and continued from about 1800 to 1300 B.C. with a succession of incursions from the West, produced various pottery types in northwestern India. Shahi Tump ware, known chiefly by a number of badly made pots and shallow bowls from a cemetery, indicates the arrival of the earliest invaders in Baluch Makran. A people with a similar equipment destroyed and occupied the settlements at the sites of Jhukar, after which they have been named, and Chanhu-daro in Sind. They produced a buff-slipped ware with boldly executed patterns in black and red, including leaf forms, checkered squares, a ball-and-stem motif, and a series of converging loops as a rim pattern for dishes. Pottery with cream slip and broad bands of red found at Periano Ghundai may derive

from Jhukar. Polychrome wares such as that of Trihni in Sind and apparently allied shards found in the Zhob help in part to fill the period 1400–1200 B.C. With these should be associated pottery called after the site of Jhangar in Sind, a handmade gray ware, having no slip and a simple incised decoration. Though this industry consists mostly of undistinguished small bowls, a form of triple jar links it with Shahi Tump and with Sialk in Iran, and so with the period of invasions (FIG. 294).

A ceramic type of this period, Ravi ware, comes from a post-Harappan cemetery at Harappa in West Punjab (Panjab); it is a red-slipped ware with elaborate decoration in black. This decoration, which includes peacocks, bulls, stars, fish, and arrowhead birds, shows sufficient Harappan influence to indicate some actual contact with that people. Shapes are quite different, with the exception of dishes on stands, which show the connection with the Harappa culture. At the sites of Rupar and Bara in East Punjab a ceramic has been found in the upper part of levels classified as late Harappan, which, however, has no connection with that culture; but motifs such as "arrowhead between horns" and large irregular stars link it with Ravi types.

In addition to pots, bowls, and dishes for household use, potters made small terra-cotta figurines of men and animals. On the present evidence there is little doubt that this practice was introduced by the Harappans. Figurines of oxen have been found at considerable depth at Mohenjo-daro in Sind, while none can so far be associated with the stages of the earliest hand-made pots or with that of Kechi Beg-Amri. Though some of these figures were without doubt toys, the bulk of them must be of a votive character connected with a mother goddess and cattle cult.

Sites of the Kulli culture in southern Baluchistan have produced similar figurines of mother goddesses and oxen. The former are crudely modeled with arms akimbo and hands on hips, which are splayed out in pedestal form; they are ornamented with a number of applied necklaces. The oxen are painted with dark stripes. Fragile cream-colored goddess figures, modeled with applied wiglike headdress and necklaces, come from the Zhob in northern Baluchistan and spread southwest to sites around Quetta. In addition bulls painted in the Kulli manner and what may well be a horse come from the Quetta area. So far no terra-cotta figurines can be associated with the period of invasions.

There has recently come to light, throughout west-central India, a style of painted pottery which is potentially of the greatest historical value, coming as it does in that dark period prior to the invasion of Alexander. The site of Maheshwar, at the age-old crossing of the Narmada, provides the main link in a chain of sites producing this ware, from Jorwe on the upper Godavari in the south to Rangpur in Gujarat in the north. The bulk of this pottery consists of small shallow open bowls, wheel-thrown with a slip in shades of red, orange, and tan, with simple geometric patterns of hatched and solid triangles and diamonds, and parallel slanting lines. Contemporary at Maheshwar there is also a ware with a cream slip with rare decoration of men and animals; trough or channel spouts are an equally rare feature in this ware. The dating is still uncertain; but a likely range is 1400–300 B.C. The first date is that of the Rangpur culture, which spread to the upper Godavari by 1150 B.C. and survived in that area until the beginning of the 3d century.

Excavation in northern India, undertaken in an attempt to fill the gaps in our knowledge of the period 1550–350 B.C., has provided useful material, the precise dating of which is still very controversial. Small fragments of a coarse-to-medium pale red ware with a roughly applied ocher surface, which may be a postfiring wash, found at Hastinapura, may be of importance, as they appear at other Ganges valley sites in possible association with notable copper hoards. Following on this ware, and possibly to some extent contemporary, comes a painted gray ware of considerable importance. This is a wheel-thrown fabric of finely levigated clay, uniformly fired to a pale gray or whitish body with a darker gray surface. This surface, often having a glossy slip, is painted with patterns consisting of groups of vertical lines, bands of sigmas, concentric circles, pothook

spirals, and arrangements of dots and dashes. East Punjab is full of sites producing this ware. This pottery introduces shapes, particularly dishes with flat or slightly rounded bottoms, that are characteristic of the early historic period. Both painted gray ware and the contemporary black pottery are close precursors of northern black polished ware, widely known as "N.B.P.," and, though the dates are still in dispute, they were probably made in the period about 700–400 B.C.

*b. Early historic and medieval period.* Toward the start of the earlier half of the 1st millennium B.C. we see the approach of a horse-riding people who brought the use of iron for the first time to the borders of India through Iranian and Baluch Makran. They also brought a distinctive pottery known as "Londo ware," handmade and tempered with crushed potsherds and decorated with pothook spirals, horses, and birds; an allied ware with large volutes as decoration; and squat flasks.

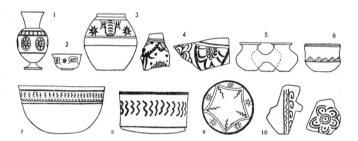

Protohistoric Indian types. (1–3) Terra cottas from Ravi, ca. 1800–1100 B.C.; (4) fragments of terra cottas from Trihni, ca. 1800–1100 B.C.; (5, 6) terra cottas from Jhangar, ca. 1800–1100 B.C.; (7–10) gray terra cottas from Maheshwar, ca. 1100–400 B.C.

Associated with the first arrival of iron in that area is the important south Indian red-and-black pottery. This ware, some of which seems to have been wheel-thrown and some handmade on a *tournette*, has a burnished slip and is black inside and for some distance down from the rim on the outside — an effect produced by the firing. This pottery is also associated with megalithic cists and pot burials, both enclosed in stone circles. The point from which it spread is unknown. The claim that similar ware comes from the general area of Kathiawar, Gujarat, and southern Rajputana would not exclude the possibility of coastal spread southward to what is now Dravidian-speaking India, where this culture probably met with less resistance than in the tougher, more civilized north.

*Northern black polished ware* is of the greatest consequence, for it provides a readily recognizable feature linking the immediately pre- and post-Mauryan periods. This is a highly characteristic gloss ware, the shapes, body clay, and even to a certain extent the surface treatment of which derive directly from painted gray ware. It is wheel-thrown and is fired to a pale or whitish gray and has an intensely black or purplish-black glossy surface.

A number of shards from the middle Ganges valley, notably from Rajghat, have red-on-black decoration, the color and technique of which indicate a process similar to, if not identical with, that of Attic red-figure ware. Though probably originating in Uttar Pradesh about 400 B.C., this pottery was spread far and wide, but it is only its occurrence at the Bhir mound at Taxila that has so far provided any real dating evidence. Here the belief that this site was abandoned at the time of the invasion of the Bactrian Greeks in 180 B.C., in conjunction with dates assigned to three hoards, has conditioned chronology. (It is improbable, however, that the Bactrian Greeks settled at Taxila before about 145 B.C.; in any case, the terra-cotta figurines testify that the Bhir mound was occupied by the local population until the beginning of the 1st century B.C.) The hoards contain coins dating from 319 to 248 B.C., but these may well have been buried at the time of the Bactrian invasion. This is the oldest known setting for this ware, and it is doubtful whether the excavations at Kausambi (Kosambi) in Uttar Pradesh can provide a date that is appreciably earlier.

Though terra-cotta figurines were a common feature of the Harappa culture, the number recorded that can be placed unequivocally within the period 1500–300 B.C. may, optimistically, be counted on the fingers of one hand. Various sites in northern India and West Pakistan have produced — notably at Sar Dheri, 10 miles northeast of Peshawar — crude "timeless" terra cottas that cannot be fitted into any chronological phase because of their limited artistic range. The Sar Dheri figures, found throughout a wide area, are naked but for necklaces and girdles; similar examples from Mathura (Muttra), Ahichchhatra, Patna (Pataliputra), and other sites show like characteristics. These archaic terra cottas, with their pinched-out noses, their eyes applied or roughly incised, and their form peg-shaped or spade-shaped, or with crude rudimentary legs, have from time to time been assigned to the 2d and 3d millenniums B.C., but in fact none can be dated earlier than 350 B.C. They occur throughout the life of the site at Sar Dheri (ca. 300 B.C.–A.D. 300). Whereas the making of crudely modeled figurines was in all probability the unaided work of the potter, those partly or wholly produced from a mold depended for their artistic superiority on the ability of professional mold makers. In early types, late Maurya or early Śunga, only the face is the product of the mold and the stylized body is the work of the potter. In the earlier molded figures the clothing and ornaments either are very plain or are applied and decorated with incised or stamped patterns. From 150 B.C. to some time in the 1st century of our era this type of figurine, designated "Śunga" for convenience, improved in technique; poses became less frontal and more sophisticated.

Figurines from Mathura in gray terra cotta show the earlier characteristics, with molded faces and applied ornament on crudely modeled bodies. At many sites — Taxila, Mathura, Ahichchhatra, Kausambi, Patna, and Tamluk — we find a female figure with molded face and body, and with applied headdress, large hemispherical earrings, a heavy necklace, and a three-knobbed bracelet; all these figures are of about 180 B.C. Red terra-cotta plaques molded with men and women either singly or in pairs are common on all the sites of northern India. The molds were probably made directly in intaglio, as the fine ornamental work can be produced far more easily by this method.

After painted gray ware ended, painted pottery did not reappear until the close of the 2d century B.C. in the upper levels of the Bhir mound at Taxila. From this time, certainly until the 7th century of our era, red wares painted with designs in black are common on sites throughout northwestern India. The earlier examples are simple patterns and conventionalized plant forms, the later being far more naturalistic. Among the latter are those of Rangmahal in Bikaner, which are of the Gupta period or later. For the most part these designs are in black or dark brown paint on medium-sized globular pots and flat dishes, applied direct to the pot or to a red-slipped surface.

The practice of decorating pottery with incised patterns occurs quite early. In Harappan times incised wavy lines, impressed intersecting circles, and rouletting appear. During the Kushan and Gupta periods a great variety of stamp patterns, including rosettes, leaf forms, fish, cowries, swastikas, and *triratnas*, were applied to red-slipped wares. In early medieval times decoration employing raised patterns came into fashion.

The evidence from the excavated sites of Ahichchhatra and Hastinapura in regard to the period A.D. 50 to 300 is so unsatisfactory, and that of Taxila so meager, that recognition of figurines as belonging to that time is largely subjective and based on stylistic grounds. To this period belong large molded tiles (such as those in Mathura and those with which the monastery at Harwan in Kashmir is paved), stamped with designs of archers on horseback, deer, fighting cocks, and people on balconies.

Gupta figurines once seen are for the most part readily recognized. Heart-shaped faces with broad forehead and pointed chin, a somewhat sharp prominent nose, and a full lower lip are the main characteristics. A girl in a swing from Rajghat, a part of old Benares, is an example of Gupta work in terra-cotta at its best. The tradition of making terra cottas was carried on into medieval times, but few of any merit date later than A.D. 650. At Akhnur in Jammu and Ushkur in Kashmir fine terra-cotta heads were unearthed at monastery sites of the 7th century. Large terra-cotta panels from Rangmahal, Ahichchhatra, Bhitargaon, and Paharpur formed part of the decoration of brick temples; they cover the period from Gupta times to the 8th century.

A finely levigated pottery with highly polished slip is common in western India from Kathiawar to Kolhapur. It can be dated in the first three centuries of the Christian era by reason of association with Greco-Roman antiquities of that date and of its similarity with Roman pottery. High, narrow necks and sprinklers are outstanding features, the former obtaining throughout northern India in Kushan and Gupta times. Jars with rims folded flatly downward, shallow open bowls, and globular pots with purple and white painted bands are also found in this ware.

Sites in southern India have not produced terra-cotta figures to the same extent as those of the north. South of the Narmada the chief sources are Kondapur and Maski in Hyderabad State, and the Nilgiri burial cairns, which have yielded many funerary figurines. Excavations at Nasik, Paithan, Brahmapuri, and Brahmagiri have produced only about a dozen specimens among them. From the Sātavāhana site of Kondapur a number of small molded figures of caparisoned horses and bulls, a lion, and human figures which may represent yakshas and yakshis have been unearthed. They are of a creamy white color, having been coated with kaolin before baking. The female figurines of Maski are all of types that can be dated in the first three centuries of our era, including two with a high "kalathos" style of headdress. Parallels with this kind of headdress, dwarf figurines, and facial types from northern sites all confirm this dating. Vast quantities of buffalo figurines were deposited in the Nilgiri burial cairns, and human and animal figures form a decoration surmounting the lids of the burial urns. These are all very crude and stylized and are made of gritty, grayish brown, badly fired pottery. They date from the first half of the 1st millennium of our era.

*c. Islamic period.* Apart from undistinguished wares of village potters, this period is characterized by the introduction of Islamic glazed wares (see *Late antiquity and the Middle Ages: Islam*). At very few sites has the presence of Islamic glazed wares been recorded in a clear archaeological context. The earliest examples are those found at Brahminabad-Mansura in Sind, occupied by the Arabs in 730 and deserted probably early in the 14th century. Here fragments of Mesopotamian luster and lead-glazed wares and Samarkand slip-painted ware occur. At Adilabad, part of the city complex of Tughlakabad near Delhi, glazed pottery of the Islamic period has been found in some quantity, and the very brief period of occupation dates this exactly in the first half of the 14th century. In the upper levels also of Hastinapura, glazed pottery of this type, late imported Timurid ware of the second half of the 13th century and local imitations of the 14th century, have been found. It is clear that rather inferior copies of Iranian glazed wares were made throughout northern India.

*d. Modern times.* Within the period 1880 to 1940 we have record of plain, painted, and glazed pottery, all of which perpetuate to some extent the traditions of the past. The plain expendable products of the village potters call for little comment. In the majority of households, the receptacles for cooking and serving food are of metal, while pottery is used for water storage. What is with little doubt a survival of the production of painted wares does continue and has been observed at Balreji in Sind, Gujargarhi in the North-West Frontier Province, Rawalpindi and Harappa in West Punjab, and further south at Nowgong in Vindhya Pradesh. In his *Industrial Arts of India*, Birdwood praises the glazed wares of Sind, the Punjab, and Madura. These are glazed in the old Islamic tradition in turquoise blue, dark green, dark purple, and golden brown. They are ornamented with blooms on a stem (in compartments or dispersed over the whole surface) and knop and flower patterns (divided by various running patterns in bands).

Crude "timeless" terra-cotta figurines of mother-goddess type are still made in Bengal, showing how little such features as pinched-out noses and cylindrical bodies can be relied on as dating criteria. Highly colored clay images are turned out

in large numbers for festivals, but these have little in common with the early figurines. Terra-cotta toys were made for European children about 1870–90 (e.g., a soldier with tunic and haversack from Sar Dheri and an ayah, or nurse, from Peshawar). On the whole, recent figurines are of better-levigated clay than the early ones and are hollow, being produced by joining molded portions. An interesting range of terra-cotta animals is made by Gujars in western Punjab. The date of some terra cottas, such as female heads with gold-painted crowns from Mardan in northwestern Pakistan, is still problematic, but they and similar ones from the Jumna valley may well prove to be of the 10th to 12th century.

Douglas H. Gordon

*China. a. Neolithic and Shang-Yin period (1523–1028 B.C.).* The traditional chronology is 1766–1112 B.C., the revised one, 1523–1028 B.C. The first find of neolithic pottery was made by the Swede J. G. Andersson in 1921 at Yang-shao in Honan province, and the name of this site has been given to the whole range of wares of which this is the prototype. Very soon, however, Andersson found — and further systematic excavations conducted by the Chinese confirmed — that the center of this culture called "Yang-shao" was in reality much more to the west, in Kansu province. Here Andersson distinguished, in the same cultural context, a variety of painted pottery named for the sites of Ma-ch'ang, Pan-shan, and Ch'i-chia-p'ing. This last has been found in graves containing small bronze vessels from the time of the Shang dynasty (which in the last period adds its name to that of Yin). The potter's wheel not yet being in use, the wares of Yang-shao were made by coiling the clay on a turntable; the thin necks are skillfully formed. Characteristic is a type of burial urn with a long and narrow neck (but at Pan-shan some urns have a shorter and wider neck), with ring handles at the widest diameter of the body (PLS. 120, 219) and a kind of tripod that later, in its bronze derivatives, was to be called *li-ting.* Domestic vessels were made up of types with handles, narrow mouths, or everted lips and conical lids. The decoration, in red and black, although highly stylized, includes animal elements (e.g., claws and horns) spread over the whole surface. In this, and in general make, the Yang-shao pottery recalls the painted pottery of western Asia and some south Russian sites (Tripolje; see ASIATIC PROTOHISTORY); this painted pottery extends at least into Shensi as well as Honan, and also into Manchuria, and the chronological limits — still uncertain — provisionally can be fixed from 2000 to 1000 B.C.

The only other important group of neolithic pottery in northern China is the one named after the town of Lung-shan in Shantung. Typical examples of this pottery, a fine black ware, have been found in the coastal regions of Shantung and Kiangsu and inland in Honan, which thus shares in two neolithic cultures. From the stratified sites of Honan it was possible to establish that Lung-shan pottery is later than Yang-shao but earlier than Shang-Yin. The Lung-shan culture levels show a common gray pottery decorated with beaten striated patterns from pads or with incised chevrons. The typical shapes are big urns on small flat bases, with straight or slightly everted lips; cooking vessels with rounded bases and flat shoulders; and a tripod vessel with separately formed feet, luted onto the rounded body (the prototype of the bronze *li-ting*); also a wide-bowled vessel on a high splayed foot, prototype of the bronze *tou.*

The area of northern Honan where the Yang-shao and Lung-shan pottery overlapped seems to have been the center of the first Bronze Age culture of China. The traditional date for the beginning of the Shang dynasty is 1766 B.C., but no site which can be attributed with confidence to so early a period has yet been found. It is claimed by the excavators that the Shang habitation site of Chêng-chou (Chengchow) in Honan shows two strata earlier than the level contemporary with the last capital of the Shang at An-yang (1300–1028 B.C.). The *li-ting* is again found in pottery, and also two other smaller tripods, the beak-spouted wine cup, *chüeh,* and the tall vessel for heating wine, *chia,* both with flat bases suggesting bronze prototypes. In the stratum immediately before the An-yang

period a hard gray stoneware was found decorated with chevrons and in shapes known in later bronze vessels, the *kuei, p'an,* and *hu.* In fact all that is at present known of these earlier Shang levels suggests that the culture was homogeneous with the later period, e.g., in the An-yang region (PL. 220), and that experiments had already begun with both hard porcelaneous wares and with feldspathic glaze. It is now established that a green to greenish-brown glaze, fitting well to the body and evenly applied, was the principal innovation of this culture. The second innovation was a white ware made of kaolin and fired at a temperature of about 1000°C. This was a scarce and, no doubt, a highly prized ware found also at Hui-hsien, always fully decorated with impressed designs of stylized animal forms tending to a chevron pattern. Only two complete pieces are known. The Shang period brought a new departure in pottery shapes, the most important being shouldered vases, generally sharply contoured; a squat form of the *li-ting* with the body almost confounded in the legs; the other bronze shapes, *tou, p'an,* and *kuei,* and a *hu* vase with tubular handles and knobs in the foot rim to take a cord. At Chêng-chou, but apparently not at An-yang, a striking beaker was found with very large curled handles. Pottery kilns have been found that consist of a two-tiered oven with fire below stoked from the front and with holes in the floor of the upper chamber to carry the draft through to a vent in the roof around the vessels placed in it. The whole was small and implied local production.

*b. Chou period (1027–256 B.C.).* The long period of the Chou dynasty is relatively poor in pottery; what has come down to us is mainly grave pottery, which at first was not very different from the Shang forms. From a Lo-yang grave of Western Chou date (1027–771 B.C.) are vessels imitating bronze forms (*yu, tsun, ting, kuei, chüeh, chih*); other pieces continued to have feldspathic glazes, but at late Chou sites no glazed pottery has been found.

In the last phase of the Chou dynasty, the Warring States period (480–221 B.C.), one innovation is the painting of broad designs in pottery. This painting is in strong colors, red and yellow with black or white outline, on white ground; it is clearly a cheap substitute for inlaid bronze, characteristic of the 4th century B.C. In the same period a fine style of decoration was produced by burnishing designs in linear chevrons and spirals on a fine gray pottery. This so-called "graphite" decoration (from its resemblance to pencil work) is reported to have been found at Lo-yang and certainly in controlled excavations at Hui-hsien, where shapes include a low tripod bowl with feet in the form of men. But it must be stated that no figurines or pigmented miniature vessels with burnished or lacquered surface have been found in these or any other controlled excavations, and the dancing figurines in many Western and Japanese collections are not authenticated by archaeology.

At Shou-chou (mod. Shou-hsien) in Anhwei excavation has revealed finely potted ware decorated with simple impressed designs of spirals or stylized birds in zones, sometimes covered by a thin feldspathic glaze on the shoulder. Wares of this type appear widely distributed, and toward the beginning of the Han dynasty (206 B.C.) they are found in other shapes, especially ewers with spouts of "chicken-head" shape. This feature seems to connect them with the earliest products of the Yüeh kilns in Chekiang.

*c. The Han period (206 B.C.–A.D. 221) and that of the Six Dynasties (220–589).* This period saw the development of a considerable industry in the Yüeh district of Chekiang for the production of a high-fired fully glazed stoneware. The lead glaze was probably derived from Western sources with which China was in touch at this time through her expansion to the limits of Turkistan and active trade thence through Iran to the Mediterranean. The resulting range of glaze from a yellow buff to a deep green served for low-fired vessels and for animal and human figurines (PL. 172) and models of buildings and utensils made as tomb furniture. The earliest Yüeh ware (Yüeh-yao; *yao* means "ware") belongs to Han graves (Shanghai provincial depot), and some of the commonest shapes copy

contemporary bronze forms. The shapes of these early Yüeh wares are heavy, with broad unglazed bases, slightly concave, and without foot rims. Ewers and vases have heavily flanged mouths, high handles, and loops on the shoulders, often square in section (PL. 165). Decoration consists only in hatching or applied masks of bronze style from molds. The body is gray, burning purple where exposed in the kiln.

Stoneware of Yüeh type in the 6th century has been found in graves at Ching-hsien in Hopei dating between 521 and 565. They are vases of unusual type and are probably from a local kiln. The elaborate molded decoration is derived from Sassanian silverware, but the presence of large lotus petals suggests a Buddhist intermediary, perhaps in Central Asia.

The green-glazed stoneware (PL. 236) of Chekiang established such a reputation that imitations were made in both northern and southern China. In Hunan, perhaps at Yo-chou near Ch'ang-sha — mentioned in the literature as a center of ceramic production — was produced a rather inferior ware, not porcelaneous, whose brownish-green glaze does not adhere well to the body (II, PL. 14).

At T'ing-kuan-hsien, in Shensi, a kiln making celadon ware has been found with an inscription indicating activity between A.D. 345 and 357, but the finds are not older than Sung (960–1279).

*d. Sui period (581–618).* During this period the Yüeh kilns continued to be active; and from a find in a tomb dated 603 at An-yang, it can be established that the shapes had begun to change into those of the succeeding T'ang period. This intermediate stage is characterized by double-loop handles below the neck of vases and piecrust lips on bowls. An ovoid vase with small mouth is a favorite shape; this also sometimes has a piecrust zone around the middle. The glaze — mainly a brownish green or a grayish blue — is inclined to run in streaks and is often crackled.

*e. T'ang period (618–906).* In this period the production of high-grade stoneware developed into an important industry, supplying many distant markets in southeastern Asia, Iran, the Persian Gulf coast, Mesopotamia, and Egypt. It is known that fine white porcelain was made at this time in the Hsing-chou district, Hopei (the famous Hsing ware, Hsing-yao, praised by the *Ch'a-ching*, a text of ca. 9th cent.), and white porcelain bowls are known that, on the evidence of shape or archaeology, must be of T'ang date; but the Hsing-chou kilns have not been found. The only T'ang kilns known at present are those in the Yüeh district near the Shang-lin-hu in Chekiang.

The existence of a white porcelain at least as early as the 9th century has been certainly known since the publication by F. Sarre (*Die Keramik von Samarra*, Berlin, 1925) of the finds of the German expedition to Samarra on the Tigris, which was a palace city of the Abbasside caliphs from 836 to 883 (see ABBASSIDE ART). It has since been found on other Near Eastern sites, such as Susa in southwestern Iran, where stratification indicates a 9th-10th-century date for it. This Samarra ware, as it has come to be called in the West, has a hard white body, is highly vitrified, with a milky glaze forming greenish-white drops near the base. The foot can be broad and flat with a recessed center, the edge trimmed with a knife and cutting back at more than 90°, or with a higher and narrower rim beveled on the outside but only roughly finished on the inner surface. The first type of foot was imitated in the pottery of eastern Iran and in the contemporary white porcelain of both southern Iran and Syria, which, like much other T'ang pottery, was influenced by metalwork; the other is found on the more heavily potted bowls which often have lobed sides and occasionally a foliate edge. It is not known where this ware was produced. On the other hand, kilns have been found in the Ting-chou area, in a village called Chien-t'zǔ-ts'un (Hopei) which have been identified, first by F. Koyama (1949) and afterward also by Chen Wan-li, as the kilns of the famous Sung Ting-yao (see below). These kilns appear to have been in operation at least as early as the Five Dynasties period (907-60), for fragments resembling the Samarra type with

recessed base and rolled lip have been found. It seems likely therefore that the Samarra ware is a primitive Ting-yao, made by the same kiln which afterward developed the fine ware used in the Northern Sung imperial palace. White wares were undoubtedly made elsewhere in China under the T'ang dynasty, but examples which have been found in tombs in Hunan and Szechwan have more earthy bodies and a colder white glaze, and may be classed as imitations of Hopei products.

The Yüeh ware of T'ang date — from which two kilns have been identified in Chekiang, one in Yu-yao-hsien near the Shang-lin-hu and the other in Yao-tzu-hsien — has carved decoration of wave or lotus patterns, phoenixes, dragons, or flowers (PL. 166). The gray body is now completely covered by the glaze; the rather high, well-formed, and outward-splayed foot rims required support in the kiln by five or six piles of clay, traces of which remain embodied in the glaze. The principal shapes are shallow bowls carved with lotus petals outside and incised phoenixes within; deep bowls with wave patterns outside and dragons among waves inside; conical tea bowls with lobed mouth and nearly straight sides on a slightly recessed foot; vases with ovoid bodies and expanding mouths, or tall necks and vertical flange to support the cover.

Best known today of all the T'ang wares is the *san-t'sai* ("three-colored") glazed pottery which was freely buried with the dead. The principal glazes employed are a chalky blue, an orange-red, a spinach green, and a lemon yellow; they are usually laid on a white slip, often being allowed to run, but sometimes controlled to some extent by incised designs. Favorite shapes are the covered globular vase, the offering tray with slightly upturned rim and usually three low feet, the tripartite vase with tall trumpet mouth and often with high splayed feet. Some more elaborate ewers closely imitate metal forms derived from the gold and silver ware in that post-Sassanian style which flourished in central Asia in the 7th century. The offering trays usually have incised designs in the center (PL. 167), most frequently a lotus but also occasionally a goose in flight among lotus plants. Applied ornament is found on the vases and generally derives from metalwork and is often of clear Middle Eastern origin.

The *san-t'sai* glazes were continued in northern China and Manchuria by the Liao dynasty (907-1125). The blue glaze does not seem to have been used, but the orange-red and green persist, and a white glaze was introduced. There were some new shapes, most typical being a bottle imitating a leather flask and a tall-necked vase with funnel-shaped mouth. Unlike their T'ang predecessors the Liao vessels are often decorated with incised flowers under the glaze, sometimes filled with other glazes, while molded ornament is much less common. A find of a Liao kiln at Lin-huang has recently been reported by Li Wen-hsin (*Chinese Journal of Archaeology*, 1958, no. 2).

*f. Sung period (960–1279).* Both incised and molded decoration is found on fragments from the Ting kilns of this period (see above), but the incised predominate. Favorite designs are lotus, fish, or ducks. Apart from examples of the cream-white glaze, there are a fair number of fragments of a similar ware with a black glaze. Much rarer are a spinach-green and a purplish-brown (persimmon) glaze, the latter perhaps to be identified with red or purple Ting mentioned in literature. Typical Ting shapes are deep basins and shallow straight-sided cups with everted lips and often foliate rims, ewers and vases with slender necks, tall-shouldered vases with narrow mouth, plates whose flanges, often lobed, are turned sharply inward, and stemmed cups with a rather short foot.

A finer quality of Ting ware, destined probably for the imperial palace, has a highly translucent body showing orange by transmitted light; foot rims are small but carefully formed; the bowls were usually fired resting on their lips, which are themselves bare of glaze and have often been sheathed in copper. The ideogram *kuan* ("official"), incised in a cursive character under the glaze of a fragment found by Chen Wan-li and a complete piece in the Percival David Foundation of Chinese Art in London, confirms the supposition that this ware, though produced in the common kilns — that of Ju (1107) was the

first devoted to the production of palace ware — was made by imperial order.

During the Northern Sung period (960–1127) the tradition of green-glazed (iron oxide) wares was carried on in various places in northern China and in Korea, where the earliest datable native celadon is said to have been found in a tomb of 993. It is probable that there were "northern celadon" kilns in Hopei, for shape and decoration seem to connect many pieces with the Ting ware of this province, but the only kilns that have been identified at present are in faraway Shensi in the northwest, about 50 miles north of Sian; they are known collectively as Yao-chou.

The products are among the best northern celadon types, with highly vitrified glaze, generally but not always inclining to olive green. The commonest shapes are small bowls and dishes, with molded allover floral designs inside but often with freely carved lotus petals outside; plain open bowls with foliate lips; tripod incense burners; and small ewers of depressed globular shape freely carved with floral sprays around the body and lotus petals on the shoulder.

Another important center of pottery production was Tz'ŭ-chou in southern Hopei; from there comes the carved or painted stoneware, covered with a transparent or green glaze, that must have been the principal everyday pottery of the period (PLS. 166, 258, 259). The light body is covered with a slip and then decorated either by carving through this slip or by painting on it with a brush. After the carved pieces are covered with a transparent glaze, they appear with white designs on a gray to biscuit-color ground. The black painted designs may be further decorated by cutting or incising into the black glaze. The commonest shapes are tall vases with narrow mouths (the *mei-p'ing*, or vase for displaying plum blossom); the squat, square-based bottle, and the pillow. Large open-mouthed jars were probably not made before the 14th century. The Japanese expert F. Koyama has identified an important kiln producing these wares at Chiao-tso in Hsiu-wu department of northern Honan (*Bijutsu Kenkyu*, no. 161, Dec., 1950), and most Japanese scholars attribute the finest Sung Tz'ŭ-chou pieces to this so-called "Hsiu-wu kiln." In the West, however, the old label of Tz'ŭ-chou is still applied to the whole group, although some of the finest pieces were made in Honan.

Koyama shows that the various types of Sung pottery were not produced exclusively in the locality from which they derive their name. This is certainly true also of Chün-yao, which takes its name from Chün-chou in Honan, south of Kaifeng, but was produced in several other localities. This also is a

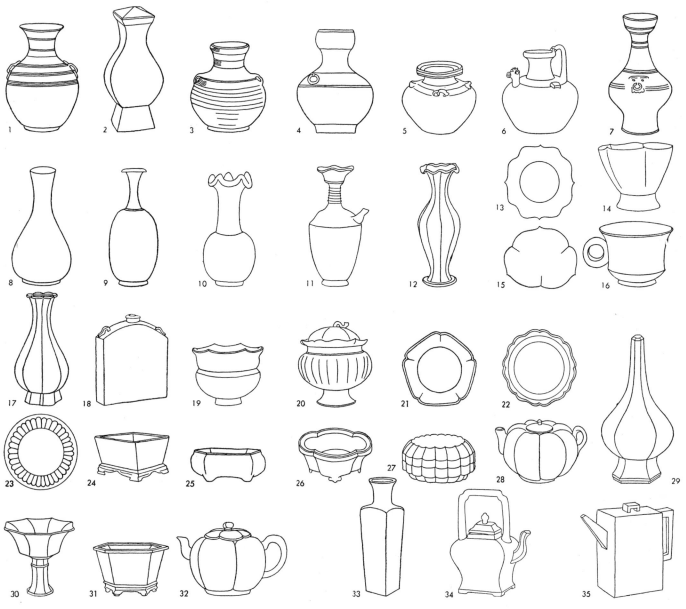

Typical forms of Chinese ceramics, Han to Ch'ing periods: (1–7) 3d cent. B.C.–6th cent. of Christian era; (8–16) T'ang period (618–906); (17–28) Sung period (960–1279); (29–32) Ming period (1368–1644); (33–35) Ch'ing period (1644–1912) (*from T. Dexel, Die Formen chinesischer Keramik, Tübingen, 1955*).

stoneware, rather heavily potted and covered with a flocculent blue glaze, often rather full of bubbles. There are often partings and marks in red, produced by brushing traces of copper on the body before glazing. The blue is due to the presence of iron in the glaze.

A special kind of Chün-yao, evidently made in reducing air, is green — a characteristic walnut-skin color due to ferrous oxide. These pieces are often of superior quality, glazed all over, and show the traces on the base of the four, five, or six "spurs" that supported them in the kiln. But the glaze is dense and opaque, and therefore quite different from that of the most distinguished member of the group, convincingly identified by Sir Percival David as examples of the classic Ju-yao, imperial ware of the best years of Northern Sung before the capture of the emperor Hui-sung by the Tartars and the flight to the south in 1127. The Ju pieces (PL. 166) are more finely potted and generally have a slightly splayed and delicately formed foot, which was supported in the kiln by spurs, generally four in number, that left traces like sesame seeds in the glaze. On some small pieces, however, there are only three such spur marks, and one cup stand at least is without them. Shapes are generally purely ceramic and even when they derive from silver models, they sometimes echo Ting-yao shapes (e.g., the paper-beater vase formerly in the Chinese Imperial Collection in Peking and the Clark bottle). Ting-yao is said by Lu Yü to have been superseded for imperial use by Ju-yao because of the scratches in the Ting glaze. This view is also implied by Hsü Ching's report on Korean celadons (1124), which are said to have been mainly copied from Ting shapes but are also like the new Ju wares. Ju-yao is a buff or pinkish-yellow stoneware with a rather soft body and dense greenish-blue glaze, smooth but not wholly opaque, sometimes but not always crackled. Only 30 pieces are known to survive, but if the evidence of an inscribed trial ring in the Percival David Foundation of Chinese Art is accepted, the kiln was opened only in 1107 and so had a life of not more than 20 years. Ju-yao was not imitated during the Southern Sung period (1127–1279) or later. The only wares which approach its quality are some of the Korean celadons (see KOREAN ART).

The other official (kuan) wares of the Northern Sung have not been conclusively identified. Two varieties are distinguished: Tung-yao, of which there remain rare examples of uncertain authenticity, was made for the court of the Later Liang dynasty (907–22) in the premises of the palace at Kaifeng, the winter or eastern (tung) capital. Ch'ai-yao, reputed to have been made at Chêng-chou in Honan in the mid-10th century for one of the emperors of the Five Dynasties period, is even less known than Tung-yao, and its identification with a fine celadon ware regarded as a northern kuan product is problematical.

Two other types of ware undoubtedly made during the Northern Sung period in a number of different areas remain to be mentioned. These are the black-glazed wares and the wares with pale blue glazes descriptively known as ch'ing-pai ("blue-white") or ying-ch'ing ("misty blue"). It seems likely that the black glazed ware was developed especially for tea drinking: certainly the earliest kiln near Chien-ning in northern Fukien specialized in tea bowls. Thousands of wasters were found on a kiln site 30 miles north of the city by J. M. Plumer in 1935, and it was from this coast that the wares were exported to Japan in large quantities. They apparently took their Japanese name of temmoku from a mountain near Hangchow, which was the port of shipment. Chien bowls (PL. 167) have a dark body, nearly purple where exposed, and a very thick viscous glaze. The main color ranges from a very dark blue to a dark brown but is hardly ever uniform, the iron having oxidized in streaks or patches. The glaze is usually full of bubbles, and if these have burst in the kiln, the surface shows a constellation of silvery markings producing the "oil-spot" effect. The foot is well formed and usually bare, and the glaze has frequently parted from the lip, which is therefore sheathed in copper or, more rarely, silver.

Before the end of Northern Sung this black glaze was imitated in the north. The more common imitation was a pottery — made especially in Honan, but also in Hopei —

whose glaze was thinner and better controlled, so that it was possible to regulate the rust-colored markings where the iron had oxidized through the local application of a fluxing agent. The shapes are usually not unlike those of other northern wares, especially Ting-chou and Tz'ŭ-chou, and may well have been produced in the same kiln centers (PL. 169).

Black ware was also made near Ch'i-chou in the province of Kiangsi, which was to become the greatest ceramics factory district. The light gray body was more thinly glazed than the Chien type; special attention was given to pattern, which sometimes took the form of flowers or tortoise-shell markings or even of Chinese written characters. A charming effect was produced by laying a natural leaf inside a bowl: it served as a fluxing agent and left its ghostly outline in the glaze.

In Kiangsi was found the largest center of kilns producing the high-fired ware ch'ing-pai. Great mounds of kiln waste have been found at Hu-t'ien, near the later ceramic metropolis of Ching-tê-chên. It is not known when production started here, but probably not before the 12th century. It continued into the early Ming period. A similar ware was also made in southern China from the beginning of the 14th century. The body of ch'ing-pai is more sugary in appearance and coagulative in structure than the other early porcelains, and it consequently permits a sharper finish and more intricate forms. This is seen both in shape, where lips and foot rims are thinner and perforation possible, and in decoration, as in the small covered boxes, often of flower shape. Some pieces continue the Yüeh tradition with dragons carved inside bowls or allover flower scrolls on the high-shouldered vase (mei-p'ing). Others again show combed designs akin to Ting, but the foot rims are higher and thinner, and the execution less refined and less carefully finished.

In the south the ceramic industry flourished in Chekiang, near the capital Hangchow, during the period of Southern Sung (1127–1279). At Chiao-t'an ("Suburban Altar") the kiln — one devoted to palace production — has been identified and wasters have been recovered, from which it is possible to identify many pieces. The leading characteristics of this ware are the thiness of the body and the even density of the glaze, which was applied in successive coats, each coat being allowed to dry before the next one was applied. The variety of color and decoration is much reduced, ranging from a watery green to a deep violet-blue, and the glaze is partly translucent and often crackled, an effect admired at the time. Bronze and jade shapes were imitated. The lines are less marked and the several parts — neck, handles, lip — less sharply differentiated. This was in accord with contemporary taste, which valued above all the smooth, opalescent, jadelike glaze, in which some lime in suspense gave an added quality of mystery, while closely fitting the form of the vessel. Corresponding to these palace wares and hardly less beautiful are other types of celadon made in Chekiang, especially that from Lung-ch'üan. It has a light gray body which, being ferruginous, burns orange-red where exposed; its glaze is very smooth, dense, close-fitting, and generally uncrackled. This ware won a high reputation wherever it was carried throughout Asia and North Africa and was largely exported until the early Ming period, when the kilns were transferred to Ch'ü-chou, farther north in the same province. Two special types have been highly valued in Japan, a shouldered vase of paper-beater or mallet form (kinuta), and a spotted kind (tobi), made by local application of excess iron or fluxing agent. These are rare, but many thousands of fragments of other wares from these kilns have have been found on the beaches of Japan, testifying to the volume of imports in the 12th and 13th centuries; the political hostility to the Mongols after 1280, however, put an end to importation.

g. Yüan period (1260–1368). Although the Mongols had no ceramic tradition of their own, their widespread empire developed or opened up trade routes across Asia and made possible the exchange of ideas and merchandise between China and Iran, Tibet and India, and renewed contacts in southeastern Asia and the Indian Ocean. Most notable in ceramic history was the introduction of pure cobalt ore (Mohammedan blue) together with the idea of painting designs under the glaze.

Marks and symbols on Chinese ceramics. (*A*) Reign marks of the Ming dynasty: (1) Hung-wu (1368–98); (2, 3) Yung-lo (1403–24); (4, 5) Hsüan-tê (1426–35); (6–8) Ch'êng-hua (1465–87); (9) Hung-chih (1485–1505); (10) Chêng-tê (1506–21); (11) Chia-ching (1522–66); (12) Lung-ch'ing (1567–72); (13) Wan-li (1573–1619); (14) T'ien-ch'i (1621–27); (15) Ch'ung-chêng (1628–43). (*B*) Reign marks of the Ch'ing dynasty: (1, 2) Shun-chih (1644–61); (3, 4) K'ang-hsi (1662–1722); (5, 6) Yung-chêng (1723–35); (7–9) Ch'ien-lung (1736–95); (10, 11) Chia-ch'ing (1796–1820); (12, 13) Tao-kuang (1821–50); (14, 15) Hsien-fêng (1851–61); (16, 17) T'ung-chih (1862–74); (18, 19) Kuang-hsü (1875–1908). (*C*) Symbols and emblems: (1) Swastika (*wan*); (2) incense burner (*ting*); (3) one of the "12 ornaments" (*fu*); (4) lotus (*lien hua*); (5) palm leaf (*chiao yeh*); (6) "fungus of immortality" (*ling chih*); (7) prunus (*mei hua*); (8) hare (*t'a*). (*D*) Probable marks of merchants and workshops: (1) mark, perhaps of a European merchant, on *famille-verte* and blue-and-white wares; (2) mark on blue-and-white ware; (3, 4) marks, perhaps of workshops, formed by indecipherable characters that appear to have been invented on late Ming and Ch'ing export wares.

Analysis has shown that the blue of the earliest Chinese blue-and-white has the same impurities as the cobalt ore of Iran. These beginnings cannot be closely dated but are unlikely to have occurred before or much after 1300.

The only officially sponsored ware under the Yüan was the *shu-fu* (a term meaning "central palace," and hence "privy council"). This ware is transitional between the *ch'ing-pai* and the blue-and-white. It has a hard white body covered by a smooth slightly bluish-white glaze, and decoration consists of the characters *shu fu* or others expressing wishes for long life and prosperity, among floral scrolls in slip under the glaze. There may also be some combed ornament on the outer surface. This ware was probably made near Ching-tê-chên, but wasters have not yet been found at these kilns. All these types must be placed in the first half of the 14th century.

The next secure date is 1351, which occurs in identical inscriptions on two tall vases decorated with dragons and phoenixes among clouds and with symbols of auspicious objects around the high and hollow base (Percival David Foundation of Chinese Art). Both potting and design are accomplished, and these vases have now been shown to serve as a center of a group of some hundred examples, much the greater number of which have been preserved in the old Ottoman imperial collection in the Topkapi Palace in Istanbul, or in the gift presented to the shrine of Sheikh Safi at Ardebil in 1612 by Shah Abbas I the Great of Persia (now transferred to the Teheran Museum). They are decorated with a wide range of floral, animal, bird, and fish subjects, and the dishes often have scalloped edges with a wave design, all entirely Chinese and owing nothing to Western influence. Nearly all the shapes too are Chinese, including the plum-blossom (prunus) vase (*mei-p'ing*), double-gourd vases, and jars. The only Western shape is a form of the pilgrim flask. Chinese blue-and-white vessels are depicted in Persian miniatures from the end of the 14th century.

Throughout the 14th century the northern kilns continued to make black-glazed wares, Chün types, and the Tz'ŭ-chou stoneware. The only innovation here occurred during the 13th century, when overglaze enamels were first applied to some smaller Tz'ŭ-chou pieces; but the green, red, and yellow enamels are seldom successfully fired, while the decoration is of the simplest. Overglaze enamels were not taken any farther until the 15th century. Experiments were also made with copper red in underglaze decoration exactly parallel to the early blue-and-white. Copper proved more difficult to control, and the desired red color was seldom fully achieved.

*h. Ming period (1368–1644).* During this period came the development of a great ceramic industry in Kiangsi around Ching-tê-chên and the establishment there of an imperial factory. This district was favored with an abundant supply of kaolin and petuntse, the two ingredients of the very hard translucent white porcelain and the brilliant clear glaze. But the very success of these factories led to the decline of the celadons and other surviving Sung wares. The only factories still competing with Kiangsi at the end of the period were in the south, in Fukien around Tê-hua, where cream-glazed porcelain figurines were developed as the specialty of a considerable industry; and in Kwangtung, where several heavier and coarser types were made for both domestic use and export.

The basic product of the Ching-tê-chên industry at all times was underglaze blue-and-white, but it appears that the earliest imperial wares were the plain white pieces of the Yung-lo period (1403–24), the so-called "bodiless" (*t'o-t'ai*) porcelain; these had decoration either in slip or incised designs with dragons or phoenixes and with incised marks under the glaze, all so difficult to distinguish, except by transmitted light, that Chinese connoisseurs refer to it as *an-hua* or "secret decoration." Meanwhile the blue decoration had been improved, and in the reign of Hsüan-tê (1426–35) it was ordered for the palace and received the imperial mark on vessels and dishes of superlative quality, decorated in refined taste with subjects that were similar to those of the earlier wares but more sparingly and discreetly used (PL. 280). The mark of this classic reign was used on later replicas of imperial quality and also on copies made in later centuries for collectors. The imperial factory was closed from 1435 until the Ch'êng-hua period (1465–87), and it is hard to identify any wares made in the interregnum. The Ch'êng-hua imperial wares were much less varied than the early-15th-century types; they are decorated in a paler blue and less firmly handled, but they include new types of great elegance, especially the small "palace" bowls, decorated with fruit or flowers, and the small wine cups. No doubt production of ordinary blue-and-white continued on a large scale throughout the century, though foreign trade declined because of restrictions on Chinese merchants' going abroad.

Monochrome-glazed wares were also made at Ching-tê-chên, especially copper red and turquoise at the beginning of the century and imperial yellow from the Hsüan-tê period onward. Copper red was also used at this time, in conjunction with underglaze blue and also alone in isolated motifs of fish or peaches on small white pieces. Yellow enamel was also used to wash in the background of some pieces previously decorated in blue under the glaze (PL. 168). Other overglaze enamels, often in addition to a blue outline, began to be used in the 15th century, at first sparingly; the earliest were green and iron red; turquoise and yellow were added in the Ch'êng-hua period. A characteristic style of this period, called *tou-t'sai* or "contending colors," was used to enhance a design carried out in blue with an effect quite different from that obtained later by allover enamel decoration, when the ground was also enamel, or by picking designs of dragons or clouds out of the enamel. Another way of using colored enamels is known as *san-t'sai* or "three-color," in which the designs were outlined with threads of clay, like the cloisonné of enamel on metal. The glazes of lead silicate in turquoise, dark blue, manganese purple, and yellow were fired at a medium temperature. It is not known where this type was made or when production started: no pieces bear dates earlier than the reign of Chêng-tê (1506–21), but they are reputed to have been made from the later 15th century. Bulb bowls, large vases, and garden seats of barrel shape are typical products.

In the 16th century underglaze blue remained the largest product. In the Chêng-tê period special pieces of fine quality with Arabic and Persian inscriptions were made for the Mohammedan eunuchs, who were powerful in the administration. The Chia-ching period (1522–66) was remarkable for the depth and brilliance of the blue from the pure imported cobalt. Orders for the palace at this time were on an enormous scale, from 30,000 to 100,000 pieces in a single year. Such porcelains continued to be used in later reigns, as was shown when the large fish bowls found in the tomb of the emperor Wan-li (d. 1619), opened in 1958, proved to be of this period (*ILN*, no. 6253, Apr. 11, 1959, pp. 616–17). By this date the imperial resources had declined so far that the best wares were being made for private clients, who preferred a more individual and painterly style of decoration. It is the beauty of the drawing which gives the blue-and-white of the first half of the 17th century, known as the "transition period," a special place in Chinese ceramics. The later Ming enameled works are richly decorative, excelling in a brocade effect on a colored ground or in a combination of bright enamels with underglaze blue outline on the white ground. Blue-and-white made for export at several provincial centers began to appear in the European market from the late 16th century on. One other late Ming factory made pottery in Chinese taste, but nonetheless exported large quantities to Europe in the 17th century: that of Yi-shing at Yang-hsien in Kiangsu province, near Soochow. Here teapots were made in a red or buff stoneware with mat or low-gloss surface in shapes often copied from natural objects, such as bamboo or gourd, but also plain except for the poems inscribed in the clay with a stylus. The Yi-shing ware was imitated in several European centers in the early 18th century, most notably by Böttger at Meissen, but earlier in Holland and England.

*i. Ch'ing period (1644–1912).* In the first half of the 18th century fine wares continued to be made for the imperial palace.

Blue-and-white remained the largest export, but enameled wares, growing in popularity, finally ousted it from first place.

It is characteristic of the K'ang-hsi (1662–1722) style of decoration that it covers the whole surface of a dish or vessel, a principle already established in 1672. Tsang Ying-hsüan, (under whose direction the factory at Ching-tê-chên, destroyed by rebel forces in 1675, was reconstructed in 1683) improved the quality of both the body and the blue, which is unrivaled for its brilliance and luminosity; also he introduced mass-production methods and division of labor, so that a single piece might pass through 70 hands before firing. The interest of the Emperor in European science, including perspective, is reflected in the decoration of the porcelains — as can be seen in the dishes traditionally called "birthday plates," and believed to derive from a great service ordered in honor of K'ang-hsi's birthday, in 1713. The borders are of coral color obtained with iron red, while the field is decorated with slightly modeled human figures or birds. Another red introduced at this time at the imperial factory was rose pink, made from gold chloride, an invention of a Netherlander, Andreas Cassius, about 1650. First considered a foreign color (*yang-t'sai*), it was not employed on porcelain before about 1720. In the reign of Yung-chêng (1723–35) the most beautiful and characteristic use of this pink was as a monochrome on the underside of saucer dishes, contrasting effectively with the many-colored, finely drawn pictorial decoration of the front. These two types of enameled porcelain were given in 19th-century France the names of *famille verte* and *famille rose* (PLS. 289, 297).

Another type highly valued in the West 50 or 75 years ago is the *famille noire*, in which the background is covered with a brownish-black pigment of cobalt and manganese, overlaid by a thin greenish enamel (PL. 170). Although most examples of this ware were no doubt made in the 19th century, the type probably originated under K'ang-hsi, when there was a much better black glaze, known as "mirror black," a jet black monochrome with a lustrous tone (PL. 298). Much more important were the monochromes with colored glazes derived from copper, of which the most famous is *lang-yao*, the oxblood-colored glaze, deep and luminous, which demanded great skill from the potter in regulating the draft in the kiln, since the main firing had to be done in a reducing atmosphere but had to conclude with a strong oxidizing period, during which the outer and thinner glaze was bleached and only particles of copper remained in the lower strata. If this oxidizing process was carried farther, bleaching continued and greenish specks appeared; the finished glaze is known as "peach bloom." Because of the difficulty of achieving this glaze, it is found mainly on smaller pieces intended for the writing table, while the *lang* wares are often large vases.

Finally mention must be made of a special type of enamel ware reputed to have been developed under the auspices of the imperial palace in Peking during the K'ang-hsi period and in use until the mid-18th century. Whatever the origin of this ware (called *kiu-yüeh*), it is obvious that it is a refined white porcelain, very thin and translucent and decorated in a semi-European style, though evidently rare and not intended for export. The suggestion that it was produced under the direction of one or another of the French and Italian Jesuits established in the palace is supported by the brocade designs in French taste covering the ground of some pieces of the landscape in the modified Chinese style associated with the Italian Giuseppe Castiglione (1698–1766), who took the Chinese name of Lang Shih-ning.

Basil GRAY

*Japan. a. Jōmon period.* The high esthetic and technical quality of Japanese pottery and porcelain has secured them an eminence comparable only to that of Chinese ceramics. At intervals progress was stimulated by the effort to reproduce Chinese and Korean wares, but the product was individual. Particularly through its association during the last four centuries with the quasi-religious estheticism of the tea ceremony, pottery has enjoyed a special cult. In Japan taste inclined toward pottery — toward recognition of the diverse qualities of partic-

ular kilns, awareness of the material and its touch to the hand, appreciation of the work of individual potters (PL. 172).

The earliest pottery found in Japan is the Jōmon ware of the Neolithic period (see above: *Protohistoric "ceramic cultures"*...; see also ASIATIC PROTOHISTORY), extending from an unknown antiquity until about the 2d century B.C. It is thick, poorly fired coarse ware, handmade (often by coiling strips) and generally covered with the impressions of a toothed stamp or of cord wound on a stick (II, PL. 16). It belongs to a primitive tradition extending across northern Asia, represented in northern Europe in the Neolithic and the Early Bronze Age; but peculiar to Japan is the elaborateness of its ornament. Urns with small flat bottoms or on pedestals are the dominant shapes. Specially ornate, spouted vessels are among its latest and most exotic creations.

*b. Yayoi culture.* The pottery of the Yayoi culture, which succeeded the Jōmon and spread through habitable Japan in the period from 200 B.C. to about A.D. 250, is totally different: light red in color, wheel-turned, almost entirely free of plastic encumbrance, the ornament being confined to cord-impressed and incised chevrons, triangles, etc.; the chief shapes are an urn with a tall flaring neck and a *tazza* on a tall foot (PL. 171). Although pottery of this kind is not clearly recognizable on the continent, the presence in southwestern Japan of bronze weapons and bells (the *dōtaku*), deriving ultimately from Chinese models, shows that influences reaching Japan via Korea were decisive factors in molding Yayoi culture, and it is likely that in germ at least the potter's methods came from the same quarter (II, PL. 16).

*c. Tumulus period.* The Yayoi tradition continued into the earlier part of the Tumulus period (mid-3d–mid-6th cent.), during which the Japanese state took shape and its leaders came to be buried in the vast and often richly furnished mausoleums from which the period takes its name. The vessels show a simplification of shapes, some degeneration of the paste, and an unexplained substitution of round bases for the earlier flat ones.

In this later stage the ware is termed "Haji" from the name of the "guild" of potters mentioned in the Japanese dynastic annals. In the latter part of the Tumulus period, however, perhaps from about 400, an important technical advance was made, the introduction of the climbing-passage kiln (*noborigama*). Hitherto pottery had been fired on an open hearth or in a shallow covered pit with flue. The climbing-passage kiln, exactly resembling the form in use contemporaneously in Korea, was a short tunnel excavated on a hillside about 15 to 35 ft. long, inclined upward from the mouth at a slope seldom exceeding 15°, with a flue at the upper end. In later times the passage was subdivided. In principle the Japanese kiln has not changed to the present day. The so-called "Sue ware" (formerly called "Iwaibe") of the Tumulus period technically and stylistically is a simple transplantation of a Korean tradition, from whose products it is often hard to distinguish. It is thin, gray, wheel-made, fired at about 1000°C, in hardness ranking as stoneware.

Another important result of the new kiln was the formation of a feldspathic "kiln glaze" on the shoulder and upper part of the Sue vessels. The Yayoi-Haji tradition survived alongside the Sue. The famous *haniwa*, primitive and vigorous figures of warriors, servants, and animals are modeled in red earthenware resembling this pottery; they were buried on the perimeter of the burial mounds and inside them.

*d. Nara and Heian periods.* The history of Japanese ceramics during the Nara (A.D. 645–793) and Heian (A.D. 784–1185) periods is still little known. The chief evidence for the former period is provided by the vessels stored in the Shōsōin of the Tōdaiji Temple in Nara. They are part of a treasure dedicated in perpetuity by the widow of the emperor Shōmu in 786 and were probably used in ceremonies following his death. Most important are the "three-color wares." Of these vessels only five (two bowls, a cup, a drum body, and a model of a pagoda) are actually glazed in the three colors, green, white, and yellow; of the rest, 35 are white and green, 13 green, 3 brown, and 1 white. The colors are in low-fired lead glaze, green predomi-

nating over the irregular mottling of white and yellow when these colors are present. The paste is buff and somewhat softer than stoneware. It was long debated whether this pottery could be Japanese or an import from T'ang China. The argument for China at first seemed strengthened by the apparent absence of the ware outside the Shōsōin, but recent discoveries on temple sites in Kyoto, Nara, and Otsu and kilns near Kyoto have shown that it was in general use in the district around the imperial capital. The greater part of it however, was glazed in green only. It is possible that the manufacture of this ware, and with it the introduction of a soft lead glaze, was first in the hands of Chinese immigrants.

Certainly the soft-glaze tradition was entirely extinct before the end of the Heian period (PL. 171). The future lay rather with the hard feldspathic glaze — the "ash glaze" of Japanese writers. At some date unknown, but thought to be only a little later than the Shōsōin three-color ware, means were found to apply deliberately and to the whole surface of a vessel an even glaze resembling the irregular "kiln glaze" already present on some vessels of the Sue period. Ten "medicine jars" (covered vases) stored in the Shōsōin, of characteristic Buddhist shape, have still the grayish-green accidental glaze on the shoulders and a gray body of Sue type. The deliberate ash glaze varied in color from green to light brown. It was used at kilns in the Mino and Owari districts of Gifu Ken (ken signifies "prefecture"), mainly on small plates and bowls. The plain shallow bowls achieved fame later with tea masters as "mountain (i.e., rustic) tea bowls" — yamachawan — though it is doubtful if that was their original use. With the decline of the temple patronage that potters in western Japan had experienced in the lavish days of the Nara and Early Heian periods, the production of the green-glazed wares of both kinds declined. Lacquered wooden vessels were coming increasingly into use.

The wares at the so-called "six ancient kilns of Japan" were intended merely to meet the needs of their peasant users. The kilns have many traits in common, all making as their stock form tall storage jars up to 2 ft. in height, in a coarse, dark red, gritty ware, seldom with any suggestion of deliberate glazing and devoid of ornament. Such wares had a rustic beauty and an uncompromising presentation of their material that appealed to the cultivated puritanism of tea masters from the 16th century onward. The Tokonabe group in the Chita peninsula in Aichi Ken numbered over a hundred kilns. Their jars have a narrow foot, a high, relatively sharp shoulder, tall neck, and molded lip. The body is generally composed of several turned segments. The surface is hand-smoothed, fragments of the grits projecting in places. Besides the jars a few bottle shapes were made, as well as tiles and the shallow yamachawan, these last also frequently covered with the olive-colored glaze. Decoration consists only of three sets of horizontal grooved cordons on the jars ("three-groove jars") and a variety of repeated stamped marks following the edges of the segments of the body and placed there to seal the joins; the marks are simple geometric figures or characters. The kilns were active in the later Heian and the Kamakura periods (ca. 11th–14th cent.). Tokonabe jars are the kind most frequently found in the "sutra mounds," in which they were buried; they contained Buddhist texts, some of which are dated.

Wares analogous to those of the Tokonabe kilns were made in Fukui Ken of Echizen province, in the Tamba region of Hyogo Ken, in Shiga Ken (Shigaraki ware), and Okayama Ken (Bizen ware). Bizen ware acquired a smoother, dark red surface. Its tradition of strong, simple potting continued to modern times. Its cylindrical vases, gourd-shaped bottles, water jars, and handled trays in the 16th and 17th centuries enjoyed special favor with the tea masters. The tea caddies of Tamba were prized.

The most varied and promising wares however, were those from Seto, in Owari province, the most important of the ancient ceramic centers, where the tradition of wood-ash glazing persisted from early times. From the 11th century green-glazed bowls and dishes with a foot rim were made in imitation of Chinese celadon (Owari celadon); after a period of decline caused by civil disturbance, the activity of the Seto kilns began again in the second half of the 13th century. The effort to copy Chinese wares continued. The addition of iron to the constituents of the ash glaze produced an allover glaze in two varieties: one varying from light yellow to apple green with a tendency to flake away from the body, and another dark brown and adhering closely. These glazes were applied to tall vases with high shoulders and narrow mouth — the most characteristic products of the Kamakura age at Seto — modeled on the mei-p'ing form of Sung China. Bottles with narrower shoulders and breadth toward the bottom, or with vertical neck and outturned wavy lip, also copy Sung forms. Floral decoration in flowing scrolls was incised in the paste before the application of the glaze or stamped in separate units. The darker glaze is often irregular, appearing translucent or opaque according to its thickness, and variegating the surface with the interplay of the glaze and the incised pattern underlying it. These handsome jars mark the climax of the older tradition of Japanese potting. Their debt to Chinese models is superficial: the attempt at a sophisticated ornament does not diminish an engaging rusticity quite Japanese in feeling. The same glaze and technique of grooved or incised ornament are found in small lidded bowls used as tea caddies. In the same ware there are figures of lions, probably made, like many of the vessels, to furnish temples. By the beginning of the 14th century the quality of the large vases declined and the kilns stagnated.

*e. Seto group.* About 1500 the requirements of the tea cult first made themselves felt at Seto, and the kilns rose again to a new level of prosperity and intense activity, which has lasted to modern times. The term seto-mono became colloquially equivalent to pottery itself. Kilns now regarded as belonging to the Seto group were founded in the neighborhood of Kujiri in Mino province, a short distance from Seto. The passage kiln was enlarged. New amber and yellow glazes are found in use at both the Seto and the Mino kilns, the most popular of these being a thin, lusterless variety with a surface rough to the touch, like a salt glaze. The simple floral decoration associated with the thin glaze is incised and often covered with a splash of green derived from iron or copper. Tea bowls, small covered boxes, and saucerlike dishes are the commonest forms found in this Ki-seto (yellow Seto) ware. In shape Ki-seto tea bowls either follow the shallow earlier type of the yamachawan or have vertical sides with a slight offset at the center. The elegance of the latter shape seems to owe nothing to foreign models, but the tea bowls for which Seto became famous from the 15th century (and which were copied in other parts of the country) are a frank attempt to reproduce the Chinese tea bowls of Chien ware. Known in Japan as temmoku, these were being imported in large quantities from ports on the Fukien coast. The Seto shape closely follows the Chinese, even to the precise bevel of the foot rim; but the habit of scraping the part of the side just above the base with a knife after turning on the wheel is a Japanese peculiarity. The Seto potters failed to reproduce the "hare's fur" and "oil-spot" variegation found in the Chinese glaze and were content to imitate it rather remotely by applying two layers of glaze, of lighter and darker brown color, achieving a pretty effect of their own. A "temmoku ordering house" was opened in Kyoto in the 16th century to meet the demand for the ware in tea ceremony.

The celebrated tea master Senno Rikyu is said to have prized some of the Seto ware in the earlier 16th century. By the end of that century the tea masters and their powerful devotees in army and government had become the chief arbiters of ceramic taste in both central Japan and Kyushu. In particular their influence was predominant at the Mino kilns, where in the last quarter of the 16th century two famous wares were invented, later named after the tea masters Shino Soshin and Furuta Oribe (late 16th–early 17th cent.). The characteristic glaze of Shino ware is thick, viscous-looking, translucent, clouded white in color, with a tendency to produce large bubble pits or craquelure on the surface. It is feldspathic and hard, but with a softly lustrous surface. A red tinge appears where the glaze runs thin. Figured decoration is executed in brown

under a more transparent glaze or incised through a brown underglaze slip to reveal the white paste, the slip turning the white glaze to a light gray (Nezumi-shino). The use of a reddish paste under the same translucent glaze produced the brownish-red Aka-shino. The tea bowls assumed what was henceforward to be a characteristic Japanese shape: a cylindrical form $2^1/_2$ to 4 in. high, with vertical sides. The glaze stops short of the foot. The thick sides, irregular lip and profile, and even the foot have all the appearance of manufacture by hand, although the first shaping was on the wheel. Oribe ware delights in light and bluish greens achieved by adding copper to the feldspathic glaze. The green is used alone, to cover incised decoration or to fill the spaces around a design painted in iron brown, when the whole is finally covered with a hard, transparent white glaze. The principal Shino forms are tea bowls, water jars, and simple trays and dishes. Oribe forms are more varied: trays in the shape of baskets or fans, animal-shaped incense burners, and even figurines of Dutchmen. The molded pieces often have a surface marked by the weave of a textile which was placed between the form and the clay. Besides floral decoration, Oribe ware makes use of quasi-abstract geometric shapes, inspired in many cases by brocaded and woven textiles. Rendered in limpid colors of glaze and clay, such pieces achieve the richest decorative effect ever produced by the application of glazes on a relatively soft body. The absence of craquelure enhances their pristine freshness.

*f. Karatsu ceramics.* Second only to Seto as a great pottery center is Saga Ken in Kyushu, the former Hizen province, where productivity continued into modern times. Its principal ware is called "Karatsu," after the town where the products of the widely scattered kilns were gathered for sale. Karatsu ware must date back no farther than the last decade or two of the 16th century, having been introduced at that time by Korean potters brought to Japan in the train of Hideyoshi's expeditionary armies. The form of passage kiln and the fast, foot-turned wheel brought into use were of the latest Korean type. The commonest Karatsu, particularly in the earlier period, is decorated with iron-oxide pigment beneath a thin colorless or whitish glaze, generally with a fine craquelure, in a manner closely resembling the corresponding ware of Mino. Milk-white and dark brown opaque glazes, both feldspathic, were soon introduced, and in combination with different clays, they were used to produce red- and black-surfaced pottery, again in imitation of the Mino kilns. The brushed surface called *hake-me* and the inlay of small decorative motifs in white on a darker ground, termed *mishima*, are Korean techniques inherited by the Karatsu potters. Like the Mino and Seto pottery, the products of the Karatsu kilns enjoyed great popularity with the tea masters. Besides a variety of tea-bowl shapes, including both the Korean and Japanese types, Karatsu wares comprise tea-jars, bowls, water jars, flower vases, and plates, all of which could find a place in the tea ceremony. The deliberate distortion of shapes, after turning them on the wheel, by denting the side or bending the lip is as common in Karatsu as in the products of Mino.

Other Kyushu kilns worked in the same technical and artistic tradition as the Karatsu potters, producing individual wares in a narrower range. In Fukuoka Ken the Takatori kilns, famous for their tea caddies, favored a thick glaze of yellow or amber diversified with splashes of white; at Agano white spots were scattered on a copper green ground of glaze. The kilns of Kagoshima Ken produced wares collectively termed "Satsuma," making much use of the white opaque glaze. The *dakatsu* ("serpent's skin") glaze of white over black was the specialty of the Ryumonji and Tateno kilns of the Satsuma group. White, amber, and black glazes were applied to tea bowls, the white sometimes decorated with simple designs in brown iron paint. Later the Tateno kiln, copying a Kyoto fashion, adopted the "brocaded" style, decorating in low-fired colored glazes over the hard white glaze. The activity of the Kyushu kilns continued from their founding in the late 16th or the 17th until the 19th century, and some of them survive in pottery production until the present time. From the 17th century on-

ward the esthetics of the tea cult, the guild tradition, and the attention of men of outstanding artistic gifts combined to make of pottery an individual art.

INDIVIDUAL POTTERS. *The raku masters*: *Tanaka Chōjirō*, son of a Korean or Chinese potter, founded the celebrated line of the raku masters in Kyoto between 1570 and 1590. His tea bowls, favored and established by the tea master Senno Rikyu, represent the Japanese form par excellence. They are handmade, with thick vertical walls, simple vertical rim, hand-smoothed and slightly irregular; the foot rim is about one-third of the width of the mouth; the black lead-glazed surface is slightly dimpled, of a leathery appearance, gleaming but not glassy. The porosity of the ware makes it a nonconductor of heat, as befits tea bowls. The forms are balanced without being geometrically exact. The main surviving work of Chōjirō consists of seven bowls certified (as was the practice) by inscriptions on their boxes by Rikyu himself. His only signed piece now surviving is a lively lion intended for a ridge tile. After his death in 1592 Chōjirō was succeded by his son (or younger brother) *Jōkei*, who had bestowed on him by Hideyoshi the privilege of marking his tea bowls with the character "raku." (Some, however, hold that the first to use the seal was the third master.) Little of Jokei's work is now identified, possibly because it is confounded with Chōjirō's. His bowls are said to be thicker and heavier. *Dōnyū* (also known as "Nonko"), the third master (1574-1656), is regarded as the greatest of the line. He made a greater variety of shapes in vases and censers and added a red glaze, sometimes decorating the surface of his bowls with combing. *Ichinyū* (d. 1696), the fourth and last of the "great raku masters," relied mainly on reproducing the style of the founder, adding as his own contribution a black glaze with red variegations. The 13th raku master died in 1945. The potters *Dōraku* (17th cent.), *Honami Kōetsu* (1558-1637), also a painter, and the latter's grandson *Honami Kūchū* (1601-82) are regarded as collaterals of the raku line. – *Nonomura Ninsei* is associated with all the tea ware other than raku manufactured in Kyoto and referred to as "Kyo." Born in Tamba province toward the end of the 16th century, he is said to have received his early training from a Korean potter. Toward 1650 he is found active as a potter in Kyoto, residing near the Ninnaji Temple (from which he takes the first syllable of his artist's name, Ninsei). Before his arrival tea ware manufactured in the capital had been in the style of Seto, being in the hands of potters who had come from that center. Ninsei made tea bowls, water jars, tea caddies, the small boxes called *kōgō*, and censers, these last often in the shape of birds. He made lavish use of low-fired glazes, handling them as a painter, creating landscape, floral, and geometric designs in a range of bright, opaque colors. Light blue, with gold and silver, and bright colors over a dark brown ground were favorite combinations. He imitated lacquer work, raising the forms into low relief. His effects are sometimes cloying to Western eyes, but the technical virtuosity is astonishing. – *Ogata Kenzan* (see OGATA), brother of the painter Kōrin, was less experimental in his methods. His pottery resembles the grayish or cream-colored ware characteristic of the Awata kilns in the vicinity of Kyoto. The decoration consists mainly of summary painting with the brush in iron-oxide pigment, usually combined with brown and white slip. Kenzan's best work is associated with the period of his studio at Izumiya, near the capital. His painted figures and landscapes, often accompanied by poems in powerful calligraphy, appear mostly on square or oblong trays with sloping rims. His plates display a dreamlike medley of leaves and water, swaying curves and boatlike shapes, water wheels, and the like, executed in combinations of black, green, red, and blue, with the lightest possible touch. Many of the pieces were designed and executed with his brother Kōrin, to whom is perhaps due the decorative and allusive vein of the painting.

*g. Porcelain.* The introduction of porcelain into Japan is also a result of the settlement of Korean potters in Kyushu following Hideyoshi's campaigns (late 16th cent.). Although China had made porcelain for centuries before, the secret of its manufacture had not previously leaked out. But porcelain could not be made before China clay was available. This was discovered in 1616 at Izumiyama in Hizen province, by the Korean Ri Sampei. With the whole of his village of Korean potters, some 900 individuals, he moved to Sarayama, in the vicinity of Arita, near the source of the clay, and founded the industry which flourishes to the present day. The earliest Arita ware is white, clear-glazed, with decoration in cobalt blue under the glaze. Its simple linear and floral designs resemble those on contemporary Korean porcelain, but they are also not unlike contemporary provincial porcelain in China; influences from both quarters may be considered. Japanese

blue-and-white porcelain was exported by the Dutch from their factory at Nagasaki and in 1653 is recorded as appearing in the apothecaries' shops in Batavia. The decline of Chinese production at Ching-tê-chên between the advent of the Manchu dynasty and the reorganization of the kilns in the 1680s stimulated the demand for Japanese porcelain. A little after the opening of the Arita kilns others were founded at Mikawachi and exported from the port at Hirado. Hirado ware shared in the general improvement of paste and glaze in the mid-17th century and competed with Arita for the export trade.

The potter subsequently known as Kakiemon I, the founder of a line surviving until the present, is credited with the introduction in 1644 of the technique of enameling, whereby decoration in colored glazes was added over a hard glaze in a second firing. This innovation was probably in response to the demand by the Dutch traders and their European customers for colored ware like that formerly imported from China. The new colored porcelain — "five flasks with red and green painting" — is first recorded in the Batavian registers in 1659.

Much of the enameled porcelain was exported from the small port of Imari. This "Imari ware" is the "Old Japan" of the English 18th-century inventories. The majority of it, and the type to which the term "Imari" is now confined, was decorated with red enamels and gold together with underglaze blue. Sometimes there were touches of turquoise, leaf green, *aubergine*, or yellow enamels. The ornament commonly depicts flowers, figures, ships, etc. In Europe the excellence of the other two great divisions of Japanese colored porcelain, Kakiemon and Kutani, continues to be extolled. Indeed, both belong to the highest ceramic achievement.

The paste of the Arita porcelains is on the whole less white and less smooth than that of the Chinese ware of Ching-tê-chên. The variation in its quality reflects the individual standards of a multitude of small independent kilns. The glaze used in the 17th and 18th centuries is covered with minute holes. The paste of the high-grade wares made at the Kakiemon kiln is of a milk-white color, superbly smooth. The delicate potting is of a perfection hardly ever surpassed in the history of ceramics, the glaze smooth and flawless, the elegant painted ornament executed with consummate artistry. The chief Kakiemon enamels are a soft orange-red, grass green, and lilac blue; of less frequent occurrence are pale primrose yellow, turquoise green, gold, and occasionally underglaze blue. The painting is sensitively disposed on the white ground, of which it occupies only a small part. Its restraint is in utter contrast with the riot of Imari. Tradition claims that the Kakiemon potters were active from 1644, but the Japanese confess themselves unable to distinguish the work of the first three holders of the name, that is, of the founder and his two sons, whose products are never marked. A plausible hypothesis is that the typical refined Kakiemon was not perfected before the 1670s, since the paste and glaze made in the early decades following the discovery of kaolin in Japan cannot from the start have so far outstripped the Korean tradition in which its makers were trained. Enameled pieces of more primitive appearance, characterized by less perfect paste, a somewhat different range of lower-toned colors, and a freer, broader painting style, have been claimed to represent the earliest Kakiemon manner; but the grounds for doing so, or at least for attributing such pieces exclusively to the Kakiemon, are not satisfactory. Most probably earlier-looking enameled ware reflects the average product of a number of kilns, including the Arita group and Akaemachi.

Out of the same generalized early style of enameling of Hizen province arose the tradition of Kutani porcelain. Kilns were founded in the mid-17th century at Kutani Mura in Ishikawa (Kaga province, west Honshu) by a member of the Maeda family of hereditary feudatories. Their products were for the special use of the Maeda clan. A potter is said to have been dispatched to Arita to learn the art of porcelain and enameling. The earlier Kutani porcelains are remarkable for the power of their brush painting and the somber intensity of their palette of yellow, dark purple, and bluish green. The influences traceable in Kutani designs, apart from that of Arita, come possibly from the Shonzui blue-and-white porcelain (a ware supposedly of Chinese origin, though surviving only in Japan) and from the enameled Chinese ware of the T'ien-ch'i period (1621–27). A "red-enameled" style is distinguished from "green Kutani," the latter having only yellow, purple, and blue-green enamels, the last often forming the ground. The shapes cover the same range as Kakiemon: plates and trays, simple and double-gourd bottles, boxes, baskets, teapots. The decoration may be summed up as flowers, birds, landscape with figures, and geometric pattern and diapers taken from textiles. The early phase of the Kutani kilns ends, it is thought, in the late 1670s or 1680s. They were thereafter quiescent until revived by the Yoshida family for a short period from 1823, when reproductions of the old types were made in large quantities, to the confusion of some modern collectors.

Among the great 17th-century porcelain traditions remains that of the Nabeshima kilns. Noble feudatories of that name founded a factory at Okawachi, near Arita, in the early 18th century. Its products were reserved for the use of the Nabeshima clan, and only a relatively small quantity of the early pieces have found their way into modern collections. If anything, the paste is a little finer and a little harder than that of Kakiemon, the glaze flawless. The colors include a distinctive red and recall the tones and combinations found on Chinese *tou-t'sai* enamelled ware of the Ch'eng-hua period (1465–87). In ornament the Nabeshima potters were immensely inventive: flowers, fruit, birds, streams, palisades, bridges, mostly on a large scale, a single unit often filling the field. The stock shape is a plate raised on a ring foot, the latter often decorated with the "Nabeshima comb-tooth pattern." The enamel colors are regularly combined with design in underglaze blue. Sometimes outlines in blue under the glaze are doubled by an enamel line of red over it. Some use was made of tracing: the design drawn with "gourd charcoal" on thin paper being rubbed repeatedly on the dish in the biscuit state. For the past century Japan has been the world's largest exporter of porcelain. However banal the ornament applied to much of this factory product, its technical quality remains very high. In Japan itself pottery production by small kilns in family hands is still economically possible in Hizen, the Seto district, and Kyoto, but it is doubtful if it can continue much longer. Amateur and studio pottery flourishes, encouraged in part by the activities of the Folk Art Museum in Tokyo.

William WATSON

BIBLIOG. *General*: A. Brougniart, Traité des arts céramiques ou des poteries, 2 vols. and atlas, 3d ed., Paris, 1877; T. Kerl, Handbuch der gesamten Thonwaren-Industrie, Braunschweig, 1907; E. Hannover and B. Rackham, Pottery and Porcelain: A Handbook for Collectors, 3 vols., London, 1925; G. Ballardini, E. Bassani, and G. Giovannoni, EI, s.v. Ceramica; G. Liverani, Il museo delle ceramiche in Faenza, Rome, 1936; B. Rackham, A Key to Pottery and Glass, London, Glasgow, 1940; W. B. Honey, The Art of the Potter: A Book for the Collector and Connoisseur, London, 1946; A. Lane, Style in Pottery, London, 1948; M. Korach, Definizione tecnologica del termine ceramica, B. del Mus. Internazionale delle Ceramiche, XXXV, 1949, p. 118 ff.; W. B. Honey, European Ceramic Art from the End of the Middle Ages to about 1815: A Dictionary of Factories, Artists, Technical Terms, etc., London, 1952; T. Emiliani and G. Vecchi, Intorno ad una classificazione sistematica dei prodotti ceramici, B. del Mus. Internazionale delle Ceramiche, XXXIX, 1953, p. 187 ff.; T. Emiliani, La tecnologia della ceramica, Faenza, 1957.

*Protohistoric and primitive cultures*: L. Franchet, Céramique primitive: Introduction à l'étude de la technologie, Paris, 1911; G. Frankfort, Studies in Early Pottery of the Near East, Royal Anthropological Inst., Occasional Paper, VI, London, 1924; H. S. Harrison, Horniman Museum Handbooks: Evolution of the Domestic Arts, II, Baskets, Pottery, etc., 2d ed., London, 1924; T. A. Joyce and H. Braunholtz, Handbook to the Ethnological Collections, British Museum, 2d ed., London, 1925; H. S. Harrison, Pots and Pans: The History of Ceramics, London, 1928; A. O. Sheppard, Ceramics for the Archaeologist, Carnegie Institution, pub. 609, Washington, 1956; R. Pittioni, Zur Chronologie der Bronzezeit Mitteleuropas, ActaA, IX, 1958, p. 191 ff. *a. Africa*: R. Kandt, Gewerbe in Ruanda, ZfE, XXXVI, 1904; Annales du Musée du Congo, Ethnographie et anthropologie, La céramique, series III, vol. II, 1, 1907; W. S. and K. Routledge, With a Prehistoric People: The Akikuyu of British East Africa, London, 1910; F. Stuhlmann, Handwerk und Industrie in Ostafrika, Abh. des Hamburger Kolonialinstituts, X, 1910; N. W. Thomas, Pottery-making of the Edo-speaking Peoples, S. Nigeria, Man, X, 1910; A. J. N. Tremearne, Pottery in N. Nigeria, Man, X, 1910; P. A. Talbot, In the Shadow of the Bush, London, 1912; A. Eichhorn, Beiträge zur Kenntnis der Waschambaa, BA, II, III, 1913; G. Tessmann, Die Pangwe, 2 vols., Berlin, 1913; H. Meyer, Die Barundi, Leipzig, 1916; F. Staschewski, Die Banjangi, BA, VIII, 1917; G. K. Lindblom, The Akamba,

Stockholm, 1920; E. W. Smith and A. M. Dale, The Ila-speaking Peoples of N. Rhodesia, I, London, 1920; J. W. Crowfoot, Further Notes on Pottery (Nuba Tribes), SNR, VIII, 1925; P. A. Talbot, The Peoples of S. Nigeria, III, Oxford, 1926; R. S. Rattray, Religion and Art in Ashanti, Oxford, 1927; W. E. Nicholson, The Potters of Sokoto, N. Nigeria, Man, XXIX, 1929, XXXI, 1931; H. J. E. Peake and H. J. Braunholtz, Earthenware Figure from Nigeria in Newbury Museum, Man, XXIX, 1929; G. Caton-Thompson, The Zimbabwe Culture, London, 1931; Ling Roth, Unglazed Pottery from Abeokuta, Nigeria, Man, XXXI, 1931; J. W. Crowfoot, Pot-making in Dongola Province, Sudan, Man, XXXIII, 1933; T. P. O'Brien and S. Hastings, Pottery-making among the Bakonjo, Uganda, Man, XXXIII, 1933; E. J. Wayland, M. C. Burkitt, and H. J. Braunholtz, Archaeological Discoveries at Luzira, Uganda, Man, XXXIII, 1933; H. J. Braunholtz, Wooden Roulettes for Impressing Patterns on Pottery, Man, XXXIV, 1934; W. E. Nicholson, Bida (Nupe) Pottery, Man, XXXIV, 1934; W. E. Nicholson, Brief Notes on Pottery at Abuja and Kuta, Niger Province, Man, XXXIV, 1934; R. P. Wild, Stone Age Pottery from the Gold Coast and Ashanti, JRAI, LXIV, 1934; R. P. Wild and H. J. Braunholtz, Baked Clay Heads from Graves at Fomena, Ashanti, Man, XXXIV, 1934; J. M. Culwick, Pottery among the Wabena of Ulanga, Tanganyika Territory, Man, XXXV, 1935; L. H. Wells, Ornamental Motives from Bantu Pottery, Man, XXXV, 1935; R. P. Wild, An Ancient Pot from Tarkwa, Gold Coast, Man, XXXV, 1935; H. J. Braunholtz, Archaeology in the Gold Coast, Antiquity, XL, 1936; D. Shropshire, The Making of Hari (Clay Pots), Watewe Tribe, Man, XXXVI, 1936; R. P. Wild, Funerary Equipment from Agona-Swedru, Winnebach District, Gold Coast, JRAI, LXVII, 1937; P. G. Harris, Dakakari Peoples of Sokoto Province, Nigeria, JRAI, LXVIII, 1938; R. de Z. Hall, Pottery in Bugufi, Tanganyika Territory, Man, XXXIX, 1939; H. R. Palmer, Stone Circles in the Gambia Valley, JRAI, LXIX, 1939; M. D. W. Jeffreys, A Musical Pot from S. Nigeria, Man, XL, 1940; G. Vieillard, Sur quelques objets en terre cuite de Djenné, NIFAN, 1940; R. D. T. Fitzgerald, Dakakari Grave Pottery, JRAI, LXXIV, 1944; W. Fagg, Preliminary Note on a New Series of Pottery Figures from N. Nigeria (Nok), Africa, XVIII, 1945; W. Fagg, Archaeological Notes from N. Nigeria (Nok), Man, XLVI, 1946; G. Duchemin, Tête en terre cuite de Krinjabo NIFAN, XXVI, 1946; R. Mauny, Jerres funéraires, NIFAN, XXX, 1946; M. D. W. Jeffreys, Ogoni Pottery, Man, XLVII, 1947; L. S. B. Leakey, Dimple Based Pottery from Central Kavirondo, Coryndon Museum, Occasional Paper, II, Nairobi, 1948; R. B. Nunoo, Report on Excavations at Nsuta Hill, Gold Coast, Man, XLVIII, 1948; F. Addison and O. G. S. Crawford, The Wellcome Excavations in the Sudan, vols. I-II, Jebel Moya, vol. III, Abu Geili, Oxford, 1949–51; W. Fagg, New Discoveries from Ifé, Man, XLIX, 1949; R. Mauny, Statuettes de terre cuite de Mopti, NIFAN, XLIII, 1949; M. Aris, Fouilles de tombeaux anciens à Tienra, NIFAN, XLVII, 1950; M. W. D. Jeffreys, Carved Clay Tobacco Pipes from Bamenda, British Cameroons, Man, L, 1950; J. P. Lebeuf and A. Masson-Detourbet, La civilisation du Tchad, Paris, 1950; M. Cardew, Nigerian Traditional Pottery, Nigeria, Lagos, 1952; E. C. Lanning, Some Vessels and Beakers from Mubende Hill, Uganda, Man, LIII, 1953; M. Trowell and K. P. Wachsmann, Tribal Crafts of Uganda, London, 1953; G. Szumowski, Résultat des fouilles à Fotoma, NIFAN, LXIV, 1954; K. C. Murray, The Art of Ifé, Nigerian Museum, Lagos, 1955; H. Cory, African Figurines: Their Ceremonial Use in Puberty Rites in Tanganyika, London, 1956; G. Smolla, Prehistorische Keramik aus Ostafrika, Tribus, VI, Lindenmuseum, Stuttgart, 1956; R. B. Nunoo, Excavations at Asebu on the Gold Coast, J. of the West African Science Assoc., III, 1 1957, pp. 12–44; Anonymous, A Terra-cotta Head Excavated at Ifé, Man, LVIII, 1958, G. Szumowski, Pseudotumulus des environs de Bamako, NIFAN, LXXVII, 1958; Mensch und Handwerk: Die Töpferei, Museum für Völkerkunde, Basel, 1959. *b. Southeast Asia and Oceania*: E. H. Man, On the Aboriginal Inhabitants of the Andaman Islands, JRAI, XII, 1883; E. H. Man, Nicobar Pottery, JRAI, XXIII, 1894; C. G. Seligman and T. A. Joyce, On Prehistoric Objects in British New Guinea, Anthropological Essays Presented to E. B. Taylor, Oxford, 1907; F. von Luschan, Zur Ethnographie des Kaiserin-Augusta Flusses (Sepik), BA, I, 1911; R. Neuhauss, Deutsch Neu-Guinea, I, Berlin, 1911; O. Reche, Der Kaiserin-Augusta Fluss, Ergebnisse der Südsee Expedition, 1908–10, II, Ethnographie, A, Melanesien, I, Hamburg, 1913; J. W. Layard, Degree-taking Rites in Southwest Malekula, JRAI, LVIII, 1928; E. Mackay, Painted Pottery in Modern Sind, JRAI, LX, 1930; A. C. Haddon, A Prehistoric Sherd from the Mailu District, Papua, Man, XXXII, 1932; B. Blackwood, Both Sides of Buka Passage, Oxford, 1935; K. Roth, Pottery-making in Fiji, JRAI, LXV, 1935; A. Aiyappau, Handmade Pottery of the Urali Kurumbars of Wynad, S. India, Man, XLVII, 1947; L. Dumont, A Remarkable Example of S. Indian Pot-making, Man, LII, London, 1952; J. H. N. Evans, Bajan Pottery, Sarawak Mus. J., VI, 5, 1955; T. Harrison, Distribution and General Character of Native Pottery in Borneo, Sarawak Mus. J., VI, 5, 1955; A. Morrison, Murut Pottery, Sarawak Mus. J., VI, 5, 1955; E. W. Gifford and D. Shutler, Jr., Archaeological Excavations in New Caledonia, Anthropological Records, XVIII, 1, 1956. *C. The Americas*: W. H. Holmes, Origin and Development of Form and Ornament in Ceramic Art, Bur. of Am. Ethn., Ann. Rep., IV, 1886; P. Kelemen, Mediaeval American Art, New York, 1946; G. H. S. Bushnell and A. Digby, Ancient American Pottery, London, 1955. (1) *North America*: F. H. Cushing, Study of Pueblo Pottery, Bur. of Am. Ethn., Ann. Rep., IV, 1886; W. H. Holmes, Pottery of the Ancient Pueblos, Bur. of Am. Ethn., Ann. Rep., IV, 1886; W. H. Holmes, Ancient Pottery of the Mississippi Valley, Bur. of Am. Ethn., Ann. Rep., IV, 1886; G. Nordenskiöld, The Cliffdwellers of the Mesa Verde, Southwestern Colorado, Stockholm, 1893; J. W. Fewkes, Archaeological Expedition to Arizona in 1895, Bur. of Am. Ethn., Ann. Rep., XVII, 2, 1898; W. H. Holmes, Aboriginal Pottery of the Eastern United States, Bur. of Am. Ethn., Ann. Rep., XX, 1903; J. W. Fewkes, Two Summers' Work in Pueblo Ruins, Bur. of Am. Ethn., Ann. Rep., XXII, 1904; C. E. Guthe, Pueblo Pottery-making: A Study at the Village of San Ildefonso, Phillips Academy, Andover, Papers of the Southwestern Expedition, no. 2, New Haven, 1925; A. V. Kidder and A. O. Shepard, The Pottery of Pecos, vol. II, Phillips Academy, Andover, New Haven, 1936; H. M. Wormington and A. Neal, The Story of Pueblo Pottery, Denver Museum of Natural History, Denver, 1951. (2) *Mexico and Central America*: W. H. Holmes, Ancient Art of the Province of Chiriquí, Bur. of Am. Ethn., Ann. Rep., VI, 1888; C. V. Hartman, Archaeological Researches in Costa Rica, Royal Museum, Stockholm, 1901; G. C. MacCurdy, A Study of Chiriquian Antiquity, New Haven, 1911; T. A. Joyce, Mexican Archaeology, London, 1914; T. A. Joyce, Central American Archaeology, London, 1916; T. W. F. Gann, The Maya Indians of Southern Yucatan and Northern British Honduras, Bur. of Am. Ethn., B. 64, 1918; F. Boas and M. Gamio, Estudio de la cerámica Azteca, Publicaciones de la Escuela Internacional de Arqueología y Etnología Americana, Mexico City, 1921; W. Staub, Pre-Hispanic Mortuary Pottery of the Huaxtecas, El México antiguo, I, Mexico City, 1921; E. Noguera, Algunas características de la cerámica de México, JSAm, XXII, 1925; S. K. Lothrop, Pottery of Costa Rica and Nicaragua, Museum of the American Indian, 2 vols., New York, 1926; T. A. Joyce, Maya and Mexican Art, London, 1927; T. A. Joyce, The Pottery Whistle-figurines of Lubaantum, British Honduras, JRAI, LXIII, 1933; S. Linné, Archaeological Researches at Teotihuacan, Mexico, Statens Etnografiska Museum, N.S., no. 1, Stockholm, 1934; D. Brand, The Distribution of Pottery Types in North-Western Mexico, AmA, XXXVII, 1935; W. D. Strong, Archaeological Investigations in the Bay Islands, Spanish Honduras, Smithsonian Misc. Colls., XCII, 14, 1935; R. E. Smith, Ceramics of Uaxactun: A Preliminary Analysis of Decorative Technics and Design, Carnegie Institution, pub. 473, Washington, 1936; O. G. Ricketson, Jr., and E. B. Ricketson, Uaxactun, Guatemala, Carnegie Institution, pub. 477, Washington, 1937; S. Linné, Zapotecan Antiquities, Statens Etnografiska Museum, N.S., no. 4, Stockholm, 1938; J. E. Thompson, Excavations at San José, British Honduras, Carnegie Institution, pub. 506, Washington, 1939; S. K. Lothrop, Coclé, an Archaeological Study of Central Panama, part 2, Memoirs, of the Peabody Mus., VIII, 1942; S. Linné, Mexican Highland Cultures, Statens Etnografiska Museum, N.S., no. 7, Stockholm, 1942; C. W. Weiant, Ceramics of Tres Zapotes, Bur. of Am. Ethn. B. 139, 1943; A. V. Kidder, Excavations at Kaminaljuyú, Guatemala, Carnegie Institution, pub. 561, Washington, 1946; A. O. Shepard, Plumbate, a Meso-American Trade Ware, Carnegie Institution, pub. 573, Washington, 1948; G. C. Vaillant, The Aztecs of Mexico, 2d ed., Middlesex, 1950; A. L. Smith and A.V. Kidder, Excavations at Nebaj, Guatemala, Carnegie Institution, pub. 594, Washington, 1951; A. Caso and I. Bernal, Memorias del Instituto Nacional de Antropología y Historia, II, Mexico City, 1952; P. Drucker, La Venta, Tabasco: A Study of Olmec Ceramics and Art, Bur. of Am. Ethn., B. 153, 1952; J. M. Longyear III, Copan Ceramics, Carnegie Institution, pub. 597, Washington, 1952; M. N. Porter, Tlatilco and the Pre-Classic Cultures of the New World, VFPA, XIX, 1953; H. Berlin, Late Pottery Horizons of Tabasco, Mexico, Contributions to American Anthropology and History, no. 59, Washington, 1956. (3) *South America*: W. Reiss and A. Stübel, The Necropolis of Ancon in Peru, 3 vols., Berlin, 1880–82; J. P. Ambrosetti, Los cemeterios prehistóricos del Alto Paraná, Buenos Aires, 1895; M. Uhle, Pachacamac, Report of the William Pepper Peruvian Expedition, Philadelphia, 1903; J. W. Fewkes, The Aborigines of Porto Rico and Neighboring Islands, Bur. of Am. Ethn., Ann. Rep., XXV, 1907; S. A. Lafone-Quevedo, Tipos de alfarería en la región Calchaquí, Revista del Mus. de La Plata, XIV, 1907; F. F. Outes, Alfarerías del Noroeste argentino, Anales del Mus. de La Plata, I, 5, 1907; E. Boman, Antiquités de la région andine de la République Argentine, Paris, 1908; T. A. Joyce, South American Archaeology, London, 1913; M. Uhle, Die Ruinen von Moche, JSAm, N.S., X, 1913; M. H. Saville, The Antiquities of Manabí, Ecuador, 2 vols., New York, 1917; B. W. Merwin, Dutch Guiana Pottery, The Mus. J., VIII, 3, Philadelphia, 1917; R. and M. d'Harcourt, La céramique ancienne du Pérou, Paris, 1924; W. E. Roth, An Introductory Study of the Arts, Crafts and Customs of the Guiana Indians, Bur. of Am. Ethn., Ann. Rep., XXXVIII, 1924; A. L. Kroeber, W. D. Strong, and A. M. Gayton, The Uhle Pottery Collections from Moche, etc., Univ. of Calif. Pubs. in Am. Archaeol. and Ethn., XXI, 1–8, 1924–27; S. Linné, The Technique of South American Ceramics, Göteborg, 1925; A. L. Kroeber, Archaeological Explorations in Peru, I, Ancient Pottery from Trujillo, Field Museum of Natural History, Anthropological Memoirs, II, 1, Chicago, 1926; M. Schmidt, Kunst und Kultur von Peru, Berlin, 1929; R. Larco-Hoyle, Los Mochicas, 2 vols,. Lima, 1938–39; R. Larco-Hoyle, Los Cupisniques, Lima, 1941; W. D. Strong, G. R. Willey, and J. M. Corbett, Archaeological Studies in Peru, 1941–42, New York, 1943; B. J. Meggers, The Archaeology of the Amazon Basin, HSAI, III, 1948; A. Kidder, Jr., Venezuelan Archaeology, HSAI, IV, 1948; W. C. Bennett, The Gallinazo Groups, Viru Valley, Peru, Yale Univ. Pubs. in Anthropology, XLIII, 1950; G. Kutscher, Chimu, Berlin, 1950; E. Becker-Donner, Die nordwestargentinischen Sammlungen des Wiener Museums für Völkerkunde, Archiv für Völkerkunde, V–VII, 1950–52; G. H. S. Bushnell, The Archaeology of the Santa Elena Peninsula in South-West Ecuador, Cambridge, England, 1951; H. Baldus, Tonscherbenfunde in Norparaná, Archiv für Völkerkunde, VI–VII, 1951–52; H. Ubbelohde-Döring, The Art of Ancient Peru, London, 1952; J. A. Billbrook, On the Excavations of a Shell Mound at Palo Seco, Trinidad, B.W.I., Yale Univ. Pubs. in Anthropology, L, 1953; W. C. Bennett, Ancient Arts of the Andes, Museum of Modern Art, New York, 1954; J. C. Cubillos and C. and V. A. Bedoya, Arqueología de las riberas del río Magdalena, Espinal-Tolima, Rev. Colombiana de Antropología, II, 2, 1954; G. Reichel-Dolmatoff, Investigaciones arqueológicas en la Sierra Nevada de Santa Marta, Rev. Colombiana de Antropología, II, 2, 1954; G. and A. Reichel-Dolmatoff, Momil, Excavaciones en el Sinú, Rev. Colombiana de Antropología, V, 1956.

*The ancient world. a. Civilizations of the ancient Near East*: H. Frankfort, Studies in Early Pottery of the Near East, I–II, London, 1924–27; M. Welker, The Painted Pottery of the Near East in the Second Millennium B.C. and Its Chronological Background, Philadelphia, 1948. (1) *Egypt*: H. Wallis, Typical Examples of the Art of the Egyptian Potter, London, 1900; W. M. F. Petrie, The Arts and Crafts of Ancient Egypt, 2d ed., London, 1910, chap. 12; W. M. F. Petrie, Corpus of Prehistoric Pottery and Palettes, Lon-

don, 1921; J. Vandier, Manuel d'archéologie égyptienne, I, Paris, 1952. (2) *Mesopotamia*: E. Douglas van Buren, Clay Figurines of Babylonia and Assyria, New Haven, 1930; W. Andrae, Assur farbige Keramik, Berlin, 1933; Du Mesnil du Buisson, A propos du décor céramique de haute antiquité à Baghouz (Syrie), Mél. Martroye, Paris, 1940, pp. 1–25; P. Delougaz, Pottery from the Diyala Region, Chicago, 1952; A. Parrot, Archéologie mésopotamienne, II, Paris, 1953; B. Hrouda, Die bemalte Keramik des zweiten Jahrtausends in Nordmesopotamien und Nordsyrien, Berlin, 1957. (3) *Syria and Palestine*: E. Saussey, La céramique philistine, Syria, V, 1924, pp. 169–85; L. H. Vincent, La peinture céramique palestinienne, Syria, V, 1924, pp. 81–107, 186–202, 294–315; M. Dunand, Remarques sur la céramique archaïque des pays cananéens, Berytus, III, 1936, pp. 141–47; G. E. Wright, The Pottery of Palestine from the Earliest Times to the End of the Early Bronze Age, New Haven, 1938; W. F. Albright, The Archaeology of Palestine, Harmondsworth, 1949; V. R. Grace, The Canaanite Jar, The Aegean and the Near East, Studies Presented to H. Goldman, New York, 1956, pp. 80–109; S. J. Saler, Ez-Zalihiyye in the Light of Ancient Pottery, Liber Annuus, VII, 1956–57, pp. 53–63. (4) *Anatolia*: H. de Genouillac, Céramique cappadocienne, Paris, 1926; H. T. Bossert, Altanatolien, Berlin, 1942; H. Goldman and J. Garstang, A Conspectus of Early Cilician Pottery, AJA, LI, 1947, p. 370 ff.; H. H. von der Osten, Buntkeramik in Anatolien, Orientalia Suecana, I, 1952, pp. 15–37. (5) *Cyprus*: E. Gjerstad, Cypriot Pottery, Classif. d. Cér. Ant., 1931; C. F. A. Schaeffer, Missions en Chypre, 1932–35, Paris, 1936; E. Gjerstad, Swedish Cyprus Expedition, The Cypro-Geometric, Cypro-Archaic and Cypro-Classical Periods, Pottery, IV, 2, Stockholm, 1948, pp. 48–91; E. and J. Stewart, Vounous 1937–38, Lund, 1950; C. F. A. Schaeffer, Nouvelles missions en Chypre: Enkomi-Alasia, Paris, 1952. *b. The Aegean and Greece.* (1) *General*: Furtwängler-Reichhold; E. Pfuhl, Bilder griechischer Vasen, 13 vols., ed. J. D. Beazley and P. Jacobsthal, Berlin, Leipzig, 1930–39; E. Buschor, Griechische Vasen, Munich, 1940; A. Lane, Greek Pottery, London, 1948; F. Villard, Les vases grecs, Paris, 1956. (2) *Bronze Age*: British School at Athens, Excavations at Phylakopi in Melos, London, 1904; C. Tsountas, Αἱ προϊστορικαὶ ἀκροπόλεις Διμηνίου καὶ Σέσκλου, Athens, 1908; A. J. B. Wace and M. S. Thompson, Prehistoric Thessaly, Cambridge, England, 1912; C. W. Blegen, Karakou, Boston, New York, 1921; M. Demargne, Céramique de la Crète préhellénique, Classif. d. Cér. Ant., 1921; A. Evans, The Palace of Minos at Knossos, 6 vols., London, 1921–36; C. Dugas, Céramique des îles de la mer Egée, Classif. d. Cér. Ant., 1923; L. Rey, Céramique de la région macédonienne, Classif. d. Cér. Ant., 1923; S. Xanthoudides, The Vaulted Tombs of Mesara, Liverpool, 1924; E. J. Forsdyke, Catalogue of Vases in the British Museum: Prehistoric Aegean Pottery, I, 1, London, 1925; C. W. Blegen, Zygouries, Cambridge, Mass., 1928; F. Chapouthier, J. Charbonneaux, R. Joly, and P. Dermargne, Fouilles executées à Mallia, par l'Ecole française d'Athènes, 5 vols., Paris, 1928–53; J. Hazzidakis, Les villas minoennes de Tylissos, Paris, 1934; L. Pernier and L. Banti, Il palazzo minoico di Festòs, 2 vols., Rome, 1935–51; W. Lamb, Excavations at Thermi in Lesbos, Cambridge, England, 1936; H. T. Bossert, Alt Kreta, Berlin, 1937; C. W. Blegen, Prosymna, Cambridge, England, 1937; W. A. Heurtley, Prehistoric Macedonia, Cambridge, England, 1939; J. D. S. Pendlebury, The Archaeology of Crete: An Introduction, London, 1939; C. F. A. Schaeffer, Ugaritica, 2 vols., Paris, 1939–49; A. Furumark, The Mycenaean Pottery: Analysis and Classification, Stockholm, 1941; A. Furumark, The Chronology of Mycenaean Pottery, Stockholm, 1941; H. van Effenterre, Nécropoles de Mirabello, Paris, 1948; A. J. B. Wace, Mycenae: An Archaeological History and Guide, Princeton, 1949; C. W. Blegen, J. L. Caskey, M. Rawson, and J. Sperling, Troy: General Introduction, 3 vols., Princeton, 1950–53; F. A. Stubbings, Mycenaean Pottery from the Levant, Cambridge, England, 1951; C. Zervos, L'art de la Crète néolithique et minoenne, Paris, 1956; C. Zervos, L'art des Cyclades du début à la fin de l'âge de bronze, 2500–1100 avant notre ère, Pairs, 1957. (3) *Archaic*: E. Pfuhl, Der archaische Friedhof am Stadtberge von Thera, AM, XXVIII, 1903, pp. 1–288; K. F. Kinch, Fouilles de Vroulia, Berlin, 1914; K. F. Johansen, Les vases sicyoniens, Paris, Copenhagen, 1923; E. R. Price, Pottery of Naucratis, JHS, XLIV, 1924, pp. 180–222; C. Dugas, La céramique des Cyclades, Paris, 1925; H. G. G. Payne, Cycladic Vase-painting of the Seventh Century, JHS, XLVI, 1926, pp. 203–12; P. N. Ure, Boeotian Pottery of the Geometric and Archaic Styles, Classif. d. Cér. Ant., 1926; E. R. Price, East Greek Pottery, Classif. d. Cér. Ant., 1927; A. Rumpf, Chalkidische Vasen, 3 vols., Berlin, Leipzig, 1927; P. N. Ure, Sixth and Fifth Century Pottery from Excavations Made at Rhitsona in Boeotia, Oxford, 1927; H. G. G. Payne, Early Greek Vases from Knossos, BSA, XXIX, 1927–28, pp. 224–98; C. Dugas, Exploration archéologique de Délos, X, Paris, 1928 (also eastern Greece); T. B. L. Webster, A Rediscovered Caeretan Hydria, JHS, XLVIII, 1928, pp. 196–205; E. Buschor, Kykladisches, AM, LIV, 2, 1929, pp. 142–63; H. G. G. Payne, Necrocorinthia: A Study of Corinthian Art in the Archaic Period, Oxford, 1931; D. Levi, Lo stile geometrico cretese, ASAtene, X–XII, 1931, pp. 551–623; J. D. Beazley, H. G. G. Payne, and E. R. Price, Hellenic Cretan Vases, CVA, Oxford, Ashmolean Mus.; fasc. 2, 1931; C. Blinkenberg and K. F. Kinch, Lindos: Fouilles et recherches 1902–14, IV, Paris, 1931–41; H. R. W. Smith, The Origin of Chalcidian Ware, Berkeley, 1932; H. G. G. Payne, Protokorintische Vasenmalerei, Berlin, 1933; R. Eilmann, Frühe griechische Keramik im Samischen Heraion, AM, LVIII, 1933, pp. 47–145; E. Pottier, Fragments d'une hydrie de Caeré, MPiot, XXXIII, 1933, pp. 67–94; R. M. Cook, Fikellura Pottery, BSA, XXXIV, 1933–34, pp. 1–98; C. Dugas and C. Rhomaios, Exploration archéologique de Délos, XV, Les vases préhelléniques et géométriques, Paris, 1934; E. Kunze, Jonische Kleinmeister, AM, LIX, 1934, pp. 81–122; J. M. Cook, Protoattic Pottery, BSA, XXXV, 1934–35, pp. 165–205; W. Lamb, Excavations at Kato Phana in Chios, BSA, XXXV, 1934–35, pp. 138–64; C. Dugas, Exploration archéologique de Délos, XVII, Paris, 1935 (also eastern Greece and Crete); R. Eilmann and K. Gebauer, CVA, Berlin, Antiquarium, Band 1, 1938; N. Plaoutine, CVA, Louvre, fasc. 9, [ca. 1938]; R. S. Young, Late Geometric Graves and a Seventh Century Well in the Agora, Hesperia, sup. II, 1939; W. Kraiker and K. Kübler, Die Nekropolen des 12. bis 10. Jahrhunderts, Kerameikos, Ergebnisse der Ausgrabungen, I–IV, Berlin, 1939–43; P. Kahane, Die Entwicklungsphasen der attisch-geometrischen Keramik, AJA, XLIV, 1940, pp. 464–82; H. G. G. Payne, Perachora, Oxford, 1940; M. Robertson, The Excavations at Al-Mina Sueidia, IV, The Early Greek Vases, JHS, LX, 1940, pp. 2–21; S. S. Weinberg, What Is Protocorinthian Geometric Ware?, AJA, XLV, 1941, pp. 30–44; G. Nottbohm, Der Meister der grossen Dipylon Amphora in Athen, JdI, LVIII, 1943, pp. 1–31; S.S. Weinberg, Corinth: The Geometric and Orientalizing Pottery, VII, 1, Cambridge, Mass., 1943; D. Levi, Early Hellenic Pottery of Crete, Hesperia, XIV, 1945, pp. 1–32; P. Devambez, Deux nouvelles hydries de Caeré au Louvre, MPiot, XLI, 1946, pp. 29–62; J. M. Cook, Athenian Workshops around 700, BSA, XLII, 1947, pp. 139–55; W. A. Heurtley and M. Robertson, Excavations in Ithaca, V, The Geometric and Later Finds from Aetos, BSA, XLIII, 1948, pp. 1–124; R. J. Hopper, Addenda to Necrocorinthia, BSA, XLIV, 1949, pp. 162–257; D. Feytmans, Les Pithoi à reliefs de l'île de Rhodes, BCH, LXXIV, 1950, pp. 135–80; K. Kübler, Altattische Malerei, Tübingen, 1950; M. Santangelo, Les nouvelles hydries de Caeré au Musée de Villa Giulia, MPiot, XLIV, 1950, pp. 1–43; W. Kraiker, Aigina: Die Vasen des 10. bis 7. Jahrhunderts, Berlin, 1951 (also includes Attic pottery); R. Desborough d'Arcy, Protogeometric Pottery, Oxford, 1952; R. M. Cook, A List of Clazomenian Pottery, BSA, XLVII, 1952, pp. 123–42; J. Boardman, Pottery from Eretria. BSA, XLVII, 1952, pp. 1–48; T. J. Dunbabin and M. Robertson, Some Protocorinthian Vase Painters, BSA, XLVIII, 1953, pp. 172–81; J. L. Benson, Die Geschichte der korinthischen Vasen, diss., Basel, 1953; K. Kübler, Die Nekropolen des 10. bis 8. Jahrhunderts, Kerameikos, V, 1954; S. S. Weinberg, Corinthian Relief Ware: Prehellenistic Period, Hesperia, XXIII, 1954, pp. 109–37; L. W. Kraiker, Ornament und Bild in der frühgriechischen Malerei, Festschrift Schweitzer, Neue Beiträge zur klassischen Altertumswissenschaft, 1954, pp. 36–47; K. Kunze, Bruchstücke attischer Grabkratere, Festschrift Schweitzer, Neue Beiträge zur klassischen Altertumswissenschaft, 1954, pp. 48–58; R. M. Cook, CVA, London, Br. Mus., fasc. 8, 1954; J. K. Brock, Fortetsa, Cambridge, England 1957; W. Schiering, Werkstätten orientalisierender Keramik auf Rhodos, Berlin, 1957; T. J. Dunbabin, Perachora, II (to be published). (4) *Attic and Boeotian*: A. Fairbanks, Athenian Lekythoi, 2 vols., New York, 1907–14; P. N. Ure, Black Glaze Pottery from Rhitsona in Boeotia, Oxford, 1913; W. Riezler, Weissgrundige attische Lekythen, 2 vols., Munich, 1914; Beazley, VA; G. M. A. Richter, The Craft of Athenian Pottery, New Haven, 1923; E. Buschor, Attische Lekythen der Parthenonzeit, Münch. Jhb. der bildenden K., II, 1925, pp. 167–99; P. Jacobsthal, Ornamente griechischer Vasen, 3 vols., Berlin, 1926–27; J. D. Beazley, Greek Vases in Poland, Oxford, 1928; L. D. Caskey and J. D. Beazley, Attic Vase-painting in the Museum of Fine Arts, Boston, 2 vols., Boston, 1931–54; D. M. Robinson, Excavations at Olynthus, V, Mosaics, Vases and Lamps Found in 1928–31, Baltimore, 1933; K. Schefold, Untersuchungen zu den Kertscher Vasen, Berlin, Leipzig, 1934; G. M. A. Richter and M. J. Milne, Shapes and Names of Athenian Vases, New York, 1935; C. H. E. Haspels, Attic Black-figured Lekythoi Paris, 1936; J. D. Beazley, Attic White Lekythoi, Oxford, 1938; H. Bloesch, Formen attischer schalen von Exechias bis zum Ende des strengen Stils, Bern, Bümplitz, 1940; R. Lullies, Zur boiotischen rotfiguren Vasenmalerei, AM, LXV, 1940, pp. 1–27; P. Wolters and G. Bruns, Das Kabirenheiligtum bei Theben, Berlin, 1940; Beazley, ARV; J. D. Beazley, Potter and Painter in Ancient Athens, Proc. of the Br. Acad., XXX, 1945; G. M. A. Richter, Attic Red-figured Vases, New Haven, 1946; P. E. Corbett, Attic Pottery of the Later Fifth Century from the Athenian Agora, Hesperia, XVIII, 1949, pp. 298–351; D. M. Robinson, Excavations at Olynthus, XIII, Vases Found in 1934–38, Baltimore, 1950; J. D. Beazley, The Development of Attic Black-figure, Berkeley, Los Angeles, 1951; G. M. A. Richter, Attic Black-figured Kylixes, CVA, Met. Mus., fasc. 2, 1953; Beazley, ABV. *c. Italy and pre-Roman Europe*: O. Montelius, La civilisation primitive en Italie (with pls.), 5 vols., Stockholm, 1895; T. E. Peet, The Stone and Bronze Ages in Italy and Sicily, Oxford, 1909; M. Mayer, Apulien vor und während der Hellenisierung, Leipzig, Berlin, 1914; E. M. W. Tillyard, The Hope Vases, Cambridge, England, 1923; D. Randall MacIver, Villanovans and Early Etruscans, Oxford, 1924; P. Ducati, Ceramica della penisola italiana, Classif. d. Cér. Ant., 1924; F. von Duhn, Italische Gräberkunde, Heidelberg, 1924; B. Pace, Ceramiche della Sicilia, Classif. d. Cér. Ant., 1926; P. Ducati, Storia dell'arte etrusca, 2 vols., Florence, 1927; N. Moon, Some Early South-Italian Vase-painters, BSR, XI, 1929, pp. 30–49; G. M. A. Richter, Polychrome Vases from Centuripe, Metropolitan Mus. Studies, II, 2, 1930, pp. 187–205; IV, 1, 1932, pp. 45–54; P. Ducati, Pontische Vasen, Berlin, 1932; G. Q. Giglioli, L'arte etrusca, Milan, 1935; B. Pace, Arte e civiltà della Sicilia antica, I-III, Milan, Genoa, Rome, 1935–46; A. D. Trendall, Paestan Pottery, London, 1936; A. D. Trendall, Frühitaliotische Vasen, Leipzig, 1938; J. D. Beazley and F. Magi, La Raccolta Benedetto Guglielmi nel Museo Gregoriano Etrusco, I, Vatican City, 1939; C. Quarles van Ufford, Les terres-cuites siciliennes, Assen, 1941; J. D. Beazley, Groups of Campanian Red-figure, JBS, LXIII, 1943, pp. 66–111; Beazley, EVP; Ars Hispaniae, Madrid, I, 1947, pp. 262–84; A. D. Trendall, Paestan Pottery: A Revision and a Supplement, BSR, XX, 1952, pp. 1–53; A. D. Trendall, Vasi italioti ed etruschi a figure rosse: Vasi antichi dipinti del Vaticano, Vatican City, 1953–55; L. Bernabò Brea, Sicily before the Greeks, London, 1957; P. Bosch Gimpera, Todavía el problema de la cerámica ibérica, Mexico City, 1958. *d. Hellenistic, Roman, and Provincial*: J. Déchelette, Les vases céramiques ornés de la Gaule romaine, 2 vols, Paris, 1904; W. Ludovici, Stempel-Bilder und Stempel-Namen römischer Töpfer von meinen Ausgrabungen in Rheinzabern, I–V, 1901–27, 5 vols., Munich, 1905–28; C. H. Chase, Catalogue of the Loeb Collection of Arretine Pottery, New York, 1908; R. Pagenstecher, Die Calenische Reliefkeramik, Berlin, 1909; F. Behn, Römische Keramik mit Einschluss der hellenistischen Vorstufen, Mainz, 1910; A. Merlin, B. Archéologique, 1910, p. ccx; 1912, p. ccxv; 1913, p. ccxvii; 1914, pp. clxix–cliii, cxcix–ccii; 1915, pp. clxxvii–clxxx; 1916, pp. cxxiv–cxxix; 1917, pp. ccix–ccxv; 1918, pp. clxxiv–clxxxi; 1921, pp. cxviii–cxix; J. Curle, A Roman Frontier Post and Its People: The Fort of Newstead, Glasgow, 1911; R. Forrer, Die römischen Terra Sigillata Töpfereien von Heiligenberg-Dinsheim und Itten-

weiler im Elsass, Stuttgart, 1911; J. P. Bushe-Fox, Wroxeter, I–III, 1912–14; F. Haverfield, Conspectus of Potters' Stamps on Plain Samian Ware Found at Cambridge 1906–14, Archaeologia Aeliana, series III, XII, 1915, pp. 273–86; G. H. Chase, Catalogue of the Arretine Pottery in the Boston Museum of Fine Arts, Boston, 1916; R. Knorr, Töpfer und Fabriken verzierter Terra Sigillata des ersten Jahrhunderts, Stuttgart, 1919; F. Oswald and T. D. Price, An Introduction to the Study of Terra Sigillata, London, 1920; H. Sumner, Descriptive Account of the Roman Pottery Made at Ashley Rails, London, 1921; F. Courby, Les vases grecs à reliefs, Paris, 1922; P. Barocelli, Albintimilium, MemLinc, XXIX, 1923, pp. 5–146; B. Kuzsinszky, A legrégibb terra-sigillata edények Pannoniában, Archaeologiai Értesítő, XL, 1923–26, pp. 88–113; T. Knipowitsch, Untersuchungen zur Keramik römischer Zeit aus den Griechenstädten an der Nordküste des Schwarzen Meeres, I, Die Keramik römischer Zeit aus Olbia in der Sammlung der Eremitage: Materialien zur römisch-germanischen Keramik, IV, Frankfort on the Main, 1929; K. Kübler, Spätantike Stempelkeramik, AM, LVI, 1931, pp. 75–86; F. Oswald, Index of Potters' Stamps, Liverpool, 1931; B. Kuzsinszky, Das grosse römische Töpferviertel in Aquincum, Budapest Régiségei, XI, 1932; A. Oxé, Arretinische Reliefgefässe vom Rhein: Materialien zur römisch-germanischen Keramik, V, Frankfort on the Main, 1933; A. Oxé, Römische-italische Beziehungen der früharretinischen Reliefgefässe, Bonner Jhb., CXXXVIII, 1933, pp. 81–98; N. Glueck, Explorations in Eastern Palestine I, Annual of the Am. Schools of Oriental Research, XIV, 1933–34; H. A. Thompson, Two Centuries of Hellenistic Pottery, Hesperia, III, 1, 1934, pp. 311–480; P. Hermet, La Graufesenque (Condatomago), Paris, 1934; A. Oxé, Frühgallische Reliefgefässe vom Rhein: Materialien zur römisch-germanischen Keramik, VI, Frankfort on the Main, 1934; N. Glueck, Exploration in Eastern Palestine, II, Annual of the Am. Schools of Oriental Research, XV, 1934–35; G. Juhasz, Die Sigillaten von Brigetio, Dissertationes Pannonicae, Budapest, 1935; A. U. Pope, A Survey of Persian Art, I, Oxford, 1935, p. 646 ff.; H. Comfort, A Preliminary Study of Late Italian Sigillata, AJA, XL, 1936, pp. 437–51; R. E. M. and T. V. Wheeler, Verulamium, Oxford, 1936; A. Westholm, The Temples of Soli, Stockholm, 1936; F. Oswald, Index of Figure Types on Terra-sigillata "Samian Ware," Liverpool, 1936–37; J. H. Iliffe, Sigillata Ware in the Near East, PEQ, VI, 1937, pp. 4–53 (with bibliog.); K. Kiss, Die Zeitfolge der Erzeugnisse des Töpfers Pacatus von Aquincum, Laureae Aquincenses, I, Dissertationes Pannonicae, series II, X, 1938, pp. 212–28; J. A. Stanfield and G. Simpson, Central Gaulish Potters, Oxford, London, 1938; H. Comfort, RE, sup. VII, 1940, s.v. Terra sigillata, col. 1295 ff. (with full bibliog.); W. Schwabacher, Hellenistische Reliefkeramik in Kerameikos, AJA, XLV, 1941, p. 182 ff.; N. Lamboglia Terra sigillata chiara, R. Ingauna ed Intemelia, VII, 1941, pp. 7–22; C. Alexander, Arretine Relief Ware, CVA, Met. Mus., fasc. 1, 1943; L. Vásquez de Parga, Estado cultural del estudio de la terra sigillata, Archivio Español de Arqueología, L, 1943, p. 123 ff.; W. Drack, Die helvetische Terra Sigillata, Schr. des Instituts für Ur- und Frühgeschichte der Schweiz, II, 1945; N. Glueck, Explorations in Eastern Palestine, IV, Annual of the Am. Schools of Oriental Research, XXV–XXVIII, 1945–49; J. M. Bairrao-Oleiro, Elementos para o estudo de terra sigillata em Portugal, Revista de Guimarães, LVIII, 1948, pp. 81–111; E. Delort, L'atelier de Satto, Vases unis, 3.000 marques, Mém. de l'Acad. Nationale de Metz, XVII, 1948; H. Dragendorff and C. Watzinger, Arretinische Reliefkeramik mit Beschreibung der Sammlung in Tübingen, Reutlingen, 1948; P. de Palol Salellas, La cerámica estampada romano-cristiana, Crónica del IV Congreso Arqueológico del Sudeste Español, Elche, 1948; W. Drack, Die römischen Töpfereifunde von Baden-Aquae Helveticae, Schr. des Instituts für Ur- und Frühgeschichte der Schweiz, V, 1949; I. A. Richmond, Excavations at the Roman Fort of Newstead, 1947, Proc. of the Soc. Ant. Scotland, LXXXIV, 1949–50, pp. 1–38; N. Lamboglia, Gli scavi di Albintimilium e la cronologia della ceramica romana, Bordighera, 1950; A. Arribas Palau, La terra sigillata emporitana, Crónica del II Congresso Arqueólogico Nacional, Madrid, 1951, Saragossa, 1952, pp. 475–83; P. de Palol Salellas, Un vaso de terra-sigillata de fábrica hispánica, Crónica del II Congresso Arqueológico Nacional, Madrid, 1951, Saragossa, 1952, pp. 463–72; R. Knorr, Terra-Sigillata Gefässe des ersten Jahrhunderts mit Töpfernamen, Stuttgart, 1952; G. Simpson, The Aldgate Potter; A Maker of Romano-British Samian Ware, JRS, XLII, 1952, pp. 68–71; E. Delort, Vases ornés de la Moselle, Nancy, 1953; M. A. Mezquiris, Sigillata hispánica de Liedena, Príncipe de Viana, XIV, 1953, pp. 271–307; F. O. Waagé, The Roman and Byzantine Pottery, Hesperia, II, 1953, p. 279 ff.; P. Karnitsch, Liste der Töpfer und Töpferstempel auf verzierter und glatter Sigillata, Forsch. in Lauriacum, II, I–IV, 1954; C. Martínez-Munilla, Terra sigillata hispánica, AEArq, XXVII, 1954, pp. 227–31; R. J. Charleston, Roman Pottery, London, 1955; F. Braemer and A. Aynard, Les fouilles de La Graufesenque en 1950, BAFr (1952–53), 1955, pp. 34–38; G. Chenet and G. Grandson, La céramique sigillée d'Argonne des II$^{e}$ et III$^{e}$ siècles, Gallia, sup. VI, 1955; P. de Schaetzen, Index des terminations des marques des potiers gallo-romains sur terra sigillata, Latomus, XXIV, 1956; R. H. Rowland, Greek Lamps and Their Survival, Princeton, 1958; A. Stenico, EAA, s.v. Aretini, vasi (with bibliog.); Catalogue des musées et collections archéologiques de l'Algérie et de la Tunisie: La Blanchère et Gauckler, Catalogue du Musée d'Alaoui, 236, nos. 206–11.

*Late antiquity and the Middle Ages*: *a. Early Christian, barbarian, and Byzantine*: O. von Falke, Majolika, Berlin, 1896; O. M. Dalton, Catalogue of Early Christian Antiquity, British Museum, London, 1901; H. Wallis, Early Italian Majolica, London, 1901; J. Clédat, Mém. de l'Institut Français d'Archéologie Orientale du Caire, 1904, p. 66; J. Strzygowski, Koptische Kunst (general cat.), Vienna, 1904; E. von Stern, Theodosia und seine Keramik, Odessa, 1906; H. Wallis, Byzantine Ceramic Art, London, 1907; Cabrol-Leclercq, VIII, col. 1086; O. Wulff, Altchristliche und mittelalterliche byzantinische und italienische Bildwerke, I, Berlin, 1909, p. 243; J. Ebersolt, Catalogue des poteries byzantines et anatoliennes du Musée de Constantinople, Constantinople, 1910; C. M. Kaufmann, Die Menasstadt, Leipzig, 1910; W. von Bode, Die Anfänge der Majolika Kunst in Italien, Berlin, 1911; K. Schumacher, Altertümer und heidnische Vorzeit, V, Mainz, 1911, p. 128; W. Unverzagt, Materialien zur römisch-germanischen Keramik, III, Frankfort on the Main, 1919; G. A. Soteriou, Deltion, Archaiologikon, VII, 1924, p. 188; H. Wollmann, Roma aeterna, 1924, p. 87; O. M. Dalton, East Christian Art, Oxford, 1925, pp. 345–49; F. Sarre, Die Keramik von Samarra, Berlin, 1925; A. J. Butler, Islamic Pottery, London, 1926; P. Toesca, Storia dell'arte italiana, I, Turin, 1927, p. 1136; G. Migeon, Manuel d'art musulman: Arts plastiques et industriels, 2d ed., Paris, 1927; K. Kübler, Athen. Mitt., LIII, 1928, p. 183; A. Grabar, Recherches sur les influences orientales dans l'art balkanique, Paris, 1928; G. Gerola, Felix Ravenna, 1930, p. 11; D. Talbot Rice, Byzantine Glazed Pottery, Oxford, 1930; W. F. Volbach, Mittelalterliche Bildwerke aus Italien und Byzanz, 2d ed., Berlin, 1930; F. J. De Waele, The Roman Market North of the Temple at Corinth, Am. J. of Archaeol., XXXIV, 1930, p. 432; G. Ballardini, Faenza: R. di Studi Ceramici, B. del Mus. Internazionale delle Ceramiche di Faenza, 1931, p. 4; D. Talbot Rice, Burlington Mag., 1932, p. 281; G. Ballardini, BArte, XXV, 1932, p. 551; Geschichte des Kunstgewerbes, V, Berlin, 1932 (including W. F. Volbach, Das christliche Kunstgewerbe der Spätantike und des frühen Mittelalters im Mittelmeergebiet, II, Keramik, pp. 77–81; W. Zoloziecky, Das byzantinische Kunstgewerbe in der mittelalterlichen und spätmittelalterlichen Periode, pp. 192–96; H. Kohlhaussen, Gotisches Kunstgewerbe, Keramik, pp. 466–72); G. Ballardini, "Corpus" della maiolica italiana, I, Rome, 1933; F. Sarre, Forsch. und Fortschritte, IX, 1933, p. 422; N. C. Debevoise, Parthian Pottery from Seleucia, Ann Arbor, 1934; N. C. Debevoise, B. of the Am. Ceramic Soc., 1934, p. 293; L. Hussong, Frühmittelalterliche Keramik aus dem Trierer-Bezirk, Trierer Z., XI, 1936, p. 75; K. Miatev, Die Keramik von Preslav, Sofia, 1936; W. F. Volbach, BArte, XXX, 1936–37, p. 345; R. Ettinghausen, Survey of Persian Art, I, London, New York, 1938, p. 646; M. Alison Frantz, Hesperia, VII, 1938, p. 429; F. Deichmann, Berliner Museen, 1938, p. 62; G. Bellardini, La maiolica italiana dalle origini alla fine del Cinquecento, Florence, 1938; H. Fuhrmann, Römisches Mittelalter, 1940, p. 92; G. Chenet, La céramique gallo-romaine d'Argonne du IV$^{e}$ siècle, Mâcon, 1941; P. de Palol Salellas, La cerámica estampada romano-cristiana, Crónica del IV Congreso Arqueológico del Sudeste Español, Elche, 1948, p. 450; J. Chompret, Répertoire de la majolique italienne, Paris, 1949; E. Gose, Gefässtypen der römischen Keramik im Rheinland, Kevelaer, 1950; Toesca, Md; H. T. Bossert, Geschichte des Kunstgewerbes, V, Berlin, 1952; C. Cecchelli, Vita di Roma nel medioevo, I, Rome, 1952, p. 3; J. Ainaud de Lasarte, Ars Hispaniae, Cerámica y vidrio, X, Madrid, 1952; F. Tischler, Der Stand der Sachsenforschung, no. 35, Bericht der R. G. Kommission, Frankfort on the Main 1954, p. 41; D. Talbot Rice, Byzantine Polychrome Pottery: A Survey of Recent Discoveries, CahA, VII–VIII, 1954–56, p. 69; E. Coche de la Ferté, L'antiquité chrétienne, Paris, 1958, p. 115; G. Liverani, La maiolica italiana (sino alla comparsa della porcellana europea), Milan, 1958 (Eng. ed., Five Centuries of Italian Majolica, New York, 1960). *b. Iran*: De Morgan, Mém. de la Délégation française en Perse, 13 vols., Paris, 1900–12; R. Pumpelly, Explorations in Turkistan, Washington, 1908; W. Andrae, Hatra nach Aufnahmen von Mitgliedern der Assur Expedition der Deutschen Orient-Gesellschaft, I–II, Leipzig, 1908–12; G. Contenau, Manuel d'archéologie orientale, 4 vols., Paris, 1917–47; F. Sarre, Die Kunst des alten Persien, Berlin, 1925; O. M. Dalton, The Treasure of the Oxus, 2d ed., London, 1926; R. Dussaud, Observations sur les céramiques du II mill. a.C., Syria, IX, 1928; A. Godard, Histoire universelle de l'art, I, Paris, 1932; A. Hertz, L'âge de Suse I et II, RA, XXXV, 1932; F. R. Wulsin, Excavations at Turang Tepe near Astarabad, sup. to B. of the Am. Inst. for Persian Art and Archaeol., 1932; V. Gordon Childe, Notes on Some Indian and East Iranian Pottery, Ancient Egypt, 1933; W. Andrae and H. Lenzen, Die Partherstadt Assur, Leipzig, 1935; G. Contenau and R. Ghirshman, Fouilles de Tepe Giyan, Musée du Louvre, Paris, 1935; E. Herzfeld, Archaeological History of Iran, London, 1935; A. Stein, An Archaeological Tour of the Ancient Persis, Iraq, III, 1936; M. Rostovzeff, Dura and the Problem of Parthian Art, New Haven, 1936; E. F. Schmidt, Excavations at Tepe Hissar-Damghan, Philadelphia, 1937; R. Ghirshman, Mad-i-Alì, RAA, XIII, 1938; A. U. Pope and P. Ackerman, A Survey of Persian Art, 6 vols., Oxford, 1938; R. Ghirshman, Fouilles de Sialk, Paris, 1938–39; A. Stein, Old Routes of Western Iran, London, 1940; G. Contenau, Les éléments de l'art perse, RA, XXXVII, 1940–41; E. Herzfeld, Iran in the Ancient East, London, New York, 1941; D. E. McCown, The Comparative Stratigraphy of Early Iran, Chicago, 1942; G. Contenau and R. de Mecquenem, Mém. de la Mission Archéologique en Iran, Paris, XXIX, 1943; A. Christensen, L'Iran sous les Sassanides, 2d ed., Copenhagen, Paris, 1944; D. H. Gordon, Sialk, Giyan, Hissar and the Indo-Iranian Connection, Man in India, XXVII, 3, 1947, pp. 195–241; R. E. M. Wheeler, Iran and India in Pre-Islamic Times, Ancient India, IV, 1947–48, pp. 85–101; C. F. A. Schaeffer, Stratigraphie comparée et chronologie de l'Asie occidentale (III et II mill.), London, 1948; G. Contenau, Arts et styles de l'Asie antérieure, Paris, 1948; R. Ghirshman, L'Iran, des origines à l'Islam, Paris, 1951 (Eng. ed., Iran, Harmondsworth, 1954); V. Gordon Childe, New Light on the Most Ancient East, London, 1952; V. Gordon Childe, L'Orient préhistorique, Paris, 1953; H. Frankfort, The Art and Architecture of the Ancient Orient, London, 1954; G. Contenau and R. Ghirshman, Village perse-achéménide, Mém. de la Mission Archéologique en Iran, Paris, XXXVI, 1954; U. Monneret de Villard, L'arte iranica, Milan, 1954; M. Bussagli, Catalogo della Mostra d'arte iranica, Milan, 1956. *c. Islam*: D. Fouquet, Contribution à l'étude de la céramique orientale, Cairo, 1900; F. Sarre, Denkmäler persischer Baukunst, Berlin, 1901–10; J. Gestoso y Pérez, Historia de los barros vidriados sevillanos desde sus orígines hasta nuestros días, Seville, 1903; F. Sarre, Die spanisch-maurischen Lüsterfayencen des Mittelalters und ihre Herstellung in Malaga, Jhb. der königl. preussischen K. Samml., XXIV, 1903, pp. 103–30; A. Van de Put, Hispano-Moresque Ware of the 15th Century, London, New York, 1904; J. Font y Guma, Rajolas valencianas y catalanas, Vilanova y Geltrú, 1905; A. Van de Put, Supplementary Studies..., London, 1911; H. Rivière, La céramique dans l'art musulman, Paris, 1913; M. Pézard, La céramique archaïque de l'Islam et ses origines, Paris, 1920; G. Migeon and A. Sakisian, Les faïences d'Asie Mineure, Rev. de l'Art Ancien et Moderne, XLIII, 1923, pp. 241–52,

353–64, XLIV, 1923, pp. 125–41; G. Migeon, Nouvelles découvertes sur la céramique de Damas, Rev. de l'Art Ancien et Moderne, XLIV, 1923, pp. 383–86; G. Contenau, Syria, V, 1924, p. 105; E. Kühnel, Islamische Kleinkunst, Berlin, 1925; F. Sarre, Die Keramik von Samarra, Die Ausgrabungen von Samarra, II, Berlin, 1925; F. Sarre, Keramik und andere Kleinfunde der islamischen Zeit von Baalbek, Berlin, Leipzig, 1925; E. Kühnel, Daten zur Geschichte der spanisch-maurischen Keramik, Jhb. der asiatischen K., II, 1925, pp. 70–180; G. Migeon, Manuel d'art musulman: Arts plastiques et industriels, II, Paris, 1927; R. Koechlin, Les céramiques musulmanes de Suse au Musée du Louvre, Mém. de la Mission Archéologique de Perse, XIX, Paris, 1928; E. Cohn Wiener, Turan, Islamische Baukunst in Mittelasien, Berlin, 1930; A. Bahgat and F. Massoul, La céramique musulmane de l'Egypte, Musée arabe du Caire, Cairo, 1930; R. L. Hobson, Guide to the Islamic Pottery of the Near East, British Museum, London, 1932; E. Kühnel, Die abbasidischen Lüsterfayencen, Ars Islamica, I, 1934, pp. 149–59; H. Ritter, J. Russka, F. Sarre, and R. Winderlich, Orientalische Steinbücher und persische Fayencetechnik, Istanbuler Mitt. no. 3, 1935; R. Ettinghausen, Evidence for the Identification of Kashan Pottery, Ars Islamica, III, 1936, pp. 44–75; M. Bahrami, Recherches sur les carreaux de revêtement lustré dans la céramique persane du XIII^e au XV^e siècle, Paris, 1937; R. Mayer-Riefstahl, Early Turkish Tile-revetments in Edirne, Ars Islamica, IV, 1937, pp. 249–81; R. Ettinghausen, The Ceramic Art in Islamic Times: Dated Faience, A Survey of Persian Art, II, 1667–96, Oxford, 1938–39; A. U. Pope, The Ceramic Art in Islamic Times: The History, A Survey of Persian Art from Prehistoric Times to the Present, II, 1446–1666, 6 vols., London, New York, 1938–39 (see also review by F. D. Day, Ars Islamica, VIII, 1941, pp. 13–58); N. Wilber, The Development of Mosaic Faience in Islamic Architecture in Iran, Ars Islamica, VI, 1939, pp. 16–47; A. Lane, Guide to the Collection of Tiles, Victoria and Albert Museum, London, 1939; K. Otto-Dorn, Das islamische Iznik, Istanbuler Forsch., XIII, 1941; M. Dimand, A Handbook of Muhammadan Art, II, Metropolitan Museum, New York, 1944; M. Gonzales Martí, Cerámica del Levante español, Siglos medievales, I, Loza, Madrid, 1944; A. Lane, Early Islamic Pottery, London, 1947; A. W. Frothingham, Lustre-ware of Spain, Hispanic Society of America, New York, 1951; M. Gómez-Moreno, El arte árabe español hasta los Almohades, Ars Hispaniae, III, 1951, pp. 310–23; M. Gonzales Martí, Cerámica del Levante español, Siglos medievales, II, Alicatados y azulejos, III, Azulejos, socarratas y retablos, Madrid, 1952; J. Ainaud de Lasarte, Cerámica y vidrio, Ars Hispaniae, X, 1952; A. Lane, The Ottoman Pottery of Isnik, Ars Orientalis, II, 1956; A. Lane, Later Islamic Pottery . . . , London, 1957.

*The West in modern times. a. Europe*: For the early bibliog., see EI, s.vv. Ceramica (1931), Maiolica (1934), and Porcellana (1935); G. Morazzoni, Le porcellane italiane, Milan, 1935; E. Campos y Cazorla, Cerámica española, 1936; G. Ballardini, La maiolica italiana (dalle origini alla fine del Cinquecento), Florence, 1938; T. d'Albisola, Ceramica futurista, Savona, 1939; M. Laeuger, Keramische Kunst, 1939; B. Leach, A Potter's Book, London, 1940; B. Rackham, Victoria and Albert Museum Catalogue of Italian Maiolica, London, 1940; Ä. Stavenow, Ceramiche svedesi, Domus, 1942, p. 438 ff.; E. Neurdenburg, Oude Nederlandsche Majolica, 1944; M. Escrivà de Romani, Historia de la cerámica de Alcora, Madrid, 1945; G. Fontaine, La céramique française, Paris, 1946; J. Helbig, La céramique bruxelloise, Brussels, 1946; S. W. Fisher, English Blue and White Porcelain of the 18th Century, London, 1947; R. G. Haggar, English Pottery Figures (1660–1860), London, 1947; C. Sempill, English Pottery and Porcelain, London, 1947; W. A. Stachelin, Bibliographie der schweizerischen Keramik vom Mittelalter bis zur Neuzeit, Basel, 1947; A. Sancho Corbacho, La cerámica andaluza, 1948; W. B. Honey, European Ceramic Art from the End of the Middle Ages to about 1815, Illustrated Historical Survey, London, 1949; E. Rosenthal, Pottery and Ceramics, London, 1949; J. Chompret, Répertoire de la maïolique italienne, 2 vols., Paris, 1949; G. Polidori, La maiolica antica abruzzese, Milan, 1949; W. B. Honey, English Pottery and Porcelain, London, 1949; A. Brougniart, Traité des arts céramiques, Paris, 1950; G. Morazzoni, La maiolica antica ligure, Milan, 1951; W. B. Honey, European Ceramic Art: A Dictionary of Factories, Artists, Technical Terms, etc., London, 1952; B. Rackham, Italian Maiolica, London, 1952; B. Siepen, Herman Gretsch, Stuttgart, 1952; E. Tilmans, Porcelaines de France, Paris, 1952; G. Savage, 18th Century English Porcelain, London, 1952; W. J. Rust, Nederlands Porselein, 1952; Céramiques des maîtres de la peinture comtemporaine, Lausanne, 1953; P. Verlet, S. Grandjean, and M. Brunet, Sèvres, Paris, 1953; D. Billington, The Younger English Potters, Studio, 1953, p. 78 ff.; W. Mankowitz, Wedgwood, London, 1953; A. Lane, Italian Porcelain, London, 1954; G. Dorfles, Ceramic Art in Italy Today, Studio, 1954, p. 83 ff.; E. Tilmans, Faïence de France, 1954; H. Rissik Marshall, Coloured Worcester Porcelain, London, 1954; G. Morazzoni, La maiolica antica veneta, Milan, 1955; N. Ragona, La ceramica siciliana dalle origini ai nostri giorni, Palermo, 1955; E. Meyer-Heisig, Deutsche Bauerntöpferei, Munich, 1955; B. Therle Hughes, English Porcelain and Bone China, 1743–1850, London, 1955; E. Hiort, Modern Danish Ceramics, Copenhagen, 1955; Porsilin, 3–4, 1955; B. Zilliocus, Ceramic Art in Finland, Studio, 1955, p. 736 ff.; S. Ducret, Unknown Porcelain of the 18th Century, Frankfort on the Main, 1956; A. Lesur-Tardy, Les poteries et les faïences françaises, Paris, 1957; R. Marlow, Pottery and Decorating, London, 1957; D. C. Towner, English Cream-coloured Earthenware, London, 1957; H. P. Fourest, Les faïences de Delft, Paris, 1957; K. Hüseler, Deutsche Fayencen, 3 vols., 1958; G. Liverani, La maiolica italiana (sino alla comparsa della porcellana europea), Milan, 1958 (Eng. ed., Five Centuries of Italian Majolica, New York, 1960); W. Chaffers, Marks and Monograms on Pottery and Porcelain, London, n.d.; A. Schönberger, Meissener Porzellan mit Höroldt Malerei, n.d.; W. B. Honey, German Porcelain, London, n.d.; W. B. Honey, French Porcelain of the 18th Century, London, n.d.; A. Lane, French Faïence, London, n.d.; G. W. Ware, German and Austrian Porcelain, London, n.d.; W. B. Honey, Old English Porcelain, London, n.d. *b. United States*: E. A. Barber, The Pottery and Porcelain of the United States: An Historical Review of American Ceramic Art from the Earliest Times to the Present Day, 2d ed., New York, 1901; E. A. Barber, Marks of American Potters, Philadelphia, 1904; A. W. Clement, Our Pioneer Potters, New York, 1947; J. Ramsay, American Potters and Pottery, New York, 1947; Design Quarterly, nos. 42–43, 1958 (special issue on contemporary American pottery). *c. Folk art*: F. A. Schaeffer, L'origine de la céramique populaire d'Alsace, spécialement des ateliers de Soufflenheim et de Betschdorf, Art populaire, travaux artistiques et scientifiques du I^er Congrès international des arts populaires, Prague, 1928, I, Paris, 1931, p. 226 ff. (including V. Scerbakivskyj, La céramique peinte contemporaine des paysans ukraniens, p. 228 ff.; J. Ferrandis, La céramique de mariage de Valence, p. 233; R. Navarro, La céramique populaire de Palencia, p. 234; J. Martínez Cabrera, La céramique populaire dans la province de Tolède, p. 235; M. Gómez-Moreno, La faïence de Fajalauza, Grenade, pp. 236–37; K. Cernohorsky, L'art populaire de la faïence en Tchécoslovaquie, p. 237 ff.); F. Carreras y Candi and others, Folklore y costumbres de España, I, Barcelona, 1931; G. Cocchiara, Le lucerne siciliane a figura umana, Archivio Storico Siciliano, N.S., II, 1936, III, 1937; C. Calò, I figuli di Grottaglie, Noci, 1937; T. Toschi, Saggi sull'arte popolare, Rome, 1945; R. Weiss, Volkskunde der Schweiz, Erlenbach, Zurich, 1946; J. Saavedra Menéndez, Enciclopedia de la cerámica, Buenos Aires, 2 vols., 1947–48; P. L. Menon and R. Lecotté, Au village de France, 2 vols., Paris, 1954; L'arte populaire hongrois, 2d ed., Budapest, 1955; L'art populaire en Roumanie, Bucharest, 1955; B. Valenzuela Rojas, La cerámica folklórica de Pomaire, Archivos del Folklore Chileno, 1955, nos. 6–7; K. Šourek, L'art populaire en images, Prague, 1956; J. Vydra and L. Kunz, Malerei auf Volksmajolika, Prague, 1956; B. Valenzuela Rojas, La cerámica folklórica de Quinchamali, Archivos del Folklore Chileno, 1957, no. 8.

*The Asiatic world. a. India and southeastern Asia*: G. C. M. Birdwood, The Industrial Arts of India, London, 1880; H. Hargreaves, Excavations in Beluchistan, Archaeological Survey of India, Memoirs no. 35, 1926; A. K. Coomaraswamy, Archaic Indian Terracottas, IPEK, 1928; A. Stein, Archaeological Tour in Waziristan and Beluchistan, Archaeological Survey of India, Memoirs, no. 37, 1929; A. Stein, Archaeological Tour in Gedrosia, Archaeological Survey of India, Memoirs, no. 43, 1931; J. Marshall, Mohenjo-daro and the Indus Civilization, London, 1931; R. L. Hobson, A Guide to the Islamic Pottery of the Near East, British Museum, London, 1932; N. G. Majumdar, Explorations in Sind, Archaeological Survey of India, Memoirs, no. 48, 1934; V. S. Agrawala, Mathura Terracottas, J. of the United Provinces Hist. Soc., 1936; A. Stein, Archaeological Reconnaissances in North-western India and South-eastern Iran, London, 1937; E. Mackay, Further Excavations at Mohenjo-daro, Delhi, 1938; S. Kramrisch, Indian Terracottas, JISOA, VII, 1939; M. S. Vats, Excavations at Harappa, Delhi, 1940; V. S. Agrawala, Rajghat Terracottas, J. of the United Provinces Hist. Soc., 1941; D. H. Gordon, Early Indian Terracottas, JISOA, XI, 1943; E. Mackay, Chanhu-daro Excavations, New Haven, 1943; D. H. Gordon, Early Indian Painted Pottery, JISOA, XIII, 1945; A. Ghosh and K. C. Panigrahi, The Pottery of Ahichhatra, Ancient India, I, 1946; H. Waddington, Adilabad, Ancient India, I, 1946; S. Piggott, Prehistoric India, Harmondsworth, 1947; E. J. Ross, A Chalcolithic Site in Northern Beluchistan, INES, V, 1947; R. E. M. Wheeler, Harappa, 1946, Ancient India, III, 1947; V. S. Agrawala, The Terracottas of Ahichhatra, Ancient India, IV, 1947–48; A. Ghosh, Taxila (Sirkap), 1944–45, Ancient India, IV, 1947–48; R. E. M. Wheeler, Brahmagiri and Chandravalli, 1947, Ancient India, IV, 1947–48; D. H. Gordon, Present Day Painted Pottery, J. of the Indian Anthropological Inst., N.S., II, 1948; B. de Cardi, On the Borders of Pakistan, Indian Art and Letters, XXIV. 1950; M. G. Dikshit, Excavations at Rangpur, B. of the Deccan College Research Inst., XI, 1950; J. Marshall, Taxila, London, 1951; H. D. Sankalia and M. G. Dikshit, Excavations at Brahmapuri (Kolhapur), 1945–46, Poona, 1952; B. Subbarao, Baroda through the Ages, Baroda, 1953; B. B. Lal, Excavations at Hastinapura (all periods), Ancient India, X–XI, 1954–55; D. H. Gordon, The Pottery Industries of the Indo-Iranian Border, Ancient India, X–XI, 1954–55; H. D. Sankalia and S. B. Deo, Excavations at Nasik and Jorwe (all periods), Poona, 1955; W. A. Fairservis, Excavations in the Quetta Valley, West Pakistan, Anthropological Papers, no. 45, American Museum of Natural History, New York, 1956; B. Subbarao, The Personality of India, Baroda, 1956. *b. China*: J. G. Anderson, An Early Chinese Culture, B. of the Geological Survey of China, 1923; B. Rackham, The Earliest Arrivals of pre-Ming Wares in the West, Transactions of the Oriental Ceramic Soc., III, 1923–24, pp. 10–16; J. M. Plumer, A Note on the Chien-yao (Temmoku) Kiln-site, OAZ, XI, 1935; G. Hedley, Yi-hsing Ware, Transactions of the Oriental Ceramic Soc., XIV, 1936–37, pp. 70–87; P. David, A Commentary on Ju-ware, Transactions of the Oriental Ceramic Soc., XIV, 1936–37, pp. 18–69; J. M. Plumer, The Origin of "Secret Colour" Ware, ILN, Mar. 13 and 20, 1937; F. Koyama, Shina Seiji Shi-ko (History of Chinese Celadon), Tokyo, 1943; W. B. Honey, The Ceramic Art of China and Other Countries of the Far East, London, 1945; A. Hetherington, Chinese Ceramic Glazes, South Pasadena, 1948; Cêng Tê-K'un, Szechwan Pottery, Apollo Annual, I, 1948, pp. 27–32; J. M. Plumer, The Ting-yao Kiln-sites: Koyama's Significant Discoveries, Archives of the Chinese Art Soc. of Am., III, 1948–49, pp. 61–66; F. Koyama, The Story of Old Chinese Ceramics, Tokyo, 1949; O. Karlbeck, Early Yüeh Ware, Oriental Art, II, 1949, p. 3 ff.; O. Karlbeck, Protoporcelain and Yüeh, Transactions of the Oriental Ceramic Soc., XXV, 1949–50, pp. 33–48; G. Sayer, Ching-tê-chên T'ao lu, or the Potteries of China, London, 1951; B. Gray, Early Chinese Pottery and Porcelain, London, 1953; G. St. G. M. Gompertz, Some Notes on Yüeh Ware, Oriental Art, N.S., II, 1956, pp. 3–8, 109–16; Chê'n Wan-li, Chung-kuo ch'ing-tz'u-shih-lüeh (Brief History of Chinese Celadon), Shanghai, 1956; W. Willetts, Chinese Art, II, Harmondsworth, 1958, pp. 393–500. *c. Japan*: G. Knuttel, Japans aardewerk ten dienste van de theeceremonie, The Hague, 1948; T. Mitsuoka, Ceramic Art of Japan, Japan Travel Bureau, Tokyo, 1949; Pageant of Japanese Art, IV, Ceramics and Metalwork, Tokyo, 1952–54; S. Jenyns,

Japanese Porcelain, Catalogue of an Exhibition Held by the Oriental Ceramic Society, London, Mar-Apr., 1956; S. Toju Zenshu, Kawade Shobo, Tokyo, 1956–57.

Illustrations: PLS. 120–173; 18 figs. in text.

**CEYLON.** The English spelling of the Singhalese Sēlān, derived from the Sanskrit Siṃhala (Pali, Sīhala), perhaps alluding to the lions (siṃha, sīha) once abundant in the island. In Indian literature Ceylon is also called Laṇkā and Tāmra-parṇī (Tambapaṇṇi), whence the Ταπροβάνη of classical sources. Its geographic location has made Ceylon, separated from the Indian subcontinent only by a narrow stretch of sea (the Straits of Palk), open to influences originating in India (see CEYLONESE ART). Occupied in part by the Portuguese in the 16th century and later by the Dutch (17th–18th cent.), at the beginning of the 19th century it had come under British rule as a colony. Declared independent in November, 1947, in February of the following year it was granted the status of a Dominion within the British Commonwealth. Divided into nine provinces, it had a population of 8,929,000 in June, 1956, distributed over an area of more than 25,000 square miles. The art monuments of Ceylon consist for the most part of the sculptures of Buddhist religious edifices (stupas and viharas). There are also, however, notable examples of Hindu religious art (Ämbakke Devāle, Devundara, Jaffna, Polonnaruva, Tirukkovil) and of secular architecture (Anuradhapura, Kandy, Panduvas-Nuvara, Polonnaruva, etc.). There are also traces of the Dutch occupation (Galle, Jaffna) and one prehistoric construction (Padavigampola).

The ancestors of the great majority of the present population of Ceylon emigrated from India and, no doubt, introduced to Ceylon the art and architecture with which they were familiar in their homeland; the island was open to cultural influences from India throughout the centuries. The position of Ceylon athwart the maritime trade route from the West to the East made the influence of the principal seafaring nations of the world felt in the island in matters of art and architecture as well as in economics and politics.

From the earliest times the Singhalese originating in northern India (whose name eventually came to be applied to all the inhabitants of Ceylon), had to contend with the Tamils from southern India for the possession of the island, and on several occasions a Tamil prince occupied the throne of Anuradhapura. But it was only in the 8th century that a shrine in southern Indian style was built in Ceylon; this, too, not in the capital city but in an out-of-the-way place in the Central Province. Architectural monuments and works of art dating from the period when the island was a province of the Chola empire (see ANDHRA; DRAVIDIAN ART) in the 11th century are found at Polonnaruva, the medieval capital.

Owing to recurrent invasions from southern India and internal strife among the Singhalese themselves, the regions that had witnessed the flowering of Singhalese culture began to be depopulated in the 13th century, a process hastened by malaria. Architectural monuments, sculptures, and paintings after the 13th century are mostly to be seen, therefore, in the central and southwestern areas. The monuments of the Portuguese and Dutch occupations of the maritime provinces are naturally met with at the principal seaports, such as Matara, Jaffna, Galle, and Trincomalee; those in Colombo, however, were sacrificed for the modern development of the city.

As in doctrine, so also in art, the people of Ceylon have been conservative; but certain architectural and artistic features — for instance, the circular temple, the vaulted brick shrine, and the moon stone — underwent elaboration in Ceylon.

In the 18th century, after a period of decline, the Buddhist religion was reestablished in the island by missionaries who were invited from Siam. Along with religion, images and other sacred objects of considerable artistic merit were brought to Ceylon from Siam and are still preserved in temples in and around Kandy. In more recent times, Buddha images and other religious objects have been imported from Burma. Modern Buddhist temples on the seaboard have been influenced to some extent by Burmese Buddhist architecture.

National art forms suffered an eclipse under British rule, throughout the greater part of which the fashion among the Ceylonese was to imitate the ways of life of the ruling race. With the upsurge of national feeling at the beginning of the present century, there was a tendency to imitate Indian art, particularly that of Bengal. On the other hand, modern European art trends have also exerted considerable influence on the work of many artists.

The protection of the artistic heritage is not being neglected. The Archaeological Department has occupied itself actively, if

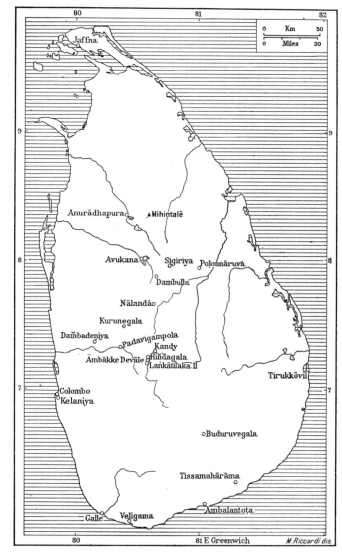

Ceylon: principal centers of archaeological and art interest.

a little spasmodically, with the preservation of monuments since the last decade of the 19th century. One section of the Colombo Museum is dedicated exclusively to the preservation of ancient objects found in that locality; there are local archaeological museums at Anuradhapura and at Dedigama. The Kandy Museum specializes in work of the period during which it was the capital of the Singhalese Kingdom. That of Jaffna contains antiquities found in the northern section. A recently founded school of art in Colombo trains its students in the art techniques of both East and West.

PRINCIPAL SITES AND MONUMENTAL COMPLEXES. The sites of major art interest are the following:

The Abhayagiri. Second largest among the ancient stupas of Ceylon, north of the walled city of Anuradhapura, it was built by Vaṭṭagāmaṇī Abhaya in the 1st century B.C. and enlarged by Gaja-

bāhu I in the 2d century of our era. It has a diameter of 355 ft. at the base, and its present height, with the upper part of the spire missing, is 245 ft. When entire, it is said to have been 140 cubits (350 ft.) high. The paved platform on which the stupa stands is 587 ft. square. The frontispieces (*vāhalkaḍas*) projecting from the base of the stupa date from about the 2d century, and on the steles flanking them are interesting figure sculptures and plant motifs which are among the earliest sculptures known in Ceylon.

The Ämbakke Devāle. A shrine dedicated to Skanda, about 7 miles southwest of Kandy. On the wooden pillars supporting the roof of the pavilion, in front of the main shrine, and on the members of the woodwork of the roof there are carvings representative of the best Kandy style work of this class. The construction of the roof gives an idea of the methods of early Ceylonese architects.

Ambalantota. Site of an ancient Buddhist monastery, close to the mouth of the Valave River in the Hambantota District. Contains Buddha images and bodhisattva figures, more or less fragmentary, which may belong to the early centuries of the Christian era. A slab of southern Indian marble has also been found there containing a bas-relief of the Buddha renouncing the pleasures of life and embracing asceticism.

Anuradhapura. Now the capital of the North Central Province, the city was the capital of the Ceylonese kings from the 4th century B.C. to the end of the 10th century. In and around this city were built the earliest Buddhist shrines, among which particular mention may be made of the Bo-tree shrine, the Thūpārāma, the Mahā-thūpa (Ruvanväli), the Mirisavāṭi, the Dekkhiṇathūpa, the Abhayagiri, the Jetavana, and the site now called Isurumuniya. To the west of the city were the meditation houses now referred to as "palaces." Extensive monastic establishments surrounded the walled city and their ruins extend for three or four miles. Stylobates and stereobates of edifices with beautifully sculptured flights of steps giving access to them are a common sight. Noteworthy are the remains of the palace within the citadel and the pleasure garden of the king, by the embankment of the artificial lake, Tisaveva, constructed in the 3d century B.C. There are numerous stone-faced bathing pools, among which the most magnificent is the pair known as Kūṭṭam Pokuṇa. The small museum contains antiquities unearthed in Anuradhapura and sites in the neighborhood.

Avukana. About 2 miles from the Kalaveva embankment, one of the greatest of the Ceylonese irrigation works constructed in the 5th century; site of an ancient Buddhist monastery of about the 2d century B.C. On a rock face here is carved a colossal standing image of the Buddha measuring 42 ft. in height, including the lotus pedestal. Enclosing the image was an 8th-century shrine, the lower part of which was constructed of massive slabs of well-cut granite.

Buduruvegala. In the heart of the forest 7 miles southwest of Vellavaya in Uva Province. Carved on the steep face of a rock is a group of huge figures of great artistic merit, a Buddha image over 50 ft. high, attended on either side by two bodhisattvas, each of whom is accompanied by his spouse and another divinity. The images, which on grounds of style may be ascribed to about the 9th century, are of Mahayana character.

Dambadeniya. In the Kurunegala District; capital of Ceylon during the 13th century. At the site are architectural fragments and figure carvings representative of the art of that period.

Dambulla. A site in the Matāle District dating back to pre-Christian centuries. A large cave, below the drip ledge of which is a Brahmi inscription, contains stucco and wooden images of the 12th century, painted over at a later period. On the walls and roof of the cave are paintings in the late Kandy style of the 18th century.

Dedigama. In the Kegalla District; the birthplace of Parākramabāhu I (reigned 1153–86). A very large stupa was built here to mark the room in which he was born. During excavation of the monument many interesting objects that were deposited in the relic chambers were brought to light; particular mention should be made of a hanging lamp with an automatic device to replenish the oil from a reservoir formed of the belly of a carved elephant. The lamp is also remarkable as a work of art. The antiquities are preserved in a small museum on the site.

The Degaldoruva. A shrine in the Kandy District partly hewn out of rock, on the walls of which are fairly well-preserved paintings of the 18th century.

Devangala. In the Kegalla District; has a history going back to the 12th century, but its interest for the student of art is the discovery in a 16th-century stupa of bronze Buddha images and reliquaries representative of that period.

Devundara. At the extreme south of the island, in the Matara District, Devundara was the center of the cult of Upulvan, the national god of the Singhalese. A small 7th-century shrine of simple and graceful outline is one of the very few examples of Singhalese stone architecture. Architectural fragments and carved stones of about the 14th and 15th centuries, a Buddha image in archaic style, and several images of Hindu gods have been found here.

Dimbulagala. An extensive ancient site in the Tamankaduva District of the North Central Province. In a rock shelter at a place called Puligoda-galge in the vicinity are the remains of paintings of the 12th century.

Gadala. In the Kandy District; has a well-preserved stone shrine in the Dravidian style (see DRAVIDIAN ART) of the 14th century. On the pillars and stylobate of the building are sculptures characteristic of the style and the period. In the shrine is a bronze Buddha image, a little over a foot high, in a style reminiscent of the Nalanda images.

Galabedda. Ancient Udundora, a royal seat of the 12th century in Uva Province. A beautiful stone bathing pool is its most important architectural monument.

Galle. Capital of the Southern Province; has a well-preserved Dutch fort, within which are several buildings, including a church.

Galmaduva. In the Kandy District; has a shrine of the 18th century built in the form of a pyramidal tower enclosed by a wall with openings formed by perfect arches.

The Gal Vihara, Polonnaruva. Noteworthy for the colossal images of the Buddha, two seated, one standing, and another (the largest) in a recumbent posture, carved on the face of the rock. One of the two seated images is within an excavated cave, on the walls of which are remnants of paintings. The images date from the 12th-century reign of Parākramabāhu I.

Hindagala. Six miles southwest of Kandy. High up on the rock roof of a cave, which is at least as early as the 7th century, there are considerable remains of paintings which are stylistically similar to the later work at Ajanta (q.v.).

Isurumuniya. An ancient Buddhist site beside the embankment of the Tisaveva in Anuradhapura. At this site are the well-known man-and-horse rock relief, in Pallava style; a bas-relief depicting an amatory couple in Gupta style; and a number of other sculptures of considerable artistic merit.

Jaffna. Present capital of the Northern Province; was seat of the Tamil kings who ruled the northern districts from the 13th to the 16th century. The inner shrine of the Nallūr Kandaswāmy Temple dates from the 15th century. Has the most perfect example of a Dutch fortress to be seen in Ceylon. Within the fort is one of the largest Dutch churches in the island. A small museum in the town contains objects of artistic interest discovered in the area.

The Jetavana. Built by Mahāsena in the 4th century, this stupa, situated southeast of Anuradhapura, in the largest in Ceylon. It is 370 ft. in diameter at the base, and its broken spire rises 231 ft. above the pavement. At the frontispieces facing the cardinal points are sculptures in a mature style.

Kandy. Present capital of the Central Province, it was the last capital of the Ceylonese Kings. The Temple of the Tooth Relic, one of the holiest shrines of Ceylon Buddhists, is a good example of the wooden architecture of the 17th century. Opposite the Temple of the Tooth Relic is the Nātha Devāle, dedicated to Avalokiteśvara, which is of stone construction and dates from about the 14th century. The Audience Hall of the Ceylonese kings has delicate carvings on its wooden pillars.

The Kaṇṭaka Cetiya (chaitya), Mihintale. A fairly large stupa, built in the earliest days of Buddhism in Ceylon and enlarged in the 1st century B.C. The architectural details of an early stupa can be studied best at this monument. It also possesses the best-preserved frontispieces to be seen anywhere in the island. The steles flanking the frontispieces have bas-reliefs in a very archaic style, some in a more developed style.

Kelaniya. Near Colombo, the modern capital of Ceylon; has one of the earliest Ceylonese stupas, which, however, is not seen in its old form, having been restored in the 18th century. In a shrine adjoining the stupa are paintings of that period with a very effective color scheme.

Kokebe. Site in the Anuradhapura District of a group of cists.

Kurunegala. Present capital of the Northwestern Province; was the capital of the island in the first half of the 14th century. Stone sculptures of that period were found on the old palace site.

The Laṇkātilaka, near Kandy. A shrine of brick construction with a vaulted roof and side arches, dating from the middle of the 14th century; situated 7 miles southwest of Kandy.

The Laṇkātilaka, Polonnaruva. A 12th-century brick building with a vaulted roof, dating from the reign of Parākramabāhu I, this is the most imposing edifice built by ancient Ceylonese architects.

Mahiyangana. At this site in Uva Province was one of the earliest stupas in Ceylon. In a relic chamber of later date wall paintings, bronze figures, and other objects of art from the 11th century have been discovered.

Medirigiri. Ancient Mandalagiri, in the Tamankaduva District of the North Central Province. The shrine here is one of the best preserved specimens of the circular chaitya to be seen in Ceylon. It dates from the 8th century. The special feature of this monument is the screen wall imitating a railing, in line with the outermost of the three concentric circles of stone pillars which supported the domical roof of wood.

Mihintale. A hill 8 miles east of Anuradhapura. In addition to the Kaṇṭaka Chaitya separately noted, there are various other remains dating from the 3d century B.C. to the 10th century. Paintings have been discovered in the relic chamber of one stupa, and golden reliquaries and Buddha images in another. A bath adorned with sculptures and a rampant lion are also noteworthy.

Mulgirigala. A site in the Hambantota District dating from pre-Christian centuries. In a shrine from the 18th century are found paintings of that date.

Nalanda. In the Matale District; possesses the only example in Ceylon of a stone-built shrine in the Pallava style of architecture. Sculptured stones are to be seen in the debris formed by the collapse of portions of the shrine, which is of Mahayana type.

Nilligkama. In the Kurunegala District; noteworthy as the site of an 8th-century *bodhighāra*. The doorframes are decorated with creeper designs, and the upper platform is also carved.

Padavigampola. Near Rambukkana, in the Kegalla District, has the only known example of a dolmen in Ceylon.

Panduvas-Nuvara. Ancient Parakramapura, in the Kurunegala District. The remains of the palace of Parākramabāhu, unearthed at the site, furnish a complete ground plan of a medieval palace.

Pankuliya. Site of an ancient Buddhist monastery, north of Anuradhapura. In a ruined shrine at the site is a colossal seated Buddha image with the hands in the protection (*abhaya*) attitude, the only one of this type known in Ceylon.

Polonnaruva. The capital of Ceylon in the 11th and 12th centuries, it is today the capital of the district of the same name. The city is called Pulastipura in the Pali chronicles (see CEYLONESE ART). The oldest building of note preserved today is the Śiva temple in the Chola style of architecture. Remains of the royal palace and Buddhist religious edifices to be seen here are important for the study of Ceylonese architecture and arts of the 12th century. The Gal Vihara, the Potgul Vihara, the Laṇkātilaka, the Tivaṇka, the Thūpārāma, and the Vaṭadāgē are among the principal edifices and are listed separately.

The Potgul Vehera (Vihara), Polonnaruva. A colossal statue carved on the face of a rock here, traditionally believed to be a representation of Parākramabāhu I, is very probably the figure of a king bearing the yoke of sovereignty.

The Ridī Vihara. A Buddhist site in the Kurunegala District dating back to pre-Christian times. Noteworthy are a shrine in the Pāṇḍya style with a later addition in Vijayanagar style, and paint-

ings on the walls of a shrine of the 18th century. The doorframe at the entrance is decorated with carved ivory panels.

The Ruvanväli (Ruvanveli, Ruwanweli), Anuradhapura. Called the Mahāthūpa in the Pali chronicles (see CEYLONESE ART), it was built in the 2d century B.C. and is the third largest dagoba in Ceylon. In addition to the sculptures at the frontispieces, which are fragmentary and scattered about, four huge Buddha images and a bodhisattva figure have been found.

Seruvila. In the Eastern Province; has one of the most venerated stupas in Ceylon. A Buddha image of stone, seated on the coils of the serpent Mucalinda and protected by the serpent's hood, is the best image of this type found in Ceylon.

Sesseruva. In the Kurunegala District; notable for a great image of the Buddha carved in high relief on the face of a rock.

Sigiriya. In the Matale District; famous for the paintings found in a pocket on the western face of the rock, on the summit of which a palace was built by a king of the 5th century.

Situlpavu. In the Hambantota District; site of an ancient Buddhist vihara. An image of a bodhisattva in the Pallava style has been found here.

The Thūpārāma, Anuradhapura. First stupa built in Ceylon. The stone pillars with carved capitals arranged in four concentric circles round the stupa supported a domical wooden roof.

The Thūpārāma, Polonnaruva. The best preserved, though the smallest, of the vaulted brick buildings at Polonnaruva.

Tiriyay. Ancient Girikandi Vihara, in the Trincomalee District. The remains of the circular shrine here are of interest for the study of ancient Ceylonese architecture, and the "guard stones" (stone guardian figures) at the entrances date back to the 8th century.

Tirukkovil. In the Batticaloa District; has a well-preserved Hindu temple built in the Pāṇḍya style.

Tissamaharama. Ancient Mahagama, capital of the principality of Rohana, in the Hambantota District. Among the extensive ruins are a number of early sculptures.

The Tivaṇka, Polonnaruva. A vaulted brick shrine named from the *tribhaṅga* pose of the image (flexed at three points). On the walls are 12th- and 13th-century paintings depicting Buddhist stories.

The Vaṭadāgē (circular shrine), Polonnaruva. Dating in its present form from the 12th century, this is the most elaborate example of a circular shrine enclosing a stupa found in Ceylon. The screen wall connected with the outermost circle of pillars is decorated with a design of four-petaled flowers. The four Buddha images against the base of the stupa, facing the cardinal points, are noteworthy for the sculptural treatment of the hair, resembling a skull cap.

Veligama. In the Matara District; noted for a colossal sculpture carved in high relief on a rock. The image, popularly known as "The Leper King," is a representation of Avalokiteśvara.

BIBLIOG. See CEYLONESE ART.

Senarat PARANAVITANA

Illustration: 1 fig. in text.

## CEYLONESE ART.

The origins of Ceylonese art are linked with the introduction of Buddhism to the island, according to local chronicles (see *Sources*), by Mahendra (Mahinda), son or younger brother of the Indian emperor Aśoka Maurya (ca. 268–233 B.C.). Buddhism (q.v.), still the prevailing religion of Ceylon, has been the main source of art inspiration; second to it, Hinduism (q.v.), introduced by a wave of Dravidian immigrants from southern India (see ANDHRA; DRAVIDIAN ART), has produced the most significant art expression. Secular art is seen only in the royal palaces and perhaps in the construction of certain bathing pools, though these, considering the ritual character of the bath in Ceylon as well as in India, should

rather be treated as examples of religious art. Affected by Indian cultural currents but withdrawn by its geographical position from the complex events of the history of the subcontinent, Ceylon preserved its inheritance of Indian art (q.v.) long after the elements had vanished from their original home, while evolving and elaborating a character of its own.

SUMMARY. History (col. 331). The stupa and religious architecture (col. 332). Secular architecture (col. 334). Sculpture (col. 334). Painting (col. 337). Minor arts (col. 338).

HISTORY. The Singhalese, who form about 70 per cent of the population of Ceylon, are descendants of Aryan-speaking immigrants from northern India who settled in the island some five centuries before the beginning of the Christian era. The Tamils, who at present inhabit the northern and eastern parts of the island, constitute an overflow of the Dravidian-speaking population from southern India. Apart from a minority that has been converted to Christianity, the Singhalese profess Buddhism, which was established as the religion of the kings and people of Ceylon as a result of the missionary enterprises of the great Indian emperor Aśoka in the 3d century B.C. The majority of the Tamils are Hindus, and their art and architecture are the same as those of their brethren in southern India. The art that is distinctive of the Singhalese, though ultimately of Indian origin like their language and religion, has developed during the centuries in accordance with their national individuality and has preserved until very recently many motifs that became obsolete in India itself at a rather early date. It is therefore in the art and architecture of the Singhalese that Ceylon can make a special contribution to the study of Indian art as a whole.

Devānampiya Tissa, the Singhalese contemporary of Aśoka, gave an enthusiastic welcome to the missionaries dispatched by the Maurya emperor and embraced the religion preached by them. Acting on their advice he established monasteries and built shrines dedicated to his new faith at his capital, Anuradhapura. A few decades after the establishment of Buddhism as the state religion of the island, invaders from southern India established Tamil dominion at Anuradhapura that lasted for about half a century until Singhalese sovereignty was restored about 150 B.C. The period that followed up to the 4th century, in spite of occasional inroads by Tamils from southern India and domestic distrurbances now and then, saw the flowering of the early civilization of the Singhalese. The embellishment of the stupendous Buddhist shrines built during this period gave a strong impetus to the development of the arts of painting and sculpture.

The great achievement of the 5th century was the building of Sigiriya, in which rare artistry was combined with a bold engineering feat. In the period from the 6th to the 10th century, new influences from India modified the architectural and artistic motifs that either were brought by the Singhalese when they originally settled in the island or were introduced as a result of cultural contacts with Mauryan India.

The conquest of Ceylon early in the 11th century by the great Chola emperor Rājarāja was catastrophic to Singhalese political institutions as well as culture and art. For over half a century Ceylon was a province not only of the Chola empire but also of Dravidian culture. Saiva shrines in Dravidian style were built at Polonnaruva, the Chola capital, in the 11th century. Although Singhalese sovereignty was restored by Vijayabāhu I in 1070, the ancient capital, Anuradhapura, was supplanted by Polonnaruva as the center of political and artistic activities. The accession of Parākramabāhu I in 1153 inaugurated a great era of building activity. The arts of painting and sculpture were assiduously cultivated in the second half of the 12th and the first decade of the 13th century. But this brilliant period came to an end with a southern Indian invasion in 1213. When the Portuguese arrived in Ceylon in 1505, driving the inhabitants to the hills, the arts in Ceylon were in decadence. This process was accelerated by the continuous struggle maintained by the Ceylonese against the Portuguese and against the Dutch and the British who supplanted them.

THE STUPA AND RELIGIOUS ARCHITECTURE. A study of the remains of the earliest Buddhist monuments in Ceylon reveals that the indigenous art of central India, represented by the monuments of Bharhut, Sanchi, and Bodhgaya, furnished the inspiration and models for these shrines. The court art of the Mauryas, containing within it elements of Persian and other foreign origin, had no influence in the development of art and architecture in the island.

Most enduring of the early religious monuments built in Ceylon were the stupas — solid hemispherical mounds of earth or brick for enshrining corporeal relics of the Buddha or the saints. The stupa was of pre-Buddhist origin; in course of time, however, it came to be considered as the characteristic Buddhist shrine and the principal Buddhist architectural form.

The original simple form developed, in the course of centuries, into elaborate designs as the faith spread into lands far removed from its place of origin. In the time of Aśoka and for two or three centuries after him, the Indian stupa consisted of a hemispherical dome rising from one or three terraces, with a railing at the summit. An octagonal pillar of wood or stone was built into the center of the dome, rising from the cistlike relic chamber placed on the level of the topmost terrace and projecting above the railing on the summit. An umbrella, the symbol of sovereignty in ancient India as well as Ceylon, made of wood or of stone, surmounted the monument to indicate that the Buddha, symbolized by the stupa, is the Lord of the World. A railing encompassed the monument at the base; in some stupas there was a railing on the basal terrace also. A torana (Skr., torana), or gateway, gave access through the railing; in larger stupas there were four gateways. The monument was decorated with banners at the top and garlands of flowers around the dome.

The stupas that were built in Ceylon during the early period of Buddhism are not found today in their original form. They were reduced to ruins, and some have been restored more than once. But the descriptions of these shrines found in the ancient literature indicate that they were of the same pattern as the stupas of ancient India. This conclusion is confirmed by the discovery of a number of golden reliquaries that are miniature stupas, identical in form with those at Sanchi.

In Ceylon, as in India, the piety of devotees added to the number of umbrellas surmounting a stupa. Instead of one, as used originally, there was a series of umbrellas, one over the other. The upper umbrellas gradually diminished in size, the topmost being of very small diameter. In course of time, this series of umbrellas was translated into brick masonry, in the form of a conical spire with moldings, and was crowned with an umbrella of wood or metal. In a brick contruction the shaft of the series of umbrellas had to be less slender than in a wooden or metal one, and it developed into a cylindrical feature ornamented with pilasters between which were figures of guardian deities. Before this development of the spire the square railing above the dome had become a solid cubical structure of brick masonry, ornamented with a railing pattern on all four sides. In the middle of each side of this cubical structure was placed the figure of a sun. Apart from this development in the upper portion of the stupa, which had taken place before the 8th century, the form of this typical Buddhist shrine underwent little change in Ceylon. In some of the smaller stupas built by the Mahayanists the dome was elongated, not bubble-shaped as in earlier monuments, and the terraces at the base were reduced to a series of moldings, one above the other. An unusual type of stupa in Ceylon, of which the best preserved example dates from the 12th century, is in the form of a stepped pyramid of seven stages.

The largest of the colossal stupas of Anuradhapura, the 4th-century Jetavana, has a diameter of 370 ft. at the base and was originally about 400 ft. in height. Projecting from the base and facing the four cardinal points are offsets or frontispieces, the lower portions of which are faced with limestone to form a series of molded horizontal stringcourses separated by vertical bands. These frontispieces have been compared to the projections at the cardinal points in the stupas of the Andhra country (see ANDHRA) and seem to have developed

in Ceylonese stupas about the beginning of the Christian era. Each frontispiece (*vāhalkada*) of the Ceylonese stupa is flanked by steles surmounted by figures of bulls, elephants, horses, or lions according to the direction in which the structure faces. The earliest extant sculptures in Ceylon are those ornamenting the steles of the frontispieces.

The smaller stupas were enclosed within circular shrines whose dome-shaped roofs, constructed of wood, were supported by stone pillars. The domical shape of the roof was obtained by the use of curved rafters or ribs that were fitted to a circular base at the top and held in position by the pressure from both sides. A circle of pillars planted a few feet away from the base of the stupa supported the roof above it. There was a lower roof shaped like a cyma curve, supported on two or three concentric circles of pillars extending out on all sides of the central domical roof. Between the two outer circles of pillars there was also a brick wall giving additional support to the lower roof. Early examples of these circular shrines enclosing stupas (*cetiyāghāra*, Skr., *caitya*) appear to have been constructed entirely of wood, hence no remains of them are found today. In about the 8th century several of these circular shrines were built with stone pillars, for example, those at the Thūpārāma and the Laṅkārāma at Anuradhapura and at Mandalagiri (mod. Medirigiri). In the most developed example of a shrine of this type, the Vaṭadāgē at Polonnaruva, a low screen wall of stone slabs decorated with four-petaled flowers is connected to the outermost circle of pillars (PL. 176). At Medirigiri the screen wall occupying a similar position imitates the familiar Buddhist railing found at Sanchi and other early sites in India. Ornamental flights of steps give access to the shrine at the gates facing the cardinal points.

A sculpture at Bharhut, another at Nagarjunakonda, and the rock-cut chaityas at Guntupalle and Junnar attest to the existence of the circular type of shrine in India during the early Buddhist period, but in later times in India the apsidal type of temple for enclosing stupas became more common. In Ceylon, however, the ancient type persisted down to the 15th century and underwent an evolution that was lacking in the land of its origin. Some of the most impressive ancient monuments in Ceylon are shrines of this class — for example, the Vaṭadāgē at Medirigiri.

In the early period of Buddhism the cult of the Bo tree (*Ficus religiosa*) shared with the stupa the devotion of lay believers, and a type of shrine called *bodhighāra* came into being in connection with the sacred tree. This consisted of a pillared pavilion with an ornamental roof surrounding all four sides of the platform on which the sacred tree was planted. The most important shrine of this class in ancient Ceylon was the Bo-tree shrine at Anuradhapura, which is, however, a restoration. Substantial remains of a *bodhighāra* of the 8th or 9th century have recently been identified and conserved at Nillakgama in the Kurunegala District.

Residences for royalty and for religious dignitaries, as well as monastic buildings, were largely of wood in ancient Ceylon. Their descriptions given in the chronicles indicate that they were of considerable size and grandeur and were richly ornamented. During the early centuries of the Christian era, stone began to be used for pillars and flights of steps of the more sumptuous edifices, and the molded stylobates were faced with brick or stone. The moldings generally favored were the ovolo, cyma, and torus. The flights of steps were flanked by stones carved into the shapes of the *makara*, a fabulous composite animal. At the terminals of these were placed slabs of stone with rounded tops, bearing representations in bas-relief of vases filled with flowers or of anthropomorphic serpent deities.

While the majority of the ancient buildings had a superstructure of wood, there was also a type of edifice which was entirely of brick construction, apart from the flights of steps and doorframes, which were of stone. The earliest datable example of this type of shrine, which is referred to in Ceylonese literature as *geḍigē*, belongs to the 8th century. The roof of a building of this type was constructed as a brick vault. There is evidence to establish that the true arch was known to Ceylonese architects as early as the 8th century; but in the construction of vaults and arches they generally adopted the method of corbeling.

The *geḍigē* type reached its utmost elaboration in the Laṅkātilaka of Polonnaruva built by Parākramabāhu I in the 12th century. Even in its present ruined condition the Laṅkātilaka is an imposing edifice. The north wall, now standing to a height of 55 ft., must originally have been not less than 100 ft. in height. The length is 124 ft. from front to back, and the maximum breadth is 66 ft. at the square shrine, within which is a colossal image of the Buddha in stucco and an antechamber, with an entresol between the two. The broad entrance is flanked by polygonal piers; there is an arched side entrance on the northern façade. In its exterior aspect the edifice rises from a heavily molded base; the façade, divided into tiers by horizontal moldings, is ornamented with models of shrines between pilasters.

The ancient Ceylonese apparently tried to develop a style of stone architecture sometime in the 7th century. The result is the small shrine at Devundara in the extreme south of the island, which is noteworthy for the simplicity and harmony of its form and its balanced proportions. This attempt to create lithic forms in architecture was not continued, perhaps because of lack of suitable building stones, but the shrine now known as the Haṭadāgē at Polonnaruva, intended to house the Tooth Relic, was of stone construction up to the level of the upper story. The Dravidian type of stone architecture, which originated in the 7th century in southern India and in which edifices of great complexity and magnitude were created in later centuries, was also known in Ceylon. The earliest building in this style is a Mahayana (or rather, Vajrayana) shrine at Nalanda in the Central Province. It is in the late Pallava style, as attested by the form of its corbels and of the *kūḍu*. A Saiva shrine (Śiva Devāle No. 2) at Polonnaruva in the Chola style was built in the first half of the 11th century when the island formed a province of the great Chola empire. Another shrine, Śiva Devāle No. 1, at the same capital, is in the Pandya style.

SECULAR ARCHITECTURE. Among secular monuments, the most spectacular was the palace built on the summit of Sigiriya rock by Kassapa I in the 5th century, together with the galleries which gave access to it along an almost unscalable precipice (PL. 176). The rock with the palace and gardens on its summit formed the central feature of a large walled city, within which were well-laid-out gardens containing ponds, pavilions, and fountains. There are substantial remains of royal palaces at Anuradhapura, Polonnaruva, and a number of other places in the island. The pavilion, or Hall of Public Audience in the royal palace at Polonnaruva, built on a high platform of three tiers and ornamented with friezes of elephants, lions, and dwarfs, contained four rows of elegantly carved stone pillars that supported the ornamental wooden roof. There are also beautiful stone baths within royal precincts as well as in monastic dwellings.

SCULPTURE. Ancient Ceylonese buildings were often ornamented with sculptures. In the shrines there were images of the Buddha, of gods, and of other supernatural beings who were worshiped by the faithful. In the ornamentation of buildings, however, the ancient Ceylonese architects, unlike their compeers in many parts of India, exhibited commendable restraint. The sculptural ornamentation is so disposed as not to interfere with the architectural form. As a rule it is set against a plain background which further emphasizes the ornamentation and heightens its effect. But in later periods, perhaps owing to the influence of Dravidian architecture, sculptural ornamentation was applied, particularly to the doorways, with greater exuberance and less discrimination.

Just as the architecture of the earliest stupas of Ceylon followed the lines of the monuments of Sanchi and Bharhut, so the earliest preserved specimens of sculpture in Ceylon remind us of similar work at those ancient Buddhist sites in India. As already noted, the earliest examples of sculpture in Ceylon are found on the frontispieces of the great stupas at Anuradhapura and Mihintale. Some of the figures carved on the steles at the Kaṇṭaka Cetiya of Mihintale are in the archaic style of

the Bharhut sculptures. The early sculpture of Ceylon, like that of central India, was conceived frontally; the figures are flat and appear as silhouettes. The headdress of the figures is of the type found at Bharhut and Sanchi (PL. 179).

A very common decorative motif in the steles of these frontispieces is a stem springing from a vase; on either side of the stem are prancing addorsed beasts — lions, bulls, elephants, and horses — alternating with figures of Erotes. The figure of a deity seated on a flower or some other religious symbol crowns the stem. This *kalpavṛkṣa* (tree of life) motif is reminiscent of similar decorative designs on the pillars of some of the gateways at Sanchi. There is enough similarity to establish a common origin for sculptures of this class found at Sanchi and in Ceylon. The *kalpavṛkṣa* of Singhalese art, however, in keeping with its general tone, is more restrained in the elaboration of details than the examples at the central Indian site, and much more so than those at Amaravati.

Side by side with these sculptures of a distinctively archaic character, we find at the frontispieces figure sculptures exhibiting a much more mature art, in which the third dimension has been fully mastered. The human figure is modeled with great skill in easy and graceful postures, and drapery is treated with a very effective linear rhythm. These characteristics show the influence of the art of the Andhra country. Furthermore, a number of pieces of sculpture have been discovered, including a life-size Buddha image in the round, which must have been imported to Ceylon from the Andhra country; this is apparent not only from their style but also from the material used for them: the type of marble, not available in Ceylon, from which the sculptures of Amaravati, Nagarjunakonda, and other ancient Buddhist sites in the Kistna Valley were fashioned. The art originally introduced from central India into the island had thus been profoundly modified by its contact with the more mature art of the Andhra country.

The earliest standing Buddha images of the island agree in all details with the freestanding statues of the Buddha belonging to the last phase of the Amaravati school. (In Ceylon there are no locally produced bas-reliefs of the period in which the image illustrates a religious narrative.) The earliest known images, life-size or more than lifesize, were set up in shrines for veneration. As in similar Buddha images of the Andhra country, they have the right shoulder bare and the robe drawn to the left side of the body, making a heavy swag at the bottom hem. These images are of dolomite, a limestone which, among local stones, is the closest approximation to the marble in which the sculptures of the Andhra country are executed. An image of the Buddha, 6 ft. in height, of southern Indian marble has actually been found in Ceylon. It is reasonable to assume that artists from the ateliers in the Andhra country, invited to Ceylon, not only carved Buddha images out of locally available stone but also trained local artists to fashion the sacred images then being introduced all over India.

Belonging to this early phase of art, in addition to figures of nagas and other supernatural beings, are a number of statues in princely attire. These are also of limestone and are generally taken to be representations of the Buddha before his renunciation of worldly life.

Architectural features that received sculptural embellishment during this early period are not preserved in a condition adequate for purposes of esthetic evaluation. There is an obvious relationship between the early sculptures of Ceylon and those of Sanchi and Amaravati. Yet the artists of the island have given expression to their national characteristic in the eschewing of crowded compositions, in the less expressive facial features, and in the restraint that is always noticeable in their work.

The Andhra influence on the art of Ceylon becomes less and less noticeable and finally disappears in about the 5th century. From that time until the 12th century not a single piece of sculpture in Ceylon can be accurately dated on the basis of direct evidence. Only comparison with Indian sculpture gives any understanding of the development of Ceylonese sculpture during this period.

A colossal seated image of the Buddha on the Outer Circular Road at Anuradhapura, attributed to about the 5th century, is universally acknowledged to be one of the outstanding achievements of Ceylonese art. The drapery is without folds, and one shoulder is bare. In general appearance the seated image seems to be related to the Mathura type of the Buddha (PL. 181).

The refinement of form and serenity of expression characteristic of the art of India during the Gupta epoch are noticeable in a number of Buddha and bodhisattva heads in the museums at Colombo and Anuradhapura and also in a bas-relief showing an amatory couple, now preserved at the ancient site called Isurumuni in Anuradhapura.

Also at Isurumuni is another famous sculpture typical of a further development in the art of the island. Carved in sunken relief on the face of a large boulder, at a height of about 15 ft. from the ground, is a human figure with a serious and thoughtful facial expression, seated in what is known in Indian art as the royal pose (*mahārājalīla*). Behind the figure of the man is the head of a horse emerging from the rock. Coomaraswamy identifies the figure of the man in this sculpture as the sage Kapila, but the royal pose is against that identification. The author believes that the human figure represents Parjanva, and the horse's head, Agni, the fire god. Whatever the subject, there is no doubt that the sculpture has stylistic affinities with the art of southern India under the Pallavas. The cold severity of the face, the economy in the representation of the bodily form, the comparative lack of ornament, and the elongated limbs all attest the relationship. A bodhisattva figure from Situlpavu in southeastern Ceylon and an image of a deity found at Kurukkalmadam in the Eastern Province are obviously works of the same school.

Assignable to the later Anuradhapura period are the best preserved and most representative examples of two types of sculpture characteristic of Ceylonese art: the figures of naga kings in human form guarding the entrances to shrines and known therefore as "guard stones," and the semicircular slabs of stone rather inaccurately called "moon stones," which are placed at the foot of flights of steps (PL. 180). In the examples that can be assigned to the close of the Anuradhapura period (10th cent.) there is exquisite refinement of details, with emphasis on technical finish and virtuosity of carving and modeling. These characteristics, which also distinguish Pāla art, are found, for instance, in the guard stones at the entrance to the Ratnaprāsāda in Anuradhapura. The influence of Pāla art on that of Ceylon during the 9th and 10th centuries is attested by a find of miniatures, obviously products of this school brought to Ceylon from northeastern India.

The moon stones of Ceylon in their fullest development are ornamented with a half-lotus in the center and concentric bands in which are creeper motifs, rows of *haṃsa*s (geese), processions of the four beasts — lion, elephant, horse, and bull — and a conventionalized flame forming the outermost band. The rhythmic intricacies of the creeper and the naturalistic modeling of the bulls and elephants are noteworthy. It is generally admitted that the sculptural details of the moon stones are not purely decorative but symbolic of spiritual ideals. A bas-relief from Amaravati shows a moon stone at the entrance to a stupa, and actual examples have been found in front of shrines at Nagarjunakonda. Moon stones have for centuries occupied a special place in the art and architecture of Ceylon and continued to be elaborated in the island even after they went out of vogue on the mainland after the 5th century.

Buddha images of colossal size, carved in high relief on the faces of rocks, are also a feature of the art of this period. The image of the Buddha at Avukana, which, with the lotus pedestal, is 42 ft. high, is at least as early as the 9th century (PL. 181). At Buduruvegala in the south-central part of the island there is an impressive group of rock-hewn images: a central Buddha, over 50 ft. high, attended by two bodhisattvas, one on either side. Each of the bodhisattvas is, in turn, attended by a divine being on each side, one being his consort. The iconography of the images leaves no doubt of their Mahayanistic character.

Like its architecture, the sculpture of the Polonnaruva period (12th cent.) was a continuation and a development of that of the preceding epoch. There was a falling off in quality in some directions; for instance, the moon stones and

guard stones that can definitely be assigned to the 12th century are frigid forms without the suppleness and grace of the earlier work. The most stupendous works of sculpture of the 12th century are four gigantic Buddha images carved on the face of a rock at the site known as Gal Vihara, in Polonnaruva. The rock relief at Potgul Vehara, in Polonnaruva, is in a class by itself. It is popularly believed to be a representation of Parākramabāhu the Great. The figure breathes dignity and has a calm and majestic expression. Unlike most Indian sculptures, it does not appear to delineate a type; the artist has attempted to portray individual characteristics. It may therefore have been a portrait, perhaps of a king. Worthy of note also, from the 12th century, are some Buddhist bronzes (PL. 183).

The sculptural work produced after the 13th century is of little artistic merit compared with the work of earlier centuries. The Buddha images, as a rule, are devoid of grace; they are turned out in accordance with rules of proportion from which the artists dared not depart. Hindu images of this period are equally devoid of artistic worth. At Yapavu and Horana there are friezes of dancers and musicians with swaying limbs in violent movement.

In addition to the Saiva bronzes already referred to, probably of southern Indian origin, images in metal (gold, silver, copper, and bronze) have been found dating from the 4th century and later, generally following the lines of those fashioned from stone. A nearly life-size bronze of Pattinī Devī, now in the British Museum, is a remarkable work of art. Mention may be made also of an image of Maitreya found at Anuradhapura, now in the Colombo Museum. Figures in terra cotta and stucco were common in architectural decoration.

PAINTING. Though it can be inferred from references in literary works that painters practiced their art in Ceylon from about the 3d century B.C., the earliest paintings preserved are the well-known Sigiriya frescoes from the 5th century. Pictures were painted on wooden boards and on cloth as well as on the walls of palaces and shrines. The *Cūlavaṃsa* refers to picture galleries in parks attached to royal palaces in the 12th century. The caves that served as abodes of Buddhist recluses in pre-Christian centuries and were later converted into places of worship were adorned with paintings (PL. 178).

The Sigiriya paintings are in a cave beneath the overhanging western face of an almost unscalable rock, on the summit of which Kassapa I, 5th-century king of Ceylon, built a palace resembling the abode of Kubera, the Indian Pluto. Twenty-two figures of females bedecked in costly garments and rich jewelry, some in pairs, others single, are all that now remains of a large number of similar figures that adorned an extensive area of the rock face, so that the rock of Sigiriya appeared like the Kailāsa on which Kubera had his abode. The female figures are represented as rising from clouds, the lower limbs not being depicted, like the apsarases (nymphs) who hover about Kailāsa. Some of the figures are of golden complexion, while others are dark-skinned. They are holding flowers in their hands or raining them down. The female forms, with the faces in three-quarter profile, are drawn with great skill, the sensitive lines of the hands and figures being particularly worthy of mention. In comparing these paintings with those of the same period in India, it is apparent that their drawing and coloring have more robust strength than those of the mainland. The palette of the artists was limited to red, yellow, and green. Though the art is mainly one of line, shading was used in modeling the limbs. The pigments were prepared from minerals, and the technique appears to have been fresco. As in Indian art, the figures adhere to a canon of abstract beauty, with swelling rounded breasts, slender waists, long eyes like those of the fawn, and sensuous lips, but the physical type, with oval faces, must have reflected Ceylonese taste of the time.

The very fragmentary remains of paintings to be seen in a cave at Hindagala, 6 miles southwest of Kandy, are of the same period as the paintings of Sigiriya or perhaps a little later. The pigments used are the same as at Sigiriya; the drawing is excellent, and the composition (which uses the method of continuous narration, like the bas-reliefs of Bharhut and Sanchi) is well balanced. The figures, with rounded faces, resemble those of Ajanta, both in type and in the linework, more than the Sigiriya figures do. The scene depicted appears to be the visit of Indra to the Buddha in the Indraśāla cave.

The paintings found in the relic chambers of stupas could not have been intended for esthetic enjoyment or religious edification, for they would not have been seen by human eyes after the dome of the monument was completed. Such paintings must have been considered necessary to impart to the stupas their sacred character as symbolic representations of the universe. In the lower relic chamber of a stupa at Mihintale have been discovered representations of divine beings, drawn in outline, among clouds. These sketches, which date from about the 8th century, are interesting because they show us the methods adopted by the artist in his works. The central line, drawn in red paint, that guided him in arranging the figures in a balanced composition is still to be seen. The paintings in the relic chamber at Mahiyangana, assignable to the 11th century, are finished products with expressive linework and effective color schemes.

In the shrines anciently known as Tivanka-patimā-ghāra there are considerable remains of the numerous paintings that adorned the walls of the palaces and shrines of Polonnaruva in the 12th century. These indicate that the ancient pictorial tradition was still vigorous in Ceylon in the 12th or 13th century, although it had lost its vitality in India itself. The paintings in the Tivanka shrine depict religious scenes, episodes from the previous lives of the Buddha as well as from his last earthly career. Many of the paintings at Polonnaruva compare favorably with the artistic output of the classic period in India.

Painting shared in the general decline of Ceylonese civilization that set in after the middle of the 13th century. Literary works contain references to paintings executed on walls and on cloth in the period between the 13th and 15th centuries, but of these nothing has been preserved. It is from the 18th century that we once again come across paintings in the service of religion. But the school of painting that flourished in the 18th century and later does not appear to have had its roots in the art of Sigiriya and Polonnaruva. This art is two-dimensional and the coloring is flat. The human figures are generally stiff and lack grace, though there is a certain humorous quality in the drawing at times. The color schemes are effective, and the decorative designs, which are different from those in vogue during the earlier centuries, are abstract in form and often beautiful (PL. 177). This school, both in its motifs and in its technique, obviously derived inspiration from the contemporary art of southern India and the Deccan, but the subject matter is almost exclusively Buddhist, for it was the 18th-century Buddhist revival that gave impetus to it.

Paintings in this style continued to be executed on walls of Buddhist shrines up to the closing decades of the 19th century. The influence of the colonial art of the British on the educated Ceylonese made them look down on the products of the traditional school, and a vulgar naturalistic style, imitating cheap prints imported from Europe, was adopted as the symbol of progress. The influence of modern trends in art on present-day Ceylonese painters has made many educated people look at the works of the past, including the art of the 18th century, with greater appreciation of their merits, and inspiration is often drawn from them in the laudable efforts that are being made today to create an art expressing the spirit of the land and the people.

MINOR ARTS. Ivory was used very early, not only for sacred images but also for objects for personal use. A 3-in. ivory figurine of a nude female wearing a necklace and a girdle of beads at the waist, found inside a reliquary in the south frontispiece of the Ruvanvāli dagoba in Anuradhapura, dates from the 2d century. Its nearest parallel is an ivory statuette of Indian workmanship found at Pompeii. The arts of the jeweler and the lapidary were practiced with varying degrees of skill throughout the historical period.

Ivory carving of great delicacy was produced in the 18th century. The plaques ornamenting some of the carved wooden

doorjambs of Buddhist shrines and the handles of fans used by Buddhist monks are particularly worthy of mention. Metalwork and lacquered woodwork of this period are also of great merit; but these arts were abandoned for want of patronage. An effort is being made today to revive these ancient skills, but it may have come too late.

SOURCES. The oldest sources for the history of Ceylon and its culture (and in fact, the first examples of historiography in all Indian literature) are two chronicles compiled in the central-Indian language of Pali. They are the *Dīpavaṃsa* ("history of the island"; ed. and trans., H. Oldenberg, London, 1879) written by unknown authors in the 4th and 5th centuries, which covers the period up to the reign of Mahāsena (first half of the 4th cent.); and the *Mahāvaṃsa* ("great history"; ed. and trans., W. Geiger, 2 vols., London, 1908-12), written by Mahānāma at the end of the 5th century, which treats the same period as the earlier work but more comprehensively and rigorously. The *Mahāvaṃsa* is continued in the *Cūlavaṃsa* ("little history"), the first part (ed. and trans., W. Geiger, London, 1925), written by Dhammakitti, extending to the reign of Parākramabāhu I (1153-86) and the second part, by Tibboṭuvāve, to the time of King Kittisirirājasiṃha (1747-80). See also H. W. Codrington, *A Short History of Ceylon*, London, 1927; and B. C. Law, *On the Chronicles of Ceylon*, Calcutta, 1947.

BIBLIOG. J. Fergusson, History of Indian and Eastern Architecture, London, 1877; J. G. Smither, Architectural Remains of Anurādhapura, Ceylon, Colombo, 1877; A. K. Coomaraswamy, Arts and Crafts of India and Ceylon, Edinburgh, 1913; A. K. Coomaraswamy, Bronzes from Ceylon, Colombo, 1914; A. K. Coomaraswamy, History of Indian and Indonesian Art, London, 1927; V. A. Smith, History of Fine Art in India and Ceylon, 2d ed., rev. by K. de B. Codrington, Oxford, 1930; J. P. Vogel, Buddhist Art in India, Ceylon and Java, Oxford, 1936, pp. 75-89; B. Rowland, The Wall Paintings of India, Central Asia and Ceylon, Boston, 1938, pp. 83-87, PLS. 24-28; S. Paranavitana, The Stūpa in Ceylon, Colombo, 1946; S. Paranavitana, Sinhalese Arts and Culture, J. Royal Soc. Arts, XCVIII, 1950, pp. 588-605; S. Paranavitana, The Statue near Potgul Vehera at Polonnaruva, Ceylon, Artibus Asiae, XV, 1952, pp. 209-217; M. Levi d'Ancona, Amarāvatī, Ceylon, and Three Imported Bronzes, AB, XXXIV, 1952, pp. 1-17; W. E. Ward, Recently Discovered Mahiyaṅgana Paintings, Artibus Asiae, XV, 1952, pp. 108-113; S. Paranavitana, The Sculpture of Man and Horse near Tisāvāva at Anurādhapura, Ceylon, Artibus Asiae, XVI, 1953, pp. 167-190; S. Paranavitana, Art and Architecture of Ceylon, Polonnaruva Period pub. by Arts Council of Ceylon), n. p., 1954; S. Paranavitana, The Significance of Sinhalese Moonstones, Artibus Asiae, XVII, 1954, pp. 197-231; A. C. Lothian, A Handbook for Travellers in India, Pakistan, Burma and Ceylon, London, 1955, pp. 566-604; S. Paranavitana, Saṁkha and Padma, Artibus Asiae, XVIII, 1955, pp. 121-127; A. K. Coomaraswamy, Mediaeval Sinhalese Art, 2d ed., Broad Campden, 1956; B. Rowland, The Art and Architecture of India, 2d ed., Harmondsworth, 1956, pp. 209-223; M. B. Ariyapala, Society in Mediaeval Ceylon, Colombo, 1956; W. Rahula, History of Buddhism in Ceylon, The Anurādhapura Period, Colombo, 1956; see also: Reports of the Archaeological Survey of Ceylon, 1890-1955; Memoirs of the Archaeological Survey of Ceylon, I-VI; Ceylon Journal of Science, Section G, Archaeological Summaries, I, pp. 1-14, 43-60, 91-100, 143-164, II, pp. 1-16, 73-98, 149-174.

Senarat PARANAVITANA

Illustrations: PLS. 174-183.

CÉZANNE, PAUL. Cézanne was born in Aix-en-Provence on Jan. 19, 1839. His family appears to have been of Italian origin (Cesana Torinese, at the French frontier on the slopes of Monginevro) and to have settled in France in the 16th century. At the beginning of the 18th century they were already established in Aix. Paul Cézanne's father, Philippe Auguste, returned to Aix from the nearby town of Saint-Zacharie and in 1848 became a cofounder of the Cézanne and Cabanol banking firm. The future painter's surroundings therefore were those of a well-to-do bourgeois family: he had neither to worry overmuch about his future nor later to depend for a living on the sale of his work.

Cézanne first went to school in Aix from 1844 to 1849, in the Rue Epinaux, then to the Pensionnat St.-Joseph, and in 1852 to the Collège Bourbon, from which he was graduated. It was at the Collège Bourbon that Cézanne formed intimate friendships with Emile Zola and Baptistin Baille, which were important for his future development as an artist. Zola was then living with his widowed mother in Aix. After moving to Paris in 1858, Zola recalled this friendship in some of his works (e.g., *L'Œuvre*); it is further documented in a voluminous correspondence (Rewald, 1939).

"We were," Zola wrote (*Documents littéraires*, chapter on Alfred de Musset), "three friends .... On holidays, on days we could escape from study, we would run away on wild chases cross-country .... And our loves at that time were, above all, the poets. We did not stroll alone. We had books in our pockets or in our game-bags. For a year Victor Hugo reigned over us as our absolute monarch. He had conquered us by his powerful demeanor of a giant, he had delighted us with his forceful rhetoric." (In connection with Cézanne's early work it is important to note this youthful preference for one aspect of romanticism.) Later these three young men were joined by Numa Coste, the sculptor Philippe Solari, Henri Gasquet, Anthony Valabrègue, Paul Alexis, Marius Roux, and others; gradually they moved away from the romanticism of Victor Hugo to that of Alfred de Musset. "I think," Zola continued (*Documents littéraires*), "that Musset seduced us first by his swagger air of a gamin of genius. The *Contes d'Italie et d'Espagne* carried us into a world of mocking romanticism, which allowed us to drop, without regret, the serious romanticism of Victor Hugo." It was within the framework of this romantic spirit that Cézanne continued to develop his vocation of painter.

The first fruit of this romantic period — somewhere between Hugo and Musset, touched by memories of Edward Young and Jean Paul Richter — was the poem "Une terrible histoire," which Cézanne sent to Zola (who was already in Paris) on Dec. 29, 1858. The correspondence which ensued between the two friends, incidentally, was interspersed throughout on Cézanne's part with lines of verse and poems as well as drawings and water colors.

In 1856 Cézanne began to attend the drawing courses of Joseph-Marc Gibert at the Ecole des Beaux-Arts in Aix; many of his drawings of that time show how he was mastering the academic style, but as yet there was nothing personal or revolutionary in his work. In 1858, in order not to go against the wishes of his father, Cézanne enrolled in the Law School of the University of Aix. It was approximately at this time, however, that he decided to dedicate himself to painting. While still continuing with his law studies, he enrolled at the end of 1858 in the School of Design in Aix, where he remained until 1861. Meanwhile he tried, unsuccessfully, to overcome his father's opposition to painting as a career and to secure parental permission to settle in Paris. Finally, in April, 1861, aided by his mother and sister, he succeeded in carrying out this wish. In Paris he frequented the Académie Suisse and the society of a fellow townsman, Villevieille. At the same time, in the Salon of 1861, his attention was attracted to Meisonnier, Cabanel, and Gustave Doré — that is, to precisely those painters against whom the polemic of the new generation was beginning to be directed. However, Cézanne also studied Caravaggio and Velázquez at the Louvre, perceiving immediately the profound differences which separated them from the minor baroque masters in the churches of Aix. Perhaps indeed it was this discovery which brought on an inner crisis — a feeling that he had no real ability. At any rate, he decided in September, 1861, to return to Aix and enter his father's banking house.

As soon as he reached his native city, Cézanne obstinately and remorsefully began again to think of painting and enrolled once more in the School of Design. He remained in Aix until November, 1862, when nothing could keep him from returning to Paris; he stayed there for a year and a half and — very important for his development — saw the Salon des Refusés in 1863 and in the following year the great exhibition of Delacroix, who finally, in spite of the Academy, was acknowledged as a master. The year 1863 was important for Cézanne also as the date of his meeting with Pissarro.

The jury of admission for the Salon of 1863 had been so rigidly attached to academic concepts that even Napoleon III felt that it was desirable to let the rejected artists show their works in another wing of the Palais de l'Industrie, and his decision was announced in the *Moniteur* of Apr. 24. But the Salon des Refusés was not a triumph for the artists concerned, and the derision with which Manet's *Déjeuner sur l'herbe* was received is well known. While this very scorn brought many of these artists nearer to one another, Cézanne felt himself more attracted, at the moment, to Courbet and Delacroix, although he admired Manet.

The experiment of the Salon des Refusés was not repeated because it was alleged that public order would be jeopardized, and so to the Salon of 1865 Manet sent the *Olympia*, which had the same *succès de scandale* as the *Déjeuner sur l'herbe* had had two years before. Meanwhile in 1864 Cézanne had returned to Aix, not as a result of an inner crisis this time but simply from a distaste for city life which was recurrent with him. His pictures were sent to various salons and they were regularly refused; in 1866 he sent a famous letter to Nieuwekerke, the *intendant* of the Beaux-Arts: "I cannot accept the judgment of colleagues whom I have not myself appointed to estimate the merit of my paintings. I am writing you therefore to press my request. It seems to me that my wish is not extravagant and if you will inquire of any painter who finds himself in my position, he will tell you that he protests against the jury, that he wishes to participate in one way or another in an exhibition open to every serious working painter" (Venturi, 1936, p. 21).

In this letter Cézanne was speaking also for all those painters whom the jury had turned down in spite of the zeal that Corot and Daubigny (who were jury members) had displayed in defending them. Manet, Cézanne, and Renoir were not allowed to exhibit. Zola wrote *Mon salon* primarily in defense of Manet, arguing with an adroitness for which, it seems, Cézanne himself was largely responsible.

In 1865 Zola published *La Confession de Claude*, a novel which he had begun to write during a summer's stay at Aix and which he dedicated to Cézanne and Baille. Marius Roux, another of the friends at Aix, introduced it to the readers of his own town in an article in which, at the express request of Zola, he devoted a good deal of space to the fellow citizen to whom the book was dedicated. "Cézanne," he wrote (Rewald, 1939, p. 95), "is one of the excellent pupils whom our school at Aix has given to Paris .... A great admirer of Ribera and Zurbarán, our painter is autonomous and his works have always his own stamp, and if I cannot predict for him the brilliant success of those he admires, yet I am certain of one thing, that his work will never be mediocre."

Meanwhile Cézanne continued in his search and indeed began to find a means of expressing his ideals in his painting which academic training had not provided; as a result he created a style which he himself described as *couillard* (wanton). This style appears at the same moment as his revolt against the Academy and its preconceptions — the letter to Nieuwekerke is the consequence.

As we have seen, Cézanne alternated his stays at Aix and Paris. In Aix he often took refuge at the Jas de Bouffan, a country house nearby, owned by his father, one of the joys of which was a beautiful walk of chestnut trees. When in Paris, he frequented those painters who were later called the "impressionists" and, above all, Pissarro. His paintings continued to be refused at the salon, and matters were not improved by the fall of the Second Empire in 1870. While in Paris in 1869 he met Hortense Fiquet, with whom he lived for a while (without his father's learning of it) and whom he married later, in 1886. During the war of 1870 the painters separated. A few, such as Monet and Pissarro, went abroad; Cézanne spent the whole time at Aix and at L'Estaque, a village on the Bay of Marseilles, without any further contact with his friends until after the war. Then the friendship with Pissarro grew; the latter's color researches influenced Cézanne, who fully comprehended the value they had for his own purposes. Cézanne even went in 1872 to Pontoise, where Pissarro and others were living, fully convinced of the importance of painting "en plein air, sur le motif." Cézanne, with Hortense and their son Paul (born that year), lodged in a hotel there and also went to nearby Auvers, where Dr. Gachet had a house. Gachet was one of the few amateurs interested in the new painting and had bought some impressionist canvases. Cézanne spent two years at Pontoise and Auvers-sur-Oise, where he did some prints on the suggestion of Gachet, who had fitted up a printing workshop. Here also he simplified his palette. "Our Cézanne," says Pissarro, writing Guillemet from Pontoise (Rewald, 1939, p. 196), "has great promise and I have seen, and indeed I have at my house, a painting of his of remarkable strength and vigor."

It was above all at the urging of Pissarro that Cézanne exhibited in 1874 at Nadar's, in the first exhibition of the artists who called themselves the "Société anonyme des artistes peintres, sculpteurs et graveurs." This was the exhibition in which a painting of Monet's gave rise to the coining of the term "impressionist." Among other things, Cézanne exhibited two of his most noteworthy paintings, *A Modern Olympia* and *The House of the Hanged Man at Auvers-sur-Oise* (PL. 187; both in the Louvre). These paintings — and the others also — aroused the laughter of the public. When the impressionists had their second exhibition two years later, Cézanne did not wish to exhibit with them, but after having continued to work at Pontoise and Auvers, he consented to show some of his work in 1877 at the third exhibition. To this he sent 16 paintings without obtaining on this occasion, any more than on the last, the approval either of the public or of the critics, with the exception of some favorable remarks by a young man named Georges Rivière. Once more living in seclusion at L'Estaque, Cézanne continued to send to the official salons paintings which were invariably refused, until 1882 when finally he was accepted as "a pupil of Guillemet" and so labeled. However, the salons of the succeeding years again refused his works.

In 1886 the long friendship with Zola came to an end. Zola had just published *L'Œuvre*. The hero of this novel, Claude Lantier, was a painter who could have been modeled on either Cézanne or Manet but who more particularly resembled Cézanne. The painter was represented as a failure. For some time Zola had been growing cooler toward the impressionists, and in *L'Œuvre* his real judgment on Cézanne appeared: an aborted genius ("un génie avorté"). Cézanne wrote Zola a cool letter which proved to be the last of their long correspondence. No open rancor was shown and no judgment was passed on the book: "My dear Emile: I have just received *L'Œuvre* which you were kind enough to send me. I thank the author of the *Rougon-Macquart* for this kind token of remembrance, and I ask him to allow me to clasp his hand while thinking of the old days. Ever yours, under the impulse of past times" (Venturi, 1936, p. 19). The letter was written from Gardanne on Apr. 4, 1886. Cézanne and Zola never met again, not even when Zola went to Aix 10 years later.

The fact was that Cézanne no longer particularly wished to see his old friends. From time to time he interrupted his stay in Provence to make some little journey, and in 1890 he went to Switzerland. In this same year he began to suffer from diabetes. In 1897 his mother, to whom he was much attached, died, and in 1899, as part of the arrangements for entering upon his inheritance, he was obliged to sell the Jas de Bouffan. In the meanwhile, however, his works had begun to arouse some interest, and his friends had not forgotten him. In 1895 Pissarro, Monet, and Renoir induced Ambroise Vollard to hold a Cézanne exhibition, and they were supported by others. But the artist was not satisfied even with the favorable criticisms, for they indeed showed little understanding of his work. The public itself began to show some interest, however, and finally in 1899 Cézanne sent several pictures to the Salon des Indépendants and again in 1901 and 1902. Thanks to Maurice Denis (who had in 1900 painted his *Homage to Cézanne*), he participated in the famous Exposition of 1900 in Paris. In 1904 a whole room in the Salon d'Automne was reserved for his works, and he exhibited there again in 1905. On Oct. 15, 1906, when he was painting outdoors, he was overtaken by a storm, and perhaps as a result of this, his health suddenly worsened. He died at Aix on Oct. 22.

Cézanne studied for several years under Joseph-Marc Gibert at the École des Beaux-Arts of Aix, where he learned academic design. In his first works, particularly in those before 1866, Cézanne showed also that he had assimiliated something from local Provençal painters. Logically one would suppose it would be through impressionism that he would attain maturity, but between the first and second journeys to Paris he developed a manner which recalls in part the works he had admired in the Louvre — Marius Roux wrote of his fondness for Ribera and Zurbarán — and in part things seen in Provence. The first painter who seems to have had any influence on him was Emile

Loubon, who, born in Aix in 1809, had been successively in contact with Decamps and Troyon in Paris. Later he settled in Marseilles as head of the School of Drawing, introducing his own romantic taste. Cézanne's technique between 1865 and 1870 shows evidence of Loubon's influence.

One of the most important Provençal painters, who undoubtedly shows an affinity to Cézanne, is Paul Guigou, an artist who died in 1871 at the early age of 37, a friend of Monticelli and like him a protégé of Loubon.

Another Provençal painter — and this time a great artist — was to exercise a considerable influence over Cézanne: Daumier. As an artist Daumier had had a Parisian education, but he was Marseillais by birth. Cézanne took certain subject matter from him, *The Ass and the Robbers* and *The Assassination*, both from before 1870, but it is above all in their attitude to the world and to life that an affinity between the two painters is to be found. If one wishes to consider Delacroix as a romantic and Courbet as a realist, then Daumier is a synthesis of both these attitudes, while he is also a Provençal full of emphatic gestures and passions.

As for Cézanne, he was too much a poet to rest content with Courbet's realism and too *sauvage* to assimilate Manet's way of looking at things. And so it was that, from his youthful works on, Cézanne created the bases for the development of his style and of his lyrical quality. This poetic world of his was concrete and rooted in his native soil, but he invested it with romantic passion and fantasy and created an altogether imaginative realm. To find a bridge between this his personal world and the means of expressing it, Cézanne had to create a style much more complex than that of his youth, which had been based on contrasts of light and shade and forced preexpressionistic adumbrations of reality. His palette therefore became richer and his color took on those vibrations which only the discoveries of impressionism had made possible. The lesson of impressionism once assimilated, Cézanne was able to create a truly monumental style while adhering to the familiar motif of an "architecturally" conceived Provençal landscape.

At any rate we may say that two other great painters fascinated Cézanne: Delacroix and Courbet. We find Cézanne even in middle and later life making copies of Delacroix in water color; for example, *Medea* (1879; Venturi, 1936, no. 867) and *Hagar in the Desert* (1899; Venturi, 1936, no. 708). Indeed, the example of Delacroix was of great benefit to Cézanne. From him he learned to break the "closed" classic form and to construct with light in a chromatic rhythm open to all the effects which color can produce. Of course, the romanticism of Delacroix would naturally fascinate the young Provençal. Joachim Gasquet (1926, p. 180) tells of a conversation which he had with Cézanne about Delacroix in which Cézanne observed, "One can speak of him in the same breath as Tintoretto and Rubens without blushing.... He remains the finest colorist France has ever had, and nobody in our country has had, more than he, charm and pathos at one and the same time, no one has had a more vibrant color. We all paint differently because of him, just as we write differently because of Victor Hugo."

The influence of Courbet was probably greater, if less direct, and probably served as a corrective to any possible excess of romanticism on Cézanne's part. It is clear that paintings such as *The Promenade* (1868–70; Venturi, 1936, no. 116) and *The Conversation* (1870–71; Venturi, 1936, no. 120) were inspired by him. Very often, when Cézanne painted in shadow without losing intensity, he is reminiscent of Courbet. For all that, the two masters had a differing pictorial sense, as can be seen in paintings of about 1865 which seem to be like Courbet, but which on closer examination show a mastery of color of quite a different sort.

The impetuosity, the *brio*, of Cézanne about 1865 was noticed by his friends, and Valabrègue tells us that a portrait which Cézanne did of him was painted "not only with the knife but with a pistol." He adds that when Cézanne painted the portrait of a friend, "it seemed as if he wished to avenge himself for some secret injury." And indeed it seemed as if Cézanne was in revolt against everything.

Between 1865 and 1869 Cézanne painted a series of portraits of his uncle Dominique, the best of which is probably that in the Minneapolis Museum. The Minneapolis *Uncle Dominique* justifies the passage from Valabrègue quoted above. It is not just a question of the thickness of the brushwork but of the actual use of a palette knife to intensify the color and give the impression of volume. At the same time the artist uses no contrasts of light to bring about this impression and no contrasts of light and shade to bring out relief. Although the portrait is, as it were, emphatic and the spatial problem absent (at least considered as a problem of color used for purposes of space creation), the image has a consistency and monumentality of the kind which Cézanne was to attain in the fullest degree after 1880. During this period Cézanne believed he could achieve volume by density of paint, in which Courbet influenced him, but he also believed that he could render every effect of light by a sensitive use of paint, in which he differs from Courbet. The same problem appears in even more spectacular paintings of the same period, exacerbated by an even greater sensuality, such as *The Orgy* (1864–68) and *The Temptation of St. Anthony*. *The Orgy*, which was inspired by Veronese, lacks Venetian color, and the richness of the paint is unable to convey either light or atmosphere. Cézanne here was too involved with his subject matter and lacked detachment and contemplation. The nub of his difficulties was his relation to reality. As we have said, he believed he was a realist and he made every effort to be one. His preferences in painters of the past (Zurbarán) and of his own day (Courbet) were consistent with his conscious aims. But we are tempted to ask: what was realism for Cézanne at this moment? It was certainly not that of Courbet, whose realism consisted in looking at nature with the aim of seeing how it could be rendered in painting. The realism of Cézanne is at bottom amorphous, a superstructure built upon strongly personal and emotional tendencies; it is the romantic transformation of reality. To attain this end, Cézanne needed some of that same devotion to reality which the impressionist painters felt. There is no doubt that the path was traced between 1865 and 1870; it was then with the Uncle Dominique series that he began to disregard his previous academic instruction and his early preferences for Cabanel and Meissonier and to understand the meaning of light as a method of construction. This is to be seen in a still romantic painting, *Melting Snow at L'Estaque* (ca. 1870; Venturi, 1936, no. 51), much better organized than the *Pastoral* of the same time (Venturi, 1936, no. 104); no structure of design in the ordinary sense supports the composition, but the construction is equated with the chromatic whole. Cézanne was now prepared to accept the entire impressionist lesson, to see color as a constructive element; and what is more, not just to use color for tonal contrast but also to fuse and disintegrate color in patches so as to lend greater reality to his rendering of volume. Hence not the thickness of the impasto but color construction reveals the nature of his vision.

A first success in this manner is *The Black Clock* (1868–71; Venturi, 1936, no. 69), which, although still painted "thickly," is nevertheless the product of the brush, not of the palette knife, and in which therefore the colors are more transparent and a greater chromatic unity is achieved. Here, too, there is more "life" in the color and in the atmosphere, and the treatment of space has the same pictorial intensity, and hence the same emotional intensity, as every other particular of the painting. The color, it is true, is not clear in all its range, and some of the dark tones contrasting with the whites of the tablecloth in the foreground seem to predominate, but the light with which these are filled makes them brighter and richer than usual. In the case of *The Black Clock* the interest lies also in the fact that the emotion is inherent in the form rather than, as it was before, in the romantic brushwork.

The years between 1863 and 1870 saw the emergence of the first major impressionist works after impressionism had left the experimental stage and achieved a style in its own right. Certainly one cannot say that *The Black Clock* is one of these, but it is affected by the new style.

The war of 1870 dispersed the artists, but they came together again immediately after the Commune. Cézanne went to Pon-

toise and to Auvers-sur-Oise and worked outdoors in close contact with Pissarro, in a landscape filled with light and rich atmospheric qualities. Without doubt Cézanne once again owed much to Pissarro, who taught him that reality could be observed with a certain detachment and might be rendered as seen through the artist's temperament, in a moment's fleeting apperception — without his incorporating in this rendering all the aversions and attractions which he might feel as an ordinary individual. The drama — if this is required — should reside in the light and shade, not in the literary associations evoked by the subject matter. Pissarro had a maturing effect on Cézanne and pushed him farther along the path which had brought him good results in *The Black Clock*. Greater liberty of treatment and greater richness of color were needed. And Pissarro was precisely the one artist among the impressionists who had a feeling for structure, who in fact sought a structural synthesis of light itself. For this reason he was probably the nearest to Cézanne and his wish to be "monumental."

The view of the *House of the Hanged Man* (PL. 187) well illustrates Cézanne's new direction and anticipates later influences other than impressionism. Space is no longer formless; in spite of the continued thickness of the impasto, the vibration of the light lends the space a certain compactness so that, with its passages of great delicacy, a weightless but fullbodied mass results. The light which achieves this synthesis of volume and space gives what is represented a sense of permanence or, to use a word which can be applied to the later works of Cézanne, a sense of continuation. Here, Cézanne fused his conception of monumentality and grandeur with his desire for structure fortified by Pissarro, but he went farther in that he was not content with a purely "optical" effect and was already in search of a means (through form) of conveying emotional content. This accounts for the mistaken notion (beginning with Emile Bernard) that Cézanne was the restorer of a neoclassic order or that Cézanne was not an impressionist. Such misconceptions cannot be justified, because Cézanne achieved structure and volume through a use of color unknown to him before his contact with the impressionists; further, he achieved a detachment from reality, transforming it from subject into motif, which was one of the great accomplishments of impressionism.

In 1874 Cézanne took part in the first impressionist exhibition. He was therefore in the middle of the antiacademic movement, but there was already a difference between him and the other painters, who accepted him only at the sinisterce of Pissarro. However, it is true that Renoir and Monet, to cite only two of the most important impressionsts, held Cézanne in considerable esteem. Comparing his work with the work of the other impressionists of those same years, and of Pissarro himself, one realizes that Cézanne was immersed in the movement and accepted its methods and its way of looking at things; he nevertheless arrived at rather personal results, the difference lying in the fact that he went beyond physical appearance. Objects imposed themselves; and he felt their inherent greatness, their durability as facts. It is enough to look at the *Still Life* of the same time as the Auvers landscapes (1873; Venturi 1936, no. 185) or the *Vase of Flowers* (1873–75; Paris, Louvre; Venturi, 1936, no. 183) to be persuaded that Cézanne was not engaged in undoing form by his luminous color; on the contrary he was rendering it tightly, tilting the planes so as to bring out the volumes.

Cézanne refused to exhibit at the second exhibition of the impressionist group in 1876, but this did not mean a breach, for he again exhibited with them in 1877. Later, when he no longer took part in group exhibitions, he justified his abstention : "I had decided to work in silence until the day when I should be able to defend my attempts theoretically" (letter to Maus, Nov. 25, 1889; Venturi, 1936, p. 42). Even when his style had moved far from impressionism and when the impressionist painters themselves had somewhat changed direction, Cézanne cherished the old lesson. His slogan about redoing Poussin according to nature was doubtless due to his impressionist inclinations.

Probably the Impressionist Exhibition of 1877 was the best

of the series; it was the last complete one. Cézanne was represented by 16 works in all, including both oils and water colors, but they were not understood even by those sympathetic to impressionism. Georges Rivière was decidedly alone when he wrote on Apr. 14 (Venturi, 1936, p. 29), "M. Cézanne is the artist most attacked by both the press and the public for the last 15 years. There is something of the finest period of Greece in his work; his canvases have the heroic serenity of antique painting and pottery, and the ignorant visitors who laugh when they find themselves in front of the *Bathers*, for instance, seem to me like barbarians criticizing the Parthenon. Those who have never held a brush or a drawing pencil in their hands say that he cannot draw and have reproached him with imperfections which are in fact refinements only reached by an enormous practice and knowledge." The comparison with antiquity was of course not meant by the writer in a literal sense but as a comparison of quality only, and he emphasized the knowledge which Cézanne possessed and which we have already noted above. It was Matisse who later declared, "There were so many possibilities in Cézanne that, more than most people, he needed to put his ideas in order" (Venturi, 1936, p. 44).

*The Enclosure Wall*, painted about 1876 (Venturi, 1936, no. 158), shows that Cézanne had acquired not only a way of seeing characteristic of the impressionists, but also their technical methods. Colors are put on in small unconnected touches and in varying directions. The wall is violet with the reflections of trees in blue, the field is green, the earth yellow-green, the trunks of the trees are gray or gray-brown, the foliage green with one yellow branch, the roofs of the houses red, and the sky gray; space in depth is attained almost entirely by color or, less often, by atmospheric gradations. In short, everything in this painting is consistent with impressionism, and not even Cézanne's sense of greatness contradicts it.

In his impressionist period Cézanne naturally tended to give first place to landscape painting, but as we have seen, still life was not missing and this indeed was what enabled him to improve his vision of objects to the point of perfection. There were also portraits and in that of Victor Choquet (Venturi, 1936, no. 383; PL. 184), which was done in 1876–77, the human values Cézanne had absorbed from impressionism emerge. The gray-blue hair, beard, and jacket, the blue-white shirt, the reddish flesh tones are shown against a clear green background. The scheme therefore is dark on light. The brush strokes too, even though heavy in color, vary so that the light can shimmer and itself give form to what is portrayed. From this perfect fusion of form and color emerges the semblance of the man, of the patron dear to Cézanne as he was to Renoir, sensitive, serious, unhappy, willful, with an independent inner life. The work of art and the representation of a life harmonize because of the interest that Choquet had for Cézanne and because of the latter's capacity to see not only objects in nature but spiritual values also.

The decade following 1877 saw Cézanne striving toward a new constructive dimension — a structure of the image, whether human, still life, or landscape — which stressed volume more and more while it also became increasingly abstract. Here his inner search for the painting's true dimension in space and time anticipated the clarity of his late works. Cézanne, isolated since the failure of the impressionists' third exhibition and no longer exchanging ideas with other painters, created in his solitude something that was to be a major contribution to 20th-century art: he now subordinated everything to a heightened sense of the structure of the pictorial image — an aim apparent not only in his works but also in his criticism of Gauguin, whom he reproached for his "Chinese" images, evidently without understanding them. His judgment of Monet, whom he defined as an "eye" (though not meant disparagingly, since he added "What an eye!"), was along the same lines. Cézanne was not satisfied only with a feeling for things themselves, nor did he aim for coloristic abstraction that would intensify emotion through color. For him the abstract was concerned with volume and image, intensified in their essence which he achieved through strict formal control rather than expressionism — for by this

time he had outgrown the forced romantic-expressionistic manner of such paintings as *Melting Snow at L'Estaque.*

As late as 1873–77 Cézanne had painted pictures of romantic inspiration such as *The Temptation of St. Anthony* (Venturi, 1936, no. 241), in which there was perhaps a certain contradiction between the subject and the impressionist technique, but it is also true that paintings like these anticipated in a sense some of the *Bathers* series.

After 1877 Cézanne was in full reaction against official art. After his return to L'Estaque he reacted strongly to the discouragement following the failure of the impressionist exhibition. Nonetheless he continued to send paintings to the official salons, although certain that they would be refused; he did this not out of a desire to be conciliatory, but to emphasize the validity of his ideas and, as a consequence, the error of others. At L'Estaque Cézanne had always before him the landscape which he loved, and he had learned from impressionism the importance of working directly from nature.

Cézanne's structural aims are clearly revealed in several paintings with Provençal motifs which he did toward 1878 after his return to Provence. Above all there is a water color worthy of notice in this connection (1875–78; Venturi, 1936, no. 839). In a landscape in traditional perspective, two trees emerging from the color masses are solid, delimiting forms. The mountain in the background is not a backdrop but rather serves to gather and limit in a compact space, all vibrant with color, the entire landscape and the emotion which it arouses. Everything is built with color; there is not a single closed, defining line, nor any light and shade effects. The work does not consist of form filled with color but of the direct use of color areas to build up form. Here again is proof of the importance of impressionism for the development of the artist. Furthermore it reveals not that the change is either sudden or violent but rather that Cézanne retained and expanded what he had previously learned.

Even when he left Provence, as he did between 1879 and 1882, Cézanne found in northern landscapes the same motifs suggesting constructive order. The motif of a winding road is developed in several paintings of this period (Venturi, 1936, nos. 329, 330, 334): it is still a rising path, but it is not the chief element of the composition; the slopes, the trees, the houses are presented as volumes which press in upon it. The unity of the style is founded on contrasts.

But Cézanne's constructionism asserts itself most clearly after his return to Aix. During that period, between 1883 and 1887, he rarely left Provence and remained in constant touch with the southern landscape, its light, and its particular contrasts. He kept aloof from the impressionists and did not take part in their new investigations. Though, as he himself stated, he sought a theory, he endeavored to identify theory with painting rather than to create a purely intellectual superstructure to it. Later he admitted to Emile Bernard (Venturi, 1936, p. 53), "I confess that I am afraid of too much technical knowledge and that I prefer naïveté." This liking for the primitive is well realized in such paintings of 1883–85 as the well-known *Houses at L'Estaque* (Venturi, 1936, no. 397; PL. 184). Following a principle which Pissarro had already investigated, he reduced all the openings, the doors and windows of the houses, so that the walls present an unbroken surface and allow greater play to the light. But when Pissarro had painted houses in this manner as early as 1867, in the *Edge of the Jallais at Pontoise,* his preoccupation had been mainly with color; the volumes were less pronounced, or at least spread on one plane. Here too for Cézanne the problem was essentially one of construction. The planes of the earth and of the rocks are accentuated, but it is the geometric scheme, the structural idea, which is brought home to us by the direct sensation that we have of each individual element. The resultant impression is so intensified and so unadorned that it amounts to something akin to primitivism. This painting has the same revelation of the essential forms in rocks and houses and the same exclusion of all irrelevancies that Giotto gave the frescoes of the story of Joachim in Padua. A major difference lies in the treatment of light and shade, which is much more complex in Cézanne.

Through light and shade, through simplification, Cézanne reached the essence of things. The "theory" which he adopted was based on his critical perceptions rather than on intellectual constructions, and allowed his vision to appear to be composed of pure sensibility.

One effect of this return to the primitive is the identification of the painting with the motif. It was between 1882 and 1887 that Cézanne created some of his most celebrated landscape motifs, such as that of Mt. Sainte-Victoire, a mountain that he had drawn since his youth and continued to paint all his life. But it was at this period that for the first time he identified the motif of the mountain with his painting. The *Mt. Sainte-Victoire Seen from Gardanne* (1885–86; Venturi, 1936, no. 435) shows Cézanne to be in full command of his habitual volumes and of their distribution in space and depth. Houses and rocks, all are treated with the same distribution of light and shade, of clear rose and blue tones beyond the green field, with the purpose of creating a volumetric mass seen against the sky. Viewed from Gardanne, Mt. Saint-Victoire is nothing but a rocky slope, and Cézanne, in his pursuit of simplification and monumentality, turned to advantage the very aridity of the motif.

Seen from Bellevue, however, Mt. Sainte-Victoire appears to tower over the valley of the Arc, as for instance in the *Mt. Sainte-Victoire* with two pines (1885–87; Venturi, 1936, no. 455; PL. 191). In this painting Cézanne did not represent the scene as it actually appears, but brought the mountain nearer in order to give it volumetric consistency and adapt it to the concave shape of the valley. Here we may say that the organized form distorts in order to express an underlying truth that does not emerge clearly in the natural vision itself. This kind of truth made Cézanne force the depth of the space to the surface, emphasized by the pine trees framing the scene. The decorative intention is clear; but we have here a kind of decorative character which assumes a distribution of pictorial elements on the surface — without, for that reason, altering the realization of depth, which indeed is accentuated by the contrast. The representative energy, the passionate undercurrent that exists in the *Mt. Sainte-Victoire* with two pines shows the direction of Cézanne's imagination and presages the paintings he did at the end of the century.

Another pictorial motif favored by Cézanne was that of the Bay of Marseilles seen from L'Estaque; in one of the numerous versions of this scene (New York, Met. Mus.; Venturi, 1936, no. 429; PL. 190), done between 1883 and 1885, the painter imposed on himself the same space problems as in the Mt. Sainte-Victoire painting. In reality the mountains of the background seen from L'Estaque are several miles away and are normally seen somewhat vaguely. In order to indicate their structure, Cézanne brought them nearer. But he preserved the space relationship between near and far by making the first plane more distant that it would be in reality. To both the first plane and the background he gave positions different from those they actually occupy and excluded the place which he himself occupied, thus avoiding any subjective references. Similarly he treated the surface of the sea as though seen from a fairly high point so that it appears to rise and gives the impression of a considerable volume. This concentration of the surface of the sea is still more evident in another picture of the same subject (Venturi, 1936, no. 493), later by some years (1886–90), in which the artist worked on the assumption that this volumetric mass of water was also a mass of color, thus giving it a still more dramatic significance. It is the mass of water which makes the distance of the background convincing even though the mountains have the volumetric density of a close-range view. Cézanne thus organized an objective relation between village, mountain, and sea — objective not in relation to nature but in terms of the picture and of art.

It was not only the Provençal landscape that Cézanne identified with his world. Everything he painted assumed a character of permanence and understated monumentality, whether it happened to be a still life, a vase of flowers, or a portrait. *Vase of Flowers and Apples* (1883–87; Venturi, 1936, no. 513) is an example. The colors are intense and simplified. The plane

on which the vase rests seems to tilt in order to emphasize the volume of the objects, but the volume does not weigh down the composition; indeed, the composition is articulated by the contrast of colored planes, and the whole space is compact and organic. In a portrait of his wife (ca. 1885; Venturi, 1936, no. 521) the image is both lightly handled and clearly defined; its decidedly volumetric treatment is relieved by dashing brushwork from which its air of grace derives. Cézanne here reached the culminating point of his constructionism, and after 1887 he was able once again to invent more freely, simultaneously achieving a stricter formal synthesis. Henceforth he was to identify the emotion with the total compositional space rather than with structure alone, thus creating a synthesis between the multiplicity of planes and the constructed images. A new geometric and expressive order was to result from every contact with landscape, objects, and the human figure alike.

In Cézanne's last period he did not detach himself from the stimulus of nature although he treated it with a greater degree of abstraction. Also, he was aware that "a new era in art is being prepared" (letter to Camoin, Jan. 28, 1902; Venturi, 1936, p. 44). However, the whole new process is spontaneous, not contrived. It seems as if Cézanne discovered his abstract forms one at a time and that he was astonished at his own discoveries. This was the moment when he succeeded in imposing a new order on his sensations, and as soon as the order was found, the sensation itself acquired validity. An example is a painting of 1888, *The Bridge on the Marne at Créteuil* (Venturi, 1936, no. 631), in which Cézanne developed the space in depth and accentuated its synthetic character to obtain an effect of monumentality. The equilibrium between voids (the sky and the water where it is without reflections) and solids (including the reflections) is perfect. The latter have the necessary transparency, yet are so ordered that they have value as volume as well. The colors also, even though varied — yellows, reds, greens — are inserted into the general harmony of contrasts and of hazy blues. Unity of vision, even in the variety of elements, is perfectly realized, and the vision is absolute, concrete, certain, and noble.

In *The Kitchen Table* (1888–90; Venturi, 1936, no. 594; PL. 185), as Erle Loran has shown (*Cézanne's Composition*, Berkeley, 1946), the basket of fruit is seen at a level different from that at which the table is seen, and the left side of the table cannot connect under the tablecloth with the right-hand side. Cézanne purposely distorted objects to show them from various points of view and worked around them, so as to accentuate their volumetric nature and to bring out, by means of this distortion, the vital energy of the objects. The universally recognized beauty of his still lifes resides precisely in the fact that he could persuade us that the distortions are "truer" than what the average person sees in reality.

All this leads to a consideration of the position of Cézanne in the last 20 years of the century and his enormous influence on the development of later taste. It is clear that Cézanne always kept, and meant to keep, the appearance of physical reality, while he altered this reality to conform to an emotion of either a spiritual or a sensory nature. In this his painting is logically distinguished from what the cubists did a few years later, but on the other hand it is evident that the principles of cubist taste are to be found in Cézanne. There is a famous letter (1904) on this subject to Emile Bernard (Rewald, 1937, p. 259): "You must see in nature the cylinder, the sphere, the cone, all put into perspective, so that every side of an object, of a plane, recedes to a central point. The parallel lines at the horizon give the extension, that is a section of nature, or, if you prefer, of the spectacle which the *Pater omnipotens aeterne Deus* spreads before our eyes. The perpendicular lines at the horizon give the depth. Now to us nature appears more in depth than in surface, hence the necessity for introducing into our vibrations of light, represented by reds and yellows, enough blue tones to make the atmosphere perceptible."

Cylinders, spheres, and cones are not to be seen in pictures by Cézanne; his words merely expressed an ideal aspiration and looked to an organization of form transcending nature — nothing more. The phrase can be read also in the light of

another of his: "The method to be pursued becomes clear when one is actually in the presence of nature. It develops according to circumstances. It consists of looking for the proper expression of what one feels, and in organizing sensation in terms of one's personal esthetic" (Rewald, 1937, p. 348). And according to Emile Bernard (*Souvenirs sur Paul Cézanne*, Paris, n. d., p. 273), "The transposition made by the painter in his own optical system gives a new interest to the reproduction of nature. He expresses in painting what has not yet been painted. Thus he becomes a painter in the absolute sense, that is to say, the painter of something other than reality. This is no longer sheer imitation."

Years later, in 1923, Juan Gris wrote, "Pictorial mathematics leads me to the physical representation." This seems at first glance an idea analogous to Cézanne's but is seen to be different when one reads Gris's premise: "The world from which I draw the elements of reality is not visual, but imaginative" (D. H. Kahnweiler, *Juan Gris*, Paris, 1946, p. 272). The world of Cézanne was still visual and sensory precisely because he had been through impressionism and even now wished to make of impressionism "something solid and durable like the art in museums" ("une chose solide et durable comme l'art des musées"). If he anticipated certain things which later would be to cubist taste, it was because he strove for an ever-greater synthesis of emotion and form and even of emotion and space. Thus, as in *The Kitchen Table*, he distorted traditional perspective and created various perspectives from various points of view, thereby identifying space with a succession of visual images echoing in his consciousness and producing that identity of space and time that Bergson called "real duration." All this, of course, took place in Cézanne without any theoretical preconception and without his having read Bergson.

In spite of what has been said, sensation was the base of all Cézanne's work. "All the rest is only scaffolding. His forms are always sought in nature" (Simon Lévy, *Cézanne*, Paris, 1923). However, sensation does not mean a neglect of pictorial compositional order. A painting by Cézanne was always the product of meticulous formal organization and therefore nearer to abstraction than to realistic representation. Cézanne had found in impressionism a corrective to the second-hand realism which had constituted his stock in trade when he arrived in Paris. When he abandoned his impressionist friends, it was to make new researches into abstraction. A letter of Jan. 25, 1904, written to Louis Aurenche (Rewald, 1931, p. 257), reveals something about Cézanne's progress from nature to style. "You speak in your letter of the realization in my art. I do think I am getting nearer it every day, though not without difficulty. For if a strong feeling for nature — and I certainly have it, and deeply — is the necessary basis of every conception of art and on it rest the grandeur and beauty of future work, no less essential is the knowledge of the means of expression, and that is acquired only by long experience." In the last years of his life Cézanne was acutely aware of the disparity between the objective appearance of reality and his own sensory perceptions of reality. The abstract intermediary of style, even at the expense of fidelity to appearance, was required to translate the perceptions into emotion and to make those perceptions living and eternal in the idiom of painting.

Another *Mt. Sainte-Victoire* was painted between 1894 and 1900 (Venturi, 1936, no. 665). Here the mountain no longer closes off the wide valley; it is experienced in all its power and grandeur and even becomes threatening. The summarily treated first plane moves toward the rocky mass, and the simple forms of the rocks have potential movement, even struggle. Passion prevails once more over contemplation. The expression of forces liberated from their earthly prison replaces the former calm and ample vision.

At the same time an ever-increasing sense of the volume in the objects represented did not bring the artist to the point of renouncing color; on the contrary, color too became ever more intense and more structural in function. In this sense Cézanne reached beyond the cubists, for his example in this matter was to be taken up again many years later, toward 1940, by a younger generation of painters. Typical of this luminous

constructivism are the various landscapes showing the black château, such as that of the Reinhart Collection in Winterthur (Venturi, 1936, no. 667), painted between 1894 and 1896. Impressionism, in the sense of luminous vibration, has here become a solid thing, and the appearance of reality has not been dissolved by division into touches of color, but is based on a structure built up of light. Although the trees still act as coulisses, in reality there is no true background because all is reduced to a single plane. What is more important for future painting is not the thing represented, which has been broken down for expressive intensity, but the light itself. There is here a perfect coincidence, an identity indeed, of form and color.

If in the years 1882–88 the attention of Cézanne seems to have been drawn above all to landscape as a means of expressing order in sensation, from 1890 to the end of the century his masterpieces mostly represent human figures. The *Portrait of Paul Cézanne* (1890–94; Venturi, 1936, no. 578) is perhaps the most human image of himself which he has given us. The conjunctions of the facial planes are as energetic as those of the rocks of Sainte-Victoire mentioned above, and they immediately force on us the impression of the face of the man himself, of his good nature as well as of his acute, penetrating glance. The portrait is perfectly placed in the space and has the effect of a sudden and powerful apparition.

An expression of easy grace, frankness, and natural dignity is that of *Madame Cézanne in the Greenhouse* (ca. 1890; Venturi, 1936, no, 569). The continuous defining line of the forehead, the insertion of the oval of the face in the concavity formed by the hair, the formal regularity of nose, mouth, and chin, reveal the geometric ideal of the artist. Yet this ideal takes on life through the delicacy with which the tones are rendered, the flesh lighted with yellow, rose, and red and shadowed with green and blue. The tone is truly serene, the grace of the face emerges like a flower from the blue of the dress, and similarly the blues and browns of this form emerge from the touches of red, green, and yellow of the background.

The solidity of a monumental tower, on the other hand, is the impression conveyed by *Woman with a Coffeepot* (1890–94; Venturi, 1936, no. 574; PL. 189), seen in an uncompromising frontal pose. However, the position of the figure in the space and the manner in which the surroundings are treated give absolute unity to the whole picture. The intense blue of the dress, laid in facets around the bulk of the body, constructed from light as was the volume of the *Black Château*, contrasts with the delicate gray-rose of the background and with the orange tones reflected in the flesh.

One of the most famous compositions of Cézanne is that of *The Cardplayers*. Cézanne used this subject several times, with a greater or lesser number of players, but one in particular (1890–92; Venturi, 1936, no. 556; PL. 185) is perhaps the most successful. The color effect lies in the contrast between the blue-violet of the left-hand player's jacket and the yellow with blue shadows of the right-hand player's and between these tones and the reds of the background and of the flesh tones and the yellows of the table. A thousand gradations of these tones give volume to the figures and objects represented. Their solidity and their character, the evident truth of their action, the solidity of the unified composition show that the intensity of color does not detract from, but rather enhances, the whole. A continous contour line might, one would have thought, have involved the danger of isolating the figures. It does not do so because this outline, like the table and the background, is composed of zones of color. Cézanne may be said to have substituted modulation, a rhythmical arrangement of zones, for modeling. Each pictorial fragment is attached to another, according to the relation of the planes. As Cézanne himself said to Larguier, "Painting does not consist in copying the given object mechanically; it is a question of harmonizing a number of relationships." And the unity which derives from these relationships is not physical but spiritual; that is why the character of the two peasants, not merely their image, is given. "To look at things according to nature, that means to bring out the character of one's model." And again, as he said to Borely, "I love above all the aspect of those people who

have grown old without having done violence to custom, and who have simply yielded to the natural action of time. See that old coffeehouse keeper — what style!"

After 1890 the favorable reaction to impressionism and later the response to symbolism caused the younger painters to fix their attention on Cézanne. However, they were able to know his work reasonably well only after 1895, when Vollard held his first exhibition devoted entirely to the master. Despite the persistently hostile reactions of the public and of the critics in the daily newspapers, Cézanne's fame continued to spread. Although at first he was annoyed by this, as if it were an affront to his loneliness, toward 1900 he began to understand that the young men were in earnest, and when they came to Aix on pilgrimage, he received them kindly and was generous with his counsel. Meanwhile Cézanne, who like Zola had been a convinced anticlerical, felt himself drawing nearer to Christianity, in order perhaps to have some support against all the humiliations which he had suffered; and a new religious sense resulted, too, from his study of nature. While it is true that in these last years Cézanne expressed his thoughts on art verbally and in writing, his painting grew away from his theory and increasingly became an emotional extension of his feeling for all creation. In 1904 an exhibition of his works in the Salon d'Automne definitely established his success, and Cézanne was deeply pleased by it; he returned to Aix to work until his death. In this period the unity of style arrived at in his earlier years was further intensified and filled with passionate feeling. Cézanne's absolute independence of style became increasingly apparent both in terms of subject matter, which he constantly and exhaustively reexamined, and of form, regularized and abstracted according to his theoretical speculations.

Sometimes these procedures gave his pictures a tragic tone. Such is the case with the *Still Life* (1895–1900; Venturi, 1936, no. 736). The transformation of the fruit, drinking glass, and jug into light and shade, into blue-violet, reds, orange-yellow, is so complete that one does not look at the objects as such but feels instead the vehemence of the color tones which are filled with an intense and tumultuous life of their own. The care in the execution, the discontinuous touches of the kind which once distinguished light and shade, have given way to wide brush strokes of fused color which occasionally leave unfilled spaces on the canvas. A further development of technique might have entailed the loss of the original emotional impulse, but Cézanne checked himself in time.

In 1896 he went to Talloires, where he painted the *Lake Annecy* (Venturi, 1936, no. 762). Here the unity of vision is so well conceived that the waters of the lake appear to merge with the trees, the houses, and the mountains. They all seem to become a fusion of blue (blending occasionally into rose and green) which creates the light as well as the shade. Chaos is no longer ordered by divine agency according to natural laws but by an artist according to the demands of his painting. In the last years of his life — that is, 1904–06 — Cézanne looked at his beloved Mt. Sainte-Victoire with eyes as fresh and youthful as they had been at the beginning of his artistic career. He saw the mountain now as distant and imposing, no longer because of its volumetric mass but because of its spiritual light as it rose from earth to sky; it was an immense area in which orange and green and blue-violet tones symbolized the things of this world. The ever-freer touch of the brush, as in the water colors, created an increasingly intense color. We follow the shadow into light from the valley to the mountain, from earth to sky. The light is tenuous and distant.

Some of the greatest works of the later years are the water colors to which we have alluded above. It seems as if, in portraying his gardener Vallier in 1906, whether in oil (Venturi, 1936, no. 718) or in water color (Venturi, 1936, no. 1102), Cézanne was portraying himself. The solidity of the portrait and the extreme vivacity of light and of touch reveal the old man facing the nearness of death. Precisely because the drawing does not delimit the form, it more freely suggests the spirit.

In his later years Cézanne often painted scenes of bathers (PL. 186). In some large oil canvases he devoted himself to the architecture of the scene with an exceptional sense of the

possibilities of grandeur inherent in it, but in some of the water colors he treated the same subject in lighter, more improvised, and more intimate ways, as in the *Bathers* (1904–06; Venturi, 1936, no. 1105), which is a continuous stream of atmospheric masses and dreamlike figures, closer in effect to music than to architecture.

Thus in his last years Cézanne revived the romantic sentiments of his early youth without relinquishing the harmonious equilibrium between explosive passion and the vision of color and form to which he had clung from the earliest years of his impressionist work. The study of light and color, of planes and volumes, of space and its relation to the object, and especially the need to imagine a world of art distinct from that of nature allowed Cézanne to create a large number of works which have their own kind of perfection and at the same time permitted him to inaugurate a new era in the history of art.

When Cézanne died in 1906, Picasso had already begun to paint *Les Demoiselles d'Avignon*, and in the following year Braque went to L'Estaque, where he began to paint those landscapes which were to lead him to cubism. The lessons which Cézanne's work contained, however, go beyond cubism and are still valid for today.

His art has been greatly admired in our century, and the bibliography is extensive; and even in the 19th century there were exceptions to the rigidly negative verdicts of the critics. Particularly toward the end of the century, some of the young painters recognized him as a master.

We have already seen how Zola changed his position from admiration to carping and unimaginative criticism of his friend's work; in fact, it was not just a matter of Cézanne: Zola's whole attitude toward impressionism changed, and his later writings on the subject were very different from those he had earlier devoted to Manet. At bottom Zola realized that he had "arrived;" the public which liked his novels cared little for impressionism and still less for Cézanne, whom the critics, even those friendly to the impressionists, constantly needled. At first this occasioned doubts in Zola's mind — not so much about the ideas of his friends as about their capacity to realize these ideas. When writing *Le Ventre de Paris*, he had wanted to convey in his descriptions of Les Halles a sense of color and had evidently been inspired by Cézanne. In *L'Œuvre* he wrote of Claude Lantier, the same painter who appeared among the vegetable stalls at Les Halles in *Le Ventre de Paris*, as a failure ("un raté"). *L'Œuvre* appeared as an appendix to the newspaper *Gil Blas* in 1886; however, nine years earlier, at the time of the third impressionist exhibition, in 1877, there had already been mention — and in enthusiastic terms — of Cézanne. Georges Rivière had already written in *L'Impressioniste* of Apr. 14, 1877, that Cézanne was a great painter. He compared him to the Greeks. To be sure it was not, strictly speaking, a critical article; it was more the spontaneous expression of a young enthusiast who felt the beauty of the paintings he saw. In an article which appeared in *Le Journal* of Mar. 25, 1894, and then again in his *Histoire de l'impressionisme* of the same year, Gustave Geffroy did no more than repeat Zola's verdict: "It is obvious that the painter frequently leaves things unfinished, that he has not been able to overcome some particular difficulty, and that the inability to bring his conception to fulfillment is there for all to see."

At the same time Geffroy initiated a serious critical error which persisted for a long time in the assessment of Cézanne's work: "Cézanne has become a sort of precursor of the symbolists, and it is certain that there is a direct and well-established relation between the painting of Cézanne and that of Gauguin, Emile Bernard, Van Gogh, etc." It is probable that another misinterpretation, this time made by Gauguin in 1885, contributed to the tendency to see Cézanne as a precursor of the symbolists: "See how Cézanne is misunderstood: he has the essentially mystical nature of the East (his features resemble those of an old Oriental); under his formal expression he shows his love for the mystical and for the heavy tranquillity of a man who has gone to sleep in order to dream" (Venturi, 1936, pp. 13–14).

Obviously Gauguin was distorting the meaning of Cézanne's work for his own purposes; he saw in it what he himself wished to express, but it is enough to look at the works of the two men to see Gauguin's mistake. Gauguin had, however, bought a picture by Cézanne for his own collection.

Aside from Gauguin and the symbolists, the divisionists and neoimpressionists also wished to feel that they derived from Cézanne. In 1899 Signac wrote, "Cézanne's touch is the link between the technique of the impressionists and that of the neoimpressionists." This is a criticism which lacks precision but serves to reaffirm the impressionist origin of Cézanne. On the other hand, a notion first expressed by Emile Bernard, which has gradually spread and is decidedly misleading, is that of Cézanne as a classicist and a restorer of order. This rests on a misconception of both his painting and his theory of painting as revealed in the letters of his last years. Cézanne himself was aware of this error and in several letters he expressed himself somewhat adversely on the painting and ideas of Emile Bernard, describing him as "a distinguished esthete whom I regret not having under my influence so that I could suggest to him the sane, the comforting, the accurate notion that a development of art is only possible through contact with nature" (letter to his son Paul, Sept. 8, 1906; Venturi, 1936, p. 45). He continued in the same letter, "I can hardly read his letter, though I think it full of sense, but the excellent man turns his back in practice on all that he says in his writings. When he draws he produces only old stuff, which suggests his dreaming about art and what he has seen in museums rather than any emotion which he may have felt when confronted with nature. Even more, it reveals that philosophizing spirit which comes to him from too great a knowledge of the old masters whom he admires." A little later Cézanne returned to the same theme and called Bernard "an intellectual stuffed with museum memories." Bernard's interpretation was accepted because it coincided with a "return to the Academy" (a movement represented by artists such as Bernard himself and Maurice Denis) and a return also to literary symbolism, which had nothing in common with either impressionism or the symbolism of Gauguin.

The first to react against the idea of Cézanne as an artist "who didn't finish things," an idea promulgated by Zola, Geffroy, and many others, was Thadée Natanson in an article in the *Revue Blanche* of 1895 on the occasion of the exhibition arranged by Vollard: "His mastery captures the charm of nature rather than rearranging it." Nevertheless fashionable criticism continued to deny the merit of the artist, and as late as 1905 in the *Revue* of Dec. 15 Camille Mauclair had the temerity to write, "As for M. Cézanne, his name will remain attached to one of the most memorable artistic jokes of these last 15 years. It required that 'cockney impudence' of which Ruskin spoke to ascribe 'genius' to this worthy old man who paints for pleasure in the provinces and produces paintings that are heavy, ill-constructed, and conscientiously nondescript — still lifes rather crude in color if beautiful in texture, leaden landscapes, and figures which a journalist has recently described as 'michelangelesque,' but which are really the formless efforts of a man who has been unable to make good will take the place of knowledge."

Naturally with the revolution of taste which took place in the first decade of the 20th century, the attention given to Cézanne was constantly on the increase, even though some wished arbitrarily to make the significance of his art fit their own theses. So it was that just as certain people wished to make Cézanne a restorer of neoclassic order, others wished to see him as a forerunner of cubism, a point of view which had a certain amont of truth in it but which tended *ipso facto* to diminish his own art and make of him nothing but the precursor of the modern movement. A large number of monographs dedicated to the master began to appear: Julius Meier-Graefe published one in Munich in 1910; the same year saw two others, by Rivière and Elie Faure; and in 1914 Vollard published his reminiscences of Cézanne, which contained some critical comments on his work as well. The monograph brought out by Joachim Gasquet in Paris in 1926 was in the nature of a literary evocation of the man who had been his personal friend; it did not pretend to be a critical contribution.

The first serious systematic criticism of the works of Cézanne came from the pen of Roger Fry (1927). This critic drew attention to the formal values of Cézanne's work, stressing its abstract character. The importance of Fry's study lay in the fact that he reconstructed the personality of the painter through certain paintings, although he made no attempt to consider all the paintings individually. Fry's error lay in neglecting the importance of impressionism for Cézanne. It was perhaps precisely because the author wished to emphasize the structural and abstract character of Cézanne's art that he failed to see how impressionism had taught Cézanne to construct with color, which in turn had revealed the possibility of constructing organically and not just illusionistically as in the times of Provençal realism. Fry wished to see impressionism not in terms of structure but rather as luminous vibration.

Lionello Venturi reacted against this mistaken bias (1936), insisting on the necessity of taking Cézanne's impressionist experience into account for his subsequent development, and in general the author questioned every excessively abstract interpretation of the master of Aix. Along with the 1936 critical essay there appeared a catalogue of Cézanne's work, and subsequently more articles on him in which Venturi reiterated his ideas on the painter; he attempted to make them more precise in his volume *Da Manet a Lautrec* (1950).

A notable contribution to our knowledge of Cézanne has been provided by John Rewald in various works: *Cézanne et Zola* (1936; subsequently enlarged, this volume became *Cézanne, sa vie, son œuvre, son amitié pour Zola*, 1939) and *Paul Cézanne, Correspondance recueillie* (1937). In these works Rewald has collected numerous documents which allow us to follow not only the life of the painter but also the development of his artistic personality.

The volume of Fritz Novotny and Ludwig Goldscheider (*Cézanne*, 1937) is important for the question of space relations in the work of Cézanne. The spatial problem is examined in all its aspects. It is considered not merely from the standpoint of illusionary and perspective effects but also in its capacity for generating emotion.

In this century Cézanne's fame has steadily increased, and there have been many exhibitions since the one of 1895. Recognized in all the criticisms as the master who gave the initial impetus to modern art, Cézanne has continued to exercise an influence on even the youngest artists. As Pierre Francastel has said in his book *Peinture et société* (1952), "The destruction of the Renaissance idea of space made a great step forward with Cézanne.... It is no longer enough to destroy; a new sense of space, different from the old, is being created." Since modern painting has had to reconquer space, developing a new set of spatial values, which is above all a sense of space color, the example of Cézanne remains valid and indeed unique.

BIBLIOG. Articles on the death of Cézanne in the newspapers of Aix-en-Provence and Marseilles appeared in La Provence Nouvelle, Le Mémorial d'Aix, Oct. 23, 1906, Les Tablettes Marseillaises, Oct. 28, 1906, Le Radical, L'Eclair de Montpellier. For a complete bibliography and catalogue of works, see L. Venturi, Cézanne, son art, son œuvre, 2 vols., Paris, 1936; B. Dorival, Cézanne, Paris, 1948. Here only the principal references are given: M. Roux, La Confession de Claude par Emile Zola, Mémorial d'Aix, Dec. 3, 1865; E. Zola, Mon Salon (with dedication and appendix), Paris, 1866; P. Mantz, L'Exposition des peintres impressionnistes, Le Temps, Apr. 22, 1877; G. Rivière, L'Exposition des impressionnistes, L'Impressionniste, Journal d'Art, Apr. 14, 1877, p. 2; T. Duret, Les Peintres impressionnistes, Paris, 1878; E. Zola, Le Naturalisme au Salon, Voltaire, June 12, 18, 21, and 22, 1880; J. K. Huysmans, Trois peintres: Cézanne, Tisson, Wagner, Cravache, Aug. 4, 1888; E. Bernard, Paul Cézanne, Les hommes d'aujourd'hui, VIII, 1892, p. 387; G. Geffroy, Cézanne, Le Journal, Mar. 25, 1894; T. Natanson, La Revue Blanche, IX, second half-year, 1895, pp. 253–54; P. Signac, D'Eugène Delacroix au néo-impressionnisme, La Revue Blanche, XVI, 1899, pp. 13, 115, 357; G. Lecomte, Paul Cézanne, La Revue d'Art, Dec. 9, 1899, pp. 81–87; R. Marx, Un Siècle d'art, Paris, 1900; H. von Tschudi, Die Jahrhundert-Ausstellung der französischen Kunst, Die Kunst für Alle, Munich, 1900–01; M. Denis, Exposition François Vernay, L'Occident, Mar., 1902 (reprinted in Théories, Paris, 1913); E. Bernard, Paul Cézanne, L'Occident, VI, July, 1904, pp. 17–30; J. E. Blanche, Notes sur le Salon d'Automne, Mercure de France, LII, 180, 1904, pp. 672–90; P. Cézanne, Quatre lettres sur la peinture à Charles Camoin présentées par G. A. (Guillaume Apollinaire), Les Soirées de Paris, II, 1904, pp. 43–47; C. Mauclair, L'Impressionnisme, son histoire, son esthétique, ses maîtres, Paris, 1904, chap. 7, p. 152; J. Pascal, Cézanne et Renoir au Salon d'Automne Paris, 1904; R. Marx, Le Salon d'Automne, GBA, Dec., 1904, pp. 458–74;

M. Denis, Cézanne, L'Ermitage, Nov. 15, 1905; C. Mauclair, La Crise de la laideur en peinture, La Revue, Dec. 15, 1905; C. Morice, Aquarelles de Cézanne, Mercure de France, LVI, 193, July 1, 1905, pp. 133–34; L. Vauxcelles, Cézanne, Le Gil Blas, Mar. 18, 1905; C. Morice, Enquête sur les tendances actuelles des arts plastiques, Mercure de France, LVI, 195, Aug. 1, 1905, and LVII, 197, Sept. 1, 1905 (cf. the numerous replies to the fourth question; How important do you consider Cézanne?); T. Duret, Histoire des peintres impressionnistes, Paris, 1906; G. Moore, Reminiscences of the Impressionist Painters, Dublin, 1906; X (C. Morice), Mort de Paul Cézanne, Mercure de France, LXIV, 225, Nov. 1, 1906, p. 154; E. Faure, Paul Cézanne, Paris, 1910; J. Meier-Graefe, Paul Cézanne, Munich, 1910; C. Morice, Exposition d'œuvres de Cézanne, Mercure de France, LXXXIII, 304, Feb. 16, 1910, p. 726; R. Fry, The French Post-impressionists, preface to the Catalogue of the Second Post-impressionist Exhibition, Grafton Galleries [London], 1912, reprinted in Vision and Design, London, 1920, also New York, 1956; F. Burger, Cézanne und Hodler, Munich, 1913; A. Dreyfus, Paul Cézanne, ZfBK, XXIV, pp. 197–206; A. Gleizes, La Tradition et le cubisme, Montjoie, Feb., 1913; G. Kahn, Aquarelles de Cézanne, Mercure de France, CVI, 396, Dec. 16, 1913, p. 882; A. Vollard, Paul Cézanne, La Vie, II, 48, Nov. 29, 1913, pp. 253–58; Cézanne, Paris, 1914 (writings of Octave Mirbeau, T. Duret, L. Werth, F. Jourdain, Bernheim-Jeune and letters of Cézanne to Bernheim-Jeune); Sedici opere di Cézanne, Maestri moderni, La Voce, 1914; A. Vollard, Paul Cézanne, Paris, 1914; G. Coquiot, Cézanne, Paris, 1919; E. Bernard, La Méthode de Paul Cézanne, Mercure de France, Mar. 1, 1920; L. Henraux, I Cézanne della raccolta Fabbri, Dedalo, 1920, pp. 285–86; W. Barth, Paul Cézanne, Basel, 1921; C. Camoin, Souvenirs sur Paul Cézanne, L'Amour de l'Art, Jan., 1921, pp. 25–26; J. Gasquet, Paul Cézanne, Paris, 1921, 1926; M. J. Friedländer, Über Paul Cézanne, Die Kunst, Feb., 1922, pp. 137–45; J. Meier-Graefe, Cézanne und sein Kreis, Munich, 1922 (Eng. trans., London, 1929); H. von Wedderkop, Paul Cézanne, Leipzig, 1922; P. Muratov, Cézanne, Berlin, 1923; G. Rivière, Le Maître Cézanne, Paris, 1923; A. Salmon, Cézanne, Paris, 1923; W. Pach, The Masters of Modern Art, New York, 1924; E. Bernard, Sur Paul Cézanne, Paris, 1925; L. Larguier, Le Dimanche avec Paul Cézanne, Paris, 1925; W. George, Les aquarelles de Cézanne, Paris, 1926; A. Nuerenberg, Paul Cézanne, Moscow, 1926; L. Venturi, Il gusto dei primitivi, Bologna, 1926, pp. 321–25; A. Vollard, Paul Cézanne, New York, 1926; R. Fry, Cézanne, a Study of His Development, London, 1927; F. Novotny, Paul Cézanne, Belvedere, XII, 1929, pp. 440–50; E. D'Ors, Paul Cézanne, Paris, 1930; R. M. Rilke, Briefe aus den Jahren 1906 bis 1907, Leipzig, 1930; D. Le Blond-Zola, Zola et Cézanne, d'après une correspondance retrouvée, Mercure de France, 781, Jan. 1, 1931, pp. 39–58; F. Novotny, Das Problem des Menschen Cézanne in Verhältnis zu seiner Kunst, Zeitschrift für Ästhetik und Allgemeine Kunstwissenschaft, XXVI, 2, 1932, pp. 268–98; H. Granville Fell, Cézanne, a Pioneer of Modern Painting, London, Edinburgh, n.d. [1933]; G. Rivière, Cézanne, le peintre solitaire, Paris, 1933; N. Javorskaia, Paul Cézanne, Milan, 1935; G. Mack, Paul Cézanne, New York, 1935; L. Venturi, Paul Cézanne, L'Arte, May-Sept., 1935; E. Faure, Cézanne, Paris, 1936; R. Huyghe, Cézanne, Paris, 1936; L. Larguier, Paul Cézanne ou le drame de la peinture (La Galerie des illustres), Paris, 1936; J. Rewald, Cézanne et Zola, Paris, 1936 (reprinted with numerous additions and retitled Cézanne, sa vie, son œuvre, son amitié pour Zola, Paris, 1939; Am. ed., Paul Cézanne: A Biography, trans. M. Liebman, New York, 1948); M. Raynal, Cézanne, Paris, 1936; G. Wildenstein, Cézanne, avec une bibliographie des ouvrages suscités par l'exposition à l'Orangerie, GBA, II, 1936, pp. 134–36; F. Novotny and L. Goldscheider, Cézanne, New York, 1937; F. Novotny, Cézanne, Vienna, 1937; L. Venturi, The Early Style of Cézanne and the Post-impressionists, Parnassus, Mar., 1937, pp. 15–18; P. Cézanne, Correspondance recueillie, ed. Rewald, Paris, 1937 (Eng. ed., Letters, ed. J. Rewald, trans. M. Kay, London, 1941); R. Goldwater, Cézanne in America, AN, Mar. 25, 1938; W. Pach, Queer Thing, Painting, New York, 1938; F. Novotny, Cézanne und das Ende der wissenschaftlichen Perspektive, Vienna, 1938; R. Cogniat, Cézanne, Paris, 1939; L. Venturi, Les Archives de l'impressionnisme, Paris, 1939; L. Venturi, Cézanne, Water Colours, London, 1934; R. M. Rilke, Lettres sur Cézanne, trans. and preface by Maurice Betz, Paris, 1944; E. A. Jewell, Cézanne, New York, 1944; P. M. Auzas, Peintures de Paul Cézanne, Paris, 1945; G. Schildt, Le Comportement psychologique de Cézanne, interprétation de son art et de sa personnalité, Stockholm, 1946; J. Rewald, The History of Impressionism, New York, 1946; J. Rewald, Paul Cézanne, New York, 1948; A. Lhote, Cézanne, Lausanne, 1949; L. Guerry, Cézanne et l'expression de l'espace, Paris, 1950; L. Venturi, Da Manet a Lautrec, Florence, 1950, pp. 107–21; F. Jourdain, Cézanne, Paris, 1950; J. Rewald, Paul Cézanne, Carnets de Dessins, Paris, 1951; G. Schmidt, Aquarelles de Paul Cézanne, Basel, 1952; H. L. Scherman, Cézanne and Visual Form, Columbus, 1952; B. Dorival, Cézanne, Paris, 1952; M. Schapiro, Cézanne, New York, 1952; T. Rousseau, Cézanne, Paris, 1954; M. Raynal, Cézanne, Geneva, 1954; L. Venturi, Four Steps toward Modern Art, New York, 1956, pp. 61–75; K. Badt, Die Kunst Cézannes, Munich, 1956; H. Perruchot, La Vie de Cézanne, Paris, 1956.

Lionello VENTURI

Illustrations: PLS. 184–191.

**CHAGALL, MARC.** Russian painter (b. Vitebsk, July 7, 1889; often given mistakenly as 1887). Between 1907 and 1910, Chagall studied at the Imperial School of Fine Arts, St. Petersburg, and then with Leon Bakst. His most important formative years, however, were 1910–14, when he lived in Paris in close contact with the cubist painters and with such avant-garde poets as Blaise Cendrars, Guillaume Apollinaire, and Max

Jacob. Although he exhibited regularly at the Salon des Indépendants, his first one-man show was not held until 1914, at the gallery of Der Sturm, Berlin. In that same year he returned to Russia, where he married and remained until 1923. During these revolutionary years, Chagall was appointed Commissar of Fine Arts in Vitebsk and provided teaching posts for other Russian modernists such as El Lissitzky and Kazimir Malevich. In Moscow, in 1919, he executed mural paintings, sets, and costumes for Granovsky's Jewish State Theater, including designs for three one-act plays by Sholom Aleichem. Between 1923 and 1941 the artist lived mainly in France, traveling also throughout Europe, Egypt, and the Near East. From 1941 to 1947 he resided in the United States and Mexico and designed sets for the Ballet Theater productions of *Aleko* (1942) and *Firebird* (1945). In 1947 Chagall returned to Europe, where, in 1950, he settled in Vence, in southern France. Such characteristic paintings as *I and the Village* (1911), *The Birthday* (1915), and *Time Is a River without Banks* (1930–39) may be found in the Museum of Modern Art, New York. His most important book illustrations are those for Gogol's *Dead Souls* (1948), La Fontaine's *Fables* (1952), and the Bible (1956; II, PL. 296), all three projects commissioned by the dealer Ambroise Vollard.

With De Chirico, Chagall was one of the first 20th-century masters to explore the fantastic world of symbols and memory images, thereby prefiguring the surrealists' more concerted effort to investigate subconscious experience. His pre-1910 work already attempted to transcend a realist viewpoint in its somewhat primitive and expressionist style and in its occasional juxtapositions of separate spatial and temporal events. Moreover, the work of this period established Chagall's characteristic interest in the fundamental human themes of birth, love, marriage, and death, as witnessed in the Jewish quarter of his native Russian village. His contact with cubism, however, was decisive in providing a pictorial technique that could enlarge the imaginative freedom he had searched for in Russia. Liberated by the fragmented, air-borne world of the cubists, Chagall's poetic fantasy was extended to create a new gravity-defiant realm of childhood recollections and exuberant emotions that parallel the descriptive liberties of children's art itself.

Often, too, Chagall introduced a more intricate symbolism that depended upon Yiddish folklore as well as a highly personal blending of traditional Jewish and Christian iconography. Stylistically the artist's work after the mid-1920s has tended to move from the taut, angular structure of cubism to more softened and fluid relationships of color, shape, and space.

WRITINGS. *Ma vie*, 1st ed., Paris, 1931, new ed., Paris, 1957.

BIBLIOG. J. Sweeney, Marc Chagall, New York, 1946 (bibliog.); L. Venturi, Chagall, Lausanne, 1956 (bibliog.); W. Erben, Marc Chagall, New York, 1957; J. Lassaigne, Chagall, Paris, 1957.

Robert ROSENBLUM

## CHAM, SCHOOL OF.

The kingdom of Champa, established at the end of the 2d century and lasting until the 17th century, gave rise to a style of art known as the Cham school. It appeared along the eastern coast of Annam from the border of Cochin China in the south, reaching northward to the so-called "Annam portal." The continual relocation of Champa's capital and the resultant stylistic changes in Cham art warrant separate treatment for the work of this school as against the artistic output of centers such as Khmer (q.v.), which spread Indian influence.

SUMMARY. Introduction (col. 357). Chronology of the styles (col. 358): *Style of Mi-sön E₁, or early style (8th cent.); Style of Hoa-lai (8th–9th cent.); Style of Dông-düöng (last quarter of the 9th cent.); Style of Mi-sön A₁; Style of Binh Dinh (11th–13th cent.); Late style (14th–17th cent.).*

INTRODUCTION. Owing to the investigations of P. Stern, great progress has been made during the past 20 years not only in the classification of Champa monuments and sculpture

into various schools but also in determining their chronology. However, all the problems created by Champa's history of continual destruction and reconstruction are not entirely resolved in detail. Earlier studies have been invalidated by the mistaken belief that the tower of Mi-sön A₁ (PL. 193) and the sculpture of Tra-Kiêu (dated from the 7th century; see PL. 196) predated the other Cham monuments. Among the earlier studies was the work of H. Parmentier, who prepared a detailed catalogue of the known isolated sanctuary towers and separate brick structures. He proposed (erroneously) the following classification and chronology based on the architecture: Originally two types of architecture appeared simultaneously, although their origins and subsequent development were different. In the first type — the "primitive art," which appeared in the 7th century — structures previously made of perishable material were transposed into brick. The primitive art was fully developed in the Mi-sön tower A₁. The other type of architecture — the "cubic art" — is characterized by its squat proportions, and can be seen in the towers of Po Dam, Hoa-lai (PL. 192), and the monastery of Dông-düöng (PL. 192; FIG. 359). The two architectural types later blended in the "mixed art" encountered in the towers of Mi-sön A₈₋₉, ₁₁₋₁₃, and B₂. Both primitive and mixed arts disappeared in the 9th century, when the Chams withdrew toward the south. Parmentier holds that this first period, which he calls "primary" (ending with the move to the south), was followed by a secondary period, which embraced the "classic" art of the 11th-century towers of Binh Dinh. The classic forms repeat in a simplified way the forms of the primitive and the mixed art, finally distorting them to the point of decadence. Straddling the primary and secondary periods, there was a "pyramidal" art (so called from the appearance of its superstructures), represented by the towers of Ban An and Hüng-thanh.

Parmentier's classification suffers from the serious drawback of placing two such different styles as the primitive and the cubic in the same period. This was pointed out by P. Stern, who proposed a more satisfactory classification and chronology. Stern used a method based on a minutely detailed examination of the evolution of decorative motifs, which has had remarkable results in the study of Khmer art. Analysis of the decorative motifs makes possible greater precision of dating than does a study of the architecture, which is so often rebuilt and in which variations of form are much less apparent. Stern's work was based on the following elements of Cham decoration: (1) the arch, including (*a*) the large arches crowning doors or blind doors, or framing the figures represented between the pilasters, and (*b*) the small arches adorning the base of the pilasters and the foundation; (2) the pilaster, embellishing the main body of the structure by dividing the walls and extending from the foundation to the cornice; (3) the frieze of garlands running under the cornice to the tops of the pilasters and between the pilasters themselves; (4) the small columns which frame the doors and blind doors; (5) the cornice and the base (the study of which is often difficult, since the former is high overhead and sometimes mutilated, the latter often buried or covered with thick vegetation); (6) the accentuating sculptural projections at the corners of the towers' upper levels; (7) the corner crowns (actually miniature temples) placed at the four corners of each story to fill the space left by the setback; (8) the lintel, an element of secondary importance, used only in cases where there is a tympanum to be supported, since the arch does not entail the use of a lintel.

CHRONOLOGY OF THE STYLES. The chronology and classification proposed by Stern, using these elements as a basis, are as follows:

*Style of Mi-sön E₁, or early style (8th cent.).* From the architectonic point of view, the extant material (a pediment and a fragment of a small column) is insufficient to give an idea of the whole. The decoration, however — particularly that of a superb pedestal from the tower of Mi-sön E₁ — betrays a fairly recent Indian origin as well as an unmistakable kinship with the early periods of other currents of Indian art as they

appeared in southeast Asia. On a relief of dancers and a representation of Viṣṇu, the influence of Indian art of the Gupta period (with reminiscences of the naturalism of the Sanchi area) is especially marked. The Mi-sön E₁ style, characterized by the flattened shape of the arch, the isolated decoration against a plain background, and the circular form of the small columns, offers, according to Stern, the remarkable union of an intense realistic vitality with a complete, idealized harmony.

At the present time, the transition between the early style and its successor is represented by a single Cambodian monument probably built by Cham architects: the Prasat Damrei Krap of Phnom Kulên (beginning of the 9th cent.). Its great arch, as well as certain details of the pilasters and small colonette, foreshadow the style of Hoa-lai.

*Style of Hoa-lai (8th–9th cent.).* This style, which was found almost exclusively in the south, coincides with the

emerges in anatomic details such as heavy lips, flattened nose, and jutting brow ridges. From these traits of the sculpture as well as the all-pervasive, exuberant decoration characterized by the vermiculated vine tendrils, there emanates an impression of barbaric vitality. In the art of adjacent countries, this vitality is a particular manifestation of native resurgence after a period of Indian influence. But in Champa, where the Indian influence lasted beyond the 9th century, there are too many indications which place the art of Dông-düöng between the Hoa-lai and Mi-sön A₁ (PL. 193) styles to allow a date much later than the end of the 9th century. Its originality stems from factors which elude us; only the results are clearly evident. The salient traits of the Dông-düöng style are the vermiculated rinceaux, or twisting foliate ornament, which pervade the entire decoration and the form of the small arches; the arches are composed completely from the lines of this rinceau. A typical arch consists of a large central cluster and two raised sections at

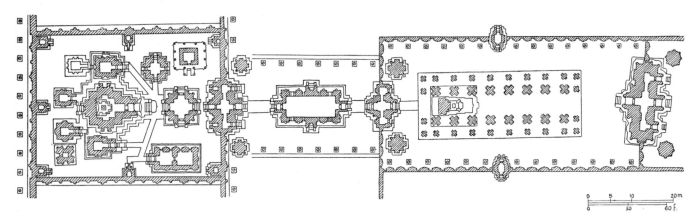

Dông-düöng (Vietnam), Buddhist monastery of Lakṣmīndra-Lokeśvara, ground plan, 9th cent. *(from Parmentier).*

transfer of the capital of Champa to Panduranga (Phanrang) in the middle of the 8th century. Monuments in this style are still standing and are virtually intact. They are characterized by a decoration of branches that covers the large and small arches and by a particular type of pilaster composed of a vertical strip of dentate foliage that runs between two plain surfaces. The decoration of the frieze on the wall under the cornice and above the shafts of the small colonette is common not only to this style but also to the preceding one and to the initial period of the style following. The decoration consists of a double, triple, or crossed garland, drooping in rounded loops, which encloses flowers and foliage; it also includes pendants of flowers or fabric. The colonette is octagonal. The red-brick sanctuary tower of Hoa-lai (PL. 192) represents both the fusion and contrast of the grandeur and dignity of the pilasters and the elaborate and luxuriant decoration of the arches. In the southern tower (the earliest) the superstructure displays an arch whose branches emerge from the mouth of a monster's head which is enclosed within a cornice. This motif is virtually identical with the *kūḍu* (small arched niches decorating stories in temple buildings, common in the Dravidian art of southern India in the 8th century). The same characteristics recur in the monument of Po Dam, which seems to be a small-scale reproduction of the tower of Hoa-lai and of the tower of Mi-sön A₂. In the Hoa-lai style, the decoration of the pilaster, the type of frieze, and the octagonal form of the colonette are prototypes of the following style.

*Style of Dông-düöng (last quarter of the 9th cent.).* This style, known chiefly through the ruins of the Buddhist monastery of Lakṣmīndra-Lokeśvara (PL. 192; FIG. 359), is contemporaneous with the rise in 875 of a new dynasty at Indrapura in the north. By that time the style was already far from its Indian origins, of which there remains only a leaning toward overelaborate ornament and foliate decoration. In full round or relief renderings of the sculptured human figure, the basic native character

each side, also composed of floral clusters. The pilasters of this style have decorated sides and a relatively broad, undecorated central band, which is reduced to a mere slit in the succeeding style. The frieze consists of a double garland of jagged leaves.

The following period, which is reminiscent of the 8th century in its classic harmony, marks an abrupt change — a kind of reaction against the underlying native stratum. This does not, however, interfere with the general arrangement, the combination of the pilasters, the shape of the arch, or the details of the frieze (PL. 193). There are also monuments belonging to this post-Dông-düöng period that represent the transition from the Dông-düöng style to Mi-sön A₁; the tower of Mi-sön A₁₀, for example, still exhibits some of the excesses of the Dông-düöng epoch. But it is at Khüöng-mi (PL. 193), in the decoration of the pilasters, that innovations are apparent which foreshadow the style of Mi-sön A₁, particularly in the spaces between the pilasters; the spaces have relief borders with a wide slit between them which extends into the frieze. Other innovations seem to be due to foreign influence: the lozenge-shaped decoration of the central space between the pilasters is similar to that of the Khmer towers of Prah Kô (879); on the external faces of the pillars the rounded, leafy rinceaux with rounded moldings and without vermiculation are similar to those of Candi Kalasan in Java (778).

*Style of Mi-sön A₁.* According to Stern, the following are the essential traits of the Mi-sön A₁ style (PL. 193; FIG. 361): decoration with coiled, leafy rinceaux (Javanese influence); coupled pilasters, with a cleft or slit which extends into the frieze; a space between the pilasters, with raised moldings or figures carved in relief; a projecting double cornice, done in openwork (*à jour*); the light, sculptured accents, also done in openwork; small columns, curved or countercurved; balustrades. A further detail reveals Javanese influence: the small arch enclosing a *kālamakara* (a type of decorative motif containing

the head of a monster, characteristic of Javanese art), which is also found on the pedestal of the principal tower of Po Nagar at Nhatrang (FIG. 362). Mi-sön A₁, which according to early chronological studies had no apparent antecedents, now seems to be the result of a long evolution. The sculpture of this epoch is known chiefly through specimens from the excavations at Tra-Kiêu — male and female dancers (PL. 196), elephants, and rearing lions. The figures are graceful and sinuous, their realism contrasting with the exaggeration of Dông-düöng sculpture. The chronology of the Tra-Kiêu sculpture, originally placed at the dawn of Cham art, becomes quite clear when compared with the figures in the niches of the tower of Mi-sön A₁. We find the same tiered headdresses, the same smile on the faces of those statues which are obviously portraits of deified beings, the same delicate brow ridges tracing in relief two separate arcs, the same protruding, almond-shaped eyes. In short, the Tra-Kiêu sculpture shows the same reaction to the Dông-düöng style as does the architecture.

The transition from the previous style to Mi-sön A₁ was as abrupt as the transition from Mi-sön A₁ to its successor was gradual. The political decline of Champa and the removal of the capital southward to Vijaya (Binh Dinh), the first time in 982, brought about a decadence in its art, marked by a coarsening and impoverishment of the forms. The porportions of the buildings became less harmonious, and the ornamentation

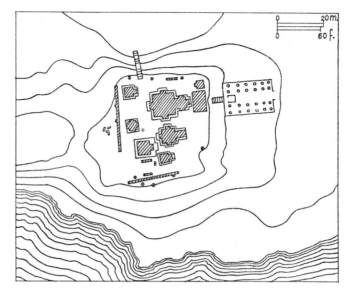

Nhatrang (Vietnam), sanctuaries, general plan, 11th cent. (*from Parmentier*).

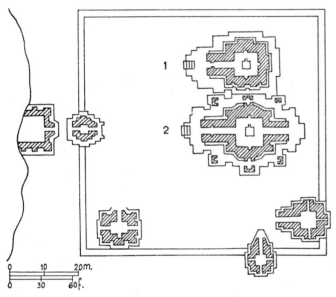

Mi-sön (Vietnam), temples in group A, ground plan, 9th cent.: (1) Temple A₁; (2) temple A₁₀ (*from Parmentier*).

gradually disappeared. The transition can be observed in the Po Nagar tower at Nhatrang, which, in its present state, seems to be no earlier than the 11th century and among the earliest monuments of the Binh Dinh style.

*Style of Binh Dinh (11th–13th cent.).* The royal court of Champa was permanently transferred to Vijaya in A.D. 1000. This resulted in the construction of numerous monuments in the Binh Dinh region, the earliest of which seem to be Binh-lâm and the "Silver Towers." In this style the arch assumed a pointed horseshoe shape which was close to the lancet arch. The pilaster lost its slit, which had extended as far as the frieze without penetrating it. In the space between the pilasters, the two sides of the border molding drew closer together until they fused. The frieze displayed a continuous simple garland or at times a series of smaller garlands. The projecting sculptured accents were no longer executed in openwork, and their points became hook-shaped. The corner crowns were not, as formerly, small-scale reproductions of complete buildings, but only reproductions of the superstructure. The towers of Binh Dinh were often built on hills. The Khmer influence, which was particularly significant during two successive Khmer oc-

cupations in the 12th century, explains the individual features of the superstructure of the tower of Hüng-thanh, reminiscent of the style of Angkor Wat; the typical Khmer motif of the Garuḍa — half man, half bird, with upraised arms — occurs on the corners of Hüng-thanh. The Khmer influence also explains the plan of the "Ivory Towers," clustered in threes along a single axis; the profile of their superstructures, with its rounded form, lacks both the projecting sculptured accents and miniature corner crowns. In style, the architraves of the Ivory Towers closely resemble those of the Bayon temple of Angkor Thom.

The three monuments most representative of the Binh Dinh style are Thü-thiên, the "Copper Tower" (PL. 194), and the "Golden Tower," which combine the characteristics noted.

In the sculpture, particularly that of Thap-mam, there is also clear evidence of foreign influence, both Khmer and Vietnamese; however, we find as well a resurgence of the basic native element, evident in a taste for exaggeration previously noted in the Dông-düöng epoch (PLS. 195, 196).

*Late style (14th–17th cent.).* This style is marked by a decline owing to an exhaustion of the sources of inspiration. The earliest monument of the late style, Po Klaung Garai (14th cent.; PL. 194, FIG. 362), still retains several traits common to the Binh Dinh style: the arch with an acute point, the pilasters without decoration or molding, the projecting central area in the space between the pilasters. Po Klaung Garai also shows characteristics of the late style, such as the massive corner crowns with their continuous curvilinear external outlines. The small arch, in this style, repeats the profile of the corner crowns, and the sculptured accents become heavier; the pilasters grow progressively simpler until, as in the monument at Po Romé (17th cent.), they disappear, except for

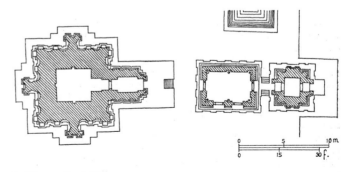

Po Klaung Garai (Vietnam), the temple, ground plan, 14th cent. (*from Parmentier*).

the pilasters at the corners. Sculpture degenerates to a simple head or torso projecting from a block. Finally it is reabsorbed gradually into the stone, until it becomes a mere stele.

BIBLIOG. H. Parmentier, Les monuments Čams de l'Annam, Paris, 1909; H. Parmentier, Les sculptures chames, Ars Asiatica, IV, Paris, Brussels, 1922; P. Stern, L'art du Champa (ancien Annam) et son évolution, Toulouse. 1942.

George Cœdès

Illustrations: PLS. 192–196; 4 figs. in text.

**CHAMPAIGNE**, PHILIPPE DE. Painter of the French school (b. Brussels, May 26, 1602; d. Paris, Aug. 12, 1674). Champaigne was trained in Brussels, chiefly under Jacques Fouquières. In 1621 he moved to Paris, where he became in 1629 a naturalized French citizen. With the patronage of Marie de' Médicis (to whom he was named official painter in 1628), Louis XIII, and later Cardinal Richelieu, his work was soon much in demand. After 1629 it became necessary for Champaigne to maintain an atelier, where he employed assistants in the execution of his large compositions. One of the original members of the Academy of Painting and Sculpture, founded in 1648, he later was named professor, then rector, of that body. In 1643 the painter came strongly under the influence of the ascetic doctrines of Jansenism and thereafter maintained close relations with the Jansenist establishment at Port Royal, near Paris. Despite this association, which was extremely important in the development of his later style, Champaigne continued to provide paintings, mural decorations, and tapestry designs for the crown, for Richelieu, and for the Jesuits, who were eventually responsible for suppressing the Jansenists.

Of Champaigne's many mural decorations, only those in the Church of the Sorbonne remain in their original places. Among the most important of his larger compositions are *Assumption*, 1628 (Grenoble, Mus. des Beaux-Arts); *Vow of Louis XIII*, 1638 (Caen, Mus. des Beaux-Arts); and *Echevins of the City of Paris*, 1648 (Paris, Louvre). Champaigne will perhaps be best remembered as a portraitist. His official portrait style, a restrained interpretation of the formulas of Rubens and Van Dyck, can be seen in *Cardinal Richelieu*, 1636 (Paris, Louvre). The *Unknown Man*, 1650 (Paris, Louvre), and *Jean-Baptiste Colbert*, 1655 (New York, Met. Mus.), reveal the somber and intimate portrait style of his later period. The masterpiece of Champaigne's late years is *Two Nuns of Port Royal: Ex-voto of 1662* (Paris, Louvre; II, PL. 213), which was presented to the convent at Port Royal. Champaigne successfully adapted the baroque of his native Flanders to the more sober requirements of French taste. His straightforward compositions, restrained color, and often penetrating realism reflect — as do paintings of his more famous contemporary, Poussin — the rationalism of French thought in the 17th century. See BAROQUE, II, col. 340.

BIBLIOG. B. Dorival, Philippe de Champaigne (Cat. of the exhibition at the Orangerie), Paris, 1952; A. Gazier, P. et J. B. de Champaigne, Paris, 1893; A. Mabille de Poncheville, Philippe de Champaigne, Paris, 1938.

John W. McCoubrey

**CHAO MÊNG-FU.** Chinese academic painter, born in 1254 at Ho-chou of a noble family related to the first Sung emperor. He was educated in the Imperial University at Hangchow and followed an official career until the fall of the Southern Sung dynasty in 1279. It was not long before Chao Mêng-fu became what in modern terminology would be described as a collaborationist. He offered his services to the Mongol court in 1286 and served brilliantly, not only as administrator but also as court painter to Kublai Khan. He held a number of important government positions, and after his death in 1322 was given the posthumous title of Duke of Wei. Like Rubens, he was at once a courtier, an administrator, and the most distinguished painter of his day. Chao Mêng-fu was also renowned as a calligrapher, particularly for his "small

model characters" (*hsiao k'ai*). In this field his performance was based on classic precedent, particularly the writing style of Mi Fei (q.v.). He was, in fact, equally skilled in "seal" characters, "official" script, and "cursive," or "grass," writing.

Chao Mêng-fu was always described as a model of Confucian virtues (see CONFUCIANISM), and this sober attachment to tradition is reflected in his painting, based almost entirely on classical models. As a painter he was extremely versatile in subject and technique. Among his models were some of the great names of the T'ang and Sung periods (see CHINESE ART). It is said that Wang Wei (q.v.) provided the inspiration for Chao Mêng-fu's landscapes. In the painting of horses, his real specialty, he imitated Han Kan and Li Lung-mien (q.v.). Although Chao Mêng-fu modestly deprecated any comparison with the great T'ang master, he was quite happy to believe that he had surpassed Li Lung-mien. Chao Mêng-fu prided himself on having expressed the spirit or character of his equine subjects, and some of his contemporary critics claimed that his paintings of horses in their freedom of spirit symbolically portrayed the official enjoying freedom from his labors and duties.

There are scores of paintings bearing the signature of Chao Mêng-fu in both European and Far Eastern collections, but it is doubtful that more than a handful of these can be accepted as genuine. More often than not we are forced to rely on later copies to judge his subjects and styles. A picture formerly in the Stoclet Collection in Brussels is typical of his style as found in numerous specimens attributed to him (PL. 198). The two horses represented on the silk reveal a style of drawing that blends the archaic linear manner of Han Kan with something of the more realistic immediacy associated with Li Lung-mien. The arrangement of the two forms on a diagonal is another archaism; there is, however, a sense of aliveness and implied movement in the fleeting poses that is quite different from the static arrangements of Chao's predecessors and is perhaps to be recognized as typical of that more intimate everyday naturalism which typifies the work of so many Yüan painters, both in animal painting and in landscape.

Another scroll attributed to Chao Mêng-fu, in the Freer Gallery of Art, Washington, D.C., represents horses at a ford, in the same style; it shows the animals moving in the spatial ambient of a landscape, which is painted with the same concern for the texture and articulation of the trees that marks the naturalistic drawing of the horses. Although not all critics are agreed that this work is actually by the master's hand, it is at least an early and faithful copy of a lost original (PL. 199).

Chao Mêng-fu's manner of painting horses is essentially a linear one like that of his predecessors. His animals lack the statuesque rigidity of Han Kan and Li Lung-mien. At first the emphasis on contour makes the forms strike the eye more as moving silhouettes than actual three-dimensional shapes. But the use of light ink wash to reinforce the outlines, as in the Washington scroll, serves to suggest a certain solidity and texture. This abstract modeling, a variety of *mu-ku-hua*, or "boneless painting," contrasts with the lively, crisp brush drawing of the water and tree trunks, in which the richness of the ink is a factor in suggesting both texture and color. On the whole Chao Mêng-fu's style in animal drawing is one of rather precise, dry realism, with some suggestions of archaic models that remind us of the drawings of Pisanello in the combination of formalism and naturalism. There is always the greatest mastery in the presentation of difficult poses and in the suggestion of animation.

Still another remarkable painting, certainly one of the finest scrolls ascribed to Chao Mêng-fu, is also in the collection of the Freer Gallery (PL. 200). In its combination of realism and sophisticated ink drawing it is more in the style of the period. The subject is a sheep and a goat, drawn in monochrome ink, with a short explanatory note by the artist that may be translated as follows: "I have often painted horses, but very seldom sheep. When Chung Shin asked me to paint, I amused myself by making a picture from life; and though I could not equal the men of old, the painting does achieve spirit harmony." What the artist meant by saying that his creations were filled with spirit harmony (*ch'i-yün*) was that he had been able to

imbue these commonplace animals with the pose and movement and form that we recognize instinctively as completely appropriate to their species: from the point of view of structure, texture, and characteristic attitude, the sheep is completely sheeplike and the goat satisfyingly goatlike. The ability to suggest an appropriate vital movement or aliveness through appropriate articulation rather than by attempting to copy outward appearance has always been the first principle of Chinese painting. In Chao Mêng-fu's painting the animals are drawn as though prepared for imminent movement. They are drawn with the greatest economy of brush stroke, a technique that, in its combination of ink wash and dry brush, suggests both texture and structure. The result is due not only to consummate mastery of the medium but also to the artist's ability so to fix in his mind the essentials of natural forms that he can re-create them in painting and endow them with life. The painted forms on the paper are beautifully balanced by the colophon in the painter's incomparable and expressive calligraphy.

A beautiful landscape scroll generally accepted as by Chao Mêng-fu's hand is the *Autumn Colors of the Ch'iao and Hua Mountains* (Palace collection, formerly in Peking). This is, to be sure, again a traditional classic subject, but its treatment is different from the handling of earlier painters. The artist presents the mood of a place, rather than its exact topography. It will be noted that the perspective is more normal from the Western point of view. The landscape is filled with many kinds of trees, some of which have a resemblance to the austere, iron-hard drawing of pines and cypresses by Li Ch'êng. Mt. Ch'iao, instead of being represented as a vast pinnacle towering to the summit of the panel, as in Northern Sung landscapes, is a dark hump on the horizon, only partially seen through the groves of trees across the lake. Notable are the textural interest inherent in the variegated quality of the ink — now heavy and moist, now dry — and the studied contrasts of brush strokes, sometimes thick and dense, sometimes feathery in thinness. At first glance there is something almost casual about the brushing of the clumps of weeds in the foreground and the middle distance. But it will be seen that these forms are really a repeated theme or *leitmotiv* uniting and animating the different portions of the surface. As in the scroll of horses in the Freer Gallery, the artist has made a suggestive pattern of the tongues of land breaking the shore line of the lake.

Another picture in the Palace collection, entitled *Bamboo Garden by the Murmuring Waters*, represents a clump of bamboo growing behind a large irregular rock that shelters the tiny figure of a seated recluse. The composition is a type of outdoor still life — an intimate view of a rockery with plants — also treated by Wang Yüan and in the 17th century by Shên Chou and Wên Chêng-ming (q.v.). Of special interest in this picture are the varied textures of the ink, appropriately defining the different objects in the arrangement.

Also attributed to Chao Mêng-fu are several versions of a painting entitled *Itinerant Tea Vendors*, which is believed to stem from an original by the famous T'ang figure painter Yen Li-pên (q.v.). These, too, are close copies of a classic original and reveal little of the artist's personal style. The same can be said of his copy of Wang Wei's famous Wang Ch'üan landscape in the British Museum and his *Return of Lady Wen-ch'i*, in Berlin, another exercise in the T'ang style.

Chao Mêng-fu's copies of horses by Han Kan and his landscapes after Wang Wei are often original in much the same sense as Turner's exercises in the manner of Ruisdael or Poussin are original creations inspired by these famous prototypes. There is a quality of immediate realism that makes the horses appear almost as representations of individual steeds and the landscapes suggest the character of actual scenes within the framework of classic landscape composition.

Another work attributed to Chao Mêng-fu is *The Starved Horse*, a copy of which by Kuan Tao-shêng, formerly in the Del Drago Collection, New York, shows an emaciated foundered steed grazing by a solitary pine tree (PL. 197). Although the drawing and spacing are certainly not up to Chao Mêng-fu's standard, the intensity of the rather brutal realism is typical of Yüan art (1260-1368). The subject as treated by other

painters, such as Kung K'ai, is believed to refer symbolically to the retired official, forgotten and forlorn, in the cold evening of life.

Chao Mêng-fu's style was perpetuated by his son, Chao Yung. In his *Horse and Groom*, in the Freer Gallery of Art, the subject is a rather literal reworking of one of the famous *Tribute Horses* by Li Lung-mien. The drawing is harder and less sure than Chao Mêng-fu's handling of similar themes, and the painting is distinguished mainly by the vividness of the color contrasts between the silvery gray of the stallion and the brilliant crimson of the attendant's robe.

Benjamin ROWLAND

SOURCES. Chang Ch'ou, Ch'ing-ho shu hua fang (Barque of Paintings and Books of the Ch'ing-ho), 1763; Y. Saitō, Shina gaka jimmei jiten (Biographical Dictionary of Chinese Painters), Tokyo, 1900, 2d ed., 1912; Sōraikwan Kinshō: Chinese Paintings in the Collection of Abe Fusajiro, Osaka, 1930, pl. 31; Chao Mêng-fu, Album published by the Palace Museum, Peiping, 1933; Chung-kuo hua-chia jên-ming ta tz'ŭ-tien (Biographical Dictionary of Chinese Painters), Shanghai, 1934; O. Sirén, Chinese Painting, Leading Masters and Principles, VII, London, 1958, pp. 102–4 (with complete œuvre catalogue).

BIBLIOG. L. Binyon, A Landscape by Chao Mêng-fu, TP, I, 1905; S. Taki, Chao Tzŭ-ang a hachi-shun-zu ni tsuite [Concerning the Painting of Eight Stallions by Chao Tzŭ-ang (Chao Mêng-fu)], Kokka, no. 435, 1927, pp. 35–9; O. Sirén, Histoire de la peinture chinoise: II, L'époque Song et l'époque Yüan, Paris, 1935, pp. 113–17; W. Cohn, Chinese Painting, London, 1948, pp. 80–1; L. Sickman and A. C. Soper, The Art and Architecture of China, Harmondsworth, 1956, pp. 149–51; O. Sirén, Chinese Painting, Leading Masters and Principles, IV, The Yüan and Early Ming Masters, London, 1958, pp. 17–29.                    * *

Illustrations: PLS. 197–200.

**CHARACTERIZATION:** PSYCHOLOGICAL, PHYSIOGNOMICAL, AND ETHNIC. Ascribing specific characteristics to various human types and classes has remote religious and psychological origins, and has been investigated in ancient and modern treatises on astrology, physiognomy, the temperaments, and the passions. Particularly important is the application of theories of characterization to the representational arts. The theories have always been a source of artistic inspiration, even though their influence is not always easy to isolate.

The representation of either traditional or sporadic "characterized" or "characteristic" figures would seem, at first glance, to result from an interest in the appearance of reality; for within a given culture characterization is generally accompanied by an interest in portraiture (q.v.), genre scenes (see GENRE AND SECULAR SUBJECTS), and so forth. But actually the study of human character in art derives from a secondary, more indirect view of reality, permeated with experiences drawn from cultural tradition. Thus the formal expression of character frequently involves stylization or distortion in drawing or color.

SUMMARY. The concept of character in treatises on the representational arts (col. 366). Virtues and vices, the planets, the four temperaments (col. 369). Convention, decorum, costume (col. 371). Physiognomy (col. 373). Individual characterization as an element of style (col. 374). Characterization in the Asian world (col. 375). Aspects of characterization other than European and Asian (col. 378): *Pre-Columbian America; Benin.*

THE CONCEPT OF CHARACTER IN TREATISES ON THE REPRESENTATIONAL ARTS. The word "character" faithfully preserves the Greek χαραχτήρ from the verb χαράσσω ("to engrave"). Originally "character" meant an instrument for making a distinctive and indelible sign, that is, for drawing, incising, or stamping coins or seals. In the representational arts, however, the word designates descriptive features, especially the intellectual and moral qualities of an individual or the traits that distinguish him as a personality. The concept has been examined in a body of treatises of Greek origin. Aristotle, dealing with the six elements of tragedy, maintains that character should reveal a clear moral bent, must be justified by reality and legendary or historical tradition, and must be self-consistent. He considers the abstract side of characterization, the tendency to styliza-

tion, and fidelity to nature: "The poet may well follow the example of good portrait painters, who, while reproducing the particular features of an individual, draw a portrait that does not depart from likeness but is nevertheless more beautiful than the original" (*Poetics*, 15). Aristotle may have had in mind Lysippos' attempt to reconcile the direct study of nature with the canons of proportion laid down by Polykleitos. This effort to harmonize art and life occurs especially in tragedy. Aristotle also touches on the problem of broad type classifications: "Each class of men, each natural type, will have an appropriate manner of showing its true appearance. By 'class' I mean the differences in age — the child, the mature person, the old person; in sex, male or female; in nationality, Spartan or Thessalian, for example" (*Rhetoric*, iii, 7). Although Aristotle's concern is less with imitation of nature than with decorum and regard for traditional standards, his statements provide valuable insights and theories that anticipate an important evolution within Hellenistic art.

Reliefs and statues of the earliest Mediterranean civilizations and the ancient Near East generally make no attempt to characterize individuals or distinguish them according to social or human categories. Exceptions sometimes occur in the representation of foreigners (PL. 212), old men, etc.; otherwise bodies and faces are undifferentiated and interchangeable. The generic terms *kouroi* ("youths") and *korai* ("maidens"), referring to archaic Greek statues of nude male and draped female figures, indicate certain traits shared within each group, whether the figures represent gods, mortals, or shades. Individual persons are distinguishable only by variations of style, artist, or workshop. Even the male and female types resemble one another: women have flat bosoms and heads that could be masculine. Often the general category of a statue can be determined only by the place where it was found: if in a necropolis, it is a deceased person; if in a temple, a god. "I am Chares," reads the dedicatory inscription on one of the statues from Miletus, in no way differentiated from the others.

Although the 5th century B.C. largely abandoned the conventions of the archaic period, traces of an indeterminate quality in statues still remained. Since the prevailing ideal was the male athlete, his body fully developed through exercise, female faces and figures of this era seem masculine. There was still no distinction between man and god; the *Apollo* from the west pediment at Olympia is no more than a handsome athlete. There have been many discussions regarding the identity of the *Diadoumenos* and the *Doryphoros* of Polykleitos; is the youth a victorious athlete, Apollo, Achilles? On a black-figured vase of the period, two gods advance side by side, identical in features, posture, dress, and beard. There would be nothing to differentiate them if one god did not bear lightning, a scepter, and a crown of olives (representing Zeus) and the other the thyrsus and wreath of ivy (representing Dionysus). Statues of athletes of the 5th century are distinguished mainly by their individual activities: some hurl the discus, some hold the lance, some crown themselves or bind on their foreheads the garlands of victory; these figures refer to one victor or another at the games.

There are, however, in the 5th century various postures and gestures (other than those assigned to athletes) which indicate certain basic human categories. A seated position on a throne or bench is reserved for superior beings, while kneeling figures denote humility or inferior rank. There is a whole language of gestures, such as that of the orants and the mourners. To indicate fertility a goddess may place her hand on her breasts or her genitals.

Waldemar DEONNA

The art of the 4th century and the Hellenistic period, in frank opposition to the classical idealization of human and divine figures, manifested a strong interest in individualized types, emotions, ages, and sexes, particularly in sculpture. Rendering of expressions and gestures was carried to an almost exaggerated degree of virtuosity (PL. 210), and there was a corresponding intense study of anatomy. It is worth noting that Pliny considered this entire period as a barbarous age which produced no art — just as, for analogous reasons, neoclassical criticism was to depreciate mannerism and the baroque. Yet the 4th century and Hellenistic era saw the rise not only of characterization in art but also of portraiture and genre scenes. It should be observed, however, that even during the Hellenistic period characterization did not distinguish sharply between individual personalities; it defined a small number of types or social classes, and within these categories the remarkable uniformity of rendering indicates an idealizing rather than a naturalistic intention. This same tendency may also be perceived in the treatises on characterization during the period. Theophrastus (d. 287 B.C.), whose *Characters* is the first work to reach us in which a systematic classification of human types is attempted, reduced them to a few categories based mainly on their vices, social behavior, and temperament. It was a pessimistic, almost ironic concept of character, and it showed, among other things, the lack of a true interest in mankind. At the same time it indicated the significance characterization had for literature and controversy; often the only purpose was to serve as an intentional and comic contrast to the prevailing or idealized standards.

The categories established by Theophrastus and Aristotle, and listed by Horace in his *Ars poetica*, became quite popular among teachers of rhetoric through the centuries. The categories came to serve more as a stylistic convention than as a formula for interpreting the reality of life and the variety of men. Theophrastus' categories recurred in classical comedy, and, through the works of Menander, Plautus, and Terence, were transmitted to Renaissance Italy, Elizabethan England, Spain of the golden age, and France of the baroque era. At times the characters became so highly stylized in the theater that they could be adequately indicated by masks. Thus the original mimetic impulse gradually gave way to abstraction and idealization. The principal outcome of this change was an idealization of the ugly and an exaggeration of characteristics.

The most fruitful fields for characterization are always in comedy (see COMIC ART AND CARICATURE) and genre scenes rather than tragedy (see THE SUBLIME) or historical painting. The manner of characterization reflects various theories of what is comic. In the transition from antiquity to the medieval and modern world, characterization became extremely complicated, probably owing to the reemergence of earlier concepts rather than conscious formulation. Partly through contact with the pagan world, a new element in the concept was introduced: the somewhat magical interrelation of human and animal types with an exchange of moralizing or even demonic attributes (see DEMONOLOGY). These attributes may have had their source in religion or caste distinctions in an archaic era. Astrology made another highly important contribution to the diversity of character traits and has interesting survivals in popular art.

Characterization underwent two main phases in Western representational art. In the Middle Ages and to some extent in the Renaissance, character was regarded as a sign of predestination and was therefore connected with the moral scheme of the virtues and vices. Most frequently it depended on the influence of the planets, which governed the four temperaments. In the 17th and 18th centuries, character was considered the result of upbringing and was connected with concepts of decorum and habit. It thus lost some of its emotional and demonic significance and became instead one aspect of culture, to be observed with historical accuracy. However, the relation of character to the passions became a matter of special interest. The famous treatise by Charles Le Brun (or Lebrun, 1619–90), which was published in many editions, is particularly relevant in this connection (PL. 206). Le Brun's concept was influenced by the definitions in Aristotle's *Poetics* and in Horace's *Ars poetica*, where character is regarded as a tendency of the soul. Connected with these concepts of character is a theory of esthetics which recurs, sporadically but persistently, in every period of Western culture: beauty is the visible image of inner harmony and the reflection of an objective order in the cosmos.

Parallel to this runs another phase of characterization in Western representational art — an opposite concept of character which emphasizes the special case or the exception

from the norm and equates character with ugliness and derogatory imitation; the polemic implications of this attitude survive in romantic realism. Thus the use of the term "character" frequently remains ambiguous. From the moral point of view, character can have either a positive or negative significance. It can be attributed either to the object represented or to the work of art as a whole. It may vary according to the manner of representing the subject and to changes in the esthetic. Nevertheless, character follows a clearly determined historical course, and even the changes in theoretical definitions reflect distinct evolutions in style or taste. Character may therefore be interpreted as the manifestation or representation of emotions (A. Possevino, Charles Le Brun, Roger de Piles) or as the distinguishing quality of an individual or an object (C. A. Dufresnoy, C. du Cange); it may be considered as a defect to be corrected or respected (Dufresnoy) or as a desirable distinction (Quatremère de Quincy). In any case, character always — even in the Orient, when connected with astrological concepts — reveals the artist's attempt to overcome literal representation and to depict reality by abstracting its most significant elements. This selective process is particularly noticeable in the Middle Ages and the Renaissance. It is accompanied not only by the revival of representational art but also by a heightened awareness of the relation between images and ideas.

Eugenio BATTISTI

VIRTUES AND VICES, THE PLANETS, THE FOUR TEMPERAMENTS. Medieval thought probably provides the clearest expression of the complex cultural affiliations of characterization. It added to the type characterization found in literature, especially classical comedy, a classification by virtues or vices in accordance with moral theology. The iconography of virtues and vices generally consisted of personifications of moral attributes (PL. 211). Sometimes, however, these symbolic figures were identified with historical personages regarded as incarnations of specific virtues. For example, in a 12th-century Flemish manuscript (Valenciennes, Bib. Municipale, no. 512, fol. 4v) illustrating the life of Gregory the Great, the four Virtues who "exalt him above his transitory existence" characterize Gregory as one who especially exemplified these virtues.

This manner of characterization through attributes, symbols, and associated images lasted a long time in medieval art and later developed into the so-called "moralized" or mythological portrait, in which the background elements have symbolic meaning and the figure is often represented in the guise of a Christian saint or a god or philosopher of antiquity. In any event it was the human virtues of the saint or god rather than the superhuman qualities that were portrayed as reincarnated.

Romanesque and Gothic art frequently represented a class, social stratum, or profession without individual characterization, especially when showing the months and their occupations, as in the tympanum of Vézelay. In a French manuscript of about 1390 (Paris, Bib. Nat., fr. 400) the virtues and vices are connected with classes of society; they appear as figures riding symbolic animals and are differentiated according to sex, age, and social position: Pride is associated with kings, Avarice with merchants, Envy with monks, Intemperance with youths, Wrath with women (Mâle, 1925).

With the development of historical allegory, medieval artists often exemplified moral concepts by historical persons in what was almost an inversion of the classical theme of the mythological portrait: Abraham was Obedience, Moses was Cleanliness, Job was Patience, Judith was Humility (e.g., the Bamberg Apocalypse; *Speculum Virginum*, reproduced in Katzenellenbogen). Vices sometimes appeared overcome by their opposite virtues; for example, in a 14th-century manuscript reproduced by Mâle, Nero is at the feet of Justice, Holophernes at the feet of Fortitude, and Epicurus at the feet of Temperance. Assigning definite physical features to symbolic or allegorical images was very significant for the development of characterization. For example, Wrath was shown with hair standing on end (Giotto, Padua, Arena Chapel; PL. 211) and Foolishness by a smile, as in numerous representations of the Foolish Virgins.

When, in the late Middle Ages and Renaissance, evil persons were depicted as ugly — for example, the henchmen in the Passion of Christ — or when the facial characteristics of the Jews were caricatured, the allegorical reference gave way to a more direct connection between moral and physical qualities.

Two related doctrines served as a guide for the classification of psychological types in the late Middle Ages and the Renaissance: the astrological theory and the theory of the four temperaments. According to the first, the birth of a man under the ascendancy of a given planet determined not only his character but his social status and profession as well. In Islamic culture seven professions were subordinated to each planet (frescoes of Kuseir 'Amra). This theory penetrated into the West in the 13th century by way of Spain, to merge with the Western traditions of representing the professions, which were derived partly from the concept of the four seasons and partly from the so-called "mechanical and liberal arts." The oldest and one of the most important cycles in which this synthesis is already complete is that of the Palazzo della Ragione in Padua (14th century, but repainted at the beginning of the 15th). In the graphic arts of the 15th and 16th centuries in Italy and the north, even the landscape is "characterized," although always in relation to human activities. Thus work in the fields is governed by Saturn, war by Mars, love by Venus, the arts and trades by Mercury, etc. The various classes of society are represented on 15th-century playing cards (the poor man, the servant, the artisan, the merchant, the nobleman, the knight, the doge, the king, the emperor, the pope; PL. 201); social classes may also be seen in Jost Amman's popular *Ständebilder* (representations mainly in prints of all ranks shown exercising their crafts and professions) and in Holbein's *Dance of Death*.

According to Arabic sources of the 9th century, astral divinities were connected with the four temperaments: Venus or Jupiter with the sanguine temperament, Mars with the choleric, the moon with the phlegmatic, and Saturn with the melancholic. The temperaments were illustrated either by a typical scene or by a figure (PL. 203); in figures there was an attempt to distinguish visually between the psychological and physical characteristics. In German prints of the second half of the 15th century, "the sanguine temperament is represented by a youthful, fashionable falconer who walks on a band of clouds and stars which indicates his congeniality with the element of air. The phlegmatic . . . appears as a fattish burgher who stands in a pool of water, holding a rosary. The choleric is a warlike man of about forty, briskly walking through fire; to show his irascible temper he brandishes a sword and a stool. The melancholic, finally, is depicted as an elderly, cheerless miser standing on the solid ground. Leaning against a locked desk the top of which is nearly covered with coins, he gloomily rests his head on his right hand while with his left he grasps the purse hanging from his belt" (Panofsky, 1948). When the temperaments are represented by scenes, the iconography of the virtues and vices is frequently adopted: Luxury provides the pattern for the sanguine temperament, discord for the choleric, despair for the melancholic. In the Renaissance, when the theory of the temperaments entered the field of emblems (see EMBLEMS AND INSIGNIA; PL. 202), the faces of saints, apostles, and prophets were temperamental types; there are abundant examples of this in north European art, such as sculpture by Nicolaus van Leyden, Lorenz Luxberger, and Jakob Kaschauer (Hartlaub, n. d.). Dürer's *Four Apostles* (Munich, Bayerische Staatsgemäldesamml.) provides the most famous example: St. John is sanguine, St. Mark choleric, St. Paul melancholic, and St. Peter phlegmatic. Here, in a reversal of medieval thought, Dürer used the saints not to exemplify a general concept of virtue but rather to represent the four temperaments and "by implication . . . four basic forms of religious experience" (Panofsky, 1948).

These iconographic traditions persisted until the 18th century or even longer. In his *Treatise* of 1584, Lomazzo particularly stressed the connection between character, temperament, and astrological predestination and drew specific conclusions regarding coloring, physiognomy, gestures, and

the general form and proportions of the body. Baroque art, with its great interest in the representation of the passions, also relied heavily on these traditions; some sculptures by Bernini are particularly famous in this connection (PL. 207). Henri Testelin in his essay *Sur l'expression générale et particulière* (1675) and Antoine Coypel in his lectures *Sur l'esthétique du peintre* (1721) still made use of this old theory of the temperaments (Jouin, 1883).

CONVENTION, DECORUM, COSTUME. From the 15th century on, when theories of rhetoric greatly influenced the art of the Renaissance and the baroque, the doctrine of the appropriateness of form to content that was developed by Aristotle and other ancient theoreticians assumed increasing importance. The doctrine had two aspects, often closely interrelated: (1) The figures should accord with the traditional characterization of the historical or legendary heroes represented; (2) the form should be suited to the subject matter. Alberti, in his consideration of the appropriate form and proportions to be given to figures (*Della pittura*, ed. H. Mallè, Florence, 1950), draws upon classical sources: "It would be absurd if the hands of Helen or Iphigenia were old and Gothic, or if Nestor had a soft breast and delicate neck." With respect to costume: "It would be unsuitable to dress Venus or Minerva in a burlap sack." This principle of expressing the passions in a manner appropriate to the character and dignity of the person depicted was reaffirmed by Daniello in his *Poetica* (1536; Lee, 1940) and in the treatises of Dolce (1557) and Lomazzo. It finally gave rise to the academic concept of expressions (set forth notably in the famous lecture delivered by Le Brun on Poussin's *Gathering of the Manna*) and to the well-known maxim of Boileau: "Conservez à chacun son propre caractère. / Des siècles, des pays, étudiez les mœurs, / Les climats font souvent les diverses humeurs /" (*L'art poétique*, III, Paris, 1674, pp. 113–15). Roger de Piles (*Dissertations*, Paris, 1681) stresses the same theme; Abbé Dubos (*Réflexions critiques*, Paris, 1719) and Antoine Coypel (*Discours*, Paris, 1721) also return to it. As late as 1771, Sir Joshua Reynolds discussed the equation between character and decorum: "Each person should also have that expression which men of his rank generally exhibit; the joy or the grief of a character of dignity is not to be expressed in the same manner as a similar passion in a vulgar face" (*Discourses*, IV, London, 1769–91).

Two slightly different ideas converged in the concept of decorum: (1) the appropriate representation of various aspects of human life and (2) conformity to what was considered decent and proper in morality, religion, and taste. In Biblical representations, decorum entailed strict adherence to scriptural narrative. In theatrical representations, it required scenery fitting the character of the play; we have precise instructions such as those given by Serlio (PL. 204). The notion of decorum also involved certain aspects of costume (q.v.), already discussed by Benedetto Varchi as a necessary element of tragedy in order to show "whether those who speak are good men, kings, misers, or spendthrifts, whether they love or hate . . ." (*Quattro lezioni sulla poesia*, Florence, 1553). The continuing relationship between the theater and the visual arts led to descriptions of what were regarded as true and appropriate models for iconography and characterization; Lomazzo offered a whole series of this sort.

Henri Testelin (*Sentiments des plus habiles peintres sur la pratique de la peinture et sculpture mis en tables de préceptes*, Paris, 1680) proposed a systematic use of specific proportions for different types of individuals. This was not a new idea; early in the 16th century, Albrecht Dürer had elaborated a range of proportions intended to provide the artist "not with one canon, but with specimens and methods which would enable him to produce . . . all possible kinds of figures: noble or rustic; leonine, canine, or foxlike; choleric, phlegmatic, melancholy, or sanguine; wrathful or kindly; timid or cheerful" (Panofsky, 1948). Testelin, however, differentiated the proportions even more precisely according to the characters and the context in which they appeared, establishing differences according to age, sex, and subject matter: In rustic themes, coarse-spirited men

with soft, "watery" temperaments should be heavily proportioned; they should have flaccid muscles, large heads, short necks, high shoulders, narrow chests, thick legs, and clumsy feet; for serious historical themes, proportions should be beautiful and pleasing, with bodies slender; for heroic subjects, proportions should be chosen from different models to form perfect figures; all gods, heroes, and giants should be larger than the surrounding figures. Action and movement should be appropriate to the age, sex, and condition of those represented. (Persons of dignity are more controlled; the vulgar give way to their passions.) The most interesting feature of Testelin's treatise is the establishment of a connection between characterization and style: rustics should be drawn with an undulating, coarse, and hesitant line; important personages with a noble, well-rounded, firm line; heroes with broad, strong, and decisive strokes; gods or saints with a powerful, austere line that has no superfluity (Jouin, 1883).

Following Testelin, M. F. Dandré-Bardon in his *Traité de peinture* (Paris, 1765) established six types of outline and form according to the following subjects: (1) common and rural persons, (2) important and respectable persons, (3) heroes, (4) pagan gods, (5) strong and awe-inspiring types such as Hercules, and (6) pleasing types such as Helen. Bardon, like Daniel Webb in *An Inquiry into the Beauties of Painting* (London, 1665), added specific advice on colors and their suitability with respect to the character of various subjects and persons.

The question of the relation between characterization and style has remote origins. The starting point is once again Aristotle, with his three degrees of imitation (i.e., better than, equal to, or worse than, reality). Coypel applied this to the history of art: Raphael and Michelangelo render men better than they are, the Venetians just as they are, the Germans and Dutch worse than they are. From this classification (corresponding to the classification of literature into tragedy, comedy, and satire) arises the concept of the *grand caractère*, as well as its opposite — the vulgar, the simple, and the pastoral (Gombrich, 1953). The transference of character to style or form was facilitated by the importance that the concept of character had in architectural theory, where physiognomy, movements, and action did not enter into the question. The psychological character of forms, already indicated by Vitruvius (*De architectura*, ix, 4), was emphasized by Alberti (*De re aedificatoria*, 1485, ed. J. Rykwert, London, 1955) and S. Serlio (*Sette libri dell'architettura*, Venice, 1537), who required a correspondence between not only the architectural character of the temples (strong, gentle, etc.) and the gods or saints to whom they were dedicated but also between the character of civil buildings and those who commissioned or occupied them (Doric for warriors, Ionic for scholars, Corinthian for "honest and pure persons," etc.). In addition, Serlio specified the psychological character of each individual form. His ideas recur, with greater or lesser emphasis, in all the mannerist and baroque theorists from Lomazzo to the neoclassic Milizia. Gradually the concept of character ceased to be a "principle of individuation" or a valid criterion for the analysis and interpretation of reality and entered into the more complex realm of human nature. It became an essential factor of a work of art and as such was connected with manners and even stylistic modes. Two styles, or rather two artistic currents, the picturesque (q.v.) and the sublime (q.v.) in the 18th century, depended on the classification of objects and aspects of nature according to their character: familiar and attractive in the picturesque, imposing and awe-inspiring in the sublime. This classification became a contrast not only between the pictorial and the plastic but also between moving, flowing lines and firm, incisive contours; it became as well a contrast between variety and movement, on the one hand, and solemnity and stability, on the other.

The stylistic concept of character is connected with the development of symphonic music rather than with theories of literature or drama. As the pathos of a musical selection may be revealed to us by its sonorous rhythm, so the emotional theme of a picture is revealed through the general rhythm of its forms and colors. This idea, already mentioned in a letter from Poussin to Chantelou, is elaborated by Testelin

(*Sentiments des plus habiles peintres*, 1680): "If the subject is war, everything should be turbulent, full of terror and agitation; if it deals with joy and peace, everything should appear pleasant and calm; if serious and grave, everything should breathe greatness and majesty." The idea was echoed by A. Coypel: "Every picture should have a distinctive manner. The whole will then be either bitter or sweet, sad or gay, according to the character of the subject one wishes to represent. In this, one can follow the charming art of music." Similar ideas are found in the English theorists of the 18th century, such as Daniel Webb and Sir Joshua Reynolds, who single out Van Dyck and Rubens as the artists who have best achieved a unity and immediacy of characterization. De Piles applies these ideas to a more systematic type of criticism; he finds in Titian the quality of gracefulness, in Veronese truth, and in Rubens (*Fall of the Damned*, Munich, Alte Pin.), chaos and despair. The thesis that character is what distinguishes the work of art or its general effect (which is in turn dependent on the analysis of detail) obviously had its greatest influence on romanticism. Delacroix seeks this concetrated harmony of form, movement, and color in all his works; Whistler, proceeding from the detailed analysis of his portraits to the pure and directly emotional coloristic effects of atmosphere, finally established the poetic accent of a landscape which lacked not only all distinct details but even the essential outlines.

PHYSIOGNOMY. Two separate approaches to representations of the physiognomy may be distinguished historically: the general and the particular; both are derived from the ancient theory of character. The latter consitutes the realistic aspect of characterization (see REALISM), the basis of which is the principle that the physiognomy corresponds exactly to the individual's spiritual and moral make-up. The realistic movement reached its peak in the 18th century. Swift advised Hogarth to represent men without resorting to caricature because the face reveals the soul; Goethe said that "a man's aspect is the best guide to whatever can be found out or said about him" (Steinbrücker, 1915); Johann Sulzer (*Allgemeine Theorie der schönen Künste*, Leipzig, Berlin, 1771–74) asserted that the body is the soul itself made visible.

All physiognomic studies are ultimately derived from antiquity; even the ecclesiastical authors evoke the authority of Greek treatises by Pseudo-Aristotle, Polemon, Adamantis, and others. The theories of all these ancient writers have in common the following points: (1) deduction of character from expressive movements and parts of the body, especially the face and eyes; (2) parallelism between men and animals; and (3) classification of types according to (a) sex and age, (b) temperament, spiritual and physical make-up, and professional group, and (c) ethnic characteristics. The major exponents of these theories as applied to art are Pomponio Gaurico (*De sculptura*, Florence, 1504, ed. Brockhaus, Leipzig, 1886); G. B. della Porta (*De humana physiognomia*, Vico Equense, 1586; PL. 205); Rubens in his sketches (*Théorie de la figure humaine*, Paris, 1773); and Charles Le Brun (*Méthode pour apprendre à dessiner les passions*, Paris, 1698, Augsburg, 1732; PL. 206). The subsequent connection of this theory with early ideas about evolution by P. Camper (*Dissertation sur les variétés naturelles qui caractérisent la physiognomie des hommes de divers climats*, 1791–92, *Oeuvres de P. Camper*, Paris, 1803) had special influence on 18th- and 19th-century caricature (see COMIC ART AND CARICATURE). Somewhat different theories of physiognomy flourished between the end of the 18th and the early 19th century, propounded by Johann Kaspar Lavater (1741–1801), with whom Goethe at one time collaborated (*Physiognomische Fragmente zur Beförderung der Menshenkenntnis und Menschenliebe*, 1775–78), and by his adversary G. C. Lichtenberg (1742–99; *Polemik mit Lavater*, Göttingischer Almanach, 1773). Lavater maintained that character can be ascertained from the structure of the head, especially the forehead. Lichtenberg in his "pathognomics" ridiculed Lavater, claiming that it was the muscles, modeled by habitual gestures and expressions, which provide the guide to character; this thesis, incidentally, in contradiction to those based on astrology and the theory of temperaments,

had already been proposed by Leonardo in his *Treatise on Painting*. The more dynamic interpretations of physiognomy, in contrast to the static determinism later to be formulated by Lavater, had special success in England, where similar ideas were expressed by James Parson (*Human Physiognomy Explained*, 1746) and in the outline for the *Second Characters* by the third Earl of Shaftesbury (1671–1713). Lavater's ideas, however, were widely diffused in the first half of the 19th century; though Gavarni ridiculed them ("a nose is an accident and not an indication of character"), Girodet took the ideas seriously in his poem "Le peintre" ("The painter [who is] . . . a talented student of the wise Lavater attentively observes the bearing, the form, the color of the face and distinguishes a lunatic from a stupid man, the senseless one from the wise"; quoted in Levitine, 1954). Girodet used these theories in his historical paintings to define faces. It is precisely the attempt to portray individual character that differentiates his historical pictures from those of David and leads to the romantic quest for the expressive. Character thus stands at the opposite pole to the norm of ideal beauty.

INDIVIDUAL CHARACTERIZATION AS AN ELEMENT OF STYLE. "Character," as we have been using the term, is something inherent in the subject and constitutes its singularity, which the artist perceives. However, "character" also has a meaning which applies to the artist — his personal style. Hogarth used "character" in the latter sense, differentiating it from "caricature," in his print *Characters and Caricaturas* (1743; PL. 208) and in the inscription added in 1753: "Being perpetually plagued, from the mistakes made among the illiterate, by the similitude in the sound of the two words 'character' and 'caricatura' I ten years ago endeavoured to explain the distinction by the above print." On another print, *The Bench*, he wrote: "There are hardly any two things more essentially different than 'Character' and 'Caricatura,' nevertheless they are usually confounded and mistaken for each other" (Nichols, Stevens, and Ireland, 1900). The best definition of character in Hogarth's sense is that given by De Piles: "There is only one important thing in drawing . . . I cannot express it better than by the word 'character.' This character is implicit in a painter's manner of imagining things and is the distinguishing imprint which he gives to his works as the vivid picture of his own spirit."

The use of the term "character" to denote an author's personal style occurs frequently in classical studies of rhetoric. Dionysus of Halicarnassus wrote of the "character" of Thucydides, and Cicero used the term in *De oratore*. Character as the artist's style, according to De Piles, derives from innate talent (*caractère du génie*) and habitual practice (*caractère de la pratique*) — in other words, invention and execution (*L'idée du peintre parfait*, Paris, 1699). In the hands of A. Coypel and others, this thesis became fundamental for the concept of art as the expression of the artist's personality. Coypel (*Discours*, 1721) said that Guido Reni was "a sweet and temperate spirit and his manners were noble and great: this is the spirit of his pictures." The concept of art as an expression of personality led to an appreciation of whatever was done rapidly and with few corrections. Such works had "spirit and character." De Piles cited Rembrandt's drawings, among others, to illustrate this point.

In this context, the artist's character influences his choice of subject matter. Shaftesbury (ed. Rand, 1914) described "an Italian, or Spaniard, an odd figure wrapt in a ragged cloak, but with formal mien, the shrug, or strut. So a country peasant, or boor, a Jew. One of Salvator Rosa's cut-throat figures, shaberoons, ragamuffins, moss-troopers, knights of the post, jilts, drabs, eavesdroppers, gamesters, sharks, players, musicians, mountebanks, quack doctors, sharpers, *ambubaiarum collegia* [Syrian dancing girls]. All these the more pleasing as more secret, mysterious, difficult and withal instructive in manners and of real use in life and towards the knowledge of mankind in the world." The attitude revealed here corresponds to the category of derogatory imitation, already stressed by Bellori in his life of Caravaggio (*Le vite de' pittori, scultori ed architetti*,

Rome, 1672). But Shaftesbury stresses a particular awareness on the part of the artist, whose choice of subject matter in turn influences his manner of painting; this manner should render everything in a lively and spirited way.

Another new theme was knowledge of mankind and the world, which explains the predilection for the unusual and the exotic. In late Gothic art and in the Renaissance, the figures of Jews, Negroes, and various foreign types (PL. 212) were introduced into historical or religious paintings to indicate that the events took place in the Orient. Later these interpolations lost their precise significance (for example, the famous jesters and halberdiers which Veronese was called on to justify before the tribunal of the Inquisition). Exotic types were increasingly employed for no other reason than variety (see EXOTICISM). Still later, as in Rubens, Rembrandt (PL. 212), and Castiglione, these character figures indicated a curiosity regarding unusual motifs. The most important factor was the artist's determined, active, and systematic role in the discovery of new character types.

The so-called *têtes de caractère*, more or less connected with the ancient theme of famous men, remained a part of the artist's studio repertory for a long time and even influenced the psychopathic creations of F. X. Messerschmidt in the 18th century (Kris, 1932) and the studies of Géricault (1791–1824) of the insane (Miller, 1940–41). In these works, the artist is not interested in the subject because it has a certain character, but rather because it allows him to develop a characteristic manner or style of his own, free from convention; thus once again the concept of character, here regarded as a stylistic quality, appears in diametric opposition to the classical criteria. The historical continuity of the concept of character and characterization — and, as we have seen here, the extreme difficulty of defining it precisely — suggests a contrast, at times perhaps subtle, with canons of absolute beauty. Thus the concept of characterization forms a steppingstone, if not the foundation, in the development of the romantic or modern theory of art.

Jan BIALOSTOCKI

(The author acknowledges with thanks the suggestions of Professors Erwin Panofsky, E. H. Gombrich, and Meyer Schapiro).

CHARACTERIZATION IN THE ASIAN WORLD. In the East, theories of characterization did not have so great an influence on representational art as in the West. Visible evidences of the theories appear to be less systematic and more sporadic because of the variety of types depicted and the many different philosophic, religious, and magical attitudes toward the human condition. The development, however, is not completely different. Efforts at characterization relied primarily on the most obvious variations in costume and only secondarily on the depiction of individual features. Thus the rows of donors and conquered peoples represented in reliefs of the apadana at Persepolis (the audience hall built by Darius I) are individualized by ethnic groups; a specific incident is here related to the people as a whole, in allusion to the power, expansion, or even universality of the Achaemenid dynasty. Within the fundamental unity of a group characterization, individuals are differentiated only by slight variations in posture or in the offerings they bear. The same may be said of ancient Egyptian reliefs (PL. 212), though here it is less apparent. An inscription at Naqsh-i-Rustam explains the purpose of such scenes: "If you ask how many countries King Darius rules, look at the images of those who carry his throne, and you will know. You will realize that a Persian's sword has reached to distant lands. You will realize that a Persian has fought far away from Persia" (cf. G. Kent, *Old Persian Grammar*, New Haven, 1953, p. 40 ff.). This is echoed by the title borne by Darius and other Achaemenid monarchs: "King of countries of every race and tongue." The subject matter of Achaemenid reliefs is made clear through identifying costumes (the enthroned king with crown and beard, the priest with tiara, the bodyguard with bow and arrows, etc.), which reflect actual ceremonies and costumes designating rank. These ceremonies and costumes were attentively studied by the artists so that beholders could

recognize them quickly. In some Sassanian (Persia) commemorative reliefs, such as those of the time of Shapur II, Romans are indicated by their characteristic costume — a pleated dress which was a variation of the toga. True physiognomic rendering of portraits did not exist in the Sassanian world. To indicate a ruler, the emblem of the crown was used, which varied from one sovereign to another. Similarly, other emblems differentiated noblemen (see EMBLEMS AND INSIGNIA).

The same conventions were found in Central Asia, where the various ranks of the nobility could be recognized by their costumes (for example, the donors in the partially Sassanian paintings of Kucha). Although the faces and weapons are almost always identical in works of this area, one sometimes finds figures individualized by characteristic emblems on the crests of their helmets. This, however, does not exclude attempts at ethnic characterization through physical features (such as red hair and blue eyes) and the individualization of special groups. Outside Persia and central Asia, works under strong Persian influence (such as the terra-cotta bricks from Harwan in Kashmir, probably Sassanian rather than Parthian) vividly characterize the nude hermits of the Indian forests by their coiffure — hair falling over their shoulders. This, however, is only the representation of a type, not a true portrayal of a person and also has analogies in the West (PL. 211).

In India, the costume generally had great importance, even when there was an attempt to portray the features. The prevailing religious aim in works of art gave rise to a series of types representing important personages (the king, the hero, the queen, etc.) easily and quickly recognizable by the faithful. In these figures the expressive quality was stressed more than the anatomic structure, and individual features were portrayed only to indicate foreigners or cripples. The expressive quality was accentuated by the fact that the artist could represent specific emotions through the code of hand gestures derived from the dance. Constant use of an established canon of beauty for female figures made them all sensual and voluptuous.

The law of karma and the cycle of birth and death gave man a special position in creation, a sense of brotherhood with other creatures, even though man could impose his will on the gods through sacrifice (Veda) and was closer than other beings to enlightenment (Buddhism). There was no attempt to find images to express specific virtues or vices in physical terms for two reasons: the relative indifference to good or evil and the lack of a tragic sense (no separation or solution was ever final, since everything occurred within the infinite circle of existences). Astrological predictions in India were not associated with iconographic concepts; only the superior being (*mahāpuruṣa*) was characterized. The texts give us a list of physical and physiognomic characteristics comprising 32 major signs (*lakṣana*) and 80 minor ones, which enabled the sages to recognize the glorious destiny of the future buddha at his birth. Should the buddha choose the worldly life, he would become a universal sovereign (cakravartin); should he choose the contemplative life, he would become an Enlightened One. The artists took from the astrological physical description of the Buddha only a few elements such as the *uṣṇīṣa* (the protuberance on top of his head, which becomes a kind of topknot and undergoes many strange transformations) and the *ūrṇā* (the point between the eyebrows). The hair was transformed into stylized spirals (see MATHURA), which suggested to some that the Buddha had woolly hair and a Negro origin. The monk's dress, the absence of jewelry (later corrected), and earlobes deformed by heavy earrings complete the image, undoubtedly a fine example of a characterized figure. If exceptional physiognomic features appear, for the most part quite unreal, it should be borne in mind that the representations of buddhas and bodhisattvas tend to assume the ethnic characteristics of the people who create them; they become Chinese in China or Japanese in Japan, just as barbaric bodhisattvas with Kushan features are typical of Gandhara art. In Gandhara it should be noted that the Buddha is also represented with the characteristic gesture of the classical philosopher.

Many types of characterization may be recognized in the various phases of the Gandhara school: monks with shaved

heads and distinctive garb, sometimes with accentuated eyebrows and deeply wrinkled faces; half-naked Brahman ascetics with long, pointed beards and hair gathered into a knot, carrying a stick and a vessel for alms; female dancers; workers; the *mahānagna* (professional assassin); and so forth. Figures with distinctive ethnic features or other physiognomic characteristics are particularly abundant in the stuccoes of Taxila (Pakistan) and Hadda (Afghanistan). We find a great variety of human types: hermits, soldiers, Westerners, members of caravans from the north, foreigners of every race, and the like. The variety resulted from actual observation — highly diverse peoples mingled in this region — and from an affirmation of the universality of Buddhism. This universality, proclaimed by thousands of representations adorning the sides of stupas, accounts for the diffusion into Central Asia of an assortment of characterized types. Although as a result of the comparative industrialization of metalwork in central Asia there are stereotyped images mechanically repeated by impressions taken from a matrix (as at Tumshuk), there are also grotesque images like caricatures; racial characterization is so exaggerated as to produce truly demonic figures (see DEMONOLOGY). Some are literally terrifying, while others have astonishing or ridiculously monstrous aspects, such as those which had already appeared in Gandhara.

The mingling of different races in Central Asia had, during the T'ang period, a profound influence on China, which ruled these regions for a long time. Many of the characteristic funerary terra-cotta figurines (*ming-ch'i*) of this period show definite ethnic characterization. Armenians, Iranians, Chorasmians, Sogdians, Indians, Javanese, Khotanians, Kucheans (or Tokhari), Arabs, Semites, Turks, and others are clearly recognizable by their physical features and costumes (PL. 212). Sometimes ethnic characteristics are linked with special professions: the Armenians are wine merchants, the Kucheans musicians, the Turks falconers. Within the various ethnic groups there are also recurrent types, such as the member of the caravan or the serving maid. The curiosity indicated by the large number of these figurines gave rise to the phenomenon of exoticism (q.v.), which is associated with imperial expansion and a definite interest in different human types. Exoticism in Chinese civilization, however, treated human representations in a somewhat unusual way. As O. Sirén (1934) has pointed out, the human form in Chinese sculpture was not a very important motif because Chinese works of art were never "the glorification of individual beauty, of physical movement, or of motifs based only on material experience." They were often conceived almost like symbols "offering a more general and typical idea." Since Chinese sculpture was, like medieval art in Europe, "essentially conventional," this interest in the costume and physiognomy of foreign peoples was really a product of characterization. Beside the characterization necessary to make the compositions intelligible (the soldier clad in his armor, the musician with his instrument, the king and queen with their retinue) and the conventional self-portrait of the artist with his brush (as in the scroll paintings of Tun-huang), the Chinese also attempted characterization according to moral traits. This is proved by the saying of the ancient philosopher Ts'ao Chih (192–232) quoted by Chang Yen-yüan in his work, *Li-tai ming-hua-chi*, written in 847: "When one sees pictures of the Three Kings or the Five Emperors, one cannot help assuming an attitude of respect and veneration, and when one sees pictures of the San Chi [the sovereigns inspiring sadness], one can only feel sad. When one sees portraits of rebels or ungrateful sons, one can only grind one's teeth. When one sees pictures of men of high principles and great wisdom, one forgets to eat. When one sees portraits of faithful subjects dying as victims of their duty, one can only feel exalted, and so on. Thus we realize that painting serves us as a moral guide." The philosopher here refers to wall paintings now lost. They were not true portraits but more or less fanciful and certainly effective evocations of historic personages, to either inspire or serve as examples to be avoided. It is apparent that the characterization of moral qualities or defects was widespread and carefully studied, and was even carried to the point of transforming certain persons into examples of virtues or vices. Probably the vast majority

of now-lost ancient Chinese paintings depicting human beings must have had a moral significance; thus they belong to the realm of characterization. Further indication of the characterizing aspect of these ancient works is provided by some statements of the famous 4th-century painter Ku K'ai-chih. In addition, through a series of documents beginning as early as the Chou dynasty, H. Doré (IV, 1917, p. 327 ff, and passim) has clearly demonstrated the existence in China of ideas analogous to those in the West regarding astrological influences on character and the interpretation of physiognomy. It is interesting to note that a preliminary examination of features and bony structure was required for some emperors of remotest antiquity before they were entrusted with the burdens of state. There are, however, energetic refutations of the theory that character may be deduced from the features: for instance, Sün-ch'ing (also called Sün-tzŭ), referring to literary sources, denies that the emperors Chieh (Hsia period) and Chou (Shang-Yin period) could have had a physical appearance corresponding to their moral corruption; actually Chieh and Chou were two of the San Chi, the sovereigns inspiring sadness.

In the decorative carvings of the Han period, other sorts of characterization appear — often lively genre scenes of hunters or peasants at work, easily recognizable by their costume, tools, and the job they perform. They may be seen again in the Tun-huang wall paintings, where the great number of character types is especially notable. Frequently recurring types are the schoolmaster and the damned in the underworld. In Japanese representations, the damned are clearly differentiated by their features; in China, their crimes are differentiated by the penalty exacted and the presence of the various supreme judges (called *wang*, or king) who preside over their execution. Occasionally one finds representations of a lohan, or arhat (a personage in Hinayana Buddhism comparable to a saint), derived from the type of Gandhara monk previously mentioned. The features and the emaciated, almost skeletal anatomy sometimes give the arhat a highly grotesque appearance (e.g., the arhat painted in color on silk by Kuan-hsiu, in the National Museum, Tokyo); at other times the arhat is only a particularly expressive picture of a monk characterized by dress, pose, and in some cases specific attributes.

After observing that throughout Asia Europeans became exotic character figures, as the Central Asian barbarians became for the T'ang empire, we should mention that the various types of Japanese prints (from the old *sumi-e* to the *nishiki-e*) provide other examples of characterized types, such as the refined and gentle courtesan who personifies that ephemeral world which inspires the style of Ukiyo-e (q.v.) and, above all, the reciting actor. It is the actor's mask, either profoundly incisive in its effect or graceful and gentle, that interests the artist. The use of this accessory, which could indicate a spiritual attitude or an intense emotion, gave rise to an intellectual investigation of types and a study of the harmony or the discord, always slight, between the movements of the body and the fixed, immobile mask.

Mario BUSSAGLI

ASPECTS OF CHARACTERIZATION OTHER THAN EUROPEAN AND ASIAN. In the art of primitive people, certain formal characteristics occur repeatedly in the representation of human and animal figures. Tendencies toward stylization, geometrization, symbolism (in which portrayals have a ritualistic quality), stereotyped caricature (New Caledonian masks), and a kind of idealization in proportions (sculpture of Ife, Nigeria) can be distinguished. These tendencies often exist simultaneously within the same culture. Without exception they all further a conventional, artificial kind of representation. Only rarely, and to a limited extent, do primitive figures suggest a real interest in portraiture. Essential physical features, mainly those that differentiate the sexes or the human from the animal, are repeated. In Melanesian masks and the wood sculpture of the Maori (New Guinea) and the Congo, tattoo marks and other bodily decorations are faithfully reproduced, as are deformities, ornaments, headdress, and traditional costumes. In all these cases, however, the characterization applies to the entire tribal group and never to an individual.

Along with this tendency to symbolism and stylization, there are a few localized cultures which have developed a predilection for individual characterization, which sometimes attains a high artistic level, as in Mochica and Chimu ceramics (see ANDEAN PROTOHISTORY, I, cols. 370–371, 380–381), the pre-Columbian sculpture or architectural carvings, and the Benin sculpture of Nigeria.

*Pre-Columbian America.* On Mochica vases, which originated in the northwestern coastal area of Peru and later spread north and south, painted designs and bas-reliefs show persons differentiated by details of dress rather than features; but in high reliefs or sculpture in the round, faces are rendered with sensitivity and realism (see I, PLS. 176–180, 185–189, 193, 194). An obvious portrait intention is evident in the differentiation of posture and the physiognomy with incisive features. This differentiation is accompanied by a careful portrayal of each person's social condition and rank: nobles wear sumptuous costumes; warriors wear heavy armor; the priest wears a ceremonial dress; the prisoner is shown nude. Contrasting with these realistic portrayals are symbolic or fantastic figures inspired by myths: Warriors are sometimes depicted with animal heads or bodies, members of the upper class by symbolic predatory creatures (pumas, foxes, owls, serpents). The mythical god Ai-pec (see DEMONOLOGY) is frequently represented in human form, with cat's paws, thus linking portraiture, costume, and symbol. The range of subjects is exceptionally wide: figures of chieftains characterized by austere aristocratic bearing, strong soldiers, musicians, fishermen, simple artisans, weavers displaying their wares, blind men, persons wasted by illness with faces and chests covered with festering boils. Animals are also characterized: a frog staring fixedly upward with heavy eyelids seems to anticipate danger; an owl holds a struggling shrew in its beak; a starling eats an ear of corn. Mochica ceramics, exceptional among fairly conventional geometric styles, give the picture of a strongly organized state and a highly stratified society with many social classes and professions.

In the same northern coastal zone of Peru, the Mochica style is continued in Chimu ceramics. In this pottery, frequently monochrome, individual physical characteristics are often rendered in high relief; low-relief or painted decorations follow conventional canons. Themes are, for the most part, a continuation of those found in Mochica art. In certain figures, a tendency toward caricature can be seen in an exaggeration of the features: the face of an old man is excessively wrinkled; an obese man has layers of fat on his face and neck. But we also find intensely realistic figures such as a sleeping warrior, a blind man with his features contorted in a grimace, a sick man with bent head and pock-marked skin, a drunkard with wan face and stupefied expression, supported on the arms of two companions. Realism of this sort, derived from certain Mochica works, alternates with such representations as sailors, a llama herdsman, a doctor or an instructor with a boy, a blind flutist.

From the occasionally rather crude modeling and somewhat coarse technique, the stereotyped repetition of Mochica themes, and the restricted color range, we have the impression that Chimu ceramics represents a derivative phase of art, approaching the decadence of mass production. Yet despite these inadequacies, it remains one of the outstanding manifestations of realistic art in pre-Columbian America.

In Mexico, tendencies toward geometrization and stylization generally prevail. An exception is the Olmec culture (also called "La Venta" after the main site of the archaeological excavation). Olmec flourished toward the end of the classical Mayan period. Highly refined sculpture in the round, carved from semiprecious stones (jadeite, serpentine, diopside), shows a careful study of anatomy and a masterly and dynamic treatment of the human body. Facial expression is accurately rendered, with attention given to the smallest details. Besides male and female figurines, Olmec sculpture includes marble masks and animal figures, among which the figure of the jaguar with protruding fangs, hollow eyes, and tongue hanging out is especially notable.

The Olmec interest in characterization occasionally spreads to other cultures in this region, where as a rule the opposite tendency prevails. The basalt or onyx heads of the classic art of Veracruz are of special interest: Although small, they strikingly reproduce human heads with a disconcerting effect of immediacy. The features differ from one to another, but the various examples have uniform elements — swollen, half-open lips, the sleep of death with closed eyes, hair gathered into a ritual knot on top of the head. Sculptures in marble and other hard stones display striking elements of realism and emotion, which are in strong contrast to the tendency of Aztec art toward conventionalized form. For example, in a scapolite sculpture the goddess Tochi is represented nude in the act of childbirth, crouching and convulsed with effort, her eyes wide open and an anguished grimace on her face.

In classical Mayan art, the clay statuettes of the Isle of Jaina and the Usumacinta River Valley are specially noteworthy for their characterization. Round or hollow (some served as whistles), with richly polychromed decoration, they represent naturalistically a series of persons or groups distinguished by their headdresses and gestures. The orator is shown with outstretched arms addressing the crowd; the nobles wear their superb headdresses and ornaments, the warrior his shield and helmet; an old man embraces a young girl. These statuettes represent a completely secular art.

One may say of pre-Columbian art in general that an interest in the representation of certain types and classes (rather than individual personality) is apparent predominantly in cultures with a highly developed social stratification and is usually accompanied by an effort to differentiate the various social strata and professions.

*Benin.* A tendency toward characterization also appears in the Benin art of south-central Nigeria. This art flourished from the 16th to the 17th century, and the greater part of the surviving bronze or ivory works belong to this period. Yet at an even earlier date (1350–1500) there seems to have been a production of magnificent bronze portrait heads. Indigenous artists in the service of the court executed relief plaques, bronze masks and earrings, heads, statuettes, groups in bronze or ivory, ivory cups with relief decoration, etc. The Benin style differs from the neighboring Ife art (see GUINEAN CULTURES) by its intentional and specific characterization of the social status of the persons represented; in Ife art, however, a single model is repeated in a uniform manner. Personal variations in physiognomy or psychology are never portrayed, and faces are rather conventional, uniform, and inexpressive. Types are differentiated by their characteristic costumes, headdress, ornaments, postures, actions, gaits, etc. Themes include the sacrifice of animals; warriors pompously astride their horses; trumpeters with necklaces and bracelets — their helmets, jackets, and skirts decorated with geometric motifs; European soldiers aiming their rifles; hunters alone or in groups, on horseback or on foot; priests officiating with two assistants at their sides; kneeling chained prisoners dragged by two guards; busts or heads of high dignitaries; noblemen of the court (characterized by their helmets and wide necklaces); enthroned kings held aloft between two kneeling attendants; the impressive entrance to the royal palace, protected by guards; drummers and sistrum players; a serpent devouring a native; and so forth. Benin art is predominantly aristocratic and courtly. The artists are concerned with showing, through a great variety of details, social status rather than personalities.

In African art in general, characterization is achieved through conventional, purely symbolic means, as for example in the royal portrait statues of the Bushongo (see BANTU CULTURES) or the wooden statues of the Congo, where we frequently find a seated or kneeling mother holding a child. Though the posture expresses mother love, the features of the figures remain intentionally stereotyped and uniform.

Vittorio LANTERNARI

BIBLIOG. H. Jouin, Conférences de l'Académie royale de peinture et de sculpture, Paris, 1883; H. Jouin, Charles Le Brun et les arts sous Louis XIV, Paris, 1889; H. Morley, Character Writings of the Seventeenth Cen-

tury, London, 1891; U. L. L. Robert, Les signes d'infamie au Moyen-Age: Juifs, Sarrazins, hérétiques, lépreux, cagots et filles publiques, Paris, 1891; F. Lippmann, The Seven Planets, London, 1895; J. Nichols, G. Stevens, and S. Ireland, Life and Works of William Hogarth, III, V, VIII, Philadelphia, 1900; G. L. Hendrickson, The Origin and Meaning of the Ancient Characters of Style, American J. of Philology, XXVI, 1905, pp. 249–90; H. Klaiber, Leonardo da Vincis Stellung in der Geschichte der Physiognomik und Mimik, RepfKw, XXVIII, 1905, pp. 213–339; H. Doré, Recherches sur les superstitions en Chine, 10 vols., Shanghai, 1905–25; W. Wätzoldt, Die Kunst des Porträts, Leipzig, 1908 (Die Darstellung des Charakters, p. 24 ff.); F. Baldensperger, Les théories de Lavater dans la littérature française, Etudes d'Histoire Littéraire, series II, 1910, pp. 51–91; A. Shaftesbury, Second Characters, or The Language of Form, ed. B. Rand, Cambridge, England, 1914; L. Planiscig, Alessandro Magnasco und die romantisch-genrehafte Richtung des Barocco, Monatshefte für Kunstwissenschaft, VIII, 1915, pp. 238–48; C. Steinbrucker, Lavaters Physiognomische Fragmente im Verhältnis zur bildenden Kunst, Berlin, 1915; E. Panofsky and F. Saxl, Die Entwicklung der Planetendarstellung: Dürers Melencolia, I, Leipzig, Berlin, 1923, pp. 121–36; E. Faral, Les arts poétiques aux XIIᵉ et XIIIᵉ siècles, Paris, 1924; G. M. Fess, The Correspondence of Physical and Material Factors with Character in Balzac, Philadelphia, 1924; A. von le Coq, Bilderatlas zur Kunst- und Kulturgeschichte Mittel-Asiens, Berlin, 1925; E. Mâle, L'art religieux de la fin du Moyen-Age en France, 3d ed., Paris, 1925; F. Tupper, Types of Society in Mediaeval Literature, New York, 1926; Encyclopaedia Britannica, 14th ed., s.v. Character; J. Barthoux, Les fouilles de Haḍḍa: Figures et figurines, Paris, 1930; F. M. Barbado, La physionomie, le tempérament et le caractère, d'après Albert le Grand et la science moderne, Revue Thomiste, XXXVI, 1931, pp. 314–51; E. Kris, Die Charakterköpfe des F. X. Messerschmidt, JhbKhSammlWien, VI, N.S., 1932, pp. 169–228; E. Wind, Humanitätsidee und heroisiertes Porträt in der englischen Kultur des 18. Jahrhunderts, Bibliothek Warburg, Vorträge 1930–31, Leipzig, Berlin, 1932, pp. 156–229; P. Alfassa (A. Blunt), L'origine de la lettre de Poussin sur les modes d'après un travail récent, B. de la Société de l'Histoire de l'Art Français, 1933, pp. 125–43; H. Brockhaus, Ein edles Geduldspiel: "Die Leitung der Welt oder der Himmelsleiter," die sogenannten Taroks Mantegnas vom Jahre 1459–60, Miscellanea di storia dell'arte in onore di I. B. Supino, Florence, 1933, pp. 397–416; R. D. Löwenberg, Der Streit um die Physiognomik zwischen Lavater und Lichtenberg, Z. für Menschenkunde, IX, 1933, pp. 15–33; W. R. Juynboll, Het komische Genre in de Italiaanische Schilderkunst, gedurende de 17de en de 18de Eeuw, Leiden, 1934; O. Sirén, La scultura e la pittura cinesi, Rome, 1934; H. W. Janson, A. Mythological Portrait of the Emperor Charles V, Worcester Art Museum Annual, I, 1935–36, pp. 19–31; J. Landquist, Temperament- och Konstitutionsforsking från antiken till romantiken, Festschrift G. Castrén, 1938, p. 171 ff.; J. Evans, The Theory of the Temperaments: Taste and Temperament, New York, 1939; A. Katzenellenbogen, Allegories of the Virtues and Vices in Mediaeval Art, London, 1939; S. N. Das Gupta, L'intimo aspetto dell'antica arte indiana, Rome, 1940; C. N. Greenough, Character of Nations, Massachusetts Historical Society, Proceedings (1932–36), LXV, 1940, pp. 475–92; R. W. Lee, Ut pictura poesis, AB, XXII, 1940, pp. 197–269; A. Locke, The Negro in Art, Washington, 1940; M. Miller, Géricault's Paintings of the Insane, Warburg, III, V, 1940–41, pp. 151–63; J. Schmidt, Physiognomik, Paulys Real-Encyclopädie der classischen Altertumswissenschaft, XXXIX, 1941, pp. 1064–74; P. Frankl, The Earliest Jewish Portrait, Historia Judaica, V, 1943, pp. 155–64; V. Hall, Decorum in Italian Renaissance Literary Criticism, Modern Language Quarterly, IV, 1943, pp. 177–83; F. D. Klingender, Hogarth and English Caricature, London, New York, 1945; W. Deonna, Du miracle grec au miracle chrétien, 3 vols., Basel, 1945–48; J. Reider, Jews in Mediaeval Art: Essay on Antisemitism, 2d ed., New York, 1946, pp. 93–102; B. Boyce, The Theophrastan Character in England to 1642, Cambridge, Mass., 1947; R. Krautheimer, Tragic and Comic Scene of the Renaissance: The Baltimore and Urbino Panels, GBA, series VI, XXX, 1948, pp. 327–46; E. Panofsky, Albrecht Dürer, 3d ed., Princeton, 1948; A. Niceforo, La fisonomia nell'arte e nella scienza, Florence, 1952; E. H. Gombrich, Renaissance Artistic Theory and the Development of Landscape Painting, GBA, series VI, XLI, 1953, pp. 335–60; E. Kris and E. H. Gombrich, The Principles of Caricature, in E. Kris, Psychoanalytic Explorations in Art, London, 1953, pp. 189–203; G. Auriti, Compendio di storia della cultura giapponese, Rome, 1954; E. H. Gombrich, Leonardo's Grotesque Heads, Leonardo, Saggi e ricerche, Rome, 1954, pp. 197–219; G. Levitine, The Influence of Lavater and Girodet's "Expression des sentiments de l'âme," AB, XXXVI, 1954, pp. 33–44; E. Tea, Leonardo e il costume, Raccolta Vinciana, XVII, 1954, pp. 63–79; A. Rubens, A Jewish Iconography, London, 1954; W. Hogarth, The Analysis of Beauty, ed. J. Burke, Oxford, 1955; G. Krien, Der Ausdruck der antiken Theatermasken nach Angaben im Polluxkatalog und in der pseudoaristotelischen "Physiognomik," Jahreshefte des österreichischen archäologischen Instituts in Wien, XLII, 1955, pp. 84–117; E. Forssman, Säule und Ornament, Stockholm, 1956; S. Gunasinge, La forme féminine dans la sculpture pré-Gupta, Arts Asiatiques, III, 1956, pp. 98–124; J. von Schlosser, La letteratura artistica, 2d ed., Florence, 1956; G. Widengren, Some Remarks on Riding Costume and Articles of Dress among Iranian Peoples in Antiquity, Arctica: Ethnographica Upsaliensa, XI, 1956, pp. 228–76; J. Baltrusaitis, Physiognomie animale, Aberrations, Quatre essais sur la légende des formes, n.p., 1957, pp. 7–46; R. Ghirshman, Notes iraniennes, VII: A propos de Persépolis, Arts Asiatiques, XX, 1957, pp. 265–78; H. Ingholt, Gandhāran Art in Pakistan, New York, 1957; R. Spencer, Ut rhetorica pictura, Warburg, XX, 1957, pp. 26–44; G. F. Hartlaub, Kunst und Physiognomik: Fragen an die Kunst, Stuttgart, n.d., pp. 183–91; J. G. Malher, The Westerners among the Figurines of the T'ang Dynasty of China, Rome, 1959; E. H. Gombrich, Art and Illusion, New York, 1960.

Jan BIALOSTOCKI

Illustrations: PLS. 201–212.

**CHARDIN**, JEAN-BAPTISTE-SIMÉON. French painter (b. Paris, Nov. 2, 1699; d. Paris, Dec. 6, 1779). First-born son in the large family of a Parisian cabinetmaker, Chardin had to earn his own living from an early age and could not, as he would have wished, devote himself to literary studies. At eighteen he was a student of the painter of "histories" Pierre-Jacques Cazes, whose works he copied, as was the custom. Haillet de Couronne in his "Eloge de Chardin," delivered in 1780 before the Academy of Rouen, says that the artist's father arranged for his enrollment in the Academy of St. Luke; however, his name does not appear in the list compiled by J. J. Guiffrey in his *Histoire de l'Académie de St. Luc* (Paris, 1915).

For a short time Chardin worked with Noël-Nicolas Coypel. During this period he painted a huge wooden signboard for a surgeon who was a friend of his father; it represented "a man wounded by a sword transported to the office of the surgeon, who examines the wound to treat it, surrounded by numerous onlookers." The signboard itself, which measured 14 ft., 7 ⁵/₈ in., by 2 ft., 4 ¹/₂ in., is now lost, but the Goncourt brothers, who engraved an anonymous sketch of it, found in it "the spirit and the fire of the late Venetian masters." Chardin was perhaps imitating Watteau, who had depicted on a signboard the shop of the art dealer Gersaint.

After the period with Coypel, Chardin participated in the restoration of the frescoes by Primaticcio and Il Rosso at Fontainebleau, under the guidance of Jean-Baptiste Vanloo. In 1728 he sent several paintings, including *The Rayfish* (Louvre), to the open-air exhibition of young painters in the Place Dauphine, an annual event held on Corpus Christi. His friend the engraver Charles-Nicolas Cochin tells us that to obtain judgment on the quality of his own painting Chardin invited several important people and showed them his works intermixed with those of other artists; Nicolas de Largillière admired his paintings and attributed them to a "good Flemish painter."

On Sept. 25, 1728, Chardin presented several of his paintings before the Academy of Painting (Académie Royale de Peinture et de Sculpture), which selected *The Rayfish* and *The Buffet* (PL. 216) and forthwith accepted him as a member; the record of the session described him as "a genre painter of animals and of fruit." He did large paintings in the manner of Alexandre-François Desportes and Jean-Baptiste Oudry, among them the still life with a duck hanging on a wall and a lemon on a table, mentioned by Mariette (P. de Chennevières and A. de Montaiglon, eds., *Abecedario de P.-J. Mariette*, I, Paris, 1851–53, p. 536), the *Spaniel* of 1730 (Coll. Wildenstein), and the *Running Dog*, now in the S. Marina Collection, Buenos Aires; subsequently he did many smaller studies of rabbits hanging on a wall with kitchen utensils in the manner of Jan Fyt or Frans Snyders. Other compositions of this sort are the two in the Louvre, *Menu de maigre* and *Menu de gras* (both dated 1731); a *Kitchen Table*, dated 1733, is in the Museum of Fine Arts in Boston.

On Jan. 26, 1731, Chardin married the twenty-two-year-old Marguerite Saintard; their son Pierre-Jean (b. Nov. 18, 1731) also became a painter. The well-known painting *Woman Sealing a Letter* (Berlin, Staat. Mus.), although it carries the date 1733, probably depicts his wife at the time of their engagement. At the exhibition in the Place Dauphine in 1732 Chardin showed two decorative panels depicting instruments and trophies of music, painted for the Comte de Rottembourg, as well as a small painting of the Duquesnoy bas-relief showing eight children playing with a goat (Paris, Mus. Jacquemart-André), which was bought by his former master Vanloo.

During the early 1730s Chardin's style underwent a profound transformation. His technique matured, he treated new subjects, described as "in the manner of Teniers"; for the most part these genre scenes depict the modest life of the *petite bourgeoisie*. But little by little Chardin lost his taste for anecdote and detail; simplifying his subjects, he ultimately achieved a grandeur and severity comparable to that of the Le Nain brothers or Pieter de Hooch. Among the first paintings of this period were *The Washerwoman* and its companion piece, *The Water Urn* ("La Fontaine," 1733), both in Stockholm (Nat. Mus.). He also painted some portraits, doubtless at the suggestion of his friend

the painter Jacques-André Aved, whom he represented in a large painting entitled *The Prompter* (Louvre), signed and dated 1734. The model for several versions of *Soap Bubbles* and for the first versions of *House of Cards* (1735) was his little son.

In 1735 Chardin was refused the coveted position of professor in the Academy of Painting. (In this year too he suffered a tragic personal loss, the death of his wife and two-year-old daughter.) However, two years later (1737), when his works were exhibited at the Salon, he began to know success. He had simplified not only his subjects but also his technique; he experimented with the densities of whites, achieving tones that Decamps later despaired of being able to reproduce: "These whites of Chardin's! They elude me." His impasto was now rich and thickly applied, with relief and luminosity, power and precision. The works of this period are among his most remarkable, and his success led him to make numerous replicas. Noteworthy examples are the *Little Girl with Cherries* and its companion piece *The Little Soldier Boy* (both formerly Rothschild Coll.); *The Tavern Boy* and *The Kitchen Maid* ("L'Ecureuse") (both 1738, private colls.; versions in Glasgow, Hunterian Mus.); *The Girl Scraping Vegetables* ("La Ratisseuse," 1738; formerly Vienna, Liechtenstein Gall.); and *The Maid Returning from Market* ("La Pourvoyeuse"), of which there are versions in Ottawa (Nat. Gall. of Canada), in the Louvre (PL. 215), and in other collections.

Chardin's genre paintings, although modest in size and subject matter, attracted the attention of great collectors whose taste had been formed by the art of Watteau and Boucher (qq.v.); among these were the Comte de Tessin (who bought for the King of Sweden), the Prince of Liechtenstein in Vienna, the court of Russia, and great Parisian "amateurs" such as the Chevalier de la Roque, the Comte de Vence, M. de la Live de Jully. Chardin did portraits of the children of the jeweler Charles Godefroy, the *Young Man with a Violin* and the *Child with Top* (both in the Louvre; PL. 218); the latter, exhibited in the Salon of 1738, is one of the most beautiful of his portraits of children, the illuminated face radiating intelligence and sensitivity. At Versailles in 1740, Philibert Orry presented Chardin to Louis XV, to whom he showed two paintings, *The Grace* (PL. 214) and *The Industrious Mother* (Louvre), both of which the King kept for himself. In these two paintings, which were meant to be hung symmetrically, the compositional lines are subtly counterbalanced, the tones delicately harmonized. The engravings made after them by the talented and famous Cochin indicate their success. Chardin, in fact, owed a measure of his popularity to engravers (Cochin, Pierre Louis de Surugue, Bernard Lépicié), who made his works known to the general public. In 1743 Gautier Dagoty put up for sale colored engravings of *The Tapestry Worker* and *The Draftsman* (both Stockholm, Nat. Mus.). It was Dagoty who first recognized the modernity of Chardin's technique: "All his objects reflect one another, and there results a transparency of color that enlivens everything his brush touches."

In 1740 Chardin exhibited two paintings with unusual subjects taken from fables, *The Monkey of Philosophy* ("Le Singe de la philosophie," or "Le Singe antiquaire") and *The Monkey-Painter* (versions of both of which are in the Louvre and other museums). Alluding to the human comedy, they are a good-natured satire on official academicism. This kind of subject, rare in decorative painting, had been used by Watteau and was later to be exploited by Jean-Baptiste Huet. However, this was not an area in which Chardin excelled, and he limited himself to a few conventional renditions.

In 1741 Chardin's production slowed down; in fact the critics reproved him for showing only two works, the *Morning Toilette* (Stockholm, Nat. Mus.) and the *Portrait of M. Lenoir's Son Making a House of Cards*. The former work, commissioned by the Comte de Tessin, was praised by these very critics for its fine pictorial qualities. It is probable that Chardin was at this time very busy making copies of his own paintings because they were in such demand; further, the fact that in January, 1742, Cochin and Jean-Baptiste Jouvenet inquired after him on behalf of the Academy of Painting would seem to indicate that poor health was interfering with his work. In 1743 the

artist lost his mother, who had been living with him; the next year he married the widow of Charles de Malnoë, Françoise-Marguerite Pouget, by whom he had a daughter. Two paintings for the Comte de Tessin, now in the National Museum of Stockholm, are of this period: the *Amusements of Private Life* (Salon of 1746) and the *Woman Checking Her Accounts* ("L'Œconome," Salon of 1747); Surugue's engravings made them known immediately to the public. He also painted two life-size portraits, one of M. Levret of the Academy of Surgery. Critics were increasingly favorable to him, deploring only the fact that his best pictures were being sent abroad; many, as we have seen, went to Sweden, and *The Attentive Nurse* ("La Garde attentive," or "Les Aliments de la convalescence"), companion piece to *The Governess*, painted in 1739 (now in Ottawa, Nat. Gall. of Canada), entered the collection of Prince Liechtenstein in Vienna.

Charles-Antoine Coypel, a nephew of Noël-Nicolas, obtained for Chardin, through M. de Tournehem, director of the royal works, the commission for a painting that figured in the Salon of 1751 under the title *The Bird Organ* ("La Serinette," or "La Dame variant ses amusements"; New York, Frick Coll.). Evan H. Turner in 1957 showed beyond doubt that the young woman represented in this painting is Chardin's second wife and not Mme Geoffrin, as has sometimes been stated. Chardin continued to do intimate genre scenes, but almost all were copies of his already well-known works. He also painted still lifes and portraits; among the latter the most moving is *The Blind Man* ("L'Aveugle des Quinze-Vingts," formerly Rothschild Coll.), exhibited in the Salon of 1753, touching in the sobriety of line and color and far removed from contemporary sentimentality. Several of the attributions of portraits are questionable: for example, the beautiful one of Rameau in Dijon (Mus. B.A.) seems to be in a spirit and of workmanship different from Chardin's. In 1755 Chardin was named treasurer of the Academy of Painting, with the task of arranging the paintings of the Salon. Until the time (1757) when he was given lodgings in the Louvre, in one of the apartments reserved by the king for artists, he exhibited little, although he painted numerous still lifes. He sought those effects of light so well described by Gautier Dagoty; when Bachaumont speaks of his technique one seems to hear the reproaches leveled a hundred years later at the impressionists: "His manner of painting is singular; he places colors one next to the other without mixing them, so that his work seems somewhat like mosaic."

Chardin's still lifes are difficult to date because of the copies executed in different periods. It is only after 1756–58 that there appear compositions ordered by patterns of light. In these, objects of silver and crystal reflect carefully arranged fruit, or sometimes a white vase illumines the objects placed around it. Among many such paintings are the *Bowl of Olives*, *Grapes and Pomegranates*, *Still Life with Pipe* (all in the Louvre), and the *Bowl of Plums* (Washington, Phillips Coll.). In a more refined technique that recalls Boucher are *Preparations of a Meal* (Carcassonne, Mus. B.A.) and its replica dated 1763 (Louvre).

Diderot, who was among the admirers of Chardin's still lifes at the Salon of 1763, wrote, "It is difficult to comprehend this kind of magic. Thick layers of color are applied one upon the other and seem to melt together. At other times one would say that a vapor or a light foam had breathed on the canvas.... Draw near, and everything flattens out and disappears; step back, and all the forms are re-created."

Through Cochin, who continued to be one of his protectors, Chardin received a commission from the Marquis de Marigny to paint three overdoors for the Château de Choisy: *Attributes of the Arts*, *Attributes of the Sciences*, and *Attributes of Music*. These were exhibited at the Salon of 1765, where they were a great success. Removed in 1792, they were placed in the Monastery of the Petits Augustins; two of them, the *Attributes of the Arts* and the *Attributes of Music* (PL. 213) are in the Louvre; the third has disappeared. Satisfied with these decorations, Cochin proposed to the Marquis de Marigny to decorate the music room of the Château de Bellevue "with

two overdoors by M. Chardin; this artist achieves a degree of perfection unique in this genre." At the Salon of 1767, Chardin exhibited two paintings of various instruments of military and domestic music (Paris, private coll.).

In 1765 Chardin, who, through his wife, had connections with Normandy, requested admission to the Academy of Rouen to fill the place left by the death of Michel-Ange Slodtz. After 1770 the health of the artist worsened, and he was saddened by the disappearance of his son, who was taken prisoner by pirates in Italy. Furthermore his popularity began to decline with a public that now preferred the moralizing subjects of Greuze. Nevertheless, he continued to produce small, intimate scenes, repeating themes he had painted 40 years before. Other factors contributing to his depression were the departure of his protector Marigny, whom Louis XVI replaced with the Comte d'Angiviller, and the disgrace of Cochin. In addition, Chardin was a victim of a change in administrative personnel; Jean-Baptiste Marie Pierre, the new court painter, did not spare him.

Several of Chardin's biographers believe that it was failing eyesight that led him to begin to use pastels. And in fact the artist himself wrote to D'Angiviller in 1777 that his infirmities interfered with his painting in oil: "For this reason I have begun to work in pastels." It was perhaps in these latest works, when the artist was no longer hampered by material preoccupations but could single-mindedly follow his inspiration, that he reached the climax of his art. Simple and severe, these paintings have great power of suggestion. Such works as the *Self-portrait* (PL. 216), the *Portrait of Madame Chardin*, the *Self-portrait with Eye Shade* (all three in the Louvre), are treated with a broad and rhythmic technique of large parallel strokes of color superimposed and reflecting one another. The critics recognized the mysterious beauty of these pastels: "M. Chardin," wrote one, "reminds me of the athletes who, after a terrible combat, summon up all their strength to go and die in the arena."

In the last year of his life, though weakened by a painful illness, Chardin exhibited several pastels, one of which, the head of a boy ("Un Jacquet, petit laquais"), was acquired by the King's aunt, Mme Victoire, who gave the painter a gold snuffbox. Several months later, on Dec. 6, 1779, Chardin died in his apartment in the Louvre  The paintings and drawings found in his studio were sold at auction at the Hôtel d'Alègre, Rue St. Honoré, on Mar. 6, 1786.

That Chardin died in poverty is probably not true. He was one of the few painters who at a fairly early age knew, if not celebrity, at least a certain renown. Moreover, as we have seen, he had patrons of high rank, the King, princes, great financiers; he even numbered artists among his admirers: the painters Vanloo, Aved, Jean François de Troy, the engravers Laurent Cars, Jacques-Philippe Le Bas, the draftsman Nicolas Charles de Silvestre, the sculptors Jean-Baptiste Lemoyne and Jean-Baptiste Pigalle, the architects Pierre Boscry and Louis-François Trouard, and the goldsmith Jean-Nicolas Roettiers.

A number of Chardin's followers were more successful than the master, perhaps because their scenes with moralizing content made a greater appeal to the public taste. Among them were Etienne Aubry; Louis Aubert, remembered for his *Salad Washer* ("L'Eplucheuse de salade," 1743); Jérôme-François Chantereau, who imitated Chardin, although he was a student of Jean-Baptiste Pater, Michel Nicolas Lépicié, Roland de La Porte, and Mme Vallayer-Coster (all of whom imitated Chardin's still lifes); and Michel-Honoré Bounieu, whose signature on the painting *Preparations for the Stew* (Louvre) was covered by that of the master (see H. Adhémar, "Une Nature Morte de M. H. Bounieu, autrefois attribuée à Chardin," *B. du Laboratoire du Musée du Louvre*, June, 1956). Also in the Chardin tradition, when they painted intimate and familiar scenes, were Françoise Duparc and Martin Drolling; still later there was Meissonier.

Imitators and copyists of Chardin have long made the problem of attribution difficult, but it is only very rarely that a style cannot be distinguished from that of the master. Chardin's technique seems at first glance simple and facile. His colors are sober and without much variation, although the surface

is often laboriously worked with various tones superimposed to create a harmonious effect. Anticipating Cézanne, Chardin sought to render form by means of light and the reality of matter by means of thick and rich impasto. He imbues his effects with a soft glow that contributes to the charm of the whole while softening the contrasts.

Chardin has a distinguished place among the painters of his period. Unquestionably he was the greatest master of still life in the 18th century. His originality, grounded in simplicity and good taste, and his immense talent as a painter have won him ever greater recognition. His paintings form a striking contrast to the elegant works of the followers of Watteau: he is justly called "the painter of the French *bourgeoisie*." Not even in the 19th century did the French middle class find an artist who better depicted its simple and humble occupations. The pastels, which collectors and amateurs have valued from the beginning, entailed great labor, and Chardin was obliged, despite his modest way of life, to set high prices on them. Unable to satisfy all his commissions, he made much use of engravings and perhaps also of copies. Although he was esteemed by connoisseurs and the public, the official critics constantly complained about his not treating noble subjects such as history and mythology.

The sources on the life and works of Chardin are meager; the few pages about him that appeared in the various critiques of the Salons where he exhibited from 1737 to 1779 are generally severe (J. G. Wille, *Mémoires et journal*, pub. by Duplessis, 2 vols., 1857). One can follow him from year to year in the meetings of the Academy of Painting, which he attended regularly. The information is rarely significant, however, for he was reticent, usually limiting himself to expressions of approval. Chardin wrote little; we have the record of some words addressed to Diderot and noted by him in his review of the Salon of 1765, complaining that the training of artists was too long, laborious, and academic. The instruction, said Chardin, was restricted to copying from plaster casts, no attention being given to the study of nature. Several inventories and notarized statements compiled after the death of his first wife (Wildenstein, 1933, pp. 64–67) in connection with the wardship of his son yield information on his finances, his works, and his mentality.

Pierre-Jean Mariette gives the facts of Chardin's life in his 1749 manuscript notices on painters and engravers ("Notice sur Chardin," in P. de Chennevières and A. de Montaiglon, eds., *Abecedario de P.-J. Mariette*, I, Paris, 1851–53, pp. 355–60). The "Eloge de Chardin" delivered in 1780 by Haillet de Couronne before the Academy of Rouen, based on the "Mémoires" furnished by Cochin, was published, from the manuscripts preserved in the Ecole des Beaux-Arts, by L. Dussieux, E. Soulié, P. de Chennevières, P. Mantz, and A. de Montaiglon in the *Mémoires inédits sur la vie et les ouvrages des membres de l'Académie royale de peinture et de sculpture*, II, 1887, pp. 428–41. The original "Mémoires" by Cochin and a letter written by him to Haillet de Couronne, commenting on the "Eloge," were published by C. de Beaurepaire in *Précis des travaux de l'Académie des sciences, belles-lettres et arts de Rouen*, 1875–76, reedited by C. Henry in 1891 and in 1931 by A. Pascal and R. Gaucheron.

In the 19th century the Goncourt brothers wrote some excellent pages on Chardin, followed by an ambitious catalogue that is unfortunately useless because of the errors of attribution it contains (E. and J. de Goncourt, *L'art au XVIIIᵉ siècle*, Paris, 1873).

In 1876 E. Bocher sketched a *Catalogue de l'œuvre de Chardin* (Paris, 1876). In 1908 J. Guiffrey produced his *Catalogue de l'œuvre peint et gravé* (Paris, 1908), and in the same year a catalogue was published by A. Dayot and L. Vaillat (*L'Œuvre de J. B. S. Chardin et J. H. Fragonard*, Paris, 1908), slightly modified by E. Herbert and A. Furst (*Chardin*, London, 1911). A. Pascal and R. Gaucheron in 1931 published for the first time a number of documents in *Documents sur la vie et l'œuvre de Chardin* (Paris, 1931).

The point of departure for research on Chardin remains the monograph by G. Wildenstein (*Chardin*, Paris, 1933). In

this fundamental work were published for the first time the archival documents and a catalogue of works classified by subjects, indicating engravings, sales, collections, and doubtful works. A new edition (in preparation) classifies the paintings in chronological order. Earlier monographs of importance were those written by G. Schéfer (*Chardin*, Paris, 1904), E. Pilon (*Chardin*, Paris, 1909), and A. de Ridder (*Chardin*, Paris, 1932).

The specific problems that remain to be treated are chiefly the origins of Chardin's style and the definition of the elements that relate him to the Dutch painters and those that separate him from them (this question has been touched upon by De Ridder). Pertinent here is the judgment of André Gide before Chardin's paintings in the Louvre: "In studying Chardin I had rather be expositor than critic — let style go by the board, experience perceptions to my own wonderment, then get to the bottom of them for myself. There is always a gain to be had from taking, before a great figure, an attitude of receptive humility" (*Journal*, May 4, 1893).

BIBLIOG. For sources and bibliography up to 1933, see G. Wildenstein, Chardin, Paris, 1933 (2d ed. in preparation). W. Pinder, Gesammelte Aufsätze aus den Jahren 1907–35, ed. L. Bruhns, Leipzig, 1938, pp. 21–28; T. Rousseau, Jr., A Pastel Portrait by J. B. S. Chardin, B. of the Fogg Art Mus., IX, 3, 1940; B. Denvir, Chardin, New York, 1950; T. Rousseau, Jr., A Boy Blowing Bubbles by Chardin, BMMA, III, 1950, pp. 221–27; H. Shipp, A Chardin Still Life, Apollo, LV, 1952, p. 142; C. Sterling, La nature morte, Paris, 1952; R. S. D[avis], Institute Purchases a Great Still Life by Chardin, B. of the Minneapolis Inst. of Arts, XLIII, 1954, pp. 50–51; M. Proust, Chardin: The Essence of Things, AN, LIII, 1954, pp. 39–42; N. Wallis, Chardin, the Superlative Craftsman, The Connoisseur, CXXXIII, 1954, p. 3; E. H. Turner, La Serinette by J.-B.-S. Chardin: A Study in Patronage and Technique, GBA, IC, 1957, pp. 299–310; F. Jourdain, Chardin, Paris, n.d.

Hélène ADHÉMAR

Illustrations: PLS. 213–218.

**CHARONTON,** ENGUERRAND. French painter of the school of Provence (b. Laon, France, ca. 1410–15; still active in 1466); his real name was Quarton. Nothing is definitely known of his origins or training except that he migrated to Provence from the diocese of Laon in Picardy. In 1444, when Charonton's name first appeared in a document, he was living in Aix-en-Provence and was already referred to as a "master." His style indicates that he carried with him to the south strong impressions of northern Gothic, especially the sculpture of the great cathedrals. There are also stylistic reminders of the Flemish school in his painting, particularly of Robert Campin (q.v.). In February, 1446, Charonton was living in Arles, but by August of the following year he had transferred to nearby Avignon, where he can be followed until July, 1466.

There are two documented and authentic works by Enguerrand Charonton, painted respectively in 1453 and 1453–54. The first is the *Virgin of Mercy*, commissioned by the son of Jean Cadard for a chapel in the Church of the Celestins at Avignon, today in the Musée Condé at Chantilly. In painting this picture Charonton collaborated with an artist named Pierre Villate, called "Malebouche." The other documented painting is the great retable of the *Coronation of the Virgin* (V, PL. 384; Hospice of Villeneuve-lès-Avignon), commissioned in April, 1453, with the requirement that it be completed for the feast of St. Michael in September, 1454. The contract, discovered by the Abbé Requin, records the artist's agreement with Jean de Montagnac to paint the retable for the Church of the Chartreuse of Villeneuve-lès-Avignon. With its many stipulations about the subject and the arrangements for payment, the contract is one of the most detailed plans that has ever survived for an existing work of art and provides an unparalleled source of information about art commissioning in 15th-century France. Although a careful itemizing and listing of figures was included in the contract, a wide margin of choice and interpretation was left to the judgment of the artist. It has been suggested that the beautiful *Pietà* of Avignon in the Louvre (V, PL. 383) is another work by Charonton. See also FRENCH ART.

BIBLIOG. Abbé Requin, Réunion des sociétés des beaux-arts des départements, 1889, documents inédits, pp. 132–35, 176–83; L. Labande, Les primitifs français, peintres et peintres-verriers de la Provence occidentale,

Marseille, 1932, pp. 77–78; C. Sterling, Le couronnement de la vierge (Chefs-d'œuvres des primitifs français), Paris, 1939.

Margaretta M. SALINGER

**CHASSERIAU,** THÉODORE. French Creole painter (b. Samaná, Hispaniola, Sept., 1819; d. Paris, Oct., 1856). In 1822 his family moved to Paris, and from 1830 to 1834 he worked in Ingres's studio. His *Suzanna in Her Bath* (Louvre, 1839) and *Vénus Anadyomène* (Louvre, 1839) define his heroine, with long, sensual, oval face, full lips, large and languid almond eyes, and tawny skin. *Christ in the Garden of Olives* (Cathedral of St.-Jean-d'Angély; 1840), with its composition and technique inspired by Delacroix, shows Chassériau as a partisan of not only the romantic Delacroix but also the classicist Ingres. These two painters were, at that time, leaders of rival schools of painting, and for the rest of his life Chassériau oscillated between the two opposing influences in both subject matter and style.

Chassériau executed two important commissions: frescoes (in the Ingres tradition) on the life of St. Mary the Egyptian for a chapel in the Church of St.-Merri, Paris (1842–43), and representations of Commerce, War and Peace, etc., for the Paris Cour des Comptes (1844–48). From 1836, with his sketches of Bedouins at Marseilles, Arab themes were prominent in his work: the dramatic series of engravings for *Othello* in 1844, the *Caliph of Constantine* in 1845 (Mus. Nat. de Versailles), the melancholy scenes inspired by his voyage to Algeria in 1846. In 1853 Chassériau produced his great *Tépidarium* (Louvre), which showed nudes set in an archaeological décor. His portraits are varied and much admired: Adèle and Aline Chassériau appear in the Louvre painting *Two Sisters* (1843). Falling within the Ingres concept of the portrait, though more nervous and impetuous, are his lively pencil drawings of the Princesses Belgiojoso and Marie Cantacuzène (later Mme Puvis de Chavannes) and his beloved Alice Ozy. Gautier said of Chassériau's art that it was a mixture of Hellenic purity and oriental exoticism.

The heirs to the Chassériau tradition are Puvis de Chavannes (q.v.), Gustave Moreau, and Odilon Redon (q.v.). See also FRENCH ART.

BIBLIOG. V. Chevillard, Une peinture romantique, Théodore Chassériau, Paris, 1893; H. Marcel and J. Laran, Théodore Chassériau, Paris, 1911; L. Bénédite, Théodore Chassériau, sa vie et son oeuvre, 2 vols., Paris, 1932; J. Adhémar, Inventaire du fonds français, Paris, 1949 (prints). Catalogues of exhibitions: L. Bénédite, Paris, 1897; C. Sterling, Orangerie, Paris, 1933; R. Bacou and M. Sérullaz, Louvre, 1957.

Norman SCHLENOFF

**CHILE.** The territory of Chile, a republic since 1818, consists of an extremely narrow, elongated strip between the Andean cordillera and the Pacific Ocean. Easter Island, or Rapa Nui, in the Pacific Ocean, is an administrative dependency of Chile, but geographically it belongs within the province of Polynesia (q.v.).

Throughout Chile are found settlements of indigenous tribes, whose artistic production is limited in both quantity and quality. A characteristic trend in the post-Conquest period has been the local adaptation, especially in architecture, of art forms derived from a European heritage.

SUMMARY. Pre-Columbian epochs (col. 388). Colonial and modern art (col. 391): *Principal centers.*

PRE-COLUMBIAN EPOCHS. The monuments revealed by excavations partially fill the gaps in our knowledge of pre-Conquest history. From the artifacts found at various levels of the great *conchales* (mounds of mollusk and crustacean shells) in the northern area, four successive strata have been differentiated.

The first two strata date from a widely diffused and remarkably uniform preagricultural culture, lacking pottery but possessing a few crude fishing tools. In the mounds in Arica, Pisagua, and Taltal similar articles have been found in the lowest strata: fishhooks of

shell, either single or compound, harpoons with a detachable head, stone scrapers, and similar primitive instruments. More careful preparation of tombs has been noted in the second stratum: they contain modest tomb furnishings, and the bodies, placed in extended position, are covered with woven reed mats; mummies of children wear wigs, and the faces are covered with a masklike clay covering. The third and fourth strata, much more recent, testify to the presence of more highly developed tribes, agriculturists who drove out the original inhabitants and settled in the northern valleys of Chile. In chronological order, these tribes were the so-called "El Molle" people, the Atacameños, and the Diaguitas. The El Molle culture, which extended over a wide area of northern Chile, was discovered and studied in the 1930s (Cornely, 1956). It is named after El Molle, where the most important and oldest burial grounds were found. Additional ones were discovered in the area occupied by the Diaguitas. Further, between El Molle and Almendral, in a hilly region on the southern bank of the Río Elqui, stand the ruins of a fortress, impregnable on three sides, whose important tombs are intact. The chief relics of the El Molle culture are the vases, characterized by great thickness and brilliant coloring. They have stirrup handles and geometric designs and are in tones of buff, black, and white.

The Atacameños settled near the Río Loa and pushed south from there, occupying the oases in the Atacama desert — that of Calama in particular — as far as the Río Copiapó. Because of the poor soil, as well as for reasons of defense, they did not build large cities, but settled in small communities scattered about in the most fertile spots. They were intelligent builders, and in this respect resemble the Peruvians. They built two characteristic types of towns, known locally as the *pucara* and the *pueblo viejo*.

The *pucara* is a fortress, generally in a hilly area, surrounded by high walls of rough stone erected without cement, called *pircas*, reminiscent of the first phases of Inca architecture. Within the ring of walls are one- or two-storied houses, granaries, and ovens laid out in no fixed order (e.g., the *pucara* of Turi, with its labyrinthine plan). A typical element of this structure is the window, which perhaps originated in the area before the Inca period. From the present ruins it would appear that the original *pucaras* were those of Lasana, San Pedro de Atacama, and Turi. In times of danger the agricultural tribes took shelter in these fortresses, which were placed at the edge of their cultivated fields.

The plan of the more common *pueblo viejo* is quite varied. There are no fortifications or surrounding walls, and the houses, larger than those in the *pucara*, are separated from one another. The ruins of Zapai are a typical example.

Atacameñan pottery consists chiefly of vases of considerable height, with a flat or conical base, sometimes with handles; the ground is red with white or black decoration, in some cases in slight relief. Two types or styles of decoration can be distinguished: one, a simpler style, tending to darker tones, the other influenced by Peruvian styles, employing polychromy and geometric decorative motifs, especially triangular designs. The tombs of this phase have yielded many wooden objects, including bells with wooden clappers, decorated boxes, and carved tablets for ritual and secular purposes. In the Calama oasis objects have been found whose fabric clearly shows their Tiahuanacan origin (see BOLIVIA; ANDEAN PROTOHISTORY, cols. 386–87), as well as pottery similar to the Chincha ware of southern Peru.

The Diaguitas, who occupied the valleys between the Copiapó and Choapa Rivers, are linguistically and anthropologically related to the Andean tribes of the same name in northern Argentina. Their pottery displays a variety of forms, with three consecutive stylistic periods: archaic, transitional, and "classical."

Among the more popular types, dating from the earliest period, are the *jarro zapato* — a vase in the form of a shoe, with a characteristic lateral prolongation — urns with a large, often widely flaring collar, *jarros patos* ("duck vases"), and several kinds of anthropomorphous dishes and vases. The colors include red — usually for the background — black, and white. In the last phase Peruvian typological influences (the aryballus) and decorative ones may be observed. Other interesting objects are the urns, which have features in common with those of the San José and Belén types of the Argentine. The Diaguitas understood metallurgy and produced outstanding jewelry of copper, bronze, and later, under Inca influence, gold and silver.

In various regions of the territory occupied by the Diaguitas, rock engravings have been found: at Llanos, Pibra, Chañaral, Cachiyuyo, and El Cuyano. On the rocks at Incahuasi, stylized men and llamas are depicted, and hunting scenes in which dogs and stars appear.

The artistic contribution of the more southern tribes, probably of Araucanian stock, was slight, being limited to useful forms.

The Picunches (or "people of the north," settled between the Choapa and Itata Rivers), the Mapuches ("people of the earth"), and the Huilliches ("people of the south," living south of the Río Toltén) produced scantily decorated pottery. The true Araucanians settled in southern Chile, between the Itata and Toltén Rivers, perhaps as early as the 14th century. They show points of contact with Polynesia, particularly in sculpture and wood carving (ceremonial axes, etc.).

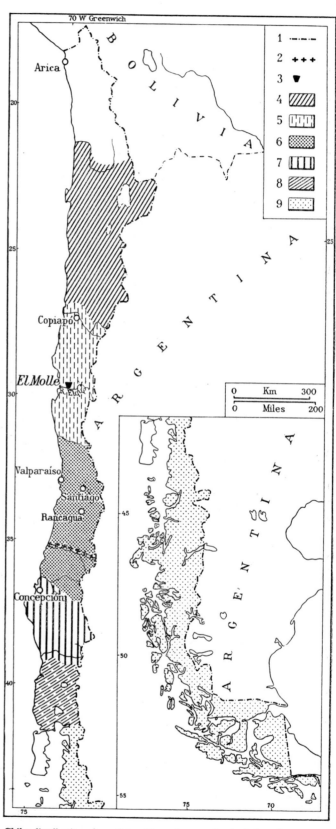

Chile: distribution of pre-Columbian cultures and principal modern centers. *Key*: (1) Political boundaries; (2) southern limit of Inca expansion; (3) region of El Molle archaeological explorations; (4) Atacameñan culture; (5) Diaguita culture; (6) Picunche culture; (7) Mapuche (Araucanian) culture; (8) Huilliche culture; (9) Tehuelche (Patagonian) culture.

Bibliog. J. T. Medina, Los aborígenes de Chile, Santiago, 1882; M. Uhle, Los indios atacameños, Revista Chilena de Historia y Geografía, III, 5, 1913, pp. 105-11; R. E. Latcham, La prehistoria chilena, Santiago, 1928; R. E. Latcham, Arqueología de la región atacameña, Santiago, 1938; J. B. Bird, Excavations in Northern Chile, APAmM, XXXVIII, 1943, pp. 171-318; W. C. Bennett, The Atacameño, HSAI, II, 1946; J. B. Bird, The Cultural Sequence of the North Chilean Coast, HSAI, II, 1946; J. M. Cooper, The Araucanians, HSAI, II, 1946; G. Mostny, Ciudades atacameñas, Santiago, 1949; P. Rivet, Los orígenes del hombre americano, Cuadernos Americanos, no. 5, Mexico City, 1953; G. Mostny, Culturas precolombinas de Chile, Santiago, 1954; S. Canals Frau, Las civilizaciones prehispánicas de América, Buenos Aires, 1955; F. L. Cornely, Cultura diaguita chilena y cultura de El Molle, Santiago, 1956 (reprint of study published in 1938).

COLONIAL AND MODERN ART. Owing to the frequency of earthquakes, Chile has few colonial monuments. Inestimable losses occurred with the severe earthquakes of 1960. Interest centers chiefly in the early ground plans of the cities, which even today determine the plans of some of them. In the south interesting mid-16th-century ruins of structures built for defense against the Araucanians remain. The forts of Amargos and Niebla, built as defenses against Dutch and English pirates, date from 1600. Chilean colonial architecture of the 17th and early 18th century was characterized by simplified and impoverished Iberian styles. Domestic architecture remained on a rather provincial level: adobe houses, low, stuccoed, with small patios, enriched in the 1700s with columned doorways and rounded tympanums decorated in the center (e.g., the Casa Sànchez Fontecilla in Calle Las Agustinas, Santiago), with wooden loggias and wrought-iron railings of Basque origin. The oldest churches had sparsely decorated façades and single-aisled interiors with the wooden beams showing.

Toward the middle of the 18th century Bavarian rococo forms were introduced by architects and craftsmen summoned by the Jesuits, particularly through the initiative of Father Carlos Haymhausen, the founder of the so-called "Calera de Tango" school, of which scarcely any examples survive. After the Jesuits, the Italian Joaquín Toesca y Richi (1745-99), trained in Rome and Madrid, played a dominant role; in several public buildings in Santiago he substituted a moderate neoclassicism for Spanish American baroque. This manner continued to dominate Chilean architecture until about 1850, when it was displaced by Restoration and Louis Philippe styles, imported by Raymond A. Q. Monvoisin (1790-1870) and the architect Claude François Brunet de Baines (1799-1855), who in 1850 founded the School of Architecture in Santiago. Also active were other foreign architects, including the Roman Eusebio Chelli, Jesse L. Wetmore from the United States, and the English architect W. Hovenden Hendry. The 19th-century taste for "revivals" was spread by such local architects as Fermín Vivaceta and Manuel Aldunate. Art Nouveau (q.v.) was introduced in Santiago in 1910 by Italian craftsmen. In 1916 the artistic cultural group known as "Los Diez" ("The Ten") was founded. After 1920 a cultural renaissance took place. Modern architecture, less widespread than in other Neo-Latin countries, nevertheless attained a rather high level. Noted architects are Sergio Larrain, of the Catholic University of Santiago, Emilio Duhart Harosteguy, Jaime Bellalta, and Jorge Costabal.

Spanish influence predominated in the painting and sculpture of the 16th and 17th centuries, but only a few names — for example, the Dominican De los Reyes (early 17th cent.) and Pineda y Bascuñán — are known. About the middle of the 17th century the school of Cuzco predominated, with such rather ingenuous paintings as those in the Monastery of S. Francisco at Santiago. The portraitist José Gil de Castro ("El Mulato") was active. The baroque style was introduced by the Jesuits; the schools of Bucalemu, Olleria, and Calera de Tango produced elegant silverware, engravings, woodcuts, and paintings. Also important in the artistic development of Latin America in general was the initiative of the Bavarians Carlos Haymhausen and J. Pitterich, who were responsible for the sumptuous decorations of the S. Miguel Church in Santiago. Proponents of neoclassicism in sculpture were Ignacio de Andía y Varela (1757-1822) and Ambrosio Santelices (1734-1818). After Chile attained independence, various European artists (from Bordeaux, Liverpool, and elsewhere) arrived. Outstanding among the first romantic painters were Antonio Smith (1832-77), a landscapist, and Manuel Antonio Caro (1835-1903), who painted scenes of popular life. With Nicanor Plaza (1844-1917) and Pedro Lira (1845-1912; also active as a publicist and organizer of exhibitions) there was a transition to realism. In sculpture, the path opened by Nicanor Plaza and José Miguel Blanco was followed by Virgilio Arias (1855-1941). Academic tendencies were replaced in the late 19th century by the symbolism of Carlos Lagarrique, Guillermo Córdova, Sergio Montecinos Montalva, and Israel Roa Villagra; a remarkable and original personality was that of Roberto Matta, who was also active in Europe. The truly Chilean school, whose roots remained Spanish despite

French influence, favored landscape and portraiture. It is represented by three artists in particular: Alfredo Valenzuela Puelma (1865-1909), Alberto Valenzuela Llanos (1859-1925), and Juan Francisco González (1854-1933). About 1920, reflections of the rather different styles of Cézanne and the Fauves were apparent in Chile. Among the many artists of note, some of whom are associated with the Academy of Fine Arts in Santiago or in Viña del Mar, are Gregorio de la Fuente, Pedro Lobos, Mario Pérez de Arce Lavin, and A. Poblete.

*Principal centers.* Arica. This city on the northern coast may have been founded by the ancient Peruvians; it was occupied by the Spanish in 1556 and was several times destroyed and rebuilt. It has a reticulated ground plan. Early in the 20th century the prefabricated Church of S. Marcos, designed by Gustave Eiffel, was erected.

Concepción. It was founded in 1550 on the seashore, on a symmetrical plan. Destroyed by an earthquake in 1751, it was rebuilt on its present site with rectilinear streets. Severe damage was suffered again in 1960. Since 1924, it has been the seat of a university.

Copiapó. Founded in 1540 under the name of San Francisco de la Selva, it consists of small one-storied houses. Vicente Cumplido built an elegant theater in 1848, now destroyed.

Rancagua. Its plan is similar to that of Santiago, with two dividing main boulevards which intersect at the central plaza. Among the few colonial survivals are several parts of the Casa de Pilastras.

Santiago. Founded in 1541 under the name of Santiago del Nuevo Extremo, it was built according to a perfectly rectilinear plan, with square blocks of 420 ft. and streets 33½ ft. wide. On each block four buildings were erected. A plaza, with the governor's palace and a church, was laid out in the center of the city. From its original plan, consisting of ten east–west streets and eight north–south streets, Santiago grew in all directions; the houses were mostly low and broad, with Spanish-type patios. The Church of S. Francisco with one aisle is the sole monument (now remodeled) left from the late 16th century. In the main cloister of the monastery attached to the church are many paintings of the 17th century illustrating the life of St. Francis. In the center of the ancient city is the quadrangular Plaza de Armas, flanked by the most important colonial public buildings: the Cathedral, begun in 1541, rebuilt (with nave and two aisles) in 1560, further rebuilt in 1647 and 1679, and completed by the architect Toesca in 1780; the City Hall, formerly the Intendencia, by Toesca and Melchor de Xara Quemada; the Archiepiscopal Palace; and the Post Office. Also by Toesca are the churches of La Merced and S. Domingo, the Mint (begun in 1780), and other lesser buildings. Dating from the colonial period are the Posada del Corregidor (1750-67) and the Casa Colorado. José Gandarillas (1810-53) erected buildings in Neo-Gothic and colonial styles; more interesting are his activities as conservator of ancient monuments and founder of the Museo Nacional de Bellas Artes, together with the Frenchman Pierre Dejean. The architect Brunet de Baines in 1850 founded the first school of architecture; he was responsible for some beautiful classicizing buildings, including the Municipal Theater (1853; destroyed in 1870). Lucien A. Henault began construction of the University in 1863. Eusebio Chelli built the present seat of the Brazilian Embassy; also active was the Englishman W. Hovenden Hendry as well as the German Teodor Burchard, who worked in a Neo-Gothic style. In the beginning of the 20th century, the central plaza was enriched by the construction of public buildings, including the Cousiño Palace, the Church of the Sacramentinos, the Palace of Fine Arts (1910), and the Tribunal, in the style of Art Nouveau. The city has many famous avenues and parks, such as "Las Delicias," and fine examples of local architecture, such as the Casa de Duhart by Emilio Duhart Harosteguy (1946) and the Casa Costabal by Jorge Costabal (1955), as well as homes built in the prevailing "California style."

Valparaíso. Founded in 1536, Valparaíso, which is situated on a broad bay, is the oldest Chilean city. It was destroyed by an earthquake in 1730 but was quickly rebuilt and has continued to develop since 1830. In the lower section are the commercial quarters with broad thoroughfares and imposing public buildings; the old upper city is residential. Nothing is left from the colonial period. In the late 19th century the city gained a homogeneous appearance through the work of architects either English or of English origin, such as John Stevenson and Ricardo Brown, or architects from the United States, such as John Brown.

Bibliog. Colección de historiadores de Chile y de documentos relativos a la historia nacional, 45 vols., Santiago, 1861-1923; V. Grez, Les beaux

arts au Chili, Paris, 1889; T. Child, the Spanish American Republics, New York, 1891; B. Vicuña Subercaseaux, La ciudad de Santiago: Planos y las transformaciones, Selecta, V, 1910; T. Guevara Silva, Historia de Chile: Chile prehispano, 2 vols., Santiago, 1929; R. Toro y Toro, Toesca: Ensayo sobre su vida y obras, Boletín de la Academia de Historia, II, 3, Santiago, 1934; A. Benavides Rodríguez, La arquitectura en el Virreinato del Perú y en la Capitanía General de Chile, Santiago, 1941; F. Violich, Cities of Latin America, New York, 1944; A. Benavides Rodríguez and M. Bianchi, The Art of Chile, The Studio, 1950, p. 139; A. Romera, Historia de la pintura chilena, Santiago, 1951; R. Montandón, Chile: Monumentos históricos y arqueológicos, Mexico, 1952; E. Secchi, La casa chilena hasta el siglo XIX, Cuadernos del Consejo de Monumentos Nacionales, Santiago, 1952; H.-R. Hitchcock, Latin American Architecture Since 1945, New York, 1955; E. Pereira Salas, La arquitectura chilena en el siglo XIX, Cuadernos de la Universidad de Chile, n.d.

Romolo Trebbi del Trevigiano

Illustrations: 1 map in text.

# CHINA

**CHINA.** Roughly speaking we may say that China consists geographically of the area between the Gobi Desert on the north, the Yellow Sea and the South China Sea on the east and southeast, the plain of the Red River (Songkoi, Coi) on the south, and the Tibetan massif on the west and southwest. Nevertheless, China's political boundaries have undergone great changes in the course of history. The territories that, about 400 B.C., made up the Middle Kingdom (Chung Kuo), namely, the kingdoms of Ch'i, Lu, Sung, and Ch'in, extended over part of the loess region crossed by the middle reaches of the Yellow River (Huang Ho, Hoang-ho) and over almost all the Great Plain (Chinese, *chung-yüan*, central plain), the vast settling bed for the silt carried along by the Yellow River. Here was the starting point, in the 3d century B.C., for the unifying movement which, under King Ch'êng of Ch'in, known to history by the title of "August First Emperor," led to the founding of the first integral Chinese state. Thus, the Ch'in dynasty (or Ts'in) became the first Chinese imperial dynasty, and it is significant that it was from the name of these rulers, as shown by P. Pelliot ("L'origine du nom de 'China'," TP, XIII, 1912, pp. 727–42), that our name "China" was introduced into usage.

Today, as the People's Republic of China, proclaimed Oct. 1, 1959, China is a political unit enclosing approximately 3,760,181 square miles including, in addition to the area of Chinese culture proper, a certain number of territories inhabited by ethnic minorities, such as Manchuria, Inner Mongolia, and Sinkiang, which have been considerably influenced by Chinese culture as well as by other great cultural and artistic traditions (see ASIA, CENTRAL; MONGOLIA; MONGOLIAN ART; ORDOS; STEPPES CULTURES). The present Chinese government claims sovereignty over the regions of Tibet as well, although this area can be considered foreign to Chinese culture, having been more influenced by that of India; Tibet, therefore, is treated in separate articles (see TIBET; TIBETAN ART).

Further discussion of many of the sites described below is to be found under CHINESE ART. In addition, the architectural sections of that article, especially *Later architecture*, describe a number of monuments which have not been duplicated below.

SUMMARY. The geographical setting of Chinese civilization (col. 394). Administrative divisions of China (col. 395). The regional aspects of Chinese civilization and art (col. 397): *Archaeological excavations; The spread of Chinese culture over the territory of modern China; Regional differentiations in Chinese art.* Anhwei and Kiangsu (col. 406): *Survey of geography and art history; Monuments and archaeological sites; Kiln sites.* Chekiang and Fukien (col. 409): *Survey of geography and art history; Monuments and archaeological sites; Kiln sites.* Honan (col. 412): *Survey of geography and art history; Monuments and archaeological sites; Kiln sites.* Hopei (col. 420): *Survey of geography and art history; Monuments and archaeological sites; Kiln sites.* Hunan, Hupeh, and Kiangsi (col. 429): *Survey of geography and art history; Archaeological sites; Kiln sites.* Kansu (col. 431): *Survey of geography and art history; Cave temples.* Kwangtung and Kwangsi (col. 436): *Survey of geography and art history; Kiln sites.* Manchuria and Adjacent Regions (col. 438): *Survey of geography and art history; Monuments and archaeological sites; Kiln sites.* Shansi (col. 443); *Survey of geography and art history; Monuments and Archaeological sites.*

Shantung (col. 447): *Survey of geography and art history; Monuments and archaeological sites.* Shensi (col. 451): *Survey of geography and art history; Monuments and archaeological sites; Kiln sites.* Sinkiang (col. 455): *Survey of geography and art history; Monuments and archaeological sites.* Szechwan (col. 458): *Survey of geography and art history; Monuments and archaeological sites; Kiln sites.* Yunnan and Kweichow (col. 462): *Survey of geography and art history; Monuments and archaeological sites.* Formosa (col. 465).

THE GEOGRAPHICAL SETTING OF CHINESE CIVILIZATION. The territory which received the main impact of Chinese culture, and which throughout the course of history was inhabited and dominated either politically or culturally by the Chinese, extends over a vast territory of the Asian continent in which the climatic and geographic differences are considerable. The manner in which Chinese culture was diffused from the plains of present-day northern China, where it began, was determined partly by the nature of geographical conditions.

The area of Chinese culture is bounded on the northeast by the wooded mountains of Manchuria and on the north by the vast steppes and deserts of Mongolia. On the northwest it is confined by the deserts of Central Asia, which are pierced by two routes of communication, following the chain of oases bordering the deserts and linking China with the western regions of the Asian continent. To the west and southwest, the Tibetan plateau forms an almost insurmountable barrier, while the sea which washes the southern, eastern, and southeastern coasts constitutes a well-defined boundary.

That this geographically determined isolation has been broken through on several occasions during the millenniums of continuous Chinese civilization has been of prime importance to the development, not only of the culture of China proper, but also of the cultures of the neighboring countries. The Chinese, either by land or by sea, emigrated abroad as explorers, conquerors, or bearers of culture. On the other hand, foreigners reached China in the role of conquerors, traders, Buddhist missionaries, or students of Chinese culture. For many centuries, the cultures of Japan and Korea (see JAPANESE ART; KOREAN ART) depended largely on that of China, as did those of Mongolia, Central Asia, and Indochina (see ASIA, CENTRAL; CHAM, SCHOOL OF; MONGOLIAN ART; STEPPES CULTURES; VIETNAMESE ART).

Within the natural boundaries of China, several geographically well-differentiated areas may be discerned. The Kunlun chain (K'un-lun) and the ridge of the Chinling (Ch'in-ling) divide China, climatically, into a northern and a southern part. North and south of this chain, the basins of two of China's largest rivers, the Yellow River and the Yangtze (Yangtze Kiang, Yang-tze-kiang), which created the great alluvial plain of eastern China, divide the country into northern, central, and southern regions.

The mountains of northern China, with their plateaus and slopes furrowed by rivers, are covered with an extremely fertile layer of loess, the yellow earth of China. The plateau of the present-day province of Shansi slopes gently southwest toward the gradually broadening valley of the Fen (Fên) River and the Yellow River, while the latter, approaching from the north, is obliged by the mountain ranges running from the west to the east to turn sharply eastward. To the east and southeast, the Shansi plateau is separated from the alluvial plain by mountain ranges, while on the north the steppes form the boundary. At its great bend, the Yellow River is joined by the Wei River, which, flowing from the west, follows the southern edge of the loess region. The southern part of the Wei valley is bounded by the Chinling Mountains. The narrow valleys of the northern tributaries are difficult of traverse, so that the fertile Wei valley and Shansi are both protected regions in which independent communities could be easily established. Farther east, the Yellow River valley broadens even more until it becomes a vast plain. In the region of the east coast the Yellow River meets an obstacle in the mountainous region of Shantung, particularly the impressive Mount T'ai (T'ai-shan, Tai Shan).

Many times the Yellow River has changed its course and forced a new passage to the north or the south of the mountains of Shantung, inundating the plain. The water, thick with loess, flowed into the sea through a multichanneled and swampy delta in the vicinity of Tientsin or followed the course of the Huai River, blocking the natural outlet of this river by raising the level of the river bed with its sediment of loess. The uninterrupted alluvial plain extends from the mountains of Shantung to the south until it merges gradually with the plain of the Yangtze River. This region, in which the Huai River flows, links the northern with the central zone of China.

While the Yellow River is scarcely navigable along most of its course and so cannot serve as a means of communication of any importance between eastern and western China, navigation on the Yangtze is easy, and this fact made it possible for the latter to become an important artery of communication and transport. In the Yangtze basin a unified area was easily established, separated from the Wei basin on the north by mountains, and accessible from the north only

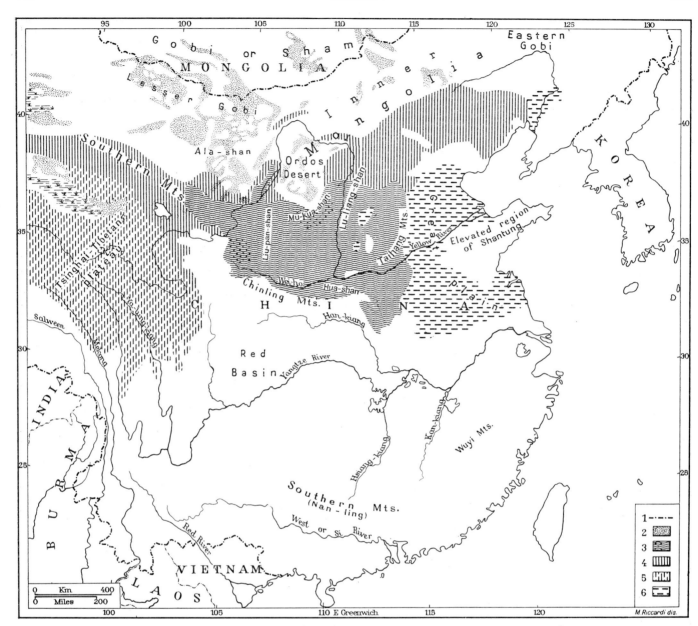

Geographical and geological setting of Chinese culture. *Key:* (1) National boundaries; (2) desert; (3) loess deposits; (4) loess in mountainous regions (5) plateau predominantly loess; (6) loess and alluvial terrain.

across the eastern plain. It was further linked to the northwest and the south by river transport via the Han and Hsiang tributaries.

Along the upper course of the Yangtze River, the Red Basin of Szechwan forms a geographic unit surrounded by mountains. Because of its fertility and its easily defended access, this area played a strategic role of paramount importance in Chinese history.

The topography of southern China, that is, the regions lying south of the Yangtze, is different from that of central and northern China. In the western part, the mountain ranges run from north to south, bounding the Tibetan plateau and forcing the Salween and Mekong Rivers to flow southward. Farther east and south, except for the inaccessible plateau of Kweichow, the mountains become lower. In these regions the rivers form, toward the sea, the basin of the West or Si River (Hsi-kiang), which serves as a main artery of communication. The coastal provinces of Fukien and Kwangtung are completely oriented toward the sea, and their coasts are indented with numerous inlets and natural harbors.

Bibliog. F. von Richthofen, China, 4 vols., Berlin, 1877–1912; G. B. Cressey, China's Geographic Foundations, New York, 1934.

ADMINISTRATIVE DIVISIONS OF CHINA. China proper is divided into 18 provinces, and this administrative structure has varied only little in modern times. More frequent changes occurred in the north,

northwest, and western regions. Six of the 18 provinces of China proper can be considered as belonging to the north: Kansu, Shensi, Shansi, Honan, Hopei (formerly called Chihli), and Shantung. Belonging to central China are Szechwan, Hupeh, Anhwei (Anhui), Kiangsu, Hunan, and Kiangsi. Making up south China are Kweichow, Yunnan, Kwangsi, Kwangtung, Fukien, and Chekiang. Under the government of the People's Republic of China, the boundaries between the provinces of China proper have been shifted several times, but, especially since several of these changes have been rescinded, the present subdivision is, in its main outlines, what it was in the past.

On the other hand, the People's Republic has instituted important changes in the surrounding regions, and has considerably reduced the number of provinces in comparison with the years preceding World War II. Manchuria then consisted of four provinces: Jehol, Liaoning, Kirin, and Heilungkiang. The first of these was abolished in 1956 and split up among Inner Mongolia, Liaoning, and Hopei. Inner Mongolia became an autonomous region consisting largely of territories of the abolished provinces of Suiyuan and Chahar, as well as zones once belonging to Jehol and Heilungkiang. The northern province of Ninghsia was added in 1954 to the territory of Kansu province. In the west the provinces of Tsinghai (Chinghai) and Sinkiang (which includes the area often referred to as Chinese Turkistan) have been retained, but the eastern part of Sikang prov-

ince (Hsikang) has been merged with Szechwan as far as the upper course of the Yangtze (which there is called the Chin-sha-kiang) and the remainder incorporated into Tibet (q.v.).

In the topographical sections the toponymy outlined above has been followed whenever necessary, but, in order to avoid confusion, references to the numerous autonomous regions created within the provincial boundaries since 1949 have been omitted. Familiar spellings have been used for names of provinces, major geographical units, and the larger cities, with variants shown in the sections below. The name "Peking," or "northern capital" (which was called Peiping when the capital was removed to Nanking in 1928), has been retained in connection with art history. Archaeological and art sites, on the other hand, are more strictly transliterated. Names ending in -ssŭ temple, -t'a, pagoda, -ts'un, village, -hsien, district, -shan, montain, -ho or -kiang, river, -hu, lake, etc., are here uniformly hyphenated; practice varies, and such endings may be capitalized.

BIBLIOG. T. Shabad, China's Changing Map, New York, 1956.

THE REGIONAL ASPECTS OF CHINESE CIVILIZATION AND ART. Archaeological excavations. In any study of the regional aspects of Chinese culture and art an important preliminary reservation should be made. Without underestimating the highly important achievements of many Chinese, Japanese, and Western scholars, we must admit that our knowledge of regional aspects of Chinese art is in no way proportionate to the enormous quantity of objects of archaeological and art-historical interest which have spread throughout the world the fame of ancient Chinese art. By far the great majority of the Chinese art objects preserved in public and private collections are of unknown provenance. In some cases the source has been purposely concealed; other pieces have come from clandestine excavations or chance finds and reached their final destination through many intermediaries, who either had good reasons to suppress the archaeological and topographical data or had no interest in these facts. Despite the wealth of material, it has therefore not often been possible to gain a clear insight into the chronology, spread, and distribution of art forms, styles, and techniques over the territory of Chinese civilization.

The number of archaeological excavations carried out in China and neighboring countries in the years before World War II is small if compared to those carried out in countries of the Near East, south and southeast Asia, and Japan.

With the active support of the government, the many archaeological institutes and study groups which have been organized in the People's Republic of China have carried out extensive excavations during the 1950s. The earthwork necessitated by widespread industrialization as well as the building of river dams and roads has increased the number of chance finds, which are now properly investigated by trained archaeologists. Apart from a number of spectacular discoveries which yielded art objects of great artistic importance, there have been a great number of less sensational finds which may give us valuable clues to problems previously unsolvable. So far, only a small part of these new finds have been made public in detail. Although special attention to some of the most important finds is given, many conclusions are bound to remain tentative until more information is forthcoming.

*The spread of Chinese culture over the territory of modern China.* The bronze culture of the late Shang period (1300–1028 B.C.), as we know it from the material excavated at An-yang, in Honan province, is a descendant of various neolithic cultures which flourished in the Great Plain of northern China (see ASIATIC PROTOHISTORY). These cultures are known from sites on the periphery of the Great Plain, where they occur in their pure form, unmixed with elements from one of the other cultures. The closer we come to the fertile Great Plain, however, the more we discover an increase in the number of mixed sites.

In a vast area extending from northern Manchuria across Inner Mongolia into Chinese Turkistan (in Sinkiang province), artifacts have been found of a microlithic culture which is known as the Gobi culture, after the Gobi Desert, where many remains of this culture have come to light.

In western China there prevailed a neolithic culture which is called the Red Pottery culture, after the color of its most characteristic pottery, or the Yang-shao culture, after the village where the first traces of it were discovered. The vestiges of this culture are extremely abundant, especially in Kansu and in the valleys of the Wei and Fen Rivers, and it can be traced throughout the provinces of Honan and Hopei into Manchuria, where it mixed with the microlithic Gobi culture.

In the coastal zone from northern Hopei through the region of Hangchow (Hang-chou), remains have been found of the Black Pottery culture, also called the Lung-shan (Lung Shan) culture after

the important site in Shantung (near Ch'êng-tzŭ-yai) where it was first discovered. This culture, of which a black pottery is a characteristic product, extended over the Liaotung Peninsula and far into Honan. Even in Shensi some sites have been located.

In the Yellow River plain, these cultures merged to give birth to the Gray Pottery culture, which is associated with that of the Shang people.

All over the rest of China cultural remains and artifacts of other neolithic cultures have been found. Some of these cultures date from the 3d and 2d millenniums B.C., others from a time when northern China had already entered the Bronze Age. At our present state of knowledge, it seems probable that the neolithic cultures of the Yangtze basin had little or no influence on the culture of the Shang people, although recent finds indicate, according to some, that the glazed pottery shards which were found in the ruins of An-yang may be the remains of a ware imported from the south (see below, *Anhwei*). The bronze culture of the Shang and of the following Chou period (1027–221 B.C.) gradually spread over other parts of the country. In the early Chou period it had already spread into Kansu, Hopei, Hupeh, and Kiangsu. Although several neolithic cultures were gradually being superseded by the bronze culture of northern China, the Stone Age lingered on for a considerable time in the more inaccessible parts of the country.

The Shang or Yin culture probably spread over a much wider territory than was previously supposed. Chêng Tê-k'un, who has mapped all finds up to 1956, mentions 84 different sites. The majority are in Honan (54), 12 were found in Shantung, 7 in Hopei, 4 in Shansi, 5 in Shensi, 4 in Anhwei, and only 1 in Kiangsu. This last site, in the district of Ch'in-chiang, is the most southerly and is the only site south of the Huai River. The site farthest north was in the Ch'ü-yang area of Hopei, the farthest west in the Pin-hsien district of Shensi. The distribution of the sites indicates that the Shang culture was generally limited to the alluvial plains and that its penetration into the surrounding "barbarian" regions followed the valleys of the rivers Fen and Wei.

During the long Chou period, many of these "barbarians" of different stock were incorporated into the Chinese cultural sphere, but the central plain remained the heart of the kingdom, coveted by the parties contending for power. The north of China had disintegrated into a great number of small states, while, in the south, other states with mixed cultures comprising both Chinese and southern elements had assumed the real power. The coastal states of Wu and Yüeh, although at one time very powerful, were probably less important for the formation of the culture of the late Chou period than was the state of Ch'u, the influence of which reached as far north as the northern part of the province of Anhwei.

Although there was certainly a northward penetration of cultural elements from the south, there was also a very important expansion of the northern Chinese culture to the south. This southward penetration of the Chinese had already begun during the Shang and early Chou periods, but was intensified later, especially during the unification of China by the state of Ch'in, which was to establish the first unified Chinese empire toward the end of the 3d century B.C.

One of the first regions to be completely conquered and colonized was the Red Basin of Szechwan, a fertile agricultural area which provided Ch'in with the prosperity and power to conquer the remaining so-called "Warring States" (Warring Kingdoms). During the Ch'in and Han periods the expansion in a southerly direction continued. From Szechwan, Chinese emigrants penetrated into Yunnan, a province which for many centuries continued to have a predominantly non-Chinese population. All over southern China the Chinese advanced, occupying the areas best suited for agriculture and pushing the natives back into the inaccessible mountain areas. In such provinces as Chekiang and Fukien, the native population was completely absorbed or expelled; in Yunnan, Kweichow, Kwangtung, and Kwangsi there still remains a sizable nucleus of non-Chinese inhabitants, and the process of Sinification is still continuing at present.

In later times, Chinese emigration to the south was stimulated by conquests of part or the whole of northern China by foreign invaders. During the period of the Six Dynasties, and later when, in the 12th century, the Khitan and Jurchen tribes conquered parts of northern China, many Chinese retired behind the protection of the rivers in the south, leaving the plains, which could easily be conquered by enemy cavalry.

One of the results of the Chinese southward move seems to have been the displacement of the Tai (Thai) tribes, who crossed the mountains of Yunnan province into Indochina and Thailand. Today these form the nucleus of the population of Thailand (q.v.). Along China's northern borders, the evolution of history presents a totally different picture. There were no extensive agricultural areas defended by non-Chinese tilling the land. The steppes and deserts of Mongolia and the plains and forests of Manchuria were inhabited by tribes of herdsmen, who moved about freely in search

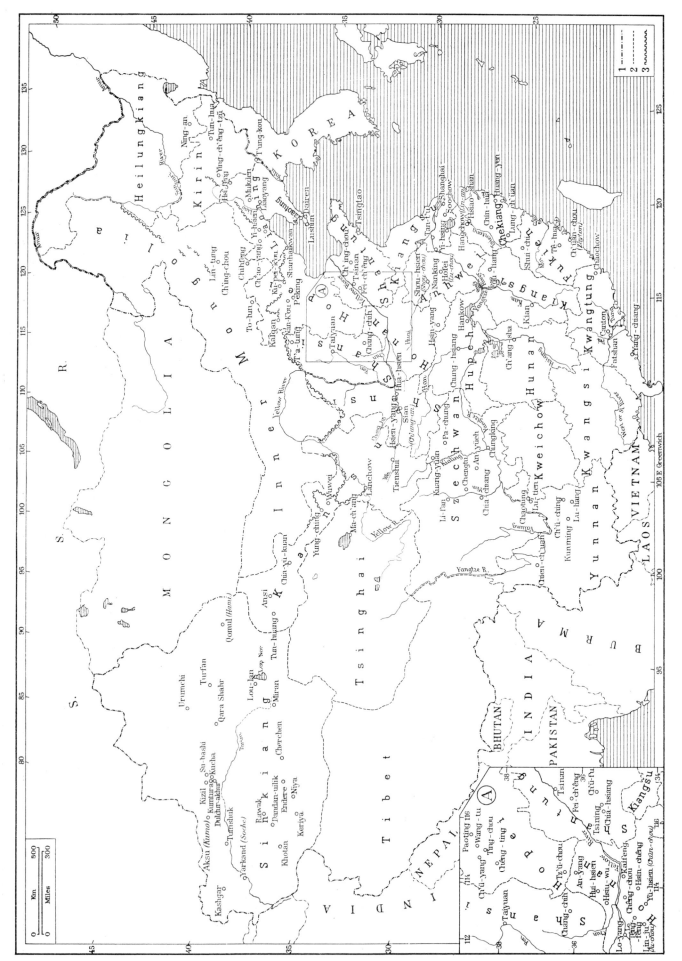

Principal centers of diffusion of Chinese civilization. *Key:* (1) National boundaries; (2) provincial boundaries of the People's Republic of China; (3) Great Wall.

of pastures for their cattle and sheep. Their main strength came from their mobility and from their early adoption of cavalry warfare as the type most suited to their environment. It seems that they began to use the horse about the 5th century B.C., and that their horsemanship was very soon taken up by the Chinese who came into contact with them.

The history of the many wars fought out along China's northern borders is known almost exclusively from Chinese historical records, and we can easily imagine that these accounts present a somewhat one-sided picture of what really happened. From these we are led to regard this region as an inexhaustible reservoir of barbaric tribes, whose main interest was to invade China to grab its riches, and who could be warded off only by the construction of such chains of fortifications as the famous Great Wall or be defeated by swift Chinese counterattacks. In reality, however, the history of China's northern frontiers must have been far more complicated.

One of the main obstacles to a clear understanding of the political and cultural history of the northern frontier region is the baffling variety of tribes and peoples, of widely different race, language, and customs, which came to be recorded in the Chinese annals. Some of these may have come from as far away as Lake Baikal. Many of them have disappeared without leaving any trace, and we have therefore no idea what language they may have spoken or to which race they may have belonged. The Chinese nomenclature for these barbarians is extremely confusing, and several tribes may have been given different names during the successive dynastic periods or may have reentered the historical picture at a place far removed from the frontier posts where they came into contact with the Chinese for the first time.

Although the historical picture is thus characterized by great variety, the historical process which took place remained practically the same throughout the ages. Sometimes the non-Chinese tribes came into contact with Chinese civilization at a time when a strong dynasty was able to maintain its authority, either through direct control from the imperial capital or by indirect control over tribes and autonomous states. The attraction of the benefits of the superior Chinese material culture was strongest for those tribes who lived around the periphery of the territory under Chinese control. It often happened, when the central power was weakened, that these tribes, which had adopted certain techniques from the Chinese, led the less Sinicized tribesmen from the interior in the attack against China. Although as a rule quite inferior in numbers, the tribes made up for this deficiency by their mobility, to such a degree that in numerous instances their efforts to conquer China were crowned by at least partial success. Although many tribes managed to carve a small territory out of the large Chinese empire there were only a few that succeeded in gaining a more or less lasting victory. Some (Toba, Jurchen) succeeded in conquering large parts of the central plain, but only two conquered the whole of China, the Mongols and the Manchus. The rivers and mountains of southern China formed a terrain unsuited for cavalry warfare, and only the strongest achieved the momentum to overcome this powerful obstacle.

If their surprise attack met with success, the barbarians usually settled for good within the Chinese borders. The fact that many of the conquerors strove to maintain their tribal organization has caused some authors to suggest that the Sinification of these invaders was only minimal (e.g., K. A. Wittfogel and Fêng Chia-shêng, *History of Chinese Society*, Liao, New York, 1949). However, if we put less stress on the sociological aspects of Sinification, it becomes evident that Chinese culture had such an absorbing influence that no restrictive measures aimed at retaining the original customs and language could prevent its final victory. Even so, if there remained a relatively large number of tribesmen in the homeland who were isolated from the influence of Chinese culture, this acculturation could be kept in check for a long time. This was especially the case with the Khitans and the Jurchen, perhaps the only peoples who managed to develop a culture that retained distinctively non-Chinese characteristics.

Although it sometimes happened that the occupation of China came to an end through a decisive defeat of the conquerors in their original homeland (e.g., as with the Khitans), the Chinese were more often than not their own "liberators." By the time the Chinese desire to be governed by a native dynasty was manifested in a successful revolt, a considerable part of the descendants of the original conquerors had often been already absorbed by intermarriage.

It is difficult to estimate the importance of the influence of these foreign invasions upon the development of Chinese culture. Perhaps their importance is overestimated if we look only at the monuments which bear testimony to their presence, for often the foreign dynasties were fervent protectors and patrons of Buddhism, and many of the great Buddhist monuments of northern China were built at their instigation and under their régime.

Emigration and the conquest of a large part of southern Manchuria and northern Korea during the Han period brought Chinese culture to the Korean peninsula, which has remained ever since under strong Chinese cultural — and at times political — influence (see KOREA; KOREAN ART). From Korea began the penetration of Chinese culture into Japan (see JAPANESE ART). A corresponding penetration is apparent in the south, where Chinese culture exerted a profound influence upon the culture of parts of Indochina (see CHAM, SCHOOL OF; VIETNAMESE ART).

While Chinese culture exerted its influence far beyond the borders of the country, there are within the borders of present-day China many peoples who have been influenced by Chinese culture only to a negligible degree. Some of these have, on the contrary, appreciably influenced certain aspects of Chinese culture, as have, for example, the Tibetans (see TIBET; TIBETAN ART). Tibetan culture cannot be regarded as a part of the Chinese heritage, but the Tibetan type of Buddhism, known as Lamaism, spread to China during the reign of the Mongol Yüan dynasty (1260–1368), and the influence which it exercised over large parts of northern China, especially during the Manchu reign, has been of the greatest importance.

The Mongols, too, succeeded in retaining their own culture, quite different from that of the Chinese (see MONGOLIAN ART). That part of Mongolia which does not form part of the independent Mongolian People's Republic (Outer Mongolia) has now been placed almost entirely under the jurisdiction of the autonomous territory of Inner Mongolia. Although a considerable number of remains of Chinese settlements and fortifications have been located in this territory by archaeologists, it seems quite certain that the number of Chinese who lived there was always quite small.

The present-day population of Chinese Turkistan (in Sinkiang) is only in a very small part formed by the descendants of those who created the great Buddhist monuments of that region (see ASIA, CENTRAL; below, *Sinkiang*). It contains a large percentage of Uigurs and Kazakhs who have scarcely been Sinicized at all.

*Regional differentiations in Chinese art.* The considerable differences between the climate of northern and southern China, and the differences in the way of life which were the result of these climatic conditions, sometimes manifest themselves in differences in regional art styles. It is obvious that these differences are most clearly felt in the field of Chinese architecture, in which construction was adapted locally to the climatic conditions prevailing. The excavations of the last ten years have brought to light a considerable number of small model houses which were placed in the tombs during the Han period. The models of watchtowers (which have been known for many years) are clearly the product of the north, where real towers of this type were built to warn against the surprise attacks of the Hsiung-nu and other invaders. The models of houses, which have been excavated in such southern regions as the province of Kwangtung, are of a distinctly different type. Built on high poles, the houses are obviously intended for a watery region, and the flimsy walls permit a maximum of ventilation in a humid climate.

If we compare the oldest wooden temple building of China, the main hall of the temple Fo-kuang-ssŭ on Wu-t'ai-shan (Mount Wu Tai) in Shansi province, with almost contemporaneous Japanese monuments which have obviously been derived from an architectural style of a more southern Chinese region, we notice immediately some important differences. In the northern Chinese building the space between the outer columns was closed with thick brick walls, whereas the Japanese monuments show no such solid protection against the cold winds. Yet the adaptation to the requirements of a cold climate does not seem to have affected the essentials of the architectural construction: the brick walls have no weight-bearing function, but have been treated structurally just like screen walls of more southerly buildings too weak to carry the weight of the roof, even though the brick walls should have been adequate to support a significant structural load. Apart from these differences there are many others for which no such obvious explanations can be given, e.g., the pronounced curvature of the roofs, which is a stylistic characteristic of southern Chinese architecture, or the distinctions between northern and southern memorial gates (*p'ai-lou*).

Several regional distinctions which appear in ancient Chinese art may be connected with particular developments in Chinese political history. The pyramidal structure of Chinese government organization often resulted in the capital being not only the political, but also the cultural heart of the empire. Although this metropolitan culture often diffused out into the adjacent regions, those at the periphery of the empire hardly participated in it. In those far-off regions where favorable conditions existed for the development of a culture of a distinctly regional type, we are sometimes fortunate in having numerous monumental remains (e.g., in Szechwan). As a rule, however, those territories which at some time during the course of history housed the capital of the empire for a longer period are often much richer in monuments of importance for art history than the territories of the periphery. Often a direct connection can be established be-

tween the presence of important monuments and the existence in the vicinity of an ancient capital. Such is the case with the cave sculptures of Lung-mên, Yün-kang, Hsiang-t'ang-shan, and at Hang-chow. In the case of imperial mausoleums (near Nanking, Sian, Peking, and Mukden) the connection is even more obvious.

At the present stage of our knowledge it is often extremely difficult to recognize in the artistic products of certain remote regions the survival of specific stylistic traits which had been fashionable in the capital long before. An art form in which this phenomenon can be observed clearly is the plastic art of making tomb figures. Whereas in the Han period several regions (Szechwan and Kwangtung) developed distinctly regional styles of tomb figures, the southern tomb figures of later periods are often local, outspokenly provincial types, derived from an earlier style prevalent in the regions surrounding the capital.

One of the strictly regional styles which may be observed in

were built there at the same time that such surviving monuments as the rock temples of Yün-kang, Lung-mên, and many other sites were being constructed in the north under the T'o-pa (Toba) Wei dynasty. These sources indicate that the Buddhist art of southern China was certainly not lagging behind the great achievements of the north, even though extensive complexes of rock sculptures were probably quite rare. The fact that hardly any monument of importance antedating the monuments of the 10th-century Wu-Yüeh kingdom has survived should be ascribed to purely coincidental factors and is in no way an indication of the absence of a flourishing tradition of Buddhist art.

The same holds true for the Buddhism of the T'ang (618–906), Sung (960–1279), and Yüan dynasties (1260–1368). Although there are many temples which have preserved the famous names of monasteries mentioned in ancient Chinese sources, most of them have little more in common with these monuments than their names.

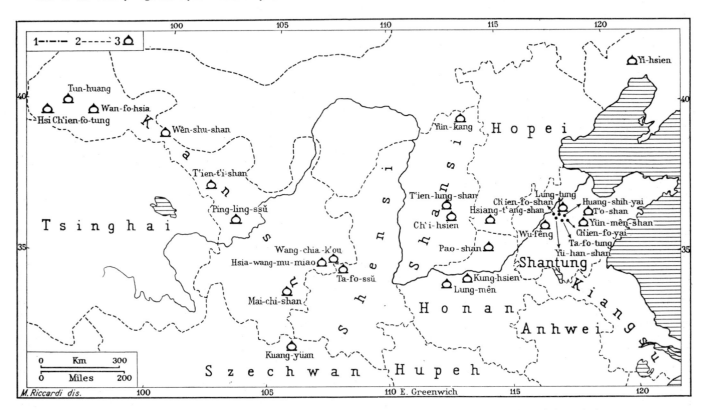

Area comprising Buddhist rock-cut architecture. *Key*: (1) National boundaries; (2) provincial boundaries; (3) sites.

different aspects of culture is that of the Khitans, who ruled over Manchuria and northern China during part of the Sung period. Although it is often extremely difficult to distinguish their culture from that of the succeeding Jurchen, the differences from Chinese civilization are often clearly visible. The culture of the Khitans and the Jurchen shows a considerable degree of Chinese influence, and it is evident that they often used Chinese craftsmen for the construction of their monuments and the production of their pottery. Yet the type of pagoda which is characteristic of the Khitan Buddhists is found only in Manchuria and in the part of northern China which they occupied. In architecture in wood these characteristics are much less apparent, probably because so little of the contemporaneous purely Chinese architecture has survived. Quite distinctive from pottery of the Ting-yao style, which was produced in kilns operated by potters from the Ting-yao kilns, the Khitans developed ceramics of another type, a fact which clearly demonstrates their cultural independence. True to their nomadic traditions, they copied their forms from leather vessels, while the elements of floral decoration are based on the flora of their homeland Manchuria.

Although numerous monuments of architecture and sculpture which survived the ages give us an idea of regional styles, the distribution of these monuments over the whole of the Chinese territory presents a rather misleading picture. The relatively small number of monuments of cultural interest which are to be found in southern China is first of all the result of the destruction caused by the Taiping rebellion of the mid-19th century, and only partially caused by the area's long-time remoteness from the heart of the empire. Today only literary sources can give us some idea of the many monuments which

An uneven distribution also affects our knowledge of Chinese bronzes, funerary sculpture, and other types of tomb offerings. The first discoveries of tomb figures were made in the region surrounding the ancient northern Chinese capitals. Thus the attention of archaeologists and grave robbers came to be focused on those regions where the chances of finding valuable funeral offerings were best. The huge cemeteries outside each of the ancient imperial capitals were larger and more likely to contain richly furnished tombs; therefore it was in these regions that the excavation activities, illegal as well as legal, were concentrated. The result is that the funerary art which we have come to know from the multitude of objects in private and public collections outside China is most often that of the central provinces. As has been pointed out already, it is probable that these finds often represent the highest form of art, but the pieces which have gone abroad do not give us a true picture of Chinese funerary art in all of its regional characteristics. The tomb figures which were made in the region of Szechwan in the Han period are only seldom represented in our collections (there are two heads in the Museum für Völkerkunde in Munich), and the Kwangtung type is also almost entirely absent.

The same situation holds true to a certain extent for Chinese bronzes. These were sought after mainly in the northern Chinese territory which was known to have played a role of importance during the Shang and Chou periods. The type of early Western Chou bronzes which has been excavated in the Anhwei-Kiangsu region during the last few years is hardly represented in our collections (a possible example of this style is reproduced by O. Sirén, *Kinas Konst under Tre Artusenden*, Stockholm, 1942, pl. 32B). The

possibility exists that this regional type of bronzes will always remain extremely rare, but we should take into account the possibility that its almost complete absence in our collections is due to pure coincidence. The vessels which can be attributed to certain regions on the basis of the style and content of the inscriptions would seem to support this argument.

The form of art which at first glance might seem most suitable to study in its regional aspects is painting. In no other form of Chinese art is the use of regional classification and grouping of masters so widespread and so generally accepted. Yet closer study of the regional problems of Chinese painting reveals that the terminology fails to live up to its promises and often does not correspond to real regional differences in style.

The distinction between a northern and a southern school of Chinese painting, which was introduced by the art historians Mo Shih-lung (second half of the 16th century) and Tung Ch'i-ch'ang (1555–1636), was based upon a distinction made between different schools of Buddhism and has no regional art implications at all.

A great number of later Chinese painters are grouped together under such names as the Eight Masters of Chin-ling (i.e., Nanking), the Eight Eccentrics of Yang-chou, etc. Often, however, such classifications, popular among Chinese art historians, have little real value, as the masters thus grouped under one heading have often little in common and almost never a common style or program.

But even though these regional distinctions are sometimes of little significance, there are certain regional aspects of Chinese painting which are as evident as they are surprising. First of all there is the unquestionable fact that Chinese painting of the Ming and Ch'ing periods is mainly a product of the regions bordering the lower basin of the Yangtze River, and almost all great Chinese painters came from the provinces of Chekiang, Kiangsu, or Anhwei. How one-sided the distribution of painting genius was can be demonstrated best by grouping the places of birth of about 350 of the best-known painters from the 14th century onward: 193 come from Kiangsu, 83 from Chekiang, 27 from Anhwei, and 15 from Fukien. From all other provinces come no more than 40 painters, several of whom left their native provinces to work in Kiangsu or Chekiang during the rest of their lives.

Although there are a few notable exceptions, including the famous 17th-century monk-painter Tao-chi (or Shih-t'ao), most of these artists who where born outside the above-mentioned provinces were court painters.

It would seem that this interesting phenomenon began to manifest itself during the Southern Sung period. Earlier painters of name had come to the capitals from all over China. It is clear that, with the rather limited contact between northern and southern China during the occupation of the north by the Khitans and the Jurchen, the number of artists from the north who came to be mentioned in the annals and biographies became smaller.

After the occupation of the whole of China by the Mongols, the traditions of the Sung Academy at Hangchow were preserved by painters living in the area where once the capital of the Sung had been established. With the restoration of native imperial power under the Ming and the revival of the Academy by the Ming emperors, the painters from the province of Chekiang were in majority at court. Opposed to this so-called "Chê school" were the literati painters of Wu, in Kiangsu, the province which was to remain the center of unorthodox painting for the next few centuries.

No change of capital could influence the growth and spread of literati painting, which was never officially connected with the government. After the establishment of the Ch'ing capital at Peking, Nanking became a kind of artistic center for the unorthodox painters, who, if tied to anything, adhered to the vanished *ancien régime*.

With regard to ceramics, too, the transfer of the capital of the Sung to the south seems to have had a lasting effect. Although the south had been an important, if not the most important, producer of ceramics for many centuries, northern China produced a great variety of wares during the Northern Sung period. Although production continued there after the withdrawal of the Chinese government and the potters of the north exerted a strong influence on the wares made by the invaders, it seems that the production declined. Apparently no new spectacular innovations and techniques were developed, at least if we are to assume that the application of overglaze enamels in Tz'ŭ-chou (see below, *Hopei*) had already been introduced before the tragic turn of events. Production of the same wares continued far into the Ming period, and in some places even to the present day, but the wares lost their supremacy.

The influx of potters from the north brought about a considerable enrichment of the production in the south. It is quite possible that the contact and mixing of these divergent ceramic traditions is one of the reasons for the surprisingly many-sided development of ceramic art in the south, which, as in painting, was to remain forever the real artistic center.

ANHWEI (Anhui, An-hui) AND KIANGSU (Chiang-su). *Survey of geography and art history.* South of the mountains of Shangtung there is a vast area where the alluvial plains of the Yellow River and the Yangtze River come together. This area is bounded on the southwest by the hills which separate it from the middle Yangtze basin and on the south by the mountains running south of Hangchow.

The northern part of Anhwei and Kiangsu includes the basin of the Huai River. Toward the end of the 12th century, the Yellow River, seeking an outlet to the sea farther south, turned into the lower course of the Huai River; subsequently its sediment raised the river bed so much that the Huai lost forever its natural outlet to the sea. The numerous attempts to end the inevitably resulting floods were crowned with success only in recent times. Farther south lies the area formed of alluvial material from the Yangtze; the process of silting is still going on and has shifted the river's mouth farther east. The plain is traversed by many canals and has numerous lakes, the largest being the T'ai-hu ("great lake"; Tai Hu).

In the flood plain of the lower Yangtze River several neolithic sites have been discovered belonging to the Black Pottery or Lungshan culture. In southern Anhwei and Kiangsu there are also many sites of another neolithic culture, which Chêng Tê-k'un has called the culture of the Yangtze Mound Dwellers, but which other archaeologists call the Hu-shu culture, after the village Hu-shu-chên, about 20 miles southeast of Nanking, where there is an important archaeological site. The pottery associated with this culture is usually a hand-shaped, sandy-red ware, sometimes decorated with impressed or incised designs. This culture came under the influence of that of north China at the end of the Shang or the beginning of the Chou period. Shang bronzes of a purely northern Chinese style have been discovered at Fu-nan in Anhwei (*Wên-wu ts'an-k'ao tzŭ-liao*, 1959, no. 1). In southern Anhwei and Kiangsu, however, bronzes of a Western Chou date have been found which show marked regional characteristics. Most important are the bronzes from Tan-t'u and Yen-ch'êng in Kiangsu (*Wên-wu ts'an-k'ao tzŭ-liao*, 1959, no. 4) and the recent spectacular discovery of bronzes and glazed pottery at T'un-chi in Anhwei. Although it is yet too early to draw definite conclusions from these finds, it would seem as though the bronze style of the late Chou period had been strongly influenced by the local style of the "barbarian" state of Wu, to which these remains should be attributed. The vessel types typical of the Shang and early Western Chou periods sometimes appear with a decoration which has the air of a later period, but which could very well be the precursor of the late Chou style of decoration.

The Huai River valley is one of the most important areas where bronzes of the late Chou period are found. Here they are so abundant that Karlgren has called the late Chou style the "Huai style," but this term has been criticized by many scholars. Virtually all excavations before World War II were clandestine and illicit. Thanks to the work done by O. Karlbeck, we do know something of the provenance of many of the objects which thus came into European and American collections, but no definitive account has ever been published of the very important discoveries made before the last war in the Li San-ku mound south of the village of Chu-chia-chi, near present-day Shou-hsien (formerly Shou-chou) in Anhwei. The excavations there turned up a great many very fine bronzes which were in all probability buried shortly before the end of the Ch'u kingdom which reigned over this part of China during the late Chou period.

Karlgren's assumption that the area of Shou-chou, the last capital of the Ch'u kingdom, had already been an important center of bronze casting at an earlier time has been confirmed by excavations. The 5th-century B.C. tomb of a marquis of the small state of Ts'ai, discovered in 1955, contained many beautiful bronzes from a period a little earlier than the Ch'u bronzes. Moreover, Shou-chou was also, as Karlgren has demonstrated, an important center for the manufacture of mirrors, an art which continued its uninterrupted course up to the Han period along clearly traceable lines.

Besides these Shou-chou mirrors, the Han period has left us few art objects which may be called characteristic of this region. The Han tombs recently discovered in the district of T'ung-shan in the northern part of Kiangsu province, near Hung-lou-ts'un, Miao-shan, and Chou-chuang (*K'ao-ku t'ung-hsin*, 1957, no. 4), are decorated with stone reliefs; these should be considered as derivations of a cultural tradition centered in what is now Shantung province.

After the Han period, the southern part of Anhwei and Kiangsu provinces gained in importance because of the founding of the city now called Nanking, capital of six consecutive dynasties which from A.D. 265 to 589 dominated the region southwest of the Chinling Mountains and southeast of the Yellow River. The monuments from these times which remain today are few but of great importance. These are the colossal sculptures erected near the tombs of the emperors of the Liu Sung dynasty (420–79), those of the Southern Ch'i (479–502), the Liang (502–57), and the Ch'ên (557–89). They represent winged lions and other fantastic animals, usually

called chimeras in Western literature on the subject. In many cases it is difficult to establish the identity of the emperors or members of the imperial family near whose tombs these sculptures were placed, a problem which has caused great confusion among Western students, though this has been partially dispelled by the conscientious work of Chu Hsi-tsu and his colleagues. There is equal uncertainty as to the origin of the practice of erecting such sculptures in pairs near the mound. The stone lions of Szechwan and Shantung, dating from the Han period, clearly show that this custom goes back farther in the past. The monuments of Tan-yang and Nanking, mostly sunk into the ground but now being reerected at ground level, are the pinnacle and at the same time the end of a tradition which was to revive later in quite different form and to decline ingloriously with the funerary sculpture of the tombs of the Ming and Ch'ing emperors.

Few important Buddhist monuments remain in the region, despite the prestige enjoyed by Buddhism in the Six Dynasties period (220–589) and later in these parts of the country.

Although the kilns of Shou-chou and Fêng-yang-hsien are mentioned already in T'ang texts, the region of Anhwei and Kiangsu, except for the southern part, cannot be considered an important center of Chinese pottery. As the find at T'un-chi indicates, however, it may have been of great importance in early Chou times.

Among the other crafts mention must be made of silverwork. In 1955 a treasure was discovered consisting of more than a hundred objects of gold and silver. The pieces were probably made, according to inscriptions on the silver, at Lu-chou (now Hofei) about 1333.

BIBLIOG. Chu Hsi-tsu et al., Liu-ch'ao ling-mu t'iao-ch'a pao-kao (Report on the Investigations of the Tombs of the Six Dynasties), Monumenta Sinica, I, Nanking, 1935; B. Karlgren, Huai and Han, BMFEA, XIII, 1941, pp. 1–125; O. Karlbeck, Selected Objects from Ancient Shou-chou, BMFEA, XXVII, 1955, pp. 41–129; Yin T'iao-fei, Kuan-yü Shou-hsien Ch'u-ch'i (Ch'u Vessels of Shou-hsien), K'ao-ku t'ung-hsin (Kaogu Tongxun), 1955, no. 2, pp. 21–4.

*Monuments and archaeological sites.* Yen-tun-shan. In 1954 on this mountain, about 18 miles east of Tan-t'u, in Kiangsu, 12 bronze vessels came to light accidentally during digging by some farmers. Unfortunately it was not possible to establish later whether the bronzes came from only one tomb or from several, for in the vicinity other bronzes too were found.

Among the more important objects, all made in a manner typical of the early Western Chou period, are two bronzes of the *kuei* type with four handles (also known as *chiu*), one of which bears a long inscription that enables us to date the piece at the beginning of the Chou period (reign of Chêng Wang). Very curious are a bronze of the *hsi-kuang* type in the form of a quadruped, a type from which the Ming imitations are derived, and two libation cups or horns. These are the oldest bronzes found south of the Yangtze River and are therefore of great importance. The style of the decoration of some bronzes is very similar to that of vessels found at T'un-chi (see below).

BIBLIOG. Wu-shêng ch'u-t'u chung-yao wên-wu chan-lan t'u-lu (Illustrated Catalogue of Important Objects Excavated in Five Provinces), Peking, 1955, figs, 11–19.

Shou-hsien (former Shou-chou). In 1955 an excavation near the west gate of the city of Shou-hsien, in Anhwei, brought to light a tomb which was later called that of the Marquis of Ts'ai. It contained a great number of bronze vessels and other bronze objects, and, in addition, more than fifty pieces of jade. All the objects bore decorations characteristic of the late Chou period.

In the tomb were found three series of bells. One of these was a series of *yung-chung* (bells with oblong handles), consisting of 12 pieces, 4 of which had, however, been broken during the digging. Another series of bells of the *po* type may have consisted originally of 8 bells, 6 of which were recovered intact. Completely intact was one series consisting of 9 pieces. Several fragments found in the tomb may have belonged to a fourth series.

Many pieces bear inscriptions, but it has not been possible to establish which Marquis of Ts'ai it was who was buried in this tomb. Though this makes dating uncertain, the interpretations of Chinese experts establish 493 B.C. as the earliest and 447 B.C. as the latest possible date.

BIBLIOG. Wu-shêng ch'u-t'u chung-yào wên-wu chan-lan t'u-lu (Illustrated Catalogue of Important Objects Excavated in Five Provinces), Peking, 1955, figs. 37–60; Provincial Museum of Anhwei, ed., Shou-hsien Ts'ai-hou-mu ch'u-t'u i-wu (Objects Excavated from the Tomb of the Marquis of Ts'ai at Shou-hsien), Peking, 1956.

T'un-chi. In March, 1959, a team of Chinese archaeologists excavated two tombs which are thought to date from the Western Chou period, situated about 3 miles west of T'un-chi, in southern Anhwei. The tombs yielded more than seventy pieces of hand-shaped, brown and green glazed pottery in shapes often resembling those of bronze vessels (*ho, kuan, p'an, tou,* and *tsun*). The find of such a quantity of early glazed pottery vessels intact is the first of its kind.

In both tombs a number of bronze vessels were found, all of well-known Shang-Yin and Western Chou shapes. One bears an inscription of Shang or early Chou type. The decoration, which in some respects, resembles the interlacery, resembles that of the late Chou period, is highly unusual. A comparison with vessels from other finds in Anhwei and Kiangsu suggests that parts of this find represent a hitherto unknown local bronze culture.

BIBLIOG. K'ao-ku hsüeh-pao (Kaogu Xuebao), 1959, no. 4, pp. 59–90.

Ch'i-hsia-ssŭ. In the grounds of the temple Ch'i-hsia-ssŭ at the foot of Shê-shan, northeast of Nanking in Kiangsu, stands a stone pagoda, the Shê-li-t'a, five stories and almost 50 feet high. On a richly sculptured octagonal base, on top of which a sculptured lotus throne is placed, stands a high shaft. The sides of the shaft are decorated with bas-reliefs, two representing lokapalas (celestial guardians), one representing probably Mañjusrī, and one Samantabhadra. The others are decorated with false doors. The shaft is surmounted by five blind stories, separated by projecting stone slabs sculptured in the shape of pent roofs. The stories and roofs diminish in size as they rise. On each side of the stories are bas-reliefs representing a seated Buddha.

Especially noteworthy are the eight panels of bas-reliefs, separated by sculptured pilasters, which form part of the base. These panels, of extremely fine quality, represent the eight principal moments in the life of Śākyamuni: his descent from the Tushita heaven, his birth, the Four Encounters, the flight from the palace, the temptation of Māra, the Enlightenment, the First Sermon, and the Parinirvāna.

The pagoda, built of gray marble, was erected on the site of an earlier building, dating from the 7th century. The present building dates from the years between 923 and 933.

BIBLIOG. D. Tokiwa and T. Sekino, Shina Bukkyō Shiseki (Buddhist Monuments in China), IV, Tokyo, 1926–38, pp. 8–12; Sekai Bijutsu Zenshū (Arts of the World), XIV (China, III), Tokyo, 1951, pl. 6.

Soochow (Su-chou). Soochow, the ancient capital of the kingdom of Wu and the provincial capital of Kiangsu, has played an important role in the cultural history of China, especially during the Ming period. In and around this town lived almost all of the great literati painters of the Wu school, as well as important professional painters.

Though it suffered much damage during the Taiping rebellion, Soochow seems to have been somewhat better preserved than such important centers as Yang–chou, Hangchow, and Nanking. Situated on the Grand Canal close to the northern shore of the T'ai-hu, the city was built on an almost rectangular ground plan and is completely surrounded by moats and walls, penetrated by six gates and five water gates. As in most other ancient towns the streets intersect at right angles, and there are many canals and bridges. The axial north–south road (the Huo-lung-chieh) connects the grounds of what was formerly the temple Pao-ên-ssŭ in the north with the temple dedicated to Confucius in the south.

Among the ancient monuments which have been preserved is the San-ch'ing-tien, hall of the Taoist temple Yüan-miao-kuan. This large building, measuring about 150 by 85 ft., is a rare example of architecture in wood of the Southern Sung period. It probably dates from the late 12th century but must have undergone many changes and repairs. Of all extant wooden buildings it comes closest to the rules laid down in the architectural manual *Ying-tsao fa-shih*.

In the grounds of the Pao-ên-ssŭ stands the tall Pei-t'a (northern pagoda), about 250 ft. high, which dates from 1138 and is one of the most impressive architectural monuments of China. It has nine stories and is built on an octagonal ground plan, with an inner core around which the outer wall was built. Each story is surrounded by wooden balconies and pent roofs, which have been frequently restored, although probably in the original style.

There are three more ancient pagodas within the city walls: the "Twin Pagodas" in the eastern part of the town, six stories and about 75 ft. high, dating from 1135, and the pagoda of the temple Jui-kuang-ssŭ in the southwest, which has seven stories and is supposed to date from the Hsüan-ho era (1119-26).

Soochow was an important center of garden culture, and despite the drastic changes of the 19th century some of the gardens are still of great beauty. They show interesting combinations of decorative stones, lotus ponds and lakes, ancient trees, pavilions, "moon gates," and zigzag bridges. One of the most famous is the Shih-tzŭ-lin (the Lion Grove), which was constructed about 1340 and shortly afterward immortalized in a masterpiece of the great painter Ni Tsan (National

Palace Museum, Taichung). Other famous gardens are those of the great Ming painter Wên Chêng-ming, the Cho-chêng-yüan, and the Liu-yüan, situated west of the town.

On the famous Hu-ch'iu, or Tiger Hill, 3 miles to the northwest overlooking the town, most of the present buildings are of recent date, but the pagoda of seven stories, over 130 ft. high, has fortunately been preserved. The construction of this pagoda started in 959, and the sixth story was completed during the early years of the Sung period. During the last years of the Ming a seventh story was added and measures were taken to stop the sagging. The leaning pagoda always threatened to collapse until it was completely restored in 1956.

BIBLIOG. O. Sirén, A History of Early Chinese Art, IV: Architecture, London, 1930; D. Tokiwa and T. Sekino, Shina Bukkyō Shiseki (Buddhist Monuments in China), II, Tokyo, 1926-38, pp. 9–12; E. Boerschmann, Die Baukunst und religiöse Kultur der Chinesen, III: Pagoden, Berlin, Leipzig, 1931, pp. 160–74, 214–22; O. Sirén, Gardens of China, New York, 1949, pp. 93–101; Sekai Bijutsu Zenshū (Arts of the World), XIV, (China, III), Tokyo, 1951, pp. 14–7; L. Sickman and A. Soper, The Art and Architecture of China, Harmondsworth, 1956, pp. 264–5; S. E. Lee, Some Problems in Ming and Ch'ing Landscape Painting (Views of Tiger Hill), Ars Orientalis, II, 1957, pp. 473–6; Wên-wu ts'an-k'ao tzŭ-liao, 1958, no. 1, p. 81.

Hofei (Ho-fei, formerly Lu-chou). In 1955 workmen felling a huge old tree near Hofei, in Anhwei, found among the roots a jar of thick pottery containing 10 gold objects and 91 silver ones of 11 different types. In addition to a great number of plates, cups, and flasks, the forms of which are strongly reminiscent of Sung and Yüan pottery, there was found a beautiful silver box with an engraved decoration of flowers and birds. One of the pieces, a vase with cover, is inscribed with a date corresponding to 1333. Five of the vases bear the artist's signature, while four cups bear inscriptions giving Lu-chou as the place of their manufacture.

BIBLIOG. Wên-wu ts'an-k'ao tzŭ-liao, 1957, no. 2, pp. 51–8: Arch. Chin. Art Soc. Am., XI, 1957, pp. 80–1.

*Kiln sites.* Yi-hsing. The source of the reddish-brown stoneware called Yi-hsing-yao (Yi-hsing ware), is, as the name implies, the district of Yi-hsing on the shores of the T'ai-hu in Kiangsu. The identification of this ware is certain because it has been manufactured up to the present day in a good many kilns in this region. The tradition which names a certain Kung Ch'un as the potter of the first pieces of Yi-hsing-yao, early in the 14th century, may be correct, but the dating of the many signatures found on specimens of this ware is made difficult by the many false dates and signatures.

BIBLIOG. G. Hedley, Yi-hsing Ware, Tr. O. Ceramic Soc., XIV, 1936, pp. 70–87.

CHEKIANG (Chê-chiang) AND FUKIEN (Fu-chien). *Survey of geography and art history.* The coastal region of Chekiang south of Hangchow, the entire province of Fukien, and the eastern tip of Kwangtung consist almost entirely of mountainous terrain which has determined the formation of a highly indented coastline abounding in inlets and gulfs. The mountains run mainly northeast to southwest and parallel to the coast. Their height decreases as they approach the coast. This conformation is interrupted, however, by the river valleys, the largest of which is that of the Min. In the northern sector, the Tsientang (Fuchun, Ch'ien-t'ang) River follows the direction of the mountains and flows northeast into Hangchow Bay.

Chekiang and Fukien, with inhabitants who undoubtedly were not of Chinese origin, played a role of little importance during the Shang and Chou periods because of their inaccessibility. Chinese immigrants from the north settled here, and gradually the aborigines moved away or were assimilated, unlike their counterparts in the southern provinces, leaving no trace at all.

During the Six Dynasties period (3d to 6th centuries), the province of Chekiang rose to prominence. Buddhism, one of whose sects, the T'ien-t'ai, was named perhaps after a mountain in south Chekiang, flourished here, but no Buddhist monuments of that period remain. The Buddhism which we see displayed in the monuments of this region was that of the Five Dynasties (10th century) and the Sung and Yüan periods. The beginning of this renaissance coincides with the secession of the coastal area south of the Yangtze about the end of the T'ang period (618–906), and with the formation of the independent state of Wu-Yüeh, which was to be reunited with the Chinese empire only in 978 under the central authority of the Sung. The rock sculptures in the vicinity of Hangchow give a clear picture of the later development of the T'ang style in the period of the Wu-Yüeh kingdom and under the Sung, a development to be followed by a radical change brought about by the arrival of Lamaist Buddhism during the rule of the Mongol dynasty.

Decisive for this region was the catastrophic defeat suffered by the Sung in their encounter with the Jurchen, following which the Chinese were obliged in 1127 to shift their capital from Kaifeng, in Honan province, to Hangchow (then Lin-an). For the first time in China's history, Chekiang found itself changing from a peripheral area to the center of the empire; this caused a great influx of population. The increment of manpower made it possible to develop the region's natural resources and to establish seaports to provide for an ever-growing maritime trade which put the country in contact with overseas nations. A large part of Chinese export pottery was manufactured in Chekiang and Fukien; however, it would be wrong to consider this rapidly expanded production, and the technical perfection attained, as direct consequences of the arrival of the many northern Chinese who, after the fall of Kaifeng (1127), fled the north together with the officials of the government. The potters who worked at Hangchow to produce the wares for the use of the imperial court, the Kuan-yao (Kuan ware), continued techniques that had been developed in the imperial kilns of Kaifeng in the north, but this type of pottery, the superb qualities of which have so impressed Western collectors, was not the only type produced in this region, and certainly not the oldest.

There is a multitude of evidence of international contacts in the Chinese port regions, which developed as a result of the growing trade with foreign lands. Many Arabic tombstones have been found in the vicinity of Tsinkiang (formerly Ch'üan-chou, the Zayton of Marco Polo), which was the most important port before the development of Foochow and Amoy, but it cannot be said that Chinese art was appreciably influenced by these foreign communities.

Except for some pagodas built of brick and therefore resistant to fire and the wear and tear of time, little remains of the architecture of the Sung period. The pair of stone pagodas at Tsinkiang (Ch'üan-chou) are typical of the prevalent local style and were constructed in their present form in the mid-13th century. The beautiful curvature of the roofs, which lightened the profile of these rather squat pagodas, remains to this day one of the most important characteristics of the southern Chinese architectural style.

BIBLIOG. G. Ecke and P. Demiéville, The Twin Padogas of Zayton, Cambridge, Mass., 1935; D. Tokiwa and T. Sekino, Shina Bukkyō Shiseki (Buddhist Monuments in China), V, Tokyo, 1938; W. B. Honey, The Ceramic Art of China and Other Countries of the Far East, London, 1945.

*Monuments and archaeological sites.* Vicinity of Hangchow (Hangchou, formerly Lin-an). In the vicinity of Hangchow and the Western Lake (Hsi-hu), rock sculptures and a certain number of natural caves decorated with sculptures are to be found at several places. Most of these go back to the period of the Five Dynasties, or to the Sung and Yüan dynasties. At the time of the Wu-Yüeh kingdom the production of these sculptures had already begun, and it was intensified after the seat of the central government came to Hangchow during the Sung period. The numerous pieces of sculpture made during the Yüan period, particularly on Fei-lai-fêng, were executed on orders from a local official of the Mongol government. The following are the principal groups:

Chiang-t'ai-shan. On this mountain, which is part of the Phoenix Hill, stands a group of sculptures dating from the Five Dynasties and the Sung periods. An extremely large group, the tallest of which is about 11 ½ ft. high, consists of a trinity of Amitābha flanked by two standing bodhisattvas, and two lokapalas, or Buddhist guardians. The inscriptions indicate that the group was carved during the reign of the emperor Jên-tsung (1023–63) of the Sung dynasty. In a smaller niche stands the image of the pilgrim Hsüan-tsang flanked by two female figures.

Shih-wu-tung. This natural cave, about 8 ft. deep and about 20 ft. wide, situated at the foot of the mountain Nan-kao-fêng on the southwest side of the Western Lake, has cut into its walls three altars containing almost seven hundred sculptures with figures of Buddhist saints which, at some later time, were covered with a layer of gilding. Some pieces are dated, the oldest 944, the latest 974. The sculptures are rather crude and grotesque; their artistic value is not very great.

Yen-hsia-tung. In this deep, tapering natural cave on the southern slopes of Nan-kao-fêng are to be found many large Buddhist images carved from the living rock. These include 18 lohans (Skr. *arhat*), an Avalokiteśvara, a Mahāsthāmaprāpta, and several other figures. Also carved from the rock is an unusual model of a seven-storied octagonal pagoda. The cave walls surrounding the pagoda model are covered with smaller figures in bas-relief representing high-ranking officials. An inscription found there some time ago indicates that the cave was designed under the patronage of Wu Yen-shuang, brother-in-law of Wen-mu, king of Wu-Yüeh.

Fei-lai-fêng. On the face of this mountain and on the walls of the four natural caverns found in it, there are a great number of sculptures carved from the rock, dating from the Five Dynasties,

Sung, and Yüan periods. The many sculptures of varying sizes, among which are several fine pieces, may be said to constitute a compendium of the iconographic and stylistic changes which occurred in Chinese sculpture from the 10th to the late 13th centuries. The oldest dated sculpture of these caves was carved in 951. A large number of sculptures were executed during the last years of the Chih-yüan period (1264–95) of the Yüan dynasty.

With the Mongols appeared a completely new style and iconography, completely eliminating that of the Sung period, itself derived from the style of the late T'ang dynasty. Tantric representations became predominant, showing a strong Tibetan influence. Especially noteworthy is the appearance in sculpture of Maitreya in the form of Pu-tai (P'u-t'ai), a figure in the Buddhist pantheon which was to become much more widespread in later times.

BIBLIOG. O. Sirén, Chinese Sculpture, London, 1925, I, pp. cxiii–cxiv, IV, pls. 601-8B; E. Boerschmann, Die Baukunst und religiöse Kultur der Chinesen, III: Pagoden, Berlin, Leipzig, 1931, pp. 301–3; D. Tokiwa and T. Sekino, Shina Bukkyō Shiseki (Buddhist Monuments in China), V, Tokyo, 1926–38, pp. 99–109; Wên-wu ts'an-k'ao tzŭ-liao, 1956, no. 1, pp. 9–26, no. 12, pp. 28–30.

Chin-hua. The hexagonal Pagoda of the Ten Thousand Buddhas (Wan-fo-t'a) at Chin-hua, in Chekiang, so called after many Buddhist figures molded one to each brick, suffered destruction during the hostilities in 1942. In its foundations an underground chamber was discovered in 1956 which, although already despoiled by thieves, still contained many objects. These serve to illustrate the Buddhist art of the beginning of the Sung period in the Chekiang region. A hexagonal stone lantern, almost 57 in. high, is one of the largest objects; it bears a Buddhist text and a date corresponding to 1062. It is probable that this is both the date of the building of the pagoda and that of the year in which the objects were placed in the crypt; an iron chest in which the objects were probably kept also bears an inscription of that year. The most interesting part of the collection consists of some sixty bronze and iron statuettes of buddhas and bodhisattvas. The majority of these figurines have a nimbus with openwork decoration. As a whole they are important because they form an integral and datable group of small Buddhist figures of a late date. Especially interesting is the archaistic style of several pieces which recalls that of the Six Dynasties period.

BIBLIOG. Wên-wu ts'an-k'ao tzŭ-liao, 1957, no. 5, pp. 4–14; Chin-hua Wan-fo-t'a ch'u-t'u wên-wu (Cultural Relics from the Wan-fo Pagoda at Chin-hua), Peking, 1958.

Kiln sites. During the years since about 1930 several scholars have located kiln sites where the Yüeh-yao (Yüeh ware) was made (PLS. 165, 166). Several kilns seem to date back to the Han period, but most are of the Six Dynasties and the T'ang periods. The following kiln sites are the most important:

Tê-ch'ing. In these kiln sites, about 25 miles north of Hangchow, which were discovered by Yonaiyama Tsuneo in 1930, several types of early Yüeh-yao were found, including pieces in the shape of Han bronzes and the well-known ewers with spouts shaped like chicken heads. Some are covered by a blackish-brown glaze instead of the greenish-gray of the common Yüeh-yao type. In 1956 Chinese archaeologists reinvestigated several kiln sites near Tê-ch'ing. Although some of the kiln sites may date back to the Han period, most are from the Six Dynasties and T'ang periods.

Ch'iu-yen. This site, about 30 miles southeast of Hangchow and Hsiao-shan, is the most renowned of the ancient Yüeh-yao kiln sites. It was discovered by Matsumura Yūzō in 1936 and visited by Brankston one year later. The bowls and jars of porcelaneous stoneware, similar in body to the pieces from Tê-ch'ing, often have a molded decoration of diamond diaper, flowers, and masks, as well as incised designs. The glaze is mostly a grayish olive green. Most kiln sites seem to date from the Six Dynasties period.

Shang-lin-hu. These kiln sites, in the district of Yü-yao, had already been inspected by Bishop Moule in 1890. Nakao Manzō and Kaida Mantarō, who investigated the sites in 1930, found among other things a fragment bearing a date corresponding to 978. The sites, which have since been investigated by several scholars, are quite numerous; they are found along the slopes of the mountains surrounding the lakes. Recent Chinese investigations have unearthed several more dated fragments (850, 922, and 978). The period of greatest activity occurred under the Wu-Yüeh kingdom, 10th cent.

Yü-wang-miao. The kiln sites of Yü-wang-miao, near Shaohsing, were investigated in 1944 by Yoneda Shigehiro, but no shards have been collected to identify Yüeh-yao in collections outside China as coming from these kilns.

Shang-tung. In 1954 a kiln site was discovered near the village of Shang-tung, on the banks of the river Yung-hsing-ho, southwest of Hsiao-shan. The ware from these kilns is almost identical with that of the Ch'iu-yen kiln sites listed above.

Huang-yen. A few years ago, eight kiln sites were discovered about 9 miles south of Huang-yen in central Chekiang. The shards were similar to those found at Shang-lin-hu.

BIBLIOG. J. M. Plumer, The Origin of the "Secret Colour Ware," ILN, Mar. 13 and 20, 1937; A. D. Brankston, Yüeh Ware of the "Nine Rocks" Kiln, BM, LXXIII, 1938, pp. 257–62; Wên-wu ts'an-k'ao tzŭ-liao, 1955, no. 3, pp. 66–73; G. St. G. M. Gompertz, Some Notes on Yüeh Ware, O. Art, N. S., II, 1956, pp. 3–8, 109–16; G. St. G. M. Gompertz, Chinese Celadon Wares, London, 1958; K'ao-ku t'ung-hsin, 1958, no. 8, pp. 44–7; K'ao-ku hsüeh-pao, 1959, no. 3, pp. 107–20.

Lung-ch'üan. The remains of kilns where, in the Sung, Yüan, and Ming periods, the vast majority of Chinese celadons were made (see CERAMICS) are located in the vicinity of the city of Lung-ch'üan, in Chekiang, scattered along the Wei River and its tributaries. The investigations conducted by Ch'ên Wan-li in 1928 and again in 1934 contributed greatly to the dating and location of the various kilns recorded in literary texts. Thirty-odd of them have been discovered.

The earliest kiln sites date from the Sung period, but it is possible that production had already begun at the time of the Five Dynasties. The site of Liu-t'ien, which according to local historical sources was probably the most important production center during the period of the Southern Sung, is identified by Ch'ên Wan-li with the Ta-yao (Great Kiln) in the southwest of the district of Lung-ch'üan, near the sources of the small river Hsia-mei. Although, as the T'ao-lu affirms, in the early Ming period the manufacture was transferred to nearby Ch'u-chou, experts suppose that production continued at Lung-ch'üan during the Ming period.

BIBLIOG. J. M. Plumer, Long-lost Chekiang Kiln Sites..., ILN, Mar. 13, 1937; K. Fujio, Shina Seiji Shikō (A History of Chinese Celadons), Tokyo, 1943, pp. 209–60; Ch'ên Wan-li, Chung kuo ch'ing-tz'ŭ shih-lüeh (A Short History of Chinese Celadons), Shanghai, 1956; G. St. G. M. Gompertz, Chinese Celadon Wares, London, 1958, pp. 50–65.

Shui-chi. J. M. Plumer in 1935 discovered the kilns of Chien-yao (Chien ware) near Shui-chi, in north Fukien, and proved the authenticity of the old information concerning the origin of this type.

In 1954, a group of Chinese archaeologists under the direction of Sung Po-yin examined the site; thus it was possible to locate kilns of Chien-yao to the east, northeast, and southeast of the village of Ch'ih-tun, south of Shui-chi. Seven kilns were found near Lu-hua-p'ing where, among other objects, a sagger was found, bearing an inscribed date corresponding to 1142. One other kiln site was found near the village of Ta-lu and three near Niu-p'i-lun. The body and glaze of fragments from all the kilns were virtually identical.

BIBLIOG. J. M. Plumer, A Note on the Chien-yao (Temmoku) Kiln-site, OAZ, XI, 1935, pp. 193–4; J. M. Plumer, The Place of Origin of the World-famous Chien Ware Discovered, ILN, Oct. 26, 1935; J. M. Plumer, Saggars of Sung, I: The Wares of Chien, Oriental Art, I, 1948, pp. 83–6; Wên-wu ts'an-k'ao tzŭ-liao, 1955, no. 3, pp. 50–65.

Tê-hua. It has long been known that Tê-hua, in Fukien province, was the source of the blanc de chine which became so famous in Europe, but still unknown are the exact whereabouts of the kilns and the date when production of this white porcelain began. Malcolm Farley has found fragments with cream, blue, and white glaze as well as shards of the Ying-ch'ing type. Several years ago Sung Po-yin, during the investigation of four sites near Tê-hua, found a great number of fragments, none of which were of the Ying-ch'ing type. Near Shih-p'ai-ko he found both saggers and fragments. Local tradition has it that the potter Ho Ch'ao-tsung, who was widely known because of the many seals bearing his name on blanc de chine, worked here. He probably lived toward the end of the Ming period. Sung Po-yin found, near Shih-p'ai-ling, several fragments of porcelain decorated in underglaze blue which sometimes has the written mark "yüeh-chi." So far it has not been possible to prove that white porcelain was already being made here during the Ming period.

BIBLIOG. M. F. Farley, The White Ware of Fukien and the South China Coast, Far Eastern Ceramic B., VII, 1949, IX, 1950; Sung Po-yin, T'an Tê-hua-yao (A Talk on Tê-hua Porcelain), Wên-wu ts'an-k'ao tzŭ-liao, 1955, no. 4, pp. 55–71.

HONAN (Ho-nan). Survey of geography and art history. The territory of this province belongs mainly to the alluvial plain of the Yellow River, which flows from east to west across its northern part. To the west, the valley of the Yellow River is restricted between the ranges of the Chinling Mountains on the south and the plateau of Shansi to the north, while farther east it broadens gradually. The

Shansi plateau shelters the plain from the cold north winds blowing from Central Asia in winter.

The high bed of the Yellow River causes it to have only a few tributaries, the most important being the Chin River, which rises in Shansi, and the Lo River, which flows from behind the Mang-shan. The eastern part of the province consists of the basin of the rivers which empty into the Huai River, while the watercourses from the southwest empty into the Yangtze River farther south. Honan is separated from the middle course of this stream by highlands.

Except perhaps for Shansi, no province has played a role in Chinese history comparable to that of Honan. The Great Plain, called the Central Plain (*chung-yüan*) by the Chinese, has from earliest times formed the center of the Chinese nation. The neolithic cultures were attracted from the north (the microlithic Gobi culture), from the west (the Yang-shao culture), and from the east (the Lung-shan culture) and became established in this rich agricultural region. (The Yang-shao culture takes its name from the site in western Honan where J. G. Andersson first found traces of it in 1921). Here these cultures united and mingled and came to flower, only to be superseded by the Gray Pottery culture. Here, buried deeply, lie the remains of the cities and settlements of the Shang and Chou dynasties. Many of the early emperors established their capitals here, and the region remained the center of the Chinese empire until the disastrous defeat suffered by the Sung in 1127, which delivered the capital Pien-ching (modern Kaifeng) to the invading Jurchen; after that the capital was transferred to the south, never to return to this region again. (See CHINESE ART, *Neolithic* and *Shang-Yin*.)

The province of Honan, with the great cities of Loyang (Lo-yang) and Kaifeng (K'ai-fêng), is a region in which many artistic monuments, together with countless ruins and archaeological sites, recall a glorious past. There are abundant remains dating from the earliest times. The site of the Great City of Shang (Ta-yi Shang), near An-yang, which was the last capital of the Shang sovereigns, aroused much interest at the time of its discovery and excavation, but now it is no longer the only site where material for the study of the culture of this period can be found. The remains of an ancient city discovered near and partly below the modern city of Chengchow (Chêng-chou) are identified by some with the Shang capital Ao, the center of Shang civilization before the transfer to An-yang. The clear stratification of the sites has provided possibilities for tracing the history of the Shang people even farther back into the past.

During the Chou period two important cities were built on the north bank of the Lo river: Wang-ch'êng to the west and Ch'êng-chou (not to be confused with Chêng-chou, or Chengchow, mentioned above) to the east of the river Ch'an. The exact boundaries of these two towns have not yet been established, but a recent survey by archaeologists of the Academia Sinica has brought to light sections of an Eastern Chou city wall which seems to belong to the ancient city of Wang-ch'êng (*K'ao-ku hsüeh-pao*, 1956). When the Chou rulers were expelled from their western capital, they established their court at Wang-ch'êng (771 B.C.), moving in 509 B.C. to Ch'êng-chou and returning again to Wang-ch'êng in 314 B.C. Although their power by that time was little more than nominal, as the real leadership had been taken over by successive rulers of various of the Warring States, the present territory of Honan remained the heart of the Chinese nation.

Remains from the period of the Warring States and from the whole late Chou period are numerous in Honan. Finds dating from the first half of the Chou period are much less frequent than those of the Shang and late Chou periods. Perhaps this can be explained by the fact that the center of power was farther west, but there is also the possibility that bronze casting at the time when the middle Chou style flourished was not only technically but also quantitatively inferior to the preceding and following periods.

Evidence of the flourishing art of bronze casting toward the end of the Chou period is nowhere else to be found in such abundance as in Honan province. The region around present-day Loyang, where in olden times the cities of Ch'êng-chou and Wang-ch'êng were located, contains innumerable sites. It has been possible to locate definitely the provenance of only a small number of the objects discovered before World War II. Notable among these are the famous furnishings from the tombs of the Han family at Chin-ts'un, which have attracted widespread attention because a large number of them found their way to Western collections.

The provenance of many pieces being unknown, it is difficult to connect certain of the stylistic traits of the late Chou bronzes with any particular locality, nor can they be related to one or another of the Warring States which dominated parts of Honan. The Han family tombs, with their furnishings, and the group of mirrors of Loyang described by Karlgren, show how the area including Loyang must have been a center of great artistic activity during the late Chou period. Very likely this activity had no connection with the reign of the Chou kings, nominal rulers of the kingdom. Instead, one may imagine it to have been stimulated by the flourishing of the state of Han (not to be confounded with the regime which gave its name to the Han dynasty), which in the last years of the Chou dynasty ruled over a long strip of territory south of the Yellow River. In the case of finds such as the discoveries at Chang-t'ai-kuan, which show great similarity to the art of Ch'ang-sha (see below, *Hunan*), it is obvious that the objects must be attributed to the Ch'u kingdom.

In the present cities of Loyang and Kaifeng, which in the course of histor yhave at various times been capitals of China, the only ancient remains are a few isolated architectural monuments. However, of these, a most imposing and important Buddhist monument may be connected with Loyang's function as a capital. After the transfer of the capital of the Wei dynasty from Shansi province to Loyang in 493, work began on the great complex of sculptured caves at Lung-mên, which continued to be enlarged until the T'ang period and which is one of the most extensive in all China. In other localities of the same province, at Kung-hsien and on Pao-shan in the vicinity of An-yang, cave temples have been preserved, but their size is small in comparison with that of the complex of Lung-mên.

In addition to the Shang and Chou bronzes, a large share of the products of another Chinese craft, that of the potter, must be ascribed to the territory of Honan. Various types of pottery were manufactured under the rule of the Sung emperors in the region surrounding the capital Kaifeng. Although ancient Chinese sources provide few reliable data on pottery, it is certain that in the Kaifeng area, either north or south of the Yellow River, there existed numerous thriving centers, which were closed in part or transferred to the south after the fall of the capital in 1127.

*Monuments and archaeological sites.* Chêng-chou (Chengchow). In 1950 the chance finding of a gray shard of the Shang period attracted the attention of Chinese archaeologists to the city of Chengchow (in archaeology, usually Chêng-chou), thought to be a site where Shang relics could be found. In 1952, excavations were started within the city and its environs; these have revealed the ruins of a city of the Shang period, identified by some with the Ao mentioned in the ancient annals, supposed to have been founded by the tenth king of the house of Shang and to have been the capital for one or two centuries before King P'an-kêng transferred it to Hsiao-t'un, near An-yang, some time between the dates 1384 B.C. (chronology of Tung Tso-pin) and 1300 B.C. (chronology of Karlgren).

The results of numerous excavations have made it possible to establish that the modern city was built upon the remains of the Shang city and that it covers only two fifths of the ancient capital; the ruins extend more than a mile to the east and somewhat less than a mile and a quarter north and south. The city was surrounded by a wall of rammed earth. In many places were found pits with walls of rammed earth which served as dwellings or storage places, although house foundations similar to those of An-yang were also found. A remarkable quantity of pottery was discovered almost everywhere. Also brought to light were a pottery kiln, a bronze foundry, a workshop for the manufacture of bone objects, and a great number of tombs.

The paramount importance of the Chêng-chou excavations, however, lies in the fact that it has been possible to distinguish clearly the various cultural strata in many sites. Although the strata are not the same everywhere, they have given us a better knowledge of the development of Shang culture, and have clarified problems which had previously been exceedingly obscure. At both Êrh-li-kang, south of Chêng-chou, and Pai-chia-chuang, a village less than a quarter of a mile northeast of Chêng-chou, two strata have been distinguished under the surface layer. In the People's Public Park (Jên-min Kung-yüan), on the bank of the river north of the city, three distinct strata have been found. The uppermost of the three contained cultural remains resembling those of the Shang strata of An-yang; the lower two correspond to the two strata of Pai-chia-chuang and Êrh-li-kang. Only the lowest contains no bronze objects.

At Êrh-li-kang a great number of oracle bones have been found, only two of which, however, bear inscriptions. One, closely related to those found at An-yang, came from the upper stratum; the other, found at a lower level, bears only one (undecipherable) character.

The chronology based on this stratification is confirmed by the stylistic development of the pottery and bronzes found in these strata. It is now possible to follow the successive stages by which, for example, the hollow tripod *li* was transformed from a true tripod resting on three pointed feet to a low standing vessel ending in three points. Similar phenomena can be observed in the other types of pottery and bronzes. The latter are clearly differentiated from the better-developed types of An-yang by simpler forms and decoration.

BIBLIOG. Chêng Tê-k'un, The Origin and Development of Shang Culture, Asia Major, VI, 1957, pp. 80–98 (with references to Chinese reports): Chêng-chou Erh-li-kang (Report on the Excavations at Êrh-li-kang). Peking, 1959.

An-yang. The remains of the great city which was the capital of the Shang kings from 1300 to 1028 B.C. (or 1384 to 1111 B.C., according to Tung Tso-pin's chronology) are located along the banks of the Huan River north and northwest of the city of An-yang in the northern part of Honan province. In 1899 some bones excavated by chance in this area, several bearing inscriptions in archaic characters, aroused the interest of Chinese archaeologists. These were soon identified as oracle bones from the Shang period and caused a great sensation at that time among epigraphists. The first excavations, which yielded spectacular results, were carried out between 1928 and 1937. These were terminated when the Japanese invasion forced the Chinese archaeologists to suspend digging. World War II and its aftermath prevented an immediate resumption of the excavations as well as the publication of full results of the earlier work. Digging was resumed at Hsiao-t'un and Ta-ssŭ-k'ung-ts'un in 1950.

Excavations have been carried out so far at 11 sites on both banks of the Huan River. Although from T'ung-lo-chai in the west to Hou-kang in the east the terrain investigated is slightly more than 3 miles long, it has not yet been possible to determine the boundaries of the ancient city. The sites lie within a mile and a quarter of the banks of the Huan River.

The following excavations have been carried out on the north bank. At T'ung-lo-chai, three strata are clearly distinguishable, representing the Red Pottery (Yang-shao) culture; the Black Pottery (Lung-shan) culture, and the Gray Pottery (Shang-Yin) culture. At Kao-ching-t'ai-tzŭ, the same three strata were found, and on the Northwest Hill (Hsi-pei-kang) at Hou-chia-chuang, a great necropolis was discovered containing royal tombs. Here the famous white pottery was discovered (PL. 220). At Hou-chia-chuang, where there are many Yin tombs, there were discovered seven large tortoise shells used for divining. At Wu-kuan-ts'un Nan-pa-t'ai, two strata have been identified, one belonging to the Lung-shan culture and the other to the Shang-Yin culture. This site was originally the continuation of that of Ssŭ-p'an-mo on the south bank, from which it was separated when the river changed its course. Finally, at Ta-ssŭ-kung-ts'un, both before and after World War II, a great number of Shang-Yin tombs were discovered.

The following excavations were carried out south of the Huan River: at Fan-chia-chuang, so far investigated only superficially; at Ssŭ-p'an-mo, where both a cemetery and dwellings were explored; at Wang-yü-k'ou, and Huo-chia Hsiao-chuang, where a cemetery of the Shang-Yin period was found. Hsiao-t'un is the most important and the central site, with two strata, one representing the Lung-shan culture and the other the Shang-Yin culture. The majority of the oracle bones with inscriptions come from Hsiao-t'un, where many dwellings were also found. In Hou-kang, the succession of the three strata (Yang-shao, Lung-shan, and Shang-Yin) was recognized for the first time.

The excavations along the banks of the Huan River have made it possible to reconstruct in part the history of the region. The first known inhabitants whose remains have been found brought the Yang-shao culture there and settled on the banks of the river. At present we know three of their dwelling places. After them came the representatives of the Lung-shan culture, who probably at first inhabited the same centers as their predecessors, but who later spread out to new settlements in the immediate vicinity. The foundations of their huts have been located at five sites. The burial places of the Yang-shao and Lung-shan peoples have not yet been located.

The Shang-Yin people, who later lived in this region, came perhaps from Chêng-chou and brought a highly developed culture, which thrived remarkably during the three centuries in which it dominated this area. However, since the occupation lasted without interruption until the end of the Shang-Yin period, when the city was destroyed, the differentiation of the various Shang-Yin strata is rather difficult. Some experts have advanced the theory that the period of the houses with rammed-earth foundations must have been preceded by another during which the predecessors of the Shang-Yin people from Chêng-chou lived there in dwelling pits. The major building activity should then have coincided with the arrival of King P'an-kêng and his people in 1300 (Tung Tso-pin, 1384) B.C. The significance of certain peculiar trenches, found in many places, is still rather in doubt: some scholars believe they were used for drainage, others think they served as primitive water levels for the construction of foundations. On the basis of the partly deciphered inscriptions on the many oracle bones found here, as well as the numerous finds of bronzes, marble sculptures, jades, pottery, and other objects, it is possible to reconstruct with some accuracy the cultural life of the people of this great city.

BIBLIOG. Preliminary Reports of Excavations at Anyang, Academia Sinica, Peiping, 1929–33; W. P. Yetts, The Shang-Yin Dynasty and the An-yang Finds, JRAS, 1933, pp. 657–85; W. P. Yetts, Recent Finds near An-yang, JRAS, 1935, pp. 467–74; Chêng Tê-k'un, The Origin and Development of Shang Culture, Asia Major, VI, 1957, pp. 80–98; Li Chi, The Beginnings of Chinese Civilization, Seattle, 1957; M. Loehr, The Stratigraphy of Hsiao-t'un (Anyang), Ars Orientalis, II, 1957, pp. 439–57.

Hui-hsien. The village of Ku-wei-ts'un in the district of Hui-hsien has enjoyed since 1929 the reputation of being one of the most important sites for Yin and Chou relics. (An example is shown in II, PL. 15.) Only in 1937, however, did the Academia Sinica first attempt to excavate a number of tombs in that vicinity. These excavations, the results of which were never completely published, were interrupted by the Japanese invasion. Karlbeck has given a report as an eyewitness of an excavation begun by the local inhabitants. In 1950 excavation work was resumed, and in the three-year period 1950–52 excavations were made in the following places:

Liu-li-ko (less than 2/3 mile east of Hui-hsien). In the north and south sectors were discovered the remains of many hut foundations and tombs dating from the Shang-Yin, Chou, and Han periods. The total number of Shang-Yin tombs is 53. It was demonstrated on the basis of the stratification that the 16 tombs in the southern sector were of a later date than the others, which antedated the An-yang period. The Yin tombs yielded many pottery fragments, a small number of bronzes of chüeh and ku type, objects of jade, and uninscribed oracle bones. In addition to 28 tombs dating from the late Chou period, there was also found a trench in which 19 chariots together with their horses were buried. This discovery was extremely important because of the knowledge it provided of the chariots and the exact position of the bronze ornaments. Nearly all the tombs had been despoiled long before.

Ku-wei-ts'un (about 2 miles east of Hui-hsien). Here was found a gigantic mound containing three large and two small tombs. A fourth tomb of large dimensions was found nearby. According to Karlbeck, these had all been partly pillaged before World War II. Nevertheless, a great number of interesting objects were discovered in them, including a horse's head with gold and silver incrustation, part of the ornamentation of a chariot, a bronze basin with a decoration depicting a ritual dance, a terra-cotta bowl with a base in the shape of three human figures, a richly decorated jade pendant, and many other objects.

Chao-ku-ts'un (11 miles southwest of Hui-hsien). Here a number of neolithic remains and seven tombs of the late Chou period came to light. The tombs contained much pottery and several fine bronzes.

Ch'u-ch'iu-ts'un (about 12 miles west of Hui-hsien). Here ashpits were found containing objects from the Shang-Yin period, 15 late Chou tombs and 9 tombs of the Han period.

Po-ch'üan-ts'un (about 2 miles north of Hui-hsien). In a tomb were discovered a group of tomb figurines of the Han period, remarkable for their highly realistic style.

BIBLIOG. O. Karlbeck, Notes on a Hui-hsien Tomb, Röhsska Konstlöjdmuseet Arstryck, 1952, pp. 40–7; J. F. Haskins, Recent Excavations in China, Arch. Chin. Art Soc. Am., X, 1956, pp. 46–8; Hui-hsien fa-chüeh pao-kao (A Report on the Excavations at Hui-hsien), Peking, 1956.

Chin-ts'un. In the vicinity of the village Chin-ts'un, near Loyang, were discovered in 1929 the tombs of the rulers of the Han state which dominated the region from 450 to 230 B.C. The tomb furnishings, rich and varied, were excavated by the local inhabitants and were scattered throughout the world. Although there had been no scientific supervision, many data on these excavations were collected by Bishop W. C. White, from oral communications by the townspeople and the merchants. Among the many articles found in these tombs (jades, bronzes, mirrors, lacquer objects, and weapons), especially famous are the bells. The inscriptions on the so-called Piao bells cannot be dated exactly. The dates suggested vary from 550 to 380 B.C. One characteristic of this find which aroused particular interest is the frequency of gold and silver incrustation on bronze vessels and other objects.

BIBLIOG. W. C. White, Tombs of old Loyang, Shanghai, 1934; S. Umehara, Rakuyō Kinson Kobō Shūei (Collection of the Best Specimens from the Ancient Tombs of Loyang), Kyoto, 1937; B. Karlgren, Notes on a Kintsun Album, BMFEA, X, 1938, pp. 65–81.

Hsin-chêng. In 1923 there were found here more than a hundred objects, including 93 bronzes. The tripods of the ting type (19) and the small bells (17) are especially numerous. Among the objects, all kept in the museum of Kaifeng, one bears an inscription referring to an event which occured in 575 B.C. The vessels are partly in middle and partly in late Chou style, indicating different dates.

BIBLIOG. C. W. Bishop, The Find at Hsin Chêng Hsien, Artibus Asiae, nos. 2 and 3, 1928–29, pp. 110–21; Kuan Po-i, Hsin-chêng ku-ch'i t'u-lu (Illustrated Catalogue of the Vessels from Hsin-chêng), Shanghai, 1929; Sun Hai-po, Hsin-chêng i-ch'i (Relics from Hsin-chêng), Shanghai, 1937.

Chang-t'ai-kuan, in the district of Hsin-yang. During the digging of a well in 1956 a large tomb (29 × 25 ft.) was discovered, built of wood and consisting of an antechamber, a central room, a rear chamber, and four lateral chambers. Despite the rather considerable damage caused by the digging, it was possible to extract from the tomb a large number of objects in good condition, some of which are unique and of a type hitherto unknown.

Among the most interesting objects recovered from this tomb are a number of lacquered wooden objects, tomb figures, pieces of furniture, and musical instruments. There is one large wooden figure of a fabulous beast with a long tongue and a deer's antlers on its head. A pair of sculptures in the shape of tigers together form a drum stand. These objects, as well as a table and a complete bed, are all decorated in a style similar to that of the Ch'ang-sha lacquers, and should therefore be attributed to artisans of the Ch'u people.

Of the bronzes a set of 13 bells is especially noteworthy, because it was found in such perfect condition that the musical scale could be recorded. That the 13 bells constitute a complete set is proved by the inventory of the tomb, which was written on bamboo strips, and in which the number is mentioned. The largest of the bells has an inscription which Kuo Mo-jo connected with a historical event mentioned in the chronicle Ch'un-ch'iu ("Spring and Autumn Annals") for the year 525 B.C. The ornament of the bronzes is characteristic of the late Chou period.

When a second examination of this tomb was made in 1957, another tomb of similar structure was found 30 ft. away from it. Although it had been looted at some earlier time, a few objects were found in it. Here too was found a figure with antlers of the same type as the figure in the first tomb. Among the many lacquered objects was an especially remarkable pair of phoenixes standing on a stylized tiger which served as a pedestal or drum stand; this pair is comparable to the cranes in the Cleveland Museum of Art (PL. 226).

BIBLIOG. K'ao-ku t'ung-hsin, 1958, no. 11, pp. 79–80; Wên-wu ts'an-k'ao tzǔ-liao, 1957, no. 9, pp. 21–33, 1958, no. 1, pp. 15–28.

Lung-mên. These cave temples are located on the steep banks of the Yi River 15 miles south of Loyang. The oldest probably date from the period immediately following the transfer of the Wei dynasty capital to Loyang (A.D. 493); the latest are from the mid-8th century. There are numerous caves on both sides of the river, more than forty in all; but during the period of the Wei, temples were constructed only on the western bank, where are situated also the most important monuments of the Sui and T'ang periods. The caves on the western bank form two groups: one group to the north, of which 6 monuments are noteworthy, and 15 to the south. Only one of the first group, the Pin-yang cave, dates from the Wei period, whereas the southern group has at least 7 caves from the same period, the oldest of which is the Ku-yang cave. The caves on the eastern bank are all of the T'ang period, but are generally of less interest because of their poor state of preservation.

While dated inscriptions are rare at Yün-kang (see below, Shansi), they occur frequently at Lung-mên. They contain the names of the founders and the expression of their pious wishes and enable us to follow the gradual growth of this complex of caves.

Work on the Ku-yang cave (PL. 255), the most ancient, seems to have been started soon after or even before the transfer of the capital to Loyang in 493 and to have continued for a long time. The more important additions seem to date from before 525. The walls of this vaulted rectangular cave are crowded with niches of varying size. Against the rear wall there is a Buddha over 13 ft. high, seated on a pedestal over 6 ft. high, with a halo decorated with flames and small buddhas in bas-relief. The figure is flanked by two bodhisattvas. The Ku-yang cave with its numerous figures of cross-legged bodhisattvas continues the last phase of the Yün-kang style, but it does not yet show the clear deliberate planning of some of the later caves.

The finest cave of all is the Pin-yang cave (No. III), hewn out by order of the emperor and already completed perhaps by 523. Standing against the rear wall is a group composed of a cross-legged Buddha flanked by two disciples, Ananda and Mahākāśyapa, and two bodhisattvas. The principal figure is a typical example of the Wei style, which served as a model for the sculptors of the Japanese Tōri school when, in the 7th century, they executed the bronze triad in the Golden Hall of the temple Hōryūji near Nara (see JAPAN; JAPANESE ART). There are also sculptured trinities on both side walls. The inner side of the façade was once covered with four superposed series of bas-reliefs on both sides of the entrance. The emperor, empress,

and their retinue were once portrayed there, but the beautiful bas-reliefs were detached during the 1930s and have since been scattered over the world. Fragments of the bas-reliefs of the empress have been collected by the Nelson Gallery of Art in Kansas City and partially reunited, while the Metropolitan Museum of New York has been able to gather together many fragments of the bas-relief of the emperor. During the Wei period the original plan of excavating here a series of three caves, one alongside the other, was not carried out, but the project was resumed during the Sui period and completed under the T'ang.

Cave XIII, known as the Lien-hua-tung (Cave of the Lotus), derives its name from a large relief on the ceiling representing a lotus surrounded by flying apsarases. The cave was completed about 520, but several dated inscriptions indicate that enlargements were made in the period of the Northern Ch'i (550–577) and also in the T'ang period. In this cave also the damage is considerable.

During the T'ang dynasty (618–906), sculptural activity again reached a new culminating point; it was then that the majority of the sculptures and the caves of Lung-mên were executed. Besides the alterations in already existing caves, new ones were created (Caves I, V, VII–XII, XVI). There are here also two very important groups carved on the cliff walls. On the north side of the western bank there is a partially completed group (No. VI) consisting of a triad with a seated central figure 13 ft. high, flanked by four figures: two bodhisattvas and two lokapalas (divine guardians of the world). The great Vairocana with minor figures, situated on the south side of the western bank, is one of the most impressive sculptures of Lung-mên. Work on this group, consisting of a colossal figure of the Buddha Vairocana, two disciples, two lokapalas, and two bearers of the vajra (sacred thunderbolt), was probably begun, according to an inscription, in 670 and may have been completed in 675. The figure of Vairocana, including the pedestal and nimbus, is about 50 ft. high. The other figures vary from 30 to 36 ft. in height. The huge figures are carved out in a niche which is about 100 ft. wide and 120 ft. deep, and were probably once protected by a large canopy which has completely disappeared. Recently, several proposals to protect the sculptures with a new structure have been put forward.

BIBLIOG. E. Chavannes, Mission Archéologique dans la Chine Septentrionale, I, Paris, 1915, part 2, pp. 320–561; O. Sirén, Chinese Sculpture, I, London, 1925, pp. 20–25; D. Tokiwa and T. Sekino, Shina Bukkyō Shiseki (Buddhist Monuments in China), II, Tokyo, 1926–38, pp. 55–99; S. Mizuno and T. Nagahiro, Ryūmon, A Study of the Buddhist Cave-temples at Lungmen, Honan, Tokyo, 1941.

Kung-hsien. Along the Lo River, several miles northwest of the city of Kung-hsien, are the caves of Shih-k'u-ssǔ. These have been hollowed out of the mountain face on Mang-shan, and the Chinese name means literally "rock cave temples." There are five caves, one of which, the fourth, may be subdivided into two parts. The first three, close to one another, are on the east side, while the fourth and fifth, on the west, are divided by a triad of standing Buddhist figures of large size. The inscriptions found in the caves prove that the earliest sculptures date from about 500, while the majority are later and date from the period of the Eastern Wei (534–50) and that of the T'ang. This latter group, however, which is different from the earlier works, is of scant importance. The second, third, and fifth caves have a heavy central column such as is found in other cave sites. The fifth cave, which belongs to the Wei period, is the largest and contains a large number of sculptures of great artistic merit. Highly successful artistically and thoroughly representative of the Kung-hsien sculptures are the numerous reliefs depicting processions of the founders, carved in superposed ranks on the walls, and the reliefs of apsarases and lotus flowers on the ceiling. The stone of Kung-hsien is a rather soft, bluish-gray sandstone, and the sculptures have badly eroded. They have also suffered greatly from the loss of the many reliefs and heads that have been removed.

BIBLIOG. E. Chavannes, Mission Archéologique dans la Chine Septentrionale, I, Paris, 1915, part 2, pp. 562–76; O. Sirén, Chinese Sculpture, London, 1925, I, pp. xlvii–l, 26–7, II, pls. 98–104; D. Tokiwa and T. Sekino, Shina Bukkyō Shiseki (Buddhist Monuments in China), II, Tokyo, 1926–38, pp. 101–10.

Ling-ch'üan-ssǔ. On two peaks of Pao-shan, 23 miles west of An-yang, are two caves belonging to the temple Ling-ch'üan-ssǔ: the Ta-liu-shêng-k'u and the Ta-chu-shêng-k'u. The first cave, containing a Buddhist trinity, dates from the period of the eastern Wei (546), while the second, larger cave dates from the Sui period and is a fine example of the style of this period (589). On the façade at the entrance are carved reliefs depicting Nārāyaṇa and Kapila. The cave contains three trinities with Vairocana, Amitābha, and Maitreya respectively as the central figures, flanked by lohans and bodhisattvas. The four corner pillars of the cave have religious scenes and small buddhas in bas-relief.

BIBLIOG. D. Tokiwa and T. Sekino, Shina Bukkyō Shiseki (Buddhist Monuments in China), III, Tokyo, 1926–38, pp. 81–9.

Sung-yüeh-ssŭ. The pagoda of this temple on Sung-shan is the earliest of the many brick pagodas in China. Literary evidence points to a date in the third decade of the 6th century.

The pagoda is built on a dodecagonal ground plan. The high, plain ground story is separated from the main story by a cornice of corbeled bricks. The corners of the main story are accentuated by hexagonal columns. The main story is crowned by a series of 15 corbeled eaves, diminishing in size as they rise, giving the monument an elegant profile.

The ground story once had entrances on the sides facing the cardinal points. The main story has arched recesses on the sides facing the cardinal points. The other sides have a brick relief consisting of a small single-story pagoda with an arched entrance, placed on a base decorated with oval niches containing crouching lions. The 14 blind stories are decorated with square windows and arched doors. The finial which crowns the top is considered to be of a later date. Originally the whole monument was plastered, but hardly any trace of the plaster now remains.

The style of this impressive monument is nowhere repeated in any of the surviving pagodas in China. There is a possibility that it was copied from some Gupta Indian prototype, but whether it was of a unique structural type at the time it was built can no longer be established.

BIBLIOG. D. Tokiwa and T. Sekino, Shina Bukkyō Shiseki (Buddhist Monuments in China), II, Tokyo, 1926–38, pp. 132–4; O. Sirén, A History of Early Chinese Art, IV: Architecture, London, 1930, p. 61.

T'ieh-t'a (Iron Pagoda). To the temple of Yu-kuo-ssŭ at Kaifeng, otherwise vanished, belonged the so-called "Iron Pagoda," an octagonal monument of 13 stories, built of brick. This monument gets its name, not from the building material, but from the color of its brick. The pagoda was restored several times, as may be gathered from many inscriptions on tiles and cast-iron figures preserved within it, but the original structure seems to date from about 1044.

The pagoda's outer walls are covered with glazed tiles decorated with Buddhist figures. The brackets of the cornices and roofs also have glazed tiles, all this giving the monument a most colorful appearance. For its height — more than 150 ft. — the tower is extremely slim, the width being only about 30 ft. The pagoda was erected with a solid core, around which a narrow turning staircase was built. The vault of the staircase connects the inner core with the shell of the façades. Each story has arched windows on the cardinal points, except on the south where niches with yellow-glazed Buddhist figures were installed in 1936. Despite the many alterations and extensive repairs, this pagoda is one of the finest and most graceful monuments of Sung architecture.

BIBLIOG. O. Sirén, A History of Early Chinese Art, IV: Architecture, London, 1930, pp. 46–7; E. Boerschmann, Die Baukunst und religiöse Kultur der Chinesen, III: Pagoden, Berlin, Leipzig, 1931, pp. 231–7; D. Tokiwa and T. Sekino, Shina Bukkyō Shiseki (Buddhist Monuments in China), V, Tokyo, 1926–38, pp. 48–50.

Fan-t'a. The Fan pagoda (PL. 273) which belonged to the temple Kuo-hsiang-ssŭ in Kaifeng (K'ai-fêng) was built in 977; later destroyed, it was rebuilt in 1384, and again restored in 1649. Since only three stories of this hexagonal pagoda were rebuilt, it has a squat, truncated profile, far different from the original. The whole pagoda is encased in square bricks, each containing a concave medallion with a seated Buddha in relief. Originally all the bricks were enameled green. Although this double-walled pagoda is now only a fragment of the original, it still is an interesting example of the decorative style of pagoda building during the Sung dynasty.

BIBLIOG. O. Sirén, A History of Early Chinese Art, IV: Architecture, London, 1930, p. 47; E. Boerschmann, Die Baukunst und religiöse Kultur der Chinesen, III: Pagoden, Berlin, Leipzig, 1931, pp. 61–9; D. Tokiwa and T. Sekino, Shina Bukkyō Shiseki (Buddhist Monuments in China), V, Tokyo, 1926–38, pp. 46–8.

Kiln sites. Lin-ju-hsien. The present-day district of Lin-ju (formerly called Ju-chou), south of the Yellow River, is the place where the Ju-yao (Ju ware) mentioned in many Chinese sources was produced.

In 1931 the Japanese Harada Gentotsu visited the villages Chang-hsieh-li, Ku-i-li, and Kuei-jên-li, where he located six kiln sites and from which he took home a great number of shards, mainly of the so-called "northern celadon" type, but also of the Chün and Tz'ŭ-chou types. This investigation, which was rather hasty because of unfavorable local conditions, has led the Japanese to suppose that the Ju-yao mentioned in Chinese sources is identical with the so-called "northern celadon." This opinion, shared by some Amer-

ican and Chinese scholars, is quite different from that of Sir Percival David, who has identified as Ju ware a certain buff stoneware covered with an opaque, slightly crackled glaze of a soft bluish-gray color. His identification is based on a testing ring (dated 1107), some shards reported to have come from the site, and the rather conflicting evidence to be culled from Chinese sources. Sir Percival's Ju-yao is actually quite similar to the finest quality of Chün ware. So far no new investigation of the kiln sites, which might clear up this extremely complicated problem, has been undertaken.

BIBLIOG. P. David, A Commentary on Ju Ware, Tr. O. Ceramic Soc., 1936–37, pp. 18–69; J. Ozaki, Sōgen no Tōji (Ceramics of Sung and Yüan, Eng. trans. R. T. Paine, Jr.), Far Eastern Ceramic B., Sept., 1948, and Mar., 1949; Sekai Tōji Zenshū (Ceramic Art of the World), Tokyo, 1955, X, pp. 180–5; P. David, Introduction, Catalogue of the Exhibition of Ju and Kuan Wares, London, 1952; G. St. G. M. Gompertz, Chinese Celadon Ware, London, 1958, pp. 26–39.

Yü-hsien (formerly Chün-chou). Chün-yao (Chün ware), a stoneware of light gray or buff color, covered with a lavender or blue-green glaze, sometimes with purple splashes, is named after the district of Chün-chou, the present-day Yü-hsien. Kiln sites have been located in the village of Shên-kou-chên within the ancient Chün district, but finds of shards both north and south of the Yellow River's present course suggest that Chün ware was made at several places, among them Chiao-tso and Tang-yang-yü, both north of the river (see following section).

BIBLIOG. Sekai Tōji Zenshū (Ceramic Art of the World), X, 1955, pp. 185–6; O. Karlbeck, Notes on the Wares from Chiao-tso Kilns, Ethnos, VIII, 3, 1943, (repr. Far Eastern Ceramic B., IV, 1952, pp. 8–16); O. Karlbeck, On Reported Kiln Sites near Lin-hsien, Far Eastern Ceramic B., IV, 1952, pp. 8–16.

Hsiu-wu. The remains of kilns at Tang-yang-yü and Chiao-tso, a few miles northwest of Hsiu-wu, were discovered in 1933 by R. W. Swallow, and later examined by O. Karlbeck and F. Koyama. Apart from a comparatively small number of shards of the Ting and Chün types, fragments of the Honan Temmoku type were found. The largest group, however, consisted of shards of the Tz'ŭ-chou type. These shards were mostly of an extremely fine quality. Japanese scholars have succeeded, by means of these shards, in identifying several pieces in Japanese collections as products of Hsiu-wu kilns.

BIBLIOG. R. L. Hobson, Ceramic Documents from Honan, BMQ, VIII, pp. 70–1; O. Karlbeck, Notes on the Wares from Chiao-tso Kilns, Ethnos, VIII, 3, 1943 (repr. Far Eastern Ceramic B., 1952, pp. 8–16); Wên-wu ts'an-k'ao tzŭ-liao, 1954, no. 4, pp. 44–7; Sekai Tōji Zenshū (Ceramic Art of the World), X, Tokyo, 1955, pp. 227–35.

Pei Hsiang-t'ang-shan. The caves of Hsiang-t'ang-shan, situated at the Honan-Hopei border in both provinces, are discussed under Hopei, below.

HOPEI (Hopeh, Ho-pei). *Survey of geography and art history.* Up to the time when this province (formerly called Chihli) received parts of the abolished provinces of Jehol and Chahar (1953–56), all the territory composing it was virtually one large unit because of its geographic configuration. It consisted almost entirely of the alluvial plain of the numerous rivers flowing seaward from the mountains, the chief of these being the Yellow River, which has often changed its course flowing through the swampy region north of the mountains of Shantung. The northern, western, and eastern frontiers are sharply marked by the mountains and the sea: in the north, the Yen Mountains cut off the Manchurian plain, save for a narrow coastal strip, which is the natural gateway to the north. In the west, the Taihang Mountains rise abruptly from the plain and form the boundary with the Shansi plateau.

Considering the role played by Hopei in the history of Chinese culture, we are wont to overstress the importance of Peking. Indubitably great as was its importance as imperial capital, it must not be forgotten that the growth of this city is a comparatively recent phenomenon, whereas the importance of the region as a whole goes back to a much earlier period.

The plain of Hopei came into the Chinese sphere quite early. On the other hand, the narrow coastal strip has made possible contacts with the inhabitants of the Manchurian plain. This point, which throughout the ages has always been a keystone in Chinese strategy, served, on the one hand, as an exit for the armies of the strong dynasties when they were preparing to attack Manchuria and Korea, but was, on the other, a weak point against which the northern peoples concentrated their forces in attacking the Chinese defensive cordon. As a result of this strategic position, the province has had a turbulent history, reflected to some extent in its still-existing monuments.

As early as the Shang period the influence of the bronze culture extended to the northern limits of the alluvial plain; the discoveries

made at Ch'ü-yang (Pai-chia-wan) in this province prove how far north the Shang culture extended. During the middle Chou period, there arose in northern Hopei the state of Yen. In the late Chou period, this state seized control of all of southern Manchuria and had a defensive chain of walls built far beyond Shanhaikwan (Linyu). After the Chinese were temporarily driven back inside their natural frontiers under the brief Ch'in dynasty, this region again became the bridgehead for the attacks of the Han emperors, who subjugated areas of Manchuria and Korea, partially colonized them, and occupied them for several centuries. One of the most interesting finds is a tomb near Wang-tu dating from the Han period, which affords the earliest evidence of the existence of mural paintings in China proper.

The late 3d century, when the flood of northern tribes rose against the weak Chinese dynasties, marked the beginning of a very turbulent period for this province. The Hsiung-nu, Hsien-pi, and Mongol peoples ruled the north of China for a short while, then had to yield briefly to a Chinese dynasty (the Northern Yen, 409–36). The latter in its turn was forced to relinquish this territory for a very long time to the "barbarians." It was then that the powerful Northern Wei dynasty (386–535) first took possession of Hopei. In general, foreign dynasties favored Buddhism. The oldest dated specimen of Buddhist sculpture in China, a gilt-bronze figurine of the year 338, was made, according to its inscription, in the Hsiung-nu state ruled by the Chao dynasty. From the modest beginning represented by this figurine, which clearly shows its derivation from foreign styles, that of Gandhara (q.v.) in particular, there was created a tradition of great importance in the history of Chinese Buddhist art. In the region around Paoting (Tsingyuan) and Ting-chou there was to develop an important center of Buddhist sculpture recognizable not only from its local material (white micaceous marble), but also from its distinctive style, which developed quite independently of the more central regions of the realm.

Although too great importance should not be attached to the fact that the oldest specimen of gilt-bronze sculpture comes from this region, inasmuch as it is not possible to determine whether the survival of this single piece is a coincidence or not, the qualitative difference between the stone sculptures (e.g., a votive stele of A.D. 516 now in the University Museum of Philadelphia) and the bronze sculptures (including a Buddha of A.D. 536 in the same museum) is striking. In comparison it seems as if stone sculpture had not yet reached its full maturity. It may be expected that the great discovery of sculptural fragments at Ch'ü-yang in 1953 will, as soon as the reports on it are published, enable us to get a clearer idea of the sculpture of the Northern and Eastern Wei dynasties in this region. Among the dated pieces there are 12 from the Northern Wei period, dated between 520 and 533. If we consider the statistical data from this collection, consisting of 237 dated pieces, as a true reflection of the development of Buddhist sculpture in this area, then we may conclude that the development was very rapid after a somewhat hesitant start. No less than 43 dated pieces are from the extremely brief dynasty of the Eastern Wei (534–50), a quite significant number.

The downfall of the Eastern Wei placed Hopei under the rule of the dynasty of the Northern Ch'i, who established their capital at Yeh in Honan, just beyond the present provincial border. This dynasty reigned for only 27 years, but during this period Buddhist sculpture attained its first great affluence in this region, perhaps because the imperial house favored the Buddhists and persecuted the Taoists. This period marks the beginning of work on the caves of Hsiang-t'ang-shan, two great groups of temples, the most important sculptures of which were executed during the period of the Northern Ch'i. In this group the great standing figures of the Buddha and bodhisattvas are for the first time completely detached from the walls. Ting-chou, where a school of sculptors passed through the initial stage of their development, was perhaps the birthplace of the first great sculptures completely in the round and not destined for caves. Alongside the monumental standing figures of Buddha and bodhisattvas there are also many smaller sculptures, including groups of buddhas, bodhisattvas, and lohans against a background of trees, of a sort numerous among the Ch'ü-yang discoveries. By comparing the sculptures of the Northern Ch'i kingdom with those of the centers farther west, we can see clearly that it was the Northern Ch'i dynasty which set the standard and that a very important role was played by the workshops of Hopei. The discovery of the sculptures of Ch'ü-yang, containing 95 dated pieces from the brief dynasty of the Northern Ch'i and 77 from the equally brief period of the Sui dynasty (581–618), proves beyond all doubt that Buddhist sculpture occupied an important position in the art of that time. There is no doubt that during the T'ang dynasty Hopei lost its preeminence as a center for sculptures. In the period from the beginning of the T'ang to about 750, that is, up to the time when the temples of Ch'ü-yang were destroyed, there were few sculptures executed there. Only ten of these are dated.

It is probable, however, that the tradition of Buddhist sculpture in Hopei never completely died out, so that when the Khitans, who like the Wei before them favored Buddhism, arrived on the scene, there must still have existed a climate propitious for a remarkable renaissance of the antique styles. Everywhere in this province the religious activity of the Khitans is apparent. On Fang-shan, where there had long been a Buddhist center, but where the work of carving Buddhist sculptures in stone had been interrupted in 809, activities were resumed again in 1027. The Yün-chü-ssŭ was enlarged by the addition of several buildings, including two large pagodas. Pagodas in the pure Liao style, as found in Manchuria, are rare in Hopei. The style is here obviously influenced by contemporary Chinese architecture. As in other regions dominated by the Liao, very important monuments of architecture in wood have survived in Hopei. The most important of these are the gate and the Kuan-yin hall of the temple Tu-lo-ssŭ at Chi-hsien, and the main hall of the temple Kuang-chi-ssŭ at Pao-tu-hsien. These buildings, which doubtless owe their origin to the religious zeal of the Khitans, were, however, built in an area inhabited entirely by Chinese. The lack of an adequate number of surviving monuments from preceding periods or from the areas under Chinese domination, with which to make a comparison, renders it impossible to judge to what extent we may speak of Khitan influence on Buddhist architecture in this region. In other realms of art and culture too, a strong Chinese influence, as well as the strong admiration of the Khitans for Sung culture, is evident. From the kilns of Ting-chou, where the famous Ting-yao (Ting ware) was made, the Khitans took away a great number of potters when they invaded this region during the hostilities that preceded the Sino-Khitan treaty of 1005. These potters were put to work in various kilns in Manchuria and introduced into Liao pottery the ever more frequent use of a white glaze along with the three-colored technique which had been taken over indirectly, probably via contacts with the kingdom of P'o-hai. The official (kuan) pottery of the Liao (see below, Manchuria) was very much like the Ting-yao, clear evidence of the high esteem in which the Liao held Chinese pottery.

During the fairly long-lasting peace with the kingdom of Liao, the line of demarcation between Liao territory and the Sung realm divided the province of Hopei into two parts. The region north of the frontier passes, which the Liao quickly subjugated, remained solidly in their hands, and it was near the present-day city of Peking that their southern capital was founded. The Jurchen, conquering nearly all of northern China, also conquered Hopei, thus beginning a foreign domination of this province which the Mongols, in their turn, were to extend all over China.

How important China was to the great Mongol empire is evident from the fact that Kublai Khan, in contrast to the ancient custom, had himself proclaimed emperor in 1260 not at Karakorum but at the Chinese frontier. In 1264 he proclaimed Peking, which he called Khanbalik (i.e., "city of the Khan," the Cambaluc of Marco Polo), the capital of the Mongol empire. The description of the capital given by the famous Italian traveler does not, however, depict the city as it is known today. The Ming dynasty, which put an end to the Mongol domination, in the early days preferred Nanking as its capital, but at the ascension of Yung-lo to the throne in 1420, Peking again became the capital city. For Hopei it was important that Peking was to remain the capital until the end of the Chinese empire. At the time of the Manchu conquest (1644) the northern part of the city, which surrounds the inner Imperial City, was assigned to the Manchu banners; it retained, however, the character given it by Yung-lo, because of the rapid acculturation of the Manchus.

The recent administrative changes have brought within the territory of Hopei the part of former Jehol province which contains the city of Chengteh (Ch'êng-tê, formerly Jehol). This city with its many architectural monuments in the Tibetan style (see CHINESE ART, Later architecture) is perhaps even more characteristic of the style and grandeur of the Ch'ing emperors than the capital of Peking.

*Monuments and archaeological sites.* Wang-tu. While a mound was being leveled east of this city in 1952, a tomb built of brick was discovered. One of its chambers contained a series of interesting wall paintings dating from the Han period. The tomb, perfectly symmetrical in plan, has seven chambers. An antechamber, a central room, and a rear chamber are arranged from north to south, as is customary in such tombs, and connected by passageways, while the antechamber and central room both have lateral chambers on the east and the west side. The northern wall of the rear chamber, in which the coffin was placed, has a niche. The low, pointed arches of the corridors and of the vaults rest upon masonry walls in which horizontal and upright courses of brick alternate. The structure of the arches is like that of several other tombs of the same province and the same period, but here the walls of the antechamber and the corridor leading from it into the central room are covered with

wall paintings. The outlines are done in black and the surface areas in mineral colors, red, yellow, and green. Each wall is divided into two parts by a horizontal line 15 in. from the floor. The lower part is decorated with pictures of animals; the upper bears a number of portraits of petty officials, in which the features are strongly characterized. These portraits are accompanied by inscriptions indicating the rank and office of each. In the corridor leading from the antechamber to the western chamber, there is a poem in praise of the deceased, written in red on the wall, from which it appears that he lived during the Han dynasty. Some Chinese archaeologists date the tomb about the beginning of the Christian era, on the basis of the style of the script. Others, however, identify the deceased as Sun Ch'êng, marquis of Fou-yang, who died in A.D. 132. In view of the rarity of wall paintings in Han tombs found within the boundaries of China proper, this discovery is of paramount importance, in spite of its slight artistic merit.

BIBLIOG. Wang-tu Han-mu pi-hua (Wall Paintings of a Han Tomb at Wang-tu), Peking, 1955. K'ao-ku t'ang-hsin, 1958, no. 4, pp. 66–71.

Ch'ü-yang (Pai-chia-wan). In 1953, during the course of work near the pagoda southwest of the city where the temple Hsiu-tê-ssŭ once stood, a large number of damaged sculptures and small steles were dug up. The excavation of two wells located under Sung foundations has turned up no less than 2,659 sculptures, not too badly damaged, 237 of which have dated inscriptions. The earliest is of the year 520, the latest 750. A fair number are from the period of the Eastern Wei (43 pieces), the Northern Ch'i (95 pieces), and the Sui (77 pieces). The destruction is supposed to have occurred shortly after 750, during the fighting connected with the rebellion of An Lu-shan. Although only a small number of the sculptures are intact, this find, owing to the great number of dated pieces, is interesting; it provides us with a better understanding than was possible heretofore of the schools of sculpture in Hopei. Only a few specimens have so far been published.

BIBLIOG. Lo Fu-i, Ho-pei Ch'ü-yang-hsien ch'u-t'u ch'ing-li kung-tso chien-pao (Brief Report on the Excavations at Ch'ü-yang, Hopei), K'ao-ku t'ung-hsin, 1955, no. 3, pp. 34–8.

Hsiang-t'ang-shan. This mountain lies in the west of Hopei and in the north of Honan. In 1921, the Japanese D. Tokiwa discovered in two sites on this mountain a group of temples forming two complexes called Pei (northern) and Nan (southern) Hsiang-t'ang-shan. The former consists of three large and four smaller caves, plus a small number of niches. The system of numbering used by the Chinese (followed in this article) differs from that adopted by Sekino and Tokiwa, as well as from that of Mizuno and Nagahiro. Nos. III, IV, and VI (Sekino, Nos. II, III, IV, also called the south, central, and north caves) date from the Northern Ch'i period, 550–77. The excavation of these caves can be connected with the establishment of the capital of this dynasty at Yeh in Honan. The other caves are from the Sui period (Nos. I and II) or much later (e.g., No. V, dated 1524). Cave III has along all three sides a series of seven Buddhist figures: in the center, a seated buddha, flanked by two lohans, two bodhisattvas, and two Pratyeka buddhas (the name given to those buddhas who do not communicate their teachings to others). The sculptures are remarkable for their full round forms; they are carved out of the walls, but are virtually freestanding in the round. Visible above their heads are many small reliefs of buddhas in rows. Cave VI is the largest of the group. Here, too, a rectangular pillar, richly carved, has been cut out of the rock. Along the walls are huge images of buddhas, flanked by two bodhisattvas.

Nan Hsiang-t'ang-shan has two groups of caves; Nos. I and II are at a lower level, and Nos. III–VII are located higher up the mountain. No. I serves as the warehouse of a newspaper, while No. II is completely walled up. The neighboring Hsiang-t'ang-ssŭ is now the office of a local newspaper. The caves are very similar to those in the northern group in plan and in the reliefs adorning them. Of the great sculptures, now largely vanished, it is probable that three are those in the University Museum, Philadelphia (PL. 243). The very fine bas-reliefs of small figures which once filled the caves have for the most part been removed. Some are in foreign collections, as, for example, the magnificent Western Paradise (Sukhāvatī), now in the Freer Gallery of Art in Washington, D.C.

BIBLIOG. D. Tokiwa and T. Sekino, Shina Bukkyō Shiseki (Buddhist Monuments in China), III, Tokyo, 1926–38, pp. 41–58; S. Mizuno and T. Nagahiro, Kyōdōzan Sekkutsu (The Cave Temples of Hsiang-t'ang-shan), Kyoto, 1937; Lo Shu-tzu, Pei-ch'ao shih-k'u i-shu (The Art of the Cave Temples of the Northern Dynasties), Peking, 1955, pp. 187–217; L. Sickman and A. Soper, The Art and Architecture of China, Harmondsworth, 1956, pp. 54–7.

Yün-chü-ssŭ. This temple, standing on Fang-shan, was very famous in the history of Chinese Buddhism because of the *sūtras* incised there on stone slabs first during the Sui and T'ang periods,

from 605 to 809, and later again during the Liao period, from 1027 to 1094. About 2,700 of these slabs are at present conserved in the caves on Shih-ching-shan, an eastern crest of Fang-shan.

On each of the five summits of Shih-ching-shan (also known as Hsiao-hsi-t'ien or "Little India"), a pagoda has been erected. The one on the central summit is a one-story structure, nearly cubic in shape. It is covered by a tiled roof with a richly sculptured acroterium. The rectangular entrance opening to the interior is flanked by two bas-reliefs of lokapalas and is framed by a pointed arch.

There are a great number of pagodas in this locality, some dating from the T'ang, others from the Liao period. On the southern summit of Shih-ching-shan is a nine-story pagoda built of limestone slabs on a square ground plan. Its structure is very similar to that of the pagoda on the central summit. The main difference is that the cubic first story is surmounted by a series of blind stories, accentuated by cornices of projecting stone slabs. Buildings of this type, of which several are found in the grounds of the temple Yün-chü-ssŭ, are not really architectural monuments, but are rather models on a reduced scale of larger brick pagodas. Four of these miniature pagodas, dating from the second and third decades of the 8th century, are placed at the corners of the terrace on which stands the large Pei-t'a ("northern pagoda"), dating from the Liao period. Some contain other sculptures besides the bas-reliefs executed on the walls.

The Pei-t'a, also called Hung-t'a ("red pagoda"), represents a style seldom met with in Liao architecture, and one distinct from that of the Nan-t'a in this complex, which is of the usual Hopei Liao type. The lower part consists of a high shaft divided into two stories and has an octagonal ground plan. It stands on a richly sculptured, lotus-shaped foundation. The façades which face the cardinal points of the compass have arched doors or arched recesses, while the intervening façades have window frames and pilasters. The building is crowned by an unusual superstructure, consisting of a dome and spire, reminiscent of lamaistic architecture. The date usually accepted for this monument is 1117, the same as that for the Nan-t'a. Although the structure of the two-story shaft is similar to that of other Liao monuments, the possibility that the upper parts were later rebuilt in a different style should not be excluded.

The Nan-t'a ("southern pagoda"; PL. 273) in this complex is of a Liao type which is found again elsewhere in Hopei. Its main difference from the Manchurian pagodas is that the first story is left without sculptural decoration. It has been reported that several of the monuments here were damaged during World War II.

BIBLIOG. O. Sirén, A History of Early Chinese Art, IV: Architecture, London, 1930, pp. 47, 50; D. Tokiwa and T. Sekino, Shina Bukkyō Shiseki (Buddhist Monuments in China), III, Tokyo, 1926–38, pp. 59–72; Wên-wu ts'an-k'ao tzŭ-liao, 1955, no. 9, pp. 48–53; L. Sickman and A. Soper, The Art and Architecture of China, Harmondsworth, 1956, pp. 240, 272, 274.

Lung-hsing-ssŭ. This temple, situated in the eastern section of the city of Chêng-ting, was founded on its present site in 971. It consists of a considerable number of buildings of architectural and sculptural importance.

Of paramount interest is the Fo-hsiang-ko, a large, three-story building of Sung date, extensively restored in 1703, and already almost reduced to ruins before World War II. Inside this building a colossal bronze figure of Kuan-yin, over 40 ft. high, stands on a stone pedestal. It is of the same date as the building which was erected around it and is likewise in poor condition. The head of the statue has been restored, and all but two of the separately cast arms, which originally numbered 42, have been lost. The front of the pedestal is sheathed in richly sculptured marble. High reliefs in clay, probably dating from about 1000, were made on the walls of the Fo-hsiang-ko. The scene on the east wall, representing the Bodhisattva Samantabhadra traveling through the air with a host of celestial beings, is the best preserved. The beautiful Kuan-yin which formerly adorned one of the walls (see Sirén, loc. cit. below, pl. 3, 1) seems to have disappeared.

Behind the Fo-hsiang-ko there are two pavilions of similar architecture, a *sūtra* library and the Maitreya hall. Both are provided with a balcony on the second story, which is protected by an extra pent roof. The revolving bookcase contained in the *sūtra* library is an interesting example of the reproduction of architectural details, such as the elaborate bracketing system, in a miniature model. Its date is somewhat uncertain; Soper places it in the 11th century, whereas Sekino and Tokiwa consider it to be of the Ch'ing period.

The last of the important early buildings of this temple is the square Mo-ni-tien (Maṇi hall), which according to Soper may antedate the Fo-hsiang-ko, but which Japanese experts have dated about 1050. The fact that it has an entrance on all four sides is its most unusual architectural feature.

The main hall, which had fallen into ruins when Sekino and Tokiwa visited the temple, and which stood on a line with the Mo-ni-tien and the Fo-hsiang-ko, has now been completely torn down, like the bell and drum towers, which were only recently demolished.

BIBLIOG. D. Tokiwa and T. Sekino, Shina Bukkyō Shiseki (Buddhist Monuments in China), IV, Tokyo, 1926–38, pp. 82–8; O. Sirén, Chinese Sculptures of the Sung, Liao, and Chin Dynasties, BMFEA, XIV, 1942, pp. 45–65; L. Sickman and A. Soper, The Art and Architecture of China, Harmondsworth, 1956, pp. 261–4.

Wu-t'a-ssŭ (Temple of the Five Pagodas). The official name of this temple, standing near Peking, is Ta-chêng-chia-ssŭ. It is notable for its unusual architecture, inspired by that of the Mahābodhi temple at Bodhgaya, in India. The building, which is named after the five pagodas standing on top of it, was built in 1437 at the suggestion of the Tibetan monk Paṇḍita. The five pagodas, surrounded by a balustrade, stand on a square terrace foundation about 50 ft. long and 38 ft. high, which consists of a plinth surmounted by five superimposed friezes of equal height, accentuated by straight cornices. The five friezes are formed of rows of sculptures in relief, representing seated Buddhist figures, separated from one another by decorated columns. In contrast with the temple of Bodhgaya, in which the central pagoda is much higher than the other four, here the central pagoda with its 13 stories rises only slightly higher than those standing at the corners, which are 11 stories high. The pagodas, built like the Bodhgaya prototype on a square ground plan, are covered with reliefs. Another building of almost identical architecture near Peking, at the Pi-yün-ssŭ, is of later date (1748).

BIBLIOG. D. Tokiwa and T. Sekino, Shina Bukkyō Shiseki (Buddhist Monuments in China), V, Tokyo, 1938, pp. 157–60.

The Chü-yung-kuan (gate). This gate (PL. 279) stands near the town of Nan-k'ou, where the main highway from Peking to Kalgan crosses the Great Wall. The round arch frame on the façade is decorated with reliefs. The walls and ceiling of the vault, however, have been leveled off so as to form three flat planes which have been adorned with reliefs covering the entire interior of the gate passage. This type of vaulting, also found in Chinese bridges, makes this gate of great architectural interest, and the reliefs make it a monument of supreme importance in the art of the period, since, together with the sculptures of Hangchow, in Chekiang, they are the best known of the few remaining examples of Yüan sculpture. In perfect agreement with the trend of Buddhism in those times, these sculptures are strongly influenced by Tantric Buddhism (see BUDDHISM). The reliefs of the arched frame represent figures familiar from Tibetan and Nepalese art (qq.v.). In the center we see a Garuḍa (mythical bird) flanked by nagas (Skr., nāga, water spirit), a pair of makaras (fantastic aquatic animals), and two elephants. In the passage there are a great number of Buddhist images in relief. These representations terminate at the two exits of the gate in four panels depicting the four lokapalas, which are really the masterpieces of this monument. On the ceiling are four mandalas (magic diagrams) and numerous inscriptions in Sanskrit, Chinese, Tibetan, Tangut, and Uigur, as well as a number of dhāraṇīs (magic formulas) written in Phags-pa script. The monument was probably built in 1345, as one inscription suggests. In Chinese sources, however, it is stated that 1326 was the year in which the dhāraṇīs were inscribed. Originally there was a stupa on top of the gate, surrounded by balustrades of carved marble at the edge of the wall; today only the latter remain.

BIBLIOG. D. Tokiwa and T. Sekino, Shina Bukkyō Shiseki (Buddhist Monuments in China), V, Tokyo, 1938, pp. 148–52.

The Great Wall. Under the reign of the first emperor of China, Shih Huang-ti of the Ch'in dynasty (221–206 B.C.), the walls which had been built in the late Chou period by the smaller northern states as a defense against barbarian invasions from the north were joined together into one great system. The impressive monument (PL. 285) in existence today is not, however, the same as that erected by the great emperor, nor can it boast of such great age.

From Shanhaikwan on the Hopei coast to Chia-yü-kuan in the western part of Kansu province, the Great Wall has a length almost equal to the distance from Paris to Istanbul. Intended to protect several strategic points, trade routes, and frontiers, it follows a highly irregular course. North of Peking, near Nan-k'ou, there is a northern branch which extends into northern Shansi. At present it follows the borders of the Ordos region beyond the Yellow River, but formerly there was still another system of walls north of the great bend of the Yellow River (see below, Shansi). At the points crossed by great trade routes gates were set up. The largest of these gates are: near Shanhaikwan (Shan-hai-kuan) on the route to Manchuria; near Ku-pei-k'ou on the road to former Jehol; the Chü-yung-kuan (see above) on the road to Kalgan; on the road to Urga; the Yên-mên-kuan on the route to Mongolia via Shansi; and, lastly, the Chia-yü-kuan on the road to Central Asia.

The structure, the building material used, and the state of preservation of the wall vary greatly from one place to another because the transportation problem required the builders to avail themselves of local materials or those available within a short distance. In several localities, particularly in western China, there is simply an earthen wall, but elsewhere, particularly in Hopei, the sand and rock filling of the wall are sheathed in brick reinforced with a plinth of square stone blocks. On top of the wall a paved road was built, 16 ft. wide, between battlements about 5 ft. high. At the base the wall is about 20 ft. thick. Towers placed at irregular intervals rise about 13 ft. above the walls. In view of the somewhat different architectural structure of these towers, it has been conjectured that they had been built as fortified strong points before the construction of the walls and were later joined together. It is probable that the best-preserved parts of the wall date back to the early Ming period (14th century).

BIBLIOG. W. E. Geil, The Great Wall of China, London, 1909; L. N. Hayes, The Great Wall of China, Shanghai, 1929; O. Sirén, A History of Early Chinese Art, IV: Architecture, London, 1930, pp. 3–6.

Peking (Pei-ching; officially named Peiping in 1928). The city of Peking, capital of the Chinese empire after the Ming emperor Yung-lo transferred his residence from Nanking to the north in 1420, was constructed upon the remains of many earlier cities. The oldest of these, the location and extent of which it has been possible to determine with some accurancy, is the T'ang city of Yu-chou, which was relatively small in extent. Its northern part was probably situated in the southwestern corner of what is called the "Tartar City." Nan-ching, the southern capital of the Khitans, embraced the western part of the present "Chinese City" as well as an area which is now completely outside the walls of Peking. Under the domination of the Jurchen, when the central capital (Chung-tu) was located here, the city extended toward the east until it occupied all of the Chinese City and a large area to the west and south of the present walls. After the annihilation of the Jurchen by the Mongols (1264) a new capital was built, occupying the larger part of the present Tartar City and a broad area north of it.

When the emperor Yung-lo established his imperial capital here, it marked the beginning of a period of great progress and architectural activity for Peking. In the early days of the Ming dynasty the town occupied the area of the Yüan city, but during this period many people settled upon the remains of the Jurchen and Khitan capitals south of the walls. In 1564 this part was at last fortified with a system of walls and incorporated into the city, which thus attained the limits it has maintained up to the present day. At the time of the arrival of the Manchus the original city, i.e., the northern part, was completely reserved for the Manchu banners (hence the name "Tartar City"), while the southern extension became known as the "Chinese City."

As a result of its history of erratic growth without planning, the city of Peking does not have that rigorously symmetrical layout on an axis familiar to us from such cities as Ch'ang-an (see below, Shensi). Despite its lack of such symmetry, the northern quarter, or Tartar City, has a predominantly square plan, determined by the three concentric rectangles formed by (1) the outer walls, (2) the imperial enclosure, forming the so-called "Imperial City," and (3) the walls of the imperial compounds, which were closed for centuries to foreigners and hence called the "Forbidden City." This complex of walled palaces, audience halls, and gates is not situated, as was the case in Ch'ang-an, on the northern side of the residential center, but a little to the south of it. The road leading into it, running north and south, with imposing gates, is not exactly in the center but slightly west of the central north–south axis of the city.

A wall divides the Tartar City from the Chinese City. The latter developed only half as far as the former in a north–south direction, but extends farther east and west.

In the Chinese City two altars are to be found which played an important role in the annual Imperial Rites. Within two enclosures (roughly 4 miles and 3 miles in circumference respectively) stands the Altar of Heaven (T'ien-t'an), surrounded by double walls, the outer one square, the inner one circular. Richly decorated gates of honor (p'ai-lou) give access by roads running in the direction of the four cardinal points to the altar itself. This consists of three round terraces, one above the other, each more than 5 ft. high and respectively about 210, 151, and 92 ft. in diameter. These terraces are covered with marble slabs and surrounded by sculptured balustrades. The altar, where the emperor annually offered sacrifices to heaven, was erected by Yung-lo about 1420, but owes its present form to a radical restoration effected under Ch'ien-lung in 1754. North of the Altar of Heaven, on a marble terrace, is the Ch'i-nien-tien (Hall of the Annual Prayers), a round temple rebuilt early in the 20th century, with a triple roof covered with blue tiles. This structure, which many have erroneously considered to be the Temple of Heaven itself, is really unimportant, despite its imposing size, from either the ritual or architectural viewpoint. West of the Temple of Heaven, inside a similar enclosure, stands the complex of buildings known

as the Temple of Agriculture (Hsien-nung-t'an), where each year the emperor performed the ritual plowing.

The Altar for the Adoration of the Earth, the counterpart to the Altar of Heaven, is situated outside the north wall of the city. Laid out on a quadrangular plan, it consists of a terrace with steps, on two levels, about 105 ft. and 56 ft. in length.

The western wall of the Imperial City extends farther west than perfect symmetry would allow. This irregularity may perhaps be explained by the desire to include three artificial lakes and their

The Ch'ien-mên provides access to the Tartar City, whence a road interrupted only by the Chung-hua gate leads to a wide square. From there, entrance into the Imperial City is gained by crossing five marble bridges over a small stream and passing through a gate, the T'ien-an-mên. To the right and left, concealed behind high walls, were the T'ai-miao and the Shê-chi-t'an. The latter, the Altar of Earth and Agriculture, is now a park, but the T'ai-miao, where ancestor worship was practiced, is still a grandiose architectural complex. After its reconstruction in 1464, it seems to have undergone

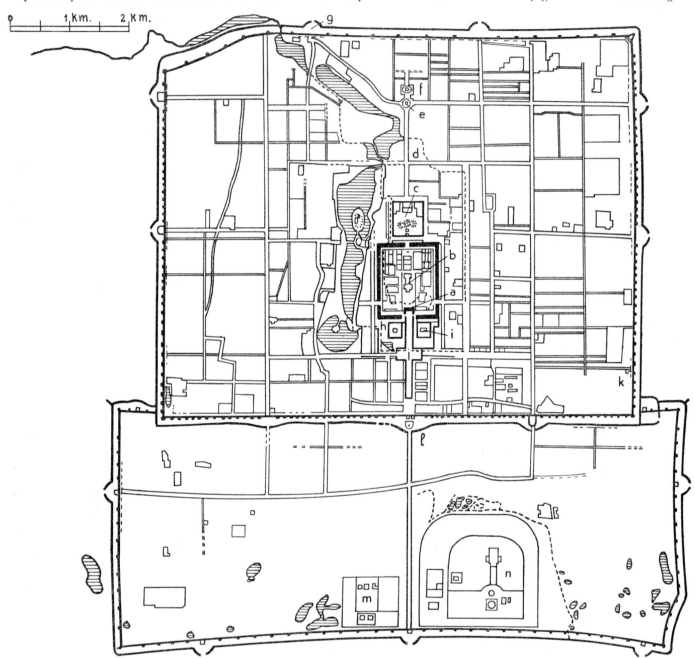

Plan of present-day Peking within the walls of the 15th and 16th cent. Forbidden City: (*a*) Wu-mên, entrance gate; (*b*) San-ta-tien; (*c*) Prospect Hill. Tartar City: (*d*) Hou-mên; (*e*) Drum Tower; (*f*) Bell Tower; (*g*) Tê-shêng-mên; (*h*) Central Park (formerly Shê-chi-t'an); (*i*) Working People's Palace of Culture (formerly T'ai-miao); (*j*) T'ien-an-mên square; (*k*) Observatory; (*l*) Ch'ien-mên, entrance gate. Chinese City: (*m*) Temple of Agriculture; (*n*) area of the Temple of Heaven (*after Willetts*).

islands within the imperial enclosure. Under the Manchus a part of this area was not completely closed to the public, as was the Forbidden City, the heart of the Imperial City and of the entire empire.

From the Yung-ting gate (Yung-ting-mên), in the southern part of the Chinese City, to the Bell and Drum Towers in the northern section of the Tartar City, Peking is crossed by a main north–south axial road, interrupted only by the buildings of the Forbidden City and the so-called "Prospect Hill," which is supposed to protect it against the maleficent influences from the north. Access to the various quarters traversed by this artery is cut off by imposing gates.

few alterations. It is laid out like a palace with three buildings standing on a north–south axis.

The Wu-mên, a monumental gate with two salient wings massively constructed, surmounted by five buildings, gives admittance to the Forbidden City itself. The plan of this gate is a repetition of the others previously noted. The visitor then passes again over the small Chin-shui-ho via five small bridges, and through the T'ai-ho gate, to reach the most grandiose and representative architectural group of buildings in Peking, the San-ta-tien, or "three great halls," which date from the late 18th century. The largest of these buildings,

which stands on a marble terrace, is the T'ai-ho-tien, a pavilion for audiences. The square central hall, or Chung-ho-tien, is much smaller. The building farthest north is the Pao-ho-tien, for imperial guests.

The architecture of the Ming and Ch'ing periods in Peking (PL. 293) is so impressive, particularly in the Forbidden City, that its architectonic decadence, easily seen when each building is studied by itself, is not at first glance apparent. Peking, created by Yung-lo and transformed later, particularly by K'ang-hsi (1662–1722) and Ch'ien-lung (1736–95), today gives an impression of truly imperial magnificence. The ensemble of palaces, gates, and buildings, beautiful in its variety and studied effects, and the impressive scale of the official buildings and palaces effectively mask the weakness of the stagnant architecture of the period. The decorations, the balustrades of sculptured marble, and the dazzling colors of the tiles distract us and temper our judgment.

Not only inside the city but outside it as well (PLS. 285, 286, 294) are many monuments commemorating the glory of the great Ming and Manchu emperors. Toward the north, not far from Nan-k'ou, stand the tombs of 13 Ming emperors, particularly famous for the colossal animal sculptures lining the road of approach. Very recently the tomb of Wan-li was opened, yielding numerous objects of great importance. For further detail see CHINESE ART, *Later architecture*.

BIBLIOG. G. Bouillard, Pékin et ses environs, Peking, 1922–25; O. Sirén, The Imperial Palaces of Peking, Paris, Brussels, 1926; D. Tokiwa and T. Sekino, Shina Bukkyō Shiseki (Buddhist Monuments in China), V, Tokyo, 1938; O. Sirén, A History of Early Chinese Art, IV: Architecture, London, 1930; L. C. Arlington and W. Lewisohn, In Search of Old Peking (guide with bibliography), Peiping, 1935.

*Kiln sites*. Ting-chou. This was the center where the renowned Ting-yao (Ting ware), a white porcelain with incised or molded decoration, was produced. Remains of kilns dating from the Sung period have been located by F. Koyama near the villages Chien-tz'ŭ-ts'un and Yen-shan-ts'un, north of Ch'ü-yang. The Ting-yao discovered in the first of these villages is superior to that of the second in quality. Koyama's investigations have also demonstrated the existence of the Red and the Black Ting ware mentioned in Chinese sources, which probably refer to types of Ting ware coated with a blackish-brown and a red-brown glaze and sometimes retaining traces of gold decoration, as found here. After the Khitan invasion some of the potters moved to Ch'i-chou in Kiangsi. Most of the fragments found by Koyama bear incised decoration. Molded designs are so rare that the specimens which have such decoration may perhaps be attributed to southern Chinese kilns.

During the Liao dynasty potters from the Ting-yao kilns were put to work at the kilns of Manchuria, as is evident from the great quantity of fragments of excellent imitation Ting-yao found there.

BIBLIOG. Sekai Tōji Zenshū (Ceramic Art of the World), X, Tokyo, 1955, pp. 210–6; J. M. Plumer, The Ting-yao Kiln Sites: Koyama's Significant Discoveries, Arch. Chin. Art Soc. Am., III, 1948–49, pp. 61–9; S. E. Lee, Sung Ceramics in the Light of Recent Japanese Research, Artibus Asiae, XI, 1948, pp. 166–7.

Tz'ŭ-chou (Tz'ŭ Chou). This is the center for production of the Tz'ŭ-chou-yao (Tz'ŭ-chou or Tz'ŭ Chou ware), a type of pottery covered with a slip and decorated in widely varying ways. This ware was probably manufactured, not only in Tz'ŭ-chou, which is still today a very busy ceramic center in southern Hopei, but also in many other places in northern China under the Sung, Yüan, and Ming dynasties. (See CERAMICS; PLS. 166, 169, 258–260.) In 1941 F. Koyama visited the village of P'eng-ch'eng-chên in the district of Tz'ŭ-chou, where there is a group of kilns. There he discovered the remains of a Sung kiln with many fragments, but the material collected was largely lost in Tokyo during the war.

BIBLIOG. Sekai Tōji Zenshū (Ceramic Art of the World), X, Tokyo, 1955, pp. 224–6; S. E. Lee, Sung Ceramics in the Light of Recent Japanese Research, Artibus Asiae, XI, 1948, pp. 169–70.

HUNAN (Hu-nan), HUPEH (Hupei, Hu-pei), KIANGSI (Chianghsi). *Survey of geography and art history*. This territory, which is traversed from west to east by the Yangtze River, consists of the basins of three great rivers which all flow together here, the Han River in Hupeh, the Hsiang in Hunan, and the Kan in Kiangsi. The area is surrounded by hills and mountains and is divided into three parts corresponding to the basins of these three rivers.

At a very early period this region, through its excellent waterways, came within the sphere of Chinese cultural influence. Even before World War II, many relics of antiquity had been discovered in the marshes near the city of Changsha (in archaeology, usually transliterated Ch'ang-sha), providing a glimpse into the culture of the Ch'u kingdom, which, during the late Chou period, ruled over a large part of the present-day provinces of Hunan and Anhwei. Some of the distinctive traits of the Ch'u culture were already known

from literature, but that the arts and crafts of this region had such a special local character was first apparent from the discoveries of the years 1936–37.

It is highly probable that Ch'u culture arose from the mingling of northern and southern cultures. The Shang and Chou peoples must have contributed to its formation, probably through the immigration of Chinese from the north. It seems probable that this influence was exerted also during the reign of the Shang and not only under the Chou, considering the finds made in 1957–58 in the vicinity of Hankow and Wuchang, in Hupeh. The bronzes found there are very similar to the Shang bronzes from Êrh-li-kang (see above, *Honan*), which date from the pre-An-yang period. Unfortunately the circumstances under which this find was made are not quite clear. The bronze bells of the early Chou period which were found in the environs of Chung-hsiang, on the banks of the Han River, clearly demonstrate the early date of the importation of the bronze culture into this area and make clear that it preceded by many centuries the flourishing of bronze casting during the late Chou period. Ch'ang-sha in its heyday was an important center of Ch'u art and from many points of view can be considered at least equal in artistic standing to the centers in northern China. The fall of the Ch'u state, shortly before the unification of China under the aegis of Shih Huang-ti (3d century B.C.), did not, however, signify the end of the artistic influence of Ch'u. It is apparent today that it played an important part in the formation of Han culture.

In neither Hunan nor Hupeh have many important cultural remains from later ages been preserved. This is at least partly due to the devastations attending the Taiping rebellion.

Kiangsi province, on the contrary, was extremely prominent in the annals of Chinese ceramics. Its fame was not due solely to Ching-tê-chên, the great porcelain manufacturing center, which is located there. In sources as early as the T'ang period mention is made of the various types of Kiangsi ceramics then existing. The great development and expansion of the kilns began first, however, under the Sung dynasty. With the arrival of potters from north China after the fall of Kaifeng (1127), this development was given great impetus.

BIBLIOG. W. B. Honey, The Ceramic Art of China and Other Countries of the Far East, London, 1944; S. E. Lee Sung Ceramics in the Light of Recent Japanese Research, Artibus Asiae, XI, 1948, pp. 166–8; Chiang Yuen-yi, The Ch'u Tribe and Its Art, Shanghai, 1949–50; K'ao-ku t'ung-hsin, 1958, no. 1, pp. 56–8, no. 9, pp. 72–3.

*Archaeological sites*. Ch'ang-sha (Changsha). Numerous tombs dating from the Chou period and later were discovered at Ch'ang-sha and its vicinity, in Hunan, in 1936 in the course of excavations. Among the material found in these tombs was a great quantity of exquisite lacquer work, several fine wooden sculptures, jades, and bronzes, mostly dating from the late Chou period, at which time this region was still a part of the Ch'u kingdom.

Among the spectacular discoveries made before World War II is a wooden object, probably a drum stand, consisting of two cranes standing upon two intertwined serpents (PL. 226), now in the Cleveland Museum of Art. In the spring of 1949 a truly sensational find was made in the southeastern suburb of the modern city, where a fragment of a painting on silk was recovered in quite good condition; this depicts a female figure accompanied by a phoenix and a dragon and is without doubt the oldest Chinese painting on silk in existence. It may go back to as early as the 5th century B.C. and is not later than the 3d century B.C.

Beginning in 1951 extensive archaeological exploration was carried out in and around Ch'ang-sha. The work concentrated, especially in 1951 and 1952, on the area around Wu-chia-ling, slightly north of the city, and in Yang-chia-ta-shan and Shih-tzŭ-ling to the southeast. During these excavations, continued in successive years, more than a thousand late Chou tombs were found for historical and art-historical research.

Because of the extremely damp climate prevailing in this region, most tombs were found to be in a poor state of preservation. Sometimes, however, the outer coffin of the tomb had been sealed off with a fine white clay, and in these tombs most objects were almost perfectly preserved. The various *ming-ch'i* (funerary objects) usually were deposited between the inner and outer coffin, both of which in most of these tombs were solidly constructed in a technique showing a highly developed carpenter's craft.

Among the funerary objects there was a great quantity of plain and painted pottery, usually of such poor quality as to have been unsuitable for daily use. The number of bronze vessels, swords, and mirrors, the last mostly of Karlgren's Shou-chou types (see CHINESE ART, *Chou peiod*) was considerable. Swords and halberds were numerous. Two of the spearheads found were inscribed with a great number of archaic characters (as yet for the most part undecipherable), often repeated in rows. Very unusual is a bronze with an engraved design on the inside composed of birds, trees, and fig-

ures. Although the design is well known from other excavated pieces, this is the first instance of inside decoration found so far. A great quantity of lacquer work was found, including such objects as an armrest, a 23-stringed musical instrument of the *sê* type, tables, shields, and boxes for cosmetics. Of great historic interest is the find of a Chinese brush, by far the oldest discovered to date. These excavations are of great importance for establishing the chronology of Ch'u art, because the construction of the tombs often offers a clue to their approximate date.

BIBLIOG. J. H. Cox, An Exhibition of the Antiquities from Ch'ang-sha, Gallery of Fine Arts, Yale University, New Haven, 1939; Chiang Yuen-yi, The Ch'u Tribe and Its Art, Shanghai, 1949–50; Ch'ang-sha fa-chüeh pao-kao (A Report on Excavation at Ch'ang-sha), Peking, 1957; Ch'ang-sha Ch'u-mu (The Ch'u Tombs of Ch'ang-sha), K'ao-ku hsüeh-pao, 1959, no. 1, pp. 41–60.

*Kiln sites.* Yung-ho. Brankston's investigations proved, shortly before World War II, that the Sung pottery known by antique dealers as "Kian Temmoku" came from Yung-ho, near Kian (Ch'i-an) in central Kiangsi. He found a multitude of fragments of a light-brown or gray hard pottery having a "hare's fur" glaze with a stenciled decoration of flowers, phoenixes, medallions, and leaves.

Ching-tê-chên. According to some sources, as early as the Han period potters worked in this ceramic center near Fou-liang, in Kiangsi. The fragments found by Brankston in the vicinity of Ching-tê-chên, at Hsiang-hu, Hu-t'ien, and Nan-shan, show that in the T'ang period a type of pottery resembling the Yüeh-yao was manufactured there. At that time the kilns were in all probability located very close to the best clay deposits in the hills outside the city. According to some sources, early in the 11th century (1004–07) pottery was manufactured which was intended for the imperial court, but the great imperial factory of porcelain, which throughout the entire Ming period dominated all Chinese pottery production, was not built before 1369. This was located on the Pearl Mountain (Chu-shan), in the center of modern Ching-tê-chên. Everywhere, both within and without the village, a great quantity of porcelain fragments have been found, and in the village itself fragments of imperial blue-and-white were discovered, with marks of the Chêng-tê and Hsüan-tê periods. Near Hu-t'ien, Brankston discovered several dumps of potsherds. The more westerly dumps contained many blue-and-white shards, as well as fragments of the Ying-ch'ing ware. Farther east, the blue-and-white shards were scarcer, while the Ying-ch'ing fragments increased. Near Nan-shan, adjacent to the deposits of Ying-ch'ing fragments, other fragments of the bluish Shu-fu porcelain of the Yüan period have been found. Through these discoveries the provenance of this pottery, made on official order, was established.

BIBLIOG. A. D. Brankston, An Excursion to Ching-tê-chên and Chi-an-fu in Ksiangsi, Tr. O. Ceramic Soc., XVI, 1938–9, pp. 19–32; Ching-tê-chên t'ao-tzŭ shih-k'ao (A History of the Pottery from Ching-tê-chên), Peking, 1959.

KANSU (Kan-su). *Survey of geography and art history.* In the region between the Tibetan mountains and the Mongolian steppes there is a series of parallel mountainous ridges, the Southern Mountains (Nan-shan). On reaching the Ordos plateau one range veers northeast while the other continues to the east to form the Chinling Mountains. Between the Tibetan plateau and the borders of the Mongolian steppes winds a natural highway which follows the valleys between mountains and connects the plains of northern China with the Tarim Basin in Central Asia. This province of northeastern China, which on one side belongs to the loess region and on the other forms part of the Mongolian steppes and is traversed by mountains, is particularly important because of the routes of communication which cross it, and is also remarkable for its extremely interesting monuments. In the eastern part of the present Kansu province, in the upper reaches of the Wei River and its tributary the Ching-ho, there flourished the neolithic Red Pottery culture or the Yang-shao culture, so called after the site in Honan where it was first found. The distribution of this culture extended from Kansu deep into the central plain of northern China, where it contributed to the formation of the culture of the Shang kingdom. (See CHINESE ART, *Neolithic.*)

Archaeology has been unable to answer the question as to whether the Chou people had their origin in this region. During the long Chou period, and the following Ch'in empire, only the eastern part of Kansu came within the Chinese cultural sphere. In 1955 there was unearthed at Kan-ch'üan-hsiang, in the Tienshui area, a fine bronze of the *kuei* type dating from the early Chou period, but no other bronzes of that period have so far been discovered in this area. In many sites along the Wei River, however, Chou pottery has been found.

The Great Wall of Shih Huang-ti put a large part of Kansu outside the Chinese cultural sphere and left the territory in the hands of the barbarians, the Hsiung-nu, whose descendants (the Huns) were later to ravage the Western world. During the Han period the Kansu corridor acquired great military and strategic importance because of the Chinese expansionist policy. The Hsiung-nu were the strongest enemies of the Han armies. They expelled the blue-eyed Yüeh-chih (Yuechi) and drove them westward so that they came to play an important role in the history of India as well as China.

The victorious armies of the Han emperors brought Kansu into the Chinese community. Chinese colonies within and around the military garrisons were transformed into centers along the trade routes uniting China with India and the Middle East via Central Asia. The Great Wall of China (see above, *Hopei*) had been completed and now protected the road traversing the whole of Kansu against attacks from the north.

In the turbulent centuries following the downfall of the Han empire, the various ruling houses succeeded one another with astonishing speed. During this period Buddhism became established in China. In Kansu this religion has left an abundance of monuments of great cultural interest, of which numerous cave temples are the most impressive. Whereas the cultural history of other provinces has to be reconstructed by studying a great variety of remains, we can follow the history of Kansu simply by looking at the colorful wall paintings of the cave temples. Not only the variance in styles, but also the continual changes in the costumes and appearance of the accurately portrayed Buddhists bear witness that in the shifting political history of the region the Buddhist sanctuaries always remained centers for the pious believers in the common faith.

Literary evidence proves that the first cave temples originated in the late 4th century, but the oldest group that is well preserved and can be accurately dated is of a considerably later period. Cave temples were built on a large scale throughout all northern China and were decorated with paintings and sculpture during the reign of the Northern Wei dynasty (386–535). Recent researches have shown that some early caves in Kansu may date from the Western Liang period (401–21). Cave temples existed throughout Kansu, from Tun-huang, in the far west, to the Wang-chia-k'ou group on the Shensi border.

Compared to similar temples in other places farther east, at Yün-kang in Shansi, Lung-mên in Honan, and many other places, most of the Kansu cave temples show traits that give them a typically regional character. In part this special character can be explained by the close contacts of Kansu with the monastic communities located along the Central Asian caravan routes. The cave temples of Central Asia evidently served as models for the Buddhists of Kansu.

Decisive for the architecture of cave temples was the fact that in Kansu, as in the Tarim Basin, there was a dearth of stone suitable for executing sculptures in the round or in relief as in Yün-kang and Lung-mên. The extremely soft sandstone made it possible to hollow out caves, but the sculptors could in most cases only cut out the rough shape of the sculptures, which were later finished with clay, and utilize molds, with or without wooden armatures. Both artistically and quantitively, sculpture remained on a subordinate level in Kansu. Painting was more important. The natural material was ideally suited for this, inasmuch as the soft walls could easily be smoothed off.

The oldest caves with wall paintings in Kansu probably date from the 5th century, but the first small groups of cave temples, which later developed into gigantic complexes, were begun even earlier in many places. The style of the paintings was highly reminiscent of Central Asian models, with many stylistic elements derived from the Buddhist art of Gandhara (q.v.).

The Sui period (581–618) was quickly followed by the rise of the T'ang dynasty (618–906), which dominated not only Kansu, but also a large part of Central Asia, and the golden age for these temples began. China not only welcomed and adapted foreign styles in the decoration of these caves but extended as well the influence of its own art, as is unmistakable from the paintings in the cave temples of the monastic communities of Turfan (q.v.).

When the T'ang dynasty declined, the Tun-huang complex had already nearly reached its largest development; succeeding generations demonstrated their faith only through embellishment of the existing caves. The Tungus (Hsi-hsia kingdom), who held a large part of Kansu under their sway from the end of the 10th century till the arrival of Genghis Khan, were very devout Buddhists, but their contribution to the art of the cave temples was very modest. When in 1227–28 Genghis Khan and his Mongolian horsemen put an end to the reign of the Hsi-hsia, the Tantric Buddhist cult quickly invaded the temples, and the mandalas of Tantric Buddhism (see BUDDHISM) made their first appearance along with the first application of the true fresco technique.

It seems that with the coming of the Hsi-hsia the Chinese monks were forced to flee, hiding their books and pictures. This signified the end of the golden age of Tun-huang, and elsewhere the decline came almost simultaneously. Although not all the temples were abandoned at that time, their importance as religious centers declined.

After Tibetan Buddhism (Lamaism) definitively replaced the other religious sects, leaving its imprint all over north China with its ubiquitous stupas, Islam infiltrated Kansu. One of Kublai Khan's nephews, a governor of Kansu who greatly favored the new religion, lost his life in an attempt to seize the imperial throne (1307). Nevertheless, Islam continued to be an important factor from that time on, without, however, leading to the appearance of new art forms.

During World War II the study of Tun-huang was intensively encouraged and since then has gone forward at an ever accelerating pace. Also of great interest are the discovery and description of several vast complexes which, although not comparable with Tun-huang as to their state of preservation, have still provided important material for art history.

BIBLIOG. A. Stein, Ruins of Desert Cathay, Personal Narrative of Exploration in Central Asia, 2 vols., London, 1912; A. Stein, Serindia, 5 vols., Oxford, 1921.

*Cave temples*. Tun-huang. (See also the article TUN-HUANG.) On the boundary between China proper and Chinese Turkistan (Sinkiang), 13 miles southeast of the town of Tun-huang, on the flanks of Ming-sha-shan, there is a complex of caves which is called Ch'ien-fo-tung (Cave of the Thousand Buddhas) or Mo-kao-k'u. It is the largest and, in part, the oldest of the groups of cave temples extant in China. The brittle rock here does not lend itself to sculpture; therefore, a type of mold sculpture employing a wooden armature and a mixture of clay and straw predominates. The chief interest in these temples lies in the many series of wall paintings (see PLS. 237, 238, 244, 249; II, 390). The oldest of these that can be accurately dated was painted during the Wei period (520-24).

As almost the only remnants of Buddhist-inspired early Chinese painting these caves are extremely valuable. They form for us an irreplaceable link in our reconstruction of that chain of pictorial styles running from India through Central Asia to China.

The Mo-kao-k'u cave temples were discovered by Przevalsky early in the 20th century. The discovery in 1900 by a Taoist monk of a vast collection of documents and paintings, which in all probability had been walled up in Cave 16 since early in the 11th century, promptly aroused the attention of Sir Aurel Stein, who acquired a large share of the treasure (1907). In 1908 P. Pelliot also visited Tun-huang and took back to Europe a large part of the remainder of the archives, books, and paintings. For Sinology and for the study of Buddhism this find, the materials of which are preserved mostly in London, Paris, and New Delhi, is of immense value.

The most recent and complete numbering of the caves (followed here) is that of the Tun-huang Research Institute, established in 1943, which has undertaken a systematic investigation of the complex.

The most ancient caves are located in the center of the flank of the mountain, almost the entire surface of which is pitted by the entrances to the temples. These caves, Nos. 251, 254, 259, and the small group including Nos. 266-275, are very close together. All of these are on the second and third levels of construction.

Cave 248, southward, is the earliest one of the Wei period, while the one farthest north dating from that period is No. 428. Between No. 458 and No. 442, there is a small section of the mountainside where no Wei caves are to be found. Since the Wei caves which are situated farthest from the center happen also to be the most recent, the assumption is justified that during the Wei period the complex of caves was extended outward in both directions from the center. The absence of Wei caves between No. 458 and No. 442 must be attributed to a landslide caused by one of the frequent earthquakes that throughout the ages have afflicted the region. It is possible that the anterooms of these caves may have been interconnected by piercing the walls or by building passageways along the façade of the rocky wall, in the manner still to be seen in the complex of Yü-lin-k'u (see below). Following the earthquakes, however, these structures would have collapsed, while the halls in the caves escaped, being on a deeper level. The various types of caves and courtyards are adaptations of the Indian vihara (a Buddhist monastery, originally a court, on the four sides of which were the monks' cells) and the *caityagṛha*, a Buddhist temple, which contained a stupa.

The caves dating from the Sui period are nearly all aligned along the third level of construction and extend northward from No. 428 (end of the Wei caves) to No. 330 and southward above the Wei caves to No. 264. South of the whole Wei group only Caves 247 and 244 date from the Sui period, while much farther south, beyond the nine-story wooden façade dating from the Ch'ing period, Caves 203 and 204 are also attributed to the Sui.

During the T'ang period (618-906), the complex was extended northward and southward, so that at the end of that period it was virtually at its present size. Following the natural calamities which destroyed part of the complex, and because of the lack of room to dig new caves, work during the Sung period was concentrated increasingly on restoration, alteration, and expansion of the ones already existing. Four more caves were built under the Hsi-hsia and nine more under the Mongols. One of the noteworthy achievements under Sung rule was the execution of a gigantic wall painting which covered a part of the mountain face, but this has now disappeared.

Even later are a number of wooden façades which were erected in front of the cave entrances to prevent landslides. One of these may date from the late T'ang period (No. 196), while three others are of the 10th century (No. 427, dated 970; No. 431, dated 980; and No. 444, dated 976). These early structures are interesting architecturally, unlike the later ones, which almost all date from the Ch'ing period. Almost everywhere on the rock can be found traces of wooden passageways, which today have practically disappeared.

According to the latest chronological data, the inventory of the Tun-huang complex is as follows: 23 caves from the Wei period or somewhat earlier; 95 from the Sui; 213 from the T'ang; 33 from the Five Dynasties; 98, Sung; 4, Hsi-hsia; 9, Yüan; and 5 of later date. A recent inventory of the sculptures has provided the following figures:

| Period | Number | Badly damaged | Restored | Intact |
|---|---|---|---|---|
| Wei | 268 | 31 | 1 | 236 |
| Sui | 444 | 5 | 197 | 242 |
| T'ang | 661 | 33 | 393 | 235 |
| Five Dynasties | 36 | 1 | 24 | 11 |
| Sung | 225 | — | 171 | 54 |
| Hsi-hsia | 5 | — | — | 5 |
| Yüan | 8 | — | 8 | — |
| Ch'ing | 631 | — | — | 631 |

Such precise dates are not available for the paintings. During World War II, Hsieh Chih-liu drew up an exceedingly summary inventory, which was published only recently. Although the text of P. Pelliot's publication, which was supposed to accompany the photographic reproductions published by him (1920), has never appeared, his reproductions of the wall paintings have been invaluable as the only available material for study. Besides the paintings in the caves themselves, the scrolls preserved in the library are also important, not so much for their artistic merit, but more because many of them are dated and enable us to follow the development of the different iconographic themes. Although their technique is quite different, their close iconographic affinity with the wall paintings gives us some idea of the paintings from these distant sanctuaries, which comparatively few scholars have been able to visit.

About 20 miles southwest of Tun-huang, on the north bank of the Tang River, there is a group of temples known as Hsi Ch'ien-fo-tung, i.e., the Western Cave of the Thousand Buddhas. The river, by undermining the mountainside, has caused several landslides which have seriously damaged the complex. Today only 19 caves remain. These were inventoried and numbered by Chang Ta-ch'ien during World War II (Nos. 1-19, from west to east) and were further investigated in 1953 by the Tun-huang Research Institute. Two of these caves (Nos. 4 and 5) date from the Wei period and it is thought by some that they antedate the earliest caves at Tun-huang. The others date mostly from the T'ang period, except for Nos. 3 and 12, which are from the Sung and Hsi-hsia periods respectively.

BIBLIOG. P. Pelliot, Les grottes de Touen-Houang (6 portfolios of plates), Paris, 1920-24; A. Stein, Ancient Buddhist Paintings from the Cave of the Thousand Buddhas on the Westernmost Frontier of China, London, 1921; A. Stein, Serindia, Oxford, 1921, II, pp. 791-1,088, III, pp. 1,392-1,431; A. Waley, A Catalogue of Paintings Recovered from Tun-huang by Sir Aurel Stein, London, 1931; E. Matsumoto, Tonkōga no Kenkyū (A Study of the Paintings of Tun-huang), Tokyo, 1937; Wên-wu ts'an-k'ao tzŭ-liao, 1953, nos. 33-34, pp. 122-8, 1956, no. 2, pp. 39-76; Hsieh Chih-liu, Tun-huang yi-shu hsü-lu (Descriptive Catalogue of the Art of Tun-huang), Shanghai, 1955 (on Hsi Ch'ien-fo-tung in particular, pp. 421-40); B. Gray and J. B. Vincent, Buddhist Cave Paintings at Tun-huang, London, 1959.

Yü-lin-k'u. About 40 miles south of the city of Ansi (An-hsi) there are several groups of caves, located opposite each other in two steep cliffs on the banks of the Yü-lin River. All together they form the Yü-lin-k'u or Wan-fo-hsia. These caves were first inspected by Sir Aurel Stein, and later by Langdon Warner. During World War II, Chang Ta-ch'ien visited the site and drew up an inventory of the caves. The Tun-huang Research Institute in a later investigation discovered an even larger number of caves. There are at this site 42 caves in all, of which 31 are on the east side and 11 on the west; 3 date from the T'ang period, 8 from that of the Five Dynasties, 13 from the Sung, one from the Hsi-hsia, 7 from the Yüan, and 9 from the Ch'ing. Just when the first cave was excavated is uncertain, but in some caves it has been found that a second layer of painting covers earlier pictures from the beginning of the T'ang period. In Caves 17 and 28, paintings from the T'ang period have been found intact.

The system of passageways connecting the caves of the upper part of the eastern side with one another is of considerable architec-

tural interest. Inscriptions and the vestiges of paintings found on the walls seem to confirm the assumption that the construction of these passageways does not antedate the Yüan period.

The paintings in the courtyard of Cave 15 and Cave 25, in particular, are of exceptionally fine quality. Those in the latter cave were described in detail by Langdon Warner; according to recent reports, they have since been severely damaged. In No. 25 we find on the northern wall a mandala of Vairocana, on the eastern wall a representation of the Sukhāvatī or Paradise of Amitābha and on the western wall a depiction of the Tushita Paradise, probably dating from the 9th century. (An inscription made by a visitor is dated 901.) All the pictures show a close affinity with those of the corresponding period in Tun-huang. In Cave 3 are wall paintings from the Mongol period, which show the distinct influence of Tantric Buddhism.

On two facing rock walls, situated at Shui-hsia-k'ou, between Ansi and the cave temples of Yü-lin-k'u, there is a small number of cave temples. These were investigated during the last war by Chang Ta-ch'ien, who listed in his inventory a single cave on the north wall and five on the south. Although almost all of the existing paintings are from the Sung period, the architecture would seem to indicate that the complex was partly of the Wei period.

BIBLIOG. A. Stein, Serindia, III, Oxford, 1921, pp. 1,108–14; L. Warner, Buddhist Wall-paintings, A Study of a 9th Century Grotto at Wan-fo-hsia, Cambridge, Mass., 1938; Hsieh Chih-liu, Tun-huang yi-shu hsü-lu (Descriptive Catalogue of the Art of Tun-huang), Shanghai, 1955, pp. 441–96, 497–9; Wên-wu ts'an-k'ao tzŭ-liao, 1956, no. 10, pp. 9–21; Tun-huang Yi-shu hua-k'u, IV: Yü-lin-k'u, Peking, 1957.

T'ien-t'i-shan. On this mountain, about 30 miles south of the city of Wuwei, there is a group of cave temples, explored by archaeologists in 1952. An inscription dated 1444 proves that at that time there were 26 temples, of which only 13 still exist. Eight of these contain wall paintings or reliefs. In 1927 there were still 18 caves at this site, but a violent earthquake later buried 5 of them under a landslide.

Of the 13 remaining caves, 2 date from the Wei period. Just as in the case of the caves constructed during the Sui and T'ang periods, these too were altered and restored under the regime of the Hsi-hsia. Cave XIII contains a seated Buddha about 85 ft. high, flanked by two lohans, two bodhisattvas, and two lokapalas. All these figures are partially carved into the wall, the details having been finished in clay. During the investigation of the site, fragments were found of a painting on silk from the early 7th century and fragments of Buddhist manuscripts, the oldest of which are of late Wei date.

BIBLIOG. Wên-wu ts'an-k'ao tzŭ-liao, 1955, no. 2, pp. 76–96.

Yung-ching. Situated some 15 miles northwest of Yung-ching, on the flanks of the mountain Hsiao-chi-shih, is a group of cave temples known as Ping-ling-ssŭ. Although frequented by Lamaist monks ever since the Mongol period, the site was rediscovered by archaeologists only in 1951. It was first described by Li Tao-yüan (d., 527) in the Shui-ching-chu. The earliest inscription so far discovered, recording the construction of one of the caves, dates from 513, but this does not exclude the possibility that some of these caves may be even older. In all, the complex consists of 36 caves, 10 of which are from the Wei period, 21 from the T'ang, and 5 from the Ming. There are also 88 niches in the cliff wall, including 2 of the Wei period, 85 of the T'ang, and 1 of the Ming period. The group of archaeologists who made a provisional reconnaissance of this site in 1952 numbered the caves north to south from 1 to 124. Although many of the caves were restored and remodeled during the Ming and Ch'ing periods, the group as a whole is in good condition.

The niches numbered 1 and 2 are at a short distance from the others. No. 1 is noteworthy for a large trinity of standing figures, modeled during the Ming period. On the northern flank the complex is dominated by a huge seated Buddha of the T'ang period, about 80 ft. high. This figure was carved in the same way as the Buddhas in the earliest Yün-kang caves (in Shansi) and the Bamian statues (see AFGHANISTAN). Among the outstanding characteristics of this complex are the numerous stupas in bas-relief, which Chinese experts attribute to the T'ang period.

BIBLIOG. China Reconstructs, no. 4, July-Aug., 1953, pp. 25–7; Ping-ling-ssŭ shih-k'u (The Rock Caves of Ping-ling-ssŭ), Peking, 1953; Wên-wu ts'an-k'ao tzŭ-liao, 1953, no. 29, pp. 21–9.

Mai-chi-shan. On the steep flanks at the summit of this mountain about 37 miles south of Tienshui, a great number of caves, thoroughly examined only in 1953, were constructed. These temples, hollowed out of soft rock, underwent numerous restorations in the Sung, Ming, and Ch'ing periods that have particularly affected the sculpture. Nothing is known as to the exact date of the construction of the first caves; it is presumed that they go back to the late 4th century. The complex is mentioned in literature as early as 420, but the earliest dated votive inscription (Cave 115) is of the year 502. In Cave 190 a small sculpture in black stone was found which, according to some experts, may date from the 4th century.

To date, 188 caves have been counted; among them are 12 that date from the early Wei period, 70 from the middle, and 25 from the late Wei period; 11 date from the Northern Chou (557–81), and 6 from the Sui period. (See PL. 251.)

BIBLIOG. Mai-chi-shan shih-k'u (The Rock Caves of Mai-chi-shan), Peking, 1954; Wên-wu ts'an-k'ao tzŭ-liao, 1954, no. 2, pp. 3–50 (including a report of the investigations), no. 3, pp. 108–13, no. 4, pp. 101–4, no. 5, pp. 86–95, no. 6, pp. 95–107 (inventory of the caves).

Ching-ho valley (in Kansu and Shensi). Along the valley of the Ching-ho on the border of Kansu and Shensi at least five cave temples were located by the China expeditions of the Fogg Art Museum (1923–25). Two of the sites are within the boundaries of the present province of Shensi; the other three are in Kansu. These sites are:

Hsüeh-lien-tung (in Shensi). The caves of this site (exact number unknown) have all been restored in recent times. The original sculptures may have been of pre-T'ang date.

Ta-fo-ssŭ (Temple of the Colossal Buddha, in Shensi). The name of this site is derived from a huge sculpture, about 40 ft. high, representing a seated Buddha and two smaller standing attendants (bodhisattvas). According to a local tradition the temple was founded in the first year of the T'ang period, and the large sculptures, which have undergone several restorations, probably date from about that time.

Lo-han-tung (Cave of the Lohans, in Kansu). The site consists of several caves constructed at different levels in the face of the cliff. The main cave has a central pillar. The sculptures, most of which have been crudely restored, may partly date from the early 6th century.

Hsia-wang-mu-miao (in Kansu, near Ching-chou). A cave with a central pillar has a new masonry façade of three stories. The richly sculptured pillar is comparatively well preserved and shows many stylistic and iconographic parallels with the sculptures of Cave VI at Yün-kang (see below, Shansi). The cave, which has interior bas-reliefs depicting the life of the historical Buddha, may date from the late 5th century. Several heads broken from sculptures, now preserved in the Fogg Art Museum, are of a somewhat later date.

Wang-chia-k'ou (or perhaps Shih-ch'ü-ssŭ, in Kansu). A large cave, the entrance of which is flanked by bas-reliefs of guardian figures, contains 23 large sculptures, 7 of which may represent the buddhas of past kalpas. There is a smaller cave, also flanked by guardians. Two large caves are completely undecorated. A stele, now placed in the Confucian temple at Ching-chou, on which an inscription mentions the date 512, may have come from this site.

BIBLIOG. Fogg Art Museum Notes, April, 1924; H. F. Jayne, The Buddhist Caves of the Ching Ho Valley, Eastern Art, I, 1929, no. 3, pp. 157–73, no. 4, pp. 242–61; Wên-wu ts'an-k'ao tzŭ-liao, 1956, no. 10, pp. 27–8 (discussion of Ta-fo-ssŭ).

KWANGTUNG (Kuang-tung) AND KWANGSI (Kuang-hsi). *Survey of geography and art history.* The region of the "two Kwangs" (Liang-kuang) is the southernmost part of China. Extending along the northern border is the chain of the Nan-ling (or Nan-shan, Southern Mountains) separating this region from the area around the middle course of the Yangtze River.

Three rivers cross this region, all emptying into the sea in the vicinity of modern Canton: the Hsi-kiang (West or Si River), the Pei-kiang (North River), and the Tung-kiang (East River).

Shortly after the first Ch'in empire had subjugated northern China, the troops of Shih Huang-ti marched against the territory south of the mountains (Ling-nan), which was completely conquered between 221 and 214 B.C., along with a part of Indochina. These areas, where very few Chinese were settled, soon afterward regained much of their independence. However, during the Han dynasty, the kingdom of Nan-yüeh (the center of which was probably not far from modern Canton) was again incorporated into the Chinese empire and Chinese immigration increased. The south of present-day China passed permanently into Chinese hands, and so, for a long time, did a part of Indochina. The northern part of Indochina, conquered by the Chinese in 214, 111, and 42 B.C., has remained within the sphere of Chinese culture, which left its ineradicable imprint on the region.

Under the T'ang dynasty, the number of Chinese in the southern provinces was still small (if population statistics are to be believed), compared to that of Chinese in the north. The aborigines now passed into the minority. Such tribes as the Miao-tzŭ (Miaotse), the Chuang, and the Yao were gradually expelled from the more fertile areas.

To some extent they mingled with the Chinese, whose culture was far superior to their own.

We can only conjecture as to the cultures of the peoples encountered in this area by the Chinese immigrants of the Han period. The rock drawings to be seen in places in Kwangsi are attributed by some authorities to the Han period, but it is entirely possible that they date from a later time or are only a few hundred years old.

A drum of the Đông-So'n type, excavated a few years ago in a tomb of the early Han period near Kuei-hsien in Kwangsi, proves that the remarkable bronze culture typified by these drums (see ASIA, SOUTH; ASIATIC PROTOHISTORY), was diffused not only in Yunnan but throughout southern Chinese territory.

A great number of Han tombs, mostly built of brick, have been excavated in recent years around Canton. Their furnishings give the impression of a distinctly local culture; although there are among the *ming-ch'i* a considerable number of objects which were probably imported (particularly among the terra-cotta tomb figurines), there are many of a style quite different from that of the northern types. The houses represented in the Cantonese Han models differ markedly from those of northern China. Often huts standing on high poles are represented.

A mixture of Chinese and foreign traits is discernible in the figures of dancing girls and tomb guardians. Among the latter there is a human figure with a long, protruding tongue, which is reminiscent of the monsters of Ch'ang-sha (in Hunan). The "drooping hands" attitude is clearly derived from Chinese choreographic gestures and is also found in figures from the north. But such exotic, star-bedecked headdresses as those of the Cantonese dancing girls have never been found in the north. A ship model found appears to represent a houseboat rather than a seagoing vessel.

Toward the end of the Han period, this coast came to play an important role in China's overseas contacts, and Canton, with its ideal location in relation to the hinterland, became a port to which people of different languages and races came from distant lands, including many Moslems. This city had a large foreign colony composed of Arabs, Persians, Syrians, Moslems, Central Asian Nestorians, and Jews. No T'ang monuments have survived to recall this "international" period in Canton's history, perhaps because the city was destroyed twice during the T'ang period, in 759 and 859. At the time of the second destruction, by the rebel Huang Ch'ao, many foreigners were killed, if credence is to be given a contemporary Arab account. Despite this, Islam persisted around Canton, particularly among the non-Chinese inhabitants of the area. Here, as in other parts of China, Islam failed to become a source of inspiration for new and significant art forms. The prestige and vitality of the ancient Chinese culture were too strong. Still, a most unusual monument is the minaret of the mosque of Huai-shêng (Huai-shêng-ssŭ) in Canton, probably built about 1120 and one of the oldest Islamic monuments in the Far East. No important monument of the other foreign religions has survived in Canton.

The scarcity of ancient monuments in the entire Canton area is due in part to the Taiping rebellion of the 19th century, but the destruction it caused throughout all the territory south of the Yangtze River is not the only factor. Another is that the region south of the mountains was too peripheral ever to have been the seat of a capital, even though it was predestined by its location to become the last stronghold of those dynasties retreating from the north.

*Kiln sites.* Although Kwangtung and Kwangsi are admittedly less important in the history of Chinese pottery than was neighboring Fukien province, several types which obviously developed in the area around Canton have become generally known.

One of these, a type of reddish-brown pottery, coated with a thick *flambé* glaze in blue, yellow, gray, and red, is usually known as "Kwangtung pottery." Some believe the manufacture of this ware began during the T'ang period, but actually all the specimens so far discovered probably date from the 17th and 18th centuries and were made around Yang-chiang and Fatshan near Canton. They have a superficial resemblance to Chün-yao, which was probably the inspiration for the potters, although the workmanship is much cruder.

The kilns of Chaochow (Ch'ao-chou), in eastern Kwangtung, are comparatively little known, but were probably very important during the Sung period. In a tomb a few miles southwest of this city, on Yang-p'i-kang hill, were discovered (1922) four Buddhist statuettes in white porcelain and a censer. All these objects bore long inscriptions with the place and date of manufacture and the potters' names. The dates correspond to the years 1067–69, and the kiln was specified as that of Shui-tung. The Chaochow kilns have been investigated by Malcolm Farley, John Galbin, Jao Tsung-yi, and most recently by Ch'ên Wan-li. On the mountain Han-shan and in the environs, at least a hundred different kilns have been found. White and ivory-glazed porcelains and hard pottery of Ying-ch'ing and *temmoku* types have been found. It is believed that these kilns were destroyed

at the time of the Mongol invasion, and that production was resumed only during the Ming period.

BIBLIOG. M. F. Farley, The White Wares of Fukien and the South China Coast, Far Eastern Ceramic B., VII, 1949, IX, 1950; Wên-wu ts'an-k'ao tzŭ-liao, 1955, n. 6, pp. 61–7, 1957, no. 3, pp. 36–9; K'ao-ku t'ung-hsin, 1956, no. 4, pp. 18–20; Sekai Tōji Zenshū (Ceramic Art of the World), X, Tokyo, 1955, pp. 222–3.

MANCHURIA AND ADJACENT REGIONS. *Survey of geography and art history.* The provinces of Heilungkiang (Hei-lung-chiang), Kirin (Chi-lin), and Liaoning (Liao-ning) form a geographic entity bounded by mountains, rivers, and the sea. Extending along the western frontier are the high Khingan Mountains (Hingan, Hsing-an) and on the east the Changpai range (Chang-pai-shan). On the north are the Little Khingans and the Amur or Heilung (Black Dragon) River, which form the boundary with the Soviet Union, while on the southeast the Yalu River marks the boundary with Korea. To the south the Liaotung Peninsula extends into the Yellow Sea, which bathes the southern frontier. The region, lying between two mountain ranges, consists partly of hills and mountains, partly of a great plain in which the watercourses ultimately empty into either the Amur River or the Yellow Sea.

In the 20th century the frontiers of Manchuria have undergone several changes, due particularly to the eventful political history of the region. The most important change which took place in the 1950s was the dissolution of the province of Jehol, which was partitioned among Hopei, Liaoning, and the autonomous territory of Inner Mongolia. The western portion of Heilungkiang province, inhabited by Mongols, was transferred also to Inner Mongolia (see MONGOLIAN ART). In order to round out the discussion below (particularly for the Liao period), some sites outside the present boundaries of Manchuria have been included.

Politically, Manchuria has been of prime importance in China's history, for it has been the country of origin of various peoples who have gone on from there to the total or partial conquest of China. At various times, however, it has been under the rule of the Chinese, traces of whose cultural influence are almost omnipresent throughout the region. Neolithic finds in great numbers have been made, although the lack of clearly distinguishable strata has made it hard to date them. In southern Manchuria, vestiges of the microlithic Gobi culture mingle with those of the Yang-shao culture originating in the Great Plain, while numerous remains of the Lung-shan culture are found on the Liaotung Peninsula.

No remains have so far been identified of the Shang bronze culture. The use of bronze apparently came into Manchuria during the Chou period, when the area north of and surrounding Peking was part of the kingdom of Yen. This kingdom gradually extended its influence northward, protecting its frontiers with a Great Wall which, at the start of the 3d century B.C., when Yen's power reached its zenith, probably extended to the vicinity of the present Korean boundary.

Considerably earlier than this wall, which has completely vanished, are several bronzes discovered by chance in 1955 in the Ling-yüan area, formerly in Jehol province, but now in Liaoning. In all, the find consists of 13 virtually intact vases and fragments of 2 others. The types of bronzes were already known from discoveries elsewhere, but the *tsun* type in the shape of a goose is exceptional. The style is that of the very early Chou period.

Under the Ch'in dynasty southern Manchuria temporarily escaped from Chinese influence. The emperor Shih Huang-ti ordered the various sectors of the Great Wall to be joined in a single system, but in the territory formerly belonging to the state of Yen, the wall extended only to Shanhaikwan, which even today marks its terminus. Under the sway of the Han emperor Wu-ti, China extended its rule to southern Manchuria, and during this period also occupied northern Korea. At that time, the most important Chinese colony was in the vicinity of the present town of Pyongyang, in Korea, and the tombs of Lo-lang, which aroused such interest when excavated by the Japanese, were then constructed (see KOREA; KOREAN ART).

The territory included in modern Manchuria has also yielded many important finds dating from the Han period. The tombs with wall paintings which were discovered by the Japanese at Ying-ch'êng-tzŭ (on the tip of the Liaotung Peninsula) and at Liao-yang (south of Mukden) are extremely important for the history of Chinese art, since they provide material for the study of painting in a hitherto virtually unknown period. As a whole this painting is pervaded by a typically provincial air, only to be expected in a region so remote from the center of Chinese culture. The mortuary gifts were often imported from China, as were, for example, those found in the so-called "Tomb of the Painted Basket" in Korea. These are often of superior quality.

The political and cultural situation as it existed in those areas peripheral to the territory occupied by the Chinese is strikingly il-

lustrated by the mingling of relics of Chinese and nomadic types found in the cemetery of Hsi-ch'a-kou in the district of Hsi-fêng, Liaoning province, which has unfortunately been devastated by inexpert digging. Han coins have been discovered alongside ornaments in the Ordos (q.v.) style. The finds of lacquer ware and Chinese textiles of the Han period, made during excavations at Noin-ula, north of Urga in Mongolia (see ASIATIC PROTOHISTORY), and several discoveries in Siberia prove to what remote places Chinese art objects were carried by the nomadic tribes.

After the fall of the Han dynasty (221) there followed a period of great political unrest in northern China. Three states contended for the legacy of the Han. The more northerly, the kingdom of Wei, emerged the victor in the struggle and for a fairly long time was able to maintain its hegemony over southern Manchuria. Before the waves of tribes of Turkish, Mongol, and Tungusic origin, which for periods of varying length managed to gain control of various areas in northern China, the Chinese prevailed culturally rather than politically, although the Chinese Northern Yen dynasty (409–36) succeeded briefly in maintaining its own rule until it was overthrown by the T'o-pa (Toba) tribe. The glorious epoch of the T'o-pa (or Wei) dynasty, to whom we owe the most beautiful cave temples of northern China, has also left its traces in Manchuria in the badly damaged temples of Wan-fo-tung, in Liaoning province.

During the period of separation from China, some of the territory which today is part of Manchuria ultimately came under the control of a state which never exercised any power over China, the Korean kingdom of Koguryo, which was deeply affected by Chinese cultural influences. The capital of this state toward the end of the Han dynasty was Huai-jên (near modern Huan-jên) on the Hun-kiang, a tributary of the Yalu. The capital was transferred in the 3d or 4th century to T'ung-kou, in the vicinity of Chi-an on the western bank of the middle Yalu, and in 427 to the vicinity of modern Pyongyang in northern Korea (q.v.). The ruins of T'ung-kou, investigated by Japanese archaeologists, are of great interest. The wall paintings in the tombs, like those in the Manchurian Han tombs, are the work of a provincial school. The Chinese inscription on the stele of the king Kwanggaet'o is of great historic value as a source for our knowledge of Korean history.

Few monuments of any importance have been found belonging to the Sui and T'ang periods, during which Manchuria was again under Chinese influences as far as the Nonni and Sungari Rivers. The pagoda at Ch'ao-yang, in Liaoning province, extensively restored later, is thought to have been built during the expedition of the T'ang armies against Korea or soon afterward.

As the power of the T'ang dynasty declined, two new states arose in Manchuria, one of which was to play an important role in Chinese history. From 713 to 926, part of Manchuria was under the sway of the kingdom of P'o-hai, which, following the Chinese example, constructed five capital cities. The remains of the eastern capital (Lung-ch'üan-fu), east of the Heilung River in Heilungkiang province, give us a fragmentary idea of its culture. On the mountain Niu-ting near Tun-hua, in Kirin province, a long inscription from the kingdom of P'o-hai was the first important epigraphic discovery in this territory.

The Khitans were nomads related to the Hsien-pi, who supported themselves by cattle breeding. They came into contact with Chinese culture in southern Manchuria and, during the 10th century, extended their domain, first occupying the kingdom of P'o-hai, which they decisively defeated in 926. The ensuing war with the Chinese indirectly brought about the rise of the Sung dynasty, which was proclaimed by the general sent against them. For some time the Khitan princes (Liao dynasty, 907–1125) ruled over Manchuria and parts of northern Shansi and Hopei. From the contact with the Chinese an art and culture different in many respects from those of the T'ang and Sung developed among the Khitans. Two of the five capitals founded by the Liao lay in what is now Inner Mongolia: the principal capital, Lin-huang-fu (now in the territory of the Jo-oda banner, near Lin-tung), and the central capital, Ta-ting-fu (now in the Chahar banner, near To-lun). The eastern capital, Liao-yang-fu, was situated at modern Liao-yang, in Liaoning province. Within China proper, Ta-t'ung, in Shansi, and a town near the present Peking functioned as the western and southern capitals.

Among the numerous Buddhist monuments built by the devout Khitans there are a number of pagodas remarkable for their peculiar style. In Manchuria alone there remain at least some twenty of these octagonal pagodas, usually 7 or 13 stories high. Of the wooden structures from the Liao period, only one is in Manchurian territory, but this is the largest and most impressive of all. It is the Ta-hsiung-tien of the temple Fêng-kuo-ssŭ at Yi-hsien (I-hsien) in Liaoning province, built in 1020; it contains a group of figures also dating back to the same period.

The painting of this period is represented by the wall paintings in tombs of the sixth, seventh, and eighth emperors of the Liao at the ancient city of Ch'ing-chou (see below). The most original creation of the Khitans was their pottery, which first attracted the attention of Japanese and Western scholars about 1935; until that time it had been thought to be a provincial type of T'ang pottery. While it is true that Liao pottery, glazed in three colors, is in many respects similar to and derived from T'ang models, shapes are quite original. The so-called "cockscomb" bottle or vase, ch'i-kuan-hu, is derived from the shape of the leather bottles of the nomads. A whole series of dated tomb finds now makes it possible to trace the stylistic development of this pottery, and a number of kilns have been located.

Many of the Liao traditions were adopted by the Jurchen who succeeded them. Except for several pagodas, the spires of which have a slightly more austere profile, no other important monuments in Manchuria can be attributed to the Chin dynasty (1115–1234). The period of the Mongol Yüan dynasty (1260–1368), which reigned over all Manchuria, left few monuments of interest.

The reign of the Chinese dynasty of the Ming was overthrown when, near the end of the 16th century, the Manchus, descendants of the Jurchen, revolted against the Chinese imperial power. They captured Mukden in 1625 and a few years later opened a path through the Great Wall. A series of bloody campaigns was to seal the sovereignty of the Manchurian Ch'ing dynasty over all of China in 1659. Of all the many monuments recalling the Manchu domination, the outstanding are the palaces of Mukden (Shenyang), which go back to the beginning of the Ch'ing dynasty, and the two mausoleums of the first Manchu emperors. (See CHINESE ART, Later architecture.) The Ch'ing sought to protect the land from Chinese immigration and thereby contributed to the preservation of ancient monuments. Under their rule began the spread of Lamaism and, to a lesser degree, Islam. Lamaism in particular definitely influenced the architecture, which no longer was local in character, but had what in general might be called a northern Chinese and Tibetan flavor. This was also true of the civil architecture. The best example of the latter is the Summer Palace in Chengteh (Ch'êng-tê, now in Hopei), begun under K'ang-hsi and enlarged by Ch'ien-lung. As the power of the Manchus waned, a contributing factor to the loss of typically Manchu cultural character was the mass immigration of Chinese.

BIBLIOG. T. Sekino and T. Takejima, Ryōkin Jidai no Kenchiku to sono Butsuzō (Architecture of the Liao and Chin periods and Its Sculpture), Tokyo, 1925 (plates), 1944 (text); R. Nakamura, Manshū no Bijutsu (The Arts of Manchuria), Tokyo, 1941; M. Igarashi, Nekka Koseki to Chibetto Bijutsu (Monuments of Jehol and Tibetan Art), Tokyo, 1943; J. Murata, Manshū no Shiseki (Monuments of Manchuria), Tokyo, 1944; L. Sickman and A. Soper, The Art and Architecture of China, Harmondsworth, 1956; K'ao-ku hsüeh-pao, 1956, no. 1, pp. 29–42 (on Han and pre-Han archaeology); Wu-shêng ch'u-t'u chung-yao wên-wu chan-lan t'u-lu (Illustrated Catalogue of Important Objects Excavated in Five Provinces), Peking, 1958, pls. 20–7 (the bronzes of Ling-yüan).

*Monuments and archaeological sites.* Dolmens. In the region lying between the Liao and Yalu Rivers there have been discovered more than twenty tombs built of megalithic stone, of the type generally called "dolmens." The "Liaotung Peninsula type," found here, is related to that of northern Korea but is somewhat different from the south Korean and Kyūshū types, and hence is described by Japanese archaeologists as the "northern" type. These dolmens nearly always consist of three flat slabs planted upright in the earth and surmounted by a block, the ends of which extend beyond the supporting slabs. Some Japanese experts date them between the 3d century B.C. and the 4th A.D.

BIBLIOG. T. Mikami, Dolmens in Manchuria (text in Jap.), Kokogaku Zasshi, XXXVIII, 1952, pp. 52–74; K'ao-ku t'ung-hsin, 1956, no. 2, p. 30.

Ying-ch'êng-tzŭ. In 1931 on the tip of the Liaotung Peninsula between Dairen (Ta-lien) and Lushun (Port Arthur), two brick tombs were discovered which very probably date from the Han period. One of them, which has well-preserved wall paintings, consists of an anteroom, a chamber, and a lateral room, with ogival vaults. Of special interest is the construction of the central room, which contains a mortuary chamber of the same shape, but smaller, built under the large vault. The plastered walls bear paintings in black, with red added in places. The painting on the north wall of the interior central chamber is noteworthy for its representation of the worship of an ancestor who appears as a spirit, perhaps that of the person entombed here. This theme, which recurs in other places, is treated here with extraordinary verve.

BIBLIOG. O. Mori and H. Naito, Ying-ch'êng-tzŭ, Kyoto, 1934.

Liao-yang. The tombs in the vicinity of Liao-yang, attributed to the Han period, are of a type built entirely of slabs of slate. The one found near Pei-yüan is the best preserved. Quadrangular in shape (17 × 16 ft.), it includes a central mortuary chamber surrounded by a gallery on all four sides. On the north, south, and east sides it has respectively one, two, and three lateral chambers. On the west side

is an entrance. The stone walls are completely plastered. Four of them are decorated with polychrome paintings, in contrast to the almost monochrome paintings of Ying-ch'êng-tzŭ. Among the representations is a procession of chariots with parasols, a theme which was apparently highly esteemed in the Han period. The scene depicting sacrifice to an ancestor, noted in the tomb of Ying-ch'êng-tzŭ, is also present here, although handled in a less spectacular fashion. Japanese experts date this tomb within the first three centuries of the Christian era.

BIBLIOG. W. Fairbank and K. Masao, Han Mural Paintings in the Peiyüan Tomb at Liao-yang, South Manchuria, Artibus Asiae, XVII, 1954, pp. 238–64.

Wan-fo-tung. This complex of cave temples on the rocky banks of the Ta-ling River, about 5 miles north of Yi-hsien in Liaoning province, consists of two groups of seven caves. In the eastern group, Caves IV and V contain sculptures from the Wei period, executed after 499. The state of preservation here is deplorable in comparison with that of northern Chinese cave temples. Cave I of the western group, which is quadrangular and has at the center a column with decoration in relief carved out of the rock, still contains, despite repeated restorations, several decorated niches and sculptures in relief that are stylistically reminiscent of those at Yün-kang, in Shansi.

BIBLIOG. R. Nakamura, Manshū no Bijutsu (Arts of Manchuria), Tokyo, 1941, pp. 38–55; J. Murata, Manshū no Shiseki (Monuments of Manchuria), Tokyo, 1944, pp. 396–409).

Lung-ch'üan-fu. The ruins of this capital of the kingdom of P'o-hai are located in the district of Ning-an, in the northeast of Heilungkiang province. Although the kingdom had five different capitals, this one, founded in the 8th century near Tung-ching-ch'êng, remained inhabited for a longer time than the others and thus had a greater number of public buildings, palaces, and temples. The investigations of J. Murata established that the city was patterned after the T'ang capital Ch'ang-an, in Shensi, on a reduced scale of one-eighth. The northern section included an inner Imperial City, within which the Forbidden City formed yet another closed complex. Only the foundations of palaces and temples remain, but an octagonal stone lantern 17 ft. high still stands in the grounds of a neighboring temple, the Lung-hsing-ssŭ, rebuilt under the Manchus. Among the finds are a great quantity of bricks bearing floral motifs, tiles, pottery fragments, a stone lion's head, and a cast-iron Buddha. All these works are closely related to T'ang styles. Subsequently the city was again used as a temporary capital by the Khitans and Jurchen at a time when the center of their power still lay in these northern regions. Later, however, it was virtually razed to the ground.

BIBLIOG. J. Murata, Manshū no Shiseki (Monuments of Manchuria), Tokyo, 1944, pp. 141–72; Sekai Bijutsu Zenshū (The Arts of the World), VIII (China, II), Tokyo, 1952, pp. 19–22; Hei-lung-chiang-shêng chi-ch'u wên-wu i-chi (Some Monuments of Heilungkiang Province), Wên-wu ts'an-k'ao tzŭ-liao, 1957, no. 11, pp. 59–60.

Ch'ing-chou. This ancient Liao city, now a deserted ruin, was situated near the present town of Pai-t'a-tzŭ (formerly in Jehol province, now in Inner Mongolia). The mausoleums of the Liao emperors Sheng-tsung (983–1030), Hsing-tsung (1031–55), and Tao-tsung (1055–1101) were discovered at this site in 1920 by J. Mullie. The excavations brought to light first a number of mortuary steles with inscriptions, partly in Khitan script, and then a collection of tomb furnishings.

The eastern tomb, i.e., the Ch'ing-ling (ling = tumulus), which was that of Emperor Sheng-tsung, contains wall paintings of paramount significance for the study of Liao painting. The tomb consists of an anteroom and a central chamber with five lateral chambers interconnected by a series of passageways. The domes of the mortuary chambers are perhaps an imitation of the tents of the nomads. The walls are covered with portraits, remarkable for their realism and extraordinary individual characterization. Altogether there are over seventy persons depicted, not only high officials and warriors, but also simple fishermen, some in Khitan costume, others in Chinese. Painted on the four walls of the central chamber is a series of landscapes depicting the Four Seasons. The style shows many similarities to a well-known pair of paintings of deer from the Palace collection of Peking (now in the National Palace Museum, Taichung, Formosa).

Near the mausoleums stands the Pai-t'a (white pagoda), which is octagonal and has seven stories. Its style is quite different from that of the usual Liao pagodas. It is plastered white and has a gradually tapering profile. Each story has doorways on four of its sides and rises to a cornice of projecting stones which form a slanting roof. The bracketing system is faithfully imitated in brick. The themes depicted in relief on the walls are different on each story. On the lowest story we find lokapalas, elephants (perhaps as a symbol of Samantabhadra), lions (perhaps as a symbol of Mañjuśrī), and small pagodas.

BIBLIOG. T. Sekino and T. Takejima, Ryōkin Jidai no Kenchiku to sono Butsuzō (Architecture of the Liao and Chin periods and Its Sculpture), Tokyo, 1925 (plates), 1944 (text), pp. 173–82; R. Nakamura, Manshū no Bijutsu (The Arts of Manchuria), Tokyo, 1941, pp. 69–72; J. Tamura and Y. Kobayashi, Tombs and Mural Paintings of Ch'ing-ling, Liao Imperial Mausoleums of the Eleventh Century A.D. in Eastern Mongolia, Kyoto, 1952–53; L. Sickman and A. Soper, The Art and Architecture of China, Harmondsworth, 1956, p. 274.

Ch'ao-yang. The Pei-t'a (northern pagoda) of this city, in Liaoning province, is quadrangular, with 13 stories. Thought to have been built during the T'ang period and to have been restored under the Liao (about 1050), it is decorated with reliefs on the slightly tapering shaft. It is thought that the Nan-t'a (southern pagoda), which is also quadrangular (highly unusual for pagodas from the Liao period), was built during the Liao period in imitation of the Pei-t'a. On each side reliefs depict a seated Buddha on a richly decorated lotus throne, flanked by attendant figures, apsarases (celestial nymphs), and stupas.

BIBLIOG. T. Sekino and T. Takejima, Ryōkin Jidai no Kenchiku to sono Butsuzō (The Architecture of the Liao and Chin periods and Its Sculpture), Tokyo, 1925 (plates), 1944 (text), pp. 196–212; R. Nakamura, Manshū no Bijutsu (The Arts of Manchuria), Tokyo, 1941, pp. 86–98; L. Sickman and A. Soper, The Art and Architecture of China, Harmondsworth, 1956, p. 272.

Fêng-kuo-ssŭ. In the northeastern part of the city of Yi-hsien (I-hsien), in Liaoning province, stands the Fêng-kuo-ssŭ, the most ancient wooden temple remaining in Manchuria. The hall (called Ta-hsiung-tien) is 9 bays wide and 6 deep (about 160 × 80 ft.). The interior is divided into an anterior and a posterior nave, each obtained by eliminating a row of 6 columns. In the posterior nave there are 7 large statues of Buddha accompanied by bodhisattvas. Like the building itself, these statues date from 1020, but they were extensively restored during the late Ming period. The complex system of brackets supporting the purlin under the eaves of the projecting roof is very similar to that of the pavilion of Kuan-yin of the Tu-lo-ssŭ (984), in Hopei.

BIBLIOG. T. Sekino and T. Takejima, Ryōkin Jidai no Kenchiku to sono Butsuzō (The Architecture of the Liao and Chin Periods and Its Sculpture), Tokyo, 1925 (plates), 1944 (text), pp. 47–70; R. Nakamura, Manshū no Bijutsu (The Arts of Manchuria), Tokyo, 1941, pp. 56–69; L. Sickman and A. Soper, The Art and Architecture of China, Harmondsworth, 1956, pp. 277–278.

Ta-ying-tzŭ. Of the many Liao tombs excavated during the mid-20th century, that of Ta-ying-tzŭ, near Chihfeng (Ch'ih-fêng) in Inner Mongolia, discovered in 1953, is in many respects the most important. Constructed, as shown by the mortuary inscription, in 959, it is the tomb of the son-in-law of an emperor of the Khitans. It consists of five vaulted rooms built of brick. There were found in this tomb many funerary objects showing how highly the Khitans esteemed horsemanship. Among these are two gilt-silver saddlebows adorned with repoussé representations of phoenixes and dragons chasing a flaming jewel. In the same tomb many ornaments of silver and parcel-gilt silver, a fine intact silver teapot, an iron helmet, and a pair of stirrups, as well as a quantity of the famous whistling arrows were found. There were also two white porcelain bowls, similar in body and glaze to those of the Ting-yao type, which have the character kuan (official) incised in the bottom under the glaze. Also among the finds were white porcelains of a somewhat different type, including several cockscomb bottles (ch'i-kuan-hu), providing perhaps a clue to the development of the shape of this type of Liao pottery, slightly modified forms of which are found in tombs of later date.

BIBLIOG. Wu-shêng ch'u-t'u chung-yao wên-wu chan-lan t'u-lu (Illustrated Catalogue of Important Objects Excavated in Five Provinces), Peking, 1958, pls. 104–21.

Kiln sites. Lin-huang-fu. In 1940 the remains of a kiln were found within the walls of the Imperial City of Lin-huang-fu, near Lin-tung in Inner Mongolia. The Japanese who conducted the excavations there believe that the imperial porcelain was manufactured in this kiln, but this theory is considered unfounded by the expert Li Wên-hsin, who in 1958 finally published a complete report of the excavations. Probably these kilns were in operation for only a few years about 1075. The artisans who worked there had probably been brought from the northern Chinese kilns where the Ting-yao was manufactured. The vast majority of the fragments found are of a white porcelain with incised decoration much like the Ting-yao ware. Much rarer were fragments of a black-glazed pottery almost always made of a very similar clay. Fragments of a green-glazed pottery were also found.

In the immediate vicinity of Lin-huang-fu the remains of two other kilns have been found. One, a small kiln, is on Nan-shan, where a type of pottery with a three-colored glaze and another with a light pink body covered with a white glaze were manufactured.

The other kiln site is near a place called Pai-yin-ko-lê, where fragments were found of a hard pottery, with a black or "tea-dust" glaze.

BIBLIOG. Li Wên-hsin, The Kiln-sites Found at the Ancient Lin-huang City of Liao Dynasty (text in Chinese), K'ao-ku hsüeh-pao, 1958, no. 2, pp. 97–109.

Kang-wa-yao-t'un. Near this village, about 44 miles west of Chihfeng (Inner Mongolia), there were, during the Liao period, kilns of vast size. The types of pottery manufactured were imitations of Ting-yao — pottery of light pink body with a three-color glaze, and pottery with a dark green glaze.

Chiang-kuan-t'un. Near Chiang-kuan-t'un, east of Liao-yang, on the south bank of the Taitze (T'ai-tzŭ) River, remains of many kilns probably dating from the Liao period have been found. One kiln, located slightly to the north, dates back to Mongol times (pottery with black glaze), and an inscription on an ink stone found during excavations has led the archaeologists to suppose that part of these kilns had already been used during the Jurchen period. Besides the types of Liao pottery already mentioned, an imitation of Tz'ŭ-chou-yao was made here.

In addition to the kilns mentioned above, Japanese experts have found other kiln sites in the environs of Chengteh, Fu-shun in Liaoning, Chihfeng (where the so-called Chien-wa-yao was made), and Kirin (Yungki). The reports of these investigations have been published only in Japanese journals which are not easily accessible (cf. the bibliography in Sekai Bijutsu Zenshū, X).

BIBLIOG. Li Wên-hsin, Liao-tz'ŭ chien-shu (A Short Account of Liao Ceramics), Wên-wu ts'an-k'ao tzŭ-liao, 1958, n. 2, pp. 10–20; G. Kuroda, Pottery and Porcelain of the Liao and Chin Dynasties (text in Jap.), Sekai Tōji Zenshū (Ceramic Art of the World), X, Tokyo, 1955, pp. 239–58.

SHANSI. *Survey of geography and art history.* The territory of this province forms a distinct geographic unit. To the east and south the frontier is formed by mountain ranges that separate it from Honan and Hopei provinces. The south-flowing Chin River links it with the fertile plain. Part of the southern and all of the western frontier are formed by the Yellow River. In the north, the plateau that forms a large part of the province is bounded by the steppes.

From many points of view, Shansi possesses the necessary geographic conditions for the development of an independent state and a true local culture. Traces have been found of the Red Pottery (or Yang-shao) culture along the Fen (Fên) and its tributaries, along the Chin River, and as far as the northern part of the province, where these remnants occur in conjunction with vestiges of the microlithic Gobi culture. Vestiges of the Shang culture are found along the Fen River, but it probably extended only within the fertile valleys, while the "barbarians" continued to live in the mountains and on the plateau.

During the Chou period, the state of Chin was established here, between the Fen valley and the Yellow River. This state gradually extended its territory to include a large part of modern Shansi and the so-called "Ho-hsi" region west of the Yellow River in Shensi province. Rivalry for the control of the latter region caused an agelong conflict with the rival state of Ch'in. The role which Chin played in Chinese politics, particularly in the 7th and 6th centuries B.C., was so important that this period is called that of the "Chin hegemony." During the final centuries of the Chou dynasty, however, Shansi lost most of its importance. In 376 B.C., Chin was split into three states, Han, Wei, and Chao. The decline and fall of Chin was perhaps one of the most important factors in the rise of the state of Ch'in, which found the way opened to the Great Plain and was consequently able to proceed to the conquest of the central part of the country.

Dating from this period of virtually uninterrupted civil strife are the fine bronzes and *ming-ch'i*, found in large numbers in Shansi. The find of Li-yü (1923), in the northern part of the province, and those made in the 1950s, for example, at Chang-chih in the Fen valley, prove the existence of a highly developed bronze culture there, although there is no evidence for the existence of a typical local bronze style.

During the Ch'in and Han dynasties, which permanently incorporated Shansi into the Chinese empire, the northern frontiers were protected from foreign invasions by means of a long wall which united other already existing fortifications into a single defensive system. Apparently it ran somewhat north of the present Great Wall. Where the latter curves southward west of Tatung (Ta-t'ung), the older wall once curved northward and shielded the entire bend of the Yellow River. The territory enclosed within this bulwark was inhabited by Chinese, as is made clear by the Han remains that lie just within the narrow strip between the Yellow River and the Han wall (which runs parallel to the river in an east–west direction, somewhat to the north).

Although protected by the wall, after the decline of the Han dynasty this area came more than once either completely or partially under foreign domination. Except for several monuments which the T'ang built here (T'ien-lung-shan, Wu-t'ai-shan, etc.), the largest and most impressive monuments date from periods in which Shansi was controlled by non-Chinese peoples. In 386 the T'o-pa, a branch of the Hsien-pi tribe, founded their capital at modern Tatung, in northern Shansi. During their rule (Wei dynasty) Buddhism, after surviving the initial persecutions, became very powerful. It also became a prime source of artistic inspiration, evidenced in the complex of cave temples at Yün-kang, which were begun about 460–70. Although some of the Kansu caves are older, the highest development of early Chinese Buddhist sculpture was attained with the harmonious blending of Chinese and Indian elements in the cave temples of Shansi.

The feverish large-scale building activity that took place in the vicinity of Tatung halted abruptly when the Wei transferred the capital to Loyang, in Honan, in 494. Shansi sculpture took on new life in the late 6th century when the province was partitioned between the Northern Ch'i dynasty in the east and the Northern Chou dynasty in the west, although the tradition had never been interrupted. Several of the sculptures discovered during excavations made in 1954 and 1955 in the environs of Taiyuan bear inscriptions from the years 540–45 (Eastern Wei dynasty).

The founder of the Northern Ch'i dynasty was a native of Taiyuan. Although Yeh, in northern Honan, was the capital of his short-lived dynasty, his native city continued to play a significant role. The most important complexes of Northern Ch'i sculpture are located in the earliest cave temples of T'ien-lung-shan, near Taiyuan, and of Ch'i-hsien, farther south. During the succeeding Sui and T'ang periods, the importance of Shansi further increased, and although there are many centers of T'ang sculpture in remote parts of China, such as Szechwan and Shantung, hardly any of them seem to have attained the artistic level of T'ang sculpture at T'ien-lung-shan.

With the decline of the T'ang empire, the stone sculpture of Shansi also declined rapidly. Probably it was never able to recover from the severe blow inflicted by the anti-Buddhist persecutions and the iconoclasm of the mid-9th century. The monasteries on Wu-t'ai-shan, that important goal of pilgrimages and the center of the cult of Mañjuśrī, were razed to the ground. The main hall of the temple Fo-kuang-ssū, which was rebuilt soon after and is the only existing wooden structure of the T'ang period, gives us some idea of the original magnificence of the site. When we see the Wu-t'ai-shan complex of temples as they were depicted in the wall paintings of Tun-huang in Kansu, we can realize how different it was from its present appearance.

Because northern China was spared the destruction of the Taiping rebellion (19th cent.), many wooden structures still exist there Many of these date from the periods when the Khitans and Jurchen controlled most of Shansi, though there are no examples extant here of pagodas of the Liao-Chin type (which occur in their purest form in Manchuria). The Hua-yen-ssū and P'u-ên-ssū at Tatung are among the most interesting specimens of the wooden architecture of the Liao and Chin dynasties in Shansi. It is difficult to discover to what extent this architecture had a character of its own; the few existing examples of Sung architecture in wood suggest that in Shansi the Chinese exerted a guiding influence upon the development. A few buildings from the early 11th century, such as the Shêng-mu-miao at Ch'in-tzu, near Taiyuan, and the hall of Mañjuśrī in the Fo-kuang-ssū, on Wu-t'ai-shan, date, perhaps, from before the Khitan invasion.

During the reign of the Liao and Chin, sculpture flourished anew with, on the one hand, a purely archaizing tendency seeking to revive the Wei, Northern Ch'i, and T'ang styles (the most impressive example of which is the colossal Buddha in Yün-kang Cave III) and, on the other hand, a new style. The latter, much more important, is related to a fundamental change in the material used by the sculptors, for in northern China, from that time on, wood almost completely replaced stone. The style of this wooden sculpture is a derivation from that of the T'ang and can be traced back to the last years of that dynasty. In its new form it had such vitality that it was only in the 14th and 15th centuries that signs of decadence became evident. Even though only a small number of the wooden sculptures in American and European collections can be definitely attributed to Shansi (including the Avalokiteśvara and the Mahāsthāmaprāptā, dated 1195; Toronto, Royal Ontario Mus.), many have remained in their original place. These prove that the center of this new school of sculpture must have been in Shansi. The clay-modeled figures of the Hsia Hua-yen-ssū at Tatung (1038) and of the Kuang-shêng-ssū near Chao-ch'eng-hsien (ca. 1150) are, because of their excellent state of preservation, a valuable aid in dating the wooden sculptures. In the Fen River valley there are numerous wall paintings and sculptures, many of which represent Kuan-yin (Avalokiteśvara).

A curious complex of cave temples on Lung-shan, near Taiyuan, dates from the first years after the Mongol expulsion of the Jurchen, and is particularly noteworthy because it is inspired by Taoism rather than Buddhism.

Tantric Buddhism entered Shansi with the Mongols. The extensive complex of temples on Wu-t'ai-shan became one of the great Tantric centers in China. The Tantric movement put an end to the more rigid style which had come to prevail in wooden sculpture, and the Tibetan element ultimately prevailed over the Chinese.

*Monuments and archaeological sites.* Chang-chih. In 1954–55 excavations laid bare some tombs of the late Chou period just north of Chang-chih, on the ridge of a hill on the Fen River. Of these tombs Nos. 12 and 14 contained many objects of interest, including several of great artistic merit. The furnishings of Tomb 14 included 8 bells, varying in height from 12 $^3/_4$ to 7 $^1/_2$ in., and 2 sets of musical stones, one of 7 and the other of 9 pieces. The most spectacular discovery in this tomb, however, was a series of 12 small pottery figures of the much discussed Hui-hsien type (see above, *Honan*). These are distinguished from the current faked pieces by their more rigid, primitive forms, completely alien to the grace and dynamic character of most of the spurious figurines. This discovery proved for the first time the existence of an authentic late Chou prototype of the known imitations.

BIBLIOG. Wu-shêng ch'u-t'u chung-yao wên-wu chan-lan t'u-lu (Illustrated Catalogue of Important Objects Excavated in Five Provinces), Peking, 1958, pls. 61–70.

Li-yü. In 1923 a group of late Chou bronzes (PL. 230) was discovered at Li-yü, on the north flank of Hêng-shan, following a landslide. Of these, 20 pieces were acquired by the Parisian antiquarian L. Wannieck, placed on exhibit at the Musée Cernuschi, Paris, in 1924, and later dispersed among various American and European collections. Another 18 pieces are now in the provincial museum of Shansi. Two swords from this group (Mus. Guimet, Paris, and Freer Gall., Washington) bear inscriptions which some experts believe establish these pieces as dating from 228 to 222 B.C. Even if this interpretation is correct, it cannot serve to date the entire group of bronzes, and several pieces may be considerably earlier. The style of decoration, typical of the late Chou period, is characterized chiefly by stylized animal motifs, interlace patterns in low relief, and rope patterns. These bronzes must be connected with the state of Chao, which ruled over this part of Shansi in the late Chou period.

BIBLIOG. G. Salles, Les bronzes de Li-yu, RAA, VIII, 3, 1934.

Yün-kang. On the steep slopes of Wu-chou-shan, about 10 miles west of Tatung in northern Shansi, is the famous complex of cave temples of Yün-kang. The terrain consists of horizontal limestone strata, well suited for cave digging and sculpture in the living rock. Over a distance of slightly under two-thirds of a mile, 20 large and 20 smaller caves were hollowed out, as well as many statuary niches. The most important caves in the complex are clustered in four groups in three sections of the hill.

The earliest caves are Nos. XVI–XX, all five having been sculptured at the instigation of the priest T'an-yao and under imperial patronage in the years after 460. The carved figures in these caves are so closely crowded within the confines of the walls and vaults as almost to seem cramped. From the exterior, the figures are only dimly visible through the arched doors and windows, except for Cave XX (II, PL. 382), where the roof and façade have fallen away.

The seated figure in Cave XIX, 55 ft. high, is flanked by two seated figures in individual side niches, one of which is visible because of the collapse of the façade. The technique used in hollowing out these caves was evidently inspired by that of Bamian (see AFGHANISTAN). Despite the gigantic scale, the proportions have been well maintained in general, and the large statues are neither squat nor too heavy.

The "five caves of T'an-yao" are followed by Caves VII, VIII, IX, and X, carved out in pairs. They differ from the preceding caves in having an anteroom (PL. 245) and a rear chamber, the walls and ceilings of which are covered with niches and figures in relief. The façades of Caves IX and X are almost completely open, supported by pillars carved out of the rock.

When additional caves were made later, the architecture of those already existing was copied. Cave XII follows the model of Nos. IX and X, and Cave V, in turn, imitates the earliest caves of T'an-yao. Undoubtedly one of the most beautiful caves is No. VI, thought to have been the last to be constructed under imperial auspices before the transfer of the Wei capital to Loyang in 494 put an end to the intense activity here. In this cave, as in Nos. V and VII, located in the area of the Shih-fo-ssŭ (Temple of the Stone Buddhas), a massive pillar at the center of the square room has been cut from the rock

and chiseled into the shape of a pagoda. The temple walls and the sides of the pillar are completely covered with sculptures, both inside and outside the niches. There are a great number of very beautiful bas-reliefs (PL. 240), including the well-known depictions of the life of Śākyamuni. This cave dates from about 490 and admirably illustrates Chinese progress in the adaptation of Central Asian styles.

Between 500 and 535 a number of smaller caves were sculptured here, together with many niches. It is interesting to compare these with the Lung-mên caves of the same period, near the new capital at Loyang, particularly because these sculptures are better preserved.

Cave III is the only one which was left unfinished. Japanese experts at first considered its great Buddha trinity to be of the Sui period. From the detailed investigations conducted by the Japanese scholars Mizuno and Nagahiro during World War II, it was concluded that these sculptures probably date from the Liao period (10th–11th cent.). The Chinese do not concur in this date. However, since many traces have been found, in the vicinity of Tatung and elsewhere, of the renaissance of sculpture under the Khitans, Mizuno's hypothesis is probably correct.

BIBLIOG. T. Shinkai and T. Nakagawu, Unko Sekkutsu (Rock Carvings from the Yün-kang Caves), Tokyo, Peking, 1921; D. Tokiwa and T. Sekino, Shina Bukkyō Shiseki (Buddhist Monuments in China), II, Tokyo, 1926–38, pp. 13–50; O. Sirén, Chinese Sculpture, London, 1925, I, pp. xi–xiv, 8–18, II, pls. 17–66; S. Mizuno, Archaeological Survey of the Yün-kang Grottoes, Arch. Chin. Art Soc. Am., IV, 1950; S. Mizuno and T. Nagahiro, Yün-kang, The Buddhist Cave Temples of the Fifth Century A.D. in North China, Kyoto, 1952–55; Lo Shu-tzu, Pei-ch'ao shih-k'u (Cave Temple Art of the Northern Dynasties), Shanghai, 1955, pp. 7–82.

T'ien-lung-shan. This complex of cave temples, discovered by the Japanese scholar T. Sekino in 1918, consists of two groups of caves on the southwestern slope of T'ien-lung-shan, 15 miles southwest of Taiyuan. Several Japanese scholars, as well as O. Sirén, visited, studied, and photographed this complex before it was despoiled of many of its sculptures by purveyors to unscrupulous antiquarians about 1923. The pillaging took place, unfortunately, at two different times. First the heads were stolen, and later the bodies, so that the figures now in various museums are almost all headless.

Most of these 24 caves, which are constructed on a rather small scale, date from the period of the Northern Ch'i and the T'ang. From the first period are Caves I–III on the eastern hill, and Nos. X and XVI on the western. Cave VIII is of the Sui period, very probably dating from 584. Caves IV–VII, XI–XV, and XVII–XXI are from the T'ang period, while No. IX is attributed to the Sung or Liao period.

The entrances of the caves of the Northern Ch'i period have a decoration derived from wooden architecture. In some cases the entrances are flanked by two stone guardians. In the caves, the sculptures (PL. 256) in high relief often consist of a seated Buddha and two standing bodhisattvas on each wall. Each group is contained within a leaf-shaped niche. The bas-reliefs on the walls represent monks and buddhas, and the trapezoidal panels of the ceiling, tapering toward the top central square with its lotus rosette, all bear very beautiful reliefs of apsarases. Caves II and III are probably somewhat earlier than Nos. X and XVI. The latter two contain a larger number of figures, two disciples of the Buddha and two lokapalas having been added to the trinities, while in Cave XVI the lotus-shaped decoration of the throne and the plinth of the base on which the principal figure stands show a later development in ornamentation. This cave also has a portal, supported by two hexagonal columns, on which rest a series of imitation roof brackets in relief. In the portal stand two fine lokapalas.

Cave VIII, dating from the Sui period, is the largest of the complex and also the only one with a center square pillar left in the rock when the cave was excavated. On the walls of the cave and on the sides of the pillar sculptures were carved, many of which were already seriously damaged at the time of their discovery.

The first sculptures of T'ien-lung-shan are artistically inferior to works of other cave temples of the same period, but this is not true of the T'ang sculptures, which, through both their artistic qualities and their number, show this to have been a period of artistic affluence. The lack of T'ang inscriptions makes it impossible to date the caves of this period accurately. O. Sirén makes a distinction between an earlier and a later group, the first consisting of Caves IV, V, VI, and XIV, and the second of Caves XVII–XXI. He dates the later group between 800 and 820 and the other some twenty years earlier. Japanese scholars are inclined to date the two groups respectively between 700–30 and 700–40. In their opinion the work on this complex was discontinued about the middle of the 8th century.

In the T'ang caves the high reliefs are almost sculpture in the round. Cave XIV, from which most of the sculptures have been removed (two are in the Mus. Rietberg, Zurich, one in the Mus. van Aziatische Kunst, Amsterdam, and one in the Nat. Mus., Tokyo), is one

of the most representative examples of the mature T'ang sculpture of T'ien-lung-shan.

The T'ang sculptures here form a group apart among the sculptures of this period. The graceful, full, often almost sensual forms, and the dynamic posture reminiscent of the *tribhanga* of Indian sculpture, are only examples of many aspects revealing a powerful Indian influence. The exceedingly soft sandstone was admirably adapted to the execution of this style and probably heightened its effect.

BIBLIOG. T. Sekino, Tenryūzan Sekkutsu (The Grottoes of T'ien-lung-shan), Kokka, no. 375, 1921; S. Tanaka, Tenryūzan Sekkutsu (The Grottoes of T'ien-lung-shan), 1922; O. Sirén, Chinese Sculpture, 4 vols., London, 1925, pls. 206–29, 293–9, 485–504: D. Tokiwa and T. Sekino, Shina Bukkyō Shiseki (Buddhist Monuments in China), III, Tokyo, 1926–38, pp. 17–35; S. Yamanaka, Tenryūzan Sekibutsu (The Stone Buddhas of T'ien-lung-shan), Osaka, 1928.

**Wu-t'ai-shan** (Mount Wutai). The monasteries and temples of this mountain were from the earliest times the center for the veneration of the Avataṃsaka Sūtra and the bodhisattva Mañjuśrī. The five peaks (*wu t'ai*, i.e., five terraces) from which the mountain gets its name, surrounded by a great many monasteries, were associated with that mythical locality where, according to the Buddhist scriptures, the bodhisattva Mañjuśrī is supposed to have resided. Subsequently, the five peaks were particularly connected with the five Tathāgatas in accordance with the doctrine of esoteric Tantric Buddhism which in ancient times was preached at the monasteries of these mountains. (See BUDDHISM.)

With the passage of time these monasteries have experienced many vicissitudes. During the anti-Buddhist persecutions of the mid-9th century, the temples, which are mentioned at great length in the diary of the Japanese pilgrim Ennin, were almost all destroyed. An early Sung wall painting in Cave 61 at Tun-huang (P. Pelliot, op. cit., under *Kansu*, pl. 117), depicting a panorama of Wu-t'ai-shan with its temples, is helpful in reconstructing the approximate appearance of this pilgrimage site at that period. Visible in the painting are no less than 67 large and small temples, 28 pagodas, many bridges, walls, etc. Before World War II there still existed some hundred temples and monasteries here, but as a result of repeated restoration nearly all the present temples have only the name in common with the ancient structures mentioned in the accounts of pilgrims. For many centuries most of the monasteries have belonged to the Lamaist sect, a fact clearly apparent in the Tibetan style of architecture of the numerous stupas.

The sole exception among all these structures of late date, going back at the most to the Ming dynasty, is the Fo-kuang-ssŭ, of which the main hall dates from the second half of the 9th century, as Chinese archaeologists were able to establish in the 1940s. This is the oldest wooden building extant in China.

BIBLIOG. D. Pokotilov, Wu-t'ai, Its Former and Present State (in Rus.), St. Petersburg, 1893; E. Chavannes, Mission Archéologique dans la Chine Septentrionale, VI: Wou-t'ai-chan, Paris, 1909; W. Fischer, The Sacred Wu-t'ai-shan, 1925; D. Tokiwa and T. Sekino, Shina Bukkyō Shiseki (Buddhist Monuments in China), V, Tokyo, 1938, pp. 1–38; S. Ono and C. Hibino, Godaisan (Wu-t'ai-shan), Tokyo, 1942.

**Lung-shan.** On the eastern face of this mountain are eight caves containing Taoist sculptures. Caves I, II, and III (Sekino and Tokiwa's numeration) are located toward the south, one above the other. Side by side to the north are Nos. VII and VIII, and in between are Nos. IV, V, and VI. Except for Caves III and VII, they seem to have been built under the auspices of the Taoist Sung P'i-yün in 1234–39. This famous Taoist personage is portrayed in a sculpture located in Cave VII, which is dedicated to him and seems to have been constructed during his lifetime.

The iconography of the sculptures is strongly influenced by that of Buddhism. This is clearly evident in the arrangement of the trinities, as well as by the presence of halos, temple guardians, and so forth. The persons portrayed are famous Taoists or such legendary Chinese figures as Shên-nung, Huang-ti, and Fu-hsi.

BIBLIOG. O. Sirén, Chinese Sculpture, London, 1925, I, p. 165, IV, pls. 609A–612B; D. Tokiwa and T. Sekino, Shina Bukkyō Shiseki (Buddhist Monuments in China), III, Tokyo, 1926–38, pp. 35–41.

**SHANTUNG.** *Survey of geography and art history.* This province, originally an island, was joined to northern China by silting of the Yellow River. It consists of two distinct parts: the western part belongs to the flood plains of the Yellow River, from which the T'ai-shan, the sacred mountain of China, rises. Farther east, on the other hand, the mountains form a series of hills that march toward the sea and that were once connected with the mountains of the Liaotung Peninsula of Manchuria. The Yellow River found its course obstructed by the T'ai-shan and over the years has many times changed

direction, seeking an outlet now to the north and now to the south of the mountains.

Found distributed over nearly the whole province of Shantung are remains of the neolithic Black Pottery or Lung-shan culture, which may have spread from this area to the north, south, and west, and which must have contributed greatly to the beginnings of the bronze culture of the Shang people. The type site of this culture at Ch'êng-tzŭ-yai (Lung-shan) is located to the northeast of Tsinan (Chi-nan). Traces of the Yang-shao culture are virtually absent.

In the vicinity of Tsinan (the modern provincial capital), Ch'ü-fu, and Tsingtao (Ch'ing-tao) there are remnants of the Shang culture.

The great age in the history of this province was no doubt the period of the Chou, when Shantung was part of the territory of the states of Lu and Ch'i. The greatest Chinese philosopher, Confucius, was a native of Lu, and his tomb is venerated to this day at Ch'ü-fu. The houses of his descendants, the temple erected in his honor, and an abundance of commemorative steles, mostly of the Ming and Ch'ing periods, occupy considerable space within the walls of his native city. (Cf. PLS. 438, 439.) However, no trace of a monument of the period of Confucius himself has survived.

The monuments of Shantung are mainly of two types. The first consists of a group of Han mortuary monuments. Small offering shrines were erected near the burial mounds, built of heavy stone slabs and decorated in various techniques. These have been known for centuries, through rubbings made by Chinese scholars, and on Hsiao-t'ang-shan one of them has been preserved almost intact. Almost all the decorated stone slabs from the small temples that once stood near the Wu family tombs (the famous Wu Liang-tz'ŭ) have also been preserved. The recent find of a large tomb at Yi-nan, decorated with similar designs although treated in a rather different manner, has added greatly to our knowledge of Han art. The local character of the style becomes more noticeable if it is compared with the art of Szechwan, where many finds of the same kind have been made. The Yi-nan find revealed that the carefully arranged, somewhat static reliefs of the Wu Liang-tz'ŭ are not truly representative of the Han reliefs of Shantung as a whole, and that the differences between the reliefs of the Wu Liang-tz'ŭ and the much livelier, but less systematic Szechwan art are slighter than was once thought.

Like Szechwan, Shantung has many noteworthy Han stone sculptures. If the date assigned to the Wu Liang-tz'ŭ (147–80) is also applicable to the pair of large stone lions standing in the immediate vicinity of the mounds, these are the oldest of their kind. Also, the two stone guardians near the tomb of Lu Wang at Ch'ü-fu (146–56) and several other "stone men" are among the extremely rare examples of Han stone sculpture. Comparison with the earlier sculptures of the tomb of Ho Ch'ü-p'ing (in Shensi) shows, however, hardly any trace of stylistic development. The colossal mass of stone still continued to prevail over the sculptured forms.

Another group of great monuments of a quite different character was inspired by the Buddhist sacred scriptures. Among these there are some dated steles, bearing inscriptions from the years around 520. At about the same time work must have been started on the cave temples, as is apparent in the inscriptions of the severely damaged Huang-shih-yai and in an isolated figure carved in the rock near the cave temple of Lung-tung.

From this modest start during the rule of the Northern Ch'i there developed later in the Sui and T'ang periods an important local tradition of Buddhist sculpture. Near Tsinan, in particular, and farther east near Yitu (Ch'ing-chou), several groups of cave temples are found. The great development of this school during the Sui period has made of this province a veritable storehouse of Sui sculptures, far superior to many from the other provinces. Since the Shantung stone is harder than that of Shansi, many of the sculptures here are better preserved.

This sculpture reached its zenith in the T'ang period. Sculptures of later date, such as the great Buddha of the K'ai-yüan-ssŭ (1036) near Li-ch'êng, and a sculptured niche (1318) near the cave temple of Lung-tung, prove that the great tradition declined considerably.

A few pagodas of the Sung period also remain, for example the octagonal pagoda of the Hsing-lung-ssŭ (982 or 1063) at Yen-chou, and the Iron Pagoda (1105) of Tsining (Chi-ning). The most important and imposing complex of Ming and Ch'ing architecture is in the city of Ch'ü-fu.

BIBLIOG. E. Chavannes, Mission Archéologique dans la Chine Septentrionale, I, Paris, 1913, part 1; T. Sekino, Shina Santōshō ni Okeru Kandai Fumbō Hyōshoku Fuzu (The Decoration of the Han Tombs in Shantung Province), Tokyo, 1916; O. Sirén, Chinese Sculpture, 4 vols., London, 1925; D. Tokiwa and T. Sekino, Shina Bukkyō Shiseki (Buddhist Monuments in China), I, Tokyo, 1926.

*Monuments and archaeological sites.* Hsiao-t'ang-shan. On this mountain, 25 miles southwest of the city of Fei-ch'êng, stands an offering shrine belonging to a burial mound, sheltered by a small

temple which was built entirely over it. It is important inasmuch as these stone structures have disappeared almost everywhere else. It was built of limestone slabs on a square ground plan. The sloping roof is made of four large slabs, which make the structure about 13 ft. wide. The façade is open, creating a wide entrance divided in two by an octagonal pillar standing on a plinth in the center. The pillar has a capital supporting a heavy stone beam, further supported on the two ends by similar pillars (of a later date) and by two rectangular columns. The side walls consist of one slab, and the rear wall of two, all smoothed off and decorated with scenes and ornaments in intaglio.

The succession of scenes in clearly demarcated zones and the penchant for certain historical and mythological subjects are closely reminiscent of the reliefs of the Wu Liang-tz'ŭ, but the decorative technique is very different. Among the representations is one showing Shih Huang-ti fishing up the Chou tripod, a theme known from similar representations elsewhere. There are also hunting scenes and processions, characteristic of Han reliefs and paintings.

A dated inscription made by a visitor establishes the monument as earlier than 129. The tradition attributing the erection of the shrine to the pious Kou Chü probably is of much later date.

BIBLIOG. T. Sekino, Ancient Chinese Stone Shrines, Kokka, no. 225, Feb., 1909, pp. 229–41; E. Chavannes, Mission Archéologique dans la Chine Septentrionale, I, Paris, 1913, part. 1, pp. 62–94; W. Fairbanks, The Offering Shrines of Wu Liang-tz'ŭ, HJAS, 1941, pp. 16–19.

Wu Liang-tz'ŭ. Chao Ming-chêng (1081–1129), a famous archaeologist of the Sung dynasty, mentions in one of his writings the existence of a temple where offerings were made at the burial mounds, near Chia-hsiang, where certain members of the Wu family were buried between 147 and 180. Shortly afterward, Hung Kua (1117–84) published rubbings of the reliefs adorning the stone slabs of the walls in this temple, and Chinese archaeologists since then have frequently referred to the Wu Liang-tz'ŭ (offering shrine of Wu Liang) in their writings. In the 18th century there were unearthed in the same locality numerous reliefs that apparently belonged to several similar shrines. Huang Yi (1744–1801) assembled all these reliefs in a building where, except for a few pieces, they are still preserved today. In 1941 W. Fairbanks published a proposed reconstruction, generally accepted today, of the reliefs from the four shrines. The figures, shown against a background of vertical striations, display a great variety of lively scenes. In many cases the artist has explained the subjects, which are superposed in rows, with brief inscriptions. The themes, drawn from official histories and also from apocryphal texts and legends, have been the subject of many studies. Until a few decades ago, the Wu Liang-tz'ŭ reliefs were almost the only material from which Han painting could be reconstructed, and for the study of Han folklore they remain a highly valuable source.

BIBLIOG. E. Chavannes, Mission Archéologique dans la Chine Septentrionale, I, Paris, 1913, part 1, pp. 94–221; W. Fairbanks, The Offering Shrines of Wu Liang-tz'ŭ, HJAS, VI, 1941, pp. 1–36.

Yi-nan. In March, 1954, a tomb was discovered here, still concealed under its original mound, so that the architecture of its eight rooms had remained completely intact. The entrance is on the southern side, from which one enters the three main rooms, located one behind the other and accompanied by two side chambers on each side. The symmetry of the ground plan is broken by a long, rectangular chamber behind the side chamber on the east side. The entire structure is 25 ft. wide by 29 ft. deep; 280 stone slabs were used in constructing it, 42 of which bear incised or bas-relief decoration. In general, the themes are similar to those of the Wu Liang-tz'ŭ, but the style is considerably different, for here the figures and scenes were incised in the stone in thin lines. An Chih-min has suggested a date of 220–313 for this tomb, while other scholars prefer to place it in the Han period, shortly before 193.

BIBLIOG. K'ao-ku t'ung-hsin, 1955, no. 2, pp. 12–16, 16–20; Tsêng Chao-chü, Yi-nan ku-hua-hsiang shih-mu fa-chüeh pao-kao, Peking, 1956; Chêng Tê-k'un, Ch'ih-yu, the God of War in Han Art, O. Art, N. S., IV, 2, 1958, pp. 45–54.

Huang-shih-yai. In a natural cave and in sculptured niches on the northwest face of Li-shan, south of Tsinan, there are about 75 carved figures, all dating from the 6th century. The earliest votive inscription is of the year 522, the latest, 540. The style of the sculptures is characteristic of the Wei period. Unfortunately the heads of nearly all the statues have been carried off.

BIBLIOG. D. Tokiwa and T. Sekino, Shina Bukkyō Shiseki (Buddhist Monuments in China), I, Tokyo, 1926, pp. 75–7; Wên-wu ts'an-k'ao tzŭ-liao, 1955, no. 9, pp. 22–39.

Lien-hua-tung. This cave is dug in the flank of Wu-fêng, 25 miles south of Fei-ch'êng, and takes its name, "Cave of the Lotuses,"

from the relief decoration on the slightly arched ceiling, which is completely covered with stylized lotus flowers. There is also a sculptured group consisting of a seated Śākyamuni flanked by two disciples and two bodhisattvas, with approximately 150 small niches containing reliefs of the Buddha. One of these bears a votive inscription dated 560. No exact date can be determined for the cave itself because of the damage suffered by the principal inscription (which may be from 562), but it seems very likely that it was indeed constructed about that time.

BIBLIOG. O. Sirén, Chinese Sculpture, London, 1925, I, pp. 70–1, IV, pl. 264; D. Tokiwa and T. Sekino, Shina Bukkyō Shiseki (Buddhist Monuments in China), I, Tokyo, 1926, pp. 80–2.

Ch'ien-fo-shan (Mount of the Thousand Buddhas). This rock face, a part of the Li-shan, almost 2 miles southeast of Tsinan, contains many niches and sculptures. In contrast to Yü-han-shan, all the figures are Buddhas and Maitreyas, which, to judge from the inscriptions, were all executed between 581 and 598. Recently all the sculptures here were completely repainted.

BIBLIOG. E. Chavannes, Mission Archéologique dans la Chine Septentrionale, I, Paris, 1915, part 2, pp. 574–6; D. Tokiwa and T. Sekino, Shina Bukkyō Shiseki (Buddhist Monuments in China), I, Tokyo, 1926, p. 91; Wên-wu ts'an-k'ao tzŭ-liao, 1955, no. 9, pp. 26–8.

Ch'ien-fo-yai (Rock of the Thousand Buddhas). On a rocky slope southwest of the Shên-t'ung-ssŭ, 30 miles southeast of Tsinan, more than 70 niches and 5 caves have been carved out. The great majority of the sculptures date from the 7th century.

The most important cave is No. II, which consists of two chambers separated by a pillar in the center of the façade. In each of these there is a seated Buddha against a back wall, on which are small figures in relief. The main figures, identified as Amitābha and Śākyamuni by the inscriptions, date from 618. Other figures in this complex date from 644 and 657. These were executed upon the order of the monk Ming-tê, master of the renowned pilgrim Yi-ching (7th cent.). Sirén has supposed on stylistic grounds that some figures belong to the period of the Northern Ch'i, but those bearing dated inscriptions are without exception from the 7th or the early 8th century. The Ch'ien-fo-yai has suffered little damage.

Near the Shên-t'ung-ssŭ are several pagodas, including the Ssŭ-mên-t'a (Pagoda of the Four Doors), which takes its name from the doors on each side of the square structure. It has only one story, and the roof, crowned by a peak ornament, is supported by a cornice of layers of projecting stones. According to some, it dates from 544 and contains sculptures from the period of the Eastern Wei or the Northern Ch'i period. However, these have suffered considerable damage and have been badly restored.

Of somewhat different structure is the Lang-kung-t'a or Lung-hu-t'a (called "Lung-hua-t'a" by Sirén), a tripartite building with a square ground plan. The base is divided by three cornices, in the form of slabs projecting widely on all sides. The shaft, provided with niches, is of special interest because of the rich decoration in relief. The upper section consists of two low stories, both with two series of brackets which formerly supported the roofs, but which have disappeared. The pagoda probably dates from the late T'ang period (9th and 10th cent.).

BIBLIOG. O. Sirén, Chinese Sculpture, London, 1925, I, pp. 69–70, III, pls. 260–3; D. Tokiwa and T. Sekino, Shina Bukkyō Shiseki (Buddhist Monuments in China), I, Tokyo, 1926, pp. 54–63; O. Sirén, A History of Early Chinese Art, IV: Architecture, London, 1930, p. 50; E. Boerschmann, Die Baukunst und Religiöse Kultur der Chinesen, III: Pagoden, Berlin, Leipzig, 1931, pp. 278–83, 367–70; Wên-wu ts'an-k'ao tzŭ-liao, 1956, no. 3, pp. 62–4, no. 10, pp. 28–36.

Lung-tung. Located about 12 miles southeast of Tsinan, this temple consists of two natural caves and a number of niches with reliefs dating from the 6th century to the Yüan dynasty. The largest cave, divided into two parts, contains 28 sculptures of great size, the largest being about 16 ft. high; they reveal an unmistakable Sui style, but the softness of the rock has caused great erosion. The earliest sculpture in this temple is a standing Buddha in Wei style, near the entrance to the largest cave. Tokiwa and Sekino have identified this Buddha with an image recorded in local gazetteers as bearing an inscription of 537. A niche with a votive inscription of 1318 contains a very interesting group of figures, among them Śākyamuni and his disciples Mahākāśyapa and Ānanda, as well as the bodhisattvas Mañjuśrī and Samantabhadra seated upon their symbolic mounts, the lion and the elephant. The niche is a fine example of Yüan work.

BIBLIOG. O. Sirén, Chinese Sculpture, 4 vols., London, 1925, p. 95, pls. 356–60; D. Tokiwa and T. Sekino, Shina Bukkyō Shiseki (Buddhist Monuments in China), I, Tokyo, 1926, pp. 82–7.

Yü-han-shan. On an overhanging cliff of the southern face of this mountain, about 10 miles southeast of Tsinan, there are five rows

of niches with Buddhist figures. The lowest row includes five large niches, in each of which is a Buddhist trinity. The second row has 27 figures about a foot high. The third has 11 sculptures, one of which bears an inscription of 584. The fourth row contains 17 sculptures, and the fifth, a group of quite large figures. The total number of sculptures is 92. On the basis of the inscriptions, we may suppose that the figures were executed between 584 and about 600, except for the Amitābha, which dates from 759, and a Maitreya, from 837. Despite the serious damage caused by erosion, the high quality of these sculptures is still unmistakable.

BIBLIOG. O. Sirén, Chinese Sculpture, 4 vols, London, 1925. p. 94, pls. 351–5; D. Tokiwa and T. Sekino, Shina Bukkyō Shiseki (Buddhist Monuments in China), I, Tokyo, 1926, pp. 87–90; Wên-wu ts'an-k'ao tzŭ-liao, 1955, no. 9, pp. 26–39.

Yün-mên-shan and T'o-shan. On both these peaks, lying opposite one another 2½ miles from Yitu (Ch'ing-chou), caves and sculptures are carved in the rock. Yün-mên-shan has five caves. Nos. I and II (according to Sekino and Tokiwa's numbering) contain important sculptures of the Sui period (PL. 245). In Cave I, there is a trinity consisting of a seated Buddha and two standing bodhisattvas. On the back wall there are small reliefs, thirty-odd of the Buddha and the rest of Amitābha. The donors' votive inscriptions indicate that they date from 596–99, and the trinity is probably of the same period. In Cave II only one of the very beautiful bodhisattvas that once accompanied the principal figure remains.

The other caves are of the T'ang period and were built between 727 and 753. A remarkable group is that of a seated Buddha accompanied by four attendants (ca. 727), carved from a wall completely covered with small figures of buddhas.

On the T'o-shan, close to the summit, are six cave temples. Nos. II, III, and IV contain important sculptures of the Sui period, which, although somewhat stiffer and heavier, reveal a close stylistic kinship with the figures of the Yün-mên-shan. In both No. II and No. III, the central figure is a seated Śākyamuni. Here, too, the wall behind the principal figure and the attendant bodhisattvas is covered with small standing buddhas in relief. A donor's votive inscription indicates that this cave was sculptured between 577 and 594. According to the inscriptions, Cave I dates from 702–03; it contains some fine T'ang sculptures.

BIBLIOG. O. Sirén, Chinese Sculpture, 4 vols., London, 1925, pp. 90–3, pls. 334–50; D. Tokiwa and T. Sekino, Shina Bukkyō Shiseki (Buddhist Monuments in China), IV, Tokyo, 1926–38, pp. 56–61; Wên-wu ts'an-k'ao tzŭ-liao, 1957, no. 10, pp. 30–3.

SHENSI (Shen-hsi). Survey of geography and art history. The territory of the present province of Shensi consists of various geographic units differing sharply one from another. The cultural and economic center is the valley of the Wei River, crossing the province from west to east and emptying into the Yellow River. The northern part of Shensi borders on the desert of the Ordos (q.v.) and is separated from it by the Great Wall.

In the remote past, the valleys of the Wei and the Ching-ho (King River) belonged to the area of the Red Pottery or Yang-shao culture, very numerous remains of which have been found in recent years, including a complete village (Pan-p'o-ts'un) located east of Sian. During the Shang dynasty, the bronze culture of the Great Plain must have spread here. This is attested by the finds made near Nan-sha-ts'un (Hua-hsien) in the Wei valley and at Pin-hsien in the Ching-ho valley. Several important bronzes of the early Chou period have also been found.

The Wei valley played a decisive role in the history of China at the time that the state of Ch'in was founded here. In a strategically favorable position, Ch'in contended with the state of Chin (see above, Shansi) for the possession of the Ho-hsi territory, and, after the downfall of Ch'in, found an outlet toward the Great Plain, conquered Szechwan, and soon afterward won control over the entire country.

The capital of the first empire was built in the territory of the conqueror, at Hsien-yang in the Wei valley. This established a tradition, for other princes and dynasties subsequently established their capitals in this area, in the vicinity of the modern city of Sian (Hsi-an). One result of this was that Shensi, today outside the political and cultural center of China, was for centuries the heart of the Middle Kingdom, and enjoyed consequently a typically metropolitan culture.

The Han dynasty established here its capital, Ch'ang-an, which, from an agglomeration of official buildings and dwellings, was transformed into a metropolis more than 3½ miles square. Nothing remains except the vestiges of walls and foundations, but a critical study of these has made it possible to reconstruct roughly the outlines of the city. Only to the southeast and northwest did the builders depart from an almost perfectly square ground plan. This city developed gradually, so that there was no precise symmetry in the placing of the markets and most important buildings. Three gates on each

side provided access to the city, the walls of which were almost precisely aligned with the four cardinal points. The remains of the Han city are located about 6 miles to the northwest of present-day Sian. (Both "Hsien-yang" and "Ch'ang-an" are viewed as ancient names of Sian, but the capital actually shifted to the southeast with the centuries.)

Under the rule of the usurper Wang Mang (A.D. 9–23), efforts were made to heighten the government's prestige by constructing several buildings that from ancient times were associated with royalty, the Ming-t'ang and the Pi-yung, traces of which are believed to have been found recently south of the Han city. This once-powerful city was subsequently reduced to a group of small villages, linked together by what had been the streets of the former Imperial City.

One single monument in the Wei valley can provide some idea of the grandeur of the Han dynasty. This is the tomb of the general Ho Ch'ü-p'ing, for whose mortal remains a great burial mound, surrounded by large stone sculptures, was built in 117 B.C. Ségalen's archaeological expedition first drew attention to these sculptures. The best-known is that of a horse trampling a barbarian, which, despite the obvious unfamiliarity of the artist with the technique of sculpture in the round, can be considered a fine example of primitive sculpture. The others (of the 16 known pieces) are merely crude blocks of stone handled in primitive fashion to portray various animals. The recent find of a similar sculpture near Hsien-yang (now in the provincial museum of Shensi) proves for the first time that the products of this primitive school of sculpture were not confined to the funerary monument of Ho Ch'ü-p'ing.

The best of the Shensi tomb sculptures were to be found in the old imperial province. Along the "Spirit Road" (Shên-tao) leading to the tomb of the T'ang emperor Kao-tsung (d. 683) were erected many gigantic stone sculptures. The horses, lions, and imposing high officials among them are all rather massive and of a stiff monumentality; by contrast, one of the group, a very beautiful Celestial Horse with stylized wings, can well stand comparison with the winged lions of the earlier imperial tombs near Nanking. On the other hand, the figures near the tomb of the mother of Empress Wu (684–705) already reveal the weakness which was to appear so obviously in the Ming tomb sculptures: a lifeless, stiff heaviness.

The ostriches standing near the tomb of Kao-tsung were executed in high relief, a technique already successfully adopted in other instances, for example, in the oldest T'ang imperial funerary monument. The reliefs for this monument were ordered about 637 by the emperor T'ai-tsung, founder of the dynasty, and intended for a doorway or gate leading to his mound. The plans are attributed to the painter Yen Li-pên, but it is not clear in what order the reliefs were arranged. (Two are now in the University Museum, Philadelphia, and four in the provincial museum of Shensi.)

The T'ang dynasty established its capital at Ch'ang-an, where the preceding Sui dynasty had settled in 583. This new city was somewhat south of the former Han capital of Ch'ang-an. In building it from scratch, without having to take into account already existing palaces, temples, and residential complexes, the planners were able to improve upon earlier capitals, such as Loyang and Yeh, both in Honan. The ground plan of Ch'ang-an displays the checkerboard plan so much favored by the Chinese. The streets intersected one another at right angles in the north–south and east–west directions, and the eastern, western, and southern walls each had three gates. In the northern section was the Imperial City with the many buildings of the palace; a new quarter of palaces (Ta-ming-kung) was added outside the walled rectangle on the north during the T'ang dynasty. Fire and destruction have left little of this beautiful T'ang city except the characteristic street system. Because of the anti-Buddhist persecutions of the mid-9th century, all the temples have been lost, together with the marvelous paintings and sculptures which were described at length in the Li-tai ming-hua-chi (847) of Chang Yen-yüan. (All wall paintings of the T'ang period found in this province come from tomb excavations.) On the frontier with Kansu, in the Ching-ho valley, there are some small temple complexes which, being located on the caravan road leading from the capital to Central Asia, must have enjoyed a long period of prosperity, but their sculptures, much restored, cannot give us any accurate idea of those that stood in the capital. The same is true of the cave temples in the district of Lin-yu.

Despite the destruction, the high artistic level of metropolitan sculpture is attested by the sculptures from Ch'ang-an now scattered around the entire globe, including those originally from the Pao-ch'ing-ssŭ. The Sian style of sculpture is perhaps derived from that which, during the period of the Northern Chou, had its center here, and one of the finest creations of which is an Avalokiteśvara (ca. 570) now in the Boston Museum of Fine Arts. A few pagodas, the most famous of which is the Ta-yen-t'a, are an impressive, if isolated, reminder of the golden age of Buddhism and of the life of the great pilgrim Hsüan-tsang in particular.

While the great city was sacked and demolished, the extensive cemetery, expanding over the centuries in the surrounding countryside, retained a large part of its treasures. Although the interest awakened in T'ang funerary sculpture about 1910 attracted many grave robbers, who have scattered through the Western world the contents of many of the tombs, many virtually intact tombs continue to be excavated by Chinese archaeologists. According to the wealth and the rank of the deceased, the tombs contained either costly hand-modeled figures or simple, cheap molded pieces. These figurines represent people of widely different races, quite in keeping with the cosmopolitan life in the T'ang capital.

Until the end of the dynasty of the Northern Sung (1126–27), Ch'ang-an and the Wei valley retained their importance, although the capital was moved several times. The emperors preferred Loyang (in Honan) as their residence, although they often returned to Ch'ang-an. With the fall of Kaifeng, however, and the southward emigration, Ch'ang-an lost forever its position as China's political center, and this meant inevitably the end of its cultural life.

BIBLIOG. O. Sirén, Chinese Sculpture, 4 vols., London, 1925; K. Adachi, Chō-an Shiseki no Kenkyū (Researches on the Historical Remains of Ch'angan), Tokyo, 1933; R. B. Acker, Some T'ang and Pre-T'ang Texts on Chinese Painting, Leiden, 1954; Wên-wu ts'an-k'ao tzŭ-liao, 1957, no. 3, pp. 5–12, no. 4, pp. 5–9, and 1958, no. 5, p. 80, no. 11, pp. 65–6.

*Monuments and archaeological sites. Hsing-p'ing.* In the Wei valley, in the district of Hsing-p'ing, stands a high mound which, according to tradition, was built over the tomb of the famous general Ho Ch'ü-p'ing, who died in 117 B.C. The monument, important for the very large stone sculptures surrounding it, dates from the 2d century B.C. In all, 16 pieces (including some found in 1957) are known. The best known is that of a standing horse trampling on a recumbent barbarian archer. The natural form of the rock almost prevails over the work of the sculptor, who has taken the maximum advantage of the original shape. Some sculptures have a crude, almost unfinished appearance.

The 7 sculptures recently discovered have been described as an elephant, 2 fishes, 2 monsters, a frog, and an unrecognizable animal. The sketchily sculptured elephant may possibly have been inspired by the animal which, a few years before Ho Ch'ü-p'ing's death, was offered to the emperor in tribute. Of great interest is the fact that on one of the pieces there is an inscription of three characters bearing the name of the Ministry of Public Works (Tso-ssŭ-k'ung), while another inscription, partly illegible, records the name of this district in the Han period.

BIBLIOG. V. Ségalen, JA, V, 1915, pp. 471–4; V. Ségalen, G. de Voisins, and J. Lartigue, Mission Archéologique en Chine, I, Paris, 1923–24, pls. 2, 3; J. Lartigue, Au tombeau de Houo K'iu-ping, Artibus Asiae, II, 1927, pp. 85–94; Wên-wu ts'an-k'ao tzŭ-liao, 1955, no. 4, pp. 11–18, 1958, no. 11, pp. 62–3.

**Ch'ang-an.** The sites at Ch'ang-an, capital during the Han, Sui, and T'ang dynasties, are described under the survey above.

**Ta-yen-t'a (Great Gander Pagoda).** This pagoda (PL. 273), which forms part of the temple Tz'u-ên-ssŭ near Sian (Hsi-an), was built under the guidance of the famous pilgrim Hsüan-tsang in 652. The building as it now stands is the result of many radical changes and partial reconstructions. The last two of the present seven stories were added before the mid-10th century. The pagoda, of brick, is almost square in ground plan (about 82 ft. square) and is almost 200 ft. high. Each story, diminishing in size, is separated from the next by a cornice of projecting stones and has four arched windows. The upper stories are reached by means of a central stairway. On the ground floor, which has a solid core, four corridors lead to the central room (22 ft. square). In the pagoda's southern wall are two niches containing imperial steles. The carving on the stone plinth of the western entrance depicts a Buddhist temple, which until a short while ago was almost the only source for the study of Chinese wooden architecture of the T'ang period. The name of the pagoda seems to have been taken from that of a pagoda of Magadha in India which Hsüantsang saw during his journey and which probably served as a prototype for this monument.

BIBLIOG. D. Tokiwa and T. Sekino, Shina Bukkyō Shiseki (Buddhist Monuments in China), I, Tokyo, 1926, pp. 5–10; E. Boerschmann, Die Baukunst und religiöse Kultur der Chinesen, III: Pagoden, Berlin, Leipzig, 1931, pp. 39–52.

**Pao-ch'ing-ssŭ.** Until the beginning of this century there were kept in this temple, at Sian, a number of exquisite T'ang sculptures, which had been brought here from the temple Kuang-chai-ssŭ. Some were originally part of the decoration of the Ch'i-pao-t'ai (Terrace of the Seven Treasures, or Jewels), which was built at the command of the usurping Empress Wu (reigned 684–705). These

sculptures were first installed in the pagoda of the temple Pao-ch'ing-ssŭ, but after a restoration of the pagoda (1723), some pieces were put into the pagoda walls and others were inserted into the brick walls of the main temple hall. The 19 pieces in the main hall (17 trinities and 2 statues of the eleven-headed Kuan-yin) were taken to Japan by Hayazaki in 1906. Other pieces, of which 5 represent the eleven-headed Kuan-yin (PL. 254), are now in various private and museum collections (Mus. of Fine Arts, Boston; Freer Gall. of Art, Washington; Hara Coll., Yokohama). Some of the sculptures have dated inscriptions (A.D. 703, 704, and 724). As a whole, they may be divided stylistically into three groups: an early T'ang group, a series made during the reign of the Empress Wu for the Ch'i-pao-

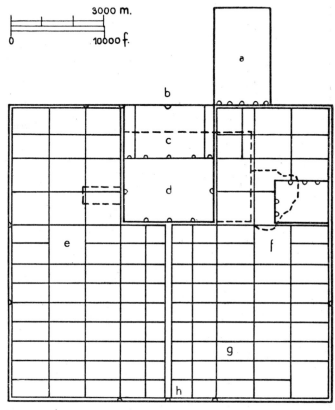

Plan of Ch'ang-an in the T'ang period (A.D. 618–906); modern city limits shown by broken line. (a) Ta-ming-kung; (b) An-li gate; (c) T'ai-chi palace; (d) Imperial City; (e) west market; (f) east market; (g) Ta-yen-t'a; (h) Ming-tê gate (after Willetts).

t'ai, and a series dating from the beginning of the K'ai-yüan era (712–41). All of these were carved in high relief and placed in deeply carved niches, broad for the trinities and narrow for the standing Kuan-yin figures. They represent the best quality of T'ang sculpture in the capital area.

BIBLIOG. O. Sirén, Chinese Sculpture, 4 vols., London, 1925, pp. 391–7; D. Tokiwa and T. Sekino, Shina Bukkyō Shiseki (Buddhist Monuments in China), I, Tokyo, 1926, pp. 23–30; T. Fukuyama, Grouping of the Buddhist Reliefs of the Pao-ch'ing-ssŭ Temple in Hsi-an, China, Ars Buddhica, IX, Oct., 1950.

**Ching-ho valley.** For cave temples in this valley, see above, *Kansu.*

*Kiln sites.* Around the village of Huang-pao-chên, on the railway halfway between Tungchuan and the present town of Yao-hsien, many shards and saggers have been found which prove that this was once an important center of pottery production. Sung sources indicate that the ware made here was called Yao-yao (Yao ware) after the district of Yao-chou, to which the village at that time belonged. The shards are of the well-known "northern celadon" type, and the ware is therefore closely related to that of kilns in nearby Honan and Hopei. An inscription of 1105, found by Ch'ên Wan-li in the ruins of a small shrine dedicated to the tutelary deity of the potters of Tangyang-yü (in Hopei), mentions the previous founding of a similar shrine here, at Yao-chün. A stele commemorating the founding of this shrine was found at Huang-pao-chên. It bears a date corresponding to 1084 and thereby proves the Sung date of the kilns.

At Huang-pao-chên only two complete pieces of Yao ware were found, but 45 intact pieces were discovered (1954) in a hole dug

into a cliff beside the Huang-lung-ho, in nearby Pin-hsien. The pieces, among which were many lotus-shaped bowls, had probably been hidden there by monks of the local monastery in the middle of the last century.

Bibliog. Wên-wu ts῾an-k῾ao tzǔ-liao, 1954, no. 4, pp. 44–7, 1955, no. 4, pp. 75–8; Yao-tz῾ǔ t῾u-lu (An Illustrated Catalogue of Yao Ware), Peking, 1956.

Jan Fontein

Sinkiang (Hsin-chiang). *Survey of geography and art history.* This province embraces a vast area bounded on the west and northwest by the Soviet frontier from the Pamirs to north of the Altai, on the northeast by the Mongolian People's Republic, on the east by the western sections of the provinces of Kansu and Tsinghai, and on the south by Tibet. It includes Chinese Turkistan, which until about the year 1000 was known as Serindia.

Sinkiang province was established in the 18th century, taking in the territories wrested by the Manchus from the Dzungars, or Kalmucks, in the northern part of the region, and from the small Moslem kingdoms in the Tarim Basin. At that time the province extended north as far as Lake Balkhash, and the small Moslem kingdoms located west of the Celestial Mountains (T῾ien-shan) were also considered tributary countries. It was only during the second half of the 19th century that the frontier between the Manchu empire and the Russian empire was stabilized.

Within the province lie immense desert and mountain regions which are largely uninhabited. In general it can be said that the regions north of the Celestial Mountains and their extension are inhabited by nomadic Turkish and Mongol peoples, while the arable regions are occupied by Chinese who are predominantly Moslem; the more northerly regions, on the other hand, are populated by Turkicized Moslem Indo-Europeans and by Turkish peoples. For an explanation of this ethnic distribution see Asia, Central.

The Chinese Turkistan of today consists essentially of the basin of the Tarim River and the territory northeast of this, including the regions of Turfan and Qomul (Hami); it is surrounded by high mountains on most of its perimeter, and the great Takla Makan Desert occupies its central part.

The population of eastern Turkistan is largely made up of fixed tribes of Indo-European origin in whose midst elements of Turkish origin have established themselves, imposed the Turkish language, and modified the physical type to a degree that varies according to the region.

A complex of cultural centers grew up along two great trade routes which, as early as the Neolithic Age, ran between the Far East and that region the Chinese called by the generic term of "Hsi-yu" ("the western countries"), a term at first applied particularly to Serindia and later extended to include Iran, the eastern Mediterranean, and even the western borders of India. One of these roads, starting in Kansu, passed by Qomul, Turfan, and the cities north of the Celestial Mountains, reaching the Land of the Seven Rivers; from there one branch led to the steppes north of the Caspian and the Black Sea and another veered south and west to Sogdiana, Khwarizm, and northern Iran. The second and far more important trade route likewise started in Kansu. It was later to be known as the "Silk Road." It, too, was split into two branches, one passing to the north and the other to the south of the Tarim Basin, which were reunited in the western reaches and, after crossing the Pamirs, ultimately reached eastern Iran. Two other routes, less important commercially but highly significant culturally, led from southwestern Serindia to Kashmir and Gandhara and from the Khotan region across the Ladakh and Karakoram ranges to Kashmir.

At an early date there grew up along the Silk Road several urban centers which were the capitals of small independent states. These alternately fell to the Chinese during periods of expansion and recovered their autonomy when China was obliged to relinquish its colonial empire, until about the time of the Moslem conquest (1000). At that time the small states farther west were subjugated by the Turks and later, in the 13th century, by the Mongols, who controlled all of Serindia. During this period the Buddhist culture disappeared, though it persisted in the eastern sector until the 15th century, when it, too, was conquered by Islam. This explains why most of the sites in the western part — Kashgar, Yarkand, and Khotan on the southern route, and Aksu and Tumshuk on the northern route — suffered irreparable damage, whereas the more easterly localities — Kucha and Qara Shahr (Karashahr), on the northern route, and Cherchen on the southern route — are comparatively better preserved. The same is true of the Turfan (q.v.) group and, no doubt, for that of Qomul, which, unfortunately, it has not been possible to study. Some localities were spared by the Moslems because they had been abandoned earlier, some at the time of the Han, or later — for instance, several in the Khotan region, Niya, and Miran — and others, such as Endere, at the time of the Tibetan invasion.

Thus there exists a series of cultural centers of varying importance, some of which are still rich in archaeological material, while others are almost entirely destroyed.

Despite the spectacular finds of the expeditions that have worked there, Serindia (or Turkistan) must be considered a region which has been only superficially investigated and where extraordinary discoveries are possible.

The southern route links two cultural areas, that of Khotan and its environs and what might be called the "southeastern area," corresponding to the former realm of Shan-shan, with Cherchen and Miran; Lou-lan constitutes a separate site, of purely Chinese culture, in which, however, western influences developed. The northern route traverses four centers: Kashgar and Yarkand, Aksu and Tumshuk, Kucha, and Qara Shahr. Last, the more northeasterly section includes the centers of Turfan and Qomul.

Bibliog. F. Grenard, Haute Asie (Géographie Universelle, VIII), Paris, 1929, pp. 287–333; see also bibliography Asia, Central.

*Monuments and archaeological sites.* Khotan (Chin., Hotien). The locality which probably was the ancient capital of the realm of Khotan from early in the Christian era until it was destroyed by the Moslems in the 11th century is called Yōtkan and is known only from Chinese sources. The only objects known to survive from there were discovered by natives looking for gold on the sites of Buddhist temples and rulers' palaces. (See I, col. 828 and Khotanese Art).

Rawak (Ravaq), northeast of Khotan, is a large monastic complex whose oldest parts probably date back to the 3d or 4th century and whose more recent parts date from the 8th century. There is a three-storied stupa of great dimensions, surrounded by a wall decorated both inside and out with colossal statues. (See I, col. 829.)

Dandan-uilik, northeast of Khotan, is also a monastic city composed of a group of temples and dwellings; the temples consist of a cella and a corridor, in perishable materials, probably dating from the end of the T῾ang period (9th–10th cent.). (See I, col. 828.)

Niya, on the river of the same name, east of Khotan, is much more elaborate. Numerous buildings have been found, outstanding among which is a small sanctuary of the same type as those of Dandan-uilik, but of the 3d century at the latest, when the Han rule in this region came to an end. Documents show that some houses may date from the beginning of the Christian era. (See I, col. 829.)

Endere, farther east, can be associated with the Khotan group. The remains consist of a circular enclosure embracing monastic dwellings standing near a temple, a stupa, and houses for the garrison. The shrine is of the same type as those of Dandan-uilik; the complex may date from the late 8th century. (See I, col. 830.)

Bibliog. A. Stein, Sand-buried Ruins of Khotan, London, 1903; A. Stein, Ancient Khotan, 2 vols., Oxford, 1907.

Southeastern area. This region, extending from Cherchen to Lop Nor, is notable mainly for the site of Miran. A neolithic specimen of painted pottery acquired at Cherchen indicates that at some remote time a center of importance must have existed there.

Essentially Miran consists of the ruins of a temple formed of a massive quadrangular structure enclosing a rotunda where a stupa stood; the walls are adorned with paintings, and documents preserved in the walls place it in the 3d or early 4th century. (See I, col. 827.)

Lou-lan is a complex standing north of Lop Nor and consisting primarily of a cemetery where numerous relics of predominantly Chinese influence have been discovered. It probably dates from about the beginning of the Christian era to the 3d century, at the latest, when the site was abandoned. (See I, col. 836.)

Kashgar is the most westerly region of former Serindia; it was the first to be destroyed by the Moslems, and little remains but badly ruined traces, such as some stupas (the Maurī-Tim and the Tōpa-Tim farther southeast; see I, col. 830). Perhaps systematic excavation will uncover the ancient cities which preceded Kashgar and Yarkand and the monastic complexes.

Aksu (Chin., Kumo) and Tumshuk lie north of the middle Tarim River. The city bearing the Turkish name of Aksu was perhaps earlier called Bharuka and may overlie the ancient site, of which nothing has yet been found. Tumshuk, farther west, is memorable for the ruins of a monastic city. It comprises several temples of the Gandhara type overlooking the Tarim Valley from the nearer mountain spurs; within them were found many archaeological vestiges from the ruined stupas and shrines; remains of houses and terraces show

traces of what may have been at least two monasteries. (See I, col. 830 and PLS. 472, 476, 477.)

The Kucha (q.v.) complex may be subdivided into two main groups: the temples and monastic cities built in the open, and those in caves hollowed out of rock. The most important of the first are found at Duldur-akhur, southwest of Kucha; others, less important, such as Qum-Arïq, have been found on the route from Kucha to Kirish. A greater wealth of archaeological material has been preserved from the second group; the principal ones are those of Kizil and Kumtura in the Muzart Valley west of Kucha, and those of Ačiğ-Iläk and Sim-Sim, the first located south and the second northwest of Kirish; Kirish is northeast of Kucha. Also notable are the rock temples of Su-bashi. Other less important sites include Kizil-Karga, or Kizil-shahr (northwest of Kucha on the road to Kizil), Hisar, Tajzik Karaul, and Tonguz-bash, all only superficially explored.

The vast ensemble of Kizil ranges over four centuries; the earliest shrines date from the late 4th century, the most recent from the late 7th century. (See I, col. 831 and PLS. 471, 474, 475, 478-481, 483, 489.)

Kumtura includes a smaller number of rock shrines and a small temple built in the open; many shrines are of approximately the same period as those of Kizil; a few are perhaps late 8th century. (See I, col. 832.)

Ačiğ-Iläk and Sim-Sim are smaller complexes; the former may date from the late T'ang period (10th cent.) and the latter from the 7th-8th century to the middle of the 9th.

Duldur-akhur and Su-bashi are the most important "constructed" (as opposed to rock-cut) monastic communities in the region and may date from the 5th to the 8th century. (See I, col. 833 and PLS. 473, 482.)

Qum-Arïq probably belongs to the same period as the two above.

Qara Shahr (Karashahr) is especially noted for the sites of Shikshim and Shorchuk, to use the names given them by the archaeologists who have investigated them: it includes constructed temples and rock shrines; several of them date from the 8th century, while others are in all probability earlier, perhaps from the 6th century; still others are much later, perhaps from the middle of the 9th century. (See I, col. 833.)

Turfan is a complex containing sites of widely varying dates. The most important are the ruined cities of Idikut-shahri and Khocho (Chin., Kao-ch'ang), which are the ancient capitals of the kingdom of Turfan, and the cemeteries of Astana and Qoshgumbaz. A few miles northeast of these cities lies the gorge of Senghim (Senghim-aghïz), which contains numerous monasteries and temples built of brick or cut into the mountainside (I, PL. 490). The gorge gives access to the monastery of Bezeklik, which includes constructed temples and rock shrines. About three miles north of Bezeklik is Murtuk, with rock shrines and brick buildings, and about six miles from Murtuk is a site with very ancient temples, Čiqqan-köl. About 10 miles east of Khocho, the little village of Toyuk still has the ruins of two vast monasteries combining a system of rock shrines with brick structures, as at Murtuk. Finally, two sites must be added to this list: that of Bulayïk, a village north of Turfan, near which only a great many manuscripts have been found, and that of Hasa-shahri, where, in the center of a sandy desert, Von Le Coq has essayed the excavation of the ruins of a monastery. (See I, col. 834.)

Qomul (Hami) has not yielded any important discoveries, although some ruins exist a few miles north of the city. The ruins are Indian in style, approached by large stairways.

These cultural centers have all been influenced by the great civilizations surrounding them. Chinese influence, for instance, was exerted on the southern route as far as Khotan from the beginning of the Christian era and was several times felt along the northern route, particularly during the T'ang dynasty (7th-10th cent.) as well as later. Indian influence was exerted through Kashmir both in Khotan and at Kucha and as far as Turfan, especially through the medium of the Gupta (q.v.) art of northern India (4th-5th cent.). The Indian influence was probably first manifested in these regions at about the beginning of the Christian era; much later (8th-10th cent.) all Serindia as far as Turfan was permeated by Tantric Buddhism in the Tibetan form it had taken on after spreading from Kashmir. The Greco-Buddhist art of Gandhara (q.v.), however, had the strongest influence; from the 4th century on it was especially apparent in Tumshuk, Kucha, and Qara Shahr; subsequently there were additional influences from Sassanian Iran and the eastern Mediterranean. Hellenistic motifs seem to have arrived via Khwarizm and Sogdiana (qq.v.) along the routes coming from north of the Black Sea, whereas the routes leading from the steppes bore motifs typical of the animal art of those regions. Thus Serindia was a crossroads to which the principal civilizations of Asia brought the essentials of their art concepts; from the interpenetration and blending of these there issued, not an art, but a style that was typically Central Asian and may be considered, according to the time and place, as a manifestation of now one, now another art culture.

BIBLIOG. See ASIA, CENTRAL.

Louis HAMBIS

SZECHWAN (Szechuan). *Survey of geography and art history.* The heart of this province consists of a basin surrounded on all sides by mountains, called the "Red Basin" because of the abundance of red sandstone. It lies at a higher level than the central plain of the Yangtze River, but considerably lower than the Tibetan plateau in the west, parts of which have belonged to Szechwan since the dissolution of Sikang province in 1955. The western boundary is now formed by the Chin-sha-kiang (the upper reaches of the Yangtze). From north to south the province is crossed by rivers that all discharge into the Yangtze along the southern frontier. The geographic conformation of this Land of the Four (ssŭ) Rivers (ch'uan) was very favorable for its inhabitants; it had the fertile soil and sheltered location of the Red Basin, while the routes of communication with Kansu, Shensi, and Yunnan, as well as the navigation on the Yangtze River, prevented it from becoming too isolated.

Szechwan's great importance in Chinese history is attested by its monuments and by historical sources. The facts that Szechwan lacquer ware of the Han period has been found thousands of miles distant from the source of manufacture, and that the earliest development of printing took place here, are only examples of the cultural importance of this province. Nothing in the art of this region displays a provincial character in the derogatory sense of the word, although certain local traits, particularly in sculpture, are evident.

Many prehistoric finds (those made before and during World War II having been studied by Chêng Tê-k'un) prove that Szechwan was inhabited from the very earliest times. The kingdom of Shu (the ancient name of the Szechwan area) is mentioned in the oracle-bone inscriptions of An-yang (in Honan) in the late Shang period. To the north, in the area of Li-fan, bronzes have been found showing stylistic relationship with those of the Ordos region, while in many places bronze objects, mainly weapons, of the late Chou style have been found. Some of these may have been imported into Szechwan, but it is obvious that a native bronze culture had already been created in this province before that time. The use of iron was also known. Near Tung-sun-pa, on the northern bank of the Yangtze, many late Chou tombs were excavated in 1954-56.

In 316 B.C., Szechwan was conquered by Ch'in generals, who began their campaigns from Shensi and then made this province the base for the conquest of other states until the first Chinese empire was established. During the Han period, immigration completely changed the demographic composition of Szechwan, which became, and permanently remained, a Chinese province.

The number of funerary monuments of various types from the Han period is very large. Even before World War I the French expedition under Victor Ségalen had found and studied several. Many winged lions and decorated stone pillars, which traditionally flanked the path leading to the burial mounds, were preserved up to modern times. The "stone men," of the type found also in Shantung, are of slight artistic merit, but the lions are very fine, and the decorated pillars even more so. The latter are distinguished from similar monuments in Shantung by their superior and more animated workmanship and by more complex architecture.

The pillars of the Shên tomb (2d cent.), near Ch'u-hsien, and the tomb of Kao Yi (209), near Yaan in former Sikang province, are the best-preserved specimens of imitations in stone of wooden watchtowers. Resting on a rectangular column is an ingenious system of beams and brackets, supporting a richly decorated frieze and a roof covered with imitation tiles. Altogether about twenty pillars and a dozen sculptures of winged lions have survived in Szechwan.

Carved into the rock along the Yangtze, Kialing (Chia-ling), and Min Rivers are countless tombs which were very early reopened and used as shelters or living quarters. Several archaeologists have already studied some of them. These tombs are particularly numerous along the Min River from Ipin (Yi-pin, Suchow) to Loshan, and near the towns of P'êng-shan and Hsin-chin, respectively south and west of Chengtu (Ch'êng-tu). The caves of Loshan (Chia-ting), ranging in depth from slightly more than a yard to about 80 ft., are often grouped together with a common vestibule. On the walls of the vestibules (which may be compared in function to offering shrines such as those on the Hsiao-t'ang-shan, in Shantung), reliefs are carved. Those representing watchtowers and winged lions indicate that the arrangement of the cave tombs is substantially the same as that of tombs in the open air, with the various architectural and sculptural elements represented here in relief in order to adapt them to

cave construction. The great "sarcophagi" carved from the rock floor served as a repository, not for the remains of the deceased, but for the tomb furnishings. In the vicinity of Hsin-chin the tombs are much simpler in architecture; the wall decorations are omitted, and here the coffins, carved separately and placed within the tomb, bear the reliefs. The composition of the reliefs and their distribution over the surface is generally not as well organized as in Shantung, but the conception is ampler and the scenes are less rigidly stylized. The repertory of subjects is in many respects similar.

Another aspect of Han art in Szechwan is found in the decorated slabs with which the walls of many tombs were covered. The largest specimens, almost always individual pieces, display surprising vivacity and a penchant for movement, songs, dances, and games. Many of these slabs, the finest of which come from a tomb on the Fêng-huang-shan (Mount of the Phoenix) near Chengtu, are of high artistic merit; they are also informative as to the daily life of the time. The smaller pieces are inferior in quality, having been generally mass-produced by means of molds. If these slabs are compared with those from the central provinces (such as those collected by W. C. White), it is hard to escape the impression that the art of Szechwan has an individuality and merit all its own.

The human type represented in the Han mortuary sculpture differs greatly from that of the central provinces, both in facial expression and dress. The most sensational find made since World War II is that of a horse, 40 in. high, with a chariot. The type of horse, much heavier than is usually found in sculpture, funerary or otherwise, may belong to a different breed from those represented in the tomb art of the central provinces.

The fame of Szechwan lacquer ware during the Han period spread far beyond the boundaries of the province. Since pieces found elsewhere, as in Korea, bear inscriptions, it has been possible to assign the majority of these refined products to workshops in the vicinity of modern Chengtu. To date, no pieces of lacquer ware definitely attributable to these shops have been found in Szechwan.

It is clear that the tradition of Szechwan Buddhist sculpture is of ancient date, even if we are unwilling to assign to the late Han period some Buddhist sculptures in caves subsequently used for other purposes, for example, those of Ma-hao, near Chia-ting. Excavations near the ruins of the Wan-fo-ssŭ, in the western suburbs of Chengtu, have already yielded about 200 sculptures that, although badly damaged, indicate a tradition of the highest quality. The pieces bearing the earliest dates are from the Liang period (6th cent.), to which belong also the earliest sculptures found by Ségalen, namely those carved on Han pillars at P'ing-yang. The oldest dated Buddhist sculpture so far discovered anywhere in the province is of the year 483.

Within the borders of this province, reliefs and niches containing sculptures, as well as rock sculptures, have been found on mountain slopes in 125 different places. In 63 of these sites the sculptures date from the Sui and T'ang periods, but outstanding complexes were also executed under the Five Dynasties and the Sung, for instance, in the vicinity of Ta-tsu. The art reached its zenith during the T'ang period, and the later sculptures lack the strength of the T'ang pieces; however, the Sung sculptors, who had a penchant for the realistic, the sentimental, and the narrative, produced many fine statues. Traces of Tantric Buddhism are comparatively scarce here.

One of the most important finds made in Szechwan is the tomb of the "emperor" Wang Chien (847–918), an adventurer of shady reputation who, one year after the official end of the T'ang dynasty, had himself proclaimed emperor and reigned briefly over Szechwan.

By the late 9th century, various books, including dictionaries and geometric texts, were being printed at Chengtu with the use of xylographic plates. Here, too, another necessity, paper money, was provided by printing. With the conquest of Szechwan by the Later T'ang (929) printing spread to other regions and at an early date was of great benefit to scholars and students of the scriptures.

Bibliog. V. Ségalen, G. de Voisins, and J. Lartigue, Mission Archéologique en Chine, 2 vols. (atlas), Paris, 1923–24; V. Ségalen, L'art funéraire à l'époque des Han, Paris, 1934; W. Franke, Die Han-zeitlichen Felsengräber bei Chia-ting, West Ssuchuan, Studia Serica, VII, 1048; R. C. Rudolph and Wên Yu, Han Tomb Art of West China, Berkeley, 1951; R. Edwards, The Cave Reliefs at Ma-hao, Artibus Asiae, XVII, 1–2, 1954; T. F. Carter, The Invention of Printing in China and its Spread Westward, ed. by L. C. Goodrich, New York, 1955; Chêng Tê-k'un, Archaeological Studies in Szechwan, Cambridge, 1957; Liu Chih-yüan, Ssŭ-ch'uan Han-tai hua-hsiang-chuan i-shu (Decorated Tiles of the Han Period from Szechwan), Peking, 1958.

*Monuments and archaeological sites.* Wan-fo-ssŭ. Near Chengtu, where this temple stood during the Ming period, sculptures, all without heads, were dug up in the late 19th century. Along with many fragments and detached heads, there were also found some pieces with dated inscriptions. Some pieces seem to have been sold abroad, but the museum of Szechwan still has a considerable number. It is calculated that more than 200 sculptures have been found altogether, of which a hundred or so are in Chinese public collections. Although they cannot compare in numbers with those of Ch'ü-yang in Hopei, the sculptures of Chengtu are far superior in quality. The oldest are of the Liang period and bear dates corresponding to 522, 529, 533, and 548. Pieces of the period of the Northern Chou (dated 562, 566, and 567) and of the T'ang (728, 737, and 847) have also been found. The red sandstone in which the sculptures were executed proves that they were made locally. Of importance are some standing Buddhas and a lokapala, all probably dating from the late 6th century. The inscriptions indicate that from the earliest times there was a temple here which, over the centuries, several times changed its name. Only in the Ming period did it acquire the name Wan-fo-ssŭ (Temple of the Ten Thousand Buddhas), evidently derived from the presence of a great number of sculptures. The temple was destroyed during the hostilities at the end of the Ming period.

Bibliog. Fêng Han-chi, Ch'êng-tu Wan-fo-ssŭ shih-k'o tsao-hsiang (The Stone Images from the Wan-fo-ssŭ at Chengtu), Wên-wu ts'an-k'ao tzŭ-liao, 1954, no. 9, pp. 110–20; Liu Chih-yüan, Ch'êng-tu Wan-fo-ssŭ shih-k'o i-shu (Stone Sculptures from the Wan-fo-ssŭ, Chengtu), Peking, 1958.

Lung-hsing-ssŭ. To the west of Ch'iung-lai (southwest of Chengtu), on the Ta-nan River, is the temple Ta-fo-ssŭ, where a great number of fragments of Buddhist sculpture have been found. It appears that the original name of the temple was Lung-hsing-ssŭ and that sculptures continued to be made here after the anti-Buddhist persecutions of the mid-9th century. Up to 1948 more than 200 pieces had been deposited in the Chengtu museum, while later another 170 pieces were excavated. Among them are a great number of *sūtra* pillars, some inscribed with datable inscriptions, all from the T'ang period. Although there is one sculpture bearing a date corresponding to 681 and another from 795, the datable *sūtra* pillars are all from the 9th century (842, 849, 858, and 859). Among the sculptures, which are all of red sandstone and therefore definitely a product of this region, there are only a few statues which are not completely disfigured. Especially noteworthy is a standing lokapala clad in armor, which is of the same type as the well-known group in the Tōji temple in Kyoto, Japan.

Bibliog. Fêng Kuo-ting et al., Ssŭ-ch'uan Ch'iung-lai T'ang-tai Lung-hsing-ssŭ shih-k'o (T'ang Stone Sculptures from the Lung-hsing-ssŭ at Ch'iung-lai in the Province of Szechwan), Peking, 1958.

Huang-tsê-ssŭ. This temple is located on the western bank of the Kialing River west of the city of Kuang-yüan. The complex of cave temples nearby consists of 6 caves and 28 niches. It is not known when work was begun on them, but from the style of the sculptures and from the only inscription (Cave XXXI, A.D. 826), it would seem that most of them were begun in the T'ang period. In two caves, Nos. IV and VII, the latter with a central pillar carved from the rock, there are some very fine and well-preserved T'ang sculptures. Just over 3 miles north of the city, there once stood a monument known as the Rock of the Thousand Buddhas, with many T'ang sculptures, but the caves and most of the niches were almost completely destroyed during construction work on a road.

Bibliog. V. Ségalen, G. de Voisins, and J. Lartigue, Mission Archéologique en Chine, Paris, 1923–24, II, pls. 92, 96–7; Wên-wu ts'an-k'ao tzŭ-liao, 1956, no. 5, pp. 56–60.

Pa-chung. In the immediate vicinity of this city there are sculptures in five mountain sites. Four of the complexes derive their names from the cardinal points of the compass, and one from the temple Ta-fo-ssŭ (Temple of the Great Buddha), the name of which comes from a gigantic Buddha of recent date, about 5 miles north of the city. The sculptures are nearly all ruined or badly damaged by weathering.

The most important group is that located on Hua-ch'êng-shan, not far from the city. It consists of three different parts, but most of the niches are grouped near the so-called Fo-yeh-wan. Out of a total of 130 niches, a compact group of 46 date from the T'ang period, as is evident from the style of the numerous sculptures and several inscriptions (A.D. 735 in No. 69, 846 in No. 93, and 877 in No. 65). The niches, rather shallow and provided with two decorated pillars, are so close together that the pillars of one are immediately next to those of another. The artistic quality of the sculptures is far superior to that of most of the other rock niches in this province.

Bibliog. V. Ségalen, G. de Voisins, and J. Lartigue, Mission Archéologique en Chine, Paris, 1923–24, II, pls. 98–104; Wên-wu ts'an-k'ao tzŭ-liao, 1956, no. 5, pp. 51–5.

An-yüeh. In this inaccessible district sculptures and niches, mostly of modest size, have been found in more than 15 mountain sites. The majority are near the so-called Ch'ien-fo-chai, situated about 2 miles from the city of An-yüeh. There, on the northern and

southern parts of the cliff face, are two groups of niches, almost 70 in all, containing about 1,800 sculptures. The dress and the head-dresses of the figures are characterized by elaborate ornamentation, which indicates that they may date at the earliest from the late T'ang period. In No. 4, a niche which in turn contains numerous small niches, there is an inscription of the T'ien-pao era (742–55), but there are a great number of Sung niches as well, for example No. 5 (dated 1203).

Another group in this area, 1 1/2 miles south of the city, comprises four large niches and a cave, all containing Buddha statues ca. 16 ft. high. Unfortunately the cave, Yüan-chiao-tung, which must originally have contained many sculptures, is very severely damaged. Many sculptures were restored and polychromed in later times.

BIBLIOG. Wên-wu ts'an-k'ao tzŭ-liao, 1956, no. 5, pp. 47–50.

Ta-tsu. Rock sculptures have been identified in 19 sites in the vicinity of this city. The most important complexes of niches are on Pei-shan, 2 miles north of Ta-tsu; on Nanshan, 1 1/2 miles south; and on Pao-ting-shan, 15 miles northeast.

On Nan-shan is the Taoist monastery Yü-huang-kuan, where there are four caves with Taoist sculptures, all of the Sung period, strongly reminiscent of the Buddhist sculptures of this region.

In several places on Pei-shan, there are niches carved into the rock, which, except for the so-called Fo-wan, have been greatly damaged by weathering. The Fo-wan (Bay of the Buddhas) is a rocky wall in the form of a bay, on which sculptures have been carved in three places. In all, there are 290 niches containing about 7,000 figures. The earliest date from the late 9th century, but the vast majority are from the Sung period. Often the sculptors display a sentimental realism, typical of many Sung stone sculptures, but the series of figures in Caves 125 and 136 show that the Buddhist sculpture of that period could at times reach a very high artistic level.

On a peak facing the Pei-shan stands a Sung pagoda, the interior of which is decorated throughout with reliefs. An important recent find is that of a stone-engraved copy of a painting by the famous master Shih-k'o (10th cent.) depicting the debate between Mañjuśrī and Vimalakīrti.

The caves and niches on Pao-ting-shan, which, according to tradition, were carved out at the suggestion of a certain Chao Chin-fêng about the end of the 12th century, form an imposing and cohesive unit, completely covering a rock face 65 ft. high and 650 ft. wide. Among the scenes depicted are the life of Śākyamuni, with a noteworthy large representation of the *Parinirvāṇa*, a number of Jātakas, and many other *sūtra* subjects. Many of them are accompanied by explanatory inscriptions.

BIBLIOG. Wên-wu ts'an-k'ao tzŭ-liao, 1956, no. 5, pp. 66–9, 1958, no. 4, pp. 26–8; Hsien-tai fo-hsüeh (A Study of Present-day Buddhism), 1957, no. 9, pp. 18–22; Ta-tsu shih-k'o (Rock Sculptures of Ta-tsu), Peking, 1957.

Chia-chiang. A few miles south of this city, on the bank of the Ch'ing-i-kiang, some 200 niches have been carved into the rock. They vary in height from 13 ft. to 20 in. and contain many sculptures. On the basis of inscriptions, this complex, usually called the Ch'ien-fo-yen (Rock of the Thousand Buddhas), dates for the most part from the 7th, 8th, and 9th centuries. Several caves can be dated, for example, No. 63 (857), No. 62 (859), and No. 78 (776). Among the more interesting niches are Nos. 69, 132, and 152, in which there are large sculptures representing the Western Paradise of Amitābha. Represented on the front part of the dais in this group are 18 celestial figures playing musical instruments and dancing. The same scene is to be found repeated some ten times in one type of niche (e.g., Nos. 52, 120, 121, 128, and 173), enclosing a Buddhist trinity flanked by Mañjuśrī and Vimalakīrti; here the celestial figures number only 10. This type of niche is rare elsewhere in Szechwan. A niche with figures representing the colloquy between Mañjuśrī and Vimalakīrti (No. 2) seems to be unique in the sculpture of this area. Cave 64 is very important as perhaps the only one in the complex to show the influence of Tantric Buddhism, but its artistic merit is slight.

BIBLIOG. V. Ségalen, G. de Voisins, and J. Lartigue, Mission Archéologique en Chine, Paris, 1923–24, II, pls. 128–44; Wên-wu ts'an-k'ao tzŭ-liao, 1958, no. 4, pp. 29–31.

Jên-shou. Among many sites in the area south and southwest of Chengtu, the most numerous, and the most important artistically, are located a few miles northeast of Jên-shou on Shih-chü-shan, near the Wang-o-t'ai (terrace from which one can gaze at the sacred mountain O-mei). There are two parts in the complex, one with 20 niches and the other with 7. The groups of sculptures in the niches, the height of which varies from 8 ft. to 40 in., nearly all represent the Buddha flanked by two disciples, two boddhisattvas,

and two lokapalas. On the rear walls there are reliefs of the Eight Classes of Superhuman Beings, while on the base are figures in relief of celestial musicians, reminiscent of those of the Ch'ien-fo-yen in Chia-chiang. Most of the niches are of the T'ang period. An inscription gives a date corresponding to 790.

BIBLIOG. Wên-wu ts'an-k'ao tzŭ-liao, 1957, no. 10, pp. 37–40.

Tomb of Wang Chien (near Chengtu). This large-scale tomb was discovered in 1939 and excavated in 1942–43, on a hill where, according to tradition, the poet Ssŭ-ma Hsiang-ju (200–118 B.C.) supposedly played his lute. Measuring 131 ft. long, 33 ft. wide, and 33 ft. high, with vaults and 14 arches, it consists of an anteroom, a mortuary chamber, and a rear chamber, separated by doors. The anteroom was found empty, but in the rear chamber, before a statue presumed to be that of the deceased, i.e., the usurper Wang Chien (847–918), was found a jade book with inscriptions.

In the central room of the tomb, which lies on a north–south axis, is a platform on which lay the coffin, which had been almost completely destroyed by grave robbers. This platform consists of a plinth with lotus pattern, above which are a frieze and a cornice adorned with bas-reliefs of dragons and cloud motifs. The frieze consists of alternate panels in high relief (women dancing and playing instruments) and in bas-relief (phoenixes), the panels being separated by square columns. At the ends of the long (east and west) sides of the platform there are beautiful figures of guardians who seem to support the podium with their hands. These figures, depicted from the waist up as though they were rising out of the ground, together with the excellent craftsmanship of the pedestal, make this tomb unique in Chinese tomb art. Robbers had despoiled the tomb of much of its rich furnishings, among which were pieces of pottery of the type manufactured at Liu-li-ch'ang, near Chengtu, and objects of jade, bronze, and silver. It has been possible to reconstruct a few pieces.

BIBLIOG. Chêng Tê-k'un, The Royal Tomb of Wang Chien, HJAS, VIII, 1944–45, pp. 235–40; M. D. Sullivan, the Excavation of a T'ang Imperial Tomb, ILN, XX, Apr., 1946; Fêng Han-yi, Discovery and Excavation of the Yung Ling, Arch. Chin. Art Soc. Am., II, 1947, pp. 11–20; Sinologica, II, 1949, pp. 1–11; K'ao-ku T'ung-hsin, 1955, no 3, pp. 49–53; Wên-wu ts'an-k'ao tzŭ-liao, 1955, no. 3, pp. 91–111, no. 7, 1957, pp. 24–7.

*Kiln sites.* Ch'iung-lai. On the west bank of the Ta-nan River southwest of Chengtu, near Ch'iung-lai, D. C. Graham, O. H. Bedford, and Chêng Tê-k'un found (1936) remains of some kilns. On the basis of inscribed fragments from the periods of the T'ang (754, 823, and 874–79) and the Northern Sung (1117), it is thought that production of this pottery, which has many T'ang characteristics, continued into the Sung period, but that the kilns were abandoned soon afterward. Although the Ch'iung-lai pottery, sometimes glazed in several colors, never acquired national fame, the discovery of these kilns identified the source of part of the pottery found in the tombs in this region.

Liu-li-ch'ang. The remains found in this region near Chengtu belonged to kilns which probably were active in the Sung period. The pottery found in the tomb of Wang Chien has been identified as a product of these kilns, thus proving that they were already in operation in the late T'ang period, but several dated pieces are of the Sung period (e.g., 1117, 1219, and 1276). The most recurrent type of pottery is reminiscent of the brown or green glazed ware. Particularly noteworthy is a green-glazed imitation of Shu-fu ware (Yüan period).

BIBLIOG. Chêng Tê-k'un, Szechwan Pottery, Apollo, 1948; Chêng Tê-k'un, Archaeological Studies in Szechwan, Cambridge, 1957.

YUNNAN (Yün-nan) AND KWEICHOW (Kuei-chou). *Survey of geography and art history.* The southwestern part of China, divided administratively into Yunnan and Kweichow, includes a plateau that gradually slopes downward, and also the mountainous, bleak region separating China from Tibet and Burma. Waterways are almost totally lacking, so that all trade is carried on via land routes. This is the reason for the agelong isolation of this region.

The history of these provinces consists primarily of repeated attempts by the ruling dynasties in China proper to subjugate the area, and of local efforts, repeated with equal frequency, to form small independent kingdoms. These kingdoms nominally always remained under Chinese suzerainty. Chinese culture began to penetrate as early as the end of the Chou period, and during the Han dynasty Chinese immigration increased. About 10 million non-Chinese still live in Yunnan and Kweichow, and the Chinese have never made up more than 70 per cent of the population. The ethnographic composition of the non-Chinese inhabitants is very diverse, with great variety in origin, language, and culture.

The intensive infiltration of Chinese as early as the period of the Eastern Han is proved, not only by statistics in historical works, but also by the numerous so-called Liang-tui mounds in the areas around Kunming and Chaotung, and near Ch'ü-ching, Lu-liang, and Lu-tien. Archaeological investigations have shown that these mounds contain various types of brick tombs, mostly dating from the first four or five centuries of the Christian era. In structure and furnishings they are closely akin to the Szechwan tombs. The earliest tomb found so far which can be dated (by its inscriptions on brick) was built A.D. 266-78, but many others can be assigned to the Han period on the basis of inscriptions on bronzes and by their architecture. The Chaotung tombs contain bronzes which all date from the period of the Eastern Han. In general, these tombs are slightly earlier than those in the Kunming and Ch'ü-ching areas.

A base carved from red sandstone found, according to its discoverers, in a Liang-tui mound, is believed by some scholars to be the pedestal of a Buddhist statue. This hypothesis seems to be invalidated, however, by the date of the inscription, A.D. 84. Some efforts have been made to establish a connection between this find and the frequently postulated existence of a trade route between India, Szechwan, and Yunnan, but better proofs are needed before the existence of Buddhist art in Yunnan at so early a date can be accepted.

The attention of scholars has long been focused on the curious bronze art of this region, which displays unmistakable Chinese influence, but also a strong local character. A find on Shih-chai-shan, west of Chin-ning, caused a great stir in recent years; it not only verified the attribution to Yunnan of certain types of weapons, but also yielded an extremely rare collection of objects that may throw new light on the Dông-So'n culture known from Indochina. The only tomb found intact contained drums of the known Dông-So'n type, some Chinese mirrors from the 2d century B.C., and several very odd bronze objects. The most extraordinary of these were two drum-shaped vases on the lids of which were fastened several separately cast figures of animals and human beings. One group represents an offering scene, in which several men are being sacrificed beside a column around which two snakes are coiled and on top of which there is a tiger. This relic confirms the tradition, several times cited in Chinese sources, that the veneration of a column existed in this region. However, it is not as yet clear who the representatives of this culture were, or whether it is permissible to associate them with the Dông-So'n culture. Since the principal personage in the two scenes, a woman of ferocious appearance armed with a cudgel, has a hairdress compared by archaeologists to that of the Miao-tzŭ (Miaotse) tribe, this culture is thought to be related to that of certain ethnic groups still found in that area. It is called by its discoverers the Shih-chai-shan culture.

During the T'ang period, under the leadership of Sinicized Tai (Thai) elements from the population, an independent Buddhist state was formed which lasted until the arrival of the Mongols in 1253, and a Buddhist culture with a strong local color arose. The most important specimens of Buddhist art of this so-called Nan-ch'ao kingdom are of three types. Scattered among American and European collections are a group of bronzes, closely related to one another, depicting a standing Kuan-yin. The somewhat uniform character of the pieces, identified by H. B. Chapin as having originated in Yunnan, indicates a frequent repetition of this iconographic type. The important role played by Kuan-yin in Nan-ch'ao Buddhism is explicable by the fact that Avalokiteśvara was the tutelary deity of the Tuan family, who ruled over Yunnan from 937 to 1253 and subsequently acted as governors under the Mongols. The dating of these figures is not certain. The specimen in the Fine Arts Gallery of San Diego is proved to have come from Yunnan and can be dated 1147-72. Testing of the ashes preserved in one of the figures by the C14 (carbon 14) method bore out Chapin's supposition that some figures might be considerably earlier. This supposition was based on stylistic comparison of the figures with the few Yunnanese paintings which have been preserved. Among the latter is a copy, probably of the 12th century, of a scroll painted in 898-99, in which Kuan-yin was portrayed in a manner similar to that of the bronzes.

Stylistically very close to the bronzes and to these scrolls is a third group of works which pertain to the Nan-ch'ao period and its Buddhism, namely, the sculptures and cave temples on Shih-chung-shan, 6 miles south of the city of Chien-ch'uan in northern Yunnan.

This curious Buddhist culture probably received a severe blow when the Mongol Uriangkatai occupied the region in 1253 in order to launch his invasion of southern China. Among the Mongol officials who exercised actual power (jointly with the Tuan family, which continued to rule nominally) the most important was the Moslem Sayid Ajall, a native of Bukhara who was in Yunnan from 1274 to 1279; he was famous for the hydraulic works, and for the first mosque, which he had built in this region. His sons, who continued the family traditions, made Yunnan a veritable bulwark of Islam. During a Moslem uprising (1856-73), many treasures of the Nan-ch'ao

period, including a large statue of Kuan-yin cast in the 8th century, were lost.

Yunnan was the last province to be won by the victorious Ming armies from the Mongols (1382) and was also the last to remain faithful to the Ming dynasty. The last heir to the Ming throne fled from here across the Burmese frontier in 1659, together with his court, which had been converted to Catholicism.

Even after the fall of the Nan-ch'ao kingdom, the sculptural traditions of Yunnan were not completely lost, as is proved by a stele dated 1470 and by many later sculptures. The wooden sculptures of the 17th and later centuries, executed by artists of several ethnic minorities, are manifestly influenced by the ancient Nan-ch'ao tradition.

BIBLIOG. H. B. Chapin, Yünnanese Images of Avalokiteśvara, HJAS, VIII, 1944-45, pp. 131-86; B. Gray, China or Dong-so'n, O. Art, II, 3, 1949-50, pp. 99-104; K'ao-ku t'ung-hsin, 1957, no. 3, pp. 1-7; A. G. Wenley, A Radiocarbon Dating of a Yünnanese Image of Avalokiteśvara, Ars Orientalis, III, 1957, p. 508; Wên-wu ts'an-k'ao tzŭ-liao, 1957, no. 11, pp. 47-8.

*Monuments and archaeological sites.* Shih-chai-shan. On this hill, west of the city of Chin-ning in Yunnan province, many bronzes were excavated in 1954, casting new light on the culture of this region in the Han period. One tomb was intact and from it came some very interesting objects, among them the following:

(a) A bronze drum, filled with cowrie shells, decorated with combed ornament, with circles, birds, "feathered men," etc.; it is of a Dông-So'n type well known from excavations in Indochina (see ASIA, SOUTH).

(b) A bronze vase with 4 feet and 2 tiger-shaped handles, also filled with cowrie shells; on the lid are separately cast figurines representing 6 oxen around a miniature drum.

(c) A drum-shaped vessel filled with cowrie shells, the cover of which is decorated with 18 separately cast figurines from 1 to 2 3/8 in. high. (See IV, PL. 452.) They represent 3 men and a number of women along with a taller female figure placed on a small pedestal and surrounded by servants. She seems to be watching over the others who are working, some of them weaving. The lid on which the figures are fastened is decorated with engraved peacock ornament.

(d) A similar vessel having at least 40 figurines standing around a column which is surmounted by a tiger and entwined by two serpents. The scene seems to represent the sacrifice of a human being to the column.

(e) A bronze female figure, armed with a cudgel and standing more than 16 in. high, found placed upon the drum first mentioned.

Highly important in establishing the chronology of these finds is the fact that the tomb also contained three mirrors of Karlgren's type K (see CHINESE ART, Chou), that is, of the 2d century B.C.

The excavations were resumed late in 1957 and at that time some 90 bronze tomb figurines of an extraordinary style came to light. A seal was also found bearing the inscription: "Seal of the King of Tien [Yunnan]." Unfortunately, there has been only a very brief notice concerning these new excavations, and it does not specify even in which tomb the seal was found. The publication of a monograph on the extremely rich finds — more than 3,000 objects from 19 tombs — has been announced.

BIBLIOG. Excavations of Early Dwelling Sites and Tombs at Shih-chai-shan, Chin-ning, Yunnan, K'ao-ku hsüeh-pao, 1956, no. 1, pp. 43-63; Wên-wu ts'an-k'ao tzŭ-liao, 1957, no. 4, pp. 56-8.

Chien-ch'uan. In three different sites on Shih-chung-shan, 3 miles southeast of Chien-ch'uan, in northern Yunnan, there are several caves, niches, and sculptures from the period when this area belonged to the Ta-li kingdom (Nan-ch'ao). The largest group of figures is that of the Shih-chung-ssŭ, where there are eight caves hollowed out of the steep rocks. Besides a Buddhist trinity curious representations of the sovereigns of Ta-li with their entourage should be mentioned. The figures are very much like those in a scroll painted by Chang Shêng-wêng (1180) in the Palace collection, formerly in Peking, and in the *Nan-ch'ao t'u-ch'üan*, which was probably recopied in the 12th century from an original of 899. The oldest dated inscription of the Shih-chung-ssŭ complex (1179) was inscribed on the richly ornamented façade of No. 8, a niche from which the principal figure has been removed.

Among the sculptures scattered on the cliff wall of the Shih-tzŭ-kuan and in the environs of the village of Sha-têng, an important group of reliefs recently brought to light includes one of a king, a queen, and a young prince with their entourage, as well as a standing Kuan-yin of the type noted in the bronzes. In a niche near Sha-têng there is an inscription from 841. Despite the marked range of dates there seems to be hardly any evolution in the style of the sculptures. Many of them are well preserved. The remarkable number of unfinished pieces may indicate that the work was interrupted abruptly, perhaps by the Mongol invasion.

BIBLIOG. Sung Po-yin, Chien-ch'uan shih-k'u (The Caves of Chien-ch'uan), Peking, 1958; Wên-wu ts'an-k'ao tzŭ-liao, 1957, no. 4, pp. 46–55, 1958, no. 4, pp. 32–3.

FORMOSA or TAIWAN (T'ai-wan). The island of Taiwan, opposite the southern coast of China, is best known in the West by the name of Formosa, from the Portuguese word for "beautiful" given to it by the 16th-century navigators. Its area is about 14,000 square miles and it is crossed from north to south by the Central Range, a forbidding range of mountains that occupies almost half the area of the island. Only the western coast is fairly flat, and it is in this

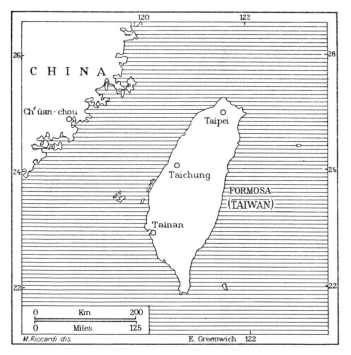

Formosa. Principal centers.

region that the greater part of the population is settled. Although crossing the Formosa Strait was not without dangers, especially because of the uncertain weather conditions, the distance which separated the island from the Chinese mainland was small enough to allow a constant infiltration of settlers.

Some archaeological work was initiated during the Japanese occupation (1895–1945), and the archaeologists who came here after the Nationalist Chinese established their government in Formosa in 1949 have contributed much to the solution of the problems connected with the early history of the island.

Though excavations have not yet been carried out on a very large scale, the prehistoric finds indicate that there must have been contacts between the prehistoric cultures of the lower Yangtze River basin and those of Formosa. Probably these prehistoric cultures lasted longer and are of somewhat later date than those on the mainland, as may be expected from an insular culture. At several sites it has been possible to establish a clear sequence of strata between several different cultures, e.g., Yüan-shan in northern Formosa. Who the bearers of these cultures were is difficult to establish, though it has been noted that some of these peoples extracted their eye-teeth and incisors, a habit which still exists among some Miao tribes of the mainland.

The development of Formosa parallels in some respects that of south China, but the gradual infiltration of Chinese settlers and the subsequent Sinification went on here at a much slower pace, not only because of the natural barrier of the Formosa Strait, but also because of the primarily continental orientation of the Chinese empire.

Among the early Chinese settlers who drove such tribes as the Ami, Bunu, Tayar, Tsowu, Saishet, and Yami from the fertile plains in the western part of the island, the Hakka were in the majority. About three centuries ago the immigration of Chinese increased considerably, mainly because of the conquest of southern China by the Manchus.

At that time Formosa was already a factor of some importance in the political history of the Far East. The Dutch East India Company had secured a foothold in the island in 1624, and fortresses were built at the present city of Tainan. The Spaniards established a trade settlement in the northern part of the island soon afterward, but

were ousted by the Dutch in 1642. In 1661 the famous pirate Cheng Ch'eng-kung, better known as Koxinga (a corruption of his title Kuo-hsing-yeh), who had sided with the surviving members of the Ming house, succeeded in driving out the Dutch. Although the supporters of the *ancien régime* maintained themselves on Formosa for some time, the Manchus finally managed to conquer it (1683), making it administratively part of the province of Fukien, whence most of the Chinese population at that time had come. During the Manchu period, immigration continued, though the immigrants now came mostly from Kwangtung rather than Fukien. The original inhabitants of the island, who were then living at a neolithic cultural level, were either absorbed by the immigrants or escaped assimilation with the Chinese civilization by seeking refuge in the mountains. These aborigines have not disappeared altogether and still represent a minor fraction of the population. Their cultural traits, now threatened with annihilation through increasing contact with the outside world, are being extensively studied by the Institute of Ethnology (established in Formosa in 1955), which publishes a *Bulletin* and maintains exhibits.

Formosa, even after its submission to the Manchus, remained an outpost of the empire and contains few outstanding monuments. The finest temples, such as the Lung-shan-ssǔ near Taipei, belong to the reign of Emperor Ch'ien-lung (1736–95).

Of major interest, however, is the fact that the core collections of the National Palace Museum and the National Central Museum (both formerly in Peking) are now housed in the small center of Pei-kou (near Taichung) in central Formosa. The former Palace collection of Peking, probably the most important single assemblage of Chinese art in existence, was built up largely by the Emperor Ch'ien-lung in the 18th century, though it was later modified by both additions and losses. Before the Japanese occupation of Peking in 1937 the choicest objects were removed to safety by the Chinese government, ultimately finding their way to Formosa.

The collections kept at Pei-kou are extremely rich in paintings, particularly of the Sung, Yüan, and Ming periods, as well as in calligraphic works. Notable groups of tapestries, jades, porcelain, and metalwork are also preserved. A selection of the objects is shown on a rotating basis in a gallery erected at nearby Wu-feng.

The Academia Sinica, reestablished at Nankang, near Taipei, preserves objects of the early period of Chinese history, including the bulk of the archaeological material recovered from An-yang, the Shang capital. The National Historical Museum, in Tapei, contains collections formerly in the Honan provincial museum at Kaifeng, notably a series of objects from excavations of Shang dynasty sites.

BIBLIOG. C. Imbault-Huart, L'Ile Formosa, Paris, 1893; W. Campbell, Formosa under the Dutch, London, 1903; A. Lippe, "Art Journey to Formosa," Arch. Chin. Art Soc. Am., IX, 1955, pp. 9–19; A. Lippe, The Hidden Treasures of China, Met. Mus. of Art B., XIV, 1955, pp. 54–60; Chêng Tê-k'un, Archaeology in China, I: Prehistoric China, Cambridge, 1959, pp. 130–2; Wang Shih-chieh, ed., Three Hundred Masterpieces of Chinese Painting in the Palace Museum, 6 vols., Taichung, 1959.

Jan FONTEIN

Illustrations: 6 figs. in text.

**CHINESE ART.** The art of China was the first of any Far Eastern land to be discovered and to be highly appreciated by the West, and yet it had already a history of more than two millenniums behind it at the time when Europeans first became aware of it. To be sure, Chinese silks were known in classical times, having reached the Roman empire by the overland routes through Central Asia, the so-called "Silk Road." It was said that these silks came from the land of the Seres, but of China and the great Han empire then flourishing there was only the vaguest knowledge. So far as we know, there was no direct contact at all between the two great empires which together dominated most of the ancient civilized world. The West and the East formed two distinct cultural spheres and led almost completely separated existences, totally unaware of each other's traditions, values, and history.

During the ascendancy of the Mongols, various European travelers, among them the Venetian Marco Polo, succeeded in penetrating into China. The accounts of their adventures, however, had little or no effect upon the almost completely ethnocentric vision of the West. In particular, the account of Marco Polo was regarded until modern times as a fantastic exaggeration, interesting to read, but unworthy of serious belief. The soberer reports of other travelers, such as Giovanni da Pian del Carpine and Guillaume Rubruquis, received less wide circulation; but nothing could have made the civilized world of the West at that

time accept the idea that other great cultures and civilized states existed outside of Europe and the territory immediately touching the Mediterranean, the *orbis terrarum*. The Chinese, for their part, were incapable of regarding the inhabitants of other parts of the world as more than barbarians whose sole function was to pay homage and tribute to the emperor of the Middle Kingdom.

During the 15th century the Chinese flotillas reached the east coast of Africa, but these expeditions were soon discontinued, with the result that the maritime trade routes between Europe and Asia were to be discovered by the Europeans rather than by the Chinese. In the 16th century the Portuguese reached southern China. From that time on, the products of Chinese artistry began to reach the Western world more directly and in appreciable quantities. The import of Chinese porcelain was at first limited; in particular, that porcelain manufactured for the Portuguese trade, the first *chine de commande*, is extremely rare. In Europe, the real vogue for Chinese export porcelains began in the 17th century, when the various East India companies brought huge quantities of blue-and-white porcelains, as well as lacquer work, to the European markets. Although the quality of these wares was inferior to some of those made for the Chinese market, and to the 14th- and 15th-century export porcelain which we now know to have been sent to the Near East and Indonesia, it was, from the technical point of view, vastly superior to anything which could be produced in Europe at that time. In Europe the technique of porcelain manufacture was long to remain a mystery, and after its final rediscovery at Meissen it was kept for some time a closely guarded trade secret. The imported Chinese art objects profoundly influenced Western arts and crafts, and there arose a trend toward exoticism (q.v.) in European art and a vogue for *chinoiserie* that dominated European applied arts for a time. The faithful copying of Chinese models soon gave way to a more playful and fanciful approach; various elements from widely different sources were confused and blended, and the imitators made no clear distinctions, for instance, between Chinese and Japanese themes and techniques.

The influence of China upon the culture of Europe and the early penetration of Western ideas in China, both of which were results of trade relations and missionary activity, have been the subject of many specialized studies. Nevertheless, many difficult problems pertaining to cultural relations still remain unsolved, and the analysis of European connoisseurship and of Western collecting depends to a considerable extent upon their solution. In general, however, it may be said that the interest of the 17th- and 18th-century European collectors centered upon contemporary Chinese export art, or (especially in the 18th century) upon those types of objects which had accumulated in Europe since the establishment of trade relations with China. The very existence of the art of Chinese antiquity was virtually unknown, although Europeans had been already impressed by the long history and continuity of Chinese cultural traditions.

In the second half of the 19th century, when such pioneers as Stanislas Julien (1856), Sir Augustus Franks (1877), Du Sartel (1881), and Stephen Bushell (1897–99) published their first treatises and catalogues of Chinese art, the only known types of porcelain were the Ch'ing and the late Ming wares which had earlier been imported. Even the ancient Chinese bronzes which were exhibited by the Chinese government in Paris in 1900 attracted very little attention. Since that time, however, there has been a radical change both in collecting, in critical connoisseurship, and in the methods of historical research. The English scholar and connoisseur R. W. Hobson, whose book *Chinese Pottery and Porcelain* appeared in 1915, was the first to establish the tradition of critical appreciation which made England the treasure house of Chinese pottery and porcelains. The abundance of mortuary ceramics and tomb figures which came to light during the construction of the Chinese railway system attracted the attention of English and French collectors, and even before the beginning of World War I antiques of the Han, T'ang, and Sung periods had reached the Western art markets in considerable quantities. In this

way, the names of the Chinese dynastic periods, before then known only to the few professional Sinologists, became commonly accepted as designations for various kinds of pottery and porcelain.

The range of the European view of Chinese art has been extended again and again by the inclusion of new fields. During the twenties and thirties of this century, Chinese bronzes, Buddhist sculpture, jades, and ancient lacquer work successively came to the attention of Western collectors. Large public and private collections were formed in Europe, the United States, Canada, and Japan. Extensive historical research, making ever-increasing use of Chinese sources, greatly augmented our knowledge of the setting in which the great art of China had been produced. Art-historical studies relied to a large extent on stylistic methods, for although some important field work had been done, archaeological exploration lagged far behind. Gradually a coherent picture was built from the fragments of knowledge contributed by the various branches of art scholarship. An excellent example of what could be achieved under the circumstances is Karlgren's chronological and stylistic classification of bronze art, which, in spite of its shortcomings, brought order to utter chaos by a clever combination of stylistic and epigraphical analysis. This was achieved in a period when only a few scattered "closed finds" of bronze vessels were known. Although Chinese archaeological science was to remain in its infancy for a long time to come, several scholars distinguished themselves in the pioneer field work. Favored by the political situation, the work of greatest importance was often done by Japanese. The same circumstances forced Chinese archaeologists to discontinue or interrupt their activity in the central provinces, but encouraged them to concentrate on previously neglected areas in western China, with the result that such remote sites as Tun-huang in Kansu province were given the attention hitherto lavished only on the rich finds of documents and texts taken home by British, French, and Japanese expeditions to that region.

The greatest step forward in our comprehension of the complex of Chinese art may be said to be the realization of the vast difference between the products designed primarily for Western markets and those, much more typically Chinese, which were never intended for export and accordingly came to the attention of art historians and collectors outside China only after the dispersal of important ancient Chinese collections.

The most recent discovery of the Western art world is Chinese painting. Except for a few scattered masterpieces which had been acquired more by luck than by design, the great Western collections had never acquired paintings equal as a whole to their bronzes, sculpture, and porcelain. Western connoisseurship relied mainly on the prejudices of traditional Japanese critical taste. Thus, often, copies with only a remote resemblance to originals of the Southern Sung academic school were regarded as China's most significant achievements in painting. Painting of the Sung period was considered to represent the last great flourishing period, after which an unavoidable decline was thought to have set in. More recently attention came to be focused on later Chinese painting, in particular the works of the so-called *wên-jên-hua* (see below, *Ming*). Museums and collectors in the United States, especially, have formed important collections of later Chinese painting. The Western study of Chinese painting based on firsthand reference to original materials has at last begun to make some progress.

Next to the progress in the study of Chinese painting, the most remarkable postwar development is the rise of archaeological science in China and the concentration of Chinese universities and scholars on systematic exploration of known and suspected sites. The results of this activity have been augmented by the extraordinary number of chance finds occurring in the course of civil engineering work and industrial excavation, saved in many cases just in time for proper investigation. The problems solved by these finds, often dated and of precisely known location, are many, but it will take considerable time to assess their proper significance in many cases, and we may expect them to remain the focus of scholarly attention for many years to come.

Many of the sites, monuments, and wares referred to below are located and further described under CHINA. In that article will be found also maps and alternate spellings of various place names. See also the articles on the various art forms, especially CERAMICS and LACQUER.

SUMMARY. The Neolithic period (col. 469): *Ceramics; Sculpture; Architecture.* The Shang-Yin period (col. 472): *Centers of Shang culture; Shang bronzes: a. Types of bronze vessels; b. Decorative motifs; Sculpture; Jades; Architecture.* The Chou period (col. 480): *Chou bronzes; Ceramics; Sculpture; Painting; Other arts.* The Han dynasty (col. 490): *Sculpture; Painting; Mirrors; Bronzes; Ceramics; Lacquer.* The period of the Six Dynasties (col. 498): *Early Buddhist art; Funerary sculpture; Painting; Mirrors; Ceramics.* The Sui and T'ang dynasties (col. 506): *Painting; Sculpture; Ceramics; Minor arts; Architecture.* The period of the Five Dynasties (col. 519): *Painting; Ceramics.* The Sung dynasty (col. 524): *Painting; Ceramics; Architecture.* The Yüan dynasty (col. 538): *Painting; Ceramics, silverwork, lacquer.* Later sculpture (col. 545). The Ming dynasty (col. 549): *Painting; Ceramics; Lacquer, metalwork, minor crafts.* The Ch'ing dynasty (col. 561): *Painting; Ceramics and export art; Jades.* Later architecture (col. 570).

THE NEOLITHIC PERIOD. During the millennium before the advent of the Shang culture, as we know it from the excavations at An-yang in Honan, various related neolithic cultures flourished in the loess region and in the basin of the Yellow River, or Huang-ho, which are designated with names derived from the color of their characteristic pottery or from the place where traces of them were first found. In the hilly, eroded loess region in northwest China, the dominant tone was set by the Red Pottery culture, also known as the Yang-shao culture, after the place (Yang-shao-ts'un in Honan province) where, in 1921, the Swedish archaeologist J. G. Andersson discovered for the first time traces of China's neolithic past. Subsequently, Andersson discovered further evidence of this culture in many other places. He tried to establish a chronological order for the various neolithic cultures in Honan and Kansu, beginning with the Ch'i-chia-p'ing culture, which he placed between 2500 and 2200 B.C., and ending with the Sha-ching, between 700 and 500 B.C., which may be regarded as a neolithic culture surviving far into the Chinese Bronze Age. As a result of the many discoveries made in recent years by Chinese archaeologists the chronology of these cultures has had to be radically revised, although this in no way detracts from the great contribution made by Andersson. (See also ASIATIC PROTOHISTORY.)

*Ceramics.* Andersson's most spectacular discovery was the existence in China of a neolithic pottery industry on a remarkably high technical level, employing geometrical decorations of exceptional beauty and variety. The early stages of the Yang-shao culture (3000-2200 B.C.) are represented in the lowest stratum of various sites in the neighborhood of An-yang (see CHINA, *Honan*), where this culture may be seen in its pure state, in contrast to the mixed cultures of many sites in Honan such as that at Yang-shao-ts'un.

The middle stage of the Yang-shao culture is represented in the neolithic village excavated a few years ago at Pan-po-ts'un (see CHINA, *Shensi*), east of Sian. One of the pottery finds is a shallow bowl decorated with fish and with remarkable stylized designs believed by some Chinese archaeologists to be human figures and by others to represent insects. Some of the most beautiful and highly developed forms of decorated pottery were collected by Andersson from the graves at Pan-shan in Kansu (PLS. 120, 219). Round funeral urns were found with either short, broad-mouthed necks or long narrow necks, both types having two handles attached to the middle part of the belly. The decoration was applied to the upper half of the urn only and never extends below the handles. Almost as varied as the different forms — N. Palmgren (1934) was able to distinguish some forty — are the geometrical patterns in red, black, and brown. Sometimes the decoration consists simply of a number of alternating red and black horizontal lines, with a border of regular undulating lines underneath. A more striking and constantly recurring pattern, however, is the spiral in which black and red lines curve counterclockwise

inward around small circular centers. Among the other patterns are the saw-tooth (which, according to Andersson, who calls it the "death pattern," is found only on funeral urns), the lozenge, the triangle, and even the "double gourd," which was to become so popular in later Chinese art.

The theory exists that there is a direct link between Chinese neolithic pottery and that of western Asia and the Black Sea region (see ASIATIC PROTOHISTORY). The most serious objection to it, apart from the great distances that would have had to be traversed, is the fact that the people of the Yang-shao culture were not nomadic and were indeed in some cases settled as agricultural communities for many centuries in a single place.

Some of the dates proposed by Andersson, based exclusively on comparisons between the styles of the painted pottery ware (apparently only a small proportion of the pottery found), cannot be accepted without further investigation. His dates for Ch'i-chia-p'ing, for instance, are too early and those for Ma-ch'ang (PL. 219) are altogether uncertain. However, there can be hardly any doubt that the approximate dates he suggests for the Hsin-tien culture (south of Lanchow), based on a clear difference between strata, are correct.

This culture (which was probably contemporaneous with the bronze culture of Chêng-chou, ca. 1500 B.C.) is a striking proof of the rapid decline of the Yang-shao culture. Not only has the quality of the pottery deteriorated, but the oval-shaped urn with its gradually tapering neck flaring out again somewhat at the rim is more primitive in conception. Moreover, the geometrical patterns, such as zigzags, meanders, spirals, and saw-tooth patterns, are much simpler and less rhythmical.

Though not all of the Yang-shao pottery was turned, the use of the wheel became general in the Black Pottery culture, also known as the Lung-shan culture from the site at which it was first found. This culture, which must have been widespread along the north China coast, in the Liaotung Peninsula and Shantung province, made its influence felt as far south as Hangchow and merged in the northern Chinese plain with that of Yang-shao. It flourished particularly between 2500 and 1500 B.C., and the remarkably thin, hard-baked black pottery often has a fine luster and is of exceptionally high quality. It differs markedly from the pottery of Yang-shao both as regards ornamentation (the Lung-shan ware is not painted at all) and in shape.

The Lung-shan pottery was gradually replaced by the gray pottery of the Hsiao-t'un culture (near An-yang, which is associated with the cultural remains of the Shang people). This gray pottery appears to be closely related in form to the Lung-shan pottery, but its quality is superior to the gray ware which both the Lung-shan and the Yang-shao cultures produced in addition to their own characteristic red and black wares. The types of vessels which the Lung-shan and Hsiao-t'un cultures have in common are those found later in the Bronze Age: the tripod *ting*, the hollow tripod *li*, the steamer *hsien*, and the beaker-shaped *ku*. (See ASIATIC PROTOHISTORY, I, FIG. 15; and below, *Shang-Yin period.*)

From the merging of the three great northern Chinese neolithic cultures, characterized by the red, the black, and the gray pottery, in which process the gray gradually absorbed the other two, there developed in north China the Shang culture, which marks the beginnings of the Chinese historical period. Elsewhere in China a number of other neolithic civilizations persisted for a considerable period of time, but they could not be compared with the Shang bronze civilization, as the excavations in Honan show, once this had attained its full development. (See also CERAMICS.)

*Sculpture.* Owing to the small number of scientifically conducted excavations, little is known as yet about Chinese neolithic sculpture. The only pieces which can with any degree of confidence be reckoned among the earliest specimens of Chinese sculpture are some remarkable disk-shaped earthenware objects which would seem to have served as lids for an unknown kind of pot of the Yang-shao culture in Kansu. They are convex in shape, with indented edges, and in the center there is a stylized representation of a human head with the

eyes and mouth indicated by small round holes. They are decorated in red and black; in a single case this decoration represents the eyes, nose, and beard of a human face, although the ornamentation is usually purely abstract.

In 1955, a clay figure was discovered at Shih-chia-ho, near Tien-mên in Hupeh, which belongs to a mixed neolithic culture. It is a very rough and primitive representation, 3 in. high, of a seated human figure. In the same site was found a 2-in.-long figure of a bird, which may already have in it something of that "primitive naturalism" which Salmony considered a characteristic of neolithic sculpture. The marble and jade pieces that he ascribes to this period are, however, in no way similar in style.

An interesting piece of sculpture executed in this primitive naturalistic style, said to have been found in a site near Taiyuan

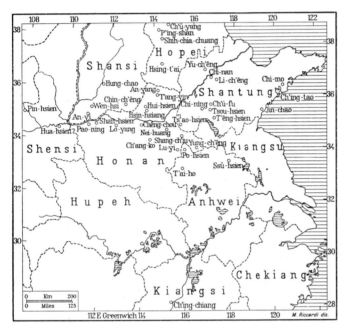

Area of the Shang culture, 2d millenium. B.C. (*after Chêng Tê-k'un*).

in Shansi, may be seen in the Nelson Gallery of Art in Kansas City. In this case, however, the execution is so primitive that it is difficult to say whether it is intended to be a bird or a tortoise. A figure much more characteristic of this naturalistic style is a buffalo in the Toronto museum, said to have been found in An-yang. Apart from the above-mentioned specimen of clay sculpture, scarcely any pieces can be definitely attributed to the Chinese Neolithic period.

*Architecture.* As a result of the discovery and careful excavation, in 1953 and the years following, of the neolithic village of Pan-po-ts'un, east of Sian (see CHINA, *Shensi*), we have at last been able to learn a little about the neolithic architecture of China.

Remains of different types of dwellings have been found, some square or rectangular and others round. The two types seem to have existed side by side, but the strata in which these dwellings are found are difficult to distinguish from one another, as the site was continuously inhabited for a very long time, and it has therefore not been possible to determine which kind of dwelling is older.

The round dwellings had a diameter of about 16 ft. Outside the walls, which were between 1½ and 3 ft. thick, were holes for the wooden posts which supported the roof. The shape of the roof cannot be determined with any degree of certainty; some hold that it was conical or resembled a beehive, others that it was flat and that the ceiling was supported by rafters. Sometimes there is only one hole, in the middle of the dwelling, which suggests that the roof was supported by one upright pole. The floors and the inside walls of both types of

houses were plastered. In the middle of the room was the stove, probably separated from the rest of the room by two screens. The entrances face south; in the case of the square or rectangular dwellings the floor is often 3 ft. lower than the ground and is reached from the outside by means of steps.

The largest building discovered, which the Chinese archaeologists have assumed to be a "clan house," covers an area 65 × 40 ft. The earthen floor is surrounded by a low wall of stamped earth 20 in. high and 3 ft. thick. In this wall rested 12 pillars which probably served both as a framework for the walls and as supports for the roof. In the middle of the hall traces were found of 2 pillars, deeply sunk into the ground at a distance of 15 ft. apart, which must have supported the ridge beam.

Despite the scantiness of these archaeological data, we already recognize in this village — which is believed by some to have belonged to the middle Yang-shao period and to have been built in part about 2500 B.C. — some essential characteristics of later Chinese architecture, especially in the use of pillars and in the southern orientation of the buildings.

THE SHANG-YIN PERIOD (1558?–1028? B.C.). For a long time Western scholars, generally skeptical of ancient Chinese historical traditions, believed that the earliest dynasties mentioned in the Chinese chronicles were mythical rather than historical. It is true that none of the many recent excavations has shown the least trace of the first of these dynasties, the Hsia, which according to varying Chinese chronologies is said to have ruled from 1989 to 1558 B.C., or from 2205 to 1766 B.C. On the other hand, there is no longer any question as to the historical status of the Shang dynasty, and the names of many of its rulers, as recorded in the ancient chronicles, have been confirmed by inscriptions. Its chronological limits, however, still remain uncertain. Traditional Chinese chronologies place it between 1766 and 1122 B.C., or 1558–1050 B.C., but other dates have been suggested. The Chinese scholar Tung Tso-pin, for instance, believes that the Shang dynasty came to an end in 1111 B.C., a date differing by less than a century from those advanced by other scholars, such as Karlgren. The dates shown in the heading above (1558–1028), and for the Chou period, below — though by no means certain — reflect the opinions of the later scholars.

As far back as 1899, near An-yang (see CHINA, *Honan*) animal bones and tortoise shells were discovered with clear marks of human workmanship. Some of these were inscribed in an archaic script, the elements of which were later recognized as the prototypes of the Chinese characters. It was already known from historical sources that the Chinese had employed bones and tortoise shells in divination; the practice was to smooth the surface and reduce its thickness by boring in some places, after which a bar of red-hot iron was brought close to the thin places, thus producing cracks to be interpreted by the diviner. In many cases the questions, and the answers of the oracle, were engraved on the bones. The archaic form of Chinese writing used in these oracle-bone inscriptions has been partly deciphered since their discovery, so it may be said that we are now acquainted to a certain extent with the life and culture of the Shang period. Among other things, the oracle bones have given us the names of some of the ancient rulers, confirming those furnished by traditional historical texts.

These inscriptions, extremely important for our knowledge of Chinese history, aroused such interest in archaeological circles that large-scale systematic excavations were begun on the main site where oracle bones had been discovered. These excavations brought to light the remains of a great city, the last capital of the Shang kingdom, on the banks of the Huan River near An-yang and Hsiao-t'un in Honan.

*Centers of Shang culture.* The capital at An-yang must have been the residence of a dozen Shang sovereigns between the years 1300 and 1028 B.C. (or 1384–1111 B.C., according to Tung Tso-pin). The excavations carried out on its site have yielded a large quantity of oracle bones and many other highly significant objects. The extent of the city, though still uncertain, is indicated by traces of the great number of pits used as dwellings or

as storage places and by the foundations of buildings made of stamped earth. Nearby a huge necropolis has come to light. In the tombs, some of which are extremely large and thus are probably the burial places of royal personages, there have been found richly decorated bronze vessels, large sculptures in stone, jade ornaments and emblems, large quantities of gray pottery and a small quantitiy of white ware (PL. 220), as well as a variety of other objects and fragments, all attesting the surprisingly high cultural and artistic level reached in the Shang period.

The excavations made between 1928 and 1937 have also shown that the area along the Huan River had been inhabited even before the late Shang period. At different sites three strata of remains have been clearly identified; the lowest of these contained remains related to the Yang-shao (Red Pottery) culture, while those in the next stratum belonged to the Lung-shan (Black Pottery) culture. The relics of Shang culture were always found above these two strata.

The discovery of this stratification, although of the greatest importance for chronological sequence, has misled some scholars into the belief that the highly developed culture of the late Shang period derived directly from the neolithic cultures. These scholars have tried to explain the sudden appearance of a perfect technique of casting bronze (which characterizes late Shang culture) as an exotic importation, and the high quality of the decoration on these bronzes as an adaptation to metalwork of techniques previously applied to vessels of less durable material, such as bone or white earthenware. This hypothesis no longer seems necessary.

The discovery that a more ancient Shang city, representing a preceding stage of this same culture, had existed elsewhere in the same province brought back to its true proportions the significance of the An-yang stratification. In 1950, a fragment of earthenware, found by mere chance near modern Cheng-chow (Chêng-chou), gave Chinese archaeologists the clue which led to this discovery. In the following years, a great many excavations were carried out in this area (see CHINA, Honan), revealing the site of a city which may have been the capital for several centuries before King P'an-kêng moved with his people to An-yang. Here too several strata of remains were found, differing somewhat from those of An-yang. At Êrh-li-kang and in Pai-chia-chuang there were only two strata; in the People's Public Park (Jên-min Kung-yüan) north of the modern city, two comparable strata were found and, in addition, a third with remains apparently contemporaneous with some from the An-yang Shang strata. From this evidence it was established that the finds of Chêng-chou were to a great extent older than those of An-yang.

This relative age was further confirmed by a careful comparison of bronze and earthenware vessels found in different places and in different strata, which revealed a definite sequence in the stylistic development of the forms and the decoration. The lowest strata of these three sites yielded no bronzes at all, but an astonishing development of bronze casting is apparent if we compare, for example, Chêng-chou tripods of the chüeh type with bronzes of the same type brought to light in An-yang. Specimens of chüeh have been found also at Liu-li-ko in Hui-hsien in strata which suggest that they too belonged to the pre–An-yang phase of Shang culture. That the decoration of the most ancient pieces lacks refinement may be due to a difference in the quality of the particular pieces found, rather than to a chronological development in technique. The fact, however, that these pieces have a flat bottom, a form much easier to cast than the round-bottomed forms of the chüeh from An-yang, and the inferior quality of the bronze alloy used, convincingly show us that the Chêng-chou bronzes represent an earlier, more primitive stage of Chinese bronze art. The scholars Chou Hêng and Chêng Tê-k'un have pointed out similar stylistic phenomena in the other types of vessels and utensils.

A corresponding development in the oracle bones must also be noted. In Chêng-chou only two of these bones bearing inscriptions have been found; one of these, with an inscription similar to those of An-yang, was found in the top stratum; the other, in a deeper stratum, had an inscription consisting of only one character. On the other hand, in An-yang about 100,000 oracle bones have actually been found. A great many of these, being pierced, must have been strung together or stuck on some sort of file spindle; they seem to have formed an archive, which was located at the elbow of the Huan River, near Hsiao-t'un.

Scholarly opinions differ as to the subdivision of the Shang strata in the various sites excavated at An-yang. This is partly due to the difficulties of working on prewar material, but more particularly to the fact that in the late Shang period An-yang was inhabited for centuries without interruption, which increases the difficulty of distinguishing one stratum from another. Some scholars believe that they can identify two Shang strata in Hsiao-t'un and suppose that the Shang people already lived there before the capital was transferred. The remains of the original city are supposed to lie beneath the foundations of pounded earth, which are presumed to date from the time when the capital was established there. Chou Hêng, who distinguishes three phases in the development of Shang culture in An-yang, judges — by comparison with the finds of Chêng-chou — that the most ancient phase of the An-yang Shang culture is later than that of Chêng-chou II and earlier than Chêng-chou III. Although the last word has not yet been said on the chronology and sequence of the remains of Chêng-chou and An-yang, it is already clear from finds at Chêng-chou that the origin of Bronze Age culture in China can be explained without any hypothesis of importation.

*Shang bronzes.* Bronzes are the best-known products of all Shang art because of the enormous quantities which have come to light during the excavations in northern China. The forms and styles of these bronzes, which were probably used mainly for ritual purposes, vary considerably. The study of the forms, decorative motifs, and inscriptions of these bronze vessels has a long tradition in China which seems to have begun in the 11th century with the antiquarians of the Sung dynasty. An approximate idea of the chronology and stylistic evolution has been achieved only very recently, but we now know that in a great many cases the dates assigned to various pieces by Chinese scholars of the past, on the basis of historical events or personages mentioned in the inscriptions, were substantially correct. In this field pioneer research has been carried out by the Swedish Sinologist Bernard Karlgren, who, having interpreted the inscriptions, on the one hand, and having analyzed the decorative motifs, on the other, was able to give a chronological order to the styles of the bronzes. Although some of his ideas have found few adherents, his work has vastly improved and systematized our knowledge of the stylistic evolution, especially bringing a certain order into the dating of bronzes, which before that time was in most cases quite confused.

The art of bronze casting was modified after the fall of the Shang dynasty, at the end of a long period. Karlgren described a transitional style, the so-called "Yin-Chou style," but it is not recognized by many as such and does not, in comparison with the preceding and following styles, display many elements which can be said to typify it. (See below, Chou dynasty.)

Already within the Shang style, however, clear stylistic differences had made their appearance both in the types of vessels and in the decorative elements. There is a clear difference between the bronzes from Chêng-chou and those from An-yang, as well as between some of the An-yang bronzes and innumerable others of unknown origin. Karlgren identified 33 different elements in the decoration of Shang bronzes. These he grouped into three classes, designated A, B, and C, assigning 6 elements to the first class, 11 to the second, and 16 to the third. While the elements of Class C are found in combination with those of A and B, those of the two latter classes are never found together. Karlgren accordingly formulated this hypothesis: In the Shang bronzes there are two distinct styles, one, designated as Style A (formed by the elements of Classes A and C), which is earlier, and a second, Style B (formed by the elements of Classes B and C), which is chronologically later. An extremely important difference observed by Karlgren between pieces of Styles A and B is that in the former the decoration

covers almost the entire surface (*uni-décor*), while in the latter some areas are normally left undecorated. In Style A, the predominant motif is the one called *t'ao-t'ieh* by Sung antiquarians, which consists of the stylized figure of a fantastic animal, occurring with many variants (see ASIATIC PROTO-HISTORY, I, FIG. 26). In Style A, the *t'ao-t'ieh* appears against a background of geometrical motifs; in Style B, it almost completely disintegrates into geometrical elements.

Karlgren's classification has met with numerous objections, from, among others, Max Loehr, who classes Shang bronzes on purely chronological standards. His five groups (An-yang I–V) are each characterized by steps in the gradual improvement and refinement of the casting technique and the decoration. The chronological differences claimed by Loehr, however, cannot (like the stylistic differences between the Chêng-chou and the An-yang bronzes) be checked on the basis of the An-yang stratification, so that Loehr's method affords a lesser degree of certainty. His method differs further from that or Karlgren in that, while Karlgren analyzes the largest possible number of bronzes, Loehr bases his stylistic classification on the "general impression" received when each piece is looked upon as a unity of form and decoration. Proceeding in this manner, Loehr sometimes reaches conclusions completely opposed to Karlgren's, going so far as to consider the latter's Style A as the last stage of the Shang style. The contradictory conclusions of these two eminent scholars clearly show that the stylistic development of Shang bronzes is far from self-evident and that the problems set by these bronzes have not yet been solved at all.

In addition to vessels many other types of bronze objects have come down to us, among them being daggers, knives, halberds, axes, and other weapons — partly for ritual use — as well as bells of various shapes and numerous bronze ornaments, the use of which is as yet mostly unknown. These objects represent a far from negligible percentage of the great quantity of Chinese bronze pieces scattered among museums and art collections throughout the world. Their function in Chinese culture can be established only for those pieces found in the course of scientifically conducted excavations, and even then exact evidence for their use is rare. There are also sculptured animals in bronze (see below).

*a. Types of bronze vessels.* The Shang bronzes appear in a considerable number of standard forms, each of which has certain minor variants. Although a large number of pieces are known which cannot be easily classified, generally speaking most classical bronzes may be assigned to one or another typological class. Each traditional type-form bears a name, in some cases the same as that used at the time when the bronze was cast, as known from inscriptions. In other cases, where the original name is doubtful, the nomenclature is that coined by the Sung antiquarians, who attempted, on the basis of ritual texts of the Chou period (see below), to identify the use to which each type of vessel was put.

In some cases the function of vessels of a particular type-form is rather uncertain; nevertheless, there is no doubt that a very large part of the vessels known to us were used for purely ritual purposes and that certain forms corresponded to certain uses. Some of the most frequent type-forms go back to the remotest phase of bronze casting, others appear only in the final phase, and preferences for particular forms vary according to the stylistic period.

According to the function of each type, as the Sung scholars supposed it to be, classical bronzes fall into three classes: (1) food vessels, divided into vessels for cooking and vessels for serving or preserving food; (2) wine vessels; and (3) water vessels. The vessels for cooking or preparing food include, among others, the following type-forms: the *ting* (PL. 228), a cauldron with three or four legs, usually with two handles, which often in the oldest variety is square in form (*fang*) with four cylindrical feet and is called the *fang-ting*; the *li* (II, PL. 15), a vessel with hollow feet, derived from a prehistoric earthenware prototype; an intermediate type between the preceding two, called by its modern designation the *li-ting*; and the *hsien*,

a sort of double boiler for steaming food with the top part shaped like a *ting* without feet and the bottom like a *li*. The most common of the serving vessels is the *kuei* (II, PL. 14), a deep round basin occurring both with and without handles, and sometimes standing on a high square base.

Wine vessels are subdivided into vessels for warming wine, and drinking vessels or storage containers. The *chüeh* tripod (cf. II, PL. 15, of the Chou period), belonging to the first group, has both a handle and a spout and, to judge from the Chêng-chou excavations, is one of the most ancient types known. To the second group belong: the *ku* (PL. 227) a deep beaker with flaring rim; the *tsun* (a name also applied to various other types eluding an accurate classification), which is less slender and contains a greater volume than the preceding type; the *hsi-tsun*, made in the shape of a bird, often an owl, or an animal, often a ram or an elephant (cf. PL. 224, of the Chou period); the *kuang* (PL. 222), resembling a gravy boat with a lid in the shape of an animal's head and back; and the *yu*, which usually has a lid of broad oval form.

Water vessels, the third type, occur in two common shapes, the *p'an*, a broad, shallow bowl, usually with handles and a high foot rim, and the *yi*, which, like the *kuang*, resembles a gravy boat, but lacks the lid and stands on three, or four, feet.

There are many other types besides those listed above (e.g., PL. 221) and it has been possible to classify a total of about forty.

*b. Decorative motifs.* In the decorations on the bronzes of the Shang period, which cover the whole surface of the piece or a part of it, we find a few geometric motifs (including interlocking T's and a beautiful background spiral, the *lei-wên*, or thunder pattern) and a great many more or less stylized animal motifs. Karlgren distinguished over thirty different design elements; a certain number of these, however, can be reduced to stylistic mutations of a single animal, evidently fanciful, which, following the Sung antiquarians, we usually and probably inappropriately call the *t'ao-t'ieh*, or "glutton," a name taken from a text of the 3d century B.C. (see ASIATIC PROTO-HISTORY, I, FIG. 26; cf. II, PL. 10, a Chou example). This animal can be recognized by a characteristic persisting through all changes of style and degrees of stylization, that is, the absence of the lower jaw. The frequency of the *t'ao-t'ieh* as a decorative motif suggests that this animal played an important role in the religious life of the Shang period. Although many hypotheses have been put forward, it is impossible to ascertain exactly what the *t'ao-t'ieh* may have been, for it has not yet been identified in the oracle-bone texts, if it is indeed mentioned.

In his studies, Karlgren starts from the premis ethat the most naturalistic form of the *t'ao-t'ieh* is also the most ancient, and that, through an increasing stylization, those ultimate forms were derived in which only the monster's prominent eyes can be recognized, its head having otherwise completely fused into the geometric design. Loehr rejects this theory and thinks that the completely stylized *t'ao-t'ieh* appears at an early date in Shang bronzes (his style An-yang II).

While certain indications incline us to recognize in the *t'ao-t'ieh* a forerunner of the Chinese dragon, so popular as a motif in later periods, there are also some forms of the *t'ao-t'ieh*, such as that in which this fantastic animal is shown with buffalo horns, which rule out such an identification. Moreover, another imaginary animal more closely resembling the dragon also appears in many variations on these bronzes. The cicada is also represented, as well as various types of birds clearly based on nature and of a less fanciful character than the animal motifs.

The entire decorative repertory of the bronzes, both geometric and animalistic, the latter inspired by mythical as well as existing animals, actually consists of a very small number of motifs. The smallness of this repertory, however, is camouflaged by the variety of combinations and by the refined taste presiding over the choice of the motifs and their adaptation to the different shapes of the bronzes. The outstanding difference between Karlgren's A and B styles, as noted above, is the different extent to which the decoration is allowed to occupy the surface of the piece. In the case of Style A, the artist

seems to have succumbed to a *horror vacui* and has covered the entire surface of the vessel, filling up the spaces between decorative elements in bold relief with a continuous network of geometric motifs. With Style B, on the other hand, only a portion of the surface is decorated and the differences in depth of relief are smaller; in some cases the decoration is limited to a band or a frieze.

To explain the origin of the obvious stylistic differences in the Shang bronzes, the Chinese archaeologist Li Chi has suggested that their decoration is derived from wood carvings, the existence of which was ascertained during the An-yang excavations. Li Chi also seeks the origin of some motifs in the west, e.g., in Mesopotamia, although he discerns, on the other hand, affinities with the art of other Pacific peoples, such as the superimposition and repetition of the same motif and the convention of splitting an animal profile into two symmetrically placed halves. Li Chi interprets the latter as an attempt at dimensional representation in relief. He tries to explain the two degrees of decoration, "total" and "partial," with the hypothesis that bronzes of a square or rectangular shape, which he associates with total decoration, are derived from wooden prototypes, while the partially decorated bronzes, distinguished by their rounded shapes, are derived from earthenware prototypes. Many difficulties, however, arise as soon as we try to derive the decoration of bronzes from decoration in other materials, even if we admit that lost prototypes once existed in a perishable material. There is no doubt that wood carvings existed in An-yang — the finds prove this — but they belong to a period in which the art of bronze casting was already fully developed. The same may be said of objects in other materials suggested by still other scholars as possible antecedents of bronze. Certainly Chinese bronzes are greatly indebted for their shapes to the final phases of prehistoric pottery, above all to the black pottery of Lung-shan, but their decoration, to the best of our knowledge, did not originate from this culture. The carved bone objects of An-yang do not impress us as having been executed before the bronzes found there; and the same may be said of the white An-yang pottery (PL. 220), which has sometimes (probably erroneously) been considered a forerunner of the bronzes.

Even the most superficial study of the fanciful fauna appearing in the decoration of Chinese bronzes must lead to the conclusion that the endless repetition of these animals has a significance going far beyond any mere decorative function. That human and animal sacrifice was practiced in this period has been proved, for An-yang at least, beyond any possible doubt, but we have no direct light on the complex of conceptions and beliefs which might explain the ritual symbolism of the animal motifs. The riddles so tantalizingly presented by this problem have naturally evoked many attempts at solution. In general, two approaches have been taken, sometimes in combination. In what we might call the philological approach, an attempt has been made to identify and explain the themes on the basis of ancient Chinese literary sources. These were, in the vast majority of cases, recorded at a period when Shang times had already faded in memory or been perhaps forgotten, so that an interpretation based on them is fraught with hazard. In the other, the ethnographic approach, a solution has been sought in parallels with other cultures both in Asia and farther afield. It is not yet possible to assess adequately the results thus obtained, but neither of these methods satisfies present-day scientific standards. It is still possible that the further decipherment of oracle-bone inscriptions or the results of new excavations may yield new knowledge of the religious life of the people and of the significance of Shang art.

*Sculpture.* One of the most sensational discoveries made by Chinese archaeologists during the An-yang excavations was that of the large marble and limestone sculptures found at Ssŭ-p'an-mo, Hsiao-t'un, and Hou-chia-chuang. The most impressive of these sculptures, and the best-preserved, come from the great tomb (No. 1001) of the Northwest Hill (Hsi-pei-kang) at Hou-chia-chuang; it belongs to that series of tombs which Pelliot was the first to call, probably correctly, the "royal tombs." The shape and decoration prove that these sculptures are contemporary with the bronzes. The most surprising characteristic of the sculptures — some of which are almost 16 in. tall — is a well-balanced and well-developed structure, with full-round modeling far superior to that of the crude statues sculptured a thousand years later near the tomb of General Ho Ch'ü-p'ing (see CHINA, *Shensi*).

The fanciful beasts of the bronzes appear again in the sculptures, and parallels with jade carvings (see below) are not infrequent. These bizarre animals have a weird and sometimes even gruesome appearance. Of the mythical fauna, the best-known representatives, found in the royal tombs, are a kneeling tiger-headed monster and a monstrous bird resembling an owl or some other bird of prey. There are also other more realistic and recognizable animals, such as elephants, buffaloes (e.g., in the Sedgwick Collection in London, PL. 229), and frogs. In some exceptional instances we see a trend (so far not observed in any of the pieces coming from scientifically conducted excavations) toward angular, cubic shapes, reminding us somewhat of certain modern Western sculpture. Some consider these pieces, for instance, one in the Seattle Art Museum, as going back to a pre–An-yang or neolithic phase, but this is rather uncertain. In representations of human beings a predilection for kneeling or seated figures is to be observed.

In this sculpture both the forms and the decorative motifs show a high level of technical skill. The engraved or thread-relief surface decoration, produced by abrading the background, consists of simple geometric motifs, which accentuate the animal's form or supply details not sculptured, such as eyes, mouth, and teeth. With the exception of the larger pieces already mentioned, all the marble and limestone sculptures known from this site are small. According to somewhat vague reports, however, the remains of sculptures of monumental size have also been discovered at An-yang.

The most remarkable fact about this Shang sculpture is that it appeared like a comet of intense splendor only to disappear again at once, swallowed up in the darkness. We feel ourselves in the presence of an entirely mature art which must have developed over the course of centuries before reaching its climax here. Perhaps some information on the antecedents of the Shang sculpture can be filled in from our still very imperfect knowledge of the pre–An-yang culture. As to the successors of the Shang civilization, while Chou bronzes (see below) are very often discovered, so far no trace of a Chou sculpture in stone has been found, and it must be concluded that the bright light of Shang sculpture went out with the disappearance of the culture that produced it.

Shang bronzes in the shape of animals are works of art no less notable than the sculptures in stone. Here we have a tradition perhaps even earlier than that of stone sculpture, and one which, unlike the latter, continued under the Chou. Some of these zoomorphic bronzes appear to have been conceived in the first place as vessels, rather than as images of animals, as for instance, the owl of the Holmes Collection, which greatly resembles the marble "owl" of the royal tomb at Hou-chia-chuang. The famous elephant of the Camondo Collection (Musée Guimet, Paris) and the rhinoceros of the Avery Brundage Collection (Chicago) show a purer zoomorphic treatment. The elephant, whose physical details are summarily represented, but nevertheless easily recognizable, is completely covered with the decorations typical of this period, i.e., chiefly *t'ao-t'ieh* designs and spirals. At the same time the rhinoceros is modeled in a much more naturalistic style, so that not even the second horn (indispensable for an exact zoological identification) has been left out, but decoration is entirely absent. Here the representation of the animal is primary, notwithstanding the fact that this piece was also used as a vessel. It was found more than a century ago in the province of Shantung and bears an inscription which assigns it to the reign of the last Shang ruler.

*Jades.* White marble sculpture in the round seems bound up with the Shang culture, while jade work, which became at the same time an equally flourishing art, preserved its own tradition throughout the centuries and enjoyed a spectacular

rebirth in the 18th century. From a mineralogical point of view, neither the Chinese word *yü* nor the European term "jade" is an adequate designation for the material with which we are concerned here, unless *yü* and "jade" be understood as generic names covering the different qualities of a number of similar semiprecious stones and minerals. The most important are nephrite (calcium-magnesium silicate) and jadeite (sodium-aluminum silicate); besides these two, the Chinese used to include as *yü* softer minerals, such as chloromelanite, amphibole, and serpentine. The ancient jades are normally of nephrite, found in comparatively small pebbles in Sinkiang and in Siberia (see ASIATIC PROTOHISTORY), while the 18th-century jades are of jadeite, obtained in much larger blocks from Burma and the neighboring areas of Yunnan (see GEMS AND GLYPTICS). The great variety of forms and colors naturally occurring were often cleverly exploited to produce a surprising variety of effects in the sculptures. In spite of the great technical difficulties involved in carving jade, because of its hardness, this material had for centuries the greatest attraction for Chinese artists. Magical properties were attributed to it, such as the ability to prevent the decomposition of corpses, so that jade objects acquired an important place among tomb ornaments.

Our knowledge of early jade carving, in contrast with our

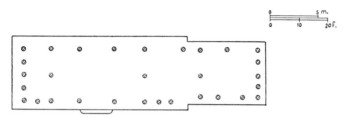

Plan of a large hall at An-yang, Honan, late Shang period, 1300–1028 B.C. (*after Sickman and Soper*).

knowledge of bronzes, is extremely uncertain, and we can in many cases only conjecture as to the use for which particular objects were made and the significance — probably ritual and symbolic — of the various types. This is partly because inscriptions, frequent on bronzes, are almost never present on jades. Since almost all pieces have come from unsupervised excavations about which no archaeological data are available, attempts to establish a plausible chronology of early jades have been based primarily on the decorative motifs, which are sufficiently linked with those of the bronzes to furnish a fairly dependable standard. The problem of chronology has been studied especially by Alfred Salmony, whose conclusions appear in his *Carved Jade of Ancient China* (1938), based mainly on decorated pieces, and *Archaic Chinese Jades* (1952), which presents an ample study of the pieces in the Sonnenschein Collection. In the latter work, he considers, besides stylistic elements, the technical characteristics of Chinese jades and traces of working methods to be observed on them.

Although dependable data on jade work during the neolithic period are extremely scarce, we are probably safe in assuming that Shang jade art developed at least in part out of the neolithic. Very little has been published on the jades found in An-yang and elsewhere; nevertheless, there is a group of pieces which, thanks to Salmony's stylistic research, can be assigned with considerable certainty to the Shang period. Notwithstanding their different forms, the pieces in this group appear quite homogeneous from the point of view of decoration. Among these Shang jades, knives, axes, and ritual weapons in the form of spades and chisels have an important place. Some types seem related to neolithic stone tools, others to bone or bronze objects. Some pieces are large enough to indicate that they were actually used, if only in ritual; others are so extremely small that we may suppose they served merely as badges of office and rank.

Already in the Shang period those peculiar flat round disks, pierced in the center, which we suppose to have been a symbol of heaven and which are termed *pi*, appear as a very common form. Throughout this period and the succeeding early Chou,

the *pi* are without decoration (II, PL. 31). Some scholars believe these disks to be derived from the ferrules or the round tip of the scepters which were once the insignia of office of high dignitaries, and which later came to be a symbol of the "mandate of heaven" and thus of imperial power; on this point no common opinion has yet been reached. The counterpart of the *pi* is the *ts'ung*, which symbolizes the earth and takes the form of a prism pierced lengthwise. This particular shape cannot easily be related to any object in common use, so we are inclined to claim a purely ritual origin for it. However that may be, it seems fairly certain that the most common form of the *ts'ung*, the long cylindrically pierced prism, was not yet in use in the Shang period.

The workmanship of Shang jades reveals a complete mastery of the material, and the range of subjects represented is closely akin to that found in the decoration of bronzes and in marble sculpture. The figures are not usually engraved; instead, the background is abraded, producing a design in shallow thread-relief. One of the finest pieces of this type assignable with certainty to the Shang period is a musical stone, 33 in. long, found soon after excavations were resumed (1950) in the village of Wu-kuan-ts'un near An-yang. What most impresses us in this stone, even more than the beautiful stylization of the tiger which is represented, is the elegant manner in which the animal's profile is contained within the shape of the stone. The shapes and decoration of these jades are based on predominantly animalistic themes, in which the tiger has a preeminent place. Whereas the fauna of the bronzes is nearly always greatly stylized, that of the jades is not only more varied but can be more easily identified. Many of the zoomorphic jades, which, having holes bored into them, possibly were used as pendants, may date from the early Chou period. There are, however, a small number of decorated animal silhouettes which have been excavated at An-yang — among them one representing a mythical owl-like animal, also known from bronze and marble reliefs. In Hou-chia-chuang, tiger silhouettes in jade have been found which are about 3 in. long and which have only very summary decoration or none at all.

*Architecture.* First at An-yang and later at Chêng-chou many foundations of pounded earth have come to light, attesting to large-scale building activity at these sites. In An-yang the remains of ditches appeared under the foundations. Some believe these to have been used as primitive water levels in the construction of the foundations; others think they formed a system of sewers. Sockets have been found in the foundations for columns which must have supported the roof. These columns seem to have been symmetrically placed at regular intervals and to have rested on disks of stone or bronze. Even though we do not know how the roofs were constructed, it is clear that, as in the neolithic houses of Pan-po-ts'un (see above), several of the essential characteristics of Chinese architecture are already present. For the reconstruction of Shang architecture, there are also pictographs of houses and towers engraved on the oracle bones, but often we do not know whether these pictographs represent the ground plan or the elevation of the buildings.

THE CHOU PERIOD (1027?–221? B.C.). The long Chou period is clearly marked by two phases. In the first phase, the rulers of Chou, a state occupying the Wei valley in modern Shensi, overthrew the Shang dynasty (either in the year 1122 B.C. or in 1050 B.C. according to two different traditional Chinese chronologies or, according to modern scholarly opinion, either in 1111 or 1027 B.C.). After destroying the Shang capital, they set up a new capital of their own in the vicinity of the modern city of Sian (Hsi-an), in Shensi province, and granted various districts of the country in fief, perpetuating the feudal system which had grown up under the Shang. In the 8th century B.C., after a period of unrest with gradual weakening of royal power, one of the feudal lords was able to seize and destroy the capital with the help of the Hsiung-nu, a barbarian tribe living on the borders of the kingdom. The weak sovereign then on the throne lost his life in the holocaust. His successor

abandoned the ruined city and established a new capital farther west, situated near the modern city of Loyang (Lo-yang) in the valley of the Lo River in Honan (771 B.C.), thus inaugurating the second phase of Chou history. The new capital was in a safe and sheltered position, but unsuited to defend or wield power over the land, so that from that time on, the rule of the Chou sovereigns was almost wholly nominal. The actual power passed to the many small city states, which formed into larger groups, each trying to dominate the others.

Thus the period of the Chou dynasty is usually divided, according to where the capital was situated, into a Western Chou period from 1027? to 771 B.C. and an Eastern Chou period from 771 to 256 B.C. (or to the beginning of the Ch'in dynasty, 221 B.C.). Chinese scholars also recognize two traditional subdivisions falling within the Eastern Chou period: the Ch'un-ch'iu (Spring and Autumn) period, called after the "Spring and Autumn Annals" attributed to Confucius, which recount the events in the state of Lu from 722 to 481 B.C., and the *Chan Kuo* (Warring States, or Warring Kingdoms) period, a designation which aptly characterizes the period between the 5th century (various exact dates are used) and 221 B.C. The application of this time-honored, but perhaps somewhat arbitrary, periodization to artistic styles, as some Chinese and Japanese archaeologists do, is a practice frowned upon by most Western scholars.

The Eastern Chou period as a whole is characterized by continuous changes in power relationships between the many small states and groups of states which all nominally recognized the sovereignty of the Chou rulers. Toward the end of this period, a number of powerful states on the periphery of the Chinese cultural area began the struggle for the domination of China. First the state of Ch'i (in Shantung and Hopei), then Chin (in Shansi) won supremacy. Gradually, however, the Ch'in kingdom, centered in Shensi, gained access to the central plains and with this (particularly after Chin split up into three separate states in 376 B.C.) acquired control of the whole country. The Ch'u kingdom, which had originally centered in Hupeh and had steadily extended its hold over the northern agricultural areas, remained one of the last redoubtable opponents of Ch'in. In 256 B.C. the last Chou ruler was deposed, but it was not until 221 B.C., when all opponents had been overcome, that the ruler of Ch'in became the first emperor (Shih Huang-ti) of a unified China.

Though the Chou period represents a continuous succession of civil wars, it is nevertheless the "Classical Age" of China. Scarcely one hundred and fifty years after the reign of the last Chou ruler, with memories of that dynasty already growing dim, the Chinese had begun to idealize the Chou period and to see it as the embodiment of their ideals. It was indeed the time of China's famous philosophers, who propounded their philosophical and political ideas at the courts of the various states, large and small. They left behind them a wealth of literature which, even though not always handed down to us in its original form, provides a vivid picture of an exceptionally highly developed cultural life.

As the result of a custom which gave rise to heated discussions among the philosophers, that of lavishly furnishing the graves of the dead so that the spirit would have familiar and pleasant surroundings, we are fairly well informed about the art forms realized in more durable materials, although not everything excavated from tombs is necessarily representative of the arts and crafts of the living, all traces of which have entirely disappeared.

*Chou bronzes.* Archaeological excavations have not yet revealed a clear dividing line between the bronze art of the Shang period and that of the early Chou. While the level of Chou civilization was probably lower than that of the inhabitants of the Great City of Shang, it may be assumed that the changes in government did not immediately affect the styles of the ceremonial bronzes. The bronze vessels which we are able to assign to the period of the first Chou rulers, on the basis of the content and style of their inscriptions, do not differ greatly in shape and ornamentation from the ceremonial vessels which

have been found in the An-yang excavations and which can therefore definitely be attributed to the Shang period. It is clear that the bronze art of the early Chou period is derivative in character and that the emergence of a new style about 900 B.C. marks the beginning of a true Chou art with its own characteristics. Karlgren, in his first great study of Chinese bronzes (1936), noted four differentiative criteria which he regarded as characteristic of a transitional Yin-Chou style (see above) of the early Chou period. However, not long afterward two of these stylistic criteria were recognized in pieces excavated at An-yang, suggesting a Shang date since this capital had been razed by the Chou conquerors. The only remaining difference between bronzes of the Shang-Yin and Karlgren's Yin-Chou style is to be found in the treatment of the flanges, which are formed as an uninterrupted segmented ridge in the Shang bronzes, but are broken up into hooked projections in the early Chou. This, however, is hardly adequate to provide characterization for a whole style. We may say, accordingly, that the bronze style of the early Western Chou period may be regarded as a continuation of the Shang bronze style.

A great number of vessels bear inscriptions indicating that they were made under the Chou regime. An exact dating of these bronzes by their inscriptions, however, meets with various difficulties. For the first centuries of the Chou period the chronology is still rather uncertain, and the Western dates given for the cyclical dates occurring in the inscriptions often vary considerably according to the authority consulted. The interpretations of the long Chou inscriptions also are far from consistent, and it is often not entirely certain to which reign the piece should be attributed, except when the name of a Chou king or a recorded historical event is mentioned. Even so, many pieces which originally belonged together, but which have been dispersed after a clandestine excavation or chance find, can be regrouped on the basis of formal identity or similarity of inscriptions. Such is the case, for example, with the important group of Ch'ên-ch'ên bronzes, which are thought to have been found near Lo-yang in 1928. This group consists of about 35 vessels, many of which are signed by an official named Ch'ên-ch'ên.

Even if an inscription can be attributed with reasonable certainty to a particular date, it does not supply proof for the date of other vessels from the same site. This holds true especially for such cemetery sites as the one at Hsin-ts'un (about 12 miles southwest of An-yang), where the Academia Sinica, in 1932–33, brought to light some 90 tombs of greatly varying age, dating from the early Western Chou period down to Eastern Chou times. Of three important bronze finds made in recent years, not one yielded bronzes of a completely homogeneous group. In two cases, at Ling-yüan and Tan-t'u (see CHINA, *Manchuria* and *Kiangsu*), the circumstances under which the bronzes were found are uncertain, and it is possible, therefore, that they may have come from more than one tomb. A tomb at P'u-tu-ts'un, near Sian in Shensi, yielded a *ho* with an inscription which mentions King Mu (947–928? B.C.) as a living person, but other pieces from the same find could be earlier or somewhat later. Apparently some bronzes were kept as family heirlooms for a considerable time before being buried in a grave. If the style changed during the period in which the vessels were kept, the heterogeneous character of the find is easily detected (see below, the Hsin-chêng find), but as long as the stylistic changes were negligible, a considerable difference in date may go undetected. Thus, notwithstanding an abundance of epigraphical and art-historical material, the date for the change to a new bronze style has not been definitely established. In view of the length of the Chou period and of the obvious fact that the style could hardly have changed overnight, it is hardly of importance whether this change had been completed by 950 or 875 B.C.

Though there may be differences as to the date, the change in style itself is so striking that we can speak of an almost revolutionary development. Although the coming of the new style was relatively sudden, and we do not find many pieces in a "transition style," this development was not a kind of delayed-action time bomb which was set at the time of the col-

lapse of the Shang state and went off a century or more later. The characteristics of the earlier period were not completely lost, but the craftsmen created something entirely new by consciously working on and changing the old forms. The name given by Karlgren to this style, namely, the "middle Chou style," is considered by other scholars to be misleading. The term "Second Phase," used by Yetts, is more neutral and perhaps more exact.

Almost all the old classical types of vessels disappear and are replaced by new, occasionally rather squat and heavy ones. The *t'ao-t'ieh*, which played such an important part in Shang art, loses its prominence, and the *lei-wên*, or thunder pattern, disappears completely. Replacing these, we have new forms and new ornamentations, which Karlgren classifies under 12 main headings. The bell of the *chung* type, the *fu* type of box, with its two exactly equal halves, and the *i* resembling a sauceboat are among the new vessel types, while the curved legs of the tripod, the vertical stripes and "fin flanges" of the *li* tripods, and the frequently occurring scale bands are among the more striking stylistic innovations. An important new feature of the ornamentation, which is often robust and sometimes heavy, is that decorative elements are sometimes interlaced, giving an effect of greater relief to the ornamentation. Recent finds in southern Anhwei suggest, however, that this element may be of a somewhat earlier date and of southern origin.

Bronze finds belonging to the middle Chou period (PLS. 223, 225) are considerably fewer in number than those of the Shang-Yin and of the early and late Chou periods, and the number of more or less controlled excavation sites is extremely small as well. Before World War II the only known bronzes of this period were those excavated at Hsin-chêng in Honan province in 1923. Some of these pieces have unmistakable middle Chou characteristics, but others are typical examples of the late Chou style. One inscription has been the subject of much study, as it seems to give some indication, albeit by no means certain, of the date. The opinion of the Chinese scholar Wang Kuo-wei that this inscription dates from 575 B.C. has been accepted by many. However, this does not provide a date for the whole find, as is clearly indicated by the differences in style between the various pieces. The only known large find of bronze vessels belonging exclusively to the middle Chou period was made in 1952 in the village of T'ai-p'u-hsiang, near Chia-hsien in Honan. It consists of 22 vessels of common middle Chou types and a large number of smaller bronze objects.

Though the middle Chou style may not have the subtlety and refinement characteristic of the Shang period and may even sometimes be somewhat crude and clumsy, the best pieces excel in vigor and monumental quality, features not hitherto found in such degree. One of the most impressive examples is the pair of tigers (PL. 223) in the Freer Gallery in Washington, discovered in 1923 in the neighborhood of Fêng-hsiang in Shensi. There is nothing suggestive of feline litheness about these animals; instead they have a massive and angular appearance which is particularly striking when viewed from the front, when the dominant impression is that of grimly stylized rows of sawlike teeth.

It is not yet possible to say with any certainty when the middle Chou style was replaced by what Karlgren calls the "Huai style" from the name of one of the most important regions of provenance, but which could probably better be termed the "late Chou style." It is certain that the new style had already made its appearance in many areas in the 6th century B.C., though the middle Chou style from which it developed may have lingered on in places for a considerable period. Some late Chou pieces bear inscriptions referring to historical events, and in the case of about ten vessels this has led to a more or less definite dating. Here the change in style seems to be far less sudden than that from the Shang style to the middle Chou, and it seems to have been accompanied by a further refinement in casting methods. The somewhat heavy though dynamic qualities of the middle Chou are replaced by something less monumental, lighter and more delicate. This tendency to perfect what immediately preceded is accompanied by a return to motifs of a much earlier period, which is difficult to

account for, though quite unmistakable. The ornamentation of the Shang and early Chou bronzes, which had disappeared with the advent of the middle Chou period, now reappears, although in a modified form. Even the *t'ao-t'ieh*, the fabulous animal of the Shang bronzes, returns to the scene, though in its new "baroque" guise it has lost its magic quality. The mythological animals are no longer depicted for mysterious religious purposes, at which we can only guess, or for their symbolical significance, but for purely decorative purposes. The geometrical patterns of the Shang period, the interlocked T's, for example, now recur, side by side with plaited bands and cord patterns which are entirely new in the bronze art of China. Some of these new features have been attributed to the influence of the art of the Central Asian steppes (see STEPPES CULTURES); the mirrors, which appear for the first time, and the swords characteristic of this period (perhaps related to the *akinakes* of the Scythians) are also said to have their origin in the steppes.

The phenomenon of the appearance of certain decorative elements of the Shang-Yin and early Chou period in the bronze art of the late Chou period has not yet been sufficiently explained. In the case of middle Chou vessels the number of states mentioned in inscriptions is relatively small, and the area in which pieces have been excavated is so far considerably less extensive than that in which early and late Chou vessels have been found. This would seem to point to the possibility that the middle Chou style flourished only in a small area and that both the middle and late Chou styles are direct derivatives of the Shang-Yin and early Chou styles. There are, however, several arguments which can be brought against such a hypothesis. First of all, the transition between middle Chou and late Chou styles is gradual, and many transitional pieces do exist. Moreover, there are two inscribed vessels of the middle Chou style that, on epigraphical evidence, are attibuted to the state of Ch'u, which we would expect to be free from middle Chou influence. The strongest argument, however, against a common source of both middle and late Chou styles is the fact that in the late Chou period the decorative elements alone, but not the vessel types, seem to have been taken over from an earlier source, whereas vessel types continuing the middle Chou style frequently occur.

The problems concerning the origin of the late Chou style can be solved only — if ever — by evidence from new finds, which may give us a better idea of the geographic distribution of Chinese bronze styles. This possibility is demonstrated by the recent find at T'un-chi, in southern Anwei; here the presence of bronzes apparently of the Western Chou period, which have preserved Shang-Yin shapes but have in various cases a decoration strikingly similar to the late Chou style, seems to upset our previous notions. The southern location of this site may be of great significance for the explanation, not only of the peculiarities of these pieces, but of the provenance of the late Chou style.

The finds made before World War II which are of the greatest importance for our knowledge of late Chou art are those at Li-yü (in northern Shansi, 1923), Hsin-chêng (in central Honan, 1923), Chin-ts'un (near Loyang, Honan, 1925), and Shou-chou (modern Shou-hsien in Anhwei, 1933 and 1938). None of these was excavated under expert supervision, but they are all more or less "closed finds." Information on the last-mentioned find was, however, very scanty until details of recent excavations were published. The same is true of the sites at the modern city of Changsha (Ch'ang-sha) in Hunan province and at Hui-hsien in Honan, first excavated in 1936 and after 1929, respectively.

The numerous finds made in the 1950s, which have in many cases been excavated under the supervision of professional archaeologists who have published reports, have yielded invaluable additional information about late Chou art. The grave of the Marquis of Ts'ai near Shou-hsien (1955), the two graves at Chang-t'ai-kuan (near Hsin-yang, Honan, 1956–57) and the complex of graves at Ch'ang-sha are among the most noteworthy discoveries. Of great interest also is the find of bronzes at T'ang-shan in Hopei.

Though Karlgren's choice of the term "Huai" for the late Chou style has been criticized, the new finds have borne out once more the importance of the Huai River valley during the late Chou period as a center for the art of bronze casting. Shou-chou, now Shou-hsien, was the capital of the state of Ch'u during the decline of the Chou dynasty. Ch'u had extended its territory northeastward from Hupeh and was in conflict with its old enemy, Ch'in. Shou-chou became the capital when the Ch'u state was nearing its downfall, and it was just at this time of political weakness that the bronze art reached its culminating point. The richest find of bronzes, from Chu-chia-chi near Shou-hsien (1933 and 1938), about which little definite information has been published, can on the basis of an inscription be linked with the period of the last Ch'u ruler (237–228 B.C.). There can be no doubt that the Ch'u state exerted a very strong influence on the bronze art of the late Chou period, just as it was destined to have a strong influence on Han art (see below).

Part of the regular furnishings of a ruler's grave in the late Chou period included a series of various kinds of bells. Some have cylindrical handles, while others have a handle in the form of two animals facing each other. None shows any trace of having had any kind of clapper. Attempts have been made to reconstruct the tone scale of the late Chou period through a study of bells which had been dispersed in various museums and collections, but which had originally formed part of one series. This had come to seem impossible, because none of the series is complete and many of the bells are in imperfect condition. Now, however, a perfectly preserved series of 13 bells has been found in a grave (No. 1) at Chang-t'ai-kuan, which, judging by their inscriptions, probably date back to 525 B.C.

The influence of the nomadic art of the steppes and Sino-Siberian styles on the bronzes of the late Chou period is particularly interesting (see ASIATIC PROTOHISTORY). It can be seen in the adoption by the Chinese of a number of ornamental motifs which do not appear in the older Chinese bronze art, such as plaited bands and cord patterns and fine granulations arranged in rows or as ground filling. Karlgren has noted the Chinese adaptation of the most characteristic feature of the nomad "animal style," namely, the practice of depicting an animal with its body in profile and with the head turned. This feature may be seen, for example, in the knoblike bodies and turned heads of the Li-yü bronzes from northern Shansi (see above). A group of bronzes depicting hunting scenes, obviously inspired by the steppes art, is particularly beautiful; the repetitive pattern was stamped on and consists of friezes divided from one another by bands. The hu form of these vessels is typically Chinese, and the bases of a number of them have purely Chinese ornamental motifs, such as the band of triangles and whorls. Another unmistakable Chinese feature is the t'ao-t'ieh mask (II, PL. 10). On the other hand, the scenes of the chase, which depict men armed with spears, swords, and bows and arrows, on foot and in horse-drawn chariots, hunting tigers, wild buffaloes, and flights of birds, have a surprisingly lively quality which appears for the first time in Chinese art. It marks the end of the old notions of rigidity and symmetry and introduces in their place a greater freedom and a new vitality.

Another enrichment of bronze art occurred in the late Chou period with the introduction of the practice of inlaying bronzes with various materials. Malachite and turquoise had already been used for inlay in the Shang period, but inlaying acquired a new and much greater importance during the Chou period, when it was applied to the surface of bronze vessels as an integral part of the ornamentation to accentuate the design. The use of gold and silver incrustation to ornament bronzes became particularly common in the Loyang vicinity, as is clearly shown by numerous pieces said to have come from Chin-ts'un, where the state of Han ruled between 450 and 230 B.C. Inlay was often used on small and graceful objects of daily use such as belt hooks. Incrustation was also used, though not so extensively, on mirrors; there are examples of inlaid mirrors in what became known as the Chin-ts'un style in the Freer Gallery of Art, in Washington, and in the Hosokawa Col-

lection. In one piece, a very intricate geometric ornamentation is remarkably combined with a naturalism which far surpasses even that of the hunting scenes. Between whorl complexes resting on dragons' legs, we suddenly see a horseman raising his sword to strike at a fearsome snarling tiger, which lifts its great paw in a last desperate effort to defend itself. This combination of striking naturalism with the most refined geometric decoration may be seen again in later lacquer.

Mirrors (IV, PL. 262) have a special importance in the bronze work of the Chou period. The oldest ones, which were made about 600 B.C., are often square, in contrast to the later round types, and consist in some instances of two bronze plates fitted together. The top plate may have a decoration in openwork or relief or be incrusted with turquoise or some other semiprecious stone. The circular ornaments occasionally to be seen at the four corners of the square mirror are a reminder that originally the two plates were held together by means of nails. A cord passing through a pierced knob was used to hold the mirror. No handle was attached as an integral part of the mirror before the time of the Five Dynasties (see below). The decoration on the reverse side of these mirrors appeared just about the time when Chinese bronze casting entered upon its last great phase.

The center of origin of this new art form is not certain, but it seems to have spread very rapidly. Through the centuries mirrors went through a number of remarkable evolutions in style. There is a fairly gradual transition from the Chou to the Han period (see below) so that they form, as it were, a bridge between the bronze art of the two periods.

As in the case of bronze vessels, the phases in the development of mirrors were first recognized by Karlgren, who proposed a classification, chronologically and according to style, into 11 groups. His first group (A) is the only one not based on clear style characterization; we shall do better to accept as the first group the early "two-layer" type which A. Salmony correctly described as the earliest form of Chinese mirror. Five other groups (Karlgren's B–E and G) can be ascribed to the late Chou period. In the mirrors of the B type (6th and 5th cent. B.C.), the rim is still quite flat and the decorated area is separated from it by a grooved circular band. The knob with the hole for the cord is small, as is the case with all late Chou types of mirrors. In the mirrors of the C type (5th–3d cent. B.C.), the various parts are more clearly differentiated: the concave rim curving up into a high ridge, and a smooth band standing out in relief around the small, bare central field mark off the decorated area. Against a background of comma patterns we see such motifs as quatrefoils emanating from the central field, slanting T's executed as broad, slightly concave bands, or zigzag lozenges, sometimes combined to form stars and executed in the same technique.

Whereas according to Karlgren the C type is found mainly around Shou-chou (Shou-hsien, Anhwei), the somewhat later D type (4th–3d cent.) is associated with Loyang and its vicinity. The thin mirrors of this type often have a concave rim with a flat outer part or a star-shaped flat margin. The knob is surrounded by a small, often decorated central field, which may be square, round, or in the shape of a quatrefoil or star. The principal background patterns consist of various types of lozenges, and volutes and triangles. Most striking is the decoration of graceful animals, as a rule quite different from that on bronze vessels of the period.

In the E type (second half of 3d cent. B.C.), also of the Shou-chou region, the band bordering the central field is always circular and larger than in the preceding categories. It is usually set off by a rope pattern. The rim is always concave with a high outer ridge. The principal decoration consists of dragons, partly dissolved into an inexhaustible variation of beautiful arabesques and often combined with zigzag lozenges.

The G type has a concave rim and a central band set off with a rope pattern. A frequently occurring element is a star-shaped, smooth concave band running through the decorated area. This again is essentially a Shou-chou type and probably dates from the 3d century B.C., although it seems to have been much less popular than the E type.

With the mirrors of the F type, on which for the first time inscriptions occur, we enter the Han period. This type, however, still shows clearly its derivation from late Chou types. About 100 B.C. an entirely new style of bronze mirror emerged which is quite independent of the late Chou styles described above.

*Ceramics.* The Shang and Chou periods formed the age of bronze in China. Vessels for religious and ceremonial purposes were made of bronze, whereas the simpler vessels for daily usage were probably mostly of pottery. But within the pottery there was a clear difference between fine and coarse wares. The gray ware found in great quantities in Shang sites was of a much coarser and simpler type than the rare white pottery (PL. 220) of which, so far, few intact pieces have been found. In this white ware, the influence of bronze art is clearly felt, the decoration being quite similar to that of certain types.

The glazed ware which made its first appearance in Shang sites (at An-yang) is in most cases partly covered with an incidental ash glaze. The recent discovery of about seventy pieces of glazed pottery in two tombs of the Western Chou period at T'un-chi, in southern Anhwei, opens up the possibility of a southern origin for the technique of applying glaze. These pieces, all made without the wheel, mostly imitate the shapes of bronzes (*tou*, *tsun*, *p'an*, and other types). All have a greenish or brownish glaze. The brown glaze seems to have been applied with a brush, whereas the green-glazed vessels were dipped and are therefore glazed inside as well as outside. The incised decoration is simple, consisting of horizontal lines, rope patterns, and hatched zones.

The pottery of the late Chou period is artistically more attractive. A beautiful urn with a lid, covered with an olive-green lead glaze (PL. 230), said to have been found in the graves of Chin-ts'un, shows great similarity with bronzes in the geometric ornamentation of the bands. Objects with such a high standard of execution are on the whole rare, but they give us a good idea of the precursors of the Han pottery, which were still largely based on bronze forms. Opinion is strongly divided on the beautiful models of bronzes said to have been found in Hui-hsien, since they have not been found in any site excavated by expert archaeologists. However, authentic figurines of animals and dancing girls have been excavated (see below). An interesting bowl, found in the Hui-hsien district, on a raised foot and supported by three kneeling human figures, was obviously not inspired by bronze art.

The black pottery of the Lung-shan culture was succeeded in the late Chou period by another form of black polished pottery, though there is no demonstrable connection between the two. This pottery is decorated either with incised figures or with a burnished geometric design. Not only the green lead glaze but also the so-called "protoporcelain" with a feldspar glaze would seem to have been produced in the late Chou period. The resemblance of the Yüeh-yao (see CERAMICS) to bronzes of the late Chou period is so striking that we must assume that the history of this ware had already begun at this time.

*Sculpture.* According to one theory, Chinese funerary sculpture of the Han and T'ang periods (see below) owes its origin mainly to the abandonment of the practice of human sacrifice at funerals. Although there is no doubt that such sacrifices were made in the Shang period, as has been clearly proved by the excavations at An-yang, there is so far no proof that the practice continued under the Chou dynasty. In the Shang period chariots had been buried together with their horses and drivers; in the Chou period chariots and horses continued to be buried (they occur, for example, among the extensive finds at Liu-li-ko near Hui-hsien), but without the drivers. The fact that Confucius — in a saying attributed to him — expressed approval of the use of straw dummies at funerals, but rejected that of "tomb figures" (*yung*) because they were too reminiscent of human sacrifices, would seem to show that such sacrifices were no longer made during his lifetime. The practice of substituting objects made solely for burial purposes, known as *ming-ch'i*, or tomb objects, for real articles of daily use goes back to the Chou period. Generally speaking, the quality of the *ming-ch'i* is inferior to that of their counterparts in ordinary daily use. At Ch'ang-sha, for example, nearly all excavated pieces of pottery are of such poor quality as to be actually incapable of being put to practical use. Confucius, indeed, is quoted as saying that the utilitarian objects and musical instruments placed in the tomb should be unfit for real use. With the appearance of the *ming-ch'i* we also find the first models of chariots and boats, and these models now replaced the real chariots in the tombs. The use of figures of horses instead of the sacrifice of live horses is, moreover, mentioned in texts of the Han period. The word *yung*, used in classical texts for tomb figures, is explained by later commentators as meaning a tomb figure with movable limbs. A number of figures of men with movable arms are known from Han finds, and a clay funerary figurine of the late Chou period representing a duck with movable tail and wings has been found near Chêng-chou at Êrh-li-kang. Wooden funeral figures of human beings appear for the first time in tombs of the Ch'u state during the late Chou period. These rigid, strongly stylized wooden figures have been dug up in very large numbers, particularly in Ch'ang-sha. They are often found in pairs, representing a man and a woman, inserted in the space between the inner and the outer coffin.

A few figures of the Ch'ang-sha type, which belong to the Chou period, have been found in the two graves at Chang-t'ai-kuan near Hsin-yang, Honan. One of these is a very simple standing figure with both arms folded over the breast. The face and clothing have flowing and rounded lines, and there is no trace of the stylized angularity characteristic of the usual Ch'ang-sha figures. In other figures from the graves of Chang-t'ai-kuan the arms and long sleeves are made of separate pieces of wood and attached to the body. The treatment of the features is very summary. The figures of the "guardian of the tomb" found in both graves at Chang-t'ai-kuan are particularly interesting. They represent monsters with long protruding tongues and with real antlers of deer mounted on their heads. The standing phoenixes and recumbent tigers found in these graves, which seem to have served as stands for drums, can be compared with the beautiful pair of cranes from Ch'ang-sha in the Cleveland Museum of Art (PL. 226). It is clear from the easy flowing forms of these figures, which show perfect control and strong imaginative approach in execution, that the sculptors of the Ch'u state had developed a lively and characteristic sculptural style of their own. The rigidity of the wooden human figures is in such striking contrast to the grace of these animal figures that one is led to assume that this rigidity is deliberate rather than due to the inexperience of the artist.

Since World War II much attention has been given to the figurines of men and animals said to have been found in graves in the Hui-hsien district, and there has been a good deal of controversy about their authenticity, though the discovery of similar figurines at Chang-chih (see CHINA, *Shansi*) shows that, at any rate, a late Chou prototype for these pieces did exist. These figurines are in some ways related in style to the erect wooden figure found in a grave (No. 2) in Chang-t'ai-kuan. The figures of female dancers in European and American collections, which are so striking because of their dramatic dancing postures, are probably for the most part not authentic Hui-hsien sculptures. Those few of certain authenticity are rigid and stylized in form, with summarily rendered hands and arms protruding stiffly from the body; they look as though they had been cut out of cylindrically shaped pieces of clay.

An entirely independent group is that of the kneeling bronze figures which are believed to have come from the tombs of Chin-ts'un and elsewhere. Judging by the hollow tube which the figures are holding, they must have served as decorative sockets for some object of unknown purpose. These figures are heavy in form, with disproportionately large heads and broad flat faces. The bodies are squared-off, angular, and massive. Far more lively, though clearly belonging still to the same group, are the almost comical figures of a pair of wrestlers or acrobats in the Spencer-Churchill Collection (Gloucestershire) and a small boy dancing on a tortoise in the C. T. Loo Collection (New York).

*Painting.* Some years ago the oldest known brush, dating from the late Chou period, was excavated near Ch'ang-sha. In the same area a fragment of a painting on silk was discovered in 1949, in a tomb at Ch'ên-chia-ta-shan. It represents a female figure, above which hover a dragon and a phoenixlike bird, and it is painted in a simple and cursory manner.

Besides this fragment, a few other specimens of Chou painting are known. One consists of a group of primitive figures painted around the edge of a still partly undeciphered piece of writing — possibly an exorcist's formula — also found in Ch'ang-sha. From about the same period date some of the rare painted bronze mirrors. Somewhat better preserved than these, however, is a painting on two shells, in the Cleveland Museum of Art. On one of these a hunting scene is depicted in astonishingly vivid detail. In the foreground there is a falling deer, brought down by two arrows, with two hunters in lively motion running toward it. Farther back we see a chariot drawn by four horses, three in front view, with only two legs visible, and the fourth represented in semiprofile. The whole scene, framed in a red line which follows the shape of the shell, is surrounded by fleeing animals and birds. In spite of the almost microscopic dimensions of the scene, the painter has succeeded in recreating the suspense and action of the situation in the most convincing way. We can draw some further conclusions — albeit somewhat one-sidedly — about the artistic achievement in Chou painting from the traditional decoration of lacquer work (see LACQUER).

An indirect source of information on the art of painting in the late Chou period is the decoration on bronze vases, such as that from the Jannings Collection, which depicts a large number of figures in considerable detail. The scenes depicted include an archery contest, women picking mulberries, a bird hunt in which the archers use arrows with lines attached, a fight between two ships, and the storming of a wall. The scenes depicted on an *i* in the Seattle Art Museum and a *hu* in the Musée Guimet in Paris are less lively and the figures are more rigid.

*Other arts.* The jade work of the Chou period can often be dated by comparing the ornamentation with that of contemporary bronze pieces. While it is difficult to differentiate between the bronzes of the Shang and early Chou periods, the difficulty becomes even greater in the case of jades, where there are practically no inscriptions and no controlled excavations to give any indication of dates. Thus the conclusions reached in even such detailed studies as those of A. Salmony are still somewhat hypothetical. However, generally speaking, the same developments would seem to have occurred in the early Chou period in jade art as in bronze. The old Shang style persisted for some time, but gradually lost its vigor. The decoration in relief was maintained for a considerable time, but the thread-relief of the Shang period was eventually replaced by a plain surface, and there was a gradual decline from the amazingly high level of craftsmanship which gave the Shang jades their perfection. Contours and lines were constantly repeated and became conventional and uniform. The earth symbol, the *ts'ung*, now appeared, probably for the first time. Side by side with the annular disks known as *pi* (II, PL. 31), which at this period began to be decorated for the first time — an example is the *pi* in the Seattle Art Museum, which has a symmetrical stylized animal design — annular disks of the *hsüan-chi* type with serrated edges began to appear. According to Henri Michel, these disks, combined with jades of the *ts'ung* type, must have formed an astronomical instrument, but this highly ingenious theory is not generally accepted. A. Salmony is inclined to think that the *hsüan-chi* was used to fasten ropes around bales of silk.

A frequently found type of jade object dating from the early Chou period is the amulet in the form of an animal silhouette. Among the clearly recognizable specimens of the fauna of northern China represented are the tiger, occasionally the elephant, the deer (including the *Elaphurus davidianus*, clearly recognizable by its antlers), the buffalo, the hare or rabbit, the fish, the tortoise, various birds, and even the silkworm, this being carved usually in the round.

In the middle Chou period jade art reached a low ebb, with marked technical decline and reduction of the repertory to a few stereotyped patterns. This decline was only temporary, however, for during the late Chou period there was a great revival of jade art, together with that of bronze casting. As was the case with bronzes, we see here borrowings from the art of the Shang and the early Chou period. Here, too, the symbolical ornamentation to which mysterious magic qualities had been attributed acquired a purely decorative function. A particularly striking characteristic is the ground filling in the form of innumerable varieties of comma patterns brought out in relief by carving out the background. The dragon, the only mythical animal to survive through the ages as a symbol of fertility and as a rainmaker, is depicted in innumerable variations in the jades of this period (PLS. 229; II, 15) as a graceful silhouette of bends and curves in sharp contrast with the angular and stiff creatures of the archaic period.

The refinement of the technique of jade carving, which during this period undoubtedly reached its highest level, with gracefully interlaced designs and decorative openwork, gave to many of the Chou jade pieces the appearance of precious stones. Jade had not entirely lost its symbolical significance; besides being a utilitarian object and an ornament for the living, it was much used as an offering to the dead, mainly because it was said to prevent the decomposition of the corpse. It was also used as an inlay material for bronze. A beautiful girdle hook inlaid with three jade disks was found a few years ago at Ku-wei-ts'un (in Honan), but several other examples of the late Chou period already were present in Western collections.

The girdle or belt hook, which is believed to have been taken over by the Chinese from the art of the steppes during the late Chou period, is met with in a great variety of shapes, ornamentations, and techniques. All forms have a hook, and a stud on the back, both of which are functionally essential; apart from these indispensable characteristics there is a great variation in shape and also in size (ranging from less than 1 to 12 in. in length). They are cast and sometimes gilded, sometimes inlaid with glass or jade, or beautifully incrusted with gold or silver. Often they are made in three parts, a hooked part, a long, rectangular, grooved middle part, and a *t'ao-t'ieh* mask forming the end. Sometimes the whole girdle hook looks like a bent and rounded miniature scepter. It may also have an openwork design of intertwined animals or represent, as in the case of the girdle hook in the Jean Coiffard Collection (Musée Cernuschi, Paris), a tiger silhouette, which in this piece is decorated with a motif strikingly reminiscent of the middle Chou scale band pattern. The high level of artistic achievement which characterized the belt hook in the late Chou period continued well into the Han period.

THE HAN DYNASTY (206 B.C.–A.D. 221). Apart from a short interruption about the beginning of the Christian era, the Han dynasty ruled for more than four centuries over a large part of the present territory of China and, in addition, extended its rule over foreign peoples far beyond the natural Chinese boundaries. The Han period may be divided into two parts, the Western (or Former) Han period, from 206 B.C. to A.D. 8, and the Eastern (or Later) Han period, from A.D. 25 to 221. No other period has been equal to this in importance for the creation of the traditional culture of China. In many respects the Chinese of later epochs are truly "Sons of Han," as they proudly call themselves, for it was this dynasty more than any other which was responsible for the continuity of Chinese civilization. The social and political system built up by the short-lived Ch'in dynasty (221–206 B.C.) from the confusion the Chou sovereigns had left behind them continued to exist during the Han period. At the same time there developed a clear general tendency to idealize the more remote past of the Chou period, which was held in the highest esteem and was the inspiration of a new culture. The originality and vitality we observe in the relics of the Han period combined with many elements of the old Chinese civilization to form, in spite of outside influences, the enduring core of Chinese national culture. Politically the Han empire showed strong expansionist tendencies. Within the

Chinese borders, unification of the ethnically and culturally non-Chinese regions was actively pursued; abroad, the Chinese armies fighting the Huns penetrated deep into Mongolia and Central Asia. The southern part of Manchuria, a considerable part of the Korean peninsula, and a part of Indochina came under Chinese rule and were partly settled by Chinese colonists.

Though Buddhism penetrated into China during this period, it did not yet acquire a prominent position. Only after the fall of the Han dynasty, when the empire split up into a number of independent states, did Buddhism extend and flourish throughout Chinese territory.

*Sculpture.* The art objects of the Han period which have come down to us through the ages or have been recovered by archaeological excavation are not those with which the Chinese of Han times normally surrounded themselves. They consist almost exclusively of objects which were produced, in accordance with ancient tradition, to placate the spirits of the ancestors. Practically all known Han art is directly connected with the well-cared-for tomb which every important personage had built for himself or his relatives. Because they were despoiled by grave robbers, we have no knowledge of the contents and furnishings of the tumuli of the old emperors and their families, though the possibility cannot be excluded that an intact tomb may some day come to light. However, the tombs of less illustrious personages have in some cases been preserved complete, and these give us an extremely vivid picture of the funerary art of the Han period.

The sculptures which have been preserved may be divided into three groups. First, there are the stone sculptures representing men and animals, often of large size, which were ranged along the so-called "Spirit Road" (Shên-tao) that led up to the burial mound. Secondly, there are the much smaller funerary sculptures (*ming-ch'i*) consisting of human and animal figurines, models of houses, carts, ships, etc., which were placed in the grave to be used by the spirit of the deceased. Then, lastly, there are the bas-reliefs which decorate the walls of the burial chambers or of offering temples near the mound. Monumental sculpture in the round, which seems to have vanished after the time of the Shang rulers of An-yang, came into prominence again during the Han period after a disappearance of about one thousand years.

One of the few monuments which can be attributed with reasonable certainty to the first half of the Han period is a tomb at Hsing-p'ing (see CHINA, *Shensi*), which is generally accepted as the resting-place of the famous General Ho Ch'ü-p'ing, who died in 117 B.C. This attribution is strengthened by the discovery in 1957 of two inscriptions, one of which shows that the tomb was built on official order. The monument consists of a mound around which are placed a number of large stone sculptures. Some of these sculptures are little more than very superficially carved boulders; others may be regarded as real sculptures in the round. The sculpture that was first discovered and is also the best of the group represents a horse trampling on a fallen warrior, a subject well in keeping with the career of the general who is believed to lie buried here. Though it is evident that the artist was not entirely at home in his craft, and the shape and proportions are somewhat clumsy, an impressive and monumental sculptural effect is achieved, whereas in the other sculptures, the artist almost invariably failed to free himself from the shape of the stone. A number of the sculptures are nothing more than bas-relief imposed on the natural form of the stone block; however, the more familiar bas-relief technique produced results that are surprisingly vivid. Some experts have attributed this sudden appearance of monumental stone sculpture and the practice of placing figures near tombs to a tradition imported from western Asia, which would also explain the limited experience of the artist in this medium. Though such an explanation is certainly possible, these sculptures (unlike the later winged lions) are so obviously Chinese, and some of them, particularly the horses, are so obviously related to finds in tombs of the late Chou period, that it seems inadvisable at present to accept the hypothesis. The information published about a new find in 1957 shows that the Ho Ch'ü-p'ing tomb was not a unique monument. In the vicinity of Hsien-yang, also in Shensi province, a similar summarily carved boulder has been found which is now generally accepted as belonging to the Western Han period.

The number of sculptures which have survived from the Eastern Han period is considerably larger. Nearly all are to be found in two provinces remote from each other, Szechwan in the west and Shantung in the east (see CHINA). Most of the sculptures which can be dated fairly accurately belong to the 2d century, though there are indications that some may date from the first century. (We may therefore assume that the tradition exemplified by the Ho Ch'ü-p'ing monument continued without interruption until the appearance of these monuments of the 2d century.) No clear evolutionary trend can be observed in the earliest dated monuments. The rigid ceremonial figures at the temple of Chung-yüeh-miao in Têng-fêng (Honan province) and at the tomb of a king of Lu near Ch'ü-fu (Shantung), dating back to about 118 and 146–56 respectively, are all somewhat primitive in execution. They are only roughly hewn stone pillars, more massive than beautiful, but their rigidity may have been deliberate and not entirely due to lack of skill. The wooden figures found in and around Ch'ang-sha have the same rigidity, which is not found in any other funerary object of the period. It has been suggested that these figures follow a special "ancestral" style for purely religious reasons apart from artistic considerations.

In this connection it is most unfortunate that the stone animal figures which are said to have been erected at the tomb of the king of Lu have all disappeared. The animal sculptures which, if the suggested dates are correct, were made only a short time after the sculptures of Têng-fêng and Ch'ü-fu already have a much freer and more lively style. This is true not so much of the large stone lions of the Wu Liang-tz'ŭ (see CHINA, *Shantung*), which probably date back to 147, as of the lion in the Museo Nazionale d'Arte Orientale in Rome, which is usually thought to date from about the same time. The monumental sculptures of a winged, horned, and tigerlike mythical creature, sometimes called a "chimera" (PL. 241), show to what extent the Han monumental sculpture had developed in the later days of the dynasty. The sculptor seems to have hesitated, when depicting this mythical animal (which was probably of foreign origin) between a naturalistic method of flexible lines and the stylized linear forms so characteristic of Han art.

Besides this type of stone sculpture, about ten examples of which are to be found in Szechwan, we have a different type of tomb monument in the stone pillar shaped like a watchtower which marked the point where the "Spirit Road" crossed the fence around the burial mounds. Since the finest and architecturally most advanced specimens are in Szechwan province, some experts have thought that these pillars may have been imported along the route from India into Szechwan. However, these are not real architectural structures and may be a very free imitation in stone of wooden architecture. The fundamental form of the watchtower, as known from models found in graves and representations on tiles, has been maintained; we can recognize on the rectangular shaft the beams and brackets that support the hipped roof, and the roof tiles are carefully imitated in stone. A sculptured frieze has been added, however, which suggests to some experts a comparison with Persian architecture, though it may have been a purely decorative addition. The pillars of Shên in the Ch'u-hsien area (probably 2d cent.) have rectangular shafts decorated with beautiful bas-reliefs, including some of animals which represent the points of the compass. The monster's head pushing between the lowest beam ends and the Atlantean figures on the four corners of these pillars are in high relief. Whereas the bas-relief work marks a transition between rigidly stylized forms and a free and lively naturalism, the embellishments in high relief had already developed further in the direction of naturalism.

However, we are better able to study the naturalism of the Han period in the many examples of funerary sculpture that have come down to us. We are tempted to neglect this abundance of Han funerary statuary because of its almost childlike

and anecdotal character when compared with the imposing sculpture in stone. It owes a special charm, however, to the fact that the tradition of providing the dead with familiar surroundings was still living and meaningful. The figurines (PL. 172; IV, PL. 460) of men and animals, the models of houses and rice fields, the boats and vehicles are of interest not merely because of the information they provide (on everyday life, on architecture, on ship building, etc.), but also because of their unprecedented realism and exuberance. Although the wooden models of earlier centuries still occur in the Han period, it had become general practice to make funerary figurines and models of clay. The gray and reddish pottery was sometimes covered with a green lead glaze characteristic of this period, and in many cases the figures were painted over a thin coating of slip. The hands often have two holes in which it is thought that wooden objects were held, though no such objects have so far been found. The difference between the figurines which were individually modeled and those produced by molds (which is so striking later in the T'ang period) is, judging by what has been found so far, less pronounced in the Han dynasty. There can be no doubt that many of the human and animal figurines found in the Han tombs were mass-produced, for large numbers of identical specimens are known to exist. The stylized forms of these figures were perhaps specially designed for easy mass production. The great degree of uniformity observed in many collections, however, is to be attributed only partly to mass production. It is also due to the fact that most of the figures have come from the same area, namely, from around the old capitals of northern China. In the provinces of Szechwan and Kwangtung new types, hitherto practically unknown, have now been found. In Kwangtung, special local characteristics were derived from population groups which were not Chinese and had not yet been assimilated. The models of houses are different from those usually encountered, because they reproduce dwelling types that were adapted to the local climate. The tomb figurines from Szechwan represent a style which can hold its own with, and is quite different from, that of the central and northern provinces. (This phenomenon is also to be observed in other branches of Han art, for example in monumental sculpture.) Among the most striking finds that have been made since World War II are a pottery horse and chariot, about 3 ft. high, found in a tomb near Chengtu, and a stone sculpture representing a man on horseback, about $2\frac{1}{2}$ ft. high, discovered in 1957 and believed to date back to 182. In this case the potter, using a far more workable medium, has left the stone sculptor far behind him.

The human figure in the funerary sculptures of Szechwan is very different from that of the central and northern provinces; the faces are flatter and less expressive, but there is sometimes an ease and grace not found again until the T'ang period. It is possible that a number of these figures are of later date, and that the Han style continued in Szechwan after it had been replaced in northern China by the Wei style.

As far back as the Sung period Chinese antiquaries discovered the bas-relief sculpture of the Han period, which has also received much attention in Western works on Han art. These reliefs, too, are mainly found in the provinces of Szechwan and Shantung; recent finds made in Kiangsu, north of the Huai River, and in Shensi, cannot compare in importance with those of the other two regions. They also have their origin in the tradition of veneration for the dead. Sometimes carved directly out of the rock face or on flat stone slabs, they serve as decorations for a burial chamber or sacrificial chamber.

The reliefs from Shantung province have been found mainly in small shrines built of heavy stone slabs and situated close to the grave mound. Since World War II a number of finds have shown that in Shantung the tombs themselves were likewise often decorated with reliefs. Most of the monuments that have been preserved belong to the 1st or 2d century. The earliest datable monument is the shrine near the grave of General Chu Wei, which was built about A.D. 50, but which has lost much of its artistic value as the result of later recarving. The only intact offering shrine, one which now stands sheltered beneath a temple on Hsiao-t'ang-shan in Shantung, is of a slightly later date. It bears an inscription made by a visitor in 129 and must therefore have been built before that time.

On Liang-ch'êng-shan in Shantung, a number of scattered slabs with reliefs have been found, one of which (PL. 232), now in the Rietberg Museum in Zurich, is dated 114. A tomb of great importance was discovered a few years ago at Yi-nan, in which some fifty decorated stone slabs were found, though there has been much controversy about the date. Some Chinese experts place this monument between 220 and 313, but most authorities regard it as belonging to the Han period. A monument that has been known for many centuries is the shrine of the Wu family near Chia-hsiang in Shantung, known as the "Wu Liang-tz'ŭ" (see below).

A large number of stone reliefs have been found in the neighborhood of Chia-hsiang. Wilma Fairbank has shown that these reliefs, now housed in a special building, belonged to three offering shrines built near the tombs of the Wu family, the earliest probably in 147 and the last in 168. Apart from these monuments, there are many others of lesser importance.

The monuments with bas-reliefs in Szechwan must have been made at about the same time as those of Shantung. The inscriptions show that here too this art flourished during the 2d century; however, the reliefs are not found in chambers made of stone slabs or in offering shrines, but in tombs dug out of the red sandstone on the mountain faces. The numerous cave tombs found along the Kialing and Min Rivers are of two kinds. In the neighborhood of the city of Loshan (Chia-ting) the tombs lie at the end of a horizontal shaft penetrating deep into the rock. The approach to this shaft is through an entrance hall, also hewn out of the rock and probably corresponding to the offering shrines of Shantung, and it is in this entrance hall that the bas-reliefs are found. In the neighborhood of Hsin-chin, however, the tombs are constructed without an entrance hall, and the reliefs are carved on a heavy stone coffin, resembling a sarcophagus, which lies in the funeral chamber, but probably was not meant to contain the remains of the dead. The execution of these reliefs may vary a great deal according to the locality. The outlines of the subject may be engraved on the slabs of stone which have been rubbed smooth, or they may be in intaglio throughout, so that they stand out against a plain background. In other cases the scenes are rendered in very low relief against a striated background. Or again, in some pieces the figures have been left untouched and their outlines hatched in.

The subjects, which vary considerably and give us a striking picture of the complexity and richness of the Han culture, may be divided into three groups: everyday life with its occupations and amusements; the historic past, often idealized and treated as a subject for moral edification; and Chinese folklore and popular beliefs. The subjects based on everyday life provide invaluable information on the history and material culture of the period. Processions of horses and chariots, often with canopies, and hunting scenes are very common. The innumerable figures provide a great deal of information on dress, military garb, and weapons.

Everyday life is reproduced in an even more lively and sometimes more artistic manner in the tiles that were sometimes used to decorate funeral chambers. In Szechwan particularly beautiful specimens of such tiles are found, although fine pieces have also come to light in Honan, as a publication of W.C. White reveals. In Honan the ornamentation was stamped into the clay, but in Szechwan the tiles were made in molds, so that the ornamentation stands out in low relief. The examples published by Richard Rudolph and Wen Yu, which were not mass-produced like the more ordinary tiles, are among the finest. In all Han art, there is little that can compare with these tiles in liveliness and realism (PL. 231). The lines with which the artist suggests the swift movements of dancers, acrobats, and hunters, the frenzied tension of the gambler, and the disciplined concentration of the archer show a wonderful strength and control which we see again only on rare occasions at a much later stage in Chinese pictorial art.

The second group of subjects, dealing with historical events, reflects the Confucian moralizing trend predominant at the

time. It is noteworthy that there was a clearly demonstrable connection between the written and the pictorial edifying story, as E. Chavannes has shown. The "Gallery of Famous Women" (*Lieh-nü-chuan*), written by the author and critic Li Hsiang (79–78 B.C.), and the parallel work, "Gallery of Devoted Sons," and even the famous chapter in the "Historical Memoirs" (*Shih-chi*) by Ssŭ-ma Ch'ien (135–87 B.C.) dealing with well-known murders, have all been depicted in stone bas-reliefs. Obviously both literature and art were likely to reproduce the stories that were current at the time, but the very close relationship between the art and literature of this period is nonetheless remarkable. A striking description of a battle fought between the Chinese and the Huns (Hsiung-nu) of Central Asia, which has come down to us in the official chronicle of the Western Han period (*Ch'ien Han-shu*) is based on a picture of the event available to the chronicler, a stone-carved version of which may be seen among the reliefs on Hsiao-t'ang-shan. A favorite historical subject is that of the attempt on the life of China's first emperor Shih Huang-ti (227 B.C.), whose memory was execrated by the Confucianists of the Han period because he caused all classical books to be burned. This episode is depicted both in Shantung and in Szechwan bas-reliefs. One of the Szechwan versions of the event corresponds so closely to that shown in the Wu Liang-tz'ŭ reliefs that Rudolph thinks they must have had a common prototype. Slight differences between the versions depicted on various tiles correspond in a remarkable manner to the differences between the various known texts relating this incident. As might be expected, the artists often preferred the more dramatic or exaggerated version of the event. The dagger thrown by the assassin Ching K'o at the fleeing emperor is thus made to pierce a bronze pillar in his palace instead of merely grazing against it.

In contrast to the subjects with a strong moral and Confucian tendency, we have a whole group of fantastic, mythological, and supernatural themes centering around legendary emperors. Gods of the wind and the rain and Hsi-wang-mu, the Queen of the West, who became so familiar a figure in later times, appear on the scene for the first time. It is evident that Confucianism (q.v.), the philosophy of the Han intellectual elite, was unable to oust an entirely different tendency which was strongly influenced by Taoism (q.v.).

Though the Szechwan tiles may mark the peak of artistic achievement in this form, in general the Shantung reliefs far surpass those of Szechwan, particularly in composition. Whereas the latter mostly represent only one scene, the slabs of Shantung are covered from top to bottom with rows of different scenes, separated by plain bands. The reliefs of Hsiao-t'ang-shan still belong to a relatively early stage, whereas those of Wu Liang-tz'ŭ (see CHINA, *Shantung*) have clearly reached a peak of artistic development. The great reputation these reliefs have acquired, as a result of widely circulated rubbings (PL. 233) and of the works of such experts as Chavannes, has, however, led to the belief that they represent the dominant style of the period. In reality, in the reliefs of the Yi-nan tomb, which probably are somewhat later, the delicate hatching which frames the flat figures and their far more dynamic execution are just as characteristic.

*Painting.* Excavations carried out in that region of Manchuria which formed a part of the Chinese empire during the Han period, and an occasional discovery in the territory of China proper, have now given us some direct knowledge of Han painting. Just as there was some analogy between bas-reliefs and literature, so was there between these reliefs and painting. Here, again, our knowledge is based on tomb monuments, though many passages in the literature of the Han period show that the walls of imperial palaces and the houses of persons of high rank were adorned with paintings.

In 1952 a tomb of the Han period was discovered in the neighborhood of Wang-tu in Hopei province (q.v., CHINA) in which a number of wall paintings had been preserved. In this tomb the wall is divided by a horizontal line into two parts, a lower part which has paintings of animals and birds, and an upper part which has 24 full-length portraits of persons whose ranks are stated in the accompanying inscriptions. They are not persons holding high office, but mostly petty officials. It is as if the antechamber was regarded as the office of the deceased in the life hereafter, where, rather than in the actual tomb chamber, he would be surrounded by the constables, bailiffs, and clerks who had served him when he was the local representative of authority on earth. The paintings were executed on whitewashed brick walls, the surface of which had not been smoothed. The outlines first were done in black, after which the surfaces were painted in with red, yellow, and green mineral paints. In connection with the themes represented, it may be noted that (according to the *Ch'ien Han-shu*) in 51 B.C. the emperor Hsüan-ti ordered paintings to be made in one of the halls of his palace, depicting 11 ministers and generals who had rendered great services to the Han dynasty; some decades later the poet Yang Hsiung was ordered to provide one of these portraits with eulogies. It is quite possible that in this remote part of the empire a local official should have been inspired by such an example to have his tomb decorated with murals depicting his own faithful retainers. The fact that the portraits of his subordinates are strikingly individualized suggests that such painting had not yet become stereotyped.

Two of the tombs discovered in Manchuria should be noted: that of Ying-ch'êng-tzŭ at the southern extremity of the Liaotung Peninsula, and that of Pei-yüan, near Liao-yang (see CHINA, *Manchuria*). In the first of these, under the pointed arched vault of the central chamber is a smaller chamber of the same shape and construction, on the walls of which are some highly interesting paintings. The mural on the northern side, i.e., the side associated with the realm of the dead, is of great iconographic importance, since its subject, known from other mural paintings and stone reliefs, is that of the relations between the living, on the one hand, and the dead or supernatural beings, on the other. In the foreground three figures hold a ceremonial tablet, one standing, another kneeling, and a third prostrating himself before a sacrificial table, on which is a round box or vessel between three small-eared cups of a well-known Han type. Directly above this, a dignitary with a sword stands on a small cloud, attended by a servant and in conversation with an old man. It is to be supposed that this latter scene is taking place in a higher supernatural sphere, for the chief figure is standing on a stylized cloud, and around the figures are stylized cloud motifs, a bird, a feathered ghost, and a dragon, all closely resembling similar representations on lacquer, mirrors, and bas-reliefs of the Han period. It seems reasonable to assume that the painting depicts a sacrifice made to the dead (perhaps to the dignitary with the sword). The three men offering the sacrifice may represent three generations of descendants, or may depict one man during three different stages of the ceremony. The latter interpretation seems the more likely one, for in the stone reliefs we find often a chronological succession of events combined into a single picture. Though the painting is somewhat primitive and provincial, as might be expected in view of the location, the treatment of the subject is most extraordinary.

The tomb of Pei-yüan differs completely from that of Ying-ch'êng-tzŭ. It is constructed entirely of stone slabs, used not only for the walls, but also for the ceiling and the supports. On some of the plastered walls murals have been painted. Some of the subjects are already familiar to us, for example, processions of horses and chariots (in which we note attempts to experiment with perspective and to achieve spatial effects), meetings with the ghosts of ancestors, and performances by acrobats. Whereas in the Ying-ch'êng-tzŭ paintings there is an almost entire absence of color, those in the Pei-yüan tomb are polychrome. The Japanese experts who discovered the tombs consider them to have been built between the 1st and 3d century. Stylistically the murals of Pei-yüan are the forerunners of a group painted in the 4th and 5th centuries in the tombs of the kingdom of Koguryo, on the Chinese–north Korean frontier and thus even farther removed from the heart of Chinese culture. (See KOREA; KOREAN ART.)

Our knowledge of painting in the capital and in areas closer to the main stream of Chinese culture is even more fragmentary.

The painted tiles in the Boston Museum of Fine Arts (PL. 234), which are believed to have come from Honan, resemble the murals of Ying-ch'êng-tzǔ in some respects, but represent a much higher artistic level. The free and flowing lines of these paintings, in which the first traces of something resembling a calligraphic technique are already discernible, the diversity of facial expressions and of posture, and the tendency to paint figures in well-composed and natural groups are all unmistakable signs of an art that has evolved beyond the purely decorative stage. As for the subject matter, we find, in addition to typical genre paintings, others which have as their theme the Confucian doctrines and legends.

*Mirrors.* About the end of the 2d century B.C., during the reign of the emperor Han Wu-ti (140–87 B.C.), new types of ornamentation began to be applied also on the bronze mirrors, which by this time had lost all traces of the Chou style. The backs of the mirrors were now covered with decorative elements grouped with mathematical precision around a large knob which developed out of the former pierced eye provided for the cord. This characteristic decoration, seen for the first time in the mirrors classified by Karlgren as the F type (2d cent. B.C.), was gradually refined until it reached its highest point in the first half of the 1st century B.C Besides the first appearance of inscriptions, the most striking feature in this ornamentation comprises concave bands in the form of the letters T, L, and V, known as the "TLV" pattern. The types showing this pattern, which has a number of variations, generally have a heavy central boss in the middle of a four-petal pointed rosette, which in turn forms the center of a square of concave bands. Along the inner edge of this square are 12 protruding round studs separating the characters of the Chinese zodiac. From the middle of each side of the square, more concave bands extend outward in the shape of the letter T. These are flanked on each side with rosettes. Directly opposite the corners of the square the concave bands form a V shape, and directly opposite the T's an L shape. The V's and L's reach to the first of a series of concentric bands which frame the entire design. One of the bands bears an inscription, while the others are hatched, or have a serrated or stylized cloud pattern. On the surface bounded by the square and the circular rims, within which occur the T, L, and V patterns, there are also representations in thread-relief of the Black Tortoise, the Scarlet Bird, the Blue Dragon, and the White Tiger, i.e., the symbols of the north, south, east, and west. The exceptional precision of these designs and the systematic way in which they are arranged reflect the fact that, as the inscriptions reveal, magic powers were attributed to them. There can be no doubt that these mirrors and perhaps other types, too, have a definite connection with Han astronomical and cosmological lore. W. P. Yetts sees a connection between them and sundials, while Schuyler Camman regards the pattern as a cosmic symbol.

Toward the end of the Han period, the White Tiger and the Blue Dragon on the mirrors were replaced by the legendary figures of Hsi-wang-mu, the Mother Queen of the West, and Tung-wang-kung, the Father King of the East, deities much venerated in Taoism (q.v.). This change marks the beginning of a new style of mirror which reached its full development during the period of the Six Dynasties.

*Bronzes.* With the coming of the Han Dynasty and the social and religious changes that accompanied it, the remarkable ornamental styles of the bronzes, which for many centuries had played a dominant part in Chinese art, practically disappeared, with the exception of the painted ornamentation sometimes found, for example, on the inside of the lids of gilt-bronze caskets of the *lien* type, and the ever-present *t'ao-t'ieh* masks. There is a considerable variety of forms, including cylindrical caskets of the *lien* type, with three legs shaped like bears, vases reminiscent of the *hu* of the late Chou period, and lamps shaped like a ram or with a stand in the shape of a goose's foot (*yen-tsu-têng*). The cylindrical caskets and the incense burners, the bottom part of which is reminiscent of the *tou* of Chou bronze art, sometimes have a lid in the form of weirdly shaped mountain peaks, which some consider to represent P'êng-lai-shan, the Island of the Immortals in Taoist mythology (see ESCHATOLOGY), while others see in them a representation of the Chinese conception of the world — a central mountain surrounded by peaks marking the four cardinal points.

*Ceramics.* There is a striking similarity between the Han ceramic and bronze forms, particularly in the case of the *lien* and the *hu*. The soft gray or brick-red pottery is nearly always covered either by a lead glaze occurring in many shades of green (PL. 165; II, PL. 14) or a coating of slip which has been painted over in unfired colors (PL. 231). A steadily increasing number of vases bear inscriptions, so that it is often possible to date them accurately. (See CERAMICS.)

*Lacquer.* The Han styles of lacquer work were undoubtedly strongly affected by the lacquer art of the Ch'u state, as is evident by comparison with the finds made at Ch'ang-sha, the capital of Ch'u in the late Chou period. Many of the Han lacquer pieces found by Russian and Japanese expeditions on the outer fringes of China have inscriptions which make it possible to date them fairly accurately, as well as to determine their place of origin in relation to their technical characteristics. A considerable proportion of them come from two imperial factories in Szechwan. These include oval cups with two handles, many rectangular and cylindrical caskets, and deep bowls of different shapes and sizes. The decoration, in red, yellow, green, and blue, consists of a great variety of patterns, the most important of which is the "cloud scroll," a pattern of strangely curving lines from which emerge the limbs and heads of birds and animals. This design, with its rhythmic movements repeated in endless variations, gives Han lacquer its characteristic archaic and dynamic quality. But we also find, as in other Han art, the representation of morally edifying historical figures and scenes based on the teachings of Confucius. An example of such lacquer painting may be seen on the celebrated basket found in the Tomb of the Painted Basket in Lo-lang (a Chinese colony in Korea, q.v.), which dates from the 1st century. The figures, placed within a narrow frieze framed with geometric patterns, are nearly all seated and can be identified by the names written beside them. The faces of old and young are clearly differentiated, but impersonal in other respects, in contrast to the individualized portraits in the wall paintings at Wang-tu (see above), which date from about the same period. (See LACQUER.)

THE PERIOD OF THE SIX DYNASTIES (A.D. 220–589). The period between the fall of the Han dynasty and the unification of China again under a Chinese dynasty (the Sui, see below) is generally known as the period of "the Three Kingdoms and the Six Dynasties," although the number of states and ruling houses which existed for more or less brief periods of time was much greater than this title indicates. The period of the Three Kingdoms or San Kuo (220–77) derives its name from the three states which contended for supremacy: Wei in northern China, Shu in western China, and Wu in southeast China. Wei eventually prevailed, and for a while China was reunited under the dynastic name of Chin. But with the advent of the 3d century a new danger appeared in the shape of the "northern barbarians." Various Turkish, Mongolian, and Tungusic peoples took advantage of the weakness of the Chin dynasty, drove the Chin rulers southward at the beginning of the 4th century, and occupied parts of northern China. The numerical weakness of these people was more than compensated for by the boldness and rapidity of their tactics. Their rule was political and military only. The language, the customs, and the economic and social structure remained largely unchanged, whereas the conquerors tended after a few generations to merge with the Chinese. During the 4th and 5th centuries more than a dozen foreign dynasties held sway in the north of China. In the end, the Northern Wei or T'o-pa (Toba) dynasty (386–535) gained the upper hand throughout the north. Southern China, which had Nanking as its center, was ruled, after the collapse of the Eastern Chin in 420, by four successive

dynasties: the Liu Sung (420–79), the Southern Ch'i (479–502), the Liang (502–57), and the Ch'ên (557–89). In 535 the Northern Wei dynasty split up into the Eastern and Western Wei, but the territories ruled by them were soon divided between two new dynasties, the Northern Ch'i (550–77) in the east, and the Northern Chou (557–81) in the west. Finally, the first sovereign of the Sui dynasty succeeded in reuniting the whole of China under one rule.

With all this confusion of wars, political discord, and palace revolutions, the great religious, cultural, and social changes that took place tend to be relegated to the background. However, the literary and artistic treasures that remain from this chaotic period show how great an importance it had for the enduring culture of China, an importance fundamentally far greater than that of the dynastic changes.

*Early Buddhist art.* During the 1st century Buddhism (q.v.), advancing along the great caravan routes of Central Asia, had gradually moved eastward until it had penetrated China. It reached China also by sea from the south and, according to some authors, along the trade route from India which ended in Yunnan and Szechwan. At an early date, foreign missionaries began to translate the Buddhist scriptures into Chinese. During the 2d century a number of small Buddhist communities sprang up in various parts of China, though a considerable span of time was yet to pass before Buddhism was to play an important role. The collapse of the Han empire and the bloody struggles that ensued damaged the prestige of Confucianism, and the wretched plight of the people made them turn, at first, to neo-Taoism. After the conquest of northern China by the Hsiung-nu (316) and the flight of the Chin dynasty to Nanking, the political and social changes cleared the way for a great dissemination of Buddhism. The greatest advance was made during the Wei dynasty. In the south, because Buddhism became prevalent gradually, and perhaps also because there were fewer foreign missionaries, Buddhism became more strongly Chinese in character than was the case in any other part of the land.

The few examples of Buddhist art which are known to date from the time when Buddhism began its expansion in China are already Chinese in appearance or show a Chinese influence. In view of the high level already achieved by Chinese sculpture and painting, the esthetic and stylistic ideas as well as the traditions which Buddhism brought to China were bound to undergo a transmutation. The classicism of the Han period, which had made the Chinese conscious of their ancient traditions, played an important part in this process. Both in doctrine and in art, Indian Buddhism had to adapt itself to Chinese tastes and ideas, although the descriptions of buddhas and bodhisattvas given in Buddhist texts provided a certain guarantee of iconographic conformity. It must also be remembered that only on the rarest occasions could a Chinese artist see the monuments of Indian Buddhist art with his own eyes; except for easily transportable pictures and small sculptures, he had to make do with the descriptions of returning pilgrims and of missionaries, who were usually acquainted only with the art of a particular region. The preference of each Buddhist sect for some special figure from the Buddhist pantheon, the nature of the local population, and the materials locally available are only a few of the factors which led to the great variety of Buddhist art in China. As long as Buddhism remained a living religion in India, Indian Buddhist art exerted a strong influence on that of China, but it is difficult to define exactly how that influence was exerted or to determine along what routes and at what time the various iconographic and stylistic elements reached China. Our knowledge is, moreover, limited by the fact that many of the ancient Buddhist monuments, including all those in southern China, have been destroyed, and we have to rely in many cases solely on literary records.

The earliest Buddhist art found in China consists of representations of Buddha, apsarases, and (somewhat later) Buddhist trinities on the backs of Chinese mirrors of the 3d and 4th centuries. Until that time the figures on such mirrors had been Taoist, and the Buddhist figures have a Taoist air about them. Some of these mirrors have been discovered in Japan, where they must have been imported at an early date. The earliest known Chinese gilt-bronze statuette of the Buddha (Brundage Coll., Chicago) bears a date corresponding to 338 and comes from a small state set up in what is now Hopei under Hsiung-nu rule. It is strongly reminiscent of the Gandhara (q.v.) style, but is clearly different in some respects; particularly, the folds of the robe are not arranged in easy flowing lines, but form, on the contrary, a rigidly symmetrical pattern. The number of dated gilt-bronze pieces of the 4th century is very small, and the authenticity of some of the inscriptions has been contested. The number of 5th-century pieces is larger. A list of 55 images (16 in stone), dating from 390 to 501, was published by B. Rowland in 1937. These images are still rather primitive, and their iconographic repertory remains very limited. A Chinese innovation would seem to be the leaf-shaped mandorla with the flaming edge.

During the 5th and early 6th centuries, cave temples were built throughout northern China from the farthest west (Tun-huang) to Manchuria (Yi-hsien) in the east. The Wei rulers are often said to have built the first of these temples, but the oldest ones preceded the Wei period; built in Kansu in the west, they were modeled on the cave temples found along the caravan routes of Central Asia (see CHINA, *Sinkiang*). Owing to the sandy nature of the stone in that region and frequent earthquakes, the earliest cave temples have all disappeared. According to literary sources, however, the first is said to have been built in Tun-huang in 366. The first cave temples that can be accurately dated by inscriptions belong to the early years of the 6th century.

During the Northern Liang dynasty (prior to 439) work was begun in Kansu on the recently rediscovered caves of Wen-shu-shan, now almost entirely in ruins, where two pillars inscribed with *sūtra*s and dated 429 and 434 were found. The T'ien-t'i-shan group, which is also in ruins, probably dates back to about the same time, while the Ping-ling-ssŭ complex must already have been quite extensive at the beginning of the 6th century, if we are to believe the historical records. The earliest date established in the Mai-chi-shan group is 502, but here too the first construction must be earlier. (See these sites under CHINA, *Kansu.*) After the Wei rulers had subjugated the Northern Liang in 439, they appear to have moved a large number of craftsmen to their capital at Tatung, in Shansi province, and it is possible that this mass transfer of craftsmen was connected with the building of the Yün-kang caves.

The architecture of the earliest caves follows Central Asian models and clearly reveals its Indian origins (see BUDDHIST PRIMITIVE SCHOOLS; INDIAN ART). The Indian vihara and chaitya, which are themselves derived from earlier forms of architecture in wood, are clearly recognizable. The central pillar carved out of the rock in the Chinese cave temple is an imitation of the apsidal stupa in the Indian chaityas, while the horseshoe arch of the entrance to the cave and the lantern roof are also obviously inspired by Indian architecture.

The first series of caves at Yün-kang, XVI-XX (see CHINA, *Shansi*), which were begun at the instigation of the priest T'an-yao in 460 under the patronage of the Wei sovereigns, are particularly reminiscent of the sculptures at Bamian (see AFGHANISTAN). Through the windows and doorways hewn out of the rock wall the sculptors hacked their way into the stone and carved out gigantic images of Buddha, which, as at Bamian, the hollowed-out caves seem scarcely able to contain (PL. 245). Caves continued to be made at Yün-kang far into the 6th century, but the peak of activity had already been reached at the time of the transfer of the Wei capital to Loyang in 494. The huge round-faced Buddhas of Yün-kang (II, PL. 382), with their sharp-cut features and clearly delineated drapery folds, may owe their strongly linear treatment partly to the fact that they had to be distinguishable in the semidarkness of the caves. The treatment of the draperies is neither that of Gandhara nor that of the Gupta school (qq.v.), at that time already flourishing in India, but seems based on Central Asian models from Kizil or thereabouts (see ASIA, CENTRAL).

The ornamental designs around the doors, windows, and niches are still somewhat reminiscent of the so-called Greco-Buddhist art. The impressive sculptures represent a hybrid form of art, as yet only partially Sinicized; nevertheless, in caves V and VI (PL. 240), the first symptoms of a new trend (destined to reach its full development at Lung-mên) are already visible. The face is slimmer, while the drapery folds, concealing the lines of the body, spread out in straight lines to a beautifully arranged border of pleated folds and points, treated in a purely linear manner. The use of flatter and slimmer lines gives the Chinese Buddha image an entirely new appearance. It shows that the example of other Buddhist centers is not being followed and symbolizes the Sinification of Buddhism.

After 494, Lung-mên, in Honan province, replaced Yün-kang as the imperial center of Buddhist art. (For fuller description, see CHINA, Honan.). It was only to be expected that the flat treatment of the smaller sculptures at Lung-mên (PL. 255) would lead to a revival of bas-relief sculpture. The confirmation of this expectation is provided in the relief showing the processions with the emperor and empress in the Pin-yang cave at Lung-mên (first quarter of 6th cent.), in which both the movement of the group and the individual figures are very effectively handled. If these scenes are compared with those from the life of the Buddha in Cave VI at Yün-kang (PL. 240), which are only a few decades older, it becomes clear how rapid was the advance from the experimental stage to full mastery of the art of bas-relief.

From the beginning of the 6th century it is possible to follow the stylistic evolution of Chinese sculpture step by step for several centuries from dated stone and gilt-bronze sculptures. A gilt-bronze shrine of the Buddha and Prabhū-taratna (Peytel Coll., Musée Guimet, Paris) is an example of the first Buddhist style in China at its highest level. The robes falling in rigid folds like ornamental draperies on a throne and ending in points, the fine hands and feet, the soft features, and the beautiful leaf-shaped mandorlas edged by flames, with halos in the form of a lotus flower surrounded by concentric circles, are all characteristic of this style. The inscription establishing the date of this shrine as 518 is now illegible.

The first stage in the Buddhist sculpture of China (PL. 242), called the "archaic" period by Sirén, represents the period of transformation of a foreign into a Chinese art form (II, PLS. 389, 391). The extreme rapidity with which Buddhist art spread (large Buddhist monuments are to be found in Manchuria and Shantung as well as in the more central provinces by the first half of the 6th century) is undoubtedly one of the main reasons for its diversified character at this stage.

When the Northern Wei dynasty was split up in 535, artistic activity under imperial patronage was interrupted for a while, but a revival occurred when the Northern Chou and Ch'i dynasties gained supremacy in northern China shortly after the mid-6th century. Sirén has suggested that the period between the collapse of the Wei and the beginning of the T'ang dynasty should be known as the "transition" period, i.e., the period of transition from the "archaic" style of the Wei period to the mature style of the T'ang. The most representative works of the Northern Ch'i are the first caves of T'ien-lung-shan (PL. 256) and the two Hsiang-t'ang-shan groups of caves (PL. 243), while at least 11 of the caves at Mai-chi-shan (PL. 251) can be attributed to the Northern Chou (see CHINA, Shansi, Honan, and Kansu, respectively). Sculptural activity must have been concentrated mainly in the eastern part of the country, for sculptures of the Western Wei are much rarer than those of the Eastern Wei, and Northern Ch'i sculptures are much more numerous than works of the Northern Chou. The sculptures now tend to assume a greater plasticity; in some of the cave temples they are detached from the wall to become sculptures in the round. The noticeable differences between the Northern Chou style and that of the Northern Ch'i can be attributed to the influence of Indian Gupta sculpture, which acted as a strong new stimulus to the latter. This Indian influence is particularly noticeable in the caves of Hsiang-t'ang-shan, where the drapery folds cling to the body so as to reveal its forms. The round halos decorated with flowers

and the endless repertory of ornaments on the walls, pedestals, and pillars can be clearly traced to Indian or Sassanian forms.

It is difficult to say when this foreign influence reached its peak. In the earliest caves of T'ien-lung-shan (II and III) there are relatively few signs of it, and the groups of sculptures, each composed of a Buddha carved in high relief with a bodhi-sattva on either side in lower relief, seem to represent a somewhat archaistic style (PL. 256). All the Northern Ch'i caves have exceptionally fine ceilings in the form of a truncated pyramid decorated in low relief. The flat center has a lotus carved on it, around which, in the four trapezoid panels of the ceiling, apsarases and other celestial beings hover. Another interesting form of bas-relief work under the Northern Ch'i dynasty is that found on "funerary couches." Numerous fragments, minutely decorated as if they were ivory ornaments, reveal both in subjects and style the strong influence of the Middle East, from which the doctrine of Zoroaster penetrated into China at this time.

Two fine sculptures in the round found in the Northern Chou territory are the standing bodhisattva (Avalokiteśvara?) in the Eumorfopoulos Collection (Victoria and Albert Mus., London) and the standing Avalokiteśvara from Ch'ang-an in the Boston Museum of Fine Arts. Despite their common origin, these two statues are markedly different. The first one is devoid of the profusion of jewelry, including ropes of pearls, which covers and accentuates the forms of the other.

In the meantime, another school of Buddhist art was emerging in Hopei. This school made use of a white micaceous marble found in the neighborhood of Ting-chou and Paoting, an almost ideal material for the sculptor. The recent discovery of a large number of fragments of sculpture in the ruins of Hsiu-tê-ssŭ near Ch'ü-yang (see CHINA, Hopei) shows that this school was already in existence during the Eastern Wei period and had reached its maturity in the time of the Northern Ch'i. Apart from smaller sculptures and steles, monumental sculptures in the round have also been found in Hopei. There is a delicate smoothness and a flatness about the figures which contrasts with the rounded forms of the head. The drapery folds, which cling to the body, fall in subtle and gracefully flowing lines. A sculpture that should be noted is the enormous standing Amitābha in the British Museum in London, found in the neighborhood of Ting-chou. It bears a date corresponding to 585 and still has all the characteristics of the Northern Ch'i period.

Toward the end of the 6th century, a period of great though short-lived artistic activity took place in Shantung, a region which had until then played only a minor part in the production of Buddhist art. Several fine monuments such as those on T'o-shan, Yün-mên-shan, and Yü-han-shan were erected in rapid succession in this region (see CHINA, Shantung).

During this brief period, the Gupta elements seem to have been almost entirely absorbed, and the sculptures become more Chinese in appearance. Though the large Buddha and bodhi-sattva figures lose some of their grace, they acquire a greater dignity. The last traces of the "archaic smile," which since the Wei period had imparted an air of mystery to these sculptures, now disappear. The bodhisattvas are richly attired, with an abundance of ornaments, the most characteristic of which at this period is a richly adorned crown. The smaller figures, such as those of Yü-han-shan, have a certain opulent beauty and grace, in contrast to the large and stately Buddhas.

*Funerary sculpture.* It might have been expected that when Buddhism and with it the idea of reincarnation gained a firm foothold in China, the old Chinese tradition of equipping the funerary chambers with objects needed in the life beyond the grave would disappear. The contrary is the case, however, and this tradition persisted even during the centuries when Buddhist influence was at its strongest. Because of the lack of datable evidence no clear picture can be formed of the development of this funerary art between the Han and the Wei periods. Some of the funerary figures which archaeologists attribute to the Chin dynasty (3d cent.) are deceptively similar to those of the Han. The familiar Han objects reappear, for

## 503

CHINESE ART

example the cart drawn by an ox, figurines of dogs, farmyard animals and horses, and the martial figure of a man brandishing a lance (IV, PL. 460), perhaps an exorcist (*fang-hsiang*).

The objects of a somewhat later date found in Tomb M 229 near Jen-chia-k'ou (in the vicinity of Sian, Shensi), which is dated 519 and was discovered in 1955, are of special interest. On either side of the entrance to the vaulted funerary chamber stood, at the time of discovery, two figures of tomb guardians in military regalia, each having beside him a fabulous beast with sharp spines protruding from its back. Though devoid of artistic significance, these animals are important in that they clearly represent an intermediary stage, as it were, between the rhinoceros tomb guardian of the Han and Chin periods with the three-pointed protrusions on its back, and the monsters, the so-called "Earth Spirits," which guard the entrance to the T'ang tombs.

An entirely new kind of funerary figure appears during the Wei period. Notwithstanding the Buddhist religious zeal of this non-Chinese reigning house, many of the princes of the dynasty had their tombs furnished with numerous figurines in the ancient Chinese manner. The contents of two of these tombs, dated respectively 523 and 525 (the only dated tombs of artistic importance from this period), are now in the Royal Ontario Museum at Toronto. They show that although the Wei funerary sculptures may be derived to some extent from the Han sculptures, their treatment is very different. Among the animal figures the horse is the most important, as is to be expected under a dynasty of nomad origin. The type of horse is very different from that of the Han sculpture; it is here a graceful racing type with slender legs and a long neck, often with a wide saddlecloth and fine ornaments on the chest and hindquarters. The human figures are tall and slender and wear long robes, sometimes with a girdle fastened very high around the waist, and characteristic high hats. The soldiers have leather jerkins and wide trousers fixed with straps below the knees. All these strongly resemble the garments depicted on the stone reliefs of Lung-mên and evidently represent the normal T'o-pa clothing.

Judging by some forty statues and pieces of pottery found in 1955, in a tomb dated 559, near K'ung-p'o in the neighborhood of Taiyuan, in Shansi, a "transition style" is also to be found in the funerary wares. These objects have numerous features characteristic of the Wei period, but their execution already shows affinity with the subsequent Sui-T'ang style.

*Painting.* The changes in the art of painting during the period of the Six Dynasties are of great importance. To begin with, the artist emerged from anonymity and for the first time became an individual with a name and an identity. This fact, though it should not be overstressed, assumes special significance when viewed against the background of the ideas prevailing during that period. Another important development is the emergence of a new form of literature which discusses the merits of the artists and the criteria to be applied to the art of painting. This literature was preceded and influenced by critical works on poetry and calligraphy (q.v.). The most important of the early works on Chinese painting is the *Ku-hua p'in-lu* ("Ancient Chronicle of the Classification of Painters") of Hsieh Ho, written in the late 5th century, in which are set out the famous "Six Principles" of painting, which were to play such an important part in numerous later works on the subject. The interpretation of these principles has given rise to much discussion among the students of early Chinese painting. The picture we are able to form, with considerable difficulty, of the history of Chinese painting from the time when critical works on art begin to appear (second half of the 5th cent.) has in it numerous gaps. What is more, it is two-sided. On the one hand, literary sources provide us with the names of painters and controversial estimates of their work or unanimous praise of their genius, as well as numerous colorful anecdotes. On the other hand, the few paintings, often much restored or painted over and in poor condition, which have later been attributed to the famous masters mentioned inspire little confidence. Almost all of them are copies and it is often impossible to

decide at what period they were painted. Hsieh Ho's advice to painters to practice their art by copying the work of the old masters has often been followed and has made it possible to reconstruct to some extent the style of some of these masters with the help of authentic ancient copies. However, in such cases little of the true genius of the original comes through.

We have as a source of information numerous murals such as those from the Tun-huang cave temples (see below) and the tombs of the Koguryo kingdom (see KOREAN ART), but these are all works from the periphery of China and of definitely provincial origin. In the central provinces, where the great masters must have worked, practically nothing has been found so far except scenes engraved on stone, which tell us little about actual painting.

However, despite the great gaps and all the uncertainties and contradictions in the information at our disposal, a few works of art have been preserved of such great historical and in some cases artistic value that they deserve close study, if only as the only known examples of a great and ancient school.

One of the first and, according to nearly all accounts, the greatest of the ancient masters was Ku K'ai-chih (q.v.), who lived from about 345 to 405. Hsieh Ho, the first critic to mention him and the one who may be regarded as best qualified to give an opinion on his work, does not speak too highly of him. Hsieh Ho has been much reproached for this by subsequent critics. The few works which are traditionally attributed to Ku K'ai-chih, all of which are represented only by copies made at a considerably later date, differ so much from one another in execution and composition that it is impossible to form a clear idea of his style. (It should be noted here that the theme of a picture was an important criterion at a later period for determining its authorship, especially when a given theme was known to have been painted by a certain master.) The most famous of Ku K'ai-chih's paintings is represented by the great horizontal scroll (PL. 235) in the British Museum, entitled *Admonitions of the Instructress to the Court Ladies* (*Nü-shih-chên*). It consists of a series of scenes interspersed with the edifying verses which the scenes illlustrate. The work is remarkable for the delicacy and firmness of its brushwork, though the colors have largely been spoiled as a result of subsequent repainting. Significant details, for example the shading of the curtains of the canopied bed in the famous "bed scene," suggest that certain painting methods have been used that became current only in the T'ang period, a technical anachronism introduced in the copying. For this reason it is difficult to decide what importance must be attached to the most striking feature of these scenes — the extraordinary way in which the facial expressions have been captured and the emotional character of the situations has been recreated. The movement with which the emperor dismisses his concubine, in the seventh scene, clearly suggests the very human quality of the situation depicted, even without reference to the fine verses in defense of polygamy which have been illustrated here. Another painting attributed to Ku K'ai-chih illustrates a poem by Ts'ao Chih (3d cent.) entitled *The Nymph of the River Lo* (*Lo-shên-fu*), late copies of which, probably made during the Sung period, are in the Freer Gallery of Art in Washington and in the former Palace collection of Peking (now mainly in Formosa). Here we have a single scene set in a rustic landscape. A somewhat forced and anachronistic style emphasizes the impression, more so than in the case of the *Nü-shih-chên* scroll, that this work is a copy.

The only other great master of the period of the Six Dynasties whose name can be linked to a still existing painting is Chang Seng-yu, who painted at Nanking in the first half of the 6th century. One of the paintings attributed to him in the *Hsüan-ho-hua-p'u* (the catalogue of the imperial collection, early 12th cent.) is entitled *The Five Planets and Twenty-four Constellations*. An incomplete scroll on the same subject in the Osaka Municipal Museum in Japan (Abe Coll.) is widely attributed to this painter, although this attribution has been questioned since the earliest times by Chinese connoisseurs, and there is every reason to suppose that the scroll was, in fact, painted during the early T'ang period.

The outlines of the human and animal figures which symbolize the planets and constellations are carefully but unimaginatively drawn and do not reveal the hand of an artist of genius. The text, however, written in seal characters (see CALLIGRAPHY), has been highly praised by calligraphers of later generations.

The other important relics of the painting of this period are the wall and ceiling paintings in the caves of Tun-huang (PLS. 237, 238, 244; II, 390) and other cave temples in the province of Kansu (q.v. under CHINA). Despite the destruction by the frequent earthquakes which have afflicted this region, about twenty of the caves which were built during the Northern and Western Wei periods have survived. The walls are covered with a series of murals which constitute a unique monument of early Buddhist painting. The paintings were rendered in tempera — no fresco paintings appear in Tun-huang before the Yüan period — and the dulling of the strong colors through the ages has certainly not added to their beauty, but it is probable that the colors were never particularly subtle or refined even in their original state. The heavily outlined figures have a stiff and wooden appearance. The faces, the pointed folds of the garments, and the somewhat awkward posture of the figures, with feet wide apart, suggest Central Asian influences that were only partially assimilated. An interesting feature is the close connection, noticeable even in the earliest caves, between the murals and the sculptures. The main figure in a particular group, for example, may be either painted or sculptured in relief; where it is rendered in relief, the subsidiary figures and the halo and mandorla may be painted on the wall behind. The themes treated in the earliest caves cover only a rather limited range of subjects. In the principal groups the Buddhas and bodhisattvas are surrounded by long superimposed rows of seated Buddha figures, forming what is known as the "Thousand Buddha" theme (*ch'ien fo*) and filling a large part of the available wall space. Scenes from the *sūtras*, which became common in the later cave decoration, are here still rather scarce. Much more popular were themes taken from the Jātakas, i.e., stories of the Buddha in his earlier incarnations (see AJANTA; BUDDHISM). The successive scenes of these tales are depicted in horizontal panels having a common background of mountain scenery so arranged that each stage of the narrative has its own separate space. The order of these scenes is from left to right, a Central Asian convention which was soon abandoned in favor of the Chinese right-to-left order. Though the paintings in the oldest caves of Tun-huang may represent a primitive and still somewhat crude stage of Chinese Buddhist painting, the Chinese feeling for rhythm, movement, and fantasy is already sensed in the wall paintings of some of the earliest dated caves. Cave 285, for example, which dates from 538–39, has a ceiling decorated in an exceptionally lively manner with purely Chinese scenes drawn from Taoist legends. The well-known scenes depicting the conversion of the robbers are painted in a vivid manner which shows a new and freer approach on the part of the artist to his subject — a tangible proof that at this time Buddhist art was becoming increasingly Chinese in character. A subject which begins to appear conspicuously in Tun-huang shortly before the beginning of the Sui period is the discourse of Vimalakīrti and Mañjuśrī. Vimalakīrti, the personality in Buddhist literature who realizes most completely the indigenous Chinese ideal of virtue and saintliness, has always held a place of special honor in Chinese Buddhist iconography, and this theme recurs innumerable times in Chinese art through the ages.

*Mirrors.* During the 3d century, the small state of Wu (221–80), located near what is now Shaohsing in Chekiang province, became important as a center for the production of mirrors. The decorations on the mirrors from Wu usually had as their subject one of the legends of Taoist folklore, though occasionally the king of Wu is himself depicted, a clear indication of the special ties that existed between the house of Wu and the bronze casters.

*Ceramics.* During this period, a hard, resonant stoneware covered with an olive-green, brown, or blue-green feldspar glaze (PL. 236) was developed in the old Yüeh district, in Chekiang. This is the well-known Yüeh-yao (Yüeh ware), the origins of which may go back to the Chou period, for O. Karlbeck has shown that certain wares technically similar to the Yüeh-yao bear a fairly close resemblance in form and ornament to the late Chou bronzes.

The earliest wares from the kilns of Ch'iu-yen and Tê-ch'ing (see CHINA, *Chekiang*) resemble those studied by Karlbeck in some respects, and it seems probable that the pieces he attributes to the late Chou period came from kilns in this region. It is still very difficult to date the early Yüeh-yao, but during the last few years many specimens have been found in tombs and some of them can be dated by inscriptions. (See CERAMICS, text and PL. 165.)

THE SUI (581–618) AND T'ANG (618–906) DYNASTIES. The Sui dynasty lasted only a short time; nevertheless, it was the precursor of the much more powerful and long-lived T'ang dynasty, which succeeded in reestablishing the prestige of China at home and abroad at the level of Han times, and it has an importance far out of proportion to its duration, as a result of the achievement of its founder Yang Chien in uniting the realm again under one dynasty. Ch'ang-an and Loyang (Lo-yang) became again the western and eastern capitals of a united kingdom and were restored by the Sui emperors in all their spendor and magnificence.

The energetic early emperors of the T'ang dynasty forestalled the threat of the Tartars on their northern borders by several quick military expeditions which penetrated into the heart of Mongolia. The T'ang empire became a power to be reckoned with even in far distant regions. The might of the Chinese armies was felt as far away as Lake Balkhash, and even the petty states in the Indus Valley accepted Chinese suzerainty. The capital of the realm became a cosmopolitan center to which merchants came from all parts of Asia as well as Buddhist pilgrims from many lands.

In the course of the 8th century, during the reign of Minghuang (also known as T'ang Hsüan-tsung), the first signs of decadence began to appear in the Chinese empire, which had by this time become in every sense a great world power. During the first half of this century, the Chinese were still able to hold in check the rebellious peoples along their long frontiers. Probably, however, the turning point came with the defeat of Kao Hsien-chih on the Talas River in 751, which enabled Islam gradually to force Buddhism out of Central Asia. Soon the empire was obliged to draw back its borders drastically. Under pressure from the Tibetans in the west and the Uigurs in the northwest, China lost its corridor to Central Asia, while the Tungus kingdom of P'o-hai and the up-and-coming Khitans gobbled up Manchuria, the neighbor of the ever-unconquered Korea. The political chaos which the T'ang rule left behind set the stage for a new invasion, this time from Manchuria.

Even during the rule of the T'ang, anti-Buddhist persecutions had put an end to the magnificent temples which had adorned the Chinese capitals. We find, however, a clear reflection of the varied international contacts of the period in the cosmopolitan character of T'ang art. Exotic influences are to be observed, not only in the field of Buddhist art (which had been turned into new channels by a renewed Indian influence), but in fact everywhere.

*Painting.* The glorious, yet for China also very precarious period of T'ang rule produced many great painters. The literary sources, which, in comparison with those of earlier centuries, pour forth an abundant stream of documented information, give us a variegated picture of highly talented artists busy enriching the temples of the capital with wall paintings, of foreign artists introducing new viewpoints and techniques, and of court painters depicting the life of the capital and the palace in all its splendor and exuberance. By 847, however, when Chang Yen-yüan, the foremost chronicler of painting in the T'ang period, put on paper his famous work, *Li-tai ming-hua-chi,* "The Chronicle of Famous Painters of All Ages," he was unable to suppress an undertone of grief for what had already

been lost, even though political considerations forced restraint upon him. Even before his work was completed, the hard facts of history had overtaken him: the wall paintings in the temples of the two capitals Ch'ang-an and Loyang, the masterpieces of China's greatest painters, were practically without exception destroyed during the anti-Buddhist persecutions of 842–5. In spite of this tragic loss, if (as Matsumoto Eiichi has done in his iconographic studies) we compare the Buddhist repertory represented on the temple walls of the capitals, as given by Chang Yen-yüan, with the paintings preserved at Tun-huang, we can be convinced that our picture of the iconography of Buddhist painting is fairly complete. Without doing any injustice to the beauty of some of the paintings at Tun-huang, however, we may be certain that in these specimens of the art of the time, preserved in the remote wilderness of Kansu, we can find no adequate reflection of the mastery of China's greatest painters.

Nor do the copies of their works on silk and paper do these masters any honor. In the case of the greatest, Wu Tao-tzŭ (700–70; cf. PL. 281), so numerous are the anecdotes about his inspired and obsessed brushwork that we cannot doubt the great artistic mastery to which these stories from diverse sources so clearly attest. Neither the rubbings from stone reproductions of his monochrome drawings nor the dubious copies associated with his name (Jungkung Coll., Chicago, and Abe Coll., Osaka Municipal Mus.), however, can possibly be thought worthy of his talent. The wall paintings of the Hōryūji temple in Nara (Japan), which shortly after World War II were destroyed by fire, were probably the last remaining works to approximate the art of the great T'ang masters.

Even though most of the famous T'ang artists are now represented only in copies or in paintings by imitators — and it is impossible to distinguish from this latter category the works of the early art counterfeiters, who followed like shadows the rise of respectable artistry — we find ourselves on somewhat more easily surveyable terrain than was the case with earlier painting. There is indeed a series of portraits of priests in the possession of the Tōji temple in Kyoto from the hand of Li Chên, an artist of secondary importance, which was actually taken to Japan during the T'ang period and which we may accordingly regard as authentic. The short span of time that intervened between the active lives of the great masters and the creation of the oldest copies which have come down to us is also perhaps significant.

It is possible to form some idea of the style of Yen Li-pên (q.v., active ca. 630–70) from the horizontal scroll painting with imperial portraits in the Museum of Fine Arts, Boston. The 16 emperors, beginning with Wên-ti of the Han period and ending with Yang-ti of the Sui, are all represented somewhat monotonously, full length in very similar poses, with no great variation either in their state robes or in their retinues. However, in the facial expressions we can recognize truly striking differences which form the most interesting trait of this otherwise not very inspired work. It is for the greatest part a probably rather accurate but somewhat scholastic copy. From the point of view of art history, it is of the greatest importance that this painting was already ascribed to Yen Li-pên as early as the 11th century. In the same museum there is another work attributed to Yen Li-pên, a horizontal scroll painting representing a group of five literati charged with the study of the classical texts. The scholars, seated on a platform, are surrounded by numerous attendants. In contrast with the scroll of imperial portraits, the figures here have all been assembled in a group, forming a masterful composition. The tradition ascribing this work to Yen Li-pên, despite its venerable antiquity, is extremely doubtful, even more so since there exists a second version of the middle group of figures (Nat. Palace Mus., Taichung) ascribed to the 10th-century master Ch'iu Wên-po. There is, however, a possibility that both paintings are derived from a still older example.

Though our knowledge is scanty indeed, the most important phenomena which characterized the development of Chinese painting during the T'ang period are to some extent visible. It is completely apparent, not only in the literature, but also

from the few preserved works, that an enormous revolution had taken place since the development of such individual masters as Ku K'ai-chih. Landscape had appeared from time to time in earlier paintings, as a background against which human activities could be depicted, but had not yet claimed full attention for itself in a pure art of landscape painting. It is true that certain famous mountains were painted time and again, but only because of the historical or religious associations which every cultivated Chinese felt upon regarding their image. During the T'ang period we see the development of the landscape and its establishment in Chinese art as an independent theme, completely or almost completely equal with figure painting. That this development in China led so early (in contrast to European painting) to the definite supremacy of the landscape is to be explained by the Chinese orientation toward nature. At the same time this love for the landscape, which once awakened never cooled in ardor, inevitably pushed the art of figure painting into the background, so that it was never again to grow in comparable fashion.

Li Ssŭ-hsün (q.v.; 651–716) and his son Li Chao-tao (ca. 675–730), the best-known representatives of a great family of artists, appear to have played an important role in this development. At the same time they were the first artists of note to make popular a completely new technique. This consisted of the combination of fastidiously minute brushwork (*kung-pi*) with polychrome coloring in which green and blue malachite colors and gold predominated. Their style found adherents even as late as the Ming period and is associated by the Ming painter and art theoretician Tung Ch'i-ch'ang (q.v.; 1555–1636) with a "northern school" which he distinguishes as one of the main streams in the ancient art of painting. It is no longer possible for us to form directly an idea of the work of Li Ssŭ-hsün. The style of his son, however, can be reconstructed to some extent on the basis of a number of extant copies, of which three (from the Palace collection of Peking) are now to be found in the National Palace Museum at Taichung, Formosa. Two of these paintings, which are obviously only different versions of the same work, picture a traveling party in a mountain landscape. The title declares this to be the party of the T'ang emperor Ming-huang in the mountains of Szechwan. Steep cliffs, between which the mountains in the background loom up half hidden by clouds, dominate the entire picture with their strongly accented dolomite-like structure. In the more horizontally built-up version of this picture red plays an important role, second only to green and blue in the palette of the copyist. The entire landscape breathes an almost supernatural atmosphere, and it is just this style with its strongly decorative color effects which was chosen by later masters to depict "Dream Landscapes," "The Island of the Blessed," and other fantastic landscapes. Even though the landscape here begins to play a dominant role through the effect of the high-rising, angular, and split mountaintops, the human personages, painted with an eye for minute detail, are not condemned as in later landscape painting to play a completely subordinate role. The column of travelers proceeding slowly along winding paths and through mountain passes, pausing to let the transport animals rest in the first open place, commands our attention too strongly to be regarded as secondary, which is not surprising in view of the title of this painting. The masters of the Li school were certainly not the first to apply themselves to landscape as an independent branch of painting. The development took place gradually, reaching with these masters the first phase in an evolution which would lead in the 10th century to complete domination by the landscape. They also exerted a significant influence on such later painters as Chao Po-chü (Sung) and Ch'iu Ying (Ming).

The renowned poet-painter Wang Wei (q.v.; 699–759), whom Tung Ch'i-ch'ang proclaimed to be the first master of the so-called "southern school," was a man of great erudition and a poet to be reckoned among the most important even in this period of China's greatest poets. He remained an example for later generations of literati painters and was a personality who accorded completely with their ideals. In opposition to the style of the Li masters, which was later to contribute to

the so-called "academic" styles, Wang Wei was a proponent of the monochrome ink landscape painted in his "broken ink" technique (*p'o-mo*), recognizable from the strongly calligraphic outlines and the expertly brushed-in shadings which bring out beautifully the structure of mountain masses. At least this is what the literature has to say about his work, and we have no alternative but to believe it, since the copies associated with his name, of which only a very small number exist, reveal no trace of all this. The finest of the copies of his figure paintings is a small horizontal scroll painting representing the literator Fu Shêng (3d cent. B.C.). Still, it is strongly to be doubted that this masterpiece (Osaka Municipal Mus., Abe Coll.) is in fact a representative specimen of Wang Wei's art. At best, one might compare the conceptions of perspective which underlie the representation of the round mat upon which the scholar is seated with the handling of the walls in his best-known work, the landscape scroll in which he depicted the surroundings of his country residence Wang-ch'uan. There are innumerable copies of the latter. The complicated pedigrees of these copies, which are conspicuous for their utter lifelessness, indicate that in the most fortunate cases they come to us third or fourth hand. The rubbings from stone engravings of his work are probably somewhat closer to the originals. None of these reveal a really fundamental difference from the work of the Li masters as we know it, although the figures and buildings (still given emphasis by Li Chao-tao) here occupy a subordinate position.

Perhaps the indirect form in which this great art has come down to us causes us to underestimate the importance of T'ang landscape painting and to regard it merely as a forerunner of the better-preserved schools of the 10th century. In the T'ang period figure painters continued to play an extremely important role. They did not as a group choose (Wu Tao-tzŭ being an exception) the Buddhist religion with its inordinately large pantheon of buddhas and bodhisattvas as a predominating theme. The paintings of such artists as Chang Hsüan (first half of 8th cent.), known through the copy of his work *Women Preparing Silk* ascribed to the Sung emperor Hui-tsung (Mus. of Fine Arts, Boston), are, in spite of the grace and charm of the figures, little more than pictorial counterparts of the funerary sculpture of this period. The same holds for that painter of the life of the nobility and the court, Chou Fang (late 8th–early 9th cent.), who owes his great reputation to a number of paintings of court ladies, of which probably no more than one or two actually come down to us from his time.

Han Kan, a court painter from the time of the emperor Ming-huang (712–56), who was famous for his paintings of horses, has an especially great significance, since the possibility exists that he is the only painter of his time of whom some authentic works have been preserved. One of these, representing a horse tied to a post (Coll. Sir Percival David, London), illustrates convincingly the new style Han Kan is said to have created through observation of the horses of the imperial stables. Even those of his works with less spectacular speed and rhythm, for example the polychrome horizontal scroll painting in the Musée Cernuschi (Paris), display sharp observation and accurate characterization of the fine horses, which we are able even to identify by name from the harness details.

A completely different aspect of T'ang painting is revealed in the wall paintings of this period. Although the paintings found in tombs are fewer than in the previous period, such finds as that in a tomb dated 710 at Ti-chang-wan, near Hsien-yang in Shensi, are of great importance in that they come, not from the periphery, but from the very heart of the Chinese cultural area. The published reproductions of these unfortunately fragmentary wall paintings suggest that Chinese archaeologists could scarcely have exaggerated their quality when they compared them with the unpreserved works of Wu Tao-tzŭ. The portrait of a man, especially, though fragmentarily preserved, is of such rare expressiveness and individuality as is seldom met with in painting and which is extremely surprising in a burial crypt where one might expect a certain shoddiness.

For the great Tun-huang (q.v.) complex of cave temples in Kansu, the coming of the T'ang dynasty and the accompanying stimulation of traffic on the caravan routes meant the climax of a centuries-long development (see the preceding section). Approximately half of the wall paintings which have so far been investigated seem to date from the T'ang period, although a part of the caves in which they are found must have been in existence before that time. Toward the end of the T'ang period, it would seem, the complex attained its greatest possible extension, and activity concentrated on providing the existing temples with new wall paintings or otherwise enlarging and embellishing them. As the number of foreign visitors to Tun-huang increases, and the literature about this site grows, the point of view steadily gains currency that, even though the successive Tun-huang styles are not altogether representative of the art of painting in the central provinces, these wall paintings deserve our attention, not only for their iconographic, but also for their artistic characteristics.

Iconographically and stylistically the Tun-huang wall paintings of the T'ang period (PL. 249) display great differences from those of earlier times (cf. PLS. 237, 238, 244). The color scheme is extended, and landscape and figure painting, in even more complicated compositions with numerous figures, come to their full development. The displacement in the choice of themes is conspicuous and has a direct connection with the manner in which Buddhism developed in China. The Jātaka tales and the scenes from the life of the Buddha recede into the background to make place for paradise scenes: the Western Paradise of Amitābha, the Eastern Paradise of Bhaiṣajyaguru, and the Paradise of Maitreya. The Western Paradise of Amitābha, depicted according to descriptions in two of the *sūtras*, was especially popular in Tun-huang and is represented more than a hundred times — the two others more than fifty times. In general, the many figures of celestial beings and musicians which populate the paradise scenes are placed in a landscape in which architecture plays a predominant role, pushing into the distant background the hills and cliffs which functioned both as the connecting and as the dividing element in the early wall paintings. Of the texts which had earlier been represented, only the story of Vimalakīrti retained its popularity until the end of artistic activity at Tun-huang, when the Uigurs and Hsi-hsia made themselves masters of the complex.

*Sculpture.* Though our knowledge of sculpture during the T'ang period (PLS. 245, 252–256; II, PL. 391) is perhaps not so fragmentary as that of the art of painting, it is highly one-sided. The variety of plastic techniques, which we can still detect, for instance, in the Japanese Buddhist art of the Nara and Heian period, and which were undoubtedly entirely of Chinese origin, is not to be seen at all in the Chinese works which remain from that time. The bronze, clay, wood, and lacquer sculptures have almost without exception been lost, so that only the stone sculpture remains for us today. These sculptures, the only surviving evidence of the greatness of the proud capital city Ch'ang-an, are now spread over the entire world. The same is true of the finest of China's cave-temple complexes, T'ien-lung-shan, which was rediscovered in this century and systematically despoiled to benefit the commercial art dealers; fortunately, in this case, scientific investigators were able to study the now widely dispersed statues while they were still *in situ*.

Although both religious and secular sculpture was produced during the entire T'ang period, one can point out within this span of time not only periods of great affluence for the plastic arts, but also a time of deep decay. Mizuno, on the basis of dated inscriptions from the cave temples at Lung-mên, which were considerably extended during the T'ang period, believes that only between 630 and 640 did the Buddhist sculptors begin to show signs of increased activity. He believes that the high point of this activity fell approximately in 660–70, that it declined sharply during the reign of the famous emperor Ming-huang (712-56), and thereafter came to an almost complete stop. It is questionable how far this single complex of cave temples can be called representative for all of China. Mizuno's analysis would seem to be correct for the north of China, but the development of sculpture in stone in the province of Szechwan displays a completely different picture. In that

region, just in the second half of the 8th century, an entirely new school began to rise which produced innumerable cliff sculptures and smaller cave temples. While in the center of the country anti-Buddhist persecutions (mid-9th cent.) dealt a death blow to a flourishing artistic tradition, one can find no trace in Szechwan of a similar abrupt interruption, and work on the numerous cave complexes was carried on without break into the period of the Five Dynasties and the Sung period. The cave complexes of Kansu in some cases received their most extensive additions during the T'ang period (Tun-huang, Ping-ling-ssŭ), while other complexes (Mai-chi-shan) were not added to at all. The mature T'ang style of Buddhist sculpture, which quite justifiably received great admiration outside China, cannot be better characterized than in the words of the great Buddhist Tao-hsüan (died 667), who felt obliged to complain that the sculptors gave their Buddhist figures the appearance of dancing girls, as a result of which the dancing girls were tempted to think that they looked like bodhisattvas. However one-sided this judgment may be, it evokes the somewhat voluptuous realism of the T'ang style.

The caves of T'ien-lung-shan (PLS. 252, 256), which date from before 750 (according to Mizuno; Sirén dates Nos. 17–21 in early 9th cent.), display a clear influence from the late Gupta (q.v.) styles. The faces, otherwise the least successful element of these sculptures, acquire strongly naturalistic features, while serene tranquility makes way for a controlled rhythmical movement obviously based on the Indian *tribhaṅga* attitude. The treatment of the draperies, the proportions, and anatomical details become more natural. Especially in the last statuary groups of T'ien-lung-shan, the buddhas and bodhisattvas acquire an almost satisfied earthly appearance that reminds us no longer of the spiritualized and refined sculptures of earlier centuries. This tendency toward an extreme realism, which turns into a sweet sentimentality only in its very last examples, is, however, by no means present everywhere. The specimens which are the most interesting artistically are the sculptures from the Terrace of the Seven Treasures (Ch'i-pao-t'ai) of the temple Kuang-chai-ssŭ at Ch'ang-an (see CHINA, *Shensi*). All that remains of this terrace are a number of sculptures in high relief which were first transferred to another temple and from there have been dispersed over the entire world. The trinities, which largely date from the early 8th century, have a somewhat stereotyped composition which reminds us of paintings with similar themes from Tun-huang, though they are artistically on a much higher level. An even more severe modeling is displayed in the small niches with representations of the eleven-headed Kuan-yin (PL. 254). Such details as the halo with its lotus arabesque decoration and flaming border, as well as the treatment of the draperies in which even the sash falls symmetrically, testify to a strict, careful mode of working which, rather than being in any way rigid, strikes us as truly inspired. Only the overlong arms, one extended, the other raised in a gesture characteristic of the Kuan-yin figures of this time, disturb the perfect, stiff harmony, which is far removed from the mobility of the early T'ang sculptures of T'ien-lung-shan (Caves 4, 7, 11, and 14) and is not to be reconciled in any way with the sculptures from the last caves of this complex (Nos. 17–21).

Taoist sculpture, which had already made its first appearance during the period of the Six Dynasties, was never, in this land which had had such an enormous variety of Buddhist sculpture, able to develop into an independent art form. Iconographically, it maintained a perfect monotony from the very beginning, repeatedly representing either the Taoist supreme being, the Emperor of the Mysterious Origin (Hsüan-yüan Huang-ti), or the philosopher Lao-tzu, depicted in a sitting position, flanked by two attendant figures. In the accompanying inscriptions, as well as in the technical terms used, we are struck by the frequent use of expressions which are borrowed directly from Buddhism and betray an utter poverty of original or independent ideas. (See TAOISM.)

The situation with regard to other non-Buddhist sculpture is rather different. The best-known work is beyond a doubt the famous relief representing the six favorite chargers of the

T'ang emperor T'ai-tsung, the actual founder of the dynasty. These reliefs, which were located in a building near the burial tomb of the emperor, and two of which are now in the University Museum in Philadelphia, were, according to an old tradition, carved after a design by the famous painter Yen Li-pên. If this tradition is correct, this is a remarkable example, rare in the history of Chinese sculpture, of cooperation on a high artistic level.

Although the names of innumerable painters have come down to us, practically all the Chinese sculpture known is anonymous or was carved by masters whose names have not been preserved. Only in the T'ang period does something like individual identification of the artist appear to have arisen. The most famous of these masters, all of whose works, as far as is known, have been lost, was a certain Yang Hui-chih, a contemporary and schoolmate of the famous painter Wu Tao-tzŭ. Despairing of ever being able to equal the latter, he was said to have devoted himself to sculpture and to have established in this art a reputation corresponding to that of Wu in painting. The *Li-tai ming-hua-chi*, a well-known survey of the temples in the two capitals before the anti-Buddhist idol-breaking and destruction of the mid-9th century, gives the names of various other sculptors. The anecdote about Yang Hui-chih's motivation for taking up sculpture, which probably originated at a later date, can scarcely be considered a proof of the equality of sculpture and painting, either during the T'ang period or later. The art of sculpture never achieved such a distinguished position. In all of Chinese literature, which is so richly endowed with critical works on painting and calligraphy, there is no text devoted exclusively to sculpture.

In the funerary monuments of the later T'ang emperors, sculpture in the round takes the place of reliefs, though here and there relief is reverted to in the gigantic animal carvings, e.g., in the representation of the extraordinary ostriches which occur here. In contrast with the fantastic chimeras and winged lions of the southern dynasties, the T'ang sculptures lack vivacity and inspiration. Except perhaps for the winged horses, these colossal monuments are heavy, lumbering, and lifeless, already the terminal product of a development which survived statically well into the Ming and Ch'ing periods.

For no single form of Chinese plastic art is the qualification "naturalistic" so appropriate as in the case of funerary sculptures (PLS. 172, 239, 246; IV, PL. 460). During the T'ang period, this remarkable art form attained its high point and began also unmistakably upon its decline. The elegant life of the court and the cosmopolitan character of the capital are expressed more clearly and more tangibly here than in any other art form of the period. The charging horses ridden by polo players, the ensembles of ladies playing musical instruments (PL. 246), and the acrobats all show us the sport and recreation of the inhabitants of the imperial cities. The exotic bearded camel drivers with their heavily laden pack animals, merchants of many different races and from many different lands — these give us a picture of the lively commerce which was carried on along the caravan routes pacified by Chinese garrisons, while the stately dignitaries represent the wise administrators, and the armored warriors the heroic defenders of the world state that was T'ang China.

This extraordinarily decorative, but even in its best moments somewhat superficial funerary sculpture is so emphatic in its material ostentation that we cannot compare it in any respect whatsoever with Buddhist sculpture. Even more, it would seem, than in earlier times, there is a conspicuous difference in the quality of the various sculptures, probably because the custom of furnishing tombs with figures diffused downward from the top through the precisely delineated strata of the hierarchy. The tombs of the highest personages in the land were fitted out with great series of individually modeled figures, which were put on ostentatious display upon the beginning of the funeral rites. Those lower on the hierarchical ladder had to be satisfied with less finely modeled figures or with standardized types made in great quantities by means of molds. Under the ordinances of the T'ang state, various officials occupied themselves with the regulation of these class differences. The

sumptuary regulations prescribed both the dimensions and the number of figures to correspond to the rank of the deceased. The augmented numbers prescribed by each of the successively revised sumptuary ordinances lead us to believe, however, that the restrictive stipulations were unable to withstand the tendency to make ever larger and more expensive tomb figures, sometimes even from precious metals.

Inasmuch as the extremely numerous tomb figures in collections are practically without exception from the loot of grave robbers, we lacked until a short time ago clear-cut evidence as to the number of figures that were placed in each tomb, as well as the fashion in which figures were arranged within the tomb. Several score of finds during the 1950s, however, have shed more light on this question. Among the necessary fixtures in the tomb of a high official of the T'ang regime were the figures of two fantastic monsters, generally called "earth spirits" (t'u-kuei), which indeed do appear to represent an "earth spirit" and the "spirit of the ancestors." These figures were erected at the entrance to the grave chamber and were accompanied by two tomb guardians, often rather close copies of the Buddhist lokapalas. These four figures are almost without exception larger in size than the other figures in the tomb, as appears from the texts of the sumptuary ordinances, as well as from comparison of the pieces found in any given tomb.

Fairly general during the T'ang period was the practice of placing in the grave a series of 12 standing figures with the heads of the animals of the zodiac (IV, PL. 460). Horses and camels occur practically always in pairs and are frequently accompanied by their grooms. Dancing girls, musicians, soldiers, and the stately high dignitaries occurring practically always in pairs, as well as innumerable animal statues (PL. 250), are also an important part of the inventory of tomb furnishings.

With regard to technique, one can distinguish two types of T'ang funerary sculpture. One is unglazed and decorated with motifs executed in cold painting; the other displays the well-known three-color glaze of T'ang ceramics. The blue glaze, which is frequently found in pottery, is, however, rather rare in the funerary sculpture.

In the tomb figures we are able to recognize, through the extremely faithful reproduction of the details of the costumes, a clear-cut reaction to changes in fashion. The chronological order of these changes is not yet completely clear, but it seems well established that during the 8th century, especially, the ideal of feminine beauty was conceived as round and plump, in contrast with the preference for a slenderer type in the preceding century. It has been suggested that this fashion was induced by the reportedly well-filled-out figure of the favorite of the emperor Ming-huang, the notorious Yang Kuei-fei. The "Yang Kuei-fei type" of tomb figure displays a surprising likeness to representations of court ladies in painting, for example, in works in the Yakushiji in Nara, in the ethnographic museum (Statens Etnografiska Mus.) in Stockholm (found by Sven Hedin in Turfan), and also in the decoration on a piece of lacquer in the Low-Beer Collection.

What actually caused the striking decline in the artistic quality and the use of tomb figures during the later T'ang period is not yet entirely clear. One might seek the cause in Buddhism, but this was also for Buddhism a time of decline. The opposition of certain censorious officials to the wasteful extravagance of elaborate funerals was generally based upon an arsenal of arguments which all dated from before the actual flourishing of funerary sculpture. There is a very good possibility, however, that an increasing preference for cremation, not from religious, but from financial and economic reasons (among others, the shortage of land available for cemeteries), caused funerary sculpture almost completely to disappear.

The discovery of the tombs of two members of the imperial family of the Southern T'ang state (10th cent.) reveals that the funerary sculpture was not even a faint reflection of the extremely refined artistic life at the court of these unfortunate rulers. The figures strike us as rustic and primitive. Characteristic of this late funerary sculpture, as appears also from other finds, are the heavy pedestals upon which the animal sculptures were placed.

In the border areas of China the tradition of funerary sculpture still continued for a considerable space of time. In the British Museum there are tomb figures from a tomb in Szechwan dating from the year 839. Recently, near Chengtu, a tomb dated 1147 was found with a great number of tomb figures of a type hitherto unknown. Wooden tomb figures, as well, are known from the Sung period. It is, accordingly, altogether possible that the tradition was able to survive into the Mongol period, at which time one may speak of a marked revival. Regardless of how interesting these specimens from a later period may be, there can be no doubt that the artistically important funerary sculpture disappeared for good from the stage of Chinese art about the 9th century.

*Ceramics.* The most important development in the field of Chinese ceramics in the centuries between the fall of the Han and the rise of the T'ang dynasty was that of the Yüeh-yao. This development continued during the T'ang period, partly in different kilns situated in the old Yüeh area in Chekiang — among other places at Shang-lin-hu, which seems to have displayed the greatest activity in the 10th century. While the period of the Six Dynasties saw few spectacular changes, except in funerary sculpture, we find during the T'ang dynasty a great variety of ceramic products which, like the tomb figures, reflects the trend of these times (PLS. 166, 167, 246, 247, 250).

The ceramic wares intended principally for funerary purposes (PL. 165), like the tomb figures, usually show a white, somewhat rose-tinted body. The use in the decoration of green, yellow, amber, blue, and black glazes is very striking. These are all frequently employed as monochrome glazes, but occur as well in combinations of three different colors. In the latter case, they are usually separated by a modeled or stamped design. In both shape and design we find numerous reminders of exotic forms and decorative motifs. In the egg-shaped vases with narrow ringed necks and two handles in the form of dragons' necks, we recognize the Greek amphora, while all sorts of variations on the rhyton also occur. The extraordinary combination of all sorts of exotic motifs of Hellenistic and Sassanid origin (to which the European interest in T'ang ceramics can be ascribed to a considerable extent) is undoubtedly in part a consequence of the extensive foreign contacts of the T'ang empire. When we consider, however, that adaptation of foreign decorative motifs had already been going on for several centuries in Buddhist sculpture, and that other motifs regarded as of exotic origin, such as the horses in the "flying gallop," had already been completely naturalized in the art of the Han period, the development during the T'ang period appears less abrupt than is often suggested. These exotic influences are still more conspicuous in the art of working precious metals, and this, in turn, perhaps influenced ceramics; the close relationship between these two forms of Chinese handicraft continued in the Sung and Yüan periods. A ceramic technique which is typical of the T'ang period is the so-called "marbled pottery," produced by mixing clays of different colors; after baking it was covered with a light-yellow glaze, and the various colored "veins" display a remarkable resemblance to marble.

Broken fragments of various kinds of T'ang pottery, among others the Yüeh-yao as well as white porcelain (associated by G. Lindberg with the Hsing-yao pottery mentioned in literature), have been found far beyond the borders of China. The best-known site of these finds is Fostat (near Cairo), which was founded in 641 and laid waste in 1169. Much T'ang pottery has been found at Samarra on the Tigris, while also at Brahminabad (India), which was destroyed by flood about the beginning of the 11th century, broken fragments of Chinese stoneware have been found. (See CERAMICS.)

*Minor Arts.* The personal possessions of the Japanese emperor Shōmu, which were offered in 756 to the Tōdaiji temple in Nara and have since been preserved in the Shōsōin repository, form as a whole a completely unique collection of the finest 8th-century objects of handicraft from China and Japan. Which of the objects are of Chinese origin cannot always be determined (the pottery which was formerly regarded as Chinese is beyond

any doubt Japanese); however, objects which may have been produced in Japan betray the influence of the styles and techniques which prevailed at that time in the T'ang empire. Furniture, musical instruments, lacquer inlaid with mother-of-pearl, silver, and ivory reveal to us a technical perfection and a refined beauty which one might have imagined from the descriptions in literature, but could scarcely have believed were it not for this imperial collection.

The influence of western Asia on the art of the T'ang period is nowhere so evident as in the art of the gold- and silversmith. Historical sources repeatedly describe the close relations between the Chinese court and the princes of Sassanid Persia, who were under threat from the Arabs. After the fall of the Sassanid empire, many Persians appear to have fled to China and to have established themselves in Ch'ang-an and in Hangchow, among other places. Beyond any doubt, the Chinese

were applied to the ceilings of the burial chamber, so that the symbols for east and west had to be interchanged with respect to the north-south axis. Moreover, when, in the course of the 7th century, silvered mirrors of a type incorrectly called "sea-horse and grapes" by Sung antiquarians came into vogue, a fifth animal appeared in the place of the knob which is thought to symbolize the center of the universe. In this type the knob is replaced with the figure of a reclining monster rendered in rather high relief, the surrounding surface being covered with a decoration in which grapevines and fantastic animals are worked together in one congested, intertwined configuration. It has been assumed that this type has a connection with Manichaeism, which was flourishing in China in the T'ang period. Since both lions and grapes, which play a prominent role in this decorative type, are of foreign origin and are designated in Chinese with assimilated loan words (*shih*, lion

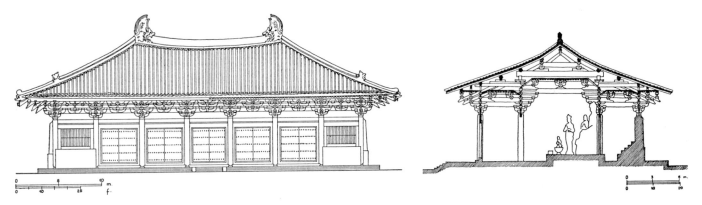

Main hall of the temple Fo-kuang-ssŭ on Wu-t'ai-shan, Shansi (mid-9th cent.), elevation and section (*after Sickman and Soper*).

gold- and silversmiths profited greatly from the arrival of their extremely adept Persian colleagues. Their influence appears not only in technique but also in decoration. The silver basins, cups, dishes, and ornaments, which are sometimes partly gilded, were decorated in various ways — by chasing, by hammering in relief, and sometimes also by engraving. Frequently the pieces were built up of several sections soldered together.

In the chased decoration, more often than not applied against a background of small round studs, hunting scenes with archers and galloping horses as well as innumerable variations of flowering branches with birds and animals play a prominent role. In a number of these pieces, which can be dated with certainty in the T'ang period — since a pair of large silver vases in the Shōsōin, Nara, Japan, have an inscription of the year 767 — the influence of the Sassanid goldsmiths has been very strong indeed. Various pieces, however, display a much more Chinese decoration.

Special mention is due the tomb figures in silver, which, in spite of the fact that their manufacture was expressly forbidden in the sumptuary ordinances of the T'ang regime, seem nevertheless to have been produced. The number of known specimens is at present limited, and while the objections to their authenticity are probably unfounded, it has not yet been confirmed by scientific excavation. The standing figures, which are of a very common T'ang tomb-figure type, and also the oxen, of which a few specimens are known, are all made by soldering together two separate halves. The finest of all these figures, a horse from the Kempe Collection (Ekolsund, Sweden) is much more complicated, having been built up of a large number of pieces and supplied with a beautiful decorative harness.

*Mirrors.* In the Sui and T'ang variation of the TLV decoration on mirrors (see above, *Han*), the T's and L's vanish and the V's opposite the corners mark off the four areas in which the animal symbols of the four points of the compass are placed. To judge by the inscriptions, this decoration was maintained until approximately 650. The positions of the animals with respect to each other are frequently changed, because the mirrors

< Per., *sir*; *p'u-t'ao*, grape <Gr., *botrus*), this supposition does not seem far-fetched.

A completely separate category is formed by the mirrors which were used in the wedding ceremony. These usually, but by no means always, have a lobed shape. Birds especially were depicted in relief because of their propitious symbolism: the Chinese phoenix (*fêng-huang*), peacocks, mandarin ducks, and magpies. We frequently see these birds holding in the beak a cord symbolizing the marriage bond.

A radical departure in decorative technique is displayed by mirrors inlaid with silver and gold in lacquer on a bronze underground. The T'ang date of this type is not only to be deduced from the style of the decoration, but is confirmed by archaeological discoveries and the presence of such pieces in the Shōsōin.

*Architecture.* The splendor of the palaces and temples of the two capitals of the T'ang empire, which we know from extensive descriptions in contemporary sources, vanished long ago, leaving as its only trace the checkerboard pattern of the street plan of Ch'ang-an (see CHINA, *Shensi*) and that of the other towns which were modeled after the T'ang metropolis. Except for one building on a modest scale, the main hall of the temple Fo-kuang-ssŭ on Wu-t'ai-shan (FIG. 515), no wooden structure of the T'ang period seems to have survived. Of the less perishable pagodas built of brick and stone, several have come down to us. The best-known is the so-called Great Gander Pagoda (Ta-yen-t'a) at Sian (see CHINA, *Shensi*), which was built at the request of the famous pilgrim Hsüan-tsang (652). The present structure (PL. 273) differs considerably from the original, which seems to have been based on an Indian prototype and was therefore a monument of unique type, in an architectural style probably somewhat unusual even at the period in which it was built.

In the vicinity of Sian there are also to be found the Small Gander Pagoda, built between 707 and 710, and the tomb pagoda of Hsüan-tsang, built in 669 (extensively restored in 828). Several examples of pagodas of the T'ang period exist

on Fang-shan (see CHINA, *Hopei*). Whereas the only major example of a pre-T'ang date, the pagoda of the Sung-yüeh-ssŭ on Sung-shan (see CHINA, *Honan*) rises from a dodecagonal plan, most T'ang pagodas are square in ground plan. Some of them, like the Ssu-mên-t'a of the temple Shên-t'ung-ssŭ (see CHINA, *Shantung*), consist of a square structure surmounted by a roof which is supported by several layers of corbeled bricks. A more complicated type consists of the same cubic structure crowned by seven stories of corbeled bricks or projecting stone slabs. Usually there are no true stories, but a series of closely set eaves, without any trace of a floor between them. Although no wooden pagodas of the T'ang period are left, their influence is almost omnipresent. The imitation of wooden architectural elements in stone seems to have increased during the T'ang period and reached its greatest development during the Sung and Liao. In this period there was also a tendency toward profuse sculptural decoration, and bas-reliefs can be seen on the various types of pagodas, for example, those on Fang-shan. The most elaborate decoration is to be found on the Lang-kung-t'a of the temple Shên-t'ung-ssŭ (see CHINA, *Shantung*).

southern façade and almost never at one of the gable ends. Most buildings, with the exception of the pagodas, consist of one or two stories. More often than not, the second story has a purely decorative function.

Just as the construction of buildings by means of columns and beams is less rigid than that in which the walls must bear structural weight, the steeply sloping, curving roof, which is characteristic of Chinese architecture, is supported by structures of a more flexible nature than those traditional in the West, which are primarily designed to prevent sagging of the roof. The transverse beams bear a framework of vertical posts and horizontal beams, rising step by step to the required height of the ridge beam and thus forming a suitable support for the curving roof. In regions where earthquakes are frequent, this flexible type of construction offers great advantages.

In order to provide the maximum amount of protection against the scorching sun and the pouring rain, the Chinese architects constructed widely projecting, deeply overhanging eaves. In order to carry the heavy weight of these eaves, it was necessary to stay the purlins. The simplest method was to lengthen the transverse beams, which then had to run

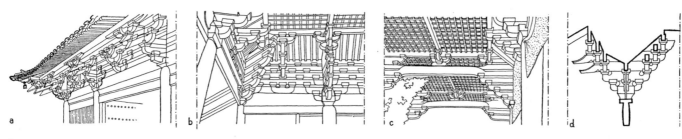

Examples of architectural construction: (*a, b, c*) the temple Fo-kuang-ssŭ on Wu-t'ai-shan, Shansi (mid-9th cent.), detail of exterior eaves and two interior details; (*d*) eaves brackets of the San-ch'ing-tien of the Taoist temple Yüan-miao-kuan, at Soochow, Kiangsu (prob. 12th cent.), section (*after Sickman and Soper*).

Until about the year 1940 Chinese architecture in wood (the first traces of which were discovered in the neolithic remains near Pan-po-ts'un described above, and of which many vestiges have been found in the ruins of An-yang) could only be hypothetically reconstructed from architectural survivals in Japan, where a number of temple buildings following the Chinese T'ang style have been preserved. From these the general principles were sufficiently familiar, especially since Chinese architecture never underwent such radical changes as characterize, for example, European architecture since the Renaissance. Although much of the history of Chinese architecture will always remain unknown, there is every reason to believe that the basic concepts have remained more or less the same through the ages.

One of these basic architectural concepts, already apparent in the neolithic remains, is the use of columns as supports for the roof and the structure of buildings, the walls of which have almost exclusively a protective function. The walls constructed between the columns serve only as a screen, being of insufficient strength to bear the heavy weight of the roof. The material used for these screen walls may differ according to the climate of the region. In the northern parts of China it was usually brick; in the warmer regions of the south flimsier materials were often employed. The heads of the columns carry the weight of the superstructure. Sunk into a platform of pounded earth or stones and resting on bronze disks or flat stones, the columns are tied by transverse beams, which span the nave of the building, and by longitudinal beams, which constitute the architrave. The width of the nave and the intercolumnar bays depends therefore on the length of the available timber, a factor which has forced the Chinese to reduce the size of their buildings — especially in modern times after extensive deforestation made large-size timber extremely rare. The depth of a building may be increased by erecting extra rows of columns; large buildings usually have four longitudinal colonnades, not counting an extra colonnade for a portico. The entrance is always in the middle of the

straight through the columns and project outward to reach the lowest purlin. Later these simple, single horizontal stays were elaborated into a system of bracket arms, projecting from the head of the column and consisting only partially of transverse beams. In this way an elaborate system of superimposed bracket arms of gradually increasing length spanned the distance between the columns and the purlin of the eaves. Its most elaborate development is to be found in Japan rather than in China, where the horizontal bracket arms did not exceed five, according to the architectural treatise *Ying-tsao fa-shih* of the Sung period. In order to increase the structural stability, longitudinal brackets providing support for the purlins in the plane of the wall and intercolumnar brackets also came into use. This multiplication of the elements of the bracketing system, further complicated by slanting bracket arms incorporated into the transverse and longitudinal brackets and running in the same direction as the rafters, is one of the most interesting features of Chinese architecture. The bracketing system of each period and style had a character of its own. It continued to be an essential element of architecture in wood until the Ming period, when it lost its tectonic function to become merely a decorative element. It also inspired the architects of stone pagodas, who often imitated its characteristics in stone.

All these main features of Chinese architecture can be observed in the oldest existing wooden building in China, the main hall of the temple Fo-kuang-ssŭ on Wu-t'ai-shan (FIGS. 515, 517; see also CHINA, *Shansi*), which dates, according to an inscription, from the mid-9th century. Although extremely valuable as a historical monument, it can hardly be regarded as a perfect specimen of the great architecture of the T'ang period; it was built only a short time after all important buildings of this large Buddhist center were razed, during the anti-Buddhist persecutions of the Hui-ch'ang era, and typifies only the first timid attempts at reconstruction. The main hall, consisting of seven to four bays, is single-storied and covered by a hipped roof. The ends of the ridge beam are decorated with two

acroteriums. The southern façade has doors in five bays, the remainder being protected by brick walls. The overhanging eaves of the roof are supported by a bracketing system far more complicated than that which is illustrated in the depiction of a Tʻang temple engraved over the door of the Ta-yen-tʻa (see CHINA, *Shensi*). It shows already a system of double slanting bracket arms running parallel, anticipating the Sung style, but not yet fully developed. The intercolumnar bracketing is simpler. In many respects the building is similar to the *kondō* of the Tōshōdaiji at Nara (Japan), as Soper demonstrated.

THE PERIOD OF THE FIVE DYNASTIES (907–60). The downfall of the Tʻang dynasty ushered in an era of utter chaos. In different parts of the country, adventurers and generals proclaimed themselves "emperors," but only five of the ephemeral dynasties they established were later considered worthy to be reckoned in the naming of this period. They are generally designated as the "Later" or "Posterior" Liang, Tʻang, Chin, Han, and Chou. These five dynasties all had Kaifeng (Kʻaifêng) in Honan province as their capital, although their authority extended only over a small part of the previous Tʻang empire. Elsewhere, other small states played an important role in the cultural life of the period: the state of Shu in the province of Szechwan, which had Chengtu (Chʻêng-tu) as its capital, the Southern Tʻang state (937–75) around Nanking, and the kingdom of Wu-Yüeh (907–78), which had established its capital at Hangchow (Hang-chou).

This period of almost continuous civil war was of such great importance in the cultural history of China that it deserves separate treatment, notwithstanding its short duration. The courts at Chengtu and Nanking attracted the outstanding artists of that time; and it was during this period that one of China's greatest contributions to civilization, the invention of printing, spread from Szechwan over the whole of China and from there to the neighboring countries. At the court of Nanking, over which the great poet and connoisseur Li Yü presided, there arose a kind of genre painting which is an impressive relic of the *fin de siècle* atmosphere prevailing in those luxurious and refined surroundings. There also the custom of mounting Chinese paintings on brocades seems to have had its beginning. The kings of the Wu-Yüeh state fervently devoted themselves to Buddhism — in the year 955 no less than 84,000 miniature pagodas were cast, many of which have been preserved. At their command, new cave temples and rock sculptures were hewn out of the mountains near Hangchow, and under their patronage the kilns of the famous Yüeh-yao produced some of their finest wares.

But the weakness and dissension of the Chinese had already attracted the attention of the neighboring powers. From the north the Manchurian Khitans began an invasion of Chinese territory, and shortly thereafter the Tangut Hsi-hsia conquered the province of Kansu. A general sent to combat the Khitans, a certain Chao Kʻuang-yin, made use of the opportunity to proclaim himself emperor of China. Unlike his many predecessors, he maintained his power, and 19 years later the whole of China was reunited under his dynasty, that of the Sung.

*Painting.* The turbulent 10th century witnessed a remarkable revival of painting, during which the foundations were laid for the general trends in this art during the next centuries. If we add the information culled from many literary sources to the evidence of the few surviving authentic paintings from this period and the somewhat more numerous reliable copies, there emerges a picture of an extremely varied and surprisingly original art form. One cause of the variety may be the fact that the center of culture was no longer concentrated in one central capital, but that the artists were attracted to several different parts of China. Although the development of the styles in the different capitals did not run parallel, these various centers did not by any means lead an isolated and separate artistic life. The biographies of some of the greatest painters of this period show that several of them visited more than one of the artistic capitals. Though the "unconventional" or "untrammeled" style (see below) seemed to prevail in Szechwan,

and the "decadent" genre painting is closely connected with the court at Nanking, the local color of these styles should probably not be stressed too much.

By far the most striking developments in Chinese painting of the 10th century are: the rise of a monochrome style which was to some extent influenced by the ideas of the Meditative Buddhists of the Chʻan (Zen) sect (see BUDDHISM); the maturing of an extremely refined genre painting; the marked interest of some artists in the "birds and flowers" theme; and the first flowering of pure landscape painting.

Huang Hsiu-fu, author of the work *I-chou ming-hua-lu* (second half of 10th cent.), which gives many details on the lives of the painters from Szechwan, proved by his new system of classification of painters — ever since Hsieh Ho the favorite pastime of many Chinese art critics — the great importance attached to the new developments in monochrome painting. Instead of the usual three classes, which had been given different names by various authors, he proposed a new category superior to all three, the so-called "unconventional" class (*i-pʻin*), the members of which were withdrawn from judgment by the usual criteria because of their completely different views and methods. These were the masters who expressed their artistic inspiration with complete spontaneity in the medium of the Chinese ink, directly transmuting their ideas into a new form. The followers of Wu Tao-tzǔ's style, who stressed the importance of strong calligraphic contours, were numerous, but gradually there emerged a variation in which the contours were filled with a complex of various types of brush strokes and washes. These new techniques have been designated by Chinese critics as *pʻo-mo*. This term is a romanization of two different technical terms (one meaning "broken ink" and the other "splashed or spilled ink") which have caused much confusion among Western art historians. It seems that the meaning of the two terms has shifted in the course of the centuries and that their usage in China has not always been strictly differentiated. The "broken ink" method is used generally to denote that in which shading and modeling are effected by means of *tsʻun* ("wrinkles") within the contours; the "splashed ink" method is one in which contours are neglected in favor of heavy strokes and splashes. Both methods were much in favor during the 10th century.

The personification of Meditative Buddhism, with its stress upon a strongly individualistic experience of Enlightenment, is the lohan (Skr., *arhat*), the disciple of the Buddha who has reached the state of Enlightenment (see BUDDHISM). It is hardly surprising that the 16 lohans which Buddhism of the 10th century acknowledged (later two more were added to this group) were a favorite theme of the Chʻan Buddhist painters. How unconventional the representations of these holy figures were may be judged from the early series of paintings which are attributed to Kuan-hsiu (832–912; II, PL. 393). Best known is that in the Japanese imperial collection (formerly in the Takahashi Coll.). In this series the lohans are seated among or upon rocks of extremely bizarre shape. Their equally bizarre, pseudo-Indian countenances seem to mimic the shapes of rocks, while their arms and bodies assume the warped shape of old pine trees. These exotic, almost grotesque and caricatural faces are painted in a style which strongly reminds us of rubbings from engravings on stone. However, it seems that these paintings were not actually made after rubbings, but that the opposite is the case. The inscription on the painting which looks most "Chinese," and which has consequently been regarded as a self-portrait of Kuan-hsiu, has been deciphered with the aid of an engraved version of the painting; if the inscription is authentic, the whole series could be dated between 880 and 894. Kuan-hsiu is often regarded as a typical Szechwan painter, which is, however, only partially correct, as he lived only the last 12 years of his life in that province.

Completely different is the work of the painter Shih-kʻo (second half of 10th cent.), of which only two heavily restored paintings (II, PL. 393) are known. They are probably copies made in the Southern Sung period. Both represent meditating or sleeping patriarchs, one seated in a meditative pose, the other leaning with his right elbow on a sleeping tiger. This reduced

version of the subject which is usually called the "Three Sleeping Figures" (with two additional sleeping disciples) brings us to a theme and a painting technique which are characteristic of Ch'an Buddhist painting. (The theme is well known in Japanese Zen painting and has even been copied in Persian miniatures.) In this pair of paintings by Shih-k'o the heads and the bare upper part of the body of one of the figures are painted in light gray with an occasional dark accent on the mouth and the bracelets. The outlines of the clothes are depicted in a much more spontaneous, almost impulsive way, with a few rapid strokes resembling grass-script characters (see CALLIGRAPHY), filled with a light-gray wash. Just as Ch'an Enlightenment comes after a long period of spiritual exercise, the painter seems to have grasped suddenly the right inspiration and poured it out onto his paper in a few rapid brush strokes. The result bears a superficial resemblance in technique to the "sketches" made in Western art, but too many experiments and failures have preceded these masterpieces to permit drawing a direct parallel. On the whole this "sketchy" technique in Shih-k'o's work would seem somewhat too mature for the period. Both paintings have been cut out and pasted onto another paper, on which were painted an incorrectly copied (or forged) signature and date, together with imitation seal impressions. The recent discovery of a stone-engraved copy of a painting by Shih-k'o (see CHINA, Szechwan) may make it possible to decide with more certainty the characteristics of his style. Whatever it may have been, the connection with Ch'an Buddhism and the "unconventional" technique seems to be well established. The same can be said of the painter's connection with Szechwan, for unlike Kuan-hsiu he lived most of his life in that province, leaving it only after the establishment of the Sung capital at Kaifeng.

The artistic climate of Nanking, the capital of the Southern T'ang state, was like that of another world. There can be hardly any doubt that the unfortunate Li Yü (937–78), great poet and collector and last prince of his dynasty (who was taken captive when his capital was conquered by the Sung armies in 975), contributed positively to the remarkable artistic activity at his court. The paintings attributed to his circle are like his poetry: the work of an exquisitely refined genre school which chose the pleasures of court life as its main theme. The atmosphere evoked by the few surviving works is one of preciousness, effete charm, and an attitude of *après nous le déluge*.

The most famous of Li Yü's court painters was Chou Wên-chü. Only copies of his works seem to have survived. Among them is a long scroll (PL. 268), painted about 1140, which has been cut up into several parts; fragments of it are to be found in the University Museum (Philadelphia), the Fogg Art Museum (Cambridge, Mass.), and the collections of Sir Percival David (London Univ.) and the late Bernhard Berenson (Florence). Although parts of this scroll display exquisite brushwork, the general impression is very much that of a copy. Perhaps somewhat truer to the original of Chou Wên-chü is a scroll in the Art Institute of Chicago showing a high official seated on a screened-off platform, listening to an orchestra of court ladies. The expressions of concentration on the faces of the listeners have been rendered in a most convincing fashion.

It is a point of great interest that the high official looks exactly like the principal personage in another painting which is one of the best-preserved works of this period. This is the famous hand scroll called *The Night Revels of Han Hsi-tsai* (Hui-hua-kuan, Peking); it is an original by or an exact and early copy after the little-known painter Ku Hung-chung. The original of this scroll, which depicts the surprisingly harmless nocturnal amusements of the minister Han Hsi-tsai in a way which is psychologically as penetrating as it is reticent in its pictorial representation, had to be explained by a moralizing story. It is said to be a kind of secret report in pictorial form made at the order of the emperor, who wanted confidential information on the conduct of this minister. In scenes separated by screens and beds we see the principal figure, the minister Han Hsi-tsai, repeated each time in a different situation; in one scene he is surrounded by guests listening to a female orchestra, and elsewhere he is beating the drum to accompany

a dancing girl. The painter has succeeded in creating the impression that we are peeping at the minister from a hidden place between the screens. He has concentrated more on facial expressions than on the movements of the figures, and the principal figure, instead of being a debauched *bon vivant*, looks as stiff as a poker, almost a stranger in his surroundings. The excellent composition of the groups of figures, the lines of the draperies, much more complex than on the copies of T'ang works, as well as the extremely delicate coloring characterize the painter as a great artist.

Next to figure painting, the theme which is often called "birds and flowers" played an important role in the painting of the Five Dynasties. Of the two greatest masters, Huang Ch'üan, active at the Szechwan court, and Hsü Hsi, at the court of the Southern T'ang, no genuine works seem to have been preserved. This is all the more regrettable because, according to literary sources, there existed a considerable difference between the styles of these two masters. Huang Ch'üan is said to have stressed the importance of coloring, suppressing heavy outlines, whereas Hsü Hsi worked mainly in strongly accentuated contours. During the Sung period, when painters from all corners of China flocked to the new central capital seeking an appointment to the newly founded Imperial Academy, the so-called "boneless" method of Huang Ch'üan became the accepted style. How complete this victory must have been can be demonstrated by the fact that Hsü Hsi's son Hsü Ch'ung-ssŭ adopted the style of his father's opponent, suppressing even the last vestiges of black contours in his own work. In this respect he was probably even more drastic than Huang Ch'üan himself. Even though these masters are now little more than names, they were of great importance as precursors of the great masters of flower and bird painting of the Sung Academy.

The high artistic level of the 10th-century painters of plants and animals is demonstrated by two anonymous paintings from the former imperial collection in Peking. (This collection, commonly referred to as the "Palace collection" below, is now for the most part in Taichung, Formosa, q.v. under CHINA.) Both paintings, probably forming a pair, represent deer in a forest of maple trees, painted after keen observation of the living animal and with a great devotion to nature; one of them is pervaded with an atmosphere of peaceful quiet, whereas the other, in contrast, shows the same animals in a startled tense attitude. The thick vegetation which covers the entire painting, the minute details, and the rich coloring remind us of realistic miniature art. The theme and the style of these two works can be compared with a wall painting representing Autumn, one of the Four Seasons found in the tomb of the Liao emperor Sheng-tsung in Inner Mongolia (ca. 1031). These wall paintings, which combine strong, clear outlines with a bright polychromy, are certainly not of the same high artistic level, but probably represent a provincial offshoot of a central Chinese style which flourished almost a century earlier in the heart of the empire.

The influence which the 10th-century painters of figures, flowers, and birds exerted upon the painters of the Sung period may have been considerable, but it is small in comparison with the lasting influence of the 10th-century landscape painters, for these epoch-making artists actually set the styles for many centuries to come. It was during the 10th century that the landscape became a completely independent theme, and not merely a useful setting for groups of figures. The polychrome landscape in which the groups of figures formed a narrative element was now replaced by a largely monochrome scene with high soaring peaks surrounded by mists and clouds, in which a personage, if introduced at all, was a small solitary figure that stressed the gigantic proportions of the world surrounding him. These mountain landscapes were certainly not completely fantastic or removed from nature; the masters, each in his own part of China, had studied the shape and structure of mountains, the twisting of rivers and paths, and the effect of changing seasons and weather. But they then tried to recreate these familiar forms and effects into a visionary landscape art, more ambitious than merely topographical representation. Per-

spective in the European optical sense is lacking entirely. The landscapes are rather the expression of the totality of impressions gathered during wanderings through the mountains. It is as if the spectator, led by the hand of the artist, climbs the mountains and visits their temples or waterfalls, or other beautiful spots, set amid strangely shaped pine trees or fantastic rocks.

The Chinese attitude toward nature did not set the human being apart; man was seen as one of the many creations of the interacting great cosmic forces. Although fear of certain natural phenomena is a characteristic of mankind, in China the fear of mountains (which disappeared in Europe only with the romantic movement) is conspicuously lacking. The painter strove to capture the essence (ch'i) which was thought to pervade all nature. The fact that he often expressed himself in terms borrowed from the Chinese philosophy of nature has sometimes given the misleading impression that Chinese landscape art is a disguised form of deeply religious, magic art. This interpretation neglects the purely secular pronouncements of the artists themselves, which may be found interspersed among poetic, fantastic, and cosmological speculations.

The unique position which Chinese landscape art was to enjoy is due to the great masters of the late 10th and early 11th century. Within one century there lived and worked a great number of truly original and outstanding artists, who have been regarded ever since as the greatest Chinese painters. Ching Hao, Kuan T'ung, Li Ch'eng, Tung Yüan, Chü-jan, and Fan K'uan are the best known and the most imitated. Of these the latter four are classified as Sung masters (see below), but the transfer of dynastic power had no effect upon the continuity in the evolution of Chinese landscape painting in this first great phase of development. With these names the long list of important masters is far from exhausted. Some are important as pioneers, others because of their great influence upon later generations. Their works have been copied innumerable times, and their different renditions of the structure of rocks and mountains have served as examples for almost all later generations. Original works of these masters, however, are extremely rare. Several early copies, in many cases impressive works of art, as well as the extremely interesting literary remains which attest their genius, can only partially compensate for this loss.

Ching Hao, active during the first half of the 10th century, is the first of these early landscapists. Probably all of his genuine works have been lost, and the few extant paintings attributed to him (e.g., Palace coll.; Freer Gall., Washington) show considerable stylistic differences. Also attributed to him is an early treatise on landscape painting entitled Pi-fa-chi ("An Account of Brush Method"), which consists partially of a discussion between a young man (presumably the artist) and an old sage. In a polished and beautiful, but often somewhat obscure literary style it states the ideals of the early landscapists, and for the first time discusses the Chinese attitude toward nature in relation to landscape painting. The artist, we learn, does not seek a true likeness to nature, because he considers the external form superficial. He strives rather to render the essence of nature — not so much the landscape which surrounds him as the forces which created the universe and give it its constantly changing appearance. It is not surprising that the author favors the "unconventional" painters, who had in other themes already turned their backs on mere visual reality.

Ching Hao was a northern Chinese, and so was his younger contemporary Kuan T'ung, pupil of a certain P'i Hung, but apparently influenced by the older master too. The only work which may with some confidence be tentatively attributed to Kuan T'ung is a landscape Ford across the Mountain Stream in the Palace collection. The whole composition is dominated by a high, steep mountain in the center, composed of piled-up rocks and crowned by forests. At the left, mountain ranges disappear into mists in the distance. In the foreground two waterfalls come together and pour into a broad stream which stretches out to the right. This method of connecting background and foreground was later to become a cliché usually connected with the so-called "high distance" composition scheme, in which the eye of the spectator wanders from the

flat foreground into high soaring mountains. The artist has carefully built up the structure of the rocks with solid and firm brush strokes, in all shades of gray and black, and has created a well-planned arrangement of trees and shrubs. A few sketchily painted houses and a man with a donkey stress the grandeur of the landscape.

To judge from the few surviving works, a contemporary painter, Kuo Chung-shu, seems to have produced landscapes in which architectural elements played a much more prominent role. A copy after this master (Osaka Municipal Mus.) represents a minutely drawn imperial palace with many of the smallest architectural details. The large buildings do not, however, seem to fit into the landscape rising up behind it.

*Ceramics.* The 10th century seems to have been a period of great activity in the manufacture of the famous Yüeh-yao. To judge from a number of pieces which can be dated by inscriptions, the production of some of the kilns at Shang-lin-hu and Yü-wang-miao (see CHINA, *Chekiang*) continued until the end of the 10th century. The Yüeh-yao kilns were within the domain of the kings of Wu and Yüeh, prior to their defeat by the Sung armies in 978, and from their reign dates the famous "private color ware" (*pi-sê-yao*) mentioned in later literary sources. It may have been the defeat of this local dynasty which caused the center of ceramic production to move to the district of Lung-ch'üan (also in Chekiang), where the famous Sung celadons were later made. (See CERAMICS.)

THE SUNG DYNASTY (960–1279). The first emperor of the Sung dynasty, who reunited China, was still unable to extend his authority over all the territories which had belonged to the sphere of direct Chinese influence. Parts of Shansi and the part of Hopei surrounding Peking had already fallen into the hands of the Khitans, whose rulers had presumed to call themselves equal to the emperor of China and who had established their own dynasty (Liao) in 907. The Chinese barely managed to withstand the Khitan attack upon their capital (Kaifeng) in 1004, but one year later a treaty was concluded between the Chinese and the Khitans which ushered in a century of lasting peace along the northern borders. In the Ordos region and Kansu, however, the Chinese were compelled to concede territory to the Buddhist Hsi-hsia (Tanguts). In 1126, the Jurchen, who had replaced the Khitans along the northern borders after defeating the Liao a few years earlier, overran large parts of northern China. Emperor Hui-tsung was carried off to Manchuria with most of his family, the capital was pillaged, and soon a large-scale exodus to the south began; there, in Hangchow, a member of the imperial family ascended the throne, safe behind the natural barrier of the Yangtze River where the cavalry of the invaders was at a disadvantage. After several abortive attempts to regain the lost territories the dynasty accepted the inevitable, leaving large tracts of northern China in the hands of the "barbarians." When in the early 13th century the Mongols appeared at the Chinese frontiers, the Sung dynasty committed the imprudence of conspiring with the Mongols against the Jurchen. The Jurchen were defeated in 1234, but this did not save the Chinese from a fate even worse; after years of tenacious resistance they had to surrender the whole of their territory to the Mongols.

The cultural history of the Sung dynasty is as splendid as its political history was tragic. The leaders of wrangling political factions at court, as well as the emperor Hui-tsung himself, were great calligraphers, painters, and poets. Although the fall of Kaifeng meant the loss of the large imperial collections of paintings, calligraphs, and ancient bronzes, the traditions transplanted to more southerly soil survived and even thrived remarkably. In the north, although the invaders celebrated their victory by throwing the imperial collection of ancient bronzes into the ponds of the palace, they were not as barbarian as they have sometimes been depicted by Chinese historians. The artistic activity which had not been directly connected with the Sung court went on almost without interruption, though sometimes on a more modest scale. Both the Khitans and the Jurchen favored Buddhism in a way com-

parable to that of the ancient T'o-pa of the Wei dynasty. The Khitans developed a culture which, in spite of many elements derived from Chinese prototypes, had a pronounced independent character, especially in pottery and architecture. Perhaps the most convincing argument against their barbarism is their remarkable sculpture in wood, which we have always regarded as purely Chinese, but which developed in the northern territories occupied by the Khitans and Jurchen.

*Painting*. The great masters of the Chinese landscape in the early Sung period (PLS. 262, 269) followed in the footsteps of the previous generation. Li Ch'eng, Hsü Tao-ning, Yen Wên-kuei, Tung Yüan, Chü-jan, and Fan K'uan are the most famous names of this period. For posterity, Tung Yüan and Chü-jan may have been of most importance, but Fan K'uan was regarded by most of his contemporaries as the greatest of them all.

The works of Li Ch'eng (active second half of 10th cent.) and his follower Hsü Tao-ning are clearly related. Autumn and winter were their favorite seasons, and a cold, deserted, somber atmosphere often pervaded their paintings. In Li Ch'eng's work for the first time the warped and grotesquely shaped old pine trees descended from the distant mountains to take their place in the foreground; though snowy peaks were still the principal theme in some cases, elsewhere attention was concentrated almost entirely on these fantastic creations of nature, which were to fascinate painters from that time on. In Hsü Tao-ning's work these pine trees appear again. His sparsely wooded mountains have a gently sloping profile which sharpens near the top. The repetition of this landscape element in the long hand scroll *Fishing in a Mountain Stream* (PL. 262) produces an undulating horizon and mountain shapes that look like a row of fishing nets drying on poles. In a hand scroll in the Yūrinkan Museum (Kyoto) a limitless panorama is suggested by mists in a light-gray ink tint, which hide the distant mountains from sight. Instead of the bulky monumentality represented in the mountains of Ching Hao and Kuan T'ung, who adopted the "high distance" scheme (see above), this master chose the so-called "level distance" method, which gives the impression that we are overlooking a distant mountain landscape from the top of a range on the other side of a river; the river is often represented in the foreground to facilitate a smooth transition from one part of the composition to the next. It is supposed that Li Ch'eng was the first master to adopt this type of "perspective," which was admirably suited to the long horizontal hand scroll; however, in those of his works handed down through copies no composition of this type is to be seen.

The last of the Sung masters in the north was Fan K'uan (active till about 1030). In two works in the Palace collection attributed to him, a high mountain dominates the composition. This required a clear structural elaboration of the mountain formations, which Fan K'uan achieved by covering the weather-beaten surface with dots of greatly varying density. These two works are so similar in composition that we must probably regard them as two versions of an original, or as a copy and an original. Yet the great differences in brushwork suggest that, in at least some early copies, only a rough imitation of the original composition has been preserved — and that any conclusions about the stylistic peculiarities of each of these masters must be only hypothetical.

Two masters who influenced the work of the later literati painters were Tung Yüan (second half of 10th cent.), and Chü-jan, a somewhat younger painter who followed his example. With these southerners, the landscape of southern China found its place in painting. Their critics tell us that their landscapes were built up of rough brush strokes which made their paintings seem most satisfactory if looked at from a certain distance. Especially successful is the effect which Tung Yüan created by means of clouds, which slip through the valleys between the high mountain ranges, thus strongly enhancing the illusion of depth and distance. A hand scroll attributed to him, the authorship of which has often been doubted, but which is of undeniably high quality, belongs to the Boston Museum of Fine Arts. This fragmentary work unites in one painting almost everything that the early landscapists of the previous century had tried to do. It demonstrates a perfect mastery of the brush which dispenses with superfluous or empty brush strokes, but which makes every stroke full of meaning. Using all the different shades from light gray to dark black which Chinese ink can produce (with only incidentally some faint colors) the artist combined the impressive steep mountain ranges, the wide expanse of water, and the horizon receding into misty vapors into a perfectly harmonious composition.

Chü-jan's style seems to have been somewhat less impressive and powerful, for his landscapes are imbued with a lovelier, softer atmosphere. The works attributed to him show a remarkable homogeneity of style, with mountains built up of many small, rounded, superimposed hills and a completely natural vegetation, ranging from clearly identifiable trees in the foreground to carefully spaced black dots in the background.

Kuo Hsi (ca. 1025–75) was evidently influenced by Li Ch'eng, but his work has strong individual qualities. Kuo Hsi is also one of the artists about whom we are best informed and was apparently one of the most interesting personalities. His works are as rare as those of the other masters, but his pronouncements on the ideals of landscape painters, which were compiled and edited by his son, give such an excellent description of his ideas and methods that we can almost visualize his paintings. The Palace collection contains several works, including one which is signed and bears a date corresponding to 1072; all show the pine trees which he had adopted from Li Ch'eng, but the composition and brushwork vary considerably, and it is almost impossible to decide which works reflect accurately the style of the master. Two important hand scrolls attributed to Kuo Hsi are in American collections: One is entitled *Clearing Autumn Skies over Mountains and Valleys* (Freer Gall., Washington), the other is a short hand scroll showing a pavilion surrounded by bare trees and set in a wide, open landscape with distant views (Coll. of John M. Crawford). Though neither work is signed, the paintings are of a quality which presupposes an artist of great capacities. The transition from delicate brush strokes to hazy washes, from dark colors in the foreground to light gray in the distant parts, and from high mountain ranges to wide plains and lakes is effortless and completely natural. The rendering of atmospheric effects is highly sensitive and romantic. His work, when compared with that of Hsü Tao-ning, who was also a follower of Li Ch'eng, lacks the almost supernatural visionary atmosphere and seems to be somewhat more realistic, imbued less with awe than with love of nature.

Kuo Hsi's ideas were certainly not revolutionary, but the notes which were compiled and edited by his son constitute the most important of the early treatises, and the clearest expression of what J. F. Cahill has labeled the "primary concept" of Chinese painting. Although the early treatises differ on many points, and the abstruse and mystical terminology often makes it difficult to decide what is meant (see CRITICISM), the general idea which underlies their opinions seems to have been roughly shared by all. The use of traditional forms, composition formulas, and brush techniques, which may sometimes have been disastrous for mediocre artists but never enslaved China's greatest masters, was almost universally accepted.

There gradually occurred, however, a change in the ideas about the function and the meaning of painting. These new ideas, which may be referred to collectively as the "secondary concept," were born in a coterie of artists of the Northern Sung period, who all belonged to the intellectual elite of China, and among whom such versatile artistic personalities as Huang T'ing-chien, Su Shih, and Mi Fei (Mi Fu) were the most creative. The artistic expression of these new ideals took form in the so-called "literati painting," first called *shih-ta-fu-hua* ("gentleman painting"), but now commonly known by its later name *wên-jên-hua* (see below). Some of these concepts were taken over from theories about the art of calligraphy, with which these artists were intimately familiar. For example, it was a commonly accepted idea that the artist could express

his emotions in the abstract forms of separate strokes or characters and that the spectator, in turn, could read in calligraphic writing the true character of the artist. Taken over by painters, this led to the theory that the quality of expression in a picture is not so much determined by the artist's response to the object as by his personality, and that there need not be a connection between the expressive and representational content of a work of art. This new stress on the personality of the artist, and the gradual change in ideas which occurred, can best be demonstrated by the shift of meaning which seems to have taken place in the expression *ch'i-yün* ("spirit resonance") — a term used by art critics ever since Hsieh Ho had coined it some centuries earlier. Although the exact meaning of this term has been variously explained, it is clear that in the early texts it is used to describe a quality of the object to be represented, whereas now it seems to denote a quality inherent in the artist himself.

It is hardly surprising that artists who regarded the expression of the personality as of primary importance put the technique of painting in second place. For this they were severely attacked by their opponents, and some of this criticism has survived to the present day. The literati painters have been described as "arrogant" because of their air of haughtiness and as "dilettantes" because they painted for pleasure, not for a living.

The early literati painters were primarily calligraphers who merely tried to lift painting to the same level of artistic individual expression which calligraphy and poetry had earlier attained. To what extent they were able to achieve their lofty aims is difficult to determine, because few of the early works have been preserved. A favorite theme, one which began at this time to play a role of great importance in Chinese painting, was the bamboo. The bamboo was a symbol of the ideals of the literati: the regularity of its joints, its hollowness ("empty soul," a Taoist ideal), and its resilience were associated with the noblest characteristics of the true gentleman. The silhouette of the bamboo, drawn in strong brush strokes reminiscent of calligraphic techniques, became the specialty of many literati painters. The bamboos of Su Shih (Su Tung-p'o, 1063-1101), who followed the style of Wen T'ung (second half of 11th cent.), were highly praised by his friends, but no representative authentic specimen seems to have survived.

Mi Fei (q.v., 1052-1107), or Mi Fu, was one of the first of the true literati painters to paint landscapes. According to his own statement he did so only during the last seven years of his life, and not one authentic work seems to have survived. He adopted the "unconventional" technique of building up mountains by means of thick dots and splashes. His style was often imitated, first of all by his own son, Mi Yu-jên (1086-1165), and we therefore have a general idea of what his works must have looked like. Of Mi Fei's writings, several have been handed down, in which he is revealed as a poet of little more than mediocre talent, but as a connoisseur of surprising astuteness and a critic with as sharp a tongue as China has probably ever known. Although in later sources his many connections with the imperial collections are repeatedly mentioned, it is extremely doubtful whether he was ever fully appreciated in court circles. His deprecating comments about ancient and contemporary masters who were greatly in vogue in his lifetime, and especially his sarcastic remarks about the small number of existing authentic paintings by certain ancient masters to whom dozens of paintings in the imperial collections were attributed, seem to indicate that his taste differed considerably from that of most of his contemporaries. In the cultural climate of the Northern Sung period the spirit of the *wên-jên-hua* could hardly thrive. Mi Fei's genius as a calligrapher was universally recognized, but none of his paintings entered the imperial collections, and not before the last part of the Yüan period did the landscape painting of the literati become generally admired.

Already in earlier times Chinese court painters had been brought together in institutes known as Hua-yüan ("Academy of Painting"), where they could maintain contact with each other and with their imperial patrons. In this respect the Sung dynasty followed the example of the provincial courts

of the period of the Five Dynasties, but the great interest displayed by some of the Sung emperors in this institution considerably augmented its importance. To the Imperial Academy of the Sung court belonged a great number of artists, graded into a hierarchy of several ranks. In establishing the criteria for admission and promotion the opinion of the emperor played an important part. Especially during the reign (1101-26) of Emperor Hui-tsung, who was an artist of great talent himself, the imperial influence upon the work of the academicians must have been a decisive factor.

The style created by Huang Ch'üan, who had come to Kaifeng from Szechwan at the beginning of the Sung period, for many years remained authoritative for painters of flowers and birds. The more dynamic and spontaneous style of his southern Chinese rival Hsü Hsi (see above, *Five Dynasties*), with its strong calligraphic contours, could not maintain the prestige it had enjoyed before the Sung period. Yet the decorative, naturalistic, polychrome style of painting which now prevailed was not of such orthodox character as to remain unaffected by change. (The lack of a sufficient number of authentic works makes almost any attempt to determine the stylistic development extremely hazardous.) Chao Ch'ang, an artist from Szechwan of the early 11th century, seems to have undergone the influence of both Hsü Hsi and his son. In the eyes of the artists of the Academy he remained an outsider, but he was to exert a strong influence upon later masters. I Yüan-chi, who is famous for his paintings of monkeys, never was attached to the Academy, but was called to the capital (ca. 1064-67) to decorate the walls of a palace building. According to a malicious anecdote told by Mi Fei, he was poisoned by the academicians, who were jealous of his talents. Within the Academy Ts'ui Po, who was appointed during the reign of Sheng-tsung (1068-85), and his pupil Wu Yüan-yü seem to have set the style. Of neither artist have important authentic works been preserved, but some echo of their style may perhaps be found in the work of Emperor Hui-tsung, who studied with Wu Yüan-yü.

It is only logical that later Chinese artists should have extolled the painting genius of Hui-tsung since he was the reigning monarch. The works which bear his signature are comparatively numerous, and it is generally thought that at least a few of them may be authentic. These are of such importance that the eulogies of later critics seem fully justified. The works which have been accepted as authentic by several art historians are painted in two different styles. The first group consists of delicate, minutely drawn polychrome paintings on silk representing birds, some without ink contours (as in the work of the younger Hsü), others with a combination of thin contours and bright colors. The best-known works represent a dove seated on a peach-blossom branch (Inoue Coll., dated 1107), a quail and narcissus (Asano Coll., possibly a school work), and a five-colored parakeet on an apricot tree (Mus. of Fine Arts, Boston). The latter was probably not painted by the emperor himself, but the inscription in his thin and elegant handwriting seems to be authentic. These paintings bear witness to a careful study of ornithology (although one sometimes gets the impression that stuffed rather than living birds served as the source of inspiration). They have an atmosphere of distinction and polychrome finesse, but there is also an unmistakably static element in them. Among the works attributed to Emperor Hui-tsung which are possibly authentic, but less certain, there are a number of monochrome bird paintings. Here the somewhat rigid and refined immobility of his polychrome paintings is replaced by a more dynamic conception. In the monochrome landscapes attributed to him, of which the autumn landscape in the Palace collection is the most convincing example, the brush technique and the composition are closely related to the works of such masters as Li Ch'eng and Kuo Hsi, although the traditional theme seems to be rendered with less poetic feeling; unfortunately, few of these works seem to have survived.

Another Northern Sung master was Li Kung-lin (1040-1106), better known as Li Lung-mien (q.v.), who enjoyed such a high reputation that Mi Fei says he dared to start painting

only after Li Lung-mien was incapacitated by rheumatism. Although Li Lung-mien belonged to the circle of the literati, he was the only one among them who was primarily, if not exclusively, a painter. Like Mi Fei, he filled various official posts, but he never rose to high office as Su Shih had done. With that eccentric connoisseur he also shared an interest in antiques, especially in ancient bronzes. In a time when the academic tendency was to suppress calligraphic contours, he revived the traditional T'ang style of monochrome outline drawing, and most of the works attributed to him are monochrome *pai-miao* ("contour") paintings, often on Buddhist themes. One of the few authentic masterpieces, representing five tribute horses, was lost during World War II. His great reputation was due to his Buddhist figure paintings.

The fall of the capital Kaifeng and the arrest and deportation of the emperor, followed by the occupation of northern China by the Jurchen, made its influence felt in all spheres of Chinese cultural life. Kao-tsung (1127–62), who established the "temporary" capital at Hangchow, made an energetic and successful effort to revive the Imperial Academy. Several painters went south and were reunited under imperial patronage. Some of these masters had already enjoyed a great reputation at the Northern Sung court, others were new members, some being descendants of former court painters.

The first director of the new Academy was Li T'ang (VI, PL. 81), who was already of advanced age when he was appointed and should consequently be regarded as a Northern Sung master. The only exactly dated work from his hand is a landscape in the Palace collection called *Pine Winds in Endless Valleys* (1124), which displays a striking resemblance to the work of the early landscape painter Fan K'uan. Along with the dotting technique of Fan K'uan, however, he developed a quite different brush technique known as "big-ax wrinkles," which gives his high mountains the stratified appearance of diagonally slanting layers of stone. The same technique is found in a pair of landscape paintings in the Daitokuji temple in Kyoto, on one of which a hidden authentic signature was rediscovered only a few years ago. These are probably the remaining half of a series representing the Four Seasons, and both have lost much of their compositional balance by later trimming. This drastic cutting may partly account for the absence of the imposing grandeur which characterizes the scroll in the Palace collection, but these two paintings are quite different also for other reasons: The influence of Fan K'uan and his dotting technique is altogether absent, and a more dynamic treatment is evident, especially in the crooked shapes of the trees and the rushing water. This may point to a somewhat later date. Li T'ang acquired a great reputation as a painter of water buffaloes and cowherds, a theme so common (cf. PL. 267) in the Southern Sung period that we may suppose it had a deeper meaning — possibly derived from Meditative Buddhism or Taoism — than appears at first glance. The same theme was painted by the Taoist monk Fan Tzǔ-min (13th cent.), e.g., in a long hand scroll in the Art Institute of Chicago.

Li Ti, like Li T'ang, was a court painter who had originally worked in the Northern Sung Academy. A pair of paintings in the Yamato Bunkakan Museum are perhaps the best of his works. Using ink, brown, white, and a little red, the painter created two variations on the theme "Home-coming in the Snow." The returning hunters, one carrying a rabbit and the other a pheasant, have been drawn to the smallest detail with a very fine brush; they form a striking contrast to the well-balanced landscape background with snow-covered trees. A painting of chickens (in the Hui-hua-kuan, Peking) shows even greater attention to such small details as the soft down; yet this miniature has been definitely lifted above the level of mere ornithological illustration by the natural movements of the birds, which have been admirably rendered. This trend toward a greater interest in movement is also visible in the work of other bird painters of the Southern Sung Academy, such as Sung Ju-chih.

Another academician who survived the transfer of the Academy was Li An-chung. His *Eagle Pursuing a Pheasant* (PL. 266), dated 1129, has a movement and a quality of suspense rarely found in academic bird paintings. An album leaf dating from before the transfer (Severance A. Millikin Coll., Cleveland) represents a landscape of autumn trees in the mists; it shows that the highly exact representation of birds could very well he combined with a much more romantic and visionary style in the landscape. The theme of domestic animals such as dogs and cats was the specialty of Mao I (ca. 1170), whose father Mao Sung had been a member of the Northern Sung Academy.

Generally speaking, the stylistic development of the themes of flowers, birds, and animals was not very spectacular during the Southern Sung dynasty. Quite the opposite is the case, however, in landscape painting. Here a new tendency, in which the members of the Ma family and the master Hsia Kuei played the most prominent role, came into being. It may have been influenced by the circumstance that the not very orthodox Li T'ang was the first to direct the Imperial Academy of Hangchow, for Ma Yüan, the greatest artist of the Ma family, was greatly indebted to this master. Perhaps also there was an infiltration of ideas from the "unconventional" schools such as those of the literati painters and the Ch'an monks, even though the various schools often led each a separate life. The style of landscape painting created by the Ma and Hsia school exerted its influence on many later orthodox painters, but it suffered a decline in prestige with the rise of literati painting. In Japan, however, the works of the Southern Sung Academy attracted the attention of collectors as early as the Ashikaga period and have since been avidly collected there.

Five generations of the Ma family served in the Imperial Academy of the Sung period. Ma Fèn — whose name will always, though probably incorrectly, be connected with the magnificent hand scroll *The Hundred Geese* (Honolulu Acad. of Arts) — was the first of this line. He served in Hui-tsung's Academy in the north until the fall of Kaifeng, and his son was a member of the Southern Sung Academy during the reign of Kao-tsung. Of the two sons of this master, Ma Kung-hsien and Ma Shih-jung, the first is by far the best known. His signature appears on a painting in the Nanzenji temple at Kyoto (PL. 264) which represents a discussion between the poet Li Po and the hermit Yao-shan. The most striking feature of this painting is not the gesticulating figures by the table, but the huge pine trees under which the table is placed. In the sharply drawn, almost zigzag branches, projected over the wide-open space of the background, we notice the first example of a technique for which the school was to become renowned. Ma Shih-jung was a little-known master, but his son Ma Yüan is considered the greatest artist of the family, only rivaled by his son Ma Lin.

Ma Yüan (q.v.) became a member of the Imperial Academy during the reign of Kuan-tsung (1190–94) and remained a member until his death about fifty or sixty years later. Although he took Li T'ang as an example, he must have undergone also the influence of his father and uncle. In his work we notice a new type of composition which, although certainly not the artistic invention of this master, from now on begins to assume greater importance. Departing from the classical schemes of landscape painting, he concentrates his rocks, pine trees, and figures in the lower part and toward the side of the picture. Thus the accent is put completely on one side, and a wide space is created on the other. Yet the composition is never awkwardly lopsided; angular, horizontal pine branches traversing the empty upper area bring it into balance again. The rendering of space is even more accentuated when a seated human figure is placed at the foot of the picture. A perfect example of this type of composition is *Scholar Contemplating the Moon* (PL. 265); the placing of the figure and the direction of the scholar's gaze almost automatically lead the attention of the spectator into the broad expanse of space. An earlier picture, formerly attributed to Emperor Hui-tsung, but now generally considered a late Northern Sung academic picture (Konchiin, Kyoto), shows the same type of composition in reverse. In this case the gazing figure's attention is fixed on two birds high up in the sky. (The birds are so small that they have sometimes been overlooked by scholars studying

reproductions.) This landscape, together with a companion piece, demonstrates that Ma Yüan's "one-sided" composition scheme and his placing of figures was taken over from earlier academic painters. In the structure of rocks and cliffs Ma Yüan often shows his indebtedness to Li T'ang, but he painted the more distant mountain ranges only as light-gray silhouettes, with little or no indication of structure, thus strengthening the illusion of distance and depth.

It is said that Ma Yüan's son Ma Lin (PL. 270) was only a mediocre imitator of his father's style and that the father sometimes signed his works with the name of the son in order to enhance the latter's prestige. Such stories often occur in Chinese sources and it is difficult to say how reliable they are. But even if this story be true, there is no point in trying to detect among Ma Lin's signed works some which might be attributed to his father, because the influence is evident in any case. In the catalogue *Kundaikan Sayuchōki* (ca. 1500) Ma Lin is placed in a higher category than his illustrious father, probably because the Japanese compilers happened to have seen better works by him. Whatever the reason for this somewhat surprising classification, the number of paintings purported to have been painted by Ma Lin and handed down in Japanese collections is considerable. The stylistic differences among them, and especially between works in Chinese and in Japanese collections, seem to indicate that a considerable number of attributions are incorrect. Ma Yüan must have had a great number of academic pupils, and here, as in so many other cases, later connoisseurs have attributed most of their unsigned works to the two great masters.

Ma Lin's *Evening Landscape* (PL. 270) bears an inscription of two lines of poetry written by Emperor Li-tsung (1254), an early instance of a poetic inscription on an academic painting. The painting is an excellent example of a style in which depth and distance have been effectively suggested with the utmost economy of pictorial means. The mountain range merges imperceptibly into the wide expanse of water, which has been summarily indicated by a few wavy lines in the foreground. Four swallows skim over the gently rolling waves, and the far horizon is hidden in a thin evening mist colored red by the setting sun. Along with Ma Yüan's *Angler in a Boat* (Nat. Mus., Tokyo) this landscape represents the pinnacle of what might be called the "pineless" style of the Ma family; an extremely subtle suggestivity has been reached with simple brushwork and a quiet restraint.

The only artistic personality of equal standing in the academy was Hsia Kuei (q.v., ca. 1200, PL. 263). The two great painters Ma Yüan and Hsia Kuei have several things in common, as might be expected of contemporaries and fellow-academicians — for example, the influence of Li T'ang (seen in the structure of Hsia Kuei's rocks) and the use of the one-sided composition. In Hsia Kuei's work, also, two different styles may be observed. The horizontal scroll *Clear View over Rivers and Mountains* exemplifies a style in which the brushwork is extremely detailed, except for the use of powerful "big-ax wrinkles" in the rock formations. Steep cliffs and angular rocks, wooded with beautifully composed forests, alternate naturally with rivers and lakes spanned by bridges and overshadowed by the characteristic "Ma-Hsia" pine trees. The great variation in the landscape offers an almost complete compendium of the pictorial elements of this school. This painting seems much more convincing than the celebrated *Ten Thousand Miles of the Yangtze River* in the Palace collection, which is now considered to be an excellent work in the master's style. The *Landscape in a Rainstorm* (formerly Kawasaki Coll.) represents the master at his best in a quite different style, which is characterized by a more fluid, sweeping brush technique, a much more generous use of ink, and a greatly simplified structure. The one-sided composition scheme is no longer followed strictly: the mountains in the background, indicated by a few wet strokes, have been placed in the center of the picture. The wildly sweeping trees and the small figure on the bridge with an umbrella pressed against his body create an extremely vivid impression of a rainstorm. The heavy black blotches, the vigorous outlines of the trees, a few swift long strokes, and the richness in tone values make this work one of the best examples of Chinese monochrome painting. A comparison with the rendering of the same theme by Ma Yüan (Seikadō Foundation, Tokyo) shows that the two painters could sometimes be very different.

There existed in Southern Sung China yet another school of painting which was saved from utter oblivion only by the interest of Japanese travelers. This is the painting which flourished in the monasteries of Meditative Buddhism (Chin., Ch'an; Jap., Zen). It has been highly appreciated by Japanese art historians of all periods and has in recent times received much attention in the West. The works of this school are often regarded as the greatest paintings in the history of Chinese art. As is so often the case, this new school of artists, most of whom were Buddhist monks, was not an abrupt phenomenon. The early "unconventional" painters, such as Shih-k'o (see above) and the Northern Sung literati painters, had prepared the ground for it.

The connection between the religious and artistic ideas of these Ch'an monks is not always as obvious as many authors have taken it to be, but there are some characteristics which both spheres of thought seem to have in common. The spontaneous and almost simultaneous expression in painting of a sudden inspiration reminds us of the suddenness of the Enlightenment which the Ch'an monks sought to attain. The absence of a Buddhist pantheon depicted according to canonical prescriptions is conspicuous; in its place we notice a predilection for portraits and for historical as well as legendary figures associated with the Ch'an sect. Such everyday subjects as plants, fruits, and animals, which are also frequent, are quite in keeping with the simple way of life of the Ch'an monks. There is also a certain resemblance between their abstruse way of transmitting their spiritual experiences and their style of painting. Neither relies on a detailed rational description, but chooses instead to hint rather than to demonstrate.

Ch'an painting does not have a uniform style. Some paintings, especially the landscapes, owe much to the influence of Mi Fei and Mi Yu-jên. And, just as the academicians came to adopt certain characteristics of the literati school, the "unconventional" Ch'an painters were not completely untouched by influences from the Academy. Actually, the first great Ch'an painter, Liang K'ai (q.v.), made his reputation as a member of the Academy, from which he later resigned to live in the temple Liu-t'ung-ssŭ near Hangchow, which was the artistic center of the Ch'an school of painting. During the period in which he worked in the Academy he was strongly influenced by the *pai-miao* ("contour") style of Li Lung-mien. This influence is quite evident in his most "academic" masterwork, representing Śākyamuni returning from the mountains (private coll., Japan), which was painted for the emperor when Liang K'ai was still a member of the Academy. The landscape setting is quite elaborate in comparison with his later works, and the use of red for the Buddha's clothes and a flesh-colored paint for the bare parts of the body, as well as the carefully drawn folds of the garment, still have an academic flavor. On the other hand, the portrait of the emaciated Indian ascetic, lost in meditation, has a dramatic quality lacking in academic painting. Completely in accord with the philosophy of Ch'an, the Buddha is no longer the remote, supernatural being into whom he had been transformed during centuries of Buddhist painting, but has become again a historical person of the highest spiritual level, whose exemplary life can be a personal example. It is almost as if the claim of the Ch'an Buddhists that their doctrine had been handed down orally directly from the Buddha himself has in this painting a pictorial parallel.

In Liang K'ai's supposedly later works we notice the so-called "abbreviated brushwork" (*chien-pi*), a method in which the number of strokes is drastically reduced, as in grass script (see CALLIGRAPHY). This method is applied most effectively in the portrait of the T'ang poet Li Po (IV, PL. 282). A few vigorous contour lines indicate the long robe, and a few dark strokes, forming a vivid contrast with the gray tones of the contours, indicate the feet, beard, and hair of the poet. The artist has completely eliminated the surroundings, and the brushwork

expresses a refined, poetic quiet. These works demonstrate that Liang K'ai was certainly one of China's greatest artists. He was a pupil of the Ch'an master Wu-chun, who was an amateur painter of probably mediocre quality, but a great calligrapher.

To judge from his works, almost all of which have been handed down to us in Japanese collections, Mu-ch'i was one of the most versatile Ch'an artists. He painted figures, animals, flowers, and fruits, as well as landscapes. Three of his greatest masterpieces are the paintings representing monkeys, a crane, and a white-robed Kuan-yin (Daitokuji, Kyoto). The restrained brush technique, totally removed from the impetuousness of the "ink-play" paintings, shows traces of the influence of the academic styles, especially in the way the rocks have been rendered. It is not certain whether these three paintings originally belonged together; if they did, the grouping of two pictures of animals with an image of Kuan-yin may have a symbolical meaning. In any case the three pictures form a perfect harmony, with the background mist facilitating the transition from one painting to the other. The animals have been depicted in characteristic poses, the crane proudly walking from the bamboo bush, the monkeys clinging together on a branch in the chilly mist. The Kuan-yin has been depicted strictly in accordance with the iconographic rules of the period, which called for a white robe. The robe is painted in soft, fluid lines and left blank, thus creating a contrast with the various tones of gray which must have been much stronger when the painting had not yet darkened. The tree on which the monkeys are sitting reminds us of some of the works of Liang K'ai. The same holds true for the magnificent *Myna Bird on a Pine Tree* (Coll. Matsudaira), which may, however, be the work of a pupil.

Although Liang K'ai and Mu-ch'i are by far the best-known masters, many other painters worked in a similar technique and style. Of some the names are known, e.g. Lo-ch'uang, Li Ch'üeh, and Yü-chien (a name used by two masters). Because almost all of the existing works have been handed down in Japanese collections, and the Ch'an masters were often imitated there, it is not only difficult to distinguish between the different Ch'an masters, but it is sometimes almost impossible to determine whether a painting is Chinese or Japanese.

Apart from the paintings of birds, flowers, and figures, some Ch'an masters also excelled in landscape painting. Whereas Liang K'ai's landscapes are influenced by the work of such early masters as Fan K'uan, Mu-ch'i's landscapes show strong influences of *wên-jên-hua* painting, especially that of Mi Yu-jên. Very popular was the theme "Eight Views of the Rivers Hsiao and Hsiang," which represents the southern Chinese landscape in different seasons. A long hand scroll by Mu-ch'i treating this theme was cut up into eight parts, four of which have been preserved. These are misty panoramas in which the sketchy, roughly drawn landscape elements, reduced to a few strokes and blotches, are connected into one harmonious, organic unity by wide expanses of water and fog. The spontaneous brushwork creates an atmosphere of gentle charm, whereas the variations of Yü-chien on the same theme were painted with a much more impulsive stroke, which makes a rougher, wilder impression.

The unconventional ideas and techniques of the Ch'an painters left little or no imprint on the work of later generations of Chinese artists. It enjoyed great prestige only among a small coterie which produced no great poets or statesmen to impress the Chinese cultural elite. Although the tradition of "ink play" continued far into the Yüan period, the Ch'an masters were soon almost completely forgotten, and it was only in Japanese art (q.v.) that they exerted a great influence.

*Sculpture.* See below, *Later sculpture.*

*Ceramics.* The new shapes, decorative techniques, and glazes which characterize the magnificent Sung ceramic art did not suddenly come into being without roots in the past. The technical proficiency which enabled the Chinese to produce a gray porcelaneous stoneware and white translucent porcelain had already come to full development. Celadon, in all its variations,

is obviously derived from the Yüeh-yao, which had been produced for centuries. And one may presume — on the basis of the great quantity of black-glazed pottery shards found in such Yüeh-yao kilns as Tê-ch'ing (see CHINA, *Chekiang*) — that the ceramics subsumed under the vague collective name *temmoku* also had a history of respectable length behind them.

The Sung style in ceramics, i.e., that of the porcelain, pottery, and stoneware the beauty of which is determined primarily by the form and the color of a monochrome glaze, may well have continued locally until far into the Ming period; however, as a whole it may be clearly distinguished from that of the earlier T'ang and also from the later developments under the Ming (characterized by the triumph of underglaze cobalt blue and a series of completely new shapes). Various Sung types, such as the *mei-p'ing* vase (see CERAMICS), survived the Yüan period to acquire a place in the Ming repertory.

The great reputation of Sung ceramics in Europe has given rise, incorrectly, to the belief that in China as well this form of art was regarded as one of the most important. Beside the noble arts of painting and calligraphy, the Chinese acknowledge no other form of equivalent artistic level. Although the Sung emperors reserved the loveliest products of a few kilns for themselves, the potter and his art were held only in low regard, and the extensive Sung literature includes no works in which ceramics are viewed as a form of art.

The many types of Sung ceramics are usually classified by names which for the most part indicate the provenance of the type concerned. For some types both the ancient designation and the precise identity and origin are established, but for others this is not the case. The methods employed to identify the various types diverge greatly. The Chinese, with designations which they have used traditionally, have never chosen to give a sharply defined technical description of any particular type at all. English scholars, like Sir Percival David, attempt primarily to reconcile the contradictory descriptions and nomenclature found in Chinese literature and to connect them with types in Western collections. Japanese scholars have placed the investigation of the kiln sites before everything else and have come sometimes to remarkably divergent conclusions — for example, with regard to the so-called Ju-yao (Ju ware). The very mixed remains frequently found in the kiln sites seem to indicate a danger in restricting the provenance of a particular type to a particular locality. After the fall of Kaifeng in 1126, the center of gravity moved southward from the great flourishing centers of north China, and it is not always clear to what extent the north Chinese forms survived the transplantation. The ceramic types originally associated respectively with north (see Liao examples, PLS. 169, 248) and south display marked differences.

Certain types of Sung ceramics have no applied decoration of any sort and thus the pieces owe their beauty entirely to the combination of form and glaze. This is the case, among others, with the imperial (*kuan*) types, with the Chün-yao (Chün ware), where bright red spots in a lavender-colored glaze form a striking effect, and also with the imperial variant of this porcelain called Ju-yao (PL. 166) by Sir Percival David. The light crackle effect of David's Ju-yao reappears in the Kuan-yao of Hangchow in much stronger degree, on pieces which, again, are otherwise left undecorated. Surpassing the virtuosity of even the Chün-yao, if that is possible, are the glaze effects of the Chien-yao and the Kian (Chi-an) Temmoku, as well as the somewhat heterogeneous group of brown-black glazes included under the name "Honan Temmoku" (PL. 167). These glazes, which later admirers have called "hare's-fur," "partridge-feather," or "oil-spot," are among the most subtle and most famous decorative techniques of the Sung potters; they later played a decisive role in the development of Japanese ceramics.

In a number of other types, generally entirely monochrome, use is made of incised, molded, pressed, or engraved decoration (PLS. 166, 259, 260) which is visible on the surface through the glaze. These techniques, which are combined in all possible ways, depend for their effect on the adaptation of the decorative elements to the shape of the piece and on the strength

of the linear rendition. Perhaps the loveliest combinations are to be found on the incised Ting-yao. For instance, in the well-known type of plate with a design of ducks by the water's edge, although the birds are depicted in a stereotyped and continuously repeated posture side by side, the carefully engraved wave motif and the strongly drawn lines of the waving reeds give these pieces a restrained distinction which, regardless of the distance which separates the potter and the painter, reminds us of the bird paintings of the Imperial Academy.

The Ting-yao and the Ying-ch'ing (or so-called "Ch'ing-pai") clearly demonstrate two different conceptions of decoration. In the one (frequently incised) a very spacious decoration based upon beautiful, powerfully drawn lines prevails; in the other (frequently with molded decoration) there is a tendency toward filling the whole available surface (a *horror vacui*). In the latter it is the arrangement of the thickly packed decorative elements, such as flower motifs, birds, and geometric patterns, which determines the beauty of the design. Both conceptions outlived the Sung dynasty and the rise of a new style, and the old decorative patterns turn up again transposed into other techniques.

No other single type of Sung ceramic ware displays such amazing versatility as the Tz'ŭ-chou-yao (Tz'ŭ-chou or Tz'ŭ Chou ware, PLS. 166, 169, 258–260). The slip applied to this ware was not only utilized as a background for a painted decoration, but could also be partly cut away so as to obtain a pattern in color contrasting with the slip. This technique, designated in English by the Italian term *sgraffito*, was applied by the potters of Tz'ŭ-chou in an extraordinarily effective manner. It is characterized primarily by strongly stylized motifs. The quickly painted, sketchlike designs of written characters, plant and flower motifs, and human and animal figures that appear in the Tz'ŭ-chou-yao form in many respects the transition from the Sung to the Ming style. Tz'ŭ-chou ware also showed the first signs of a development which later dominated the entire picture of Chinese porcelain decoration, i.e., the use of painted enamel colors over the glaze — at least if the inscription on a piece in the National Museum in Tokyo dated 1201 is authentic. It was quite some time before this technique was generally accepted, and it was preceded by painted decoration in blue under the glaze. With the establishment of this decorative technique in the 14th century, the Sung style gradually lost ground and was finally superseded altogether.

Some types of Sung ceramics, such as the Chien-yao, seem to have been manufactured solely to serve for the drinking of powdered tea, which was then in general use in China, and consequently are to be found only as tea bowls. Other types present a great variety of forms, particularly the Honan Temmoku and the Tz'ŭ-chou-yao.

The overwhelming richness of forms in the Sung ceramics includes very few shapes borrowed from bronzes, which is indeed astonishing in view of the great interest which the connoisseurs of this period bestowed upon the ancient art of bronze casting. In some cases there is a clear correspondence in shape to be perceived between silverwork and ceramic ware; if imitation was involved, it is more likely to have been on the part of the silversmith than on that of the potter. Examples of metal work are shown in PLS. 274, 277. (See CERAMICS.)

*Architecture.* Probably because northern China was spared the devastation of the 19th-century Taiping rebellion, a small number of early wooden temple buildings have been preserved there which give us an excellent idea of the architecture under the Khitans (Liao dynasty) and the Jurchen (Chin). All secular buildings of the Sung period have long since been destroyed by fire or in war, and the number of Sung temple buildings is small, especially in the south, where the main hall of the Pao-shêng-ssŭ at Soochow (1013) was one of the very few survivals before it was demolished a few decades ago. Perhaps further investigations may bring to light other Sung buildings which have so far remained unnoticed. One notable recent discovery is the main hall of the Pao-kuo-ssŭ at Yü-yao (Chekiang), which probably dates from 1013 and which was at any rate built not later than 1102.

The roofs of all these buildings vary considerably in shape. As a rule they are not hipped, but are a cross between a hipped and a gabled roof, with the lower part of the gable ends covered by a pent roof and connected with the lower part of the main roof. Most roofs show a slight curve upward at the eaves. This curvature, which could be emphasized by carving the beams, is a characteristic which appears in its most exaggerated form in southern China.

The bracketing inside the buildings as well as below the eaves reached its full development during the Sung period, and the extremely complicated, but well-conceived and functional bracketing systems of the surviving buildings bear testimony to the perfection of the carpenter's craft. Whenever necessary

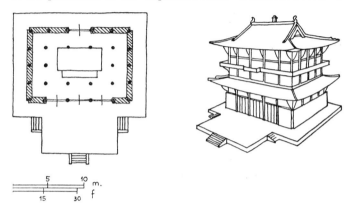

Kuan-yin hall of the temple Tu-lo-ssŭ, at Chi-hsien, Hopei (984), plan and perspective (*after Sickman and Soper*).

the double slanting bracket arm, ending in beautifully carved beaks, was used. Whereas the earlier technique, used for example in the Fo-kuang-ssŭ at Wu-t'ai-shan, left the inner end of the slanting bracket arm abutting the beams and girders and hidden by a ceiling, the bracket arms were now transformed into a true cantilever beam, so completely integrated into the beautiful structure that it could be shown. The weight of the bracketing, sometimes almost half the height of the columns, and especially that of the intercolumnar brackets later developed, called for a T section in the beam of the column head. This was an invention of the Sung period and seems to be found only in the north. The earliest buildings of the period still show a clear difference between the brackets of the column heads and the intercolumnar brackets, but this distinction gradually disappeared. In the end (after the Yüan period) the brackets, closely arranged and identical, together formed a kind of decorative cornice without structural function.

An important complex of buildings, several of which date from the Sung period, is still to be found on the grounds of the temple Lung-hsing-ssŭ in Chêng-ting (see CHINA, *Hopei*). The oldest well-preserved building there is the Mani hall (Mo-ni-tien), unusual in that it has an entrance with a hip-and-gable roof on each of its four sides. Like the main hall of the temple at Yü-yao it is a square building of seven by seven bays. It may date from before 969.

The small gate (Shan-mên) and the Kuan-yin hall of the temple Tu-lo-ssŭ at Chi-hsien (Hopei) can be dated 984 and are the earliest preserved buildings built under the patronage of the Khitans. The two-storied Kuan-yin-ko has a balcony on the second story, below which a pent roof shields the walls of the ground floor. The bracketing of the hip-roofed gate and the light pent roof is simple. The whole structure is built around a huge statue of Kuan-yin, more than 45 ft. high. Below the eaves of the hip-and-gable roof which covers the whole building the bracketing is much more intricate. It includes the double slanting bracket arm and is in many ways reminiscent of that of the Fo-kuang-ssŭ.

Several other temple buildings bear witness to the religious fervor of the Khitans: The main hall of the Fêng-kuo-ssŭ at Yi-hsien (see CHINA, *Manchuria*), dating from 1020, is the only survival in Manchuria; but in Tatung (see CHINA, *Shansi*), one

of the Liao capitals, there are several buildings of the Liao and Chin periods, including the Lower and Upper Hua-yen-ssŭ and some buildings of the P'u-ên-ssŭ (some ca. 1050, others a century later). Although there are many differences of architectural interest among these buildings, there was no marked

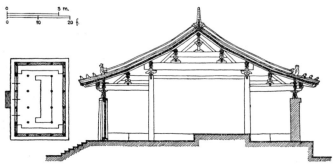

Hall of the lower temple of the Hua-yen-ssŭ, at Tatung, Shansi (Liao dynasty, 907–1125), plan and section (*after Sickman and Soper*).

development in style or technique after the Jurchen succeeded the Khitans.

A local southern Chinese style is that which received the rather misleading Japanese name of Tenjiku-yō or "Indian style." (The term, according to Ecke, is derived from the name of a mountain near Hangchow and has no connection with India.) Its most striking characteristic — one of several distinctive features — is the use of many superimposed projecting transverse brackets without the other elaborations commonly used in northern China. Hardly any wooden buildings of this style survive in China, but it became extremely popular in Japan, where a number of specimens still exist. Its main features were excellently suited for imitation in stone, as is demonstrated by the beautiful twin pagodas of Ch'üan-chou in Fukien.

The number of existing stone and masonry pagodas dating from the period of the Five Dynasties, the Sung dynasty, and the Liao and Chin periods is surprisingly large. Soper mentions a total of 60 to be associated with the native Chinese dynasties, and in the territory which was ruled by the Liao and Chin there are another 23. Some are called "Iron Pagodas" (T'ieh-t'a) after the color of their bricks; there are, however, three small Sung pagodas actually made of iron. Only one pagoda that of the temple Fo-kung-ssŭ at Ying-hsien (Shansi) is built entirely of wood. Some Japanese scholars, accepting a tradition which is based on an inscription of doubtful value, have dated this building about 1056 (according to Soper, 1058). It is a rather squat and heavy building, with a silhouette quite different from the graceful lines of most Liao masonry pagodas.

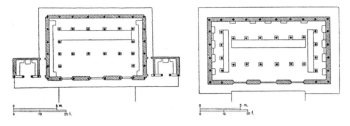

Tatung, Shansi (Liao dynasty, 907–1125). *Left*: Main hall of the Shan-hua-ssŭ (P'u-ên-ssŭ), ground plan. *Right*: Main hall of the upper temple of the Hua-yen-ssŭ, ground plan (*after Sickman and Soper*).

If it really dates from that period, it suggests that the Liao architects were much more skilled in brick than in wooden construction. As the oldest surviving example of a wooden pagoda it is a monument of great importance, whatever its esthetic merits.

The main feature of Sung and Liao pagodas is the departure from the square ground plan of the T'ang period. In the

north as well as in the south almost all are either hexagonal or octagonal, with the exception of some pagodas at Ch'ao-yang (see CHINA, *Manchuria*), where a then extant ruin of a T'ang pagoda may have served as an example. The uncompleted, truncated-looking hexagonal pagoda Fan-t'a at Kaifeng (PL. 273), dating from 977, is still of a comparatively simple construction, in which the predilection for the imitation of wooden architecture is not yet evident (see CHINA, *Honan*). One new feature is already present: a liking for colorful decoration effected by encasing the walls in tiles covered by a green glaze. Later the imitative elements became much more pronounced. Tiled roofs separate the stories, sometimes supported by wooden brackets. The colors of the roof tiles and the colored tile encasing give some pagodas an almost gaudy appearance. Others are decorated with sculptures, e.g., the twin pagodas at Ch'üan-chou, which are decorated with carefully planned iconographic bas-reliefs consisting of lohans, bodhisattvas, lokapalas, and Jātaka scenes.

The octagonal pagodas of the northern regions (PL. 273) have a rather different architectural style. They were built around a solid brick core in which no means of access to the upper stories was provided, whereas many southern pagodas could be climbed by interior staircases. On a base, profusely decorated with sculptures, rises a high shaft, decorated on all sides with bas-reliefs representing buddhas, Buddhist trinities, apsarases, and other figures. The 8 panels are bordered by pilas-

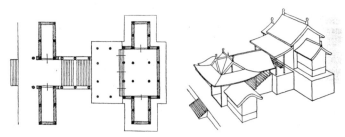

The Sheng-ku-miao at An-p'ing-hsien, Hopei (1309), plan and elevation (*after Sickman and Soper*).

ters. The shaft is crowned by a series of regularly and closely set roofs, as a rule 13 in number. The lower stories are stayed by stone brackets imitating wooden architecture, whereas the eaves of the upper stories are usually merely accentuated by a cornice of corbeled bricks. The stories diminish as they rise, forming either a regular, tapering profile or a bullet-shaped spire.

Although this type of pagoda with its many minor variations is the most common in the ancient Liao territory, there are several outstanding examples of a different architectural style, for example, the Pei-t'a ("northern pagoda") at Fang-shan (PL. 273) and the magnificent Pai-t'a ("white pagoda") at Pai-t'a-tzŭ near Ch'ing-chou (see CHINA, *Hopei* and *Manchuria*).

THE YÜAN DYNASTY (1260–1368). The conquest of China by the Mongols represents the climax of a development which had already been going on for centuries, namely, the growth of the power of her northern neighbors at China's expense. The Mongols had already seized the Peking area from the Jurchen, defeated the Tanguts, and then driven the Jurchen out of all of north China (1234). First the north and then, a few decades later, the south of China were incorporated into an extensive Mongol empire of which the Chinese nation was only a part. This part was, however, so important that Peking became the capital in 1264.

The subjugation of vast regions of Asia brought many foreign servants of the Mongol power to China. In various spheres of Chinese life the resulting exotic influence is clearly visible, but neither the Mongols nor their polyglot underlings seemed to exert any important positive influence upon the artistic life of the time. A rare example of more or less official Mongol art is to be found on Fei-lai-fêng near Hangchow (see CHINA, *Chekiang*). Many Buddhist sculptures in the Tibetan

style were carved out of the rocks on this mountain at the instigation of the hated Tibetan monk Yang-lien Chên-ch'ieh, who was in charge of Buddhist affairs south of the Yangtze River, and who forced the Taoist monks either to return to civil life or to enter Buddhist orders. These sculptures were so tainted with the bad reputation of the monk who had them carved that they fell under the outright condemnation of many Chinese authors of the Ming period. Indeed, feeling was so strong that the portrait statue of this Tibetan priest at Fei-lai-fêng was beheaded during the Ming period.

There was no longer any question of art under court patronage. The painters and calligraphers sought their inspiration in the past, especially in the Sung period or in the 10th century. When at last the Ming dynasty drove out the enfeebled and decadent Mongols, it was as though the Chinese art world was awakening from a bad dream and wanted only to forget this period as quickly as possible. What later were viewed as the great artistic accomplishments of the Yüan period were the works of masters upon whom the Mongols and their culture had no hold.

*Painting.* The Yüan period, a time of foreign domination interposed between two Chinese dynasties, lasting only about a century, was of great significance for Chinese painting. The Imperial Academy of Hangchow disappeared with the fall of the Sung dynasty; its style, however, lingered on in the south for a considerable time and survived even the reign of the Mongols.

One can roughly divide into two groups the greatest of the many Chinese artists from the Yüan period whose names and works have come down to us. In the first place, there is the group of artists who continued the traditions of the Sung Academy, which prevailed especially among painters of flowers and birds. Among them was Ch'ien Hsüan (ca. 1235-1301), a civil servant who refused to take office under the new regime. To judge by the works now ascribed to him, and by literary sources, Ch'ien Hsüan was an extremely versatile artist. His figures (VI, PL. 79) were obviously inspired by great men of the past (Yen Li-pên, Li Lung-mien, and others) while his landscapes form a continuation of the "blue and green" style of the two Lis of the T'ang period and their follower, Chao Po-chü of the Sung period. These works, inspired though they are by China's great past, hardly pe mit us to see Ch'ien Hsüan as one of China's greatest artists. Most of the works ascribed to him are paintings of flowers and insects (PL. 276), which differ strongly in style. The number of flower paintings traditionally ascribed to him, especially in Japan, is extraordinarily large. These paintings, for the most part highly refined and naturalistic, form a clear continuation of the style of the Sung Academy — not, however, that of the Southern Sung period, but that which flourished earlier during the late Northern Sung. In view of the fact that this master reverts back so far, one can perhaps better speak of an archaistic tendency than of a continuation of the work broken off by the fall of the dynasty.

A more pronounced continuation of Sung styles is represented by the landscape masters who painted in the style of the Southern Sung Academy, for instance, Sun Chün-tse (early 14th cent.). The style of the literati painters and the Ch'an monks was continued by such monk-painters as Hsüeh-ch'uang (ca. 1350), who specialized in orchids, and Tzu-t'ing (ca. 1335), who specialized in irises. Like the Ch'an artists of an earlier period, they were little appreciated in China and have come down to us only as a result of their inclusion in Japanese collections.

Probably more important were a second group of artists who endeavored to put new life into the old traditions and whose approach to painting was much more personal. The foremost master of this group was Chao Mêng-fu (q.v., 1254-1322), who is regarded by many Chinese as the greatest painter of all, in spite of the fact (later much held against him) that he was a descendant of the Sung imperial family who entered the service of the Mongol conquerors. This painter, who made a spectacular official career under the Mongols, came from a family which produced a number of artists. His brother Chao Mêng-yü and his two sons Chao Yung and Chao Lin never equaled his fame; his wife Kuan Tao-shêng (1262-ca. 1325), however, so distinguished herself as a painter of bamboos that she can probably be called the most famous woman painter in Chinese history.

Chao Mêng-fu (PLS. 197-200), rightly much esteemed as a calligrapher, is renowned as a painter primarily because of his pictures of horses. Innumerable paintings were later provided with his signature, but there are only a small number of authentic works extant. Whereas horses appear as individual animals in the work of his illustrious predecessors Han Kan and Li Lung-mien, Chao Mêng-fu often formed groups (PLS. 198, 199), grazing or running, so that he was able to combine different positions and poses. This preference for horses as a theme in painting, which seems extremely appropriate to a time dominated by the horse-loving Mongols, was not restricted to Chao Mêng-fu; Jên Jên-fa (first half of 14th cent.) almost equaled his fame in this regard. Chao Mêng-fu revealed himself in his writings as a staunch traditionalist and was modest to an extreme about the merits of his own landscapes. Yet a hand scroll like the *Landscape with Twin Pine Trees* (Coll. The Bamboo Studio, New York) clearly demonstrates his capacities as a landscape painter. In this picture, inspired by the work of the early Sung painter Kuo Hsi, he translated the ancient style into a technique closely resembling calligraphy; the trees are similar to seal script, and the rock to the *fei-pai-shu* ("flying white") style of writing (see CALLIGRAPHY).

The masters of the traditional school of the Yüan period also revived a much-loved theme of the Sung literati, namely, the bamboo. Li K'an (1245-1320), who filled various official functions under the Mongol dynasty, was not only an important master in this genre, but also left an extremely detailed treatise on bamboos and bamboo painting. It appears from this work that his bamboo paintings, of which a divided copy (Hui-hua-kuan, Peking, and Nelson Gall., Kansas City) is one of the few authentic extant masterpieces, were based not only upon a study of earlier masters, Wên T'ung, Su Shih, and others, but also upon careful observation in nature of the bamboo in all of its many varieties. Li K'an, in spite of his almost fanatical specialization in bamboo, seems also to have painted pine trees occasionally. The few examples which have been preserved indicate that this work strongly influenced that of his son Li Shih-hsing (1282-1328). A true masterpiece of this artist is the painting *Guardians of the Valley* (Fogg Art Mus., Cambridge, Mass.), in which a pair of pine trees form the principal theme, pushing the landscape, hidden in mist, completely into the background.

The bamboo theme forms a bond between certain Yüan painters who were primarily oriented toward the past and another group, who seemed to turn to the past (like all innovators in China with its rich traditions), but who in fact brought about a tremendous revolution in the art of painting. This revolution, which signified the triumph of the ideas of the *wên-jên-hua*, manifests itself most clearly in landscape painting, although several representatives of the new school applied themselves to bamboo painting as well. The new development held up for admiration the work of such early masters as Tung Yüan and Chü-jan and was accordingly later classified in the "southern school." This designation is here geographically appropriate since these literati painters worked chiefly in the lower basin of the Yangtze River. The landscape masters among them adopted types of shading and modeling (including *ts'un*) as well as other forms from the ancient landscape artists, but their attitude to this classical theme was quite different. Whereas the earlier masters had tried to capture the essence of nature, the literati painters saw the landscape as a form in which they could express their own artistic personalities. They strove to equate the arts of poetry, calligraphy, and painting, and were much more interested in the expression of personal feeling through the medium of the brush than in catching the essence of nature.

The close connection between calligraphy (q.v.) and painting which these artists brought about went farther than the use of similar materials and somewhat similar techniques.

Another result was the application to paintings of inscriptions containing more than a mere date and signature. This practice had already developed in the work of such Sung masters as Mi Fei and Su Tung-po (though its early aspects are obscure because of the paucity of authentic works extant) and was also adopted by some of the Ch'an painters. It achieved full maturity with the later Yüan literati painters, never to disappear thereafter from the Chinese art of painting. Together with the painting as a whole, the poems inscribed by the artist form an integral unit in respect to content, style of handwriting, and placement in the design. The poems are a further expression of the feelings of the artist and often give a valuable clue to his intentions. Separated from the paintings, the often mediocre quality of the poems becomes apparent, for many of the literati painters wrote little more than doggerel verse. However, in the case of a painter-poet such as Ni Tsan, who excelled in both media, painting and inscription together form a perfectly harmonious work of art.

While the Academy of the Southern Sung dynasty often gave human beings an important role in the landscape, in the Yüan literati school man, if represented at all, was again reduced to an insignificant creature, a mere dwarf among the gigantic rock formations which surrounded him. This is another characteristic which connects the new masters with the earliest generations of landscape artists in the 10th and 11th centuries.

Like the early schools, the new school also displayed a considerable variety of styles, techniques, and artistic temperaments. Later art critics have linked together four of the major talents of the new school as the "Four Great Masters of Yüan." These are Huang Kung-wang, Wu Chên, Ni Tsan, and Wang Mêng. Besides these four there are several other artists of considerable importance, among whom Kao K'o-kung undoubtedly is one of the greatest, while Fang Ts'ung-i (ca. 1340–80), Ts'ao Chih-po (1272–ca. 1360), and Shêng Mou (ca. 1310–61) are to be reckoned as painters of second rank in comparison with the enormous stature of the great masters.

The influence of the early landscape painters reveals itself most clearly in the technique of painting mountains. Both the cloud-hidden landscapes of the Ch'an masters, built up of splashes and washes, and the summary indications of the form and structure of the mountains, characteristic of some of the academic painters, gave way to mountain landscapes with rock formations and terraced masses composed as a clear-cut structural unity. These landscapes, however, usually lack the rugged, wild atmosphere of the earlier landscapes in which the artists sought their inspiration. The hills and rocks are somewhat rounder and smoother, and the trees are not usually the crooked, warped, and knotty pines of the early landscape, but straight, pruned, and more regular types reduced to standard forms.

Kao K'o-kung (1248–after 1310), who was born in a family which had emigrated from Turkistan, was one of the earliest masters of the whole group and was also an important official. In some of his works the influence of Mi Fei and his son Mi Yu-jên is clearly recognizable. His wooded mountain landscapes were built up of splashes and washes and often display very little solid structure. The effect of almost deliberate awkwardness which sometimes accompanies this technique was reduced by a more deliberate structural delineation of the mountains, in those works for which Tung Yüan is said to have been taken as the model. Fang Ts'ung-i was another artist who applied the technique of Mi Fei in his works and who often achieved through his great virtuosity a result which is considerably more convincing.

Huang Kung-wang (1269–1354), the oldest of the Four Great Masters of Yüan, never had a prominent official function. He lived the greatest part of his life amidst the landscapes which he painted, among other places in the vicinity of the Fu-ch'un-shan, which inspired his most famous works. According to the biographical notices about this master, he not only painted studio landscapes, but also worked directly from nature. Since Huang Kung-wang was of great significance later for the Ming and Ch'ing painters, his work having frequently been imitated and copied, it is often difficult to distinguish the original from the copy. The most striking instance of this is that of two

long horizontal scrolls in the Palace collection, which depict Fu-ch'un-shan and its surroundings. There are differences in style and quality between the two versions, and Sirén has assumed that the shorter version is by another hand; however, even the one which is in all probability a copy gives a fairly reliable impression of Huang Kung-wang's style. The other version, which may be regarded as authentic and which has been the property of such renowned Ming painters as Shên Chou and Tung Ch'i-ch'ang, undoubtedly had a great influence on the work of later artists. Yard on yard, as we regard this great scroll, there passes before our eyes a procession of landscape elements built up with a disciplined and versatile brush, fluently and smoothly wielded. Here there are no broad fog banks employed to camouflage the painter's inability to effect an acceptable transition from one scene to the next. Over and over again the landscape elements are repeated in new combinations which are never forced or monotonous. The mountain ridges in the background are depicted with light touches of the brush, while the frequently slanting rock formations of supple, rounded lines in the extreme foreground, interspersed with mossy spots and naturalistic groves, are surrounded by roads, water, and larger clusters of trees. This artist also found inspiration in the vertical soaring mountain landscape, and some of his vertical works seem to anticipate the remarkable terraced mountain structure which we know so well from later masters.

Wu Chên (1280–1354), who like many of his contemporaries followed the style of Wên T'ung in painting bamboos and that of Chü-jan in landscape painting, had much in common with Ni Tsan. Both went into retirement in the last years of the Yüan period and devoted themselves to painting and poetry. Their personalities, which were to appeal greatly to later generations of literati painters, are revealed not only in the few authentic paintings which exist, but also in their verse. Even though the poetic works of Wu Chên have come down to us in a very incomplete and corrupt state, they enable us to reconstruct his personality more vividly than we are able to do in the case of Huang Kung-wang, for instance, about whom we have various contemporary descriptions. From Huang Kung-wang's writings only a number of purely technical remarks about the art of painting have been preserved, forming a rather incoherent whole.

About no other Yüan painters are we so well informed as about Ni Tsan (q.v., 1301–74), who was perhaps the most brilliant of the Yüan masters. Although modern critical study may authenticate very few of the paintings ascribed to him, there can be no difference of opinion with regard to his style, which is of unmistakable originality. His vertical scroll paintings, always done on paper, which was the irreplaceable material for his manner of working, can in most cases be reduced to the same compositional formula. In the foreground there is usually an island or a projecting arm of land upon which are placed a few trees and a little house, reduced to its essential structure and amounting to no more than a pyramid roof resting on four pillars. Separated by a wide surface of water from this scene in the foreground, we see painted against the horizon a distant landscape, consisting of a few low sloping peaks or of high mountain masses painted with considerable variety. The upper margin is almost always closed by a fairly long inscription in prose ending in a verse, and many works bear also the colophons of collectors or friends of the painter. The "dry brush" that the artist employed for almost his entire composition, in which only here and there the spots of tree leaves introduce a dark note of variety, is probably the most characteristic quality of his brushwork; it gives his paintings a light, but never vague appearance and an air which is contemplative, but never uncertain or indeterminate. The verses, rich in allusions to classical or Taoist literature, are those of a man living in retirement from the world. Before the political difficulties began which ushered in the Ming era, he had given away all his possessions, among which was a rich art collection, and set off in a small boat to roam through the lake districts of the lower Yangtze. Like the other true literati painters, he gave his paintings away to people who were able to understand

and appreciate them. The verses in his elegant handwriting, which fitted his style of painting better perhaps than is the case with any other Chinese painter, have often a set beginning which indicates that he made both painting and verse for someone who had not seen him in years. In the lovely lyrics to nature we find no trace of the hard times in which the artist must have had his share. His ramblings, certainly not always as idyllic as the verses would lead us to believe, brought him constantly in contact with priests and other men living, just as he did, withdrawn from the world. It seems almost as if he painted only when someone asked him to, immediately to disappear again, like a true vagabond, from the circle of his friends. The restoration of order and peace by the Ming emperors, which he must have lived to see, had no influence upon his roving life nor upon his poetry, in which changes in the weather and in the seasons, rather than the rise and fall of princely houses, form the theme. Only in his paintings, which seem to carry an undertone of loneliness and light melancholy, can one rediscover something of the true circumstances of his life.

The last of the great Yüan masters was Wang Mêng (q.v., 1308–85), who, in violent contrast with the others, ended his life in one of the prisons of the Ming emperor. Even though he was a scion of the line of Chao Mêng-fu, which had produced numerous artists of stature among the traditionalists, and though he had received his first training from his illustrious uncle, he chose to follow the masters of the early landscape and, accordingly, the wên-jên-hua. His painting lacks the fiery élan of Wu Chên's bamboos, the cultivated reserve of Ni Tsan, and the spontaneous refinement of Huang Kung-wang. In his work, however, the fantastic image of the mountains of earlier masters is revived in a new form, which here depends upon a complicated structure built up with a rich variety of undulating brush strokes. He often reproduced architectural elements in greater detail than his contemporaries, depicting pavilions and studios occupied by a single person, a poet or a painter.

The vision and the temperament of the great masters of Yüan landscape painting differed notably, as did the pictorial effects they produced, their brushwork, and their composition. Nevertheless, the grouping of these figures under the name of the dynasty is in a sense proper, provided we do not draw the borders of the period too sharply. Wang Mêng was the only one who lived on for a considerable time under the Ming, and who thus was able to hand his style and technique on to others. The new artists who followed, however, belong to a new generation who saw the great masters of the Yüan period as predecessors and not as contemporaries.

*Sculpture; Architecture.* See below, *Later sculpture; Later architecture.*

*Ceramics, silverwork, lacquer.* The art of the Chinese potter was in some respects scarcely affected by the arrival and domination of the Mongols. Some of the earlier traditions were continued without interruption or any clear change in style (PL. 169). Ayers (*Tr. O. Ceramic Soc.,* XXIX) quite successfully tried to bring together a number of specimens of different wares which seem to date from the 14th century. Among the specimens of an unquestionably Yüan date are a vase in the Percival David Foundation, London, bearing an inscription corresponding to 1327, a stoneware pillow (1336) in the collection of C. A. Rübel, Boston, and a bottle of the Tz'ŭ-chou type with an inscription in Phags-pa script (British Mus.). This last is similar to a piece excavated by Russians at New Sarai on the Lower Volga, which was destroyed by Timur in 1395.

A distinctly new type of ceramics created under the Mongols was the so-called Shu-fu ware, which seems to have been made at Ching-tê-chên (see CHINA, *Kiangsi*) for official use. It is a fine, hard porcelain covered with a bluish or greenish glaze, usually having a molded or painted slip decoration of flowers, birds, and Chinese characters. It is sometimes regarded as transitional between the Ting-yao and the Ying-ch'ing (Ch'ing-pai) of the Sung period, on the one hand, and the 14th-century porcelain with underglaze decoration, on the other.

By far the most spectacular development in ceramics during the Yüan period was the new technique for the application of a painted decoration in underglaze cobalt blue or, to a lesser extent, in underglaze copper red. It has been assumed that the technique of using cobalt blue must have been imported from the Near East during the Mongol period. Some years ago a tomb near Canton was found to contain pieces decorated in this style supposedly dating from the Sung period, but the reliability of this evidence has been rejected by some scholars, and the pair of vases in the David Foundation in London (1351) remain the earliest datable pieces. The highly developed technique in these vases would seem to indicate that the process was not a recent development at that time. Perhaps of an earlier date are a number of small round jars ribbed in relief and covered with a somewhat bluish glaze. Of these, those with floral decoration in underglaze blue are much more common than those decorated in underglaze red; no Near Eastern prototype exists for the latter technique. There existed also in the 14th century a technique by which the design was masked out in white against a blue background. The new decorative tradition in underglaze blue was destined to predominate in Chinese ceramics for several centuries; its further development in the Ming period is treated below.

Under the Yüan dynasty great innovations took place also in the shapes of the pieces: the large dishes and bowls, which are the most common shapes encountered in 14th-century blue-and-white procelains (with the classical *mei-p'ing*), occur also in celadon. A comparison between the engraved and molded designs of the celadons and the painted decoration of the blue-and-white porcelain may make possible the more reliable dating of the celadons, which were produced without interruption throughout the Mongol period and far into the Ming. (See CERAMICS.)

The high development of the silversmith's art during the Yüan period (PLS. 274, 275) has been demonstrated in more than adequate fashion by the chance discovery of a great gold and silver hoard in Hofei (see CHINA, *Anhwei*), which on the basis of inscriptions on the pieces can be ascribed to an atelier in Lu-chou and can be dated about 1333. The forms of the vases, bowls, and plates in this treasure are visibly inspired by those found in ceramics. One piece, a silver box of lobed form, has a removable tray bearing an engraved decoration of flowers and birds. This decoration displays a certain affinity with that on a number of *sūtra* boxes in Japanese collections made by the *shên-chin* (Jap., *chinkin*) lacquer technique, in which a decoration engraved in the lacquer is filled in with lacquer covered with gold leaf. The inscriptions on two of the pieces date them in 1315 and also give the family names of the makers and the place of origin (Hangchow). The only chest of this type in a collection outside Japan (previously Staatliche Mus., Berlin) was probably destroyed during World War II. The examples in Japan (which were imported shortly after their manufacture, as is indicated by a Japanese inscription of 1358) have a closely drawn flower pattern built up of fine lines, arranged around medallions on which two birds, sometimes phoenixes, sometimes peacocks, appear against a background of stylized cloud motifs or flowers. The arrangement is not symmetrical: The tail of one of the birds always points up, while that of the other points down, and this corresponds exactly to the phoenixes on the lid of the silver box from the Hofei treasure and also to a type of decoration on 14th-century blue-and-white porcelain.

Near Hangchow, where the Sung and Chin families produced the aforementioned *sūtra* chests, the greatest center of lacquer work during the Sung and Yüan periods was established, at Chia-hsing-fu. Here two famous masters of lacquer work, Yang Mao and Chang Ch'êng, achieved great renown, especially for their application of the carved red-lacquer technique. In this technique the ground is covered with a great number of layers of lacquer, in which the design is later incised. In China and Japan as well as in Europe, a rather large number of flat round boxes made in this technique show the signature of one of these masters; how many of these pieces are really from their hands, or even from the 14th century, is

still a problem. A specimen of this type recently excavated in China, from a tomb supposedly datable between 1351 and 1359, shows remarkable similarities with previously known and published examples. This induced Sir Harry Garner to classify a small group of these pieces as of the 14th century. His classification has not yet been generally accepted, however, and has been criticized by F. Low-Beer (Oriental Art, IV, no. 1, 1958) who regards certain pieces of early 15th-century lacquer as forming the earliest clearly recognizable style group. (See LACQUER.)

LATER SCULPTURE (10th–15th cent.). Chinese Buddhist sculpture, after a remarkable flowering during the T'ang dynasty, began to show unmistakable signs of decay. The Buddhist religion had never recovered from the iconoclasm and persecutions of the mid-9th century and now unquestionably found itself in a state of decline. Nevertheless, one must not see this deterioration of Buddhism entirely as an inglorious collapse taking place over the entire Chinese empire of that time. (See BUDDHISM.)

Chinese stone sculpture after the 10th century has in general enjoyed very little attention in the West, whereas nearly all Western museums possess one or more wood sculptures generally attributed to the Sung period. Although various wooden sculptures are ascribed to the end of the T'ang or the beginning of the Sung period, precisely datable examples from the 10th century are lacking except for a single work, the famous Buddha of the Seiryōji temple in Kyoto, which, according to documents discovered some years ago in a cavity within the image, was made in 984 and taken to Japan by the priest Chōnen. It is the only extant work of artistic value representing the "Udayana" type, so called from a legend which tells how, during the life of the historical Buddha, a certain King Udayana had a likeness of the Buddha made. Purported copies of this image, which follow rather closely an early Central Asian style, were brought to China in various periods. The undulating fall of the symmetrical draperies which clothe the figure from neck to ankles is explained by reference to the legend, according to which the radiance of the Buddha was so intense that the sculptor could carve only the reflection of his form in the waters of a pond. In the hollow of the image entrails of cloth were placed, together with Buddhist texts and several remarkable documents. This image, which is still worshiped today, is no doubt one of the best-documented and most interesting wooden sculptures of the Far East; however, since it imitated as closely as possible the style of a period many centuries before, it can tell us very little about 10th-century sculpture. It lacks even the most superficial resemblance to other works ascribed to this time.

Most of the authors concerned with later Chinese plastic art have turned their attention to the monuments from the Sung, Liao, and Chin periods in north China, where, partly because the Khitans and Jurchen brought a pronounced revival of Buddhism, there are many remains of great significance. In more southerly regions practically all monuments were later destroyed; the reliquary śarīra pagoda of the temple Ch'i-hsia-ssŭ near Nanking (see CHINA, Kiangsu), with its extraordinarily beautiful representation in relief (923–33) of the life of the Buddha, seems to have survived as a unique specimen. The scenes, which are particularly detailed and minutely worked, suggest a painting transposed into relief or a wood-block engraving reinterpreted in stone. With these, as well as other sculptures in stone, one cannot escape the impression that painting, which attained under the Sung dynasty the same high level reached by sculpture under the T'ang, had exercised a strong influence on the new, more pictorial, and freer style of sculpture.

In the south, and especially in Szechwan province in the remote west, the Buddhism of the late T'ang period was able to hold its ground. The T'ang period passed imperceptibly into that of the Five Dynasties, and that, in turn, into the Sung period, without abrupt change in style. Examples of late Buddhist sculpture in stone are most numerous in Szechwan province, where extensive sculptures were carved in the living rock of the mountain faces, and the styles derived from the great

T'ang tradition continued to develop for several centuries. Before World War I the French archaeological expedition led by Ségalen, Lartigue, and des Voisins had called attention to this great multitude of monuments of late sculpture, but only in the last few years has further interest been shown in this neglected branch of Chinese art. The sentimental and facile realism characterizing the massive sculpture complexes of the 12th century near Ta-tsu forms only the last stage in this development, which gradually declined in the direction of a narrative art contrived on anecdotal effect. Since many of the stone sculptures in Szechwan bear dates, they may later permit us to date more precisely the sculptures in wood.

A great number of stone sculptures have also been preserved in the vicinity of Hangchow, the capital of the Southern Sung dynasty. The earliest ones date from the time of the Wu-Yüeh kingdom (907–78), one of the petty states which separated from the empire during the disorder marking the fall of the T'ang dynasty. Here again the development continued undisturbed when the kingdom was reintegrated under the central authority by the Sung dynasty, as well as later when the Sung capital was established here after the flight from the north (1127). The extensive complex of rock sculptures on Fei-lai-fêng, which are the most successful from an artistic point of view, was much added to even during the Yüan period, so that we can see here representatives of all the later styles of sculpture in stone brought together at one place.

In the north of China the development followed a rather different pattern, partly as a consequence of the appearance on the scene of foreign dynasties. Several notable sculptural monuments survive from the period immediately preceding the conquest of north China by the Khitans and Jurchen. In the Fo-hsiang-ko of the temple Lung-hsing-ssŭ in Chêng-ting (see CHINA, Hopei), amidst the ruins of what must have been an imposing example of wooden architecture, there stands a bronze image nearly 46 ft. high representing Kuan-yin. The image, which originally had 42 arms, but has retained only the two foremost ones, has been repeatedly restored, once during the reign of the Ch'ing emperor K'ang-hsi, at which time it was also provided with a new head. A description of its manufacture which has been preserved reveals that it was constructed of seven separately cast pieces, covered with lacquer-soaked cloth, and gilded with gold leaf. It has now fallen into deplorable condition, but it must once have been one of the most important monuments of the age. Its artistic merits are not, however, very great; it is badly proportioned, with overlong legs and too short a torso, while the stiffness of the pose is matched by the unnatural fall of the draperies and the multitude of ornamentation. The central portion of the richly decorated base probably dates from the time that the great image was constructed. Three pilasters, almost in full relief, divide the central portion into two planes; the middle pilaster is in the form of a kneeling figure; the other two are in the form of columns about which a dragon is coiled. Upon each of these are carved leaf-shaped rosettes with the figure of a musician or a dancer in relief.

This base displays a striking resemblance to that upon which the coffin was placed in the tomb of Wang Chien near Chengtu (see CHINA, Szechwan), dating from approximately the same time. There, too, musicians and dancers are depicted on otherwise undecorated panels, although the panels are narrower and phoenixes in relief take the place of the pilasters. The caryatids, in the garb of warriors, are executed in full round from the waist up and placed in the ground around the base with their faces turned toward it, so that they seem actually to support the pedestal. This richly sculptured base, preserved intact, is a remarkably fine relic of late Chinese sculpture in stone.

In the Fo-hsiang-ko, where the great Kuan-yin figure is found, there are also complicated compositions in relief composed of numerous clay figures, richly polychromed. These substitutes for wall paintings had already suffered much damage before World War II and we do not know which are still in existence; one of the finest pieces, an enthroned Kuan-yin in almost full relief, seems to have been lost. An impressive scene depicts Samantabhadra seated on the elephant and proceeding

over the clouds with an extraordinarily numerous retinue. Altogether nearly a hundred figures are drawn up in rows side by side. There is little feeling for composition, but the lakes, mountains, ships, and pavilions floating through the air, which strongly remind us of similar scenes in the painting of this period, are well integrated into the whole scene. There is a striking similarity between these reliefs and those in stone in the Ch'i-hsia-ssŭ near Nanking, which are less than a century earlier.

The transformation of Chinese sculpture in a pictorial direction is understandably most evident in the case of the modeled clay reliefs which substituted for wall paintings; however, this tendency is also observable in stone sculpture. The graceful lines and soft flowing contours of the dancing girls and the detailed representation of figures and landscapes in the stone reliefs point in the same direction.

During the 11th and 12th centuries, under the influence of foreign rulers, Buddhism came again to the forefront, just as it had before, under the Wei dynasty. Perhaps the comparison with this dynasty occurred to the princes of the Liao, for again and again we are confronted with their efforts to revive the Wei tradition. Japanese investigators have demonstrated that the colossal trinity in Cave III at Yün-kang, previously assumed to be of later date than the other sculptures in this complex (see CHINA, Shansi), must have been carved during the Liao period. The fact that this was first recognized only after many years, and has not yet been accepted by all scholars, indicates how successful the Liao sculptors were in their attempts to imitate the old styles. An important center where these deliberately archaistic pieces seem to have been produced is in the vicinity of Ting-chou, in Hopei, where in earlier times an important school of sculptors had been established. Aside from these deliberate imitations of early styles, many pieces of sculpture display an unfortunate combination of quasi-archaistic stiffness and rigid straight drapery with the naturalism characteristic of the painting of the time; however, this indicates a backsliding to primitive provincialism rather than the creation of a new style.

By far the most important art works of this period are made of wood, clay, and dry lacquer. Of the works in clay, a number of sculptural groups and individual statues have been preserved in north China and Manchuria, in temples which are themselves important by virtue of the great antiquity of their wooden architecture. These are the images belonging to the temples Tu-lo-ssŭ (984) at Chi-hsien, Hopei; Fêng-kuo-ssŭ (1012–20) at Yi-hsien, Liaoning; Hsia Hua-yen-ssŭ (1038) and P'u-ên-ssŭ (ca. 1050) at Tatung, Shansi (see CHINA, Hopei, Manchuria, Shansi).

The standing image of an eleven-headed Kuan-yin in the Tu-lo-ssŭ, the oldest of these sculptures, displays a formality and a rather awkward stiffness which suggest unfamiliarity with the material on the part of the artist; no trace of this, however, is to be seen in the later sculptures. In contrast with the sculpture in stone (likewise deriving from the late T'ang style), which as a whole began to decline from the 10th century on, the plastic arts in wood and clay began to show unmistakable signs of degeneration only during the 14th or 15th century. The round, somewhat heavy-set forms of the late T'ang period were retained, although a new, more naturalistic and human conception gave the figures a more earthly appearance. The great statuary group of the Hsia Hua-yen-ssŭ is an excellent example of this. It consists of some thirty figures modeled in clay, presumably reinforced with a wooden armature, and covered with a thick layer of gold lacquer, the whole being placed on a high base which takes up a great part of the space in the temple nave. The statues are grouped about three Buddha figures nearly 15 ft. high, each seated on a great throne with a nimbus, with Śākyamuni in the center flanked by Amitābha and Bhaiṣajyaguru. The great Buddhas are each surrounded by six bodhisattvas, two sitting and four standing, with the exception of the central image, representing the historical Buddha, which is attended by two lohans. There are also a substantial number of smaller figures. The proportions, the naturally modeled drapery, and the lively variations

in pose make of this statuary group an extraordinarily fine ensemble, although the extremely high tiaras give the figures an accent that is perhaps too strongly elongated. Sirén had assumed at one time that the sculptures must date from the reconstruction of the temple in 1140; however, Japanese specialists have shown that they are contemporary with the original construction in 1038.

The attention of Western admirers of Chinese art has been attracted primarily by the sculptures in wood. Especially from Shansi there have come a great number of wooden sculptures, produced mainly under the Chin dynasty, of which many have found their way into European and American collections. Even today in this province a great number of these sculptures still exist in local temples. It is usual for these sculptures to form a single composition, together with the wall paintings. For example, in the Parinirvāṇa scene of Cave 158 of Tun-huang (see CHINA, Kansu), the dying Buddha and several of his disciples are depicted in sculpture while other attendant personages are represented in paintings on the walls.

Only a very small number of the multitude of wooden sculptures in Western collections can be dated by inscriptions. Notable among these few are the Avalokiteśvara and the Mahāsthāmaprāpta in the Royal Ontario Museum, Toronto (1195), a standing Avalokiteśvara in the Metropolitan Museum, New York (1282), and a sitting Avalokiteśvara (1385) from the same museum. To this list of datable specimens should be added the Avalokiteśvara in the Senyūji temple, Kyoto, which according to the temple records was taken to Japan in 1255 and apparently had been made shortly before. Even these few dated sculptures indicate the great predilection of the sculptors for Avalokiteśvara (in Chinese called Kuan-yin), who played an important role in the religious life of the time. This bodhisattva, familiar to us in painting as well as in sculpture, can appear in female form — for instance, as the so-called Yü-lan Kuan-yin ("Kuan-yin with the fish basket"); even in sculptures in which he is not given a specifically female form, his features often acquire a feminine appearance. Besides the standing Kuan-yin (PLS. 272; II, 388), a particular form of sitting Kuan-yin (PLS. 257, 271) began to find general acceptance. In this pose, the Mahārājalilā, or "Repose of the Great King," he is seated with the right arm relaxed and hanging across the raised right knee, often on a rocklike pedestal or sometimes installed in a richly carved grotto symbolizing the Potalaka, the abode of Kuan-yin. In the best of these sculptures the bodhisattva retains something of his superhuman character, which, in spite of the human form of the figure, finds expression in the serene tranquillity of the relaxed, well-balanced pose. A comparison of the dated figures in Toronto (1195) and New York (1282) shows a remarkable development in style. The posture becomes looser and less bulky, and the fall of the draperies begins to play a more independent role, accentuating but not concealing the form. The end of the 13th and the beginning of the 14th century apparently marked the high point of this sculpture in wood. The Kuan-yin in the Metropolitan Museum dated 1385 represents only iconographically the Mahārājalilā pose, which has obviously now been reduced to a meaningless cliché. There is no longer an impression of relaxed serenity and calm; the clumsy, thick figure is sunk onto the lotus throne as though in exhaustion. Because of the insufficiency of dated material, it is not possible to judge how long the Sung tradition continued. It is likely that many of the numerous badly proportioned and clumsy figures are actually of later date and that the old tradition was maintained here and there locally until far into the Ming period.

Besides the Sung traditions, during the reign of the Mongols other tendencies arose in the iconography and style of plastic art. In the sculptures of the Fei-lai-fêng near Hangchow, for example, we detect the influence of the esoteric Buddhism of the Lamaistic cults, which had been introduced there with the encouragement of the Mongol governors. The form of the body, the attitude, and the iconography are all almost directly borrowed from the Lamaistic art of Tibet and Nepal (qq.v.). On a notably higher artistic plane are the sculptures in bas-relief depicting the four lokapalas, applied to the Chü-yung

gate in the Great Wall (PL. 279; see CHINA, *Hopei*). The marble tablets, which are set in a frame, are carved with a background of fine stylized cloud motifs. The lokapalas are depicted in attitudes of great agitation, with frightening expressions on their faces. A single static accompanying figure contrasts sharply with their uncontrolled gestures, accentuated by swirling scarves. The pictorial tendency, so conspicuous in earlier sculptures, here reaches its climax. In the decoration of the arch frames the influence of Lamaistic art is especially clear. Probably it is this very exotic influence which gives these sculptures, carved about 1345, a vital and fresh character at a time when sculpture in stone and wood had already fallen into decline.

The Ming dynasty sought its sculptural inspiration in the other great native dynasties of the past, but the gigantic camels, *ch'i-lin*s (fabulous beasts), elephants, and other animals which flank the way to the mausoleums of the Ming emperors lack by a great deal the beauty and power of their precursors made under the T'ang dynasty. In Buddhist sculpture as well we see only the fruitless reembroidering of old themes rigidly fixed for all time. A datable piece of sculpture, such as the gilded wooden Buddha (1411) in the Metropolitan Museum, New York, which is only a quarter of a century younger than the last dated Kuan-yin figure in the same museum, shows already the direction which sculpture was to take, namely, transition to a purely linear treatment of garments which conceal a practically formless body. The great bronze reclining Buddha in the Wo-fo-ssŭ near Peking (1469) is a well-known example of this later style.

A completely different place among late Chinese sculptures is occupied by the cast-iron figures. Some of the early, and therefore most interesting, examples of cast-iron sculpture are to be found in the Hsüan-chung-ssŭ at Shih-pi (Shansi). Along three sides of the Ch'ien-fo-ko ("Thousand Buddha Pavilion") in this temple, there are platforms of six tiers upon which a great number of cast-iron Buddhas (ca. 35 in. high) are placed. Most of them are exactly identical and they represent a somewhat rustic offshoot of the late T'ang style of T'ien-lung-shan. Dated inscriptions from 1101 to 1109 prove that the statues were produced by founders from Wen-shui, a place in the neighborhood. Iron statues found elsewhere as well seem to have been made here, where, apparently, extensive ateliers were established. Pieces of later date, for example the lohan in the Güteborg museum (1477), are distinguished by an extremely stiff and summary treatment of the garments, although various pieces display a surprisingly lovely facial expression which far surpasses the sculpture in stone and wood of this period. (See also LACQUER and, for examples of jade carving, PLS. 261, 278.)

THE MING DYNASTY (1368–1644). The revolt of Chu Yüanchang, which brought about the fall of the Mongol Yüan dynasty, began in the south of China. This was in itself no accident of history, but a symptom of the altered center of gravity of the Chinese nation, which, with the departure of the Sung emperors from Kaifeng, had shifted to the south. Even though the first national dynasty after the fall of the Mongols, that of the Ming, moved its capital to Peking in the 15th century, it was never in any sense as typically northern as were its predecessors the T'ang and the Han. Maritime commerce and voyages of discovery at this time took the place of the expansion overland into Central Asia which had previously characterized the great Chinese dynasties. The Ming emperors undertook no new adventures inland, but sought instead, through extension and reinforcement of the Great Wall, to cut China off from the neighboring lands and make her thus safe from their attacks. However, neither the long sea voyages of the Chinese, which brought them to the coast of Africa and spread their porcelain over all the Near and Middle East, nor the explorations by Europeans, who during the Ming reign first reached the coast of China, left any impression on Chinese art or culture.

In the art history of this period the south provided most of the creative ideas. Sculpture played only a subordinate role. The art of painting, which for the first time is represented by a great number of authentic extant works, displayed an important development along new lines in spite of the strong attachment to the past manifested by many of the great figures. The potter's craft, which had completely lost contact with the ideals of the Sung period, departed in altogether new directions, and other handicrafts, such as cloisonné enamel and lacquer work, flourished; in fact, it may be said that this period represents the last flowering of the traditional craft of the master lacquer workers.

As so often happened in Chinese history, a combination of bad government, economic disaster, and political weakness caused the ultimate fall of this dynasty. In the end, a revolt in north China was made the occasion to call in the help of the powerful Manchus, who had built up their nation in the Amur River region. Once inside the borders these warlike allies refused to depart and, after a struggle lasting many years, they brought all of China under their control.

*Painting* (see PLS. 281–284, 287). The tradition of the great landscape painters who lived all or part of their lives under the Mongols by no means died out with the fall of the dynasty. Wang Mêng lived long enough to cast his influence, not only through the paintings he left behind, but by personal contact with younger painters whom we may regard as true Ming masters; and that faithful disciple of the great Yüan masters, Chou Chih, of whose works only a few have been preserved, lived on until the Hung-wu era. Wang Fu (1362–1416), who gained great fame as a painter of bamboo, was never able to escape the influence of his illustrious predecessors and can be regarded consequently as the artistic heir of the Yüan bamboo painters, a qualification against which the artist himself would probably have raised no objection.

This continuation of the traditions of the Four Great Masters of Yüan was not mere sterile imitation. The artists who followed this trend had too much character of their own for that, and their artistic movement (only briefly pushed from the foreground by the rise of a new academicism) resulted in what is called the Wu school, probably the most inspired school of Ming painting. Wang Fu's pupil Hsia Ch'ang (1388–1470) left a great number of bamboo paintings, principally in horizontal format. The landscape painters Tu Ch'iung (1396–1474) and Liu Chüeh (1410–72) form the last link between the Yüan masters and the Wu school. They reached neither the level of their predecessors nor that of the later great masters of the Wu school, but they kept alive a tradition which otherwise might have disappeared under the pressure of academicism.

The first Ming emperor, who understandably, as the first Chinese ruler after a period of foreign domination, sought a restoration of the glory of the Sung dynasty, promptly followed the example of the Sung emperors by founding an Imperial Academy. An effort was also made to breathe new life into the ancient academic styles, but the attempt seems only partly to have succeeded. Only a few of the works of the early Ming academic painters have been preserved, with the result that our appreciation of the abilities of these masters must remain incomplete. Pien Wên-chin, who was attached to the Academy during the Yung-lo and Hsüan-tê eras, was according to literary sources considered the foremost representative of academicism. His bird paintings, in which he seems to have been trying to set the clock back to Huang Ch'üan, are solid and competent pieces of work but display no great talent. In Japan as well as in Europe, the work of his pupil Lü Chi has become very well known, partly because of copies and imitations by lesser academic painters, and the best of it is extraordinarily decorative; nevertheless, the effort to revive the bird-and-flower style really never achieved success.

To what the failure should be attributed is difficult to ascertain. The tyranny and censoriousness of the emperors is usually blamed in connection with the fact that certain artists signed their own death warrants by falling out of imperial favor — for example, Chao Yüan, Hsü Pên, and Wang Meng. It seems unnecessary, however, to ascribe the responsibility for the general level of art to the oppression of such emperors as T'ai-tsu (Hung-wu), regardless of how arbitrary and heavy-handed he was, according to the historical works. Emperor

Hsüan-tsung, whose reign is known as the Hsüan-tê era (1426–35), was himself an accomplished painter, to judge from the works which have come down to us, and one may very well assume that he would have promoted the revival of the Sung style, which left such a clear impression on his own work.

A proper evaluation of Ming academicism and of the Chê school (see below) is complicated by various factors. In the first place, in Europe an almost exaggerated evaluation has been placed on the works of Sung academicism, whether they were bird-and-flower pictures or landscapes in the Ma-Hsia style (Ma Yüan and Hsia Kuei). In itself this would be of little importance, had it not led to the remarkable implication that schools which developed along altogether different lines must be reckoned, even at their best, as inferior. On the other hand, in China, in those circles which opposed academicism and in which the new ideas took artistic form, no effort was spared to paint academicism black. Prejudices and differences of opinion other than those between court painters and literati, academicism and the wên-jên-hua, may have played a role; moreover, it must be remembered that usually the persons with the greatest literary prestige chose the side of the wên-jên-hua. A well-considered evaluation on the basis of extant paintings, which would seem to be the obvious solution, is rendered impracticable by the fact that the work of the most important masters of the Academy has been only fragmentarily preserved, perhaps precisely because their work was later never credited with its full value in China.

In Chekiang province, where the Sung capital (Hangchow) had been located, the style of Ma Yüan and Hsia Kuei had lingered on through the Yüan period. Needless to say, upon the restoration of Chinese power, the Academy reverted in landscape painting to the style of these masters. Many of the painters who were invited to the court in Peking were from this province or from the more southerly area of Fukien. It was by these artists and their disciples that the works in Ma and Hsia styles were produced which in Europe, and to some extent in Japan, were for a long time taken to be originals by these masters. The remarkable similarity between the original paintings of the Sung period and the copies of the Ming period, achieved by the precision of the copyists, contributed to this confusion.

Of the landscape painter Li Tsai, who was attached to the Academy during the Hsüan-tê era, only a few works have come down to us. One of these, a lovely landscape in the style of Kuo Hsi (Nat. Mus., Tokyo), reveals the influence of this early Sung master. The great Japanese painter Sesshū (q.v.), who visited China in 1468, named Li Tsai as the most important master of that time. Other artists as well underwent the influence of Kuo Hsi, but in the long run the work of Ma Yüan and Hsia Kuei seems to have made a stronger impression. This was in some measure due to the rise of the Chê school, an association both within and outside the Academy, which was not a true school in the European sense of the word. The founder of the Chê school was considered to have been the painter Tai Chin, who was invited to court and taken into the Academy during the Hsüan-tê era, but who very soon returned to Chekiang in order to live out his life of productive artistry in genteel poverty. His work, which shows markedly the influence of the Ma-Hsia style, is characterized by a more dynamic conception than would be expected of the true academicians, and it strongly influenced other artists, probably before their invitation to the court. Thus this master, who had at first been rejected in Peking, came to exercise great influence upon the work of the Academy.

The general trend in the Imperial Academy during the 15th and at the beginning of the 16th century is equivocal. There was, in the first place, a purely static element represented by what one might call the " pure " academicians, whose landscapes (in the style of Ma and Hsia) were generally left unsigned. Only a small number of signed works are known, and the signatures are often those of artists not mentioned in documentary sources. The master Wu I-hsien, whose name appears on a painting formerly in the Ostasiatische Kunstabteilung, Berlin, and now probably lost, is completely unknown

from literature. The " one-sided " composition, the placement of the trees, and the figures in a little boat identify him as a follower of the academic style of the Southern Sung school as transmitted by Tai Chin. The vivid movement with which the pouring rain is depicted shows him to be a better than average painter and disguises most effectively his somewhat static attachment to time-honored principles.

The best representatives of the Academy and of the Chê school are really those masters who are not truly characteristic of either. The painter Wu Wei (1459–1508), for instance, was the very figure of the bohemian, but in spite of his behavior he was much esteemed by the emperor Hsien-tsung as well as by Hsiao-tsung. He displayed great virtuosity and originality of brush technique, and his numerous figure paintings achieved effects which are delightfully humorous; nevertheless, his work lacks the refinement with which such masters as Tai Chin blended and tempered their expressive and powerful brushwork. Wu Wei may be reckoned among the artists who followed the Southern Sung style, but his work shows so little conformity with that of the Chê school that he has been regarded by some as the founder of a new school, named after his birthplace, Chiang-hsia.

The use of a more fluid, rougher, and livelier brush technique, which penetrated into the Academy and the Chê school in a more disciplined form through the work of Tai Chin and in a freer form through Wu Wei, is most clearly to be seen in the works of Chang Lu (1464–1538), Chiang Sung (ca. 1500), and Lin Liang (a member of the Academy ca. 1500). One of Chang Lu's masterpieces is without doubt *The Fisherman* in the Gokokuji in Kyoto. In this painting the fisherman stands ready to cast his nets from a small boat, as he and his helper drift past a soaring rocky cliff which takes up the entire right half of the composition. The strength of the brush strokes demands attention with such insistence that we are almost unaware of the complete lack of poetic atmosphere. Lin Liang was a painter of birds. In contrast to the decorative colorful paintings of his contemporary Lü Chi, the monochrome birds of Lin Liang are built up of heavy dark brush strokes, not without virtuosity and verve. However, perhaps because we are accustomed to associating the "birds and flowers" theme with decorative, polished, polychrome naturalism, his works strike us often as somewhat lacking in refinement.

In the meantime, in the ancient Wu district (the part of Kiangsu lying south of the Yangtze River) a new school was arising which, true to the ancient wên-jên-hua traditions transmitted by the literati, kept its distance from the Imperial Academy. This school, which first won adherents mainly in and around Soochow (Su-chou), was called after this district the "Wu school." The most important early master, and the one who is regarded as the founder of the school, was Shên Chou (1427–1509). Descended from an artistically talented and eminent family which had remained outside the ranks of Chinese officialdom, he sought no official career, but devoted himself wholeheartedly to painting, calligraphy, and poetry. The influence of the wên-jên-hua masters of the Northern Sung period is clearly visible in Shên Chou's style of handwriting, which was based on that of Huang T'ing-chien. On the other hand, he was strongly influenced by the painters in his family, including his uncle Shên Chên and his father. No doubt such masters as Liu Chüeh also had made a great impression on him, so that in some respects he was a direct descendant, in others a regenerator, of the style of the Four Great Masters of Yüan.

In his younger years Shên Chou, not being afflicted with the affected snobbery of many later wên-jên-hua masters, imitated artists of various schools and periods. There is even one copy after Tai Chin which has come down to us from his hand. His early work, typified by a landscape of 1464 (Abe Coll., Osaka Municipal Mus., with colophons written by various members of his family), shows a disciplined, detailed, and refined execution which indicates a reaction against the calligraphic fireworks of the Chê school. Gradually, however, he came to employ a more dynamic type of brushwork with great originality. How far he was responsible for the truly coarse work

which is ascribed to his last years is difficult to determine, inasmuch as he had many imitators and his signature was falsely used in innumerable cases. The Chinese regarded Shên Chou as a great painter even during his lifetime and, later, as one of the greatest artists in the history of Chinese painting. To some extent this fame was based, however, upon the fact that he seemed to personify the ideal characteristics of the true scholar and man of letters. Considered in the light of his own time, he was beyond any doubt a master, but when we consider how the Four Great Masters of Yüan recreated early landscape painting and how Shên Chou in his turn modified their work, the comparison results unfavorably for Shên Chou. Many of his large landscapes, except when he was working after Ni Tsan (e.g., in the landscape dated 1484, Nelson Gall., Kansas City), reveal a clear lack of ability in vertical composition. However, he shows far greater talent for landscape composition in horizontal scrolls and in album leaves (PL. 283), which were painted in series to be bound together. Here his style has a high degree of homogeneity and is extremely individual, with characteristic foliage and a particular use of "mossy points" to accent cliffs and mountains.

Shên Chou had various pupils, of whom Wên Chêng-ming (q.v., 1470–1559) was the most prominent. In contrast with his teacher, whose influence is immediately detectable in several of his paintings, the work ascribed to Wên Chêng-ming displays a much greater variety in brushwork and composition. If we may judge from the dates on his works, this variety is not due to any change in style taking place during his long life, but rather to his versatility and his ability to work in the styles of different masters. A number of works in soft colors, built up with minute brush strokes, represent the refined style of Wên Chêng-ming. Some of these, for example *The Farewell* (PL. 282), are simple in composition. In this painting, against an empty background, the artist has placed four trees, depicted in minute detail, to the left of which the painter and his guest are seated. The whole has an air that is almost academic, although this is not the academicism of the time, but a personal derivation from the Sung style of some artist such as Chao Po-chü. Other works reveal a similarity to academic landscape painters, for example *A View of the Wu-sung River* (dated 1528) with its somewhat dreary, meticulously painted waves and currents in the water. That Wên Chêng-ming did not strive only for refinement, however, is obvious from such a masterpiece as *Seven Juniper Trees* (PL. 283). Here, instead of restrained carefulness, there is an inspired effort to capture the fantastic, almost supernatural shapes of the trees. With well-planned and powerfully executed brush strokes and dots, the boughs of the trees are stretched out horizontally and divided into knotty branches with intertwined shoots and twigs growing in all directions. Although this painting occupies a unique place in the work of Wên Chêng-ming, it offers striking evidence of the genius which was later ascribed to him.

Both Wên Chêng-ming's son Wên Chia (1501–83) and his nephew Wên Po-jên (1502–ca. 1580) were strongly affected by his influence. Both seem to have had a predilection for the narrow vertical format, although Wên Chia, a painter of much less ability than Wên Po-jên, never succeeded in mastering it completely. A series of landscapes such as *The Four Seasons* (Nat. Mus., Tokyo) characterizes Wên Po-jên as one of the best literati painters of his time.

The tradition of literati painting was kept alive during the whole Ming period by a variety of artists. One of the most important pupils of Wên Chêng-ming was Lu Chih (1496–1576), who followed the delicate polychrome style of his master, painting landscapes as well as flowers. Two other pupils were Ch'ên Shun (1483–1544) and Ch'ien Ku (1508–72). Of the later generation who followed the tradition of Shên Chou and Wên Chêng-ming, such masters as Yün Hsiang (1586–1655) and Chang Hung (1580–after 1658) should be mentioned. By the time these artists had reached prominence, however, literati painting had already spread from Soochow to various other places in Kiangsu province, and several of these new branches were of considerably more importance than were the more direct heirs of the first great masters of the Wu school.

Besides the pure *wên-jên-hua* tradition, there were in Soochow other artists working in styles which are difficult to fit into any classification. Two of these artists, T'ang Yin (1470–1524) and Ch'iu Ying (first half of 16th cent.), are regarded as forming together with Shên Chou and Wên Chêng-ming the group known as the "Four Great Masters of the Ming Period." T'ang Yin, whose dissolute life and brilliant career (prematurely ended by an allegation of cheating in an official examination) were the subject of much attention both before and after his death, was excluded from the circle of the genuine literati as a result of his — probably unjust — degradation. Born in Soochow, he was one of the small group of professional artists from this district who turned to the same masters for inspiration as did the artists of the Chê school. He is consequently classed with the so-called "neo-academicians." His works, however, are in general free of the influence of the great Yüan masters, though not of that of Shên Chou. His treatment of rocky crags and mountains shows something of the angular construction and the brush technique of Li T'ang, with which he was probably acquainted through the work of Chou Ch'ên (died ca. 1535), of whom he is considered to have been a pupil.

Ch'iu Ying (first half of 16th cent.) was also a pupil of Chou Ch'ên and also active in Soochow. With him, more than with any other master, the *kung-pi* method and the so-called "blue and green" landscape style came once more to life. Ch'iu Ying, who was one of the few professional painters in the center dominated by the literati painters, and whose style departed most from that of the literati, acquired great fame in his own time with his delicate refined landscapes and figure paintings characterized by highly decorative color effects. That the literati had no snobbish prejudice against his professionalism or social origins and that they were able to recognize an undeniable talent (obscured only by a multitude of counterfeit works bearing his name) is proved by several colophons on his works. A painting in the Kurokawa Collection bears a colophon written by Wang Ch'ung (1494–1533), a pupil of Wên Chêng-ming, and several other works bear inscriptions by the great master himself. Another professional painter whom we cannot easily classify is Hsieh Shih-ch'ên (1487–after 1567). He is different from the masters of the Wu school in that the narrative element appears much more strongly in his works. His landscapes characterize him as a hybrid standing somewhere between the Chê school and the work of Shên Chou.

After the death of the Four Great Masters of the Ming Period, the literati schools became more and more predominant. The Chê school was yet to enjoy a short revival with the activity of the gifted Lan Ying (1585–1664), but otherwise literati painting achieved complete supremacy and spread from the original center in Soochow to other parts of the lower Yangtze delta. This victory was marked by the theoretical work of Mo Shih-lung (active ca. 1570–1600), Ch'ên Chi-ju (1558–1639), and Tung Ch'i-ch'ang (1555–1636). These artists, of whom only Tung Ch'i-ch'ang seems to have been of great importance as a painter, gave a new cachet to the triumph of the *wên-jên-hua* with their famous theory as to the classification of Chinese painting into a northern and a southern school. The complicated bibliographical problems which arise in a study of their many writings make it impossible to say which of these three is the source of the new system of classification. Probably each contributed his share, and a lively discussion of art-historical problems seems to have been carried on among them and a number of other artists and connoisseurs. Their theory was not — as the terminology suggests — an attempt to classify artists on a geographic basis. The terminology was borrowed from that of Ch'an Buddhism, in which Ch'ên Chi-ju especially seems to have been much interested, but the theory amounts to an ostensible separation of true masters, who are worthy of being held up as examples, from superficial painters, whose example should be avoided. The northern school, which was not very highly regarded, was traced back to the T'ang period. It started with the two Lis of the T'ang dynasty, followed by such Sung masters as Chao Po-chü, Li T'ang, Ma Yüan, and Hsia Kuei, and all those lesser artists of the Yüan and Ming periods who followed their example. The origins

of the southern school, the direct descendant of which was their own *wên-jên-hua*, were likewise traced back to T'ang times. It was supposed to have started with the poet and painter Wang Wei and then to have developed via Tung Yüan, Chü-jan, Li Lung-mien, Mi Fei, Su Tung-po, and others to the Four Great Masters of Yüan. By means of this theory the literati painters were provided with a venerable pedigree and the corresponding prestige. The haughtiness with which some of China's greatest painters were rejected, and the numerous contradictions and illogicalities in the theories, do not alter the fact that this classification achieved the greatest historical importance as a result of the authority with which it was vested. Moreover, it must be admitted that the writings expounding these theories contain numerous clever observations and often give proof of sound art-historical reasoning.

Perhaps it is partly as a result of the success of these theories that Tung Ch'i-ch'ang (q.v., PL. 284) has always been considered one of the greatest painters of the Ming period. He certainly displayed a well-developed sense for solid structure, and he never lost himself in his sometimes extremely complicated compositions. He also gave great attention to the technical aspects of painting, which had sometimes been neglected by other literati painters, and made a profound study of many of the ancient masters, as is proved by inscriptions on his works in which he states that he followed the style of one or another of the great artists of the past. His approach to this study was not very formal, however, and he almost invariably conveyed more of his own spirit than that of the masters whom he took as examples. Yet his works lack the spontaneous character of the great literati painters, and often the total effect is somewhat studied or even decidedly dull. One can hardly avoid the impression that he was first and foremost a theoretician. In some respects, especially in his insistence on careful study and technical versatility, his influence on his pupils and upon later generations of artists was no doubt beneficial. However, even if we should wholeheartedly agree with the extremely high opinion the Chinese have always had of his art, it cannot be denied that he was at least partially responsible for the formalistic attitude with which the Four Wangs were later to drain the lifeblood from the inspired works of the great Yüan masters.

Tung Ch'i-ch'ang was one, and beyond doubt the greatest, of a heterogeneous group of literati painters of greatly differing ability — and active in different centers — who have come down in history under the name of the "Nine Painter Friends." Another of this group was Li Liu-fang (1575–1629), who passed the greater part of his artistic life in Sung-chiang, where Tung Ch'i-ch'ang and his school were active; he is famous for a number of landscapes executed in heavy black tints, in which the details display strongly calligraphic brush strokes, whereas the composition — obviously reverting to that of the Yüan masters — is sometimes rather weak. Generally speaking, the literati painters of the late Ming period were most in their element when painting smaller album leaves rather than larger works; in the latter their inability to build up a complex composition — something which so little accorded with their mode of working and temperament — always threatened to recoil upon them. This was true of the Soochow painter Shao Mi (active 1629–60), who was able to achieve great distinction in his soft polychrome album leaves, although his larger landscapes are rather chaotic. Shêng Mao-hua (of Mao-yeh, early 17th cent.) was one of the greatest masters in painting album leaves with polychrome landscapes; his mastery of brush technique, also clearly to be seen in his large hanging scrolls, raises him far above most of the amateur painters of his time. A calligrapher of great stature was Chang Jui-t'u (early 17th cent.). A native of Fukien, he chose an official career which came to a premature end when he chose the losing party in a political conflict. As a result of this mistake, his merits as a painter were never fully recognized. In Japan, however, his works were very soon being collected, and there are extant in that country a great number of calligraphs in his powerful and very individual handwriting. In general, the same importance cannot be ascribed to his paintings.

Although the Chinese art critics cannot be accused of having based their judgment of paintings exclusively on the personalities of the artists, it cannot be denied that persons whose character and conduct appealed to the fancy of the critics were seldom, if ever, underrated as painters, while those who came under criticism for their actions had to belong to the ranks of the greatest masters in order to find general recognition. Three artists who won great admiration by their heroic conduct at the fall of the Ming dynasty were Huang Tao-chou (1585–1646), Ni Yüan-lu (1593–1644), and Yang Wên-ts'ung (1597–1645). It would be incorrect, however, to suppose that they owe their fame as painters to the fact that they gave their lives for the Ming cause. Even though they do not belong among the greatest of the Ming painters, their work has a personal expressiveness which raises it above the conventional landscape painting of a time in which the ideal of the *wên-jên-hua* threatened to become a stale convention. This holds true especially for Huang and Ni, in whose works pine trees play an important part. Yang Wên-ts'ung, with his subtle small landscapes in the style of the Yüan masters, was much more a follower of the older *wên-jên-hua* traditions.

With the victory of the ideals of the *wên-jên-hua*, the landscape achieved a position of dominance in Chinese painting, but this did not mean that other genres had vanished from the repertory. Such great masters as Shên Chou, T'ang Yin, and Wên Chêng-ming all applied themselves to the painting of bamboos, birds, and flowers. Bamboo painting, from the earliest times inseparably bound up with the *wên-jên-hua* tradition, was practiced by almost every literati painter at one time or another to a greater or lesser extent. The plum blossom, the chrysanthemum, and the orchid, which together with the bamboo were called the "Four Gentlemen" and were said to form the "finger exercises" of the literati painters, continued to hold their attraction, although the number of artists who specialized in these themes was, with the exception of the bamboo painters, relatively limited. Two women painters, Ma Shou-chên (late 16th–early 17th cent.) and Hsüeh Wu (1564– ca. 1637), who devoted themselves to the painting of orchids, are among the best-known of this little group, partly perhaps because women artists have never been numerous in China.

A completely isolated place in Ming painting is occupied by the bizarre works of the eccentric Hsü Wei (1521–93). If we can at all classify this unconventional figure, who demonstrated — among other ways, by murdering his second wife — that his antisocial character was not just an artistic affectation, then we must regard him as the last adherent of the tradition which was represented during the Yüan period by such masters as Jih-kuan, renowned for his monochrome paintings of grapevines. Not only the handwriting and the paintings of grapevines and banana trees, but also the landscapes of Hsü Wei display the most spontaneous brushwork to be found among the Ming masters. The few extant works which may be regarded as authentic show a combination of passionate abandon and superb control of the brush, by which deliberate coarseness is avoided and, instead, a genuine outpouring of the spirit is attained. These works approach very close to the theory of the *wên-jên-hua*, but have little in common with the civilized practices of this school. Not only the master with his peculiar conduct, but also his works with their unrestrained virtuosity must be regarded as belonging to a class apart.

The representation of the human figure during the Ming dynasty sank more and more into the background. A school or a tradition of figure painting maintained by each generation of artists, which might have provided inspiring examples to take the place of the rare masterpieces of the past, simply did not exist. Consequently, the two great figure painters of the Ming period turned back to the past, especially to the numerous rubbings from stone engravings of earlier figure paintings, which probably had more influence on their work than did the actual paintings of their predecessors. Ting Yün-p'êng (active ca. 1584–1638), one of these two, was the last artistically important propagandist of the Buddhist pantheon, which by this time was reduced to the figure of the historical Buddha and the lohans. Neither he nor Ch'ên Hung-shou (1599–1652), the

greatest figure painter of the Ming period, was capable of bringing forth such a radically new conception as marked the development of figure painting in Western art, and indeed this was never part of their intention. Within their limits, imposed by factors inherent in Chinese culture rather than by any personal lack of originality, these two masters created an extremely interesting individual style. An inescapable archaistic element infested their work, but their delicate treatment of draperies and their predilection for the grotesque, so conspicuous with Ch'ên Hung-shou especially, and so inseparably bound up with any reversion to the remote past, was not a mere lifeless and servile adherence to tradition. The expressiveness of the faces, a subtle employment of colors, and above all a power of imagination, which at times lends his figures a humorous or whimsical appearance and then again — in their carefully produced ostensible awkwardness — a true antique grandeur, all combine to confirm Ch'ên Hung-shou as one of the last great masters of figure painting in China. A rare masterpiece of this artist is the hand scroll (Honolulu Acad. of Arts) which illustrates the famous "Homecoming" of the early Chinese poet T'ao Ch'ien. Although the grotesque or the bizarre, which characterizes so many of his works, is certainly not lacking, it is here blended with a refined joy of life and a light touch of humor, completely in accord with the spirit of the text it illustrates.

Although artistic activity in the first half of the Ming period had been concentrated in such centers as Soochow, Hangchow, and Peking, with the rise to supremacy of the wên-jên-hua a number of other centers came into prominence and a great many important artists were actively involved. With little difficulty one could muster twenty artists of great ability, each of whom could be regarded as representative in one way or another of literati painting. Besides these there are a number of equally important artists who cannot without qualification be included in the literati classification.

Sung-chiang, the center of Tung Ch'i-ch'ang's movement, never achieved the position which Soochow had earlier held; nevertheless, in its vicinity was concentrated a group of masters whom the Chinese, with their love of systematic classification, have divided into the Su-sung and the Yün-chien schools. The most prominent artist of this group was Chao Tso (ca. 1600), who is regarded as the founder of the Su-sung school, which supposedly combines elements of the styles of Su (chou), or Soochow, and Sung (chiang). He was a master of the primarily polychrome landscape, in which he was able to achieve extremely beautiful pictorial effects.

In Hangchow, the ancient center of the Chê school, the Chê tradition experienced a revival, although in a form which clearly betrays the influence of the wên-jên-hua; even here the literati had secured a firm foothold. Li Jih-hua (1565–1635), who was active here, displays a strong influence from Tung Ch'i-ch'ang in his work, but lacks his careful composition, as a result of which his rather hard, sometimes almost insensitive brushwork becomes all the more conspicuous.

*Ceramics.* Long after the fall of the Sung dynasty, pottery following the Sung ideals of form and decoration was still being produced in some of the kilns where ceramic wares had been made since early in that period. The stylistic changes which occurred in such wares as the Lung-ch'üan celadons were so gradual that it is sometimes difficult to establish a basis for dating. The same holds true for some of the Tz'ǔ-chou wares and for the various glazed stonewares usually designated collectively by the Japanese name *temmoku.*

The 14th century saw the rise of a completely new technique, that of painted decoration in underglaze blue and red. By the middle of the 14th century the new style showed a radical departure from the various styles typical of the Sung period. In the first place, the decorative element, now a painted design, no longer depended upon the decorative effect of the glaze itself, with its mutations and craquelure, or upon an engraved or molded design under the glaze. In this regard, the early blue-and-white porcelain has something in common with the Tz'ǔ-chou wares. In the second place, radical changes

appeared in the shape of the pieces. In particular, the large plate was a novelty in the history of Chinese ceramics. Here there is a clear parallel between early blue-and-white and the later celadon ware, which was also exported in great quantities, as we see, for example, from the great collection of the Topkapu Saray Museum in Istanbul and the Ardebil shrine near Teheran. Perhaps there was also a certain similarity in decoration, even though the mode of application, being incised or molded in relief on the celadon, was very different.

A third point of difference, which assumes perhaps greater significance in the West than it has for the Chinese, is the fact that, from this point in the history of Chinese ceramics, porcelain drove pottery and stoneware from the scene. The fourth point, and perhaps the most important one for the further development of Chinese ceramics, was the growing concentration of the porcelain industry, if not in the immediate vicinity of the village Ching-tê-chên itself, at least in the northeastern part of Kiangsi province, where rich deposits of kaolin and petuntse were available. Beyond any doubt this concentration promoted economical production, and the Chinese potter's art developed from a handicraft carried on in a small number of potter's workshops with small kilns into an industry of gigantic proportions. The industrial organization by which enormous quantities of ware were produced in standard sizes and uniform quality brought with it naturally a division of labor, and Chinese porcelain was to acquire finally an undeniably mechanical character, even though the products retained for many centuries a surprisingly high quality and a refined distinction. A comparison with Japan, where such a concentration of workshops and kilns never took place, shows how unique this phenomenon was before the 19th century.

The new approach to painting initiated by the Four Great Masters of Yüan, and continued in the Ming period by the literati school, drew the greatest artistic talents to it like a magnet. The new conceptions in painting which were created by the intellectual elite of China (the poets, calligraphers, and painters) penetrated only with great slowness into the more conservative capital and into court circles. The vast social abyss which separated the painter and the calligrapher from the potter, the enamel worker, and the lacquerer made it completely impossible for these fresh ideas to find their way in any manner whatsoever into the handicrafts. The latter, not regarded as worthy of comparison with the arts of painting and calligraphy, existed always in cultural isolation; and, while a strong mutual influence is to be detected among the various crafts, no connection at all is to be found between the "higher" and "lower" forms of artistic expression as these are divided on the scale by the Chinese. When at last some interplay between the handicrafts and the art of the elite did manifest itself, under the Ch'ing emperors K'ang-hsi and Ch'ien-lung, it took place at exactly the moment when academic painting had reached its lowest ebb. In Japan, where this strict distinction was never made, the art of painting enriched the art of pottery over and over again; there, however, the strict code of perfectionism, which so long saved Chinese ceramics from a decline to utter spiritlessness, is lacking.

The blue-and-white porcelain of the 14th century, which belongs to the very beginning of these developments, still shows all the freshness of innovation: vigorous and harmonious shapes which make excellent use of the characteristics of the material, and a rich, varied decoration. The pieces are covered with medallions, bands, and friezes made up of closely patterned geometric, floral, and animal motifs of such naturalism that the plants and animals can sometimes be identified. A particularity to be noticed in the 14th-century pieces is the technique whereby the design in white is held back against the blue background (PL. 170).

Some of the decorative elements encountered on the 14th-century blue-and-white were permanently included in the porcelain repertory: the dragon with three, four, or five claws (PL. 280), the *fêng-huang* (a fabulous bird, usually translated as "phoenix"), the banana leaf, the lotus, and the so-called "lotus panel." However, the attractive animal figures found on the bottoms of large plates in 14th-century blue-and-white, largely

disappeared later to make way for grape clusters (PL. 280) and other conventional floral decorations. The lotus underwent numerous stylistic modifications, but held its place in the decoration of Chinese pottery to the very end, and so did the dragon, which took an ever more prominent place.

After the 14th century there arose a less crowded style of decoration which left more unembellished white space. The motifs began gradually to assume a stylized form, and the lively spontaneity apparent in 14th-century porcelain gradually stiffened into a rigid pattern of prescribed elements. The loss of this spontaneity was, however, accompanied by a remarkable improvement in techniques and a progressive refinement of the ware.

With the Yung-lo period (1403-24) appeared the application of reign marks to ceramic products (probably an indication that the Ming emperors had discovered the wares of Ching-tê-chên) and by the time of the Hsüan-tê reign (1426-35) the marked pieces show a quality which was afterward never surpassed. Yet it is not always easy to distinguish between provincial and Ching-tê-chên wares — nor between imperial wares, wares for common Chinese usage, and export wares, though most periods include a group of ceramics of such high quality that we may safely assume them to have been made for imperial use. Whatever the nature of imperial supervision was, when the imperial authority waned near the end of the Ming period, the quality of the porcelain of Ching-tê-chên also declined visibly. One of the cardinal differences between export and imperial porcelain, as we learn from the collections in Teheran and Istanbul, was that the export porcelain was generally of heavier quality. Purely commercial considerations, such as the greater breakage to be expected with more fragile pieces, may have been a factor, but the possibility that a greater number of the more fragile exported pieces have been lost over the centuries is not to be completely rejected.

Besides the use of cobalt blue, we see the appearance in the Ming period of polychrome decoration (PLS. 168, 170) as well as monochrome decoration in other colors than blue. Especially during the 14th and early 15th century, copper red was employed under the glaze, but the technical difficulties involved in obtaining a good red color prevented its use on a very large scale. A combination of cobalt blue and copper red, on the other hand, offered very attractive possibilities. Soon, however, the technique of underglaze red was abandoned and replaced by that of red enamel.

With the end of the Hsüan-tê period, the production of porcelain at Ching-tê-chên seems to have temporarily declined in quality as well as quantity, but the Ch'êng-hua period (1465-87) witnessed a marked revival, all the more notable because of the many innovations in decoration. From this time on, polychrome decoration by means of enamels assumed great importance, often in combination with decoration in underglaze blue. Perhaps the most refined examples of this new technique, which is usually called *tou-ts'ai* ("contrasting colors"), are the so-called "chicken" cups; in these the minute design was first outlined in underglaze blue, after which the outlined areas were filled with colored enamels, for example, in iron red, light green, and yellow. These exquisite cups were often imitated, and numerous later pieces pay homage to the artisans of the Ch'êng-hua period by displaying the reign mark of that period. Another technique which became fashionable was that in which a design of dragons was incised in the paste before firing and left as an unglazed area which was afterward painted with enamels of another color. In other pieces a cobalt blue underglaze decoration of flower and fruit sprays was combined with a yellow enameled background. All these new techniques, to which many more were added in the course of time by the enamelers, brought the ceramic art of the Ming period to a hitherto unknown level of technical skill and gave it a refinement which is scarcely rivaled by the ceramics of other periods.

The invention of these new decorative techniques tended to reduce the importance of the blue-and-white porcelains. Although the Hsüan-tê types had become classical and were already being copied, an increasing number of the pieces in contemporary styles showed inferior quality in the rendering of the design. In that period during which the Portuguese maintained an almost complete monopoly in the China trade, neither export procelain in the purely Chinese style nor porcelain of the sort made especially for the Portuguese market seems to have reached Europe in large quantities. However, after the Dutch East India Company had established trade relations with China, large quantities of Chinese export porcelain were exported to Europe. Although this ware enjoyed a great reputation in the West, where nothing remotely comparable in quality could be produced, it was not equal to the wares made at the same time for the Chinese market, nor to the export porcelain of the 14th and 15th centuries. In many respects the export porcelain had already begun to display the degenerative characteristics of a mass-produced article. The elements of the decoration, though not lacking in elegance, were repeated again and again with little variation, and the high standards of earlier Ming wares were abandoned. The export porcelain of this period, which enjoyed great popularity in the Near East and in western Europe, is often called "kraak" porcelain, from the Dutch version of a Spanish term designating a type of ship used in the trade with China. The same term is often erroneously applied to the somewhat later blue-and-white wares, made when the porcelain industry was suffering from the heavy damage inflicted upon Ching-tê-chên, during the wars accompanying the fall of the Ming dynasty. These wares, now usually described as "transitional," were not exported to Europe in great quantities, and for a brief period at that time Japanese wares took the place of Chinese porcelain on the European market.

*Lacquer, metalwork, minor crafts.* The lacquer workers of the Yüan period, whose names appear on many pieces made by the carved red-lacquer technique, may be regarded as the pioneers who made possible the later flowering of the art in the Ming period. This carved red-lacquer technique, together with that in which the design is cut into the lacquer and filled up with layers of lacquer of another color in such a way that the design is not lost with wear, enjoyed the ascendancy during the Ming period. Inlaying with mother-of-pearl had, in general, lost its importance. A large group of fine *sūtra* chests, sometimes cited to prove that nacre work flourished during the Ming period, are very probably of Korean origin, while what we may regard as Chinese pieces often appear to be already the predecessors of the modern mother-of-pearl bazaar wares.

A great deal of uncertainty prevails as to the dating of pieces of carved red lacquer, especially since, in contrast with porcelain wares, the possibility that the decoration and the incised date on a piece have been applied at different times is very great. It may nevertheless be assumed that there was a close relationship between the decoration of porcelain, lacquer, and even silver, and herein lies perhaps the possibility of eventually forming a general picture of the stylistic development of lacquer during the Ming period. The motif of two flying phoenixes placed opposite each other, the one with the head, the other with the tail in the air, had already appeared on the lacquer and silverwork of the early 14th century as well as on the blue-and-white porcelain. This motif appears also on the carved red lacquer of the group which Sir Harry Garner places in the 14th and 15th centuries, where it is surrounded by a lobed rosette border exactly as it is on the *chin-kin sūtra* chests. As is the case with the blue porcelain, the human figure is usually lacking in the decoration on the earlier lacquer pieces, but begins to appear more often, placed amid landscapes with trees and buildings, on the pieces with the Hsüan-tê mark. There is also a striving after polychromy which may well have been arrived at under the influence of the corresponding tendency in the ceramic arts. A background of contrasting color is achieved through the application of lacquer of another color under the layers of red lacquer in which the design is cut away, and a polychrome effect is also produced in the decoration of the painted or inlaid pieces.

In the Ming period, the technique of cloisonné enamel work came to the fore for the first time. Here, too, the dating of the extant pieces is still extremely uncertain, as a result of

which it is impossible to determine the correctness of the hypothesis that this technique may have been imported during the Yüan period. The tentative chronological classification proposed by Sir Harry Garner, based upon a comparison with the decoration on porcelain, offers many possibilities for extension and further research. His supposition that the cloisonné technique began with a relatively simple color scheme, from which it became gradually more complicated, is not only logical, but agrees with what we know about the development of taste at that time. According to the Chinese tradition, the Ching-t'ai period (1450–57) represented the pinnacle of cloisonné production, and, if so, this was certainly the only distinction of an otherwise inglorious era.

While ceramics and lacquer work both managed during the Ming period to maintain definite standards of artistic excellence, at least in those pieces where this was demanded, the imperial treasures from the recently opened tomb of the emperor Wan-li (buried in 1620) reveal the depths to which the art of working in precious metals had already sunk. Among the pieces found, the golden *chüeh*, a tripod inspired by the classical bronze type, and the ewer, which confirms the Ming dating on a similar silver piece in the Kempe Collection (Ekolsund, Sweden), are both inlaid with precious stones and jade and can only be described as examples of ostentatious splendor manifesting what was, even for those times, a remarkable lack of taste. A silver ewer in the Kempe Collection which is probably considerably older (PL. 274) is distinctly finer and more elegant in form than the one from the imperial tomb.

THE CH'ING DYNASTY (1644–1912). The Manchu emperor, who had already assumed for himself the imperial title in 1635 while the Ming dynasty still ruled, was not to be expelled once he had been admitted within the borders of the realm and into the precincts of Peking by the quarreling Chinese, and his successors, in a series of bloody campaigns, were able to complete his work by bringing all of China under their authority. However, the Chinese generals who had served as confederates in the conquest of the south revolted in 1673, and held the entire area south of the Yangtze River until the Manchus were ultimately able to suppress the insurrection.

The Manchus, who came as conquerors and were from the Chinese point of view no more than "barbarians," attempted to retain their national identity, in particular by maintaining the strict military organization of their "banners" and by forbidding marriage between Chinese and Manchus; nevertheless, they were unable to stand up against the superior traditions of Chinese culture and were not even able to avoid conversion to the use of Chinese as their colloquial language. Even before the conquest, when they dominated only Manchuria, they had displayed a deep respect for Chinese civilization, and in the end they were fully Sinicized, becoming almost more Chinese than were the Ming, and supporting the Chinese culture in its most orthodox form.

The great emperors of the Ch'ing dynasty, Shêng-tsu (reigned as K'ang-hsi, 1662–1722), Shih-tsung (reigned as Yung-chêng, 1723–35), and Kao-tsung (reigned as Ch'ien-lung, 1736–95), who had in common a sincere devotion to and serious concern for Chinese culture, did a great deal to catalogue, collect, and organize that which had been achieved in earlier periods in all fields of Chinese civilization. K'ang-hsi's name will be forever connected with the great dictionary of the Chinese language which was compiled under his patronage, while Ch'ien-lung commanded the compilation of the enormous bibliographical work which took form in the *Ssŭ-k'u ch'üan-shu*. It was also Ch'ien-lung who greatly expanded the imperial collection of paintings, calligraphy, bronzes, and other *objets d'art*. Even though this collection may have lost a considerable number of pieces in the course of the political complications following World War II, when it was moved from the National Palace Museum in Peking to Taichung on Formosa (q.v. under CHINA), the core of Ch'ien-lung's collection is still there. The great interest which the Ch'ing emperors displayed in the manufacture of porcelain contributed no doubt to the maintenance of the ancient standards of quality which long preserved this

craft from the inglorious decline which other handicrafts had already experienced.

The orientation of the Ch'ing period remained fixed upon the past and was in principle conservative. There was no longer any influx of new ideas to speak of. European civilization, with which the Chinese were acquainted through Catholic missionaries in Peking, was too remote to exercise any fertilizing influence. During this period the great current of Chinese culture, which in spite of foreign rulers had continued to flow without interruption, slowly but surely dried up. This cultural depletion may have been related to the predominating conservatism, which destroyed the attraction of the court for such original spirits of the time as, for instance, the "Individualists." The orthodox attitude of the court, however, was not necessarily the sole cause for the fact that the most significant artistic movements of the time developed in a region remote from the capital. After Chinese civilization began to apply the Confucian principle of "transmit but not create" in a drastic manner in the 18th century, it was not until modern times that new ideas touching all facets of culture were produced in China, and these are of such recent date that we still lack the distance necessary for impartial judgment.

*Painting.* Although the Manchus established their capital, after the conquest of the Chinese empire, in the city of Peking, their authority over the south of China continued for a considerable time to be somewhat insecure. In those regions remote from the capital, where from ancient times painters had lived and worked, their influence was scarcely felt, and the art of the literati continued undisturbed by their coming, except for those who had been in the government service — and not many at the beginning felt inclined to enter into the service of the new overlords. Perhaps it was a certain feeling of historical similarity between their own position and that of the great Yüan masters which led the artists of this period to a deep absorption in the Yüan works. For the painters of the Lou-tung or T'ai-ts'ang school, who were strongly influenced by the theories of Tung Ch'i-ch'ang and in some respects formed an extension of the Sung-chiang school, the emulation of the Yüan masters was not a vague sentimental movement, but a seriously conceived task which they took upon themselves with appropriate modesty. Wang Shih-min (1592–1680) and Wang Chien (1598–1677), two artists who only by coincidence bore the same family name, formed the first generation of this school. (See WANG SHIH-MIN.) The second consisted of Wang Shih-min's disciple Wang Hui (1632–1717) and his grandson Wang Yüan-ch'i (1642–1715). These painters, known as the "Four Wangs," took Huang Kung-wang and Ni Tsan as their models, and they left no stone unturned in the effort to find authentic works of these masters in order to recreate them with serious, unadulterated accuracy and with attention to the very brush strokes with which each detail was rendered. Excellent as their brushwork may be, their composition is often somewhat dry and barren. That these artists together with Yün Shou-p'ing (1633–90), the last important painter of flowers, and Wu Li (q.v., 1632–1718), who was converted to Christianity and died as a Jesuit priest without this contact with Western culture having exerted any influence on his painting, should have been viewed as the Six Great Painters of the Ch'ing Period seems at first sight astonishing. Their works are too studied, too much conceived from the point of view of art history, and too little touched by spontaneity to justify our putting these no doubt technically very competent artists on the same plane with the Four Great Masters of Yüan and the great masters of the Ming. If, however, one compares them with the painters of the revived Imperial Academy, which produced very few figures of more than average significance, in spite of the fact that Emperor Shun-chih (1644–61) was himself no mean painter and that his successors were passionate collectors, and if one considers that those who lived in retirement as monks, eccentric hermits, or gentlemen of leisure were only recognized in limited circles (not in contact with Peking and the imperial court), then this classification seems more appropriate than one might at first think. Wang Yüan-ch'i, the youngest

of the Four Wangs, held high office, and he it was who at the imperial command compiled the *P'ei-wen-chai shu-hua-p'u* (1708), the great encyclopedic work on calligraphy and painting. This is a good indication of the extent to which the court must have been biased in favor of the theories and works of the Four Wangs.

Meanwhile, even though the style of the Four Wangs and their pupils had obtained official recognition, there had arisen elsewhere movements in painting which were differently oriented. The artists involved in these movements, widely differing from one another as they certainly did, have been nevertheless brought together by the Chinese under several group names, the "Four Masters of Hsin-an," the "Eight Eccentrics of Yang-chou," and the "Eight Masters of Chin-ling," although several of the most prominent figures in this period are not included in these classifications.

Of the Four Masters of Hsin-an (in Anhwei province) the most important were Ch'a Shih-piao (1615–98) and Hung-jên (d. 1663), the religious name which the painter Chiang T'ao took upon becoming a monk. These two artists, the first a civil servant who withdrew from public life at the fall of the Ming dynasty, the second a young man who entered the monastic life in the same period, have much in common in their work. Both followed the general tendency to turn to the Yüan masters as a source of inspiration; this they did, however, in a much more spontaneous and affecting manner than their contemporaries, sometimes adopting the "dry brush" technique of Ni Tsan. While Ch'a Shih-piao was influenced by such men as Shên Chou and used a fluid brush technique producing strong contrasts, Hung-jên, who was perhaps the most original of the Anhwei masters, reinterpreted the art of Ni Tsan in the most direct fashion. Avoiding mannerisms and tricks, he made no effort to imitate the composition, but strove instead to achieve an inner relationship with the great master whom he had taken as his example. In comparison with his many surviving album leaves, the large vertical paintings of Hung-jên are small in number. In the case of many Ming artists during the early phase of the *wên-jên-hua*, the large landscapes cannot stand comparison with the horizontal scrolls and album leaves. This is no longer true in the works of Hung-jên, Ch'a Shih-piao, and a number of other masters of the Ch'ing period, probably because training in the art of painting, which had been emphasized by Tung Ch'i-ch'ang and his followers, was taken more seriously than at the beginning of the literati movement. One of the great masterpieces of Hung-jên is *The Coming of Autumn* (PL. 290), which fully testifies to the mastery this painter had developed in the large format. In detail, it shows a clear relationship with Ni Tsan, though the building up of the rock masses in flat terraces and square blocks differs completely from the method of the Yüan masters. Seldom has a work of art using different methods and a different type of composition so immediately recalled the spirit of an earlier art as does this work, with its kinship to painting of the 14th century. Hung-jên, more than any other master, realized that ideal which had been so often professed and so seldom attained — that the old masters should be emulated by "transmitting their spirit, not their external form." It is remarkable that he attracted so little attention among those who had most conspicuously flourished this principle.

The group of artists known as the "Eight Masters of Chin-ling," after the old name of the city of Nanking, had nothing in common except their supposed residence in this city, and not all, indeed, shared this. Several of the artists of this school had merits which it would be a mistake to underestimate. Among them is Fan Ch'i (1616–after 1692), one of whose finest paintings is a long hand scroll representing a river landscape (formerly Staatliche Mus., Berlin). It is painted in a surprisingly meticulous, orthodox polychrome style, reminding us of such painters as Chao Po-chü of the Sung period. The greatest artist in this mixed company is by good fortune the master whose works have been preserved in the greatest numbers, Kung Hsien (ca. 1625–after 1698). His work is that of the true individualist, having little in common with his predecessors, and not having been emulated by many of his pupils.

He worked carefully and methodically paying great attention to the technique of painting, as appears from his treatise on the art of the landscape. (His pupil Wang Kai made an important contribution to the completion of the renowned encyclopedic work *Chieh-tzŭ-yüan hua-chuan*, in which the technique of painting is dealt with in great detail.) Kung Hsien, despite elaborate structuring, was never mired down in brush strokes and composition. On the contrary, he was able to achieve something entirely new with his technical excellence and an unusual brush technique of broad, short vertical strokes which identify his works immediately. There is no place in his landscapes, any more than in those of the Yüan masters or Hung-jên, for the human figure, no matter how small and insignificant. He made use of all possible tints and shades of ink, but his preference was for the darkest tones contrasting with the white of the paper, which gave his landscapes a somber and grim aspect — like an imaginary lunar landscape — rather than the thin and melancholy loneliness of Ni Tsan and Hung-jên. In the mysterious play of light and darkness, the waterfalls and brooks stand out sharply amidst the black mountains and move like incongruous streams of lava over the carbonized black of the high, soaring mountain walls.

The group of masters whom we are accustomed to refer to collectively as the "Great Individualists" are K'un-ts'an, Shih-t'ao, Pa-ta-shan-jên, and in a certain sense also Mei Ch'ing. Their work has for a long time been highly appreciated both in China and in Japan and, more recently, has constituted one of the great "discoveries" made by Western connoisseurs. However, during their lives the extraordinary artistic talents of these artists, who lived withdrawn from society, seem scarcely to have been known outside a small circle of intellectuals who lived a similar life of retirement.

K'un-ts'an (known also as Shih-ch'i) and Shih-t'ao were referred to together as the "Two Stones," since *shih* means "stone." Both were Buddhist monks, though of somewhat unorthodox persuasion. K'un-ts'an entered a monastic order at a very early age and became later in life the abbot of the Niu-shou-ssŭ monastery near Nanking. The accounts of his life, as well as some of the inscriptions written by contemporaries on his paintings, testify to his deep religious devotion. He was undoubtedly greatly attracted by the individualistic element in the Meditative Buddhism of the Ch'an sect, and a few of his works which depict meditating figures reflect this religious interest; in general, however, it is difficult to show any clear connection between his extraordinary personality and his paintings, most of which are landscapes. His strongly individualistic conception did not bring him to such an extreme style that we are unable to place him in his time and environment, any more than his unorthodox religious convictions excluded him from the traditional monastic community. Like the masters of the Lou-tung school he constructed his enormous landscapes with the utmost care, painting every detail with punctilious precision; the aridness, however, which so often accompanies exaggerated accuracy, is completely lacking here. The movement he was able to incorporate into his landscapes is accentuated by the interplay of clouds and mist strata which intrude upon the foreground through the openings between the masses of rocks. Although he was obviously influenced by the masters of his time and his great predecessors, one cannot point to any single artist who served him as an example, since he seems to have taken nature itself as his teacher — to use an expression much beloved and much abused by the Chinese art critics. Landscapes with which he was familiar through a sojourn of years on the spot, for example the view of the Pao-ên-ssŭ (dated 1664, Coll. K. Sumitomo, Oiso, Japan), were painted with an ease and equilibrium which demonstrate fully his intimate familiarity with nature. Red-brown and blue were his favorite colors. Both horizontal and vertical scroll painting as well as the album leaf are forms in which he was at ease and which reveal him as an extremely consistent painter and a truly great master.

Buddhism takes a much less prominent place with the second of the Two Stones, Shih-t'ao (Tao-chi). As a distant family relation of the Ming imperial house, he became a Buddhist

monk at the fall of the dynasty in 1644. Apparently, however, he never retired to the isolation of a monastery, but mostly led a roving life. He knew personally the other three Great Individualists, but on the whole the members of this group seem to have exercised very little influence on each other. He began very young to paint and dedicated himself at first especially to plants, among others the orchid and the bamboo, as in the piece dated 1662 in the Cleveland Museum of Art; only later did he turn to landscape painting. The great landscape inspired by Li T'ai-po's poem on Lu-shan, a mountain which Shih-t'ao knew very well, has the largest dimensions of any remaining work (Coll. K. Sumitomo, Oiso, Japan). It shows clearly that Shih-t'ao was much less at home from a technical point of view with a large format than with a small album leaf, where the virtuosity of his sometimes extremely minute brushwork was much more effective. The structure of the mountain, which rises up to a great height and is partly concealed from view by mist, is not successfully executed; however, the two figures in the foreground, who stand on the edge of a deep precipice contemplating a waterfall, accentuate the height of the mountain and the depth of the ravine, giving the necessary balance to the vertical movement in this extraordinarily large painting.

The true genius of Shih-t'ao is displayed most convincingly in his album leaves (PL. 292) and hand scrolls. There is no trace in these of the gloom and melancholy of Hung-jên or Kung-hsien, and the human element so conspicuously lacking in the works of those painters is almost always represented. Some of his album leaves are in monochrome, painted with a fluid brush and a rich variation of tones, but Shih-t'ao was even more a virtuoso with polychrome album leaves, sometimes rendered in a technique closely resembling that of European water colors. Blue and brown were his favorite colors and were often applied in washes over which the black outlines were painted while still wet, so that the contours lost their sharp delineation. Shih-t'ao was extremely versatile, and his paintings show a great variation in theme as well as in technique and style. Landscapes are by far the most numerous, although he also painted bamboos and flowers, and even left a self-portrait. He sometimes used a fine brush, rendering elaborate and complex details in the construction of rocks and mountains; in other paintings he used a sweeping wet brush. Some paintings were executed with such spontaneous verve that we might almost call them "coarse" — which is indeed the proper epithet for the later imitations, provided with poetical inscriptions in a bad counterfeit of Shih-t'ao's fine handwriting. In the treatise *Hua-yü-lu* (full German translation by V. Contag), Shih-t'ao set down, in a brilliant but extraordinarily difficult style, the essence of his artistic credo. This work is the principal source of information about his personality and reveals him as an individualistic and original virtuoso of the highest order. Yet, saturated as it is with Taoist and Buddhist allusions, it sometimes seems less a sincere outpouring of the artist's heart than a literary tour de force, a play with words. The same holds true for some of his paintings, which are touched with humor, for the games he played with the great masters of the past, and for the self-conceit which he sometimes assumed and which was in all probability no more than a pose.

Chu Ta, better known as Pa-ta-shan-jên (q.v.), was, like Shih-t'ao, a distant relative of the Ming imperial family who withdrew into retirement at the fall of the dynasty. If we may believe the numerous anecdotes concerning this artist, his eccentricity was not merely a pose, but the direct consequence of a complicated and pathological character. Album leaves make up a great number of his paintings, usually in monochrome, representing landscapes, flowers, birds, and fishes rendered in a sketchy, spontaneous manner. His extraordinary talent for composition and his mastery of the monochrome technique remind us of the early Ch'an masters, and especially of the equally eccentric Ming painter Hsü Wei, who is perhaps closest to him in personality and whose paintings he frequently copied. The brushwork of his masterpieces (e.g., the album in the Coll. K. Sumitomo, Oiso, Japan) has a power and a certainty of intention which is rare in the history of painting, even in a country where the power of the brush was from ancient times a criterion of beauty and character.

It is quite probable that there is a hidden symbolism behind some of the work of Chu Ta, such as his sometimes bizarre combinations of fishes, birds, and rocks, and his delightfully painted animals. The hand scroll representing rocks, plants, and fishes in the Cleveland Museum of Art is an example. The spontaneous "ink play" of this painting is accompanied by inscribed verses which, though abstruse and full of dark allusions, seem to suggest heaven, the faded glories of the Ming past, and Buddhist immortality in three symbolic scenes. A leaf in the Sumitomo Collection (1694) representing two quails by a rock has in common with this hand scroll a pun on the word "yellow," the imperial color, evidently an allusion to the imperial descent of the artist. The large landscapes of Chu Ta (PL. 290), often painted in a wild impulsive manner, seem to be truly the creations of a mad genius, but the chaos of strokes and dots which seems to reflect the chaotic spirit of the artist becomes much more methodical when the paintings are looked at from a distance. An artist like Chu Ta, who was scarcely understood as a personality during his own lifetime, and whose poems were a problem even for the great literati of that time, will probably always remain a mystery. It seems safe to conclude, however, that there was more method in his madness than has usually been supposed. A letter which has come down to us, written to him by Shih-t'ao, seems to point to that conclusion.

Mei Ch'ing (1623–97), who came from Anhwei and who was, therefore, at home in the same environment as Hung-jên and Ch'a Shih-piao, departed radically from the style of those artists. In spite of his relationship with the Yüan tradition in the work of Wu Chên, for example, he created a completely new and personal style which broke so sharply with convention that we should do best to regard him as one of the Individualists, especially in view of his contacts with Shih-t'ao. The Huang-shan, a famous mountain in Anhwei near which he had spent much time, inspired him, as it had Shih-t'ao, to paint some of his best works. Most of his paintings repeat the particular type of pine tree characteristic of this region, which has full spreading branches and no peak. In Mei Ch'ing's paintings the pine forests become one close-packed, prickly whole, and in his subtly painted album leaves (PL. 291) we have almost the impression of looking, not at a chain of pine-covered mountaintops, but rather at a rotten tree stump covered with a luxuriant growth of moss. In other works he demonstrates a somewhat rougher and more emotional brushwork.

The style which had been created by the Four Wangs, Wu Li, and Yün Shou-p'ing, on the basis of that of the Sung-chiang school led by Tung Ch'i-ch'ang, became one of the official styles of the Ch'ing period. In general, however, after the Six Great Painters of the Ch'ing Period, their school brought forth very little great talent. Such court painters as T'ang Tai (active, first half of 18th cent.), who left evidence of his technical competence as well as of his lack of artistic inspiration in his treatise on the technique of painting and in his relatively few extant paintings, and Li Shih-cho (ca. 1750), who was a highly polished artist, are unable to stand comparison with the groups from Anhwei and Nanking, not to speak of the Individualists. Most of these artists had technical competence, but the Lou-tung school declined in significance after the time of the Great Six in spite of the imperial favor which it received.

One of the most interesting figures of the Ch'ing period and one who stood out far above the other painters of the court circle was Kao Ch'i-p'ei (1672?–1734, PL. 288). He was the most important master of finger painting, a somewhat out of the way technique which, it would seem, was initiated by the first Manchu emperor himself. In the history of Chinese painting we repeatedly encounter artists who tried to replace the brush by another instrument, by a lotus stem, for instance; for the most part these efforts amounted to little more than playful experiments and very quickly passed into oblivion. This was not the case, however, with the art of finger painting, in which the tips of the fingers and the long nails of the literator (who demonstrated his repugnance for manual labor by

letting them grow as long as possible) served in place of the brush. The painters who applied this new technique made no strict principle of adhering to it and did not hesitate to resort to the brush in order to paint in with water colors the lighter areas, and perhaps for this reason it became something more than a vain game of virtuosity. Kao Ch'i-p'ei's nephew Chu Lun-han as well as a number of lesser masters followed his example, and finger painting, which later found exponents in Korea and Japan as well, enjoyed a certain popularity for a considerable time.

Among the painters at the court of Ch'ien-lung (1736–95), the Italian missionary Giuseppe Castiglione (1688–1766) won a special fame under his Chinese name Lang Shih-ning. He was certainly not the only European, nor was he the first, to be active in China as a painter. Chinese interest in European painting, which especially concentrated on the representation of perspective, had developed much earlier, but reached its high point with the popularity of Lang Shih-ning. In view of the predilection of Western orientalists for subjects and personalities which seem to form a bridge between East and West, it is understandable that his work soon attracted European attention; however, it breathes a hybrid spirit which awakens on our part more curiosity than admiration.

The emperor Ch'ien-lung must be assessed very highly as a collector, even though he deprived many of the most beautiful old paintings in his collection of much of their effect by inscribing overlong and extraordinarily uninteresting poems and colophons on them. Nevertheless, he was not particularly original in his taste for the painting of his own time. Such representatives of the imperial taste of the Manchu period as the painter of birds and flowers Chiang T'ing-hsi (1669–1732) or Chin T'ing-piao (active ca. 1720–60) fail to command our admiration. However, we should perhaps not be too harsh in our judgment, for it is doubtful whether Ch'ien-lung had any knowledge at all of the many more interesting movements in painting which took place outside the vicinity of the capital.

A group of independent figures known together as the "Eight Eccentrics of Yang-chou" close the series of interesting personalities in which Chinese painting through the centuries has been so extraordinarily rich. The common denominator of this group seems to be mainly the fact that these artists all resided for a shorter or longer period in Yang-chou (Yang-chow, in Kiangsu). With the exception of Lo P'ing, their period of activity was largely during the first half of the 18th century. Probably the most interesting members of this school are Chin Nung (1687–1764), Chêng Hsieh (1693–1765), Lo P'ing (1733–99), Hua Yen (1682–after 1760), and Huang Shên (1687–ca. 1768). The first two are famous not only as painters, but also as calligraphers, Chin Nung having been by far the more versatile of the two. There can be no doubt that his angular thick handwriting enormously enhances the beauty of his copies of the Buddhist *sūtras* and that there was no writing more perfectly suited than his for reproducing the Buddhist texts. This master painted not only plum blossoms, likewise a specialty of Lo P'ing, and bamboos, the great favorite of Chêng Hsieh, but also horses and, especially, Buddhist figures. All these masters seemed to feel keenly the fact that they were the bearers of an ancient tradition. It was still the practice to declare that they had taken a particular master from the past as their example; however, while the academic artists were slowly crushed under the weight of tradition, this was not the case with the independent artists.

In Li Shan we find something similar to Hsü Wei, though he lacks the enormous impetuosity of that artist. His studies of rocks, plants, flowers, and insects are set down on paper with powerful brush strokes in a few accurate, telling lines and black dots. In the case of Chêng Hsieh and Lo P'ing, who also painted primarily in black and white, the influence of their calligraphic training is clear; the latter artist in particular, by the sensitive brushwork in his figure painting and his perceptive psychological treatment of the human face, is characterized as a painter of truly great merit. On the other hand, neither the figure painting of Huang Shên, which displays a cheerful but not very profound vision, nor his hand-

writing, which can rank as one of the most illegible hands of any Chinese artist, are very impressive. The work of these painters, especially that of Chêng Hsieh, was influenced by Shih-t'ao, who is said to have passed the last years of his life in Yang-chou. This group of artists, who were the last representatives of the great Chinese tradition, never achieved the heights which had been reached by the early Individualists, but their originality cannot be denied.

*Ceramics and export art.* The coming of the Manchu dynasty, which sounded the rapid and inglorious decline of most of the Chinese handicrafts and degraded both carved red lacquer and cloisonné, which was still being produced in great quantities, to a lifeless and tasteless mass product, gave surprisingly a new and a last great stimulus to the ceramic arts in China. The porcelain which was produced during the reigns of K'ang-hsi, Yung-chêng, and Ch'ien-lung shows, on the one hand, an effort to revive some of the many techniques which had been developed during the Ming period and, on the other hand, an incessant search for new technical possibilities to extend polychrome decoration (PL. 170) and to add new and rare tints to the repertory of monochrome decoration. There was also a sort of renaissance of the Sung styles which was closely connected with the interests of the emperors, especially Ch'ien-lung, in the Kuan-yao produced in the Southern Sung capital Hangchow. A considerable number of pieces of this ware were in the imperial collection, and some had inscriptions engraved by Emperor Ch'ien-lung with his own hands, expressing his admiration for the Sung ceramics. This attitude toward the ceramic arts was unique on the part of the emperor, though his predecessors had indeed concerned themselves seriously with the ceramic industry. Whereas earlier the line of demarcation between porcelain intended for imperial use and that intended for export is often difficult to determine, there appear in this period a number of pieces which, from the marks applied to them, were beyond a doubt produced at the order of the emperor and for the use of the court. The technical and artistic characteristics of these pieces clearly excel those of other similar pieces.

The adherence to previous decorative techniques and the revival of Ming styles is manifested by copies in the Yung-chêng period of Ming blue-and-white and by the reanimation of the *tou-ts'ai* technique of the Ch'êng-hua period. During the entire K'ang-hsi period the technique of underglaze decoration in cobalt blue was maintained at a high level, while also during the reign of Ch'ien-lung fine pieces were produced in this style. However, the creative genius of the Chinese porcelain decorator found another possibility for development. This was the technique of enameled porcelain, which under the patronage of the Ch'ing dynasty became a triumph of the potter's art.

The Ch'ing period porcelain with polychrome decoration which was exported to Europe is generally roughly divided into four groups according to the main color of the decoration. These are the so-called *famille verte* (PL. 289), *famille noire* (PLS. 170, 298), *famille rose* (PL. 297), and *famille jaune*. A great deal of the *famille verte*, which was produced in great quantities especially during the K'ang-hsi period, was exported to Europe. The differences in style within this group were relatively slight; the pieces themselves, however, differ considerably as to quality. In contrast with the rather overloaded decoration of the export porcelain, the pieces made for the Chinese market show a less crowded ornamentation much better adapted to the form of the piece, painted generally in a much more refined and delicate style. Elegant female figures, branches of flowers, butterflies, and birds in the decoration display an unmistakable relationship to the styles of academic painting. While academic painting was completely subordinate in importance to the work of the Individualists, transmuted in the hands of the enameler, the style came fully into its own in the art of porcelain decoration. The pinnacle of this development was reached when rose as an enamel color, which had at first occupied only a very modest position, completely replaced green, and the *famille rose* (PL. 297) resulted. The

Ku-yüeh-hsüan porcelain, the finest ware decorated in the *famille-rose* style, which seems to have been produced exclusively for the Chinese market and especially for the court, represents the ultimate point in technical perfection and refinement, slowly acquired through long effort. On pieces in the *famille-rose* style, the design, applied with rare feeling for line and color, together with the carefully calligraphed lines of verse and the red seals, though adapted to the round surface, closely correspond to the manner of the accomplished professional paintings of the Imperial Academy.

The inevitable decline was long in coming; a centuries' old tradition of highly developed, perfection-seeking craftsmanship can maintain itself for a long time in a country such as China, where, at that time, almost ideal conditions prevailed for the maintenance of tradition. However, under Ch'ien-lung the potter departed from those objectives which he had earlier conceived so clearly and had so directly approached. A lapse into repetition and a freezing of decoration through monotonous repetition, rather than any notable technical decline, are the characteristics of the decay which began at that time and thereafter became ever more conspicuous. The imitations in ceramics of lacquer work, cloisonné enamel, and jade are clever tricks of virtuosity which amaze us with their deceptively accurate mimicry of materials so different from porcelain, but the very quantities in which they were produced suggest that the mentality of the potter and of his patrons as well had greatly changed.

The last great director of the imperial porcelain factory at Ching-tê-chên was T'ang Yin, who assumed his office with the ascent to the throne of Ch'ien-lung and remained responsible for the production of imperial porcelain until either 1749 or 1755. It appears that decay set in shortly after his departure. The porcelain of the Chia-ch'ing period (1796–1821) is nevertheless often difficult to distinguish from the Ch'ien-lung porcelain unless the marks on the piece ensure the accuracy of the dating. The following period (1821–50) was marked by a conspicuous decline in quality. The great Taiping rebellion, which afflicted China about the middle of the 19th century and brought great devastation to Ching-tê-chên and the surrounding areas, represented, in spite of later efforts to revive the ancient handicraft, the final end of a very ancient tradition, the fruits of which more than anything else had made the name of China known over the entire world.

During the K'ang-hsi period, when the productivity of Ching-tê-chên, which had been drastically reduced at the time of the fall of the house of Ming, had again begun to rise appreciably, important quantities of blue-and-white porcelain (PL. 289) were shipped to Europe. Obviously well aware of the commercial possibilities of porcelain export, the Chinese, in the efficient and businesslike manner which characterized in every way the management of Ching-tê-chên, adapted themselves to satisfy the demands of their foreign customers. As a result, there grew up, especially in the port city of Canton, a thriving center for a sort of hybrid handicraft to produce goods intended exclusively for the European market.

A great part of the Chinese export porcelain of the K'ang-hsi period shows scarcely any European influence. Occasionally we see that in the shape some special European requirement was taken into consideration, and porcelain copies were made of European glass, silver, earthenware, and porcelain. There are also a number of pieces which betray their European destination in their decoration, notably those showing the heraldic arms of various countries or provinces or of innumerable prominent European families. Besides this group, the so-called Jesuit porcelain was decorated with pious Christian motifs. Originally the exotic decoration, often reproduced from engravings or drawn designs, was applied in Ching-tê-chên; during the Yung-chêng period, however, the porcelain to be enameled was usually taken to Canton, especially after that city had become an important center for what we now call "Canton enamel," as a result of the importation by missionaries of the technique for applying enamel to metal.

Within the framework of Chinese art as a whole these hybrid, commercialized forms of handicraft were scarcely representative of Chinese culture of that time. Probably the Coromandel screens, which were so much admired in Europe, form an exception to this. Incorrectly named after a transshipment area on the coast of India, these specimens of later Chinese lacquer work, which were probably manufactured in north or central China, are by no means typical mass-produced export products. Among the finest examples there are several which depict purely Chinese scenes on one side and on the other represent Europeans hunting or aboard ship. Considering the repertory of themes rather than the style, which is purely Chinese, one might be inclined to regard these pieces as export products, but the Chinese were themselves interested in the Europeans who came to China and were wont to depict these strange barbarians on porcelain or lacquer for their own use. The Coromandel screens, together with several rare examples of porcelain not intended for export and bearing representations of Europeans, may form the Chinese counterpart of the *chinoiserie* which developed in Europe.

A special technique which the Chinese learned from the Europeans and which was especially practiced in Canton was painting on glass. In this technique the painting was executed in reverse on the back of the material, with the details and shadows painted in first and the large areas later. It was widely applied in China for the production of knickknacks for export, but seems to have attracted little attention in China itself and never attained a high artistic level, except perhaps in the decoration of small snuff bottles painted on the inside in the *églomisé* technique. To permit the application of the water colors which were used for this purpose, it was necessary to etch the surface of the glass with a corrosive acid. Since this technique first became known in China about the end of the 19th century, these ingeniously decorated snuff bottles could not have been created before that time. (See CERAMICS; LACQUER.)

*Jades.* While Chinese sculpture in stone and wood showed in general a steadily progressing decline from the 14th century on, the art of jade cutting held its own through the centuries (PLS. 261, 278) and rose to a spectacular pinnacle during the 16th century. Our knowledge of Chinese jades, which begins with the Han period, is extremely sketchy as a result of the paucity of datable pieces. A few definite data are provided by the finds in the grave of Wang Chien (10th cent., Szechwan), two pieces from the Ardebil shrine near Teheran, and various other scattered pieces which have an engraved name or date; but these are insufficient to establish a chronology of later Chinese jade working. It seems quite certain, however, that the discovery of great quantities of jadeite in Burma and its subsequent import into China on a large scale began with the 18th century. A few specimens which, on the basis of inscriptions, can be dated in the Ch'ien-lung period provide evidence of the flourishing of this handicraft in the 18th century. Among these pieces, besides human and animal figures, a great number copy the classical forms of Shang and Chou bronze vessels, emblems, and *ju-i* scepters. We find also great jade boulders, far larger than the nephrite boulders which were usually imported from Central Asia, which were carved to represent cliff landscapes complete with groves of trees, pavilions, and human figures. One of the largest examples, perhaps, is the approximately 6-ft.-high boulder erected in the Lo-shou-t'ang ("Hall of Happy Longevity") in the Forbidden City of Peking. This enormous jade mass has been carved to depict the hydraulic works of the legendary emperor Yü, and an imperial inscription dates it in 1788.

LATER ARCHITECTURE. Of all Chinese architecture, only that of the Ming and Ch'ing periods can be observed in an abundance of existing monuments of greatly varying style, size, and function. Considering the whole history of Chinese architecture, however, this is perhaps the least interesting period. The great architecture in wood had been characterized by inventive resourcefulness, clearness of conception, and a sense for functional construction combined with artistic vision, all of which are displayed in high degree in the few surviving Sung and Liao monuments, although these are certainly no adequate

reflection of the Sung architecture that once existed in the capitals of the empire. To this great tradition of architecture in wood the Ming and Ch'ing architects added little or nothing.

The study of certain types of painting and ceramics has demonstrated that it is hazardous to stress the decadent character of Ming and Ch'ing art as a whole, because those art forms which were in decline were often in the course of replacement. In architecture we lack these compensations to relieve the general picture of stylistic deterioration. Judged by the standards of Sung architecture in wood, the Ming and Ch'ing periods constitute an age of decline, if not of downright decadence. However, the architecture has a grandeur which is quite unique in character. This quality may already have existed in the lost monuments of Sung times, but it is completely lacking in the architecture of Japan, which never adopted the Ming and Ch'ing styles.

The first significant change to strike the eye in this later period of Chinese architecture is the steadily increasing use of stone and brick. Li Chieh, the author of the standard work on Sung architecture, the *Ying-tsao fa-shih*, completely ignored the use of brick and stone in the construction of many of the pagodas of that time. Building in brick was completely subordinate in prestige to building in wood, and the brick buildings abound with artificial, nonfunctional, and purely decorative imitative elements, a phenomenon which can be observed both in buildings on the surface and in subterranean structures (e.g., the Sung tombs at Pai-sha, Honan). Brick was mainly used in China because of its greater durability and strength.

The important position of brick and stone in Ming architecture is aptly represented by the most impressive and gigantic building project of the Ming emperors: the Great Wall (PL. 285; see CHINA, *Hopei*). Actually, however, the Ming emperors did little more than restore and connect dilapidated sections of previous wall systems, and, moreover, only small sections of the Great Wall present the impregnable appearance familiar to us from pictures.

During this same period many cities were provided with new, stone-sheathed defensive walls and fortified gates. The common plan for the gates of large cities involves a double fortification. In the middle of a U- or crescent-shaped counterscarp there is a heavy, multistoried gate tower to protect the vaulted tunnel entrance. Right behind this gate tower, which is usually built of brick and must have been altogether impregnable before gunpowder came into common use, there is a second one, usually of wood and likewise multistoried, erected on the main city wall just above the vaulted gate entrance. Sometimes, as at the P'ing-tzŭ-mên of Peking, the passage through the counterscarp is not centered below the gate tower, but is placed quite near the main city wall.

The vaulted gate passages, often with a square recess in the middle to accommodate the swing of the heavy gates, must have come as a surprise to earlier generations of Western art historians, who had never seen the interior of a Chinese tomb and who could not therefore have been aware that the principle of vaulting had been known to the Chinese since Han times. The extremely rare cases in which the Chinese applied this principle in the building of temples have been connected by some scholars with the activities of Western missionaries, a theory which archaeological evidence now definitely seems to have refuted. On the sacred mountain O-mei in Szechwan province, there is a temple hall with a large cupola built of brick. This is thought to have been constructed during the Wan-li period (1573–1619). Also of early 17th-century date are the so-called "beamless halls" (*wu-liang-tien*) of some other temples, such as that of the Yung-tsu-ssŭ at Taiyuan, built in 1611, that of the K'ai-yüan-ssŭ at Soochow (1618), and the *sūtra* hall of the Ling-ku-ssŭ near Nanking. In all of these, barrel vaulting is accompanied by a façade construction which carefully and minutely imitates architecture in wood.

In the construction of pagodas, it seems that the architects of the Yüan and Ming periods continued to follow the style established by their predecessors of the Sung and Liao periods. The pagoda at Pa-li-chuang near Peking, which was built in 1576, is an almost perfect copy of the Hopei Liao type, which is represented by the pagoda in the nearby T'ien-ning-ssŭ (PL. 273). The resemblance is so striking that we are led to suppose that the pagoda at Pa-li-chuang is a carefully reconstructed or restored Liao pagoda.

Although little is known about the early types of gates, it seems that the vaulted passages of gate towers first appeared in the early Ming period. Whether the unusual flattened shape of the vaulted passage of the Chü-yung-kuan (PL. 279), a gate of the Great Wall near Nan-k'ou (see CHINA, *Hopei*) which dates from the Yüan period, was common at that time is difficult to establish. The whole structure is so much a product of foreign influences that we can hardly connect it with other Chinese monuments. At the same time, another distinctly foreign type of monument appeared which was to change the landscape of northern China — the stupa of the Lamaist Tibetan type. One of the earliest examples is the *śarīra* stupa of the temple Ch'ing-ming-ssŭ near Taiyuan, built in 1385. Perhaps even earlier is the plastered *Pai-t'a* ("white pagoda") of the Miao-yin-ssŭ at Peking, which may date from 1279. On Wu-t'ai-shan there are several stupas dating from the early Ming period, and thousands of later stupas are found all over northern China and Manchuria.

At the capitals construction was undertaken on a truly impressive scale. The first of the Ming emperors had built palaces and official buildings at Nanking, but these were almost all razed to the ground in later times. In Peking, which again became the capital in 1421, many buildings remain from the Ming period, though for the most part in the somewhat modified reconstructions of the Ch'ing period. The building style of the capital was one of imposing grandeur, quite in keeping both with the magnificence of the court and the outlook of the emperors. (See PLS. 286, 293, 294.) The conventional formula of symmetrical halls centered on an axis, separated by wide courtyards, the whole embellished by the lavish use of sculptured balustrades, bridges, monumental sculptures, and brightly colored tiles, is nowhere more effective and successful than in the Imperial City and the Forbidden City of Peking. The planning of the town was much less rigidly symmetrical than had been the case in previous capitals, partly because the Ming emperors kept a part of the Mongol capital intact, and this slight deviation perhaps saves the total effect from monotony. The gay colors of the glazed tiles and the wooden elements of the architecture, together with the richly sculptured stone columns and balustrades, succeed in dissimulating the architectural shortcomings of this style of building, which was primarily intended to create a majestic effect. A closer study of monuments not built for the emperor and his capital, which do not have this same impressive size, reveals the essential mediocrity of Ming and Ch'ing architecture. The Chih-hua-ssŭ at Peking, completed in 1444, is considered by many to be one of the best examples of Ming architecture and also one of the most typical, since it did not undergo drastic repairs during the Ch'ing period as was the case with so many other temple buildings. This temple shows the traditional layout of gates and buildings centered on an axis, with a drum tower, a bell tower, and two halls (Ta-chih-tien and the *sūtra* hall) placed to balance symmetrically on the east and west side. Compared to the imperial buildings, the scale is modest. The two-storied Ju-lai-tien, the cupola of which has been removed and is now on display at the Nelson Gallery, Kansas City, shows all the characteristics of later Chinese architecture.

The bracketing system, one of the great assets of earlier architecture, gradually lost its structural function, which was taken over by beams. The proportions of the bracketing sets diminished and the deeply overhanging roof disappeared. From this time on the brackets were to assume a purely decorative function. Brackets of the same type appeared in the roof construction, so closely set together all along the roof as to form a kind of decorative cornice. In general the art of carpentry in this later period shows an unmistakable decline.

The Manchu emperors followed the example set by the Ming emperors and commanded projects which resulted in great activity in building. Even before they took Peking they had already had suitable quarters built for themselves at Muk-

den, to which they had moved their capital in 1625. The old palace of Mukden consists of three groups of buildings, partly built before the moving of the capital to Peking, partly dating from a later time. The eastern section consists of the octagonal Ta-chêng-tien, flanked by two rows of six smaller buildings. This group of modest-sized buildings, erected about 1637, was the center of the military government at the beginning of the Manchu era. The octagonal ground plan of the main building is seemingly reminiscent of the architectural style of the Jurchen, the ancestors of the Manchus. In the center lies the complex of buildings of the Imperial City, with the Ta-ch'ing-mên, the Ch'ung-chêng-mên, the Phoenix Pavilion, and the Ch'ing-ning-kung placed on the north-south axis and a multitude of other buildings disposed on the east and west sides. The western part of the palace consists of a garden in which the most important building is the Wên-yüan-ko; it formerly housed a copy of the great anthology of books called the *Ssü-k'u ch'üan-shu*, compiled 1773–82. Although the layout of the buildings of the Mukden palaces shows already the strong influence of Chinese town planning, the whole complex aptly symbolizes the modest beginnings of the Manchu imperial reign. With the removal of the capital to Peking, building activity came to a sudden stop, to be resumed only much later during the reign of Ch'ien-lung.

In Peking, the Manchu emperors retained the complex of buildings which the Ming emperors had left behind, restoring and rebuilding such monuments as the Wu-mên (1647), the T'ai-ho-tien (1669), and the T'ai-miao (1799). They also erected many new buildings, however, including such widely known monuments as the Pai-t'a (1654), built on a hill on the island in the Northern Lake of the Imperial City. The beautiful scenery to the northwest of Peking attracted the emperors K'ang-hsi and Ch'ien-lung, who had their summer palaces built there (PLS. 286, 294). In the first half of the 18th century, the buildings of the Yüan-ming-yüan (V, PL. 196) and the Ch'ang-ch'un-yüan were constructed as a Chinese experiment in baroque style, undertaken as a result of the influence of European missionaries. Just as the works of Lang Shih-ning (Giuseppe Castiglione) can scarcely be considered typical of Chinese painting, so must the curiously hybrid style of these buildings, now reduced to ruins, be regarded as in no way representative of Chinese architecture. (See EXOTICISM.)

Quite different are the buildings of the Pi-shu shan-chuang ("Sans Chaleur") at Chengteh (Ch'êng-tê), now in Hopei province (formerly Jehol). The terrain in which these summer residences were built is hilly and was formerly covered with beautiful forests. Numerous small summerhouses in Chinese style, mostly in the southeastern corner of the walled enclosure, housed the emperor and his retinue during hunting parties. In the mountains farther to the north a number of temples were erected. One of these, the Yung-yu-ssŭ, has a fine octagonal, nine-storied pagoda (1764). To the north and east of the imperial residences are a number of temples which display a completely different style of architecture, having been built toward the end of the 18th century after Tibetan prototypes.

The P'u-t'o tsung-ch'êng chih-miao was built after the model of the palace of the Dalai Lama at Lhasa, the so-called Potalaka, whereas another, the Hsü-mi-fu shou-miao, was built in imitation of the Tashilumpo monastery at Shigatse. On top of the massive, squat buildings with brick façades, which remind us of the outer gate towers of the walled cities, pavilions were built. Often canopies of glazed tiles were let into the walls above the windows. But even though these attempts to relieve the monotony of the massive brick construction demonstrate the Chinese liking for variation and color, the Tibetan style never was quite assimilated. One of the most interesting buildings at Chengteh is the pagoda which was erected behind the imitation of the Tashilumpo monastery. The lowest story was built on a square foundation, surrounded by an octagonal gallery, surmounted by a balcony. The seven higher stories, sheathed in glazed tiles, are also octagonal. Like the rest of this monument in Tibetan style the pagoda was built to commemorate the visit to Peking of the third Panchen Lama, who died there during a smallpox plague. Besides these huge monu-

ments, there are several other buildings and monuments in a foreign style, such as the marble pagoda of the Hsi-huang-ssŭ (Peking, 1779), a curious mixture of Chinese and Tibetan architecture, and the Wu-t'a-ssŭ (see CHINA, Hopei), built after the temple of the Mahābodhi at Bodhgaya, India. Building activity here continued almost to the end of the Ch'ing period. The Hall of Annual Prayers (Ch'i-nien-tien), belonging to the complex of the Temple of Heaven (PL. 286), which is one of the most widely known Chinese buildings, was built as late as 1896.

A separate category of buildings and sculptures are those belonging to the imperial mausoleums (PL. 285). The recent excavation of one of the 13 Ming tombs, that of Wan-li, gave for the first time an idea of the arrangement and architecture of a great imperial tomb. The technical difficulties which the excavators faced when trying to find the entrance to the tomb make it practically certain that all Ming tombs are still intact, preserving behind their marble subterranean gates the remains of the deceased and the lavish funerary gifts with which he was surrounded.

Because of the interest of the emperors in foreign styles, Chinese architecture of the last centuries displays a much greater variation than did that of earlier epochs. Not in all respects, however, can it be said that the willingness to imitate resulted in an enrichment of Chinese culture, since, for the most part, these foreign styles were never assimilated and always kept a distinctly exotic character, contributing little to the rapidly declining native architectural art.

BIBLIOG. *General.* O. Kümmel, Die Kunst Chinas, Japans und Koreas, Wildpark, Potsdam, 1929; O. Sirén, A History of Early Chinese Art, 4 vols., London, 1930; O. Sirén, Kinas Konst under tre Årtusenden, 2 vols., Stockholm, 1942; Sekai Bijutsu Zenshū, (Arts of the World), VII, VIII, XIV, XX (China, I-IV), Tokyo, 1950–53; J. Buhot, Arts de la Chine, Paris, 1951; R. Grousset, La Chine et son art, Paris, 1951; M. Paul-David, Arts et styles de la Chine, Paris, 1951; L. Sickman and A. Soper, The Art and Architecture of China, Harmondsworth, 1956; W. Speiser, Die Kunst Ostasiens, Berlin, 1956; E. Consten, Das alte China, Stuttgart, 1958; W. Willetts, Chinese Art, 2 vols., Harmondsworth, 1958.

*Neolithic period.* J. G. Andersson, Children of the Yellow Earth, London, 1934; Li Chi et al., Ch'êng-tzŭ-yai, Nanking, 1934 (Eng. trans., K. Starr, New Haven, 1956); N. Palmgren, Kansu Mortuary Urns of the Pan-shan and Ma-ch'ang Groups, Peiping, 1934; A. Salmony, Carved Jade of Ancient China, Berkeley, 1938; G. D. Wu, Prehistoric Pottery in China, London, 1938; J. G. Andersson, Researches into the Prehistory of China, BMFEA, XV, 1943, pp. 1–304; J. Haskins, Pan-po, A Chinese Neolithic Village, Artibus Asiae, XX, 2/3, 1957, pp. 151–8; Chêng Tê-k'un, Archaeology in China, I: Prehistoric China, Cambridge, 1959.

*Shang-Yin period.* W. P. Yetts, The George Eumorphopoulos Collection, 3 vols., London, 1929–33; H. G. Creel, The Birth of China, London, 1936; B. Karlgren, Yin and Chou in Chinese Bronzes, BMFEA, VIII, 1936, pp. 9–154; B. Karlgren, New Studies on Chinese Bronzes, BMFEA, IX, 1937, pp. 9–119; A. Salmony, Carved Jade of Ancient China, Berkeley, 1938; C. Hentze, Die Sakralbronzen und ihre Bedeutung in den frühchinesischen Kulturen, Antwerp, 1941; F. Waterbury, Early Chinese Symbols and Literature: Vestiges and Speculations, New York, 1942; B. Karlgren, Weapons and Tools of the Yin Dynasty, BMFEA, XVII, 1945, pp. 101–44; J. E. Lodge, A. G. Wenley, and J. A. Pope, A Descriptive and Illustrative Catalogue of Chinese Bronzes, Freer Gallery of Art, Washington, D.C., 1946; H. Hansford, Chinese Jade Carving, London, 1950; A. Salmony, Archaic Chinese Jades, Chicago, 1952; M. Loehr, The Bronze Styles of the Anyang Period, Arch. Chin. Art Soc. Am., VII, 1953, pp. 42–53; Chêng Tê-k'un, The Carving of Jade in the Shang Period, Tr. O. Ceramic Soc., XXIX, 1954–55, pp. 13–31; M. Loehr, Chinese Bronze Age Weapons, Ann Arbor, Mich., 1956; Chêng Tê-k'un, The Origin and Development of the Shang Culture, Asia Major, N.S., VI, 1957, pp. 80–98; Li Chi, The Beginnings of Chinese Civilization, Seattle, 1957.

*Chou period.* S. Lemaître, Les agrafes Chinoises jusqu'à la fin de l'époque Han, Paris, 1925; W. P. Yetts, The George Eumorphopoulos Collection, 3 vols., London, 1929–33; G. Salles, Les bronzes de Li Yu, RAA, VIII, 3, 1934, pp. 146–58; B. Karlgren, On the Date of the Piao-Bells, BMFEA, VI, 1934, pp. 137–51; W. C. White, The Tombs of Old Loyang, Shanghai, 1934; J. G. Andersson, The Goldsmith in Ancient China, BMFEA, VII, 1935, pp. 1–38; B. Karlgren, Yin and Chou in Chinese Bronzes, BMFEA, VIII, 1936, pp. 9–154; S. Umehara, Etude des bronzes des Royaumes Combattants, Kyoto, 1936; B. Karlgren, New Studies on Chinese Bronzes, BMFEA, IX, 1937, pp. 9–119; S. Umehara, Rakuyō Kinson Kobō Shūei (Selected Relics from the Tombs at Chin-ts'un, Loyang), Kyoto, 1937; B. Karlgren, Notes on a Kin-ts'un Album, BMFEA, X, 1938, pp. 65–81; A. Salmony, Carved Jade of Ancient China, Berkeley, 1938; W. P. Yetts, The Cull Chinese Bronzes, London, 1939; B. Karlgren, Huai and Han, BMFEA, XIII, 1941; A. Salmony, On Early Chinese Mirrors, Art in Am., XXX, 3, 1942; T. Nagahiro, Die Agraffe und ihre Stellung in der altchinesischen Kunstgeschichte, Kyoto, 1943; J. E. Lodge, A. G. Wenley,

and J. A. Pope, A Descriptive and Illustrative Catalogue of Chinese Bronzes, Freer Gallery of Art, Washington, D.C., 1946; Chiang Yuen-yi, Chang-sha, The Chu Tribe and Its Art, Shanghai, 2 vols., 1949–50; E. Consten, A Hu with Pictorial Decoration, Arch. Chin. Art Soc. Am., VI, 1952, pp. 18–32; A. Salmony, Archaic Chinese Jades, Chicago, 1952; S. Umehara, Painted Bronze Mirrors of the Period of the Warring States, Bijutsu Kenkyu, no. 178, Nov., 1954, pp. 153–72 (text in Jap.). Chʻüan-kuo chi-pên chien-shê kung-chʻêng-chung chʻu-tʻu wên-wu chan-lan tʻu-lu (Archaeological Finds at Construction Sites), Shanghai, 1955; J. F. Haskins, Recent Excavations in China, Arch. Chin. Art Soc. Am., X, 1956, pp. 42–63; Yang Tsung-ying, Chan-kuo hui-hua tzŭ-liao (Materials on Painting during the Period of the Warring States), Peking, 1957.

*Han period.* E. Chavannes, La sculpture sur pierre en Chine au temps des deux dynasties Han, Paris, 1893; B. Laufer, Chinese Pottery of the Han Dynasty, Leiden, 1909; E. Chavannes, Mission Archéologique dans la Chine septentrionale, 2 vols. text, 3 vols. plates, Paris, 1913–15; B. Laufer, Chinese Clay Figures, Chicago, 1914; V. Ségalen, G. de Voisins, and J. Lartigue, Mission Archéologique en Chine, Atlas, 2 vols., Paris, 1923–24; Y. Harada, Lo-lang, A Report on the Excavation of Wang Hsü's Tomb in the "Lo-lang" Province, an Ancient Chinese Colony in Korea, Tokyo, 1930; O. Fischer, Die Chinesische Malerei der Han-Dynastie, Berlin, 1931; Y. Harada, The Tomb of the Painted Basket of Lo-lang, Keijo, Seoul, 1934; O. Nori and H. Naitō, Ying-chʻeng-tzu, Kyoto, 1934; V. Ségalen, G. de Voisins, and J. Lartigue, L'art funéraire à l'époque des Han, Paris, 1935; F. Low-Beer, Zum Dekor der Han Lacke, Wien. Beiträge zur K. u. Kulturgeschichte Asiens, XI, 1937, pp. 65–73; O. Maenchen-Helfen, Zur Geschichte der Lackkunst in China, ibid., pp. 32–64; J. Prip-Møller, Kinas Bygningskunst, Arkitekten, XXIX, 3/4, Copenhagen, 1937; H. C. Hollis, Cranes and Serpents, B. Cleve. Mus., Oct., 1938; J. H. Cox, An Exhibition of Chinese Antiquities from Chʻang-sha, New Haven, 1939; W. P. Yetts, The Cull Chinese Bronzes, London, 1939; O. Janse, Archaeological Research in Indo-China, 2 vols., 1947–51; S. Camman, The "TLV" Pattern on Cosmic Mirrors of the Han Dynasty, JAOS, LXVIII, 1948, pp. 159–67; S. Mizuno, Chinese Stone Sculpture, Tokyo, 1950; Corpus des pierres sculptés des Han, 2 vols., Peking, 1950–51; R. Rudolph and Wen Yu, Han Tomb Art of West China, Berkeley, 1951; Sekai Bijutsu Zenshū (Arts of the World), VIII (China, I), Tokyo, 1951; R. Edwards, The Cave Reliefs at Ma Hao, Artibus Asiae, XVII, 1, 2, 1954; W. Fairbank and M. Kitano, Han Mural Paintings in the Peiyüan Tomb at Liaoyang, Southern Manchuria, Artibus Asiae, XVII, 3/4, 1954, pp. 238–64; S. Camman, Significant Patterns on Chinese Bronze Mirrors, Arch. Chin. Art Soc. Am., IX, 1955, pp. 43–62; Chʻüan-kuo chi-pên chien-shê kung-chʻeng-chung chʻu-tʻu wên-wu chan-lan tʻu-lu (Archaeological Finds at Construction Sites), Peking, 1955; O. Sirén, Chinese Painting, I, London, 1956; Chʻên Wan-li, Tʻao-yung (Pottery Figurines), Peking, 1957; Shensi Po-wu kuan-tsang shih-kʻo hsüan-chi (Selected Sculptures from the Shensi Provincial Museum), Peking, 1957; Wên-wu tsʻan-kʻao tzŭ-liao, 1957, no. 12 (cover illustration); W. Willetts, Chinese Art, 2 vols., Harmondsworth, 1958.

*Six Dynasties period.* O. Sirén, Chinese Sculpture, 4 vols., London, 1925; O. Sirén, A History of Early Chinese Art, III: Sculpture, London, 1930; B. Rowland, Notes on the Dated Statues of the Northern Wei Dynasty and the Beginnings of Buddhist Sculpture in China, AB, XIX, 1, 1937; S. Umehara, Shao-hsing Kokyō Shūei (Selected Mirrors from Shao-hsing), Kyoto, 1940; H. Münsterberg, Buddhist Bronzes of the Six Dynasties Period, Artibus Asiae, IX, 4, 1946, X, 1, 1947; Sekai Bijutsu Zenshū (Arts of the World), VII (China, I), Tokyo, 1952; W. R. B. Acker, Some Tʻang and Pre-Tʻang Texts on Chinese Painting, Leiden, 1954; S. Matsubara, White Marble Buddhist Statues in "Hanka Shiyui" Pose in the Eastern Wei to Northern Chʻi Dynasties, Bijutsu Kenkyu, no. 181, May, 1955, pp. 25–38 (text in Jap.); O. Sirén, Chinese Painting, 3 vols., London, 1956, part 1; S. Matsubara, A Typical Example of Buddhist Bronzes of Hopei Style in the Chêng-kuang Period, Northern Wei, Bijutsu Kenkyu, no. 198, May, 1958, pp. 11–33 (text in Jap.); N. Kumagai, Three Buddhist Bronzes of the Earliest Age in China, Bijutsu Kenkyu, no. 203, March, 1959, pp. 240–8 (text in Jap.); S. Matsubara, Eastern Wei Sculpture, Its Characteristics and Its Connection with Japanese Tōri Style Sculpture of the Asuka Period, Bijutsu Kenkyu, no. 202, Jan., 1959, pp. 17–33 (text in Jap.).

*Tʻang period.* P. Pelliot, Les Grottes de Touen-houang, 6 vols., Paris, 1914–24; S. Omura, Shina Bijutsushi, Chōsohen (A History of Chinese Art: Sculpture), 3 vols., Tokyo, 1915; R. L. Hobson, The George Eumorphopoulos Collection: Catalogue of the Chinese, Corean, and Persian Pottery and Porcelain, I, London, 1925; O. Sirén, Chinese Sculpture, 4 vols., London, 1925; D. Tokiwa and T. Sekino, Shina Bukkyō Shiseki (Buddhist Monuments in China), 5 vols., Tokyo, 1926–38; J. Harada, Catalogue of Treasures in the Imperial Repository Shōsōin, Tokyo, 1932; E. Matsumoto, Tonkōga no Kenkyū (A Study of the Paintings of Tun-huang), 2 vols., Tokyo, 1937; H. Ingram, Why Tʻang?, Röhsska Könstslojdmuseets Årstryck, Göteborg, 1946, pp. 35–41; G. Lindberg, Hsing Yao, Attempt at an Interpretation of the Tʻang Hsing Chou Ware, O. Art, II, 2, 1950, pp. 149–55; H. Münsterberg, Chinese Buddhist Bronzes of the Tʻang Period, Artibus Asiae, XI, 1/2, 1948, pp. 27–45; O. Ceramic Soc., Wares of the Tang Dynasty, exhibition cat., London, 1949; B. Gray, Early Chinese Pottery and Porcelain, London, 1953; S. Camman, The Lion and Grape Patterns on Chinese Bronze Mirrors, Artibus Asiae, XVI, 4, 1953, pp. 265–91; B. Gyllensvärd, Chinese Gold and Silver in the Carl Kempe Collection, Stockholm, 1953; W. R. B. Acker, Some Tʻang and Pre-Tʻang Texts on Chinese Painting, Leiden, 1954; J. L. Davidson, The Lotus Sūtra in Chinese Art, New Haven, London, 1954; S. Camman, Significant Patterns on Chinese Bronze Mirrors, Chin. Art Soc. Am., IX, 1955, pp. 43–62; G. Lindberg, Hsing-yao and Ting-yao, BMFEA, XXV, 1955, pp. 19–71; O. Sirén, Chinese Painting, I, London, 1956; Los Angeles County Museum, The Arts of the Tʻang Dynasty, exhibition cat., Los Angeles, 1957; B. Gyllensvärd, Tʻang Gold and Silver, BMFEA, XXIX, 1957, pp. 1–230; W. Willetts, Chinese Art, II, Harmondsworth, 1958, pp. 415–500, 689 ff.; Shensi-shêng chʻu-tʻu Tʻang-yung hsüan-chi (Selected Tomb Figures of the Tʻang Period Excavated in Shensi), Peking, 1958.

*Five Dynasties period.* O. Sirén, Early Chinese Painting, I, London, 1933; S. Sakanishi, An Essay on Chinese Landscape Painting, London, 1935; S. Shimada, Ihin Gafu Ni Tsuite (On I-pʻin, the "Extraordinary Style"), Bijutsu Kenkyu, no. 161, 1950, pp. 20–46; B. Rowland, Early Chinese Paintings in Japan: The Problem of Hsü Hsi, Artibus Asiae, XV, 3, 1952, pp. 218–32; Y. Yashiro, Again on the Sung Copy of the Scroll "Ladies of the Court" by Chou Wên-chü, Bijutsu Kenkyu, no. 169, 1952, pp. 157–62 (text in Jap.); L. Sickman and A. Soper, The Art and Architecture of China, Harmondsworth, 1956, pp. 103–20; O. Sirén, Chinese Painting, I, London, 1956; Nanking Museum, Nan-tʻang Êrh-ling (Two Burial Mounds of the Southern Tʻang Dynasty), Nanking, 1957; Chin-hua Wan-fo-tʻa chʻu-tʻu wên-wu (Objects Excavated from the Wan-fo Pagoda at Chin-hua), Peking, 1958.

*Sung period.* Ku Teng, Chinesische Malkunsttheorie in der Tʻang- und Sungzeit, OAZ, N.S., X, 1934, pp. 155–75, XI, 1935, pp. 28–57; G. Ecke, Structural Features of the Stone-built Tʻing Pagoda, Monumenta Serica, I, 1935–36, pp. 253–76, XIII, 1948, pp. 331–65; O. Sirén, The Chinese on the Art of Painting, Peiping, 1936; W. C. White, Chinese Temple Frescoes, A Study of Three Wall-paintings of the Thirteenth Century, Toronto, 1940; A. C. Soper, The Evolution of Buddhist Architecture in Japan, Princeton, 1942; M. Aoki, Chūka Bunjinga Dan (A Discussion of Chinese Literati Painting), Tokyo, 1949; L. Bachhofer, Maitreya in Ketumatī by Chu Hao-ku, India Antiqua, Leiden, 1949, pp. 1–7; B. Rowland, The Problem of Hui-tsung, Arch. Chin. Art Soc. Am., V, 1951, pp. 5–23; Sekai Bijutsu Zenshū (Arts of the World), XIV (China, III), Tokyo, 1951; A. C. Soper, Kuo Jo-hsü's Experiences in Painting, Washington, D. C., 1951; S. Shimada and Y. Yonezawa, Painting of Sung and Yüan Dynasties, Tokyo, 1952; W. Speiser, Ma Lin, Festschrift Eduard von der Heydt, Zurich, 1952; S. Yorke Hardy, Illustrated Catalogue of Tung, Ju, Kuan, Chün, Kuang-tung and Glazed I-hsing Wares in the Percival David Foundation of Chinese Art, London, 1953; Wen Fong and S. Lee, Streams and Mountains without End, Ascona, 1955; Sekai Tōji Zenshū (Ceramic Art of the World), X, Tokyo, 1955; Musée Cernuschi, L'art de la Chine des Song, Paris, 1956; L. Sickman and A. Soper, The Art and Architecture of China, Harmondsworth, 1956; O. Sirén, Chinese Painting, II, London, 1956; I. Tanaka, The Art of Liang Kʻai, Bijutsu Kenkyu, no. 184, Jan., 1956, pp. 129–49 (text in Jap.); A. G. Wenley, "Clearing Autumn Skies over Mountains and Valleys" Attributed to Kuo Hsi, Arch. Chin. Art Soc. Am., X, 1956, pp. 30–41; Yü-yao Pao-kuo-ssŭ Ta-hsiung-pao-tien (The Main Hall of the Temple Pao-kuo-ssŭ at Yü-yao), Wên-wu tsʻan-kʻao tzŭ-liao, 1957, no. 8, pp. 54–9; R. Edwards, The Landscape Art of Li Tʻang, Arch. Chin. Art Soc. Am., XII, 1958, pp. 48–60; W. Willetts, Chinese Art, II, Harmondsworth, 1958; J. Cahill, Chinese Paintings, XI–XIV Centuries, New York, 1959.

*Liao period.* O. Sirén, A Chinese Temple and Its Plastic Decoration of the 12th Century, Etudes d'Orientalisme publiées par la Musée Guimet à la mémoire de Raymonde Linossier, Paris, n.d., pp. 499–505; E. Boerschmann, Pagoden im Nördlichen China unter fremden Dynastien, Der Orient in Deutscher Forschung, Leipzig, 1944; Sekai Bijutsu Zenshū (Arts of the World), XIV (China, III), Tokyo, 1951; Sekai Tōji Zenshū (Ceramic Art of the World), X, Tokyo, 1955; Wu Hsing-han, Liao-tzʻŭ chien-shu (A Brief Account of Liao Wares), Wên-wu tsʻan-kʻao tzŭ-liao, 1958, no. 2, pp. 10–23; Wu-shêng chʻu-tʻu chung-yao wên-wu chan-lan tʻu-lu (Illustrated Catalogue of an Exhibition of Important Objects Excavated in Five Provinces), Peking, 1958, pls. 104–21.

*Yüan period.* W. Speiser, Die Yüan-Klassik der Landschaftsmalerei, OAZ, N. S., X, 1935; L. Sickman, Wall-paintings of the Yüan period, Rev. Arts Asiatiques, 1937, pp. 57–67; V. Contag, Schriftcharakteristiken in der Malerei dargestellt an Bildern Wang Mengs und anderen Malern der Südschule, OAZ, N. S., XVII, 1941; E. A. Lippe Biesterfeld, Li Kʻan und seine "Ausführliche Beschreibung des Bambus," OAZ, N. S., XVIII, 1942–43; M. Aoki, Chūka Bunjinga Dan (A Discussion of Chinese Literati Painting), Tokyo, 1949; H. Franke, Two Yüan Treatises on the Technique of Portrait Painting, O. Art, III, 1950, pp. 27–32; Sekai Bijutsu Zenshū (Arts of the World), XIV (China, III), Tokyo, 1951; S. Shimada and Y. Yonezawa, Painting of Sung and Yüan Dynasties, Tokyo, 1952; R. Edwards, Chʻien Hsüan and Early Autumn, Arch. Chin. Art Soc. Am., VII, 1953, pp. 71–83; Sekai Tōji Zenshū (Ceramic Art of the World), XI, Tokyo, 1955; Chieh-shao An-hui Ho-fei fa-hsien-ti Yüan-tai chin-yin chʻi-min (An Introduction to the Yüan Gold and Silver Vessels Discovered at Ho-fei, Anhwei), Wên-wu tsʻan-kʻao tzŭ-liao, 1957, no. 2, pp. 51–9; A. G. Wenley, "A Breath of Spring" by Tsou Fu-lei, Ars O., II, 1957, pp. 459–69; J. Cahill, Chʻien Hsüan and His Figure Paintings, Arch. Chin. Art Soc. Am., XII, 1958, pp. 11–29.

*Later sculpture.* O. Sirén, Chinese Sculpture, 4 vols., London, 1925; D. Tokiwa and T. Sekino, Shina Bukkyō Shiseki (Buddhist Monuments in China), 5 vols., Tokyo, 1926–38; O. Sirén, Studien zur Chinesischen Plastik der Post-Tʻangzeit, OAZ, XIV, 1927; L. Bachhofer, Two Chinese Wooden Statues, BM, Oct., 1938, pp. 142–6; L. Bachhofer, Two Chinese Wooden Figures, AQ, Autumn, 1938, pp. 289–98; O. Sirén, Chinese Sculpture of the Sung, Liao and Chin periods, BMFEA, XIV, 1942, pp. 45–64; A. Priest, Chinese Sculpture in the Metropolitan Museum of Art, New York, 1944; T. Takejima, Ryōkin Jidai no Kenchiku to sono Butsuzō (Architecture of the Liao and Chin Periods and Its Sculptures), Tokyo, 1944; Sekai Bijutsu Zenshū (Arts of the World), XIV (China, III), Tokyo, 1951, XX (China, IV), Tokyo, 1953; R. B. Hawkins, A Statue of Kuan-yin:

A Problem in Sung Sculpture, Record of the Art Mus., Princeton Univ., XII, 1, 1953, pp. 3–36.

*Ming period.* R. L. Hobson, The Wares of the Ming Dynasty, London, 1922; V. Contag, Tung Ch'i-ch'ang's Hua Ch'an Shih Sui Pi und das Hua Shuo des Mo Shih-lung, OAZ, N. S., VIII, 1933; L. Reidemeister, Ming Porzellan, Berlin, Leipzig, 1935; A. D. Brankston, Early Ming Wares of King-tö Tchen, Peiping, 1938; S. Jenyns, Chinese Lacquer, Tr. O. Ceramic Soc., London, 1939/40, XVIII, pp. 11–34; V. Contag and Wang Chich'uan, Maler und Sammlerstempel aus der Ming- und Ch'ingzeit, Shanghai, 1940; A. L. Hetherington, Introduction, Catalogue of the Exhibition of Monochrome Chinese Porcelain of the Ming and Manchu Dynasties, London, 1948; M. Aoki, Chūka Bunjinga Dan (A Discussion of Chinese Literati Painting), Tokyo, 1949; J. P. Dubosc, Great Chinese Painters of the Ming and Ch'ing Dynasties, XV to XVIII Centuries, New York, 1949; R. G. Sayer, Ching-tê-chên t'ao-lu, London, 1949; R. T. Paine, Jr., The Ten Bamboo Studio, Arch. Chin. Art Soc. Am., V, 1951, pp. 39–54; V. Elisséeff, Notes sur l'histoire des lacques, Et. d'Outre-mer, Dec., 1952, pp. 393–400; J. A. Pope, Fourteenth Century Blue-and-white, Washington, 1952; H. Trubner, Chinese Ceramics, Los Angeles, 1952 (exhibition cat.); S. Jenyns, Ming Pottery and Porcelain, London, 1953; Sekai Bijutsu Zenshū (Arts of the World), XX (China, IV), Tokyo, 1953; H. Garner, Oriental Blue and White, London, 1954; Tseng Hsien-ch'i and R. Edwards, Shên Chou at the Boston Museum, Arch. Chin. Art Soc. Am., VIII, 1954, pp. 31–45; Tseng Yu-ho, "The Seven Junipers" of Wên Chêng-ming, Arch. Chin. Art Soc. Am., VIII, 1954, pp. 22–30; S. Jenyns, The Wares of the Transitional Period, Arch. Chin. Art Soc. Am., IX, 1955, pp. 20–42; Sekai Tōji Zenshū (Ceramic Art of the World), XI, Tokyo, 1951; Tseng Yu-ho, Hsüeh Wu and Her Orchids in the Collection of the Honolulu Academy of Arts, Arts Asiatiques, II, 1955, fasc. 3, pp. 197–209; The Arts of the Ming Dynasty, Tr. O. Ceramic Soc., 1955–56, 1956–57; J. A. Pope, Chinese Porcelains from the Ardebil Shrine, Washington, 1956; Tseng Yu-ho, Notes on T'ang Yin, O. Art, N. S., II, 3, 1956, pp. 103–8; H. Vanderstappen, Painters at the Early Ming Court (1368–1435) and the Problem of a Ming Painting Academy, Monumenta Serica, XV, 1956, pp. 259–302; D. Gure, The Arts of the Ming Dynasty, Artibus Asiae, XX, 4, 1957, pp. 309–20; A. Migot, Les temples bouddhiques du Mont O-mei, Arts Asiatiques, IV, 1, 2, 1957; F. Low-Beer, Lacquer of the Ming Dynasty, O. Art, N. S., IV, 1, 1958, pp. 12–17; Hsia Nai, Opening an Imperial Tomb, China Reconstructs, VII, 3, Mar., 1959, pp. 16–21.

*Ch'ing period.* P. Pelliot, A propos du Keng Tche T'ou, Mémoires concernant l'Asie Orientale, Paris, 1913; O. Sirén, The Walls and Gates of Peking, London, 1924; E. Boerschmann, Chinesische Architektur, Berlin, 1925; O. Kümmel, Ostasiatisches Gerät, Berlin, 1925; O. Sirén, The Imperial Palaces of Peking, 3 vols., Paris, Brussels, 1926; O. Sirén, A History of Early Chinese Art, IV: Architecture, London, 1930; G. Ecke, Zur Architektur der Landhäuser in den Kaiserlichen Gärten von Jehol, Architectura I, 6, Berlin, 1933, pp. 3–12; H. Maspero, R. Grousset, and L. Lion, Les ivoires religieux et médicaux chinois, Paris, 1939; V. Contag, Die Sechs berühmten Maler der Ch'ing Dynastie, Leipzig, 1940; F. D. Lessing, Yung-ho-kung: An Iconography of the Lamaist Cathedral in Peking with Notes on Lamaist Mythology and Cult, Stockholm, 1942; M. Igarashi, Nekka Koseki to Chibetto Bijutsu (Monuments of Jehol and Tibetan Art), Tokyo, 1943; J. Murata, Manshū no Shiseki (The Monuments of Manchuria), Tokyo, 1944; W. Fuchs, Rare Ch'ing Editions of the Keng-chih-t'u, Studia Serica, Chengtu, 1947; C. Lancaster, The European Style Palaces of the Yüan Ming Yüan, GBA, Oct., 1948; F. Koyama, The Story of Chinese Ceramics, Tokyo, 1949; O. Sirén, Shih-t'ao, Painter, Poet and Theoretician, BMFEA, XXI, 1949; V. Contag, Die beiden Steine, Braunschweig, 1950; M. Jourdain and S. Jenyns, Chinese Export Art, London, 1950; S. Jenyns, Later Chinese Porcelain, London, 1951; Ch'iu K'ai-ming, The Chieh Tzu Yüan Hua Chuan, Arch. Chin. Art Soc. Am., V, 1951, pp. 55–69; S. Hummel, Beiträge zu einer Baugeschichte der Lamapagode, Artibus Asiae, XVI, 1/2, 1953, p. 111 ff.; Sekai Bijutsu Zenshū (Arts of the World), XX (China, IV), Tokyo, 1953; H. Franke, Zur Biografie des Pa-ta-shan-jên, Festschrift Friedrich Weller zum 65. Geburtstag, Leipzig, 1954, pp. 119–30; R. Goepper, T'ang Tai, ein Hofmaler der Ch'ingzeit, Munich, 1956; A. Lippe, Kung Hsien and the Nanking School, O. Art, N. S., II, 1, 1956, pp. 21–9, IV, 4, 1958, pp. 159–70; Sekai Tōji Zenshū (Ceramic Art of the World), XII, Tokyo, 1956; L. Sickman and A. Soper, The Art and Architecture of China, Harmondsworth, 1956, pp. 188–201, 283–8; S. Camman, Chinese "Eglomisé" Snuff-bottles, O. Art, N. S., III, 3, 1957, pp. 85–9; M. Kitano, Yang-chou School of Painters, Kyoto, 1957.

The literature referring to specific monuments and archaeological sites has been listed below each entry under CHINA.

Jan FONTEIN

Illustrations: PLS. 219–298; 1 map and 7 figs. in text.

**CHIRICO**, GIORGIO DE. Italian painter (b. Volos, Greece, July 10, 1888). In 1906, after artistic training in Greece, he traveled with his family to Munich by way of Italy and studied at the Munich Academy for two years. In 1909 he returned to Italy. By 1911 De Chirico had moved to Paris, where he made the friendship of Guillaume Apollinaire, and exhibited at both the Salon d'Automne (1912 and 1913) and the Salon des Indépendants (1913 and 1914). Stationed with the infantry regiment at Ferrara in 1915, De Chirico two years later met Carlo Carrà,

with whom he founded the short-lived *scuola metafisica*, an informal school of painting which asserted the fantastic, so-called "metaphysical" viewpoint. In 1919 De Chirico began to write for the magazine *Valori Plastici* and to study and imitate the old masters; he also began at this time to reject his art of the preceding years in works that offer a tepid neoclassicism or a recreation of such diverse masters as Raphael, Rubens, and Courbet. Returning to Paris in 1925, he had somewhat vexed relationships with André Breton and the surrealists, who considered him both a forerunner of their movement as well as a traitor to its principles. He returned to Italy in 1940.

Such characteristic paintings as *The Nostalgia of the Infinite* (1913–14), *The Evil Genius of a King* (1914–15), and *The Sacred Fish* (1919) may be found in the Museum of Modern Art, New York. De Chirico also designed for the theater, executing the *décor* for Savinio's play *The Death of Niobe* (1926), the Ballets Russes de Monte Carlo's *The Ball* (1926), and a Berlin production of Křenek's opera *The Life of Orestes* (1930).

Stimulated by the antirealist esthetic of Nietzsche and the *fin-de-siècle* imagination of such artists as Böcklin (q.v.), Von Stuck, Klinger, and Kubin, De Chirico was one of the pioneers of 20th-century fantastic art and a major influence on surrealism. He created, shortly after 1910, his characteristic dream world in which an uncanny clear light, depopulated Renaissance buildings, irrational spaces, ominous statues, and enigmatic juxtapositions of objects evoke an aura of stagnation, silence, and mystery. While these melancholy and arid "dreamscapes" have provoked Freudian interpretations, they have also been considered a personal symbolization of the industrial backwardness of Italy, heir to a moribund classical civilization. Accurate information about De Chirico has been obscured by the artist himself, who has not only decried his early surrealistic achievements but also deliberately misdated his own works and painted in a style he had previously abandoned in order to suggest an earlier execution. See also EUROPEAN MODERN MOVEMENTS; V, PL. 133.

WRITINGS. Hebdomeros, Paris, 1929; Commedia dell'arte moderna, Rome, 1945; Memorie della mia vita, Rome, 1945.

BIBLIOG. G. Lo Duca. Dipinti di Giorgio de Chirico, Milan, 1936 and 1945; R. Carrieri, Giorgio de Chirico, Milan, 1942; I. Faldi, Il primo de Chirico, Venice, 1949; J. Soby, Giorgio de Chirico, New York, 1955; J. Sloane, Giorgio de Chirico and Italy, AQ, XXI, Spring, 1958, pp. 3–22.

Robert ROSENBLUM

**CHOREOGRAPHY:** POSE, GESTURE, AND GROUPING. The dance has been an important factor in the development of the representational arts. Defined broadly to include nearly all group activities with arranged scenic effects (e.g., ritual and religious rites, formal parades, games), the dance presents the painter or sculptor with material already conceived esthetically; well-defined patterns and movements, executed by human beings in a given three-dimensional area (see SPACE AND TIME), suggest rhythmic and compositional motifs that can be translated by the artist into ornamental vocabularies (see ORNAMENTATION). The activities subsumed under dance may also serve as a primary source for esthetic ideals; this is particularly true in civilizations dominated by tradition and ceremony.

SUMMARY. Primitive society (col. 578). The ancient world (col. 580). Asiatic civilizations (col. 581). Europe from the Renaissance to modern times (col. 585).

PRIMITIVE SOCIETY. In many primitive societies, dance engages the entire tribal group in a magic and ritual, rather than a purely recreational, function. As such, dance is related not only to myths, from which subject matter, characters, and groupings are taken, but also to ceremonial art and its associated activities. Pictorial representation of the dance is widespread among primitive cultures; subject matter and execution are constantly inspired by magical-religious beliefs and practices. Frequently primitive dances are accompanied by an immense variety of decoration — a wealth of costumes, fantastic and capricious

hairdress and masks, and colorful symbolism in the painting of faces and bodies; as a result it is often difficult to distinguish the representational and decorative elements from the choreographic.

The underlying ceremonial themes in works of art are not always obvious when regarded outside their cultural context. An example of this can be found in the aboriginal Australian art (see AUSTRALIAN CULTURES) of colonial times, continuing to the present day in remote northern groups in Australia, particularly in Kimberley and Arnhemland. In certain places within this area, and during periodic religious ceremonies, tribe members execute schematic rock paintings and engravings representing mythical personages, animals, monsters, or totemic ancestors and their mythological lives; simultaneously these beings and events are reevoked in dances and dramatic pantomimes. Thus we have further evidence that art and choreography are functionally linked.

In the widely diffused rock art of southern Africa, attributed to the Bushmen, the depiction of masked dances is frequent. The dancers imitate animals or insects, such as the mantis, whose propagation or capture the rite is meant to further. It is assumed that ritual dances existed in prehistoric times. In the early Paleolithic rock engravings of the Addaura cave near Palermo, a ritual dance seems to be represented, with numerous elongated figures rhythmically agitating their raised arms and apparently moving in a circle around two recumbent male figures. Rock paintings in eastern Spain show similar subjects. However, the greatest amount of primitive material related to choreography is offered by pre-Columbian and contemporary indigenous American cultures.

Among choreographic themes in primitive art, the dancing shaman beating the drum is especially interesting; the theme is frequently found in Eskimo cultures (q.v.), but it is also prevalent in other Arctic cultures such as the Koryak of the Kamchatka Peninsula. Other ritual dances appear in Eskimo ivory carvings on utensils such as pipes, arrow straighteners, and drills, schematically but effectively disposed within the small space available. The Plains Indians of North America colorfully adorned their tepees, drums, and shields with scenes of religious ceremonies such as the sun dance, corn dance, buffalo dance, and pine-tree dance. The figures were shown arranged in a circle, half circle, or line, dressed in multicolored costumes, marching with solemnly liturgical or elegantly dexterous movements. The Plains Indians' numerous representations on leather of running horses and hunting scenes also fit into the category of choreography; the eurythmy of these groups is so great that the whole gives the impression of a parade proceeding in coordinated movements.

Although geometric ornamentation prevails in the basketry of the natives of North America, in some work from California a circle of alternating male and female dancers is presented on a round basket (M. Covarrubias, *The Eagle, the Jaguar, and the Serpent*, New York, 1954, pl. 25, above). A specialty of the Pueblo IV period was great polychrome wall frescoes placed in the kiva (half-underground ceremonial house used as a temple). Some of the best of these frescoes are found at Awatobi (Hopi area, Arizona), representing sacrificial ceremonies; the style is similar to that of the modern Pueblo Indians. In the middle of one Awatobi fresco there is a masked figure of a girl in dancing posture; she is large in scale, compared with two smaller lateral figures who offer two fowls for sacrifice. The flat color, line of the drawing, and dynamic symmetry of the figures create an expression of rhythm characteristic of this culture. An imaginative sense of color and a more decisive tendency toward geometry of line are found in the sand paintings of the Navaho, made for healing rites by special shamans.

Interesting examples of choreography in pre-Columbian cultures occurred in the painted Mochica and Chimu pottery of ancient Peru (see ANDEAN PROTOHISTORY). Here, too, the subject matter was mythical and ritual. Recurrent themes such as dances, processions in honor of a divinity, and runners in ritual games were transmitted from the Mochica to the Chimu culture. Of particular interest is the depiction on hemispherical jugs of noble warriors in multicolored costumes, completely armed and adorned with the most variegated decorations; they march single file in the manner of a continuous frieze.

Especially outstanding among the painted processions of Peru is that of the moon god Si, the highest Chimu deity, on a vase in the Museum für Völkerkunde in Berlin (Kutscher, 1950, pp. 36–37, fig. 37). The god is borne forward on a litter by a pair of carriers; a crown of rays emanates from his person. He is followed by a procession of armed demons with animal heads, accompanied by smaller figures of animals. On another Chimu vase (Kutscher, p. 30, fig. 32) we find a group of four musicians — two flute players and two trumpet players.

The theme of the dance of death is frequent. On a vase from Trujillo, Peru, a row of spirits is shown engaged in an orgiastic feast (Kutscher, p. 31, fig. 33). On another vase (Kutscher, p. 32, fig. 34), the dead, appearing as skeletons, abandon themselves to a wild dance accompanied by flutes; two skeletons in the foreground indicate the rhythm with sticks equipped with rattles. In a third death dance the skeletons hold one another's hands in dance movement.

In the painted decoration of the Chimu vases, we find rows of runners following one another; frequently the rows are very small. They may consist of men (Kutscher, p. 35, fig. 36, pp. 38–39, fig. 38) or demons (Kutscher, pp. 52–53, fig. 50; p. 58, fig. 54) with animal heads, carrying bags of beans in their hands (Kutscher, fig. 38). In some instances the choreographic theme has a wholly or predominantly decorative function, as in examples showing figures placed symmetrically; the decorative value is similar to that found in Peruvian textiles.

Three-dimensional figures of dancers, either alone or in groups, are frequent in the art of the Mayas, Aztecs, and other Mexican cultures; they are either modeled in terra cotta (PL. 299) or carved in stone.

Vittorio LANTERNARI

THE ANCIENT WORLD. The large figures from the great Mesopotamian palaces (PL. 301) as well as the reliefs and paintings of Egypt have a strong ceremonial element in their solemnly rhythmical disposition. Rows of soldiers, priests, tribute bearers, prisoners, and slaves are distinguishable one from another only by exterior marks such as costume and hairdress; the major fact — the act of homage, or the religious reverence — depends on the rhythmic disposition or movement of the figures. Walking figures are well illustrated in Iran in the Tripylon of Persepolis and the audience hall of the Palace of Darius I (H. Frankfort, *The Art and Architecture of the Ancient Orient*, Harmondsworth, 1954, pls. 178–79, 181–83); in the latter, the alternation between figure groups and ornamental bands shows a rhythmic equation of figure and ornament. This tendency, however, is much older than the Palace of Darius; the pottery of Samarra in Mesopotamia shows figures of female dancers in a circle transformed into a geometric motif (A. Parrot, *Archéologie mésopotamienne*, II, Paris, 1953, pl. 3). The group in wood of small Egyptian soldiers walking in a parade (Cairo, Eg. Mus.) similarly relates to choreography; this is also true of the phalanx of Eannatum (I, PL. 506), which has, however, a practical rather than esthetic purpose. Other rhythmical representations of scenes, especially those which almost seem to reproduce a ballet, can be called choreographic with even more justification. Among these are certain pantomimes depicted in Egyptian grave paintings of the Middle Kingdom; the subject matter is allegorical, with such themes as the impetuous wind or Pharaoh striking down an enemy.

Similar developments can be traced in the Cretan-Mycenaean world. Theseus' and Ariadne's famous dance to celebrate the victory over the Minotaur is remembered in literature; sculptured dancers appear in the terra-cotta group of Palaikastro (PL. 299), in a Cypriote group (IV, PL. 91), and in the representations of snake goddesses (or priestesses with serpents) who are actually sacred dancers. The famous Daedalic *choros* of this region should be understood rather as a group of dancers than as an indication of a place.

During the Geometric period (see GEOMETRIC STYLE), the choreographic sources of iconography (e.g., dance scenes in the round) are submerged in a general tendency to place hu-

man figures in a rhythmic pattern alternating with ornamental motifs (II, PL. 32), as can be seen in some manifestations of true primitive art. Furthermore, a sense of processional rhythm dominates the rows of animals in the Orientalizing representations.

In archaic and classic art (when figures again become dominant) it is difficult to distinguish faithful representations of iconographic themes inspired by the dance from a mere taste for rhythmic repetition. The interest in rhythmic repetition was carried over to classic and Hellenistic art from the decorative and additive traditions of archaic art (e.g., dance schemes on Greek vases and in tomb paintings from Tarquinia, Ruvo, and other sites in Italy; PL. 299). Rhythmic repetition appeared also in the dancing maenads attributed to Kallimachos and in Neo-Attic works such as the relief portraying the Curetes in the Vatican Museums. The motif of rhythmic repetition was particularly appreciated in the Roman period because it was a means of suggesting a whole crowd with only a few figures; we see this in the marching and parading troops on the columns of Trajan and Marcus Aurelius in Rome (2d cent. of our era) and even more in the scenes of imperial ceremonies on late-antique reliefs. The concept of divine majesty, shown by a figure's frontality, was combined in this period with an ordered, rhythmic, and repetitive disposition of the court officials, which occasionally violated the laws of linear perspective (as in the Arch of Constantine) or reversed them (as in the Theodosian reliefs from the Hippodrome in Constantinople; late 4th cent.). Rhythmic balance was encouraged in ancient art by a court ceremony that prescribed in detail the acts and movements required of the emperor and dignitaries for each occasion, as well as their precise place in the hierarchy.

In Byzantine civilization this taste for ordered movement or prearranged disposition of figures was applied to religious imagery; outstanding examples can be found in S. Apollinare Nuovo, Ravenna, in the rows of virgins and martyrs (PL. 301), or in the evangelists, apostles, and symbols arranged like the spokes of a wheel in the dome of the two baptisteries. This style was petrified in the imagery of peripheral cultures, for example, Coptic (see COPTIC ART), where patterns were created which continued unchanged for centuries.

Even though there was no medieval choreography which can be strictly connected with that of the preceding centuries, traces of choreography can be found in medieval court and church ceremony (in the liturgy it is obvious) as well as in mystery plays. Through these sources, choreography as a motif was adopted in art, especially in manuscript illumination and in tapestries; it is particularly evident in symbolic representations such as those of paradise, where the figures in repetitive or hierarchic composition seem to resemble stage productions.

One can discover reflections of the ancient ceremonial spirit even in architecture: in the great stairways of Mesopotamian palaces or the large inner courts of the Cretan palaces, in halls for the celebration of mystery rites (e. g., that at Eleusis in Greece), in the complexes of porticoes, halls, atria, and tribunal areas of late Roman palaces and circuses, as well as in the long naves of Christian basilicas and the wide inner squares or large regular courtyards of medieval castles and Renaissance palaces.

Michelangelo CAGIANO DE AZEVEDO

ASIATIC CIVILIZATIONS. The importance of the dance and its relation to the representational arts varied in Asia according to the values of the great civilizations which dominated the continent with their religious and artistic schools. In the ancient Near East, the whirling motif seen on the pottery of Samarra (4th millennium B.C.; H. Frankfort, *The Art and Architecture of the Ancient Orient*, Harmondsworth, 1958, fig. 1) exploits the emotional possibilities of the simplest geometric figures to express the movement of men and animals. The whirling motif is also known in the Indo-Iranian cultures, where fragments of vessels show human figures holding hands, their faces clearly drawn. As in Samarra, movement is implied by the wind-blown hair and the circular dance. In the pottery of Tell Arpachiya (near Nineveh), figures standing close to one another

with clasped hands form a continuous frieze which is soon transformed into abstract ornament; in Iran, rows of curved dancers hold one another by the shoulders in a different type of rotating movement. Motifs inspired by battle dances appear later in Iran (Sialk, IB).

At Harappa in the Indus Valley, one of the two most important works of sculpture — a torso (now mutilated) in gray stone (New Delhi, Mus. of Central Asian Ant.) — is connected with the dance. If the reconstruction is exact, the torso indicates a stylized choreographic step that is a dance of Śiva; the rhythm symbolizes the flow of life that oscillates between creation and destruction. In India the dance as such was regarded as an imitation of nature because it mirrored the rhythm of creative flux. The representation of human figures in Indian art often takes inspiration from the dance. Various technical texts advise the painter to learn the art of dancing so as to tell long and complicated stories such as the entire *Rāmāyaṇa*.

In sculpture as well as in painting cycles human and divine figures often assume dancing postures (PL. 300). Not only the characteristic posture of the *tribhaṅga* (the threefold flexion of the body) but the anatomy seems to be inspired by male and female dancers. The smallest gesture has a precise significance; the same is true of the mudra and the asana (positions of hands and body connected with yoga technique), which, like the dance, have their mimic codification. Births of Indian heroes, whether Buddha, Kṛṣṇa, or Rāma, are accompanied by dances of celestial nymphs. Moreover, there are many death dances. The characteristic postures of dancers are transformed into decorative motifs for the sculptural decoration of the temples. Even actions completely foreign to choreography, such as drawing a bow, are sometimes transformed into dance steps; and with the development of tantric symbolism the representations of divinities accompanied by their female energies, or *śakti*, assume poses similar to those of the dancing Śiva. When Tantric Buddhism began to develop along parallel lines with Saiva Tantrism, the pattern of the cosmic dance was transmitted outside India and gave rise in Nepal to images of singular elegance and in Tibet to the terrifying figures of divinities.

In Gandhara (q.v.) we find few iconographic reflections of the dance, either because in this culture the human figure had different functions in art and choreography or because there was a tendency to reduce movement in art. Some groups of dancing and music-making young men or women do appear, however, in scenes probably unrelated to Buddhism. The girls swirl in their veils and beat their hands on their knees [relief, 3d cent. (?); Rome, Mus. Naz. d'Arte Orientale]. The gestures and movements of the men, completely foreign to India, appear on a relief of three dancers with Scythian costume and Phrygian caps (2d–3d cent.; Cleveland Mus. of Art), who in pose, costume, and coordinated movements seem to be almost a prefiguration of the mosaic of the three Magi in the left-hand nave of S. Apollinare Nuovo in Ravenna. These Gandhara themes are probably of Iranian origin, for they are not to be found in India proper. Probably also of Iranian origin is the theme of minor divinities represented in flight as if in a dance free of all earthly gravitation. It spread from Gandhara to classical India, Central Asia, China, and even to Japan (wall paintings of Hōryūji, near Nara).

Official Iranian art of the Achaemenid period reveals scanty and indirect connections with the dance; in the depiction of ceremonies, a pictorial order and rhythm is imposed on groups symbolizing the various peoples of the empire. The recurrent motif of the dancer in rigid frontality, holding her veil with both hands, appears in minor works of the Parthian period, on terra-cotta sarcophagi and plaques. Such Parthian images as well as the veil motif are found in the Gandhara school in examples that have no direct connections with the dance. Iran and the Central Asian regions under its influence developed the veil motif widely in the Sassanian period; as in Gandhara, it is often used to enliven human representations.

Wherever Buddhism spread — even in China and Japan — figures of celestial dancers and devas emerged as secondary, almost decorative, divinities; the graceful effects of floating veils and scarves proved inexhaustibly inspiring to artists. Sassanian

Iran reelaborated the old motif of young dancing and music-making girls already seen in Gandhara; the motif extended even to the post-Sassanian period, as is proved by three silver cups recently discovered in the Mazanderan district, now in the Archaeological Museum of Teheran. Despite the flat relief and strong stylization of the cups, the artists succeeded in effectively representing on them a circular dance movement. Other more complicated dance steps are to be found on a post-Sassanian silver plate (Paris, Bib. Nat.), undoubtedly religious but of uncertain interpretation.

The interest in sacred and secular dance in Sassanian Iran was almost as great as the interest in music; the rather static representations on silver plates of lightly veiled dancing girls were numerous. In the mosaics of Bishapur, a group of dancers stylistically close to Hellenistic or Roman "impressionism" are more heavily clothed; but in their lively dance movements they resemble the girls on the silver plate in the Bibliothèque Nationale. The motif of the relatively static dancer covered with veils appears also in the terra-cotta tiles of the temple of Harwan in Kashmir. The style is clearly Iranian, with scarcely any Indian elements.

Several motifs such as the acrobatic dancers so characteristic on Sassanian silver spread into Central Asia. Wei-chih I-sêng, a Central Asian painter from Khotan, active in China in the mid-7th century, seems to have produced the most brilliant version of a girl swirling in the dance; a scroll belonging to the Berenson Foundation (Florence, Italy) in which a Central Asian dancing girl faces a Chinese partner may well be by his hand. The female dancer recurs in two paintings representing Vaiśravana (Bishamon), the guardian of the north, one preserved in the Freer Gallery of Art, Washington, the other formerly in the Palace collection, Peking. The latter painting seems to bear the signature of Wu Tao-tzǔ, but both are copies of an original by Wei-chih I-sêng. This Khotanese artist, who had a liking for exotic subjects, wanted to represent the whirling movement of the dance found in the paintings of Khotan and in the frescoes of Cave 220 (A.D. 642) at Tun-huang (q.v.), western China, where the dancers tread on a small oval rug. The veils, the strange mantilla, and the general position of the body and the limbs of the dancing girl express the rapidity and power of rotation without spoiling the gracefulness of the movement; the effervescent treatment of the dress goes back to a prototype in Sassanian silver. The dance of the Chinese dancer of the Berenson scroll is of a different kind: the long sleeves are similar to those of the dancing-girl figurines from the T'ang tombs; probably this dance is a variation of the dance of the flying swallows mentioned in T'ang texts. In the wall paintings of Tun-huang the compositional rhythm of the long rows of donor deities often suggests the movement of a dance.

Macabre elements which first appeared at Hadda (Afghanistan) spread through Central Asia. At Kizil, near Kucha, we find in a vast Buddhist composition what is almost an anticipation of the Western dance of death; a lightly clothed female dancer is backed by a grinning skeleton. The motif probably derives from a Hellenistic prototype. The anatomy of certain grotesque Dharmapāla dancers is so stylized as to reveal the skeleton without divesting it of flesh. Couples of dancing skeletons appear on late Tibetan tankas. Dances with no religious connotation are represented in the wall paintings of Tun-huang, as in the festival procession of Chang I-chao in Cave 156.

Mario BUSSAGLI

In China suggestions of the dance can be found in the Hui-hsien figurines, ascribed by some experts to the late Chou period and by others to a much later time. Certain funerary tiles of the late Han tombs, expressing a particular trend in taste, rendered the sword dance and the rhythmic drum dance (po-hsi) in an exciting manner; but generally the dance was not a frequent theme in China, and the tradition of the painting schools excluded it from the repertory of the greater artists. Exceptions to this restriction on choreographic decoration were the funerary terra-cotta statuettes, frequent in the T'ang period but no longer used when cremation took the place of burial, as well

as the Li Lung-mien (q.v.) scroll (late 11th cent.) entitled Chi-jang t'u ("Beating the Ground"), showing musicians, dancers, and beggars.

Jan FONTEIN

The poses of T'ang funerary statuettes, some of which are masterpieces, correspond generally to descriptions in contemporary literature. Among the statuettes are youthful male dancers, believed by J. G. Mahler to be foreigners from the south, and acrobatic dancers with grotesque faces similar to the masked dancers of the Kucha reliquary (Tokyo, priv. coll.). Mahler stressed the role that Hu-hsüan dancers played in Chinese literature; their swirling dance was, as the verses of Po Chü-i and Yüan Chên prove, introduced into China about A.D. 720, perhaps from Sogdiana.

Mario BUSSAGLI

The theme of the dance was frequent in Korean painting of the late 18th century. The outstanding masters here were Kim Hung-to, Kim Tuk-sin, and Sin Yun-pok. In the gay life of the Yi period, courtesans and dancing girls (kisaeng) played an important role; some of their dances, such as the sword dance, with its persistent rhythm and whirling movements, could be caught in a few quick brush strokes.

In Japan, the dance has been an ever-recurring artistic theme, playing an important role in early mythology, religion, and the theater. In paintings of the earlier periods, religious and court dances occurred with some frequency. The art of the Ukiyo-e (q.v.), or "floating world" school, favored the popular dances of the amusement districts, depicting dancing girls, courtesans, and actors of the Kabuki stage.

The hand scrolls of the Kamakura period (13th–14th cent.) and more especially those of the E-den type (illustrated biographies) afford an intimate view of daily life in the temples and monasteries of the Buddhist sects, as well as a precise documentation of their ritual dances. An interesting example of the period is afforded by the dancing scenes in the Tengū Sōshi scrolls, which satirize the solemn temple dances.

In the early 17th century a pair of two-panel screens by the painter Nonomura Sōtatsu (now in the Daigoji Monastery, Kyoto) blended three different types of Bugaku dances; the slow movements of the figures, the careful rendering of expression and miming, are unequaled when compared with later imitations by Kusumi Morikage (Tokyo, Nezu Mus.). A preference for popular dances and especially for female fan dancers existed before the Ukiyo-e. The slow and stiff movements transformed the dancing girls, even when isolated upon the screen, into decorative motifs. A pair of screens by Kanō Naganobu (d. 1654) shows a group of noble ladies performing a sword dance and a fan dance with gay, quick movements as though they were slightly intoxicated (Tokyo, Coll. Hara Kunizō). Contemporary with Ukiyo-e was the emergence of the Kabuki theater; many of its dances were represented by painters and print makers. Sharaku, for example, in his prints and rare drawings often reproduces the so-called "lion dance" and the dance of the uncovered face (kaomise). The No theater, however, inspired few artists, except for Hokusai. Although the Ukiyo-e was strongly influenced by the theater, paintings and prints in turn established conventions for gestures and poses in dance and declamation, thus helping to perpetuate a precious tradition.

Jan FONTEIN

Dance representations are rare in Islam because of an injunction in the Koran: "[The faithful] should never beat [the ground] with their feet in order to show the ornaments they are hiding" (Sura XXIV, V. 31); this statement was regarded as a clear prohibition of dancing. Nevertheless, images of male and female dancers occasionally appeared in the art of Islam, and the representation of the dance was a theme for competition among artists, as proved by al-Maqrīzī's story of the rival painters ibn-Aziz and al-Qasir (A.D. 1058), both of whom chose as their subject two dancing girls. The female dancer from Qusair 'Amra (early 8th cent.) as well as the entire pictorial decoration

of the palace still vaguely reflect Hellenistic motifs. The two dancing girls from Samarra, of the 9th century or later, appear in strict frontality and are very stylized. More harmonious and quick in movement are the two female dancers painted on the ceiling of the Cappella Palatina, Palermo; in contrast, the row of dancers in the marble bas-reliefs of Ghazni in Afghanistan seem heavy. In the wild dervish dances, represented in late miniatures, the attention of the Islamic artist was characteristically concentrated on the individuality of the dancer. In the Akbar period (1556–1605), under the influence of Hindu India, we find representations of male sword dancers, ecstatic dances, or Indian and Islamic female dancers from other lands side by side. In all cases, however, both the dance and its movement are subordinated to the interest of the general scene. Islamic dance, therefore, has no significant influence on the styles of individual artists or schools.

Wilhelm STAUDE and Mario BUSSAGLI

EUROPE FROM THE RENAISSANCE TO MODERN TIMES. In the Renaissance the dance took on a worldly and social character; it was no longer represented as a ritual but as a formal interpretation of beautiful movements and postures. European art from the Renaissance to the present is rich in all forms of dance documentation and choreographic spectacles, both literary and visual. Most interesting, from the art-historical point of view, is the influence of choreography on composition and form in works of art; artists came to understand that certain kinds of beauty can be attained through training and control of the body and its gestures. The further idea that the figure (see HUMAN FIGURE) becomes more beautiful or reveals hidden harmonies in the dance deeply influenced the artistic conception of the human body in the Gothic period. This idea continued into the 15th century, influencing not only French and Flemish painting and the Gothic art of the northern Italian courts (e.g., miniatures), but also the work of the Florentine sculptors Ghiberti and Donatello, the reliefs of Agostino di Duccio, and the paintings of Botticelli (PL. 302). The emphasis on linear rhythm originally inspired by dance became separate from the logic of movement in Agostino di Duccio and Botticelli and determined posture, gesture, facial expression, even color and costume. Thus a definite type of beauty, with great possibilities of development, came into existence with the conception of the human figure responding to the rhythm of the dance. It must be added, however, that dance was not understood as a mere spectacle but rather as an expression of an inner condition. In an almost symbolic way it could indicate beatitude (the row of blessed dancers in the *Last Judgment* of Fra Angelico, I, PL. 261), or, returning to a concept of Dante's, a state of internal harmony (the three Graces in Botticelli's *Primavera*), or popular rejoicing (dancers in the great altar of Mary by Veit Stoss, in St. Mary's, Kracow). Religious and worldly feasts and ceremonies were closely connected with the dance and therefore became a source of inspiration for the religious compositions of many Quattrocento artists including Gozzoli, Botticelli, Ghirlandajo, and Pinturicchio.

Another aspect of the influence of choreography on Renaissance art is the representation of dance in historical and legendary scenes; a typical example is the dance of Salome at the banquet of Herod. Here, however, the dancer does not perform a specific dance movement, but it is by her attitude that Salome is recognized. In Donatello's relief on the font in the Baptistery of Siena, Salome does not acquire any special gracefulness from her dance posture, but she is the fulcrum of the action (IV, PL. 242). In the same manner, the depiction of great ceremonies with many figures was doubtless a dramatic factor in the story illustrated (e.g., Donatello's reliefs for the high altar of S. Antonio in Padua) or a pretext for a rhythmic distribution of forms and colors (e.g., Gentile Bellini, *Procession in St. Mark's Square*, Venice, Accademia). Allegorical spectacles containing dances and triumphal processions, so frequent in the learned courts of the Quattrocento, inspired the frescoes of the Palazzo Schifanoia at Ferrara (II, PL. 25; IV, PLS. 1–3) and the allegorical compositions of Mantegna. The connection

between ceremonies and artistic representations is extremely close; artists were often called upon to arrange the historical or festive apparatus and to plan the choreography.

A large part of the connection between spectacles and the representational arts lies in the realm of scenography (q.v.) and is founded on perspective (q.v.). Thus the entire art of Rome in the late 16th century reflects sacred ceremonies, often introducing into them — as if to underline their theatrical character — supernatural apparitions, miracles, and allegories. The very pictorial or sculptural viewpoint of the baroque can be called choreographic because single figures and groups were distributed in space according to perspective diagonals, stepped planes, and so forth.

Pictures as well as drama followed the Aristotelian canons of unity of time, place, and action; this enabled the painter to insert into his work apparitions or miracles as real events, corresponding to the *deus ex machina* of the drama. The choreographic and dramatic element is clearly acknowledged in English theoretical writings of the 18th century. Daniel Webb insisted on the analogy of painting and theater: pictorial composition should be theatrical and dramatic. Hogarth (q.v.) said that he "wished to compose pictures on canvas similar to representations on the stage." He felt that he was obliged to treat his subjects as a dramatic author would. Painting was a stage; the men and women depicted on canvas were actors executing a pantomime with certain actions and gestures. In the romantic period, historical painting seems to have derived in large measure from stage presentations, particularly those of Shakespeare.

When the dance lost its sacred and ritual character, it acquired, as we have seen, a new importance in the development of esthetic theory. The older concept of beauty, founded on unchanging and measurable proportional relationships, implied monumentality and a complete absence of expression. In the 18th century, however, beauty in movement found an explicit theoretical justification as rhythmic development (Webb). Grace, a concept largely based on Correggio's painting, was defined as rhythmic movement separated from action, valid simply as a modulation of lines and chiaroscuro. It is easy to trace, from Correggio back to Leonardo (back in the 16th century Vasari spoke of the latter's "divine grace"), the attempt to express profound attitudes of the soul by movements of the body which, according to Giovanni Paolo Lomazzo (1538–1600), contain "the spirit and the life of art." Grace was a favorite theme of neoclassical poetry, which often equated it with classical dance. Later Stendhal called grace "romantic beauty." In our century, the historic continuity in the connection between dance and the representational arts produced attempts to translate dance (or rather ballet) into an art of movement. Cubism and futurism (q.v.) tried to represent movement concretely in terms of an interpenetration of space and time. At the beginning of the twentieth century the Russian ballet, strongly accenting the contributions of the other visual arts, aroused wide interest. Oskar Schlemmer (*Die Bühne*, Munich, 1924) elaborated a theory of choreography as organized movement of volumes and colors on the stage and used it in a theatrical production (*Triadisches Ballet*, Landestheater, Stuttgart, 1922). Contemporary artists such as Picasso and Braque in their stage settings also use this translation of choreography into art (see EUROPEAN MODERN MOVEMENTS).

BIBLIOG. R. Charbonnel, La danse, Paris, 1899; M. L. Becker, Der Tanz, Leipzig, 1901; R. S. Johnston, A History of Dancing, London, 1906; J. Dalcroze, Der Rhythmus, ein Jahrbuch, Dresden, Jena, 1911–12; S. N. Chudekov, Istoriya tantsev, 4 vols., St. Petersburg, 1913; I. Narodny, The Dance, New York, 1917; O. Bie, Der Tanz, Berlin, 1919; J. Dalcroze, Rhythmus, Musik und Erziehung, Basel, 1921; C. Sharp, The Dance, New York, 1924; M. V. Boehm, Der Tanz, New York, 1925; F. Weege, Der Tanz in der Antike, Halle, 1926; E. Freudel, Rhythmik, Theorie und Praxis der körperlich-musikalischen Erziehung, Munich, 1926; R. Steiner, Sprachgestaltung und dramatische Kunst, Dornach, 1926; L. B. Lawler, MAARome, VI, 1927, p. 69 ff.; R. Steiner, Eurythmie als sichtbarer Gesang, Dornach, 1927; H. Bulle, Untersuchungen an griechischen Theatern, Munich, 1928, p. 215 ff.; L. Curtius, Die Wandmalerei Pompejis, Leipzig, 1929, figs. 105, 107, 108, 111, 115; C. W. Beaumont, A Bibliography of Dancing, London, 1929; M. E. Perugini, A Pageant of the Dance and Ballet, London, 1930; L. Séchan, La danse grecque antique, Paris, 1930; E. Selden, Elements of the Free Dance, New York, 1930; F. Struwe, Erziehung durch Rhythmus

in Musik und Leben, Kassel, 1930; T. B. van Lelyveld, De Javanse Danskunst, Amsterdam. 1931; C. Sachs, Eine Weltgeschichte des Tanzes, Berlin, 1933 (Eng. ed., World History of the Dance, trans. B. Schönberg, New York, 1937); M. Brillant, Problèmes de la danse, Paris, 1935; L. Kirstein, A Short History of Classical Theatrical Dancing, New York, 1935; P. D. Magriel, A Bibliography of Dancing, New York, 1936; J. Sozonova, La vie de la danse, Paris, 1937; E. Brunner-Traut, Der Tanz im alten Ägypten, Glückstadt, 1938; L. Vaillat, Histoire de la danse, Paris, 1942; R. Marvell, Notes on Choreography, Dance Index, Feb., 1945; P. Michaut, Histoire du ballet, Paris, 1945; S. Lifar, Histoire du ballet russe, Paris, 1945; J. Gregor, Kulturgeschichte des Ballets, Vienna, 1946; J. Martin, The Dance, 1946; C. W. Beaumont, A Short History of Ballet, London, 1947; T. Meyer-Greene, The Arts and Art of Criticism, Princeton, 1947; P. Stern, Continuité des danses de l'Inde, L'Amour de l'Art, VI–VII, 1947, pp. 305–12; V. Lemaître, La danse, le bal, le théâtre, le cinéma, Avignon, 1948; R. von Laban, Modern Educational Dance, London, 1948; A. Chujoy, Dance Encyclopedia, New York, Toronto, 1949; G. P. Kurath, Dance, Folk and Primitive, Standard Dictionary of Folklore, Mythology, and Legend, ed. M. Leach, New York, 1949; H. Bulle and H. Wirsing, Szenenbilder zum griechischen Theater des 5. Jahrhunderts v. Chr., Berlin, 1950; G. Kutscher, Chimu: Eine altindianische Hochkultur, Berlin, 1950; D. Lynam, Storia del balletto, Florence, 1951; Various authors, L'art du ballet dès origines à nos jours, Paris, 1952; M. Wood, Historical Dances, London, 1952; R. Reyna, Des origines du ballet, Paris, 1955; G. Dorfles, Attività estetica e attività ludica, Atti del III Congresso internazionale di estetica, Venice, 1956; A. K. Coomaraswamy, The Dance of Śiva, 2d ed., New York, 1957; G. Dorfles, Il divenire delle arti, Turin, 1959; J. G. Mahler, The Westerners among the Figurines of the T'ang Dynasty of China, Rome, 1959.

* *

Illustrations: PLS. 299–302.

**CHRIST, REPRESENTATIONS OF.** See CHRISTIANITY.

**CHRISTIANITY.** Christianity has influenced painting and sculpture to the degree that images have played a part in the Christian religious experience; it has influenced architecture through buildings dedicated to worship and through the founding of religious communities. In a critical sense, it is more accurate to speak of artistic theories and practices inspired by Christianity than of Christian art as such.

For special aspects of Christian iconography, see BIBLICAL SUBJECTS; CATACOMBS; COSMOLOGY AND CARTOGRAPHY; DEMONOLOGY; DEVOTIONAL OBJECTS AND IMAGES, POPULAR; ESCHATOLOGY; HERETICAL SUBJECTS; IMAGES AND ICONOCLASM; SAINTS, ICONOGRAPHY OF; SYMBOLISM AND ALLEGORY; etc. This article deals specifically with representations of Christ, the Virgin, saints, and the Church, beginning with a historical account of the positions toward art held by the Catholic Church and by other Christian thinkers.

SUMMARY. Images and religious experience (col. 587). Architectural precepts and theories (col. 588). Medieval Christendom (col. 589). Religion and art in the Italian Renaissance (col. 591). Religion and art in the Reformation and Counter Reformation (col. 591). Recent concepts of "sacred art" and "Christian art" (col. 593). Modern Christian art. (col. 594). Christianity and iconography (col. 596): *Christ; Symbols of Christ; The crucifix; Christological groups; The Virgin; Angels; Saints, prophets, sibyls; Symbolic representations of the Church; Christian iconography in primitive civilizations.*

IMAGES AND RELIGIOUS EXPERIENCE. For the Fathers of the Church the problem of images and their role in religious experience arose from the conflict between the two traditions to which Christianity was bound, the Hebraic and the Greco-Hellenistic, which had assumed opposing attitudes with respect to the function of images in religious experience. Christianity had in a certain sense to choose between fidelity to the Hebraic interdictions and assimilation of the representationalism to which the Gentile cults were deeply committed. The first alternative would have seriously handicapped Christian proselytism; the second presented the danger of idolatry.

Rigorist hostility to images has ancient origins, having been a factor in Christian polemics against Gentile idolatry.

Without departing from this tradition St. Gregory of Nyssa (331 ?–96 ?), in his eulogy of St. Theodore Martyr, emphasized the beauty of places of worship as an element of great importance to religious experience. It was not a question of presenting divinity directly but of narrating events in order to edify the soul of the observer with examples. A fundamental role was that of paintings that portrayed the deeds of a martyr and the cruelty of his persecutors, depicting such episodes in the manner of a book, which benefits those who seek instruction from it, and adorning the walls of the temple with color. Man and human activity were to be represented, in the comprehensible events of this world. According to this view, the custom of adorning places of worship with images was sanctioned without contravening either the inner meaning of the Biblical interdictions, which forbade giving God a human appearance, or the repugnance of Christian culture of the early centuries to the anthropomorphism and idolatry of popular pagan worship.

A decisive change in the Christian concepts of representation was brought about by the work of Pseudo-Dionysius the Areopagite, in all probability a Syrian monk living in the late 5th and early 6th century, whose thought reflected the later Neo-Platonic ideas. Pseudo-Dionysius introduced into Christian philosophy the concept of "dissimilarity" as a way of "giving form to that which is formless" and "giving shape to that which has no shape." He formulated the theory of "dissimilar images" in order to justify Biblical language and its metaphors; the same concept, applied to the representational ornamentation of churches, was to provide a theoretical sanction for the use of symbol and allegory.

Thus there developed spontaneously artistic tendencies distinct from narrative that favored not only the generous use of zoomorphic motifs (see ZOOMORPHIC AND PLANT REPRESENTATIONS) but also the use of theriomorphic (see MONSTROUS AND FANTASTIC SUBJECTS) and demonic motifs (see DEMONOLOGY). There ensued acceptance of the signs of the zodiac, stars, sun, and moon, which were used allegorically (see ASTRONOMY AND ASTROLOGY), and of motifs taken from the popular Gentile, barbarian, and Eastern traditions or from esoteric doctrines, such as the labyrinth and the interlace (see MAGIC). The concept of the dissimilar image freed representation from restriction to a merely narrative function, which had imprinted on taste a realistic stamp; it tended to satisfy the desire to see, in the images adorning the church, the direct presence — and almost the participation in the acts of worship — of Christ and the saints. Thus a set formalism developed, one that was to persist particularly in the East, which favored the frontal pose and compositions according to established schemes. The favorite themes were not only acts and events in the lives of Christ and the saints but also Christ in His glory and power, the saints, still in their earthly guise, elevated to heaven, and Mary presenting the Infant Jesus to man.

The theories of the Pseudo-Dionysius were revived and propagated in the East under St. Maximus the Confessor (580 ?–662); their diffusion in the West occurred later, particularly by way of the translation and commentary of John Scotus Erigena (815 ?–877 ?). But the artistic practices that found sanction in these theories go back as far as the first centuries of Christianity; in fact, Christian thought about the representational arts reflected the conflict between two great currents: narrative-realistic and allegoric-symbolic. Images, however, whether conceived narratively or symbolically, were always considered an integral part of the environment of the place of worship, and it is impossibile to reconstruct Christian theories of art without keeping in mind the unity of the representational arts and architecture and the theories concerning the latter.

ARCHITECTURAL PRECEPTS AND THEORIES. One of the earliest documents relating to Christian architectural concepts is a passage in the *Constitutiones apostolicae*, attributed to Pope Clement I (90–99 ?) but in large part a 4th-century work, in which the principle of the basilican system is set forth. Analogously to the development of theories concerning images, this principle represented an adaptation of earlier forms to the new religion, a process not substantially different from that which occurred later in the case of central-plan constructions. In both basilican and central-plan churches great importance was given to luminosity, to the inlaying of precious metals, to mosaics glowing with gold and color, to stuccowork: architecture and image formed a single whole, and gradually, as the Church absorbed new populations, both the iconographic

repertory and the techniques of execution multiplied and were enriched. The admission of the iconographic patrimony and stylistic preferences of the new peoples who adopted Christianity is another problem which must be considered by those who wish to distinguish the elements of Christian thought that have in any way influenced artistic phenomena.

MEDIEVAL CHRISTENDOM. From the earliest years of its expansion in the Greco-Roman world, Christianity appropriated certain iconographic elements from pagan mythology; these were justified by the introduction of allegorical meanings. The same pattern was followed during and after the great migrations, as the barbaric populations gradually came to form part of Christendom. The Christian culture of Ireland, between the 6th and the 9th century, assimilated a large number of iconographic subjects and decorative themes from Celtic mythology (see ANGLO-SAXON AND IRISH ART; CELTIC ART). These subjects and themes, which were diffused throughout Christendom in the West through the efforts of St. Columban (543–615) and his followers, fostered a preference for symbolism, but not without arousing the opposition of those who maintained that only narrative painting could be reconciled with the spirit of Christianity (see IMAGES AND ICONOCLASM).

A crisis of unprecedented proportions was caused by the iconoclastic heresy that pervaded the Christian world during the 8th and 9th centuries and temporarily revived those ascetic and rigorist tendencies hostile to the introduction of any form of representation into the religious experience — tendencies that had been characteristic of the early centuries of Christianity.

The iconoclastic movement was officially inaugurated in 726 in the first declaration of the Byzantine emperor Leo III the Isaurian, who was strongly influenced against the veneration of images by Islamic monotheism. Four years later he issued a decree that forbade such veneration and ordered the removal of religious images from the churches. Leo's successor, Constantine V Copronymus, convoked a synod at Constantinople in 754 which anathematized those who venerated or produced religious images. Painting was thus condemned as a blasphemous art whenever it ventured to represent Christ, the Virgin, or the saints: only paintings of profane subjects, preferably glorifying the emperor, his family, and his court, were admissible.

The rehabilitation of images that followed the Second Nicene Council (787) was later confirmed in Carolingian texts which established that while images were not to be worshiped, neither were they to be destroyed, because in so far as their purpose was ornamental and decorative they could not be considered idols: " 'Image' and 'idol' call for very different definitions. For it is clear that images are made for the purpose of adornment or to illustrate historical events, whereas the exclusive purpose of the idol is to mislead the minds of unfortunate men by sacrilegious worship and senseless superstition. Further, the image has reference to something other than itself, the idol only to itself." Accordingly, historical painting seemed most in harmony with the position of the Second Nicene Council. But the dissemination of the writings of Pseudo-Dionysius and the philosophy of Scotus Erigena also favored the spread of symbolic art in painting and sculpture, and the internal reform of the Benedictine Order centered at the abbey of Cluny (founded in 910) contributed further to this trend.

The reform of Cluny proposed to lead the Benedictine Order back to its original austerity, but its aims also included the consolidation of monasticism as a temporal power and as a guide for society. To these ends the Cluniacs cultivated magnificence — in architecture, in the decoration of churches, in church hangings, in the liturgy and in ceremonies associated with it — as one of the principal instruments of their activity and of their ethico-religious propaganda. This was the basis of the fundamental contribution of the Cluniac reform to the so-called "11th-century renaissance" and to the diffusion of Romanesque art throughout Europe. As the Cluniac historian Raoul Glaber (ca. 985–after 1035) wrote: "In almost every part of the world, but particularly in Italy and in the land of the Gauls, churches were being rebuilt.... In fact, it was as though the world, rousing itself and putting aside its decrepit old age, was donning the gleaming white vestiture of new churches."

Pilgrimages, which were encouraged by the Cluniacs, further contributed to the renovation and enlargement of churches. The spectacular character given religious ceremonies by the Cluniacs led them to favor basilican rather than central-plan edifices. In the rich decoration of their churches they favored particularly, apart from symbolic representations, those images capable of arousing the fear of sin, divine wrath, and hell or the expectation of the Last Judgment (see ESCHATOLOGY), represented in their churches with the image of Christ as Judge.

The luxus pro Deo of the Cluniac order, however, was bound to arouse opposition and conflicts within Benedictine monasticism itself. It was in Burgundy, the center of the Cluniac reform, that the Cistercian Order arose, with the avowed aim of returning to the rectitudo regulae of St. Benedict (480 ?–543 ?), of eliminating all liturgical pomp, and of reviving the practice of retreat to abandoned and uninhabitable places in order to reclaim them by cultivating the soil. St. Bernard of Clairvaux (1091–1153), the most profound thinker and writer of the Cistercians, drew certain conclusions for esthetics from this new direction of religious thought. Bernard distinguished between episcopal churches — located in cities and open to the masses of the faithful, in which grandeur of space, opulence of decoration, and richness and variety of images are justified by the need to arouse "corporalibus ornamentis ... devotio carnalis populi" ("popular devotion through material ornamentation") — and the abbey churches. In the latter, which serve only monks who have renounced the things of this world, any grandeur, sumptuousness, or opulence would be not only superfluous but deserving of censure. Rather to be striven for were the clearly blocked-out masses that Bernard himself was to see realized in the church of Fontenay, constructed under his guidance and supervised by his brother Gerard, which was to become the prototype of Cistercian churches.

Bernard found particularly reprehensible the teratological or fantastic representations and distortions dear to the Cluniacs and to Romanesque sculpture in general. In this respect also Bernard's esthetic polemics derive from his mystical and evangelical beliefs, which dwell not on fear, as with the Cluniacs, but on a love that strives for the union of the soul with God, anticipating ideas common to the Franciscan mysticism of a century later. The ideal of architectural purity that grew out of Cistercian mysticism contributed to an interest in rational and mathematical principles of construction. Bernard's mystique of love was in harmony with the Platonic philosophy that imbued early scholasticism, with which the origins of Gothic architecture are so closely connected.

The Christian esthetics that evolved during the course of the 12th century was related especially to the interpretation of Plato's Timaeus, which was considered an antecedent of Christian revelation. The cosmic order of creation, based on the ideas of the relation of unity and multiplicity, and of nature as intermediary between man and God, formed the foundation of the new philosophical and theological ideas reflected in the new esthetics. Thus in the construction of churches great importance was given to mathematical relations as an expression of the divine reason guiding the universe. Nor were new allegorical interpretations of basilican construction lacking, such as that found in the Gemma animae of Honorius of Autun (early 12th cent.).

These concepts based on number were accompanied by the revival and reelaboration of the Platonic concept of light as the image of divine power and love, which dates back to Scotus Erigena and Pseudo-Dionysius. The revival of this idea was responsible for the dominance of void over solid in the walls of Gothic cathedrals and for the predilection for storied windows — more allegorical than narrative — which were in a sense themselves created by light. Such are the philosophical ideas that underlay the construction of the Gothic cathedrals in France and then in the rest of Europe; the basilica of Saint-Denis, reconstructed (ca. 1140) by Abbot Suger, and the Cathedral of Chartres (1134–70) are among the earliest

to reflect these new speculative and esthetic trends. The theories on the relation of art and religious experience advanced in support of Gothic art were adopted in the 13th century by the new Franciscan and Dominican Orders.

Originally the Franciscan Order labored under interdictions not very different from those of the Cistercians, which St. Francis had formulated in the name of Holy Poverty in his testament dictated in 1226. However, the Order soon had to adapt itself to the taste prevailing in the social milieu in which it functioned. But in 1260 the *Constitutiones generales narbonenses* condemned "eccentricity in paintings, carved bas-reliefs, windows, columns." This condemnation was intended not to exclude representational art but to focus attention on its narrative character in accordance with the principles enunciated by St. Bonaventure, who explicitly returned to the words of St. John of Damascus: "An image represents its prototype." Among the Dominicans, analogous theories were held by St. Thomas Aquinas, who wrote, in accordance with Aristotelian epistemological premises, that an image is justified only if it is "similitudo alterius" ("the semblance of something other than itself").

RELIGION AND ART IN THE ITALIAN RENAISSANCE. A Thomist philosopher, Blessed Giovanni Dominici, was the first among the major exponents of 15th-century devotional practices. In his *Regole del governo di cura familiare* he deals explicitly with the didactic function of sacred images, asserting that these have a place not only in churches but also in private homes, where they may be particularly useful for the instruction of children. Such images must not be adorned with "ornaments of gold and silver," however, as such ornaments may encourage idolatry. Strongly influenced by Dominici, St. Antoninus Pierozzi, bishop of Florence, wrote that it is necessary to place images of the saints in the churches not in order to offer them worship but "to impress their virtue more effectively upon the minds of men; hence they are called the books of the uneducated."

A Dominican like Dominici and Pierozzi, Fra Angelico agreed with the formulations of these men. Furthermore, like Bernard of Clairvaux, he professed and put into practice standards for two kinds of artistic production. According to him, the desired characteristics in work intended for the laity were narrative, vivid color, and a lively feeling for nature; in works intended for religious they were greater austerity of form, attenuated color, and the introduction of symbol rather than narrative as an object for meditation.

Dominici aspired to direct the Renaissance passion for works of art, conceived as objects with which to embellish private habitations, to a religious purpose, and at the same time to sanction on a religious level the evolution in taste that was beginning to reject the use of gold in painting in order to emphasize the design — that is, the pure expression of an idea — as the basis of beauty. Angelico frequently used gold in paintings intended for ordinary worshipers, but he excluded it from those destined for monastic use, in which the intellectual content was paramount.

A more radical position, toward the end of the century, was that of another Dominican, Savonarola. He maintained that the Christian religion was irreconcilable with the artistic passion of the Renaissance, which he saw as a symptom of paganizing estheticism. At the carnival of 1497 — an occasion for ceremonies intended to give a devotional direction to the love of holidays encouraged by the Medicis, who were deeply committed to that estheticism — Savonarola inspired the burning of "many panels and canvases with precious although lascivious paintings, and casts and sculptures of not indifferent beauty . . . ," an eyewitness reported. In this deed perpetrated by the followers of Savonarola we glimpse the first warning of the iconoclastic furor that was to permeate the Protestant Reformation.

RELIGION AND ART IN THE REFORMATION AND COUNTER REFORMATION. Among the causes of the Reformation must be included hostility to the Italian Renaissance and its art (for which Luther showed appreciation, on esthetic grounds).

The celebration of nature and its beauties introduced by Renaissance art into Christian worship was an element incompatible with the concept of original sin so deeply entrenched in the Lutheran conscience. The Reformation responded also to a vividly felt need for religious purification, for contact of the soul with God directly, without the mediation of images that incline men to idolatry (see REFORMATION AND COUNTER REFORMATION).

The rejection of images was supported by Calvin in the most peremptory terms, for the problem impinged upon one of the fundamental tenets of the Reformation: the universal priesthood of the faithful, which denies the distinction between the learned, to whom the Word is directly accessible, and the unlearned (called by St. Bernard "the carnal populace"), who require the mediation of images.

However, the decisions taken by the Council of Trent on December 3, 1563, concerning the problem of images were sharply opposed to the Protestant formulations: "Further, with respect to representations of Christ, the Virgin Mother of God, and the other saints — representations most especially to be placed and kept in churches — the reverence shown to them is paid to the prototype that they body forth . . . . Moreover, bishops must seriously consider that by means of the running narrative of the mysteries of our redemption, told in paintings or through the other imitative arts, the people are instructed and strengthened in their remembrance and constant prayerful contemplation of the doctrines of their faith."

In sanctioning the use of images for didactic ends, it was the purpose of the Council of Trent to confirm, in opposition to one of the fundamental tenets of the Reformation, the distinction between a teaching body, the clergy, and those to be taught, the unsophisticated laity. The mission and the theoretical justification of the arts within the sphere of Roman Catholic Christianity after the Council of Trent are summed up in these two functions: narration through images whose significance lies in the events depicted, and instruction in the articles of faith through images whose meaning lies outside themselves.

The problems posed by the Counter Reformation with regard to images also arose with regard to architecture, in which the question became that of changing church architecture to reflect visibly the division between clergy and laity. Even central-plan construction proved to be in opposition to the spirit of the Counter Reformation, in that it tended to attenuate if not to abolish the visible separation of clergy and laity and to suggest the direct presence of God without the mediation of the Church, thus potentially opening the way for the penetration of Protestantism. It was with good reason, then, that St. Charles Borromeo, archbishop of Milan, advised against the use of central-plan construction. The adoption of a longitudinal plan for the basilica of St. Peter's (1605) aptly confirmed a sanction from which the Church was subsequently to depart only occasionally.

The longitudinal plan not only served to separate clergy and laity but also satisfied the needs of preaching and of liturgical ceremony by favoring the oratorical and theatrical character introduced into church architecture in the 17th century, in part because of the impetus provided by the Society of Jesus. In the *Spiritual Exercises* of St. Ignatius of Loyola, imagination is assigned a decisive task: "To imagine Christ our Lord suffering upon the cross. . . . To see with the eye of the imagination the length, breadth, and depth of hell . . . the great fires and the souls as though with bodies aflame . . . . [To contemplate with the imagination] how the three Persons of the Trinity watched over the whole expanse or circumference of the world filled with men, and how, when it was seen that all were going to hell, it was determined that the Second Person should become man. . . . To see Our Lady and the angel who greets her, and to kneel down and derive benefit from this vision . . . ." Related to this is the precept: "Praise church ornaments and buildings; likewise images, and venerate them for what they represent," to combat the devil.

On the basis of these ideas the Jesuits accepted the esthetic ideal of the baroque and drew on its stylistic repertory to

represent, in painting, sculpture, and architecture, the war against the devil and his temptations, the triumph of faith, and the glory of the Church Triumphant. They intensified the luxurious and fantastic character of baroque art, favored by the absolute monarchs and the court aristocracies, employing it as the instrument best adapted to their aim of controlling and directing the ruling classes on the spiritual plane and, at the same time, attracting the masses through art.

The esthetic program adopted by the Society of Jesus proved effective, as a useful instrument with which to oppose the austerity of Protestantism and its appeal to inwardness, not only in that part of Europe which had remained Catholic but also on other continents, where it served the ends of the propagation of Christianity, to which the Jesuits dedicated themselves with all the intensity of their zeal and the resources of their powerful organization. The suggestive power of baroque images and architecture was in fact one of the instruments on which the missions, particularly the Jesuit missions operating in India, China, Japan, and the countries of Spanish America, relied to lead peoples away from paganism. It enabled them to make use of and to redirect both the psychological residuum of the traditions of idolatry and the local artistic traditions; the latter were frequently absorbed and assimilated by a process similar to that which took place spontaneously during the first centuries of Christianity with regard to the artistic traditions of Hellenism, Rome, and the Nordic peoples.

The Tridentine and post-Tridentine statutes, in the meantime, gave birth to the concept of "sacred art," which later became defined in Catholic theories and practices.

RECENT CONCEPTS OF "SACRED ART" AND "CHRISTIAN ART." The concept of "sacred art" held by the Catholic Church in recent times was based on the Tridentine principles of a return *ad prototypa*, to historical and allegorical didacticism, and to the exclusion of anything which might seem *profanum*, *inhonestum*, or even "unusual." Fidelity to these principles resulted in extreme caution on the part of the clergy toward representational and architectural innovations, as well as in insistence on the accepted forms in sacred images and religious architecture; it led to building in "historical styles" and to the broad use of mass-produced images in which sentimental significance prevails over esthetic quality. Some of the more recent devotional subjects, such as the Heart of Jesus, the Heart of Mary, the Madonna of Lourdes, have inspired iconographic formulas among the most popular in this standardized production. Here the difficult problem presents itself of the relation between Christian-Catholic religious experience and the traditions of modern art, which arose from principles foreign to it — if not foreign to religious experience in its generic and primitive sense, at least foreign to that type of religious experience lived within the Catholic Church. The esthetic conservatism of the Catholic Church was entirely comprehensible, as was its perplexity when confronted with the many concepts of "Christian art" formulated, from the romantic period onward, in the sphere of modern thought.

For the romantics, "Christian art" represented the antithesis of the coldness of neoclassicism against which they were struggling; it was more dramatic and more spiritual than classicizing art. Thus Chateaubriand lauded the innovations that Christianity introduced in architecture, but his vindication of Christianity as an artistic principle was also a polemic against 18th-century rationalism. Friedrich von Schlegel identified the artistic spirit of Christianity with feeling for color, which expresses the drama of the human condition. He defined painting as the Christian art par excellence, sculpture, with its purity and serenity, as the art of ancient paganism; and he exhorted the painters of his time to place their trust in Christian feeling.

For Ruskin Christian art was the authentic work of the spirit, aided according to its needs by all the lesser faculties. This esthetic concept had a polemic value in Ruskin's protest against the inheritance of the Renaissance and in his support of 19th-century Pre-Raphaelitism (see PRE-RAPHAELITISM AND RELATED MOVEMENTS) as an authentic revival of Christian art.

At the beginning of the 20th century the concept of Christian art made its appearance in the writings and militant criticism of French Catholic writers such as J. K. Huysmans and Léon Bloy. Also in France the theoretical and critical work of philosophers such as Jacques Maritain and of some religious, particularly of the Dominican Order, bear witness to a process of revision of the post-Tridentine conception of "sacred art," whose object is the admission of the creative experience of modern art into the Christian tradition.

Rosario ASSUNTO

MODERN CHRISTIAN ART. Although Christian art during the latter part of the 19th century labored under the combined disadvantage of a lack of church leadership, such as had been given during an earlier period by the Council of Trent, and the general academic situation of the arts, certain signs already pointed in a new direction. Shortly after the middle of the 19th century, in fact, a religious revival in Germany sparked by the Benedectine Order at the abbeys of Maria Laach and Beuron laid the groundwork for a movement combining Catholic theology and art, whose effects are still evident today.

In the last quarter of the 19th century various symbolist artists turned to Christianity as a source of inspiration in the Pont-Aven school led by Paul Gauguin, and such painters as Maurice Denis and Paul Sérusier produced an art filled with a strong mysticoreligious feeling. Their relatively two-dimensional formalism contrasts with the more rounded expressiveness of the work of Georges Desvallières. Already at this point the Church had begun to use serious contemporary artists such as Denis and, later, Georges Rouault (q.v.) for mural work. Symbolistically inclined artists of the late 19th and 20th centuries had recourse to Christian themes as a source for personal inspiration and expression. These works as a whole must be considered apart from art specifically designed for church use; yet there is no question that the whole range of modern art was enriched by this new interest. Thus one finds modern painters such as André Bauchant, Georges Rouault, Karl Schmidt-Rottluff, Emil Nolde, and Rico Lebrun making effective use of Christian themes apart from ecclesiastical needs. This distinction between a personal art derived from Christian inspiration and an officially sponsored Christian art is underlined by the fact that prominent Jewish artists have also dealt with this material, e.g., Marc Chagall (q.v.), Jacques Lipchitz (q.v.), and Abraham Rattner (I, PL. 124).

The important fact is that during the first half of the 20th century more and more modern artists turned to Christian art, just as the Church turned increasingly to contemporary artists. One effect of this revival, especially in the period after World War II, was the creation of a host of Catholic and Protestant churches in all parts of the world designed by outstanding architects. The figural arts (e.g., murals, stained glass, and sculpture), too, played a role in this revival, although perhaps to a lesser extent.

The revival in church architecture was apparent immediately after World War I in northern Europe, primarily in Germany and Scandinavia; after World War II the creative center shifted to the United States and France. Much of the new Christian art is Catholic, but there are also more Protestant examples than is generally realized.

The attitude of the Catholic Church toward modern art is indicated in two documents. The *Instructio de arte sacra*, issued in 1952 by the Supreme Congregation of the Holy Office, summarizes existing laws and gives general directions on the building of churches and their ornamentation but does not attempt to set styles. The encyclical *Mediator Dei* (1947) of Pope Pius XII says, "Modern pictures and statues, whose style is more adapted to the materials in use at the present day, are not to be condemned out of hand. On condition that these modern arts steer a middle course between an excessive realism on the one hand and an exaggerated symbolism on the other, and take into account more the needs of the Christian community than the personal taste and judgment of the artist, they should be allowed full scope if with due reverence and

honour they put themselves at the service of our churches and sacred rites." However individuals may interpret these statements, it is evident that the face of Catholic Christian art has changed radically in the 20th century.

Among the outstanding examples of art in Catholic churches are Notre-Dame du Raincy (1923; I, PL. 305) by Auguste Perret, a pioneer structure in which Gothic spatial ideas are preserved with prefabricated wall sections in concrete and glass; the Church of Stella Maris in Norderney, Germany (1930), by Dominikus Böhm, with its altar painting by Richard Seewald; St. Francis at Pampulha, Brazil (1943), by Oscar Niemeyer, with its magnificent concrete parabolic shells and its mural and mosaic decorations by Cándido Portinari; the world-famous Dominican convent chapel at Vence (1951), by Henri Matisse, with its wall decorations, sculptured altar, church furniture, and even vestments; Notre-Dame-du-Haut at Ronchamp (1955; I, PL. 381), built in free-form concrete by Le Corbusier; and the Benedictine Abbey of St. John at Collegeville, Minn., a long-term project by Marcel Breuer, still under construction.

Protestant architecture differs from that of the Catholic world in that emphasis is placed on the Word of God rather than on His personal presence. The minister, therefore, represents not God, as in the Catholic Church, but the congregation. Since preaching is the vital thing in Protestant churches, the Catholic differentiation between the altar zone and the nave proper is no longer needed. Generally speaking, therefore, the idea of a single room is dominant in such buildings.

Protestant churches are exemplified by Frank Lloyd Wright's Unity Church at Oak Park, Ill. (1906; I, PL. 91), a pioneer modern structure in its continuous spatial composition; the glass and steel church at Essen, Germany (1928), by Otto Bartning; the Reformed Church in Altstetten, outside Zurich (1938), by Werner M. Moser; Christ Lutheran Church in Minneapolis (1949; I, PL. 95), by Eliel Saarinen; the Unitarian church in Madison, Wis. (1950), by Frank Lloyd Wright; the University Chapel in Chicago (1952), by Mies van der Rohe; Alvar Aalto's church in Imatra, Finland (1958; V, PL. 118); and Harrison and Abramowitz's First Presbyterian Church in Stamford, Conn. (1958).

The figural arts are, by definition, more appropriate to Catholic than to Protestant worship. Many Protestant sects, however, have permitted and encouraged the use of abstract murals, stained glass, sculpture, and the like.

Among important religious sculptures are Henry Moore's *Madonna* in the church at Claydon, Suffolk (1949); Ewald Mataré's *Man of Sorrows* in the crypt of the hospital church at Köln-Hohenlind, Germany (1950); and Jacob Epstein's *Madonna* over the entrance to the Convent of the Holy Child in London (1951). Outstanding among church paintings are the Crucifixion mural at St. Matthew's Church, Northampton, Mass., by Graham Sutherland; and the fresco at the University of Notre Dame, South Bend, Ind. (1955), by Jean Charlot.

Many modern artists have designed stained-glass windows for churches, among them the painters Jan Thorn-Prikker and Fernand Léger, and the sculptor Ewald Mataré. Church tapestry includes the fine example on the altar of the church at Assy (1947), by Jean Lurçat.

Church vessels and altar furniture represent an important area of Christian artistic effort. If we contrast the so-called "St. Sulpice" style of commercialized and uninspired liturgical art with that produced or sponsored by more recent and more contemporaneously oriented organizations, the distance that church art has traveled since the 19th century is at once apparent. Organizations such as the American Liturgical Arts Society or the Swiss St. Luke's Society are among the most outstanding. Fine examples of modern church vessels are found throughout the Christian world. Enamel, silver, and gems are combined to produce simple shapes and highly abstract but symbolically meaningful decorations. Among other altar furnishings are the Matisse enamel tabernacle at Vence (1951) and Karl Schrage's silver tabernacle in the Church of the Holy Cross at Bottrop (1957).

That Christianity has found it possible to utilize modern art and architecture is due in part to the essential simplicity and austerity of the architecture itself and to the symbolical rendition of a great deal of modern painting and sculpture, which makes it congenial to both Catholic and Protestant. Henze (1956) quotes Cardinal Costantini (the Church's authority on Christian art and the organizer of the 1950 Holy Year Exhibition) as stressing "the truth that the great masters have always been the supreme representatives of their own time."

Bernard S. MYERS

BIBLIOG. J. Pichard, L'art sacré moderne, Paris, 1953; Arte Liturgica in Germania, Rome, 1956; A. Heuze and T. Filthaut, Contemporary Church Art, New York, 1956; E. D. Mills, The Modern Church, London, 1956; A. Henze, Neue kirchliche Kunst, Recklinghausen, 1958; W. Weyres, Kirchen, Handbuch für den Kirchenbau, Munich, 1956; R. Gieselmann and W. Aebli, Kirchenbau, Zurich, 1960.

CHRISTIANITY AND ICONOGRAPHY. Besides exerting a profound influence on the very conception of the arts, on critical judgment (see CRITICISM), and on the function assigned to art (see EDUCATION AND ART TEACHING; TREATISES), Christianity has also created a vast iconographic system, linked not only to sacred history (see BIBLICAL SUBJECTS) but also to the necessity of representing new subjects related to its doctrine, to the demand for new forms for existing religious and political concepts, and to the pressure of popular and devotional demands (see DEVOTIONAL OBJECTS AND IMAGES).

Until well into the 15th century, European art was invested with a prevailingly religious function. Thus its products were dedicated — at first exclusively, and from the late Gothic period onward, principally — to public or private worship. It was only with subsequent differentiation of things sacred and profane, which had reached an advanced stage by the 18th century, after the introduction of curious forms of allegorical and symbolic corruption in the baroque age, that religious art became distinct from and frequently irreconcilable with profane art with regard to subject matter and even style (see GENRE AND SECULAR SUBJECTS).

It is not surprising that the production of over one and a half millenniums should be accompanied by an extreme complexity of iconographic themes; these in turn, notwithstanding the persistence and traditionalism of religious imagery (see TRADITION), have a history full of interest and rich in unforeseen elements.

*Christ.* The fundamental problem confronted by Christian art was the representation of the deity (see DIVINITIES). As F. Michaeli observes (*Dieu à l'image de l'homme*, Neuchâtel, Paris, 1950, p. 135), the anthropomorphism of the Old Testament never completely humanizes Jehovah, even when he is described in specifically human terms. One must recognize this in order to understand the repugnance of Judaism to images which are potentially objects of worship. With the advent of Christ, however, a new factor was introduced which was compatible with anthropomorphism. The God of Israel came down to man, became man, the servant of mankind. But the limitations of human nature did not diminish His sanctity "which appears to us in the fullness of an actual living fact, and no longer in the customary language." The Son of God who descended among men was equal to the Father and was His living image. This process of humanization, this kenosis ("emptying of himself"), of divinity provided a legitimate opportunity for its representation.

But how could the divine be represented in the absence of elements which Judaic culture, by reason of its principles, could not transmit? It was necessary to turn to the conventions suggested by the Hellenistic world, all the more so as no authentic portraits existed. We may assume that the "Edessa portrait," which, according to legend, was miraculously made for Abgar, king of Osroene (179–216), represented the bearded, long-haired type generally believed to be of Eastern origin. St. John of Damascus, in the 8th century, was acquainted with a version of the legend of Abgar and the portrait, and he states that the emperor Constantine (306–37) had commissioned the reproduction in paintings and mosaics of the human visage of Christ, which St. John describes as having beautiful eyes,

joined eyebrows, a long nose, curly hair, a black beard, and a youthful appearance ("Epistola ad Theophilum," Migne, *Patrologia Graeca*, III). In the late 7th century the same characteristics were described by Andrew of Crete (ca. 660–740; J. F. Boissonade, *Anecdota graeca*, IV, Paris, 1829–33, p. 473). A number of other representations from the 6th to the 8th century reproduce this type. But we can trace it back even further, to the ampullas of Monza, Italy, which were brought from Palestine in the 6th century and which reflect compositions on monuments in that country, some of which must have dated back to the age of Constantine. This would tend to confirm St. John's report of the Constantinian use of the type.

The physical type adopted in representations of the human aspect of Christ can be correlated, then, with the legend of the "Edessa portrait," and we can postulate a probable Edessan origin for the "Eastern" type.

The existence of images of Christ from at least the 3d century onward is not surprising. According to Lampridius, an author of the 4th century, the Roman emperor Alexander Severus (222–35) placed an image of Jesus, as well as of Abraham and Orpheus, with his *lares*. We know with certainty from Eusebius (260?–340?; *Historia ecclesiastica*, VII, 18) that early in the 4th century painted icons of the apostles Peter and Paul as well as of Christ Himself were already widespread. It seems that these icons circulated even among the pagans, for whom they had an esoteric value. Eusebius also mentions a bronze group (perhaps a relief) that he saw at Paneas (Caesarea Philippi), which was said to commemorate the healing of the woman with the issue of blood. It represented a kneeling woman stretching her hands toward a standing man wrapped in a mantle, who in turn reached out toward her. The group was probably a pagan work, relating perhaps to the submission of a province or to a miracle of Aesculapius; but it is remarkable that as early as the beginning of the 4th century there existed among the Christians of Paneas an interpretation of the episode as the healing of the woman with the issue of blood. If it is true that the relief on a Christian sarcophagus of the 4th century (Lateran Mus.) is related to this iconographic type (J. Wilpert, *I sarcofagi cristiani antichi*, Rome, 1929–36), then we have further testimony concerning this representation of Christ, because here we see the Saviour erect, long-haired, bearded, in the very posture described for the statue of Paneas (PL. 304).

The "Edessa portrait" was supposedly preserved unscathed in that city through all the invasions and then transferred, after 944, to Constantinople, where it became known as the "holy mandilion" and was kept in the Chapel of the Virgin in the imperial Bucoleon Palace. It was said to have been stolen at the time of the Latin conquest of Constantinople in the Fourth Crusade (1204) and to have been sold by the emperor Baldwin II, together with other holy relics, to Louis IX of France in 1247. We know that an image, perhaps a copy of the "Edessa portrait," appeared in Genoa in the 14th century; it was a gift of Leonardo Montalto, who had received it from the Byzantine emperor John V. This is the image still preserved (beneath a rich silver cover) in S. Bartolomeo degli Armeni in Genoa; it may represent a face with a tripartite beard, like that on the so-called "Veronica's Veil" in St. Peter's.

To be grouped with the mandilion as a work in the Edessan tradition is the beautiful *Holy Face* of Laon (France), a Slavic or Slavo-Byzantine painting probably executed in the 12th century. Despite the Slavic inscription, it is thought to be of Roman provenance. Again it is a head with long, slightly wavy hair and a long beard of loose locks. The *Holy Face* recalls the description — said to have been addressed to the Roman Senate by one Lentulus, Governor of Judaea — in a Latin apocryph of the 13th century, which, however, probably depends on earlier Eastern sources. According to this description, Jesus was a little over medium height, with a face that inspired love and awe. He had nut-brown hair, rough and slightly curly, which flowed over His shoulders, and an abundant beard divided in two beneath the chin.

Another venerated image transferred to Constantinople was that of Kamuliana. This image from Cappadocia, which came to be considered a sort of guardian of Byzantium, disappeared during the iconoclastic struggles. We cannot be certain about its type; however, since Byzantine art was consistent in representing an austere face with long wavy hair and beard, it probably did not differ significantly from this ideal, which was also common in Eastern miniatures, such as the Rossano and Sinope codices (both of the 6th cent.). A unique Syrian variant, which represents Christ wearing a calotte and with thick, dark hair that does not reach the shoulders and a short beard, appears in the Syriac Gospel in the Laurentian Library in Florence (second half of 6th cent.) and in a miniature of Diyarbekir (6th cent.; Leroy, *CahA*, IX, 1957, p. 125).

What model inspired the type called "Edessan"? First of all, it draws upon the type of the teacher, i.e., the rabbi, which was widespread in the East. The Greeks were able to merge this type with their type of the philosopher, who was draped sometimes in a pallium, sometimes in an exomis, which left one shoulder uncovered, revealing the tunic beneath (in the case of the Cynics, leaving the bare shoulder exposed). It should be noted, in this connection, that Gerke (1948) has devoted a chapter to Christ the Philosopher. In the frescoes of the early 3d century in the Hypogeum of the Aurelii on the Viale Manzoni in Rome there is a shepherd Christ in the attitude of the teacher, wearing a pallium (PL. 305). This is the first appearance of the Western bearded type, and it almost certainly is of Eastern derivation.

Another Roman example, but of the late 3d century, is found in the sculpture on a fragmentary sarcophagus in the Museo Nazionale in Rome (the scene is the Sermon on the Mount). Here Jesus wears a pallium that leaves His shoulder and breast uncovered. His face is that of an old man; His curly hair does not quite reach the shoulders, and His short beard is divided at the chin. This is an unusual example, recalling, it seems to the author, less the philosopher than "Jupiter summus exsuperantissimus." In order to convey the quality of supreme divinity, the sculptor reverted to the Jovian type. The eyes, wide open and fixed, call to mind the hurler of thunderbolts. This example, unique in the period, seems to be the remote antecedent of the Christ Pantokrator ("omnipotent") of Byzantine art. An intermediary link can be recognized in the superb Christ in the apsidal mosaic in SS. Cosmo e Damiano (PL. 305; 6th cent.) in the Roman Forum. In the final analysis, even the Christ of the ampullas of Monza (and of the apse of St. John Lateran, in the mosaic reproduced from the antique original in the late 13th century by Jacopo Torriti) is a Pantokrator. This visage may well express that of the invisible Father, "the Ancient of Days" (Jesus said: "And he that seeth me seeth him that sent me"; John 12:45). Certain Byzantine authors (perhaps the earliest is Theodore Lector, in the 6th century, cited by St. John of Damascus, "Oratio III de imaginibus," Migne, *Patrologia Graeca*, XCIV, col. 1413) record the story of that painter of the 5th century in Constantinople who, perhaps in order to please some pagan, represented Christ in the image of Jupiter. But he was punished by God, and his hands withered away.

This solemn figure of Christ could well be transformed into the image of a sovereign — into the image of Christ the King, which was current particularly in the Theodosian age (379–95) — with neither regal vestments nor crown (these appear only from the late Middle Ages onward). On a sarcophagus of the 4th century in the Lateran Museums there is a representation of Christ before Pilate. Behind Christ stands a soldier who holds a crown raised over Christ's head. This is an allusion to triumph through the Passion, for Jesus, through His suffering, "conquered the world." Representations of Christ in Majesty (Maiestas Domini) in the Theodosian age and later show Christ either enthroned or standing among the apostles and other saints — who could be described as his courtiers — or occasionally among the archangels, who take their place as the *custodes divini lateris* ("guardians of the divine flank") of the sovereign.

The Christ in the apse of S. Paolo fuori le Mura in Rome is enthroned among three apostles and St. Luke; this is a work of the period of Honorius III (1216–27) and Gregory IX (1227–44), but it must substantially reproduce the design of

the earlier Theodosian mosaic. Christ is represented on a throne in the panel painting "made without human hands" (*acheiropoietos*) in the Sancta Sanctorum in Rome, a work which can justly be attributed to the 5th century (only fragments of the original remain; Cecchelli, 1956). The Saviour supports the book of the Law with his left hand, resting it on his knee. The gesture of the right hand indicates speech (the folding of the fingers has been erroneously interpreted as a gesture of benediction). Thus we are made to perceive the attribute of God as the Word (the Logos of the prologue of the Gospel according to St. John), which is embodied in Christ. A fine example is the standing Christ in the mosaic of the Confession (9th cent.) in St. Peter's in the Vatican, where on the book is written "Ego sum via, veritas et vita. Qui credit in me vivet" from the Gospel according to St. John ("I am the way, the truth, and the life," 14:6; "He that believeth in me . . . yet shall he live," 11:25). In a panel of an ivory diptych in the Staatliche Museen in Berlin (Gerke, 1948, pl. 100), the seated Christ (Logos) holds the book closed and has the face of an old man; Peter and Paul stand at either side of him (this work is thought to be of the first half of the 6th century but may date from the second half of the 5th century). Enthroned, Christ is the teacher par excellence. As sovereign He gives the law to His followers so that they may apply it. Thus in scenes of the Traditio Legis (Delivery of the New Law), Christ, flanked by the apostles Peter and Paul, gives the law to Peter, who is invested as the head of the Church (the early-5th-century sarcophagus in the Museo Nazionale of Ravenna is an example; PL. 304). Christ ideally placed in a royal palace that represents the Heavenly Jerusalem is the "King of Kings, and Lord of Lords" (Rev. 19:16).

The Christ Pantokrator appears (with clipeus and emanating sun rays) at the apex of the triumphal arch of Galla Placidia in S. Paolo fuori le Mura (mid-5th cent.). Here Christ is a true *rex tremendae maiestatis* ("king of awesome majesty"). He is shown being acclaimed by the elders, and the whole scene is apocalyptic in inspiration. We may note that while the usual bearded Christ suggests primarily the idea of the Logos, the divine teacher and bearer of the Word of the Father, the aged bearded type emphasizes the similarity to the Father.

Another type of Christ, youthful and beardless, is frequently seen in representations of the Good Shepherd, i.e., Christ carrying the lamb on his shoulders (inspired by the famous parable in Luke 15:3). Occasionally, as in the 3d–4th-century sarcophagus in the Lateran Museums (which actually may not be Christian), the Good Shepherd is shown as an old man.

The image of the youthful Christ, so frequently seen in Early Christian art, is inspired by the Hellenic ideal of the god who is beautiful and good (kalokagathia), which found its most charateristic expression in Apollo. He is the sun god who could be linked with, and at the same time contrasted to, Christ *lux mundi* ("light of the world") and who later, in the solar religion of the pagans, was proclaimed *Sol novus noster* ("our new Sun"). In the apocryphal Acts of the Apostles, which date back as far as the 2d century, apparitions of Christ in youthful form are mentioned, but these references are really to a young boy ("Acta Andreae et Matthiae," 33, in R. A. Lipsius and M. Bonnet, *Acta apostolorum apocrypha*, Leipzig, 1819–93, II, 115, no. 6; etc.). The fact that these documents are influenced by gnosticism indicates that the type of the youthful Christ may have had its roots in gnostic circles, where the ideas of the Greek world remained particularly vigorous. Appealing as this theory is, there seems to be more evidence for the relation to Apollo, particularly in the 3d century, when the solar cult took hold ever more strongly, even officially, as the unifier of the religions of the empire.

The youthful type incorporates the idea of the "young god" (*neos theos*), which was also applied to the emperors to emphasize their divine nature. The deified hero is also frequently represented as youthful. In the Hellenistic romance *The Adventures of Chaereas and Callirrhoë* (6th cent. ?), where the idea of beauty is related to virgin birth, it is said that "the beautiful are the children of the gods." Thus we

can find the true explanation for the representation of a youthful Christ in the adoption of forms in use in the Greco-Roman world to represent Apollo.

The ancient controversy over the relative beauty or ugliness of the human features of Christ should be mentioned here. Among the Church Fathers, beginning in the 2d century (St. Justin Martyr, St. Irenaeus, Tertullian, etc.), some favored the idea of physical beauty, while others rejected it. But it is clear that each opinion originated not in a portrait tradition but in a conceptual premise: the *forma Dei* ("form of God") or the *forma servi* ("form of the servant"), the latter being humble and subject to suffering, in contrast to the former. It is hardly necessary to remark that the concept of the physical unattractiveness of Christ has never taken hold among the Christian masses (Jerphanion, 1938, p. 7).

There is an image of Christ in the painting of the raising of Lazarus in the so-called "Greek Chapel" in the Catacomb of Priscilla, which has been thought to be the earliest representation of Christ; it is of the youthful type (P. Styger, *Die altchristliche Grabeskunst*, Munich, 1927, attributes it to the mid-2d cent.). In the present state of our knowledge, it would be imprudent to state whether the bearded or the unbearded type is of greater antiquity (the Edessan tradition, which argues for the former, is also very old). A well-known statuette of about the mid-4th century (or perhaps a little earlier) in the Museo Nazionale in Rome represents a very beautiful Christ of youthful aspect. He is seated on a throne and wears a tunic and pallium; He is the Son of God and the Word of God, and He is perhaps represented in the act of teaching. In a remarkable painting of the 3d century in the Catacomb of the Jordani on the Via Salaria in Rome, the apostolic council is represented on either side of an image of Christ as teacher. About a century later this theme was revived in a mosaic in the apse of S. Aquilino in San Lorenzo near Milan. In both cases Christ has a youthful appearance; in S. Aquilino the head of Christ is shown with a nimbus within which appear His monogram (chrismon) and the alpha and omega. In Early Christian art the figure of Christ was the first to be represented with the nimbus (perhaps no earlier than the 4th cent.). Later the Cross was treated in the same way, the rays becoming thicker and more brilliantly colored and sometimes jeweled.

In the 6th century the basilica of S. Michele in Affricisco in Ravenna had an apsidal mosaic (now very much restored; Berlin, Staat. Mus.) in which a youthful Christ flanked by two angels proudly bears aloft a cross and holds an open book. However, there is a bearded Christ enthroned in glory in the upper arch. Also in Ravenna, a youthful warrior-Christ (late 5th–early 6th cent.; only the upper part is original) may be seen in a chapel of the Archiepiscopal Palace. The image of Christ standing on the globe of the earth among the archangels in the apsidal *Maiestas Domini* of S. Vitale in Ravenna (6th cent.) is also of the youthful type. Finally, this category includes the striking youthful Christ enthroned on the Berlin pyxis (4th–5th cent.; Gerke, 1948, pl. 89).

The youthful beardless Christ reappeared in the 9th and 10th centuries in Carolingian and Ottonian representations; thereafter it was completely superseded by the bearded type. In Romanesque and Gothic representations Christ is almost always bearded. The Gothic period, as Jerphanion observed (1938), made of Christ an ideal type, conceiving him as the supreme doctor of the new law (for instance, the south portal of the Cathedral of Chartres), while the Romanesque period, in the frequent treatments of the Maiestas Domini, often represented him as the solemn judge, a theme that continued to appear in successive epochs (PL. 306). Baumstark has tried to identify the parallels of these compositions in Eastern art, beginning in the Carolingian period, and Berger has studied representations of Christ enthroned in Romanesque art.

Pathos was introduced into art in the 14th and 15th centuries. The head of Jesus painted by Bartolomé Bermejo (15th cent., Mus. of Vich, Spain) is a tragic image of a suffering Christ with the crown of thorns. The dead Christ was also frequently represented: the 15th-century head in the Musée de l'Oise at Beauvais is a striking example.

The Crucifixion, which will be treated here only briefly, appeared for the first time in the period of Sixtus III (432–40) on the wooden door of S. Sabina in Rome. The Christ of S. Sabina is nude except for a loincloth (*subligaculum*). Of approximately the same period is the noted ivory with leaves representing the Carrying of the Cross, the Crucifixion, and the Doubting of Thomas (London, Br. Mus.). Both at S. Sabina and in the latter work Christ is represented with long hair and beard: in the ivory, the beard is barely distinguishable, but on the first leaf, representing the Carrying of the Cross, the youthful type appears unmistakably (as well as on the leaf representing the Doubting of Thomas). The explanation of this curious alternation of types, which also occurred later in the Christological panels in the basilica of S. Apollinare Nuovo at Ravenna, is to be sought in some theological concept which we can now no longer identify, rather than in the influence of diverse prototypes.

In Byzantine art the Crucifixion is relatively rare. The famous miniature in the Syriac Gospel of the Laurentian Library (second half of 6th cent.) was conceived within the environment of Oriental monasticism. The bearded Christ is again shown with the loincloth. This representation is truly dramatic. The accentuation of the pathetic can perhaps be ascribed to a desire to emphasize the suffering of the Passion of Christ, in opposition to the Monophysite heresy which attributed to Christ a single purely divine nature not subject to suffering.

The rendering of the sacrifice of Christ in the apse of St. John Lateran (Torriti's late-13th-century version of an earlier iconographic scheme which may date from the age of Constantine) is in fact an exaltation of the triumph of Jesus ascendant over the Cross, which is both the symbol of His victory and the "sign of salvation." Representations of this kind, with the *crux florida* and the bust of Christ appearing in the sky above, are also seen on the ampullas of Monza. In the Early Christian period attention was focused more on the Cross as a symbol of salvation than on the actual suffering of the crucified Christ.

Until now we have deliberately overlooked both the scenes which narrate the events in the life of Christ and the theme of the Christ Child, which is traditionally related to the stories of the *infantia Salvatoris* ("childhood of the Saviour"; see the magnificent example on the triumphal arch of S. Maria Maggiore in Rome, 432–40). Attention should be drawn to a late icon formerly at Mount Athos (later in the Tretyakov Gallery in Moscow) representing the Christ Child asleep with eyes open (Jerphanion, 1938, pl. 6). According to Jerphanion, this is an interpretation of the sleep of the Lion of Judah (a symbol of Christ), alluding to the legend according to which the lion sleeps with its eyes open. In Byzantine and Slavic art Christ as Immanuel is frequently represented asleep on the paten, as a Eucharistic image. A subject peculiar to modern devotional art is the Sacred Heart of Jesus, inspired by the visions (ca. 1674) of the French nun St. Margaret Mary Alacoque. The theme soon became widespread after its first noted appearance in a painting (ca. 1780) by Pompeo Girolamo Batoni executed for the queen of Portugal (PL. 307). In His left hand Christ holds a flaming heart from which a great light emanates; with His right hand He makes a gesture of invitation to confide in His mercy. He has a youthful face of great beauty, long hair, and a short beard.

Carlo CECCHELLI

*Symbols of Christ.* Christian art was not limited to the representation of the human appearance of Christ. Particularly during the first centuries of the Church and during the entire medieval period, there was frequent recourse to representations of a symbolic character, derived chiefly from the Bible.

One of the most common symbols is the lamb, which appears either alone or with the Cross or the monogram of Christ or with the symbols of the Evangelists or the apostles (also represented as lambs). The lamb is often represented on the mountain of Paradise from which flow the four rivers, or else ensconced on the holy throne in preparation for the Last Judgment (Hetimasia); until the 56th synod (692) it was also repre-

sented on the Cross. Another symbol is the fish, which is sometimes represented together with the Eucharistic bread. The lion, the pelican, the griffin, and the phoenix (PL. 303) are also intermittently used to indicate the Messiah. But perhaps the Messianic emblem most characteristic of Early Christian iconography is the holy monogram (chrismon) made by crossing the first two letters of the Greek word "Christos" (XP), which adorned the labara, or standards of the army of Constantine, at Ponte Milvio (313). It is frequently represented together with the apocalyptic letters α and ω; these letters often hang from the arms of the Cross, which was the only representation of Christ permitted in the Byzantine world during the iconoclastic period. Sometimes the Cross is represented with the monogram of Christ; in other examples, grapevines or acanthus spirals grow out of the trunk of the Cross to indicate the Mystical Body of Christ.

*The crucifix.* Beginning in the Ottonian period (10th–11th cent.) representations of Christ on the Cross, both painted and sculptured, became increasingly frequent. The attitude of Christ varies in different periods: the Christus Triumphans is represented with eyes open, feet parallel and transfixed by nails, and a regal crown; the Christus Patiens (PL. 306), with head bent; the Christus Doloroso, with the crown of thorns and the tangible signs of the Passion — the diaphragm contracted with pain, the legs contorted, and the feet superimposed. This last attitude was particularly common in the Gothic period. The crucifix is often accompanied by the figures of St. John and the Virgin.

*Christological groups.* In the course of the 13th century great sculptured representations of the Deposition were produced in central Italy and the south of Spain. The use of devotional images flowered in the 14th century: the most notable are the Pietà (the dead Christ in the lap of the Virgin), the Ecce Homo and the Christ at the Pillar, the Lamentation, and, particularly in painting, Christ with the symbols of the Passion. There was a proliferation of new iconographic themes, many of which were bound up with the figure of the Christ Child. Thus we find the Holy Family, with the Virgin and St. Joseph, and St. Anne and the Virgin (a group known as "Anna Meterza" or "Anna Selbdritt"). Certain paintings include all the relatives of Christ. Frequently St. John the Baptist accompanies the Christ Child. From the 11th century on, a theme favored by the Nordic peoples was the Tree of Jesse (Isa. 11:1-2): from the body of the sleeping Abraham grow thick branches, and at the top, like a corolla, appear Christ and the Virgin. From earliest times the Redeemer was represented together with the apostles, for the most part in group scenes such as the Last Supper, the Agony in the Garden, the Ascension, and, in Greek churches, the Communion of the Apostles, but also with individual apostles, shown with hagiographical attributes. In the late Middle Ages we find many images of devotees, particularly on the fronts of sarcophagi, and later, on altarpieces, the donor often appears at the feet of Christ and the Virgin.

*The Virgin.* One of the subjects most frequently treated in Christian art is the Virgin, whose divine maternity was defined as dogma at the First Nicene Council in 325. It is true that the first images of Mary were in a sense subordinated to those of the Son. In fact, she always appeared with the Christ Child in her arms, as in the earliest examples preserved in the catacombs (Catacomb of Priscilla, Rome; ca. mid-3d cent.), which perhaps developed from representations of Isis with her son at her breast. And she frequently dominates the apse in her role as Theotokos, in accordance with a purely theological conception. The Byzantine world created several distinct types of images of the Virgin (PL. 308): the Panagia Nikopoia, the Virgin enthroned with the Child seated on her knees; the Hodegetria ("she who points the way"), the Virgin standing and holding the Child in her left arm; the Blacherniotissa, the Virgin Orans with Christ Immanuel pictured within a clipeus on her breast; the Platytera, a variant of the Blacherniotissa. While Eastern art remained faithful to these iconographic types

(to which may be added the Pelagoneotissa, or Virgin with the Child seen from the back, found in Macedonian art), in the West, particularly with the spread of devotional images in the late Middle Ages (see DEVOTIONAL OBJECTS AND IMAGES), there was much greater freedom in the representation of the Virgin. Particularly widespread was the standing Virgin dressed like a noblewoman and fondling the Christ Child, or Glykophilousa (II, PL. 483), also of Byzantine derivation; less common was the nursing Galaktotrophousa. The international Gothic particularly favored the Madonna of the Rose Garden, seated in a flower garden (the *hortus conclusus*). Other representations of the Virgin common in the 15th century were the Virgin of Humility; the Mother of Mercy, who shelters the faithful beneath her mantle, widespread especially in Italy; the Virgin of the Seven Sorrows, with seven swords driven into her heart, favored in the northern countries; and the Pietà.

Of Byzantine origin, but revived in the 16th century, is the Deësis (II, PL. 455), that is, the Virgin who, with John the Baptist, intercedes with Christ at the Last Judgment (see ESCHATOLOGY). One of the most common devotional images in the 17th century was the Madonna of the Rosary; a more obviously dogmatic image, representing the Immaculate Conception, shows the Virgin dressed in white, standing on a crescent moon and surrounded by stars, trampling on the serpent, symbol of original sin. The Assumption (PL. 310) was another common didactic theme at this time. Among the devotional images of the modern world the Madonna of Lourdes and the Madonna of Fatima, both linked to miraculous apparitions, merit notice. Naturally the Virgin also appears in scenes from the Gospels, particularly in scenes derived from the apochryphal Gospels. Thus from earliest times there were cycles of the life of Mary and the infancy of Christ. The Annunciation and the Nativity were particularly common also as isolated scenes, as was the Dormition of the Virgin (PL. 309) in Byzantine art. Beginning in the Renaissance, the Virgin and Child surrounded by saints became one of the favorite subjects for altarpieces. Of particular interest for folk art (q.v.) is the house of the Madonna, which according to legend was miraculously transported to Loreto, and which was for centuries faithfully reproduced.

*Angels.* The supernatural aspect of Christianity is underlined by the many representations of angels, usually of youthful aspect; following some initial uncertainty, they were, after the middle of the 4th century, represented with wings: cherubim, with just the head and four wings; seraphim, with six wings; and angelic choirs. Three have well-defined and recurrent attributes: Gabriel, who appears in the Annunciation with a staff or a lily; Raphael, who is connected with Tobias and is therefore shown in pilgim dress, with a fish or a medicine flask (from this derives the image of the guardian angel particularly widespread after the Counter Reformation); and Michael, who assumed hagiographical characteristics at an early date, connected, as his sanctuaries demonstrate, with the cult of the underworld and of lightning. The most famous of his sanctuaries are that on Mount Gargano, where he miraculously appeared in 492, and the one at Mont-Saint-Michel; furthermore, we know that the Emperor Constantine had a Michaelion constructed at Byzantium. Michael is a warrior angel who slays the dragon and hurls the rebel angels into hell (Rev. 12:7-9; PL. 311) at the same time he has an eschatological function as the "weigher of souls"; and as a guardian he is represented with Gabriel at the entrance to sanctuaries, cloisters, etc.

*Saints, prophets, sibyls.* Christian art gives a major place to saints (see SAINTS, ICONOGRAPHY OF), who are represented either singly or in cycles narrating their lives and miracles. Furthermore, the juxtaposition of certain scenes from the New Testament with scenes from the Old Testament interpreted as predictions of the Messiah determined a characteristic selection of Biblical personages for repeated representation (e.g., Moses, Abraham, etc.; see BIBLICAL SUBJECTS). It is unnecessary to emphasize the wide diffusion of imaginary portraits of prophets and sibyls: the latter have attributes related to those episodes

of the New Testament which they prophesied (PL. 312). During the Middle Ages apocalyptic subjects also enjoyed great popularity (see ESCHATOLOGY).

*Symbolic representations of the Church.* Representations of the Church, some of them highly symbolic (see SYMBOLISM AND ALLEGORY), were also of great importance in Christian art (PL. 314). The very structure and form of various holy edifices were assigned the significance of symbolic representations of the community of the faithful, although it is true that such elements were sometimes derived from the requirements of the liturgy or of church decoration and furnishing.

The iconographic tendencies and tastes of the later Middle Ages found expression in the numerous imposing sculpture cycles on the portals of Romanesque and, especially, Gothic churches. Here, together with certain dominant subjects related to the figure of the Redeemer (Maiestas Domini, Last Judgment, Crucifixion) and to the Virgin (Virgin and Child, Adoration of the Magi, Coronation, Assumption), there were representations of angels and personages and scenes from the Old and the New Testament, in which we see the recurrence of the typically medieval predilection — already manifested with vigor in Early Christian art — for the *concordia veteris et novi Testamenti* ("concordance of the Old and the New Testament"). Less common themes also appeared: the personification of the Church and the Parable of the Wise and Foolish Virgins. These representations sought to embrace the universe and the everyday world in a single vast rhythm *ad maiorem Dei gloriam*, with representations of the twelve signs of the zodiac, the twelve labors of the twelve months of the year, and the seven liberal arts. The multiple interweaving of themes corresponds, in the field of manuscript illustration, to the iconographic complexities, predominantly typological, of the *Biblia pauperum* and the *Hortus deliciarum* by Herrad von Landsberg (12th cent.).

Also noteworthy are the very important series of works created to serve or to commemorate the historical or religious life of the Church itself. The sculptures and paintings for the decoration of a building and its furnishings had an eminently didactic function, and the well-known subjects treated in the sculpture cycles were often enriched by various iconographical elements, such as personifications of the virtues and vices, the works of mercy (PL. 313), the dance of death, and portraits of the popes and bishops.

From the Counter Reformation on, we find the sacraments themselves (as in the famous cycle by Giuseppe Maria Crespi) and the most magnificent ecclesiastical ceremonies often transformed into genre scenes.

Not only the spiritual life of the Church but also its activity as a patron of the arts, often so enlightened as to permit the artists in its employ great freedom, was the subject of pictorial or graphic representation, as we see in the great engravings of churches, both those which accompany the city guides of the 17th and 18th centuries and those which were collected in albums. Nor should we overlook the enormous number of illustrations of sacred books promoted by religious organizations, which were often of great merit. In general, the deep penetration of the religious sense into all phases of secular life, which prevailed until a few centuries ago, brought about a high level of esthetic activity in almost every sector of handiwork and artistic production (see LITURGICAL OBJECTS), and this was in turn reflected abundantly in furnishings and utensils for nonliturgical use. Since the often declared intention of popes and of the hierarchy and clergy was, when possible, to transform the earthly Church into an effective symbol of the heavenly Church, or the Church Triumphant, there were confusions and excesses in the realm of lay taste, which were condemned by the Reformation (see REFORMATION AND COUNTER REFORMATION); but these frequently proved extremely fertile in the field of art. In fact, the enormous influence which the Church exerted on the arts was not only a consequence of its patronage or of the multiple needs that the arts were called upon to satisfy; it was more especially the result of its spiritual wealth, of its great emotional range, and of its continued power of suggestion. Thus for many centuries artists, in fulfilling their tasks, felt

themselves drawn away from the sphere of mere craftsmanship toward an expressive and moral activity to which they could also commit their consciences.

* *

*Christian iconography in primitive civilizations.* The Christian influence on primitive civilizations and the adaptation of local art to the new religious subjects introduced by the mission churches combined to produce a form of Christian art predominantly devotional. Western iconography was generally imitated, and the native element was limited to background and decorative motifs.

The Christian themes most widely diffused among native populations in every country are, first, the crucifix, then the Virgin and Child; both subjects are often treated with profound feeling. Africa offers an extensive production of Christian art: many iconographic themes are treated, including even the Stations of the Cross and the Nativity. The regions best documented are western Africa (Nigeria, Dahomey), the Congo, and Ruanda-Urundi; Kenya and Tanganyika should also be included. One of the earliest representations of Christ is the *Good Shepherd* of Benin (Rome, Lateran Mus.), a small bronze group representing a Negro shepherd bearing a lamb on his shoulders; he holds the lamb's legs together with his left hand and carries a pail in his right. This is a reinterpretation of the Christian Good Shepherd in accordance with a purely indigenous understanding: it is a shepherd bringing water to his sheep.

From Nigeria come painted wood statuettes of the Magi adorned with rich mantles and ornamental necklaces (in the style of the heads from Benin), casques, fans, etc.; these figures reproduce local pre-Christian types with the characteristic painted face, white eyes, and drooping black mustaches.

In the Congo, during the period of the kingdom of the Congo (15th–17th cent.), there developed, beginning in the earliest missionary period, an intense cult of the Cross. The numerous crucifixes found in the area bear witness to this cult. These images of Christ (*Nkangi Kiditu*) continue to have an important part in native life today, at least in respect to their magical powers as amulets, even in areas that have reverted to paganism. The face of Christ in these crucifixes in usually that of a Negro. They are cast in copper or brass from a wax mold. Small human figures representing worshipers are set above the head of Christ or kneel at His feet. Christ is never crowned but sometimes has an aureole in the form of a disk with rays. There are modern workshops of indigenous art that produce crucifixes, generally of little or no esthetic value but nonetheless distinguished by individual traits. The Christ Child in the arms of St. Anthony occupies an important place in the iconography of the Congo, where the cult of St. Anthony has been popular since earliest times.

It would be erroneous to include in this context the great flowering of religious art that took place in Latin America, for this development was due to European masters, who, even though they found a favorable soil in the fanciful and decorative local traditions, introduced their own style. From an ethnological viewpoint the most genuine interaction occurred in the great religious ceremonies and processions, but even this was not very different from the European encounter between Christianity and folklore. In general we may observe that the greater the penetration of Christian iconography as an artistic stimulus, the richer in popular appeal was the Christian Church.

Vittorio LANTERNARI

SOURCES. The Gospel according to St. John, 1:4; Revelation, passim, 20:12-15, 21:1-2; Acts of the Apostles, 17:24-29; Clement of Alexandria, Cohortatio ad Gentes, Migne, Patrologia Graeca, VIII, col. 133 ff.; Origen, Contra Celsum, I, VIII, ibid., XI; St. Gregory Nazianzen, Theologikos protos, ibid., XXXVI, col. 43 ff.; St. Gregory of Nyssa, Oratio laudativa sancti ac magni martyris Theodori, ibid., XLVI, col. 737 ff.; St. Basil the Great, ibid., XXXVII, cols. 149-50; Pseudo-Dionysius the Areopagite, De coelesti hierarchia, ibid., III. cols.1 19-340, De ecclesiastica hierarchia, cols. 369-569, De divinis nominibus, cols. 585-984, De mystica theologia, cols, 997-1048; Maximus the Confessor, Quaestiones ad Thalassum, quaestio 63 et responsio, ibid., XC, Mystagogia, ibid., XCI, cols. 657-718; Pope St. Clement I, Constitutiones apostolicae, II, LVII, ibid., I, col. 723 ff.; St. Augustine, Sermo, Migne, Patrologia Latina, XXXVIII, col. 1190, De vera religione, ibid., XXXIV,

col. 149 ff.; Paulus Silentiarius, Descriptio ecclesiae Sanctae Sophiae, Migne, Patrologia Graeca, LXXXVI, part 2, cols. 2137-38; Isidore of Seville, Etymologiarum libri xx, Migne, Patrologia Latina, LXXXII; Pope St. Gregory the Great, Epistolae, ibid., LXXVII; Pope Gregory II, Epistolae, ibid., LXXXIX; Pope Hadrian I, Epistolae, ibid., XCVI; Acta Pseudosynodi Constantinopolitani contra sacras imagines, Acta Conciliorum et epistolae decretales ac constitutiones summorum pontificum, IV, Paris, 1714; Concilium Oecumenicum VII, sive Nicaenum II, actio 6, ibid.; St. John of Damascus, De fide orthodoxa, cap. 16, De sanctorum imaginibus, Migne, Patrologia Graeca, XCIV, cols. 1167-76; Libri carolini, Capitulare de imaginibus, Migne, Patrologia Latina, XCVIII, cols. 999-1248; John Scotus Erigena, De divisione naturae, ibid., CXXII, cols. 128-29, 138-39, 827-29, 1090, passim; Raoul Glaber, Historiarum sui temporis libri quinque, ibid., CXLII, col. 651, passim; St. Bernard of Clairvaux, Apologia ad Guillemmum Sancti Theodorici abbatem, XII, ibid., CLXXXII, Liber de diligendo Deo, cols. 973-1000; St. Bernard of Clairvaux, Sermones, S. Bernardi opera, crit. ed., I, Rome, 1957; Peter Abelard, Epistola VIII ad Eloisam super sanctimonium, Migne, Patrologia Latina, CLXXVIII; Suger of Saint-Denis, Liber de rebus in administratione sua gesta, Libellus de consacratione ecclesiae a se edificatae (crit. ed., E. Panofsky, Abbot Suger on the Abbey Church of Saint-Denis, Princeton, 1946); Honorius Augustodunensis (Honorius of Autun), Gemma animae, lib. 1, Migne, Patrologia Latina, CLXXII, cols. 585-90; St. Bonaventure, Constitutiones Generales Narbonenses de observantia paupertatis, rubrica 3, Opera omnia, ed. Quaracchi, VIII, Commentarius in distinctionem: Qualiter Deus produxit hominem ad Suam imaginem, art. 1, quaestio 1, conclusio, ibid., 11; St. Thomas Aquinas, Summa theologica, I, quaestio 35, art. 1; Blessed Giovanni Dominici, Regole del governo di cura familiare, part 4, ed. Salvi, Florence, 1860, p. 13; St. Antoninus Pierozzi, Summa moralis, pars 2, XII, 3, Opera omnia, II, Florence, 1756, cols. 1534-35; G. Benivieni, Commento sopra a più sue canzoni et sonetti dello amore et della bellezza divina, Pistoia, 1500; Poesie di fra Girolamo Savonarola, G. Guasti and I. Del Lungo, eds., Lanciano, 1914, pp. 102-03; G. Savonarola, Triumphum Crucis sive de veritate fidei, lib. 4, Idolatrarum sectam omnium vanissimam esse, Leiden, 1633, p. 330 ff.; M. Luther, Tischreden, Frankfurt, 1573, p. 416: Von Mahlern, Welsche und Niederländische Mahler; Erasmus, Epistolarum D[esiderii] Erasmi, London, 1642, lib. 19, epist. 30, col. 844, lib. 31, epist. 47, col. 2049, lib. 31, epist. 59, Dilectis in Cristo fratribus Germaniae inferioris et Frysiae orientalis, col. 2095, Letter to Erasmus from Sadoleto, ibid., col. 1341; J. Calvin, Institutio cristianae religionis, lib. 1, chap. 11; St. John Strype, Annals of the Reformation and Establishment of Religion and Other Various Occurrences during Queen Elizabeth's Happy Reign, I, Oxford, 1814, part 1, pp. 260, 279-80, 281, part 2, appendix, p. 500 ff.; Concilium Tridentinum: Diarium actorum, epistolarum, tractatuum nova collectio, IX, Freiburg, p. 1078; St. Charles Borromeo, Instructionum fabricae ecclesiasticae et supellectilis ecclesiasticae, Milan, 1577, lib. 1, chap. 2; G. A. Gilio, Due dialoghi, Camerino, 1564, pp. 74-81; Monumenta historica societatis Jesu, Monumenta Ignatiana, ser. 2, Exercitia spiritualia Sancti Ignatii de Loyola et eorum directoria, Madrid, 1918, pp. 282-94, 312, 324, 326, 430, 552, passim; F. R. de Chateaubriand, Génie du Christianisme, Paris, 1885, part. 3, book 1, chaps. 3, 5, 6, 8; F. von Schlegel, Gemäldebeschreibungen aus Paris und den Niederländern, in den Jahren 1802 bis 1804, Ideen und Ansichten über Christliche Kunst, in Sämtliche Werke, VI, Vienna, 1823, Grundzüge der gotischen Baukunst, ibid.; G. W. F. Hegel, Vor lesungen über die Asthetik, XII-XIV, ed. Glockner, Stuttgart, 1939, part 2, sect. 3, Die romantische Kunst form: Einleitung, chap. 1, Der religiöse Kreis det romantischen Kunst, part 3, Das System der einzelnen Künste, sect. 1, chap. 3, Die romantische Architektur, sect. 2, chap. 3, Die verschiedenen Arten der Darstellung, des Materials, und die geschichtlichen Entwicklungstufen der Skulptur, und Christliche Skulptur, sec. 3, Die romantische Künste, Einleitung und Eintheilung, chap. 1, Die Malerei; J. Ruskin, Pre-Raphaelitism, London, 1851, The Stones of Venice, London, 1851-67, Giotto and His Works in Padua, London, 1853-60, Lectures on Architecture and Painting, London, 1854-55, Val d'Arno, London, 1874, Mornings in Florence, London, 1875-77, The Bible of Amiens, London, 1884; J. K. Huysmans, La Cathédrale, Paris, 1898; E. von Dobschütz, Christusbilder, Untersuchungen zur christlichen Legende, III, Leipzig, 1899, Trois primitifs, Paris, 1905; L. Bloy, L'invendable, Paris, 1909, Le pèlerin de l'absolu, Paris, 1914, Au seuil de l'Apocalypse, Paris, 1916, La porte des humbles, Paris, 1920; W. J. A. Visser, Die Entwicklung des Christusbildes in Literatur und Kunst in der früchristlichen und frühbyzantinischen Zeit, Bonn, 1934; J. Maritain, Art et scolastique, 2d ed., Paris, 1927; Les Cahiers du Rhône, Edition du centenaire augmentée de textes inédits, Neuchâtel, 1946, Pope Pius XII, Encyclica Mediator Dei, Acta apostolicae sedis, col. 39, pp. 543, 590-91.

BIBLIOG. F. von Schiller, Geschichte des Abfalls der vereinigten Niederlände von der spanischen Regierung, Viertes Buch, Der bildersturm, Sämtliche Werke, XII, Vienna, 1819; H. Othe, Handbuch der kirchlichen Kunstarchäologie des deutschen Mittelalters, Leipzig, 1860-64; A. Hauch, Die Entstehung des Christustypus in der abendländischen Kunst, Heidelberg, 1880; F. X. Kraus, Real-Enzyklopädie der christlichen Altertümer, Freiburg, 1882-86; H. J. Wetzer and B. Welte, Kirchenlexikon, oder Enzyklopädie der katholischen Theologie und ihrer Hülfswissenschaften, 2d ed., Freiburg, 1882-1903; J. J. Herzog and A. Hauck, Real-Enzyklopädie für protestantische Theologie und Kirche, Leipzig, 1896; F. X. Kraus, Geschichte der christlichen Kunst, vorgesetzt von Joseph Sauer, Freiburg, 1896-97, 1908; J. E. Weis-Liebersdorf, Christus und Apostelbilder: Einfluss der Apokryphen auf die ältesten Kunsttypen, Freiburg, 1902; G. Millet, Recherches sur l'iconographie de l'Evangile, Paris, 1915; G. Stuhlfauth, Die "ältesten Porträts" Christi und der Apostel, Berlin, 1918; R. Berger, Die Darstellung des thronenden Christus in der romanischen Kunst, Tübinger Forsch. Archäol. Kg., v, Reutlingen, 1926; A. Molsdorf, Christliche Symbolik der mittelalterlichen Kunst, Leipzig, 1926; Cabrol-Leclercq, s.v. Jésus Christ; Mâle, I-IV; K. Künstle, Ikonographie der christlichen Kunst, I, Freiburg, 1928, pp. 587-618; L. Bréhier, L'art chrétien: Son développement iconogra-

phique des origines à nos jours, Paris, 1928; A. Grabar, La Sainte Face de Laon: Le Mandylion dans l'art orthodoxe, Prague, 1931; C. Cecchelli, Le più antiche immagini di N.S. Gesù Cristo, Illustrazione Vaticana, III, 6, 1932, pp. 283–87; G. de' Francovich, L'origine e la diffusione del Crocifisso gotico doloroso, Kg. Jb. Biblioteca Hertziana, II, 1938, pp. 227–44; G. Jerphanion, La voix des monuments, I, Paris, 1938; J. B. Knipping, De Iconografie van de Contrareformatie in de Nederlanden, Hilversum, 1939–40; F. Henry, Irish Art in the Early Christian Period, London, 1940; L. Venturi, Georges Rouault, New York, 1940; W. Weisbach, Religiöse Reform und mittelalterliche Kunst, Einsiedeln, Zurich, 1945; J. J. M. Timmers, Symboliek en Iconographie der Christelijke Kunst, Roermond, Maeseyck, 1947; G. Auletta, L'aspetto di Gesù Cristo, Rome, 1948; F. Gerke, Christus in der spätantiken Plastik, 3d ed., Mainz, 1948; C. Costantini, L'istruzione del S. Offiizio sull'Arte Sacra, Vatican City, 1952; J. Kollwitz, Das Christusbild des dritten Jahrhunderts (Orbis antiquus, fasc. 8), Münster, 1953; G. von Simson, Die Wirkungen des christlichen Platonismus auf die Entstehung der Gotik, in J. Koch, Humanismus, Mystik und Kunst in der Welt des Mittelalters, Leiden, Cologne, 1953; G. C. Argan, Fra Angelico, Geneva, 1955; G. van Leeuw, Wegen en Grenzen, 3d ed., Amsterdam, 1955 (Ger. ed., Vom Heiligen in der Kunst, Gütersloh, 1957, pp. 161–213); P. A. Michelis, An Aesthetic Approach to Byzantine Art, London, 1955; C. Cecchelli, Iconografia del Cristo nell'arte paleocristiana e bizantina: Iconografia della Madonna e degli altri santi nell'arte paleocristiana e bizantina, Corsi di cultura sull'arte ravennate e bizantina, I, Ravenna, 1956, pp. 43–50; O. G. von Simson, The Gothic Cathedral, New York, 1956; F. Zeri, Pittura e Controriforma: L'arte senza tempo di Scipione da Gaeta, Turin, 1957, pp. 24–36, 52–60, 80–102; H. C. von Häbler, Das Bild in der evangelischen Kirche, Berlin, n.d. [1957]; G. Händler, Epochen karolingischer Theologie: Eine Untersuchung über die karolingischen Gutachten zum byzantinischen Bilderstreit, Berlin, 1958; L. Réau, Iconographie de l'art chrétien, Paris, 1958–59; J. Sauer, Die ältesten Christusbilder, Wasmuths Kunsthefte, 7, n.d.; A. Baumstark, Die karolingisch-romanische Majestas Domini und ihre orientalischen Parallelen, Oriens christianus, III, 1, p. 242 ff.

Rosario Assunto and Carlo Cecchelli

Illustrations: PLS. 303–314.

**CHRISTUS,** Petrus. Flemish painter, also known as Christi; real name Pieter Christus or Cristus (b. Baerle, date unknown; d. Bruges, 1472 or 1473). He signed many of his pictures with XPI, the Greek abbreviation of the name of Christ, in place of his own surname. The first known date in the artist's life is July 6, 1444, when he became a free master in Bruges. Ten years later it is recorded that Christus copied some works in the Cathedral of Cambrai, France. In 1463 he collaborated with another artist on a large painting of the *Tree of Jesse* for the processions of the famous Confraternity of the Holy Blood in Bruges (Chapel of the St. Sang).

The art of Petrus Christus reflects the two main trends in Flemish painting of the 15th century — the naturalistic and objective tradition of Jan van Eyck and the tradition of the Master of Flémalle, especially as the latter was passed on through the elegant, nervous, and emotional style of Rogier van der Weyden. Similarities in Christus' works to the art of Jan and Hubert van Eyck are very great; some of Christus' compositions adhere closely to Eyckian creations and, in fact, indicate that he copied their models. The *Last Judgment* (Berlin, Staat. Mus.) follows much of the arrangement of the Van Eyck *Last Judgment* (New York, Met. Mus.).

Although we have no document assuring us of Christus' presence in Bruges before the death of Jan van Eyck (1441), it seems very probable that he served an apprenticeship in Van Eyck's shop. It is fairly certain that it was Petrus Christus who completed the famous *Rothschild Madonna* (New York, Frick Coll.), planned and begun by Jan in the short time between the commissioning of the picture and Jan's death. The *St. Jerome* in Detroit (Inst. of Arts) is also apparently a joint work by the two artists. There is, to be sure, a great difference discernible in the styles of Christus and his master. Christus' works, in comparison, are pedestrian and heavy. His conception is massive and his people, set in vast airless spaces, are countrified and clumsy, with simple moving faces.

After the death of Jan van Eyck and Christus' acquisition of mastery in his own right, he showed in many of his pictures a clear tendency to draw from the Master of Flémalle, as in the *Nativity* (formerly Goldman Coll., New York), which closely recalls the Master of Flémalle's Dijon *Nativity*; there are also numerous borrowings and reflections of Rogier van der Weyden. Other important works by Petrus Christus include the *Ma-*

*donna with SS. Francis and Jerome* (Frankfurt, Städelsches Kunstinst.), the so-called *Exeter Madonna* (Berlin, Staat. Mus), the *St. Eligius* (New York, Lehman Coll.), and the two very similar *Lamentations* (Brussels, Mus. Royaux des Beaux-Arts; V, PL. 279; and New York, Met. Mus.). His portraits are often extremely fine, especially that of a pale young woman in Berlin (Staat. Mus.; V, PL. 285), the likenesses of *Edward Grymestone* (St. Albans, Earl of Verulam Coll.), and an unknown Carthusian monk (New York, Met. Mus.). Petrus Christus' major contribution in the history of painting was his determined unification of space and his formulation in practice rather than theory of the rules of perspective. See FLEMISH AND DUTCH ART.

BIBLIOG. W. H. J. Weale, Peintres brugeois, Les Cristus, Bruges, 1909; M. J. Friedländer, Die altniederländische Malerei, I, Berlin, 1924; Dictionnaire des peintres (Petits dictionnaires des lettres et des arts en Belgique), Brussels, n.d.; E. Panofsky, Early Netherlandish Painting, Its Origins and Character, Cambridge, Mass., 1953.

Margaretta M. Salinger

**CHURRIGUERESQUE STYLE.** The style is named for the Churrigueras, a family of Spanish architects and sculptors of Catalan origin but active chiefly in Madrid and Salamanca during the last quarter of the 17th century and the first half of the 18th. A phase of the Spanish baroque, this style is rooted in the ornamental forms of Catalan wood sculpture, with borrowings from the Roman baroque; it is decorative rather than inventive or extravagant. The term "Churrigueresque" is frequently applied incorrectly to works not in the style of this family and has been extended to include the more florid late baroque phase in Spain and even in Mexico.

SUMMARY. José Simón de Churriguera (col. 608). José Benito de Churriguera (col. 608). Joaquín de Churriguera (col. 609). Alberto de Churriguera (col. 609). Other architects of the Churriguera family (col. 610). Development of the style (col. 610). Critical evaluations (col. 613).

JOSÉ SIMÓN DE CHURRIGUERA (called José the Elder). It is known that José Simón, a sculptor, came before 1674 from Barcelona to Madrid, where he collaborated with his stepfather, José Rates, also a Catalan artist, on a retable for the Montserrat Hospital Church. This dramatic sculptural complex, flanked by the Solomonic (i.e. twisted) columns fashionable at the time, derived from an earlier work by Bernardo Simón de Pineda in Seville and was the prototype of many works by José Benito de Churriguera and the other sons of José Simón. José Simón died in 1679, and it is probable that his five sons were given a start in their profession by José Rates.

JOSÉ BENITO DE CHURRIGUERA. Until a few years ago it was believed that José Benito was a native of Salamanca, but documents have been found showing he was born in Madrid on Mar. 21, 1665, and baptized in the parish church of SS. Justo y Pastor on Apr. 1 of that year. His parents were José Simón and Maria de Ocaña. According to tradition he lived for some years in Salamanca and was educated in the university there. Most probably the younger José began his career as apprentice to his stepgrandfather José Rates, or possibly to another of the architect-painters of the court of Charles II, such as José Jiménez Donoso or Francisco Herrera the Younger.

José Benito's first great professional honor came in 1689, when a design of his won the competition for a funeral monument to be set up in the Church of the Encarnación in Madrid in honor of Queen Marie Louise d'Orléans, first wife of Charles II. The work is known through an engraving of Ruiz de la Iglesia published (1690) in Vera Tassis' description of the obsequies. In 1690, while making minor additions to the Monserrat Hospital Church in Madrid, José Benito was named assistant palace architect, to serve without salary until a post should fall vacant, which it did in 1696. He was also named, after 1690, architect of the Cathedral of Salamanca (Catedral Nueva), a post he held for the next 12 or 15 years while working toward its completion. The great tower at the south end of the façade was finished in 1705. It must be that José Benito's important com-

missions in Salamanca were the result of his fame in Madrid and not the other way round, as was once believed. In Salamanca, from 1693 to 1696, he built the great retable of S. Esteban (PL. 319), prototype of a series of retables designed for the Jesuits of that city, and of later retables in Madrid. From about 1699 to his death, in 1725, he worked principally in Madrid. This period, during the reign of Philip V, marked the full flowering of the Churrigueresque in Spanish art. José Benito's principal works in Madrid date from these years, when he was called the "Spanish Michelangelo" — probably a reference to the versatility of his imagination. In the neoclassic fervor of the late 18th century many of the works were altered or destroyed. The Church of S. Tomás, for instance, and the Goyeneche Palace, the present Real Academia de Bellas Artes de S. Fernando, were remodeled in 1774 by Diego de Villanueva.

José Benito's most important existing architectural work — unfortunately in poor condition — is the urban complex of Nuevo Baztán, commissioned by the Goyeneche family and dated 1722. The façade of S. Cayetano in Madrid, attributed to him, may have been based on a Roman plan; it was completed after his death by his follower Pedro de Ribera. José Benito died at his house in Madrid on Mar. 2, 1725.

JOAQUÍN DE CHURRIGUERA. Born in Madrid on Mar. 20, 1674, Joaquín collaborated with his brother José Benito as designer of retables. In 1714 he was named architect of the Cathedral of Salamanca; he supervised the building of the cupola, which was destroyed by the earthquake of 1775 and rebuilt by Sagarvinaga in a more classic style. Joaquín's surviving work in Salamanca includes the Hospedería, the College of Anaya, the magnificent College of Calatrava, finished by his brother Alberto, and, in the Cathedral, the *Altar del Cristo de las Batallas*. The so-called "College of Oviedo" was destroyed during the French invasion.

Joaquín died in 1724 at the age of 50, either in Salamanca or in Plasencia (in Estremadura), where he was engaged in his last work, the retable for the Cathedral. His style was more *retardataire* than his brothers' and remained plateresque.

ALBERTO DE CHURRIGUERA. Alberto, after his brother José Benito the most widely known architect of the Churriguera family, was born in Madrid on Aug. 7, 1676. He was once thought to be the uncle or the nephew of José Benito, but their works are contemporary, and both were engaged in building the retable of S. Sebastián in Madrid from 1710 to 1715. Before that Alberto probably completed his education in Salamanca and assisted José Benito on the great retable of S. Esteban (PL. 319), in that city. After the death of Joaquín, in 1724, the chapter of the Cathedral of Salamanca appointed Alberto to the vacant post of director of works. He completed the stalls and screen of the choir, the great tabernacle of the main altar, and the sacristy, which had probably been begun by Joaquín (PL. 315). On July 9, 1728, he was commissioned by the governor of Salamanca, Rodrigo Caballero, to construct the Plaza Mayor of that city (PL. 316), the most important public square in Spain; it was not finished until 1755, several years after his death, when his pupil Andrés García de Quiñones was director of works. In 1729 Alberto built the upper part of the façade of the Valladolid Cathedral (PL. 316). In 1733 the Cathedral of Salamanca was finished and consecrated, but in 1738 Alberto resigned his post after a disagreement with the chapter about the tower. He had already finished the College of Calatrava in Salamanca, begun by Joaquín, and, in 1731, the Church of S. Sebastián in the same city. It is almost certain that Alberto built the great chapel of S. Tecla in the Cathedral of Burgos in 1736, 11 years after the death of José Benito, to whom the work has been erroneously attributed. Alberto is also thought to have been the architect of the old chapel of S. Antonio in Madrid; the present chapel, decorated by Goya, is the work of Francesco Fontana. The time and place of Alberto's death are not known; he may have died in Orgaz (province of Toledo), where he had gone to build a church. Alberto was the most original of the Churriguera brothers, and his style, especially after José Benito's death, belongs more to the rococo than to the baroque.

OTHER ARCHITECTS OF THE CHURRIGUERA FAMILY. Little is known of José Simón's other sons, Manuel and Miguel, the brothers of José Benito, Joaquín, and Alberto. The record of Manuel's birth, on Sept. 8, 1667, is preserved in the Church of SS. Justo y Pastor in Madrid. A retable and tabernacle in the Sagrario of the Cathedral of Segovia are attributed to him, though not with certainty. As for Miguel, Mélida says that in 1726, according to an inscription, he built the Arco de la Estrella at Cáceres for the Marqués de la Enjarada.

Matías, Jerónimo, and Nicolás, the sons of José Benito, were architects like their father and their uncles; some facts are known about their lives but very little about their works, which were probably not of any great importance. They collaborated in the final work for the no longer extant church of S. Tomás in Madrid. Nicolás appears to have been the most talented of the group, since he had a part in the construction of the Plaza Mayor in Salamanca and in the "Planimetría General de la Villa de Madrid," made by royal command for Ferdinand VI and his minister, the Marqués de la Ensenada.

DEVELOPMENT OF THE STYLE. The artistic tendencies expressed in the works of the Churrigueras mark the high point of a development which began with Juan de Herrera (q.v.). Earlier architects, even such outstanding ones as Covarrubias and Machuca, had not been able to adapt the Italian style to the Spanish taste. Herrera, in the Escorial (1563–84), achieved a Spanish work in a mature Renaissance style, which expressed its monastic purpose in a sober and almost ascetic exterior. The monumental character of the design, the strongly axial and horizontal mass with towers marking the ends of the façades — these are hallmarks of the Iberian tradition. There is also a greater emphasis on planes than in French and Italian design, with the stress on the wall rather than on the openings in it. All these traits combined to give Spanish architecture the grave, forceful character it had until the 19th century.

Under Philip III (1598–1621) and Philip IV (1621–65) a profound change in taste took place. Spanish architecture became influenced by the Italian baroque — and to some extent by the Flemish — without losing its individuality, however. The baroque development began timidly with the architects of Philip III, Juan de Nates in Valladolid, Gaspár Ordóñez in Alcalá de Henares, and Jorge Manuel Theotocopuli in Toledo. These artists and others, such as the Vergaras, grafted baroque details onto the style of Herrera, but it was not until the reign of Philip IV that a true baroque style was achieved — by two architects working for the Jesuits. These were Francisco Bautista and Juan Gómez de Mora. Bautista built the splendid Cathedral of S. Isidro in Madrid, originally the church of the Colegio Imperial, and in Toledo the Church of S. Juan Bautista de Afuera. Gómez de Mora built the Clerecía, or Novitiate of the Jesuits, at Salamanca (PL. 317), one of the outstanding works of baroque architecture in Spain. In plan the Jesuit churches of Spain follow the model of their order, the Gesù in Rome; in spite of the many baroque motifs, moldings, windows, and elaborate escutcheons, there is a certain simplicity — abandoned, in the Clerecía at Salamanca, only above the balustrade, in the towers and the *españadas* (belfry gables), which belong to the Churrigueresque style. The result is a different mood, a harmonious contrast between the ornament above and the solid structure that supports it.

One can feel a development toward the Churrigueresque in the work of two other great artists of the reign of Philip IV, Alonso Cano and Francisco Herrera the Younger, each of whom excelled as painter and architect. In Cano's designs for retables the rich variation of cornices and moldings foreshadows the Churrigueras. The most important architectural work of Francisco Herrera the Younger was the basilica of El Pilar at Saragossa; as this was almost completely remodeled in the 18th century, Herrera's vigorous style can be seen only in one of the towers, whose strongly projecting ornament and exuberant use of foliage decoration also tend toward the Churrigueresque.

Another outstanding artist, almost the contemporary of José Benito in Madrid, was José Jiménez Donoso, whose most important work was the reconstruction, in 1674, of the Casa

Panadería on the Plaza Mayor (PL. 316). This building with its steep-roofed Herrerian towers is typically Spanish; its ornament is notable. Donoso was also a painter of frescoes in a manner close to the Churrigueresque. It has been thought that this style of painting was brought to Madrid by Colonna and Mitelli, two Bolognese artists who came to Spain after Velázquez' second journey to Italy. If so, we have here an important Italian influence on the Churrigueresque. But this is only a hypothesis, for the works of the Italian artists in the Alcázar and the Church of La Merced have disappeared completely.

The funeral monument for Queen Marie Louise d'Orléans, with which José Benito began his career, is theatrical in effect and shows the influence of Borromini and Dietterlin. In an age when the religious plays of Calderón were appreciated by the common man, an artist who created a work of this type was sure to find favor with both court and clergy. In the retable of S. Esteban in Salamanca (PL. 319), another major work of José Benito's, the baroque style follows the Spanish tradition, which emphasized the retable as focal point at the end of the nave. As a designer of carved and gilded wooden retables, José Benito takes his place in the development of this Spanish art.

The most characteristic element used by the Churrigueras is the Solomonic column, or *salomónica*, the twisted column named after the one in St. Peter's, which according to legend had belonged to the Temple of Solomon and which Bernini imitated in the baldachin. Bernini's great baldachin at St. Peter's was known through engravings; similar columns appear in the backgrounds of Rubens' paintings and in his tapestries at the Convent of the Descalzas Reales in Madrid. The drawings for these tapestries, now in the Prado, were brought to Madrid in 1648. Although there was an earlier use of Solomonic columns in the choir screen of the Cathedral of Sigüenza, for example, and in murals in several buildings in Madrid, José Benito was the first to sense the dynamic possibilities of this form, and he used it to integrate the retable into the church interior. The unifying element of leaf ornament appears not only around the columns, as in Bernini's work, but also on the pedestals, friezes, and acroteria. Another mark of the Churrigueresque retable is the effect of lightness. It is achieved by the use of a high plinth and a very free treatment of the entablature in which the frieze projects over the architrave and is partly covered by the brackets supporting the cornice. Drawings preserved in the Museo de la Academia de S. Fernando show two magnificent retables by José Benito which stood in the churches of La Merced and Los Basilios in Madrid but were destroyed in the 19th century. The Solomonic columns on their high pedestals are of grandiose proportions. In the retable of La Merced the cornice and base are broken by a tabernacle, or baldachin, containing an image of the Virgin. Above, under a very high arch, appears the image of Faith. These retables contain some Palladian elements, but softened by the Roman baroque, especially of Borromini, in the high pedestals and curving frieze.

In the complex of Nuevo Baztán, planned by José Benito, the church, with its steeply roofed towers and flat walls and pilasters, recalls the style of Herrera; of greater interest is the doorway of the palace, which, like the ornament around the windows, gives the effect of having been modeled by the hands of the artist. The Goyeneche Palace in the Calle de Alcalá, now the Real Academia de Bellas Artes de S. Fernando, was much altered by the chill neoclassic design of Diego de Villanueva, but the ornament around the windows is José Benito's. Originally the lower floor was rusticated in the manner Bernini used for the Montecitorio Palace in Rome and for his project for the Louvre. The façade, today devoid of interest, was similar to many of the baroque façades in Madrid. The Church of S. Cayetano, though only in part the work of José Benito, is noteworthy. According to tradition the plan came from Rome; this is possible, since the design employs the Bramantesque central plan with five domes, the one in the center supported by four piers. The façade is divided into five parts by Corinthian pilasters. The three center sections give access to the atrium through arched openings; above each portal is a niche with sculpture, so richly decorated as to be almost like an altar. The niches, capitals, and cornices are elaborately modeled in the typically baroque style of Madrid, so well adapted to the granite of the Sierra de Guadarrama.

Similar characteristics may be seen in the fine portals of Pedro de Ribera, who kept the Churrigueresque manner alive in Madrid during the first quarter of the 18th century. On the façade of the Hospicio de S. Fernando (PL. 318) the effect of metalwork given by the decoration in the center is enhanced by the graceful fall of the sculptured draperies at the side. The oval windows repeat the ornament, or rather become a part of it. None of the architectural orders are used, their place being taken by the decorative *estípite*, the inverted obelisk, sometimes a herm form, which almost entirely replaced the Solomonic column in mid-18th-century retables. The royal saint of Castile stands in a niche above the portal, and over that appears an oval window in a gable, a graceful crowning touch in the rococo style.

Another magnificent portal attributed to Pedro de Ribera is that of the Miraflores Palace in the heart of Madrid. The doorway has a boldly ornamental molding, which, on the jambs, half covers the Tuscan pilasters. The cornice is pushed up to support a balcony above. The elaborate design is crowned by an escutcheon decorated with shells and a final pinnacle.

In the sacristy of Salamanca Cathedral (PL. 315) Joaquín and Alberto de Churriguera showed great adaptability to the Isabelline Gothic style of the building. Baroque details appear only in the pinnacles above the arches and the ornamented architrave. The College of Calatrava, also by Joaquín and Alberto, is an outstanding monument of the Spanish baroque. Here the giant order of Tuscan pilasters on the façade echoes Bernini's style, but the magnificent portals decorated with escutcheons and the towers at the ends of the façade are purely Spanish. The beautiful Plaza Mayor of Salamanca (PL. 316) shows influences of the Madrid Plaza Mayor in its arched colonnades and its balconied windows, which are lower and wider than their Italian models. The buildings around the Plaza Mayor in Madrid are stuccoed, while those of Salamanca are of the local fine-grained golden sandstone, which permits a more exuberant decoration in the Royal Pavilion with its escutcheons and belfry gable crowning the façade. The pinnacles on the balustrade carry the fleur-de-lis of the Bourbon king Philip V.

In the Plaza Mayor of Salamanca the Town Hall built by Andrés García de Quiñones, the successor of Alberto de Churriguera, shows the influence of Guarini in the mass of ornament, which covers the façade instead of being concentrated in the Spanish manner around the windows and the vertical axis of the portal.

In completing the façade of the Cathedral of Valladolid, begun by Herrera, Alberto de Churriguera achieved a remarkable harmony of both structure and mood (he added the handsome upper part above the balustrade). Baroque details are found only in the great flattened volutes and the escutcheons at the sides and on the gable.

Another outstanding architect, one of a family of artists, was Narciso Tomé, who in 1715 built the façade of the University of Valladolid, the center of which imitates a retable (II, PL. 160). The giant order is similar to the one Galilei used 20 years later, in a more classic manner, for the Lateran in Rome. Both buildings recall the style of Palladio in the high plinths, thin shafts, balustrades ornamented with figures, etc. But Tomé's design has interesting baroque details, such as the curve of the entablature around the columns, following the cylindrical plan. The *espadaña* is also present — the belfry gable so typical in Spanish designs of this period.

Outside Castile there is little that can properly be called Churrigueresque, though the influence of the Churrigueras can be widely traced. In general, the baroque art of the late 17th and early 18th centuries in central and eastern Spain is characterized by a wealth of detail and a freedom that bring it closer to European rococo than to the grandiose art of the Churrigueras. In the north of Spain, Santiago de Compostela was the great artistic center for several schools of the baroque that grew up independently of the Churriguera school.

CRITICAL EVALUATIONS. The Churrigueresque style has been treated scornfully and even violently by critics ever since it was abandoned. But José Benito de Churriguera's contemporaries called him the "Spanish Michaelangelo," "the greatest artist of his day." The famous *Transparente* in the Cathedral of Toledo (II, PL. 161), a work of Narciso Tomé, was called the eighth wonder of the world in a poem by Rodríguez Galán.

Although the high point of the Churrigueresque may be placed in the early decades of the reign of Philip V (1700–46), the first Bourbon king of Spain, the coming to power of the Bourbons actually meant a reaction in taste toward a moderate classicism. Already in 1715 there was a return to the style of Herrera at Aranjuez. In the structure of La Granja near Seville it is possible to observe the transition from the indigenous manner represented by the Churrigueresque style to the French and from the French to the Italian. The rebuilding of the Royal Palace in Madrid, destroyed by fire in 1734, was entrusted to the Italian architects Filippo Juvara and his successor Sacchetti, rather than to Spaniards. These artists, along with their Spanish colleague, Ventura Rodríguez, achieved a work in the north Italian baroque manner, a style very far from the Churrigueresque. Ferdinand VI encouraged the classicizing trend by bringing foreign architects to Spain in 1746 for the founding of the Real Academia de Bellas Artes de S. Fernando in Madrid. Thus the transition from the Churrigueresque to the neoclassic in Spain was not a gradual or natural evolution but was for the most part imposed by the academies. The change in style that was in progress all over Europe was in Spain also politically motivated.

That the Churrigueresque style was favored by the last of the Hapsburgs, the enemies of the Bourbons in the War of the Spanish Succession, may explain later attacks on it by neoclassic critics and the utter lack of objectivity in the writings of otherwise reputable historians such as Ponz, Llaguno y Amírola, and Ceán Bermúdez. They and other critics and historians of the late 18th century, such as Jovellanos, mocked and belittled the Churrigueresque monuments and their magnificent stone façades. If they were less violent at times it was only when they confused the style with that of other periods.

During the first three-quarters of the 19th century the classicizing Italianate style prevailed in Spain, and most critics continued their uninformed attacks on the Churrigueresque, as did such writers as Bosarte, Madoz, and Quadrado. Even at the end of the century critics such as Mesonero y Romanos and Fernández de los Ríos, who were more aware of indigenous art, did not appreciate the monuments most typically Spanish. Menéndez y Pelayo in his monumental work *Ideas estéticas en España* (1883), pronounced the great figures of the Churrigueresque school "heresiarchs." The one 19th-century exception was José Caveda, who in 1848 gave a more objective critical analysis of the style.

At the beginning of the 20th century there was a great revival of medieval studies in Spain; however, such scholars as Lampérez y Romea, in their pursuit of the Gothic style, found nothing of interest in Madrid. But in the second quarter of the century there began a sort of neo-Churrigueresque school of architecture, influenced by Juan Moya's restoration of the façade of S. José in Madrid. Other architects, Pablo Gutiérrez Moreno, Luis Moya, and Andrés Calzada, made studies of the baroque in Spain. Otto Schubert's important scholarly work on the baroque, *Die Geschichte des Barock in Spanien* of 1908, appeared in 1924 in a Spanish translation. Its excellent illustrations and critical judgments more than outweigh the historical errors. In 1927 Elías Tormo y Monzó's *Las iglesias del antiguo Madrid* provided a valuable guide to the study of architecture in that city. In 1929 the articles of Antonio García y Bellido appeared, important studies of the Churriguera family which corrected many errors of earlier writers and supplied new biographical material. And in *Lo Barroco* of 1946 Eugenio D'Ors looked at the period from a philosophical point of view and wrote perceptively about the style called "accursed" by the neoclassicists. F. P. Verrié published his discoveries about the Catalan origin of the Churriguera family in 1947. In his *Arquitectura española 1600–1800* of 1957 George Kubler adds to the documentary evidence a long critical analysis of the works and the style of the Churrigueras.

BIBLIOG. J. de Vera Tassis Villarroel, Noticias historiales de la enfermedad, muerte y exequias de la Reina Doña María Luisa de Orleáns, Madrid, 1690; J. A. Ceán Bermúdez, Diccionario histórico de los más ilustres profesores de las bellas artes en España, Madrid, 1800; E. Llaguno y Amírola, Noticias de los arquitectos y arquitectura de España, Madrid, 1829; J. Caveda, Ensayo histórico sobre los diversos géneros de arquitectura empleados en España, Madrid, 1848; M. Falcón, Salamanca artística y monumental, Salamanca, 1867; O. Schubert, Die Geschichte des Barock in Spanien, Esslingen, 1908; J. Braun, Spaniens alte Jesuitenkirchen, Freiburg im Breisgau, 1913; J. Cavestany, Excursión a Nuevo Batzán, Boletín de la Sociedad Española de Excursiones, 1922; E. Tormo y Monzó, Las iglesias del antiguo Madrid, Madrid, 1927; J. Moreno Villa, Tres dibujos de Pedro de Ribera, Arquitectura, 1928; A. García y Bellido, Estudios del barroco español, Archivo Español de Arte y Arqueología, 1929–30; A. López Durán, El palacio y la iglesia de Nuevo-Baztán, Arquitectura, XIV, 1932, pp. 169–75; A. Calzada, Historia de la arquitectura española, Barcelona, 1933; T. L. Martin and E. Sarmiento, Masks and Monuments of the Spanish Baroque, Architectural Review, 1933; Marqués de Lozoya, Historia del arte hispánico, IV, Barcelona, 1945; E. D'Ors, Lo Barroco, Madrid, 1946; F. Chueca Goitia, La catedral de Valladolid, Madrid, 1947; F. P. Verrié, Los barceloneses Xuriguera, Divulgación Histórica, VII, Barcelona, 1949; J. A. Gaya Nuño, Madrid (Guías artísticas de España), Barcelona, 1950; F. Chueca Goitia, La Catedral Nueva de Salamanca, Salamanca, 1951; G. Kubler, Arquitectura española 1600–1800 (Ars Hispaniae, XIV), Madrid, 1957; G. Kubler and M. Soria, Art and Architecture in Spain and Portugal and Their American Dominions, Baltimore, 1959.

Manuel LORENTE JUNQUERA

Illustrations: PLS. 315–319.

**CIMABUE.** Florentine painter active in the second half of the 13th century and the first years of the 14th. Vasari's dates for the artist's birth and death (1240–1300) are based only on the rather confused information given in older sources, as Karl Frey has shown. The earliest documentary reference, discovered by Strzygowski in the archives of S. Maria Maggiore in Rome, is dated June 8, 1272, and concerns Cardinal Ottoboni Fieschi's protectorship of a S. Damiano convent; among seven witnesses appears a "Cimabove pictore de Florentia." We may conclude, therefore, that in 1272 Cimabue was in Rome and had attained his majority; hence he could hardly have been born later than 1251. The last mention of Cimabue alive appears in a registry entry by the notary Chiaro d'Andrea, dated July 4, 1302. According to this entry, the steward (*speziale camarlingo*) of the Società dei Piovuti in Pisa was entrusted with several objects belonging to members, including a tablecloth and a table mat of Cimabue's. The artist must therefore have lived beyond 1300, the date Vasari gives as that of his death. From a terzina in Dante's *Purgatorio*, Canto 11, which suggests that Cimabue was still living but neglected because of Giotto's great popularity, Brandi deduces that the artist was alive after 1315, when the canto was written. However, it should be remembered that Dante's accounts always refer to Holy Week, 1300, and not to events and persons contemporary with the writing of various parts of the poem. The fact that Dante in 1315 alludes to Cimabue may only prove what we already know — that Cimabue was alive in 1300.

Two documents from Pisa, dated Nov. 1 and 5, 1301, certify that Cimabue, together with a certain Nuchulus (Giovanni d'Apparecchiato da Lucca?) was commissioned to paint for the Church of the Hospital of S. Chiara a great *Maestà* in the form of a polyptych, with saints set in the frame and a crucifix on the gable. Either the work has disappeared or it was never executed. From the description given in the documents, Ragghianti's proposed identification of this *Maestà* with the Louvre altarpiece seems impossible. A series of payments from Sept. 2, 1301, to Feb. 19, 1302, proves that during this period Cimabue was working on the apse mosaic of the Cathedral of Pisa and had finished the figures of St. John. This is the only extant work by the master which is both documented and dated.

Cimabue's activity in the Basilica of S. Francesco in Assisi (mentioned by Billi, the Anonimo Gaddiano, and Vasari) was until recently dated either about 1280 or about 1290. The dating of 1280 was at first preferred because in the represen-

tation of St. Mark, in one of the cross vaults of the Upper Church, there is a palace, identified as the old Lateran, which bears three Orsini coats of arms; this suggests that the fresco was executed under Nicholas III (1277–80), a pope of the Orsini family. However, Brandi has pointed out that the building actually represents the Capitol. The Orsini arms, furthermore, alternate with shields bearing the initials SPQR; hence the reference is not to the reigning pope but to the senator in office. In 1288 Matteo and Bartolo Orsini were senators of Rome; and on May 15 of the same year, Nicholas IV (1288–92), the first Franciscan pope and general of the Franciscan order, published the well-known bull initiating the construction and decoration of the Basilica of S. Francesco in Assisi. Cimabue's frescoes in Assisi can therefore be assigned to some time between about 1288 and 1290. No other work by him can be dated on external evidence.

The traditional view, accepted by Vasari, that Cimabue studied with certain "Greek masters" working at S. Maria Novella no doubt contains an element of truth. However, the hypothesis that he served an apprenticeship with a nephew of one of the legendary masters from Byzantium, who had supposedly emigrated to the West as a result of the Latin conquest of 1204 (the Fourth Crusade), is unlikely. Cimabue's knowledge of the "Greek" style can be attributed, rather, to a wide acquaintance, either direct or indirect, with the far-reaching neo-Hellenistic movement of the Palaeologan renaissance in its two chief currents: the metropolitan, or courtly, with its studied and concentrated pathos, and the provincial — crude, impetuous, and tending to dramatic expressionism. Hints of the Palaeologan style of Byzantium are found in the art of Cimabue, Vigoroso da Siena, and Duccio, as well as in the anonymous altarpieces of *St. Peter* and *St. John the Baptist* in the Siena Pinacoteca. Hence icons in the purest neo-Hellenistic style were surely not unknown in Tuscany at this time (see ROMANESQUE ART). In Pisa, certainly, a vigorous current of aristocratic neo-Hellenism had been active since perhaps 1200, some decades before Giunta Pisano produced his famous *Cross* (no. 20) in the Museo Civico in Pisa. Cimabue's crucifix is clearly in the tradition of Giunta's crosses — especially the *Cross of the Monk Elia* (now lost but faithfully reflected in that of the Master of St. Francis) and the later Giunta cross in Bologna. From Giunta's crucifixes come not only the iconographical and typological motif of the Redeemer's tensely arched body but also the imposing rhythmic unity which complements it stylistically. During his stay in Rome — in 1272 or shortly thereafter — Cimabue may perhaps have admired the angels surrounding the *Christ in Majesty* at Grottaferrata; their mature Hellenistic sweetness seems to be reflected in his angels for the Assisi galleries. It is more difficult to determine where Cimabue could have become acquainted with the provincial current of neo-Hellenism. Possibly he had traveled to the Balkans; he may also have seen some of the finest provincial neo-Hellenistic works in the vicinity of Rome, in the crypt of the Cathedral of Anagni: Christ as Pantokrator, episodes from the story of Samuel, and other scenes. The dramatically expressive Balkan frescoes were the nearest prototypes of the Anagni linear energy and "impressionist" vigor of modeling. Had Cimabue no direct knowledge of Anagni, however, he may well have been influenced by the celebrated S. Martino panel at Pisa, which was in turn influenced (according to Longhi) by the Anagni Master. Cimabue probably saw the panel between 1280 and 1285, before beginning the Sta Trinita *Madonna* (PLS. 322, 323).

Cimabue's training was not exclusively Byzantine, however. His art is deeply rooted in the most Westernized aspects of the Florentine Duecento, which are exemplified by the Master of S. Michele of Vico l'Abate, Coppo di Marcovaldo, and the Florence Baptistery mosaicists, inspired in their turn by the Venetian masters (see ROMANESQUE ART). In Cimabue's Sta Trinita *Madonna* and in his *Crucifix* (PL. 320) in Arezzo may be seen the system of modeling draperies by means of a delicate network of gold highlights which Coppo di Marcovaldo, evidently attracted by mosaics, had introduced into Tuscany in such works as the *Madonna del Bordone* for the Church of

S. Maria dei Servi in Siena and his *Madonna* for the Servites in Orvieto. More important influences of Coppo, however, are his use of incisive contours (which characterize Cimabue's early works) and the dialectical relationship between a figure mass that is locked into the background plane and the elementary three-dimensionality of the throne; this relationship is responsible for much of the Sta Trinita *Madonna's* expressive power. Thus through Coppo and, beyond him, the Masters of S. Michele and S. Francesco Bardi, Cimabue draws on that current in Byzantine painting which had translated an already strongly Westernized Byzantine language into a Romance dialect. While this new vernacular was intense, imaginative, and capable of giving form to vigorous feeling, it was harsh and primitive in its vehemence. Cimabue raised it to the status of a valid artistic language, subjecting it to new standards of dignity in order to express his own religious pathos, which, while wholly Christian in content, was no less somber than Greek tragedy.

Cimabue's earliest artistic activity, so far as we know, is his participation in the cupola mosaics of the Florence Baptistery. Toesca and Salmi have traced his rather sporadic activity there in the scenes (designed by others) representing *Joseph Sold into Egypt*, the *Lament of Joseph's Parents*, and the *Naming of the Baptist*. It must have been at the same time, if not earlier, that Cimabue painted the *Crucifix* in Arezzo (PL. 320). Since he worked in Arezzo alone and with entire freedom, the *Crucifix* is of a much higher quality, but it shares with the mosaic of *Joseph Sold into Egypt* a plasticity effected by means of violent chiaroscuro and an incisive strength of contour. In the Arezzo *Crucifix* Cimabue used a Byzantine system of proportions not unlike Giunta Pisano's, but the urgency of a new approach forced him dangerously close to the extreme limit of elasticity. Whereas in Giunta's figure the melodic sweep ends with the weary rest of the head in the arc of the halo, in Cimabue's Christ an austere, sharply defined silhouette seems to prevent the form from fully emerging, while the head falls back on the shoulder with a forceful dissonance.

If this work represents the youthful Cimabue's art, then Longhi was probably incorrect in attributing to Cimabue's early activity two works in a rather different style: the little *Maestà* in the Contini Bonacossi Collection, Florence (Garrison, no. 251A; Florentine, ca. 1285–95) and four other little pictures (Florence, Coll. Longhi, no. 668; Milan, priv. coll., no. 676; Washington, Nat. Gall., Kress Coll., nos. 703, 704; Venetian, ca. 1315–35).

The Sta Trinita *Madonna*, now in the Uffizi (PLS. 322, 323), must be placed rather later, about 1285 or after. It may possibly have been done in 1285 in rivalry with Duccio, who was just then working on his *Rucellai Madonna* (IV, PL. 286) for S. Maria Novella. However, 1288–90 is more likely, for the awesome majesty of the image and its dominating power point directly to the Assisi frescoes. Key to the *Madonna's* power is the latent dynamism contained within its austere, controlled structure. The throne is depicted with only a summary indication of depth which in no way mars the compactness of the mass. The figures are held in tense immobility. They possess a sense of weight, but the relief suggested by their chiaroscuro modeling is abruptly negated by the firm, if restless, contour line. Within the symmetrical framework of the composition surges a dramatic excitement most evident in the magnificent busts of prophets on the base of the throne.

Following close upon the Sta Trinita *Madonna* are the frescoes in the Upper Church at Assisi, where Cimabue probably began working in 1288 (see above). It is now generally agreed among critics that the artist was responsible for the Evangelists in the cross vaults; for the scenes of the Apocalypse, the *Last Judgment*, and the *Crucifixion* in the left arm of the transept (PLS. 325, 326); the angels and archangels (done with some assistance) in the galleries; scenes from the life of the Virgin in the apse (PL. 324); and two episodes from the story of St. Peter in the right arm of the transept (the *Blinding of Ananias* and the *Miracle of the Lame Man*). The remaining scenes from the life of St. Peter are by an anonymous follower, as is the second *Crucifixion*, still assigned by Toesca to Cimabue. Longhi's attempt to identify the young Duccio as one of Cima-

bue's collaborators in the cycle has been rejected by other scholars (Toesca, Coletti, Brandi). An overwhelming sense of boundless, turbulent space pervades the Apocalyptic scenes, and the figures move in an abrupt rhythm of stiff, broken lines. In the *Crucifixion*, tragedy on a cosmic scale is suggested by the contrast between the void surrounding the towering Christ and the compact wall of spectators below. The tension slackens in some of the figures, however, and the group of the Holy Women and St. John is composed with a mournful, elegiac harmony of line in a remarkable synthesis of Western expressionism and muted Byzantine rhythm. A more intimate lyricism prevails in the episodes concerning the Virgin and in the two scenes from the story of St. Peter.

Another wholly authentic work, the Sta Croce *Crucifix* (PL. 321; Mus. dell'Opera di Sta Croce), shows the artist moving away from the style of both the Arezzo *Crucifix* and the Christ in the Assisi *Crucifixion*. The forms are fused in a greater unity, and the composition is broader in conception. A more convincing plasticity results from the chiaroscuro modeling no longer contradicted by linear highlights. Though a calmer work, the fresco still pulsates with intensity. These qualities can belong only to a phase later than that of the frescoes in the Upper Church of Assisi, which are characterized by a harder line and less subtly modulated plasticity. The fresco of *The Madonna Enthroned with St. Francis* in the Lower Church in Assisi (PL. 328) belongs to the time of the Sta Croce *Crucifix*, probably not before 1295; those parts least reworked by a 19th-century brush show the same dense impasto. The theory that Cimabue was then following the young Giotto in using more ample and tranquil forms must be accepted very cautiously; and Ragghianti's proposed attribution of the oldest frescoes of the Cappella dei Velluti in Sta Croce to Cimabue does not seem correct. The Sta Croce frescoes show an overlay of Cimabuesque pathos on a quiet drama suggestive of Giotto, in a spirit quite different from both the impetuous grandeur of the Florentine *Crucifix* and the cold severity of the *Maestà* of St. Francis in Pisa, now in the Louvre.

Though Longhi has proposed a later date for the Louvre *Maestà*, it cannot be very far removed from the mosaic of St. John in the Cathedral of Pisa (1301–02; PL. 327); it possesses the same tranquil design, the same controlled articulation of planes. The fact that the figure derives its sculptural modeling from Nicola Pisano, or better, Arnolfo di Cambio (cf. the De Bray *Madonna* in S. Domenico, Orvieto, 1282; I, PL. 456), gives us some inkling of its date. Its classicism is in the Roman vein and quite different from the Hellenizing classicism of the Byzantine tradition that mingles with Western vigor in the Sta Trinita *Madonna* and the Assisi frescoes. Cimabue's later works were marred by academicism and an unwonted lack of expressive vitality. In these, followed by shop and school works such as the *Madonna* of the Bologna Pinacoteca, the big Contini *Madonna* (Florence, Coll. Contini Bonacossi), and the Washington-Chambéry polyptych (Washington, Nat. Gall.), it is apparent that at the dawn of the new century the artist had indeed outlived his talent. His vain attempts to emulate the modernism of his great disciple, Giotto, by drawing inspiration from Pisan sculpture may well have hastened the moment when Giotto's ascendency was to obscure his fame.

SOURCES AND CRITICISM. Cimabue's first appearance in the literature of art is both casual and solemn. Dante's famous terzina introducing him as one example among many of the "transient glory of human power" establishes Cimabue's unique position as the patriarch of Italian painting. Nothing substantial is added by the brief references of 14th-century commentators on the *Commedia*; even the observation made in the *Ottimo Commento* concerning the painter's "arrogant" and "disdainful" character seems to have been derived from Dante, since Cimabue's name appears in the canto concerning the vainglorious (*L'Ottimo Commento della Divina Commedia*, ed. A. Torri, II, Pisa, 1828, p. 188). Cimabue's glory as the greatest master of a bygone age appears dimmed in the passage from Sacchetti's *novella* number 136, where he is grouped with Stefano, Daddi, and Buffalmacco. He is referred to again as the grand patriarch, however, by Filippo Villani, who describes him as the painter who first recalled art to the task of imitating nature, thus opening the way for Giotto. The first mention of Giotto as Cimabue's disciple is in a late-14th- or

early-15th-century commentary on Dante by an anonymous Florentine; the poetic legend of their meeting in the pastures of the Mugello Valley does not appear until later, sketched by Ghiberti and, still later, narrated at length by Vasari. In 1480 Landino repeats Villani's estimate of Cimabue as one of the earliest naturalists, with a suggestion of Humanistic rationalism (C. Landino, *Epilogo*, 1480, in K. Frey, *Codex Magliabechiano*, Berlin, 1892, p. 119).

It is not until the 16th century that a few of Cimabue's works are mentioned in the sources. In 1510 Albertini's *Memoriale* attributes to Cimabue the *Rucellai Madonna* of S. Maria Novella ("a very large painting") and the Sta Croce *Crucifix*. A little later, the *Libro di Antonio Billi* (in the older version of the *Codex Strotianus*) and the Anonimo Gaddiano, which probably derives from it, offer the following catalogue: the *Rucellai Madonna*, the panel of St. Francis in S. Francesco in Pisa, frescoes (lost) in the cloister of Sto Spirito in Florence, works (lost) in the parish church at Empoli, decorations in the Basilica of S. Francesco in Assisi. Gelli, about 1550, omits the parish church at Empoli but adds an altarpiece with a St. Cecilia. Finally, Vasari, who in the 1550 edition adds to the Anonimo Gaddiano's list the *St. Cecilia* mentioned by Gelli and a *Madonna* in Sta Croce, gives a fuller list in the separate version of 1564 and in the definitive 1568 edition. This includes, together with the works already mentioned and several more lost works (frescoes in the Ospedale del Porcellana in Florence, a panel of St. Agnes in S. Paolo a Ripa in Pisa, and a small panel of the *Crucifixion* in S. Francesco in Pisa), the Sta Trinita *Madonna*, the *Madonna* of S. Francesco in Pisa, the Sta Croce *Crucifix*, the St. Francis panel in Sta Croce, and a long series of frescoes in the Upper and Lower Churches at Assisi.

Vasari considers Cimabue a disciple of the "Greek masters," seeing the origin of his style in late Italo-Byzantine paintings; but he also acknowledges his merit in having brought "great perfection to art, eliminating . . . a large part of its awkward manner," so that Cimabue was among the first great examples of the revival of the art of painting. This — in substance, Filippo Villani's evaluation — is all the more weighty because the biography of Cimabue is the very first of Vasari's artist biographies. The evaluation is further emphasized by the dramatic note on which Vasari takes up Villani's reference to the decadence of painting.

Cimabue has maintained his position as patriarch of Italian painting up to our time, despite the attempts of 18th-century provincial scholars to diminish his fame by investigating the work of older painters in Siena or Pisa. Without denying the enriched historical framework resulting from this research, Lanzi has placed it in proper perspective. Giving due appreciation to Giunta Pisano and Guido da Siena, Lanzi nonetheless recognized in Cimabue the first great painter of the 13th century — "the Michelangelo . . . of that age" — and outlined a stylistic profile which reveals his acute understanding of the artist.

During the 19th century little was added, either factually or critically, to our knowledge of Cimabue's art until, first, the Assisi frescoes were classified stylistically by such scholars as Cavalcaselle, Thode, Strzygowski, Aubert, Frey, and Venturi, and, second, the Pisan documents were discovered, making it possible to isolate, from the mass of works handed down in the sources, a homogeneous group consistent with the documented Pisan mosaic. This group forms the point of departure for subsequent efforts to define Cimabue's personality; but the subject of the historical significance and artistic value of his work, which has attracted the attention of many major scholars stimulated by the revival of interest in the 13th century, has by no means been exhausted.

BIBLIOG. Dante, Purgatorio, can. XI, vv. 94–96, and early commentaries on the Divina Commedia; F. Sacchetti, Novelle, no. 136; L'Ottimo Commento della Divina Commedia, II, ed. A. Torri, Pisa, 1828, p. 188; F. Villani, De civitate Florentiae et eiusdem famosis civibus (ca. 1400), ed. K. Frey, Berlin, 1892; L. Ghiberti, I Commentari (ca. 1455), ed. O. Morisani, Naples, 1947; F. Albertini, Memoriale di molte statue e pitture della città di Firenze, Florence, 1510; Libro di Antonio Billi (ca. 1516–30), ed. K. Frey, Berlin, 1892; Anonimo Gaddiano, ed. C. von Fabriczy, ASI, 1892; G. Gelli, Vite (ca. 1550), ed. G. Mancini, ASI, 1896, p. 38; G. Vasari, Vite, Florence, 1568 (ed. K. Frey, I, part 1, Munich, 1911, pp. 389–462; Am. ed., trans. E. H. and E. Blashfield and A. A. Hopkins, 4 vols., New York, 1913); F. Baldinucci, Notizie, I, Florence, 1681, pp. 1–17; L. Lanzi, Storia pittorica, Bassano, 1789; G. B. Cavalcaselle and J. A. Crowe, A History of Painting in Italy, ed. L. Douglas, I, London, 1923; H. Thode, Franz von Assisi und die Anfänge der Kunst der Renaissance in Italien, Berlin, 1885; J. Strzygowski, Cimabue und Rom, Vienna, 1888; F. Wickhoff, Über die Zeit des Guido von Siena, Mitteilungen des Instituts für oesterreichische Geschichtsforschung, 1889; G. Trenta, I musaici del duomo di Pisa, Florence, 1896; L. Tanfani Centofanti, Notizie d'artisti, Pisa, 1897; M. G. Zimmermann, Giotto und die Kunst Italiens in Mittelalter, Leipzig, 1899; A. Venturi, Storia dell'arte italiana, V, Milan, 1901–39, p. 195 ff.; J. B. Supino, Arte pisana, Florence, 1904; M. Aubert, Ein Beitrag zur Lösung des Cimabue Frage, Leipzig, 1907; E. Benkard, Das literarische Porträt des Giovanni Cimabue, Munich, 1917; O. Sirén, Toskanische Maler im XIII. Jahrhundert, Berlin, 1922; Van Marle; J. B. Supino, La basilica di

San Francesco in Assisi, Bologna, 1924; A. Chiappelli, Arte del rinascimento, Rome, 1925; Toesca, Md; E. Sandburg-Vavalà, La croce dipinta italiana, Verona, 1929; C. Soulier, Cimabue, Duccio..., Paris, 1929; P. Toesca, Florentine Painting of the Trecento, New York, 1929; M. Salmi, I mosaici del "Bel San Giovanni" e la pittura del secolo XIII a Firenze, Dedalo, XXVIII, 1930-31, pp. 543-70; A. Nicholson, Cimabue, Princeton, 1932; M. Salmi, Per il completamento di un trittico cimabuesco, RArte, XVII, 1935, p. 113 ff.; E. Cecchi, Giotto, Milan, 1937; L. Coletti, I Primitivi, Novara, 1941; P. Toesca, Giotto, Turin, 1941; G. Sinibaldi and G. Brunetti, Pittura toscana del Duecento: Catalogo della mostra giottesca di Firenze del 1937, Florence, 1944; R. Salvini, Cimabue, Rome, 1946; R. Longhi, Giudizio sul Duecento, Proporzioni, II, 1948, pp. 5-55; L. Coletti, Affreschi della Basilica di Assisi, Bergamo, 1949; E. H. Garrison, Italian Romanesque Panel Painting, Florence, 1949; R. Salvini, Postilla a Cimabue, RArte, XXVI, 1950, pp. 43-60; C. Brandi, Duccio, Florence, 1951; R. Longhi, Prima Cimabue poi Duccio, Paragone, II, 1951, pp. 8-13; R. Örtel, Frühzeit der italienischen Malerei, Stuttgart, 1953; M. Meiss, Ancora una volta Duccio e Cimabue, RArte, XXX, 1955, pp. 107-113; C. L. Ragghianti, Pittura del Dugento a Firenze, Florence, 1955; S. Samek-Ludovici, Cimabue, Milan, 1956.

Roberto SALVINI

Illustrations : PLS. 320-328.

**CIMA DA CONEGLIANO.** Italian painter of the Venetian school, known also as Giovanni Battista Cima (b. Conegliano, ca. 1459, d. Venice, ca. 1517). Berenson maintains that Cima was probably a pupil of Alvise Vivarini, but Rudolf Burckhardt in his monograph on the painter argues for Bartolommeo Montagna. However, there is no question that Cima was much influenced by Giovanni Bellini (see BELLINI). The influence of Antonello da Messina in his early work and Giorgione in his later work has also been noted.

The *Madonna under a Trellis*, a tempera painting of 1489 (Vicenza, Mus. Civ.), antedates the painter's arrival in Venice, which we must assume occurred sometime between 1489 and 1492, for in the latter year, apropos of the altarpiece in the Duomo of Conegliano, he is referred to as " pictor eximius Venetiis" ("outstanding Venetian painter").

The well-known *Baptism of Christ* (Venice, S. Giovanni in Bragora) was commissioned in 1492 and probably finished in 1494. (Payments are noted in 1495.) With this painting Cima turned to the new fashionable oil technique. To the same period belongs the *St. John the Baptist with Four Saints* (S. Maria dell'Orto), so much admired by Ruskin.

In the middle period of Cima's career (1497-1509), we observe an increasing interest in light and atmosphere, but in his last years he turns again to full-bodied color. Architecture, important at the beginning of Cima's artistic activity, was gradually subordinated, along with landscape, to the role of distant decorative background to the figures. In the middle period the following paintings are noteworthy: *Madonna with Six Saints* (Venice, Accademia ca. 1496-99), *Constantine and Helena* (Venice, S. Giovanni in Bragora, 1501), and the *Madonna with Six Saints* (Parma, Gall. Naz., probably ca. 1507).

To the late period (1509-17) belong the *Madonna with Two Saints* in the Louvre (ca. 1513), the *Doubting Thomas with Magnus* (Venice, Accademia), and *Peter Enthroned* of 1516 (the last of the dated pictures; Milan, Brera).

Cima was essentially a conservative painter, entirely Quattrocento in feeling. In no sense was he a pioneer or transitional master; but he was full of charm and sunny, serene Venetian feeling and perhaps ranks first among the painters influenced by Bellini.

BIBLIOG. D. V. Botteon and A. Aliprandi, Ricerche intorno alla vita e alle opere di Giambattista Cima, Conegliano, 1893; R. Burckhardt, Cima da Conegliano, Lepizig, 1905.

Arthur McCOMB

**CINEMATOGRAPHY.** The cinema is considered here from a strictly esthetic point of view as an independent form of expression related to the representational arts. We are not concerned with the film as a technical device permitting images to be reproduced in continuous motion, with the simultaneous recording of sound, or with the special effects of which it is capable, such as accelerated and slow motion, superposition, etc. (The practical considerations are substantially the same whether the film deals with the visual arts or with scientific research and apply equally to documentaries made for cultural and for didactic purposes.) We shall no more than mention the prototypes for the cinematic medium — the various attempts made throughout the history of art to represent movement, cited in every history of the cinema: such pictorial forms of expression as Egyptian papyri, the bas-reliefs on Roman columns, medieval fresco cycles (PL. 329).

The film as an artistic language presents three main problems: (1) the influence of the representational arts on the particular idiom of the film as it evolved and became aware of its autonomy; (2) the importance of the representational arts as source and inspiration, and as a significant cultural factor affecting the personal style of the director; and (3) the relation between the language of the film and that of the representational arts, specifically with regard to documentary films on art.

To deal with such problems obviously requires an exact knowledge of the expressive means peculiar to the film, for it is through these that the film becomes what it is: narration but not narrative, spectacle but not theater, a predominantly visual art but not painting, a medium that is divided by rhythmic tempo but is not music. Nourished and taught as it is by all these other art forms, film is an independent art medium only in so far as it is able to resolve, or rather to absorb, them within itself without any perceptible residue. Moreover, it is a poetic language (an observation that will have particular relevance for our discussion of its relation to the representational arts), and thus, as Balázs (1952) has rightly observed, by its very nature it lacks the capacity of prose, understood as "non-art," to communicate abstract or purely rational concepts.

While rejecting the thesis that the cinema is one of the representational arts, we cannot deny that the visual aspect is predominant even in sound films, which inextricably combine dialogue, sound effects, and music with the image. But the film image should not be confused with the individual pictorial unit, or "frame," nor the latter with the sectional picture, or "shot," made up of a series of individual frames taken from a single point of view that produce the effect of motion when projected in rapid succession. "Still" photographs used to illustrate critical or historical essays on the motion picture are far less adequate as documentation than reproductions in art books, even where such photographs illustrate the pictorial aspects of a single film. In fact, a still which in itself is beautifully composed and lighted, to the point of resembling a masterpiece of painting, may be taken from a very mediocre film. On the other hand, a still that seems completely insignificant when seen in isolation may form part of a film of the highest artistic quality. Such paradoxes tend to perpetuate the confusion between the pictorial values of the film and its intrinsic visual qualities. Several of the early theoretical writers on film were prone, as Balázs has admitted, to fall into this confusion, applying to the cinema creative principles proper to the representational arts.

The techniques peculiar to the film are the "shot" and the "montage," or editing, that combines and assembles the shots into sequences. The total film image is dynamic because it is produced by the combining of several shots each having (usually) an internal movement that links it to the movement of the shots that precede and follow it. In the absence of such a link, that is, when no internal movement is apparent, the film image is made dynamic by editing — by juxtaposing a series of related shots, each of which appears on the screen for a given length of time. Even the filming of an actual production, such as a concert, a play, or a work of art, does not result in a mere reproduction of the original; editing has idealized the actual extent in space and duration in time. The individual shots, whose photographic values of composition and lighting are usually isolated for purposes of comparison with painting, are elements of the film image which, for all their dependence on photographic techniques, cannot be equated with photography. Because of the various camera angles from which individual shots can be taken, and the mobility of the camera, the film image abolishes the spectator's sense of detachment. But editing, continually overcoming the limitations of shots taken from a single point of view, carries the spectator into the film's own space: he gradually identifies

himself with the characters, seeing Romeo through the eyes of Juliet and Juliet through the eyes of Romeo. These possibilities for participation and identification are characteristic of the film image, which, being composed of shots projected for a given duration, divides the presentation into rhythmic sequences.

Like a painting, a film image is two-dimensional; but in addition to perspective, convergence of lines, variations in tonal values and in light and shade, it has movement to give it depth and a third dimension: the movement of the camera, which can travel through the space represented and carry the spectator along with it, and the movement of people, of objects, and of light and shade. To illustrate, for a film image resembling Pieter de Hooch's painting *The Mother* (a woman seated in shadow in the foreground beside a door opening on a lighted room in the background, from which a little girl approaches, followed by a dog) the effect of depth would be produced by the movement not only of the child and the dog but also of the ray of light falling through the open door.

To continue the comparison, the format of each frame in the film is fixed; the relation between height and width cannot be varied as in painting, to achieve more striking effects of vertical composition, and even with the use of a giant screen the shape is always a horizontal rectangle. Moreover, whereas a painting, whether framed or not, has fixed boundaries, the mobility of the camera tends to make the screen appear to extend beyond its actual dimensions.

Enough has been said on the expressive vocabulary of the film to indicate the differences between the problems of the motion picture and those of painting with regard to composition and lighting. A shot that in isolation may seem out of balance may be justified either by the movement of the camera, designed to suggest a lack of equilibrium, or by a succeeding shot that provides a deliberate contrast. Shots with a "closed," or self-contained, composition, like paintings, lack this reciprocity; the resulting film image seems shattered into a number of separate visual details. Thus it can be seen that the influence of painting on the film — as of literature and the stage — has been, and still is, negative as well as positive.

At the outset the cinema was no more than a remarkable technique for photographing and reproducing movement — a kind of side-show novelty. Any subject whatsoever (a city street with its traffic, a beach crowded with bathers, a group of workers leaving the factory) provided a pretext for turning out a few feet of film capable of exciting the public and the press. It was not until later that films of current events or important personages were taken, and the idea developed of presenting brief stories in a rudimentary form.

The fantasies made between 1899 and 1906 by Georges Méliès may be mentioned here merely as curiosities. Méliès, who had all his films colored by hand by the painter Thuillier, "certainly invented almost all the tricks or special effects of the film, but used them as a substitute for theatrical effects rather than as the expressive means peculiar to the newborn language of the film" (Paolella). The first attempts to raise the level of film spectacles were made under the influence of literature and the representational arts. Since the camera was regarded as nothing more than a mechanical means of reproduction (it was, in fact, operated from a fixed position), the film's artistic quality depended on the way in which the material was arranged and on the caliber of the photography. Thus the scene of the Last Supper in a French film, *The Life and Passion of Our Lord Jesus Christ* (Pathé, 1904), imitates Leonardo's painting. In 1905 the director Victorin Jasset produced for the Gaumont studios a life of Christ inspired by the color lithographs of the painter James Tissot, who had brought back many "artistic impressions" from a visit to Palestine; the release issued by the producer referred to the film as a plastic art "capable of creating by light and motion compositional qualities and beautiful effects not inferior to a painting by Millet or a fresco by Puvis de Chavannes." Thus in those early years the film was erroneously conceived of as pictorial because of its relation to the representational arts (PL. 330), and as literary or dramatic because of its dependence on novels, plays, or theatrical spectacles. René Clair has justly observed that if during this period more thought

had been given to the film's commercial than to its artistic aspects, it would have made more rapid progress even from the point of view of art. As a matter of fact, the film became articulate when it concerned itself, not with esthetic ideals, but with content — in other words, when it was impelled to address its public with the greatest expressive intensity. The work of the American director D. W. Griffith was highly significant in this evolution, as is best demonstrated by his film *Intolerance* (1916). But even adventure and gangster films produced with purely commercial intentions contributed, in the course of seeking effects of emotion and suspense, to the development of the film idiom.

The connection between the cinema and the representational arts is not limited to the early naïve contacts between them. Undoubtedly the film found many valuable precedents in painting. As has often been observed, it is a product of the same demands as impressionism and shows many analogies with that movement and the ones succeeding it (PL. 331). The bond between the two media is not only one of close parallels between certain stills and particular paintings — often the result of a hyperintellectual estheticism. It also involves a more diffused influence manifested in a specific "way of seeing." The "true to life" theory of impressionism, which sought to capture fleeting moments of reality by such devices as daring points of view or compositions without fixed boundaries, undoubtedly influenced film makers; it helped them discover the expressive, evocative value of shots that transformed the camera from a passive recording mechanism into an instrument of expression. The great masters of light, from Caravaggio to Rembrandt, also taught them what could be achieved through lighting. There were other ways too, in which painting exerted an influence on film, sometimes indirectly through other forms such as the theatrical spectacle (Max Reinhardt provides a significant example). As film gradually evolved its independent point of view and its own mode of expression, it outgrew imitative relations of this sort. Comparisons with the representational arts become difficult or even impossible in connection with a consummate artist such as Charlie Chaplin or important movements in film history such as Russian post-revolutionary realism or Italian neorealism. At its highest level of expression, film retains no traces of cultural precedents, for the spontaneous genius of the artist has absorbed these along with the rest of his visual heritage, and they have left on his work no imprint that can be isolated.

More direct connections with the representational arts are evident in the movement known as "avant-garde cinema," which flourished between 1916 and 1930 and combined currents from many schools of modern painting — expressionism, futurism, Dada, surrealism, abstraction, etc. In general this movement found its outlet in shorts, usually produced by painters and sculptors, frequently in collaboration with writers and poets. These experimental films made a significant contribution to the development of cinematic techniques and also served to win recognition for the film as an art form among an international circle of intellectuals.

The various currents of the avant-garde were, however, destined to exhaust themselves because the film could not absorb them. Yet the movement fulfilled a function, albeit a negative one, "since, whenever it becomes obvious that something is absurd, a limit is established that indicates a path along which it is impossible to proceed. The prudent who never look further than their own noses and never risk anything are not the ones who carry us forward" (Balázs). The course that by its very nature film had to follow lay in the direction of realism — not in the sense of a given movement or school, but in the sense that, even with editing, which can provide a certain subjective quality, film still does not involve (or even permit) the creation, alteration, or distortion of objects. This can be demonstrated clearly by the phenomenon of expressionism, the only one of the avant-garde movements to have had a direct influence on commercial films. *The Cabinet of Dr. Caligari* (1919; PL. 333), directed by Robert Wiene, is perhaps the only totally expressionist film; it marks the earliest flourishing of the art film in Germany. Actually this film presents a certain ambiguity, for its expressiveness is attained not through the camera but through the settings ("Films should be drawings brought to life," wrote the painter

Hermann Warm while he was creating the sets for *Caligari*), and through a certain distortion in the figures. This film nevertheless served to emphasize the need for expressiveness rather than for the flatly objective type of photography then in vogue everywhere, especially in Germany. Out of recognition for this need there developed the so-called *Kammerspielfilm*, of which Fred W. Murnau's *The Last Laugh* (*Der letzte Mann*, 1925), is the prime example. Following *Variety* (1925) by E.A. Dupont, whose "impressionism... shows traces of the expressionist abstraction from which it derives" (Eisner), this movement attained full maturity in "German realism."

As the film evolved, its sets and scenery came to depend more on architecture than on painting, because the movement of the camera in space gradually imposed its own three-dimensional requirements on the settings.

Surrealism, too, despite the faith of its followers ("The essence of the film is surrealism.... The film shall be surrealist" are the opening and closing statements of Kyrou's 1953 book on the surrealist film), is now extinct, although at its apogee it produced some interesting shorts. It left its traces on the commercial film, however, in dream sequences and in passages purporting to reveal the subconscious or the hidden workings of the soul. Advertising films also frequently make use of the devices of abstraction.

Faint echoes of these movements persisted in the United States, where production of avant-garde films began somewhat later than in Europe, principally as the output of refugees from Nazi Germany. Experimental films have a significant role not only because of their actual influence on the cinema but because of their frequent close connections with the representational arts; in fact, experiments made in painting often seem to find their extension in film. Avant-garde films are essential documents that must be included in any study of the evolution of modern movements in art.

A separate question is the influence exerted by the representational arts on individual directors. For some — Carl Dreyer, Luchino Visconti, G. W. Pabst, and Sergei Eisenstein, to cite only the most outstanding — it was a fundamental factor in the formation of their artistic personalities; their work reveals a refined taste and a concern with the formal values of the representational arts. In a single film one may perceive traces of Giotto, the Flemish school, Caravaggio, and Daumier, all assimilated into a coherent style that endows the work with complete unity; tracing these sources helps us reconstruct the formation of a director's personal style. The defects of such direction are not so much those of direct dependence on particular paintings or artists as of an excessive estheticism that tends to congeal portions of the film by disrupting the unity and rhythmic flow of the film image. This pictorial ambiguity is the consequence of a formalistic concept of art, which whenever it becomes apparent in film is inevitably a contradiction of the medium's true nature.

Thus the limitations of Visconti's *The Earth Trembles* (1948) are inherent in his adoption of certain pictorial devices that drain the film image of its dramatic impact. For example, in the scene that shows the fishermen's wives awaiting their husbands' return during a dangerous storm, the emphasis on the women silhouetted against the leaden sky and the white foam of the agitated sea, their black shawls blown about by the wind, breaks the tension through a labored seeking for the picturesque. The rhythm of the montage is lost. By contrast, every shot in Eisenstein's *Battleship Potemkin* (1925) has extraordinary impact; this is because the reciprocal relation of each shot to the preceding and following shots is such as to produce maximum dramatic expressiveness. The same contrast exists between Pabst's *Don Quixote* (1933; PL. 335), in which pictorialism sometimes dominates the event, and his *Tragedy of the Mine* (*Kameradschaft*, 1931), in which his vast knowledge of the representational arts is always subordinate to the requirements of filmic expression. Dreyer's *Passion of Joan of Arc* (1928; PL. 335) is another admirable example of the successful assimilation of pictorial qualities, whereas his *Ordet* (*The World*, 1955) occasionally lapses into formalism.

Aside from the innumerable films with Biblical or classical subjects modeled on color lithographs, popular prints, and other kinds of debased painting, there are many films inspired by genuine art. Painting may assist not only in obtaining authenticity (obviously the representational arts provide the film with important source material for costumes) but also in re-creating the style or atmosphere of a given period. Yet the historical film frequently manifests a dichotomy between form and content. By its very nature it cannot transmute history into current events, or the past into the present; its intrinsic character is to exist only in the present ("Pictures have no tenses," as Balázs puts it). *The Battleship Potemkin* is in some respects the greatest and best-integrated example of the historical film. One of the salient characteristics of the style of Roberto Rossellini, a director extraordinarily endowed with the cinematographic instinct, is the striking sense of authenticity that he imparts not only to contemporary subjects (*Paisan*, 1944; *Open City*, 1946) but also to events of the past (*St. Francis, Minstrel of God*, 1950).

Separate consideration should be given to films consciously drawing inspiration from the world of painting, which actually becomes the essential content; Jacques Feyder's *Carnival in Flanders* and Laurence Olivier's *Henry V* (PL. 334) may be cited as examples. Yet, though these are works of the greatest refinement, they present weaknesses from both the pictorial and the cinematic point of view. Film is not drawing or painting brought to life; nor does painting of true vitality require added allure.

Not even in connection with animated films can one speak of "painting in motion," for in these the elements of narrative invention, rhythm, dynamically resolved discoveries, and the interplay of music, voices, and sound effects take precedence over the pictorial aspects. One of the greatest creators in this field, Walt Disney, has been called the "Raphael of bad taste"; though the epithet has a certain aptness, it is essentially unjust, because it is based on erroneous standards of judgment. One need only call attention to the influence that the representational arts have had on this genre to perceive the difference between drawing and animation. For example, Gustave Doré's illustration of the animated forest in the *Divine Comedy* inspired Disney's invention of humanized trees in *Snow White and the Seven Dwarfs* (1937–38). Generally such sources are fruitful in providing isolated themes, ideas, or suggestions rather than the form itself. The animated cartoon has won recognition as an independent medium from the time of its inventor Emile Cohl (whose *Fantasmagoria* was shown for the first time on Aug. 17, 1908) to the present; it has been used by such artists as Disney, Paul Grimault, Max Fleischer, and Norman McLaren.

Folk arts have exerted their influence chiefly on puppet films; the most celebrated are those produced by the Czech Jiří Trnka (PL. 336).

All that has been said applies equally to color films. Strictly cinematic solutions to the problems of color are very rare, and, understandably enough, the most valid are found in animation films. Even in the best examples influences from painting, frequently rendered banal by technical limitations which allow the director little control over the color, tend to prevail. Here, too, the most important factors are the interior dynamics of the shot — an actor's unexpected blush, the flame that suddenly blazes forth, the varying tints of the sunset — and the relation between the isolated shots brought out by editing. In V. I. Pudovkin's *Return of Vassili Bortnikov* (1953), for example, a sequence of fine color rhythms indicates the passage of winter into spring and then summer.

The problem of films on art has assumed growing importance since World War II. The great mass of documentaries, made either for purposes of instruction or as popularizations of certain artists or works, lack value as film and display a minimum of critical sense; a few art documentaries, however, demand serious study.

The best films on art have been made by film makers, such as Luciano Emmer, Alain Resnais, and Jean Grémillon, who use works of art either for the dramatic development of the narrative content, or to portray the customs of a period, tell the story of

a celebrated personality or family, or set forth ideological or psychological conflicts. In other words, they use works of art as the plastic material out of which they construct an independent, autonomous work — the film — that has a meaning of its own closely connected with the director's artistic personality. Thus Emmer's and Enrico Gras's *Drama of the Son of Man* (1941), based on Giotto's frescoes in the Arena Chapel at Padua, is not a work of art criticism but serves to convey the emotions of the director as he contemplates these marvelous paintings. The poetry of Resnais's *Van Gogh* (1947) is a result of the director's ability to communicate the emotion he feels when confronting the work of a great master. It is natural that in such films the language of painting should be absorbed into the means appropriate to the film. The image is limited in a fresco by a wall, vault, or lunette, and in a painting by the dimensions of the canvas, and thus it becomes one object among other objects; but in the film all such spatial limitations are wiped out or annulled by the element of time (introduced by the movement of the camera and the montage), so that the illusion of a third dimension is created by specifically filmic means. The distance, or rather detachment, of the spectator from the fresco or painting is obliterated, calling to mind the old Chinese legend of the artist who became so fascinated by a mountain range in the background of a landscape he was painting that one day he entered the painting and vanished behind the mountains.

The illusion of movement can be produced by traveling shots ("panning" with a sideways motion or moving toward or away from the subject on a dolly); thus in Emmer's *Festa di S. Isidoro* (1950), based on works by Goya, the camera was oscillated to convey the motion of a seesaw. Through montage, different planes in a picture can be combined to achieve quite unexpected expressive effects. In *Van Gogh*, Resnais utilizes details taken from different paintings; for example, he cuts directly from the full figure of a peasant woman seen from behind to a shot of the same woman viewed from the front and almost in the foreground. In the same film the director shows us the exterior of the house at Arles, moving his camera forward toward a half-closed window of the artist's room until it is seen in isolation; then he cuts directly to a shot of the inside of the same window and slowly lets the camera travel backward until the whole interior is revealed — thus creating a unique effect achievable only by the film.

The effectiveness of such procedures, which, however, are often strongly and with some reason condemned by art critics, depends on the training and artistic sensibility of the director, on his taste and his capacity to understand the spirit of the artist or the work of art. Though not in a strict sense works of criticism, films on art may often be as illuminating as the felicitous metaphor of the art critic. The translation from one medium to another is always arbitrary; it is justifiable only when it is not a facile trick but a means of communicating a deep and personal emotion.

If the films on art thus far discussed tend to sacrifice pictorial elements, films of a predominantly critical character — styled "crito-films" by Carlo L. Ragghianti — must confront the problem of mastering the essential film language. This cannot be achieved by interpolating purely external devices, such as slides and photographs, though sometimes it may be necessary to use these in order to achieve results not obtainable otherwise. (We are not referring to the entirely legitimate use of these devices in documentary films such as those of U. Barbaro and R. Longhi on Carpaccio, 1947, and Caravaggio, 1948, which were made to serve as practical substitutes for slides and lectures and are marked by rigorous scholarship.)

The documentary film on art must face the serious problem of achieving a truly valid film idiom; very few worthwhile films have been produced in this genre, which, however, is capable of further development. The difficulties are many; they would appear insurmountable did we not bear in mind that the film has not the same function as a photograph or a slide in reproducing a work of art and its details. The film must arrive at critical analysis through the means peculiar to it. All too frequently knowledge and awareness of the representational arts are not combined with an equal knowledge and understanding of the medium of film. The art critic usually lacks a command of cinema techniques, while the director often lacks the necessary knowledge of art history; only in rare instances does their collaboration achieve good results.

Furthermore, the different media of painting, sculpture, and architecture each present special problems. The last two, being three-dimensional, can of course take advantage of some of film's special resources. Thus in dealing with sculpture, the film, in contrast to photography, can show many points of view in continuous progression; for architecture, the movement of the camera in panning or dolly shots can render exterior and interior space in a way not possible through other means. The difficulties encountered with painting often stem from the critical method followed by the author of the film or from the character of the work of art itself or of the painter who is the object of the critical and esthetic analysis. It is far more difficult to pursue a formalistic method of criticism than to emphasize the content of the work of art or the historical environment in which the artist worked. Thus the analysis of a representational painting would seem to be easier than that of an abstract work.

It was pointed out at the outset that the idiom of the film is a poetic one. The problem of the "crito-film," therefore, is to discover how the specific elements of film (shots, montage, camera movements, dissolves, cutting from one image to the next, etc.) can be used expressively and yet in conformity with strict critical standards. The critic who would approach a work of art through the film needs above all the sensitivity and imagination to express in cinematic terms the insights that such an approach can reveal. This suggests that even if critics were to adopt the film as a practical means for teaching or expounding their views of art, they might not all be able to avail themselves of the enormous possibilities inherent in the poetic language that is film.

Luigi Chiarini

FILMS PRODUCED BY MODERN MOVEMENTS. An important chapter in the history of contemporary art (see EUROPEAN MODERN MOVEMENTS) comprises the films produced by painters and sculptors, often in collaboration with poets and writers. Nowadays these are regularly shown to members of private film societies and presented in programs at the principal museums of modern art, which often own copies. These films (chiefly shorts), frequently allied with specific art movements, may be divided into two main categories: those that stress the rhythmic organization of invented abstract forms, or freely manipulated actual objects, and those that seek to convey subconscious content through surrealistic devices. Even when these films have narrative themes, as they sometimes do, they are in marked contrast to the realistic type of storytelling that characterizes commercial film.

As early as 1913 a sequence of abstract rhythmic designs was painted by Léopold Survage, a Russian-born cubist painter living in Paris, to serve as the basis for a film; this project, however, was never realized. In Italy in 1916 A. G. Bragaglia directed *Perfido incanto*, in which distorted objects appear amid symbolic settings; and from the same year date the manifesto of futurist cinematography and the supposed collaboration of E. F. T. Marinetti and Valentine de Saint-Point on a film now lost.

The first actual experiments in abstract film were made in Germany, simultaneously by the Swedish painter Viking Eggeling (1880–1925) and the German painter Hans Richter (b. 1888). Eggeling had evolved sequences of abstract forms, or "themes," on isolated canvases or sheets of paper, which he called *Orchestration of the Line* (1917–18), while Richter, working independently, had been engaged in similar researches in plastic expression. They began to collaborate on abstract variations arranged on long scrolls; some of these sequences were then animated as films (Eggeling's *Diagonal Symphony*, completed in 1921 after a scroll painting begun in 1919, and Richter's *Prelude*, 1920). Abandoning the principle of animating scroll drawings, Richter began to make films based on the rhythmic counterpoint of the square or rectangular shapes provided by the screen itself, and produced *Rhythmus 21* (1921) and *Rhythmus 23* (1923); *Rhythmus 25* (1925) was based on a vertical scroll painting, *Orchestration of Color* (1923), and was colored by hand. In 1922 another German painter, Walter Ruttmann, began to produce a series of films that were improvisations on abstract forms (*Opus 1, 2, 3, 4,* etc.); his experiments were later to be continued in combination with musical compositions by his pupil Oskar Fischinger.

Richter became closely associated with other artists active in the Dada movement, among them Marcel Duchamp, Man Ray, and Francis Picabia. Consistent with Dada's "anti-art" spirit and its emphasis on the automatic, the mechanical, and the accidental was a technical invention by the German artist Raoul Hausmann — the "optophone," an instrument that produces on wires a kaleidoscope of abstract colored forms which it translates into music, and vice versa. In 1925 Hausmann collaborated with Kurt Schwitters on the scenario of a Dada film now lost. Marcel Duchamp, who had abandoned painting early in the 1920s but continued to be interested in the solution of dynamic problems, created "roto-reliefs," phonograph disks on which he drew concentric lines, and "sphères tournantes," rotating spheres on which were letters that combined to form phrases. These he filmed in alternation with real objects in his *Anemic Cinema* (1926); 20 years later he used a similar system when collaborating with Hans Richter and others on *Dreams That Money Can Buy*.

A number of other artists associated with the Dada movement created films. Man Ray, photographer as well as painter, made for a Dada soiree *Le Retour à la raison* (1923), in which the movements of a paper spiral alternate with abstract and rhythmic images. In 1927 he directed another Dada film, *Emak Bakia*, which he explained "aimed at representing aspects of the outer world and seemingly everyday actions in a poetic context by releasing them from all rational logic." René Clair, in collaboration with Duchamp and Picabia, made the celebrated short film *Entr'acte* (1924), which was commissioned for the ballet *Relâche* by Rolf Maré's Ballet Suédois and had a score by Erik Satie; it incorporates a burlesque funeral procession in a spirit typical of Dada's mocking wit.

The political tinge that Dada assumed in Berlin was reflected in Richter's *Inflation* (1927–28); this film, like his *Race Symphony* (1928–29), which deals with a horse race, was semidocumentary in form. He later made films dealing with social problems, among them *New Living* (1930), on the subject of modern housing, and *Metal* (1931–33), an anti-Nazi political film, and he produced for advertising and industry a number of publicity films such as *Twopenny Magic* (*Zweigroschenzauber*), made as a promotion piece for a Cologne newspaper. The masterpiece of Richter's German period is *Ghosts before Noon* (*Vormittagspuk*, 1927–28), with a score by Paul Hindemith, in which familiar objects — hats, ties, cups, etc. — rebel against their daily routine.

Many avant-garde film makers of the mid-twenties and thereafter followed the direction in which Eggeling, Richter, and Ruttmann had pioneered, concerning themselves principally with the rhythmic interplay of abstract forms, and disregarding content; others developed the irrational aspects of Dada and paved the way toward surrealism. In *Ballet mécanique* (1924), produced by Fernand Léger and Dudley Murphy, geometrical forms drawn or painted by Léger are interspersed with photographic images whose forms and movements are so drained of human content that they become as abstract as the inanimate objects surrounding them; the artist's concern is only with their plastic beauty and rhythmically composed motion. Henri Chomette, brother of René Clair, made films in the "pure," or "absolute," cinema tradition, among them *Crystals* (1925) and *Reflections and Speeds* (1926); somewhat similar in spirit was Eugène Deslaw's *March of the Machines* (1928). The preoccupation of such films with rhythm relates them closely to musical forms; in fact, the "absolute" films made in Germany and in the United States by Fischinger manipulate simple geometrical shapes — squares, circles, triangles — in changing patterns suggested by well-known musical compositions (*Studies*, 1928–32, a series of black-and-white abstractions set to compositions such as Paul Dukas's *Sorcerer's Apprentice*; from 1933 on, color abstractions such as *Allegretto*, set to jazz, *An American March*, set to Sousa's *Stars and Stripes Forever*, and *Composition in Blue*; PL. 332). Related to these but not limited to geometric forms are the films of abstract color paintings in motion by the British artist Len Lye (*Colour Box*, 1935; *Rainbow Dance*, 1936; *Swinging the Lambeth Walk*, 1940) and those of the Canadian Norman McLaren, who draws or paints abstract sequences directly on film and synchronizes them with music (*Stars and Stripes*, 1943; *Hoppity Pop* and *Little Phantasy*, 1946; *Dots, Loops, Fiddle-de-dee*, 1948; *Blinkety Blank*, 1955; etc.). In the films made by the American brothers James and John Whitney the screen is used to articulate all the possible variations on a single motif or combination of forms, and these are completed by sound produced synthetically on the sound track through the motion of automatic devices.

The surrealist film arose as a violent reaction against the exclusively formal preoccupation and the rationalism of "pure," or "absolute," cinema; developing the irrational aspects of Dada, it reasserted the importance of poetic content and material drawn from the subconscious. As early as 1922 some *Poèmes cinématographiques* had been planned by the poet Philippe Soupault, an editor of the review *Sic*; one of these was produced by Ruttmann. The first translation

of the visual imagery of a poem into film, however, seems to have been Man Ray's *L'Étoile de mer* (1928), based on verses by Robert Desnos. Man Ray followed this with a mock adventure film, *Les Mystères du Château de Dé* (1929), enacted by masked players, and in 1935 he filmed *Essai de simulation de délire cinématographique*, now lost, on a text provided by André Breton and Paul Eluard. The poet Antonin Artaud, who was also a scenarist and a theoretician and writer on the cinema, wrote the scenario for a psychological film, *The Seashell and the Clergyman* (1928), directed by Germaine Dulac; the poet and painter Jean Cocteau in 1930 produced the surrealistic feature film *The Blood of a Poet* (PL. 332). Belgians associated with the movement include Henri Storck, who produced some short films of surrealist character (*Pour vos beaux yeux*, 1928, the story of a pair of glass eyes, and, in collaboration with Félix Labisse, *La Mort de Vénus*, 1930), and the painter René Magritte, who with Roger Livet produced *Fleurs meurtriés* (ca. 1929).

The only surrealist to occupy himself systematically with the theory of the cinema was J. B. Brunius. He exerted a great influence on the film in France by actively collaborating in a number of productions, by campaigning for the acceptance of certain types of foreign films previously disregarded in France, and by himself producing some highly original works in the surrealist manner: *Elle est Bicimidine* (1927, in collaboration with E. Gréville); *Records 37*, an early effort to synchronize creatively film images, spoken words, music, and sound effects; *Violons d'Ingres*, which includes a sequence devoted to Henri Rousseau and is the first attempt to make a painting "come to life" in film; and a series of publicity films and documentaries (*Voyage aux Cyclades*, 1931; *Author d'une évasion*, 1933; *Venezuela*, 1937; *Somewhere to Live*, 1950; etc.).

Probably the greatest of the surrealist film makers is the Spaniard Luis Buñuel. In collaboration with Salvador Dali he produced *Un Chien andalou* (1928), filled with obsessive and violent images drawn from the subconscious, and the first full-length surrealist feature film, *L'Age d'or* (1930). Equal violence, and some of the same surrealist techniques, are to be found in Buñuel's later films, such as his semidocumentaries *Land without Bread* (*Las Hurdes*, 1932; reissued in 1937), made in collaboration with Pierre Unik and Elie Lothar and dealing with the disastrous conditions in one of the poorest and wildest regions of Spain, and *Los Olvidados* (1950), made in Mexico.

The more humorous aspects of the subconscious were explored by Hans Richter, who in 1941 went to the United States and in 1944 became director of the Institute of Film Techniques in New York. From 1944 to 1946, in collaboration with the American artists Alexander Calder and Man Ray and with Marcel Duchamp, Max Ernst, and Fernand Léger, who were also at that time in the United States, he made *Dreams That Money Can Buy*, the story of seven people's fantastic visions as disclosed to a psychiatrist. Between 1956 and 1957 he produced *8 × 8*, a "chess sonata for film" consisting of eight improvisations on the game of chess enacted by a group of poets, composers, painters, and architects.

A number of the tendencies first expressed in the films of the earlier European avant-garde persist in the experimental films produced in America after World War II. Of somewhat eclectic character, these continue the pattern of drawing their inspiration largely from poetic imagery or from the subconscious; their closest affinities, however, are to poetry, music, and the dance rather than to the representational arts.

Maria Luisa CRISPOLTI

SURVEY OF FILMS ON ART. Although more than two thousand films on art have been produced during the past quarter century, and each year this number is increased by about fifty or a hundred, there is a lamentable scarcity of good ones. For the most part they are short films, one or two reels long. Despite the growing international interest in films on art, they are as a rule the result of isolated private enterprise.

Through the expressive means offered by the camera's movement and the techniques of skillful montage, the film on art can present images of its subject as no other medium can, thus providing opportunities for a special sort of critical interpretation. As a means of art instruction and art appreciation, its cultural importance is equal to that of the illustrated book or traveling exhibition, and it can often show things beyond the range of either to a greater public.

We shall not deal here with the large number of commercially made and distributed "how-to-do-it" films, which especially in the United States have increased tremendously with the growing acceptance of audio-visual education at the elementary and high-school levels; their value is essentially that of a teaching device. Our concern is with films that can interpret works of art for an adult audience and give them an art experience.

Perhaps the distinction of being the first film on art should be accorded to a Swedish production only a few feet long made early

in the century, which does no more than reproduce separate pieces of sculpture by a few disconnected shots. The first full-fledged film on art, and still one of the finest ever made, is Rudolph Bamberger's and Curt Oertel's *Stone Wonders of Naumburg* (1935); by means of superb lighting and subtle camera movement, it captures the essence of the sculpture of the famous German cathedral.

A number of other German films on art were made during the thirties for Ufa Kulturfilm but never received wide distribution outside their own country. The first films on art to receive international attention came from Belgium, and these may perhaps be regarded as outgrowths of films on travel. In 1935 Henri Storck included in his film on Easter Island a sequence showing the remarkable prehistoric carvings for which that island is famous. In 1938 Charles Dekeukeleire directed *Art and Life in Belgium* (*Thèmes d'inspiration*), drawing parallels between modern Flemish landscapes and faces and corresponding details in Flemish primitive paintings. This film was shown by the Belgian government at its pavilion at the New York World's Fair in 1939, together with two other films specially commissioned for the purpose: André Cauvin's *Memling*, showing paintings by that artist in the Musée de l'Hôpital de Saint-Jean in Bruges, and his even more remarkable *Mystic Lamb*. In the latter film, Cauvin explores with his camera details of Van Eyck's great altarpiece in St.-Bavon in Ghent, using close-ups and traveling shots just as if he were filming a living subject.

In Italy about 1940 Luciano Emmer and Enrico Gras began a noteworthy series of films of an entirely different sort. Their primary interest was in reconstructing the content of the narrative cycles rendered by great painters of the past. Using photographs rather than shooting directly from the originals, they exploited the selective powers of the camera to concentrate on details and employed the full range of montage devices to re-create rhythmically the narrative and emotional climate of the works of art. After their initial work, *Earthly Paradise* (1940; reissued 1948), the subject of which was Bosch's triptych in the Escorial, they filmed in a similar way Giotto's fresco series in the Arena Chapel at Padua (*The Drama of the Son of Man* 1941), Carpaccio's *Legend of St. Ursula* (1948), Piero della Francesca's cycle of the *Invention of the Cross* at Arezzo (1949), Botticelli's *Primavera* (1949), and other masterpieces. Though Emmer never mixed styles within a sequence, he rarely revealed a total composition, and sometimes for the sake of narrative or dramatic effect he intercut details from different paintings as if they were parts of one work — a filmic device for which he, and other film makers who followed this method, have been censured by art critics.

Still another approach was that of Curt Oertel in his study of Michelangelo, *The Titan*; he sought to re-create the life of the artist entirely from his art, without recourse to living actors or stage sets. Begun in 1939–40, this ambitious feature-length film underwent various vicissitudes as a result of World War II, and was considerably cut and reedited when it was released in America with a commentary in English in 1950. A heavily romanticized biography, it exploits the dramatic possibilities of sound, music, and camera movement.

In France, "film portraits" of living artists were made by René Lucot, in his *Rodin* (1942), and by Jean Lods, in *Maillol* (1943); both films present the artists in their own environment, show a considerable number of their works, and use photographs and documents to provide additional biographical details. A growing number of films issued later combine the biographical approach to contemporary artists with a study of their work and frequently show them in action. One of the first of these films was Thomas Bouchard's *Fernand Léger in America* (1943), an engaging document of the artist's sojourn in the United States and some of the work he did there. François Campaux's and André Leveille's *Matisse* (1946) is valuable not only for tracing the artist's development but also for showing the elaboration of a specific painting, *The Romanian Blouse*, through slow-motion studies of Matisse's brushwork and dissolving shots of the variations that the painting underwent during the many stages of its compositional development. Among several films devoted to Picasso, *A Visit to Picasso* (1950) is important because Paul Haesaerts brought to its making the authority of a trained scholar who is also fluent in the use of all devices and potentialities of cinematic technique and inventive in the explorations of new ones to suit his purposes. In 1956 the distinguished film director Henri Clouzot produced a feature-length film, *Le Mystère Picasso*, partly in color, which artfully uses every possible film trick, including animation. A wide variety of other contemporary artists have been presented through similar "film portraits": Georges Braque (André Bureau and F. Buran, 1950); Joan Miró (Thomas Bouchard, 1958); American artists from Grandma Moses (Jerome Hill, 1950) and Franklin Watkins (E. M. Benson, 1950) to Jackson Pollock (Hans Namuth and Paul Falkenburg, 1951) and Mark Tobey (Robert Gardner, 1952). The only systematic and sustained efforts in this genre, however, are the twenty or so films on British artists, made in close collaboration with the subjects, directed by John Read for the Television Service of the

British Broadcasting Corporation. Among these, two films on Henry Moore (*Henry Moore*, 1951, and *A Sculptor's Landscape*, 1958) are noteworthy as authentic presentations of the artist's work, aims, and environment; the films on John Piper (1955) and Graham Sutherland (1953) especially, draw comparision between things as they are seen in reality and as they appear in specific paintings. In his more recent films Read has used tape recordings to enable the artist to provide his own commentary.

Poetic evocations of the work of modern artists rather than factual biographies are such films as Henri Storck's *Le Monde de Paul Delvaux* (1946), which drew on the talents of the writer René Micha, the composer André Souris, and the poet Paul Eluard to re-create the imaginary visual world of the Belgian surrealist artist by means of his own paintings. Similar poetic, rather than factual, statements are Herbert Matter's *Works of Calder* (1950) and Alain Resnais's *Guernica* (1949–50). Picasso's *Guernica* was also the subject of an unfinished film that Robert Flaherty began shortly before his death; he explained that he had undertaken a film study of the painting in order "to find out why I like it."

The evocation of earlier periods through works of art is the purpose of such films as William Novik's *Images médiévales* (1950), based on illuminated manuscripts of the 14th and 15th centuries and notable for its subtle color; *Les Charmes de l'existence* (1950) of Jean Grémillon and Pierre Kast, which amusingly re-creates the mood of a period through academic French painting of the late 19th century; Victoria Mercanton's *1848* (1949), which uses paintings and graphic art of the period to tell the story of the French uprising of that year; *Lincoln Speaks at Gettysburg* (1950) by Paul Falkenburg and Lewis Jacobs, which likewise uses contemporary graphic material to set forth historic events; and Carl Lamb's *Bustelli* (1950), which makes use of small sculptures and porcelains in dramatized groups to convey the spirit of the 18th-century court at Nymphenburg.

A number of directors have turned their attention to the history of art, concentrating on particular works or artists. Their films are of special value when they show in detail works that are relatively difficult of access, as is the case, for instance, with Enrico Fulchignoni's *The Mosaics of Ravenna* (1951), George Hoyningen-Huene's *Daphni: Virgin of the Golden Laurels* (1952), and William Chapman's *Lascaux: Cradle of Man's Art* (1950). Other films constitute a record of important exhibitions; such are those documenting pre-Columbian sculpture and Mexican folk art made by Fulchignoni and shown in a major exhibition of Mexican art held in Paris in 1952. To make his film *The Drawings of Leonardo da Vinci* (1953), Basil Wright took advantage of the presence in London of some three hundred drawings by Leonardo assembled at the Royal Academy on the occasion of the 500th anniversary of the artist's birth; in selecting and grouping the drawings for the scenario, Michael Ayrton disregarded chronological sequence in order to emphasize the insatiable curiosity of the artist and the wide range of his astonishing genius. This approach may be contrasted with Fulchignoni's in *The Tragic Pursuit of Perfection* (1952), which is based on the highly romanticized biography of Leonardo by Antonia Vallentin. Perhaps the best of several films about baroque painters is Bert Haanstra's *Rembrandt, Painter of Man*. Goya has been interpreted in several films, including Jean Grémillon's *The Disasters of War*, which makes particular use of his etchings. In *Van Gogh* (1948) and *Paul Gauguin* (1950) Alain Resnais has profited from the considerable research done by the art historian Gaston Diehl but, more important, manifests his own filmic sense and daring montage.

Various aspects of peasant or folk art have been represented, for example in Mario Verdone's *Immagini popolari siciliane* and in the Canadian film *The Loon's Necklace* (1950), which uses ceremonial masks carved by British Columbian Indians (now in Ottawa, Nat. Mus. of Canada) to relate an Indian legend. Among several films on African Negro sculpture one of the most important is a color film on sculpture of the Congo region, *Sous le masque noir* (1958), by the Belgian art historian Paul Haesaerts. Children's art has been featured in the Japanese film *Pleasant Printing Work*, which captures the simple enthusiasm of child artists, and in Henri Gruel's *Martin et Gaston*, a narrative film entirely made up of the work of French school children between the ages of eight and ten.

Tracing a given theme through certain periods of the history of art is still another approach; this has been done, for example, by Carlo Castelli Gattinara in *Il demoniaco nell'arte* (1949), which concentrates on certain diabolic elements portrayed in late medieval German and Netherlandish art. A far more serious example of an art-historical essay on the screen is *Rubens* (1948), in which Henri Storck and Paul Haesaerts collaborated; a divided screen and superimposed diagrams were used to analyze the artist's style, technique, and composition. Haesaerts' *From Renoir to Picasso* (1950) is also essentially an essay in art criticism; it presents contrasting aspects of modern art as exemplified in Renoir's sensuous approach, Seurat's intellectual analysis, and Picasso's passionate distortions. Other ef-

forts to interpret the principles of modern art are *A Lesson in Geometry* (1948), in which Virgilio Sabel and Leonardo Sinigalli study the relation between abstract art and mathematical formulas, or the structures and movements of nature; and Glauco Pellegrini's *Experience of Cubism* (1950), produced in collaboration with the painter Renato Guttuso and making free use, with great originality and inventiveness, of such cinematic devices as animation, angle-shots, and superimposition. In America, the animation director John Hubley and the critic James Johnson Sweeney devised a cartoon film, *The Adventures of Asterisk* (1957), that brilliantly visualized in terms of design and characterization the clash between representational and nonrepresentational art. In 1958 an English animation artist, Richard Williams, used cartoon techniques in *The Little Island* to illustrate the relations between function, utility, and beauty.

The Italian critic Carlo L. Ragghianti has produced a number of what he describes as "crito-films" on Italian architecture and painting; he is particularly interested in the possibilities of using the cinema directly as a means of teaching art appreciation and expressing the analytical thought of the professional critic or art historian.

Art has been presented on film in a great variety of ways: that more outstanding works have not been produced in this genre is due not only to the difficulties of reconciling the aims of the creative film maker with the objectives of the art critic or historian but also to the difficulty of defining the specific audience to which such films may appeal. Aside from their use in classrooms, art films today are projected in museums and art galleries, either as part of regular programs or in conjunction with special exhibitions. The Arts Council of Great Britain maintains a mobile projection unit that shows programs of selected films throughout the country. In the United States film societies and other groups can rent art films directly from commercial distributors or from such sources as the Film Library of the Museum of Modern Art and the visual-aids department of the University of Indiana, which has built up a considerable library of selected films on art. In theaters that specialize in films of high quality, especially foreign films, films on art are occasionally shown as short subjects. The full potential of television audiences for films on art has not been realized, despite the efforts of the Educational Radio and Television Center at Ann Arbor, Mich., which besides distributing films on art, collaborated for a time with the British Broadcasting Corporation's Television Service in financing a series of films on British art.

Interest in films on art has been stimulated by a number of congresses and festivals. Special sessions of the film festivals in Edinburgh and Venice are now regularly devoted to films on art, and three international art film festivals have been held in the United States (two at Woodstock, N.Y., and one, in 1957, at the Metropolitan Museum, under the joint sponsorship of the American Federation of Arts and the College Art Association of America). There are two international organizations concerned with developing the film on art. The Fédération Internationale du Film d'Art (F.I.F.A.), founded in 1949 as an outgrowth of the Fédération Internationale des Archives du Film (F.I.A.F.), has its administrative headquarters in Paris but maintains a special information center and archives for art films at the Stedelijk Museum in Amsterdam. The International Institute of Films on Art (I.I.F.A.), also known under its French title of Comité International pour le Cinéma et les Arts Figuratifs, or C.I.D.A.L.C.), established in 1951 with headquarters at Florence, is directed by Ragghianti and serves as a central information bureau of films on art. In 1953 it issued a compendium listing more than 1,100 films on art produced in many countries, which supplanted earlier catalogues published by UNESCO. Both these organizations seek to raise standards and to cooperate with cultural authorities; they catalogue and review films on art, and in 1958 they jointly collaborated with the province of Bergamo to establish an annual international festival of films on art, with a number of awards. What is lacking, however, is a permanent national or international center for financing or producing films on art, for assembling a complete archives of such films, and for distributing films on art internationally.

John READ

BIBLIOG. *a. Technique, esthetics, and history of the film*: E. Faure, The Art of Cineplastics, Boston, 1923; V. I. Pudovkin, Film Technique (trans., I. Montagu), London, 1929 (rev. ed., 1933); P. Rotha, The Film till Now, London, 1930 (rev. ed., with R. Griffith, New York, 1950); M. ter Braak, De absolute film, Rotterdam, 1931 (Serie monografieën over filmkunst, no. 8); R. Arnheim, Film als Kunst, Berlin, 1932 (Eng. trans., P. Rotha, Film, London, 1933; selections in R. Arnheim, Film as Art, Berkeley, Los Angeles, 1957); R. Spottiswoode, A Grammar of the Film: An Analysis of Film Technique, London, 1935; J. Levy, Surrealism, New York, 1936; P. Rotha, Documentary Film, London, 1936 (rev. ed., London, 1952); E. Panofsky, Style and Medium in the Moving Pictures, Transition, XXVI, 1937 (rev. and enlarged in Critique, I, 1947); U. Barbaro, Film, soggetto e scenegiatura, Rome, 1939; The Film Index, I, The Film as Art, New York, 1941; S. Eisenstein, The Film Sense (trans. and ed., J. Leyda), New York, 1942;

R. Manvell, Film, London, 1944 (rev. ed., London, 1950); M. Deren, An Anagram of Ideas on Art, Form, and Film, Yonkers, N.Y., 1946; M. L'Herbier, ed., Intelligence du cinématographe, Paris, 1946; F. Stauffacher, ed., Art in Cinema: A Symposium on the Avantgarde Film, San Francisco, 1947; I. Barry, Film Notes, Part I: The Silent Film (B. of the Museum of Modern Art, XVI), New York, 1949; L. Chiarini, Il film nei problemi dell'arte, Rome, 1949; S. Eisenstein, Film Form: Essays in Film Theory (Eng. trans., J. Leyda), New York, 1949; R. Manvell, ed., Experiment in the Film. London, 1949; B. Balázs, Theory of the Film: Character and Growth of a New Art (Eng. trans., E. Bone), London, 1952; G.-M. Bovay, Cinéma: un œil ouvert sur le monde, Lausanne, 1952; C. L. Ragghianti, Cinema, arte figurativa, Turin, 1952; H. Richter, Easel, Scroll, Film, Magazine of Art, XLV, 1952, pp. 78–86; A. Kyrou, Le Surréalisme au Cinéma, Paris, 1953; L. H. Eisner, Lo schermo demoniaco, Rome, 1955; R. Paolella, Storia del cinema muto, Naples, 1956; The Museum of Modern Art Film Library, Documentary and Experimental Films, New York, 1959; S. Kracauer, Theory of Film: The Redemption of Physical Reality. New York, 1960. *b. Films on art*: Canada, National Film Board, The Arts in Canada and the Film, Ottawa, 1945; C. L. Ragghianti, Commenti di critica d'arte, Bari, 1946; UNESCO, Le film sur l'art, Répertoire général international des films sur les arts (Eng. ed., Films on Art), Paris, Brussels, 1949; R. Paolella, ed., Le belle arti ed il film, Rome, 1950; UNESCO, Le film sur l'Art (Eng. ed., Films on Art), Paris, Brussels, 1951; G. Amberg, Art, Films, and "Art Films," Magazine of Art, XLV. 1952, pp. 124–33; W. McK. Chapman, ed., Films on Art, New York, 1952; F. Bolen, ed., Films on Art: Panorama 1953, Paris (UNESCO), 1953; C. L. Ragghianti, ed., Le film sur l'art, Répertoire général international des films sur les arts (CIDALC, Comité International pour le Cinéma et les Arts Figuratifs, Florence), Rome, 1953; H. Lemaître, Beaux-arts et Cinéma, Paris, 1956 (Collection 7e Art); T. Bowie, Films on Art: A Critical Guide, Bloomington, Ind., 1957; T. Milani, Vie del film sull'arte, La Biennale di Venezia, no. 34, 1959, pp. 33–39.

This article was prepared with the collaboration of Helen Franc.

Illustrations: PLS. 329–336.

## CITY PLANNING. See TOWN PLANNING.

## CLASSIC ART.
As applied to a historical period, the term "classic" is used in several ways: In the broad sense it defines the civilization and art of Greece and Rome from the 1st millennium B.C. to the 5th century of the Christian era, approximately. In a more limited sense, the classic period of Greece means that period between the archaic (see ARCHAIC ART) and the Hellenistic (see HELLENISTIC ART). Within this era the truest classic phase occurred between about 460 and 430 B.C., a period that saw a vital and inimitable artistic development in Attica and the Peloponnesos. Applied to a movement throughout history, however, classic suggests a particular attitude of the spirit or the inspiration of an artistic heritage (see CLASSICISM).

SUMMARY. The concept of "classic" (col. 632): *Etymology*; *History of the concept*; *The present problem: the boundaries of classic art*. Art themes (col. 643): *Representations of gods*; *Mythological representations*; *Portrayals of daily life*; *Funerary art*. The formal development (col. 650): *The male nude*; *The garbed female figure*; *Relief*; *Hair styles*; *Drapery*. The classic in the sculpture of Greece (col. 657). The classic on the northern and western peripheries and in the Ionian towns (col. 658). The classic in architecture (col. 660). The classic in painting and ceramics (col. 666). The classic in gems, seals, and coins (col. 668). Conclusions (col. 669).

THE CONCEPT OF "CLASSIC." *Etymology*. The word "classic" is derived from the Latin *classicus*, an adjective in turn derived from the noun *classis*. Let us here confine ourselves to the meaning of *classis* as equivalent to *numerus*, or *ordo*. In this sense *classis* denotes groups of taxpayers and defines the social classes thus created. *Classicus* thus describes a Roman citizen who by his social and economic position enjoyed influence and a certain importance. Consequently the word also assumes some of the meaning of *dignitas* and *auctoritas*. In the nomenclature of those public assemblies in which the Roman people were represented by centuries (*comitia centuriata*), *testis classicus* ("witness of the highest rank") is a "rich witness" (*testis locuples*). Thus Festus (*Epitome*, ed. C. O. Müller, Leipzig, 1839, p. 113) calls " witnesses of the highest rank" those " who are worthy of a certain respect and trust." The connection of high rank with this fiscal meaning becomes increasingly loose during the imperial period. Hence when Festus (op. cit., p. 56) maintains that "those who were called witnesses of the

highest rank were those who were summoned for the signing of wills," the word means only trustworthy, important, full of authority — the connotation adopted also by Gellius (*Noctes Atticae*, XIX, 8, 15). Cicero, on the other hand (*Academica*, II, 23), refers to certain philosophers as belonging to the fifth class, *quintae classis* (implying "of the lowest rank"); these passages refer only to authors and philosophers and never to the representational arts. Apparently in antiquity the word *classicus* was never commonly used to denote intellectual facts and values, and the passages mentioned above cannot be considered the basis of our present understanding of the term. During the entire Middle Ages the word disappeared, and it was revived in the Renaissance with a different meaning, describing an author whose works were taught in the schools (implying only the Humanistic schools), and remained thus in all the lexicons until 1900.

Before the Renaissance, the ancient or contemporary writers most admired in monastic or secular schools were not termed "classic" but were rather described by the Greek word κανών ("canon"), which referred not only to the T square used by architects but also to a fixed rule, norm, and paradigm. This usage indicates how profoundly the 4th-century humanism of Christian Alexandria (that of St. Jerome and Origen) influenced the intellectual formation of the West. "Canon" was also used in the above sense for works of art in the 5th century B.C. In one document Polykleitos (q.v.) expounded the propositions on which his ideal figure, the *Doryphoros*, was based, and as early as the Roman classicism of the Augustan age the canon of Polykleitos became the norm and prototype for representing a harmonious, manly body. The statues of emperors, captured in their heroic majesty, were mostly inspired by the canon of Polykleitos, which even influenced works of the 4th century of our era. Stroux maintains that the *identity* of the concept of canon and the classic are already foreshadowed in Hellenistic writings on esthetics (Stroux, in Jäger, 1931, p. 8). Certainly in Alexandria as in Pergamon, and perhaps also in other centers of advanced culture from the 3d century on, the literary and artistic creations of the past were taken as standards or models. As in the Renaissance, manuscripts of famous writers were collected and their prices rose accordingly. The so-called *Catalogue of Those Who Have Been Illustrious in Every Form of Culture*, Πίνακες τῶν ἐν πάσῃ παιδείᾳ διαλαμψάντων — namely, the first catalogue of the classics — was composed in Alexandria, and its authors were called the ἐγκρινόμενοι, or chosen ones. In fact, whatever the Alexandrian scholars did not collect and transcribe seems to have been lost to us.

*History of the concept.* The habit of selecting works of the past as models either in form or in content is an interesting intellectual attitude whose roots we can trace to the late 5th century B.C. in Athens. It implies the belief that these works are unsurpassable and that current times are decadent. Permeating this nostalgic reevaluation of the great prototypes of the past was the intention of raising the intellectual level of the present. In the comedies of Aristophanes there are hints that the past is greater than the present. But it was Plato first and foremost (*Republic*, B, II, 6, 5) who gave philosophical form to the belief that the past was grand and noble and that the human spirit was forever striving to rediscover it (Stroux, op. cit.). This attitude was to become more insistent in Hellenistic times because of the dilution and exhaustion of the creative faculty as well as the diffusion and modification of the classic heritage caused by the intermingling of races and peoples. Eventually there emerged a refined and highly educated group who took the classic world as their model and chose to exist in its exalted spiritual climate. Most reasonably they were anxious not to let their heritage fall into oblivion or become debased. Fortunately for humanity the Ptolemies salvaged part of the intellectual patrimony of antiquity, and the most illustrious sages of the 3d–2d century B.C. — Aristarchos and Zenodotos, for example — conducted scholarly research in the Museion of Alexandria, or the Sanctuary of the Muses. This is the order of events that gave rise to what we call classical education and the cult of classicism (q.v.). Our classical heritage today would be far more extensive if the great library at Alexandria had not been burned by Caesar and the Museion by Gregory the Great. That so much has survived until our own time is due to Augustus, who realized that without culture he could neither dominate nor administer the world. He therefore founded several libraries in Rome on the model of the library of the Ptolemies. For the intellectual tradition of the West, the palace library in the Temple of Apollo on the Palatine seems to have been fundamentally important, although other later emperors liberally established new libraries.

An elaboration of the theories of esthetics and of the history of art had already existed in Greece during the 5th century B.C. (see ESTHETICS). Like Polykleitos, Iktinos had perhaps compiled a book on the laws of proportion relating to the Parthenon. In the late 5th century people tried to devise intellectual explanations for everything that had been so perfectly realized in the arts, perhaps because they were convinced that a unique period was disappearing in the disasters of the Peloponnesian War (431–404). Here we recall Plato's insistence on questions concerning the "beautiful" (καλλόν) and the "just" (ὀρθόν). His designation of ideas as the first models of being was possible only because as a genuine Greek he had tried to understand the world intellectually, departing from a purely physical vision. Hence he frequently alluded to the arts; Polykleitos was even a participant in one dialogue. Only later in his final writings Plato set off on a new ideological path and rejected the arts and poetry. We cannot say whether the problem of "perfection" and "beauty," namely, the classic problem, was later resumed by other philosophical schools in the course of the 4th century. Aristotle, at any rate, seems to have been occupied with the problem, though more from an ethical than an esthetic point of view. He preferred Polygnotos, the classic painter, to Zeuxis and Parrhasios, who, so far as we can gather, must have represented the so-called "baroque" current in post-Phidian art.

In the early Hellenistic period (3d cent. B.C.) the attitude toward the classic entered a somewhat negativistic phase. Significantly the scholar Xenocrates, nephew of Lysippos, avoiding the artist's more theoretical point of view, approached the matter from a practical angle, for he felt that either the classic was already a thing of the past or it should go out of fashion in short order. All we know about his stand as a critic points to his repudiation of the canon of beauty of Polykleitos and to his intention of promoting the acceptance of the "modern" style of Lysippos, which was indeed to become the foundation of Hellenistic art.

In later Hellenistic times (ca. 150 B.C.) the attitude toward the classic assumed a more positive character. Obviously the word "classic" was not used; perhaps "canon" was used with the same connotation as is associated with Polykleitos. Be that as it may, the late Hellenistic "classicizers," feeling that the art of their time was degenerate and tainted with Asiatic influences, were intent on its overthrow. That their attitude was dictated by a careful theory based on the study of art history may be deduced from the precise comments on late Hellenistic art — the art that they condemn. Here again our information is filtered through the writings of Roman compilers, such as Pliny, Cicero, and Quintilian. When we read the peremptory statement that after the 121st Olympiad (296 B.C.) "art ceased" ("cessavit ars deinde") and that in the 156th Olympiad "art was reborn" ("revixit deinde ars"), we can infer that about the year 293 and again in 150 B.C. some great sculpture was created and came to be so highly regarded that it was considered a landmark and established a trend; the period 293–150 B.C. is the one we call Hellenistic, and the period after 150 B.C. the one we call classicistic. Everywhere in the Greek world, in the East as in the West, the degeneration of the so-called "first baroque" and the weakening of the creative impulse can be pinpointed to 150 B.C. A figure created in late Hellenistic times no longer fills the space allotted to it, because it is diffused into its surroundings and lost in its own pathetic pose. The figures of this period lose their bulk and spatial depth and become increasingly flattened in effect, since they are designed to be viewed from a single angle (see NEO-ATTIC STYLES).

We do not know the scholar who first became aware of these facts and was able to put them into words with the acumen of a theoretician, but he was probably a product of the art-historical schools of Alexandria or Pergamon. Symptomatically, in Pergamon sculpture veered toward the classic and most probably architecture did too, from what we gather from the treatise on proportions by Hermogenes of Priene. In the works of Cicero, Quintilian, and Pliny we already find the distinction between the archaic style (the so-called "tuscanicus") the severe style, the classic style, and the postclassic style. The classic we might say, even though the word itself does not appear, was attained by Phidias, who was incomparable. In the esthetics of these writers the unattainable, the inimitable, the absolutely perfect in beauty or art, stand for the essence of the classic. Naturally the measure of the scale of values is beauty, *pulchritudo*, or the Greek κάλλος. The truth, *veritas*, the Greek ἀλήθεια, attainable by an artist, indicates the degree of development. Archaic art did not yet possess it; the severe style (αὐστηρὰ ἁρμονία) achieved it in part; and finally, it was completely attained only by the classic style (εὔκρατος ἁρμονία). In order to carry out completely this artistic stage attained by Polykleitos and above all by Phidias, the prerequisites were precision, or *diligentia* (ἀκρίβεια) of form; mastery, or *auctoritas* (ἀξιωματικόν); and seriousness of appearance. This last quality depended on the weightiness, or *pondus* (σεμνόν), or dignity of appearance in bearing and in gestures. The works of classic art, especially the creations of Phidias, possess *maiestas et pulchritudo* (μέγεθος καὶ κάλλος), or "loftiness and beauty." We shall see later that these are also the characteristics which we still today attribute to the classic.

It must have been a remarkable scholar who formulated this theory of art and criticism between 150 and 100 B.C. From him emanates all the later criticism which rhetorical teachings alone have transmitted to us. In the midst of treatises which became increasingly sparse and empty, one brief work alone sparkles: the Περὶ ὕψους, known as *On the Sublime*. We are dealing here with a practical lesson for an aristocratic disciple, written by one of those rare and deeply cultivated Greeks who could express himself perfectly in words, in the most ancient Greek sense. Among all the surviving texts, this is our most important one concerning the classic in antiquity, even if the word itself was never used, and even if it treated rhetoric rather than the representational arts.

To summarize briefly: The concept of the classic developed, taking shape and deepening increasingly throughout antiquity, from 400 B.C. on, and was applied to that which is perfect in every respect. It attained its ultimate form between 150 and 100 B.C., although the word "classic" was never used in this sense. The decisive impulse to define and evaluate the concept was provided by practical rhetoric, but by the late Hellenistic period and certainly also by the Augustan age, the arts of the 5th and 4th centuries B.C. were understood to be the classic.

The mentality of the Christian West was clearly distinguished by its desire to participate in the continuity of a tradition. During the Christian era, however, the nostalgic memory was linked with the grandeur and power of Rome because the Roman empire was, for the men of the early Middle Ages, a great deal closer than Athens in both space and time. Almost simultaneously with Constantine's transfer of the world capital to Byzantium and Rome's temporary loss of prestige, a romanticizing of Rome began to emerge. As a result, the West — unlike the Christian East, which felt its sacred duty to destroy the images and the cult places of the fallen gods — preserved and sometimes deliberately rescued from destruction the monuments of its great pagan past. When the humanistic mind of early Christianity began to speak to the grandeur of antiquity, it always imagined the power of the Roman empire and especially of the age of Augustus. It was thus throughout the entire Middle Ages, even when Rome, by then bereft of political importance, was only the city of the popes. The dominant position of the bishop of Rome above other church dignitaries led to the toleration and even to the revival of the legends concerning the eternity of Rome prophesied earlier by the sibyls. Thus the end of the world was foreseen as the day

when Rome would be demolished. From this point of view, everything that had once been understood as classic antiquity became identified with Rome.

Rome was the only city on earth where there were still splendid buildings which could be neither seen nor imitated anywhere else in the world. An even more ardent admiration probably existed for the surviving works of sculpture such as the Capitoline wolf, the *Spinario*, and the statue of Marcus Aurelius, which was moved in 1538 to the Capitoline hill. Ancient Rome remained, especially for people in the north, the most admired model for the cultivation of the human mind.

The modest compendiums of the early Middle Ages, such as the compendium by Isidore of Seville, were no longer adequate for handing down this heritage. The Middle Ages tried to imitate the beauties of classic language and architecture, the miniatures and reliefs of the Carolingian age providing obvious examples of effort and aspirations toward classic art. Some Carolingian manuscripts of astronomical texts can even be considered ancient in feeling (see ASTRONOMY AND ASTROLOGY).

The ideal of this classic antiquity was always strong in contrast to the political weakness of the West. It survived the invasions and pillagings by the barbarian hordes from the East and was carried forward by the legendary glory of the Caesars. The name of Caesar, as used during the Middle Ages, almost never meant the Divine Julius (*Divus Iulius*) but rather his great successors, above all Augustus. It was Augustus who established the reign of peace lasting 300 years, and the people of the Middle Ages looked upon him with more admiration and nostalgia, perhaps, than they accorded the poets and artists who had sung his praises.

This conscious recollecting of classic antiquity was particularly evident in Frederick II, Holy Roman Emperor who ruled in the 13th century. What we know of Frederick reveals with undeniable clarity his admiration for classic antiquity. Of the buildings constructed by him, Castel del Monte, near Bari, is sufficiently preserved to indicate a conscious evocation of Roman architecture. The adherence to Roman prototypes is revealed even more in the coins of this period, which were clearly dependent upon the gold coins of Augustus (see COINS AND MEDALS).

For the Middle Ages, classic antiquity — the central idea, if not the term — came to mean the entire ancient period which had preceded either the medieval era proper or the barbarian invasions and migrations at the close of antiquity. Although Greek antiquity had disappeared from the eyes of the West, Rome was still visible as the model. These medieval conceptions persisted even into the 14th- and 15th-century Renaissance, when antiquity began to be understood in an entirely different way. Notably in Italy the idea of Rome had its most intense expression and intellectual acme; in an Italy politically fragmented and torn by foreign domination, Rome began to appear as a national ideal, in what we might call a romantic light. Thus the image of classic antiquity was identified with ancient Rome, and thus it still survives in countries with civilizations of Latin derivation.

*The present problem: the boundaries of classic art.* Renaissance scholars saw in classic antiquity a kind of golden age, an almost divine era for humanity. By devoting themselves to elevating studies, a particular philosophical mode of existence regarded as being in harmony with ancient models, they strove to revive this ideal and also the sensual enjoyment of life itself. In harmony with the new economic and intellectual impulses in 14th- and 15th-century Italy and with the renewed passion for building, ancient statues were uncovered in Rome and greeted with as much enthusiasm as if they had been manuscripts of unknown authors. Consequently the arts began to enjoy prestige and importance for admirers of classic antiquity at least as much as literature, which up until then had been the chief object of their study (see ANTIQUE REVIVAL; CLASSICISM). Because of the scanty knowledge of Greek, the works of art uncovered were naturally regarded as Roman, especially as they had been found in the imperial palaces on the Palatine hill and in the magnificent imperial baths. With a stubbornness sometimes bor-

dering on irrepressible nationalism, Italian scholars tried long to defend their Roman origin or, for more ancient works of art, an Etruscan origin. The 16th- and 17th-century scholars of antiquity also tried constantly to explain ancient works of art by means of the histories and legends of Rome.

A problem of great interest, until now just barely formulated, would be to determine which period of antiquity was considered by enthusiasts from the 16th century on as the golden, or rather the classic, age. It would be extremely interesting to know which ancient statues were regarded as the most perfect models during the centuries following the Renaissance. The matter is further complicated because the ground covered in the first reproductions of ancient statues in publications, by De Cavallerii and De Rubeis, was continually being reworked in later publications with unimportant supplements. Nonetheless, a rigorous scrutiny of the ancient statues reproduced in publications from the 16th to the 18th century, combined with a stylistic evaluation, might reveal that the most highly esteemed works of art perhaps belonged to movements essentially parallel to artistic developments contemporary with the publications. It may suffice to remember how the *Idolino* came to Pesaro about 1530 and was hailed by Bembo in an epigram that has become famous. With its delicate sense of the body, its pose and gestures, the *Idolino* provided an undeniable analogy with many Renaissance figures. We think of the sensation and then of the revolution produced in the cultivated world by the discovery of the Laocoön about 1500 — a work in which one could not fail to recognize a note of the classic. Judging from the frontispieces of books which frequently have reproductions of ancient gods, one would say that the 17th century chose its models predominantly among the works of the so-called "Roman baroque" of the Flavian emperors and the Antonines. The 18th century, in turn, had a predilection for the sculptures corresponding to a capricious rococo taste. But these distinctions within antiquity apparently had not yet penetrated the consciousness of the people who had thus chosen their models. Classic antiquity persisted as that which was perfect and consequently as that which functioned as a model. This was in contradistinction to the viewpoint of the Middle Ages, which had denied corporeal beauty and earthly joys.

These very subtle differentiations among the works of ancient art that were particularly valued by the different periods of the Renaissance and the baroque do not seem to have been recognized. Scholars did not ask which period these most-admired works belonged to and which of their stylistic characteristics were especially valued. Such an attitude is understandable, inasmuch as a division of ancient art into periods had not yet been undertaken; and furthermore, men were little influenced by periodic changes of taste. Among ancient works of sculpture they were seeking exclusively and constantly that unique and basic quality cherished in classic antiquity and regarded as antipodal to the ideal of the Middle Ages and also, even if only tacitly recognized, to Christianity: namely, the physical beauty of the human body in the nude, its earthly, or "pagan," character, as it was then called, the art of representing it naturalistically in sculpture or in painting, and clarity of thought or architectural structure. Today we may confine what was then considered classic to the art preceding the downfall of pagan Rome — the late imperial age.

However, the word *classicus*, as we have said, was never used to describe the representational arts during the Renaissance. One spoke of the golden age of art; of the perfection of form; of the highest summit of beauty attained by artists — not, to be sure, through the imitation of nature (which obviously was to predominate) but rather through the contemplation of beauty in itself and through rendering the body in painting and sculpture.

In the 17th century, use of the word *classicus* was extended to the representational arts, particularly in France, where esthetics was firmly oriented toward fixed norms and unchanging values. About 1693 Fénelon wrote: "We have finally understood that one must write as the Raphaels, Caravaggios, and Poussins painted" ("On a enfin compris qu'il faut écrire comme les Raphaels, les Caravaches et les Poussins ont peint").

Even if today we do not approve of such parallels of writing and painting, they refer nonetheless to paintings of the highest quality — paintings later considered as belonging to the golden age. Such an age had already been spoken of as contemporary in 16th-century esthetics when, following the Reformation and the sack of Rome in 1527, it really seemed that its end had unexpectedly arrived.

Other nations also strove eagerly to establish this concept of the golden age in the framework of the burgeoning national cultures. In his treatise on the arts in his *Siècle de Louis XIV* (1751), Voltaire wrote: "The century of Louis XIV has, then, the destiny of the centuries of Leo X, of Augustus, of Alexander" ("Le siècle de Louis XIV a donc toute la destinée des siècles de Leon X, d'Auguste, d'Alexandre"). As we can readily understand, the classic in Greek had as yet no place in the concept; even the Hellenistic period, evoked by Alexander's name, remained a mere rhetorical image and did not correspond to anything tangible, although the popular conception of Alexander enjoyed an enthusiastic following. Significantly, however, from the 18th century on, the golden age came to be considered synonymous with the lifetimes of famous conquerors. Augustus was worshiped, though with little historical precision, even when Augustan sculpture was still very far from being defined. Furthermore, in a higher sense this emperor, of legendary greatness, who had brought peace and well-being to the world, was accorded a role as patron of the arts. The age of Augustus consequently was thenceforth identified with the classic. It is, moreover, extraordinarily interesting that every nation became preoccupied with discovering its own Augustan age. In England it was the period of Elizabeth I, of Anne, or of Victoria which came to rank as the Augustan age. In a famous essay, "Litterarischer Sansculottismus" ("Literary Radicalism"), Goethe lamented the difficulty, even the impossibility, of finding a classic age in Germany (E. R. Curtius, *Europaische Literatur und lateinisches Mittelalter*, Bern, 1948; Am. ed., trans. W. R. Trask, *European Literature and the Latin Middle Ages*, New York, 1953). For our own argument it is important that during the Renaissance, Rome — and more precisely the Rome of Augustus — symbolized the focal point of classicism, for the West, because it was the only accessible composite of ancient art then existing and, furthermore, continued to be illuminated with an aura of legend emanating from its own myth and from its position as the center of Christian pilgrimages. Such it remained until the 18th century, until the appearance of historicism and, above all, of Winckelmann, who was the first person to divide the existing artistic heritage into separate categories and to relate it to the scanty remnants from the history of ancient art. Thereafter the idea of an internal development began to be formulated. The concept of the sowing, flowering, and fading of art returned. With it returned the concepts of forerunners, of the exhausting and perfecting of an artistic phenomenon, which had to be enclosed within the two extreme limits. These observations led Winckelmann and his successors to realize that only Greek art, and not Roman, was truly classic. The sphere of Greek art which Winckelmann had exerted himself to elucidate belonged primarily to the 5th and 4th centuries B.C., the period to which Pliny's history of art led back. These two centuries have persisted up until the present day as the classic centuries for the majority of archaeologists. Also very significantly, Winckelmann had understood how to differentiate this classic style, which he separated intuitively rather than rationally into two phases: the "noble style" (*stile nobile*) and the "beautiful style" (*stile bello*). This nomenclature was mechanically accepted and followed until the 19th-century researches of A. Furtwängler.

It would be interesting if we could decide what contributions other European scholars have made toward understanding these problems. Similar research advanced and was carried out primarily in England, where as far back as the early 18th century a growing interest arose in Greek sculpture and architecture. This was manifested in the scholarly expeditions and artistic collections made by the aristocracy and, accompanying these, the creation of a classic style in architecture based on the Greek world. Oxford became the spiritual center of clas-

sicism understood in this sense, which afterward spread out especially to Scandinavia and also to Germany. Actually many aspects of this subject must still be examined and clarified if we are to understand the scholarly and cultural development. But one fact is still firm and undeniable: This richer and more precise, although more restricted, definition of the classic was rejected as an unhistorical postulate by archaeologists among the peoples of Latin origin — above all by Italy, France, and Spain. It was never understood by them.

In Germany scholars were able to isolate with greater exactness and rigor what should be understood as the classic. In his profound devotion to Rome, Goethe ruled out any restricted, categorical definition of the classic when he remarked that everything which is excellent is consequently classic, in whatever category it may belong (*Voss to Riemer*, 26, I, 1804). But archaeology sought an increasingly exact limitation of the classic period in the Greek world, placing it in the 5th and 4th centuries B.C., in accordance with the historiography of the final classicizing period of Hellenism. The difficulties inherent in defining these limits were pointed out in all their obviousness in the *Naumburg Journals* (Jäger, 1930). Actually all the men who were at that time participating in the discussion were so permeated by the concept of the classic that the necessary definition eluded them. They regarded it as self-evident and failed to recognize that it changed according to the taste of men and the times. Thus one meets the absurd situation of a harangue about whether Homer or Aristotle was more classic. Scholars did not want to abandon the premise of "that which is perfect in itself," but they did not concede the possibility of alternative choices, for perfection of art existed in all phases of Hellenism. Can we then say that the *Apoxyomenos* of Lysippos is still classic? Is the *Winged Victory of Samothrace* (VII, PL. 177) not perhaps an absolutely perfect creation — or the *Girl* (VII, PL. 159) from Antium (Anzio), or the *Praying Boy* (IV, PL. 203), or the Pantheon? If the term "classic" had been used for these post-5th-century works, the whole intellectual structure would have been shattered, forcing a return to the Renaissance conception that all works created before the downfall of pagan Rome were classic. The German scholars then tried to solve this dilemma by starting out from Nietzsche's interpretation of Greece, using his postulate as a basis, namely, that we must understand art from the point of view of life and life from the point of view of art, and pinpoint the phenomenon of the classic not as the esthetic perfection of form but as the artistic expression of a physical and metaphysical way of life. To some the restriction to the 5th century seemed inevitable, while those who were unwilling to relinquish the century of Praxiteles spoke of a second classic period embracing the 4th century. But then should not one speak of a later classic era in the 3d century? The 3d century created works of the highest perfection, although unfortunately only their echo survives to us through terra cottas.

Having discussed this problem, we nonetheless realize that a classic style per se does not exist, and that every age important to intellectual history has had the task of formulating an attitude toward the past and of defining as classic whatever could be considered productive (in Goethe's sense) for its particular time. We may recall that about 1920 quite a few German archaeological circles began to regard the severe style as the highest and ultimate expression of the Greek intellect and art (although they did not actually commit themselves verbally to such definition). Again not explicitly, but nonetheless clearly and irrefutably, they later began to proclaim to the neophytes that archaic art was the fundamental expression of Greek art. It was a revelation sometimes mystical, hermetic rather than illuminating, and thus not comprehensible to everyone. Inevitably also, certain critical stages of primitive art, such as the disintegration of the Geometric world or the confused decades during the Orientalizing period about 700 B.C., began to be hailed as the most creative epochs of Greek art. Psychologically we can explain the exaggerated admiration for this transitional period from the 8th to the 7th century; for like our own time, that era did not attain a genuine artistic clarification. The profound social, religious, and political up-

heavals, then as today, produced shocks and repercussions which are fascinating to modern people.

If we now abandon these narrow limits of archaeological esthetics and direct our attention to the way in which ancient art is evaluated by a larger circle of the cultivated men of our time, then undeniably we find today not the 19th-century admiration for the ancient world but rather a passion for those very cultural monuments and artistic activities which are artistically antithetical to its ideals. In fact, many men endowed with artistic sensitivity today seem to prefer Etruscan art to Greek, precisely because Etruscan art surpasses — or, more exactly, violates — all the norms established by the Greeks. The artistic creations which do not yet, or no longer, recognize realistic rendering of the human figure enjoy greater favor at the present time, whether Sardinian or Syrian figurines, Cappadocian gods, or works arising out of the decadence of ancient forms in East and West such as Sassanian, Visigothic, Mozarabic, Celtic, or Coptic.

All this leads not to a relativistic outlook but rather to a skepticism toward all surviving laws and toward all representations not genuinely full of vitality. We must not, however, think that we are giving up a lost cause or admitting defeat if we realize that the classic has always been a concept bound by its own time and determined by the necessities or aspirations of each particular period; and that those very limitations govern the choice of a model incorporating the quintessence of the ancient spirit. We should regard this interpretation as a broadening of our own field of observations and of our penetration into historical facts by considering these facts as an active force.

All these questions — about whether the 4th century is still classic and whether Lysippos should be included or barred entrance; about whether the severe style should be considered classic; about whether the classical lands are only Attica and parts of the Peloponnesos — are no longer alive today. Whenever we may be required to take an exact position about which period of Western history we regard as classic, we may answer that only the period of Pericles and Sophocles has never been denied this characterization. That epoch, in the limited area between Athens and Olympia, would represent the nucleus of what every age has regarded as the strongest, purest incarnation of classic antiquity. However, not improbably, a time may come when, because of the confusing multiplicity of cultures which the Western mind is now attempting to systematize and understand, people may once again think of ancient art as a single, quite coherent whole. Therefore the medieval definition of classic antiquity as the era stretching from Homer to Constantine may once again become commonly accepted. Even so, we shall always be able to use the term "classic," faded though it may become eventually, to distinguish it from other nonclassic periods (such as the baroque, the Gothic, or the era of paleolithic cave paintings) and to denote the acme of perfection, the most mature artistic development.

We can therefore still speak today of the 5th century as the age of the classic without its mattering whether we confine it to the second half of the century (450–400) or restrict it to the period stretching from the early years of Sophocles' activity until Pericles' death (455–430). Naturally we cannot expect to find epochs pinpointed exactly in years; and there were, of course, transitional periods at the beginning and end of even such a limited span.

All these various definitions of the classic have emanated from earlier art history, as we can readily understand, and always allude first to the more or less successful rendering of nature. Because of its positivistic point of departure, the 19th century emphasized preeminently the reproduction of nature. This conception also provides the point of departure for the 20th-century attempts at definition. The decision about the limits of the Hellenistic period was regarded as especially difficult because the period was not simply naturalistic, as was the final phase; both the early phases and the long evolutionary phases during the 3d and 2d centuries B.C. were permeated by considerations of harmony. The standards articulated during the neoclassicist period about 1900, especially by Fiedler and Hildebrandt, should therefore definitely help to clarify this

matter. Today, however, their demands seem characteristic for classicistic but not for classic works — for example, the demand for a single viewpoint for the spectator or for a self-contained gesture in a sculptural figure so that "one should be able to roll it down a mountain without its limbs' being harmed." This turn of thought also led to G. Rodenwaldt's definition in 1916 — namely, that we may call "classic" any work of art that is perfectly stylized without, however, moving far away from nature, whereby the needs both for imitation of nature

forms which may be more applicable to such currents as the early archaic age or late antiquity. They are not at all helpful in the classic Greek age, when the human body was always the fulcrum of every artistic expression, emphatically opposed to the limitations of abstract spatial categories.

At the diametrically opposite pole, E. Buschor's (1942) impassioned, sensitive intuitions define the phenomenon of classicism as a world of necessity (*Shicksalswelt*). Certainly any work of art, especially a classic one, eludes rational compre-

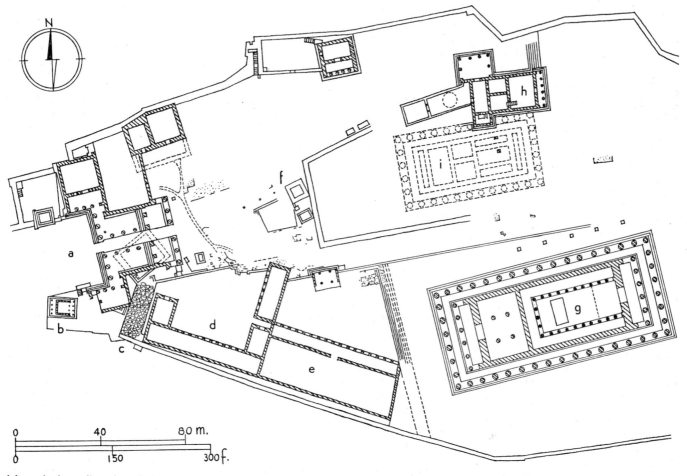

Athens, the Acropolis at the end of the 5th cent. B.C.: (*a*) Propylaia; (*b*) Temple of Athena Nike; (*c*) "Pelasgian" wall of the Mycenaean period; (*d*) Sanctuary of Athena Brauronia; (*e*) *chalkotheke* (storehouse for bronze implements); (*f*) statue of Athena Promachos; (*g*) Parthenon; (*h*) Erechtheion; (*i*) remains of archaic Temple of Athena.

and for its stylistic transformation are equally satisfied (Rodenwaldt, 1916, p. 125). Consequently, "the historical and probably also the absolute value of the classic rests in the harmony between the work of art and reality." However, these definitions are excessively vague and imprecise; even the general ideals of the Hellenistic era could thus have been considered classic. More relevantly, the definition precisely corresponds only to classicistic works (see CLASSICISM). W. Pinder speaks more clearly, defining classic art as "the yes or no to conventions," simultaneously distinguishing between "form as abandon and form as an act of will" (*Das Problem der Generation in der Kunstgeschichte Europas*, Berlin, 1926, p. 136). For Pinder, classic art represents an eternal, noble search for a balance between the yes and the no, as "the absolute in the conditional, the living form as a monumental configuration in space (which is its own controlling element)." But even here we discover immediately how these definitions are peculiarly adapted to classicistic works of art.

F. Matz (1929) tried to extricate himself from this difficulty by deepening Rodenwaldt's and Pinder's observations. Perhaps because he started out from an intellectual foundation influenced by expressionism and the abstract art following it, he sought to define the phenomenon solely by spatial criteria and abstract

hension, unless one refers to the attributes of classic art constantly alluded to and doubtless correctly recognized since antiquity: truth according to nature in anatomical rendering and movement, compactness of form, harmony and balance, an internal system of proportions, and a flowering of portraiture arising out of man's growing individuality.

We may now ask what element in the content of classic art most profoundly aroused the interest of Western civilization. From the 13th century on, the ideal of the nude and its perfect anatomical rendering were considered lost and no longer attainable. The delight that the 15th and 16th centuries experienced in rediscovering antique figures of youths revealed an enthusiasm for absolute perfection in the human body. Indeed, during the classic decades nudity and its artistic rendering had a deeper meaning than merely a portrayal of the nude as such. Anatomical precision was not the distinguishing mark, but rather the nobler attributes of the human being. (This approach, however, changed during the 4th century B.C.) The rendering of Greek gods and heroes during the 5th century lacked a certain feminine sensuality we find in the male nudes of the Renaissance and the baroque eras.

The 5th-century male figures possess as little sensual attraction as the female figures infrequently portrayed during

the classic age. The former seem to be marked by a kind of chastity and purity such as the human figure never again attained in art. This is because they belonged to the religious sphere, their nudity displaying the well-constructed body that was the highest image the 5th-century Greeks could offer their gods. Figures of men and young boys were erected in sanctuaries and were intended as votive offerings.

Representation of Greek youth in the guise of divinities gave rise to figures of such beauty as had never before been achieved, partly because the art represented not merely a rigorous esthetic concept but also a constantly changing civilization and philosophy. Greek education of the young attempted to cultivate and enhance man's physical qualities to the highest degree of perfection, as well as to enrich his religious and intellectual growth through poetry. The purpose of education was to raise man to his true level, to develop all his capacities, and to approximate in him the likeness of the gods (ὁμοίωσις τῷ θεῷ). Precisely because the representation of nudity as conceived by the Greeks did not emanate from pure admiration of the earthly form but rather from a religious dedication, we still admire the structural beauty, purity, and human perfection of Greek figures. They do not represent an esthetic hedonism of any kind but simply a bond between men and the gods. The often-vaunted idealism of Greek sculpture is thus explicable in that in his worship the Greek tended to approach the god with his whole self — in his bodily form as well as spiritually. The Greek people were illuminated with beauty at the very moment that grace flowed into them through the god's miraculous epiphany. Goethe was the first to understand this theomorphism of Greek art. By contrast to the Greek statues, the nude figures of Roman art seem to be bodies undressed. They are genuinely pagan, in the proper sense of the Renaissance and the Enlightenment.

While for modern man, ideal beauty as understood by classic taste represents something formal and removed from life, for the Greeks it represented a natural fact, not an abstraction or a visionary ideal. In the great Eastern civilizations the beauty of the human body, in the sense of a controlled physical development, did not exist. Harmonious forms had been invented long ago for animals and objects; but only in Greece did the representational arts and mythology expound the secret of the universe through the likeness of the human body, precisely because Greek religion conceived of the gods as idealized human beings rather than animals, demons, or hybrids. The god incarnate — a theme recurrent in Homer — is one of the most significant aspects of the Greek legacy.

In addition to the nudity of the human body, beauty and symmetry of features have been regarded as other essential characteristics of ancient sculpture. We often forget that the harmonious portrayal of man's physical aspect, the great goal of Western art until the middle of the 19th century, was an essentially Greek creation; this kind of beauty, however, was not typical of Greek art in its early period. The demoniac, malevolent aspect of the physiognomy disappeared only during the classic period. There are, nonetheless, various levels of beauty: What so profoundly moved the classicistic (18th cent.) critics appears today cold and schematic. The head of the *Ludovisi Juno* (Rome, Mus. Naz.), a product of Roman classicism admired so warmly by Winckelmann, seems now almost as ominous as a Gorgon's face. But this is so because today we know genuine classic Greek sculpture.

ART THEMES. *Representations of gods.* In archaic Greek art a figure of a young man had many meanings — for example, a divine image (see ARCHAIC ART, I, PLS. 346, 350); youthful figures came to be called "Apollo's" with some justification. We know such early statues of gods through references in ancient writers and through representations on Attic vases and Roman coins. These images are not different from figures of youths, except that sometimes they hold the emblems of their divine power. The same figure of a young man, however, may also portray a victorious athlete; but actually such a meaning can only be ascertained definitely if the inscription proclaiming the victory is still on the base. Furthermore, the same figure

may be intended as a portrait in the antique sense. If such portraits appear impersonal, it is because individuality was missing in the archaic world, where everything was subjected to the religious *kosmos* of the state.

Archaic statues of young men are thus not conscious works of art in the present-day sense of the word: instead they are substitutes for the vital force represented or, more precisely, the very incarnation of such a vital force. All this altered during the classic era. No longer could a single sculptural type represent alternately a god or a human being. All the classic images of the gods were unmistakably different from the representations of mortals. A god indeed could still appear in human shape during the classic era; yet even when attributes of divine power are missing, we notice immediately that a statue such as the *Apollo of Kassel* (PL. 353) portrays a being that exists on a higher plane than even a perfect man. In the classic age the sculptural image of men themselves began to be differentiated, with the statues of victorious athletes bordering on the images of the gods. It is apparent, however, despite the perfect beauty of Polykleitos' *Stephanophoros* (*The Crown Bearer*), that this is not a god who crowns himself. A particular individual was not being portrayed, but the human race, in its noblest form.

Further human differentiation can be seen in the portraits of individuals (see PL. 372), although this occurred infrequently in the 5th century. Only in the following era did the individual element in portraiture emerge, apparently correlated with the diminished importance of the city-state as a religious community and the emergence of the individual as a distinct personality. This connection seems to shed light upon an essential aspect of Greek classic art: the differentiation between the divine and the human in sculpture. The distinction, however, denotes not so much a separation as a more exact fixing of the limits of the two realms. In the following section we shall investigate certain variations, as depicted in sculpture, within the former realm — distinctions among the portrayals of the gods themselves.

It is more than coincidence that the most important cult statue — important for art as well as Greek religion, according to ancient evidence — was the *Zeus* at Olympia, a work by Phidias (q.v.). The precise descriptions of late Greek writers leave no doubt that this cult image must have surpassed all other ancient images of gods, both in its high artistic merit and its intellectual content. We possess unsatisfactory reflections of the *Zeus* in coins and even in the beautiful head discovered by J. Liegle (*Der Zeus des Pheidias im Lichte einer Neuerwerbung des berliner Münzkabinetts, Bericht über den VI internationalen Kongress für Archäologie*, 1939, p. 653 ff., pl. 76), but these do not enable us to form a sufficiently clear idea of the original. Actually the reproduction of a cult image in any nonsculptural art form, especially in coins, implies a serious transposition, not to mention differences due to the reduced size and the resulting impoverishment of forms. Our single piece of direct evidence of the Phidias *Zeus*, the only existing copy in sculpture, is the statuette from the Sanctuary of the Syrians on the Janiculum in Rome. As a work of art this statuette has little merit. Nevertheless, the god's profile reveals to us how much more μέγεθος, how much intrinsic grandeur, exists in it, compared to all the other later images of Zeus. Even such noble works as the head found in Caria, now in Boston (see PHIDIAS), reveal clearly the impoverishment of religious content and therefore also of artistic content. All the later heads of Zeus are (in the classicistic sense) merely noble, beautiful, or full of moderation, as, for example, the Otricoli head; or else they are theatrically agitated, overflowing with a pathetic air, like the heads from the height of the Hellenistic age. But only in Phidias' *Zeus* do we meet that particular classic synthesis of κάλλος ("beauty") and μέγεθος ("grandeur") — classic also in so far as it exerted a profound influence on the art of later times. The Roman *Capitoline Jupiter* can be traced back to the *Zeus* at Olympia, although it exhibits external changes demanded by the times and by the mass religion of the Roman empire. If Furtwängler's interpretation is correct, even the oldest representations of the bearded Christ were created on this Zeus model.

The differences between the 5th and 4th centuries become extremely clear in two renderings of a god, which we can re-

gard as peculiarly typical of the respective eras: the *Apollo of Kassel* (PL. 353) and the *Apollo Belvedere* by Leochares (PL. 383). Here we are confronted not so much with formal differences in a narrow stylistic sense as with differences relating to how a god lives in the artistic imagination of a creative master. We might almost speak of a religious epiphany of Apollo as the 5th and 4th centuries came to think of it. The classic master's conception was founded on the idea of κάλλος καὶ μέγεθος in stance, gesture, and form. Conversely, the conception of Leochares, whom we might consider postclassic, was based upon an emotionally aroused, theatrical, almost dancing image of Apollo. Even if these details in the *Apollo Belvedere* were emphasized through the work of the Roman copyist and later transmuted by the artistic spirit of the Renaissance (possibly through Montorsoli, one of the most remarkable 16th-century restorers), we cannot fail to recognize the deeper spiritual and sculptural differences between the two figures. Even if we limit our comparison to the manner of rendering the divine, the *Apollo of Kassel*, with its tight, compact construction and concentration of its vital forces that seem to flow back into the interior of the figure, emerges with strength and vigor; the Belvedere statue seems to spread out in all directions. In their idealization of the human body the two figures are also diametrically opposed. The classic statue (*Apollo of Kassel*) has a manly body, almost athletic in quality; the postclassic statue sets before us an almost effeminate young boy with the ambiguous character of a hermaphrodite.

Praxiteles' *Apollo Sauroktonos* (the *Lizard Slayer*; PL. 374) provides an equally forceful contrast to the *Apollo of Kassel*. Even if we ignore how much this great 4th-century master's work must have suffered at the hands of Roman copyists and restorers, and how much also it was weakened in response to the taste of later times, the two figures appear fundamentally different in pose, gesture, and religious content. Assuming that we could see a religious meaning in the slaying of the lizard, (comparable to that of the *Apollo Smintheus* by Skopas), this Apollo still does not partake of μέγεθος ("grandeur"). The figure is not sufficiently divine, if only in a sense of supreme elegance and beauty. If we did not know from ancient evidence that Praxiteles was here portraying a god, we should perceive nothing in this statue but a young man who, in a happy mood one beautiful summer day, slew a lizard with a dart. But the classic Apollo, as Homer described him in the opening passages of the *Iliad*, was like some towering cliff against which men might even be shipwrecked. The *Sauroktonos* is only a charming youth; his limbs are spread out into a fuller space, which seems to envelop and embrace him. Through this pose, which is so basically different, the distinction between the 5th-century and the 4th-century work, which is already postclassic, becomes intelligible.

We can trace a similar opposition in certain 5th- and 4th-century statues of Hermes. The *Ludovisi Hermes* (PL. 361) is a copy of a famous classic work. The firm manliness in the form of the body; the concentration of the sculptural volumes attained by bringing the legs close together; the harmony between the head and the movement of the arms; the heavy folds of the cloak, which is bunched together over the forearm — all give an energy to the figure which we seldom meet even in classic statues. Praxiteles' conception of Hermes is utterly different in these respects (see PRAXITELES). This is certainly not a cult statue, but nonetheless it is still the statue of a god. The light, playful motif of the god offering the bunch of grapes to the young Dionysos may have been demanded by the patron who commissioned the work, but the quality of smiling playfulness is assuredly a product of the artist's own imagination. Compactness and concentration of the sculptured image are replaced by an uncontrolled, expansive relaxation of the luxurious body, which is sunk in dreaming delight at its own beauty as it offers the grapes to the child. Certainly, if we understand this 4th-century statue as part of a historical development, it appears to have a maturity and richness in movement and in the handling of the whole which the 5th century lacked. The rendering of the torso is more delicate and soft, not only because of Praxiteles' own feeling for sculpture, but also because

of the 4th century's different ideal of the divine: faintly effeminate, slightly fleshy bodies began to be preferred, perhaps also because they enabled the play of light and shadow to be captured with greater virtuosity. The statue's sculptural structure is also based on principles that are diametrically opposed to the *Ludovisi Hermes*. The center of gravity is here displaced toward one side; the raised arm is supported on the trunk; the torso is expanded and relaxed: in all these details, as in the innate spiritual content, there is a difference between these two figures of gods.

The same change of taste is no less evident in the 4th century's representations of goddesses. Statues of female deities became increasingly frequent as result of the new and deeper elements in the worship of Demeter, Persephone, Aphrodite, and others; meanwhile, the images of male deities decreased in number and artistic importance until the time of Alexander the Great.

The most magnificent classic image of Aphrodite was the *Aphrodite Urania* by Phidias (q.v.). The existing replicas are quite adequate for the appreciation of its sculptural qualities. In this statue the goddess is revealed with a quality of superhuman dignity, so different from the all-too-human 4th-century images, such as Praxiteles' numerous portrayals of Aphrodite. These observations do not emanate from a modern esthetic taste or from a personal interpretation, but rather from tangible dissimilarities caused by the profound difference in the structure of sculpture during the 5th and 4th centuries. The air of majesty and the resiliency of the *Urania* are achieved by her buoyant pose and the refined, rhythmical use of the garments. Once again the body seems self-contained, with the contour centered on the axis of the figure. Her foot resting on the tortoise (the attribute of the goddess) enhances this effect, as does the way the cloak is laid over her thigh. This last motif gives a sculptural rather than linear character to the drapery. That this noble figure was considered classic is evident from its use as the model for an infinite number of later variations. Even the beautiful body and movement of the *Venus de Milo* (VII, PL. 176) depend upon the *Urania*, although they follow the formal laws of a later period. The goddess *Roma* at Ostia is represented with the same motif of the raised foot, and from Hadrian's reign on, emperors are represented thus with the foot placed on the sphere of the heavens or on the nape of an enemy's neck.

When the motif of the nude goddess became commonly accepted in the 4th century, the human aspect again triumphed over the religious. In Praxiteles' *Aphrodite of Knidos* (PL. 374) this quality is displayed in an extremely noble form, just before the decline into the eroticism of Hellenistic art. The proportions of the goddess's body are no longer classic: her head is smaller than the classic canon requires, and the proportions of the shoulders and hips are reversed, with the latter fully rounded. The delicate convex forms of the buttocks marked by dimples convey the softness of the flesh with remarkable effectiveness. The pose also reveals a richly variegated movement conditioned by a greater flexibility of the figure's axis in contrast to the concentrated, resilient effect of the *Urania*. But precisely because of such qualities the later *Aphrodite* is glimpsed in a suspended, momentary pose, her glance darting far away as if in fear — a quality quite foreign to the classic world. Praxiteles' *Aphrodite* is like a vision of a divine being who takes delight in being such; Phidias' *Aphrodite Urania* we could never summarize in any such general phrase.

We cannot perceive this kind of religious aspect in all the gods so clearly, even beyond any archaeological interpretation of form. There are gods whose images had already acquired many postclassic elements during the early classic period, in the first years of Sophocles' career (456–450). The earlier religious idea of Dionysos, for example, when he was envisaged as a bearded, majestic god, was utterly unlike the late-5th-century image of him as a young boy. But even thus changed, the seated Dionysos on the east pediment of the Parthenon still preserves a classic appearance, dignified and athletic, very different from the effeminate Dionysos of the 4th century.

Even more apparent than in Dionysos himself was the transformation of his companions, the satyrs, as early as the

first years of the classic period. Their bestial quality, which in the archaic era seemed inspired by Dionysiac frenzy, became more quiet and subdued. From the beginning of the classic period the satyr was no longer represented as ithyphallic, and the huge horse's tail became smaller. The same process of transforming animal traits into human ones was revealed in the structure of body and face; the snub nose and pointed ears still survived to distinguish a satyric from a human face, but at this point another significant change was introduced: the difference in age. At the beginning of the classic period (456 B.C.) a satyr was invariably portrayed with all the physical power of mature youth; by the end of the period we find satyrs both young and old. Then, at the close of the 5th century, there emerged satyrs with an altogether human beauty, having only the snub nose, sharp-pointed ears, and tiny tail as survivals of their former bestiality. The satyr later reached the world of Roman art, and Western art in general, as a faun. Viewed as an evolutionary phenomenon, the transformation is remarkable in that the external aspect of the creature was completed entirely within the classic period. About 460 B.C. the satyr had lost his essentially animal quality but was not yet so humbled, weak, and harmless as he appeared in the following age. It is only in late-antique art that there is found again, if only through mere exuberance of expression, an echo of his original nature.

Eros undergoes a change of form like that of the other gods. In the archaic era and the severe style, Eros was indistinguishable from any young athlete except for his wings. But with the rejuvenation in art of all the Greek gods, Eros appeared even younger. In the Parthenon frieze and on the model for the helmet (both attributed to Phidias), he is a boy. However, this is still far from the diminutive amorino that he became at the end of the 5th century (see PL. 375).

If we consider this phenomenon of the changing physical aspect of divinities as a universal process central to human consciousness, we find once again that we can pinpoint a classic period from 450 to 430 B.C., clearly separated from the 4th century. It we try to define the essence of the religious idea, we may say that during the 5th century divine beings were portrayed in human shape; but their quality was such that at first glance their very appearance raised them above mere human existence and commanded the respect of mortals. During the 4th century, however, the gods became no more than mortals. Their beauty and religious nature no longer demanded awed respect, and they withdrew into a divine realm of eternal beauty and everlasting joy, where they lived in peaceful, delighted contemplation of themselves. The gods of the 5th century, like their cult images, towered like rocks before mortals; the gods of the 4th century seemed to withdraw into the distant realm of a poetic and artistic vision. When 4th-century artists tried to portray a god with his former qualities of nobility and divine authority, they expressed this only through pathos or theatrical gestures, as in the *Apollo Belvedere* (PL. 383). Each modern spectator may understand and define differently the intellectual and religious decay of the cult image from the 5th to the 4th century; but however it is understood, we cannot deny that here we are confronted with two profoundly different ideas of the appearance of the gods.

*Mythological representations.* The representation of myth is also extremely important as far as Greek religious conceptions are concerned. It must be remembered that the joy the Greeks experienced in expressing themselves through myth had already passed its peak during the years of the severe style. The concern with mythology was decidedly on the downgrade during the 4th century. More important, beginning with the early classic period (460–450), the dramatic emphases of given myths were other than those of the archaic period. A few examples will suffice to illustrate this: In the tale of Orpheus, the horrible murder of Orpheus by the maenads was replaced by scenes of the enchanting effect of his lyre or his separation from Eurydice (PL. 363). Dionysos' thiasos, or band of followers, was rarely depicted fighting the god's enemies; instead it engaged in cult ceremonies to which the satyrs and maenads

added a tone of familiarity. In the myth of Medea the act of cooking the fatal ram was neglected in favor of the dilemma of whether Pelias' daughters should attempt the terrible rejuvenation of their father (PL. 363). Thus, from the many dramatic moments the Medea myth afforded, the 5th century selected one which permitted the portrayal of a deeper inner struggle with the least possible external theatricality.

When the 4th century adapted these myths, emphasis was placed on dramatic effects charged with erotic overtones. The sense of myth no longer lay in the pious terror of a vast decision imposed by the gods, but rather in a conflict of feelings altogether human, relating either to a triumph or to revenge for some lost prize. It is interesting to note that many myths which the archaic age seldom told suddenly emerged during the classic era and then later became rare again. One of the strangest examples of this phenomenon is the Niobe myth, which 5th-century classic art expressed in its noblest form (PL. 360), precisely because during that era the tension between men and the realm of the gods was for the first time so intensely felt. Man and the insuperable gulf separating him from the realm of the gods is most certainly the essence of this myth.

Today scholars frequently study the forms of a myth as a specific reworking of poetic material. Poetry and tragedy certainly had considerable influence on the details and the particular myths that were to be told; but perhaps the myths developed with certain details repeatedly elaborated by the tragic writers because the great classic poets were all touched by the same deep strains of the myth.

We must not confine our reflections to dramatic poetry in this present examination. The Greek myth is something almost inconceivable for us, far deeper than a mere story or a plaything of the imagination. We possess only a limited, fortuitous selection out of the vast riches of mythology, in which the theater certainly was not the only determining factor. Myth had a further function: we must remember that vases painted with mythological scenes were only very rarely functional objects for the living; most of these vases were laid in tombs, where they must have had a precise reference to the kingdom of the dead. The tremendous variety of mythical situations in which archaic art delighted appears, beginning with the earliest classic period (460–450), a little restricted, enriched by introspection, and based upon themes of spiritual decision. In the 4th-century late classic period, the mythical world appeared increasingly permeated by Aphrodite's influence. However, even when the myths began to lose their dignity because of this, they did not thereby become banal in the modern sense; they merely represented a different way of seeing and understanding.

*Portrayals of daily life.* The years 450 to 430 form a distinct period in the representations of the human realm. When we recognize the vast importance of portrayals of victorious athletes in archaic and severe sculpture, the extraordinary grandeur of the classic renderings is all the more admirable. It was then that the greatest artists, preeminently Polykleitos and his disciples (see POLYKLEITOS), tried to convey not only the athlete's physical nature but also his moral temperament or ethos. The circumspect modesty with which the victorious young man crowns himself with the victory garland had not found such an intensely spiritual expression before Polykleitos. We must also consider the sudden expansion of motifs for the victorious athlete in the 5th century — the pattern of leaning upon a pillar, the variation of stance, the distinction between the child and the grown man; all these characteristics the classic age first succeeded in ideating and rendering artistically. Fourth-century art, on the contrary, introduced no comparable inventions. And, in fact, the interest in portraying victorious athletes was no longer so intense because the religious and ethical significance that the Panhellenic games had for the entire Greek world nearly disappeared in the upheaval of all ethical values about 400 B.C. The Sophists had introduced new values, and these were beginning to dominate the Greeks' attention entirely. Athletics was restricted increasingly to the circle of professional athletes, among whom brilliant technique supplanted the creative, human purpose formerly at the core of

the athletic competition. Toward the end of his life Euripides was already bewailing the athletes' roughness and avarice. The grandeur and nobility of the older conception, and primarily of the classic image of the athlete, arose from its being interwoven with a genuine religious dedication. It was like a prayer offered by the whole civil community rather than the individual, expressed in an act of gratitude to the god. During the following epoch, however, the athlete's statue was a personal memorial, a secular image, without religious associations.

In this respect also, the 4th-century classic epoch can be unambigously distinguished from what some scholars call the second classic period and what others call the 4th-century postclassic. The decline is also very clearly revealed in the physical ideal as portrayed in sculpture. During the classic era one could speak of a εὔκρατος ἁρμονία of the ideal body: for there was certainly a harmonious balance between muscular and spiritual development. Athletic contests were held not for their own sake but rather to demonstrate the mental and physical perfecting of man through gymnastics. The moral caliber of the competition had to be very severely safeguarded. Even the high level of physical excellence in the classic period was lost because life had changed in the late 5th century, and men's bodies were also affected: the young men became weak and their muscular tissues soft and relaxed. Conversely, the professional athlete's body was now made hard and knotty in its structure, according to the taste of sports connoisseurs, to whom one can find reference as far back as the 4th century.

Perhaps this contrast between the classic and the postclassic finds especially lucid expression in the two most celebrated statues of athletes produced by the two eras: the classic *Doryphoros*, or *Spear Bearer* (Polykleitos; PL. 359), and the postclassic *Apoxyomenos* (Lysippos; PL. 382). These two works represented new directions for the artists of their own epoch and those following. *Doryphoros* is regarded as the model for the classic age and for classicism, while the *Apoxyomenos* established for its own era a new sculptural ideal of the perfect human figure which was to persist in the Hellenistic world until its decline and the classic reawakening.

Perhaps we can also discern a deeper, almost symbolic meaning, inasmuch as the *Doryphoros* is not an ordinary gymnast but Achilles, the very prototype of the Greek man, physically their ἀρχηγέτης, or "leader." Perfection in every way, deep tranquillity, dignity as if by natural right find expression here. The *Apoxyomenos*, on the other hand, presents us with a magnificent image of postclassic man, transformed by a sublime artistic sense: the new agile stance, the nervous restlessness permeating the whole figure — such is the image of man of this age who lives in a fuller sphere of existence. All classic images of human beings seem, on the contrary, as if closed within themselves.

*Funerary art.* The difference between the classic and postclassic appears even more profound in the field of funerary art, that is, art connected in any way with the world of the dead (see ESCHATOLOGY). Funerary art is exemplified by lustral vases (used for the purification rites of the dead person and his tomb), vases buried with the dead person, and the sculptured monument built over the tomb itself.

From the funerary art of 460–400 B.C. we may ascertain certain customs and standards of the era. At that time the white-ground lekythos (PL. 365) was created — a type of lustral vase which embodies the noblest expression of the Greeks' feelings toward their dead. This genre of vase as a funerary object began with the severe style and reached its peak between 450 and 430; but by about 400 the few surviving examples showed an excessively slender, curved form and elusive paintings. Characteristically, in all the scenes, the dead person was shown not as he had appeared in life but as the φάντασμα, or shade, which, according to Plato, dwells near the tomb and is sometimes visible to the living. The shade was depicted pursuing the pastimes of his earthly life — hunting, playing the lyre, conversing with friends.

An altogether different image of the dead, and of death itself, was portrayed by lustral vases of the late classic age,

about 400 B.C. The dead person appeared as he had in life, but now seated in front of his tomb with a sad expression, mourning the life he had lost and encircled by shining purple palm branches suggesting funeral torches.

Most of the extant vase specimens were discovered in tombs. From these it is sometimes possible to distinguish the dead person's belongings from the funerary trappings depicted. We are also able to distinguish certain philosophical differences tween the 5th and 4th centuries. The earlier conception, becoming increasingly rare throughout the classic epoch, was the idea that pictures dedicated to the dead person, as if through a kind of sympathetic magic, assured him of a happy existence in the other world, with all the pleasures of horses, handsome young men, music, symposiums, dicing, and sacrificial offerings to the gods. This idea gave way to an image of the dead person's life in the ethereal sphere beneath the constellations. Pictures of the stars or star divinities, such as the Pleiades and the constellation of Perseus, began to be set in the tomb with the dead person. Accordingly the extraordinary epigram written for the men who fell at Potidaea says that while their bodies rest in the earth, their psyches dwell in the ether (*Festschrift für R. Böhringer*, Tübingen, 1957, p. 420).

By the late classic era, during the Peloponnesian War (431–404), portrayals of Dionysos' cortege were more and more frequently depicted on tomb vases. Perhaps these paintings alluded to the dead person's initiation into the happy, drunken state of the bacchantes and to the abandoned languor of the wine god. During the 4th century a Dionysiac atmosphere seemed to predominate; vase paintings showing Dionysiac revels and the enchanted gardens of Aphrodite occurred more often (PLS. 375, 376). Along with these, the Eleusinian deities appear, as if to offer the initiates a happy existence after death.

THE FORMAL DEVELOPMENT. *The male nude.* The period from 540 to 430 B.C. marks an era which, both through its religious ideas and through the images conceived by its artists, raised itself thoroughly above preceding and later ages; consequently it has been considered the epoch that created the noblest forms out of its own interpretation of the visible world. Granting this, we must now see how it came about, starting from a basic element: ponderation, or the distribution of weight in the standing figure.

In the long sequence of statues of young boys and children ranging from the archaic period through the entire 4th century, the various poses and gestures reveal different artistic conceptions. The unique and vital accomplishment of the Greek classic age about 450 was that it completely freed the human body from the pompous rigidity and harsh architectural forms which had frozen the human figures in Eastern art from the 2d millennium on. The weight of the body was now divided between a supporting leg and a free-swinging leg. This scheme of the weight resting upon one leg (*uno crure insistere*) had already been recognized by historians of ancient art as the solution for distribution of weight; and in his statues of famous athletic victors, Polykleitos seems to have rediscovered the scheme about 440 B.C., thereby marking a new epoch. It was a discovery of, or rather a solution to, a problem studied for a long time and experimented with for at least two generations before Polykleitos' achievement.

About 500 we can discern the first attempts in this direction — more clearly in the designs of vase paintings than in sculpture, partly because most of the statues of young men have come down to us only as torsos rather than statues in their entirety. The vase painters Euthymides and Kleophrastes were among the first to portray figures with one leg pulled back and the other leg not exactly free-swinging, but at least differentiated and bearing less weight. In the rear view the corresponding inclination of the hips was equally apparent.

These experiments naturally enough appeared more uncertain in sculpture, in which the technical problem of the medium of construction as well as the anatomical and sculptural problems had to be dealt with. It was undoubtedly far easier to set a figure firmly on two legs so that the statue's center of gravity was between its feet. Understandably, therefore, the attempts

at changing the distribution in weight were more clearly shown in the torso than in the actual placement of the feet. The artists observed first, and tried to represent first, the varying relaxation and tension of the muscles, especially in violent movements (I, PL. 368). Their joy in discovering the use of the torso muscles explains the extremely conspicuous rendering of the muscular system appearing in late archaic reliefs such as the base from Themistokles' Wall and especially in the reliefs from the Athenian Treasury at Delphi. This newly expanded knowledge of how the body's muscular covering changes its appearance was fully reflected in relief work sooner than in completely three-dimensional sculpture; the same was true of other details as well. In the base from Themistokles' Wall, portraying the "hockey" players, we find perhaps the first example of figures with a clear rendering of the distinction between the supporting and the free-swinging leg, but in the *Youth* from Agrigento (PL. 344) we still perceive the technical difficulties of construction that its creator had to face. The two legs do not bear the weight equally; at the same time the leg that should be free is not completely so. Thus we have the rather convincing impression of a person halting in his forward motion. This figure, however praiseworthy in execution, is not the creation of a great personality but assuredly the work of a modest carver who probably transferred the image of a victorious athlete from bronze without attempting to copy it entirely, precisely because he did not know how to face the problem of the statics of a stone sculpture. The *Youth* attributed to Kritios (PL. 344), however, is a great master's work, dating from about 490 B.C. In it the free-swinging side of the body seems to have been made distinct (perhaps the right foot was slightly raised as well); there is a far sharper and more rigorous anatomical precision than in the statue from Agrigento, indicating a complete understanding and most effective rendering of muscular contraction. The buttock of the supporting leg appears rigid and tightly compressed in contrast to the relaxed buttock of the free-swinging leg. With similar effect the artist continued the tension and relaxation of the torso muscles by slightly raising the shoulder corresponding to the supporting left leg and by slightly lowering the other shoulder. An entirely frontal head, such as archaic taste demanded, would have had a displeasing effect in combination with the freedom of the pose. The artist therefore allowed the head to turn a little away from the side of the free leg, as if unconsciously and in mere obedience to the body's organic rhythm. Artistically this is such an important step for the year 490 that we cannot overestimate its significance. A feeling for the natural rendering of the body finds expression here, as has so often been pointed out, along with a more intense, exact intuition of the body's balance and counterbalances. The miraculously vivid and accurate rendering is less the result of a studious search for anatomical precision than an unconscious feeling of the power of one's own body. Here for the first time the human body was understood as a separate entity, as an individual organism capable of attaining its own freedom and self-determination by moving away from the impersonal collective images of the tyrannically governed state. The pose of the head brilliantly reveals this perception of the possibilities of greatness inherent in man, although the features as yet have no individual traits. Undeniably the breast and head of this figure have a weight and importance in the way they are joined sculpturally, found in no other statue before it.

Kritios' statue of the *Youth* is clearly one of those sculptural works which has started on the path toward perfection but cannot yet be considered truly classic. From a formal point of view the figure lacks classic serenity and harmony, and minute scrutiny reveals many details not yet classic in their anatomical rendering. The head, for instance, lacks a certain lifelike quality of emerging manly beauty appropriate to an adolescent youth. All the various shapes, including the tightly twisted curls on the crown, appear intentionally harsh and stiff; they are not yet permeated by the organic flowing quality which during the classic era subjected all the individual shapes to the superior rhythm of the body. What this statue reflects, then, is the severe style, or αὐστηρὰ ἁρμονία.

Theoreticians of style in Greece had already correctly recognized and isolated for poetry and prose a classic style, εὔκρατος ἁρμονία. The language of the archaic period had been called γλαφυρά, or "subtle, polished"; Pindar was austere, Sophocles classic. The classic style in art had its development in the magnificent new spiritual revolution resulting from the founding of the young democracies and from the Persian Wars — a revolution that had an intensive effect on sculpture, particularly the male figures, apparent in formal changes in the distribution of weight, pose, and bodily movements. These formal changes are so many steps in the whole process of social change. Assuredly the evolution during the Pentakontaetia (the 50-year period, 480–432 B.C., between the end of the Persian Wars and the outbreak of the Peloponnesian War) was not the result of the esthetic formalistic process that modern art connoisseurs have so passionately claimed it to be; it was rather a continuation, an almost biological evolution, of the total physical image of man.

Although most of the original masterpieces of these decades have been lost or preserved only through inadequate copies, we can follow the development from the severe style into the classic from 480 to 440. It must be emphasized, however, that this development did not follow some predetermined purpose, for such a purpose could not have existed. Until that time no artistic era had ever conceived of this harmonious appearance of man in art and life, and so we should regard it solely as a deep process within men, first clearly and exactly expressed, of course, in the realms of understanding, thinking, and speaking. The representational arts, in contrast to their position in other intentionally and self-consciously artistic epochs, remained, for these Greeks, barely on the periphery of the intellectual world. We may recall that during this very period the Greeks did not regard artists as intellectual beings or revealers of the beautiful and the true but as mere second-class men, or βάναυσοι ("artisans"), not even allowed to share in the freedom and full life of true Greeks. To be sure, the artist did not have time to go to school, participate in politics, or enjoy the everyday intellectual activities. The sculptor's work with hammer and chisel was rough, that of the bronze artist dirty and exhausting. We must therefore consider Greek classic art all the more magnificent for being the mere incidental fruit of an infinitely rich intellectual life, and for originating in a profession that was not highly esteemed.

We can discern several stages in the development toward the classic art of 440. The first decisive step has already been suggested by Kritios' *Youth* of about 490. If we omit sculptural works known only through copies (hence mélanges), such as the *Hero* in the Palazzo dei Conservatori, Rome, we might regard as the next stage the *Apollo* from the west pediment of the Temple of Zeus at Olympia (PL. 351), even though this work may appear from its axial composition and architectural setting to be more restricted than an individual or cult statue. This mature stage of the severe style was characterized by vigorous, full volumes found everywhere during this decade (470–460 B.C.), whether in columns, vase shapes, or ornamental forms. All the statues seem endowed with excessive physical robustness, clear not only in the physical ideal as such, but also in the almost violent idiom of gestures, suggestive of Aeschylus' and Pindar's eloquence. The human form became enriched thereby as if it had expanded, in contrast to Kritios' *Youth*. The latter, to be sure, is only a mortal and Apollo is a god, but we might meet the same phenomenon in the figures of young boys as well, if such images had survived from this period. This new quality found expression in the distribution of weight and full rendering of an organically felt rhythm. The right leg rests solidly upon the ground. The left free-swinging leg is hardly displaced, but the foot is certainly more clearly removed from the ground than in Kritios's *Youth*. The motion pervading the torso muscles arises from this stance rather than from mere external muscular expansion. The energetic tension of the head held to the side, demanded by Apollo's role in the scene of battle, vigorously enhances the spirit which dominates the enormously strong body.

Along with this powerful accentuation of physical nature,

there is a refinement and increased spirituality in the images of gods and men during the early classic period (460–450). If the *Apollo from the Tiber* (PL. 353) has a dry bodily structure, elongated like a column, it is due at least partly to the artist who created the work but still more to the artistic climate of the time. Although we know little about this artistic climate from the records of sculpture, we do know a great deal about it from vase paintings. Compared to the *Apollo from Olympia*, the *Apollo from the Tiber* has a more delicate frame, almost adolescent; but there is a similarity in the rhythm of the figure as it is derived from the distribution of weight and the placement of the feet close together. In the latter statue, a decisive step toward the classic is perceptible in the god's head, which turns not from the side of the free-swinging leg but from the supporting leg, thus producing a contrapuntal effect decisively important for the figure. This contrapuntal effect is a characteristic of all classic figures. Yet the entire development is only a preliminary attempt at portraying the figure's inner peace; it is more a promise than a complete realization. The volumes and shapes of the head of the *Apollo from the Tiber* also reveal the break with the severe tradition.

The *Apollo of Kassel* (PL. 353) marks the really decisive step toward the classic style. Here the figure already possesses the classic weightiness both in its bodily volumes and in the pose of its limbs. The placing of the feet close together contributes to the concentrated, expressive image that seems to convey Apollo's authority effectively. In contrast to early classic works, this figure seems more completely master of its own movements and limbs. Everything in it is more closely knit together, and therein lies the effect of this Apollo's intense spirituality. We observe not only the organic, functional awareness but also the way the torso is placed above the legs, which is different from preceding statues of gods. Or one can contrast the position and function of the head in the Tiber and Kassel Apollo's. Once again similar phenomena are observable in these details. To say that the purely anatomical rendering of the torso is more "correct" is thus superfluous.

The pinnacle in this field was attained by the *Doryphoros* (the *Spear Bearer*), Polykleitos' Achilles of about 440 B.C. (PL. 359). Undoubtedly many details are due to the fact that this figure does not depict a god but simply a hero, and belongs to the Argive rather than the Attic tradition. In spite of these limitations, however, we can set the *Doryphoros* in this series of statues of gods and regard it as one of the most significant examples of the entire classic development. The interrelated proportions of the human body in the *Doryphoros* border on that perfection which ancient esthetics had already recognized as inherent in the classic era. Certainly the human body achieved its most perfect sculptural rendering in this statue. No less important, the motif of the weight resting upon one leg was fully worked out here, as had already been noticed by ancient esthetic critics. This was not a pattern of movement but the tranquillity of the body completely master of its own limbs. Even the arms reflect the balance and relaxation prevalent in the whole figure: the active arm, which holds the spear, is on the same side as the free-swinging leg, and the relaxed arm balances the supporting leg. But the figure's real point of balance lies in the slight twisting of the head toward this supporting side of the body which is thus emphasized. We can judge this new, fully classic rendering of the human image better through a side rather than frontal view. For the first time, an artist was able to create a human body in sculpture, existing freely in its own radius of action. An esthetic and formalistic phenomenon, the statue revealed a complex system of balances and counterbalances between the spiritual and physical forces active in the human body that was first realized by man about 440.

A comparison of this classic image of the human body with Polykleitos' own *Diadoumenos*, which depicts not a victor, but Apollo, reveals another system of balances in a human image. There is a difference in the distribution of weight and the pose. Since the free leg of the *Diadoumenos* is still more emphatically pulled over toward the side, we have the impression that it is moving too slowly, as if it were slipping

on the ground; and instead of the figure's active ascent in an uninterrupted rhythm, there is a kind of relaxation — a weariness and almost a spiritual surrender of the soft body. The structure of the torso is noble, full, and powerful, but its surfaces are delicate and soft — decidedly too human for a god. This could hardly be judged appropriate in a classic image of Apollo, particularly among the Dorians. The body's axis follows flexibly the beautiful curve which starts out from the toe and runs throughout with unchanging strength; but the action of the hands tying the fillet suggests a weariness and almost effeminately refined, relaxed tempo.

If we reflect upon the continuous development up to the *Diadoumenos*, we cannot deny that the *Doryphoros* marked the high point and that the *Diadoumenos* betrayed the beginnings of decline. Wherever we turn our attention — even to tectonic forms such as columns, capitals, palmettes, and vases, or even to drawing — the phenomenon appeared to be general after the Pentakontaetia: clearly the vital forces which had been the decisive impulse toward classic configurations began to grow weak or to be redirected to different purposes.

How great was the break which the turn of the century marked for this development, and the consequent change in artistic tendencies, is indicated by various works of the period. We can detect certain trends common to the preceding traditions; but the static element in such works was conducive to a new solidity rather than to a harmonious suggestion of movement. The figures manifest a kind of severe style in the early 4th century. There is, however, a classic perfection in this new vocabulary of the sculptural portrayal of man. The completely three-dimensional roundness of the human body is brilliantly rendered in Praxiteles' *Satyr Pouring Wine* and in the *Aphrodite of Knidos* (PL. 374). Formalistically and esthetically these are superlative works of art, which we might safely call classic, if only the word "classic" could denote a transitional stage of an artistic development rather than the high point of a long process from which the ancients drew inspiration.

*The garbed female figure.* The representation of garbed female figures followed a development parallel to that of the male nudes. But in the female figures, especially those wearing the peplos, the progressive stages of development are even more clearly apparent. The peplos, which became fashionable in Athens about 480 B.C., was a large, broad upper garment hanging in folds, thrown over the rest of the clothing, and wrapped around the whole of the body. It was an important factor in the history of sculpture, facilitating a new vision of the blocklike construction of both male and female figures as well as their tectonic and static rendering. The statues from 480 to 470 seem to preserve the massive quality of the original material. They have a full, balanced composition, feet set apart but on the same level (instead of one foot stepping forward, as was customary), and rich harmony of drapery. Above the full, vertical, rhythmically spaced folds of the garment, the bosom appears as a solid mass, modified by only a few folds in order not to weaken the structural impressiveness of the whole. From decade to decade one can observe a growing relaxation in this sculptural composition: the slight curving of the knee, at first only a little, but later more and more firmly pressing against the garment to show the supporting and free legs through the material. At the same time there began an interplay of folds on the torso, revealing the movement of the body underneath the garment. The critical point in this evolution is evident in the structure of statues about 480, whose proportions and pose are dominated by weightiness. Next the head began to turn slightly and to incline, usually toward the side of the free-swinging leg but later (ca. 460 B.C.) toward the supporting leg. But only about 440 can one speak of an image completely subjected to and permeated by a harmonious rhythm, because then the blocklike construction of the figure was intentionally abandoned. At the same time the break between the garment on the torso and the skirt became smaller. Probably it was the Athenians who modified the peplos to harmonize with their own way of understanding the body, adding a belt over the *apoptygma* (the long overfold of peplos material that often

reached from the neck to the knees). There resulted a lighter, more elegant resiliency of the body and also a succession of richer and more varied motifs in the different parts of the garment, which was viewed as a series of units from the feet to the hem of the *kolpos* (baggy fold under the waist), then to the belt and the neck. This Attic manner of draping the Dorian cloak provided a variegated and delicate interplay of folds instead of the simple, powerful, and rich *ductus*, or lineation, of the Dorian costume. It was also extremely important that as a result of the increasingly perceptible twisting of the hip, the interplay of folds became unified. The belt no longer formed a break: the sculptural impulse permeating even the small folds overcame and covered the belt. Usually one main fold rose from the top of the foot of the free leg, arching rhythmically in a full curve, and then unfurled into many small folds, enlivening the torso and pushing upward to the neck.

For these peplos figures, then, we can trace a development reaching its acme about 440, beyond which we can no longer proceed without losing the figures' essential sculptural consistency. We can also discern the danger of such a dissolution even in a few 5th-century clothed figures. Like the *Diadoumenos*, these late classic peplos figures strike a pose with one leg placed too far to one side, so that the rhythm and all the flowing quality of the folds have a superbly springy effect, without, however, the solidity and self-containment of the classic period about 440. The new structural solidity and slight stiffening observed in figures from about 400 B.C. is just as perceptible in these figures wearing the peplos as in the male nudes. Even the figures of the early 4th century reveal a greater penetration of space than existed in the 5th century, through their distribution of weight; at the same time, they have a new sense of profundity through the movement and twisting of their bodies. In the classicism of the 4th century, particularly during the stage that produced the *Aphrodite of Knidos* and the *Satyr Pouring Wine*, statues attained for the first time a harmonious roundness and were esthetically satisfying when viewed from many angles. Solely on the basis of the evolution of both form and esthetic achievement, we might regard this new apex of sculptural excellence in the mid-4th century as the true classic; this would, of course, necessitate our excluding the 5th century from such a definition. However, on other grounds — the balance of beauty and spiritual grandeur, which even the ancient art critics had observed — the 5th century must be considered classic.

*Relief.* In classic (as opposed to classicistic) relief, the figure does not stand out in contrast to the surface of the background, but with it constitutes a unity. Relief in the classic era attained such a high sculptural value precisely because of this union of figure and background. In the 4th century, relief figures have a greater corporeality — partly because of their larger radius of action and inherently greater capacity for movement, but more because the figures are made independent of the background through the tentative but effective use of foreshortened perspective. This contrast, either actual or suggested, between the supporting background and the human image was not yet familiar to 5th-century relief sculpture. But 4th-century relief always managed to free itself, even when leaning toward classic effects, as in its early classicizing decades.

All these aspects of the development of Greek art bring us again and again to the years around 400 as the decisive period of change of the Greek spirit — a change called to mind merely by the names of Socrates and the battle of Aegospotamos. The artistic developments actually resulted from small isolated elements. The most important and also the most conspicuous were the sculptural volumes, proportions, pose, and gestures of the human figure; but even the tiny details, such as the rendering of hair and fabrics, are highly indicative of stylistic change. We could establish a syntax of these artistic forms and use it to determine the various stages of the process in order to corroborate and elucidate the developments discussed above.

*Hair styles.* The severe age (480–460) made an extremely important artistic advance when it began to represent the hair,

counterbalanced with the facial features, as a single compact mass. For some time during this period, the hair had the appearance of a skullcap, an effect relieved by the addition of painted rather than sculptured details, which, however, did not detract from the sense of cohesive volume. Sometimes the hair radiated from the crown of the head and formed a circle around the face, as in Kritios' *Youth* (PL. 344); sometimes it was knotted on the nape of the neck. In general, however, the severe age preferred long hair arranged in cohesive, well-constructed masses, in keeping with its passion for a vigorous, impressive appearance. Young men and girls usually bound their hair with a fillet and knotted it at the nape of the neck. Older fashions and other hair arrangements also occurred in the severe age; the large variety of styles clearly shows the inquiring spirit of the creative forces of the period. In the line of development of any one style, however, the heavy solidity of locks depicted from 470 to 460 (late severe style) can be contrasted with the gentle and subtle stylization of the early classic (460–450).

A new ideal of beauty that was first crystallized in the classic period was a particular arrangement of hair. The most advanced of the mature archaic works sometimes, in bold anticipation, represented this style, as we see in the head of the *Rayet Youth* with his slightly waved medium-long locks. From the late archaic era on, we find examples of other styles such as short spiral curls or separate locks arranged like fish scales or feathers. Popular among the more advanced late-6th-century Athenians was a style of short hair, falling naturally. The early classic period (460–450), with its enthusiasm for slender, graceful forms, generally preferred long hair flowing down over the shoulders and nape of the neck, at least for its statues of gods. The classic period proper (450–430), however, achieved an even greater fluidity and organic interconnection of the various elements. During the evolution of the classic *Doryphoros* type, this fluidity was so magnificently realized that each lock of hair and the total arrangement reflect the rhythm permeating the classic figure. Artists of this period for the first time fastened and arranged the hair in the particular style we see in Phidias' divine figures.

In the postclassic *Diadoumenos*, the fluidity of the hair became too soft and yielding. We might say that even in such an insignificant detail as this, only the quality of κάλλος ("beauty") remained, no longer united with μέγεθος ("grandeur"). In the classicizing tendency of the early 4th century, we observe a return to the sculptural rendering of the hair. The period tended generally to treat forms no longer as isolated details but as fused and interconnected. This treatment appears most clearly in the funerary steles and the surviving original statues of the 4th century. Those masterpieces known only through Roman copies, however, reveal instead the linear treatment favored by the classicizing Roman imperial age.

*Drapery.* The treatment of garments such as the peplos, chiton, and himation underwent a revolutionary change about 500 B.C., when artists first tried to give fabrics some sculptural value, thereby transcending the linear styles and the insubstantiality of ancient garments. Soon afterward, principally in the maidens from the Propylaia and the east pediment of Aegina, sculptors tried to make the fabric appear a tangible substance with weight and mass. This led to the dominance of pure form in the severe style (480–460), as in the rendering of hair. Through new motifs of folds they sought to make the movements independent of the soft, massed fabric (PL. 368). They consciously avoided the overflowing movements which the archaic era had always more or less resolved into ornamental patterns. The new preferred motifs were the troughlike folds, bifurcating lines, and the superimposition of part of one garment on another with folds flowing together. Even in marble sculpture, like that at Olympia, one has the impression of hand modeling, as in the clay model for a bronze. Sometimes the fabric even of the chiton resembled a layer of leather rather than fine linen. This was the passion of the age: a joy in everything solid, hard, and compact.

During the early classic period (460–450), when the taste

for slender figures was reacquired, more delicate forms in drapery were introduced, and like the flowing of the folds, the material was rendered as softer and finer. The thick eye folds or furrowed folds were made flatter and less prominent. The crude, very solid forms were beginning to be left behind, making way for the balance between the garments and the figure achieved about 440 B.C. The frieze and east pediment of the Parthenon (PL. 368) represent the highest examples of this process. Subsequently, beginning with the increasingly magnificent figures of about 430 (west pediment of the Parthenon), which were characterized by a new kind of movement, the garments flowed in cascades over the limbs. We find here no unifying rhythm but rather frequent dissonances and clashing movements, particularly in the more developed figures of the pediment (Oreithyia and Iris). The fabrics of these decades, one might say, seem to foam. Yet this effect was merely the ultimate consequence of the classic rendering of garments, perhaps grasped by none except the masters of the west pediment of the Parthenon. By the end of the 5th century, the flowing of the folds lost its torrential force, and if the movement continued, as for example on the balustrade of the Temple of Athena Nike (PL. 368), it recalled the running of a brook rather than the headlong rush of a cataract.

The trend toward softly flowing forms eventually gave an excessive pliancy to figures, and in the 4th century, or at least at its beginning, an effort was made to render even the drapery with a new solidity. Thus there was a return to classic patterns, although they failed to achieve the intimate union of figure and garments characteristic of the classic age at its peak. After 400 the fabric covering the figure was always extremely individualized. Particularly about 340 B.C. artists invented new forms to make the limp masses of drapery stand out in contrast to the figure.

Not all 5th-century artists followed the course sketched above. The theme of the archaic and constricted human figure persisted through every epoch in the East, but we have no way of knowing what it meant to the Greeks. From political and cultural history we do know of the resistance raised against those who initiated the spiritual movements of the Pentakontaetia, the 50-year period between the end of the Persian Wars and the outbreak of the Peloponnesian War. On the other hand, Euripides, even in his youthful works about 450, was a real subverter of the classic; his plays, indeed, gave expression to a new relationship between man and the the forces surrounding him. The spiritual and artistic development of the 5th century was undoubtedly less simple and unilinear than we should today like to make it appear. In certain early-5th-century works, which even at present are assigned a 6th-century date, we find an undisguised effort to cling to the external characteristics of archaic art. The so-called "hieratic sculptures" are an example; either because of the demands of the architectural setting of a temple or merely for religious reasons, these sculptures revealed a tendency to retain the old severe pose and formal archaic idiom of the garments and hair. Other examples are the *Enthroned Goddess* from Tarentum (Taranto), which we should date about 450 B.C. on the basis of the palmettes on the throne, and the *Apollo from Piombino*, which reveals the soft 5th-century forms, particularly in the back. Without retaining purely archaic forms, many other works nevertheless show a rigid adherence to earlier characteristics.

THE CLASSIC IN THE SCULPTURE OF GREECE. For a more precise knowledge of Greek sculpture, we should remember that the process of evolution traced above, with all its possible uncertainties and limitations, was worked out only in Athens and, probably, at Argos. Argive sculpture from 450 to 430 is unfortunately known only through Polykleitos' statues of athletes. This artist worked also in Athens, where his influence even before 440 is perceptible in the Parthenon frieze. As a thinker and theorist, he was concerned with an interpretation of the world of appearances, and he probably was no stranger to Socrates' circle. According to all surviving descriptions, his gold and ivory *Hera* at Argos must have rivaled the statue of *Zeus* at Olympia: this suggests that Polykleitos wanted to absorb the experience of Phidias and overcome the artistic limitations of his own native city (see ATTIC AND BOEOTIAN ART; PELOPONNESIAN ART).

At any rate, it has been impossible to identify any Peloponnesian city enjoying a continuous artistic growth up to the classic level even remotely comparable to the evolutionary process in Athens. Argive bronze statuettes which may from the distribution of weight be considered late representatives of Polykleitos' influence, and may therefore be termed classic (or perhaps actually postclassic), still reveal many archaic details, especially in the formation of the head. There is evidence of similar influence in Corinthian circles as well. Almost all the bronzes surviving to us from the classic era, such as supports for mirrors or ornaments for hydrias, are decidedly the work of craftsmen; but even up to the end of the 5th century they manifest the tenacious survival of forms from the great epoch of the severe style.

The marble sculptures of the non-Athenian Peloponnesos, such as the fragments of the Temple of Hera in Argos, do not antedate 400. Besides, the extent to which these works are due, if at all, to Argive sculptors is an open question. The patterns, however, certainly harked back to local artists, as did the sculptures in the Temple of Apollo Epikourios at Phigalia (PL. 370). If, as W. B. Dinsmoor thinks (*The Temple of Apollo at Bassae*, New York, 1933), we can assume that the Niobids from the Temple of Apollo in the Terme Museum (Rome, Mus. Naz. Rom.) and the Ny Carlsberg Glyptotek (Copenhagen) were located in the pediments, we must conclude that the artists active on the pediments were not Dorian but Ionian. The friezes of the Temple of Apollo are not Argive, as has been observed, and it would not be easy to fix the locality of the artists, for the work certainly bears no apparent relation to that from the Peloponnesos. Much the same is true of the sculptures from the temple at Selinous (Selinunte, Sicily): they are certainly neither Argive nor Sikyonian, but are related instead to the reliefs of the Delphi tholos by Theodoros of Phokaia (Phocaea).

The classic as established in Attica became diffused throughout the rest of the Greek world, although with a certain lag in time. The *Diomedes* and other works attributed to the Cretan artist Kresilas are representative in this respect; as the most complete replica of the *Diomedes*, which is in Naples, seems to indicate, they should be dated from about 420. Other works which can be judged only through Roman copies — very important products of Dorian artistic centers, such as the *Athena of Velletri* or the *Athena Giustiniani*, the so-called *Gypsy* — have a formal style assimilating them completely to the late-5th-century Attic koine, especially in their drapery and hair. In the structure of the figure, however, and in the rhythmic flow of their folds, these works unquestionably retained echoes of the severe taste of the Dorian masters about 460 B.C. But actually this well-known phenomenon of the Dorian classic, essentially reducible to the early-4th-century postclassic, has as yet been inadequately studied. The artists of this group worked primarily in bronze, and because of the harsh character of the material they could not attain the essential qualities of classic Attic art.

THE CLASSIC ON THE NORTHERN AND WESTERN PERIPHERIES AND IN THE IONIAN TOWNS. Even in the northern and eastern towns of the Greek world, the outlook, content, and forms of Attic classic art were gradually diffused exactly as the Attic dialect had been diffused during the 4th century, when it became the common language of cultivated persons and supplanted local dialects (see GREEK ART, EASTERN; GREEK ART, NORTHERN; GREEK ART, WESTERN). After the Persian Wars, Athens had become the center of the Greek world: this was why the classic ethos as a complete intellectual and artistic expression of life could flower only in Athens. All the mental energies became concentrated in that city, because only there could men with intellectual interests find a complete fulfilment of their aspirations. One calls to mind Polygnotos of Thasos, who left his own fatherland, and the Sophists, who in philosophy overthrew the classic age. The Sophists came from Abdera,

Leontini, Elea, or other distant cities, to congregate at Athens, which was for them the one possible center. The drainage of all the most important vital energies from the eastern and northern regions of the Greek world produced a definite retardation in the outlying towns; but the commercial impoverishment of Ionia was even more the result of the refined financial policy of Athens, which led eventually to the ruin of Athens itself, about the end of the 5th century, and to the end of the classic period. After the Persian Wars no more temples or sanctuaries of any importance were built in eastern Greece.

One of the most unusual aspects of the art of eastern Greece was a remarkable retardation of formal expression. When we examine the Ionian funerary steles without considering the difference in schools, we discover that the figures have great flexibility of pose and gesture. In the modeling of the hair one misses the organic composition of separate little locks crossing one another and linked together. Sometimes hair in Ionian figures has a silken consistency, as, for example, in the fragments from Candia and Megara. Elsewhere it has a rough, crude appearance, which was typical in Samos about 400. The rendering of the material and the lineation of the folds in Ionian art preserve much of the severe style, even in the late-5th century (for example, the stele of Phyllis in the Louvre). Often the figure is clothed with an ample mass of material, but sufficient elasticity of form and exactness of accent are lacking to make the curves of the great folds conform to the body's natural rhythm. Instead the tendency to reduce all the movements of folds to decorative patterns is still observable in Ionian works even from the late 5th century. Consequently it is difficult to date Ionian sculpture precisely within the 5th century. The sculptures on the Nereid monument, for example, present a certain harshness of movement atypical of the classic style; the sculptures were erroneously assigned to the middle of the 5th century until it was pointed out that the very delicate, sinuous rendering of the garments, revealing rather than covering the body, could not have occurred before the classic epoch. This strange phenomenon of a distinct Ionian ethos is clearly represented also in the *Nike* by Paionios (ca. 420; PL. 367), also once attributed to the middle of the 5th century. Stylistically the *Nike* could not have preceded the pediments of the Parthenon. Yet the composition of the figure is ingenious — possible perhaps only in Ionia and certainly foreign to classic Attica, where it would have been considered unacceptable and even offensive. Seeming hardly to touch the ground, the figure is suspended from her cloak, which is puffed out like a sail, and creates the illusion of her smooth flight from on high; the flying eagle beneath the goddess's feet intensifies the impression that she is swooping out of the clouds. This illusionistic quality, pervading the statue in a deeper sense and constituting its main effect, is the Ionian heritage which was to be further developed during the anti-classic high Hellenistic period. A more or less antistructural feeling reappeared in almost all Ionian sculpture in the round. Certainly far more Ionian terra cottas than marbles have come down to us, and even in these, the artist appears less interested in the figures than in the garments, which seem to be modeled by the wind into fluttering, feathery forms. These stylistic qualities typical of eastern Greece indicate not so much a lesser gift for expression as a different channeling of vital energy.

A still different channeling of energy is encountered in western Greece; but in Magna Graecia, material conditions were markedly more favorable than in the east, where an ever-deepening estrangement from the mother country was apparent throughout the 5th century. Southern Italy and Sicily assumed an appreciably more active role in the development of the classic. Nonetheless, the general tone of their art in the 5th and 4th centuries was always slightly provincial in spite of its external splendor. This provincialism can be attributed to the fact that the Greek colonies of Magna Graecia were always coastal cities without any sizable hinterlands; they also lacked in their internal political life the requisite continuity, by now achieved in the cities of the mother country. The succession of conquerors and tyrants in the colonies had so far destroyed the social structure that a part of the citizenry was always in exile, ready to unite with the city's enemies. Often the enemy was a barbarian people, although sometimes it might be a neighboring Greek city with a different constitution. Consequently the western Hellenic world was worn out and destroyed more rapidly than continental Greece, and with loss of substance came the real exhaustion of the civic body. These disturbed conditions were reflected in the qualities of excessive exuberance which characterized western Greek art in the 5th and 4th centuries. Instead of a classic balance, the constant tendency was toward emphasis and every kind of excess, but this very exaltation of the irrepressible impulse toward beauty, inherent in all the Greeks, became the peculiar mark of classicism in western Greece. In southern Italy an almost excessive richness and overwhelming beauty are more evident in the coins than in any other kind of art, particularly the coins from Syracuse, where the almost annual issues seem to have vied with each other in beauty and purity (PL. 384; see COINS AND MEDALS). The same tendency marked other 5th-century work, whether in reliefs or in vase painting, in which the most competent masters undoubtedly preserved an echo of Zeuxis' art. An impassioned stress on beauty ultimately diminished grandeur in works of art. There was a poverty of sculpture in the round, partly because marble was lacking in southern Italy. Soft limestone and terra cotta differ from marble in stylistic potentialities and do not constitute adequate substitutes for it. The resultant structural weakness, observable in the surviving sculpture, must have produced an unpleasing quality. The indispensable foundation for classic sculpture either was lacking in the west or did not act with the same intensity encountered in Greece itself.

An examination of the art, especially the sculptural art, of western Greece reveals that one of its distinguishing characteristics during the first classic phase (460–450) was a persistence of the severe style quite as marked as in the east. In the art of Magna Graecia the stylistic discrepancies were particularly noticeable. Here the first classic phase was practically nonexistent, while classic forms asserted themselves after the classic epoch in the mother country had already passed its zenith (430–410). Our historical picture, to be sure, cannot be exact on many points, for what is preserved represents only a very small part of what was produced. Yet the lines of development seem sufficiently clear and meaningful.

The art of Magna Graecia drifted much more rapidly than did the art of Greece proper toward the dissolution of the classic style. This is particularly evident in the coins of Syracuse, which sometimes revealed an almost poignant softness and exuberance of form; but even in the drawing of the best Tarentine painters there is a comparable enfeeblement of form. During the 4th century (the second classic period), works of extraordinary beauty were produced, but they did not have that solidity of structure indispensable to every great work of sculpture. This region lacked the intellectual quality which in the motherland was called "moderation." Works of Magna Graecia in the 4th century can scarcely be considered classic, dominated as they were by the disintegration of sculptural forms and by anticipations of the baroque.

In giving an account of classic art, it is of paramount importance to include all its manifestations throughout the entire Greek world, east and west. Only thus will it be possible to grasp the complete significance of a phenomenon which certainly meant more than the crystallization of standards pertaining to form in the era between 450 and 430 B.C. We know that the 4th and 3d centuries also possessed a beauty of form of their own and even achieved a profound expression of their spiritual and esthetic energies. Granted, however, that the limits of the classic are to some extent arbitrary, let us continue to refer to the era from 450 to 430 to symbolize the pivotal moment, the *nucleus nucleorum*.

THE CLASSIC IN ARCHITECTURE. The phenomena of historical and structural development traceable in sculpture can also be discerned in other fields of Greek art. Although Greek architecture was in no sense a reproduction of the human figure, it was conceived as an organism — a body of organized space

loosely analogous to that of the human body. This mystically held concept differs from architectural concepts in other cultures. Many scholars would perhaps be inclined to choose the Pantheon (Rome) or Hagia Sophia (Constantinople) as the highest ancient examples of architectural organization. Yet in these two buildings belonging to late antiquity we do not find

especially in the Doric temple, the space is static and broken up into parts like a human figure.

About the end of the 6th century B.C. the Doric temple, more than any other structure, achieved a fairly standardized appearance. The architectural analogies with the human form must have reached a high point precisely when the Doric

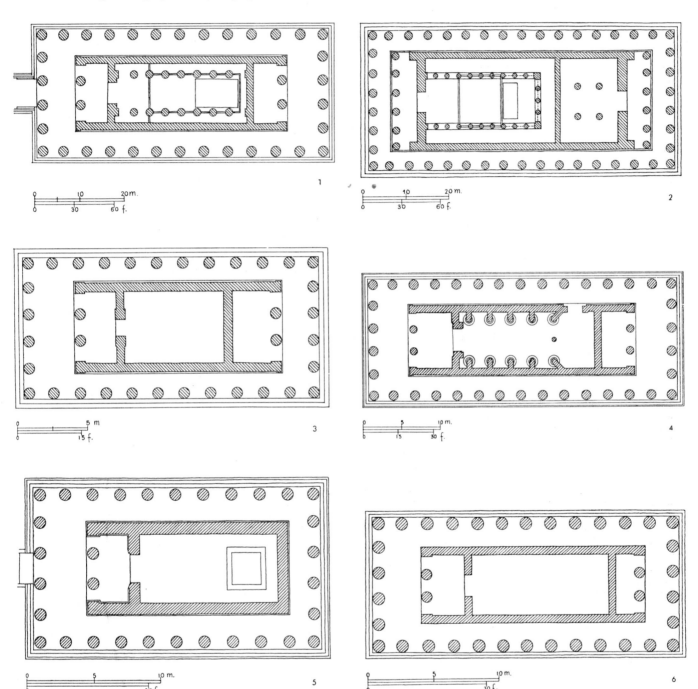

Doric temples of the 5th and 4th cent. B.C., plans: (1) Olympia, Temple of Zeus (ca. 460 B.C.); (2) Athens, Parthenon (447–432 B.C.); (3) Rhamnous, Temple of Nemesis (second half of 5th cent. B.C.); (4) Phigalia, Temple of Apollo Epikourios (ca. 420 B.C.); (5) Epidauros, Temple of Asklepios (ca. 380 B.C.); (6) Nemea, Temple of Zeus( ca. 330 B.C.).

a completely realized sculptural creation, still less an embodiment of space with characteristics of the human form. Precisely by starting with such a structure as the Byzantine Hagia Sophia, which is diametrically opposed to Greek architecture, we can grasp the meaning of the classic as we have tried to define it for sculpture. In Hagia Sophia there exists merely a spherical space, which has the appearance of being suspended, surrounding man with pure buoyancy; but in Greek architecture,

temple became clearly articulated and when the harmony of the proportions became perceptible to the senses.

In so far as we can mentally reconstruct the older buildings, they were lacking in harmonious relations between, for example, their length and breadth. Technical difficulties, especially the size of the interior space, blocked the accurate working out of such relations, but by about 500 B.C. these difficulties had been overcome. The Temple of Aphaia in Aegina (see I, PL. 332),

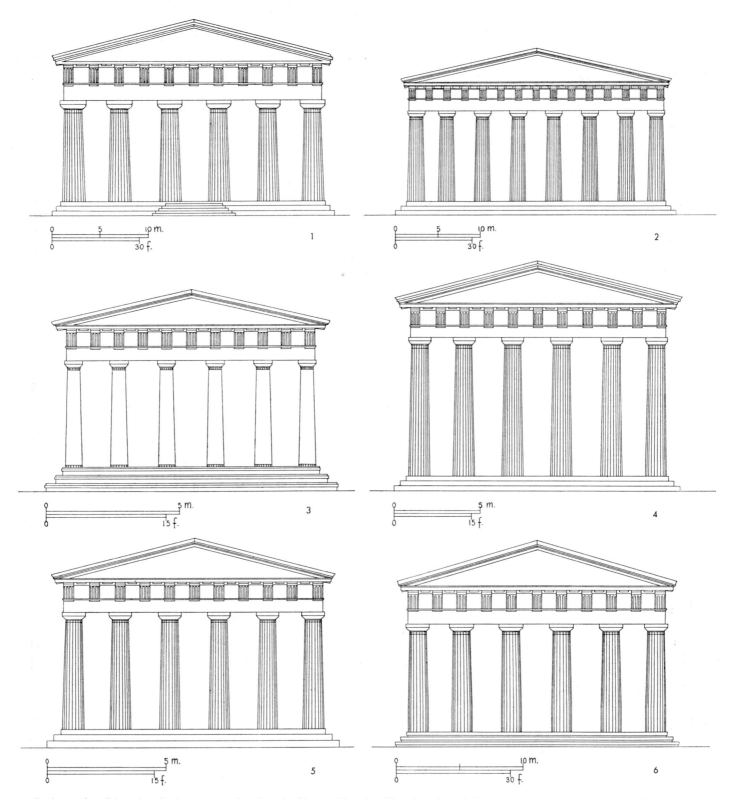

Doric temples of the 5th and 4th cent. B.C., elevations: (1) Olympia, Temple of Zeus (ca. 460 B.C.); (2) Athens, Parthenon (447–432 B.C.); (3) Rhamnous, Temple of Nemesis (second half of 5th cent. B.C.); (4) Phigalia, Temple of Apollo Epikourios (ca. 420 B.C.); (5) Epidauros, Temple of Asklepios (ca. 380 B.C.); (6) Nemea, Temple of Zeus (ca. 330 B.C.).

erected probably about 500 B.C., presents a superb example of the higher harmony of the various parts. The main characteristic of a Doric temple is the possibility of calculating all its interrelations, from the blocks in the stylobate to the proportions of metope and triglyph and the slope of the tympanum. The Doric temple can be reduced to numerically computable relationships, and marked deviations are impossible without compromising the beauty of the whole. We know today that the sublime form of a Greek temple depends on the inclination of the columns, infinitesimal irregularities in the distances between them, in the curve of seemingly horizontal lines, and in other subtle refinements. Nevertheless, the key to the unity of the structure lies in the exact mathematical relationships within it. This is best revealed in the triglyph, or what may be called the nerve center of the Doric temple. Although recent research has almost lost sight of this problem, its im-

portance was pointed out most perceptively by O. Puchstein. After a certain point in the slow evolution of forms, the triglyph became narrower and narrower as the springing quality of the columns increased. About 460, in the Temple of Zeus at Olympia and also in the Temple of Poseidon at Paestum, these relationships were adjusted at the same time as a balance for the structure's vertical proportions was being found. With these coinciding achievements, which are so clearly perceptible, the parts became connected into a unified pattern of harmonious proportions. But as early as the mid-5th century, the slenderness of the columns became so exaggerated that the building lost its compact harmony. The temple's lessening unity is also evident in the new relations between its length and breadth. Here too a sort of apex in harmony was achieved about 460 B.C., but even during the 5th century this harmony was being progressively diminished because of the increasing size of the building, as can be seen in a comparison of the Temple of Nemesis at Rhamnous with the earlier "Theseion" at Athens.

This discrepancy between the long and short sides became still more marked in the 4th century, when the spaciousness of the inner chamber gained the ascendancy, as is evident in the temples of Asklepios and Artemis at Epidauros; the late-4th-century Temple of Zeus at Nemea, however, shows a survival of the earlier proportions. Columns during the 4th century were so slender and elegant that they no longer resembled trunks, as they had during the main Doric era. The entasis, which had seemed hardly able to contain the column's flow of vital forces in 6th-century Corinth (see I, PL. 332) and Paestum (see I, PL. 333), faded away and functionally became barely discernible. Thus developed the rigid, devitalized quality typical of late Doric temples such as those of Ilion, Pergamon, and Kourno. The configuration of forces which determined the genuine beauty of Doric buildings began to disappear suddenly after 450. Perhaps in view of the course of the fatal laws governing the Doric architectural organism, Phidias and Iktinos succeeded in giving the Parthenon (mid-5th cent.) its particular perfection through an intermingling with Ionic details (PL. 337). The large number of columns in the Parthenon was also vital to its perfection, although the size of the temple did not neces-

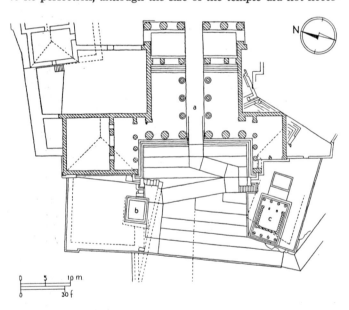

Athens, complex of the Propylaia, plan: (*a*) Propylaia; (*b*) Monument of Agrippa; (*c*) Temple of Athena Nike (*from Hesperia, XV, 1946, fig. 3*).

sarily require them. Had the usual six columns been used, the temple could never have attained such a perfect harmony.

It is difficult to trace the development of Ionic temples as we have done for Doric temples because so many of the former have been destroyed. Nevertheless, in the series of Ionic temples — the Athenian Portico at Delphi, the Temple on the Ilissos, the Erechtheion (PL. 338), the Temple of Athena Nike

(see I, PL. 392), and the temples of Athena and Asklepios at Priene — it is apparent that they reached their highest classic peak only about the end of the 4th century, with the architect Pytheos. The development of the Ionic temple illustrates the independence of the various artistic genres in Greece from the

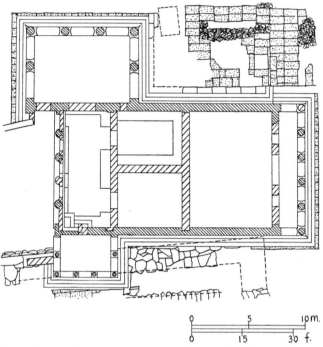

Athens, Erechtheion (421–407 B.C.), plan (the wide hatchings indicate restoration of missing elements; the dividing walls of the cella are hypothetical).

formal laws, inasmuch as the genres attained their peak development at various times.

It is noteworthy that by the end of the 5th century there was already a coexistence of more than one order in a single building: Doric and Ionic in the Propylaia (PL. 337; FIG. 665) and Doric, Ionic, and Corinthian (or foliate) in the Temple of Apollo Epikourios at Phigalia. In the latter building the Corinthian capital appears for the first time (FIG. 669). By the 4th century, theatrical (PL. 340; FIG. 667) and funerary architecture (FIG. 671) find their fullest expression.

The chronological limits discussed and established above for the Greek classic age remain valid, despite the various peaks of other artistic genres and manifestations of the spirit; no genre was so essential to the Greek world as sculpture, which had its greatest flowering in the 5th century.

THE CLASSIC IN PAINTING AND CERAMICS. If we examine Greek painting and drawing from the point of view established in the preceding discussion, it is apparent that three-dimensionality is not central to the artistic concept. Painting is an art unfolding in two dimensions: an art which sets forth three-dimensional reality illusionistically, which evokes an illusion of tangibility and physical space through the arrangement and subordination of separate forms. This was best accomplished in periods which had a less fundamental tie with the three-dimensional human body than did the 5th-century Greeks. We may infer that ancient painting developed mainly during the 6th century. Kimon of Kleonai took the decisive step by rendering foreshortenings, thereby opening the way for perspective. Mikon (q.v.) and Polygnotos (q.v.) took the second step when they gave a spatial connection to the figures, developing *obliquae imagines*, or figures seen obliquely, with foreshortenings almost correct in perspective. The most important innovation was to indicate, if not actually render, landscape. Although there were only suggestions of trees and hills, they enriched the picture pictorially and helped to establish spatially the positions of the figures. We observe a few echoes of these achievements in vase paintings. In Polygnotos' figure drawings

reconstructed from early classic vase paintings, ethos (or the noble aspect of character) is particularly emphasized; however, a less lofty conception was occasionally apparent. Polygnotos' painting must have been colored drawing like the kind found on the white-ground vases of his time; it was not painting in the modern sense, in which colors prevail with graduated values and contrasts.

Although we cannot fully ascertain the achievements in this field of the late-5th-century masters, especially Zeuxis (q.v.) and Parrhasios (q.v.), remarkable progress in placing human

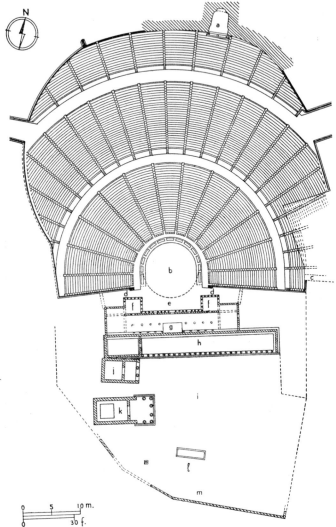

Athens, Theater of Dionysos, 4th cent. B.C., restored plan: (a) Monument of Thrasyllos; (b) "Orchestra"; (c) exit to the diazoma; (d) parodos; (e) *proskenion* (proscenium); (f) *paraskenion* (parascenium); (g) stage building; (h) portico; (i) Sanctuary of Dionysos; (j) old temple; (k) new temple; (l) altar; (m) precinct wall (*from W. Dorpfeld and E. Reisch, Das griechische Theater, Athens, 1836*).

figures in space is clearly evident, even from the small, unpretentious vase paintings of the era. For the 4th century we can infer to what extent color must have preoccupied painters of all kinds by observing how they gradually abandoned the earlier red-figured style, giving their figures a richer appearance and more spatial freedom. Like all 4th-century men, the vase painters were fascinated by the richly colored picture, and they tried to translate it, even if inadequately, into ceramics. On the basis of literary evidence, the development of color must have reached its acme in the great 4th-century painting masters, especially Euphranor, Nikias (q.v.), and Apelles (q.v.). In so far as we can ascertain by precise investigation a classic period — that is, a point of highest perfection — for Greek painting (as distinct from vase painting), we must place that period at the end of the 4th century.

For vase paintings the problem of the classic, at least as we have heretofore understood it, is entirely different. The inherent artistic possibilities do not go beyond the artisan category, even when the paintings attain the highest quality. We do not meet any great personalities in this field, as we do in sculpture. The particular laws of the craft are based on the fact that a picture on a vase is not independent, like a work of sculpture or a major painting; the vase painting and the vase form comprise a single entity. Recent research has paid too much attention to the painting alone rather than to the synthesis of vase form and image.

In some periods during the development of vase forms, the different structural parts of the vase appeared only barely differentiated. However, during the more advanced periods, such as the 4th century, the individual elements seemed to swell out and became so hypertrophied that the unity of the form was destroyed. Between these two extremes there was a period when a harmonious balance was achieved among the various parts — when the vase form as a purely sculptural image, like the figure of a man, reached its perfection; this occurred about the mid-5th century. However, there is another, perhaps more important, harmony that must be considered in the evaluation of ceramics: the balance between the vase shape as a whole and the painted design. This balance had already been achieved from 500 to 480, a period which may be considered the peak classic level of Attic ceramics. By the mid-5th century, through Mikon's and Polygnotos' pictorial works, vase figures tended to become independent, without adaptation to the vase form. During the late 5th century, when vase drawing was dominated by human bodies in spatial representations, as in the vases of Aison and Aristophanes and particularly the marvelous 4th-century painters, there was a painful disharmony between the painting and the body of the vase supporting it.

THE CLASSIC IN GEMS, SEALS, AND COINS. The very refined and artistically excellent production of gems during the 2d millennium B.C., which reached its highest level of quality about 1700 to 1600 B.C., remains outside our present inquiry. From the standpoint of quantity, the 6th century produced the greatest number of beautifully cut gems; the genre reached its first classic peak at this time. There are only a few remaining cut gems from the 5th century, although they include some works of exceptional quality. In the 4th century a new and favorable era began, later attaining a brilliant flowering during the Hellenistic age (PL. 384) and reaching a second classic peak during the 3d and early 2d centuries. The passion for the small, the delicate, and the malleable constantly led gem cutters to newer and more beautiful ways of working within the medium.

The surprising fact that gems had been quite insignificant during the century of Greek classic art is explicable in that the genre had no affinity to the 5th century's main achievements in form. Gem artists could not impose a human image on the bezel of a ring with a diameter of less than an inch and still have the image express all the qualities of the large sculpture of the period. (Similarly the tondi in late 5th-century cups never attained the beauty of the older circular pictures.) Actually the artistic milieu around 500 was extremely favorable for both gems and cup paintings. The harmonious antinomy between the flexible turning and bending of the human body (depicted with a strong two-dimensional effect) and the ring oval enclosing it must have led gem cutters to continually new and happy solutions of the problem. The fame of Theodoros of Samos, who cut Polykrates' ring, is understandable on the basis of this harmony. We do not possess any direct evidence of Theodoros' art, but a few gems in a style that stamps them as Samian suggest the quality of his output. The most exquisite gems of Dexamenos of Chios, an Ionian artist of the early 4th century, portray animals whose flexible bodies fit admirably onto the oval bezel of the ring. The gem art of the Hellenistic age drew its inspiration from his artistic advances.

The production of coins (PL. 384) must be judged quite differently (see COINS AND MEDALS). First, one must remember that the decoration of coins in all periods is secondary to financial considerations: coins must win confidence by their intrinsic

value. Like their modern counterparts, the ancient cities which enjoyed a solid financial position attached no extraordinary importance to special effects in the decoration of coins.

The reverse sides of coins usually depicted a god's head; here the standards expressed for painted Attic vases are essentially valid. A further standard is the harmony with which the design — a head, a chariot, a figure — blends with the round frame. If the design transgresses the limits proper to the genre, as occurs in the coins containing three-quarter views of faces from Ainos, Amphipolis, Syracuse, and Larisa, the artistic unity is compromised. Only in one or two dies from Klazomenai is there a perfect harmony in a three-quarter face rendered with a well-planned and restrained indication of relief.

Hellenistic age, has violently rejected it to the present day. This rejection seems to suggest a basic difference between East and West. One might say that the fundamental characteristic of Asia — the "archaic" as distinct from the "classic" in both life and art — must be explained by different, perhaps deeper, forms of spiritual life, not the least of which is the merging of the individual within his society. These differences led to different concepts of beauty; an "archaic" or Asiatic image certainly possesses its own perfection and necessity, as Goethe pointed out in a famous passage from his *Erwin von Steinbach*. The beauty of primitive art, however, is something so fundamentally at variance with that of "mature" art that it should perhaps be expressed by another word. Everything that had

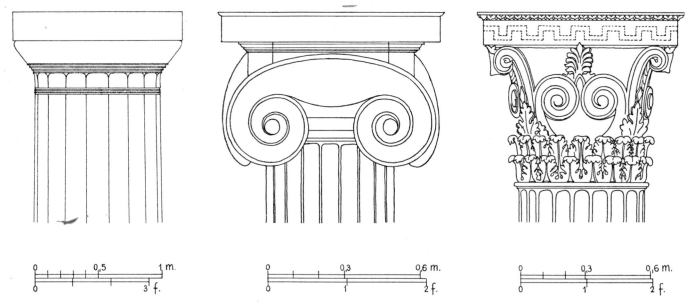

Doric, Ionic, and Corinthian capitals of the Temple of Apollo Epikourios at Phigalia (ca. 420 B.C.).

Naturally the perfection of the representation is the decisive matter in each case. If we consider the long series of identical types such as those from Tarentum, poverty of invention and carelessness in form are revealed at an increasing rate early in the 4th century. Greek coins achieved their acme of beauty precisely at the point when a softer sculptural convexity of relief was beginning to develop; at this point, about 450 B.C., the eyes began to be animated. This achievement can be seen in the coinage of Syracuse better than in any other. Here, perhaps because of the constant demand for money for commercial purposes, there was an almost yearly issuance of new coins. About mid-century, the coining of money reached its high point, through the restrained beauty of the image and through its perfect fusion with the round frame of the coin framing its border. In the "rich style," beginning about 420 B.C., the forms already began to be more complex and then more and more exuberant at the time of the victories over the Athenians (410–400). Even when designers in the 4th century tried to return to the old forms, they could not achieve the spontaneous unity of the beautiful image and the frame of the coin. A few series of Syracusan coins were, even in antiquity, considered classic because of their incomparable perfection; one even finds casts from these coins used to decorate cups or other objects.

CONCLUSIONS. From these few fragments of Greek art history, we may perhaps now deduce a standard for defining and temporally delimiting the classic age. In the eulogies of the works of Phidias, who was the creator and main exponent of the classic, two characteristics are lauded: beauty and nobility. That concept of beauty discovered and artistically embodied during the classic epoch of the 5th century B.C. today remains unchanged for Western man.

It does not seem mere coincidence that Asia, so often exposed to the Western concept of beauty, particularly during the

esthetic value during archaic times, before the classic era, arouses admiration for the natural animal quality of the human body, for its resiliently springing structure, for the delicacy of its limbs, or, in the primitive epoch, an attraction at times for details of almost savage power. Man was like a god not yet completely humanized. Only with Greek sculpture of the Pentakontaetia (480–432) did art begin to embody that grandeur and nobility inherent in the human being. But even the beginning of this era still lacked beauty such as the Greek classic age was capable of creating, precisely because of its ungovernable passion for the heroic attributes in the human image. The severe style (480–460) knew only haughtiness, pride, and nobility in appearance and feeling — not yet that classic beauty which was born only when an intellectual flame was kindled in a perfect body; when men became aware of all the limitations of human existence and of its inferiority to the divine essence. This concept recurred insistently throughout classic poetry and was articulated most purely and precisely in Pindar's last odes and Sophocles' plays. The pride typical of the early Pentakontaetia was expressed in the words, "He is wise who knows things by nature." The wisdom of the classic age was voiced as follows: "No one is wise except the man who honors god." A synthesis of beauty and nobility, of bodily and intellectual perfection, can thus be regarded as the quintessence of the classic period.

Later times were content to accept artistic images in terms of their beauty alone. Works by followers of Phidias already lacked nobility and grandeur; only beauty and grace survived in them. While in the 4th century it was possible to express verbally the concept of μεγαλοφρονεῖν, or thinking in a high-minded way, as Aristotle explained, the process had been automatic in the classic age. Just how vital and deep-seated was the classic era's awareness of this process can be indicated by its parallel in philosophy: at the high point of classic art, the

Sophists began to debate upon the union of the beautiful and the good as symbolic of man's perfection. The plays of Aristophanes and the dialogues of Plato have left us a reflection of these ideas.

Only long afterward did the Greeks become aware of this classic conception, when historical evolution had already led to other ways of life. This awareness was reflected in Aristotle's curious descriptions of magnanimity.

Perhaps we may summarize the results of our analysis of classic sculpture in this manner: Greek classic statues capture

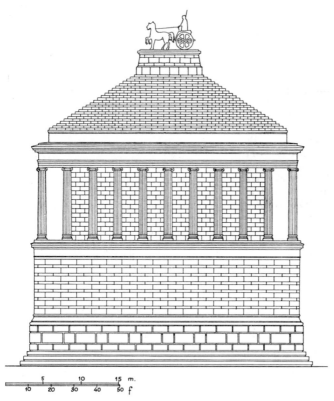

Halikarnassos, Mausoleum (ca. 350 B.C.), lateral elevation based on F. Adler's reconstruction, without the sculptural elements.

that moment in the life of a Greek man when he had the revelation of suddenly broadened human and intellectual horizons; when he was freed not only from the confined, circumscribed world of archaic existence but also, in a more external sense, from the strictures of tyrannical states, so that he could enjoy a commonly shared responsibility in government, which the state achieved in the 5th century. Orientals and barbarians never attained this level of life, even in the field of art. When the Greeks transcended their archaic life, they underwent a reawakening of human consciousness in its present, in its "here and now." For this, Ionian philosophy had prepared them. In a moment of overwhelming illumination, life became integrated, enriched, expanded, and fused. Men were released from total captivity in a life judged and ruled by gods and demons. Ionian philosophy forced a man to confront the world, the state, and other men and to recognize himself as a man. The liberation of intellectual potentialities and deeper vision of the individual became apparent in the art of the time.

The human spirit, or that which Anaxagoras called "nous," thereupon began its reign as supreme orderer. Contemporary Greek poetry was also full of this consciousness of the borders of the domains of man and the gods. Contemporary science was trying to investigate the sun, the stars, and the universe. The frequent representations of star gods give evidence of the profound impact of the newly expanded cosmological ideas. Perhaps the representation of the earth giants' assault on the heavens, on the shield of the celebrated *Athena Parthenos*, is but an allusion, veiled in mythology, to man's astrological interests. The dread of isolation of man as an individual — seen

in Thucydides' work and in Sophocles' conviction that no one may live far removed from evil except the gods — was revived as a result of events in the 5th century. Realizing their sense of destiny, we understand for the first time the seriousness, thoughtfulness, and sadness in the later classic statues.

Classic art in this later phase was no longer the serenity of a well-balanced existence but included the awareness of man's limits and a sense of responsibility toward the forces of life and death.

The human being, as he was clearly represented in classic art, was born with Kleisthenes' new constitution of the state and his liberation of the Athenians from tyranny. Through a uniting in the 5th century of fully franchised citizens and the state, democracy became for the first time a complete embodiment of the divine nomos, or order, as Solon had contemplated it. During the perfect unity between Pericles and the demos, as described by Thucydides, it was possible for sculpture to synthesize in the human body all the complex forces of human nature; man was now an organic member of the new state, not an animal in a herd such as he was at Sparta. Precisely for this reason, Sparta never had a classic period; for the individual man vitalized and spiritually enriched by the revelation of his uniqueness cannot exist under tyranny.

During the 5th century, man discovered the nobility of his fate along with the richness of his psyche, both through himself and other human beings. His nature was manifested to him as something grander than before. The Greeks of this period, ennobled by the greater depth and intensity in their own life, and realizing that their spirit distinguished them from other peoples, consciously set themselves apart from the barbarians surrounding them. Aristotle defined the barbarian as a man lacking freedom because he was a slave to his own greediness. Self-control was seen neither as a weakening nor a suppression of individual vitality but rather as a distinguishing sign of the new intellectual outlook.

It would be ridiculous, however, to think that life unfolded more gently for these men than for men in other less auspicious times. Tragic poetry and mythology surely reveal to us the abysses of life in the 5th century: it was not an innocent paradise, but rather a world of extreme tensions when life and death, action and destruction, had meaning in themselves. This concept is seen, even today, in the "Funeral Oration" that Thucydides ascribed to Pericles — a testimonial of the loftiest rhetoric, which instills a mysterious tension into the terse, simple form. The speaker told of how the fallen men had lived; he praised the city with its succession of festivals, athletic competitions, and sacrifices — that world where beauty without luxury was admired and where men toiled for a hard-won wisdom; he praised the Athenians, who did not count upon material advantages but put their faith in freedom and the state which was the educator of Greece. For such a city as this, the men whom he praised had fallen.

Any definition of Greek classicism would be inexact and incomplete if the classic were looked upon solely as a thorough intellectualization of man, contrasted to that innocent vitality of the man-animal typical of the archaic period. The 5th century was very much bound to the body, although completely aware of the limits of mortal and divine. In the following centuries the Greek gods withdrew increasingly from the affairs of men, becoming spirit elevated above the body. They were less often represented as cult images in plastic, corporeal form and worshiped more as symbols. No longer did they surround men on all sides, as in the 5th century; the gods could be reached only with toil and sacrifice. Thus profoundly had the relations changed between the human being and the divine and between the body and the psychological domain during the course of the Greeks' destiny.

A glance at the life and literature of the 4th century sheds light upon the true reasons for such representations. Political participation was no longer so intense as in the past, partly because each citizen was not habitually required to participate directly in the affairs of the state. The better kind of men alienated themselves from politics and sought to acquire virtue through wisdom rather than action, in the peaceful grove of

the hero Akademos. Against the political state, exhausted by its passions, was set an intellectual realm based on knowledge. Dramatic poetry disappeared along with the greatness of the old Attic state. Although tragedies continued to be written in the 4th century and up to the close of the ancient era, they never recaptured the magnificence of their heritage. Poetic greatness in the 4th century resided not in tragedy but in Plato's dialogues. The only dramatic form still popular was the New Comedy, which derived its vitality not from myth but from the small pleasures, misfortunes, and moods of people abandoned to the joys of refined living far removed from everyday events. Above all, the attitude toward life and the social order had changed. That self-contained realm, that way of life conditioned by cult and state which every Attic citizen had to maintain and protect through his daily actions, was destroyed in the emphasis on the isolated pursuits of philosophy, science, and rhetoric. These pursuits were already preparing the inevitable schism between men devoted to intellect and men without knowledge or moral bonds. Humanism began, nourished on the roots of a classic conception of life, but its preoccupations concerned the intellect alone; the bodily element was more and more regarded as a hindrance to the sovereign will of knowledge. The contemplative life of the 4th century was contrasted to the active life of the 5th century; the center of gravity had been moved into the intellectual sphere. Thereupon the balance of human forces, the synthesis of the two elements, was destroyed. Life could not remain on such a precipitous peak; the classic, which had come to maturity, swiftly died.

BIBLIOG. G. Rodenwaldt, Zur begrifflichen und geschichtlichen Bedeutung des Klassischen in der bildenden Kunst, Z. für Ästhetik, XI, 1916, p. 113 ff.; A. von Salis, Die Kunst der Griechen, 2d ed., Leipzig, 1922, p. 78 ff.; F. Matz, Der Begriff des Klassischen in der antiken Kunst, Z. für Ästhetik, XXIII. 1929, p. 70 ff.; R. Bianchi Bandinelli, Kunst der Antike und neuzeitliche Kritik, Groningen, 1931; W. Jäger, Das Problem des Klassischen und die Antike: Acht Vorträge gehalten auf der Fachtagung der klassischen Altertumswissenschaft zu Naumburg, 1930, von J. Stroux, W. Schadewaldt, P. Friedländer, E. Fränkel, B. Schweitzer, E. Schmidt, M. Gelzer, und H. Kuhn, Leipzig, Berlin, 1931; E. Langlotz, Griechische Klassik, Stuttgart, 1932, 1943, 1946, 1956; R. Hinks, "Classical" and "Classicistic" in the Critics of Ancient Art, Kritische Berichte zur kunstgeschichtlichen Literatur, VI, 1937, p. 94 ff.; H. Rose, Klassik als künstlerische Denkform des Abendlandes, Munich, 1937; L. Curtius, Die antike Kunst, II: Die klassische Kunst Griechenlands, Potsdam, 1938; Picard, II, 1, 1939; E. Buschor, Vom Sinn der griechischen Standbilder, Berlin, 1942; J. Charbonneaux, La sculpture grecque classique, Paris, 1943; T. S. Eliot, What Is a Classic?, New York, 1945; G. Rodenwaldt, Die Kunst der Antike, Hellas und Rom (Propyläen-Kunstgeschichte), I, Berlin, 1947, p. 30 ff.; H. Koch, Die klassische Kunst, Hallische Monographien, 2, Halle, 1948; K. Reinhardt, Von Werken und Formen, Godesberg, 1948; R. Bianchi Bandinelli, Storicità dell'arte classica, 2d ed., Florence, 1950; G. M. A. Richter, Three Critical Periods in Greek Sculpture, Oxford, 1951; W. R. Agard, What Is a Classic Sculpture?, Classical J., XLIX, 1953–54, p. 341 ff.; K. Schefold, Der Ursprung der späten Klassik, JdI, Anzeiger, LXIX, 1954, col. 289 ff.

Ernst LANGLOTZ

Illustrations: PLS. 337–384; 8 figs. in text.

## CLASSICISM.

**CLASSICISM.** According to the commonly accepted meaning of the term, "classicism" refers to a series of manifestations in which "classic" art (q.v.) — that is, the art of Athens in the 5th century B.C. — is consciously regarded as a model and source of inspiration; but it is not experienced or interpreted in any direct or original way. For this reason, classicism does not constitute a natural or spontaneous continuation of classic art. Historians of medieval and modern art have tended to narrow down (and thus to clarify) the connotation of the term "classicism" by applying it to specific and recurring traditions with which are associated certain definite motifs — stylistic, literary, psychological, religious, and political. The following discussion will show how these traditions, in a long and varied history, have a certain continuity in spite of frequent interruption and resurgence.

SUMMARY. Historical and conceptual limits of classicism (col. 674). Classicism in ancient art (col. 678). Medieval classicism (col. 682). The Renaissance and the modern period (col. 686): *The Renaissance in Tuscany; Rome; North Italy and Europe; Baroque classicism in Italy and France; Rationalism from the 18th century to the present day.*

HISTORICAL AND CONCEPTUAL LIMITS OF CLASSICISM. Classicism is a typical feature both of tradition (q.v.) and of the return to antiquity (see ANTIQUE REVIVAL) and should therefore be examined in connection with these two terms. Linguistically speaking, the meaning of the word is clear: classicism indicates the intention on the part of an artist of lending to his works and surroundings a classical imprint; more strictly, it signifies the imitation of classical antiquity for this purpose. The definition of the term arose largely as a result of the criticisms leveled by a large section of baroque culture (which regarded itself as the sole heir both of the Renaissance and of antiquity) against two separate features of 17th-century art: the naturalism of Caravaggio (accused of wanting to represent reality directly, without using the formulas consecrated by classical tradition) and the cult of the bizarre (see FANTASY). By the latter is meant the rejection of classical formulas, not for the purpose of direct imitation of nature but rather for the internal unity and autonomous nature of the art object or its function; it was a rejection in the mane of inspiration. The principal 17th-century representatives of these anticlassical tendencies were Borromini in architecture and Caravaggio and Rubens in painting. As an autonomous current of taste, classicism was represented above all by the critic Giovanni Pietro Bellori, by Poussin, and by Bernini; as a theory of art, its influence was felt not only in Italy but also in France.

The concept of classicism is fundamentally ambiguous. The extent of its application depends on the precise significance attached to the term "classic," a concept which, as we know, has not always meant the same thing in different periods of history. In addition, the successive revivals of the classical are in part reactions against intervening anticlassical periods, so that each phase of classicism has its own particular characteristics, determined by its attitude to opposing tendencies and by the compromises to which these tendencies force it. Few other terms, in fact, describe so multifaceted a phenomenon. In France, with a notable fidelity to the historical origins of the term, *classicisme* indicates the 17th and 18th centuries and, by extension (as, for example, in Hautecoeur's *Histoire de l'architecture classique en France*, Paris, 1943–57), virtually the whole period from the late Renaissance to the romantic movement. In Germany the Renaissance was of limited influence, providing in general only certain decorative motifs, and it was not until the Enlightenment and, in particular, during the discussions about rococo art (see ROCOCO) that questions of esthetics were approached with any real seriousness; in consequence, *Klassizismus* tends to mean neoclassic art (see NEOCLASSIC STYLES), that is, the movement begun by Winckelmann and Mengs, together with the period immediately preceding. In Spain, on the other hand, classicism indicates the architecture of 18th-century rationalism, especially that of Ventura Rodríguez, who only in a limited section of his work showed any deference to antiquity.

At first sight, then, the term classicism appears to be devoid of any real historical content. It seems to be applied almost casually to those periods in the history of art which, according to the stylistic development and the culture of individual countries, have seemed to later generations or contemporaries particularly dedicated to the imitation of antiquity. This dedication is usually accompanied by a conscious reaction against preceding traditions (Gothic art and mannerism in France, mannerism and rococo in Germany, the Churrigueresque style in Spain, etc.), and sometimes by a certain modernistic tendency (see MODERNISM).

Indeed, the traditional use of the term betokens an unformed empirical approach, incapable of recognizing the validity of the various movements stigmatized as anticlassical, incapable also of appreciating that these same anticlassical movements had their own genuine links with the past, often based (as in Borromini) on a careful and individual study of antiquity and on direct derivations. In any case, the concept of classicism is itself of recent date, arising, it should be remembered, when the Renaissance tradition, to which was due the most comprehensive revival of antiquity ever achieved in the West, was already in decline.

Modern criticism, however, even though it has not systematically tackled the problem of classicism, does enable us to arrive at a more adequate definition of the term. In a certain sense classicism can be described as representing a constant reaction to the baroque (D'Ors), to mannerism (Curtius, 1953), and to romanticism (Spirito). (D'Ors uses the term "classical," though "classicism" seems preferable in this context.) It is conceived rather as a continual current of taste than a historical period or intellectual attitude. This reaction, for a variety of reasons — some cultural, some historical, some political, some religious — seems to have been fairly constant in western Europe, and by the 17th century it already possessed a very long history. Various episodes in the development of medieval art, it is now agreed, are due to the impulses of classicism or of its opposite. The word "classicism" is rightly used, for instance, in speaking of the works of Nicola Pisano or of the education and taste of the Emperor Frederick II or of some remarkable late-medieval instances of architecture and sculpture that reveal a knowledge and understanding of antiquity. However, thanks to the attention devoted since the romantic period to anticlassical phases (see MANNERISM; ROMANTICISM), it is now clear that the tradition of classicism is not continuous but consists of a series of interruptions and renewals. Moreover, in addition to such ancient works as were available for study (i.e., sarcophagi, ivories, statues, and ruins), inspiration was also derived from the classicizing work of past periods, especially those immediately preceding the era in question. Thus the tradition embodies a process of successive stratifications, each revival beginning, as it were, where the previous one had left off (Bauch, 1939–40). For example, the early Renaissance discloses direct derivations from other "classical" periods, particularly the period associated with the Emperor Frederick II; 16th-century Roman art is linked to 15th-century Florentine classicism; the 17th century to Raphael, Titian, and Antonio da Sangallo; neoclassicism to Poussin and Carlo Maratti, and so on. This intermittent resurgence of classicism is made all the more dramatic by the fact that even its most splendid moments have lasted but a short time — often no more than a generation.

Equally disparate are the attitudes of classicism toward antiquity, of which certain periods had an extremely confused, not to say mythical, idea. For the Middle Ages the most fertile sources of inspiration were the monuments of Early Christian art and works in ivory; for the Renaissance, on the other hand, Roman sculpture and architecture were the chief models; for baroque classicism the ideal was Hellenism; for neoclassicism, especially in its purest form, the antiquities of Pompeii and Herculaneum, and only in its later phase the authentic Greece of the Parthenon and of Aegina.

These oscillations, which have added much richness and variety of style to the phenomenon of classicism, are mainly due to the fact that, in all its successive revivals, classicism always had a controversial aspect, was always a conscious reaction against existing tendencies, and therefore at each recurrence different themes came to be stressed. For instance, the pure color and clear proportions of Tuscan art in the 15th century are deliberately anti-Gothic, though connected with the Cistercian tradition; while the Rome of the great Humanist popes is typified by a sense of grandeur, inspired by the Theater of Marcellus, the Colosseum, and the Pantheon. Inevitably linked with the Enlightenment is the elegance of neoclassic art.

Nevertheless, an examination of all the various phases of classicism reveals that beneath these divergencies there lies a fundamental unity; and it is thus possible to use the term "classicism" not as a metaphor but as the description of a particular style, based on the constant adherence to certain theoretical, if not formal, principles.

First and foremost of the perennial features of classicism is an intense theoretical activity, as a result of which the movement has always appeared eminently rational and closely connected with literary circles. If we examine these theoretical writings, we find that they are based on a small number of ancient authorities, principally Cicero, Quintilian, Horace, and Vitruvius — all writers who attack stylistic license, the abnormal, and the fantastic. Thanks to the theoretical writings

of classicism, several passages from these classic authors formed the constant basis of all discussion on art up to and into the 19th century. For example, Vitruvius's celebrated description (*De architectura*, VII, 5) of "grotesque" decorations (see FANTASY) was used as a critical formula against arabesques and other fantastic features of medieval art, against mannerist decorations, against Borromini, against rococo art, and even against Art Nouveau; while Quintilian's distinction between Attics and Asians — the former *integri*, simple and true, the latter *inflati et inanes*, three-dimensional, suggestive, and false — underlay for more than a thousand years the rhythm of Western taste, with its oscillation between subservience to rules and artistic freedom. Just as in the imitation of ancient art classicism avoided representations of a magical or fantastic nature, so in its borrowings from ancient writings on art it limited itself, practically speaking, to the maxims enunciated by Quintilian (*Institutio oratoria*, VIII, 2, 22) : "Prima sit virtus perspicuitas" ("Let clarity be your principal virtue"); "Propria verba, rectus ordo, non in longum dilatata conclusio: nihil neque desit, neque superfluat" ("Seek the right word, the correct order; do not be verbose; let nothing be lacking, nothing superfluous").

The stylistic counterpart of these ideas is the tendency toward the impersonality of the work of art, that is, toward the rejection of all subjectivity of expression. Classicism, in general, is opposed to the personal touch, rejects freedom of composition and the uncontrolled use of elements not directly connected with the central theme (the *parerga*). Art is not fantasy or self-expression. Its purpose is to demonstrate; hence the stress laid on its didactic function, its objectivity, and the insistence on historical, heroic, educative subjects, in implicit contradiction of the Aristotelian theory of realism, whereby the skill of the artist can raise even a banal or disgusting subject to the dignity of art. Indeed, the attack on realism (see MIMESIS AND INVENTION) is one of the permanent features of classicism. We find an insistence on the necessity of a close approximation to the great models (similarity to which is often considered of itself an important virtue); a conviction that artists should have a wide historical and literary culture with which to control the imitation of nature, selecting and idealizing only what is appropriate; an emphasis on the intellectual and nonmechanical nature of the arts, with particular attention to their connections with literature and poetry.

The second essential feature of classicism is its constant connection with politics, religion, and ethics. The purely visual, the purely esthetic, never exhausts the significance of classicism, which always claims to have symbolic meaning, to express eternal and transcendental values. In its development its course ran parallel to that of the major political and religious events of Europe. In addition, it always aimed at the identification of spiritual and esthetic qualities in accordance with the Greek ideal of kalokagathia, the beautiful and the good, which harmoniously fused transcendental and human values. Various attempts to give a proportional, geometric basis to the imitation of nature are a result of this attitude. The classical tradition directly derived from Greece fused in the Middle Ages with the Hebrew, mainly on the strength of the passage from the Wisdom of Solomon 11 : 20 (Apocrypha), according to which God disposed all things by measure, number, and weight, which accounts for the frequent representations of God creating the world with the aid of a pair of compasses. The passage was annotated, commented on by St. Augustine, and passed on with the weight of his authority to the 13th century and to the Italian Renaissance. His commentary was even used by Diderot in compiling the article "Beau" for the *Encyclopédie*; the article was published separately several times after 1751. Thus the idea that beauty is essentially order, coherence, symmetry, and proportion was rooted, on the one hand, in the Pythagorean theory of numbers and, on the other, in the symbolism of the Bible; it was reinforced by the study and use of proportion and the rigorous apprenticeship to which artists were subjected (hence Curtius's theory of the late-medieval etymology of "art" from *artus*, "strictly regulated"). For thousands of years this conception of beauty helped to give the products of classicism a notable symbolic and transcendental value.

This brings us to the third and last of the essential features of classicism: its traditionalism. The history of classicism presents a marked, and sometimes excessive, uniformity of themes such as the central plan in buildings, the regal pose favored for statues (PL. 389), the alignment of columns in perspectives, and the arcaded porticoes (PL. 390); in style, too, the classical attitude leads to the same solutions, so that it is possible to apply identical standards of judgment to all periods of classicism, such as those proposed by Wölfflin, Winkler, and Worringer for classical form. In general, works of art produced in periods of classicism concentrate on drawing and relief rather than color, on repose rather than movement. In composition, they are closed and unified; in subject, they are deliberately representational. The recurrence of these characteristics led D'Ors and other theoreticians to classify them as a historical category as well as something innate in the human spirit, with a constant polar attraction. But this is not a satisfactory explanation, for the continual appearance of these features is the direct result of the links, already mentioned, which bind classicism to politics and religion. Classicism was always connected with the ideal empire and, at the height of the Middle Ages, with the Roman Church — in other words, with the two powers that claimed to derive their authority directly from the Roman empire. For Nero the classical ideal was the Hellenistic monarchy; for Constantine, the Augustan age; for Charlemagne and Emperor Frederick II it was Constantine; for the men of the Renaissance, Augustus once more; but despite these divergencies, all were at one in wanting not only to imitate but to revive the golden age of antiquity. Because of the didactic and propagandistic value constantly assigned to art, it became supremely important to imitate the imperial monuments of antiquity, especially those which had come to assume the value of real symbols of empire. (See, for example, the discussions which arose over the 12th-century frescoes in St. John Lateran, which tried visually to affirm the legitimacy of the Donation of Constantine.) But even the simple stylistic imitation of ancient art served a similar purpose, sometimes with the added function of countering "barbaric" tendencies toward stylization then in vogue. So close was this connection that one might venture to ascribe to all periods of classicism a political basis, either because they were directly promoted by the central authority or because they arose in imitation of official art (like the classicism of the Romanesque period in many provincial centers).

The three characteristics of classicism which we have mentioned, that is, its interest in theory, its symbolic value, and its sense of history, never deserted it and must be considered its essential elements. All three must coexist; otherwise it would be impossible to distinguish the true classic current from vague and episodic returns to antiquity or from later achievements in the science of perspective, construction, and architectural functionalism of the 18th century, in which classical elements are used without classical intention. At the same time classicism, thus defined, is clearly distinct from the sort of poetic re-creation of the ancient myths which we find in Botticelli or in Piero di Cosimo. These artists, in fact, because of the imaginative freedom and the emotional quality of their work, are in direct opposition to the official interpretation of antiquity, discovering in the ancient myths, as we shall see, unsuspected poetic or dramatic qualities. Indeed, the presence of mythological subjects is not of itself sufficient proof of the existence of classicism; on the contrary, classicism may well exist as a stylistic quality, quite apart from the use of ancient literary themes.

The Italian Renaissance (see RENAISSANCE), though impregnated with classical lore and possessing an essential classicizing element, should not be considered a manifestation of classicism entirely. It abounds in anticlassical elements, especially as it evolves into mannerism (q.v.), the origins of which are to be found in Leonardo, in Michelangelo, and in Raphael and his school. Furthermore, some of the Renaissance achievements, such as the landscape or the portrait, even though they have parallels in classical literature (e.g., Pliny), do not belong in the present analysis of classicism. If, however, one takes the position that the Renaissance began as early as the 12th century, it can be viewed as a direct continuation of a historical trend of classicism, coinciding in theoretical principles and artistic taste with earlier manifestations of this movement — a point of view which seems to have gained some support.

Though it may seem hazardous to pass judgment on so important and so imposing a historical trend, it follows from what has been said that classicism imposed distinct limits on the imagination and culture of artists, cutting them off from large sections of ancient tradition (i.e., from all those fantastic, extradevotional, popular, and esoteric manifestations which conflicted with the principles sanctioned by the theories of classicism). It often, too, led artists away from the imitation of nature, compelling them to copy man-made models, sometimes significant only because of their age or their supposed origin. At the same time it diverted attention from the manual execution of the work of art, from the elaboration of a personal and immediate style (so much so that important works were sometimes entrusted entirely to pupils). All these dangers, which can be summed up in the epithet "academic" — an accusation specially valid in the case of neoclassicism — were implicit in the emphasis placed by theoretical writers, both ancient and modern, on restraint, on moderation, on the rigorous imitation of the masters. It is an important merit of romanticism (q.v.) to have given this accusation a historical and definitive formulation.

Even more serious were the historical consequences of classicism. As a result of the Renaissance, classicism became most strongly entrenched in the Latin countries, particularly Italy, where it was taken up by the princely courts and ultimately led to the establishment of many conventional standards. The subject of works of art had to conform to classifications; styles and individual masters were often discriminated against. Genre paintings, picturesque landscapes, and that interest in the rendering of the transitory, impermanent aspect of the universe which is one of the great qualities of Dutch 17th-century painting, all these were indiscriminately condemned. As a consequence there gradually came about a real cultural division between the Catholic and the Protestant worlds, a division which is particularly evident in the discussions on the limits and the value of imitation, and on the principles of religious art (see REFORMATION AND COUNTER REFORMATION).

Eugenio BATTISTI

CLASSICISM IN ANCIENT ART. The use of the term "classicism" in this article to signify a series of clearly distinct cultural and historical events precludes any confusion between classicism and classic, whatever the meaning or scope given to the latter (see CLASSIC ART). We can thus safely ignore those examples, found for the most part in works of slight critical value, of the use of the term "classicism" to denote the characteristics of the classical age or even of the whole of Greco-Roman antiquity. But even when making the necessary distinction between classicism and classic, now generally accepted by archaeologists and historians of ancient art, it is still important to note some differences, or shades of difference, between phenomena usually connected with the former concept.

By classicism is meant the imitation of the classic. But this does not exhaust the problem. The works produced in the most genuine period of classic art had immediate repercussions on the contemporary world; styles persisted and were handed down; artists went back for critical or nostalgic reasons to the great models. Nor is it always clear what the classical ideal meant to the different movements which claimed to draw inspiration from it: for some it seems to have contained merely a lesson of form, for others a choice of models; sometimes it was interpreted as a program of harmony and ethos, or an inspiration embracing mythical, religious, literary, and political motifs; occasionally it was even transformed into something different from the original source, a genuine historical reality.

* *

The classic period of Greek art represents in essence a unique and unrepeatable moment in the development of the representational arts. Its most characteristic elements appeared in their entirety about 440 B.C. To contemporaries this achievement must have seemed little short of miraculous, and it is not surprising if certain artists began to regard this classic perfection as a norm, thus becoming the founders of classicism. The art to which they gave expression was a reflected art, not determined by the obscure forces of life, as was classic art (which one could almost describe as *genitus non factus*: "something born, not made by the hands of man"), but based instead on the imitation of precise models; not mastered by labor and toil but received as a gift. This can be seen, for example, in some of the metopes of the Parthenon, probably the work of an anonymous pupil of Phidias, which are harmonious and beautiful but nothing more, because they lack any intimate vital force.

A second, and in some ways more conscious, moment of classicism begins at the end of the 5th century B.C., when the creative impulse of the classic period began to lose momentum. Between 400 B.C. and roughly 370 B.C. art assumes a retrospective character. Just as Athens strove, in politics, after the terrible defeat of Aegospotami in 404 B.C., to salvage what it could from the wreck of its former greatness, so in art there are obvious signs of a tendency to return to the great models of the 5th century, to ignore the so-called "baroque" art of the war years (432–04) and imitate instead the simple harmony and noble forms of the years around 440 B.C. But conditions had altered: only in external appearances could art recover the splendor of its past beauty. As characteristic examples of this phase we may take the steles of Dexileos and Hegeso. Admittedly they may be the work of sculptors of the older generation, who in their youth had actively participated in the classic movement at its most vital. But younger artists, though equally attached to the great models of the past, no longer succeeded in reconciling the new with the old (that is, the classic), as we can see by considering their treatment of the human form and their handling of drapery. Fourth-century art really begins about 370 B.C., when, with the new political outlook, a vital impulse once more appears in the Attic spirit, re-creating classic art and infusing it with a new reality.

This return of the classic spirit in art seems to have come about almost involuntarily, to have been unplanned and unconscious. In philosophy the return was paralleled by Plato, whose conservatism and antagonism to his own times was expressed in the *Republic* and *Laws*. Plato's genius, in fact, gave him a spiritual vision which even among the Greeks has never been equaled, and his image of men in many ways embodied the ideal which had unconsciously sustained the great artists of the preceding century.

One should not forget, on the other hand, that Attic art was destined to become the depositary of classic tradition during the subsequent developments in the history of Greek art (see ATTIC AND BOEOTIAN ART). Even during the ebb and flow of the Hellenistic currents of Rhodes and Pergamon, Attic art retained its characteristics of great formal restraint and dislike of emphasis or violent expression. The Attic sense of harmony and measure was a sort of artistic constant, to which artists could always, and several times did, return. The same applies to the Attic dialect, which represents a pure and essential expression of the Greek spirit, and which became the koine, the common language and normal means of communication between educated people from one end of the Mediterranean to the other. It was to an Atticism of definite classic import that many artists returned when the formal idiom of their period began to disintegrate (see HELLENISTIC ART). Even in the frieze depicting the battle between the gods and the giants on the Pergamon altar (Berlin), this trend is evident. However, it was, above all, the masters of the Attic school themselves who opposed the most strenuous resistance to the exaggerations of the baroque derived from Asia or tried to discipline it to more classic standards.

The classic phase, which made its appearance about 150 B.C., was a deliberate return to the past, of which men of the time were conscious. "Revixit Ol. 156 deinde ars" ("Then in the 156th Olympiad art revived"), Pliny states, basing himself perhaps on the history of Greek art written by Antigonos of Karystos. Symbolic of this 2d-century revival of classicism is the fact that in the library of Pergamon — destined to preserve and hand down to posterity the noblest patrimony of the spirit of classical Greece — there was placed a replica of the *Athena Parthenos* of Phidias (PL. 385). Another outstanding example is the decision of Antiochos VI, Epiphanes of Syria, to commission for his capital, Antioch, a copy of Phidias's statue of *Zeus Olympios*, and not a work in the baroque style. Not all the works of this period, however, hark back to the classic past, but there is a trend that can be followed intermittently amidst other currents. As in all periods of decline, there is an impression of confusion, a lack of any clear sense of direction, occasioned by the many influences at work at the same time.

In time classicism tended to gain the upper hand over the other styles of late Hellenism; but this success was accompanied by a gradual impoverishment, for instead of being a conscious and deliberate movement, it became secondhand and mechanical. At this point, which coincided approximately with the Roman occupation of the Greek world, the human form began to lose its dominance in sculpture; it seemed to become void of content, its physiological and anatomical structure weakened; its treatment became two-dimensional, as if it no longer possessed the internal force necessary to prevail over space. There was a lack of solidity, a constriction about the treatment of the limbs, which created the impression of artificiality, of pose, as if the creative powers of the sculptor had been exhausted in the effort to imagine new schemes and gestures. A certain preciousness became apparent. Classic models were considered more as a point of reference than as a means of conveying the illusion of volume and weight or of expressing the forces contained in a figure, or even of endowing it with a calm and dignified appearance.

Greek sculpture after 150 B.C. showed many varied forms of this classicism. In Athens, where, as we have said, classic feeling had never really died, the transition was easy. On the other hand, in those parts of the Greek world, such as Pergamon and Rhodes, in which baroque art had been carried to its most extreme consequences, the disintegration of the prevailing style and the return to classicism were full of drama. In this process the classical models underwent modifications which anticipated the works of the 4th century.

After the end of the 2d century B.C. the return to antiquity (see ANTIQUE REVIVAL), not only to classic but also to archaic art, became a general and conscious cultural trend and is to be associated with the campaign waged in the literary field against Eastern tendencies. The classicism of the Roman age was indelibly imprinted with the work of the neo-Attic artists (see NEO-ATTIC STYLES).

Ernst LANGLOTZ

It is now usual in studies on ancient art to recognize the existence of a real period of classicism corresponding to the final phase of Hellenism and the beginnings of the age of imperial Rome. Its most characteristic phase is said to be the age of Augustus, in which classical taste was paramount in sculpture, decorative painting, bronzes, silverwork, pottery (particularly, after 25 B.C., in the productions of the potteries of Arezzo), and precious stones; at the same time Neo-Attic artists specialized in copied Greek masterpieces or elaborated upon them. Besides the classicism of the Augustan age, it is usual to note several other classic revivals during the Roman Empire. Those of the 1st century are somewhat hard to define. There was a distinct one under Hadrian (see PL. 386); others, with their own idiosyncrasies, occurred under the Severi, under Gallienus, and finally in the age of Constantine (see PL. 387). Classical touches reappear in late-antique art of the 4th and 5th centuries (PL. 391).

The problem of such manifestations is complex, and their interpretation very much a matter of opinion. From a certain point of view, they would seem to indicate the existence of periodic returns toward the great sources of inspiration found

in Greek art, with the deliberate intention of counteracting new tendencies which were inexorably making themselves felt in the arts. In this sense they provide an ever-weakening echo of the artistic revival of the 2d century B.C. (Pliny's "revixit ars," i.e.," art revived"). There is, however, an uninterrupted classical current, more or less evident, alongside the other trends that went to make up the art of Rome.

One must, indeed, remember that there are several distinct factors to be considered in the alternation between postclassic phases of innovation and periods inspired by the ideals of classicism. The classic attitude is especially apparent in official Roman art (see ROMAN IMPERIAL ART). But in popular art and in the work of dilettantes a strong local tradition naturally tended to absorb and abolish classic forms (see ITALO-ROMAN FOLK ART); in the art of the Roman provinces this was even more the case. During the Empire, however, Greece remained in one way or another faithful to her Hellenistic or Attic legacy.

It is important to bear in mind that the works of the Roman period, because of the cultural, literary, secondhand nature of their inspiration, do not possess the perfect coherence of theme, form, and spirit which had given rise to the classic art of Greece. Mythological subjects harking back to ancient compositions, themes derived from famous statues and pictures, these recur widely in all the artistic production of imperial Rome and its provinces — in architectural reliefs, sarcophagi, decorative frescoes, small bronze statues, terra-cotta work; but for all that, they do not represent or imply any conscious adherence to classical ideals. On the contrary, these borrowings from the past are often entirely absorbed in new and different concepts of form. Or sometimes, in answer to new requirements, themes which are completely foreign to the classic art of Greece strive for expression within a framework of pure Greek forms (or forms considered such), seeking to recapture the purity of 5th-century art or the spirituality of 4th-century art; this may be seen in the reliefs of the Ara Pacis (the Altar of Peace), a historical record (PL. 385), or in the statues of Antinoüs commissioned by Hadrian (PL. 386). Gradually, as time went on, the concept of classic art became wider and included not only the art of the 4th-century B.C. but also the Hellenistic. At a certain point they ceased to be distinguishable, and Hellenistic form comprising in itself all of classical antiquity stood as the symbol of resistance in the late-antique period and in the Middle Ages, counteracting the successive waves of formal abstraction which in the Western world affected artistic creation.

The simple repetition or renewal of the themes and stylistic formulas elaborated by classical Greece is not, therefore, sufficient evidence of the existence of a real classicism; what we must look for is a desire to relive the heroic world of which the great masterpieces were the artistic expression and of which their survival happily offers a more visible and tangible proof than the accounts of historians or poets. Considered in this way, artistic classicism cannot be separated from literary classicism, but is part of the general tendency of the Hellenistic and Roman world to ennoble the new by means of the old, a process involving a constant search for illustrious models and "parallels" and conceived not as the following of a recently established tradition, but as the reaffirmation of lost values. The consequence of this process was the creation of a current of ideas and symbols derived from the past, continuous in its development, but finding room for elements of reaction against contemporary or near-contemporary trends. Proceeding unevenly, with periods of greater intensity alternating with those of stagnation, this current from time to time acquired a fund of new motifs which it passed on, together with the traditional material, for the imitation of future generations.

In illustration we may take the example of the conflict between Atticism and Eastern trends which began in Greece in the 2d century B.C. It found fertile ground in Rome and was adopted and given almost an official blessing by Augustus, who opposed Hellenism in the name of a revival of autochthonous Italic traditions; from this derives the apparent paradox that the exaltation of Italic traditions, summed up in the epic of Aeneas and his followers, should assume the forms of classical

Greece. The Hellenizing emperors of the 1st and 2d centuries, on the other hand, were interested primarily in the Hellenistic monarchies. With them classicism began to mean an indiscriminate admiration for the whole of the Greek past. This can be seen in the eclecticism of the age of Hadrian, of which the Emperor's villa at Tivoli constitutes the most significant expression. But this eclecticism also embraced the essential elements of the imperial Roman ideal, as consecrated by the aspirations and achievements of the Augustan monarchy; more, it not only admitted, but deliberately cultivated and developed, new features which were more particularly Roman in origin (apparent especially in the development of architecture). This complex network of traditions, suggestions, and aspirations was handed on, as a unified ideal of ancient greatness, to the emperors of the late Roman period, inspiring the revivals initiated by Constantine and Theodosius; in the end the idea of classicism became inseparable from that of imperial Rome. Not even the crisis caused by the anti-Christian movement of the 4th century could break this unity, even though the pagan reaction spoke in the name of Rome, not Greece, and contained a certain autonomous reevocation of classic form, especially in the circle of the Nicomachus and the Symmachus families.

MEDIEVAL CLASSICISM. It is to the humanist culture of the Middle Ages that Europe owes its interpretation of classicism, thanks to which compositions were mostly planned on geometric principles and art stood for the representation of human beings and the rendering of form (see ICONOGRAPHY AND ICONOLOGY; IMAGES AND ICONOCLASM). The revival of sculpture in high relief and the monumental portrait is a consequence of this stand. Much significant information can be found in medieval treatises, which often contain pertinent remarks on the essence of classicism. Among recurrent themes we find the theory of proportions, of harmony, and of the consequent connection between the arts and music; the concept of "decorum" is enunciated, and, in the manner of Quintilian, excessive expression and ornament are condemned; the art of Athens is constantly held up as a model of purity and simplicity of style. Useful information on this point can be derived from the indexes to the works of E. R. Curtius (1948, 1953) and De Bruyne (1946). A general survey confirms the persistent presence of classicism in the art of the Middle Ages where it forms, as it were, an alternative to medieval fantasy or expressionism and sometimes even coincides chronologically with the latter. Apart from the handing down of certain representational and mythological themes (which themselves acted as a sort of incentive to return to the ancient stylistic models), antiquity also passed on to the Middle Ages some formal principles, such as the system of subdividing the face and body and probably the architectural plans of buildings on a geometric basis. In many cases, obviously, these practices were a matter of shop procedure and did not embody conceptual principles, as they did later for Brunelleschi. But the first readings and commentaries of Vitruvius, which took place at the Carolingian court and which even embraced the question of illusionistic perspective, show how, even at that early date, it was possible to compare and even to correct medieval practice by the use of ancient writings on art. Other evidence reveals the great fascination exercised by sculpture in the round, which was invested with a magic significance and valued to such an extent that statues became the emblems of various cities and were placed in the foundations of buildings to protect them against harm; in some instances they were even collected (see MUSEUMS AND COLLECTIONS). In this atmosphere of respect and conscious evocation of ancient classicism were composed the *elogia* of various cities, in which allusion was made to their antiquity, their historical importance, their monuments, and their walls.

As in all instances of a return to antiquity, it is not always easy to distinguish in these early medieval trends what is due to a specific imitation of antiquity from what is simply the result of tradition. In this case judgment is rendered more difficult by the fact that the territories which had formed part of the Roman empire seem to have contained both ateliers of a very low cultural level and a few exceptionally gifted artists,

who from time to time produced works of the highest standard. This suggests that, despite a general process of cultural transformation, there existed certain conservative circles which exercised an intelligent and refined patronage. This theory, advanced by G. P. Bognetti ("Storia archeologica e diritto nel problema dei Longobardi," *Atti del I Congresso Internazionale di Studi Longobardi*, Spoleto, 1951), is confirmed by the existence of some outstanding examples of classicism in works associated with certain nunneries. One might mention in this context the sarcophagi and the capitals in the crypt of the Abbey of Jouarre, founded about 630, where the most conspicuous monument is the memorial to the abbess Telchilde (PL. 388); or centuries later (perhaps during the Carolingian age) the stucco decorations in the "Tempietto" of Cividale. Both these works, however, probably reflect the aristocratic art of the courts. Indeed, it seems reasonable to suppose that the ruling circles not only maintained the emblems and ceremonial customs of the Roman empire but also rather casually collected works of art, thereby preserving more faithfully than other groups the traditions of ancient art.

The first classic revival of international scope, marking a break with tradition and a return to authentic sources, is provided by Charlemagne's attitude toward Constantinople and Rome. As is well known, Charlemagne aspired, even in the very title he assumed, to the inheritance of the whole Roman empire; in his writings Einhard gives the impression that Charlemagne wished to become independent of the Papacy. At his court there came into being a group of real humanists, who even adopted classical pseudonyms; one of these scholars, the poet Modoin, referred in the clearest of terms to the Emperor's intention of transforming Aachen into a second Rome, "so that the golden city, renewed, may live once more in the world" (H. Fichtenau, "Il concetto imperiale di Carlo Magno," in *I problemi della civiltà carolingia*, Spoleto, 1954, pp. 251–98; P. Lehman, "Das Problem der karolingischen Renaissance," in *I problemi della civiltà carolingia*, Spoleto, 1954, pp. 309–58). To this end, while not forgetting Byzantium, Charlemagne went back, even in the emblems of power, to ancient and thus more hallowed models: for his seals he copied a coin or medal of the 3d or 4th century; in his official dress he adopted the ancient chlamys and tunic; in his documents, a clear and monumental calligraphy. The architectural evidence is equally explicit: in its structure the Palatine Chapel at Aachen copies the Golden Triclinium of Constantinople, nucleus of the Great Palace of the Emperors built by Justinian. Charlemagne's royal palace was called the Lateran and had in front an equestrian statue of Theodoric (the prototype of the humanist monarch), clearly intended to be a counterpart to the statue of Marcus Aurelius which stood outside the Lateran in Rome and was thought to be a statue of Constantine. Thus in contemporary and later writings Charlemagne came to be compared to Constantine and to Solomon. The many scholarly treatises produced at his court reveal him as wishing to found a culture based on moderation and harmony, anxious not to exceed the golden mean, and intent on discovering the *incommutabiles regulas*, or "unchanging rules," of the perceptible word. Einhard seems to have been responsible for the classical approach to architecture in the Carolingian period. He had an excellent knowledge of Vitruvius and kept abreast of the contemporary attempts to discover the building techniques of the ancients, such as that of the Abbot Eigil, who built at Fulda a small rotunda "ad instar antiquorum operum" ("on the model of ancient buildings"). The influence of his studies and of the copies of Vitruvius which were carried out under his orders was immeasurable, and it is undeniable that Aachen contains the finest examples of German medieval architecture. As early as 926 architects were enjoined to study Euclid and Vitruvius. In the arcades of the Palatine Chapel and those of the gateway at Lorsch there is no vertical accentuation; they are distinctly pre-Renaissance in their monumentality and their kinship with Roman models such as the Colosseum. (Equally explicit references to antiquity occur in French Romanesque architecture.) The bronze window grilles of Aachen (PL. 390) and the doors, with their delicate and detailed decorative work,

are even more outstanding, both for their balanced composition and their elegance. Imitations and copies of the antique also appear in Carolingian manuscripts and ivories, though perhaps more in evidence in these works are the expressionist tendencies of the age, which reflect and exaggerate the nervous, yet vigorous, Hellenistic shorthand. Though dependent on the antique, this expressionist line is distinctly anticlassical, but in the present state of our knowledge it is difficult to say whether it came into being at exactly the same time as the classical approach to architecture or at a slightly different time. Between 816 and 834, during the episcopate of the imperial librarian Archbishop Ebbo, a typical humanist center seems to have existed in the scriptorium of Reims, where in the 13th century there was to be an exceptional flourishing of classicism in the plastic arts. Nevertheless, few works reveal the classical consistency of the bronzework at Aachen; in the illuminated manuscripts and in the best ivories the agitated line creates a sharp contrast with the deliberately precise compositions and the ever-present elaborate quotations from classic sources (see CAROLINGIAN PERIOD).

Another feature of the Carolingian era was a revival of the equestrian statue. The evidence offered by the small bronze statue of Charlemagne on horseback (Louvre; I, PL. 303) is supported by other sources such as the will of Archbishop Bruno of Cologne, which mentions a silver horse ("equitem argenteum") presented to the testator by the Archbishop of Mainz. We also have information of portraits in sculpture. The emotional power of these works is demonstrated by the curious episode of the Duke of Brittany, who defiantly caused a statue of himself to be erected on a pinnacle in order to show his independence of the Emperor. Although we are still largely ignorant of the channels through which the Carolingian renaissance was diffused, its influence was enormous. There is a clear line of descent through successive copies of the most important Carolingian works (such as the illuminations of the Utrecht Psalter, PL. 58, done at Reims in 832) to the Gothic way of seeing and representing. By the middle of the 9th century the effects of the Carolingian renaissance may be observed, for instance, in the angel in the initial "L" in a manuscript at Metz (Bib. Mun., Ms. lat. 9388, fol. 17) or in the ivories produced in Reims about 860, with their surprising mythological and historical personifications (e.g., the ivory covers of the Codex Aureus at Lorsch), or in the crystal from Lorraine in the British Museum (PL. 69), with the story of Susanna and the Elders (ca. 870). These works confirm that the Carolingian attitude veered increasingly toward classicism (A. Boeckler, "Malerei und Plastik im ostfränkischen Reich," in *I problemi della civiltà carolingia*, Spoleto, 1954, pp. 161–79).

Under the Ottonian emperors, an intentional classicism can be discerned in the manuscript illuminations depicting the emperors receiving the homage of their various provinces. A beautiful example is that at Chantilly, perhaps the work of an Italian artist, which comes from the *Registrum Gregorii* (Trier, ca. 983) and is inspired by 5th-century models. Connected with the art of this illuminator (probably active in Reichenau, Lorsch, and Trier) are some ivories which derive their delicately balanced composition from ancient prototypes (for example, the *Annunciation* and the *Nativity* in Ms. lat. 4451, Bayerische Staatsbib., Munich). The ivories of Metz and Fulda seem to be the most classical. In any case, here, as in other instances, classicism was a mere interlude in a general development that was evolving in other directions (A. Boeckler, "Ottonische Kunst in Deutschland," *I problemi comuni dell'Europa post carolingia*, Spoleto, 1955).

Important works of art based stylistically as well as iconographically on antiquity, with the intention of renewing it, appear frequently though intermittently. Outstanding among these are the Golden Altar of Basel (1002–19), perhaps from Mainz (now in the Mus. de Cluny, Paris); the bronze baptismal font of St. Barthélemy, Liège, a city known as the Athens of the North (1107–18); the bronze doors of Gniezno Cathedral, Poland (after 1127), perhaps the work of artists from Liège; and some bronzes from the Meuse Valley, now in the Victoria and Albert Museum (ca. 1180).

The close connection between history and portraiture is illustrated by two reliquaries in the form of busts, one of Pope Alexander I, perhaps by Godefroid de Huy, 1146, which is most faithful to classical conventions (Brussels, Mus. Royaux d'Art et d'Histoire), and the other of Frederick Barbarossa (ca. 1150; Hanover, Kestner-Mus.).

Roman building methods were adopted anew in Romanesque architecture: preference was given to solid masonry, rounded arches, and vaults; the use of architectural members also attempted to follow classical conventions, as may be seen in the projecting columns and decorative meanders on the façade of the Church of Saint-Gilles (PL. 390). The study of ancient sarcophagi and reliefs brought about a transition in the treatment of figures from the ritual gestures and poses of Byzantine art to a greater naturalism of representation. The rise in the political importance of the free communes was often accompanied by manifestations of classicism; thus we have the mythological reliefs carried out by Wiligelmo and his school at Modena, the apostles of St. Sernin at Toulouse (ca. 1096) and the marble decorations at Pisa and Florence. It is probable that such evidences of aristocracy and culture in the principal seats of power (where public buildings, such as the Palazzo del Comune at Verona, have the solemn character of monuments) were related to the struggle between pope and emperor, both of whom relied heavily on the classical tradition for their propaganda. One of the first artistic events to have a clear political purpose (F. Calasso, 1957) was the construction of Salerno Cathedral by Robert Guiscard, Duke of Apulia and Calabria, probably between 1080 and 1084, to celebrate his victory over the Byzantine Empire. The inscription "... Robertus dux romani imperii maximus triumphator..." ("Robert, the greatest conqueror of the Roman Empire") anticipates the policies of Roger II of Sicily. It therefore seems material that Salerno became the center of a school of ivory production in which a strong sculptural feeling was combined with vigorous composition; later reflections of this school are to be seen in ambos and pulpits of great refinement.

Intermittently during the Middle Ages some important structures had been erected in Rome, but in the second half of the 12th century many new buildings arose, probably in consequence of the reestablishment of the Roman senate (P. Brezzi, 1947). The finest examples of this activity are the basilicas, like S. Maria in Trastevere, accurately copied from early Christian models. The notion that the glories of ancient Rome were being revived was publicized by the *Mirabilia urbis Romae*, which described the remains of imperial Rome. The renaissance, or *renovatio*, of this period gave birth to a school of architecture and sculpture under the Cosmati (q.v.) which was later to merge with the classic renewal of Federick II, ultimately culminating in the frescoes and mosaics of Cavallini (q.v.).

With Frederick II, and especially with the arch of Capua (1234–39), we are on the threshold of a truly scholarly Renaissance approach. The arch contained a symbolic message of some complexity, conveyed by means of a series of allegorical representations (PL. 389), among which was the figure of Justice. This medieval material, however, was taken back to its historical origins: the sculptures (I, PL. 303) seem directly inspired by ancient models, such as the masks of the amphitheater of Capua. From later sources we gather that by virtue of its employment of ancient forms (through its style, that is, rather than by its allegorical representations), this monumental archway was intended to fill the spectator with a sense of the imperial dignity and to explain its principles and history (C. Willemsen, *Kaiser Friedrichs II: Triumphtor zu Capua, ein Denkmal hohenstaufischer Kunst in Süditalien*, Wiesbaden, 1953; Battisti, 1958). The arch was copied in the 15th century in the arch of Alfonso of Aragon, at Castel Nuovo, Naples (PL. 390). The representation of the Emperor Frederick is the most faithful imitation known to us of ancient portraiture: he is seated and wearing a toga, "extensis brachiis duobusque digitis, quasi os tumide comminacionis" ("with arms and two fingers held out, the mouth as if swollen with menace") — a gesture later to become dear to the Renaissance popes, being adopted in the statue which Julius II commissioned from Michelangelo for the

façade of S. Petronio, Bologna. It was perhaps in imitation of Frederick II that Boniface VIII caused many statues of himself to be erected during his papacy (1294–1303), thereby arousing much adverse criticism. In any case the classicism of Frederick II and his age, the consequences of which are visible in Nicola Pisano, in Arnolfo di Cambio, and ultimately in Giotto (PL. 392), led directly to the Renaissance. Its importance is further stressed by contemporary developments elsewhere in Europe; together with the spread of the Cistercian taste for simplicity and for the clear geometric treatment of space in accordance with elementary proportional schemes, we also find in various important centers an obvious revival of ancient sculpture (the Visitation group of the west façade, Reims; the front panel of the pulpit in the church of Wechselburg Castle, ca. 1220–30; the Last Judgment in the south transept of Chartres Cathedral, ca. 1205–15; the sculptures in Bamberg Cathedral, etc.; Weise, 1956). Certain heads of apostles and saints reveal a mixture of classical and later sources, which call to mind the comparisons dear to Renaissance Humanists between Christian and pagan virtues. Valentiner (1956) has quite convincingly demonstrated that this tendency to merge iconographical types was based on political motives, as, for example, in the Bamberg *Rider* (1225–35; PL. 389) and that of Magdeburg (ca. 1230) and the *Rex Justus* of Strasbourg Cathedral, all of which are presumably ideal portraits of Frederick II. Also to be included in this group is the equestrian statue of Oldrado da Tresseno (1233), which even contains the imperial eagle (Milan, Palazzo della Ragione). However, these were isolated incidents which did not outlive the peculiar historical climate that produced them, though they served as stimuli and precedents for much later generations.

In conclusion, within the complex picture of the return to antiquity, medieval classicism was distinguished by a particular propensity for volume, symmetry, order; it selected from ancient art those elements which best accorded with the treatises of rhetoric studied at the time and deliberately attached itself, for political and cultural reasons, to the courtly taste of the later Roman empire. Consequently it has a distinctly symbolic flavor, the purpose of which is to demonstrate the direct derivation of contemporary culture and political authority from the Roman empire. At the same time, because of its rejection of any form of expressive distortion and its attachment, resulting from constant reference to antique sculpture and ivories, to a decidedly three-dimensional style, medieval classicism appears to have had a naturalistic character as well. The present state of our knowledge does not justify speaking of a strict continuity: the manifestations of medieval classicism appear for the most part ephemeral and accidental. Certain centers, however (Reims, Salerno, Florence, etc.), sometimes because of external stimulus, sometimes as a result of local tendencies, revealed a particularly tenacious attachment to classicism. In general, however, precisely because medieval classicism consisted of a series of revivals rather than an unbroken tradition, its finest and most original achievements were generally to be found outside the two main centers of the classical tradition, Rome and Byzantium, at least until the time when even these two centers, especially Rome, were themselves in drastic need of *renovatio*.

THE RENAISSANCE AND THE MODERN PERIOD. For the writers of the Italian Renaissance, who had recourse to 14th-century sources, the decisive break with the Middle Ages occurred in the second half of the 13th century, with artists such as Nicola Pisano (q.v.), Cimabue (q.v.), and Giotto (q.v.). The new age distinguished itself through conscious intellectualism after centuries of devotion to simple craftsmanship. Artists were now cultured and intelligent; they had a broad education, were connected with Humanist circles, and devoted themselves, even more than the artists of the late Gothic period, to the study of ancient sculpture. Petrarch even seems to connect Giotto's ability to convey a sense of depth and volume, which scandalized the ignorant, with the artist's learning. Giotto, moreover, was attached to the papal court, and at least two of his works — the frescoes in St. John Lateran and the Navicella

in St. Peter's — had a political character. Further, the existence at Rome, perhaps in rivalry with the empire, of the will to revive at least the external appearance of ancient Rome is unmistakably shown in the intense architectural and artistic activity initiated by Boniface VIII, together with his abundant use of statues in cities under his rule, as a means of providing visible evidence of his authority.

Fourteenth-century classicism, however, was a short-lived episode. After the death of Giotto people were already speaking of an artistic decline: even the works of Giotto himself became less heroic in style after his departure from central Italy. The fresco cycle in the Upper Church at Assisi, attributed by many to Giotto, displays both a stylistic reaction against the two extremes of Gothic literalism and Byzantine distortion and a clear relation to contemporary religious struggles. (Giotto's concern with such matters is illustrated by the fact that an outspoken poem, a *canzone* against poverty, is attributed to him.) Equally important is the activity of Arnolfo di Cambio; but in this survey it is possible to call attention only to his sculpture in the round, e.g., the Virgin on the tomb of Cardinal de Braye, in the Church of S. Domenico, Orvieto (I, PL. 456), the *Dormition of the Virgin*, from the old façade of S. Maria del Fiore (formerly in the Kaiser Friedrich Museum, Berlin; I, PL. 459), and most especially the portraits, in particular the heroic figure of Charles of Anjou (Rome, Capitoline Museum; I, PL. 458).

*The Renaissance in Tuscany.* At the end of the 14th century, inspired directly by these remarkable predecessors, classicism became centered in Florence in conjunction with an intense and autonomous political reawakening (see ANTIQUE REVIVAL). In this Florentine classicism there were direct connections between artists and men of letters and Humanists such as Leonardo Bruni and Coluccio Salutati. Classicism, indeed, seemed at this point to coincide completely with the Renaissance return to antiquity, and certainly, from that time on, it was to permeate the whole history of Italian art. Nevertheless, even in Florence the evolution of classicism was not entirely smooth; see, for example, Nanni di Banco's development toward Gothic complexity of style (PL. 391), concurrent with entirely different stylistic tendencies. Consider also the fundamentally courtly spirit of the art of Ghiberti or the enormous success of Gentile da Fabriano's *Adoration of the Magi* (1423: VI, PLS. 84, 85). The fact that the Renaissance movement in Florence was led by architecture (that is, by Brunelleschi) rather than by sculpture, despite the greater accessibility of Greek and Roman models for the latter, illustrates both the substantial difference between classicism and the return to antiquity and the extremely close connection in the 15th century between classicism and religion. Wittkower has rightly pointed out that the cosmological and sacred significance attached to proportion was one of the distinguishing features of the culture of the time; his theory is supported by contemporary writings, from which it is apparent that incorrect proportions in a building devoted to religious purposes were considered to invalidate the ceremonies which took place there. Implicit here, too, was a kind of oblique Biblical reference. Many writings of the period, seemingly typical of Renaissance classicism, had their origin in ancient philosophical texts which were at that time interpreted in a religious light, such as the *Corpus hermeticum*. In the hermetic writings man was described as "a mortal god," partly because of his capacity to create for himself the image of divinity. Similarly the Renaissance treatises were often dedicated to the exaltation of man's ability to reshape his environment, lifting himself from primitive chaos to social order, and by extension these writings attributed to the architect nearly divine powers of creation and organization, thus elevating the art of architecture to an even higher moral plane than that conceded to it by Vitruvius. One of the strongest influences on Renaissance writings of this kind was that of St. Augustine, whose ideas were repeated and paraphrased. (In this connection it is interesting to note that some of the most important buildings of Florence and Rome were built for the Augustinians.) A passage from the *De ordine* (II, XI, pp. 32–34, *Patrologiae Cursus*, series I, XXXII, col. 1010 ff.) can be considered as provid-

ing a basic premise of the Renaissance theory of architecture. St. Augustine here stated that the irregular distribution of doors and windows would create a sense of uneasiness in the spectator, while their symmetrical placing "paribus intervallis" ("at equal intervals") would delight and ravish him : "unde ipsi architecti jam suo verbo 'rationem' istam vocant; et partes discorditer collocatas dicunt non habere rationem" ("whence architects themselves, using a special term, call it 'ratio', while features placed at irregular intervals are said to lack 'ratio' "). Throughout the passage St. Augustine insisted on the rational meaning of beauty and, at the same time, on the ability of reason to create a harmony of the senses, stopping short, it should be remarked, of advocating any seeking after expressive effects. This concept, described by the term *concinnitas*, was taken up by L. B. Alberti (*De re aedificatoria*, IX). No incompatibility existed, therefore, between Humanist culture and Christianity, or between reason and sense, not even in sacred art, where a "learned" architecture and a "learned" iconography were sought. Brunelleschi, with his search for the ancient *rationes*, that is, for the principles behind architectural design, attained an absolute mastery over visual reality, reconciling the logical rigor of Scholasticism with the need for emotional expression aroused by the pictorial qualities of Gothic art. In religious painting the sacred event was transferred from a legendary to a historical context — even if history did not yet mean accurate reconstruction of the past, but simply a feeling of actuality, in accordance with which it seemed legitimate to place the events of the Gospel in a contemporary Florentine setting. This feature, which gave works of Masaccio and Donatello their characteristic dramatic tone, aroused criticism and even mass reaction. On the whole Florentine classicism remained a learned movement, and its spread was very slow. Even in the nearby towns architectural classicism made little headway, and its diffusion was generally the result of personal contacts confined to a Humanist elite. In any case only Brunelleschi entirely succeeded in expressing himself in the vocabulary of classicism, without being affected by the tensions and spontaneous and forceful rebellions of a Donatello. Some of the purity and sense of objectivity that characterize Brunelleschi's greatest architectural works is due to the technical excellence of the workmanship, which does not admit of any sense of either material difficulty or effort; as a result these works rise above the sphere of craftsmanship to that of concept or pure design.

The enormous impulse which 15th-century classicism gave to all the arts, and the conflict of taste which it precipitated, are expressed in a story invented by the Florentines of a competition between Donatello and Brunelleschi for the design of a crucifix. According to the story, Brunelleschi idealized the figure of Christ so as to represent a true God, while Donatello, guided by his expressionist tendencies, so distorted the figure that it appeared that of a peasant. A comparison of the two works would show that both artists, although retaining some elements of Gothic style, had moved beyond it in opposite directions. Donatello's aim was an even more direct relation with the spectator, fraught with great emotional tension; his works, indeed, often took on the character of personifications, and these "loaded" images were suitably nicknamed by the people (such as *lo zuccone*, "the pumpkin head," an affectionate title bestowed by the Florentines on the statue of the prophet Habakkuk from the Campanile at Florence, now in the Museo dell'Opera del Duomo). Masaccio too was moving toward a form of expressionism, as in one of his late works, the *Crucifixion* in S. Maria Novella. Similarly, the work of Andrea del Castagno, another artist described as brutal by early critics, revealed in its emphatic nature clearly anticlassical directions.

Fifteenth-century Florentine classicism undoubtedly achieved revolutionary formal advances, such as the identification of pictorial vision with optical science, of religious iconography with historical fact, and of esthetic harmony with geometrical proportion and symmetry — principles which were to be the subject of constant elaboration, both stylistic and theoretical, until the advent of impressionism (see PERSPECTIVE; PROPORTION; TREATISES); at the same time, however, the theories of classicism caused crises of style for artists of dramatic intent, such as

Masaccio and Donatello, for whom the study of antiquity meant above all the acquisition of greater vigor of representation. Even some principles of classicism, such as the use of only one historical episode instead of the simultaneous representation of a number of scenes, typical of Gothic art, fell into disfavor. Despite a profound and detailed knowledge of antiquity, despite the poetic sense in which mythology was reexperienced as a significant symbolic facet of human history, even learned artists such as Botticelli can only with difficulty be thought of as classicists, and then only in a metaphorical sense. Indeed, certain important features of their work and personality, such as their preference for line rather than volume, their sense of melancholy, their lack of moral serenity, contained the seeds of mannerism (q.v.). This is particularly true in the case of Filippino Lippi, with his exuberance of decoration and his pietism, or of Piero di Cosimo, an artist whose mythological scenes, with their emphasis on the dramatic or the brutal, their sense of the tragedy of human life, imply a radically new approach to the concept of antiquity. His *Battle of the Centaurs and Lapiths* (London, Nat. Gall.) is probably the most tragic interpretation of mythology that painting has ever produced. In certain themes, on the other hand, such as the representation of Hercules, the equestrian statue, or the heroic standing figure, the spirit of classicism continued to be very strong, if episodic.

Outside Florence, however (and almost, one might say, in the wake of L. B. Alberti), classicism produced some magnificent results. Perhaps the most typical example is provided by the work of Mantegna, though in his case there is also the factor of the local tradition of Padua to be considered: witness the enthusiasm aroused in the city by the finding of the bones of Pliny, and the suggestion of the Humanist Sicco Polenton to erect a chapel in his honor. Mantegna's classicism was above all analytical and historical, motivated by a desire to re-create scenes with archaeological accuracy. All this was reflected outside Italy, where it assumed a magical, esoteric significance; and understandably so, for even in Mantegna, erudition is made to serve the purposes of a tendency toward dramatic expression and is often inclined to appear extrinsic rather than intrinsic to the style of the picture — precisely the opposite, one might say, of the classicism of Brunelleschi. The serene aspect of classicism, however, was nobly represented by Piero della Francesca. This artist's work displays not only a great restraint and a profound appreciation of the relations between color and design, but above all the capacity, even without reference to ancient prototypes, to translate the human drama into a mysterious and timeless realm. Probably no other painter has been so successful in harmonizing precept and rule with feeling and nature. His use of geometric patterns had a definite expressive function: the wrinkling of an eyebrow, the slant of an eye, the presence of an unexpected or accentuated shadow on an otherwise perfectly proportioned face, are enough to charge the regular arrangement of the composition with emotional or dramatic significance. Another aspect of the art of Piero della Francesca, also connected with the concept of classicism, is the air of mystery, the impression of aloofness, created by his images. This quality might be explainable in terms of the distinction proposed by Averroës between two types of men: the simple, the ignorant, the uninitiate, incapable of penetrating beyond the outward appearance of things, and, on the other hand, those endowed with philosophical insight and thus enabled to go beyond the letter to the inner meaning. The profound attention with which the heroic figures of the frescoes in the Church of St. Francis at Arezzo contemplate the sacred events there represented shows their ability to see beyond these events to their ultimate significance. As Ficino later wrote, nowadays we are not content with miracles; we demand a rational and philosophical confirmation. The heroic and religious fervor of Giotto and the early 15th-century Florentines was thus replaced by the Stoic ideal of spiritual moderation, coupled with a lack of interest in externals and a concentration on internal values. To Alberti this sense of poise seemed to be a reestablishment of harmony, the placing of man once more in contact with the music of the universe.

Since classicism is a spiritual attitude rather than an artistic formula, we do not find any explicit expression of these fundamental aspects of his art in Piero della Francesca's theoretical writings. Alberti, however, with whom Piero was in contact, has a phrase which could well be applied to the delicate balance of Piero's art. Beauty, he said, should be "the perfect union of different parts in a harmonious whole, in which none of them can be taken away, diminished, or altered without adversely affecting the whole." This definition, however, while being very much less rigorously formal than any which can be found in Latin writers, is somewhat superficial, and it entirely ignored the mystic feeling that fills Piero's paintings and that is emphasized by a highly individual use of light, which gives organic unity to his forms as if they were all bathed in an outpouring of divine grace. The intimate religious expression of Piero's art was developed by Giovanni Bellini, who gave it a somewhat more popular interpretation in his endearing Madonnas; Piero's perfect accord between abstract geometric structure and sensory data was brought to a heightened state of tension, particularly in portraiture, by Antonello da Messina, an artist connected equally with Italian Humanism and with the Flemish tradition. Much of Piero's spirituality can be seen in the famous Madonnas of Raphael's early years and in the delicate compositional balance still evident in Raphael's early Roman works, but already in these there is evidence of a tendency toward the physical idealization of beauty, of an interpretation of grace that is more courtly than Neoplatonic.

*Rome.* In Rome the cultural situation was such as to preclude purely stylistic experiments. Concurrent with the activities of the Augustinians (to whom are due two of the finest buildings of the period, S. Maria del Popolo and S. Agostino) and with the marked political connotations attached to art (the work of rebuilding the city, for example, was a direct consequence of the jubilee of 1450), there went the notion of a total identification of classicism with the return to antiquity. A practical instance of this was provided by the use of blocks of travertine, from the Colosseum and other ancient buildings, in structures which even in their ornamentation recalled the ancient monuments. Such a structure was the Loggia della Benedizione (later demolished) in front of St. Peter's which was imitated in the atria of several other basilicas — S. Marco, SS. Apostoli, and S. Pietro in Vincoli. This perpetuation (*translatio*) of ancient Rome in modern Rome was assisted by classical learning and by the surveying of ancient monuments, an operation for which Alberti and later Bramante constructed the necessary instruments; and it appears as a religious program in two illuminations of the *Civitas dei* (Ms. lat. 1882, Vatican Library; Ms. lat. 218, Bib. de Ste Geneviève, Paris), dating from the middle of the 15th century, in which modern Rome is equated with the Heavenly Jerusalem. Typical of this monument is the gradual suppression of a flourishing anti-Renaissance current in art, represented in 15th-century Rome not only by the presence of Lombard sculptors and architects, but also by the activities of Flemish, German, and Spanish artists. The influence of the Bible continued to be of considerable importance: the Vatican Palace was conceived as a reconstruction of that of Solomon, while a first partial rebuilding of St. Peter's was undertaken, on the basis of a passage in St. Augustine (again from the *Civitas dei*, XV, 26), with the express intention of modeling it on Noah's ark (perhaps in allusion to the unique charismatic power of the pope), and the Sistine, the papal chapel, was built to the exact measurement and plan of the Temple of Solomon. Even the splendor of the ceremonial was justified by Pius II with the aid of a remark of Solomon. Apart from the probable participation of Alberti and Rossellino (see PL. 388) in the plans of Pope Nicholas V, the artist most representative of this trend was Antonio da Sangallo. A clear indication of his genius had already been provided by the colonnaded court of the fortress of Civita Castellana, executed under Alexander VI, but his talents reached their full stature in the Church of S. Biagio at Montepulciano (PL. 390). Typically this edifice combines the monumental effect of trav-

ertine construction with an insistent rhythmic emphasis, which derives from the repeated use of the same architectural elements. Sangallo, however, had an awareness of the qualities of light and a dramatic approach which clearly separate him from his ancient models. Next to Sangallo, Bramante — despite all the orthodoxy of background and attitude which he displayed on his arrival in Rome — seems eccentric: his animation of architectural mass and his taste for pictorial effects are mannerist.

In the field of painting 16th-century Roman classicism was symbolized by the relationship between Raphael and Pietro Bembo. Giulio Mancini's *Considerazioni sulla pittura* (ed. Marucchi and Salerno, I, 1956, p. 7) states that it was Bembo who drew up the iconographical program of the famous Raphael rooms (the Stanze) in the Vatican; and mention must be made of the connections of this man of letters with the visual arts in general. Bembo was probably the foremost example of the close bond between classicism and the imitation of antiquity, which characterized this period of Roman art. His literary theory of the strict imitation of classical writers was simultaneously the direct result of his familiarity with developments in the visual arts and a powerful influence upon them. As Ulivi (1959) has observed, imitation was understood as the total absorption of a cultural background in which the highest spiritual values had already been realized, the recapturing of an experience in which the "idea" had been rendered concrete and humanized, and which constituted the nearest approach to nature itself that has been or, indeed, can be achieved. To Bembo, *imitatio* and *aemulatio* were thus interconnected; and it is not surprising that in Rome these ideas should have coincided with a purposeful exaltation of political power which resulted in the subordination of the arts to a program that was not exclusively cultural. Reaction against this situation was not long in coming, however, and the right of the artist to freedom of invention and personal idiosyncrasy in the realm of both form and content was shortly reaffirmed, largely as a result of the stylistic phenomenon represented by Michelangelo (see PL. 389), in whom the tension between the two poles of classicism and anticlassicism was ever present. By the time of the sack of Rome (1527), the cycle of Roman classicism had already drawn to a close.

*North Italy and Europe.* Despite differences of cultural and social background, the art of the Venetian mainland also in many instances tended toward classicism. In painting, Venetian classicism culminated in the *Sleeping Venus* (Dresden, Gemäldegalerie; VI, PL. 195) of Giorgione; in sculpture the decorations of 1508 by Antonio Lombardo in the private apartments of the Castle of Ferrara and a number of works by Simone Mosca are of particular importance; in the field of architecture Tullio Lombardo's Cappella del Sacramento (1516–22) in the Cathedral of Treviso and the works of Falconetto and Sanmicheli offer fine examples of the interest in classicism, as did the activities of patrons such as Giovanni Giorgio Trissino and Marco Mantova Benavides. The nature of Venetian classicism, as continued in the works of Sansovino, Titian, and Palladio, differed drastically from the Roman version, the prevailing emphasis being placed on Albertian proportional harmony and on a warm and delicately calculated equilibrium of color. The interpretation of antiquity thus produced was predominantly lyrical and evocative. Venice was one of the most important channels through which Italian classicism spread to the north, a process in which an important role was played by Jacopo de' Barbari, who was in touch with all the leading German artists of the early 16th century. The greatest representative of German classicism was, of course, Dürer (q.v.), who visited Italy on several occasions, but numerous other examples of classicism in Teutonic countries can be found; for example, the Fugger Chapel at Augsburg (1509–18), the sculpture of the Vischers and of Conrad Meit (about 1515), and such pictures as the *Allegory of Music* by Hans Baldung-Grien (Munich, Alte Pinakothek) and Cranach's nudes. As in Italy, however, German classicism did not generally outlive the first two decades of the 16th century. Dürer, for example,

underwent a real crisis about 1518–20, possibly due to the influence of Luther (F. Saxl, *Lectures*, London, 1957). Much the same situation existed in France, where the principal center of classicism seems to have been the Castle of Gaillon (Eure), residence of George Cardinal d'Amboise, patron of the most classicizing artist in France, Michel Colombe (e.g., his Louvre *St. George* relief, 1508–09). In the first decade of the 16th century other instances of classicism can be found, such as Jehan Bourdichon's illuminations in Anne of Brittany's *Book of Hours*, completed in 1508 (in which a representation of St. Sebastian recalls Perugino), or the portraits of Jean Perreal, which approach in style the art of Lombardy and the Po Valley. It is true that the influence of the Renaissance was much more widespread (see FRENCH ART; RENAISSANCE), but generally speaking, mannerism was more enthusiastically received in France, where it was grafted onto a stock of late Gothic architectural rationalism. The increasing use of regularized plans in castles built 1511–27 should not be used as an index of classicism in French architecture. However, the tomb of Louis XII at Saint-Denis (1515–31), with its direct derivations from Michelangelo's tomb of Julius II, does seem to represent an attempt to participate in the contemporary movement of Italian architecture, as do certain other isolated architectural examples, such as the unfinished, perhaps Italian-designed, Chapel of St. Michael in the Church of St. Aignan at Chartres.

In Spain the Albornoz seem to have been the first patrons conversant with newer trends, Spanish architecture at that time having been dominated by the profusely decorative style directly derived from the work of Lombard artists in Rome. However, an example of classicism is provided by Charles V's palace in the Alhambra at Granada, designed by Pedro Machuca, and the same monarch's fortress of Aquila reveals an unmistakable desire on his part to imitate the monumental style of the Augustan age. Other Spanish buildings which should be mentioned are the Sacristy (1556) of Jaén Cathedral and the Vásquez da Molina Palace at Úbeda (1562). In painting, in contrast to earlier insistently naturalistic art, pictures of Fernando Yañez de la Almedina, often strongly influenced by Leonardo (e.g., the *St. Catherine* in the Prado), were in general closely connected to early 16th-century Florentine art.

In Portugal an entire series of buildings, both religious and civil, were designed by Italian architects, but even these were chiefly mannerist.

This survey could be further extended; but enough has already been said to demonstrate that 16th-century classicism, though of great significance for all of Europe, was sporadic and short-lived. Everywhere it gave way to mannerism, a style conditioned by exacerbated subjectivity rather than a theoretical norm. This change involved not only the abandonment of the rules of proportion as well as stylistic and iconographic purity but also a taste for the undefined, the fantastic, and the instinctive free association of images.

The Counter Reformation brought a return to formal structure, but here it is perhaps more accurate to speak of rationalism or functionalism, than of classicism. The intentional simplicity of the flanks of the Collegio Romano in Rome, which reflect the rarefied geometry of Herrera's Escorial, can usefully be associated with the Jesuit prescription of 1558, whereby buildings constructed for the order "ne fiant aliquando palatia nobilium, sed sint ad habitandum, et officia nostra exercenda utilia, sana et fortia, in quibus tamen paupertatis memores videamur, unde nec sumptuosa sint nec curiosa," ("should never resemble the palaces of the nobles, but should be places to be lived in, adapted to the carrying out of our duties, healthy and strong; furthermore, that we should seem to be mindful of poverty, they should be neither sumptuous nor unusual") (Pirri, 1955). Sometimes, however, as in present-day architectural functionalism, the structural principles contained in themselves the expression of an ideal; this occurs in the Escorial, where to some exent the intervention of Italian mannerism was unfortunate, as it disrupted both the absolute geometric severity of the structure and the integrity of the scheme of recurring architectural elements — both qualities which, in Herrera's mind, carried cosmic and sacred significance.

The art of Palladio must be placed at least partly within the orbit of classicism, not so much by virtue of his use of ancient architectural elements — for here Palladio's work had an archaeological emphasis proper to mannerism — but because of his abstract sense of proportion, which is, however, strangely dissociated from the use of the traditional ancient building materials and from canonical typology; this freedom of usage permitted him without any historical justification, but with surprising stylistic coherence, to incorporate the pronaos of a temple into the design of a country villa. Of course, Palladio is not always so idiosyncratic: the double-ordered loggia of the Basilica of Vicenza was intended as an exact reference to Vitruvius, particularly in regard to the civic, representative aspect of the building. Nevertheless, in general one can concur with the opinion of Argan (1956): "For Palladio, the ancient forms are eternal forms, and the process by which they are created is a logical and grammatical process, rather than a result of the direct study of ancient monuments." Argan sees in this attitude an anticipation of 18th-century rationalism (see NEO-CLASSIC STYLES); this might explain both the vicissitudes of Palladio's reception by critics (Pevsner, 1956) and the particular success of his style in England, where the political and religious implications of classicism were less keenly felt.

*Baroque classicism in Italy and France.* It has already been remarked that the scope of classicism varied with each age; the list of ancient models was changeable, and so were the reasons for which they were revered. The 17th century also produced a form of classicism; but its distinctive flavor derived from the fact that it looked not only to antiquity for its models but to the official art of the 16th century as well. In reaction to the iconoclastic tendencies of the Reformation, the new age wished to emphasize, even in style, its intention of continuing the Renaissance. The imitation of Roman antiquity was now of secondary importance, compared with the exaltation and imitation of the Rome of Julius II and the Renaissance popes.

Seventeenth-century classicism was directed against two disparate artistic phenomena: on the one hand, mannerism — exuberant, excessive, and emotional — and, on the other, the naturalism of the Counter Reformation and of the school of Caravaggio, which seemed to imply a total rejection of tradition, even though in Caravaggio there is evidence of a knowledge and imitation of the 16th-century "classics" and of the ancients (H. Wagner, *Michelangelo da Caravaggio*, Bern, 1958). Baroque classicism was thus considerably less stringent than, for example, the classicism of the 15th century, where for Brunelleschi the repudiation of Gothic art dictated such features as the bareness of the walls, the use of calculated illumination, and the forthright statement of the pattern of load and support through a precise articulation in gray stone (*pietra serena*). There was, nevertheless, a return to compositional simplicity both in architectural plans and in historical paintings, where the role of caprice was reduced to a purely marginal and decorative one; a revival of bland naturalism was advocated in place of the distortions of fantasy and expressionism, and a return to decorum and order was proposed after a period of capricious individualism. Yet with all this, a certain dramatic and emotional element remained. To find a phrase which sums up the stylistic program of the period, we must turn to Bellori and to the theory attributed by him to Annibale Carracci of "bringing together and unifying both nature and the Idea, assimilating all the most praiseworthy qualities of past artists." This is a somewhat flexible formula and seems at first sight to include even the most exotic decoration, the stage settings, parks, fountains, and so forth — in short, all that is usually described as baroque, if not, indeed, rococo. In fact, however, for Bellori and his contemporaries the limits imposed on the "Idea" were very strict, for far from being considered as a sort of inner light, it was held to be the product of study and of culture in that it consisted of a selection from the beauties of nature. As for nature itself, this was identified, for all practical purposes, with the sensuous naturalism of Titian, the poetic scope of which is considerably narrower than that of the naturalism of Giorgione and his school. Even the concept of de-

corum, instead of conveying the sense of nobility of conception and execution, came to mean merely respect for tradition. It is thus perfectly legitimate to speak of the presence in baroque art of a current of classicism, which appeared in the decoration of the Gallery of the Farnese Palace (the most "classical" palace in Rome) by the Carracci and also in Guido Reni and in the later works of Guercino; it was supplemented by the theories of Bellori and the school of Maratta. With some important exceptions, this current dominated official taste of the 17th century and was most coherently embodied in the great architectural undertakings such as the completion of St. Peter's Square by Bernini (II, PLS. 133, 269), which, significantly, realized the plans of the Renaissance pope Nicholas V and represented the same theological concept — the universality of the Church. The impact of 17th-century classicism on architecture, the art form most closely connected to official circles, was indeed particularly marked. Disagreements in this field, such as that between Bernini and Borromini (qq.v.), were often violent, and the dislike for mannerism even led to serious and wild accusations against Michelangelo, whose architectural works were the only aspect of his art which had not already been discussed by critics of mannerism. According to Chantelou, Michelangelo had introduced "le libertinage dans l'architecture par une ambition de faire des choses nouvelles, et de n'imiter aucun de ceux qui l'ont précédé" ("license into architecture out of a desire for novelty, and to avoid imitating those who had gone before"). The greatest invention of the Counter Reformation, the large church designed for preaching, intended to serve as a vast meeting place in the city center, vaulted throughout and crowned by an impressive dome, with a monumental façade, usually of stone, was innately classical in spirit, especially when compared with the Protestant tendency toward the simplification of religious buildings and even, indeed, toward a revival of open-air preaching. This explains why, when dealing with this theme, architects and decorators, including even Bernini, tended to concentrate on the use of elements derived from Vitruvius. Another fundamentally classical theme of 17th-century architecture was the royal palace, which from ancient times had been invested with symbolic value and of which there existed some outstanding Renaissance examples, all conceived as virtually self-contained cities, such as the projects of Nicholas V and later of Bramante for the Vatican, the Ducal Palace of Urbino, and the projected development of Vigevano as a palace for Lodovico il Moro. Such examples as Bernini's unexecuted projects for the Louvre and those of Juvara and Sacchetti for the Royal Palace in Madrid clearly demonstrate that in the 17th century a classicizing style was thought suitable to this theme. In France the finest existing examples are undoubtedly the courtyard of the Invalides and the Hall of Mirrors in the Palace of Versailles (V, PL. 409), though other parts of the latter building are more related to the art of the 18th century.

One of the typical features of 17th-century classicism, whose not infrequent ambiguities sometimes lead it to express itself in ways not clearly distinguishable from the baroque, is the desire to effect a synthesis of reason and emotion differing from that of the Renaissance, in its greater emphasis on the role of the senses, a more subjective synthesis, a true merging of reason and feeling. In this sense the Wölfflinian theory of a clear-cut stylistic contrast between the two periods of art, in particular of the change from a static concept of form to one which was markedly dynamic, is valid. The 17th century restored to favor the rhetorical and didactic functions of art, while at the same time holding firmly to certain immutable theoretical principles of classicism.

Some remarks of Poussin, the artist who perhaps more than any other succeeded in reconciling a lively vein of sensualism with timeless lyrical vision, rich in Giorgionesque reminiscences, reveal to us the continuing vitality of some age-old ideas. Of the two ways in which to capture the attention of the spectator — by the use of the strange and the novel, on the one hand, and, on the other, by the observance of order — he considered the latter more consistent with his temperament: "Mon naturel me contraint de chercher et aimer les choses bien ordonnées, fuyant la confusion qui m'est aussi contraire et ennemie comme

est la lumière des obscures ténèbres" ("My natural inclinations lead me to seek out and revere things which are well-ordered, and to avoid confusion, which is as foreign and inimical to me as is light to dark shadow"). For Poussin style tended to be not a personal effusion, but the result of considered reflection: "la nouveauté, dans la peinture, ne consiste pas surtout dans un sujet non encore vu, mais dans la bonne et nouvelle disposition et expression; et de commun et vieux, le sujet devient original et neuf" ("novelty, in painting, does not consist in the treatment of a subject never before attempted, but in right and new ordering and expression; by this means, the subject, from being commonplace and familiar, becomes original and new"). Thus it is not enough merely to look at his pictures: they demand also meditation and contemplation ("le prospect"), which are rational activities. Even 17th-century landscape painting was built upon a rhetorical framework, while nevertheless remaining one of the most lyrical manifestations of the century, and by virtue of its literary associations, it always has an eschatological (and thus preromantic) significance.

*Rationalism from the 18th century to the present day.* It is not difficult to follow the disintegration of the 17th-century classical ideal in the triumph of color and touch over design and in the encroachment of ornament upon structure. Nevertheless, the decisive step came with the disappearance of the intrinsic content of the art of classicism. In the Western tradition classicism has always signified not only a formal equilibrium based on rational principles; it has also consistently appeared as the coherent expression of a universal order, to which man of his own will freely assents. For this reason we have not considered as classical the great buildings of the mannerist and baroque periods in France or the outstanding monuments of 18th-century rationalism, even if it is possible to find in them the use of a stylistic vocabulary derived from the most hallowed models or if, as especially in Italy, a classicizing current can be ascertained (for example, A. Galilei, N. Salvi, A. Pompei, etc.) or if some characteristic features, such as the dome, belong to the movement here considered. Even the Royal Palace of Caserta (I, PL. 389), which marked the height of 18th-century European rationalism, was preeminently functional and traditional in character, rather than symbolic; indeed, it can justly be regarded as one of the outstanding precursors of secular civic architecture of modern times. English Palladian architecture, too, was based above all on qualities of clarity and simplicity, with little or no symbolic intent; it is no coincidence that its buildings are all wonderfully proportioned to human needs.

The last attempt to reunite form and symbol within the framework of ancient traditions was made by the French Revolution, which clearly appreciated the didactic and edifying qualities of classicism and felt the need of using these aspects to promote the new republican government. These ideas coincided with and merged into the movement of neoclassicism (see NEOCLASSIC STYLES), which found expression at the end of the 18th century and the beginning of the 19th. Even more typical of that emotional restraint which is so integral a part of classicism are the images of Ingres, which, as it were, turn in on themselves at the precise moment or in the very situation when one would expect some emotional effusion.

With the 19th century, largely as a consequence of the attacks of the romantic movement, the peculiar synthesis of moral, religious, symbolic, and historical values that goes under the name of classicism ceased to exist, and in its place there remained merely empty academicism. With its disappearance a cultural cycle was brought to completion, a cycle whose importance in Western art is demonstrated by the crisis which has subsequently visited, and renewed, all the arts; this same crisis shows how far removed from us now are the ideals that once animated classicism. Attempts to revive classicism, confined in the main to governments of dictatorial or backward-looking tendencies, merely serve to emphasize how impossible it is to recapture these ideals.

Today, as the architect Henri van de Velde remarked at the beginning of the century, artists are seeking for a *morale*

*de raison*, not a tradition, and it is dangerous, indeed, to attempt to describe this search as a movement toward a new classical order as exemplified in the writings of M. Denis. We approach the poetry of classicism only when rationalism becomes a *mystique* of order, the expression of universal values, the visible manifestation of a cosmic principle, as in Le Corbusier and Mondrian; even then the result, within the context of a different society and a different civilization, is something utterly new.

Eugenio BATTISTI

BIBLIOG. *a. Antiquity.* For the bibliography of classicism in Greece, see also CLASSIC ART. H. Bulle, Archaisierende griechische Rundplastik, Munich, 1918; R. Delbrueck, Die Consulardiptychen und verwandte Denkmäler, Berlin, Leipzig, 1926–29; A. Merlin and L. Poinssot, Cratères et candélabres de marbre trouvés en mer près de Mahdia, Tunis, 1930; G. Becatti, Attikà, RIASA, VII, 1940, pp. 7–116; M. Squarciapino, La scuola di Afrodisia, Roma, 1943; P. E. Arias, Il piatto argenteo di Cesena, ASAtene, N.S., VIII–X, 1946–48, pp. 309–44; F. Cali, L'ordre grec: Essai sur le temple dorique, Grenoble, Paris, 1958. *b. Middle Ages and modern period.* The bibliography that follows lists only those works which have contributed directly or indirectly to the preparation of the foregoing article; for further information consult the bibliographies of HUMANISM; MANNERISM; PERSPECTIVE; PROPORTION; RENAISSANCE. Wölfflin, Renaissance und Barock, Munich, 1888 (2d ed., Munich, 1907); P. Lauer, Le Palais de Latran, Paris, 1911; A. Goldschmidt, Die Elfenbeinskulpturen aus Zeit der karolingischen und sächsischen Kaiser: VIII. bis XI. Jahrhundert, 4 vols., Berlin, 1914–34; W. Friedländer, Nicolas Poussin: Die Entwicklung seiner Kunst, Munich, 1914; H. Wölfflin, Kunstgeschichtliche Grundbegriffe: Das Problem der Stilentwickelung in der neueren Kunst, Munich, 1915 (Am. ed., trans. M. D. Hottinger, Principles of Art History, New York, 1949); G. Dehio, Geschichte der deutschen Kunst, 4 vols., Berlin, Leipzig, 1919–34; L. Planiscig, Venezianische Bildhauer der Renaissance, Vienna, 1921; J. Mesnil, Les résistances septentrionales à la conception plastique de l'espace due à la Renaissance, Atti del X Congresso del Rinascimento, 1923; P. Valéry, Eupalinos, Paris, 1923 (Eng. trans., London, 1932); E. Kaufmann, Die Architekturtheorie der französischen Klassik und der Klassizismus, RepfKw, XLIV, 1924, pp. 197–237; E. Panofsky, Idea: Ein Beitrag zur Begriffsgeschichte der älteren Kunsttheorie, Leipzig, Berlin, 1924; M. Dvořák, Kunstgeschichte als Geistesgeschichte, Munich, 1924; J. von Schlosser, Präludien, Berlin, 1927; H. Haskins, Renaissance of the Twelfth Century, Cambridge, Mass., 1927 (2d ed., New York, 1957); W. Worringer, Griechentum und Gotik: Vom Weltreich des Hellenismus, Munich, 1928; Das Problem des Klassischen und die Antike, ed. W. Jäger, Leipzig, Berlin, 1931; A. Warburg, Die Erneuerung der heidnischen Antike (Gesammelte Schriften, I and II), Leipzig, Berlin, 1932; K. M. Svoboda, L'esthétique de St. Augustin et ses sources, Brno, 1933; H. Wölfflin, Kunstgeschichtliche Grundbegriffe: Eine Revision, Logos, XXII, 1933, pp. 210–18; F. Behn, Die karolingische Klosterkirche von Lorsch, Berlin, Leipzig, 1934; E. Garger, Zur spätantiken Renaissance, JhbKhSammlWien, N.S., VIII, 1934, pp. 1–28; R. Hinks, Carolingian Art, London, 1935; W. Weisbach, Die klassische Ideologie, Deutsche Vierteljahrschrift für Geschichte, 1935, pp. 359–91; W. Pinder, Die Kunst der deutschen Kaiserzeit, Leipzig, 1935; P. Clemen and F. Baumgart, Italienische Kunst, Berlin, Zurich, 1936; A. Blunt, Poussin's Note on Painting, Warburg, 1937, pp. 344–51; T. Hetzer, Vom Plastischen in der Malerei, Festschrift Wilhelm Pinder zum sechzigsten Geburtstage, Leipzig, 1938, pp. 28–64; J. Hubert, L'art pré-roman, Paris, 1938; J. Adhémar, Influences antiques dans l'art du Moyen-Age français, London, 1939; G. Weise, Die geistige Welt der Gotik und ihre Bedeutung für Italien, Halle-an-der-Saale, 1939; K. Bauch, Klassik, Klassizität, Klassizismus: Die Kunst der Künstler, 1939–40, pp. 429–40; F. Franco, Classicismo e funzionalità della Villa Palladiana, Atti del I Convegno di storia dell'architettura, 1940; N. Pevsner, Academies of Art, Past and Present, Cambridge, England, 1940; H. Wölfflin, Schönhet des Klassischen: Gedanken zur Kunstgeschichte, Basel, 1941, pp. 28–48; G. Nicco Fasola, Nicola Pisano, Rome, 1941; U. Spirito, La vita come arte, Florence, 1941; R. Krautheimer, The Carolingian Revival of Early Christian Architecture, AB, XXIV, 1942, pp. 1–38; H. Peyre, Qu'est-ce que le Classicisme, Paris, 1942; P. Lavedan, L'architecture française, Paris, 1944 (Eng. ed. Harmondsworth, 1956); Concinnitas: Beiträge zum Problem des Klassischen, Heinrich Wölfflin zum achtzigsten Geburtstag, am 21 Juni gueignet, Basel, 1944; E. D'Ors, Del Barocco, Milan, 1945; E. De Bruyne, Etudes d'esthétique médiévale, Bruges, 1946; W. Deonna, Primitivisme et Classicisme: Les deux faces de l'histoire de l'art, Recherche, II, 1946, pp. 5–24; P. Brezzi, Roma e l'impero medioevale, Bologna, 1947; A. Viscardi, Classicismo, Movimenti spirituali, Dizionario letterario Bompiani delle opere e dei personaggi, I, Milan, 1947; H. Jantzen, Ottonische Kunst, Munich, 1947; D. Mahon, Studies in Seicento Art and Theory, London, 1947; M. Petrocchi, Razionalismo architettonico e razionalismo storiografico: Due studi sul Settecento italiano, Rome, 1947; E. R. Curtius, Europäische Literatur und lateinisches Mittelalter, Bern, 1948 (Eng. trans., London, 1953); H. Fichtenau, Das karolingische Imperium: Soziale und geistige Problematik eines Grossreiches, Zurich, 1949; F. Gerke, Die Königshalle in Lorsch und der frühkarolingische Monumentalstil in Kultur und Wirtschaft im reinischen Raum, Mainz, 1949, pp. 131–36; J. Gantner, Schönheit und Grenzen der klassischen Form: Burckhardt, Croce, Wölfflin, Vienna, 1949; G. Nicco Fasola, Ragionamenti sull'architettura, Città di Castello, 1949; R. H. L. Hamann-MacLean, Antikenstudium in der Kunst des Mittelalters (with extensive bibliog.), Marburger Jhb. für Kunstwissenschaft, 1949–50, pp. 157–250; R. Folz, Le souvenir et la légende de Charlemagne dans l'Empire germanique médiéval, Paris, 1950; W. Paeseler, Der Rückgriff der römischen Spätdugentomalerei auf die christliche Spätantike, Beiträge zur Kunst des Mittelalters, Berlin, 1950,

pp. 157–70; G. Becatti, Arte e gusto negli scrittori latini, Florence, 1951; G. Bandmann, Mittelalterliche Architektur als Bedeutungsträger, Berlin, 1951; K. Erdmann, Forschungen zur politischen Ideenwelt des Frühmittelalters, Berlin, 1951; R. Folz, Etudes sur le culte liturgique de Charlemagne dans les églises de l'Empire, Paris, 1951; H. Fichtenau, Byzanz und die Pfalz zu Aachen, Mitteilungen des Instituts für österreichische Geschichtsforschung, LIX, 1951, pp. 1–54; P. E. Schramm, Die Anerkennung Karls des Grossen als Kaiser: Ein Kapitel aus der Geschichte der mittelalterlichen "Staatssymbolik," Historische Z., CLXXII, 1951, pp. 449–515; O. H. Förster, Grundformen der deutschen Kunst, Cologne, 1952; W. F. Volbach, Elfenbeinarbeiten der Spätantike und des frühen Mittelalters, 2d ed., Mainz, 1952; R. Wittkower, Architectural Principles in the Age of Humanism, 2d ed., London, 1952; H. Eiden, Die spätrömische Kaiserresidenz Trier im Lichte neuer Ausgrabungen, Trier, 1952, pp. 7–26; H. Wentzel, Der Augustalis Friedrichs II. und die abendländische Glyptik des 13. Jahrhunderts, ZfKg, XV, 1952, pp. 183–87; J. Summerson, Architecture in Britain, 1530–1830, Harmondsworth, 1953; G. Galassi, Roma e Bisanzio, 2 vols., Rome, 1953; Humanismus, Mystik und Kunst in der Welt des Mittelalters, ed. J. Koch, Leiden, Cologne, 1953; L. Anceschi, Del Barocco e altre prove, Florence, 1954; H. Swarzenski, Monuments of Romanesque Art: The Art of the Church Treasures in Northwestern Europe, Chicago, 1954; E. Ewig, Trier im Merowingenreich, Civitas, Stadt, Bistum, Trier, 1954; Atti del V Convegno internazionale di lingue e letterature moderne (1951), Florence, 1955, pp. 165–229; G. C. Argan, Brunelleschi, Milan, 1955; D. Mahon and D. Sutton, Artists in 17th Century Rome (Catalogue of loan exhibition organized by Wildenstein and Co., Ltd.), 2d ed., London, 1955; Retorica e Barocco, Atti del III Congresso internazionale di studi umanistici, Rome, 1955; G. Francastel, Du Byzantin à la Renaissance (Histoire de la peinture italienne, ed. P. Francastel, I), Paris, 1955; P. Pirri, Giovanni Tristano e i primordi della architettura gesuitica, Rome, 1955; O. Demus, Oriente e occidente nell'arte veneta del Duecento: La civiltà veneziana del secolo di Marco Polo, Florence, 1955, pp. 109–26; E. Kaufmann, Architecture in the Age of Reason, Cambridge, Mass., 1955; F. W. Sypher, Four Stages of Renaissance Style: Transformations in Art and Literature, 1400–1700, New York, 1955; O. Demus, A Renascence of Early Christian Art in Thirteenth Century Venice, Late Classical and Mediaeval Studies in Honor of A. M. Friend, Jr., Princeton, 1955, pp. 348–61; A. Rumpf, Stilphasen der spätantiken Kunst, Cologne, Opladen, 1955; J. von Schlosser, La letteratura artistica (Die Kunstliteratur), ed. it. aggiornata da Otto Kurz, 2d ed., Florence, 1956; N. Pevsner, Palladio and Europe, Venezia e l'Europa, Atti del XVIII Congresso internazionale di storia dell'arte (1955), Venice, 1956, pp. 81–94; F. Kimball, "Classicism," Academicism, and Creation in XVIIth Century French Architecture, Scritti di storia dell'arte in onore di Lionello Venturi, II, Rome, 1956, pp.19–23; H. Keutner, Über die Entstehung und die Formen des Standbildes im Cinquecento, Münchener Jhb. der bildenden Kunst, VII, 1956, pp. 138–68; E. B. Smith, Architectural Symbolism of Imperial Rome and the Middle Ages, Princeton, 1956; W. R. Valentiner, The Bamberg Rider: Studies of Medieval German Sculpture, Los Angeles, 1956; E. Battisti, Il concetto d'imitazione nel Cinquecento da Raffaello a Michelangelo, Commentari, VII, 1956, pp. 86–104; V. Elbern, Werdendes Abendland an Rhein und Ruhr (Catalogue of exhibition in Villa Hügel, Essen), Essen, 1956; L'Italia e il mondo gotico, Florence, 1956; G. C. Argan, Borromini, Milan, 1956; Il Seicento europeo: realismo, classicismo, barocco (exhibition catalogue), Rome, 1956; G. C. Argan, L'architettura barocca in Italia, Milan 1957; E. Battisti, Postille al Seicento, Letteratura, V, 25, 26, 1957; K. M. Svoboda, Palazzi antichi e medievali, B. del Centro di studi per la storia dell'architettura, XI, 1957, pp. 3–32; V. L. Tapié, Baroque et Classicisme, Paris, 1957; J. Delumeau, Vie économique et sociale de Rome dans la seconde moitié du XVIᵉ siècle, I, Paris, 1957; A. M. Vogt, Grünewald: Mathis Gothart Nithart, Meister Gegenklassischer Malerei, Zurich, 1957; F. Zeri, Pittura e Controriforma: L'arte senza tempo di Scipione da Gaeta, Turin, 1957; F. Calasso, I glossatori e la teoria della sovranità, 3d ed., Milan, 1957, p. 146; E. Przywara, Schön, Sakral, Christlich, La filosofia dell'arte sacra, Padua, 1957, pp. 11–42; E. Battisti, Simbolo e Classicismo, Umanesimo e simbolismo, Atti del IV Convegno internazionale di studi umanistici, Padua, 1958, pp. 215–33; W. F. Volbach and M. Hirmer, Arte paleocristiana, Florence, 1958; W. Sauerländer, Les modèles de la Renaissance macédonienne dans la sculpture de Paris et d'Amiens au début du XIIIᵉ siècle, Résumés des communications, XIXᵉ Congrès international d'histoire de l'art, Paris, 1958, pp. 30–32; R. Wittkower, Art and Architecture in Italy, 1600–1750, Harmondsworth, 1958; L'Art et l'homme, ed. R. Huyghe, II, Paris, 1958; F. Ulivi, L'imitazione nella letteratura del Rinascimento, Milan, 1959.

Eugenio BATTISTI

Illustrations: PLS. 385–392.

## CLOCKS. See TIMEPIECES.

## CLODION. 
French sculptor, real name Claude Michel (b. Nancy, 1738; d. Paris, 1814). Both parents descended from families of sculptors. Clodion became a student of his uncle, Lambert Sigisbert Adam (whose style Gallicized the Berninian baroque into a lighter rococo), and a student of Jean-Baptiste Pigalle, the leading mid-century rococo sculptor. In 1759 he won the Grand Prix de Sculpture at the Académie Royale, and in 1762 went to Rome, where he remained until 1771.

He was accepted by the Académie Royale in 1773. Clodion sent to the Salon both conventional academic subjects, such as *Jupiter Fulminator*, and his more characteristic erotic statuettes of nymphs, fauns, bacchants (V, PL. 418), and cherubs. Comparing his little *Nymph and Satyr* group in the Metropolitan Museum, New York, with its prototype, Bernini's *Apollo and Daphne* (see II, PL. 272; Gall. Borghese), it is apparent that Clodion's works present no essential innovations but are rather the baroque distilled to its ultimate refinement.

The spontaneity of his modeling is captured in terra cotta, a favorite medium for these intimate little works; his surfaces seem more alive than any others in sculpture. Clodion's terracotta sculptures also radiate the hedonism, elegance, and exhilaration of the 18th century — qualities that seem the more intensified for the small scale into which they have been compressed. The medium also permitted such effortlessly prolific production that the modern scholar has unfortunately neglected these superb but almost innumerable table pieces. The few more ambitious state commissions by Clodion disclose an equal talent for monumental sculpture. In 1774 he began the marble *St. Cecilia* for the Cathedral of Rouen, for which he later made a bronze *Crucified Christ*. In 1779 he received a royal order for the large and brilliant marble statue of the seated *Montesquieu* in the Institut, Paris. After the rejection of an early nude version of the writer, Clodion finally draped him in imposing judicial robes. The lively informality of the pose — legs crossed and alert head turned — avoids the pomposity of the baroque tradition; a tradition that inspired, however, the effortless depiction of fur and fabric, complexity of the hair, cuffs, and robe border, pictorialism in the unbuttoned garment, the fringe, the broken quill, and the book binding. The statue is at once the epitome of the witty Parisian and the probing philosopher of the Enlightenment.

Clodion's model for an unbuilt memorial to a balloon ascension (1784; Met. Mus.) anachronistically eulogizes aeronautics in a style that now seems part of the remote past; swarms of *putti* such as Bernini had used to accompany religious miracles cluster about a technological miracle of science. After the French Revolution Clodion's playful *bibelots* seemed outrageous reminders of the mundane old regime. He then adopted the neoclassic style of Canova in a doleful group of the *Deluge* (1800) and in 1806 undertook reliefs for the neoclassic Colonne Vendôme and the Arc du Carrousel. See also FRENCH ART; ROCOCO.

BIBLIOG. H. Thirion, Les Adam et Clodion, Paris, 1885; H. Stein, ThB, VII, 1912.

James HOLDERBAUM

## CLOUET, JEAN and FRANÇOIS. 
Jean Clouet (known also as Janet or Jehannet) was a French painter at the court of Francis I (b. ca. 1485, according to some; d. Paris, ca. 1540). Although his birthplace is unknown, it was probably in the southern Netherlands, where the surname Clouet is common. The artist was first officially mentioned in 1516 as one of the chief painters to Francis I. However, he arrived in France before the death of Louis XII (1515), Francis' predecessor, and probably worked for Louis. Jean Clouet eventually became Francis' chief painter, with the title of Painter and Valet of the King's Bedchamber, an office that secured for him a high salary and social position. He worked in both Tours and Paris, but was never naturalized as a French citizen. Jean and his brother Pollet, a painter at the court of Navarre, were probably sons of the painter Michel Clouet, who worked in Valenciennes; very likely Jean received his earliest training from his father.

Although Jean Clouet found the tradition of the crayon portrait already established in France, he carried it to such a high point of characterization and finish that this genre became one of the dominant productions of French art. The panel portrait, as perfected in Italy during the Renaissance, also impressed him; we find in his panels certain similarities to Holbein portraits as well. No signed paintings or drawings by Jean Clouet have been preserved, but a credible body of his work has been assembled. It includes about one hundred and thirty excellent drawings of men and women of the court, most of

which are preserved at Chantilly. According to the inscriptions, the drawings were all executed during the years when Jean was chief painter to Francis I. One of them is a study for a panel portrait of Guillaume Budé (New York, Met. Mus.), which, according to a document dating from the lifetime of the painter, is certified to be his work. There are also six or seven other oil paintings and nine miniatures, including one of Charles de Cossé (New York, Met. Mus.), and eight small round portraits of Francis I and the seven heroes who fought at the battle of Melegnano, Lombardy (Paris, Bib. Nat.; London, Br. Mus.). Apparently the portrait drawings by Clouet and his followers were sketched rapidly from life and then used as a basis for the painted panels. The drawings show liveliness and observation, modified by a reticence and stylization, which made them peculiarly acceptable to the French society for which they were produced. Clouet's solution to the problems of portraiture has proved satisfactory for French painters through the centuries, down to Ingres and Degas.

François Clouet (known also as Janet; b. Tours; d. 1572) was successor to his father, Jean, at the court of Francis I. Active by 1536, François was probably trained by his celebrated parent, and most likely began his career as a member of Jean's very productive shop. On his father's death François succeeded to the title of Painter and Valet of the King's Bedchamber, serving Francis I and subsequently Henry II, Francis II, and Charles IX. François painted mythological subjects as well as portraits (V, PL. 403) and directed a large workshop that was typically Renaissance in character. The workshop produced not only drawings and oil paintings but also miniatures, designs for enamels, and plans for projects depicting the triumphal entries of royalty. See also FRENCH ART.

BIBLIOG. L. Dimier, French Painting in the Sixteenth Century, London, New York, 1904, pp. 22-49; ThB, VII, 1912, pp. 117-20; E. Moreau-Nélaton, Les Clouet and leurs émules, 3 vols., Paris, 1924; C. Sterling, A Catalogue of French Paintings XV-XVIII Centuries, Cambridge, Mass., 1955, pp. 26-30, 53-58.

Margaretta M. SALINGER

COELLO, CLAUDIO. Spanish painter of the Madrid school (b. Madrid, 1642; d. Madrid, Apr. 20, 1693). Coello was apprenticed by his father, a Portuguese bronzeworker, to the painter Francisco Ricci to learn metal chasing. Instead he became a painter and appears to have studied abroad in Italy. He collaborated with Ricci and was permitted by his friend Carreño to copy paintings in the royal collection. With José Jiménez Donoso, from whom he learned fresco, Coello carried out many decorative commissions in Madrid. He painted frescoes in Toledo and Saragossa, was named *pintor del rey* (ca. 1685), *pintor de cámera* (1686), and painter of the Cathedral of Toledo (1691). However, in 1689 he lost a competition to José de Churriguera, and it has been said that when the Neapolitan Luca Giordano was invited by the King to decorate the Escorial, Coello's rage brought on his death. Actually it now appears that Coello died less dramatically from a chronic respiratory illness.

MAJOR WORKS. *Annunciation* and other retables (Madrid, S. Plácido, 1668). - Cathedral vestry ceiling (with Donoso; Toledo, 1671). - *Triumph of St. Augustine* (Madrid, Prado, 1664). - Two Sacred Conversations (Madrid, Prado, 1669). - *S. Rosa de Lima* (Madrid, Prado, ca. 1683). - *S. Domingo de Guzmán* (Madrid, Prado, ca. 1683). - Frescoes (with assistants; Saragossa, Church of the Mantería, 1683-84). - *La Sagrada Forma* (Escorial, sacristy, 1685-90). - *Martyrdom of St. Stephen* (Salamanca, S. Esteban, 1692-93).

Outstanding Spanish painter of the late 17th century, Coello was the last of the peninsula's long line of great masters. Although the influence of Velázquez and others of Coello's predecessors can be detected, Coello derives largely from the Italian school, which he seems to have known firsthand as well as through his master Ricci and his later collaborators. He painted competently and richly a great many decorative commissions — on canvas and in fresco, both religious and secular subjects — obtained through his eminence in the court circles

of Madrid. Most famous was *La Sagrada Forma*, a large painting in the sacristy of the Escorial depicting the ceremonial installation (1684) in the sacristy of a sacramental wafer that had survived desecration by the Zwinglianists earlier in the Low Countries. Charles II, the artist, and many court notables are depicted with exceeding care by Coello, who spent five years in preparatory studies for this Velázquen composition (II, PL. 191). It seemed clear already to his contemporaries that Coello's position was seriously threatened with the invasion of Spanish painting by Giordano in 1692, an event which we can now see marked symbolically the end of Spain's golden age in painting. See also BAROQUE ART; SPANISH AND PORTUGUESE ART.

BIBLIOG. A. Palomino de Castro y Velasco, El museo pictórico y escala óptica, Madrid, III, 1724, Vida, CLXXVI, Madrid, 1947, pp. 1058-65; J. A. Gaya Nuño, Claudio Coello, Madrid, 1957.

George R. COLLINS

COINS AND MEDALS. Coins and medals constitute a special category of art objects which may be singled out from the kindred arts of metalwork (q.v.) and sculpture (q.v.) in general. In addition to their obvious paralles in size, shape, media, and techniques of production, they have in common a long history of evolution, distribution, and officially imposed iconography and style. In their commemorative purpose and in their expression of the esthetic aims of notable engravers, coins and, to an even greater extent, medals are often closely allied to the sculpture of their times. On the other hand, a distant lag behind other contemporaneous art forms has frequently existed because of the traditionalism of monetary types.

In iconography, the necessity for presenting within the limits of space and shape a variety of allusions to institutions, ideas, and political and religious events and concerns has, from their very beginning, produced on coins and medals a wealth of emblems (see EMBLEMS AND INSIGNIA) and symbols (see SYMBOLISM AND ALLEGORY). A characteristic and recurrent theme is that of the head of a ruler or other revered personage, idealized or more or less faithfully portrayed (see PORTRAITURE). The motifs on coins and medals over the centuries afford an excellent study of the conflict and exchange between literal representation and abstract symbolism.

SUMMARY. Introduction (col. 700): *Early mediums of exchange and the diffusion of coins; Techniques of reproduction; Signatures; Medals; Iconography and artistic problems; Artistic development.* The ancient world (col. 707): *Origin and diffusion of coins in the classical world; Greek monetary types; Roman monetary types; Coins in peripheral classical cultures.* Oriental coins (col. 714): *Bactria; Persis; Characene; The Parthians; The Sassanians; Indo-Greek coins; The Kushans; The Guptas; The Mongols; The Moghuls; Arab coins; The Turkoman dynasties; The Far East.* Medieval coins (col. 723): *Barbarian states (5th-7th cent.); Coins of the Carolingian period; Post-Carolingian Europe: a. Italy; b. France; c. Germany, Bohemia, and Hungary; d. England; e. Spain; Byzantine coins.* European coinage from the Renaissance onward (col. 732). Primitive societies (col. 736): *Africa; Oceania; Asia; America.* Medals (col. 739).

INTRODUCTION. *Early mediums of exchange and the diffusion of coins.* Leaving aside the oldest phases of barter and the use of cattle as a medium of exchange (of which late traces can be found in Greece as well as in Rome), we note the adoption of metal utensils for trading and, in a more advanced phase, of pieces of metal of fixed weight. Weighed metal directly preceded the introduction of coins and is an advance from the economic point of view, because of its greater practicality and adaptability. However, the use of metal instruments and the use of weighed metal do not always represent successive phases: they often occur simultaneously. Both mediums are mentioned in the Homeric poems, which give us a picture of the various premonetary mediums of barter, including cattle. In the *Iliad* and the *Odyssey* tripods, axes, and kettles often serve as gifts and prizes in such a manner as to represent a true measurement of value (*Iliad*, IX, 121, 123; XXIII, 264, 267, 702, 885). Gold and silver, too, as well as other metals appear as means of

exchange, either in the form of wrought objects or as weighed pieces (*Iliad*, VI, 48; VII, 472; IX, 128; X, 379; XXIII, 269). These primitive forms of currency are documented also outside the Homeric poems. Pausanias (X, 14, 1) mentions having seen in the Temple of Apollo at Delphi some double axes offered according to tradition by a king of Tenedos at the time of the Trojan War. In the Peloponnesos iron spits were the usual medium of exchange before the introduction of silver coinage by Pheidon of Argos; after having deprived them of their monetary character, he dedicated them to the Temple of Hera (Heraion) in Argos.

The forms that prevailed in the metal-object and weighed-metal phases are numerous and vary sometimes according to the nature of the metal. They are documented not only by literary sources but also by archaeological finds. Copper ingots of various weights but similar in form (double axes) were found at Salamis on Cyprus, at Hagia Triada (Crete), at Mycenae, at Attaleia (Pamphylia), at Kyme (Euboea), at Serra Ilixi (Sardinia; PL. 416). Egyptian paintings of the time of Thutmosis III show tribute scenes with Ethiopians and Hebrews carrying some of these ingots; other paintings of the same period show rings being weighed on a scale. Gold rings of various weights were found on Cyprus and at Mycenae and Aegina. In Ireland and Scandinavia the use of rings for exchange purposes lasted until the Middle Ages. Iron spits were found in Argos at the excavations of the Temple of Hera and in a tomb of the 8th century B.C. (*BCH*, 1957, p. 368 ff.); the objects found in a Geometric tomb at Fortetsa near Knossos (J. K. Block, *Fortetsa*, Cambridge, England, 1957, p. 202) are probably spits. The *taleae ferreae* used by the Britons for exchange together with copper and gold coins were probably small iron bars (cf. Caesar, *De Bello Gallico*, V, 12), of which examples have been found (cf. C. Fox, *A Find of the Early Iron Age from Llyn Cerrig Bach, Anglesey*, Cardiff, 1946). Copper bars going back to the beginning of the 3d millennium B.C. have been found at Mohenjo-daro in Pakistan. Gold nuggets and various gold objects were found at Troy, on Cyprus, and at Mycenae. Their use as coins is proved by their presence in the inventories of temples; tributes to the Great King, too, were often paid in pieces of gold (Herodotus, III, 94). Gold was used also in the form of jewelry (earrings, buttons, pins, links of necklaces, etc.); a large number of objects of gold and silver (mostly not intended for use), many of them very similar to those found at Troy, were discovered at Poliochnion Lemnos (*FA*, XI, 2122). Silver bars found at Troy were used even after the introduction of coins. Whole ingots or fragments of them, together with Greek silver coins, were found in Egypt, at Tarentum, and in Spain, where the use of silver as a medium of exchange is mentioned by Strabo (III, 155).

In time precious metals were cut into lozenges or pellets according to a predetermined scale of weight to make exchange easier. They were often signed by merchants or bankers with rough stampings or simple striations as though to guarantee their weight and alloy. When with the growth of trade or as a result of special political circumstances the state undertook this guarantee directly by putting its emblem on the small round pieces of metal and monopolizing the issues, the true coin in the modern sense of the word was born. A period of weighed metal preceding the introduction of coins is documented also in Italy. Rather than gold or silver, copper was used in unformed pieces (*aes rude*, diffused above all in central Italy and in Emilia) or in cast ingots with a rough imprint on their long sides (*aes signatum*; PL. 401).

The connections between the forms of premonetary mediums of exchange and the typology of coins are uncertain. The fact that the objects represented on some coins were used for exchange in premonetary phases (e.g., the double ax on the coins of Tenedos) does not seem to justify the assumption of a relationship between the typology of coins and these objects.

Coins are distinguished by three essential elements: metal, type, and weight, according to the old definition given by Isidore of Seville; if one of these elements is lacking, adds Isidore, there will be no coin ("in nomismate tria quaerentur:

metallum, figura et pondus. Si ex his aliquid defuerit nomisma non erit," *Etymologies*, XVI, 18, 12). His definition shows that the concept of the coin was well understood in antiquity.

The type, the element with which we are most concerned, is a relief (or more rarely concave) representation of a human figure, an animal, an object, or simply an inscription (in this last instance type and legend are one). One should distinguish between type and symbol; the latter sometimes appears on the field of the coin as an adjunct to the type itself, often serving to identify a mint or a magistrate or simply to distinguish one issue from another.

The characteristics of a coin depend on the system of weights and measures used in a given area at the moment of its issue and reflect political and economic conditions in the issuing state. The adoption of a definite system or the substitution of one for another is determined by the political and commercial relations of the state and its position within certain spheres of influence. At the present stage of research it is difficult to trace with certainty the regions from which the various systems of weights and measures originated, even though it may be stated with a certain degree of probability that they came from the Near East. At the point in history when coins first appeared the systems of weights and measures that were to dominate Greek coins were already established. These are the Phoenician system, that of Aegina, that of Euboea (more widely diffused than any other when it was adopted by Athens), and that of Persia or Asia Minor. In Italy there existed, besides systems adopted from the Greek colonies, local ones related to those of the Greeks; their unit of weight was the pound rather than the talent and the mina of the Greeks. The system adopted by Rome was used in the Middle Ages, surviving in the Carolingian libra, or pound.

The type of the coin is the issuing state's guarantee of its value; without this guarantee the metallic medium of exchange cannot be called a coin in the true sense of the word. Since the type was originally the imprint of the state issuing and guaranteeing the coin, it very often identifies the mint and also the period of issue, especially in ancient times.

From the first, the type has always reflected the ruling political, historical, and religious ideas in the issuing state. There are essentially religious types with figures of divinities, cult statues, or religious symbols, accompanied sometimes by inscriptions referring to the cult; such types occur not only in antiquity but also in the Middle Ages and in modern times (cf. the large number of inscriptions from the Old and the New Testament). Under religious influence the type may change entirely, as in Hebrew coins, which avoid representing the human figure, or in Islamic ones, which, with the exception of the first issues, show only inscriptions. Close to these types are those with a commemorative or political-propaganda purpose celebrating historical or contemporary personages or events. In antiquity the most significant examples are the Roman coins. The portrait on coins serves mainly a political purpose, affirming a valid and jealously defended sovereignty. The first portraits of sovereigns appear in the Hellenistic period, and in monarchies they survive to the present day. Connections with emblems can be observed in antiquity, on types identifiable with the symbol of the issuing city, and, more clearly, in the Middle Ages and in modern times, on coins bearing the coat of arms of cities (e.g., the lily on the coins of Florence), of families (e.g., the snake, *biscione*, on the Visconti coins), or popes, of independent city-states, or, most frequently in modern times, of a country (see EMBLEMS AND INSIGNIA).

The diffusion of a coin type from its place of origin into distant lands of differing cultures is a characteristic phenomenon of antiquity and the Middle Ages. A distinction ought to be made here between the diffusion of a type copied because it was popular or because the currency of the place in which it originated enjoyed international credit (e.g., the staters of Corinth and in medieval and modern times the florin of Florence, the ducat of Venice, and others) and imitation of coins among economically backward peoples without a currency of their own. The latter often led to complete deformation of a coin, making it impossible to recognize the original model, as happened when

COINS AND MEDALS

Athenian coins were imitated in southern Arabia and India and when Greek coins, especially those of Philip II and Alexander the Great, were imitated among Celtic peoples. Imitation may also lead to the adaptation of the original types to the iconography of the adopting peoples, as in Indian imitations of the Venetian ducat, in which the characteristic figures of the Redeemer, St. Mark, and the doges were transformed into Orientals. A type may also be imitated because of its artistic beauty; for example, the head of Arethusa surrounded by dolphins on the tetradrachma of Syracuse was imitated on Siculo-Punic coins.

In the diffusion of coins commercial relations obviously play an important role; they sometimes bring the coins to regions very distant from the mint of issue (Roman coins, for example, are found in India; Byzantine and Islamic ones in Scandinavia). This process does not always lead to direct imitation, but it often contributes to the knowledge in one region of pictorial representations in another with a completely different civilization, as is true for the Celtic coins mentioned above.

Sometimes several states adopt the same coin emblem to commemorate commercial or political unions. Such an agreement can be compared to that on the issue of postage stamps on the same theme by various states in our time. In fact, the propaganda once carried by the coin is now carried, though to a lesser degree, by the stamp (see GRAPHIC ARTS).

*Techniques of production.* Two ways of making coins are known from antiquity: casting and striking. The former was used only rarely in antiquity — in the first series of Roman bronze coins, in some Italic and Etruscan series (*aes grave*), and sporadically in the late Roman Empire — but it came into favor in 15th-century Italy with the development of the medal. The metal is run between two negative casting forms bearing the representation of the obverse and the reverse. The flan and the impression are thus achieved by one operation.

The ancient and more widespread system of striking coins demanded two dies — one fixed, the "anvil" die, the other movable, the "hammer" die — on which were hollowed out the representations that the blow given to the upper die impressed on the prepared flan. This system remained in use until the middle of the 16th century, when the invention of the weighted lever began the process of mechanization, which culminated in the 19th century with the adoption of the money press. It is a much discussed problem whether the ancient coiner prepared a model larger than the coin, which was then copied in a reduced scale on the die. In contrast to the modern artist, who, since incising is mechanized, only prepares a sketch, the ancient artist cut his own model on the die. From a technical viewpoint there is some similarity between the preparation of dies and working in hard stones; the materials are equally hard and require the same working instruments. It can therefore be supposed, even if there is no proof for it, that some of the great die cutters were also carvers of gems. From classical antiquity we know of only one gem carver whose name was also that of a die cutter: Phrygillos, whose identity, however, is not certain. The same type of Herakles strangling the lion depicted on gold coins of Syracuse and signed by Kimon and Euinetos is also found on an unfortunately anonymous gem of about 400 B.C. (PL. 384).

Some technical specialities should be mentioned here: the so-called "incuse square" used in archaic Greek series, made by one or more impressions of various forms (square and rectangular predominating); the incuse reverse, typical of the coins of Magna Graecia and Zankle, in which the hollow representation on the reverse is produced by another die; the blank reverse, typical of some Cypriote issues and Etruscan coins generally; bracteates, very thin coins, typical products of the medieval German mints, bearing a relief representation on only one side; the so-called *nummi scyphati*, or concave coins, issued by the Byzantine emperors from the 11th century onward; "plated" coins, with a core of base metal thinly covered with precious metal.

The various technical procedures used in the production of coins have influenced numismatic art. Casting generally produces much greater relief than striking; yet the Greek and Roman coins made by striking show noteworthy relief. In the Middle Ages the impoverishment of technical resources and the use of very thin flans almost entirely obliterated gradation of plane; the augustals of Emperor Frederick II are among the few exceptions. Relief in the Renaissance was also generally low and remained so even after the introduction of mechanization. Figures are more sharply outlined and detach themselves from the smooth background far more clearly in struck than in cast coins. The limited area provided by the coin is also of artistic consequence. Restricted space, as well as technical factors, precludes a strongly accented relief. Many details employed in heads or isolated figures are treated summarily or only suggested in groups or more complex scenes. Medals, not being bound by monetary laws to a given diameter and thickness, allow the artist greater liberty.

Photographic enlargements are of great assistance in the study of coins. They show such details as signatures of engravers often not visible to the naked eye. Photographic and other enlargements are also very useful for the discovery and study of forgeries, because they make it possible to distinguish technical and stylistic details often not perceived in any other way (see FALSIFICATION AND FORGERY).

*Signatures.* Only a few names of ancient engravers working solely on coins are known from Greek times; they occur above all in Sicily and in Magna Graecia in the short period from the middle of the 5th to the middle of the 4th century B. C. Yet we must assume from examination of the coins that outstanding artistic personalities existed before this time, sometimes not inferior to those signing coins in the following period (e.g., the demarateion of Syracuse, the unique tetradrachma of Aitnai, the tetradrachma of Naxos, etc.). Other names of engravers known only through coins are found on coins of Elis, Arcadia, Crete, and Klazomenai. Sometimes the engravers were active in several mints; Euainetos, for example, was active at Syracuse, Catana, and Camarina. Sometimes two engravers collaborated on the same coin (in Syracuse Eumenes worked together with Eukleidas, Euainetos, and Euth [. . .]; the last also collaborated with Phrygillos). The artists generally signed only their names, sometimes abbreviating them. Names of engravers do not appear on coins of the Middle Ages; it is doubtful whether the "Luteger made me" (*Luteger me fecit*) on the bracteates of Thuringia (ca. 1175) refers to an engraver. The name of the artist reappears on the medals of the Renaissance, on which the signature, often accompanied by such words as *opus* or *fecit*, is placed so prominently as to constitute an integral part of the legend. In Italy and Europe in the 16th century the signature of the artist appears on coins as well as on medals; it is usually placed in smaller letters on the lower edge of the bust or on the exergue. Various forms are used: whole signatures, abbreviations, and initials. The names of engravers are also known from documents in archives, which sometimes permit the attributions of unsigned pieces. Engravers of coins are often medalists, too: for example, Leone Leoni and Benvenuto Cellini.

*Medals.* The medal is issued by the state or private persons, essentially for commemorative purposes. The Roman pieces, commonly called "medallions," differ from modern medals in that they were issued only by the state. Not originally intended for circulation, they had an exclusively commemorative function and were given by the emperor at the beginning of the year, or on other solemn occasions, to members of his family and the highest dignitaries of the court. They were first issued under Augustus, were rare in the 1st century of our era, and became more frequent under Hadrian. The largest production of bronze medallions took place under Commodus. Beginning with Constantine gold and silver pieces, rare in the first three centuries, were struck in greater numbers; it is more exact to call them multiples of the solidus or of the siliqua, connecting them with current gold and silver coins. Medallions follow the same laws as coins so far as types are concerned, though medallion types are more complex and stylistically more elaborate; they differ from coins in weight

and diameter. Gold and silver medallions, like gold coins, were sometimes mounted and used as jewels.

Pieces similar in form to medallions called "contorniates," a modern term referring to a circular groove running along the rim, can be dated in the period between Constantius II (337–61) and Anthemius (467–72) and were both cast and struck. The types represent the effigies of emperors and empresses from Nero to Anthemius, as well as famous persons of antiquity (Alexander, Homer, Horace, Sallust), Roman monuments, divinities, scenes of games, etc. Their purpose is still under discussion. According to one hypothesis, they are meant to portray the urban life of Rome in its various aspects, especially the games (Mazzarino). Other critics emphasize the pagan character of the types and consider them instruments of anti-Christian senatorial propaganda (Alföldi).

Tokens were executed in such materials as lead, bone, terra cotta, ivory, and bronze in various forms (the bronze ones generally round) and in small size. They were used in Greece and in Rome, in the 1st and 2d centuries of our era, for the acquisition of various goods and services (the purchase of grain, admission to baths, restaurants, theaters, etc.). They were issued by private persons and by associations, and their production was continued in medieval and modern times (see SEALS).

*Iconography and artistic problems.* The engraver of coins does not always create an original work, a new type, but is often inspired by well-known works of art. Whereas the Greek artist, at least until the Hellenistic period, took his subjects from such works and reinterpreted them, the Roman artist followed his model more closely, often copying it directly and changing only minor details. Faithful reproduction is seen in the Hellenistic period, often in secondary types (Athenian coins of the new style), and still more often in Greek coins of the Roman imperial period. These coins, with their representations of cult and honorary statues and various monuments, especially temples, have a documentary value absent in Greek coins of the earlier period. Other motifs inspired by monumental art recur frequently on Roman coins in the first three centuries of our era, such as the different types of *adlocatio* (address to the troops), *adventus* (imperial arrival), *profectio* (departure), *congiarium* (distribution of food and money to civilians), and sacrifice, which appear both on imperial reliefs and on coins. There was no direct relation between works of art and coins in the Middle Ages; standardized types prevailed: symbols, monograms, etc. The 15th century saw a return to representational types and, though one cannot speak of a direct imitation of contemporary works, as in the Roman period, the problem of the relationship between works of art and coins arises once more. The portrait became dominant again; it had appeared only sporadically in the Middle Ages (the most beautiful and famous example is the portrait of Emperor Frederick II on the augustals). Architectural types reappeared, first on the medals and then on the coins of the Renaissance, especially on papal coins. They have a high documentary value. One need only mention the series of monuments of Rome and Latium on papal coins, Alberti's uncompleted Tempio Malatestiano in Rimini shown as originally planned on a medal by Matteo de' Pasti (I, PL. 52), or the basilica of St. Peter's in Rome (projects by Bramante, Sangallo) on papal models and coins.

The normally round format of the coin sets special compositional problems for the artist. These are not so obvious when the representation is a head, whose shape is easily adapted to that of the coin. Yet even here artists have sometimes tried to take up the circular motif of the border by means of accessory figures, thus creating almost a frame around the main type (e.g., the head of Arethusa surrounded by dolphins on Syracusan coins, especially the demarateion, on which dolphins form a rotating circle around the head of the nymph). The adaptation of an entire human figure is more difficult. The crouching Seilenos on the tetradrachms of Naxos in Sicily is an excellent example of compositional skill; its scheme, however, is derived from vase painting. The Greek engraver's sculptural sensibility and desire for harmony are evident in the representation of isolated figures, even within the small field of the coin. Sometimes the Greek engraver tried to neutralize the round form by creating a square to put the figures in; he achieved it by way of the inscription, which thus acquired compositional value (on Macedonian or Thracian coins, on coins of the Arsacid Parthians), or he adopted the incuse square characteristic of archaic coins (Athens, Ainos). Beginning with the middle of the 6th century B.C., the artist often found another solution through the exergue, which cuts across the field of the coin, offering the possibility of setting the figure against a straight line. The composition of a group fits the curved line more easily than does an isolated figure (among numerous examples: Herakles strangling the lion on the gold coins of Syracuse or the lion attacking the bull on the tetradrachma of Akanthos).

The problems of antiquity recur in the Middle Ages and in modern times, especially in the 15th century with the renewed dominance of the portrait; and in their solution the sensibility of the artist and the type of representation play a decisive role. It should be noted that in the Middle Ages and the Renaissance the inscription, often bounded by two circles, forms a kind of frame around the representation.

*Artistic development.* Devised as a medium of exchange, coins were intended to serve a strictly utilitarian purpose, which could be fulfilled by the state's guarantee of a piece of metal alloy of given weight. Nevertheless, from the very first they reflected the art of their time and were sometimes among the highest artistic expressions of a period. For some regions, such as northern Greece and Sicily, coins are almost the only and certainly the most authentic surviving documents of a flourishing artistic activity. From the early 15th century medals paralleled coins as artistic documents; they express in an even higher degree the taste, style, and artistic achievement of a period. Yet the production of coins, and to a lesser degree of medals, became in various periods — notably in the 20th century — a predominantly mechanical process.

Artistic development was largely determined by techniques of production, the small dimensions of the coin, and the prescribed theme imposed on the engraver. In Greece and more rarely in modern times the theme remained unchanged for several centuries (e.g., in the florin and the ducat). To mention only some outstanding examples, the head of Athena on Corinthian staters and the head of Arethusa and the quadriga on the tetradrachmas of Syracuse were repeated without change in pattern but with differences in execution in the centuries following the archaic period. In such series it is possible to observe the artistic development of a type.

The portrait, one of the constant types on the obverse of the coin, begins (except for sporadic earlier examples) with the end of the 4th century B.C. From the Hellenistic kingdoms it passed to Rome, where it acquired a realistic character; the Romans transmitted it to the barbarian kingdoms and to the medieval world. In the Hellenistic period the effigy of the ruler was isolated on the field of the coin, thus gaining a strong relief, whereas in Rome, with the exception of a few coins of Augustus and of the Constantinian period, it was surrounded by the inscription bearing his name and titles. On the more crowded Roman coins the complexity of types and the distribution of figures in various planes weaken the relief but give the scenes a spatial effect unknown in Greek coins. The introduction of a monument as architectural background sometimes contributes to this effect. The flat relief initiated in Roman coins of the Constantinian period foreshadows the almost total absence of relief so typical of medieval coins, which were predominantly linear in design. After the fall of the Western Roman Empire, Byzantine coins developed typically hieratic figures, marked by frontality, schematization, and constant repetition of types.

In the West the early Middle Ages saw a general impoverishment of numismatic art. There are a few specimens of high artistic value, notably some Gothic series of coins (gold medallion of Theodoric and bronze coins of Theodat), and one observes attempts to restore artistic dignity to coinage, as in England,

COINS AND MEDALS

where Offa, king of Mercia (757–96), had his portrait put on a penny; but these are isolated attempts rarely followed even on Anglo-Saxon coins. In some issues of the last period of Charlemagne's reign an attempt was made at portraiture, though in general coin types remained purely decorative. The human figure did not disappear completely. The so-called papal *antiquiores* bear a rough effigy of St. Peter and some rare portraits of popes. In Italy, too, the portraits of the Lombard dukes of Benevento, whose issues show some Byzantine influence, appear on their coins. The *denaro grosso*, minted in Venice at the beginning of the 13th century, spread throughout Europe in the course of the century, opening new possibilities for representation because of its larger size. The seated or standing frontal figure became common. In the 12th century a great variety of types is found on German bracteates (PL. 408).

Numismatic art in medieval Italy reached its peak in the period of artistic flowering that marked the reign of Frederick II. Characteristic are the return to soberness and to reliefs of classical form; these qualities survive in part in the real of Charles of Anjou (PL. 407). Other stages in the history of coins are represented in the issues of Philip IV of France (with the king in majesty; PL. 409), of Edward III of England with the gold noble (armed king on a ship; PL. 409), and in the second half of the 12th century of Frederick Barbarossa and Henry VI of Germany (bracteates).

The Renaissance marks a great renewal in the art of coins under the influence of the medal. Produced by the casting technique and enriched by the artistic achievement of the age, the medal introduced into the field of the coin a new feeling for relief and decoration. The portrait acquired a new dignity; an attempt was made to represent the psychological and physical characteristics of the individual. Foreshortening and perspective were effects of the new art. The coin engravers, though they employed a different idiom from that of the medalists — because of the different problems involved in the striking technique, the smaller diameter of the coin, and the much lower relief, on which light has a different effect — abandoned the abstract linear design of the preceding centuries. The field of the coin acquired a spatial expansion and depth unknown in previous coins. In the late 15th and early 16th centuries these new qualities appeared elsewhere in Europe.

With the creation of the new German silver coin, the taler, with its larger diameter and lower relief, a new style spread through Europe. This style slowly lost the simplicity and purity of Italian coins and led to grandiloquent compositions, excessive decoration, heavy design, and intricate use of heraldic decoration. All these qualities were later transmitted to baroque production, with its heavy silver pieces (scudi, piasters, large ducats; PL. 412). The process of standardization in European coins began with the reappearance of epigraphic types in the mid-18th century, and reached its apex in the 19th and 20th centuries. The neoclassic period saw the last great creation of an engraved coin: one showing the British sovereign by Benedetto Pistrucci (PL. 414). It signified a return to harmonious grouping, to the purity and compositional severity of classic art, which is known to have inspired Pistrucci directly.

THE ANCIENT WORLD. *Origin and diffusion of coins in the classical world.* Coinage as the monopoly of the state was the last phase in the evolution of metal as a medium of exchange. The use of coins did not start suddenly or in any one place but was the logical outcome not only of economic but also of social and political development. Where and when premonetary mediums of exchange gave way to coins is still uncertain. Even in ancient times there existed various traditions about the state and the people that first struck coins. Two main traditions are known from literary sources. One attributed the invention to the Lydians, the other to Pheidon of Argos. Both are reported by Pollux (*Onomasticon*, IX, 83), together with less reliable hypotheses involving mythical personalities; concerning the Lydians Pollux quotes the opinion of Xenophanes. A frequently quoted passage in Herodotus (I, 94) also claims that the Lydians were the first to strike money from "gold and

silver"; but these gold and silver coins do not seem to be the first coins that can be attributed to Lydia: coins made of an electrum alloy are well known and precisely defined by Greek authors. It is possible that Herodotus was referring to the gold staters of Croesus (Kroisos), which may rightly be considered the first gold coins of the Greek world. Whether some of the oldest series of electrum of uncertain mint were struck by the Lydian kings, according to the tradition mentioned by Pollux, or by the Greek cities of Ionia, according to some modern scholars, and which are these series is still disputed by numismatists. Robinson and Seltman ascribe the stater and coins of small denominations representing the forepart or the head of a lion to the kingdom of Lydia, before Croesus. The incuse square on these coins of small denomination, formed by two connecting squares similar to those on the last series issued by Croesus, is in favor of this attribution. The issues of some Greek cities of Ionia (Miletos, Ephesos) must be considered contemporary or almost contemporary with the Lydian series. Which of the two regions was the first to introduce coins cannot be resolved on available evidence. Probably coins were struck within a short interval in both regions, through the initiative of the Lydian kings and the Greek cities of Ionia in contact with Lydia. Their trade was facilitated by the new medium of exchange, a natural development from its predecessor, an electrum pellet without type, roughly stamped or simply striated. This pellet, actually a private coin, was found in Ionia and the Aegean region, sometimes mingled with state coins. According to studies on the finds at the Temple of Artemis at Ephesos (Robinson), the transition probably took place about the middle of the 7th century B.C.

The tradition concerning Pheidon and his first issues of silver in Aegina is mentioned not only by Pollux but by Ephoros [in Strabo, VIII, 3, 33 (F. Jacoby, *Die Fragmente der griechischen Historiker*, Berlin, 1923–58, II A, p. 72, no. 115) and Strabo, VIII, 6, 16 (Jacoby, *op. cit.*, II A, p. 94, no. 176)], by the *Chronicon parium* (*IG*, XII, 5, p. 106, 11. 45–46), and by the *Etymologicon magnum* (cf. Aristotle, *Fragmenta*, 481, ed. W. D. Ross, Oxford, 1955). The last also reports that Pheidon dedicated the ancient iron spits, the medium of circulation in the Peloponnesos before the introduction of his silver coins, to the Temple of Hera (Heraion) at Argos. Herodotus (VI, 172), Pollux (X, 179; cf. Aristotle, *op. cit.*, 480), and some of the above-mentioned sources (Ephoros, in Strabo, VIII, 3, 33; *Chronicon parium*) attribute also the introduction of a system of weights and measures to Pheidon.

Pheidon's identity and the period in which he lived are uncertain, and the texts are not in accord about his achievements. Yet there seems no doubt that the introduction of coins in Greece proper took place at Aegina, because it is at Aegina that the oldest silver coins in Greece were found. The regulation of weights and measure adopted on the island and the "Aeginetan system," to which the coins traditionally attributed to Pheidon belong, are with some probability traceable to Pheidon, even though he may not have devised them himself. The use of iron as a medium of exchange in the Peloponnesos is documented not only by various sources (Pollux, VII, 105; IX, 77 ff.; cf. Aristotle, *op. cit.*, 481; Plutarch, *Fabius Maximus*, 27, 3; *Lysander*, 17; *Etymologicon magnum*), but also by archaeological finds in the Temple of Hera at Argos, where a bundle of strongly tied iron spits was discovered (C. Waldstein, *The Argive Heraeum*, I, Boston, New York, 1902, p. 6 ff., fig. 3). A fragmentary inscription of the 7th century B.C. found in the Temple of Hera at Corinth (H. Payne, *Perachora*, Oxford, 1940, p. 256 ff.) with an offering of a drachma for something unspecified may indicate a dedication of spits.

Thus the new silver coinage originated at Aegina in the second half of the 7th century B.C., a few decades after the first issues of electrum coins in Asia Minor, and in Greece proper Aegina was the first to strike coins.

From the centers of origin in Asia Minor and Aegina coins spread throughout the Greek world and other Mediterranean regions, at first rapidly, then more slowly, until they reached the most distant places. Because of this gradual penetration, not only distant and economically backward peoples, such

as the Gauls and Britons, but also commercially advanced ones, such as the Phoenicians, adopted coins only late, often through the impact of political and military events. These peoples were familiar with the use of coins, but did not make their own because they preferred for purposes of trade the internationally known and valued coins of other states; they resorted to barter for their trade with more primitive peoples. The Greek world before the Roman conquest knew many internationally valued coins (PL. 393): the Persian daric, the staters of Corinth, the tetradrachma of Athens, and the gold staters of Alexander the Great.

The principal cities of Ionia and Mysia — Ephesos, Miletos, Phokaia, Kyzikos — began minting coins in the second half of the 7th century B.C. Their issues, like the first coins attributed to Lydia, are of electrum, the metal characteristic of the coinage of Asia Minor. Knidos (Cnidus) in Caria, whose silver coins date from the end of the century, is the exception. In Greece proper, Corinth, the greatest commercial center of the Peloponnesos, followed the example of Aegina; its first issues differing from the monetary system of Aegina can probably be assigned — although the dating is still disputed — to the last quarter of the 7th century, at the end of Kypselos' reign or at the beginning of Periander's. Athens in the last decade of the century issued the first pre-Solonian didrachmas of Aeginetan weight. About 600 B.C. or a few years later various mints became active: those of Lindos on the island of Rhodes and of Eretria in Euboea; those of Naxos, Paros, Siphnos, and Karthaia in the Cyclades; also those of some Boeotian cities such as Tanagra and Thebes. In the early 6th century B.C. coins were already firmly established in Asia Minor, the Aegean islands, and the mainland of Greece. The most important Greek mints were those of Aegina, Corinth, and Athens; the latter two, and especially that of Athens, were destined to have the most long-lived and famous coinage in the ancient world — one farspread and imitated everywhere.

During the 6th century coins spread through the whole Mediterranean basin, reaching the principal Greek cities in the East and West. In the first quarter of the century coins spread in the West as far as Kerkyra (Corfu) and Cyrene in North Africa. Smyrna in Ionia and Kameiros on Rhodes began to strike coins during the same period. All these series have some characteristics in common. They show on the reverse the so-called "incuse square," though its form and the type differ in the various mints, and with a few exceptions bear no inscription except sometimes the initials of the mints; the type on the obverse was generally considered insufficient to identify the issuing state. With the coming to power of Peisistratos, Athens began to strike a tetradrachma with the head of Athena and the owl — the first coin with a double type (on the obverse and on the reverse) in the ancient world. A short time later Croesus in Lydia issued his gold staters, the first gold coins in antiquity (PL. 393).

About the middle of the 6th century Termera in Caria, Tenedos in the Troas, Teos in Ionia, Karystos in Euboea, Heraia in Arcadia, Airaophia, Koroneia, Orchomenos, Pharai in Boeotia, the island of Thasos and, a few years later, Abdera in Thrace began to strike coins. The first series of the island of Lesbos and the first triobols of uncertain coinage in Phokis go back to the same period. In the second half of the century coins were struck in the western Greek colonies; Zankle, Himera, Naxos, and Syracuse in Sicily were the first, followed somewhat later by Akragas and Selinous. In the second half of the 6th century all the most important Greek colonies in Magna Graecia began their characteristic series with incuse obverse except Elea (Velia), which continued to use the traditional technique. In the last quarter of the century Salamis on Cyprus began to strike coins, and Darius I began to issue gold darics and silver sigloi in the Persian Empire. Between the end of the 6th century and the first years of the 5th coins spread to the north of Greece, where the main cities of Macedonia and Thrace and barbarian peoples, the Orrheskioi, Bisalti, and Derroni (PL. 393), started their characteristic silver coinage. A few years later the kings of Macedonia struck the first didrachmas and drachmas bearing their names. One can therefore conclude that at the beginning of the Persian wars coins were known in the entire

ancient world: they circulated everywhere and were minted in almost every region.

During the 5th century B.C. this diffusion of coins continued in the West and reached Marseilles about the middle of the century; in Magna Graecia coins were first struck in Cumae, then in Terina; in the second half of the century in Naples, Herakleia, and Thurii. In Sicily coins were first struck in the first decades of the century in Catana, Leontini, Gela, and Camarina. More and more mints began to operate, but some, such as those of Karystos, Tenos, and Naxos, closed because of the supremacy of Athens and its financial policy.

In the following century there began a new era for coins with the supremacy of Macedonia and the conquests of Alexander, which reached the most distant Eastern and Western borders. In the first half of the 4th century, in Greece and in the eastern Mediterranean, the end of the Athenian hegemony and the decline of the Persian Empire facilitated the opening of many mints, some of secondary importance. With the establishment of Alexander's new empire some mints were closed, but others in Greece and in the Orient were opened or grew in importance as they became mints of the empire.

The gold coins struck in great number by Philip II (PL. 396) and Alexander were widely diffused. Their staters replaced the Persian darics and became the most widely disseminated gold coins in the Greek world. The death of Alexander and the formation of the Hellenistic kingdoms led to a new diffusion of coins; even Egypt, which had never had its own coinage, started striking coins under Ptolemy with the types and name of Alexander, then with different types and Ptolemy's own name (PL. 396). Seleucus began to issue coins autonomously in Asia at about the same time. These coins came to Bactria through the Seleucid kingdom about the middle of the century and from there to India, into the so-called "Indo-Greek kingdoms," which transmitted them to the Indian kingdoms, their successors. In the first half of the 2d century coins passed from the Seleucids to the Parthians.

In the West the first issues of Emporion (mod. Ampurias, Spain) go back to about 350 B.C.; they were followed by those of Rhoda (mod. Rosas) and Gades (mod. Cádiz) a little less than a century later. Even after Roman domination some Greek centers (Thasos, Athens, Rhodes, etc.) continued the autonomous issue of silver coins in the 2d century B.C. Pergamon, Ephesos, Smyrna, and other cities in Asia Minor started striking kistophoroi (cistophori) at the beginning of the century.

In Italy, Rome began with the issues of cast *aes grave*, which was followed by the Roman-Campanian didrachma about 335 B.C. (or 50 years later according to Mattingly, Robinson, and Sydenham). In 269 B.C. (or at the latest in 187) the first Roman denarii appeared. The coins of Rome spread with the growth of Roman political influence, first in Italy and then in the whole Mediterranean and beyond. During the empire, with the permission of the Roman state, large and small mints coined copiously, but, with rare exceptions, only bronze coins. These mints disappeared slowly with the Valerians and were officially and definitively closed under Aurelian. After the fall of the Western Empire the barbarian kingdoms struck their own autonomous series, which imitated imperial coins.

*Greek monetary types.* There has been much discussion about the source of inspiration for the selection of types, and various theories have been advanced. The religious theory (Burgen, Curtius) traces all types, even such allusive or punning ones as the rose (*rhodon*) of Rhodes, the celery leaf (*selinon*) of Selinous, the seal (*phōkē*) of Phokaia, etc., to a religious principle. The commercial theory (Ridgeway) holds that many coin representations recall objects or animals which served as mediums of exchange before the introduction of the coin; this theory is certainly unacceptable for some types (e.g., wild beasts and fantastic beings). Finally, the theory of types as equivalent to seals (MacDonald) maintains that the type is always the emblem of the issuing city, even when it represents the local divinity or its symbol. This theory seems to come closest to reality, but one should not forget that the problem has numerous aspects requiring an intermediate solution.

The inspiration for the choice of types can be clearly defined only in the archaic period of Greek coins, approximately until the Persian Wars. (See I, col. 605 and I, PL. 375.) At that time the most famous and durable series of the Greek world were created, and the typology was less complex. With the later increase in the number and variety of types, it becomes more difficult to trace what prompted their choice, especially as political and economic factors also played a part in the selection of a new type or the changing of an existing one. No one source of inspiration can be singled out; a variety of influences must be taken into account. Many of the representations on Greek coins are doubtless of a religious character — not only the effigies of divinities, rare in the first phase of Greek coinage, but also such objects as the tripod and the lyre and animals, including the deer, the owl, the eagle, and the lion (also a symbol of royalty). Even the quadriga and the biga, as types celebrating athletic competitions, can be given a religious interpretation. Many other images (the shield on Boeotian coins, the ear of grain of Metapontum, the winged boar of Klazomenai, the turtle of Aegina, etc.) and the punning types do not seem to be religiously motivated but to represent the emblem of the city, the true symbol of the state.

A sometimes clearly emblematic function can be found not only in types without, or with a not immediately apparent, religious significance, but often also in representations of divinities and their symbols or of mythical heroes; the emblematic value is here superimposed on the religious value. The Pegasus of Corinth, the owl of Athens, the head of Arethusa surrounded by dolphins of Syracuse, Taras on a dolphin of Tarentum combined religious significance with an essentially emblematic character, which later came to prevail and is often documented by literary and epigraphic sources. In the present writer's opinion almost all the main types of Greek coins, especially in the archaic period, share an emblematic significance, even though their origin might have been religious or commercial. With the increased use of inscriptions the emblematic image became less important, as it was no longer needed for the identification of the issuing state, and it was given a different place on the coin or disappeared altogether. An emblematic function can be demonstrated even in later periods, when some of the most important mints coined series that preserved the old traditional types or used types that can assume an emblematic significance (e.g., the eagle on a thunderbolt for the Ptolemies).

From the typological point of view Greek coinage until the Roman Empire can be divided into three great periods: from its beginnings until the Persian Wars, from the Persian Wars to Alexander the Great, and from Alexander the Great until the end of autonomous issues. In the first period animal types prevailed; generally only the head or forepart of the body was depicted; the whole figure seldom appears. Other frequent subjects were plants and inanimate objects, as well as monstrous and fantastic beings, not often used later. The human figure is rare, especially the human figure shown in its entirety; when it appears, it is represented kneeling or standing. Groups, such as the satyr abducting a nymph, common in Thrace and Thasos, or Herakles and the Hesperides at Cyrene, or Aeneas and Anchises at Aineia, are exceptional in this period. The first heads of divinities did not appear until the middle of the 6th century B.C.; in the late 6th century human types became more frequent. A great variety of types existed besides emblematic and religious ones: types referring to the name of the city (allusive types), to the products of the soil (the ear of grain of Metapontum and the silphium plant of Cyrene), to mythical personages (Taras of Tarentum or the Minotaur of Crete), or to protecting divinities of the city (Dionysos on Naxos and Athena at Athens). On the whole, however, the typology of this period is less varied than that of succeeding ones, probably because of the characteristic Greek tendency to avoid change (especially marked in the archaic period) or because of the dominance of the incuse-square technique.

In the second period the figures of divinities constituted the majority of monetary images. Representations of the human head, which appeared late on coins but were rapidly disseminated, are found almost always on the obverse, whereas those of the entire figure, if present at all, are found on the reverse. The gradual relinquishment of the incuse-square technique brought with it an increased variety of types. For commercial reasons, in the series issued by major mints (at Athens, Corinth, Syracuse, etc.) the type of silver coins and of pieces of higher denomination remained fixed and variations occurred only in small denominations and in bronze coins. The representation of the entire human figure, generally standing or seated, became more frequent. At the end of the 5th century frontal heads were widely diffused. The Athena of Eukleidas and the Arethusa of Kimon on the tetradrachmas of Syracuse are probably the first examples.

In the third period the variety of types again increased, especially on the smaller denominations and on bronze, now coined in large quantities by almost all mints. A great innovation, after the death of Alexander the Great, was the appearance on the obverse of portraits of monarchs. The use of large, flat flans, spread by the tetradrachmas and characteristic for this time, allowed the creation of more elaborate types, often accompanied by symbols and monograms or long inscriptions. The type, even when it consisted of a human figure, was often surrounded by a crown of laurel, ivy, or oak leaves serving a purely decorative purpose.

During the empire the coins of the Greek cities that retained, or for the first time acquired, the right to strike their own coins nearly always bore on the obverse the portrait of the emperor or a member of his family, as on imperial Roman coins. Exceptions are the idealized effigy of Alexander the Great in Macedonia, the head of Athena on Athenian coins during the reign of Hadrian and of the Antonines, and the head of Demos (the people), of Boule (council of nobles), and of Synkletos (council of the people) issued by various mints, especially in the 2d and 3d centuries of our era. On the reverse appeared the most diversified types, almost all local and inspired by the cult of the region or the city; the representations include not only monuments, works of art, and famous persons whom the city of their birth wished to honor, but also notable events in the life of the city, such as games, religious feasts, visits of emperors. The coins without artistic value are important from a historical and antiquarian point of view.

*Roman monetary types.* The difference between Greek and Roman monetary typology is essentially a difference in historical background and in religious and political conceptions. Roman coinage is unitary, like the state it represents, and, except in its first period and on bronze coins until Caesar, has no fixed types. Functioning in an imperialist state, whose political expansion entailed the diffusion and imposition of its own coinage, Roman mints were not held to that stability of type to which the chief Greek mints were committed for reasons of trade. The lack of competitors in the imperial era allowed a reduction of weight and great changes of alloy, which would have had international consequences of considerable gravity for the coinage of any Greek state. In addition, the peculiar structure of the Roman state made it possible, from the beginning of the republican period, for its coins rapidly to take on an apologetic and propagandistic role, almost completely unknown in Greek coins. This role of Roman coins, especially important during the empire, and their use in commemorating and glorifying historical events and personages, are characteristic both in republican and imperial times.

The distinctive qualities of the Roman coin are apparent from the middle of the 2d century B.C., when they began to appear in the denarius with the traditional types of the first period (Dioscuri, biga of Diana and of Victory; later biga and quadriga of Juno, Mars, Apollo, Venus, etc.) — special types connected with the family history of the moneyer. These increasingly important types came to include divinities, pertaining not so much to the state religion as to the private cult of the moneyer's family. In 100 B.C. for the first time there appeared on the denarius of the quaestors L. Calpurnius Piso and Q. Servilius Caspius a type showing the coining magistrates, and not their ancestors, seated between two ears of grain. At the beginning of 44 B.C. (or at the earliest late in 45) Caesar received

from the Senate the right to place his own portrait on coins, thus starting the long iconographic series of Roman imperial coins. The functions of propaganda and historical commemoration were stressed during the civil wars and found their highest expression in the empire, when all interest was concentrated on the person and activities of the emperor and his family and on the main religious, military, and social affairs of the state during his reign; indeed, many divinities and personifications on coins were qualified by such epithets as "Augusta" and "Augusti."

The wealth of types of every kind during the first two centuries of our era, especially marked in the 2d century with a great abundance and variety of representations and rather complex scenes (political and social happenings, events connected with the family life of the emperor, such as births and marriages) gave way in the 3d century to a certain typological monotony. The figure of the emperor, divinities, and personifications now predominated, on simpler types.

In comparison with contemporary coins, medallions, especially those of the reigns of Commodus and the Antonines, offer more variegated and crowded scenes; they show greater typological wealth and complexity of representation, sometimes even details of landscapes. The emperor's military activities are stressed. In the first two centuries of our era he often appears in a toga, but from the reign of Septimius Severus onward he is almost always represented in military attire. Beginning with the tetrarchy (late 3d cent.) he again appears draped in a toga.

In the new phase that began with the tetrarchy and reached its full development under Constantine with the establishment of Christianity, Roman coins acquired the characteristics later transmitted to Byzantine coins and to the coins of the barbarian states that succeeded the Roman Empire. Starting with the tetrarchy, the number of pagan divinities declined; the surviving ones, found on the coins of Constantine, were Jupiter, Mars, Hercules, Sol, Neptune, Isis, and Anubis; under Constantine II there remained only three (Jupiter, Mars, Sol), under Constantius only one (Mars). Then they all vanished, except for a brief reappearance under Julian (Apollo, Ceres, Jupiter, Isis, Serapis, Neptune) and, together with Oriental divinities, under the Valentinians (Anubis, Isis, Horus). The figure of Rome appeared until the end of the empire, but transformed into the symbol of the city; in this new role it was occasionally accompanied, from the time of Constantine, by the figure of Constantinople. The personifications, too, gradually disappeared from coins. There were still nine under Constantine, four under Crispus (Concordia, Moneta, Pax, Securitas); Securitas survived until Constantius II. Victory, who survived until the end of the empire, from the time of Galla Placidia assumed the aspect of a Christian angel with long cross (PL. 405), an aspect she retains on Byzantine coins.

Beginning with the Valerians the representation of the emperor was limited to a few types repeated with slight variations until the end of the empire.

With Constantine Christian symbols such as the cross and the monogram of Christ appeared on coins, at first as symbols and adjuncts to other representations on small bronze coins. Under Constantius II, and later especially under the Valentinians, these symbols appeared also on gold and silver issues; beginning with the Valentinians they even constituted the type itself (e.g., the cross on the solidi of Olybrius and on gold trientes, siliquas, and small bronze coins until the fall of the empire).

*Coins in peripheral classical culture.* The spread of Greek coins led to the introduction of the practice of coinage among the Etruscans, Phoenicians, and Celts. Whereas the former two peoples developed their own monetary types, the Celts imitated Greek models circulating in international trade. The Greek colonies distributed along the shores of the Mediterranean and the Black Sea played a significant role in transmitting the concept of the coin.

The development of indigenous coinage among these peoples was a gradual process conditioned by the intensity of their contacts with the Greek world, by their economic and commercial progress, and by the evolution of their social organization. About the middle of the 5th century B.C. the Phoenicians at Tyre in the east and the Etruscans in the west simultaneously produced distinctive coin types. The Etruscans left the reverse smooth, a practice whose only precedent is found in certain Cypriote issues of the late 6th century B.C. Toward the end of the 5th century Sidon and Arados in Phoenicia also began to mint coins, while in the west the Carthaginians struck their first coins in Sicily in the course of a war with Syracuse (last decade of the 5th cent.). In the first half of the 4th century coins were minted in the Carthaginian metropolis itself.

In the late 4th and early 3d centuries the Celts in Gaul began to produce their own coinage, imitating the types of the gold staters and tetradrachmas of Philip II and Alexander the Great, but greatly modifying their formal character toward increasing abstraction (see CELTIC ART; FIG. 183).

In the period from the 3d to the 1st century coins were diffused in Arabia. In the 3d century the Sabaeans and Himyarites began issues imitating Athenian prototypes. The Nabataeans began their own coinage in the reign of Aretas III (87–62); these issues continued through the 1st century of our era. Shortly after the middle of the 2d century B.C. Simon Maccabaeus began Jewish coinage with types and legends that departed from Hellenic prototypes. The last issues of this coinage occurred during the Jewish revolt (132–35) against Hadrian. The kings of Edessa from Vael (163–65) to Abgar IX (214–16?) issued coins with their own portraits and that of the Parthian ruler Vologases III; after a few years the image of the Roman emperor replaced that of Vologases. In the 2d century of our era the kingdom of Axum began its coinage with pieces of gold and silver inscribed in Greek and Ethiopic; this continued until the 9th century.

Franco PANVINI ROSATI

ORIENTAL COINS. *Bactria.* A significant cache was discovered in the Balkh region, in 1878, containing double darics and coins of Seleucus and Antiochos I, II, and III. In 1887 near Bukhara were found heavy silver coins with, on the obverse, a horseman wearing a tunic, breastplate, and Macedonian helmet, and brandishing a spear and a sling, and, on the reverse, a man on a rearing horse charging two warriors mounted on an elephant. This represents the retreat of King Poros before the king of Taxila, an ally of Alexander; Poros was defeated on the banks of the Hydaspes (Jhelum) in 326 B.C.. The political events in this remote region made it the center of an art that was not devoid of originality, despite the fact that it was, in the beginning at any rate, wholly Greek in character and unaffected by local influences. The first Seleucids in Bactria struck coins showing a wreathed head of Zeus and Athena in a chariot drawn by four elephants with horns. Sophytes, an ally of Alexander, and later of Seleucus, against the Indian Candragupta (Sandrakottos), struck some fine coins that show his head with wreathed helmet and paragnaths (PL. 398).

The Greek princes in Bactria soon began a struggle for independence. Diodotos rebelled against Antiochos II in 248 and issued coins bearing his own effigy and name. The obverse shows his diademed head, as a young man. The reverse has on it, as a sign of independence, instead of the Seleucid Apollo, a nude figure of Zeus wielding a thunderbolt, with the eagle at his feet.

The Bactrian kingdoms, which extended as far as Chinese Turkistan and were ruled by dynasties that were sometimes at war with one another, had a succession of 37 princes in the spaces of two centuries, who left an iconographic series of coins of a high artistic level (II, PL. 84). Euthydemos of Magnesia, who was at first defeated by Antiochos III but was able to regain his independence, is represented, in classical style, with a youthful diademed head, on a coin whose reverse shows Herakles seated. An older effigy of him toward the end of his reign is strikingly realistic. He was succeeded by his son Demetrios, who was in conflict with Eukratides. The latter appears on coins with his head covered with an elephant's hide (the reverse shows Herakles standing). On silver coins may be seen

the heads of relatives of Eukratides, Heliokles and Laodike. It was only after him that Prakrit inscriptions appeared on the reverse sides of coins.

In 190 B.C. Eukratides proclaimed himself βασιλεὺς μέγας. His coins were copied by the Parthians and by Timarchos at Babylon. The only known specimen of his enormous 20-stater gold piece, weighing 2,520 grains, is kept in the Cabinet des Médailles in Paris. Because of its exceptional size and weight, it is thought to be a commemorative medal. The king is shown on the obverse without a beard, wearing a plumed helmet; the reverse represents the Dioskouroi. Another single coin is the only evidence of the revolt of Plato against Eukratides in 165 B.C. The portraits of his successors, Euthydemos II, Pantaleon (head of Dionysos and panther), Agathokles (diademed, head without beard), Antimachos, wearing a large felt hat reminiscent of the Macedonian *kausia* (Poseidon on the reverse may allude to a naval battle on the Indus; PL. 398), and Heliokles (160–120 B.C.), who struck two series of coins, one for Bactria, copied by barbarian tribes, and one for India, are all masterpieces of the coiner's art.

After Pantaleon and Agathokles, in addition to silver coins, square bronze coins were issued with inscriptions in Kharoshthi. A period of decline then set in that coincides with the invasion of the nomads about 125 B.C. Coins bearing such names as Antalkidas (caps of the Dioskouroi), Lysias, Diomedes, Archebios, Apollodotos (Athena Promachos), Strato (elephant and zebu) and his wife Agathokleia, Epander (Dionysos), Zoilos, Apollophanes, Artemidoros, Antimachos II, Philoxenos, Nikias, and Hermaios prove that the traditions of Greece were not dead; the coins, however, are but a poor reflection of a once highly developed art. It should be noted that side by side with such typical Greek divinities as Zeus holding the triple Hekate, Apollo crowning himself, Poseidon, Artemis, and Pallas wearing a short chiton, may be seen such local figures as an Indian dancing girl in baggy trousers (on coins of Pantaleon and Agathokles) and a divinity wearing a Phrygian cap (on coins of Amyntas and Hermaios).

Thus it is evident that the intercourse between different peoples entailed religious contacts as well. The Artemis depicted on the Bactrian coins was linked with the syncretic divinity that combines the qualities of the goddess of the Oxus and the Asiatic Anahita to symbolize the goddess of fertility. And Agathokles, who reigned in Arachosia and Drangiana from 180 to 165 B.C., had coins struck with what some consider a picture of a Buddhist stupa, though it is more probably only a picture of a mountain (see also BACTRIAN ART).

*Persis.* The principality of Persis had been an appanage of one of the branches of the royal line of the Achaemenids. Its rulers swore allegiance to Seleucus after Alexander's death. From 220 B.C. onward, they struck coins of the Persepolitan type. Their power was weakened by the Parthians, but they did not adopt the types of their powerful neighbors until Autophradates II, who reigned at the time of Mithradates II (123–88 B.C.) and who was the last ruler to issue coins with indigenous themes.

The portraits of Bagadat (Bagdat) I in 220 B.C. should be noted from the point of view of iconography; the ruler is shown in profile, with a short beard, long mustaches, and earrings, and he wears as a headdress the bashlyk, the symbol of the satrap, the brim of which forms a visor. Darius I wears a flat hat decorated with an eagle or a crescent; the reverse shows him seated, wearing a long robe open in front, with hanging oversleeves, under which tight-fitting real sleeves cover the arms down to the wrists. The fire temple is shown with a figure making the ritual gesture of worship, with outstretched hands; the headdress hides part of his face, as the Zoroastrian rites require. The dynasts are shown here as high priests, the heirs of the Achaemenid Magi. From Darius II, son of Autophradates II, onward, they wear the Arsacid tiara. A decline in the quality of the coins becomes apparent during the reigns of the subsequent kings: Oaxathres, Artaxerxes III, Minuchetri, Papek, and Artaxerxes V, whose portraits, fullface or in profile, are Sassanian in style. There follow the Kamnaskires, of whom

the first still presents a classical profile (on the reverse is Apollo on the omphalos). The double portrait of Kamnaskires and Queen Anzaze (PL. 398) has Zeus on the reverse. The type of the dynast evolves until he is shown wearing a royal diadem, a pointed beard, and an embroidered gown. The portraits of the last sovereigns of the Arsacid dynasty are all fullface; they are somewhat cursorily modeled and look like caricatures of the Parthian types.

*Characene.* Characene, or Mesene, was one of the small kingdoms that succeeded in resisting both the Greeks and the Persians by taking advantage of the struggle between the Parthians and the kings of Syria. An interesting coinage, which shows Seleucid influence, was developed under the first kings. There are classical portraits of Hyspaosines on silver coins, with Apollo on the omphalos on the reverse. The Greek type of Apollo appears on the coins of kings Apodakos, Tiraios I, and Tiraios II. The Chaldean ethnical traits and pointed beards of these rulers inspired more or less skillful engravers, belonging to the Greek school, to depict them in markedly bold portraits. With the subsequent kings, Themon, Attambelos I, Abinerglos, and Attambelos II (shown with an oblong face framed with thick hair), portraits became cruder (PL. 398). Still later Greek inscriptions disappeared. Under Obadas, Abinerglos, and Madabazes *potin* was the only metal used for coins; the engravers of these seem to have had difficulty in copying the Sassanian models.

*The Parthians.* When the Arsacids established themselves in Iran, they did not immediately introduce a new currency. Small silver coins with an effigy of a beardless person wearing the soft felt bashlyk and, on the reverse, an archer of a type that persists throughout the dynasty have posed a problem that is still unresolved. J. de Morgan regarded these coins as "sacerdotal money," but such a theory cannot be supported. M. Dayet thought they were coins struck by the feudal princes of Media, but this theory is hardly convincing. Other numismaticians have thought that these tetrobols, drachmas, and hemidrachmas marked the beginnings of the Parthian currency under the first three rulers and that they were meant to commemorate the founder of the Arsacid dynasty. The fact remains that nothing can be stated with certainty before the reign of Mithradates I (171–138 B.C.), whose fine coins, of an entirely Greek type, show a portrait of the king that was obviously executed by a Greek engraver, as the reverse, which is of a classical cast, bears out. His face is handsome and grave, his beard long, and his hair neatly dressed in regular wavy lines. His head is bare, except for a regal diadem ringed with a row of pearls. Phraates II (138–128 B.C.) has a short beard, a rounder face, and a larger bust; there is a Persian archer on the reverse. The portrait of Artabanus I (128–122 B.C.) and that of Himerus (124 B.C.) are classical in type, with a fine profile, and the reverse bears a woman holding a horn of plenty. The coins of Mithradates II, the Great (123–88 B.C.) show a fine effigy of the king, with a stellate tiara. A more exotic portrait shows the king wearing another tiara with pendants. There is already something Oriental in his hieratic bearing and in the impassivity of his features. (See PL. 399.)

During this period (89–88 B.C.) the cities issued their own coinage, with an effigy of their protecting divinity, Fortuna or the Greek Tyche. The same style is found during the period of Artabanus II (88–77 B.C.; not to be confused with the Artabanus II who died in A.D. 40); his hair is cut at the neck and his beard is short-clipped. Sinatroces or Sanatruces (77–70 B.C.) is an old man wearing a stellate tiara and an embroidered robe. Phraates III (70–57 B.C.) wears a headdress covered with pearls. In the reign of Mithradates III, we have a fullface portrait, with two tufts of hair framing the face. The portrait of Orodes I, (57–38 B.C.), who defeated Crassus at Carrhae, shows a trend toward rigidity. He has the fine, shrewd features of a politician. His beard is pointed and his hair semilong, arranged in curled layers. He wears the royal band and an embroidered robe. The coins sometimes show Victory crowning the king and astrological signs. The reverse side shows the usual archer

and also a group of two figures and a god seated on a throne. With Pacorus (38 B.C.) a decline sets in. The portrait becomes angular and schematic. The headdress is reminiscent of that of the kings of Edessa in Mesopotamia. The long square-shaped inscription tends to invade the field of the coin and to reduce the size of the type. On the reverse, two figures, one seated and the other standing, are holding a palm branch. Coins of Phraates IV (38–2 B.C.) show an attenuated profile and a pointed beard. Near the royal diadem a bird is depicted. The coins of Tiridates II, who replaced Phraates IV on the throne for a brief period, are similar. Phraates V, or Phraataces (3 B.C.– A.D. 4), is shown with his mother, Queen Musa, who is wearing a triple tiara. This is the first time that a woman's portrait appears on a Parthian coin. The style continued to degenerate under Orodes II (A.D. 5–6) and Vonones I, whose schematic and linear portrait is crowned by a diadem with a long buckle. Coins of Artabanus II (10–40) show him fullface with a square beard. On the reverse Victory is welcoming the king on horse-back. There is a marked contrast between the suggested might and splendor of the king and the inadequacy of the portrayal.

Mention ought to be made of the coins of some of the subsequent Parthian rulers. Vardanes I (40–45) is shown with his hair arranged in rows of small curls. Meherdates (49–50) has a fullface portrait, very cursorily executed. Pacorus II (78–82) appears as a young man. Osroes (106–30) is depicted in a conventional style; he wears a tiara, represented by graining, and a buckler, also indicated by graining, over his ears. Vologases II (77–147) is more subtly portrayed, with his hair in long curls; on the reverse is a scene with two personages. The portrait of Vologases III (147–91) is so stylized as to distort his profile; his rectangular beard and his robe are depicted by means of grooved lines. After Artavasdes (227) the Parthian rule was replaced by that of the Sassanians.

*The Sassanians.* When the Sassanians established their rule in Persia during the first quarter of the 3d century it seems as if the change in dynasty at first led to only rather superficial changes in the art of the coins. Ardashir I (211–41), who conquered Artavasdes in 227, wears above his bashlyk the Parthian tiara studded with a star. His profile, with its long wavy beard and large aquiline nose, is very striking. The effigy is well centered, framed by a regular inscription in Pahlavi. The technical level in these coins is higher than it was under the Parthian rulers, and the Greek style persists. Soon, however, specifically Sassanian motifs appeared, and Greek forms were gradually replaced by Oriental ones. This development has both a religious and a political background. A deliberate rejection of the Greco-Parthian element and of Greek religion characterized Ardashir's reign and is reflected in his coinage. Yet, in spite of this xenophobia, Greek and Roman artists were brought in from the West to direct at least the engraving of the coins, and the foreign artists only gradually accepted the style imposed on them; the compromise yielded some fine portraits (see SASSANIAN ART).

The finest Sassanian coins are those of Shapur I (PL. 399). Though his head is shown in profile, the torso is depicted frontally to set off the great breadth of shoulder. The face has fine lines, of characteristic Iranian purity, and a long aquiline nose. The heavy beard, with curls depicted by means of graining, is tied at its lower end to make it thick and round. The heavy billowing hair on the nape of the neck seems to be blown out by the wind. A fantastic headgear fits tightly over the head; it is a combination of the Persian hat with lappets and of a crenelated crown that widens to hold the celestial orb at its summit. The whole is set with gems and pearls, whose splendor the monochrome gold or silver coin suggests. The attention paid to detail and the refinement of execution do not impair the unity of style. The whole composition, which reveals the artist's great control of his material, produces an imposing effect.

Later the engraver complicated his task, with less felicitous results, by showing paired profiles of Varahran I (272–75) and his queen, who wears a peculiar form of helmet with an animal head. Facing them is a minute bust of the heir apparent.

It is interesting to note that the slow debasement of the Greek style in Iran during the Sassanian period parallels the decline in Western art that set in during the second half of the 3d century of our era and continued until the Byzantine period. Even technical factors contributed to this trend. The composition of the coins underwent similar changes in both areas. The gold pieces of Shapur were still thick like the aurei of the Roman Empire, but soon the flan became thinner and so wide that it allowed a decorative band around the type. Thickness was thus decreased partly because thin pieces of ductile metal are more easily struck than thicker ingots and also because less importance was attached to the vigorously modeled portrait and the faithful reproduction of the sovereign's features, and more to decorative effects. Engraving tended to become a graphic art. Portraits combining the majesty of a countenance with a sumptuous headdress gave way to vignettes in which the emphasis was on the pomp and trappings of power and individual character was obscured by excessive ornament. It must be remembered, however, that dress and finery serve to reflect the splendor of a dynasty and that such factors as the shape of the tiara, the placing of the side pieces, the position of the orb of the sun, and the details of goldsmith work are the only indications enabling us to identify a ruler.

The same preoccupation with decoration marks the reverses of the coins. During the early days of the Parthian Empire, the coin engravers showed the national archer seated on a cippus, like the Delphic Apollo on the omphalos, and stringing his bow, a design inspired by the Seleucid tetradrachma. But with the advent of the Sassanians this design disappeared and was replaced by a heraldic and entirely symmetrical type: a picture of the altar on which burns the sacred fire. At first only the altar is shown — a simple spare slab resting on a round pillar and supported by two pilasters. Later it is flanked by two figures; the king, who is the religious head, and the priest, or *mobed*. Both hold long lances and respectfully avert their faces from the fire, or else, facing each other over the single flame on the round altar (which symbolizes the world), they perform the rites of fire worshipers. This motif, once adopted, persisted in Sassanian coins, but the quality of the execution deteriorated more and more, until it became hardly recognizable.

The decline of this allegorical art set in very rapidly and was not connected with the economic and political prosperity of the empire. During the reign of Khosrau (Chosroes) II (590–628) coins became thin pieces of silver like the bracteates or the Byzantine *nummi scyphati*. Though the quality of the alloy remains excellent, the obverse bears only a schematic profile that has nothing characteristic about it except the special form of royal headdress, which extends beyond the circle surrounding it so that the curly locks cover the rim of the coin. On the reverse, the sketchily designed figures of the fire worshipers stand on each side engaged in some unidentifiable activity. Thus types having plastic significance were replaced by motifs which would seem to have lost their human qualities and which, apart from their pleasing design, have only a certain abstract evocative quality. Henceforth, as in the Byzantine empire, emphasis is on the majesty of the sovereign and the symbolism of his absolute power rather than on his physical person. With this type of coin the clear vision of Greek idealism comes to an end. After it came Moslem calligraphic coins, in which effigies are replaced by descriptive and religious texts (see CALLIGRAPHY AND EPIGRAPHY).

*Indo-Greek coins.* The earliest coins in India consisted of silver ingots on which a rudimentary mark, usually a rosette pattern, was stamped. British archaeologists have given them the name of "punch-marked silver." They spread to northern and southwestern India. The symbols on them are animal figures, including the rhinoceros, rabbit, fish, lion, and frog.

With the conquests of Alexander the Great and the subsequent establishment of Indo-Greek kingdoms, Greek money spread to India. Researches have shown that there existed one or two mints in Bactria, one in Paropamisus, one in Gandhara (q.v.), one in Margiana, one in Taxila, and two or three others in Indian kingdoms. From the Bactrian coinage are directly

descended all Oriental coins that bear the name, title, and effigy of the sovereign. J. de Morgan says that this custom was a source of astonishment to the first Chinese who came into contact with the Parthians. However, the influence of these coins was rather restricted. They did not affect the stylistic development of the Gandhara school. The coin engravers must thus have constituted an isolated group.

The last Greek king of Bactria was Heliokles (160–120 B.C.), who, as has already been mentioned, issued two sets of coins, one for Bactria and one for India, with considerably different portraits in each case. It was toward the end of his reign that the nomad tribes known as the Sakas (Sacae) invaded Bactria. They pushed on into India in 25 B.C. in the reign of Hermaios. The most interesting personality among this succession of kings was Menander or Melinda, who is praised both in Buddhist texts and by Plutarch. He issued numerous silver coins, many of which have been found in the neighborhoods of Kabul, Jalalabad, Peshawar, and Mathura. They bear the Buddhist emblems of the rose and the book, and the title "Soter" is inscribed on them in Greek characters.

Under the pressure of the Yüeh-chih the Sakas moved south about 130 B.C. and eventually established a kingdom that included Gandhara and Swat. Its first king was Maues, who died in A.D. 58. His coins, which bear Greek inscriptions, are superior in style to those of Hermaios, Zoilos, and Nikias. They are made of copper and bear an elephant's head, a horse, a bow in its sheath in a purely Arsacid style, Nike standing, a zebu, a lion, Herakles on horseback, and Zeus. Maues was succeeded by Azes, who is represented frontally, enthroned in state, holding the ankus, and by Azilises, Vonones, Spalisises, Heraios, diademed and with long hair, and Hyrkodes. They were followed by a dynasty whose rulers bore Parthian names. Maues and Azes had extended their rule to the Punjab, but under Mithradates II (123–88 B.C.) Parthian sovereignty had been recognized and a Parthian dynasty replaced the Sakas. Gondophares succeeded in freeing himself from this domination in 20 B.C. Many of his coins have been found at Begram. They are Arsacid in type, and the king is described in Greek as "autokrator." The coins of his successors show various influences. Those of Pakores (in Prakrit: Pakora) clearly show a Persian influence. They bear inscriptions in Aramaic characters, while the Greek inscriptions become shorter. The coins of Sanaberes and Orthagnes show similar influences. The coinage of Heraios shows mixed origins and seems to be related to that of Hyrkodes.

The Indo-Scythians, Sakas, and Indo-Parthians clearly drew their inspiration from Bactrian coins. They took over the traditional types — Zeus, the Dioskouroi, Herakles, Apollo, Artemis, Tyche, and Nike. Under Maues, Poseidon makes his appearance and, under Gondophares, turns into Śiva. Other figures are a bacchante between two shrubs, Hermes with his wand, and, during the reigns of Azes and Azilises, Hephaistos, one of the 33 gods also found on the coins of Kanishka.

Thus Indo-Scythian money draws on various sources for its subjects. Indian types begin to appear among them. An Indian dancing girl with long earrings and Oriental trousers can be seen on the coins of Pantaleon and Agathokles, Śiva (or Poseidon) on those of Gondophares, and Pārvatī, the wife of Śiva, or Lakṣmī, goddess of fortune, on those of Azes. Non-Greek or hybrid elements are frequent: a figure of a radiate sun, standing, holding a scepter, under Philoxenos and Telephos, and the head of a divinity wearing a radiate Phrygian cap, under Amyntas and Hermaios; in the reign of Maues, Tyche holding a patera and a wheel (the types are Greek but the style is barbarian), Artemis, radiate, with a veil floating around her head, a draped goddess with a crescent on her head, standing between two stars, Zeus seated and holding a human figure symbolizing the thunderbolt, and a nymph and a maenad holding two vinestalks. We may see in these examples the labors of a genuine school of art, in which the Greek teachers were able, not without great efforts, to impose a tradition and maintain their standards.

*The Kushans.* The pressure exerted by other nomads on the Yüeh-chih and the constant shifts in the political balance led to the creation of an empire that was to endure from the middle of the 1st century to the end of the 4th. It was called "Kushan," after the name of the tribe that eventually prevailed over the others. The Greek kings stood firm, however, until Hermaios concluded an alliance with the invaders, as the coins of the first great Kushan leader, Kujula Kadphises, which bear on the reverse the name Hermaios, would seem to confirm.

The most remarkable of the royal coins are those of Wima Kadphises, son of Kujula. He wears a helmet with diadem and is shown frontally seated on his throne; he holds a branch in his right hand and has his feet on a footstool; flames burst from his shoulders. On the reverse Śiva, fullface, holds a trident; his left arm is draped and flames spring from his head; in the middle distance is a zebu. Other types are the king's bust emerging from clouds, wearing a chlamys in the Greek style, and the king standing and sacrificing on the altar. The coins of Kanishka are thinner and of a less refined style. They represent Mithra diademed, Nanaia with a halo, or Buddha standing facing frontward. Huvishka's coins (PL. 400) show his bust, diademed and with a halo; he wears a conical helmet and a coat of mail, and is holding an ear of grain and a spear. On the reverse is Hephaistos, standing with a hammer and tongs. On the coins of Basodes or Vasudeva, the king stands before an altar, helmeted and with a halo, holding a sword and wearing a flared gown and pleated trousers. On the reverse Śiva is standing facing frontward and holds a crown and trident; in the middle distance is a zebu (PL. 400). Other types are the sun god, a goddess with a horn of plenty, Herakles, a divinity (Mahāsena) wearing a chlamys and holding a banner, a moon goddess fullface seated on a throne or sometimes standing, and the king riding an elephant.

The reverse of the royal effigies thus bear many types relating to various mythologies and representing the art of different nations. The Greco-Roman types depict a radiate sun god holding his scepter, the moon god, or a goddess holding a scepter ending in the figure of a horse — all these with Greek inscriptions: ΗΛΙΟC, CΗΛΗΝΗ, ΝΑΝΑΙΑ, ΗΡΑΚΙΛΟ (Herakles), ΡΑΟ-PHOPO (Ares), ΡΙΟΜ (Rome or Pallas), CΑΡΑΠΟ (Serapis), ΩPON (Uranos). The Persian types are represented by the god of fire ΑΘΡΟ (Hephaistos), the sun god ΑΡΑΕΙΧΡΟ, the horseman god ΑΡΟΟΑCΓΟ, the moon god ΜΑΝΑΟΒΑΓΟ, the god of running wind, or the god of war. Hindu figures include a female divinity, comparable to the Greek Tyche, holding a horn of plenty, ΑΡΔΟΧΡΟ, Ardhaugra or Pārvatī, or Ashis, or Lakṣmī; the god of war ΜΑΑΧΝΟ; Śiva holding a trident, or standing on a bull, his hair shaped like shells, or holding a vase, a thunderbolt, or a goat, sometimes shown with three faces; the armed divinities CΚΑΝΔΟ, ΚΟΜΑΡΟ, ΒΙΖΑΓΟ; Buddha standing and preaching or seated with his legs crossed, ΒΟΔΔΟ, ΟΔΥΟΒΟΥ, CΑΚΑΜΑ, ΓΟ ΒΟΥΔΟ.

The coins known as "Kushano-Sassanian" are similar, but they were struck on a very wide flan and their execution became ever more schematic and linear.

The Andhra dynasty in the 3d century B.C. coined money with representations of elephants or lions or with simple floral designs. The Traikutaka or Bodhi dynasty did the same, but their currencies are of no artistic interest. The Ksatrapas of the West in the 2d century B.C. were commemorated by portraits in profile in a Western style.

*The Guptas.* Much more important are the Guptas, who ruled in India from the first quarter of the 4th century in our era until A.D. 600. The Gupta era dates from the time of Candragupta (320–21), whose reign marks the beginning of a long series of coins (PL. 400).

Candragupta's coins are struck on thick globular flans and the types represent a javelin or a banner, the emblem of Viṣṇu. This sacred banner is surmounted by Garuḍa (half man, half bird), who served as a vehicle for the god. These motifs, derived from those of the Kushans, also include the king with a halo, standing and throwing incense on an altar; on the reverse is the goddess Lakṣmī, shown frontally and seated on a throne, with her feet on a lotus. Other types represent an archer, a war ax, Candragupta with Kumaradevi, to whom the king

offers a nuptial ring. On bronze coins the reverse shows Garuḍa with wings outspread, and the obverse has a bust of the king. Similar themes are found in the reign of Kumaragupta. With the Guptas, Greek and all traces of Greek culture disappear. The inscription are in a debased form of Sanskrit or Pali, which points to some kind of Hindu revival. Among coins worth noting are those showing Buddha seated in the European manner, in the same royal attitude as the Sassanian and Kushan kings. This civilization flourished until the invasion of the White Huns, or Ephthalites, in the 5th or 6th century. About 500 the coins of these barbarians show King Toromana, beardless but with a mustache, wearing a necklace and a fine embroidered headdress. A border of pearls encircles the portrait, which is a crude copy of Sassanian coins.

*The Mongols.* Among the coins that show traces of the Mongolian invasions, only a few are of artistic interest. From the 13th century onward we note the coins of Turakina, daughter-in-law of Genghis Khan, who was regent from 1241 to 1246, those of the Great Khans (1304–10), and those of the Mongols of Persia in the 13th century.

*The Moghuls.* The sets of coins that begin with Akbar (1556–1605) show the Hindu deities Rāma and Sītā, the latter with two other persons, and also animals, a falcon and a duck. An archer followed by a woman recalls the submission of the king of Bijapur, whose daughter was affianced to Prince Danigal. This coinage is very complex and comprises round and square coins as well as some mihrab-shaped ones. The emperor's effigy does not appear, except on what may be described as genuine medals, which show him holding a book, a fruit, or a goblet; a lion passant is on the reverse. These medals mark the beginning of what has been termed "Bacchanalian coins," for they allude without the slightest reticence, in fact, ostentatiously, to a marked addiction to drink on the part of Akbar and the enlightened despots who succeeded him.

The gold money of Jahangir (PL. 400) provides a picturesque series of vignettes. The emperor is shown wearing a turban with a plume and, like his predecessor, holding a goblet. On other coins he is seated on his throne, his legs crossed, a halo around his head. On the reverse are a lion and a sun. It has been said that this type shows the influence of a Christian painting, which, as has already been shown, would be in keeping with the cultivated artistic tastes of the Moghul court. According to a tradition that may be legendary, the emperor's favorite took advantage of the influence she exerted over him to have coins struck in her own name, with on the reverse one of the signs of the zodiac, Sagittarius, flanked by a tree, a stool with fringes, and a six-tiered minaret. This report does not tally with the following passage in Jahangir's *Memoirs*: "The rule of coinage was that on one face of the metal they stamped my name, and on the reverse the name of the place, and the month and year of the reign. At this time it entered my mind that in place of the month they should substitute the figure of the constellation which belonged to that month; for instance, in the month of Farwardin the figure of a ram, and in Urdibihisht the figure of a bull. Similarly, in each month that a coin was struck, the figure of the constellation was to be on one face, as if the sun were emerging from it. This innovation is my own; such a practice has never been followed until now." This is a valuable piece of evidence, showing the interest taken by the sovereign in his coins, which he does not regard merely as currency, but as works of art as well, designed to interest the people.

To this "innovation" we owe the splendid series of zodiacal gold coins struck over a period of eight years. The mint was at Agra, and Western engravers must have been called on to work there; they introduced into the designs of the delicate vignettes rhythms sometimes fairly close to those of the Renaissance (PL. 400). The coins enjoyed great popularity and were kept as jewels or talismans. For this reason many imitations of them were made for a long time after, and the number of such "false" coins is very numerous.

Among Jahangir's successors was Shah Jahan, who does

not seem to have taken as great an interest in coinage. As for Aurangzeb's coinage, which was succeeded by the coins of the great English and French companies, it is of no special interest to the art historian.

*Arab coins.* The Koranic law that forbade the representation of human and animal figures and consequently did not tolerate the art of portraiture was observed more or less strictly by believers. It is therefore remarkable that when Constantinople was taken by the Turks in 1453 the Italian medallists Matteo de' Pasti, Costanzo, and Gentile Bellini were summoned to the court of Mohammed II to portray the conqueror's features. In general, however, though Arab coins may invite study of the details of their calligraphy, which certainly has decorative qualities, they have little or nothing to do with the representational arts. They consist of thin disks, on which are inscribed passages from the suras of the Koran, with indications of where and during what reign they were struck. The influence of neighboring civilizations must not be lost sight of, however; the coinage of these civilizations was often imitated immediately after the Islamic invasions. Thus the dinars struck from the 7th century onward were copied from Byzantine coins. They show types of Justin II and Sophia, or of Heraclius, or representations of the standing caliph. At the same time silver coins of Sassanian type imitating the coins of Khosrau made their appearance. As regards genuine Islamic coins, the oldest are dirhems issued in the period 695–700. This coinage of the caliphs, because of its purely graphic character, falls almost entirely outside the scope of this article. As a result of the Arab conquests it spread as far as Spain, to the kingdom of Granada, in the 14th century, and to Morocco from the 14th to the 17th century.

*The Turkoman dynasties.* The remarks on Islamic coins apply also to the coinage of the Turkoman dynasties — the Seljuks (see SELJUK ART) in the 11th century; the Danishmends at the time of the first crusades, some of whose coins, however, do show a representational motif: a horseman with a lion; the Zengids; and the Ortokids. These last, whose dynasty was founded by Urtuk in 1084, struck dirhems which, despite the prescription of the Koran, and as a result of Seleucid, Sassanian, or Byzantine influences, depict two busts facing away from each other, a bust fullface, an archer, a horseman, a double-headed eagle, even a Christian representation of the Virgin with the name Emmanuel in Greek. The Atabeks of the Artal borrowed their monetary types from the Byzantines or from classical antiquity. In Turkey only some fine gold coins of the 17th and 18th centuries are worth noting. They show fine, elegant inscriptions carefully executed. Gold medals of a similar kind were struck in the 18th century.

*The Far East.* In China the use of some kind of money seems to go back to remote antiquity. Bronze spade-shaped coins, covered with ancient character writing (PL. 416), were reputed to be already in circulation during the reign of the legendary Emperor Yü (traditionally ascribed to the 3d millennium B.C.). These mark the beginnings of Chinese coinage. Coins took the shape of various implements and articles; trouser-coins and bells are examples. During the Chou dynasty (1027–256 B.C.) knife-money, *ch'i tao*, made its appearance. Later the ring at the end of the knife handle was separated from it and became the "cash," or "sapek," a coin pierced with a square hole (544–519 B.C.). Coins of this kind were cast during the Ch'in (221–206 B.C.) and the Han (206 B.C.–A.D. 221) dynasties, and the cash was a common coin in China until the 20th century. Chinese coins reflect other Chinese art in the casting technique, in the form of the characters used, and in their refined floral patterns. After the introduction of the dollar, or yuan, the god of longevity, shown frontally, and the dragon appeared on dollar coins. The republican coins, with portraits of Sun Yat-sen, Yüan Shih-k'ai, and other presidents of the Republic, are entirely Western in inspiration.

In Siam currency as we know it has existed only since the 13th century. It consisted, until the reign of King Rama IV

(1851–68), of doubled-up and sheared silver bars, without any engraving. Bracelets also served as currency, as in the primitive Western civilizations. It would seem that fish-shaped silver ingots were used as currency in the remote past. The nature of the currency was affected by the belief that the king's portrait must not be reproduced. This taboo remained in force until the reign of Rama V, who, in 1880, caused coins to be struck bearing his effigy in the European manner.

Among the Khmers, who established themselves in Siam about A.D. 1000, coins did not appear until the 16th century; these first coins consisted merely of oblong ingots bearing various marks. The Chinese ambassador Chou Ta-kuen, traveling in Siam at the end of the 13th century, wrote: "Payments for small transactions are made in rice, grain, Chinese articles, and cloth. Only in the more important business transactions is payment made in gold and silver."

In Japan, as in Tibet, Annam, or Korea, coins have little artistic significance. The coins known as *o-ban* issued from 1591 to 1838 were thin oval plates of gold covered with characters written with a brush. They also bore embossed seals with ornamental floral patterns. During the first years of the Meiji era, in 1870, 20-yen gold pieces were issued, showing a dragon or the rising sun surrounded by a garland of flowers.

There is little point in dwelling on the modern coinages of the Middle or Far Eastern nations that adopted European culture during the 19th century or at the beginning of the 20th century. The general trend is well exemplified by issues of coins that are no longer based on the old native traditions. Not only is the striking mechanism, like other technical inventions, borrowed from the West, but the types of the coins — the portraits and allegories — are modeled on a European art that has made its influence felt along with other aspects of European life. Thus the Negus of Ethiopia, Menelik (1889–1913), had his silver talers struck by the Paris mint and his portrait executed by the engraver Chaplain. The shah of Persia Nasr-ed-Din (1884–96), King Fuad I of Egypt (1917–36), the emperor of Japan Mutsuhito (Meiji) (1867–1912) similarly had their coinage executed abroad. The political evolution of these countries is thus closely reflected in their coinage, but the art historian finds little evidence of any original artistic expression.

Jean BABELON

NOTE: There is no consensus on the chronology of rulers of the ancient East. The dates given here may differ from those employed by other authorities.

MEDIEVAL COINS. Medieval coins may be divided into two broad periods separated by Charlemagne's monetary reform, which effected a complete break with ancient tradition for the greater part of western Europe and inaugurated a truly medieval coinage. Byzantine currency, on the other hand, was heir and successor to imperial Rome and stands apart from the evolution in the West. Its development and individual character were determined by political, economic, and religious forces in the empire.

*Barbarian states (5th–7th cent.).* Coins issued by the barbarian states in the provinces of the Western Roman Empire developed progressively, although not in a single direction, along the lines established by Roman coins. The evolution is particularly evident in Italy, where influences from the Eastern Empire were stronger, but it can also be seen in the coinage of the Visigoths and Franks in Spain and France. Types, weights, and denominations follow the Roman tradition established through the Constantinian reform.

The Heruli in Italy, and later the Goths, coined gold pieces designated as the "solidus" and the "tremissis" with the name and the image of the Eastern emperor. These coins were minted chiefly in Rome and Ravenna, less frequently in Milan and Pavia. The images are traditional ones: on the solidus a Victory holding the cross; on the tremissis the cross or Victory on a globe with a crown and the orb and cross. Bronze coins, as well as fractions of the siliqua, were also minted in the name of the Eastern emperor. By far the most important innovation,

appearing on some small silver coins of Odoacer and destined to be more widely accepted later, is the appearance of the portrait and the name of the local ruler on the obverse and of his monogram on the reverse. The most outstanding piece of this period is the gold medal of Theodoric (Rome, Mus. Naz. Romano) coined probably in A.D. 500 at the mint in Rome on the occasion of his visit to the capital. The bust of the king wearing the Roman lorica and paludamentum appears on the obverse, his right hand raised and his left hand holding a figure of Victory on a globe. On the reverse is represented Victory poised on a globe with a crown and palm branch. This is the earliest representation of a barbarian king on a gold piece, but it is a commemorative medal, not a coin in the strict sense of the term. It is unique among prevailing standardized emblems on contemporary currency, and may be linked to the finest tradition of Roman medals, for it adopts their weight and module. Exceptional for its expressive power, the medal is the most significant piece produced in Theodoric's reign and, indeed, of the entire coinage of the barbarian kings in this period.

Likewise distinct from current coinage in the choice of a portrait of a Gothic king is an issue of bronze coins by Theodat (534–36), probably minted in Rome in 536. These show on the obverse the profile bust of Theodat wearing a jeweled crown, and on the reverse a Victory on the prow of a ship with crown and palm branch (PL. 406). The head of a Goth appears for the last time before the end of Gothic rule on the demisiliquas and bronze coins of Baduila (Totila; 541–42). These show the bust in frontal or profile view as well as the king's name on the obverse. The reverse repeats the king's name or shows a standing warrior holding a staff and leaning on a shield. The latter emblem is found on bronze coins and on some copper coins of Athalaric. The mints in Rome and Ravenna issued an almost autonomous coinage during the period of Theodoric and Athalaric, the images consisting of the bust of Roma wearing a helmet and the inscription INVICTA ROMA, and of the bust with the mural crown of Ravenna and the inscription FELIX RAVENNA. Characteristic Roman figures of Victory with crown and palm branch, the eagle, the she-wolf and twins, etc., are used on the reverse of these coins.

After a brief period of Byzantine rule, the Lombards, successors to the Goths in Italy, produced imitations of Byzantine currency in their first coinage of the 6th–7th century. These were chiefly in gold, and the tremissis was the only denomination struck. With the reign of Cunipert (687–700) the last traces of the Eastern emperor's name, by now reduced to illegible letters, disappeared. On these coins, minted at Pavia, the profile bust of the king and his name are retained on the obverse, but the new image of St. Michael is used on the reverse. Indeed, the figure of St. Michael standing with shield and cross is a final transformation of the Roman Victory. The coins of Desiderius (756–74), last of the Lombard kings, are adorned simply with inscriptions and were produced by as many as eight mints. An autonomous coinage, which eliminated the king's name and bore instead only the name of the mint, made its appearance in the 8th century. When the Franks overthrew the Lombard kingdom in the north, the dukes of Benevento continued to issue the solidus in the name of the Eastern emperor (on the obverse the cross on steps), until Grimoald III (662–71) placed his name and image on the reverse.

The Burgundians and Franks coined imitations of imperial Roman currency in gold and silver during the second half of the 5th century, but Burgundian coinage terminated in 534 when the kingdom was destroyed by the Franks. The head and name of a barbarian king appeared for the first time on gold coinage (it will be remembered that the medal of Theodoric was not currency) when Theodebert I became king of the Franks (534–48). The new image was considered so revolutionary that it was mentioned by Procopius (*De Bello Gothico*, III, 33). As on Roman imperial coins, the bust of the king, placed frontally, was represented with helmet and lorica, staff and shield (PL. 409). Images on the reverse include Victory with a cross and the orb and cross, or the king with palm branch and crown trampling on a figure representing the enemy.

Imitations of Byzantine coins continued to be minted in southern France after the time of Theodebert, and the name of the Eastern emperor was retained through the reign of Phocas. Ecclesiastic currency began in the mid-6th century with coins minted by churches and monasteries in their own name or that of the bishop or abbot. At this time the minter's name was added to coins. As minters gradually became more numerous, they coined under their own name and the inscriptions included the name of the mint. The sovereign's name became increasingly rare in the 8th century; with Pepin's reign it ceased to be used. The denomination coined most frequently was the gold tremissis. Merovingian coins of the late 6th century began to dispense with representations of Victory, replacing it with the Byzantine emblems of the potent (Jerusalem) cross surmounting an orb or raised on three steps.

The Suevians in Spain coined imitations of the 5th-century Roman imperial solidus and tremissis, the obverse bearing the emblem of a cross and a crown. The Visigoths imitated the Byzantine trientes issued between Anastasius I and Justin II, with the figure of Victory on the reverse. Leovigild (ca. 569–86) was the first to put his effigy and name on the trientes. The early effigies were in profile; later the frontal bust became predominant and was repeated on the reverse. Seventh-century coins of some kingdoms present two facing busts. During the reign of Leovigild the figure of Victory on the reverse was replaced by the Byzantine image of the cross on steps. Images on the Visigothic trientes are characterized by extreme schematization, but the individual style of various mints is clearly recognizable.

Coins imitating Roman bronze pieces continued to be struck in England after the end of Roman domination, in the first half of the 5th century. Under Merovingian influence gold coinage was first minted in the late 6th century; the images imitated Frankish or Roman types and the denomination was generally the tremissis. These coins were minted until the late 7th century, when they were completely replaced by silver ones. Silver currency had not diminished even in the preceding period, and it is clear that the Anglo-Saxons were the only people who used silver from the beginning. The small silver coin called the "sceat" shows a wide variety of types. The she-wolf and twins and the two prisoners under the labarum are clearly derived from Roman coins, but the use of geometric designs on other coins is distinctly original. Names of sovereigns first appeared on coins about 650. A small copper coin called the "styca" was minted contemporaneously with silver currency.

*Coins of the Carolingian period.* Charlemagne's monetary reform was the first major attempt to establish a uniform coinage in western Europe, and although it proved to be of short duration, the principles underlying it influenced European coinage for a long time. The principal changes were the abolition of gold currency (introduced by Pepin) and a new monetary system, based on a heavier denarius, with 12 denarii to the solidus and 20 solidi (240 denarii) to the libra, whose weight was increased. The libra and solidus were moneys of account that had not been minted for centuries.

In France, gold currency had gradually diminished by the first half of the 8th century, while silver coinage had constantly increased. Pepin had abolished gold coinage altogether and replaced it with silver (which was never very abundant, however) and suppressed the name of the coiner. After conquering the Lombards, Charlemagne immediately began to coin silver denarii and gold solidi of the Lombard type in Italian mints, but having put the conquered territories on a firm foundation, he extended the abolition of gold coinage to Italy, probably in 781 with the Capitulary of Mantua. A few years later he introduced the "heavy denarius" throughout the empire. The type of the new coin, like that of its predecessor, consisted exclusively of inscriptions. After Charlemagne's coronation in 800, denarii were coined with his bust on the obverse. Following Roman models, the coins show the emperor wearing a laurel wreath and paludamentum, and they bear the inscription IMP AUG REX. On the obverse is represented a temple with a cross in the center and the inscription XPICTIANA RELIGIO, an

emblem that prevails on coins of Charlemagne's successors (PL. 409). Some extremely rare pieces coined in the mints at Arles, Lyons, Rouen, and Trier show the city gate and the name of the mint on the reverse. Coins minted at Dorestad (Holland) are decorated with a ship.

The reform did not affect southern Italy and Sicily, where Carolingian innovations were ignored by the Lombard dukes of Benevento and the Byzantines, and later by the Arabs and Normans. The discontinuation of gold currency does not mean that gold no longer circulated in the Carolingian empire and western Europe in general. To all intents and purposes, gold coins were not minted for several centuries, but some rare coins from the mint at Uzès are known from Charlemagne's reign, as are some examples of the gold solidus minted by Louis I. The solidi show on the obverse a profile bust of the emperor wearing paludamentum and laurel wreath, and the inscription MUNUS DIVINUM around a cross and crown on the reverse. However, foreign gold currency such as the Arab dinar and the Byzantine solidus was always in circulation, and gold coinage was minted regularly in southern Italy and Spain.

After Charlemagne's death the general principles of the reform prevailed for many centuries, continuing to influence various national coinages. But the strong centralization, which was a salient characteristic of Charlemagne's reform, did not survive long after his death. The denarius was the prevailing coin. Its types consist of either inscriptions (some very fine in technique and carefully arranged within the field) or temple façades, the latter persisting in Italy until the mid-10th century. Profile heads on coins were revived only during the reign of Louis I (814–40), and were used sporadically on the currency of Lothair and Louis IV. Special emphasis began to be given to the name of the mint, and, in some cases, it was the only element on one side of the coin. Louis I inaugurated a large, thin form of the denarius, characteristic of the post-Carolingian period, but its types lack the clarity and regularity of coins of normal module.

*Post-Carolingian Europe. a. Italy.* The practice of issuing papal coins, known as *antiquiores*, was begun by Adrian I (772–95) and continued until the mid-11th century. With few exceptions, the coins minted by Leo III (795–816) and his successors included also the name of the emperor. The frontal bust of St. Peter, and occasionally that of the pope, is presented rather schematically on some coins (PL. 406). Coinage of the 9th to the mid-13th century in central and northern Italy and in western Europe generally constitutes a logical development of the system and types introduced by the Carolingian reform.

In southern Italy we note the survival of Byzantine forms and images as well as influences from new Arab coins. In addition to the Byzantine type of frontal bust for dukes or princes and, chiefly on gold coins, the potent cross on steps, the images include figures of saints: St. Januarius with nimbus and Gospel book on bronze coins of the 8th–9th century from Naples; St. Maximus on the coin designated as the *follaro*, minted in the 9th century at the monastery of Casamabile; St. Erasmus on coins of Marinus II of Gaeta (978–84); St. Peter on follari coined by the dukes of Salerno Pandulfus I, prince of Capua, and his son, Pandulfus II (978–81). One of the earliest representations of the Virgin — frontal bust or standing figure with hands raised and head covered by a coif — appears on follari coined by the dukes of Salerno. The frontal bust of the Redeemer with cruciform halo appears on coins at this time, and a century later it was used by Roger Borsa (1085–1111) on a follaro minted at Brindisi. The archangel Michael in a frontal posture holding the orb and cross and the staff, is portrayed on the solidus of Sigo I coined at Benevento (PL. 406) and on 10th-century follari from Salerno. A schematic image of the city's fortifications is represented on some coins and reappears on a follaro of Gisulf I (946–77). Byzantine coins in gold and bronze were issued in Sicily until the early 9th century, when the island was conquered by the Arabs. After the conquest the aniconic gold taro was first coined and was extensively imitated in southern Italy and later by the Normans in Sicily.

Italy in the 12th century witnessed the growth of a new political system, the commune, which had noteworthy repercussions on coinage. After a long struggle with the empire to gain autonomy, the communes were officially recognized at the Peace of Constance (1183), which, however, preserved certain imperial prerogatives. As a result, numerous mints were established in the late 12th and early 13th centuries under communal and episcopal authority; many of these mints had already received the privilege of coinage from the German emperors Conrad II (1024–39) and Henry IV (1056–1106). Prior to the Carolingian period only the four mints at Milan, Pavia, Verona, and Lucca operated almost uninterruptedly under the imperial name. Their coins still carried the name of the emperor in the late 12th century, but this formality was subsequently abandoned. Except in rare instances, the types on coins of the new mints were purely epigraphic. The coins of Frederick II at Bergamo represent the bust of the emperor and a building with cupola and towers (PL. 406). A coin from Trieste bears the figure of a bishop seated frontally, holding the crosier and book; on another, St. Justus stands holding a palm branch. Coins from Aquileia portray the bishop of the patriarchal see enthroned and holding the cross.

Doge Enrico Dandolo of Venice (1192–1205) coined for the first time the *denaro grosso*, a silver coin that is heavier than the ordinary denarius and reflects the growth of trade and commerce. The new coin (also called *matapan*, perhaps because the silver was extracted from the mines of Cape Matapan in Greece) represents on the obverse a standing figure of St. Mark giving the gonfalon to the doge, and Christ enthroned frontally on the reverse (PL. 407). The grosso was imitated by mints in northern Italy (Acqui, Chivasso, Incisa, etc.) and eastern Europe (Serbia, Bosnia, Bulgaria), and was coined in the principal cities of Italy from the 12th through the 14th century. Interest in the new coin spread to other countries of Europe, and in 1266 Louis IX of France coined the *gros tournois*.

As the field of currency began to expand, new images were created, the predominant ones being figures of patron saints of cities. Many full-length figures are represented in the usual frontal posture, holding the crosier and the right hand blessing; enthroned figures and busts also occur. Among the better-known patron saints and other figures associated with particular cities are St. Ambrose of Milan (PL. 407); St. Cyrus of Pavia; St. Petronius of Bologna; St. Gaudentius of Rimini; St. Cyriacus of Ancona; the Virgin and Child for Pisa (PL. 407); the Holy Face for Lucca. Coins of Mantua show the standing figures of St. Peter and the bishop or Vergil enthroned (PL. 407); those of Volterra, a bishop standing and blessing; Roman coins (*grossi senatoriali*), the goddess Roma enthroned frontally; the gros of Avignon, the pope enthroned and blessing. The imperial eagle with wings outspread is common on the *grosso aquilino* from the mints at Ivrea, Como, Vicenza, Merano, etc.

The Normans in southern Italy and Sicily coined the taro in imitation of the Arab coin, using Kufic inscriptions on the early pieces, and ultimately adopting the cross and the inscription IC XC-NIKA. More complex images were used on bronze and silver coins as well as on the *doppio follaro*. An equestrian figure of Roger I (1072–1101) holding a standard is represented on the obverse of a doppio follaro from the mint at Mileto; the Virgin with Child enthroned appears on the reverse (PL. 406). A *trifollaro* of William I (1111–27) from the mint at Salerno has an equestrian figure of the king brandishing a sword on the obverse and a frontal full-length figure of St. Peter on the reverse. On the obverse of the silver *ducale* of Roger II (1130–54), coined at Palermo on the occasion of the tenth anniversary of his investiture as king of Sicily, the sovereign holds a double cross and stands with his son; the bust of the Redeemer appears on the reverse (PL. 406).

A coin that may be associated with imperial Rome and is distinct from all contemporary coinage, not only in style and configuration but also in weight and purity, is the augusta (a denomination mentioned in medieval sources) coined by Frederick II at the mints in Brindisi and Messina beginning in 1231. On the obverse is the bust of the king wearing palu-

damentum and laurel wreath, and the inscription CESAR AUG IMP ROM; on the reverse, an eagle with outspread wings and the inscription FRIDERICUS (PL. 407). The augustals lasted at least until the fall of the Hohenstaufen dynasty in 1266 and, judging from their great fame, may have been coined after that date. In 1266 Charles I of Anjou replaced the augustal with the real of Barletta, a coin that was identical to the former in weight and purity but now bore the bust of the king wearing the imperial crown and paludamentum on the obverse, and the Angevin coat of arms on the reverse (PL. 407). These coins were struck until 1278, when Charles I reopened the mint at Naples and initiated the coinage of the *saluto d'oro*. The Annunciation represented on the reverse of this coin was also adopted for the silver saluto (PL. 407). Charles II (1285–1309) coined the silver gigliato, which shows on the obverse the enthroned king fullface, holding the scepter and the orb and cross, and, on the reverse, the cross decorated with lilies.

The most significant change in the 13th century was the return to gold coinage in 1252 with the minting of the genovino in Genoa and the florin in Florence (PL. 407). Each had its distinctive type which remained unchanged for the duration of its coinage: a city gate and the cross for the genovino; a lily and the standing figure of St. John the Baptist holding the cross for the florin. In 1284 Venice coined the ducat, with the image of St. Mark presenting the gonfalon to the doge on the obverse, and the Redeemer in a star-studded *mandorla* on the reverse (PL. 407). The type, weight, and fineness of the Venetian ducat were preserved without change until the end of the Venetian Republic in 1797. These three gold coins of standard weight and fineness satisfied the need for gold currency, which was now generally demanded in the Western world. After 1252 other European countries attempted to produce gold coins, but a regular issue was not achieved until the 14th century. The florin and the ducat were circulated and extensively imitated throughout the medieval world, the former in France, Spain, Austria, Bohemia, and other countries of central Europe, and the latter in the Mediterranean area and in the Orient. Other cities in Italy followed the initiative of Florence and Genoa. Milan and Lucca coined imitations of the genovino and florin, as well as a gold coin with their own types; Rome coined the *ducato senatoriale*. These coins, and others issued by the dukes of Savoy, Bologna, Savona, Ancona, and Siena, anticipated the spendid series of Renaissance gold coins of the Italian seigniories.

*b. France.* Under the Capetian dynasty founded by Hugh Capet (987–96) the denarius and *obol* continued the Carolingian tradition of displaying the king's name, the mint, and the cross. Coins bearing the king's name were struck in the hereditary dominions of the dynasty or in cities outside them, but all have a distinctly local character. In addition to these, numerous issues were coined by lay and ecclesiastic feudatories, the greater number coming from the Abbey of St. Martin at Tours, which minted the *denier tournois* with a castle as emblem. When Philip II (1180–1223) took possession of the mint at Tours in 1205, he retained the type of the denier tournois. It and the royal coinage known as *monnaie parisis* now became the basis (in silver) of the monetary system. In 1266 Louis IX began an important reform in the French monetary system by coining the gros tournois and the gold écu. The emblem for the former was the traditional castle; the latter, a first attempt at a national gold coinage, without immediate consequences, however, was adorned by a shield embellished with lilies on the obverse, and on the reverse by a cross with flowers at each tip and lilies between the arms. Louis IX circulated the royal coinage throughout his domain, but imposed various restrictions, subsequently adopted by his successors. Rights of coinage were allowed the feudal lords, but circulation of the currency was limited to the territories of the lord who had issued it.

With the reign of Philip IV (1285–1314) a regular issue of gold coinage was inaugurated. The obverse shows the king enthroned on a Roman chair, or on a Gothic throne, holding a lily and a scepter topped by a lily; or else the Lamb of God

with nimbus. The reverse has a cross with lilies projecting from each arm and other lilies between the arms, sometimes set in a quatrefoil (PL. 409). The coins of Charles IV (1322–28), which represent the king standing in a Gothic niche, are distinguished by their elegant Gothic style. Those coined under Philip VI (1328–50) constitute a supreme achievement in design and execution. On Philip's gold coins the throne is transformed into an elaborate architectural form with Gothic arches and pinnacles. In some instances the king, wearing the paludamentum and holding a scepter, is seated under a baldachin furnished with curtains and adorned with lilies. Other images on coins of this period include the archangel Michael crowned, standing on a dragon and leaning on a shield; St. George on horseback slaying the dragon. On the reverse is the cross richly decorated and adorned with flowers within a quatrefoil frame (PL. 409). A new image appears on the coins of John II (1350–64): the king in armor holding a sword on a galloping horse. Types of silver coins continue the tradition of the gros tournois, but during the reign of John II a gros was issued with the kind of lily used on the florin.

*c. Germany, Bohemia, and Hungary.* The Carolingian system based on the denarius and the use of epigraphic types continued in Germany after the death of Louis the Child (911) and the advent of the Saxon dynasty. Under the feudal organization of the 10th century numerous mints were opened which produced coins for lay and ecclesiastic nobles. Some mints, such as those of the dukes of Bavaria and the archbishops of Cologne, Trier, and Mainz, were active for many centuries. The variety and number of feudal coinages permit us to do no more than cite a few examples. The king's name on the coins is often accompanied by that of the noble or bishop. In addition to types consisting of inscriptions, there were representational ones, such as those of Carolingian derivation with the general lines of a church, or simply a cupola, on the denarii of Otto I (936–73) and his successors, and those representing the emperor, the feudal lord, or the bishop holding a crosier. Figures of saints also appear: St. Simon and St. Judah on coins minted at Goslar and imitated by other mints; St. Stephen kneeling, with his hand blessing; the Virgin; lions, eagles, etc.

The bracteate, widespread in mid-12th-century Germany, is one of the most characteristic and interesting manifestations of medieval coinage in the variety of its images, in its technique, and in the vivacity and spontaneity of a style that breaks with tradition. The larger field of the coin permitted images of a hitherto unknown richness and complexity: the stoning of St. Stephen or his entombment with two angels holding a medallion of the saint (Halberstadt); the martyrdom of St. Lawrence (Merseburg); the abbess Bertha kneeling before St. Eustace enthroned (Nordhausen); the busts of St. Martin and Bishop Henry, the one on the upper, the other on the lower half of the coins, separated by a semicircle symbolizing the city walls (Erfurt). Other types represent the abbot or abbess enthroned (PL. 408), a feudal lord in armor on horseback (PL. 408), a standing nobleman in civilian dress, a lord standing with his wife, or the emperor with the orb and cross and the lily (PL. 408).

The denarius continued to be minted along with the bracteate, but Louis IV (1314–47) and his nobles followed the example of Louis IX and also coined a grossus. The German grossus adopted the type of the French gros tournois for some coins, but also devised its own images of seated or standing bishops and enthroned lords. These coins were chiefly diffused in the regions of the Rhine and the Moselle and in Westphalia.

In Bohemia, Wenceslaus II (1278–1305) coined the grossus at Prague about 1300, adorning it with a crown and a rampant lion. It was imitated by the margraves of Meissen, who adopted the rampant lion and the cross in a quatrefoil. The Meissen coins, in turn, served as models for numerous coins of Saxony, Thuringia, Hessen, etc. The lion also appears on the grossus and double grossus of Flanders. Coinage of the grossus, with increasingly elaborate images, continued throughout the 14th century, but in the first half of the 14th century Germany also began to coin the gold piece called the *goldgulden*. The types

of the latter imitate those of the florin and, to a lesser extent, of French coins. A coin of Louis IV, for example, follows French prototypes in portraying the emperor enthroned frontally. Eventually, however, foreign images were replaced by coats of arms or figures of nobles, bishops, Christ, or saints, all of which were still used in the 15th century.

The earliest coins of Bohemia date from the time of Boleslav I (936–67), who coined a rather primitive form of the denarius and adopted the image of the church from German coins. The coins of his successors carry new images: the hand of God between A and Ω; the bust in profile or frontal view; St. Wenceslaus; the prince on horseback or standing. Greater precision in execution is apparent on coins of the early 12th century; the repertory of types was enriched and even included scenes with several figures. Bracteates were first coined by Ottokar I (1197–1230) and minted throughout the 13th century, with figures of a lion, of the prince seated or standing wearing a crown, etc. As mentioned above, Wenceslaus II coined a grossus that was diffused and imitated in central Europe. The image on the first gold coins issued by John of Luxemburg (1310–46) imitated the florin, but Charles IV (1347–78) adopted the images of the king enthroned and the lion; his successors preferred the figure of St. Wenceslaus.

Coinage in Hungary began under Stephen I (1000–1038). The cross was adopted for both sides of the first issue of the denarius and was retained for a long time. Under Solomon (1063–74) the figure of the king fullface standing with arms raised made its first appearance. The repertory of types, increased in the coins of Andrew II (1205–35), includes the king, the Lamb of God, buildings, etc. Béla IV (1235–70) and his son Stephen V coined copper pieces of Byzantine derivation with the two kings standing frontally on the obverse and the Virgin on the reverse. Charles Robert of Anjou (1308–42) introduced the grossus and gold currency into Hungary with images from the florin. At the end of the century his successors substituted the figure of St. Ladislas for that of St. John the Baptist, and the native saint remained on coins until Matthias Corvinus (1458–90) adopted the image of the Virgin.

*d. England.* Ethelbert II of Kent (748–62) and Offa of Mercia (757–96), probably following Carolingian examples, began their monetary reform with the introduction of the silver penny; a national English coinage may be said to have begun at this time. The broad flat flan and the fineness of the penny reflect Carolingian prototypes, but its images are distinctive: the earliest coins already have, besides inscriptions, usually on the reverse, profile and frontal busts on the obverse. On the reverse of a rare piece coined in Ethelbert's reign, the Roman she-wolf and twins are represented. Offa's coins adorned with the head of the king constitute a supreme achievement in Anglo-Saxon coinage of this period (PL. 409). In the 9th–10th century other images were introduced: the dove, the lamb, the hand of God, and buildings of various forms. Currency produced under the Danish kings is cruder in execution; the images of the sword, the dove, the hammer, etc., are reduced to a simple outline. The king wearing a helmet on the obverse and the cross on the reverse are standard images on coins minted during the reign of Ethelred II (978–1016). On a penny of Edward the Confessor (1042–66) the king is enthroned and holds a staff and the orb and cross (PL. 409). Coinage was not affected by the Norman conquest; images such as the bust of the king and the cross remained unchanged. A penny coined by Eustace Fitzjohn represents the baron on horseback brandishing a sword. Crosses of various types prevailed on the royal penny for a long time: the "short cross" beginning in 1180 and the "long cross," with arms extended to the edge, on coins minted in 1247 by Henry III (PL. 409). The long cross with three pellets in each angle was first used in 1279. Edward I (1272–1307) adopted it for the grossus that he introduced, and it persisted on silver coinage until the reign of Henry VII. In 1257 Henry III first coined the gold penny with the figure of the king enthroned frontally on the obverse. A second attempt to produce a gold coin met with greater success under

Edward III (1327–77), who introduced the noble, with the king in armor standing on a ship on the obverse (PL. 409). The noble remained the only gold coin until 1470, when Edward IV coined the gold angel with the archangel Michael slaying the dragon on the obverse, and a ship with a cross in front of the mast on the reverse.

*e. Spain.* The Arabs in Spain at first imitated local coins, as they had done in Syria and Africa. Once they were firmly established, and after a period of transition during which inscriptions on coins were bilingual, they issued a purely Arab coinage based on the gold dinar with epigraphic types. Silver denarii were coined by the Carolingians in the mints at Ampurias, Barcelona, and Gerona. Navarre under Sancho III (1000–1035) was the first Christian kingdom to have its own coinage. Subsequently, the kingdom of Castile and León in the reign of Alfonso VI (1072–1109) issued its own coins, as did Aragon under Sancho Ramírez I (1063–94). Among the first images of these issues were figures of the king, the cross, and the monogram of Christ; later the lion was adopted for the kingdom of León. In the late 12th and early 13th centuries the Christian kingdoms issued gold coins on the model of the gold piece struck by the Almoravides. Alfonso VIII of Castile was the first to do so in 1175 with a gold coin, the marabotin, whose weight and fineness were similar to the dinar's. Although the inscription on this coin is in Arabic, the image is Christian. About the same time, Ferdinand II of León (1157–88) coined gold pieces with a figure of himself crowned on the obverse and a lion on the reverse. Alfonso X of Castile and León (1252–84) coined the gold dobla, adorned with the tower of Castile and the lion, and the silver real, decorated with a tower. Gold coinage was first produced in Aragon under Pedro IV (1336–87; PL. 408), who issued an imitation of the florin, a coin that was continued by his successors. No important innovations in Spanish currency were made until the union of the kingdoms of Castile and Aragon under the Catholic kings.

*Byzantine coins.* The Roman coin tradition continued in Byzantium after the empire ceased to exist in the West. The general line of development remained stable for almost ten centuries, that is, until the conquest of Constantinople by the Turks. Strictly speaking, Byzantine coinage may be considered as beginning with the reform of Anastasius I (498), who introduced a new denomination in bronze. This coin carried the name of the mint and the value of the piece. Silver coins were rare. A large flat silver coin, the miliarensis, was first minted by Constantine (306–37). Justinian I added the regnal year in 538 — the first appearance of annual dating on European coinage. The most important denomination was the gold solidus, which maintained its fineness until about 1000. For centuries it dominated the markets of Europe and the Mediterranean area, at first alone and subsequently with the Arab dinar. Shortly after the year 1000 the gold coin, now called the "hyperper," acquired the greater size and concave form that appeared later in bronze and silver pieces (*nummi scyphati*).

Frontality and schematization are characteristic of the types, the majority of which are strongly influenced by religious concepts. The images appearing most frequently on the obverse are the frontal bust of the emperor wearing a helmet or a crown surmounted by the cross, the emperor full-length, crowned by the hand of God, and the emperor with his wife or children. Occasionally these images appear on the reverse. The emperor may hold the orb and cross, the cross, or the scepter, or both scepter and cross. In later examples he holds a banner. Figures of the empress are most infrequent. The Roman Victory holding a cross or an orb and cross is found on the reverse of coins under Justinian (527–65). Under Tiberius II (578–82) the potent cross, on an orb or on steps, appears alone, with an inscription referring to Victory. On the coins of Heraclius (610–41) a potent cross surmounting an orb is placed on steps (PL. 408); sometimes a cross is flanked by the standing figures of the emperor and his son. On coins of Justinian II (685–95) the bust of Christ is placed frontally, the hand raised in blessing (PL. 408). Discontinued during

the iconoclastic controversy, this type was revived under Michael III (842–67).

In posticonoclastic coins Christ and the Virgin are the prevailing images. Examples of the former include the enthroned Christ shown frontally, with cruciform halo, on coins from Basil I (867–86) until the end of the empire; Christ crowning the emperor, on coins of Romanus I (919–44), or standing between the emperor and empress and crowning them, on coins of Romanus IV Diogenes (1067–71); Christ fullface standing alone, on the coins of the empress Theodora (1055–56). The bust of the Virgin Orans first appears on the coins of Leo VI (886–912) and was used for several centuries. On some coins the bust of the Virgin is represented beside the emperor Nicephorus II Phocas (963–69); on those of John I Zimisces (969–76) she crowns the emperor. A full-length figure of the Virgin crowning the emperor appears on coins from the time of Romanus III Argyrus (1028–34) onward. Beginning with the coins of Michael VIII Palaeologus (1261–82) the bust of the Virgin Orans was placed above a bird's-eye view of Constantinople. On the coins of Theodora the Virgin stands beside the empress; on those of John I Zimisces the Virgin is shown half-length holding the Child in a medallion — an image that reappears on later coins. The Virgin is seated frontally and holding the medallion on coins of Alexius I Comnenus (1081–1118). Finally, the Virgin standing with the Child in her arms is found on a silver coin of Romanus IV Diogenes.

Saints are portrayed on coins of the 11th and 12th centuries: St. George in armor standing beside the emperor John II Comnenus (1118–43); St. Theodore and St. Demetrius with haloes and the emperor holding the cross or the labarum on coins of Manuel I Comnenus (1143–80); the archangel Michael standing beside the emperor Michael VI Stratioticus (1056–57); SS. Demetrius and Constantine and the emperor Alexius III Angelus (1195–1203) holding the cross.

EUROPEAN COINAGE FROM THE RENAISSANCE ONWARD. In contrast to the 15th-century coinage north of the Alps, which remained faithful to the pattern established in the preceding century, that of Italy witnessed a far-reaching esthetic transformation affecting both style and iconography. The changes in Italian coinage were conditioned not only by Humanist aspirations, also evident in the contemporary evolution of painting and sculpture, but by political developments in the Italian states. In the political sphere the development of centralized republican states (e.g., Genoa, Venice, Lucca, and until the establishment of the Medicean dukedom, Florence) was of prime importance. New coinages were introduced as well as new denominations — the testone and the gold ducat with its multiple, the double ducat, which, by enlarging the monetary field, permitted wider scope for the inventiveness of engravers.

This new burst of activity, occurring within a Humanist tradition, brought with it the reintroduction of the antique portrait, which had made only rare appearances in the intervening centuries. This innovation was most important from an artistic point of view, as it made possible the most beautiful of Italian coin types. Indeed, the century-long flowering that began in the mid-15th century was a golden age in the history of coinage, unrivaled outside Italy or in later periods.

Among the most significant examples are the portraits (PL. 410) of Gian Galeazzo and Ludovico Sforza ("Il Moro") of Milan, Ludovico di Saluzzo of Carmagnola, the Palaeologi of Casale Monferrato, the Gonzagas of Mantua, Giovanni II Bentivoglio of Antignate, Alfonso I of Ferrara, Popes Julius II and Leo X, and Ferrante of Aragon of Naples.

Coin portraits, and coins generally, display the same characteristics as medals, which were sometimes the work of top-ranking sculptors and painters. They are distinguished by a striving after ideal form and linear precision and an interest in psychologically revealing portraiture. The execution — by hand — was such as to make of the coins works of art in their own right. The coiners were often also goldsmiths, as were, for example, Emiliano Orfini of Foligno and Benvenuto Cellini (q.v.). The

same craftsmen who were specialists in engraving for coins worked on medals and cameos.

The designs for the reverse of coins were also noteworthy, both for their artistry and for the variety of their types. Engravers, taking advantage of the larger field now offered by coins, created new types outside the medieval repertory (which, with few exceptions, had consisted of coats of arms, eagles, figures of saints, etc.), such as the typically classical equestrian figure on a testone struck by Ercole I of Ferrara, the seated Samson on a testone of Alfonso I of Ferrara (PL. 410), the Jesus and the Pharisee on a two-sequin (zecchino) piece struck by the same Alfonso, the journey of the Magi on a two and one-half ducat piece struck by Leo X (PL. 412), etc. Thereafter, subjects taken from the Old and (more frequently) from the New Testament were introduced alongside the figures inspired by classical antiquity.

Between the mid-15th and mid-16th centuries artists famous for medals and other works also executed coins: Caradosso, who engraved the double ducats and testones of Ludovico il Moro and of Gian Galeazzo Sforza in Milan; Francesco Francia, who was in the service of Giovanni II Bentivoglio; Gianfrancesco Enzola, who worked for Ercole I of Ferrara; Benvenuto Cellini in the service of Clement VII in Rome; Leone Leoni, who designed the gold double ducat of Paul III, one of the finest coins of the period.

Franco PANVINI ROSATI

Outside Italy, in the 15th century, coinage was concentrated in the hands of royal governments in the large monarchies of France, England, and Castile. In central Europe, on the other hand, coining rights were firmly held by territorial princes. The circulating medium was composed of gold coins, which served the needs of governments and of international commerce, of rather small silver coins (not over 45–60 grains), and of a range of smaller denominations in silver or billon, restricted to local transactions. The most important gold coins were the French crown, with parallel coins of French origin in Spain and in the Low Countries; the English noble, the largest of existing gold coins; the west German gold gulden with its low fineness and variegated types (hardly to be recognized as derived from its Florentine prototype); and in eastern Germany and Hungary the ducat, always true to the purity of its Venetian model. All of them retained the thin flans and the low relief peculiar to the technique of hammered coinage. The usual designs, executed in sometimes crowded late Gothic style, showed the king enthroned or on horseback, patron saints, or coats of arms on the obverse, elaborate crosses on the reverse. Legends, or inscriptions, were universally in Latin; dates and indications of value were almost entirely lacking.

In the late 15th century the development of mining north of the Alps began to bring about important changes in the circulating medium. In 1486 the first heavy silver coin, of almost 450 grains, equal in value to the gold florin, was minted at Hall in Tirol (PL. 413). Saxony in 1500 and Joachimstal in Bohemia in 1519 followed suit; before 1525, all German principalities possessing silver mines were coining large silver coins, which took the name of *Joachimstaler* (in French, *Jocondales*), soon abbreviated to *Taler* (whence "dollar").

In the course of the century the German silver taler, assuming the role formerly reserved to gold coins in international transactions, spread to eastern and northern Europe, to the Netherlands, and, in restricted measure, to England. At the other end of western Europe, Spain developed independently another heavy silver coin, the peso or piece of eight reales, struck from the yield of American silver mines from 1540 onward.

With the introduction of large silver coins the clearcut separation between international gold coinage and local silver coinage came to an end. Both metals could serve the same purpose, and gold coins as well as heavy silver coins from all countries circulated all over Europe in quantities unheard of before, in response to the needs of an expanding economy and intensified commerce. It was only the small change, consisting of thin, heavily alloyed silver coins and, for the first

time, of large quantities of pure copper coins, that remained restricted in circulation.

The revolution in coinage posed new technical and artistic problems. The difficulty of working the broad, thick flans of modern coins with the traditional methods stimulated research in the mechanization of the process. In southern Germany various devices were thought out for replacing handcraft by machines for flattening the metal, cutting the flans, and impressing the dies by water power or horsepower. Traditionalism, however, and the defects of the new tools prevented their coming into general use. In France and in England machines were introduced for a short time, but soon had to be abandoned; only in some Spanish (Segovia) and Austrian (Hall) mints did mechanization become permanent in the last years of the 16th century.

The appearance of coins underwent a profound change in keeping with the artistic ideas of the Renaissance. The example of the Italian princes who had already in the preceding century put their individual portraits on coins was followed by almost all European countries. A profile portrait of the prince with a circular legend — well known from Roman coins, which were regarded with renewed interest and collected — became the standard type for all coins. It first appeared on French testons, as it had on their Italian predecessors and on the German talers. It spread in the course of the century to most silver coins as well as to gold and copper coins, with two exceptions: Spain adhered exclusively to heraldic designs, and the cities of the Holy Roman Empire had to content themselves with patron saints or coats of arms for lack of an individual prince. The reverse of the coins continued to show shields or crosses; allegorical scenes inspired by the reverses of Roman coins remained rare outside Italy. The designing of coins was often entrusted to well-known medalists, as the coins were considered an important display of sovereignty.

H. Enno VAN GELDER

In 16th-century Italy the appearance of large silver denominations following the German example — ducatoons (the earliest was issued in 1527), piasters, and scudi — was an important innovation (PL. 412). These coins, whose weight generally varied between 375 and 525 grains, were better adapted, because of their greater area, to the representation of more complex scenes, sometimes peopled with many figures. In the papal issues figures of saints, representations of monuments of Rome and other papal cities, scenes in which the pope appears (e.g., consistories and such sacred functions as the ceremony of opening and closing the Holy Door of St. Peter's), and scenes taken from the Gospels follow one another uninterruptedly for more than a century, not only on the silver scudo but also on its gold quadruples, which appeared in the early 17th century.

In several Italian states the evolution of coinage for the most part followed the pattern of papal coining. However, Venetian types retained St. Mark and the Doge; and Genoese types referring to the Door remained unvaried until 1637, when the Virgin and Child among clouds was substituted. None of these coinages achieved the richness and variety of type of papal coins. Coats of arms remained plentiful, as did the immensely varied figures of patron saints.

Franco PANVINI ROSATI

Between 1640 and 1750 machinery came into general use in western Europe. The results are to be seen in the thickness and roundness of the flans, the neat impression, and the high relief of the design. Ornamentation or lettering on the edge was introduced in order to prevent clipping. The first steps were taken to ensure mechanical multiplication of the dies in order to increase the uniformity of coins, an objective that had proved unattainable with handmade dies.

Broadly speaking, however, the system of European coinage that had been established in the 16th century persisted without major change, and the designs of the coins remained traditional (PL. 414). The principal feature was always the head of the monarch in profile or, less often, the monarch standing or on

horseback. Even the Dutch Republic conformed to this general usage and put a nameless warrior on its coins. With few exceptions legends were still in the traditional Latin. But the religious texts of the Middle Ages began to be shortened to allow room for the elaborate titles of absolute monarchs or for national mottoes. Although the style of execution was often changed according to the latest fashion, the types themselves were seldom altered — a visible sign of the stability of money. The accession of a new monarch was the only major occasion for changing the appearance of coins. Dating them became an established practice. But indication of the value was still exceptional; the face values were more often changed than the types of the coins.

In the 20th century, after gold disappeared from circulation, a vast range of metals selected for resistance to wear, difficulty in counterfeiting, lightness of weight, cheapness, etc., came into use for coining purposes. Silver is still widely used, chiefly for its technological properties; gold and pure copper are becoming rare, while alloys of aluminum and nickel have come into the foreground.

Metal coinage having been nationalized, international commercial coins are no longer in circulation, with the exception of some few gold coinages that still play an important role in international finance though not in everyday life. The spirit of nationalism has caused the replacement of Latin by the vernacular in the legends and that of traditional designs by a wealth of emblems and allegories.

H. Enno van Gelder

In response to the requirements of commerce an unprecedented number of metal coins began to be minted in modern times. The same forces, social and economic, that decreed the virtual end of craftsmanship affected the design of coins. During the Renaissance and the baroque era coins were still produced by genuine craft artists, but later the need for mass coinage, met by the introduction of machinery, brought about a division of function between craftsman and artist with an inevitable loss of freshness and originality.

It is true that as late as the dawn of the 19th century neoclassic coin types were appearing in France, Britain, Germany, and other countries, comparable in quality to the traditional coins of earlier periods (PL. 414). The very strength of neoclassic academicism preserved a certain minimum level of technical competence until the second half of the 19th century. But the death of 19th-century academicism, however long delayed in a form as slow to change as the coin, ultimately took place; and the coins of the late 19th and 20th centuries, while attempting to retain the traditional flavor of previous periods, finally came to be designed by traditionalists without a tradition. The coins of the 20th century in the Western world have become an uninspired production on a par with official architecture and official sculpture.

* *

PRIMITIVE SOCIETIES. Among primitive peoples money is appreciated for its own sake — not merely as an economic medium but also for social and ideological reasons. At this social level a given currency functions only rarely as "general medium of exchange"; rather, its use is often confined to specific commercial transactions. Frequently money performs special functions that scarcely fall under our rationalist definition of "exchange"; for instance, when it is used as "bride price" or "blood money."

Particular types of money, although endowed with a traditional value, are used exclusively as gifts on certain ceremonial occasions such as adoptions and the conclusion of peace treaties and blood covenants. The best-known example of such ceremonial exchanges is provided by the Melanesian Kula system: two different species of objects — bracelets and necklaces, both made of shells — are exchanged by two parties, who do not become the owners but only the temporary custodians of the objects received, pending future exchanges.

Another type of money, so-called "treasure money," enhances the social prestige of its possessor but is not used as a medium of exchange. In this category are the red shells of Melanesia and the metal drums (PL. 416) and gongs of Assam, Burma, Annam, Siam, Borneo, and other Indonesian islands and the Philippines, where they are sometimes used as nuptial or ritual gifts. The perforated aragonite disks of the island of Yap, which were manufactured on the Palau islands and transported 400 miles by sea, also served as tokens of prestige.

Still another category of primitive money is commodity money, which has no intrinsic monetary character, but consists of articles that came gradually to function as money. This type of money includes various foodstuffs, such as blocks of salt (northeastern and western Africa), tea bricks (central and northern Asia), cocoa beans (pre-Columbian Mexico), cattle (Africa and Asia; cf. the Latin *pecunia*, "money," derived from *pecus*, "cattle"), cloth, articles of dress, ornaments, and tools and metals (in the form of dust, wires, and bars).

Most primitive currencies are actual commodities or clearly derived from commodities. Much smaller is the number of conventional, or symbolic, currencies without intrinsic material value, or whose material value has nothing to do with its monetary value. Whereas commodity money has a rational material value (use value) and the currency of civilized nations derives its value from the authority of the state, the value of symbolic money rests upon spiritual qualities recognized only within a restricted community. The distinction between symbolic money and commodity money is not intended by the natives; it is one suggested by the observations of students.

The magical qualities attributed to certain objects contribute to their value as money. The conventional value of drums and gongs, for example, is not derived solely from their use as musical instruments; there is much evidence to suggest that they are appreciated for the part they play in magical and ritual funcions, as well as for their metal content: metals, particularly iron (see METALWORK), play an important role in magic practices among the primitive peoples. Also the head trophies, which serve as tokens of exchange with a well-defined commercial value in Assam, Borneo, Sumatra, and New Guinea, clearly derive their value from the intrinsic qualities or presumed supernatural virtues of these objects.

As for the connection between art and the forms of currency, it is important to note that even commodity currencies are often valued on account of their outward presentation. Wrappings (as for tea, salt, etc.), colors and designs (as in clothes), may affect the validity of a currency, thus relegating to a second place the "use value" that may originally have determined the choice of the article as a medium of exchange. No systematic investigations have as yet been undertaken to determine whether the esthetic value of given currencies has contributed to the formation of their monetary value. However, the view of H. Schurtz, according to whom so-called "internal" money, that is, recognized exclusively in intracommunal trade, derives solely from ornament as a sign of high social status, must be regarded as obsolete.

It is not easy to specify which forms of currency are artistic. Of the shell currencies, diffused over large portions of the globe (Africa, North America, Oceania), only certain types have esthetic value. The same is true of metal currencies, which are also widely diffused. Beyond these two groups, particular forms of money of undeniable artistic merit have been developed by various communities.

*Africa.* Aside from cowries (*Cypraea moneta*) and other shell currencies, glass beads (the aggry beads of the Guinea coast, which the natives regard as a marvelous product of nature but which were actually imported from Europe), blocks of salt, and cattle money, metals occupy a large place in the African monetary systems; these include bars and ingots, spears and arrowheads, axes, hoes, crosses, manillas, and rings which are or were in use almost throughout the continent.

The decorative axes or hoes of the Congo (Lulua and Songe groups) are remarkably artistic (PL. 416), particularly the oldest ones, adorned with double human faces carved on the various branches of the handle, which turn back in the direction of the blade; some authors are uncertain whether they should be classified as money. Graceful or bizarre forms are also found

in the spearheads and throwing knives used as money from Gabon to Angola.

Peculiar to the Congo are the blocks of *tukula* — a red sawdust made into paste with water and imprinted with geometric motifs — which function as money, as commodity for barter, and as gifts, particularly in funerary rites. Farther north, from Nigeria to Senegal, along the entire wide curve of the Gulf of Guinea, we find brass rings (decorated in Nigeria) along with manillas, particularly on the Ivory Coast, and native fabrics printed in vivid designs. In Ghana a currency devoid of artistry — gold dust — has given rise to an interesting production — gold weights: tiny brass objects executed in the most varied forms, both abstract and naturalistic, some representing proverbs or genre scenes (see GHANA; GUINEAN CULTURES).

Passing to the east, we find the Maria Theresa taler in Ethiopia, brass bracelets in Uganda, and small perforated shell or ivory disks strung on cords more or less everywhere, not to mention cattle money, which — alongside the cowrie — is the form of currency most common in all east-central and southern Africa.

*Oceania.* No indigenous forms of currency have developed in Australia or Polynesia (and incidentally among the hunting and food-gathering peoples of Africa and among the tribes of the Arctic), even though there are currencies of the commodity type for bartering, such as boomerangs, bark, and shells in Australia and mats in Polynesia. Micronesia and Melanesia, on the other hand, offer a great variety of primitive currencies: the large perforated disks of Yap, various types of shell money, and shields, mats, animal teeth, belts, feathers, etc.; but very few are of artistic interest.

From Sagsag, in the westernmost part of New Britain, comes a characteristic currency, in the form of a broad bracelet made of tortoise shell, with engraved motifs filled in with white chalk. The so-called *navoi*, a local currency originating in New Guinea, serves as one of the principal mediums of payment of the bride price.

In Guadalcanal, in the Solomon Islands, woven shields of fine workmanship function as money, and in Kusaie Ualam (Carolina Islands), in eastern Micronesia, the most beautiful mats of Oceania are woven for use as gifts and in barter. Mussau, an island of the St. Matthias Group north of New Ireland, is known for its woven money in the form of belts; the ornamental motifs are less elaborate than those of Kusaie. In Santa Cruz the mats used as a medium of exchange are for the most part narrow and elongated, something like book markers; they are decorated with fringes and extremely varied motifs. But the most important currency of the islands is feather money (see FEATHERWORK), called *ta* or *tavan*. It consists of long woven strips rolled up in coils, to which are attached feathers of pigeons and red feathers of the cardinal honey-eater (*Myzomela cardinalis*). A scroll of about 30 ft. requires almost a year of work; its exchange value is about $35. In 1932 only about a dozen natives on the island were still capable of manufacturing the large rolls of feather money; it is a specialized trade, handed down from father to son.

In New Caledonia a peculiar form of currency, *go min* or head money, is in circulation. The best-known and most common type consists of a piece of wood in the form of a canoe, whose pointed extremities are completely covered with strips of skin of the flying fox (*Pteropus*); the middle part is sculptured in the form of a human face with a big protruding nose. This head money is probably connected with ancestor worship; it is also practical, because it is taboo for all except its legitimate owner, who is thus protected against thieves.

In New Guinea and the adjacent archipelagoes the trowels called *potuma* are used as gifts and for small transactions. They are made of bone or wood, are often elaborately carved, and sometimes studded with seeds of *Abrus precatorius*. The finest come from the Louisiade Archipelago, where they are used in payment of the bride price.

Also other ornaments, such as mother-of-pearl pendants in the form of half moons and tortoise-shell disks — the latter

executed by the Roro of Hall Sound (New Guinea) — can function as money or in barter.

*Asia.* In Asia the lack of variety in currencies is accounted for by the fact that from the borders of Europe to farthest India cattle served as money. Shell currencies and commodity currencies (salt, rice, nuts) were also widely diffused. The primitive tribes of Burma often use metal gongs of varied forms, dimensions, and values that play an essential role in the acquisition of a wife. Particularly noteworthy are the *kyee-zee* gongs of the Kari in the mountains of eastern Burma; more than a currency, they are a sign of tribal wealth, and they pass from family to family and village to village only on important occasions. They are manufactured by the Shan or Thai of southern China. Some of them are decorated with figurines (the rarer ones with cats and elephants) worked in repoussé.

In Borneo the bride price is paid in brass gongs and bells, in cannon and Chinese porcelain, as well as in implements and gold ingots. A certain type of basket, woven with a special ornamental motif, called *rejang*, from the name of the river near which the best specimens are manufactured, was an essential part of the bride price. Also bells and small cannon of Portuguese manufacture once functioned as money.

In Brunei metal buffalo bells with engraved decorations were formerly used as money; later they were replaced with a kind of cylindrical brass snuffbox with a lid.

Throughout Indonesia the characteristic serpentine dagger, the kris, with the handle shaped as a human or animal head with shoulders, serves as currency.

The most characteristic currency consists of brass drums, called *moko* or *mokko* and common in Solor, Pantar, and Allor east of Flores. Like an hourglass in shape, with four handles, these drums are decorated with geometric motifs, human faces and figures, and stylized animals and flowers. They are very precious and were used as money up to 1914. Their origin is somewhat obscure; Niewekamp thinks that the earliest specimens were manufactured in eastern Java. A great affinity has been noted between the decorative motifs of the *mokko* and those on the silver and brass gongs of Malaya as well as those on Chinese porcelain. Details of the clothing of the human figures, usually represented in crouching position, bring to mind certain mythical figures of Burmese legend and the puppets used in Siamese and Malayan shadow plays. According to Rassers, the human figures may also represent a hero of the culture who plays a part in the initiation ceremonies; this would explain why *mokko* are worshiped in connection with local cults.

*America.* The most important examples of indigenous American currencies are in the Knox Collection in Buffalo and in the Chase Collection in New York. With respect to distribution of forms of currency, the two American continents may be thought of as divided into four zones.

The first comprises the western coast from Alaska to California. The currencies predominating in the northern part of this zone were shell moneys, slaves, copper, cloth, but above all salmon; and in the southern part wild seeds. The salmon peoples (Kwakiutl, Haida, and Tsimshian) possessed a peculiar currency, the so-called "copper money": sheets of locally produced copper beaten cold into a conventionalized shape of variable dimensions. These sheets were signs of wealth rather than an effective medium of exchange and had a preponderant function in a number of tribal ceremonies. They were used as gifts, to strengthen alliances, and to pay the bride price; but they were also exchanged for slaves or distributed during the potlatch ceremonies. The upper part of this money is called the "face" and is covered with graphite on which is engraved a face representing the totem animal of the owner; each coin has its own name (PL. 416).

The second zone comprises the eastern portion of North America, from New Brunswick to Louisiana, and coincides with the zone of cultivation of corn. Here reigns a special form of shell money: wampum. This Algonquin word denotes the tubular or cylindrical shells, white or purple, of *Venus mercenaria*

and other species of mollusks, strung together in the shape of bracelets or belts, some forming ornamental or naturalistic designs. Wampum was used for ceremonial gifts, to pay fines or damages (e.g., as blood money), to make peace treaties, to send messages, to record family or tribal events, as an ornament, and, finally, as a medium of commercial exchange. Production of wampum on an industrial scale by Europeans destroyed this indigenous form of money.

In the third zone, extending from Alaska to Labrador in the north almost down to the Gulf of Mexico in the south, and comprising the area where the caribou and the bison served for food, there was no indigenous currency, although the teeth and skins of animals (especially the beaver) were used for barter. Shell money came there from the west and east coasts.

Finally, in the area of intensive agriculture, which covers about 5,000 square miles, from southern California across Central America, including Mexico and Peru, as far as Chile, the principal currency was slaves; this accounts for the absence of other, more evolved forms. In Mexico cocoa beans were used for barter, and in Peru cocoa leaves. It seems that, at least for a time, brass axes were used as money among the Aztecs of Mexico and in Peru.

Laszló Vajda

MEDALS. A medal is a piece of metal, cast or struck, generally similar in form to a coin, that commemorates in type and legend a personage or a historial event. The word "medal" derives from the Latin *metalla* and during the Middle Ages indicated the half denarius, or obol. When this coin fell into disuse, the term was applied to a coin outside circulation, so that by extension any ancient coin, especially Greek or Roman, was called a medal. Characteristic of medals, aside from peculiarities of style, technique, and types, is that they may be issued even by private persons, an attribute clearly differentiating them from coins, whose issue is directly controlled by the state. Thus the modern medal differs from the Roman medallion, whose obverse invariably bore the image of the emperor or of one of his familiars, to whom he had granted the privilege of effigy, and whose reverse carried types alluding to the undertakings of the emperor or to political, military, and religious events in the empire.

The production of medals is modern. One of the first is that cast by Antonio di Puccio Pisano, called Pisanello (q.v.), for John VIII Palaeologus in 1438 on the occasion of that emperor's arrival in Italy for the Council of Ferrara. This piece marks the beginnings of the flourishing art of the medal, which during the Renaissance gave birth to so many outstanding works. A few pieces that can be regarded as medals, since they were outside circulation and commemorative in purpose, are known to antedate Pisanello's work, but they are isolated examples with no stylistic or technical relation to the subsequent production of the Quattrocento. Such are the two gold medallions, of which old silver copies exist, mentioned in the early 15th century in the inventory of the Duke of Berry's collection. On the obverse of one of these is the portrait of the emperor Constantine, and of the other the portrait of the emperor Heraclius; on the reverses are scenes from the legend of the Cross. Far removed in style and technique from the works of Pisanello are also the medals struck in 1390 to commemorate the reconquest of Padua by Francesco II of Carrara, which on the obverse bear the portraits — strongly influenced by Roman sesterces — of Francesco I and II respectively; also the medals struck in imitation of antique models by the Sesto family, a group of engravers from the Venetian mint who copied antique coins and are believed to have created the Carrara medals.

The production of Pisanello, begun in 1438 with the medal of John VIII Palaeologus, continued for about twenty years in various Italian cities. He was at Mantua, Ferrara, Naples, where he portrayed on his medals the most famous men of the time, princes and *condottieri*, political and literary personages. Let us recall the medals of, among others, Gian Francesco Gonzaga of Mantua, Niccolò Piccinino, Lionello d'Este, Cecilia Gonzaga, Alfonso V of Aragon, Malatesta Novello (PL. 411).

A fine portraitist, Pisanello took great pains with reverses as well, showing a special fondness for animal figures, which he often boldly foreshortened.

Medals soon became popular, and many artists followed in Pisanello's footsteps, although the master did not establish an actual school. One of the best Italian 15th-century medalists was Matteo de' Pasti of Verona, active first in Ferrara (medal of Quarino Veronese) and, after 1446, in Rimini (medals of Sigismondo Pandolfo Malatesta and Isotta degli Atti; PL. 411), where he worked for many years in the service of the Malatestas (see also I, PL. 52). He is a lesser artist than Pisanello, whose influence he reflects both in portraiture and in the composition of reverse types. Only some of the more notable medalists of the 15th century will be mentioned here, grouped according to their native towns or the schools to which they belonged. Active in Ferrara were Antonio Marescotti and later Costanzo, author of a medal of the sultan Mohammed II (dated 1481). In the last decades of the 15th century and the early 16th century Pisanello had numerous successors in Mantua: Bartolomeo Talpa, Pier Jacomo Alari Bonacolsi, called L'Antico, Gian Cristoforo Romano, Bartolomeo Melioli; these artists concentrated on the members of the Gonzaga family. The best of the Mantuans was Sperandio Savelli, active at Ferrara, Bologna, and Venice. His portraits are vigorous, although frequently without grace. His compositions for the reverses are marked by a certain coldness.

Artists were at work in other cities, too: Gianfrancesco Enzola, author of the first attempts at struck medals, in Parma; Giovanni Boldù and Marco Guidizani in Venice; Giulio della Torre and Giammaria Pomodelli, active into the early decades of the 16th century, in Verona; in Florence, Bertoldo di Giovanni (q.v.), a pupil of Donatello, and Niccolò di Forzone Spinelli, called Niccolò Fiorentino, the most eminent medalist of the Florentine school, to whom are attributed some medals of Italian personages (such as the medal of Giovanna Albizi Tornabuoni; PL. 411) and certain medals dedicated to French courtiers of Charles VIII. In Rome Andrea Guazzalotti of Prato created a medallary of the popes, from Nicholas V to Sixtus IV. Also active in Rome were Cristoforo di Geremia of Mantua and his nephew Lisippo; the former was the author of a fine medal of Alfonso V of Aragon and the principal exponent of the Roman school, which in the main followed antique models. To complete this brief account of Quattrocento medalists, mention should be made of Francesco Francia in Bologna and of Caradosso in Milan and Rome, whose activity extends into the 16th century; both were authors of struck medals.

In the 16th century a general decline set in, partly owing to the abandonment of hand casting and working by hand in favor of striking, which had already found its first masters in Francia, Caradosso, and others. The art of Benvenuto Cellini also contributed to this change; as a medalist, he was important primarily for medals struck for Clement VII, the reverses of which revived antique themes. The principal Cinquecento centers were Florence, Rome, Milan, and, to a lesser degree, Venice. Active in Florence, besides Cellini, were Pietro Torregiano and Francesco da Sangallo, both sculptors, and Pastorino da Siena, Gian Paolo and Domenico Poggini, and Pier Paolo Galeotti, called Romano. In Rome striking predominated in the papal medals, because of lesser cost and greater speed of production. Gathered here from all parts of Italy to work in the papal mint were Giampietro Crivelli of Milan, Giovanni Bernardi, the Florentine Domenico Poggini, and the finest artist of the Roman school, Alessandro Cesati, called Greco or Grechetto, who was succeeded at the mint by Giovanni Antonio de' Rossi of Milan. In northern Italy the technique of casting still prevailed; the exception is the Paduan school, with Valerio Belli, known generally as Valerio Vicentino, and the famous forger of Roman coins Giovanni Calvino. Notable in the Venetian school is Andrea Spinelli. The very important Milanese school included Leone Leoni, responsible for some excellent medals (among them that of Charles V); Jacopo Nizzola of Trezzo, also in the service of the imperial court at Vienna and later of Philip II of Spain; Antonio Abondio, the school's major exponent, who was active chiefly outside Italy,

in Prague and Vienna, in the service of Maximilian II and Rudolf II.

The 16th-century tradition continued into the first half of the 17th century, especially in the works of Gaspare Mola, author of the superb Medicean and papal medals. The decline of the art after Mola's death into a purely mechanical process involved even the papal mint. Several artists working there nevertheless deserve mention: Mola's nephew Gaspare Morone Mola and the Hamerani family, medalists of German origin who worked for several generations in the Roman mint — Alberto and Giovanni Martino in the 17th century, Ermenegildo and Ottone in the following century. Some commemorative medals document various projects for monuments (e.g., the two medals for the façade of S. Maria in Campitelli in Rome; PL. 415). Francesco Travani and his son Antonio also worked in Rome, as did the brothers Giuseppe and Stefano Ortolani and Filippo Crapanese, medalist to Clement XIV. In Florence Massimiliano Soldani, author of many cast medals of members of the grand-ducal family, produced work of some distinction.

About the end of the 17th century and the beginning of the 18th the influence of French medals made itself felt all over Italy. Notable representatives of this last phase of Italian medal work were Luigi Manfredi, F. Portinari, and Giuseppe Girometti.

The art of the medal, which also flourished outside Italy from the 16th century on, was almost everywhere under Italian influence. Only Germany could boast an original and independent medallic art. In that country two schools soon formed: one at Augsburg, where the technique of casting prevailed, and the other at Nuremberg, where medals, generally struck, were often the work of goldsmiths. Belonging to the former in the 16th century were Hans Schwarz, Hans Daucher, Hans Kels the Elder, and Friedrich Hagenauer; to the latter, during the same period, belonged Mathes Gebel, Hans Reinhart (PL. 415), and others. In the 17th century the cast medal disappeared almost completely, and the medalists producing work of any importance were few: Sebastian Dadler, Johann Höhn, Georg Schweicker, Philip Heinrich Müller. The baroque period in Germany witnessed a new blossoming in the art of medals, production of which continued until the modern period.

In France, at the end of the 15th century and the beginning of the 16th, medals were issued by cities on the occasion of royal visits. Sixteenth-century French medals reflect the influence of Italian artists who were working in France. French medalists of note were Jean Goujon and, later, Guillaume Dupré and Jean Warin, who was the best of the 17th-century artists. The most important events of the reign of Louis XIV were commemorated by a medallary that was the joint work of Charles Jean François Chéron, at one time medalist to the papal court, Jean Manger, and Joseph Roettiers. Jean Duvivier worked later on official medals commemorating important personages and events, as did Simon Curé and Jean Leblanc. The medals commemorating events of the French Revolution and the Empire (PL. 415) are interesting from the documentary point of view. After a period of decadence, a revival of French medallic art occurred in the 19th century; its influence is traceable in contemporary Italian medals.

In Holland, too, the art of medals was of an Italianate cast. Sixteenth-century artists of note were Q. Metsys (q.v.; PL. 415) and Jean Second (Janus Secundus or Jan Nicolaesz. Everaerts) and, a little later, Jacques Jonghelinck. The finest artist was Stephan of Holland, whose seal "Stehf" appears on both Flemish and foreign medals. Coenrad Bloc excelled in portraits. Adrian Waterloos and Jean de Montfort were active in the 17th century.

In England medals by English artists were not struck until the reigns of Henry VIII and his successors. Foreign medalists were also working in England at this time, notably the Flemish artist Simon van de Passe, the Frenchman Nicholas Briot, and the previously mentioned Jean Warin. Among the 17th-century English artists were Thomas Rawlins and especially the brothers Abraham and Thomas Simon. With the accession of the house of Hanover in 1714, German artists arrived in England. Not until the mid-18th century does one again find

English medalists at work; the most important of these, however, was the Italian-born Thomas Parigo.

Franco PANVINI ROSATI

BIBLIOG. The bibliography of numismatics is very extensive. For reasons of space this compilation has been restricted to general works, catalogues, and monographs concerning mints or dealing with specific problems, preference being given to recent works.

*General*: L. Forrer, Biographical Dictionary of Medallists, 6 vols., London, 1904–16, sup. 2 vols., London, 1923–30; E. Martinori, La moneta: Vocabolario generale, Rome, 1915; F. von Schrötter, Wörterbuch der Münzkunde, Berlin, Leipzig, 1930; V. Tourner, Initiation à la numismatique, Brussels, 1945; F. Mateu y Llopis, Glosario hispánico de numismática, Barcelona, 1946; H. Gebhart, Numismatik und Geldgeschichte, Heidelberg, 1949; P. Einzig Primitive Money, London, 1949; A. H. Quiggin, A Survey of Primitive Money: The Beginnings of Currency, London, 1949; P. Grierson, Coins and Medals: A Selected Bibliography, London, 1954; C. H. V. Sutherland, Art in Coinage, London, 1955; A. Magnaguti, Ex nummis historia, 10 vols., Rome, 1949–59 (cat. of the author's collection). *Origin of money*: E. Babelon, Les origines de la monnaie, Paris, 1897; T. Reinach, L'invention de la monnaie: L'histoire par les monnaies, Paris, 1902, p. 21 ff.; T. Reinach, La date de Pheidon Paris, 1902, p. 35 ff.; J. N. Svoronos, Τὰ πρῶτα νομίσματα, JIAN, IX, 1906, p. 153 ff. (Fr. trans. in Rev. Belge de Numismatique, 1908, pp. 293 ff., 433 ff., 1909, pp. 113 ff., 359 ff., 1910, p. 125 ff.); H. Willers, Das Rohkupfer als Geld der Italiker, ZfN, XXXIV, 1923, p. 193 ff.; B. Laum, Heiliges Geld: Eine historische Untersuchung über den sakralen Ursprung des Geldes, Tübingen, 1924; K. Regling, RVL, IV, 1, 1926, s. v. Geld; A. W. Person, Contribution à la question de l'origine de la monnaie, BCH, LXX, 1946, p. 444 ff.; W. L. Brown, Pheidon's Alleged Aeginetan Coinage, NChr, series VI, vol. X, 1950, p. 17 ff.; E. S. G. Robinson, Coins from the Ephesian Artemision Reconsidered, JHS, LXXI, 1951, p. 156 ff.; E. Will, De l'aspect éthique des origines grecques de la monnaie, Rev. Historique, CCXII, 1954, p. 209 ff.; E. S. G. Robinson, The Date of the Earliest Coins, NChr, series VI, vol. XVI, 1956, p. 1 ff.

*Ancient coinage. A. General*: F. Lenormant, La monnaie dans l'antiquité, 3 vols., Paris, 1900–27; K. Regling, RE, XIII, 1910, s.v. Geld; K. Regling, Die antike Münze als Kunstwerk, Berlin, 1924; G. F. Hill, Tecnica monetale antica, Atti e Memorie dell'Istituto Italiano di Numismatica, V, 1925, p. 209 ff.; A. Segré, Metrologia e circolazione monetaria degli antichi, Bologna, 1928; K. Regling, Münzkunde, in Gercke-Norden, Einleitung in die Altertumswissenschaft, II, 2, Leipzig, Berlin, 1930; W. Campbell, Greek and Roman Plated Coins, New York, 1933; K. Regling, RE, XXXI, 1933, s.v. Münzwesen; W. Giesecke, Antikes Geldwesen, Leipzig, 1938; J. Milne, Greek and Roman Coins and the Study of History, London, 1939; J. Babelon, Le portrait dans l'antiquité d'après les monnaies, Paris, 1950; C. C. Vermeule, Some Notes on Ancient Dies and Coining Methods, London, 1954; C. C. Vermeule, A Bibliography of Applied Numismatics, London, 1956; A. Bellinger, Roman and Greek Medallions in the Dumbarton Oaks Collection, Cambridge, Mass., 1958. *B. Greek coinage. a. General*: P. Gardner, Types of Greek Coins, Cambridge, England, 1883; F. Imhoof-Blumer and P. Gardner, Numismatic Commentary on Pausanias, JHS, VI, 1885, p. 50 ff., VII, 1886, p. 57 ff.; G. F. Hill, Historical Greek Coins, London, 1900; G. MacDonald, Coin Types, Glasgow, 1905; L. Forrer, Notes sur les signatures de graveurs sur les monnaies grecques, Brussels, 1906; F. Imhoof-Blumer, Nymphen und Chariten auf griechischen Münzen, Athens, 1908; L. Anson, Numismata Graeca, 6 vols., London, 1910–16; B. Head, Historia nummorum, Oxford, 1911; P. Gardner, History of Ancient Coinage, 700–300 B.C., Oxford, 1918; S. P. Noe, Bibliography of Greek Coin Hoards, 2d ed., New York, 1937; M. N. Tod, Epigraphical Notes on Greek Coinage, NChr, series VI, vol. V, 1945, p. 108 ff., vol. VII, 1946, p. 47 ff., vol. VII, 1947, p. 1 ff.; H. A. Cahn, Monnaies grecques archaïques, Basel, 1947; S. L. Cesano, Numismatica antica, Doxa, Rome, 1949, p. 219 ff.; L. Lacroix, Les reproductions de statues sur les monnaies grecques, Paris, 1949; C. Seltman, Masterpieces of Greek Coinage, Oxford, 1949; L. Lacroix, Réflexions sur les "types parlants" dans la numismatique grecque, Rev. Belge de Numismatique, XCVI, 1950, p. 5 ff.; E. Gabrici, Tecnica e cronologia delle monete greche dal VII al V sec. a.C. Rome, 1951; K. Christ, Sizilien, Jhb. für Numismatik und Geldgeschichte, V–VI 1954-55, p. 179 ff.; C. Seltman, Greek Coins, 2d ed., London, 1955; P. R. Franke, Epirus, Makedonien, Jhb. für Numismatik und Geldgeschichte, VII, 1956, p. 77 ff.; H. Chantraine, Peloponnes, Jhb. für Numismatik und Geldgeschichte, VIII, 1957, p. 57 ff.; M. and L. Lanckoronski, Mythen und Münzen, Munich, 1958; H. A. Cahn, Frühellenistische Münzkunst, Basel, n.d. See the section Literaturüberblick der griechischen Numismatik in the Jhb. für Numismatik und Geldgeschichte. *b. Catalogues*: BMC, London, 1873–1937; H. Dressel and A. von Sallet, Königliche Münzen zu Berlin, Beschreibung der antiken Münzen, 3 vols., Berlin, 1888–94; G. MacDonald, Catalogue of Greek Coins in the Hunterian Collection, 3 vols., Glasgow, 1899–1905; K. Regling, Die griechischen Münzen der Sammlung Warren, Berlin, 1906; W. H. Waddington, E. Babelon, and T. Reinach, Recueil général des monnaies grecques d'Asie Mineure, 4 vols., Paris, 1908–25; R. Jameson, Collection R. Jameson, 3 vols., Paris, 1913–24; S. W. Grose, Fitzwilliam Museum, Catalogue of the McClean Collection of Greek Coins, 3 vols., Cambridge, England, 1923–29; J. Babelon, Catalogue de la collection de Luynes: Monnaies grecques, 4 vols., Paris, 1924–36; L. Forrer, The Weber Collection, 3 vols., London, 1929; Sylloge nummorum Graecorum: I, 1, The Collection of Capt. E. G. Spencer-Churchill, The Salting Collection in the Victoria and Albert Museum, London, 1931; I, 2, The Newnham Davis Coins in the Wilson Collection of Classical and Eastern Antiquities, Marischal College, Aberdeen, London, 1936; II, The Lloyd Collection, London, 1933–37; III, The Lockett Collection, London, 1938–45; IV, Fitzwilliam Museum, Leake and General

Collections, London, 1940–51; V, Ashmolean Museum, Evans Collection, London, 1951; The Royal Collection of Coins and Medals, Danish National Museum, Copenhagen, 1942–56; A. Baldwin-Brett, Museum of Fine Arts, Boston: Catalogue of Greek Coins, Boston, 1955; Deutschland, Sammlung von Aulock, Berlin, 1957. See also the sales catalogues of the principal dealers: Naville (Ars classica), Hirsch, Cahn (Münzen und Medaillen), Hess, Schulman, Santamaria, Ratto, Spink, Seaby. *c. Monographs.* (1) *The West*: J. Evans, The Coins of the Ancient Britons, London, 1864, sup., 1890; A. Heiss, Description générale des monnaies antiques de l'Espagne, Paris, 1870; A. Delgado, Nuevo método de clasificación de las medallas autónomas de España, 3 vols., Seville, 1871–79; E. Muret and A. Chabouillet, Catalogue des monnaies gauloises de la Bibliothèque Nationale, Paris, 1889; H. de La Tour, Atlas des monnaies gauloises, Paris, 1905; R. Forrer, Keltische Numismatik der Rhein- und Donauländer, Strasbourg, 1908; A. Vives y Escudero, La moneda hispánica, 4 vols., Madrid, 1924–26; R. Forrer, RVL, VI, 1926, s.v. Keltische Münzwesen; G. F. Hill, On the Coins of Narbonensis with Iberian Inscriptions, New York, 1930; G. F. Hill, Notes on the Ancient Coinage of Hispania Citerior, New York, 1931; G. C. Brooke, The Philippus in the West and the Belgic Invasions of Britain, NChr, series V, vol. XIII, 1933, p. 88 ff.; R. Paulsen, Die Münzprägung der Boier, Leipzig, Vienna, 1933; R. Pink, Die Münzprägung der Ostkelten und ihrer Nachbarn, Budapest, 1939; K. Pink, Einführung in die keltische Münzkunde mit besonderer Berücksichtigung Österreichs, Archaeologia Austriaca, VI, 1950; R. P. Mack, The Coinage of Ancient Britain, London, 1953; A. M. De Guadan, Algunos problemas fundamentales de las amonedaciones de plata de Emporion y Rhode, Numisma, IV, 1954, p. 9 ff.; L. Lengyel, L'art gaulois dans les médailles, Montrouge-Seine, 1954; K. Christ, Ergebnisse und Probleme der keltischen Numismatik und Geldgeschichte, Historia, VI, 2, 1957, p. 215 ff. (2) *Italy*: R. Garrucci, Le monete dell'Italia antica, Rome, 1885; A. J. Evans, The Horsemen of Tarentum, NChr, series III, vol. IX, 1889, p. 37 ff.; A. Sambon, Les monnaies antiques de l'Italie, I, Paris, 1903; K. Regling, Terina, Berlin, 1906; K. Regling, Zur Münzprägung der Brettier, Festschrift zu C.-F. Lehmann-Haupt, Vienna, Leipzig, 1921, p. 80 ff.; M. P. Vlasto, Taras Oikistes: A Contribution to Tarentine Numismatics, New York, 1922; S. P. Noe, The Coinage of Metapontum, 2 vols., New York, 1927–31; W. Giesecke, Italia numismatica, Leipzig, 1928; S. P. Noe, The Thurian Distaters, New York, 1935; P. W. Lehmann, Statues on Coins of Southern Italy and Sicily in the Classical Period, New York, 1946; E. S. G. Robinson, Rhegion, Zankle-Messana and the Samians, JHS, LXVI, 1946, p. 13 ff.; L. Breglia, Le "Campano-Tarentine" e la presunta lega monetale fra Taranto e Napoli, RendNapoli, N.S., XXIII, 1946–48, p. 225 ff.; O. Ravel, Descriptive Catalogue of the Collection of Tarentine Coins Formed by M. P. Vlasto, London, 1947; C. Seltman, The Problem of the Italiote Coins, NChr, series VI, vol. IX, 1949, p. 1 ff.; P. Zancani-Montuoro, Siri-Sirino-Pixunte, Archivio Storico per la Calabria e la Lucania, XVIII, 1949, p. 1 ff.; L. Breglia, Le antiche rotte del Mediterraneo documentate da monete e pesi, RendNapoli, XXX, 1955, p. 201 ff.; L. Breglia, Le monete delle quattro Sibari, Annali dell'Istituto Italiano di Numismatica, II, 1955, p. 9 ff.; H. Herzfelder, Les monnaies d'argent de Rhegion frappées entre 461 et le milieu du IV$^e$ siècle av. J.C., Paris, 1957; C. M. Kraay, The Coinage of Caulonia, New York, 1959. (3) *Sicily*: A. J. Evans, Syracusan "Medallions" and Their Engravers, NChr, series III, vol. XI, 1891, p. 205 ff.; G. F. Hill, Coins of Ancient Sicily, London, 1903; A. Holm, Storia della Sicilia nell'antichità, III, 2, Turin, 1906; P. Lederer, Tetradrachmenprägung von Segesta, Munich, 1910; L. Tudeer, Die Tetradrachmenprägung von Syrakus in der Periode der signierenden Kunst, ZfN, XXX, 1913, p. 1 ff.; K. Regling, Dekadrachmen des Kimon von Syrakus, Amtliche Berichte aus den Kön. Kunstsammlungen, XXXVI, 1, 1914, p. 3 ff.; W. Giesecke, Sicilia numismatica, Leipzig, 1923; W. Schwabacher, Tetradrachmen von Selinunt, Berlin, 1925; E. Gabrici, La monetazione del bronzo nella Sicilia antica, Atti R. Accad. Scienze, Lettere e Belle Arti di Palermo, XV, Palermo, 1927; S. Mirone, Stiela, topografia e numismatica, ZfN, XXXVIII, 1928, p. 29 ff.; E. Böhringer, Die Münze von Syrakus, Berlin, Leipzig, 1929; A. Gallatin, Syracusan Dekadrachms of the Euainetos Type, Cambridge, Mass., 1930; G. E. Rizzo, Saggi preliminari sull'arte della moneta nella Sicilia greca, Rome, 1937; G. E. Rizzo, Intermezzo: Nuovi studi archeologici sulle monete greche della Sicilia, Rome, 1939; M. Särström, A Study in the Coinage of the Mamertines, Basel, 1940; J. H. Jongkees, The Kimonian Dekadrachms, Utrecht, 1941; K. Liègle, Euainetos, Berlin, 1941; H. A. Cahn, Die Münzen der sizilischen Stadt Naxos, Basel, 1944; G. E. Rizzo, Monete greche della Sicilia, 2 vols., Rome, 1946; L. Breglia, La coniazione argentea di Alaesa-Arconidea, Archivio Storico Siciliano, series III, vol. II, 1947, p. 135 ff.; C. Seltman, The Engravers of the Akragantine Decadrachms, NChr, series VI, vol. VIII, 1948, p. 1 ff.; G. De Diccio, Gli aurei siracusani di Cimone e di Eveneto, Rome, 1957; W. Schwabacher, Das Demarateion, Bremen, 1958. (4) *Greece*: F. Imhoof-Blumer, Die Münzen Akarnaniens, Vienna, 1878; J. N. Svoronos, Numismatique de la Crète ancienne, Mâcon, 1890; Die antiken Münzen Nordgriechenlands herausgegeben unter Leitung von F. Imhoof-Blumer von der Kgl. Akademie der Wissenschaft; B. Pick and K. Regling, Dacien und Moesien, 2 vols., Berlin, 1898–1910; H. Gaebler, Die antiken Münzen von Makedonia und Paionia, 2 vols., Berlin, 1906–35; H. von Fritze, Die autonomen Münzen von Abdera, Nomisma, III, 1909; F. Münzen and M. L. Strack, Thrakien, Berlin, 1912; P. Gardner, Coinage of the Athenian Empire, JHS, XXXIII, 1913, p. 147 ff.; K. Regling, Phygela, Klazomenai, Amphipolis, ZfN, XXXIII, 1921, p. 46 ff.; C. Seltman, The Temple Coins of Olympia, Berlin, 1921; K. Regling, Mende, ZfN, XXXIV, 1923, p. 7 ff.; C. Seltman, Athens: Its History and Coinage before the Persian Invasion, Cambridge, England, 1924; J. N. Svoronos, Les monnaies d'Athènes, Munich, 1926; O. Ravel, The Colts of Ambracia, New York, 1928; O. Ravel, Les "poulains" de Corinthe, 2 vols., Basel, London, 1936–48; D. M. Robinson and P. A. Clement, The Chalcidic Mint and the Excavation Coins found 1928–34 (Excavation at Olynthus, 9), Baltimore, 1938; U. Kahrstedt, Athenische Wappenmünzen und Kleinasiatisches Elektron, Deutsches Jhb. für Numismatik, II, 1939, p. 85 ff.; J. M. F. May, The Coinage of Damastion, Oxford, 1939; B. Mitrea, La penetrazione commerciale e circolazione monetaria della Dacia prima della conquista, Ephemeris Dacoromana, X, 1945; H. A. Cahn, Zur frühattischen Münzprägung, Museum Helveticum, III, 1946, p. 133 ff.; A. R. Bellinger, Chronology of Attic New Style Tetradrachms, Hesperia, sup. VIII, 1949 (Commemorative Studies in Honor of T. Leslie Schear), p. 6 ff.; J. Desneux, Les tetradrachmes d'Akanthos, Brussels, 1949; J. M. F. May, Aynos: Its History and Coinage, Oxford, London, 1950; D. M. Robinson, A Hoard of Silver Coins from Carystus, New York, 1952; J. H. Jongkees, Notes on the Coinage of Athens, Mnemosyne, series IV, vol. V, 1952, p. 28 ff.; A. R. Bellinger, The Coinage of Potidaea, Studies Presented to David Moore Robinson, II, St. Louis, 1953, p. 201 ff.; D. Raymond, Macedonian Regal Coinage to 413 B.C., New York, 1953; C. M. Kraay, The Archaic Owls of Athens: Classification and Chronology, NChr, series VI, vol. XVI, 1956, p. 44 ff.; W. P. Wallace, The Euboian League and Its Coinage, New York, 1956; H. A. Cahn, Ein Tetradrachmon von Stagyra, Antike Kunst, I, 2, 1958, p. 37 ff. (5) *Asia Minor*: H. von Fritze, Die Elektronprägung von Kyzikos, Nomisma, VII, 1912; H. von Fritze, Die antiken Münzen von Mysien, Berlin, 1913; H. von Fritze, Die Silberprägung von Kyzikos, Nomisma, IX, 1914, p. 34 ff.; H. von Fritze, Die autonome Kupferprägung von Kyzikos, Nomisma, X, 1917; H. Gaebler, Die Silberprägung von Lampsakos, Nomisma, XII, 1923; K. Regling, Münzen von Priene, Berlin, 1927; P. Lederer, Staterprägung der Stadt Nagidus, ZfN, XLI, 1931, p. 153 ff.; J. G. Milne, Kolophon and Its Coinage, New York, 1941; W. Schwabacher, The Coins of the Youmi Treasure: Contribution to Cypriote Numismatics, OpA, IV, 1946, p. 25 ff.; W. Schwabacher, Geldumlauf und Münzprägung in Syrien im 6. und 5. Jahrh. v. Chr., OpA, VI, 1950, p. 139 ff.; H. A. Cahn, Die archaischen Silberstatere von Lindos, Charites: Studien zur Altertumswissenschaft, Bonn, 1957, p. 18 ff. (6) *Hellenistic kingdoms*: F. Imhoof-Blumer, Die Münzen der Dynastie von Pergamon, Berlin, 1884; E. Babelon, Catalogue des monnaies de la Bibliothèque Nationale: Les rois de Syrie, d'Arménie et de Commagène, Paris, 1890; H. von Fritze, Die Münzen von Pergamon, Berlin, 1890; J. N. Svoronos Τὰ νομίσματα τοῦ κράτους τῶν Πτολεμαίων, 4 vols., Athens, 1904–08; E. T. Newell, The Dated Alexander Coinage: Sidon and Ake (Yale Oriental Series, Researches, 2), New Haven, London, Oxford, 1916; E. T. Newell, Alexander Hoards, II, Demanhur (1905), New York, 1923; E. T. Newell, The Coinage of Demetrius Poliorcetes, Oxford, 1927; A. Mamroth, Die Silbermünzen des Königs Perseus, ZfN, XXXVIII, 1928, p. 1 ff.; W. Giesecke, Das Ptolomäergeld, Leipzig, 1930; E. T. Newell, The Pergamene Mint under Philataerus, New York, 1936; E. T. Newell, Royal Greek Portrait Coins, New York, 1937; E. T. Newell, The Coinage of the Eastern Seleucid Mints from Seleucus I to Antiochus III, New York, 1938; E. T. Newell, The Coinage of the Western Seleucid Mints from Seleucus I to Antiochus III, New York, 1941; G. Kleiner, Alexanders Reichsmünzen, Abhandlungen der Deutschen Akademie der Wissenschaft zu Berlin, no. 5, 1947; E. T. Newell and S. P. Noe, The Alexander Coinage of Sycion, New York, 1950. (7) *Jewish coinage*: F. W. Madden, Coins of the Jews, London, 1903; T. Reinach, Jewish Coins, London, 1903; A. Reifenberg, Ancient Jewish coins, 2d ed., Jerusalem, 1947; L. Kadman, The Coins of Aelia Capitolina (Corpus nummorum Palaestinensium, I), Tel Aviv, 1956; L. Kadman, The Coins of Caesarea Maritima (Corpus nummorum Palaestinensium, II), Jerusalem, 1957. (8) *Persia*: E. Babelon, Catalogue des monnaies de la Bibliothèque Nationale, Les Perses achéménides: Les satrapes et les dynastes tributaires de leur Empire, Paris, 1893; G. R. Kian, Introduction à l'histoire de la monnaie et histoire monétaire de la Perse dès origines à la fin de la période parthe, Paris, 1934; D. Schlumberger, L'argent grec dans l'Empire achéménide, Paris, 1953, S. P. Noe, Two Hoards of Persian Sigloi, New York, 1956; W. Schwabacher, Satrapenbildnisse: Zum neuen Münzporträt des Tissaphernes, Charites, Studien zur Altertumswissenschaft, Bonn, 1957, p. 27 ff. (9) *Africa*: L. Müller, Numismatique de l'ancienne Afrique, 3 vols. and sup., 1860–74; L. Charrier, Description de monnaies de la Numidie et de la Mauritanie, Paris, 1912; A. Anzani, Numismatica Axumita, RIN, XXXIX, 1926, p. 5 ff.; C. Conti Rossini, Monete Axsumite, AfrIt, I, 1927, p. 179 ff.; A. Anzani, Numismatica e storia d'Etiopia, RIN, XLI–XLII, 1928–29, p. 5 ff.; L. Naville, Les monnaies d'or de la Cyrénaïque, Geneva, 1951; J. Mazard, Corpus nummorum Numidiae Mauretaniaeque, Paris, 1955. *A. Roman coinage. a. General*: T. Mommsen, Geschichte des römischen Münzwesens, Berlin, 1960; A. Blanchet, Les trésors des monnaies romaines et les invasions germaniques en Gaule, Paris, 1900; G. F. Hill, Historical Roman Coins, London, 1909; H. Mattingly, Roman Coins, London, 1928. *b. Republic.* (1) *General*: E. Babelon, Description historique et chronologique des monnaies de la République romaine, 2 vols., Paris, 1885–86; M. Bahrfeldt, Nachträge und Berichtigungen zur Münzkunde der römischen Republik, 2 vols., Vienna, 1897–1900; H. Willers, Geschichte der römischen Kupferprägung vom Bundesgenossenkrieg bis auf Kaiser Claudius, Leipzig, 1909; H. A. Grueber, Coins of the Roman Republic in the British Museum, 3 vols., London, 1910; E. J. Häberlin, Aes Grave: Das Schwergeld Roms und Mittelitaliens, Frankfort on the Main, 1910; M. Bahrfeldt, Die römische Goldmünzprägung während der Republik, Halle, 1923; E. A. Sydenham, Aes Grave, London, 1926; Sammlung Ernst Justus Häberlin, Gold- und Silbermünzen der Römischen Republik, Frankfort on the Main, 1933; S. L. Cesano, I fasti della Repubblica romana sulla moneta di Roma, Studi di Numismatica, I, 2, 1942, p. 105 ff.; K. Pink, The Triumviri Monetales and the Structure of the Coinage of the Roman Republic, New York, 1952; E. A. Sydenham, The Coinage of the Roman Republic, London, 1952; A. Alföldi, The Main Aspects of Political Propaganda on the Coinage of the Roman Republic, Essays in Roman Coinage Presented to Harold Mattingly, Oxford, 1956, p. 63 ff.; R. Thomsen, Early Roman Coinage; A Study of the Chronology, Copenhagen, 1957. (2) *Special studies*: S. L. Cesano, Dizionario epigrafico di antichità romane, II, 2, 1910, p. 1623 ff., s.v. Denarius; H. Mattingly and E. S. G. Robinson, The Date of the Roman Denarius, Proceedings of the British Academy, XVIII, 1933; S. L. Cesano, La data di istituzione del denarius, B. del Museo dell'Impero Romano (appendix to BCom, LXVI), IX, 1938, p. 3 ff.; H. Mattingly, The First Age of Roman Coinage, JRS,

XXXV, 1945, p. 65 ff.; S. L. Cesano, Silla e la sua moneta, RendPontAcc, XXI, 1945–46, p. 187 ff.; S. L. Cesano, Le monete di Cesare, RendPontAcc, XXIII–XXIV, 1947–48, 1948–49, p. 103 ff.; H. Mattingly, The Various Styles of the Roman Republican Coinage, NChr, series VI, vol. IX, 1949, p. 57 ff.; L. Breglia, La prima fase della coniazione romana dell'argento, Rome, 1952; A. Alföldi, Studien über Caesars Monarchie, B. de la Société Royale des Lettres de Lund, 1952–53, p. 1 ff.; A. Alföldi, Studien zur Zeitfolge der Münzprägung der Römischen Republik, Schweiz. numismatische Rundschau, XXXVI, 1954, p. 5 ff.; T. V. Buttrey, The Triumviral Portrait Gold of the Quattuorviri Monetales of 42 B.C., New York, 1956; A. Alföldi, The Portrait of Caesar on the Denarii of 44 B.C. and the Sequence of the Issues, Centennial Publication of the American Numismatic Society, New York, 1958, p. 27 ff. *c. Empire.* (1) *General*: H. Cohen, Description historique des monnaies frappées sous l'Empire romain, 8 vols., Paris 1880–92; F. Gnecchi, Coin Types of Imperial Rome, tr. E. F. Hands, London, 1908; F. Gnecchi, I medaglioni romani, 3 vols., Milan, 1910; W. Koehler, Personifikationen abstrakter Begriffe auf römischen Münzen, Königsberg, 1910; H. Mattingly, Coins of the Roman Empire in the British Museum, 5 vols., London, 1923–50; H. Mattingly, E. A. Sydenham, and R. A. G. Carson, Roman Imperial Coinage, 7 vols., London, 1923–51; O. T. Schulz, Die Rechtstitel und Regierungsprogramme auf römischen Kaisermünzen, Paderborn, 1925; M. Bernhart, Handbuch zur Münzkunde der römischen Kaiserzeit, Halle, 1926; K. Pink, Der Aufbau der römischen Münzprägung in der Kaiserzeit, NZ, LXVI, 1933, p. 17 ff., LXVII, 1934, p. 3 ff., LXVIII, 1935, p. 12 ff., LXIX, 1936, p. 10 ff., LXXIII, 1949, p. 13 ff.; R. Göbl, idem, ibid., LXXIV, 1951, p. 8 ff.; C. H. V. Sutherland, Coinage and Currency in Roman Britain, London, 1937; L. C. West, Gold and Silver Standards in the Roman Empire, New York, 1941; J. M. C. Toynbee, Roman Medallions, New York, 1944; L. C. West and A. C. Johnson, Currency in Roman and Byzantine Egypt, Princeton, 1944; M. Grant, Roman Anniversary Issues, Cambridge, England, 1950; H. Mattingly, The Imperial "Vota," Proceedings of the British Academy, XXXVI, 1950, p. 155 ff., XXXVII, 1951, p. 219 ff.; C. H. V. Sutherland, Coinage in Roman Imperial Policy (31 B.C.–A.D. 68), London, 1951; A. Calò Levi, Barbarians on Roman Imperial Coins and Sculpture, New York, 1952; M. Grant, Roman Imperial Money, Edinburgh, 1954. (2) *Special studies*: O. Vötter, Die Münzen des Kaisers Gallienus und seiner Familie, NZ, XXXII, 1900, p. 117 ff., XXXIII, 1901, p. 73 ff.; J. Maurice, Numismatique constantinienne, 3 vols., Paris, 1903–08; L. Laffranchi, La cronologia delle monete di Adriano, RIN, XIX, 1906, p. 329 ff.; A. Merlin, Les revers monétaires de l'empereur Nerva, Paris, 1906; K. Menadier, Die Münzen und das Münzwesen bei den Scriptores Historiae Augustae, ZfN, XXXI, 1914, p. 1 ff.; A. J. Evans, Notes on the Coinage and Silver Currency in Roman Britain from Valentinian I to Constantine III, NChr, series IV, vol. XV, 1915, p. 433 ff.; L. Laffranchi, La monetazione di Augusto, Milan, 1919; L. Laffranchi, L'imperatore Martiniano e il suo tempo, RendPontAcc, III, 1925, p. 351 ff.; K. Pink, Die Silberprägung der Diocletianischen Tetrarchie, NZ, LXIV, 1931, p. 1 ff.; P. L. Strack, Untersuchungen zur römischen Reichsprägung des zweiten Jahrhunderts, 3 vols., Stuttgart, 1931–37; O. Ulrich Bansa, Note sulla zecca di Aquileia Romana: I multipli d'oro, Udine, 1936; G. Elmer, Eugenius, NZ, LXIX, 1936, p. 29 ff.; O. Ulrich Bansa, Note sulla zecca di Aquileia Romana, Aquileia Nostra, VII–VIII, 1936–37, col. 78 ff., VIII–IX, 1937–38, col. 1 ff., X, 1939, col. 37 ff., XVIII, 1947, col. 3 ff.; A. Alföldi, A Festival of Isis in Rome under the Christian Emperors of the Fourth Century, Budapest, 1937; R. Delbrueck, Die Münzbildnisse von Maximinus bis Carinus, Berlin, 1940; G. Elmer, Die Münzprägung der gallischen Kaiser in Köln, Trier und Mainland, BJ, 1941, p. 108 ff.; A. Alföldi, Die Kontorniaten: Ein verkanntes Propagandamittel der stadtrömischen heidnischen Aristokratie in ihrem Kampfe gegen das christliche Kaisertum, Budapest, 1942–43; M. Grant, From Imperium to Auctoritas. A Historical Study of Aes Coinage in the Roman Empire, 49 B.C.–A.D. 14, Cambridge, England, 1946; D. V. Hill, Barbarous Radiates, New York, 1947; O. Ulrich Bansa, Moneta Mediolanensis, Venice, 1949; M. Grant, The Six Main Aes Coinages of Augustus, Edinburgh, 1953; C. M. Kraay, The Coinage of Galba, New York, 1956; K. Kraft, Die Taten der Kaiser Constans und Constantinus II, Jhb. für Numismatik und Geldgeschichte, IX, 1958, p. 141 ff.; S. Mazzarino, EAA, II, 1959, p. 784 ff., s.v. Contorniati. (3) *Provincial issues*: G. Dattari, Nummi Augg. Alexandrini, Cairo, 1901; F. Imhoof-Blumer, Kleinasiatische Münzen, 2 vols., Vienna, 1901–02; J. Vogt, Die Alexandrinischen Münzen, Stuttgart, 1924; W. Wruck, Die syrische Provinzialprägung von Augustus bis Trajan, Stuttgart, 1931; J. G. Milne, Catalogue of Alexandrian Coins in the Ashmolean Museum, Oxford, 1933; E. A. Sydenham, The Coinage of Caesarea in Cappadocia, London, 1933; C. Bosch, Die Kleinasiatischen Münzen der römischen Kaiserzeit, Stuttgart, 1935; A. R. Bellinger, The Syrian Tetradrachms of Caracalla and Macrinus, New York, 1940.

*Byzantine coinage*: J. Sabatier, Description générale des monnaies byzantines, 2 vols., Paris, 1862; W. Wroth, Catalogue of the Imperial Byzantine Coins in the British Museum, 2 vols., London, 1908; I. I. Tolstoy, Vyzantiiskiya monety (Byzantine Coinage), 2 vols., St. Petersburg, 1912–14; A. R. Bellinger, The Anonymous Byzantine Bronze Coinage, New York, 1928; R. Ratto, Monnaies byzantines, Lugano, 1930; D. Ricotti-Prina, La monetazione siciliana nell'epoca bizantina, Numismatica, XVI, 1950, p. 26 ff.; T. Bertelé, L'imperatore alato nella numismatica bizantina, Rome, 1951; V. Laurent, Bulletin de numismatique byzantine, 1940–49, Rev. des Etudes Byzantines, IX, 1951, p. 192 ff.; H. L. Adelson, Light-weight Solidi and Byzantine Trade during the Sixth and Seventh Centuries, New York, 1957; T. Bertelé, L'iperpero bizantino dal 1261 al 1453, RIN, LIX, 1957, p. 70 ff.; M. Goodacre, A Handbook of the Coinage of the Byzantine Empire, London, 1957; J. D. Breckenridge, The Numismatic Iconography of Justinian II 685–95, 705–11 A.D., New York, 1959.

*Medieval and modern coinage. a. General*: A. Engel and R. Serrure, Traité de numismatique du Moyen Age, 3 vols., Paris, 1891–1905; A. Engel and R. Serrure, Traité de numismatique moderne et contemporaine, 2 vols., Paris, 1897–99; W. Wroth, Catalogue of the Coins of the Vandals, Ostrogoths and Lombards and of the Empires of Thessalonica, Nicaea and Trebizond in the British Museum, London, 1911; W. Jesse, Quellenbuch zur Münz- und Geldgeschichte des Mittelalters, Halle, 1924; A. Luschin von Ebengreuth, Allgemeine Münzkunde und Geldgeschichte des Mittelalters und der neueren Zeit, 2d ed., Munich, Berlin, 1926; F. Friedensburg, Münzkunde und Geldgeschichte der Einzelstaaten des Mittelalters und der neueren Zeit, Munich, Berlin, 1926; K. Lange, Münzkunst des Mittelalters, Leipzig, 1942; P. Le Gentilhomme, Le monnayage et la circulation monétaire dans les royaumes barbares en Occident (V^e–VIII^e siècles), RN, series V, vol. VII, 1943, p. 46 ff., VIII, 1944, p. 13 ff.; M. Bloch, Esquisse d'une histoire monétaire de l'Europe, Paris, 1954; C. M. Cipolla, Moneta e civiltà mediterranea, Venice, 1957; M. Bloch, Le problème de l'or au Moyen Age, Rome, 1959 p. 88 ff. *b. Italy.* (1) *General*: F. and E. Gnecchi, Saggio di bibliografia numismatica delle zecche italiane medioevali e moderne, Milan, 1889; A. Nagl, Die Goldwährung und die handelmässige Geldrechnung im Mittelalter, NZ, XXVI, 1894, p. 41 ff.; Corpus nummorum Italicorum, 20 vols., Rome, Milan, 1910–43; G. Sambon, Repertorio generale delle monete coniate in Italia e da Italiani all'estero, I (476–1266), Paris, 1912; U. Monneret de Villard, La monetazione dell'Italia barbarica, RIN, XXXII, 1919, pp. 22 ff., 73 ff., 125 ff., XXXIII, 1920, p. 169 ff., XXXIV, 1921, p. 191 ff.; La collezione Ruchat, 4 vols., Rome, 1921–23; H. Nussbaum, Fürstenporträte auf italienischen Münzen des Quattrocento, ZfN, XXXV, 1925, p. 145 ff.; R. S. Lopez, Settecento anni fa: Il ritorno all'oro nell'Occidente duecentesco, Rivista Storica Italiana, LXV, I, 1952, p. 19 ff., 2, p. 161 ff.; E. Bernareggi, Monete d'oro con ritratto del Rinascimento italiano (1450–1615), Milan, 1954; O. Rinaldi, Le monete coniate in Italia dalla Rivoluzione francese ai nostri giorni, I, Casteldario (Mantua), 1954. (2) *Special studies*: I. Orsini, Storia delle monete dei granduchi di Toscana della casa de' Medici, Florence, 1756; I. Orsini, Storia delle monete della Repubblica Fiorentina Florence, 1760; D. Promis, Monete dei reali di Savoia, 2 vols., Turin, 1841; A. Cinagli, Le monete dei papi, Rome, 1848; D. Massagli, Della zecca e delle monete di Lucca, Lucca, 1870; H. Dannenberg, Die Goldgulden von Florentiner Gepräge, NZ, XII, 1880, p. 146 ff.; A. Engel, Recherches sur la numismatique et la sigillographie des Normands de Sicile et d'Italie, Paris, 1882; C. Brambilla, Monete di Pavia, Pavia, 1883; A. Crespellani, La zecca di Modena nei periodi comunale ed Estense, Modena, 1884; F. and E. Gnecchi, Le monete di Milano, Milan, 1884, sup., 1894; E. H. Furse, Mémoires numismatiques de l'ordre souverain de Saint Jean de Jérusalem, Rome, 1885; F. and E. Gnecchi, Le monete dei Trivulzio, Milan, 1887; G. Werdnig, Die Osellen oder Münzmedaillen der Republik Venedig, Vienna, 1889; C. De Simoni, Tavole descrittive delle monete della zecca di Genova dal MCXXXIX al MDCCCXIV (Atti della Società Ligure di Storia Patria, XXII), Genoa, 1890; B. Lagumina, Catalogo delle monete arabe esistenti nella Biblioteca Comunale di Palermo, Palermo, 1892; N. Papadopoli, Le monete di Venezia, 4 vols., Venice, 1893–1919; F. Malaguzzi-Valeri, La zecca di Bologna, Milan, 1901; Q. Perini, Le monete di Verona, Rovereto, 1902; C. Serafini, Le monete e le bolle plumbee pontificie del Medagliere Vaticano, Milan, 1910–28; M. Cagiati, Le monete del Reame delle Due Sicilie da Carlo I d'Angiò a Vittorio Emanuele I, 9 fasc. and sup., Naples, 1911–16; A. Jesurum, Cronistoria delle oselle di Venezia, Venice, 1912; E. Martinori, Annali della zecca di Roma, 24 fasc., Rome, 1918–22; A. Sambon, Recueil des monnaies mediévales du sud de l'Italie avant la domination des Normands, Paris, 1919; M. Cagiati, I tipi monetali della zecca di Salerno, Naples, 1925; G. Castellani, Catalogo della raccolta numismatica Papadopoli-Aldobrandini, 2 vols., Venice, 1925; P. F. Casaretto, La moneta genovese in confronto con le altre valute mediterranee nei secoli XII e XIII (Atti della Società Ligure di Storia Patria, LV), Genoa, 1928; F. F. Kraus, Die Münzen Odovacars und des Ostgotenreiches in Italien, Halle, 1928; A. Galeotti, Le monete del granducato di Toscana, Leghorn, 1929; L. Dell'Erba, La riforma monetaria angioina e il suo sviluppo storico nel reale di Napoli, Archivio Storico per le Province Napoletane, 1932–35; E. Birocchi, Zecche e monete della Sardegna nei periodi di dominazione aragonese-spagnuola, Cagliari, 1952; P. Grierson, Cronologia delle riforme monetarie di Carlo Magno, RIN, II, series V, vol. LVI, 1954, p. 65 ff.; D. Herlihy, Pisan Coinage and the Monetary Development of Tuscany, 1150–1250, The American Numismatic Society Museum Notes, VI, 1954, p. 143 ff.; H. E. Ives and P. Grierson, The Venetian Gold Ducat and Its Imitations, New York, 1954; G. Cerrato, La zecca di Torino dalle origini alla riforma monetaria del 1754, Turin, 1956; P. Grierson, I grossi "senatoriali" di Roma (1253–1363), I (1253–82), RIN, LVIII, 1956, p. 36 ff.; V. d'Incerti, Le monete austriache del Lombardo-Veneto, RIN, LX, 1958, p. 59. *c. Spain*: A. Heiss, Descripción general de las monedas hispano-cristianas desde la invasión de los Árabes, 3 vols., Madrid, 1865–96; A. Heiss, Description des monnaies des rois wisigoths d'Espagne, Paris, 1872; F. Mateu y Llopis, Las monedas visigodas del Museo Arqueológico Nacional, Madrid, 1936; W. Reinhart, Die Münzen des tolosanischen Reiches der Westgoten, Deutsches Jhb. für Numismatik, I, 1938, p. 107 ff.; W. Reinhart, Die Münzen des westgotischen Reiches von Toledo, Deutsches Jhb. für Numismatik, III–IV, 1940–41, p. 69 ff.; F. Mateu y Llopis, La moneda española, Barcelona, 1946; G. C. Miles, The Coinage of the Umayyads of Spain, 2 vols., New York, 1950; T. Dasi, Estudio de los reales de a ocho, 5 vols., Valencia, 1950–51; G. C. Miles, The Coinage of the Visigoths of Spain, Leovigild to Achila II, New York, 1952. *d. France*: F. Poey d'Avant, Les monnaies féodales de la France, 3 vols., Paris, 1858–62; E. Caron, Monnaies féodales françaises, Paris, 1882; E. Gariel, Les monnaies royales de France sous la race carolingienne, 2 vols., Strasbourg, 1883–85; M. Prou, Catalogue des monnaies françaises de la Bibliothèque Nationale: Les monnaies mérovingiennes, Paris, 1892; A. de Belfort, Description générale des monnaies mérovingiennes, 5 vols., Paris, 1892–95; M. Prou, Les monnaies carolingiennes, Paris, 1896; A. Blanchet and A. Dieudonné, Manuel de numismatique française, 3 vols., Paris, 1912–30; L. Ciani, Les monnaies royales françaises de Hugues Capet à Louis XVI, Paris, 1926; A. Dieudonné, Catalogue des monnaies françaises de la Bibliothèque Nationale: Les monnaies capétiennes, 2 vols., Paris,

1929–32; W. Reinhart, Die früheste Münzprägung im Reiche der Merowinger, Deutsches Jhb. für Numismatik, II, 1939, p. 37 ff.; P. Grierson, The Gold Coinage of Louis the Pious and Its Imitations, Jaarboek voor Munt- en Penninggids, XXXVIII, 1951, p. 1 ff.; J. Lafaurie, Les monnaies des rois de France, I, De Hugues Capet à Louis XII, Paris, Basel, 1951; J. Lafaurie and P. Prieur, Les monnaies des rois de France, II, De François I à Henri IV, Paris, Basel, 1956. e. England: C. K. Keary and H. A. Grueber, Catalogue of English Coins in the British Museum; Anglo-Saxon Series, 2 vols., London, 1887–93; H. A. Grueber, Handbook of the Coins of Great Britain and Ireland in the British Museum, London, 1899; A. J. Evans, The First Gold Coins of England, NChr, series III, vol. XX, 1900, p. 218 ff.; G. C. Brooke, Catalogue of English Coins in the British Museum: The Norman Kings, 2 vols., London, 1916; C. Oman, The Coinage of England, Oxford, 1931; C. H. V. Sutherland, Anglo-Saxon Sceattas in England: Their Origin, Chronology and Distribution, NChr, series VI, vol. II, 1942, p. 42 ff.; C. H. V. Sutherland, Anglo-Saxon Gold Coinage in the Light of the Crondall Hoard, London, 1948; G. C. Brooke, English Coins, 3d ed., London, 1950; Sylloge of Coins of the British Isles, Fitzwilliam Museum, Cambridge, I, Ancient British and Anglo-Saxon Coins (by P. Grierson), London, 1958. f. Germany and central Europe: S. Ljubic, Opis jugoslavenskih novaca, Zagreb, 1875; H. Dannenberg, Die deutschen Münzen der sächsischen und fränkischen Kaiserzeit, 4 vols., Berlin, 1876–1905; Archiv für Brakteatenkunde, ed. R. von Höfken, 4 vols., Vienna, 1886–1906; H. Gebhart, Die deutschen Münzen des Mittelalters und der Neuzeit, Berlin, 1929; K. Castelin, Česka drobna mince, doby predhusitské a husitské (1300–1471) (Czech Money of the Hussite and Pre-Hussite Period), Prague, 1953; E. Nohejlová-Prátová, Krása české mince, Prague, 1955; R. Gaettens, Münzporträts im 11. Jahrhundert, Heidelberg, 1956.

Asia. a. Bactrian and Indo-Greek coinage: R. B. Whitehead, The Pre-Mohammedan Coinage of North Western India, Numismatic Notes and Monographs, New York, 1922; P. Gardner, The Coins of the Greek and Scythian Kings of Bactria and India in the British Museum, London, 1886; H. H. Howorth, The Eastern Capital of the Seleucidae, NChr, series III, vol. VIII, 1888; H. H. Howorth, The Initial Coinage of Parthia, NChr, series III, vol. X, 1890, p. 33 ff.; B. Head, The Earliest Graeco-Bactrian and Graeco-Indian Coins, NChr, series IV, vol. VI, 1906, p. 1 ff.; F. M. Allotte de la Fuÿe, Monnaies incertaines de la Sogdiane et des contrées voisines, RN, 1910; R. B. Whitehead, Catalogue of the Coins in the Punjab Museum, Lahore: Indo-Greek Coins, Oxford, 1914; J. Hackin, Répartition des monnaies anciennes en Afghanistan, JA, 1935; A. Foucher, Les satrapies orientales de l'Empire achéménide, CRAI, 1938; A. D. H. Bivar, Bactra Coinage of Euthydemus and Demetrius, NChr, series VI, vol. II, 1951, p. 22 ff.; M. T. Allouche-Le Page, L'art monétaire des royaumes bactriens, Paris, 1956 (Positions des thèses et des mémoires des élèves de l'Ecole du Louvre, 1945–53); G. K. Jenkins, Azes and Taxila, Actes du Congrès de Numismatique de 1953; vol. II, 1957; A. Simonetta, Notes on the Parthian and Indo-Parthian Issues of the First Century B.C., Actes du Congrès de Numismatique de 1953, vol. II, 1957. b. Characene: G. F. Hill, Cat. Arabia, etc., BMC, 1922; J. Babelon, Le trésor de Chapour, Mémoires de la délégation française sur l'Afghanistan, 1957. c. The Parthians: W. Wroth, Catalogue of the Coins of Parthia, BMC, 1903; J. de Morgan, Manuel de numismatique orientale, Paris, 1923; M. Dayet, Monnaies arsacides à bonnet satrapal, RN, 1949; B. Simonetta, Vologese V, Artabano V e Artavasde, Numismatica, 1953–54. d. The Sassanians: P. Gardner, The Coins of the Greek and Scythian Kings of Bactria and India, BMC, 1886; M. A. Stein, Zoroastrian Deities on Indo-Scythian Coins, London, 1886–87; E. Drouin, Notice sur les monnaies des grands Nouchans, RN, 1896; Furdonjee D. J. Paruck, Sassanian Coins, Bombay, 1924; J. Allan, Catalogue of the Coins of Ancient India, BMC, 1936; A. Christensen, L'Iran sous les Sassanides, Copenhagen, Paris, 1936; J. Babelon, L'art médaille sous les Sassanides, RAA, XII, fasc. I, Paris, 1938. e. China: A. E. J. B. Terrien de la Couperie, Catalogue of Chinese Coins from the VIIIth century B.C. to A.D. 621, BMC, 1892; R. Schlösser, Chinas Münzen, Werl (Westphalia), 1935; W. Kann, Illustrated Catalogue of Chinese Coins, Los Angeles, 1953. f. Japan: N. G. Munro, Coins of Japan, Yokohama, 1904; A. Fonhan, Japanische Bildermünzen, Leipzig, 1923; N. Jacobs and C. C. Vermeule, Japanese Coinage, New York, 1953. g. Siam: R. Le May, The Coinage of Siam, Bangkok, 1932. h. Annam: A. Schroeder, Annam: Etudes numismatiques, Paris, 1905. i. The Achaemenids: E. Babelon, Catalogue des monnaies grecques de la Bibliothèque Nationale, Les Perses achéménides, les satrapes et les dynastes tributaires de leur empire, Cypre et Phénicie, Paris, 1893; E. Babelon, L'iconographie et ses origines dans les types monétaires grecs, Mélanges numismatiques, IV, Paris, 1912; J. de Morgan, Numismatique de la Perse antique: Traité des monnaies grecques et romaines d'Ernest Babelon, Paris, 1933. j. Turkey: J. Ostrup, Catalogue des monnaies arabes et turques du Musée National de Copenhague, Copenhagen, 1938. k. India: V. A. Smith, Catalogue of the Coins in the Indian Museum, Calcutta: I, The Early Foreign Dynasties and the Gupta; II, Ancient Coins of Indian Types; III, Persian Mediaeval Southern Indian and Miscellaneous Coins, Oxford, 1906; E. J. Rapson, Catalogue of the Coins of the Andhra Dynasty, the Western Ksatrapas, the Traikutala Dynasty and the Bodha Dynasty, London, 1908; J. Allan, Catalogue of the Coins of the Gupta Dynasties and of Sasanka, King of Gauda, BMG, 1914; J. Allan, Catalogue of the Coins in the Indian Museum, Calcutta, IV, Oxford, 1928; J. Allan, Catalogue of the Coins of Ancient India, BMC, 1936. l. The Mongols and Moghuls: S. Lane Poole, The Coins of the Moghul Emperors of Hindustan, BMC, 1892; H. N. Wright, Catalogue of the Coins in the Indian Museum, Calcutta: III, Mughal Emperors of India, Oxford, 1908; G. Bataille, Les monnaies des Grands Mogols, Aréthuse, nos. 13–14, Oct.–Jan., 1927. m. Islamic coins: S. Lane Poole, The Coins of the Sultans of Delhi, BMC, 1884; S. Lane Poole, The Coins of the Mohammedan States of India, BMC, 1885; R. Stuart Poole, The Coins of the Shahs of Persia, Safavis, Afghans, Efsharis, Zands and Kajars, BMC, 1887. n. Iran: H. L. Rabino di Borgomale, Album of Coins, Medals, and Seals of the Shahs of Iran (1500–1948), Oxford, 1951.

Primitive money: E. Ingersoll, Wampum and Its History, American Naturalist, XVII, 1883; R. Andree, Aggriperlen, ZfE, XVII, 1885; O. Lenz, Über Gold bei Naturvölkern [Hamburg], 1895; H. Schurtz, Grundriss einer Entstehungsgeschichte des Goldes, Weimar, 1898; W. A. Nieuwenhuis, Kunstperlen und ihre culturelle Bedeutung, IAE, XVI, 1903; E. H. Giglioli, I! salemoneta dell'Etiopia, AAE, XXXIV, 1904; O. Schneider, Muschelgeld-Studien, Dresden, 1905; W. Foy, Zur Geschichte der Muschelgeldschnüre in der Südsee, Ethnologica, II, 1913; L. Pfeiffer, Die steinzeitliche Muscheltechnik, Jena, 1914; G. Thilenius, Primitive Gold, AfA, XVIII, 1921; W. C. Farabee, Recent Discoveries of Ancient Wampum Belts, Museum J. of the Univ. of Pennsylvania, XIII, 1922; A. W. Cardinall, Aggrey Beads of the Gold Coast, JAS, XXIV, 1924–25; K. Regling, RLV, IV, L, 1926, s.v. Geld; H. C. Beck, Classification and Nomenclature of Beads and Pendants, Archaeologia, LXVII, 1928; R. Schlösser, Klanggerätmünzen, Sinica, 1928; M. Heydrich, Durch die Sammlung "Das Gold der Naturvölker," Dresden, 1929; A. B. Lewis, Melanesian Shell Money in the Field Museum Collections, Chicago, 1929; A. J. Arkell, Agate Beads, Antiquity, XLI, 1936; H. G. Beazley, Notes on the Red Feather Money of Santa Cruz, JRAI, LXVI, 1936; H. Petri, Die Geldformen der Südsee, Anthropos, XXXI, 1936; R. Thurnwald, Ein vorkapitalistisches Wirtschaftssystem in Buin: Ein Beitrag zur Kenntnis primitiver Wirtschaft und Frühgeld, Archiv für Rechts- und Sozialphilosophie, 1938; C. Fox, Distribution of Currency Bars, Antiquity, XLV, 1940; R. Thurnwald, Zur Entstehung des "Geldes," Jahrbücher für Nationalökonomie und Statistik, CLII, 1940; D. Paulme, Systèmes pondéraux et monétaires en Afrique noire, Rev. Scientifique, no. 3208, 1942; E. Paravicini, Über das Muschelgeld der südöstlichen Salomonen, Anthropos, XXXVII–XL, 1942–45; R. Kaulla, Beiträge zur Entstehungsgeschichte des Goldes, Bern, 1945; M. D. W. Jeffreys, The Diffusion of Cowries and Egyptian Culture in Africa, AMA, L, 1948; P. Einzig, Primitive Money in Its Ethnological, Historical and Economic Aspects, London, 1949; A. H. Quiggin, A Survey of Primitive Money: The Beginnings of Currency, London, 1949; A. H. Quiggin, Trade Routes, Trade and Currency in East Africa, Livingstone, 1949; G. Tucci, Sistemi monetari africani al lume dell'economia primitiva, Naples, 1950; E. Dartevelle, Les "N. Zimbu," Monnaies du Royaume du Congo, Brussels, 1953; G. Odermann, Der Eingeborenenhandel in der Südsee, Annali Lateranensi, XVIII, 1955; P. Van Emst, Geld in Melanesie, Beverwijk, n.d.

Medals. a. General: F. Lenormant, Monnaies et médailles, Paris, 1884; L. Forrer, Biographical Dictionary of the Medallist, London, 1904–30; G. F. Hill, Medals of the Renaissance, Oxford, 1920; M. Bernhart, Medaillen und Plaketten, Berlin, 1920; J. Babelon, La médaille et les médailleurs, Paris, 1927. b. Italy: A. Armand, Les médailleurs italiens des XVe et XVIe siècles, Paris, 1883; A. Heiss, Les médailleurs de la Renaissance, Paris, 1883; G. F. Hill, A Corpus of Italian Medals of the Renaissance before Cellini, London, 1930; V. von Fabriczy, Medaillen der italienischen Renaissance, Leipzig, n.d.; G. Habich, Die Medaillen der italienischen Renaissance, Stuttgart, Berlin, n.d.

* *

Illustrations: PLS. 393–415.

**COLE,** THOMAS. American landscape painter of the so-called "Hudson River school" (b. Lancashire, England, Feb. 1, 1801; d. Catskill, N.Y., Feb. 8, 1848). Brought to America at eighteen, Cole lived in Steubenville, Ohio, until 1823 and painted several portraits before studying briefly at the Pennsylvania Academy of Fine Arts in Philadelphia. Living in New York in 1825, Cole was one of the founders of the National Academy and was soon to win recognition for his dramatic landscapes of the Hudson River Valley and the White Mountains in New Hampshire. From 1829 to 1832 Cole traveled in Europe and was deeply influenced by Claude Lorrain, Richard Wilson, Turner, and Jacob van Ruisdael. In Italy he sketched the ancient ruins, his romantic imagination stirred by the "poetry of decay" and his moralizing tendency stimulated by this evidence of the rise and fall of civilizations. Returning to the United States, he established a home and studio at Catskill on the Hudson. From 1841 to 1842 Cole made a second journey to Europe.

Cole's most ambitious works were a series of five allegorical scenes: *The Course of Empire*, completed in 1836 (New-York Historical Soc.), and the four episodes of *The Voyage of Life* (1839–40; Utica, Munson-Williams-Proctor Inst.; I, PL. 105). An early work, illustrating James Fenimore Cooper, was his *Scene from the Last of the Mohicans* (1827; Hartford, Wadsworth Atheneum). *The Oxbow* (1836; New York, Met. Mus.) represents his mature style. Another series, *The Cross and the World*, was never completed.

Today, Cole's naturalistic landscapes are preferred to his elaborate religious-moral allegories. He often sermonized in paint, as did his friend William Cullen Bryant in verse; both men saw nature as the visible handicraft of God and as a refuge from the ugly materialism of cities. Cole's sketchbooks show

that even his didactic pictures were based on a long and patient study of the forms of trees, clouds, and mountains. Romantic in feeling and sometimes theatrical in color and illumination, his paintings reveal a mastery of solid planes in depth and of light-filled atmosphere; whether calm or turbulent, they achieve unity in both composition and emotional expression. See also AMERICAS: ART SINCE COLUMBUS.

BIBLIOG. L. L. Noble, The Course of Empire, Voyage of Life and Other Pictures of Thomas Cole, N.A., New York, 1853; E. I. Seaver, ed., Thomas Cole One Hundred Years Later, Hartford, 1948.

Oliver W. LARKIN

**COLLECTIONS.** See MUSEUMS AND COLLECTIONS.

**COLOMBIA.** The republic of Colombia, whose boundaries were defined in 1829 and 1830 on its separation from Venezuela and Ecuador, occupies the northwest corner of South America. Its vast extent and greatly varied natural conditions gave rise, in the pre-Columbian period, to well-differentiated local cultures. After the Conquest, which followed the 1536 expedition of Gonzalo Jiménez de Quesada, the region was named the "Kingdom of New Granada" and became an artistic and economic fief of Spain. Remarkable progress, particularly in the growth of cities, was made following the organization of Colombia as a viceroyalty (1718) and its independence (1819).

SUMMARY. Pre-Columbian epochs (col. 749): *San Agustín region*; *Tierradentro region*; *Nariño region*; *Upper Cauca region*; *Quimbaya region*; *Sinú region*; *Chibcha region*; *Tairona region*. Colonial and modern period (col. 752): *Principal centers*.

PRE-COLUMBIAN EPOCHS. Archaeological research has been conducted in fragmentary fashion, owing to the vastness of the territory over which pre-Columbian cultures are distributed; however, discoveries have made possible the differentiation of eight zones (San Agustín, Tierradentro, Nariño, Upper Cauca, Quimbaya, Sinú, Chibcha, and Tairona), apparently unconnected with one another; any attempt to establish a chronology for them would be risky.

When the Spanish conquistadors arrived, several tribes (e.g., those of the Upper Magdalena) that had attained a remarkable level of cultural and artistic development had already disappeared, and the development of other groups was disrupted by the establishment of the new civilization. Most of the latter groups mingled with the conquerors, abandoning their original language, religion, and culture; their descendants, the process of intermarriage having become established from that time on, make up the rural population of many Colombian regions. Only the more isolated tribes managed to survive, as residual groups, at different stages of cultural assimilation.

*San Agustín region.* Only in this area did monumental stone sculpture develop. The culture of San Agustín, also called that of the Upper Magdalena, was established in a vast region of southern Colombia in the department of Huila. Besides hundreds of megalithic statues and the ruins of temples and tombs, excavations have yielded potsherds and a scant number of works in precious metal, obviously insufficient for reconstructing the culture of this region, for which recorded data are also lacking. The stone statuary, varying in size (some more than 6½ ft. tall), represents male and female deities, kings or caciques, warriors, and perhaps ancestor figures; frequent, too, are the representations of craftsmen, fishermen, sculptors, or high officials, sometimes identifiable from their attributes of office or profession. The diverse styles of this sculpture show that its evolution was slow and long drawn out; they range from simple sketches in which the human figure is barely recognizable to highly realistic figures. Characteristic, perhaps, of a particular style or epoch is the progressive animalization of the human figure ("jaguarization"), encountered also in other megalithic American cultures. The statues representing animals display, in addition to a close familiarity with the local fauna, religious aspects possibly derived from totemistic beliefs. Almost all the statues bear elaborate headdresses with a wide gamut of ornamental motifs (see ANDEAN PROTO-HISTORY, I, cols. 382-383, PL. 165).

The sculpture of San Agustín can, of course, be related to similar pre-Columbian work in both Central and South America; stone sculpture similar in form and technical procedures has been found at other sites, in Nicaragua, at Chavín de Huántar in Peru, at Tiahuanaco in Bolivia, and Manabí in Ecuador. Because of its geographic

location, the Upper Magdalena culture seems to be a connecting link between Central American and Andean cultures.

*Tierradentro region.* The culture of this region (located in the department of Cauca and crossed by the Río Páez) is, after that of San Agustín, the most interesting of the Colombian cultures, and perhaps one of the most ancient. Typical of this area are the subterranean tombs, the work of a people whose religion was apparently founded on a cult of the dead. They are hewn out of the bedrock and vary in form. The largest, about 16 ft., 9 in. deep, is about 20 ft., 4 in. wide, with seven burial niches separated by columns some 6 ft., 3 in. high. Walls and columns are decorated with geometric designs in black and red; in several niches there are anthropomorphous figures. As a whole, the tomb (external opening, stairs, central chamber, columns, niches, etc.) is unusually harmonious in its proportions. Some archaeologists have linked the Tierradentro

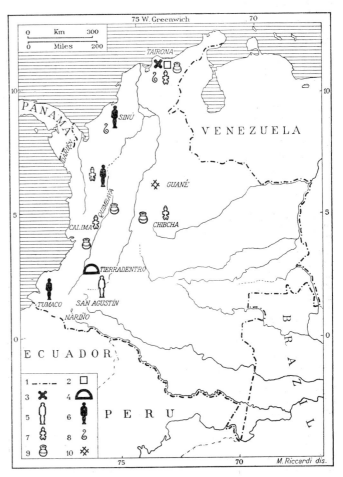

Colombia: distribution of native archaeological cultures and their artistic production. *Key:* (1) Present political boundaries; (2) temples; (3) fortresses; (4) subterranean tombs; (5) stone statuary; (6) terra-cotta figurines; (7) gold figurines; (8) metalwork; (9) pottery; (10) textiles.

culture to that of San Agustín, of which it is thought to be a later or derivative phase; on the basis of this theory an approximate chronology has been established, covering a period from the 7th to the 14th century. Actually, it is quite probable that the two cultures represent two different periods in Colombian archaeological history.

*Nariño region.* Diffused throughout the southwest of Colombia, the so-called "Nariño culture" includes, in addition to several minor ones, the Tumaco or Esmeraldas culture, located on the Pacific Coast and forming part of a large archaeological area that also extends into Ecuador. The pottery is abundant and characteristic: earthenware pots or bowls painted in two or three colors, with motifs predominantly geometric, and, especially, extremely expressive anthropomorphic or zoomorphic figurines, which offer a rich variety of racial and physiognomic types, ranging from the monstrous to the caricatural. The sense of humor revealed in certain intentional distortions, the refined stylization of animal forms, the skillful association of elements grotesque and pleasing, distorted and comic, the contrast between a subject modeled in accordance with precise canons

and a lively stylistic freedom, and, in general, the great plastic skill — all these give Tumaco pottery a fundamental importance in pre-Columbian art. The elaborate style of the figurines and the variety of techniques lead to the hypothesis of a Central American origin, perhaps of a generally Mayan character; the relationship with the cultures of Teotihuacán, Monte Albán, and Tres Zapotes in Mexico is undeniable.

*Upper Cauca region.* In this area, lying between the cities of Cartago and Popayán, emerged the so-called "Calima style" (see I, col. 394, PL. 209), examples of which were found in the tombs. Especially noteworthy is the work in precious metals. The essentially sculptural quality of the gold objects has been related to the megalithic statuary of San Agustín. The Upper Cauca pottery, which also comes principally from tombs, belongs to various types — bowls, footed jars, and globular pots; the decoration is either incised or appliquéd; painted decoration is absent.

*Quimbaya region.* The Quimbaya culture was disseminated in the central valley of the Cauca and the neighboring one of the Quindío (departments of Caldas and Antioquia); in the central and western cordilleras the pottery has refined shapes and decoration with geometric figures; anthropomorphous figures are frequent (I, PL. 173); they are either standing or seated with legs extended or flexed and are painted in two or three colors. The best Colombian work in precious metals, in gold or *tumbaga* (an alloy of copper with gold and silver), was produced in this region: necklaces, cult objects, emblems of rank, and figurines, at times grouped in composite scenes (see I, col. 393, PLS. 210–213). Such objects were made by the cire-perdue process or by hammering gold sheets, either heated or cold. Their fabric reveals familiarity with the techniques of soldering, drawing of metal, gilding, filigree, and openwork; the decoration is done with a chisel or by incising, chasing, or incrustation with precious stones.

*Sinú region.* This area, along the Río Sinú, in the department of Bolívar, has been very little studied, although at the time of its discovery it was considered one of the richest in Colombia. The few examples of goldwork found (earrings of drawn gold, filigree work, and zoomorphic figures) reveal a style akin to that of Chiriquí in Panama. The pottery style is well defined; vessels and bowls are rather thick, with incised or relief decorations representing male and female figures with astounding realism and attention to detail.

*Chibcha region.* Situated on the central plateau of the Andes in the present departments of Cundinamarca and Boyacá, on the savanna of Bogotá, this region gets its name from the Chibcha, or Muysca, politically among the most advanced peoples of Colombia, but not so highly developed artistically. The Chibcha, an agricultural people under a hereditary monarchy, were ruled by two despotic sovereigns, the Zipa and the Zaque, perennially at war over the respective kingdoms of Bacatá and Hunsa. They left no architectural monuments, nor any important sculpture, but they excelled in metalwork (openwork plaques and anthropomorphous figures, called *tunjos*; see I, cols. 393–394, PL. 212) and in the decoration of pottery, closely connected with religious or mythological beliefs (see I, cols. 367–368, PL. 173). North of the Muysca, in the present department of Santander, the Guané were settled, an industrious and skillful people who worked in gold and clay and developed the art of weaving, in which a refined decoration appears. Farther north than the Guané, the Zenú were established in a territory divided among the provinces of Finzenú, Panzenú, and Zenufana, whose conspicuous wealth deeply impressed the earliest chroniclers.

*Tairona region.* This culture, occupying the northwest of Colombia (department of Magdalena), takes its name from the Tairona, who at the time of the Conquest were established on the spurs of the Sierra Nevada de Santa Marta, and whose present-day descendants are the Kogi. The Tairona excelled in stone construction; they built temples and fortresses in an original style. Nose rings, elliptical earrings, and anthropomorphous figures are characteristic of their metalwork. The pottery found in the tombs and middens presents two distinct types: thick-walled red vases and very thin-walled black vases. Typical are the "treasure jars," some of which are decorated with curvilinear painted motifs.

The widespread diffusion of other artistic techniques (rock engravings, bone carvings, shellwork, woodwork, and lapidary work in semiprecious stones; decoration of weapons, especially for ceremonial use; painting of the body) makes attribution to any one region or definite group difficult.

BIBLIOG. L. Zerda, El Dorado, Estudio histórico, etnográfico, y arqueológico de los Chibchas, habitantes de la antigua Cundinamarca y de algunas otras tribus, Bogotá, 1883; V. Restrepo, Los Chibchas antes de la Conquista española, Bogotá, 1895; M. Triana, La civilización chibcha, Bogotá, 1922; C. L. Arango, Recuerdos de la guaquería en el Quindío, 2 vols., Bogotá, 1924; E. Restrepo Tirado, Ensayo etnográfico y arqueológico de la provincia de los Quimbayas en el Nuevo Reino de Granada, Seville, 1929; K. T. Preuss, Arte monumental prehistórico, Excavaciones en el Alto Magdalena y San Agustín, 2 vols., Bogotá, 1931; J. A. Mason, Archaeology of Santa Marta, Colombia, The Tairona Culture, Anthropological Series, Field Museum of Natural History, 1931–39; L. A. Acuña, El arte de los indios colombianos, Bogotá, 1935, Mexico City, 2d ed., 1942; G. Hernández de Alba, Colombia: Compendio arqueológico, Bogotá, 1938; J. Pérez de Barradas, El arte rupestre en Colombia, Consejo Superior de Investigaciones Científicas, Madrid, 1941; J. Pérez de Barradas, Arqueología agustiniana, Bogotá, 1943; W. C. Bennett, Archaeological Regions of Colombia: A Ceramic Survey, Yale Univ. Pub. in Anthropol., XXX, 1944; P. Kelemen, Medieval American Art, 2 vols., New York, 1944; El Museo del Oro, Banco de la República, Bogotá, 1944; P. Rivet and H. Arsandaux, La métallurgie en Amérique précolombienne, Travaux et mémoires de l'Inst. d'Ethn., Musée de l'Homme, Paris, 1946; C. R. Margain, Estudio inicial de las collecciones del Museo del Oro del Banco de la República, Bogotá, 1950; T. Arango Bueno, Precolombia: Introducción al estudio del indígena colombiano, Madrid, 1954; J. Pérez de Barradas, Orfebrería prehispánica de Colombia, Estilo Calima, Madrid, 1954; L. Duque Gómez, Colombia: Monumentos históricos y arqueológicos, Instituto Panamericano de Geografía e Historia, Bogotá, 1955.

Gabriel GIRALDO-JARAMILLO

COLONIAL AND MODERN PERIOD. The architecture of the Kingdom of New Granada during the 16th and 17th centuries was rather poor in comparison with that of the other Spanish colonies in South America and Mexico, although the religious buildings in particular were noted for the lavish decoration of interiors. The early settlements grew without any systematic planning. European influences were felt belatedly and intermittently. A rococo-baroque period of

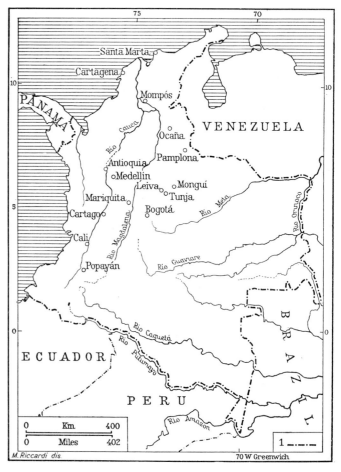

Colombia: principal modern cities. *Key:* (1) Political boundaries.

Andalusian and Castilian derivation held sway for more than two and a half centuries; it was substantially responsible for the monumental character of Colombian architecture. A neoclassic phase succeeded; the Capuchin monk Domingo de Petrés was one of those responsible for the architectural transformation that took place in

the late 18th century. A typical 19th-century eclecticism manifested itself, particularly in the Neo-Gothic style. The contribution from the Chibcha Indians was slight, except in the decoration of interiors. Various modern buildings, both public and industrial, are noteworthy.

Spanish and Italian influences were dominant in both painting and sculpture. The principal centers of painting in the 16th century were Tunja, where Fray Pedro Bedón (ca. 1556–1621) was active, and Bogotá, with its predominantly religious art. Antonio Acero de la Cruz and Bartolomé de Figueroa are regarded as the most authentic representatives of primitivism. There was a brilliant flowering in the 17th century, with Gaspar de Figueroa, Baltasar de Vargas Figueroa, and Gregorio Vásquez y Ceballos of Bogotá. Worthy of mention among later artists are Ramón Torres Méndez, the painters of the Chorographic Commission (founded 1850), and a group of miniaturists headed by Además de Espinosa.

In the 16th century the city of Santa Marta was enriched with the works of Sevillian sculptors such as Jorge Hernández (or Fernández), Martínez Montañés, Anton Sánchez de Guadalupe, and Hernando de Antezaño. Noteworthy in the 17th century are the *S. Pedro* of Pamplona, by Juan de Mesa of Córdoba, and the sacristy of S. Francisco in Bogotá; at that time Juan de Cabrera and the realist Alonso Luis de Lugo were also active in Bogotá. The sculptors of Nativity scenes — in which Oriental influences can be traced — must not be overlooked. There were many Creole decorators (e.g., Pedro Caballero), goldsmiths, and cabinetmakers. A large part of the artistic heritage, unfortunately, has been destroyed with the passage of time.

BIBLIOG. J. M. Giot, Historia eclesiástica y civil de Nueva Granada, Bogotá, 1869; V. Lampérez y Romea, La arquitectura hispanoamericana desde 1492 a 1830, Cultura Americana XI, 1922; B. V. de Oviedo, Cualidades y riquezas del Nuevo Reino de Granada, Bogotá, 1930; D. Angulo Iñiguez, Historia del arte hispanoamericano, Barcelona, 1945–50; R. Vargas Ugarte, S.J., Ensayo de un diccionario de artífices coloniales de la América Meridional. n.p., 1947; G. Giraldo-Jaramillo, La pintura en Colombia, Mexico City, 1948; E. Marco Dorta, Viaje a Colombia y Venezuela; impresiones histórico-artísticas, Madrid, 1948–51; P. Kelemen, Baroque and Rococo in Latin America, New York, 1951 (with. bibliog.); L. A. Acuña, Ambiente ciudadano del siglo XVII en el Nuevo Reino de Granada, Bogotá, 1951; G. Otero Muñoz, Apuntes sobre e arte colonial neogranadino en el siglo XVI, Academia Colombiana de Historia, VI, 1951; L. A. Acuña, El mudéjar en Colombia, Bogotá, 1952; L. Duque Gómez, Colombia: Monumentos históricos y arqueológicos, II, Mexico, 1955 (with bibliog.).

\* \*

*Principal centers.* Antioquia (Santa Fé de Antioquia). Founded by Jorge Robledo on the banks of the Tunusco. Cathedral, reconstructed several times (1547–1837), with fine sculptures; S. Bárbara, the Jesuit house; Church of Chiquinquirá; Church of Jesús Nazareno.

BIBLIOG. E. Uribe, La iglesia en Antioquia, Medellín, 1942.

Bogotá (Santa Fé de Bogotá). Monuments of the 16th and 17th centuries. *Churches*: S. Francisco, begun in the late 16th century, restored; very rich interior; famous for the works of Fray Lego, Gregorio Vásquez y Ceballos, Ignacio García de Ascucha, and others. - S. Bárbara (late 16th cent.), with works by the Figueroas and Vásquez. - La Concepción (1585), with monastery (1592). - Las Nieves, remodeled. - La Veracruz, restored in 1910. - S. Diego, with the famous statue, *Nuestra Señora del Campo*, by Juan de Cabrera. - S. Agustín (1637), with a *Flight into Egypt* by Vásquez. - Chapel of the Sagrario (1689), with paintings by Vásquez. - Third Order Franciscan church (1761–64), with baroque sculpture in wood. - La Candelaria (1686), restored. - Hermitage of Belén and Hermitage of Egypt (1653), the latter with fine paintings by Vásquez. - Chapel of Monserrate (1652–57), with works by Master Lugo and Francisco de Ascucha in the interior. - Nuestra Señora de las Aguas (1644–90), with paintings by Baltasar de Vargas Figueroa. - S. Clara (1629), by Matías de Santiago, with works by Vásquez, the Figueroas, and Acero de la Cruz. - S. Carlos (S. Ignacio; 1605), Renaissance, with works by Vasconcelos, paintings by Padre Páramo, and a painting attributed to Ribera. - Colegio Mayor de Nuestra Señora del Rosario (1651–53) with a picture gallery. - The Cathedral (1553–1678), remodeled. - New Cathedral, begun in 1572, remodeled in the late 18th century by Domingo de Petrés, restored in 1948. - S. Domingo (1577–1785–1817). *Secular structures*: House of the Marqués de San Jorge (late 18th cent.); the Mint (Casa de la Moneda, 1627), remodeled; National Archives; National Library (1774); Archiepiscopal Palace; Palace of S. Carlos; Santander Square; National Capitol (begun 1847); Colón Theater (begun 1792); La Quinta y Museo de Bolívar; Museo del Capítolo Metropolitano; Museo de Bellas Artes; Museo de Arte Colonial, in a former monastery (furniture, sculpture, goldwork, picture gallery); Museo Nacional; Museo del Seminario Conciliar; Bolívar monument.

BIBLIOG. I. P. M., Centenario del Observatorio de Bogotá, Boletin de Historia y Antigüedades, VII, 1903; J. C. García, Templos y palacios bogotanos, Boletín de Historia y Antigüedades, XVII, 1927, pp. 209–17; E. de Valencia, Fray Domingo de Petrés, Boletín de Historia y Antigüedades, XVIII, 1930; G. Hernández de Alba, Guía de Bogotá: Arte y tradición, Bogotá, 1946.

Cartagena. An important port (16th cent.) with fortifications and outer walls, in part by the Italian military architect G. B. Antonelli. Fortress of Felipe de Barajas; the Cathedral, rebuilt in 1612; Church of S. Domingo (16th–17th cent.); Monastery of S. Francisco (16th cent.); Church and Convent of La Popa (early 17th cent.); Church and Monastery of S. Pedro Claver, with decoration dating from the early 18th century; Palacio de la Inquisición (18th cent.); Museo de la Academia de Historia.

BIBLIOG. J. P. Urueta, Documentos para la historia de Cartagena-Cartagena, 1887; A. Ortega, Las murallas y los castillos de Cartagena, Boletín de Historia y Antigüedades, XII, 1918, pp. 94–96.

Monguí. Rich in colonial relics. Church and Monastery of Monguí (17th and 18th cent.), with plateresque facade, paintings by Vásquez.

BIBLIOG. R. Pizano Restrepo, Biografía de Gregorio Vásquez, Bogotá, 1936; G. Hernández de Alba, Arte en Colombia: El santuario de Monguí, Arte en América, Seville, 1949.

Popayán. Retains its colonial appearance, although several times destroyed. Clock Tower (Torre del Reloj; 1672), remodeled; Church of S. Domingo, begun in 1552, rebuilt with a monastery after 1736; Church of S. Francisco (1775); Church of S. José, rebuilt in 1736; Convent of the Carmelite Nuns (17th cent.), with richly encrusted statues; Convent of the Nuns of the Incarnation, begun 1591, rebuilt 1736; Monastery of the Camillian Fathers (1766); Monastery of the Carmelite Fathers (1684); the Hermitage, formerly the Cathedral (1585); Chapel of Belén (1679); Chapel of Jesús de la Plaza (ca. 17th cent.); Church of S. Agustín; the Cauca and Humilladero bridges.

BIBLIOG. A. Olano, Popayán en la Colonia, Bosquejo histórico de la gobernación y de la ciudad de Popayán en los siglos XVII y XVIII, Popayán, 1910; R. Negret, Guía histórico-artística de Popayán, n.d.

Santa Marta. Ancient city, destroyed in 1529, enlarged and fortified in 1665. Castle of S. Juan (1602); Castle of S. Vicente (1644); Fort of S. Antonio (1719); Fort of S. Felipe (1723–24); Cathedral (1696–1712); Bolívar's hacienda, with statue by Petro E. Montarsolo.

Tunja. A wealth of 17th-century buildings, such as the palaces of Antonio Bravo Maldonado and Governor Bernardino Mújica Guevara. Characteristic ceilings of the 16th and 17th centuries (houses of Don Juan de Vargas, Gonzalo Suárez Rendón, and Juan de Castellanos); Cathedral (1569), with Renaissance façade (Bartolomé Carrión); Church of S. Domingo (1568), with baroque Chapel of Nuestra Señora del Rosario (ca. 1680–90) and Museum of Religious Art; Monasteries of S. Francisco (1550), S. Agustín (1568–1603), and S. Clara (late 16th cent.); Church of S. Bárbara; Church of S. Ignacio (early 17th cent.); Museo del Centro de Historia.

BIBLIOG. R. C. Correa, Guía histórica de Tunja, Registro Municipal, LX, 1940, pp. 169–74; A. R. Salamanca, Guía histórica ilustrada de Tunja, Bogotá, n.d.; E. Marco Dorta, La arquitectura del renacimiento en Tunja, Revista de Indias, Madrid, 1945.

Other centers of importance: Medellín, near ancient Ana. - Marinilla, colonial in character. Chapel of Jesús, with baroque façade; Cathedral of Nuestra Señora del Tránsito. - Cartago, founded in 1540; a few remnants of the old city; Viceroy's residence; house of Don Sebastián Marisancena. - Leiva, flourished in the 17th century; houses of A. Ricaurte and of J. de Castellano, with beautiful gates; Monastery of S. Francisco and Convent of the Carmelites (restored). - In the department of Boyacá are the Monastery of El Salitre and the famous bridge of Boyacá.

\* \*

Illustrations: 2 maps in text.

**COMIC ART AND CARICATURE.** In every culture that has attained a certain level of individualism and introspection, the representational arts contain humorous portrayals of various character types, situations, attitudes, physical traits, etc. Sometimes the intention is purely comic; at other times a more satirical attitude is apparent, the joke lying precisely in the contrast between the serious, or even sacred, nature of the subject and its transformation into the ludicrous. Comic art

COMIC ART AND CARICATURE

is often related to the comic theater, particularly in its caricatures of certain stock types such as the villain, foreigner, prostitute, procurer, amorous couple, cuckolded husband, soldier, or priest. In the Western world a theory of the comic originated in relation to the drama and was subsequently applied to the visual arts. From the 17th century on, a specific genre of art — the caricature — has developed (see CHARACTERIZATION), which simultaneously combines aspects of farce, irony, and satire applied to social, political, or religious themes. Despite its intentionally popular appeal and dissemination predominantly in the graphic arts, caricature, like every kind of humorous art, has a deep and ever-increasing intellectual significance; this has made it a favorite form for some of the greatest painters and draftsmen and one of the chief sources of inspiration for contemporary art.

SUMMARY. Antiquity (col. 755). Middle Ages (col. 759). Comic art and modern caricature in the Western world (col. 760). Comic art and caricature in non-European cultures (col. 769): *India and the Far East; Islam; Primitive cultures.*

ANTIQUITY. Distortions in expression, which probably had a magical significance, are found in prehistoric art. Exaggerations of physical characteristics occur in the earliest civilizations of Mesopotamia and Egypt, where art was dominated by religious and dynastic concepts but humorous intent was basically lacking. Possibly certain statuettes of servants and dancing dwarfs from ancient Egypt (which developed a form of literary satire) may be intentionally comic, but it is more likely that they represent an attempt at realistic characterization. A limestone group of the Middle Kingdom (New York, Met. Mus.) — a squatting monkey nursing her young while being combed by another female monkey — suggests the general spirit of caricature: it is a humorous variation on a genre subject. Shells and papyri of the New Kingdom and late period show parodied actions, such as cats and mice making war or animals in the guise of musicians or chess players. A papyrus in the Egyptian Museum at Turin illustrates a hippopotamus perched on a fig tree that is being scaled by a bird with a ladder. All such scenes, however, may be regarded as illustrations of folk tales rather than as caricatures in the strict sense. On the other hand, in Assyrian reliefs of battle scenes the artist may have had, in embryonic form, the deliberately satirical intention of depicting the enemy as ridiculous.

\* \*

It was Greek philosophy that first formulated a theory of comedy. Plato condemned it as an element disturbing to the soul: "One should not be laughter-loving; when one gives way to a strong outburst of laughter, it actually produces a strong convulsion in the soul" (*Republic*, 388ᵉ). Plato tempered this general condemnation by conceding that, although laughter leads to pride and vulgarity, the comic may be justified as the foil of the serious (*Laws*, 816ᶜ), serving to establish a balance and provide harmless and suitable diversion (*Philebus*, 49ᵉ).

Proceeding from this idea, Aristotle found comedy permissible if harmless and not a cause of pain, but not if vulgar or disgusting (*Poetics*, 1449ᵃ). On principle, he objected to the comedies of Aristophanes even though he admired them; he preferred the New Comedy, "which in spite of its comic intent does not constitute invective" and is not slanderous. In contrast to Plato, Aristotle declared that comedy serves as a catharsis, inducing a happy and well-intentioned benevolence toward others; laughter establishes a balance in the soul by easing the tensions produced by repressed emotions. "Comedy imitates rather base subjects but does not deal with every kind of ugliness — only with ugly things that deserve ridicule" (*Poetics*, 1449ᵃ 32–34). Aristotle believed that comedy originated as a parody of oratory: by providing a conclusion contrary to the one anticipated and a contrast between the manner of speaking and the facts, its effect lies in the unexpected and erroneous.

Aristotle's ideas were further developed by his follower Theophrastus in two treatises, *On the Comic* and *On Comedy*. Theophrastus concluded that comedy is pure invention, as

opposed to tragedy, which is based on history and relates actual events. He defined comedy as the portrayal of characters, the creation of stock types, the analysis of individual psychology, the use of a deliberately popular mode of speech, and the representation of "everyday and private" happenings. In *Characters* he elaborated the concept of free fantasy in comedy, already pointed out by Aristotle, and gave examples for a series of stock types which were to have considerable influence during the Hellenistic period.

With the revival of the Aristophanic mode of comedy at the court of Ptolemy IV in Alexandria, Macon and Lycophron restored its power of invective. Later Cicero (*De oratore*, ii. 236) praised laughter, wit, and concise, perceptive invective as attributes of a natural disposition. About A.D. 100, Dion Chrysostomus defended the moral value of laughter and the satire of manners, declaring that "ugly things seem even uglier and hence more comic when exposed to the gaze of an entire city" (*Orations*, 2. 4). This moralistic attitude became even more pronounced in Plutarch.

While Greek philosophy was seeking to define the essential nature, moral value, and esthetics of comedy, literature beginning with Homer had already provided a rich series of instances of the comic. Derision and banter are frequent comic elements in the *Margites* ("the bobby"; a satirical epic poem, now lost, attributed to Homer) and the *Iliad*. In the latter, the impudent Thersites provokes laughter by his ugly, distorted actions and his ignominious downfall; the soft Eastern hero, Paris, is comic in his fear; there is humor in the mockery of the weak by the strong, in the wiliness of Hermes, and in the amorous intrigues of the gods. Drunkenness always provided an inexhaustible source for comedy; the ribald *kōmos* (revel) — the comic and uninhibited dance based on the movements and gestures of licentious persons — is derived from the banquet. Besides this type of comedy, clowns were sometimes brought in to divert the banqueting guests and incite laughter through their physical appearance or buffoonery. From the archaic period on, Greek literature and art found a fertile vein of comedy in striking caricatures that drew playful comparisons between men and animals or in exaggerated physical deformities and moral defects. Stock types of the comic theater such as the lame, the squint-eyed, the hunchback, the dwarf, the coward, the flatterer, the glutton, and the rustic later became intensified and elaborated in the popular theater and the farce, acquiring, however, a somewhat different emphasis (see CHARACTERIZATION).

The Romans inherited not only this entire world of Greek comedy but also the vigorous tradition of the popular Italic theater, whose comedy was probably coarser, freer, and more highly colored. There were many opportunities for comedy in southern Italy and Rome: the Saturnalia, feasts and festivals, village fairs, banquets, triumphal songs, mimes, the ancient Fescennine songs (obscene verses originating in Fescennia, Etruria, sung or recited at rustic festivals), the rude native comedies called *Fabulae Atellanae* (after the town of Atella in Osci). From the *Fabulae Atellanae* came prototypes destined to survive throughout many centuries, such as the gluttonous simpleton Maccus, the swaggering bully Buccus, the garrulous old gaffer Pappus, the scheming hunchback Dossennus, all of which projected the life of townspeople and rustics onto the stage with keen perception, realism, and vulgarity. Greek and Italian traditions gave rise to the *comoedia palliata* (ca. 250–150 B.C.; adapted from the Greek Middle and New Comedy) and the *comoedia togata* (ca. 180–170 B.C.; based on the daily life of the Romans). In the *palliata* tradition, we find in Naevius a comic spirit and biting wit; in Plautus, the lively, gay spontaneity of Italian humor; in Terence, the themes of the Hellenistic New Comedy. After Terence, however, the *togata* was to predominate in the Roman theater, as the Italic authors Afranius, Titinius, and Quinctius Atta reintroduced the indigenous rustic repertory. Under Sulla the *Atellanae* flourished again, and under Caesar the mime; while in the period of the empire a taste for all kinds of spectacles, mimes, and pantomimes continued to increase.

All these aspects of comedy, especially those represented on the stage, were reflected in the visual arts of Greece and Rome (PL. 417), which from the archaic period on portrayed

comic themes and caricatures paralleling those found in literature. Although the religious and devotional function of the major arts in Greece inhibited free expression of the comic spirit, the decorative arts exploited all types of humor, especially in vase painting, which was the product of a high level of craftsmanship and vividly reflected contemporary esthetic tastes. Scenes of the *kōmos* and the orgiastic dances of the banquets, such as the cordax, were interpreted humorously on the vases. As early as the appearance of Corinthian ware, the grotesquely padded dancers, the *komasti*, are shown in their typical contorted gesture, kicking wildly, with prominent buttocks and swollen stomachs; these are also found on Ionic and Etruscan vases and on the black-figured ware of Attica and Calchis. Some of these dances refer to Dionysiac celebrations and are sometimes satirical; more frequently, however, the *kōmos* predominates, suggesting many themes to Athenian vase painters.

Black-figured Attic vases portray the comic movements and picturesque costumes of the choruses in the primitive theater, in which people masqueraded as animals. We find humans garbed as roosters on an amphora in the Staatliche Museen (Berlin), as birds on an oinochoe in the British Museum, and, on another amphora in the Staatliche Museen, disguised as horses advancing with comical paces, causing their riders to fall backwards with hands on knees, reminding one of a chorus in Aristophanes' *Knights*. In a scene on a skyphos (Boston Mus. of Fine Arts) showing on one side men astride dolphins and on the other mounted on ostriches, the presence of a flute player is apparently a reference to the chorus of the primitive comedies with their disguises and buffoonery.

Even during the archaic period, mythology was sometimes interpreted humorously, as on a Corinthian vase showing in a subtly sophisticated manner Athena with the lame Hephaistos. The freedom and frankness of Ionic culture often found expression in a sophisticated and playful humor; one may cite two hydrias in the Louvre, showing respectively Hermes' theft of the herd of Apollo and the punishment of Tityus, where the figures and subjects are enlivened with a streak of humor; or a hydria in the Kunsthistorisches Museum, Vienna, on which the timorous Egyptians are contrasted with the strong and sinewy Herakles, while Busiris and the Ethiopians rush about like the chorus in a comic opera. Equally refined is the humor in certain Pontic vases, the best of which, in the Staatliche Antikensammlungen (Munich), represents the Judgment of Paris; in this delightful scene the artist seems to amuse himself by playfully rendering the character of the three rival goddesses, whose profiles, gestures, and demeanor are characterized most divertingly.

The comic spirit gave rise to an unbridled vitality in the nude dancers shown on the Fikellura type of vase or on the black-figured Ionic-Etruscan ware. In the Ionic ware there was also an emphasis on barbarian types such as the Negroes, who are carefully observed and whose racial characteristics and distinctive movements are rendered with lively naturalism and humor.

The scope of comedy enlarged in the 5th century B.C. to embrace not only mythology and the theater but also many aspects of daily life; a whole series of examples occurs on the red-figured Attic vases, where themes of this sort could be developed more freely than in the major arts. The humorous rendition of a mythological subject is exemplified in a kylix by Brygos, showing Hermes and Hera, the latter entrapped by satyrs in lewd postures. The whole world of the satyrs is frequently shown with great humor, animation, and vivacity in the many scenes of orgiastic dances, burlesques, masques, acrobats, and tumblers, culminating in the intense, unrestrained frenzy of the satyrs on the psykter in the Musées Royaux d'Art et d'Histoire, Brussels, decorated by the painter Douris with an extensive range of comic motifs. Banqueting scenes also continued to provide a fertile field for comic themes, and the red-figured vases jestingly portray the banqueters in various situations: in ecstasy with skyphos or kylix in hand; in an orgy accompanied by hetaerae and ephebi; even vomiting, as on a kylix painted by Brygos, or defecating, as in a revel represented on a black-figured vase by Kleisophos and Xenokles.

The masks worn in comedy may be regarded as caricatures by virtue of their stylization, expressive exaggeration of the features, and accentuation of the abnormal and grotesque. The various types created by the comic theater in Greece and Italy appear in ceramics and metalwork, while single figures as well as entire scenes from the comedies are shown in 5th- and 4th-century vase painting (PL. 417). A group of unpretentious and fragmentary 5th-century oinochoai show slaves bearing roasting spits — a motif inspired by the Old Comedy. Late-5th-century Cabiric vases, painted in the black-figured technique, parody mythological subjects, such as the apotheosis of Herakles, or Odysseus and Circe; and the numerous 4th-century vases illustrating farces provide a colorful sampling of the themes of the popular Italic comedy: the exploits of Herakles readily adaptable to farce, such as his adventures with the Cercopes and Eurystheus on a vase formerly at Catania; Apollo and Zeus on two vases at The Hermitage (Leningrad); the amatory adventures of Zeus; the birth of Helen from an egg; Chiron and the nymphs; Ares, Hephaistos, and Hera; Paris and Neoptolemos; Ajax and Cassandra; Sappho and Alcaeus — the whole realm of Mount Olympus and the heroic legends transformed into burlesque. In these representations the comedy is inherent not only in the subject and the masks but also in the parodied personages who, instead of preserving their Olympian serenity, become presumptuous and misguided mortals, timorous, confused, fainthearted, lustful, and insincere.

Side by side with this world of gods and heroes appear scenes of daily life familiar from the comic stage: the shrewish dialogues between serving-girls and termagants; the punishment and knavery of servants who are shown beaten and put to flight, recounting their misdeeds, robbing or protecting their masters; the amorous dialogues of philandering old gaffers; the fright of the miser about to be robbed; and the burlesque dances. The polychromatic, dynamic, and expressive style of the 4th-century painters of vases illustrating farces is well adapted to the comic themes which they accentuate through their own humorous spirit (PL. 417).

Throughout the Hellenistic period, the masks and characters of the New Comedy, Italic farce, and the mimes were represented in clay figurines and small bronzes. The metalworkers were especially adept at rendering the movements, gestures, and facial expressions of such stock comic figures as the fat shrew, the big-bellied blusterer, the long-winded and vapid orator, and the stupid servant and in converting them into caricatures.

Greek art also found humorous elements in other fields, such as the episodes showing the pygmies and their adventures along the Nile, fighting with storks in ambush, with huge hippopotamuses, or with terrible crocodiles. Here the comedy lies in the contrast between the grotesque, deformed, and frail little bodies of the pygmies and the fierceness or overwhelming number of their adversaries, and in the pygmies' preoccupation with disengaging themselves from surprise attacks, ambushes, and pitfalls. These rather lewd, agitated, and humorous Nile scenes, which occur throughout Pompeian paintings, mosaics, the sophisticated paintings of Palestrina and other representations, both in color and in black and white, were very popular in the Roman world; they derived from Hellenistic themes invented in Alexandria. The free spirit prevailing in the cultural atmosphere of the Hellenistic world enlarged the sphere of art, so that it no longer served merely a religious or votive function but became decorative and hence could easily assimilate types of representation inspired by laughter rather than piety. The typically bucolic and storytelling spirit of Hellenistic art gave rise to such playful and humorous little scenes, especially frequent on engraved gems, in which animals are the dramatis personae. The comedy lies in the way in which nature is turned upside down and logic reversed, so that animals are endowed with human qualities and aspects of daily life are parodied. Weak creatures become strong, slow ones swift, and slaves become the masters in a series of tiny scenes depicted with delicacy and fantasy. In the Hellenistic period we find terra cottas, bronzes, or paintings in which human figures are made into caricature by animal heads or other features in a tradition deriving from the grylli (comic combinations of animals or of animal and human forms) attributed to the painter An-

tiphilos. Literary sources also mention parodies of mythological subjects portrayed in major paintings; but since the work of the great Hellenistic painters has not been preserved and painted vases were no longer being produced, our best evidence for the comic spirit in art during these three centuries is in the small statuettes and bronzes and in the traces that survive in Roman mosaics and paintings.

Official Roman art devoted itself to imperial propaganda and to such themes as the funerary or commemorative portrait, reliefs illustrating historical, funerary, or other serious subjects, and religious or commemorative statues. In the decorative arts, however, all the motifs of Hellenistic art were elaborated and adapted to wall paintings or pavement mosaics: Alexandrian Nile scenes and pygmies, lewd and grotesque dancers, misshapen clowns, mimes, masks, simian monsters, animal disguises — all recur in Roman decoration, together with themes derived from the Italic farces. But although literature of this period created such original forms as the satire and the epigram, the visual arts invented no new types of comedy but merely repeated or elaborated the manifold Hellenistic themes. The childishly drawn graffiti, with their sketchy caricatures of gladiators, citizens, or slaves, are merely popular art at a very infantile level. While popular painting showed a tendency toward lively naturalism and facile narrative, it favored the obscene and erotic rather than the comic, and lewd little paintings abounded in houses, taverns, baths, and brothels; sometimes these were given a comic or satirical significance by means of inscriptions, as in the paintings of the Baths of the Seven Wise Men at Ostia.

Because popular art tended to artificial tales, effective advertisements, and crude obscenity, true comedy (which depends for its effects on subtle irony, mythological parody, refined licentiousness, pungent humor, sarcasm, and caricature) remained confined to the cultivated classes, who found satisfaction in the rich heritage of Hellenistic art. In the late empire, when the esthetics of comedy were transformed by Plutarch into a rigid code of morality and when Latin and Byzantine grammarians repeated the theories of Aristotle and Theophrastus, comedy tended to die out or to survive only as the increasingly hackneyed repetition of forms created by the Greeks.

Giovanni BECATTI

MIDDLE AGES. During the Middle Ages, comic art, especially as related to satire or caricature, resembled that of the Far East or primitive civilizations. Judging by the few examples that remain, medieval comic art was a relatively rare and peripheral phenomenon. Certain representations like the Gothic *drôleries* may be regarded as pure fantasy (even though some of the distortions seem to reveal a caricaturing intention) or as having a magical significance (like the designs found on weapons or coats of arms). Scenes of daily life are shown only in abbreviated form (such as the labors of the months; see II, PL. 24) and furthermore, except in a few provincial localities, are practically nonexistent before the Gothic period (see GENRE AND SECULAR SUBJECTS). The representations of nobles, clergymen, and rich people among the damned in the Last Judgment, in the *danse macabre*, or in eschatological scenes in general obviously have quite forceful satirical connotations (PL. 417), but even here the satire is indicated merely by an exaggerated type of characterization (q.v.) or is made grotesque in a manner designed to provoke laughter. Given the devotional nature of these scenes, we cannot suppose that some of the strange and obscene attributes of the demons (as similarly in the *Divine Comedy*) are the result of deliberately intended mockery.

Similarly, certain obscene representations, especially in sculpture, must also be excluded from the category of comic art, for they were probably invested with an apotropaic significance (e.g., the woman shaving herself, formerly on one of the gates of Milan). The numerous marginal representations in illuminated manuscripts, with their contorted faces and satirical allusions, should also be regarded as caprices — that is, designed purely as escapes from traditional canons of proportion or esthetic formulations.

In this connection it may prove significant to consider the relation between the scarcity of comic representations and medieval doctrines on comedy (not yet systematically edited). It should be borne in mind that according to medieval criticism, theatrical comedy had a far more profound purpose than it had in antiquity or modern times: it represented all the mores of mankind. Ancient treatises on comedy were deliberately interpreted to further this end. University courses inspired by Quintilian dealt with particular human types (not necessarily funny or satirical), such as the lovelorn youth or the paramour. Furthermore, medieval theatrical comedies (of which we have important examples dating as early as the 12th century) — even when dealing with erotic or ribald subjects — generally reveal a definite desire for idealization rather than broad humor. Only in the orbit of the universities (especially that of Pavia) can any major tendency to farce be found. Other forms of literature such as the fabliau, however, present innumerable variants of the stock characters of the comic tales: the priest, the nun, the cuckolded husband, the boastful soldier, the country bumpkin. But it is difficult to find comparable examples in the visual arts; stock characters seem to be entirely lacking in painting and sculpture. Nor can one call truly comic the many figures of minstrel acrobats illustrated in the manuscripts; these either have a documentary purpose or may be considered genre subjects, if they are not purely the result of copying classical models.

Medieval comedy, in fact, may be equated with what later came to be called "genre scenes," specifically the representation of daily life among the people. It is only in the Renaissance that these representations assumed a plainly satirical or burlesque quality or, on the other hand, under the influence of the Reformation, became naturalistic and tender. The Middle Ages had only a limited vision of the world; furthermore, to represent the world as it actually was fell quite outside the traditional role assigned to art. It is no mere accident that the fine miniatures illustrating the *Carmina Burana* are visually more related to caprice than to comic art.

Eugenio BATTISTI

COMIC ART AND MODERN CARICATURE IN THE WESTERN WORLD. Whereas in classical and medieval art caricature is restricted to relatively rare representations of a playful or ludicrous sort, in modern art caricature becomes an important problem for special critical research and esthetic theory. Although rare in major works of painting and sculpture, caricature is especially suited to printed reproduction and mass dissemination. Its close association with comedy and satire leads not only to an interchange between word and image but also to social and political criticism, this becoming an important factor in modern journalism and advertising.

Leonardo's drawings of faces with deformities or greatly disproportionate features (PL. 418) cannot strictly be regarded as caricatures but rather as caprices (see FANTASY); they transform the beautiful into the ugly, although this investigation of what constitutes individual beauty as opposed to universal beauty involves forceful characterization and emphasis on expression. Nor can the distorted faces of the henchmen in scenes of the flagellation or mocking of Christ in German and Dutch 15th- and 16th-century art (PL. 418) be considered true caricatures, for their purpose was to mirror moral deformity by its outward physical expression and generally to equate ugliness with sin, as beauty was paired with virtue. Such figures nevertheless prepared the way for the later development of caricature, as did Michelangelo's "heroic" figures, which the critics of the 17th and 18th centuries called *caricate* ("overloaded"); they were easily transformed into butts for ridicule.

The concept of caricature arose in the 17th century in the circle of the Carraccis. Caricatures by Agostino Carracci are still extant (e. g. PL. 421 and London, Oppé Coll.), but literary sources tell us that the idea of *ritrattini carichi* ("exaggerated portraits") originated with Annibale Carracci. His motives are clearly explained in Mosini's introduction to Simon Guillain's edition of the *Diverse figure* (Bologna, 1646): When nature makes a thick nose, overlarge mouth, a hunchback, or any other disproportion or deformity, she does it as a kind of playful caprice; in imitating such a subject, the artist should then fall in with the joke in order to give amusement to others, since the dispro-

portion will be doubly diverting if well imitated, and the spectator will be moved to laughter if what is already ridiculous is further exaggerated by the artist's hand. Just as Raphael and other artists who sought ideal beauty selected and combined the most perfect parts, so the caricaturist should seek to combine individual disfigurements to achieve an ultimate ideal in deformity (*perfetta deformità*). Thus arises, in antithesis to ideal beauty, the concept of "ideal ugliness," which was later to be exalted by romanticism (T. Gautier, *Les beaux-arts en Europe*, 1855).

Throughout the 17th century, caricature remained an exclusively Italian genre, with the single exception of the French artist Raymond La Fage (1656–90), who was himself a follower of the Carraccis. There are references to caricatures by Domenichino, Guercino (a notebook of his with about 200 caricatures still existed in the 18th century), Mola, and Maratti. The caricatures of Gian Lorenzo Bernini are particularly witty characterizations — no longer merely a series of physiognomic types but separate drawings characterizing the salient features of actual personages (PL. 421). Even in the 18th century, Italian artists still continued to predominate in this field (as in *"Pond's Caricaturas, Being a Collection of Twenty-five Prints"*; cf. *Print-Coll. Q.*, IX, 1922). In the hands of Pier Leone Ghezzi (PL. 422) and later of Giambattista and Domenico Tiepolo, caricature acquired an epigrammatic rather than satirical tone. As a consequence of the growing interest in physiognomy (Lavater had called portrait painting "the most natural, human, noblest and useful form of art"), the sculptor Franz Xaver Messerschmidt created his caricatured portrait heads (Vienna, Öst. Gal.); but caricatures in sculpture are always a rather isolated, side line, although practiced in the 19th century by Dantan the Younger (PL. 430) and later with masterly effect by Daumier (*Busts of Politicians*, 1832; sketches of Ratapoil, 1851).

During the 19th century caricature became an outlet of self-expression for artists whose work in general had an official, classical stamp — for example, Goya, whose caricatures as distinct from his court portraits are completely liberated from any hampering conventions. Comparable though far less expressive examples may be found in the work of Reynolds, J. T. Sergel, J. A. Koch, Hippolyte-Jean Flandrin, Adolf Hildebrand, and Puvis de Chavannes.

Romanticism not only reasserted the value of caricature as an art form (Baudelaire) but opened up a new literary field: the "layman's caricatures," noteworthy for their naïve and unconventional style (E. T. A. Hoffmann, Hugo, Baudelaire, Gautier, Mérimée, Verlaine, De Musset, George Sand, Rimbaud, Jarry, Proust, Kafka, Morgenstern, Cocteau, Lorca, Faulkner).

Despite the swift spread of caricature as an artist's caprice, it was somewhat slower to find its way into the literature of art. The verb *caricare* ("to overload") seems first to have been introduced, like the noun form, by Mosini; and in his *Life of Annibale* (Carracci), 1672, Bellori spoke of the artist's "burlesque or caricatured portraits" (*ritratti burleschi, overo caricati*). In his *Vocabolario toscano* (1681), Baldinucci defined caricature as a portrait likeness in which for the sake of jest "the defects of the features imitated are disproportionately exaggerated." Bernini introduced the term into France (1665), and soon thereafter it appeared in A. Félibien's writings (*Des Principes*, 1676) as an "exaggerated portrait" (*portrait chargé*) rendered with "three or four strokes of the pencil."

In the *Encyclopédie* of 1751, it was defined by Diderot's coeditor D'Alembert in terms similar to those of Baldinucci, but with the added comment that the artist can devote himself to this kind of "unbridled imagination" (*libertinage d'imagination*) only as a form of relaxation.

The first definition in English was given by Sir Thomas Browne (published posthumously in *Bibliotheca Abscondita* in his *Works*, 1686, and *A Letter to a Friend*, 1690): "When men's faces are drawn with resemblance to some other animals, the Italians call it to be drawn in caricatura." In 1712, John Hughes (*Spectator*, no. 537) said that "the art consists in preserving amidst distorted proportions and aggravated Features, some distinguishing likeness of the Person." We may infer that caricature was then regarded negatively as a kind of ugliness

in art from the fact that in 1751 Lord Chesterfield considered as caricatures the figures of Rembrandt, whose style even Hogarth, first and greatest of English caricaturists, regarded as ridiculous, although Rembrandt's indifference to ideal beauty never found its expression in a caricaturing style.

In the early 19th century, writings on caricature are a mélange of references to pictorial satire, illustrated pamphlets, and any other forms of art which to the taste of the time appeared "grotesque" or "caricatured." In 1792 Boyer de Nîmes compiled an anthology of caricatures relating to the French Revolution, and the French edition of Francis Grose's *Rules for Drawing Caricatures* (1788) appeared in 1802. Jaime's *Musée de la Caricature* (1834–38) brought together a long series of examples from the late Middle Ages to the 19th century. The first historical treatise appeared in 1865: Thomas Wright's *History of Caricature and Grotesque in Literature and Art* and the first volume of Champfleury's *Histoire de la Caricature*, which was to cover the whole span from antiquity to Daumier. Champfleury, a friend of Courbet's, looked at caricature from the point of view of realism and thus as a means of liberation from neoclassical idealized form; while Wright, regarding caricature as a coarse and schematic type of representation, believed it to be the first primitive and awkward manifestation of art: "Art in its earliest form is caricature."

The first to elevate caricature to the rank of a symbolic mode of expression, Baudelaire (*De l'essence du rire et généralement du comique dans les arts plastiques*, 1855), broke with two traditional concepts: the accepted classical theories of ideal beauty and the opinions of previous periods which had reduced ugliness to the realm of the comic burlesque. This positive evaluation conceived of ugliness as a revelation of demonic power and transcendent symbolism. The romantics were in fact the first to see ugliness as a manifestation of the diabolical and enigmatic aspects of existence. By thus raising ugliness in esteem (one of Langlumé's lithographs, *Pégase romantique*, carries the ironic motto, "Nothing but ugliness is beautiful; only the ugly is lovable"), they paved the way for a deeper understanding of caricature. Baudelaire's analysis of caricature as a phenomenon of civilization led him to an inquiry into the nature of comedy. He distinguished between two types of laughter, one expressive of man's sense of superiority (an idea already formulated by Hobbes, *On Human Nature*, 1650) and another mingled with the mysterious and terrifying: "The sage laughs not, save in fear and trembling." He further differentiated the satanic kind of laughter, in which man affirms his worldly pride by making whatever is beyond his understanding the butt of ridicule, and the laughter in which he seeks to come to terms with the supernatural as a means of propitiation. Baudelaire also drew a distinction between the "significative comic," which is dependent on allusions and references to the specific, and the "absolute comic" (the grotesque), which originates in fantasy and, being a form of "art for art's sake," has a creative role superior to mere imitation.

Proceeding from this recognition of a creative quality in ugliness, critics of the later 19th century tended mistakenly to regard caricature as a forerunner of modern art and to consider artists like Delacroix, Courbet, Manet, Van Gogh, and the expressionists as caricaturists, though actually there is nothing of this spirit in their distortions. In his *Kunstkritiken* (1893–94), the poet Hugo von Hofmannsthal declared that caricature had served a role in anticipating the themes and style of modern art; it had made the artists increasingly aware of the actualities of life — especially of the life of the working class, from which the major artists of the earlier 19th century had become estranged — and it had placed modern life within the orbit of art. Caricature, moreover, constitutes a kind of preparatory discipline that leads the artist to deeply penetrating characterization, and it inculcates a reverence for pure abstract form independent of content. According to Hofmannsthal, the recognition that objects exist as forms to be perceived quite apart from their conventional significance is an important artistic insight. The two roles of "closeness to life" and "stylization" which caricature plays were both to prove significant for the development of 19th- and 20th-century art.

The expressionist predilection for instantaneous and unconventional effects was to lead both to elevation of the tone of caricature and to enhancement of its demoniac aspects; and side by side with the interest in the grotesque went an interest in the world of the satanic and the fantastic (cf. W. Michel, *Das Teuflische und Groteske in der Kunst*, Munich, 1911). At about this time, E. Fuchs examined the cultural role of caricature, which he regarded as a form of illustrated social history.

In their exploration of the psychological roots of caricature as an art form, E. Kris and E. H. Gombrich (1938) postulated that in the comic aspect of caricaturing distortion, there is present a quality that goes to the root of the essential nature of things, even though it has changed with the passage of time and can no longer be fully understood in its symbolism. The satyr of antiquity, the Pulcinella of Italian comedy, the *drôleries* of the Gothic, and the figure of Don Quixote are all phenomena that have a far deeper level of interpretation than their apparent surface content. The theory of Kris and Gombrich was based on concepts of Freud, who regarded caricature as a form of degradation (cf. Baudelaire) which accomplishes its purpose "by rendering prominent one feature, comic in itself, from the entire picture of the exalted object, a feature which would be overlooked if viewed with the entire picture. . . . Where such a comical feature is really lacking, caricature then unhesitatingly creates it by exaggerating one that is not comical in itself" (Freud, 1905). Proceeding from the relationship between caricature and magical practices, Kris and Gombrich saw its prototypes in those effigies that in ancient times were pierced or burned as surrogates for an absent victim; caricature, however, dissolves the magical connection between the actual person and his image, and operates only on the latter, which it "wounds" by distorting its form.

Here we can consider only briefly the deeper significance of caricature. As may be deduced from some of the definitions cited, a period having a more positivistic outlook tends to emphasize the humorous aspects of caricature, while a restless and irrational period tends to stress its symbolical importance; from the point of view of style, caricature can be looked on either as awkwardness (as in Lord Chesterfield's *Letters*) or as a manifestation of the artist's virtuosity (Félibien). For a drawing to be called "caricatured" in the comic sense, there must be an implied contrast between the drawing and the commonly accepted canons of beauty and proportion; since the comic element lies in the contrast, caricature can develop only when a dialectic is established between beauty and ugliness. For a drawing to be satirical, however, one must know its underlying prototype (contrary to Baudelaire's idea of the "absolute comic"), since the ideal becomes the point of departure for the contrasting image that overthrows it. While caricature is a manifestation of the artist's subjectivity and creative freedom in breaking with official canons of beauty, it remains at the same time an irrevocable link to the prototype. Like every revolutionary, the caricaturist is himself part of the system he attacks.

One type of distortion is arrived at accidentally as man explores the many aspects of reality, including the supernatural, grotesque, and fantastic; but caricature is the result of a conscious, reflective, and subjective desire to mock and overthrow accepted norms. The caricature of the Carraccis arose from a tension and conflict within the artists' own experience — a welling up of a challenge to the very tenets of ideal beauty that they themselves were engaged in establishing and maintaining. When regarded merely as a playful outlet for the draftsman, caricature could detach itself from the sphere of official sanction and no longer had to be imprisoned within a rigid philosophical scheme.

From the art historian's point of view, the "invention" of the Carraccis had to be preceded by three steps: an empirical study of visual reality; the establishment of a canon of proportions, culminating in the concept of ideal beauty; and the freedom of the artist to improvise in a subjective manner. These steps were part of the evolution of esthetics during the Renaissance. The Middle Ages, concerned only with the "absolute comic" (in Baudelaire's sense) had no concept of caricature as a contrast to the beautiful.

A development preceding the emergence of caricature is represented by the physiognomic studies of Dürer and Leonardo. Despite their strong characterization, the drawings in Dürer's *Studies of Heads* (Berlin, Staat. Mus., 1513) are entirely lacking in any comic intent; they are part of the artist's researches in proportion and his quest for ideal form. Leonardo's studies are connected with attempts to establish the connection between man's soul and his outward appearance and with the significant contrast that he found between beauty and ugliness. His *Studies of Heads* (Windsor, Royal Lib.) reveals the objective spirit of the Renaissance artist's attempt to determine the rules that govern life. One must remember that during the Renaissance, man felt himself the center of the cosmos, the measure of all things, and the most fully realized of all creations. This doctrine gave him the means of measuring all created forms: "The grotesque natural forms in the animal, vegetable, and mineral kingdoms or in cloud formations are not in themselves comic, though they become so because they remind us involuntarily of related patterns on higher levels of nature and so can be interpreted as caricatures" (Eduard von Hartmann, *Aesthetik*, part II, Leipzig, n.d.). This superior attitude of man and the resultant "significative comedy" were for Baudelaire symptoms of a "discerning and jaded civilization," for in his words, if mankind were not itself a part of creation, there would be no comic sense; only man's sense of superiority makes comedy and laughter possible.

Finally the important role of mannerism should be mentioned, and the growing freedom of imaginative power that, as Kris and Gombrich (1940) pointed out, allowed the artist of the latter half of the 16th century considerable latitude for graphic improvisation. Caricature with its free distortions and variations is part of a development marked by an increase in graphic forms of art and a concept of style that has a certain mobility rather than being fixed and established. Leonardo's observations on cloud formations and the accidental stains on walls reveal his concept that the artist must begin with the coarse and crude and impose his form on this matter; the caricaturist, however, evolves his special type by abandoning the many-sided aspects of reality and instead reducing it to a few elementary strokes. But the more drastically form is reduced, the more ambivalent it becomes; the Carraccis made use of these ambiguous linear effects in their *divinarelli pittorici*. Such puzzle pictures — the enigmatic transposition of a single aspect into many possible aspects — are typical of mannerism, which delighted in producing ambiguous forms (like Arcimboldo's heads; V, PL. 240), all stressing the questionable and mocking, by their ambivalence, the dogmatic and rational.

Mannerism anticipated the concept of perfect deformity attributed to Annibale Carracci. Ignazio Danti in *Delle perfette proporzioni* (Florence, 1567) had already postulated a counter-canon, a *disordine* formed by combining elements that are entirely incompatible. Thus the Carracis, in discovering caricature, pursued the mannerist quest for plurality of forms still further. While they opposed to mannerism a classic and stabilized canon of form, suitable for "official," public art, in their private sketchbooks they gave play to complete freedom of imagination.

The stylistic evolution of caricature is determined by two forces operating in conjunction: observation of actuality and the power of abstraction. The subjective nature of a vision hastily and intuitively grasped requires that it be set down with spontaneous and sketchy means, and in order to record his momentary impressions the artist evolves a kind of symbolic shorthand or device (like the pear for Louis Philippe; PL. 429) that can be readily understood and widely popularized. Caricature combines this element of popular appeal with an esoteric quality, for it frequently requires a special knowledge of graphic relationships on the part of the observer to enable him to decipher the linear puzzle. This is quite contrary to the once-prevalent theory that caricature was a primitive form of art; yet, while it is a genre full of virtuosity and linear complexity, it also has a naïve aspect that relates it to primitive symbolism. Plate 1 of Hogarth's *Analysis of Beauty* provides an example of successive variations in the process of simplifying an antique characterized portrait. Caricature is an art that can be taught;

its formulas have long since been incorporated in "how-to-do-it" manuals that demonstrate how the elements of physiognomy may be grasped through the grouping of a few essential strokes.

Caricature's capacity for transposing form gives it an indefinable diabolical quality. When Charles Philipon was called before a tribunal because of his caricature of the *roi bourgeois* Louis Philippe (PL. 429), he laid before his judges four drawings and said: "The first resembles Louis Philippe; the last is like the first, yet — this last is a pear! Where would you draw the line? Would you condemn the first drawing? then you must also condemn the last, which resembles it and thus also resembles the King, too. You would then have to condemn any caricature portraying a head that is narrow above and broad at the bottom."

In opposition, therefore, to the fixed and definite unity of classical style, caricature is an unstable form of art, susceptible of every conceivable kind of transition or connotation. "One is lost in a world of wild jumbles in which the appearance of men mingles with that of beasts, the organic with the inorganic, and mechanical joints become parts of the body" (F. T. Vischer, *Aesthetik*, Reutlingen, 1846–57). The formal associations of the caricaturists set up a chain reaction of variations that expanded into the grotesque and the fantastic (connected with the allegories of Bosch and Bruegel, the marionettes of Bracelli and his imitators, the mannerists' puzzle pictures, the figured alphabets of the late Gothic period, and the metamorphoses of medieval handwriting). Caricature, however, as one manifestation of the "significative comic," and thus bound to its prototype, can never so distort what it represents that its formal and enigmatic relation to its subject is lost sight of. This distinguishes it from manifestations of the "absolute comic," which progress into the most extreme distortions and the fearsome realms of the illogical and completely fantastic.

Let us now consider the role that caricature has played as pictorial satire. Confined at first to the private sphere of the academies, caricature by virtue of its ability to characterize physiognomy was eventually transformed into an instrument of social criticism. This development went hand in hand with a rise in the free expression of public opinion, beginning in the 17th century with the democratically inclined northern countries (England and Holland) and reaching its ethical and esthetic apogee in the 19th century with the work of Daumier (q.v.; PL. 430). Previously satire in art had been expressed through various forms of parody and travesty, but rarely through exaggeration. During the Renaissance the transferral of human attributes and activities to animals, and vice versa, was widely used for political or religious satire or for parodying accepted works of art such as the Laocoön group ("Titian's Laocoön Caricature...," *AB*, March, 1946; PL. 423). This form of transposition is also found in the *singeries* of the 16th century, in which apes enact the roles of men (Herri met de Bles), in baroque art (Teniers), in 18th-century France (Chardin, Nicolas Huet le Vieux, Coypel), in Goya, and finally in the 19th century, as in Grandville (J. I. I. Gérard) (cf. E. Fuchs and examples in T. Panofka, "Parodien und Karikaturen auf Werken der klassischen Kunst," *AbhBerlAk*, 1851).

Anonymous denunciatory picture pamphlets filled with popular imagery abounded in the 16th century (PL. 419). Derived from the northern realism of P. Bruegel (q.v.; PL. 420), they were aimed not at social classes and their representatives but rather at all mankind, viewed as incurably deluded and hypocritical. Bruegel gave his satires the dimensions of parables and made special use of contrasting pairs [*The Rich Men's Feast* (cf. PL. 420) and *The Poor Men's Feast*]. Similarly Callot (1592–1635), in his mannerist *concetti*, used the contrast between grotesque, hybrid creatures, dwarfs, and beggars and refined, elegant dancers or acrobats (PL. 421). While Dutch painters of the 17th century gave a caricaturing exaggeration to their representations of daily life, they were expressing optimistic good humor and boundless vitality rather than social criticism (PL. 424). It was only toward the close of the 17th century that this skeptical, sensual realism passed over into satire in the work of Cornelis Dusart (1660–1704), who portrayed Louis XIV and the leaders of the League of Augsburg in numerous caricatures. The reign of Louis gave rise in France and other countries to an outburst of defamatory illustrated pamphlets; at the same time the French satirists lampooned controversies between artists or among artists, critics, and the public (Michel Dorigny, *Warning against Mansart*).

The rise of the *bourgeoisie*, the flourishing of journalism, and a heightened interest in social problems made England the chief center of satirical caricature during the 18th century. The freely handled abstract forms with which the Carraccis had invested their caricatures were united with the pungent realism of popular art, so that the style of this genre became greatly enriched and revitalized. Every manifestation of public and private life was lampooned — individual indiscretions, fashion (PL. 427), theater, manners, politics, etc. In the distorting mirror of his caricatures, William Hogarth (PL. 425), like Goya, no longer reflected individual deformities but all society in chaos, combining the previous traditions of caricature with the Dutch image of daily life. Hogarth seems to have set himself a task like that of Montaigne — observing human existence from minute to minute. In *The Rake's Progress* and *Marriage à la Mode*, he made a morality play out of human life and united the judgment of the moralist with the power of the dramatist. While reviving the medieval narrative picture, he also anticipated cinematic presentation. In caricaturing an entire situation, he frequently resorted to that play with symbols, allusions, association of ideas, and enigmas which in the esthetic of English thought constitutes one of the aspects of wit.

In this moralistic interpretation of the theme of the resemblance between human beings and beasts, English caricature tended to be coarse and violent in its form and cruel in its subject matter (e.g., Hogarth's *Four Stages of Cruelty*), as well as inclined to bitter polemic. Hogarth's predominant interest in social content was transformed by his followers Thomas Rowlandson (1756–1827; PL. 427) and James Gillray (1757–1815; PL. 428) into violent political satire, filled with patriotic zeal and directed mostly against France and Napoleon. But, still following in Hogarth's footsteps, Rowlandson and Gillray also developed the device of narrative through episodic series of pictures; these were sometimes sharply moralistic, like medieval cycles, and caricaturing in intent (e.g., Rowlandson's *The English Dance of Death*, 1816), but sometimes gentler in their narrative and humor, anticipating the picture books of the later 19th century (e.g., Gillray's *John Bull*, 1793; Rowlandson's *Tour of Dr. Syntax*, 1812). In the decades following the Napoleonic wars, noble patriotic themes gave way to caricatures of everyday life. Typical of this modified form of satire, developing out of genre and marked with a genial humor, are some works of George Cruikshank (q.v.; 1792–1878), Thackeray's caricatures, and the picture books of the Swiss artist Rodolphe Töpffer. Hogarth, Rowlandson, Gillray, and Cruikshank all gave a scenic setting to caricature, broadening it into a description of daily life and manners; in style, the sharply aggressive popular imagery of the Continent was modified but yet adapted to appeal to a wide public. Their expressive curving line was taken up by Daumier to give volume to his figures.

Before Daumier, French caricature had been an outgrowth of bourgeois realism. Debucourt (1755–1832) and Carle Vernet (1758–1832) restricted their caricaturing tendencies merely to a slight form of exaggeration. The influence of the English caricaturists was paramount, especially in the 1830s, but thereafter a counterinfluence became apparent. The outstanding satirical draftsmen were those associated with Charles Philipon (1800–62), who as editor of the journals La Caricature (1830–34) and Le Charivari (1832–42) had as collaborators Raffet, Grandville, Monnier, Traviès, Pigal, and others. When Daumier (q.v.) became associated with this group, the political cartoon was transformed from bland satire into an instrument for violent polemic. The success of his magnificent series *Le ventre legislatif* was so great that in 1835 the censors decreed that caricatures might no longer deal with political controversies, and Daumier thereafter directed his shafts against the vices, social prejudices, and conformity of bourgeois society (*Robert Macaire, Les bons bourgeois, Les gens de justice*, etc.; IV, PL. 120). During the Second Empire, in defense of democratic liberties, he resumed

his attack against obscurantists and reactionaries with the creation of Ratapoil, a Bonapartist *agent provocateur*. He ridiculed the narrow-mindedness of his contemporaries with the monumentally stupid M. Prudhomme (a figure originally invented by Henri Monnier, 1805–77, who was himself influenced by Cruikshank) and created a whole series of symbolic personages lampooning contemporary political or social types: Macaire, the hypocritical trickster, had a distant prototype in the *faux semblant*, the pious fraud of medieval satire; Daumier made him and Ratapoil incarnations of the devil. Of equal significance is his series of caricatures that constitute the first serious self-criticism of the modern city dweller; his anthology of *Les français peints par eux-mêmes* brings to mind the *Diverse figure* with which the Carraccis had portrayed the citizens of Bologna.

In the same category of those symbolic personages exemplifying the moral and political attitudes of a social class or entire nation, who were to become a constant theme in modern caricatures and humorous illustrated periodicals, are the hunchback Mayeux, whose invention has been ascribed to Traviès (1804–59), Adolf Schrödter's Herr Piepmeyer (*Thaten und Meinungen des Herrn Piepmeyer*, Frankfort on the Main, 1848–49), Rodolphe Töpffer's personages (Le docteur Festus, M. Jabot, M. Pencil), and other figures found in cartoons and comic papers, such as John Bull, Herr Biedermeyer, Uncle Sam, etc.

Other 19th-century French caricaturists were Gustave Doré (1832–83), who invested even his caricatures with a romantic sentimentality (*La ménagerie parisienne*); the mordant and scurrilous Grandville (1803–46), whose best works have a somewhat grotesque surrealist quality (PL. 429; *Un autre monde*, 1844); Paul Gavarni (1804–66; PL. 430), perceptive commentator of the humble folk of Paris who directed attention to public welfare (*Les lorettes*; *Paris le soir*); and J. L. Forain (1852–1931), who resumed some of the subjects treated by Daumier, though mitigating the sharpness of their satire and combining them in his last works with patriotic propaganda. Daumier in fact exerted a significant influence not only on caricaturists such as Forain but on expressionist artists including Toulouse-Lautrec, Van Gogh, Rouault, and Barlach; and while raising caricature to the highest level of artistic expression, he made it the mouthpiece for a new mode of thought and sentiment (cf. Baudelaire and Hofmannsthal in literature).

German caricaturists of the 19th century preferred fantasy and humor to political and social themes. Wilhelm Busch (1832–1908), pursuing the direction taken earlier by Töpffer, concentrated on picture books and children's book illustration (Max and Moritz) in an anticipation of animated cartoons and comic strips. This typically German form of humor may be found in such periodicals as *Fliegende Blätter*, founded in 1844, and *Kladderadatsch*, founded in 1848; it has its 20th-century followers in the work of A. Oberländer (1845–1923) and O. Gulbransson (b. 1873). Only toward the end of the century did a kind of violent social satire develop in Germany, to find its outlet in the satirical weekly *Simplizissimus*, founded in 1896. Among the most vitriolic of the satirical draftsmen of the German empire under the Kaisers was T. Heine (1867–1948), whose style evolved in the milieu of the *Jugendstil* (see ART NOUVEAU). In our own century the leading master of political-social satire was George Grosz (1893–1959; PL. 431), who made the picture book a powerful weapon in the class struggle.

It is certainly noteworthy that many outstanding modern artists began their careers as comic or political caricaturists (Feininger, Slevogt, Corinth, Kupka, Villon, Barlach, Gris, Calder, Orozco). This seems to indicate that the moral and social preoccupations of caricature and satire play a considerable role in leading to the distortions and abstractions of contemporary art. Yet it may also serve to explain why caricature has virtually ceased to exist as a separate genre: whereas formerly it detached itself from high art by opposing its rules, such opposition no longer exists; abstraction and distortion of the subject do not constitute a contrast to accepted formal principles but have become accepted elements within the creative process of contemporary styles. In the most recent developments of caricature, two diametrically opposed principles may

be observed: (1) the pictorial distortion that had its origins in expressionism, evoking images of striking realism and forceful satire, as in the work of Mino Maccari (e.g., his vignettes in *Selvaggio* and after the war in *Il Mondo*; see PL. 430), and (2) the more lyrical type of caricature represented by the wryly humorous and otherworldly drawings of the American artist Saul Steinberg (b. 1914; PL. 432). The art of the majority of political cartoonists in the daily press, however, frequently dissolves into mere graphic mannerism.

Werner HOFMANN

In the 20th century there are various manifestations related to the evolution of comic art, as distinguished from the more or less conventional forms of caricature found in newspapers and magazines. The most pervasive of these is the comic strip, which has become a world-wide phenomenon as an accessory of newspaper publishing. Although varying in quality, it must necessarily bow to the exigencies of mass production and daily deadlines. A variant of the comic strip is the comic book, an enlarged version of the picture narrative. Both forms appeal especially to the very young or the relatively illiterate, but in rare instances they may be more subtle in nature. Animated cartoons may be considered a film version of the comic book, although they frequently offer a more artistically imaginative and sophisticated presentation. Walt Disney is the best known of the many fabricators of animated cartoons.

In social and political caricature, the 20th century has produced a number of worthy exponents, among whom the leading master, George Grosz, has been mentioned. In Germany the period following World War I led other "New Objectivity" artists, such as Otto Dix (b. 1891) and Max Beckmann (q.v.) to express a kind of dry, harsh realism, filled with the despair of that era. These three were painters as well as graphic artists, although Beckmann's powerfully symbolic comments on the life of his time raise his paintings to the highest level of contemporary art. The graphic work of these masters is basically "fine arts" in character and not primarily designed for newspaper consumption.

In the same general graphic-arts–painting area, Mexico has produced a considerable number of important contemporary figures. The engraver José Guadalupe Posada (1851–1913), known for his biting comments on the social and political scene of his day, is the spiritual ancestor of many Mexican artists of the following generation. Of the so-called "big three," José Orozco (q.v.) is the most directly expressionist of the group in both his lithographs and his paintings; Diego Rivera (q.v.) combines the limited space of modern postimpressionism with the feeling for crowds deriving from 14th-century Italian painting; and David Siqueiros (q.v.) uses camera and motion-picture techniques to achieve the dynamic effects of optical dramatic realism. All three are noted for their profound social commentaries, but are best known for their mural painting. In all media they have produced a powerful reflection on the Mexican revolution, on which their art is based.

In the United States, graphics and painting are similarly related from the beginning of the 20th century to the present. Although in the late 19th and 20th centuries the newspaper and magazine cartoonist was still preeminent — e. g. (I, PL. 114), Thomas Nast (1840–1902) and Art Young (1866–1943) — by the end of the first decade specific individuals and groups were projecting social commentary in its fine-arts–graphic form as well as in painting. Early practitioners were John Sloan (q.v.), Boardman Robinson (1876–1952), George Bellows (1882–1925), George Overbury ("Pop") Hart, and George Luks (1867–1933). A later generation produced Peter Blume (b. 1906; *The Eternal City*, New York, Mus. of Mod. Art) and Paul Cadmus (b. 1904). More recently Ben Shahn (q.v.), Philip Evergood (b. 1901), and Jack Levine (b. 1915) illustrate the modern painter's interest in socially and politically oriented caricature (I, PL. 123). On a primarily social level, one may point to a number of sophisticated delineators of manners and customs — artists who are mainly graphic but whose extremely agile intelligence and imagination place them in a class apart. This group is exemplified by James Thurber and Robert Osborn (PL. 431).

A parallel movement has been the continuous and often very fruitful production by primarily political cartoonists whose chief outlet is the newspaper and the magazine. These are to be found in every country, and each nation has its own favorites. Among the outstanding examples are Vicky and Low in Great Britain and Fitzpatrick and Herblock in the United States. Other types of modern painters who have developed the comic or caricature point of view include the Austrian Alfred Kubin (b. 1877), whose wash drawings and pen-and-ink sketches re-create much of the terror and wry humor of the later Middle Ages in Central Europe. The Belgian James Ensor (q.v.), who is considered one of the ancestors of the expressionist movement, has produced a highly effective and symbolic kind of commentary, as represented by his *Entry of Christ into Brussels* (V, PL. 122; Knokke-le-Zoute, Casino, 1888). The extraordinary violence of Ensor's reaction against the narrow society in which he lived is reflected not only in works of this kind but in many other painted and etched allegories.

In the art of Paul Klee (q.v.) there is a tremendous range from the gently humorous to the bitterly caricatured. Every aspect of life becomes a subject for his evocative and sensitive linear art, which is universal in spirit even though derived from the restrictive circumstances of his own life and time. Klee's extreme sensitivity and delicacy have had their influence on later practitioners of comic art and caricature. If the work of such artists as Saul Steinberg is not directly influenced by Klee, it is certainly parallel in its general meaning. Picasso, who has been all things to all art forms, also occasionally indulges in the comic (PL. 431). Sometimes his allusions have a shock quality similar to that of the surrealists (see SURREALISM); sometimes his humor is contained in a kind of imaginative shorthand. Finally, in his graphic art — both drawings and prints — there is a humorous reference and economy of form completely characteristic of the comic branch of this medium.

Bernard S. MYERS

Just as "The New Objectivity" school, the American social realists, and the Mexican revolutionary artists show so many rich examples of caricature, there are other modern schools which may be related to the same development. In Dada (see EUROPEAN MODERN MOVEMENTS) and surrealism the comic impulse has received a new direction from the freeing of the unconscious as analyzed in the documents of Freud and psychoanalysis generally. The plays on words and the deliberate antisocial absurdities found in Dada may be exemplified in such surrealist artists as Dali (q.v.), Yves Tanguy, and René Magritte (b. 1898), and in celebrated incidents such as the showing, in a Dada exhibition, of a copy of the *Mona Lisa* with a painted mustache. The comic here is connected with a more strictly representational mode of symbolism, while among the more so-called "abstract" surrealists, such as Miró (q.v.) and Henri Masson (b. 1907), the comic is expressed through a free use of distortion. Analogous to the comic element of surprise in surrealism is the shock mechanism of *pittura metafisica*, especially the unexpected juxtaposition of incompatible objects, as in the work of De Chirico and Carlo Carrà (see EUROPEAN MODERN MOVEMENTS). Humor, an essential component of the antirational, post-Dada movements, has recently burgeoned in *l'art brut*, above all in the work of Jean Dubuffet, with specific references to the evocative possibilities of primitive and barbarian art (cf. M. Tapie, *Mirobolus Macadam*, Paris, 1946; J. Dubuffet, *Prospectus aux amateurs de tout genre*, Paris, 1946).

Enrico CRISPOLTI

COMIC ART AND CARICATURE IN NON-EUROPEAN CULTURES. *India and the Far East.* Although predominantly religious and commemorative, Asian art includes works with caricaturing or comic effects. In the visual arts the comic point of view corresponds to that encountered throughout Oriental literature. Both the visual arts and the drama found comic themes in daily life, and such personalities as the *vidusaka*, or buffoon, appear in these media in India, although somewhat rarely. Comic episodes occur in the widely popular fables, and occasionally may even be found in the *Jātaka* and possibly certain episodes in the life of Buddha; at least the conversion of Ananda, brought about against his own will and in spite of all resistance, seems pervaded with a genial humor. But in a cultural tradition and social order so different from our own, it is not always easy to distinguish what is intentionally comic.

In literature, comic intent that is completely comprehensible to Western understanding occurs most frequently in genre episodes (see GENRE AND SECULAR SUBJECTS). Because the Indian critics themselves held genre in such low esteem, only a few examples of the unpretentious *bhāna* ("monologues") and *prahasana* ("farces") have survived; while they exaggerate vices or the difficulties of the characters, they present a completely conventional picture of Indian life. In Eastern art, humorous episodes of daily life, with similarly commonplace figures that are comic either in themselves or in their manner of portrayal, were frequently introduced even into the most lofty or serious religious compositions (see AJANTA); but otherwise it is difficult to estimate the presumably comic intent of even such representations as the ape (PL. 417), the creature most closely related to man and almost his caricature in nature. The imitation of human actions in the ape, or its obscene postures, are evidently meant to be humorous and remain so even though we do not comprehend their exact symbolism. Typical examples occur in the Khotan terra cottas of central Asia (see KHOTANESE ART), folk artifacts far remote from commemorative and religious representations and the style of major artists. We must bear in mind that a quite different sort of symbolism may have been intended, for in Tibet, where the monkey appears in little bronzes called *ton-t'i*, the monkey is a prototype and one incarnation of sPyan ras gzigs (cf. Manibka' abum, chap. 34; rGyal rabs, chap. 7), and in the Bonpo tradition of the gÑam people the Golden Monkey (gSer gyi spren) is a fertility divinity. Representations showing apes engaged in human activities — so widely diffused in antiquity, from Egypt to Crete, Elam, Harappa (Punjab), and later in the Bronze Age culture of Siberia — are often invested with a religious significance (e.g., related to the sun god); this precludes a merely comic view of these animals. Indeed, there is wholly lacking in the East the negative estimate that made the monkey a laughable and grotesque creature to Western eyes. This does not mean that the monkey may not frequently be a comic figure, however.

The same observation may be made of the rather exaggerated characterizations found in the Chinese funerary statuettes (*ming-ch'i*), which often reproduce with particular stress the features and characteristics of certain barbarian types, especially those of central or western Asia. In attempting to emphasize the particular physical appearance of diverse ethnic types, craftsmen frequently endowed these little figures with the aspect of caricatures — an effect that is more apparent than real, though occasionally the figures seem inspired by comic intent or are a reflection of the superior attitude of the Chinese toward the barbarians — an attitude that persisted even within the cult for the exotic that prevailed at the T'ang court. Ethnic characterization was derived from the indigenous traditions of Iran and the esthetic attitudes of Hellenistic art. It was a current within the visual arts that spread widely in the regions from northwestern India to Central Asia and thence presumably into China. It is never easy, however, to determine the Central Asian artist's precise intention, especially in so completely pliant a material as stucco. Side by side with faces that by their context seem to be portraits, we find others that undoubtedly reveal a desire for the comic in their exaggerated characteristics and intentionally grotesque features. Based on actual observation and with a constant shift in values (see CHARACTERIZATION), the representation of ethnic types was the product of many different races in close proximity but with varying points of view toward each other. The transition from the portrayal of character types to true caricature (and to the comic and grotesque) was an easy one, as the evidence of the tiny Khotan terra-cotta masks attests.

The Iranian tradition attributed a caricaturelike quality to each animal or being created by the evil god Ahriman; this

may have led to an imposition of demoniac qualities on all caricatured images. Independently, in Iran, there was probably an emphasis on the terrifying aspect in art owing to the influence of local religious traditions (see DEMONOLOGY; TERROR IN ART).

With the decline of outside influence, other themes and tendencies asserted themselves in the Far East. Representations appeared which through their exaggerated characterization seem allied to caricature, though perhaps only fortuitously; examples of these are the Chinese lohan (e.g., representations of Fei K'an asleep on the tiger) and other figures (e.g., the 19th-century painting depicting Shoki putting the spirits to flight, by Kanō Hōgai, Boston, Mus. of Fine Arts) even closer to true caricatures, portraying demoniac or semidemoniac gods. With the exception of certain genre scenes, however, like the school-master mocked by his pupils or persons represented as giving way to unbridled passions, there occurs almost invariably an exaggerated form of characterization; it is almost a distortion in the artist's own soul made visible — somewhat like an expressionist work, though on a very different plane. A confirmation of this generalization may be found in the good-humored irony (but nevertheless impressive aspect) of Pu-tai, the smiling god of content; representations of this god express a different ideal within a society far removed from the Western world.

Mario BUSSAGLI

The illustrations of comic art in India (PLS. 417, 433, 434) are taken from an unpublished work by J. E. van Lohuizen de Leeuw. Selected by this author for the *Encyclopedia of World Art*, the illustrations in themselves are a significant contribution and valuable piece of research.

In Japan, caricatures and outspokenly humorous characterizations may be found in the paintings of every period. This can only partially be explained by the fact that different social conditions permitted a more overt expression of humor in Japanese art. It is sheer coincidence that in Japan many things that were not necessarily intended for posterity have survived throughout centuries of civil wars and natural disasters. We therefore have some idea of Japanese caricatures of the early Nara and Heian periods, whereas nothing comparable is known to us from China.

During the restoration of the Golden Hall (*kondō*) of the Hōryūji monastery at Nara, which probably dates from the early 8th century, a number of inscriptions and drawings were discovered on the woodwork of the ceiling. Among these drawings, which were evidently not meant to be seen after the building was completed, are several excellent caricatures of persons with long noses, the first examples of a comic type which was to play an important role in the caricatures of later centuries. These drawings may have been by the very artists who executed the large murals on the walls of the same building.

Among the documents preserved in the Shōsōin, the imperial repository of the Tōdaiji monastery at Nara, is a vast quantity of waste paper, scrap sheets, old bills, and private notes of the scribes employed in the official sutra copying bureau. These scribes, who were charged with copying the Buddhist texts of manuscripts imported from China, were among the first Japanese to have a thorough mastery of Chinese calligraphy. Among the unpretentious drawings scribbled on their scraps of paper as a pastime is an excellent caricature of a man who may represent one of the scribes himself; it is drawn on a paper with an inscription that may be dated 745, and its brushwork demonstrates the artist's skill in Chinese calligraphy.

The 12th and 13th centuries, the end of the Heian and the beginning of the Kamakura period, are the golden age of Japanese humor in art (PL. 435). The most famous painting in this genre is the *Scroll of the Frolicking Animals*, or *Animal Caricatures Scroll* (IV, PL. 282), preserved in the Kōzanji monastery near Kyoto. One of the four in this series of horizontal scrolls (*emakimono*) consists of an uninterrupted sequence of scenes depicting various animals such as hares, frogs, monkeys, and foxes competing in archery contests or wrestling matches, swimming, fighting, and participating in the funeral of a dead frog. Since there is no accompanying text, the exact meaning of the scenes and the connection between them are not always

clear. It is evident, however, that the episode which shows a frog in the guise of Buddha, accompanied by monkeys and foxes in monk's garb performing the funeral ceremony, must have been meant as a satire on Buddhist priests or doctrine. Nevertheless, it is possible that the scroll is a free variation of the so-called *Rokudō-e*, illustrations of the Six Migratory Stages through the World of Desire (in Sanskrit, *Rūpadhātu*), and, if so, is without caricaturing intent.

The close similarity in brushwork between the Kōzanji scrolls and the drawings of esoteric Buddhism indicates that the scrolls must have been executed by artists working in the monochrome style, who had been engaged by different temples to make copies of the drawings imported from China. For a long time all four Kōzanji scrolls were attributed to the priest Kakuyū, popularly known as Toba Sōjō (1053–1140); the earliest and best of the scrolls, after which the whole series has been named, might indeed date from that period, though modern criticism tends to discard the attribution to Kakuyū.

In the *Rokudō-e* one also finds another kind of humor, outspokenly macabre and grim, in the scrolls that depict the horrors of the Buddhist hells, the life of the hungry ghosts (*preta* in Sanskrit), and the miseries of human diseases. The *Handbook on Hells* (*Jigoku Sōshi*, 12th cent.) depicts with obvious relish the tortures to which the sinners are subjected, each in accordance with the nature of the crimes committed during life. Although they relied on descriptions in Buddhist texts and a widespread belief in damnation, the artists seem often, nevertheless, to have regarded hell as a subject that could be treated in a lighthearted, almost jocular fashion.

A similar taste is manifest in the *Handbook of Diseases* and the *Handbook of Hungry Ghosts*, or *Scroll of the Hungry Demons* (in Japanese, *Gaki Sōshi*, 12th cent., IV, PL. 173), which depict in explicit detail the miseries to which the unfortunate mortals afflicted by illness and the starving ghosts are subject. The cruel effect of these scenes is heightened by the presence of impervious bystanders who, far from wishing to help, seem merely to gloat in watching the misfortunes of others. Here again, however, one doubts whether the artist is to be taken completely seriously, or whether these outstanding works of the Yamato-e school ever had the moralizing effect for which they were supposedly created.

A humorous Japanese version of the Indian divinity Garuḍa, the Tengū, who symbolizes conceit, plays an important role in satirical scrolls of the Kamakura period and has remained a familiar figure in Japanese caricatures thereafter. In the *Handbook of Tengū* (*Tengū Sōshi*, late 13th cent.), long-nosed, birdlike goblins mock the behavior of Buddhist priests. This irreverence toward Buddhism and its practitioners, apparent also in some of the hell scenes, was not directed toward the priests of any particular sect, for in the *Tengū Sōshi* all priests are treated with an equally lighthearted disdain; and while in this manuscript the long-nosed Tengū are anti-Buddhist practical jokers mocking stupid priests, in the 14th-century *Story of the Demon Zegaibō* their sometimes cruel wit is directed against their Chinese counterpart Zegaibō, who loses his pride and barely escapes with his life when he is chased back to China.

The flourishing of Japanese humor is closely linked with the Yamato-e painting of the late Heian and Kamakura periods, and a lively sense of humor may be found in nearly all the horizontal scrolls of this time. Its most striking manifestation is perhaps the highly developed animal caricature. This theme was cherished by artists of many different schools and periods but found a strong revival in the 19th century in the drawings of the Ukiyo-e masters. Though the artistic level of their work cannot be compared to that of the ancient scrolls, they nevertheless show a remarkable capacity for drawing satirical parallels between animal and human actions and gestures, with a lively sense of humor that is original, in spite of its debt to earlier works.

Shinichi TANI

*Islam.* Caricature has played a rather restricted role in Islamic painting. There is even uncertainty regarding the few

known examples, for it is difficult to determine whether the artist portrayed his subject in a more or less distorted manner in order to ridicule; he may merely have intended to represent a person whose appearance was grotesque or deformed, or possibly his own awkwardness and lack of skill inadvertently appear comic to our eyes.

In the State Library at Leningrad, for instance, there is a fine miniature (Kühnel, 1922; Arnold, 1928) which Ernst Kühnel and others have attributed to Master Muhammadi (mid-16th cent.); it portrays six dancers accompanied by a musician. Three of the dancers are shown in grotesque attitudes, but obviously the artist was merely depicting a burlesque dance rather than presenting a caricature of his own invention, though he may have heightened the effect by exaggerating certain features that struck his imagination. The dancers' disproportionately large heads and coarse features are quite contrary to the accepted canons of 17th-century Persian art. This work is exceptional in both format and subject and remains unexplained by any text. Another miniature (Berlin, Sarre Coll.; Kühnel, 1922) is composed of two scenes, one above the other, by artists of two different styles; the upper portion shows travelers, the lower one blind men.

Equally exceptional is a drinking scene by the painter Sultan Mohammed (1517–40), illustrating a poem by Hafiz and apparently having a deep and probably allegorical significance (Binyon, Wilkinson, and Gray, 1933). The participants at the banquet are shown in grotesque attitudes, while three other figures — one half-submerged under a peaked hat, another covered with a monkey skin, and the third of simian appearance — seem to emphasize the miniaturist's penchant for the grotesque. There are a few other rare examples of deformed figures in Persian painting; among them are a representation signed by Dervish Husayn Naqqāsh (ca. 1530) showing an ape man (Martin, 1912), a man with an exaggerated paunch and very short legs (Coomaraswamy, 1929) by the painter Kamāl, a hunchback (1269; Martin, 1912) by Riżā-i-'Abbāsī (q.v.), who also painted the figure of a gigantic man with a birdlike head — very large mouth, tiny eyes, a small chin, and very thin nose (Pope, 1938). All these inspire the same question: are these representations of deformed people, or have the models been intentionally caricatured by the artists? The religious proscription against the portrayal of living persons would certainly have inhibited any tendency toward realism, especially an exaggerated and distorting type of realism. It was probably owing to contact with Chinese art (an influence transmitted most likely by Turkish artists of the late 15th and 16th centuries) that certain artists overcame these limitations. The masklike appearance of these grotesque faces makes them seem like surrealist compositions in a dreamlike atmosphere. Only in the case of one drawing can we assert the clear intention to render a caricature: the drawing shows a knight so thin that one can see his ribs, astride a skeletal horse and curiously reminiscent of certain representations of Don Quixote (Martin, 1912; Coomaraswamy, 1929). On the other hand, it is possible that the artist was merely portraying Majnun, an emaciated character from Nizami's poetry, suffering from unrequited love.

Wilhelm STAUDE

*Primitive cultures.* Caricature and humor are generally absent from primitive art, which in serving a primarily religious function, was an important aspect of communal life. Some primitive representations seem at first glance to be caricatures, for example, a type of wooden mask from New Caledonia which occurs repeatedly as an anthropomorphic figure with an exaggeratedly large, hooked nose and an open mouth apparently laughing. Actually these are ceremonial masks that portray mythological figures, generally water divinities. Though the exaggerated features may be monstrous or grotesque in effect, they cannot properly be regarded as caricatures, for any satirical or comic intention to portray an individual is entirely lacking.

Significant among the few examples of primitive art which appear to be intentionally comic are a group of wooden figurines by a Yoruba artist from Ijebu, found at Lagos, Nigeria (W. R. Bascom, G. Bebauer, *Handbook of West African Art*, Milwau-

kee, 1953); they portray such personages as Queen Victoria, a lawyer, and an English missionary. While the sculptor has adhered stylistically to the traditional canons of Yoruba art (see GUINEAN CULTURES), making the nose prominent and the head large in proportion to the limbs, he has exaggerated the light color of the skin and hair and has added details of costume so minutely observed that they seem satirical. When questioned, however, he denied categorically that he had intended to produce caricatures; therefore any such connotation must be regarded as the outcome of cultural contacts between the native tradition and Western civilization.

Vittorio LANTERNARI

BIBLIOG. *a. General*: J. F. Champfleury, Histoire de la caricature, Paris, 1865; J. F. Champfleury, Histoire de la caricature antique, Paris, 1865; T. Wright, A History of Caricature and Grotesque in Literature and Art, London, 1865; J. F. Champfleury, Histoire générale de la caricature, 5 vols., Paris, 1865–80 (sup. 1888); G. Arcoleo, L'umorismo nell'arte moderna, Naples, 1885; K. Überhorst, Das Komische, Leipzig, 1890–1900; H. Bergson, Le rire, Paris, 1900 (Eng. trans., C. Brereton, Laughter, New York, 1913); T. Massarani, Storia e fisiologia dell'arte del ridere, Milan, 1900; E. Fuchs, Die Karikatur der europäischen Völker vom Altertum bis zur Neuzeit, 2 vols., Berlin, 1901; E. Fuchs, Das erotische Element in der Karikatur, Berlin, 1904; F. Jahn, Das Problem des Komischen in seiner geschichtlichen Entwicklung, Potsdam, 1904; S. Freud, Der Witz und seine Beziehungen zum Unbewussten, Vienna, 1905 (Eng. trans., A. A. Brill, Wit and Its Relation to the Unconscious, New York, 1917; included in The Basic Writings of Sigmund Freud, New York, 1938); E. Holländer, Die Karikatur und Satire in der Medizin, Stuttgart, 1905; E. Fuchs, Die Frau in der Karikatur, Munich, 1906; G. A. Levi, Il comico, Genoa, 1913; M. E. Pottier, Les origines de la caricature dans l'antiquité, conférences faites au Musée Guimet en 1914, Bibliothèque de vulgarisation, XLI, 1918, pp. 193–99; G. Gori, Il grottesco nell'arte e nella letteratura, Rome, 1926; B. Lynch, A History of Caricature, London, 1926; R. Eisler, Wörterbuch der philosophischen Begriffe, I, 4th ed., Berlin, 1927, pp. 837–40; E. Kris, Zur Psychologie der Karikatur, Imago, XX, 1934, pp. 450–66 (Eng. trans. in International J. of Psycho-Analysis, XVII, 1936; reprinted in E. Kris, Psychoanalytic Explorations in Art, New York, 1952, pp. 173–88); E. Malaguzzi-Valeri, L'arte gaia, Milan, 1936; E. H. Gombrich and E. Kris, The Principles of Caricature, British J. of Medical Psychology, XVII, 1938 (reprinted in E. Kris, Psychoanalytic Explorations in Art, New York, 1952, pp. 189–203); E. H. Gombrich and E. Kris, Caricature, London, 1940; H. M. Bateman, Humour in Art, J. of the Royal Society of Arts, no. 4799, July, 1949, pp. 629–43; E. Battisti, Comedia y tragedia, Revista de Estética, 1956; W. Hofmann, Die Karikatur von Leonardo bis Picasso, Vienna, 1956 (Eng. ed., Caricature from Leonardo to Picasso, London, New York, 1957; Fr. ed., Paris, 1958). *b. Antiquity*: O. Beauregard, La caricature égyptienne historique, politique et morale, Paris, 1894; M. Bieber, Die Denkmäler zum Theaterwesen im Altertum, Berlin, 1920; G. E. Rizzo, Caricature antiche, Dedalo, VII, 1926–27, pp. 403–18; M. Bieber, The History of the Greek and Roman Theater, Princeton, 1939; H. G. Oeri, Der Typ der komischen Alten in der griechischen Komödie: Seine Nachwirkungen und seine Herkunft, Basel, 1948; L. M. Catteruccia, Pitture vascolari italiote di soggetto teatrale comico, Rome, 1951; A. Plebe, La teoria del comico da Aristotele a Plutarco, Turin, 1952; E. Romagnoli, Nel regno di Dionisio, 3d ed., Bologna, 1953; H. Kenner, Das Theater und der Realismus in der griechischen Kunst, Vienna, 1954; E. Brunner-Traut, Ägyptische Tiermärchen, Z. für ägyptische Sprache, LXXX, 1955, p. 12 ff. (on interpretation of the fables); A. Plebe, La nascita del comico, Bari, 1956. *c. Medieval and modern*: J. Grand-Carteret, Les mœurs et la caricature en Allemagne, en Autriche et en Suisse, Paris, 1885; J. Grand-Carteret, Les mœurs et la caricature en France, Paris, 1888; G. Hermann, Die deutsche Karikatur im 19. Jahrhundert, n.p., 1901; G. Paston, Social Caricature in the 18th Century, London, 1905; L. Maeterlinck, Le genre satirique dans la peinture flamande, 2d ed., Brussels, 1907; A. Blum, L'estampe satirique et la caricature en France au XVIIIᵉ siècle, GBA (52ᵉ année, 4ᵉ période), 1910, III, p. 379 ff., IV, pp. 69 ff., 108 ff., 243 ff., 275 ff., 403 ff., 449 ff.; A. Blum, La caricature révolutionnaire, Paris, 1916; A. Blum, L'estampe satirique en France pendant les guerres de religion, Paris, 1917; C. Veth, Geschiedenis van de Nederlandsche Caricatuur, Leiden, 1921; C. Veth, Comic Art in England, London, 1929; W. R. Juynboll, Het komische Genre in de italiaansche Schilderkunst gedurende de 17. en de 18. eeuw, Leiden, 1934 (doctoral dissertation); F. D. Klingender, Hogarth and English Caricature, London, New York, 1945; J. Adhémar, L'estampe satirique et burlesque en France. 1500–1800 (cat. of exhibition at the Bib. Nat.), Paris, 1950; J. Baltrusaitis, Le Moyen Age fantastique, Paris, 1955. *d. India and the Far East*: C. Netto and O. Wagener, Japanischer Humor, Leipzig, 1901; Kuno Takeshi, Notes on the Drawings and Scribblings Discovered on the Ceiling of the Main Wall, Hōryūji Monastery, Bijutsu Kenkyu, CXL, 1947 (in Japanese); M. Bussagli, Bronze Objects Collected by Prof. G. Tucci in Tibet: A Short Survey of Religious and Magical Symbolism, Artibus Asiae, XII, 1949, pp. 331–47, esp. pp. 334–36; J. Buhot, Histoire des arts du Japon, Pageant of Japanese Art, I, Tokyo, 1952 (painting); L. Sickman and A. Soper, The Art and Architecture of China, Harmondsworth, 1956. pp. 143–44; J. G. Mahler, The Westerners among the Figurines of the T'ang Dynasty of China, Istituto Italiano per il Medio ed Estremo Oriente, Oriental series, XX, Rome, 1959. *e. Islam*: F. R. Martin, The Miniature Painting and Painters of Persia, India and Turkey from the Eighth to the Eighteenth Century, 2 vols., London, 1912, pp. 8, 9, pls. 154, 158, 231; E. Kühnel, Miniaturmalerei im islamischen Orient, Berlin, 1922, pls. 66, 86; T. W. Arnold, Painting in Islam: A Study of the Place of Pictorial Art in Muslim Culture, Oxford, 1928, p. 112 ff., pl. 47; A. K. Coomaraswamy,

Les miniatures orientales de la collection Goloubew au Museum of Fine Arts de Boston, Ars Asiatica, XIII, 1929, pls. 53, 65, figs. 105, 107; L. Binyon, J. V. S. Wilkinson, and B. Gray, Persian Miniature Painting, London, 1933, p. 128 ff., pl. 75; A Survey of Persian Art from Prehistoric Times to the Present, ed. A. U. Pope, London, New York, 1938, V, pl. 921 A.

Giovanni BECATTI, Mario BUSSAGLI,<br>
Werner HOFMANN, Wilhelm STAUDE, Shinichi TANI

Illustrations: PLS. 417-435.

**COMPOSITION.** See DESIGN; INDUSTRIAL DESIGN; PROPORTION.

**CONFUCIANISM.** K'ung Fu-tzŭ (Master K'ung, Latinized to Confucius by early European missionaries) lived, according to tradition, between 551 and 479 B.C. in Lu state in the modern province of Shantung. Here, except for periods of extensive traveling to other states of the empire, he held high public offices and maintained a private school which had as its goals the conservation of tradition and resistance to the social anarchy that characterized the last centuries of the Chou dynasty (11th–3d cent. B.C.). Although Confucius probably left no writings, various works are attributed to him; at least one of these, the Analects, or Discourses (Lun-yü), in 20 books, compiled by his disciples after his death, almost certainly represents with something like the immediacy and liveliness of the dictated word the ideas and personality of the master. In it the personal characteristics of Confucius — his clothing, gesture, and gait (see especially Analects, X, 3, 4, 6, 15, 16) — are set forth for the purpose of furthering the Confucian ideal of formal perfection involving both art and social custom. At once esthetic and ethic, this ideal was both vital and productive until it degenerated into tiresome mannerism on the one side and a series of minute rules of etiquette on the other.

SUMMARY. Basic concepts (col. 775). The Confucianist Classics (col. 776). The applied arts (col. 777). Calligraphy (col. 779). Painting (col. 780).

BASIC CONCEPTS. Confucianism, a system of thought and attitudes and of social and political institutions based on these attitudes, became dominant in China in the 2d century B.C., when China's educated elite as well as the majority of her officials were counted among its adherents. Since that time it has pervaded Chinese life, shaping almost all its aspects. Most of the beliefs and teachings of the Confucianist school can be traced back to the personality and vision of its founder, Confucius (PLS. 436-439).

Confucius lived in an age when the Chinese mind was about to take another step toward self-realization (see CHINESE ART) — an age roughly contemporary with a similar development in the West. Faith in the tenets and institutions of the archaic world was on the point of dissolution, and spiritual and social traditions alike were being submitted to reflection. Confucius, like several other great teachers of this age, gave forceful expression to this change; repeatedly he affirmed his conviction that the maintenance and development of Chinese civilization were entrusted to him. His response to this vocation was an attempt to reinforce the tradition and to establish a comprehensive and integrated position within it for the human personality aware of its newly imposed responsibilities toward the civilization. Education and cultivation of the personality were thus the cornerstones of his system, and he created the ideal type of the "gentleman" (chün-tzŭ), upon whom these responsibilities would devolve. Education was not an aim in itself, and the cultivated personality was not an autonomous entity; rather, both were directed toward the maintenance and development of tradition. Service to these ends did not, however, involve technically specialized activities only; the exigencies of a constantly changing tradition could be met only by a comprehensively cultivated personality — by a man, in other words, who could assume leadership with regard to every aspect of this tradition at any level. If the gentleman was to live up to his task, he must be schooled in traditionally accepted ethics; this alone, however, was not sufficient: cultivation in nonpragmatic matters was also compulsory, the unity of ethics and esthetics being a basic tenet of Confucianism.

In the Analects (see below) this unity is expressed by the concept of wên, which referred to culture in the sense both of tradition and mores and of esthetic expression; hence its vehicle is the polite arts. Training in wên thus included proper social behavior and an attitude of respect for one's elders (I, 6). Uncultured expression (that which is of low quality esthetically) of even the best of intentions is boorish, just as overemphasis on the formal aspect of behavior is pedantry (VI, 18), the sign of a small man (XIX, 8). One of the disciples of Confucius stated this idea as follows: "Culture [refinement, wên] is identical with the matter the gentleman has to work on, and matter is identical with culture. The hairless hide of a tiger or leopard is just like the hairless hide of a dog or a sheep" (XII, 8).

Hence injunctions to expand one's learning through cultural training occur frequently in the Analects (VI, 27; IX, 11; XII, 15); such knowledge is just as important as appropriate social behavior. Only in this way can an atmosphere be created which favors the solidarity of cultivated persons endeavoring to promote the aims of humanity (XII, 24).

Confucius' own involvement in the arts is amply documented. Later Confucianism systematized his view into an educational curriculum for the gentleman, including the so-called "Six Arts": ritual and mores (li), music (yüeh), poetry (shih), writing (based on the political documents, shu), charioteering, and archery. In subsequent ages persistent attempts were made to stereotype this view of cultural training, especially by subordinating esthetics to ethics. The attempts were all the more effective since, as time went on, the basic concepts of Confucianism became progressively more rigid. Government service predominated among the gentleman's activities after the Confucianists attained a monopoly position among the competing schools of thought under the Han emperor Wu (140–81 B.C.); in this situation all the arts were frequently put to political use and the universal personality as a postulate of Confucianism was at times submerged. In all ages, however — but notably since Sung times, which were characterized by an unmitigatedly authoritarian ideology — there have been philosophers who viewed all temporal activities and their associated codes of ethics in terms of the comprehensive human being and thus reasserted the basically humanistic vision of Confucius. The one redeeming feature even of Chu Hsi (1130–1200), the great systematizer of authoritarian ideology in Sung times, was his intimate appreciation of esthetic values.

THE CONFUCIANIST CLASSICS. After Emperor Wu of the Han dynasty (206 B.C.-A.D. 221; see CHINESE ART) excluded all other schools of thought from the Imperial Academy, the writings of the Confucianist school assumed an authority as binding as that of the inspired scriptures of the various great religions. All subsequent reforms and changes had to be justified in terms of the authoritative writings, which came to be known as the Classics (ching). They consist of books that date from different ages, three of them antedating at least in part the lifetime of Confucius. One of these, the Book of Documents (Shu-ching, or Shang-shu), a collection mainly of speeches made on historic occasions, is essentially a manual of government. Another is the Book of Songs (Shih-ching, or Mao-shih), an anthology of poetry based in part on folk songs and in part on ritualistic poems and hymns and containing also emotional outpourings of tortured individuals. The third is the Book of Changes (I-ching, or Chou-i), a manual of divination couched in terminology and imagery not always easily understood, containing the oldest systematic speculations on the physical universe and man's position in the world. As divination was supposed to make man master of his fate, this has always been the favorite Classic of those who strove for the autonomy and universality of the human personality. Although it is largely composed of older strata, it contains extensive appendixes of post-Confucian date. To these three older Classics, others were subsequently added. The Li-chi, usually referred to as the Book of Rites, is a com-

pilation of late Han date only. It contains essays and stories concerning the principles of human conduct, the basic moral tenets, ceremonial and social usages, education, and music. The Spring and Autumn Annals (Ch'un-ch'iu), believed to be a rewrite by Confucius himself of the chronicle of his native state, is thought to contain in its terse wording the master's judgments on historical and political matters.

Two other works later assumed an authority equal to that of the Classics. One is the Analects, or Discourses (Lun-yü), of Confucius, a collection of anecdotes about and sayings and conversations of Confucius and his early disciples; it is our most authoritative source for his life and thought. The other is the writings of the philosopher Mencius (Meng-tzŭ), of late Chou (see CHINESE ART) date. From the ideas and formulations contained in these books, all later Confucianist thinking was derived.

THE APPLIED ARTS. Although Confucius was profoundly interested in poetry and had a deep appreciation of music, he does not appear to have had any affinity for the visual arts. The only passage in the Analects which refers to painting reads: "The business of painting follows the preparation of the plain ground" (III, 8). In later Chinese art theory this saying was generalized to mean that painting follows simplicity. The visual arts had therefore to be justified in rather devious ways.

Of the Six Arts mentioned above, it was the first, li, which provided an opening for the admission of at least one type of artistic expression into the Confucianist sphere. Li originally referred to the ritual, with the activities and implements pertaining to it. Confucius himself is known to have been eminently interested in all aspects of the ritual and to have endeavored throughout his life to conserve the traditional rituals as well as personally to observe them. He was particularly interested in the great imperial sacrifices and private ancestor worship and does not appear to have concerned himself with the rites for minor deities. Thus the maintenance of these two aspects of religious tradition became the responsibility of the Confucianists, and the observances came to be considered as Confucianist functions.

This development brought all the applied arts that served the ritual, notably bronze casting, into the Confucianist sphere. The Confucianists, however, were unable to influence the craft; the work of the craftsman was outside of the circle of accepted occupations, and his traditions remained unaffected. Indeed, by late Chou and Han times it was rather Taoist alchemists who exercised a strong influence over the craftsmen's groups. The Confucianists could, however, give the ritualistic implements a new meaning and make them convey a Confucianist message. This reevaluation of the ritualistic vessel must have taken place with the Confucianist ascendancy during the reign of Emperor Wu of Han, for it is evidenced by recorded inscriptions on sacrificial vessels. An inscription on a precious jar, attributed to Tung Fang-so (ca. 160–93 B.C.), reads: "Precious clouds emerge from the Altar of Dew, / A propitious wind arises from the Office of the Moon; / I behold the three jugs, perfect as an Imperial foot measure, / I see the eight wild geese, graceful as a coiled belt." The imagery and spirit of this inscription is still entirely Taoistic. However, the following inscription on a sacrificial cauldron on Mount T'ai, dated 93 B.C., presumably stems from the hand of Emperor Wu imself: "I climbed Mount T'ai; / Myriad ages of boundlessness, / Within the four seas everything is peaceful and quiet; / The sacred cauldron emits fragrance." Here imperial peace and order is the message which the cauldron is made to convey. Once the sacrificial vessel became the responsibility of the Confucianists, the artistry of these implements could not but appeal to the esthetic sensitivities of even the most doctrinaire Confucianist beholder. Although created by non-Confucianist craftsmen — even with imperial manufactures this tradition was never entirely broken — the object itself became an accepted part of the Confucianist world and therefore could legitimately be enjoyed and evaluated esthetically. Liu Hsiang (ca. 77–6 B.C.), an extremely orthodox Confucianist of late Western Han, had the following verse inscribed on an incense burner: "Admirable, this perfect ves-

sel, / Building up precipitously like a mountain; / Its upper part is in communication with Mount Hua; / Supported it is by a copper plate. / The central part contains the fragrance of orchids and musk, / Red-hot fire and bluish smoke. / Elegant artistry perfected its four sides, / Its top connects with the azure sky. / Embossed it is with myriad animals, / Facing each other across openwork." This inscription manifests a completely undogmatic appreciation of an object of art, describing its beauty for its own sake rather than as an expression of the Confucianist tenets with which Liu Hsiang was so much concerned. The tradition of unencumbered enjoyment of ritual objects soon gained currency and in later periods became almost universal among educated gentlemen. In this respect the principle of li, even though it did not provide an acceptable Confucianist outlet for artistic creativity, helped to establish an atmosphere of esthetic sensitivity and a tradition of art appreciation.

The principle of li was, however, responsible for bringing applied art into the purview of Confucianism much beyond the sphere of religious ritual. Even in Confucius' time the meaning of li had been broadened to include ceremonial behavior at social functions, the conduct proper to the gentleman in society, and the attitudes appropriate to him. The entire relationship of the Confucianist gentleman to his environment was thus made a function of li, including the objects with which he came into daily contact. As early as pre-Confucian times this relationship was more than merely pragmatic; the Book of Documents contains reference to an inscription on the bathtub of a semilegendary emperor indicating that its function was conceived as not merely cleansing the body but also cleansing and rejuvenating the mind. The Confucianists applied this facet of the wisdom of the ancients to every conceivable object of daily use. The book called Rituals of the Older Tai (Ta-Tai Li-chi), compiled in the 2d century, contains a collection of inscriptions on such articles, attributed to early Chou times but more probably of late Chou or Han date, which reflect the Confucianization of the gentleman's equipment. Mat and table, crockery and cutlery, and even belts and shoes are made to recall the wisdom of the ancients and to remind the gentleman to use them only in the proper Confucianist frame of mind. There is evidence that this trend reached its height in Han times, lifting these craft articles into the sphere of acceptable Confucianist pastimes. A telling example of this trend is a fan inscription by Fu I (ca. A.D. 47–92): "I use your simple roundness to fan myself, / And a clear breeze spreads. / The jadelike body of a gentleman / Relies on you for his peace of mind and comfort. / In winter you are like a submerged dragon, / In summer like a rising phoenix. / You know when to come forward and when to retreat; / At the proper time you serve or you retire." Here the fan is likened to the ideal Confucianist functionary, serving him who uses it just as the scholar serves his emperor. The image of the submerged dragon, from the Book of Changes, is applied to the fan — an image which Confucianist scholars liked to apply to themselves when unemployed — and it is credited with a knowledge of the foremost principle of the official's career, formulated, according to a tradition preserved in the Book of Changes, by Confucius himself: to serve and to retire at the proper time.

Here again, the basic unity of Confucianist ethics and esthetics asserts itself; objects that carry an ethical message can also be worthy of esthetic appreciation. This principle applies to everything within the gentlemen's reach: his buildings and gardens, for example, were creations of craftsmen, to be sure, and Taoistically oriented craftsmen. Consequently the specific implements of the scholar — brush, ink, and the ink-slab — are treated with particular love. Probably the earliest ink-slab inscriptions are by Wang Tsan (A.D. 177–217); they are not only good examples of Wang's poetic gifts but show intimately the close, almost personalized, relationship between the writer and his tools.

Unlike artistically handled ritual objects, temporal objects not only lent themselves to esthetic appreciation but also occasionally provided an outlet for artistic creativity. A piece of rhymed prose on a fan by the great scientist and poet Chang Hêng (A.D. 77–138) reads: "I selected this bamboo to make a

fan out of it. / Then I painted on it a picture full of symbolic values. / I circled the above and squared the below, / Harmonizing the dazzling colors to show the multitude of things." This painting, again, was apparently based on the symbolism of the Book of Changes, according to which heaven is round and the earth is square. There is probably no earlier recorded instance of a scholar's referring to painting as his pastime. Our knowledge of Han painting is, of course, quite extensive; for all we know, however, it may have been craftsman's painting throughout. The decoration of objects of daily use provided a situation in which painting was a legitimate activity for the scholar. Centuries passed before it came to be regarded as a liberal art rather than a craft to be practiced only in certain situations.

However, the applied arts, particularly the fields of jade, bronze, pottery and porcelain, architecture and gardening, furniture and textiles, flourished in this atmosphere, the imperial court and the great families of the gentry being sponsors and collectors of *objets d'art*. From later times we have manuals on the artistic conduct of life, the most charming being the essays of Li Yü (1611–80) on the integration of the objects of a gentleman's environment (up to and including women) into the cultivated life.

CALLIGRAPHY. In China only two of the visual arts, calligraphy and painting, eventually gained the recognized status of liberal arts, shedding the taint of craft and profession; and calligraphy (q.v.) was regarded as a more suitable artistic expression than painting for the Confucianist gentleman. His curriculum provided special training in calligraphy, and his very career was based upon the pragmatic aspect of writing, always of great importance. In addition, the very word for calligraphy, *shu*, also refers to the Classic of Documents, a textbook in political science and political history; and an essay on cultural history contained in one of the appendixes of the Book of Changes states that writing was invented for the purpose of controlling officialdom and supervising the population.

The requirement of high esthetic qualities in such useful skills as writing was asserted in the field of calligraphy through a political detour. Emperor Wu of Han is recorded to have meted out punishment to a memorialist whose poor handwriting was taken as a sign of disrespect; and there were instances of scholars' failing the imperial examinations because of poor handwriting. To write a good hand thus became a political necessity, and two eminently Confucianist virtues were required for its achievement — an unrelenting self-discipline and a reverent emulation of past masters. It is touching to read the regular diary entries of so great a statesman as Tseng Kuo-fan (1811–72) concerning his minute care in matters of calligraphic training; and even K'ang Yu-wei (1858–1927), the last great Confucianist scholar, who by temperament was a radical reformer rather than a traditionalist, said, "To learn calligraphy one must start by imitating the old masters."

Calligraphy, by its very nature, sets severer limitations on freedom of artistic expression than any other art. In no other art does the medium of expression so narrowly circumscribe the creative range of the artist. To achieve, in spite of these limitations, not only an esthetically pleasing effect but an outlet for artistic creativity, the highest degree of concentration and mastery of technique is required. It is therefore not by chance that discussions of this technique and deliberations on the creative state of mind demanded by it led to the formulation of theories of art in this field earlier than in any other, and that some of the precepts and observations to which it gave rise were then transferred to painting and even to poetry. In this way Confucianist thinking gained a degree of currency in all art theory.

Among the precepts was that of the necessity of perennial training and practice. Mastery of the technique necessitated the devotion of the craftsman; the zeal of the amateur was not sufficient. Chung Yu, a master calligrapher of the 3d century, wrote to his son: "I have studied writing for more than thirty years, and I am only now learning how to hold the brush. I cannot help thinking about it all the time; even whilst conversing, I keep drawing characters on the ground. At night when I have retired I draw with my fingers on the blanket so that by now it is worn and torn." Only by continuous concentration on the minutest details of technique could the wrist be trained to obey the creative mind without reflection.

The concept of composition was of great importance. The calligrapher distinguished the "little composition" of the individual character and the "great composition" of the entire page; the macrocosm of the completed work is composed of the microcosms of the words. The relationship between the two was for the calligrapher a perfect symbol of the functioning of the Confucianist gentleman: the cultivated individual contributing his service to produce a harmonious cultural and social unit. The important relation between the individual character and the whole must be preconceived but not necessarily consciously visualized; the genuinely creative mind will set the pattern of the whole when drawing the first stroke of the first character (Chang Shan, 14th cent.).

Much thought was given to the state of mind most conducive to artistic creation. Ts'ai Yung, a great Confucianist scholar and poet of the 2d century, said: "If you want to write you first have to drive all sad ideas out of your head; you have to be in high spirits and at ease. Before starting to write, you will first have to meditate for a certain time. If your mind is occupied, you cannot write well even with the best of brushes; but if your mind is at rest, you can give free course to your brush."

The importance of the state of mind is stressed by later theorists of calligraphy. It is, as Sun Kuo-t'ing of T'ang put it, the prerequisite to the elevation of writing from the level of mere dexterity to that of artistic creation. Only in such a state of mind is it possible to write characters "like dragons soaring into the sky and like tigers pacing the mountains," as those of Wang Hsi-chih (A.D. 321–79), one of the most famous Chinese calligraphers of all time, were described. Theories about creativity and the creative process were easily derived from such concepts.

PAINTING. Calligraphy was, however, the only one of the visual arts which from the very beginning had the status of a liberal art. The others, except for painting, always remained stigmatized as applied arts, produced by professional craftsmen. Sculpture, for example, never outgrew its link with religion, especially Buddhism and Taoism (qq.v.); nonreligious sculpture is almost entirely unknown in China, and sculptures that were put to use in a Confucianist context were regarded as objects of reverence or as guardians of tombs and mansions but not appreciated for their own sake.

The emancipation of painting from craft status and its attainment of that of a liberal art was a long-drawn-out process, and some types of painting never quite made the transition; portrait painting, for example, was from the beginning strongly influenced by the Confucianists but never practiced by them. Portraits were necessary in the Confucianist context to foster reverence for emperors and heroes and an attitude of filial piety toward ancestors; indeed, Chinese portraiture achieved its superb qualities in an atmosphere of Confucianist evaluation. It is thus not by chance that in all the centuries of its existence it remained unswayed by the artistic trends of various epochs and never ventured beyond strict realism; nor was it by chance that the current manual of portrait painting (by Ting Kao, 1818) borrowed its terminology largely from Neo-Confucianist philosophy and not from Taoism.

One attitude in particular of the Confucianists stood in the way of the acceptance of painting as a liberal art: scorn of the profit motive. For the Confucianist gentleman the only acceptable gainful occupations were public service, literary activity, and education; all other profit-yielding activities were shunned. Profit from nonscholarly occupations had been viewed as despicable only since the time of Meng-tzŭ, however, for the Book of Changes, in its unbiased way, still provided a place in its system for profit as a motivating force. It is thus not the technical perfection of the craftsman as such which the Confucianists rejected — toilsome achievement of technical

mastery was a requirement for calligraphy — but the fact that the craftsman-painter exercized his skill for profit. This is, for example, reflected in the advice given by one of the best-known court painters of T'ang to one of his disciples, warning him against becoming a painter, because the fate of the painter is not far removed from that of the slave, and urging him to take the examinations instead. And the man who was a mere painter, even a painter in an imperial academy, was still looked down upon even after painting had been accepted as an art. Occasional attempts, particularly in Sung times, to place paint-ing on the educational curriculum of the scholar-official remained eccentric and ephemeral.

The Confucianist acceptance of painting was the result of two tendencies in the system. One was the establishment of a connection between painting and another of the arts, usually poetry. Socially this meant that an artist who had established himself as a poet could practice painting as a sideline without damage to his status; conceptually it meant that ideas about poetic creativity and a generic classification of poems were transferred to painting and contributed greatly toward the evolu-tion of a theory of painting. The poet-painter is exemplified by Ku K'ai-chih (q.v.; ca. 345–406), the greatest of pre-T'ang painters, whose poetry shows outstanding color and force. In T'ang times there were Wang Wei (q.v.; 698–759), Ku K'uang (ca. 725–815), and Chang Chih-ho (ca. 745–810). Among Sung theorists such as Su Shih (1037–1101) and Huang T'ing-chien (1045–1105) the belief that poetry and painting had a common source was generally accepted. Painters such as Mi Fei (q.v.; 1051–1107) of Sung; Chao Mêng-fu (q.v.; 1254–1322) and Ni Tsan (q.v.; 1301–74) of Yüan; Shên Chou (1427–1509), T'ang Yin (1470–1523), and Wên Chêng-ming (q.v.; 1470–1559) of Ming all wrote poetry of considerably better than amateur quality.

The second tendency leading to the acceptance of painting was the bringing to bear on painting of the concepts of the least pragmatic of the Confucian Classics, the Book of Changes (I-ching). Even earlier, Wang Wei the Elder (415–43) had tried to emancipate this art from craft status by dignifying it with the concept of change, or transformation (i of I-ching); and all later theorists of painting borrowed from the Book of Changes to support their views. The eventual conceptualiza-tion of the essence of painting by Hsieh Ho (fl. ca. A.D. 500) as ch'i-yün sheng-tung was not and could not be derived from purely Confucianist thought. The first term, ch'i-yün (usually translated "spiritual harmony" or "spiritual consonance"), could, however, easily be justified by quotations from the Book of Changes. According to one of the appendixes of the Book of Changes, spiritually kindred things are in search of one another at the moment when creativity is consummated; in another appendix it is stated that "the spirits of mountain and lake communicate in order to bring about transformation and to create the myriad of things." The underlying idea of ch'i-yün and the concept of creative transformation, basic to all art, are certainly at least prefigured in these I-ching quotations.

The second term, sheng-tung (usually translated "life move-ment" or "vitality"), might have been directly derived from an I-ching passage. In the light of this passage, the term originally meant "coming to life in or through movement." The acceptance of this term opened the gates to the entire philosophy of the Book of Changes.

The outcome of these tendencies was that painting was accorded new and higher status in Confucianist thinking in early Sung times, a period which saw some of the most complex developments in the history of the Confucianist system and was immediately followed by renewed doctrinalization and rigidification. It was in this period that the great poet-painter Su Shih, also an I-ching expert, coined the term shih-ta-fu painting, usually translated "literati" painting, although the term actually means "scholar-official" and is the class desig-nation of the Confucianist. Su Shih claimed that only the Confucianist scholar had the qualifications necessary to penetrate the organic law of the universe and thus elevate painting above the mere formal accomplishment of craftsmanship. These qualifications were a high degree of organization of personality

and a "purposeless" (spontaneous) talent, of which only the Confucianist scholar could boast. Thus painting, previously regarded as unworthy of the Confucianist scholar, became not only acceptable to him but, indeed, his prerogative.

To be sure, Su's claim for the painting done by the gentle-man did not supersede the claims of professional (academic, or craftsman's) painting. His view was more influential in some schools of Chinese painting than in others; and in the art classes it especially encouraged the spontaneous (i-p'in). His term "scholar-official painting" was later modified to "the painting of cultivated personalities" (wên-jên) by Mo Shih-lung (late-16th cent.) and Tung Ch'i-ch'ang (q.v.; 1555–1636), who claimed all the poet-painters of the past as their ancestors.

In this context, then, painting was transformed from a profes-sional, or craft, art into a liberal art practiced by gentleman amateurs. This was possible technically because it used the same medium of expression as calligraphy. However, the Con-fucianist scholars who practiced this amateur art had to live with the dilemma that their art derived most of its basic in-spiration from Taoist and Zen-Buddhist concepts. Attempts were not lacking to make painting a handmaiden of Confucianist doctrine; the work of Sung Lien of early Ming is a superb example of this trend. But these attempts did not succeed in altering the new status of painting as a liberal art, since in the thinking of the Chinese intelligentsia the esthetic had long since outgrown its interdependence with the ethical.

BIBLIOG. R. Wilhelm, Der Geist der Kunst nach dem Buch der Wand-lungen, in Der Mensch und das Sein, Jena, 1931, pp. 199–245; Ku Teng, Su Tung P'o als Kunstkritiker, ÖAZ, XVIII, 1932, pp. 104–10; V. Contag, Tung Ch'ich'angs Hua Ch'an Shih Sui Pi und des Hua Shuo des Mo Shih-lung, ÖAZ, XIX, 1933, pp. 83–97, 174–88; Ku Teng, Chinesische Malkunsttheorie in der T'ang und Sungzeit, ÖAZ, XXI, 1935; O. Sirén, The Chinese on the Art of Painting, Peiping, 1936; Yang Yu-hsun, La Calligraphie Chinoise depuis les Han, Paris, 1937; V. Contag, Das Mal-lehrbuch für Personenmalerei des Chieh Tzu Yüan, T'oung Pao, XXXIII, 1937, pp. 15–90; A. C. Soper, Kuo Jo-hsü's Experiences in Painting, Washington, D.C., 1951; W. R. B. Acker, Some T'ang and pre-T'ang Texts on Chinese Painting, Leiden, 1954; J. R. Levenson, The Amateur Ideal in Ming and Early Ch'ing Society: Evidence from Painting, in Chinese Thought and Institutions, ed. J. K. Fairbank, Chicago, 1957, pp. 320–41; J. F. Cahill, Confucian Elements in the Theory of Painting, in A. Wright, ed., The Confucian Persuasion, Stanford, Calif., 1960.

Hellmut WILHELM

Illustrations: PLS. 436–439.

CONGO (former Belgian Congo). This vast territory (almost 800.000 square miles) occupies the heart of Africa; it became a Belgian colony in 1908 and a republic in 1960. Most of the population of about 14 million speak Bantu lan-guages; about two-thirds are pagan. The artistic production of the Congo is one of the richest in Africa, especially in wood sculpture.

In the first phases of contact, which began at the end of the 15th century, traditional art felt only limited European in-fluence (mainly in the lower Congo region). There is little con-temporary art of European derivation.

SUMMARY. Introduction (col. 782). The north (col. 783): *The region between the Ubangi and Congo Rivers; The region between the Bomu and Aruwimi Rivers; The central basin; The Kivu region and environs.* The south (col. 784): *The lower Congo region; The western and middle Kasai; The eastern Kasai and Katanga.* Centers of Eu-ropean influence (col. 790).

INTRODUCTION. The Congo can be divided into two regions, northern and southern, distinguished both by language and by quantity and quality of artistic production. These two main regions can be subdivided into smaller style areas (see FIG. 785).

The northern section has produced only a small number of anthropomorphically and zoomorphically ornamented utensils; other forms of applied art are scarcely represented. The sculpture gener-ally shows a derivative conception; it is thin and harsh, lacks imagina-tion, is often carelessly finished, and has few motifs. In the south, however, there is an abundance of sculpture and other art forms. The sculpture tends to be plastically conceived, less stylized, and better finished and has a great variety of motifs. No doubt, in both

areas there are exceptions, but there remains an essential difference between north and south. It should be noted that the art of the south is well represented in museums, while study of the north has hardly begun (see BANTU CULTURES; SUDANESE CULTURES).

THE NORTH. *The region between the Ubangi and Congo Rivers.* This region is inhabited by different ethnic groups, of which the most northerly tribes (Ngbaka, or Bwaka; Mbanja, or Banza; and Ngbandi) speak a non-Bantu language.

The sculpture of the region is characterized by facial tattooing in the form of dots from the middle of the hairline down to the nose, resembling a cock's comb.

Ngbaka and Mbanja sculpture are closely related. Many similar statues, masks, and cephalomorphically ornamented harps and pipes are made by both tribes. Style and finish differ: some statues have a rather fleshy appearance, while others are more angular. The few known masks, used in circumcision rites, are very simple, generally flat, and rather carelessly made. Well-decorated polychrome whistles, belts, and rods are also used in circumcision rites.

The Ngbaka make representations of the Seto and Nabo spirits and use hunting fetishes of rough workmanship in the form of small animals, the latter used also by the Mbanja. Both these tribes, as well as the Ngbandi, produce clumsily made clay funeral images.

The Ngbandi also carve ancestor figures or fetishes with a triangular carved area on the head to represent the hairdo. In their general characteristics they belong to the regional sculpture. Masks are extremely rare and difficult to differentiate from those of the Ngbaka and Mbanja. The warriors formerly wore little statuettes of wood or ivory on the upper arm and used finely woven rectangular shields decorated with geometric figures.

Very few statues and no masks are known among the tribes of the Ubangi-Shari frontier (Togbo, Gobu, Mono, and Langbase). The Togbo sculptures are strikingly massive, with the head flattened in the front and very rounded in the back.

The various small Bantu groups (Loi, or Baloi; Libinja, or Libinza; Loki, or Boloki; and Lobo), who inhabit the marshy regions between the lower Ubangi and Congo Rivers, produce well-decorated canoes and oars. Sculpture is sparse: there are a few statues in a rigid position with a bonnetlike headdress and a few cephalomorphic rods, necklaces, and whistles, but it should be noted that some of the art attributed to these groups may belong to the nearby Mbanja. Drums of well-balanced proportions in the form of antelope or buffalo are occasionally found in this region.

The southern Ngombe groups appear to have little sculpture other than a few clay pipe bowls in the form of human heads, polychrome drums with linear decoration, and some handsome stools. The small northern Ngombe group has some sculpture in the Mbanja style.

*The region between the Bomu and Aruwimi Rivers.* The artistic production of the Sudanese tribes inhabiting the basins of the Bomu, Uele, and Aruwimi Rivers (Zande, or Azande, and Mangbetu) is outstanding. Until quite recently Zande art was known only in some decorated musical instruments, pipes, and earthen jars, as well as a very few free-standing statuettes whose function is not clear. Recently, however, a whole series of sculptures in wood and terra cotta was found, which are used as so-called *yanda* images by the Mani society. The majority of these small statuettes, which are sometimes very expressive, are anthropomorphous. Some of them are well finished, others carelessly made; they are either extremely realistic or extremely schematic. There are as yet very few known Zande masks. In style these few resemble others of northern Congo, being flat and rough in appearance.

Like the Zande, the Mangbetu make pottery and stringed instruments decorated with human heads. They also produce a relatively large number of wooden statues, the exact function of which is still unclear. Their daggers, cylindrical bark boxes, and many other objects are embellished with representations of elongated heads showing typical Mangbetu cranial deformation. The Makere, Bangba, Mamvu, Popoi, and Mangbele (Ngbele), who are related to or influenced by the Mangbetu, make similarly decorated objects. Among the Bangba, especially in the village of Ekibondo, are found strikingly colorful geometric decorations on the outsides of the huts. Similar decorations are also found occasionally among the other tribes of the northern savannas.

The Boa (Babwa, Baboa), living in the southwest, produce masks with large, round, often perforated ears, and faces painted in two colors. This characteristic ear perforation is also found in the few statues attributed to the Boa. The bodies of the statues show characteristic linear tattoos.

The Binja (Binza) appear to make only a few masks, some of them in the Boa style and others with two horns on the head.

*The central basin.* Most of the various Bantu tribes inhabiting the central basin belong to the great Mongo group. They do not produce much in the way of sculpture or graphic art.

In the northwestern basin the Eleku, Injolo, and Lolungu have produced remarkable coffins, some of which are anthropomorphous while others resemble giant locusts or canoes. Most of them are painted or adorned with objects indicating the social rank or the sex of the departed. The same region also makes a few statues in a similar style.

The Nsongo (Songo) and their neighbors the Kutu (Bakutu) produce only large clay funeral statues, in either a sitting or a recumbent position. The northwestern Mongo make roughly hewn wooden images with round, flat faces, and hands on the hips.

The Kota (Bokote) appear to be the makers of a small number of gaunt images with round head, square shoulders, short arms extended in front, and fleshy legs spread apart. They are thought to be funeral statues.

Hardly anything is known of the artistic production of the Mpama-Kutu. The only two objects attributable to them are a paliform, roughly sculptured statue with typical dots tattooed on the temple (II, PL. 123), and a dagger hilt.

More primitive images with outstretched arms are probably of Lia (Lalia) origin.

Sengele production is also modest; it consists of only a few male and female images whose round heads are decorated with ridges of hair, and some wooden animal images.

More interesting are the rather numerous Mbole (Bambole) sculptures painted in ocher, white, or red, which are used in the Lilwa society. They are characterized by halolike headdress, thin trunk, and bent knees (II, PL. 102). The images used in the same society by the neighboring Yela (Boyela) resemble those of the Mbole, but they are smaller, not so slender, and rougher.

*The Kivu region and environs.* There is little sculpture in this region except among the southern Lega (Balega), who do fairly advanced work.

Among the northern Bali sculpture is poor; all that is known of their work are some clumsy images with large, rough feet and hands on hips, and a few very simply made masks.

Sculpture is more widespread among the Komo (Kumu), but equally rough and without style. Some of their images, as well as carved birds placed on the roof ridges of certain huts and some large-eyed masks, are connected with the Esumba society.

The Metoko (Mituku) make funeral images with flat, angular face, rather thin trunk, and bandy legs. They also produce some statues in the same style that are more carefully finished and decorated with linear motifs (II, PL. 102).

The Zimba make female figurines with hands on the hips. The concave face is surmounted by a protuberance suggesting a headdress or bonnet.

Lega art is the most important of the Kivu region. Many small statues and masks, which were formerly used in the Bwame society, have been found there. Most are of ivory (II, PLS. 102, 105), though some are of wood. Although in some respects the Lega sculpture is akin to that of the other northern tribes, it is not characterized by their crude, schematic portrayal of the human figure. The Lega statues with raised hands, images of snakes, Janus heads, and images with many heads or only one foot show some of the lighter sculptural concept of the southern Congo.

THE SOUTH. *The lower Congo region.* Prehistoric images have been found in this area. Excavations by Van Moortsel in the Léopoldville area have brought to light decorated pottery and a terracotta statuette, but their dates have not yet been established.

Since 1482, when the Portuguese Diogo Cão landed in the old Congo kingdom, many objects of bronze, copper, silver, and ivory have been found. Most of them are of a religious nature; some may have been imported, while others were made by the natives after European models. Some of the crosses, St. Anthony statuettes, bells, and rods show a remarkably successful combination of European and African characteristics.

The present-day art production of the lower Congo region is remarkable. Kongo (Bakongo) sculpture shows an unusual realism in human and animal representation, especially apparent in the faces of the wooden sculptures, less so in the soapstone carvings, funeral images, and masks. Human figures, kneeling or sitting, alone or in groups, are often portrayed asymmetrically, with one arm raised, the head turned to the side, a leg folded under the body, or chin on hand (II, PL. 103). Many of the ancestor images, such as the mother-and-child figures, show a more careful finish than the anthropomorphous or zoomorphic *konde*, *mpezo*, and *moganga* fetishes.

In the coastal regions, the so-called potlids carved with representations of proverbs are remarkable (II, PL. 107), as are the earthen

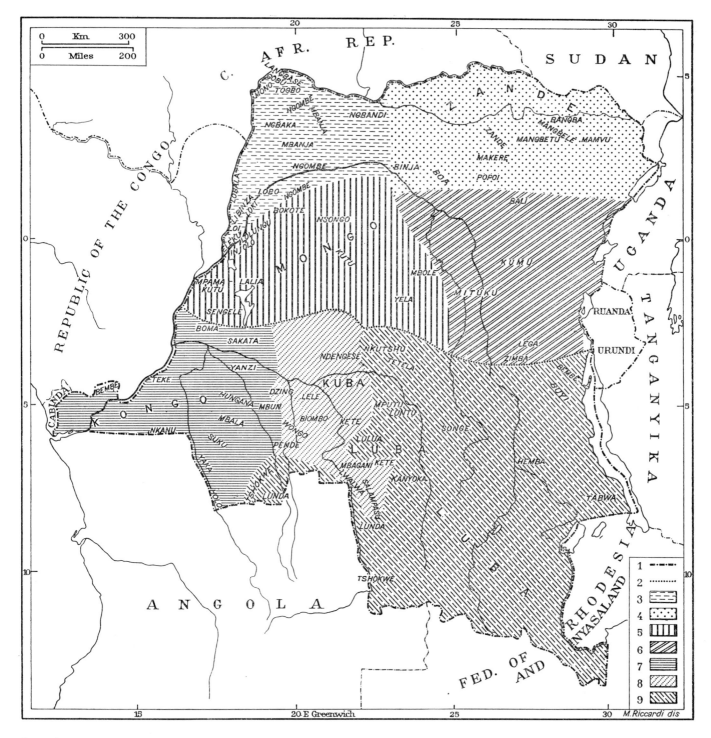

Congo: Areas of tribal styles (names of tribes in italic capitals). *Key*: (1) Political boundaries; (2) line dividing northern and southern styles; (3) region between the Ubangi and Congo Rivers; (4) region between the Bomu and Aruwimi Rivers; (5) central basin; (6) Kivu region and environs; (7) lower Congo; (8) Kasai; (9) eastern Kasai and Katanga.

jugs crowned with statuettes and the calabashes decorated with picturesque scenes.

The sculpture of the more northerly Bembe (Babembe) is confined mainly to small figures with heavily tattooed chest and stomach (II, PL. 107). The realistic representation of these statuettes relates them to the art of the Kongo tribe. Many of them carry some sort of weapon; often the eyes are indicated with bits of china.

Among the Stanley Pool tribes the Teke (Bateke) deserve special mention for their numerous fetishes, often rigidly posed, whose faces are tattooed in parallel lines. Most of these fetishes have a hole in the stomach filled with magic ingredients and closed with a pitchlike substance. The Teke also produce adzes, rods, fly whisks, and earthen jugs surmounted by human heads.

Most of the sculpture of the neighboring tribes (Humbu; Sakata; Boma, or Baboma; and Yans, or Yanzi) is related to that of the Teke.

Some Boma images, however, are distinguished by a pointed face with protuberant mouth and a high headdress. The Yans sometimes make statues with a large knot of hair on the back of the head.

The tribes of the Kwango River area have a notable artistic production. One of these tribes, the Yaka (Bayaka), makes figures with a sharply upturned nose joined to the earlobes by a line (II, PL. 109). Polychrome masks used for initiation rites often have a wide collar of raffia. Wooden masks are usually of the same style as the images, but the *kakungu* type, probably imported, has a long narrow face with heavy, rounded cheeks. Among the Yaka are also found masks in the form of animals (II, PL. 109) and some made of raffia and feathers. The small slit drums, whistles, combs, and headrests are outstanding.

Many of the polychrome panels of the Nkanu are related to the Yaka production to the southeast. This is also true of the Suku

(Basuku), whose helmet masks differ, however, from the Yaka in their anthropomorphic or zoomorphic superstructure and closed eyes. The Suku figures are distinguished by the characteristic headdress and hollowed-out temples (II, PL. 108).

Mbala sculpture can be divided into two styles. In the north are found many seated mother-and-child figures, ancestor images, and representations of musicians. The headdress is usually in the form of a helmet with straight crest. In the south the figures are more rigid, usually standing with the chin resting on the hand.

To the north, the Hungana have many sculptures resembling those of the Mbala, including some mother-and-child images. Their masks, like those of the Mbala, are closely related to those of the Yaka. The Hungana also carve ivory statuettes or pendants in low relief of a more independent design. They are carved either flat or in the round; the flat ones are sometimes double.

As yet very little is known about the statues or masks of the Mbun. A few well-sculptured rods of office surmounted by a head or bust have been found, as well as drinking vessels, sometimes in the form of a human figure. The decoration of objects of daily use has a characteristic lozenge motif.

Among the Pende (Bapende) there are two distinct sculpture styles: that of the west is related to the lower Congo, that of the east to the Kasai styles. The western Pende art production includes many red-painted masks usually used for initiation rites. Small replicas of these are made in the form of ivory pendants with a handsome patina (II, PL. 110). There are very few statues, and stools, decorated with caryatids or anthropomorphous rods, are also scarce. The wooden masks are characterized by a slightly curving forehead, eyebrows represented by a single line, wide, upturned nose, and projecting cheekbones; the headdress is covered with raffia cloth. A completely different type of mask is made entirely of raffia.

The sculpture of the Holo, though considerable and interesting, is still little known. It comprises small, horned statues with closed eyes and a sharp chin, as well as handsome bird images and slit drums resembling those of the Yaka. Most of the statues are used in magic rites, while the drums are for divination purposes. Polychrome masks in the form of buffalo, antelope, or human heads are used in circumcision rites. Musical instruments and insignia of office in the form of adzes are ornamented with heads. Remarkable framed standing or sitting figurines with arms extended, suggesting a crucifix, are used in the Nzambi society.

*The western and middle Kasai.* The Kasai region is largely dominated by Kuba (Bakuba; Bushongo) art, very important both in quantity and quality; its influence spreads far beyond the political federation of the same name. Anthropomorphous sculptures in the round are rare, with the exception of a limited number of "royal statues" — massive and realistic representations of some former Bushongo rulers (II, PL. 113) — and a few sculptures for magic rites. But there are many outstanding masks (II, PLS. 110, 115) and fine examples of carved utensils. The polychrome masks are usually made of raffia covered with cowrie shells. Some of the wooden masks have a bulging forehead; others are flatter, with a very decorative finish. Ornamental art comprises a great number of handsomely decorated objects of daily use carved with linear motifs, such as head-shaped drinking vessels, powder boxes, knives, pipes, horns, syringes, musical instruments, and adzes (II, PLS. 114, 125). There are also carefully finished animal figurines used in magical rites.

The embroidered raffia fabrics known as "Kasai velvet" (II, PL. 116) are manufactured by the Bushongo and their neighboring tribes the Lele and Nkutshu (Kutshu). The fabric is woven by men and the rectilinear motif embroidered by women. The women also make small figurines, masks, and geometric shapes of powdered camwood paste.

The artistic production of the Lele, although related to Kuba art, includes drums, pipes, drinking vessels, and a few human figures in a more formalized style.

To the west of the Lele the Dfiing-Muken have a well-developed sculpture, apparently influenced by their eastern neighbors and difficult to differentiate from their work.

The Ndengese (Dengese) masks and their excellent funeral statues with tattooed torso (II, PL. 126) are undeniably related to Kuba sculpture.

Wongo sculpture, of which only masks and decorated useful objects are known, also shows Kuba influence, as does the work of the northern Kete and Biombo. The northern Kete make polychrome statues with big heads and round, bulging eyes. Biombo art consists mainly of masks used at circumcision rites. These masks have bulging foreheads and big eyes; they are painted with alternate black and white triangular designs. The masks of the eastern Pende have a somewhat similar decoration but otherwise differ markedly from the Biombo. In addition to masks with the chin sunk in a collar — suggesting some Tshokwe (Bajokwe, Chokwe) masks — there is a flatter type, which often has a long nose and a thin chin. This type is topped by a pair of horns, a projection of some sort, or a human figure. The eastern Pende also have rather large, realistic figures which are placed on top of the huts where the symbols of authority are preserved.

Although the northern Kete are under Kuba influence, the art of the southern Kete is of a much more original character. Their relatively little-known works include masks of a heavy, ponderous type with rectangular contours, which show Tshokwe influence.

Their western neighbors, the Mbagani, make masks with sharp chin, large, white-painted eyes, small nose, and slightly bulging mouth. There are also a few statues with slightly twisted arms and hands resting on the hips or shoulders.

Only a few Lwalwa (Balwalwa; Luwa) masks have so far been discovered. There appear to be two types: one sharp-featured with a rather thin, very protuberant nose, the other less sharp with a flattened projection on top.

The wooden or plaited masks of the Salampasu are not so well finished. They are often covered with copper and may be made of resin and feathers. Sculptures, sometimes of female figures, are used in initiation rites. Musical instruments are embossed with a female figure.

*The eastern Kasai and Katanga.* The sculpture of the Tetela of the northeastern Kasai region cannot always be distinguished from that of their related neighbors, the Nkutshu. Some Tetela sculptures are as rough and crude as those of the central basin; the clear Songye (Songe, Basonge) influence in others places this art within the cultural province of the southern Congo.

The different groups known as Luluwa (Lula) and inhabiting the Luluwa basin, not only produce figures in Songye style but also have an original art of their own. Their mother-and-child statues and images of warriors are well known; other figures are pointed or stand on top of a rod. The face and body of most are plentifully tattooed in a spiral pattern and are particularly well finished (II, PLS. 111, 112), as are drinking horns, headrests, pipe bowls, and other objects of daily use. Some typical figurines sit with elbows resting on the knees. The Luluwa masks are monumental in conception and there are at least three main types.

The Mputu and Luntu sculpture is related to that of the Luluwa, but it also shows Songye influence.

Kanyoka sculpture is influenced by the Lunda and Tshokwe. Several of their sitting or standing figures, however, show the distinctive Kanyoka hairdo.

The work of the Lunda and that of the Tshokwe is so closely related that it is sometimes difficult to tell them apart. Outstanding chairs of European model, usually attributed to the Tshokwe, are covered with human figures and scenes of daily life. The same tendency toward the pictorial shows in the female figures with a mortar, in the representations of chiefs carried shoulder-high by servants, in the figure groups of musicians, and in the combs (II, PL. 124), whistles, tobacco grinders, and chiefs' scepters, decorated with human or animal figures. The number of purely zoomorphic motifs in this art is considerable.

The masks of the Lunda-Tshokwe can be divided into two categories: the well-finished wood faces of young girls, rather realistic and with a crosslike tattoo above the nose; and the more baroque specimens, made of more perishable materials such as tree bark, lianas, and raffia, and covered with a resinous substance (II, PL. 127). Most of these masks, used at initiation rites, are surmounted by large, fantastic superstructures.

Luba (Baluba) sculpture, expressive and of superior quality, dominates the production of Katanga and of the southern Kivu region. Most of the figures are female; they are shown standing or sitting, carrying a plate or serving as supports for small round stools. Female figures also appear on many objects of daily use, such as headrests, water pipes, axes and adzes, chiefs' scepters, bows, supports for arrows, divination figures, horn fetishes, and pottery. Their round fleshiness is characteristic, and much careful attention is given to the hairdo, tattooing, and other bodily features (II, PLS. 117–119).

Mask production is also important among the Luba. The style of most differs greatly from that of the figures. One type has a tattoo in parallel lines covering the whole of the face. Similar masks are found among the Songye (Basonge; II, PL. 120). Other Luba masks represent birds, buffalo, or elephant heads. Ivory is used for at least some small, stooped statuettes with hands on the breast. They are found mainly among the Luba-Hemba.

A small number of Luba statues and caryatids represent what Olbrechts called the "long-faced style of Buli" (after a village on the left bank of the Lualaba). These figures have big hands and heads, and the face is not truly negroid. The elongated head with

raised eyebrows and projecting cheekbones gives them an expression at once tragic and serene.

The Songye, who live north of the Luba region, are known as the makers of often wild-looking fetishes of horn or other materials, some of them fairly large. Most of these figures are angular with an elongated head, a protuberant stomach, and — when the statue is whole — wide, flat feet. The comparatively long neck is often composed of several layers of rings (II, PL. 122). Typically, the mouth is formed like a figure eight on its side.

The style of these figures is echoed in some types of wooden masks. Other masks of raffia have a more aggressive expression.

The sculpture of the Bembe (Wabembe) and that of their neighbors the Boyo (Buyi, Buye) are difficult to differentiate. Although they are undoubtedly related to Luba art, many Bembe-Boyo sculptures have their own characteristics such as large wide eyes, a dentellated beard, and a long and often bent trunk (II, PL. 123). The Bembe-Boyo masks, too, are distinctive: they are very flat, with big, white-painted eyes. There is also an impressive kind of four-faced mask in which the greatly enlarged eyeholes are in the form of a star, and rather small replicas of this mask, as well as stylish animal figures.

The Tabwa (Batabwa), inhabiting the southern parts between Tanganyika and Rhodesia, make a number of slender figures tattooed on the body in rows of little points. These sculptures also show Luba influence (II, PL. 123).

NOTE: The anthor has followed Boone, "Carte ethnographique du Congo belge" (Zaïre, V, 1954, pp. 451–65), in the spelling of tribal names. Variant spellings commonly used by other authorities have been added.

BIBLIOG. E. Torday and T. A. Joyce, Notes ethnographiques sur les peuples communément appelés Bakuba, ainsi que sur les peuplades apparentées: Les Bushongo, Ann. Mus. du Congo Belge, Brussels, 1910; R. P. Colle, Les Baluba, Brussels, 1913; G. F. Gregoire, Tombaux et monuments funéraires chez les Songo de la rive gauche de la Maringa, Rev. Congolaise, IV, 1913–14; E. Torday and T. A. Joyce, Notes ethnographiques sur les populations habitant les bassins du Kasai et du Kwango oriental, I, Peuplades de la forêt, II, Peuplades des prairies, Ann. Mus. du Congo Belge, Brussels, 1922; J. Maes, Aniota-Kifwebe, Antwerp, 1924; M. Planquaert, Les Sociétés secrètes chez les Bayaka, Brussels, 1930; E. von Sydow, Handbuch der afrikanischen Plastik, I, Die westafrikanische Plastik, Berlin, 1930; J. Maes, Fetischen of Tooverbeelden uit Kongo, Ann. Mus. du Congo Belge, Brussels, 1935; L. M. Bevel, L'Art de la décoration chez les Basonge, Conseiller Congolais, X, 1937; L. Bittremieux, Symbolisme in de Negerkunst, Congo Bibliotheek, Brussels, 1937. C. Kjersmeier, Centres de style de la sculpture nègre africaine, III, Congo Belge, Paris, Copenhagen, 1937; G. Hulstaert, Grafbeelden en standbeelden, Congo, I, 1938; J. Maes, Kabila- en Grafbeelden uit Kongo, Ann. Mus. du Congo Belge, Brussels, 1938; J. van Wing. Etudes Bakongo, II, Religion et magie (Inst. Royal Colonial Belge), Brussels, 1938; H. Himmelheber, Art et artistes batshiok, Brousse, III, 1939; H. Himmelheber, Les Masques bayaka et leurs sculpteurs, Brousse, I, 1939; E. Boelaert and G. Hulstaert, Les Manifestations artistiques des Nkundo (Tshuapa), Brousse, II, 1939; J. Maes, Kabila- en Grafbeelden uit Kongo, Addenda, II, Moedereerebeelden uit Kongo, Ann. Mus. du Congo Belge, Brussels, 1939; H. Himmelheber, Art et artistes bakuba, Brousse, I, 1940; F. M. Olbrechts, Stijl en Substijl in de Plastiek der Ba-Luba (Belgisch Kongo), De Kabila-stijl, Wetenschappelijke Tijdingen, V, 1940; R. Gaffé, La Sculpture au Congo Belge. Brussels, Paris, 1945; F. M. Olbrechts, Plastiek van Kongo, Antwerp, 1946; P. S. Wingert, Congo Art, Transactions, New York Acad. of Sc., IX, 2d ser., 1947; L. Zangrie, Les Institutions, la religion et l'art des Babuye (Groupes Basumba, Manyema, Congo Belge), L'Ethnographie, XL, N.S., 1947–50; G.-D. Perier, Les Arts populaires du Congo Belge, Brussels, 1948; L'Art nègre au Congo Belge, Ghent, 1950; J. Leyder, Le Graphisme et l'expression graphique au Congo Belge, Soc. Royale Belge de Géog., Brussels, 1950; A. Maessen, Un Art traditionnel au Congo Belge: La sculpture (Exposition Vaticane, Les Arts au Congo Belge et au Ruanda-Urundi), Brussels, 1950; R. L. Wannijn, Insignes religieux anciens au Bas-Congo (Exposition Vaticane, Les Arts au Congo Belge et au Ruanda-Urundi), Brussels, 1950; L'Art au Congo Belge, Les Arts plastiques, I. 5th ser., Brussels, 1951; J. van den Bossche. L'Art plastique chez les Bapende, Présence Africaine, X–XI, 1951; D. Biebuyck, Signification d'une statuette Lega, Rev. Coloniale Belge, CVC, 1953; D. Biebuyck, Function of a Lega Mask, IAE, I, 1954; D. Biebuyck, De Verwording der Kunst bij de Balega, Zaïre, III, 1954; H. Lavachéry, Statuaire de l'Afrique noire, Brussels, 1954; L. Segy, African Sculpture Speaks, 2d ed., New York, 1954; L. de Sousberghe, Cases cheffales sculptées des Ba-Pende, Bull. Soc. Royale d'Anthropologie et de Préhistoire, LXV, 1954; E. von Sydow, Afrikanische Plastik, Berlin, 1954; A. de Rop, Lilwa-beeldjes bij de Boyela, Zaïre, II, 1955; R. Verly, La Statuaire de pierre au Bas-Congo (Bamboma-Mussurongo), Zaïre, V, 1955; A. W. Wolfe, Art and the Supernatural in the Ubangi District, Man, LV, 76, 1955; Dans la Boucle du Congo, La Sculpture africaine et son destin, Namur (Grands Lacs), 1956; R. Hottot and F. Willet, Teke Fetishes, J. Royal Anthr. Inst., I, 1956; H. Huber, Magical Statuettes and their Accessories among the Eastern Bayaka and Their Neighbours (Belgian Congo), Anthropos, I–II, 1956; L'Art au Congo (cat., World's Fair, 1958), Brussels, 1958; H. Burssens, La Fonction de la sculpture traditionelle chez les Ngbaka, Brousse, XI, 1958; H. Burssens, Sculptuur in Ngbandi-styl, Een bijdrage tot de Studie van de Plastiek van Noord-Kongo, Kongo-Overzee, I–II, 1958; L. Kochnitzky, Negro Art in Belgian Congo, 4th ed., New York, 1958.

Hermann BURSSENS

CENTERS OF EUROPEAN INFLUENCE. The larger cities (Léopoldville, Elisabethville, Stanleyville) are all endowed with modern public and private buildings, tree-lined streets, and gardens; all have the character of modern colonial cities in transition. There are no traces of the Portuguese colonization (16th–17th cent.).

Léopoldville. Capital of the former Belgian colony, founded by Stanley in 1881, it is divided into industrial, commercial, administrative, and residential areas. The Museum of Indigenous Art and the sports stadiums, built according to the most modern architectural schemes, are noteworthy.

Elisabethville. Capital of Katanga, developed through exploitation of the mines of the region. It has imposing cathedrals, hospitals, and scientific establishments.

Stanleyville. Founded in 1898, it is one of the oldest cities of the Congo; the oldest residential houses date from 1909. It has a cathedral in Gothic style.

The principal collections of the art of the Belgian Congo are in the Musée Royal du Congo Belge in Tervueren, near Brussels.

\* \*

Illustration: 1 fig. in text.

CONSERVATION. See PRESERVATION AND CONSERVATION OF ART WORKS.

CONSTABLE, JOHN. Landscape painter, born at East Bergholt, Suffolk, England, 1776. The countryside around his birthplace is pastoral and gently undulating, marked chiefly by the low hills flanking Dedham Vale, along which meanders the River Stour. The artist's father, Golding Constable, owned mills on the banks of the river, made navigable by locks in the 18th century. This landscape setting of his early years had a far-reaching effect on Constable's art. His choice of subjects came to be limited to a small group of places in which his affections were deeply engaged, all sharing the pastoral quality of the scenes of his childhood, in which men pursued the traditional labors he had seen on the banks of the Stour River and in the nearby fields.

A youthful friendship with an artisan who was an amateur painter aroused Constable's own ambitions; but up to his twentieth year his work was painfully lacking in ability, and it was intended that he should follow his father's calling. Eventually, with the encouragement of the connoisseur Sir George Beaumont, of Joseph Farington, R.A., and of his mother, he went to London in 1799 to begin his formal artistic training in the schools of the Royal Academy. After searching self-criticism he resolved that he would confine himself to landscape painting and that he would avoid the direct imitation of other painters. At this time the model for landscape painting in England was still the classical ideal landscape of the 17th century. Works by Claude Lorrain, Nicolas Poussin, and Gaspard Poussin were in every large collection, and the contemporary artist was expected to conform to the principles of formal composition, lighting, and detailed finish which marked their pictures and even to imitate their tonality, distorted though this might be by a century or more of discolored varnish. Constable realized that within such limitations he could not paint the English countryside as he saw it, and in his search for more suitable methods he created his own art.

In 1802 he began the practice of sketching in oils in the open air, a form of study which he continued throughout his life. His nature sketches are dazzlingly fresh and brilliant and give direct contact with the mind of the artist, but to him they were the exercises and the raw material out of which he could create more ambitious and logically constructed landscapes. Constable's originality was soon recognized, even by men who might be expected to be hostile to it, and he received help and encouragement not only from Farington, but also from Benjamin West, the president of the Royal Academy.

During his formative period, from 1800 to 1810, Constable attempted to follow the usual practice of making sketching expeditions to a countryside of recognized romantic beauty. In 1801 he went to the Peak District and in 1806 to the Lake District. Unlike his contemporaries, he found that mountains did not exhilarate but depressed him, and he made no further sketching tours. A casual visit to a new scene could not replace for him the long process of getting to know a landscape intimately, and accordingly he went year after year from his London home to East Bergholt and Dedham or visited close friends in the southern counties. During this time, to justify his choice of a career to relatives and friends, he painted two altarpieces for local churches, but they are only feeble imitations of Benjamin West. He made strenuous efforts to succeed as a portrait painter, the chief means of earning a living then available to an English artist. Until late in his life he continued to paint portraits, but this was always an irksome task, unless his affections were strongly engaged. When he painted a member of his family or a close friend he was capable of a sympathetic likeness, as in a portrait of his fiancée, Maria Bicknell (London, Tate Gall.). Though his early attempts at portraiture led him to copy Reynolds and Hoppner for the Earl of Dysart, this technical exercise was of permanent value to him, resulting in an immediately increased facility in his landscapes. By 1810 he was producing oil sketches of the countryside of East Bergholt and Dedham in which he achieved natural color and rich atmospheric quality, free from the shackles of past formalism; fine examples are *Barges on the Stour* and *Flatford Lock and Mill* (London, Vict. and Alb. Mus.).

The years 1810 to 1815 were years of intense concentration on his painting, and also years of personal difficulty. He had fallen in love with Maria Bicknell, but her parents were opposed to her marrying a not notably successful artist. Accordingly Constable became something of a recluse, making studies in his country retreat with even greater assiduity. There are in the Victoria and Albert Museum two small pocket books which he filled in 1813 and 1814 with hundreds of free, but minutely observed, studies of the fields near his birthplace. These sketchbooks, which have all the fascination of an intimate diary, were often drawn on for the paintings he made in later years; in them he is seen to return to the same scene day after day, drawing it under varying lights and seeking for a viewpoint in which his subject formed a naturally balanced composition. The sketchbook of 1814 contains, for example, the pencil study for the composition of *Boatbuilding near Flatford Mill* (PL. 444), an oil painting now in the Victoria and Albert Museum, painted in 1815 entirely in the open air.

Pursuing his courtship with the same obstinate determination that marked his pursuit of success in painting, Constable eventually married Maria Bicknell in 1816. The 12 happy years of this marriage were also mature and productive years for Constable as an artist. Also, he began to gain some recognition. He sold his first painting to a stranger in 1814 and was elected an Associate of the Royal Academy in 1819. Having become through his marriage and the death of his parents financially independent, he felt confident enough to embark upon a series of large canvases, the subjects of which were taken from the banks of the River Stour and which he exhibited in successive years at the Royal Academy. The first of these was *Flatford Mill on the Stour* (PL. 444; 1817, London, Tate Gall.), followed by *The White Horse* (1819, New York, Frick Coll.); *Stratford Mill* (1820, Major R. N. Macdonald-Buchanan Coll.); *The Hay Wain* (PL. 441; 1821, London, Nat. Gall.); *View on the Stour near Dedham* (1822, San Marino, Calif., Huntington Art Gall.); and *The Leaping Horse* (1825, London, Diploma Gall., Royal Academy).

In 1811 Constable had formed a close friendship with John Fisher, a clergyman living in Dorsetshire and later in the cathedral town of Salisbury. This friendship was not only a great encouragement to the artist, because of Fisher's understanding of his work, but widened his choice of themes. On his many visits to Fisher's home Constable made a number of sketches, and these he used when Fisher's uncle, the Bishop of Salisbury, commissioned him to paint *Salisbury Cathedral from the Bishop's Garden* (1823, London, Vict. and Alb. Mus.), a subject he used several times (see PL. 442). His range of subjects was further extended in 1819, when he moved his wife and family for the summer months to Hampstead, a village on a hill on the northern outskirts of London, then surrounded by open country. This move became an annual custom until, eventually, he took a house in Hampstead. Here he began a long series of sky studies, based on the conviction that only one aspect of the sky was consistent with a particular kind of illumination of the objects on the ground. Many of these studies showing the foliage of bushes and trees in motion and lit by gleams from a cloud-torn sky are in the Victoria and Albert Museum and are among his most dramatic sketches. On the backs of these and other cloud studies he usually recorded the date, the time of day, and the weather conditions prevailing at the time they were painted.

At Hampstead also Constable was later to find a new type of subject hitherto unused by any landscape painter, the combination of suburban buildings with rural surroundings, as exemplified in *A Romantic House* (1832, London, Nat. Gall.).

The paintings exhibited yearly at the Royal Academy were based on such sky studies and on many oil and pencil studies of the main scene and of subordinate details. Sometimes Constable worked out his composition in a full-scale design, exactly the size of the version he was going to exhibit. These full-scale designs were naturally carried to a lesser stage of completion than the final version and accordingly preserve to modern eyes more of the immediate impact of the artist's creative genius. Well-known examples are those made for *The Hay Wain* (1821) and *The Leaping Horse* (1825, London, Vict. and Alb. Mus.).

With the exhibition of *The Hay Wain* at the Royal Academy in 1821 Constable's work became known to French artists, notably Géricault. Soon afterward two dealers, Schroth and Arrowsmith, began showing his work in Paris. Recognition outside his own country reached its climax in 1824, when *The Hay Wain* and *A View on the Stour near Dedham* were exhibited in the Salon and excited great admiration and heated critical discussion. *The Hay Wain* was awarded a gold medal, and Constable's influence over the younger French artists, in particular Delacroix, dated from this event.

In 1824 Mrs. Constable's increasingly poor health caused Constable to take her to Brighton, a fashionable seaside resort on the south coast. He found the landscape of the surrounding country unsympathetic, but he set to work on oil studies and drawings of the beach and shipping, many of which are remarkable for the atmospheric lucidity of their rendering. At this time his style of painting was changing from the serenity of the middle years of his career. He became more and more concerned with what he called "the chiaroscuro of Nature," a term covering the broken lights and accents caused by the reflection of sunlight on wet leaves and the alternation of lights and darks in the sky and the shadowed landscape. He used the palette knife increasingly and worked over and elaborated his surface incessantly to give the effect of texture in water, trees, fields, and sky. To Constable's contemporaries his painting looked unfinished, and the glazed highlights with which he enhanced them became known as "Constable's snow."

That Constable was now established as a landscape painter is shown by the number of repetitions he was called upon to make from his more popular compositions. Among the subjects he repeated most often, though always with some variation in the lighting and mood, were *Dedham Mill* (1820) and *Hampstead Heath* (first version 1828), both in the Victoria and Albert.

In 1829 his wife died, and election in that year to full membership in the Royal Academy he regarded as belated and without significance. In 1830 he began to issue a series of mezzotint engravings under the title *English Landscape Scenery*. This publication was to some extent planned in emulation of Turner's *Liber Studiorum* and was designed to illustrate Constable's range in landscapes, chosen especially with a view to recording the "chiaroscuro of Nature." Under Constable's exacting supervision the engraver, David Lucas, was remarkably

successful in carrying over the essence of his sketches into black and white.

From this time onward Constable was subject to fits of depression. He had been left with a family of seven young children and forced himself into extra exertions on their behalf. Another sorrow was the death of John Fisher in 1832. Constable had paid his last visit to Salisbury in 1829, but he made the town the subject of one more large canvas, *Salisbury Cathedral from the Meadows* (exhibited Royal Acad., 1831; Coll. Lord Ashton of Hyde). The stormy mood of this painting and, among others, *Stoke-by-Nayland* (1836–37, Chicago, Art Inst.) reflects the agitation of Constable's spirit at the time. In 1834 he formed a new friendship, with a namesake, George Constable, who lived in Arundel, and there Constable's interest was aroused in the wooded downlands of Sussex. He made many water-color and pencil sketches of this more hilly and broken scenery, but the only elaborate composition he constructed from his sketches was *Arundel Mill and Castle* (Toledo, Ohio, Mus. of Art). He was working on the picture the day he died in 1837, but it was considered sufficiently finished to be exhibited posthumously at the Royal Academy exhibition of that year. The painting exemplifies a tendency at this time to over-elaboration of detail, also seen in *Valley Farm* (PL. 440; 1835, London, Tate Gall.).

In addition to those mentioned above, important works are: *Malvern Hall* (1809, London, Nat. Gall.); *Vale of Dedham* (1811, Granville Proby Coll.); *Wivenhoe Park, Essex* (1817, Washington, D.C., Nat. Gall.); *The Lock* (1824, S. Morrison Coll.); *The Cornfield* (1826, London, Nat. Gall.); *The Glebe Farm* (begun 1826, London, Tate Gall.); *Marine Parade and Chain Pier, Brighton* (1827, London, Tate Gall.); *Dedham Vale* (1828, Edinburgh, Nat. Gall.); *Whitehall Stairs, or the Opening of Waterloo Bridge* (1832, H. Ferguson Coll.); *The Cenotaph* (PL. 440; 1836, London, Tate Gall.). For a full understanding of Constable's work it is essential to know the collection in the Victoria and Albert Museum, London, which owes its unique character to the 95 oil sketches (PL. 443), 297 drawings, and 3 sketchbooks given by Miss Isabel Constable, the painter's last surviving child.

The American-born artist, C. R. Leslie, R.A., has left in his *Memoirs of the Life of John Constable* a remarkable record, given authority by a friendship of more than twenty years. Constable was an exceptionally articulate artist, much given to pungent comments on matters which interested him, and Leslie has preserved many of his incisive sayings on his own art and that of others. He also prints passages from some lectures on the history of landscape painting that Constable delivered toward the end of his life. These reveal his detailed and perceptive understanding of the work of his forerunners, on which his own innovations were grounded. The exuberant color of the sketches produced in his early maturity was based upon the study of Rubens, in particular of *The Château de Steen* (London, Nat. Gall.), which he knew in the collection of Sir George Beaumont. Ruisdael and Claude Lorrain he particularly admired, occasionally copying works by them. Ruisdael undoubtedly stimulated Constable's study of cloud forms and of cloud shadows; while from Claude came the idea of circumambient light and atmosphere. Indeed, despite his specific rejection of the clichés of classical landscape, he owed much to Claude Lorrain and Poussin in achieving balanced and harmonious design. From Richard Wilson he learned the same lesson, and Wilson and Gainsborough pointed the way toward poetic interpretation of naturalistic detail through the handling of light. Constable is sometimes regarded as having been influenced by the theory of the picturesque, widely current in the England of his early years, which extolled careful differentiation in the form and texture of the various elements of a composition and the pictorial value of rough and rugged objects. Certainly Constable held somewhat similar views. As he himself wrote to Fisher (Oct. 23, 1821): "The sound of water escaping from mill-dams etc., willows, old rotten planks, slimy, posts, and brickwork — I love such things .... As long as I do paint, I shall never cease to paint such places .... Painting is with me but another word for feeling, and I associate 'my careless boyhood' with all that lies on the banks of the Stour. Those scenes made me a painter and I am grateful." These very words, however, indicate that Constable's approach to painting was inspired less by the concept of the picturesque than by an approach to nature similar to that of Wordsworth. In this view, every form in nature was regarded as a facet or manifestation of an all-pervasive, underlying spirit; so that study and understanding of even the simplest natural phenomenon could reveal the unity of which it formed part. This is what Constable meant when he always insisted upon a poetic approach to painting, and at the same time could say: "It is the business of a painter not to contend with nature, and put this scene (a valley filled with imagery 50 miles long) on a canvas of a few inches; but to make something out of nothing, in attempting which, he must almost of necessity become poetical" (Constable to Fisher, August, 1824).

Thus, the naturalism of Constable goes beyond the record of what the eye sees, to the use of this to express the concept of a unified nature, infinitely varied in expression, arrived at by absorbed and intense contemplation. The chief means Constable used to emphasize this variety in unity was light. Subject was unimportant, except from the point of view of awaking interest on the part of the painter. As he himself once said, "Let the form of an object be what it may — light, shade, and perspective [atmospheric perspective] will always make it beautiful." For the expression of light, he developed the use of positive color in his shadows and of a broken touch to give variety and vitality, thus to some extent anticipating the practice of the impressionists, though working in a much lower key. To the same end, expression of unity through light, is directed the dominant place Constable ultimately gave to the sky in his painting. Writing to Fisher (Oct. 23, 1821) he says: "That landscape painter who does not make his skies a very material part of his composition, neglects to avail himself of one of his greatest aids .... I have often been advised to consider my sky as *a white sheet thrown behind the objects*. Certainly, if the sky is obtrusive, as mine are, it is bad; but if it is evaded, as mine are not, it is worse .... It will be difficult to name a class of landscape in which sky is not the keynote, the standard of scale, and the chief organ of sentiment .... The sky is the source of light in nature, and governs everything."

Unity through lighting, with a vigor in handling which gives the feeling of phenomena in movement, he had achieved by 1810. Thenceforward, it was Constable's constant aim to secure these characteristics in larger works, while enriching them with undertones and overtones to prevent emptiness. His earlier large paintings, such as *The White Horse* and *Stratford Mill*, tend to be sensitively handled compilations, with formal rather than emotional unity. In such masterpieces as *The Leaping Horse* and *The Lock*, however, he attains all the vigor and unity of a sketch, with a rich orchestration of detail. It must be remembered that Constable's large paintings were mainly produced for exhibition at the Royal Academy, and apparently he somewhat tempered his own methods to suit the conventions of the day. It may well be that the large designs, exactly resembling the paintings sent to the Academy, were, in fact, Constable's idea of what a finished picture should be. In any event, in the late twenties and in the thirties, during the period of emotional stress following the death of his wife, Constable ceased to care for public opinion and produced several paintings in which every resource he possessed was directed toward an unsurpassed expression of the great forces of nature.

During his lifetime Constable's originality and uncompromising temper prevented wide recognition of his merits among both artists and the public in England, though he had devoted friends and admirers and sold a fair amount of work to private patrons. In France, however, he was quickly accepted as an important figure. After the exhibition of *The Hay Wain* at the Salon in 1824, a number of his paintings were exhibited elsewhere and several were sold in France, so that opportunity to see his work was greater than is generally realized. His influence upon Delacroix, particularly in the use of color, is well known. Equally important was his impact upon the painters

of the Barbizon school, notably on Troyon, and through them and Delacroix he came to permeate the whole approach to landscape painting in France. Any influence upon the impressionists seems to have been indirect, except in the case of Pissarro, whose work in England and for some years afterward was considerably affected by Constable's example. In England he inspired no painters of any importance, though there were a number of minor imitators, among the best known of whom was F. W. Watts, and it was not until his influence was transmitted through France back to England in the later part of the 19th century that Constable became a force in English painting. He was, however, paid the compliment of being one of the most frequently forged artists of the 19th century. There was evidently a steady demand for his works at not too high prices, and the number available for comparison in public collections was small. Thus, even before his death, imitations signed and unsigned, together with copies purporting to be versions, became frequent. Some of these entered public collections on the European Continent and in the United States, where they set false standards of authenticity; others still appear regularly in the market, a constant menace to the collector.

BIBLIOG. C. R. Leslie, Memoirs of the Life of John Constable, R. A., London, 1843, 2d ed. enlarged, 1845 (of several reprints those edited with supplementary material by A. Shirley, London, 1937, and by J. H. Mayne, London, 1951, are the most useful); C. J. Holmes, Constable, London, 1901, and Constable and His Influence on Landscape Painting, London, 1902; Lord Windsor (later Earl of Plymouth), John Constable, R. A., London, 1903; A. Shirley, The Mezzotints of David Lucas after John Constable, Oxford, 1930; P. Leslie, Letters from John Constable, R. A., to C. R. Leslie, R. A., London, 1932; H. I. Kay, The Haywain, BM, June, 1933 (important for Constable's influence in France); A. Shirley, The Rainbow: A Portrait of John Constable, London, 1949; K. Badt, John Constable's Clouds, London, 1950 (Constable's relation to nature and to scientific investigation); R. B. Beckett, John Constable and the Fishers, London, 1952 (the most complete edition of the Constable-Fisher letters, with notes); G. Reynolds, Catalogue résumé of the Constable Collection, Victoria and Albert Museum, 1959. A typewritten transcript of the artist's extant correspondence and other source material has been compiled by R. B. Beckett and deposited in the Library of the Victoria and Albert Museum under the title Correspondence and other Memorials of John Constable, R. A.

Graham REYNOLDS

Illustrations: PLS. 440–444.

**CONSTRUCTIVISM.** See EUROPEAN MODERN MOVEMENTS.

**COPIES.** See FALSIFICATION AND FORGERY; REPRODUCTIONS.

**COPLEY,** JOHN SINGLETON. American colonial painter of portraits and historical subjects (b. probably Boston, July 3, 1738; d. London, Sept. 9, 1815). His parents, Richard and Mary (Singleton) Copley, came to Boston about 1736 from Ireland. The father was a tobacconist, who, according to tradition, died on a trip to the West Indies. In 1748 the mother became the third wife of Peter Pelham, a mezzotint engraver who also taught school and dancing. Two years after Pelham's death in 1751, Copley commenced his painting career with signed and dated works. Although the mezzotint of Rev. William Welsteed (1753) remains his only known print, Copley executed more than 275 portraits in oil, pastel, and miniature before he left America. In 1766 he sent the Boy with the Squirrel (Boston, priv. coll.; see I, PL. 101) to London for exhibition. Praised by Reynolds, the picture brought Copley election to the Society of Artists of Great Britain as well as helpful letters from the American painter Benjamin West.

On November 16, 1769, Copley married Susanna Clarke, daughter of a prosperous Boston merchant. For six months during 1771 they traveled in the Colonies, going as far as Philadelphia but staying mostly in New York, where Copley painted 37 portraits. In June of 1774, fulfilling a long-debated desire to see the paintings of the European masters, Copley left America. From London he proceeded to Paris and Rome. The approach of war in 1775 caused Mrs. Copley and the children to emigrate to London, where her husband joined them

late in that year; London became their permanent home. In 1776 Copley was admitted as an associate of the Royal Academy of Arts and was elected an academician in 1779.

Despite some quarrels in which his contentious spirit was manifested, Copley had 25 years of professional success. But after 1800 he sold little work. This, together with ill health, diminished his productivity; a second paralytic stroke was the immediate cause of his death.

Copley's American work is the best painting of the entire colonial period. He quickly assimilated the influences available to him in Boston, and through most of his colonial phase availed himself freely of imported prints as source material. But his creative development was through direct study of visual actuality; he was able to organize form and color and personality, obtaining a mastery in realism superior to that found in any other pre-Revolutionary portraiture. The absence of atmosphere as well as his occasionally defective drawing were shortcomings natural to a self-taught provincial; they were, however, only incidental among the positive virtues of his mature American style, as exemplified in the Mrs. Richard Skinner (1772; Boston, Mus. of Fine Arts) and the Mr. and Mrs. Thomas Mifflin (1773; Philadelphia, Hist. Soc. of Pa.).

In Rome, Copley had begun a transformation of his technique which led to uneven results. The Mr. and Mrs. Ralph Izard (1775; Boston, Mus. of Fine Arts) shows a tendency that became intensified in his large-scale portraits — subordination of character interest to the material splendor of accessories. His religious subjects were generally inferior, but his first important effort in secular history, Watson and the Shark (1778; Boston, Mus. of Fine Arts), still asserts its authority as a splendid forerunner of 19th-century romanticism. A few later examples such as The Death of Chatham (1781; London, Nat. Gall.) and The Siege of Gibraltar (1791; London, Guildhall Art Gall.) developed the pictorial rhetoric of chiaroscuro. He executed one of his most imposing designs in The Copley Family (ca. 1780; Washington, Nat. Gall.) and achieved a surprisingly successful flamboyance in The Children of George III (1785; London, Buckingham Palace). However, Copley's increased fluency of brushwork gradually impaired the firmness of his figure construction, and before the end his compositional skill also declined. See also AMERICAS: ART SINCE COLUMBUS.

BIBLIOG. M. B. Amory, The Domestic and Artistic Life of John Singleton Copley, R. A., Boston 1882; G. Jones, ed., The Letters and Papers of John Singleton Copley and Henry Pelham, 1739–1776, vol. 71, Mass. Hist. Soc. Coll., Boston, 1914; N. B. Parker and A. B. Wheeler, John Singleton Copley, American Portraits in Oil, Pastel, and Miniature, Boston, 1938; J. T. Flexner, John Singleton Copley, Boston, 1948.

Virgil BARKER

**COPTIC ART.** The artistic production of Christian Egypt, that is, of the Christians in Egypt after the Arab conquest (called "Copts," from the Arabic Qubt, Quft, Qift, a corruption of Αἰγύπτιος), shows two main sources of derivation. On the one hand it was influenced by Mediterranean stylistic developments of late-antique and early medieval times (see LATE-ANTIQUE PERIOD; BYZANTINE ART), and on the other by the artistic tradition of Egypt itself (see EGYPTIAN ART).

The end of the Ptolemaic period and the beginning of the rule of imperial Rome saw the earliest anticipations of Coptic art, which was to reach full maturity in the 5th and 6th centuries, primarily in the monastic centers. The course of its development was checked by the Arab invasions of 640 to 642, which resulted in the institution of Islam as the state religion in Egypt; succeeding styles give evidence of a long period of decline within the closed circle of surviving Christian communities, down to the threshold of the modern age. Coptic art is characterized by a progressive evolution toward abstract design; it was influenced chiefly by Constantinople (see BYZANTINE ART), Syria (see SYRIAN ART), and, to a lesser degree, Mesopotamia and Persia.

Despite the extent of the work already done in Coptic studies, our knowledge of the development of Coptic art is still fragmentary; there is need for reevaluation of the extant

material as well as for new excavations and explorations. Unfortunately, only a small proportion of the buildings mentioned in earlier sources have survived, many having been destroyed, together with their artistic treasures, by the Arabs in the 8th century, so that essential links in the chronology are missing.

SUMMARY. Introduction (col. 797). General characteristics of Coptic art (col. 798). Emergence of the Coptic style (col. 799): *Sculpture and painting*; *Architecture*; *Minor arts*. Development of Coptic art (col. 802): *Architecture*; *Sculpture*; *Painting*; *Manuscript illumination*; *Minor arts*.

INTRODUCTION. In the first three centuries of our era, while Christianity was rapidly spreading throughout Egypt and beginning to establish an independent church there, late Hellenistic culture became concentrated in Alexandria, whose cosmopolitan culture was closely linked with the aristocratic taste of the other principal cities of the eastern Mediterranean, and whose art showed stylistic similarities to their art, especially to that of the Hellenized Syrian cities. This resemblance is seen in the porphyry and ivory carvings from the imperial workshops, and possibly in some fine silverwork which may be Alexandrian.

The farther one goes from Alexandria toward the interior of the country, the more evident appears the rejection of the cosmopolitan art of the capital, a rejection expressed by an emphasis on local characteristics and traditions. The taste of the lower classes of society seems to have been very different from, and was, indeed, sharply opposed to, the refined Hellenistic culture. Not only did they rapidly accept Christianity; they set themselves against the upper classes, initiating a truly nationalistic movement. Early manifest in the smaller provincial centers is a characteristic indigenous style that displays Coptic elements, though for a long time the administrative centers of the interior, particularly Antinoë (Antinoopolis), with Roman and later with Byzantine officials, tried to resist these indigenous tendencies. But here too the ever-increasing Orientalization of the bureaucracy, the strong influx of Byzantine, Persian, Syrian, and Armenian personnel, had its consequences for cultural development: beside the pronounced Egyptian elements in art are Persian, Syrian, and even Indian influences.

However, even in the immediate vicinity of the conservative centers, the Coptic style, emanating primarily from the monasteries, became predominant. The Egyptian monks, who in the 5th century had gathered together in large communities such as the White Monastery (Deir el-Abiad) and the Red Monastery (Deir el-Ahmar), came from the lower classes, and even the great founders of monasteries, such as St. Pachomius and St. Shenute, who were responsible for transforming the anchorites into cenobites, were adamantly anti-Hellenistic and antiaristocratic. Nevertheless, the monks had supported the Patriarch of Alexandria in the heated theological conflict over the divine and human nature of Christ; in 451 the Egyptian Church repudiated the doctrine of the Council of Chalcedon and, holding to the Monophysite tenets, became autonomous. By 500 the Coptic religion, language, and art were already clearly established in the monastic communities. From then on, a rich and well-defined religious iconography developed. Monasteries with churches and libraries were founded in great number; isolated sanctuaries, with paintings, icons, and sculptures, also contributed to the culture that was flowering at the time of the Arab invasions.

After the invasions a certain amount of cultural activity persisted, but the persecution that the Church suffered prevented any real revival. Moreover, adherence to Monophysitism set Egypt apart from the Christian East, thus bringing it more strongly under Islamic influence. This influence is evident in the churches of Cairo and in the monasteries of St. Anthony and St. Paul in the Arabian Desert and in those of the desert of Nitria. After the 8th century, Christian art in Egypt lived largely on its inheritance, repeating forms created in the three preceding centuries.

Closely connected with the Coptic Church of Egypt were the Nubian Christians (whose art has been the subject of special study by Monneret de Villard; see NUBIAN ART) and the Christians of Ethiopia, where an indigenous style had arisen (see ETHIOPIAN ART). Because of the widespread activity and traffic of Egyptian monks, the artistic interchange in territories where the Coptic religion prevailed never ceased.

GENERAL CHARACTERISTICS OF COPTIC ART. Coptic art has preserved certain constant traits throughout its history. Typical characteristics, in strong contrast to the illusionism of Hellenistic art, are its severe, almost abstract composition and accen-

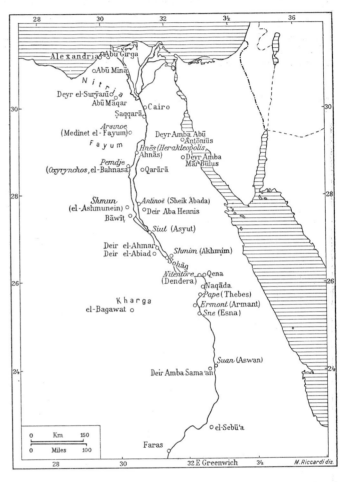

Coptic art centers. (Ancient names are generally given in the Coptic form.)

tuated stylization. From time to time, traditional Pharaonic motifs were consciously adopted, but generally speaking their reappearance was spontaneous. Thus in architecture, for example in the monasteries near Sohag, we find ground plans of the greatest simplicity and massive outer walls without any ornamentation, recalling the temples of Edfu and Dendera. The starkly frontal representations of saints completely cover the interior walls of the churches; these paintings show a characteristic system of pure colors (generally blue, red, and yellow) that continued in textiles as late as the 10th century.

Coptic religious iconography is distinctly different from that of the Byzantines. The Monophysite doctrine conditioned the type of church plan and, through its preference for cycles illustrating scenes from the apocryphal Gospels, limited the range of pictorial subjects. We generally find Christ enthroned (as at Bawit), often surrounded by angels, as the symbol of the One God, or standing in an attitude of blessing with the figure of the donor beside him (as at 'Abd el-Qadir in the Nubian desert), and we find scenes from the life of Christ: the Nativity and the Adoration of the Magi (Faras), the Baptism (Bawit, Saqqara), the childhood of Christ and the miracles (Deir Abu Hennis, near Antinoë), the Ascension (Bawit). The Virgin was frequently represented, and a special type of Virgin lactant,

reminiscent of the Mother Goddess Isis, was developed (as at Saqqara; PL. 457). On the other hand, representation of the Virgin enthroned with angels around her in a *mandorla* was very frequent during the Arab domination. The churches were generally decorated with rows of the most venerated saints, especially great anchorites, monks, and founders of monasteries. Images of soldier saints — such as St. Sisinnius, St. George, and others (as at Bawit) — are very characteristic.

EMERGENCE OF THE COPTIC STYLE. *Sculpture and painting.* The rise of the Coptic style has been linked by some scholars with the development of Alexandrian sculpture, on the evidence provided by the porphyry carvings and by the Hellenistic reliefs carved in bone discovered in great quantities in Alexandria. In both groups, however, we see a progressive decay of the plastic sense, within the context of the late Hellenistic

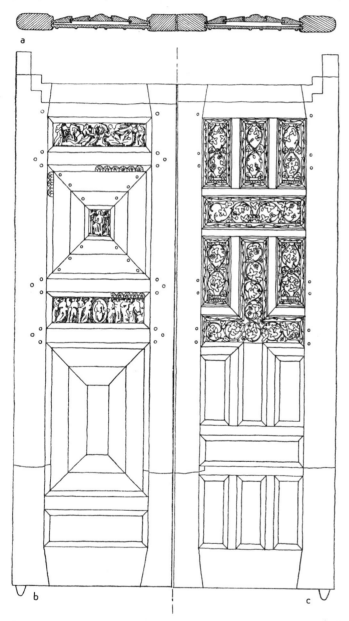

Cairo, wooden door of the Church of St. Barbara (early 6th cent.). (*a*) Cross section; (*b*) front view of one of the leaves; (*c*) rear view of the other leaf (*reconstruction by Patricolo and Monneret de Villard, 1922*).

manner, rather than the emergence of a new style. Lacking a dependable chronology, we cannot follow the evolution of bone reliefs through its various phases, and the tendency is to consider as late examples reliefs that are merely of inferior quality. Thanks to Delbrueck's studies (1931), we are better informed

about the chronology of the carvings in porphyry. For the porphyry sarcophagus of St. Helena in the Vatican Museum, Rodenwaldt (*Archäologisches Jhb.*, 1922, p. 31) insists upon an Alexandrian origin. The head of an emperor and an emperor enthroned in the Municipal Museum of Alexandria appear to have been executed in the imperial workshops. To the same group belong the emperors on the exterior of St. Mark's in Venice, the smaller figures in the Vatican, the torso in the Archbishop's Palace in Ravenna, the torso of an emperor in Berlin (Staat. Mus.), and the imperial sarcophagi and fragments of porphyry work in the Archaeological Museum in Istanbul, all belonging to the 3d and 4th centuries of our era. Two of the emperors of St. Mark's, possibly Diocletian and Maximianus Herculeus, belong perhaps among the earliest works, while the Berlin torso, judging by the type of fibula and sword, is probably from the end of the 4th century.

The bone reliefs are particularly well represented in Alexandria (Municipal Mus.), Cairo (Coptic Mus.), and Berlin (Staat. Mus.). Their motifs derive from the Alexandrian-Hellenistic repertory, and for the most part they are poor imitations intended for the decoration of furniture in the manner of such ivory work as the fine reliefs on the chancel in the Palatine Chapel at Aachen, and the Isis in Paris (Mus. de Cluny). Pagan gods, putti, and local divinities are frequently represented. Among the very few Christian subjects, the *Sacrifice of Abraham* in Berlin (Staat. Mus.) and the *Christ* in Florence (PL. 445) are of unusual quality; the iconographical similarities between the *Sacrifice* and the ivory pyxides in Berlin, Trier (Landesmus.), and Bologna (Mus. Civ.) have led some scholars to localize these ivories, too, in Alexandria, but the evidence cannot be considered conclusive. Some ivories found in Egypt, such as a comb from Antinoë (Cairo, Coptic Mus.), fragments of a pyxis (Ann Arbor, Kelsy Mus.; Mainz, Römisch-Germanisches Zentralmus.), show possible Egyptian characteristics, but the same cannot be said for numerous other Early Christian ivories, such as the diptych in Ravenna (Mus. Naz.) and the pyxides in the Vatican Museums, in Leningrad (Hermitage), Paris (Louvre, Mus. de Cluny), Bonn (Landesmus.), Tunis (Bardo), and Berlin, which have been quite arbitrarily assigned to the same group. The throne of Archbishop Maximian in Ravenna (546–56) presents one of the most disputed problems. The panels with the stories of St. Joseph reveal an affinity with the style of Egyptian art, whereas all the rest of the work is Byzantine in feeling. Probably the throne is mainly the product of a Byzantine school in Ravenna. The pyxis with Isis in Wiesbaden (Landesmus.) and that with St. Menas in London (Br. Mus.) have, chiefly because of their subjects, been considered of Egyptian origin. In none of these examples are any true characteristics of the Coptic style revealed. The close relation between the Early Christian art of Egypt and that of the other Mediterranean areas, even in the 5th and 6th centuries, is shown in the style of the wood reliefs of the door of the Church of St. Barbara (FIG. 799) of about 500 (Cairo, Coptic Mus.). The style of the rinceaux and figures, especially of the angels with the victory wreath, finds exact parallels in such five-part diptych panels as the Barberini ivory in the Louvre, in the Archbishop's throne in Ravenna, in Coptic wood reliefs such as those of Bawit, and in stone reliefs such as those of Ahnas. A more pronounced Orientalism, having affinities with Syrian art, is seen in the wood reliefs of the Church of the Muallaqa in Cairo (Coptic Mus.) showing the entry into Jerusalem and the Ascension, with an iconography similar to that of the ciborium in St. Mark's. The wood carving in high relief showing the siege of a city (PL. 445), in Berlin, is clearly related in style to the carvings in porphyry. In short, all this early sculpture is characterized by the late-antique taste of the cosmopolitan cities and is therefore markedly different from the art of the interior of the country.

Unfortunately no paintings of the Alexandrian school have survived, but we may form some idea of the style of that city by studying old copies of interesting frescoes in the catacombs of Karmuz. Among these, for example, is the *Multiplication of the Loaves and Fishes*, which reflects an age-old Near Eastern tradition; no stylistic innovation is apparent; no genuine Coptic

elements have as yet appeared. Of a later period, that is of the 4th or 5th century, are the frescoes in the mortuary chapels of El-Bagawat in Kharga Oasis; despite the distance from the capital, these are closely related to the Early Christian art of Alexandria and possibly to that of the Jewish-Christian community there. The decoration of the first chapel follows the normal iconographical cycle of the paintings in the catacombs. Thus we find the Exodus, Daniel in the lions' den, the three Hebrew children in the fiery furnace, the martyrdom of Isaiah, Jonah, the sacrifice of Abraham, Noah's ark, and other themes from the Old Testament; no New Testament miracles are represented. The scenes with the legend of Adam and the martyrdom of Thecla prove that apocryphal sources were used. Still more closely bound to the Hellenistic tradition are the frescoes of a large chapel which has a cupola decorated with concentric bands around a central disk: in the widest bands are depicted Jacob's prayer, Euche as orant, Daniel, Irene, the sacrifice of Abraham, Adam and Eve, Thecla, Noah's ark, etc. The presence of very interesting personifications of Peace, Prayer, and Justice and the allusion to the acceptance of prayers also relate this cycle to the Early Christian art of Alexandria.

A stylistic departure is apparent in the paintings of a later period, such as those of Deir Abu Hennis, in which historical subjects prevail. In these may already be seen a deliberate resistance to Byzantium, and a reflection of the rising nationalism, fostered by the Patriarchate of Alexandria beginning in the 5th century, in connection with the trend toward Monophysitism. Evident also is the influence of Sassanian art introduced from Persia with the spread of Manichaeism.

*Architecture.* Tracing a pre-Coptic phase in architecture is far from easy, since the monuments that have survived are few and have not as yet been adequately studied. The pre-Constantinian churches, which must have been very small, were destroyed during the Diocletian persecution (303), and nothing remains of the great conventual church built by St. Pachomius (320). There were also in Alexandria larger cult buildings traditionally connected with St. Helena. In her time were erected, according to Butler (1884), the Church of the Muallaqa in Cairo and the chapel at El-Baqara. Following these were large churches such as that of St. Menas (Abu Mina) in the desert near Alexandria. The saint's tomb has been destroyed, but there are still traces of the original crypt and the church of the same period built over it. Arcadius (395–408) and Honorius (395–423) built a great transept basilica on this same site. The buildings at Abu Mina conform to the Roman tradition and have affinities with various other churches, such as the basilica of Parenzo (Poreč), in the Adriatic and the eastern Mediterranean. The type of cemetery basilica found at Abu Mina was to become very common in this region; in the Monastery of Jeremiah at Saqqara the plan was copied with the addition of an enclosed tripartite narthex.

*Minor arts.* Although a variety of objects found in excavations may be identified as pre-Coptic, it is not yet feasible in most cases to order them within this general pre-Coptic phase. At Alexandria and in its immediate vicinity late Hellenistic art persisted for a long time. Excavations at the St. Menas basilica have brought to light a number of clay statuettes, some of female figures with pronounced sexual attributes. These must have been votive offerings to invoke fertility and are related to the ancient statuettes of Aphrodite (Astarte). Even the animal figures found here might be connected with this cult. Among finds from the 4th century are many clay lamps of a type widely diffused in North Africa and in Sicily, with an extremely shallow central well decorated with reliefs, and a long spout. Of the period immediately following are the very different ovoid Coptic lamps, often shaped like a frog, commonly found in Upper Egypt.

Among the bronze utensils, especially among those found in excavations in Alexandria and in the Delta region, were many late Hellenistic types; examples are to be seen in the museums of Alexandria, Cairo, Paris, and Berlin. Goblets, coffers with

figures in the classical style, bowls, censers, basins, and lamps were found in great quantity in most sites.

It is particularly difficult to date the glass objects. Many of these, especially painted ones such as the chalice in Berlin (Staat. Mus.) depicting grape gathering, and the Louvre goblet with animals, show the persistence of the antique tradition.

No less puzzling is the problem of establishing a reliable method for dating the pre-Coptic textiles that have survived. No stuffs from Alexandria or Abu Mina are extant; those found at Arsinoë (Crocodilopolis), now in Berlin (Staat. Mus.), are of a later, pure Coptic style. However, we have the pieces of woven material with late Hellenistic decoration discovered at Antinoë. Among these are large linen cloths printed in blue with mythological figures, of which there are fine examples at the Louvre and in Berlin. There is also some embroidery on wool with fishes (Lyons, Mus. Historique des Tissus; Louvre), which is purely Hellenistic. The hypothesis of Falke (1913) and some other authorities that an Alexandrian origin should be ascribed to a large group of heavy colored silks, including the famous Samson panel (the most important fragment of which is in the Dumbarton Oaks Collection, Washington) and some silks with figures of horsemen and the Annunciation from the Sancta Sanctorum in Rome (now Vatican Mus.), is not supported by the discoveries made in Alexandria. These silks are probably of Syrian origin and relatively late, in all likelihood from the 7th and 8th centuries. However, such textile fragments as the Maenad cloth in Sens Cathedral and the Nereid textile in Sion might be assigned to a late Hellenistic date on the basis of analogies with works in other media, for example, bone carvings. The earliest nub-woven cloths are still Hellenistic in style; those showing Coptic characteristics are later in date. This is true as well of the cloths woven with multicolored threads in the manner of a tapestry, showing related figural and geometric designs, such as the fragments with the large dancing women formerly in Berlin. The pictorial Hellenistic motifs are carried over into later, Coptic periods. The embroideries may be compared with the purple embroideries of Palmyra and therefore may be ascribed to the 3d century. Except in occasional early examples in which the colors are varied, the pattern is in dark colors on a light background. The subjects are for the most part putti with flowers and animals. In the 4th century a certain stylization is apparent, but with no relinquishment of the traditional motifs. Important silks of Sassanian origin are known from the earliest periods, especially from the cemeteries of Antinoë (now in Lyons, Paris, and Berlin), and these probably were the source of plant and animal motifs copied later in Egypt. Some woolen embroideries, such as the two fragments from Antinoë with a hunting scene showing the enthroned Sassanid king (in Lyons and Paris), are likewise derived from this source. The magnificently colored cloth panel in the Dumbarton Oaks Collection representing the enthroned "Hestia Polyolbos," personification of the hearth, may on the other hand reflect a late Hellenistic, or possibly Byzantine, model (PL. 446).

DEVELOPMENT OF COPTIC ART. *Architecture.* The monastic centers, which are particularly numerous in Upper and Middle Egypt, afford clear evidence of the break with the Hellenistic style of the metropolis that occurred in the 5th century. The monasteries near Sohag — especially the White Monastery (Deir el-Abiad; PL. 447), founded by Abbot Shenute about 440, according to Monneret de Villard — deliberately returned to the indigenous artistic tradition of ancient Egypt. The Abbot's intention to imitate Eastern prototypes rather than Hellenistic models is indicated by his declaration that his monastery was to "represent Jerusalem." In the White Monastery the triconch system on a cloverleaf, or trefoil, plan is used for the presbytery, which is isolated from its nave and surrounded by a number of chambers; the narthex is preceded by stairs leading to the galleries suggesting the pylons of early Egyptian temples, a resemblance enhanced by the massive surrounding walls.

The triconch plan of the presbytery is characteristic for the group of churches near Sohag. It is seen in the basilica of Naqada, which is closely related to the Church of St. John

the Baptist in Jerusalem. The Red Monastery (Deir el-Ahmar; FIG. 803), dedicated to St. Nisko, dates from the same period; the church had a three-aisled nave with galleries, and unusual freestanding columns framing hollowed-out niches in the semicircular apse. The façade has elements found in earlier Egyptian temples. Similar to these monasteries is the basilica at Dendera, provisionally assigned by Grabar (1943–46) to the end of the 4th century (most other scholars place it at the end of the 5th), which has a nave and two aisles and is preceded by a western narthex with lateral apses.

These immense buildings in the vicinity of Sohag exerted a widespread influence. At times the triconch plan of the presbytery was replaced by a cruciform transept, as in the Monastery of Jeremiah at Saqqara in Upper Egypt. At this

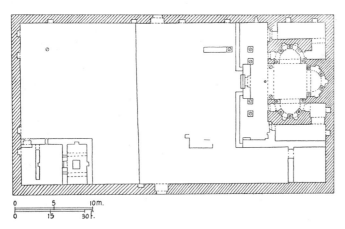

Deir el-Ahmar (Red Monastery), near Sohag, ground plan (*after Monneret de Villard, 1925*).

site four churches were built, of which two, the mortuary chapel and the principal basilica, date from about 470. The principal basilica, which has elements resembling both St. Menas (Abu Mina) and the Sohag group, has a nave terminated by a semicircular apse, and two side aisles. It is richly adorned with sculptural decoration showing fully developed Coptic traits. In Middle Egypt the major early Coptic and monastic buildings were the Church of Deir Abu Hennis, founded in the 5th century, and the important buildings of Bawit with their outstanding frescoes and sculptures; considerable excavation remains to be done. Representations of the same holy monks are found here as at Saqqara and Asyut, among them Apollo, Anoup, Phip, Jeremiah, and Onuphrius. Other monastic centers such as those in the desert of Nitria, those dependent on the White Monastery, and those situated near the Red Sea, developed an iconography and style of their own. In Upper Egypt the most important example is the Monastery of St. Simeon (Deir Amba Sama‘an), near Aswan, investigated by Monneret de Villard. The triconch presbytery persists here, and, as in most Coptic churches, there are side entrances, in this case permitting a closed western end with counterchoir.

Most of the churches that have survived, however, belong to a more recent period, dating from the 6th century or later. The *haikal*, a rectangular presbytery with three altars and a transept, is typical for these churches, as is the introduction of domes and vaulting in a basilican plan. Important later churches, sometimes incorporating earlier structures, are to be seen in Cairo, where, as a result of the transference of the Patriarchate from Alexandria, there was an important artistic flowering. Among the earliest buildings are the crypt of Abu Serga, in which it was believed the Holy Family had rested during their flight into Egypt, and the small church of Mar Mina with a nave and two aisles, restored in 793–94. The best example of a late Coptic church is the Muallaqa in Cairo, which has parts dating from the 6th century; the arches and vaults of the central nave were reconstructed in the 8th and 9th centuries. The churches of the Coptic monasteries of the desert of Nitria must have been built during the Islamic period,

for they show the strong influence of the new Islamic style, despite the persistence of the main elements of the older art.

*Sculpture.* A progressive transition to an ever more rigid Oriental stylization and an ever stronger resistance to Hellenism is also apparent in Coptic sculpture. The evolution of the Coptic sculptural style cannot be characterized, however, as a continuous one, because of the interruption of *retardataire* elements that appeared intermittently until the Islamic period, when Coptic sculpture became more consonant with contemporary styles elsewhere. Unfortunately, the monuments of the various regions have not yet been sufficiently studied to make possible the differentiation of the various regional schools. Generally speaking, the artistic centers, such as Oxyrhynchus, Ahnas, and Saqqara, which were dependent upon the old political centers remained more closely and for a longer period under the influence of late Alexandrian Hellenism than did such interior centers as Bawit, Dashlug, near Bawit, and Sohag. This fact and the multiplicity and strength of foreign influences make it difficult to establish an exact chronology. Nevertheless, just as in architecture, a national style asserted itself early.

The limestone head from Qena (PL. 448) shows in its rigid stylization the influence of Egyptian sculpture, and the sculptures of Ahnas near Heracleopolis, which Monneret de Villard assigns to the second half of the 4th century, clearly show a revival of traditional local motifs. In these and works such as the fragmentary sculptures of Oxyrhynchus preserved in the Municipal Museum in Alexandria are apparent as well the complex interrelations with the art of the Eastern provinces: with Baalbek, Palmyra, and even Transjordania (e.g., the sculptures of Khirbet el-Tannur). The Byzantine influence is clear in a comparison of, for example, the capitals of Ahnas with their acanthus foliage and those of the Golden Gate of Constantinople (425–30). It is very evident in a series of Early Christian reliefs, among them the *Virgin Enthroned* from Thebes (PL. 452), and in various decorative architectural elements, especially the basket-capitals at El-Ashmunein and Bawit, which imitated forms from Ravenna, Parenzo, or Salonika. Similar 5th-century examples, all in the Byzantine style, were found in Alexandria. Between these late Hellenistic sculptures and the first examples from Oxyrhynchus and Ahnas may be placed the sculptured decorations of the White Monastery, founded, as we have seen, about 440. Late Coptic works, especially the interesting wood carvings of the churches of Cairo and the stucco reliefs of the Monastery of Deir el-Suryani, may be dated on the basis of their similarity to contemporaneous Islamic work. Indeed, these works show a tendency away from the Coptic style, a tendency apparent for the first time in a series of Islamic-influenced Coptic wood reliefs very similar to those of the Mosque of Ibn Tulun in Cairo, of about 870.

The stylistic development of Coptic sculpture was accompanied by changes in technique. The softer style of such works as the early sculptures of Ahnas (PL. 452) was replaced by a sharper, harder working of the stone, a style particularly suitable for working in sandstone (this and wood were the preferred media). The soft sandstone permitted a deep cutting and was particularly adaptable to architectural ornamentation, as in the sculptured friezes of the White and Red monasteries (PL. 453). Characteristic of this style are the large, deeply hollowed eyes, with strongly stylized features. Deep undercutting is already found at Ahnas and more clearly in contemporaneous wood engravings, such as that of the Daniel from Bawit now in Berlin (Staat. Mus.). The tendency toward schematization and ornamentation is first seen in numerous grave steles: with representations of the dead or of orants, typical for Fayum (PL. 452); of the cross, typical for the Thebaid area; of the Key of the Nile, as in the stele from Erment (Armant) (Cairo, Coptic Mus.); of the cross encircled by a wreath (often accompanied by an eagle). These motifs were developed out of the indigenous Coptic tradition and do not appear to have any relation to similar motifs found in contemporaneous Syrian and Palestinian reliefs. At the end of the 8th century, however, this development was cut short by a return to a strict two-dimensional, planar style.

Of special interest in Coptic sculpture is its iconography. In the earlier period, in addition to the numerous steles with Christian subjects, there are, as is particularly evident in the sculptures at Ahnas, works with subjects from classical mythology. It is the prevailing popularity of mythology, and not the sensual predilections of the sculptors, as Strzygowski maintained (1904), that accounts for the repetition of the theme of Leda and the swan. The significance attached to this theme in Christian symbolism is as yet uncertain, but the image doubtless also recalled ancient local prototypes such as the union of the god Amon, in the guise of a gander, with the queen. Also of pagan origin are the lion, the frog (symbol of immortality), the ankh cross (symbol of life), the peacock, the eagle, and the dove. Classical models are closely followed in the representations of the sea goddesses and of Pan, Orpheus, Venus Anadyomene, and Dionysius, alone or seated in a chariot drawn by two oxen, as in the relief in the Dumbarton Oaks Collection in Washington, probably of the 5th century. Among the exclusively Christian figures, the soldier saints predominate. The finest example of this type is the tympanum with St. Apollo between angels, perhaps based on an antique representation of an emperor, at Dashlug. The warrior saint on foot, as in a wood relief in Berlin (Staat. Mus.), is also probably derived from a classical prototype. In this category belong the images of St. Menas, generally flanked by two camels, which appear upon innumerable earthenware pilgrim ampullas (PL. 139). These are possibly inspired by a large marble relief formerly adorning the basilica of the saint, of which a late ivory now in Milan (Castello Sforzesco) may be a version. The representations of Daniel in the lions' den are also related. The scenes of Christ are much more primitive; a typical representation of the Entry into Jerusalem is on a relief from Deir el-Abiad (PL. 452), near Sohag, now in Berlin, in which the Christ, mounted upon an ass, is reminiscent of the mounted Christ from Antinoë and the Coptic soldier saints.

Architectural decoration, although more closely dependent on Syrian and Byzantine models than the reliefs, still presents indigenous characteristics. The acanthus has given place to a typical form of flowering sprays, often enriched with animal figures. Rinceaux are also common. Nevertheless it is difficult to trace a clear stylistic development by studying these examples. So far as possible, Monneret de Villard, Duthuit, and Kitzinger have followed the general development from the 4th to the 8th century. They have demonstrated how rapidly the ornament was transformed in the course of the 6th century to an abstract, stylized form. This becomes clear in comparing the ornament of Bawit and Saqqara with the still naturalistic work of the 4th and 5th centuries from Oxyrhynchus and Ahnas.

It is now agreed that the development of Coptic sculpture was primarily a provincial phenomenon and that the influence it exerted in the Near East was much more limited than had at first been supposed. The influence of Coptic art in the West, too, has been overstated. Certainly the Coptic monuments were known through pilgrimages, but there is slight justification for attributing to these monuments any direct influence in the West — on such works as the Merovingian tomb slabs of the Rhineland, the sarcophagus of St. Adalbert in the church at Jouarre (Seine-et-Marne), and the Anglo-Saxon crosses of the 7th century.

Late medieval Coptic sculpture was decidedly ornamental in character. There are important examples in the British Museum, among them the small 8th-century reliefs with scenes from the New Testament, from the Muallaqa in Cairo, and similar reliefs from Abu Serga in Cairo, in which through Islamic influence the stylization is more pronounced. Other works, such as the wooden doors of certain monasteries in the desert of Nitria, differ from Islamic sculpture almost solely in their inclusion of Christian symbols. The most ancient of these doors are those of the monastery of Deir el-Suryani, the same period as the apse of the church (ca. 907–44).

*Painting.* The paucity of examples that have survived the destruction of churches during the Islamic era makes it difficult to trace the development of Coptic painting. As in

sculpture, we discern, rather than a uniform evolution, the rise of individual schools whose nearness to true Coptic art was in direct proportion to their geographic distance from the traditional centers of culture. The formation of a real national style began in the 5th century and reached full expression in the 6th and 7th centuries.

Some of the paintings that have come down to us are in a poor state of preservation; this group includes the paintings of the ruined monastery of Deir Abu Hennis near Antinoë, those of 'Abd el-Qadir, of Bawit, of Saqqara, of the medieval Abu Girga near Alexandria, of St. Simeon near Aswan, of the White and Red monasteries, of Esna, and of Deir el-Suryani. A few frescoes, among them those of Saqqara, have been saved by their transfer to the Coptic Museum of Cairo. In a better state of preservation are some icons, such as that from Bawit representing Bishop Abraham, now in Berlin (Staat. Mus.), which shows similarities to the frescoes of the same monastery, and to other icons in the Louvre and the Bibliothèque Nationale in Paris.

The decoration of Monophysite churches shows a certain uniformity, owing to the repetition of favored themes. The theophany, or appearance of the Godhead, constantly recurs, especially in apses; on the other hand, the scenes of the Ascension follow Syrian models. In the Biblical scenes, such as the Massacre of the Innocents, there are numerous iconographical references to the apocryphal Gospels. A favorite figure is St. John the Baptist; even more commonly represented is Zacharias, who appears in various scenes inspired by Coptic apocryphal writings. Among the stories from the Old Testament special prominence is given to those about David, drawn as well from apocryphal sources. There are also scenes from the childhood of Christ and the lives of a number of saints, hermits, and monks, such as St. Anthony, St. Macarius, and St. Pachomius, often depicted wrestling with the demons that assailed them. Very characteristic of Coptic piety is the figure of St. Sisinnius, in the act of transfixing with his lance a woman called Alabasdria, or fighting against the Manichaeans.

Among the earliest examples are the frescoes of Deir Abu Hennis, which reveal in their stylization and typical simplification of color harmonies a purely Coptic character. The fresco cycles of the great monastery of Bawit were, because of its nearness to Antinoë, particularly influenced by Byzantium (PL. 454), and in the scenes with secular subjects, such as the hunting of hippopotamuses and gazelles, we find a last echo of Hellenistic art. Most of the other frescoes, however, show an already advanced degree of rigid geometrization, as is very clearly seen in the representations of Christ triumphant and of the Virgin enthroned, surrounded by apostles and saints. They are depicted frontally and in the traditional manner, and the clear pure colors are strongly outlined. These characteristics undoubtedly indicate a 6th-century date.

In comparison with the Bawit frescoes the paintings of Saqqara, which are stylistically related to its sculptures, seem even more rigid and static. The images of Christ enthroned and of the Virgin lactant (PL. 457) are definitely two-dimensional and linear. These figures cover the entire area of the niche in typical Coptic manner.

A different style appears in the frescoes of the little church of 'Abd el-Qadir in the Nubian desert. The frescoes date from the 6th century but are closely related to Alexandrian paintings such as the frescoes of Abu Girga with the Annunciation and the legend of St. Menas. The frescoes of Athribis, which are of the 7th and 8th centuries, and those of the church of Esna (ca. 786), are characterized by a certain decadence.

The Islamic invasion did not interrupt the activity of the Coptic painters: indeed the iconography became more complicated and the composition freer. Relations with the nearest lands to the east, especially Syria, became much closer, and contacts were made with Armenia and Cappadocia. The paintings of Deir el-Suryani, with the Annunciation, the Birth, Dormition, and Assumption of the Virgin, show some Syrian influence. The decoration of the apse of the White Monastery near Sohag was begun about 1076 by an Armenian, Theodore, and finished in 1124 by another Theodore, a Copt. The paintings

of the Red Monastery were executed later, about 1301, perhaps by a master named Mercurius, and are stylistically akin to the Pantocrator of Esna. The frescoes at Abu Maqar in the desert of Nitria are of the 14th century. The panel paintings of the same monastery are closely related to Fatimid art; they reveal a progressive decline in quality. Much later, and of little artistic significance, are the frescoes in the dome of the monastery church of St. Paul (Deir Mar Bulus) with soldier saints (1713) and the similar decorations of the monastery church of St. Anthony (Deir Mar Antonius), both on the Red Sea.

*Manuscript illumination.* Most of the numerous miniatures that have survived are simple pen drawings of a style common to various regions of the Christian East, such as Armenia. The bulk of these miniatures come from the monasteries of Fayum and the desert of Nitria. Important examples are to be found in the Pierpont Morgan Library in New York, the Vatican Library (PLS. 455, 456), the Bibliothèque Nationale in Paris, and the British Museum. The influence of Early Christian art may be clearly seen in a number of these, as in the saints on a book cover in the Freer Gallery in Washington and in the Vatican Pentateuch (9th or 10th cent.).

*Minor arts.* Innumerable objects of applied art have been preserved in monasteries, churches, and burial grounds. Few civilizations have left behind a comparable wealth of utilitarian objects. Chiefly of clay, glass, or cloth, these clearly show the characteristics of the Coptic style.

Among the bronzes we find coffers, vases, bowls, censers, candelabra, and lamps; the earliest examples still show late Hellenistic forms, while later examples show more indigenous characteristics. The same may be said of the pottery, which tended toward ever more rigid and heavy forms, especially in the frog-shaped lamps found widely in Upper Egypt. Contemporary with this type is the lamp in the form of a shoe found also in Asia Minor. Lamps gradually developed from an ovoid to a pointed oval shape, and in the 8th century they assumed the Islamic form. Similar in workmanship to the North African lamps, and probably related to them, is a group of bowls and plates having, in imitation of earthenware vessels, a plastic decoration, relief-like and stylized, of Christian subject matter, generally consisting of small stamped ornaments and individual figures. Besides the relief-ornamented ware, there appears in the 5th century a simple type of painted ware in which ornament and single figures are drawn in outline; this type of painted ceramic persists into the Islamic period. Characteristic of Coptic art are large clay stands for clay pitchers, which served also to catch the water that seeped through the earthenware; these are decorated, but in an unarticulated manner.

One of the finest products of Coptic art is the textiles. Countless examples of cloth woven in various ways and for various purposes have been dug up from the hot sands that have preserved them. They have been found almost everywhere, notably at Antinoë, Saqqara, Fayum, Akhmim (anc. Panopolis), Arsinoë, and Qarara. Excellent collections are to be seen in the great museums in Cairo, Florence, Turin, Leningrad, Vienna, Lyons, Brussels, Krefeld-Verdingen am Rhein, Berlin, London, New York, Baltimore, Detroit, Washington, D.C., Cleveland, etc. (PLS. 450, 458).

The problem of the dating of Coptic textiles is of course intensified by their portability. As we have seen, the transition from purely Hellenistic to typical Coptic art occurred earliest in the provincial centers farthest removed from the cosmopolitan cities such as Alexandria and even from the smaller centers of the interior such as Antinoë. Since, as a result of the plundering of tombs, the provenance of many textiles is unknown, it is very difficult to assign dates. Moreover even the most important burial grounds, such as that of Antinoë, have not yet been scientifically studied. It seems clear, however, that in spite of the Arab conquest the designs of woollen stuffs continued in the old tradition and that the Coptic style prevailed long after the 8th century and even into the 12th.

For the most part, the stuffs came from tombs, where they had been used as burial furnishings; such furnishings

included even cushions and blankets. Surprisingly, in view of the frequent references in the *Liber pontificalis*, or "Book of the Popes," to the *vela Alexandrina* used for the decoration of churches, large pieces of stuff such as the church hanging in Berlin (Staat. Mus.) are rare. Most of the finds consist of whole or fragmentary tunics, usually with wide vertical bands and with circular or square woollen medallions inserted at the shoulders and knees. Contemporary paintings show how these were worn. They are made almost without exception of undyed linen, and the woollen pieces were usually inserted while the garment was being woven. In these Coptic stuffs the system of weaving, the manner in which the weft was passed alternately above and below the warp, is the same as that used during the ancient Egyptian and Hellenistic periods. In the so-called "purple" cloths, white threads were occasionally added with the shuttle during the weaving process. Embroidery, chiefly "flat stitching," appears in relatively late work. We have evidence also of ancient methods of weaving, with a small board, for example, used particularly for ornamental braids for clothing. Only in the cloths woven with more than one color is a real process of stylistic evolution apparent. With the spread of Coptic taste both the representation of figures and ornamental motifs underwent a change. In place of the Hellenistic ornament, Oriental motifs, possibly deriving from imported Persian and Spanish textiles, predominate. In the animals, arranged symmetrically, often flanking the tree of life, and in the figures within rinceaux, are suggestions of the contemporary sculptures of Bawit and Saqqara. The palmettes and the floral motifs are rigidly geometrical and the figures also are severely stylized. In later examples the motif of the Sassanian palmette is predominant. The cloths woven in Upper Egyptian workshops show affinities with the culture of Nubia and southern Arabia.

A similar development is seen in silks, of which we have a much more limited range of examples. Besides the pieces of genuine Sassanian origin found at Antinoë, there are many copies, especially of designs with figures of horsemen, and it is sometimes difficult to determine whether these are imported products or copies made at Antinoë. Of Sassanian origin, too, are the silks in two colors with images of horsemen, which sometimes bear the inscription "Zacharias" or "Joseph." These appear to be later in date than those of Antinoë and to have been produced in the Islamic period.

BIBLIOG. A. J. Butler, The Ancient Coptic Churches of Egypt, Oxford, 1884; H. Hyvernat, Album de paléographie copte, Paris, 1888; J. Strzygowski, Die Kalenderbilder des Chronographen vom Jahre 354, Berlin, 1888; A. Riegl, Die ägyptischen Textilfunde vom Kais.-König. Österr. Museum, Vienna, 1889; R. Forrer, Achmin-Panopolis, Strasbourg, 1891; A. Riegl, Koptische Kunst, Byzantinische Z., II, 1893, p. 112 ff.; J. Strzygowski, Die christlichen Denkmäler Ägyptens, Römische Quartalschrift, XII, 1898, p. 18 ff.; W. de Bock, Matériaux pour servir à l'archéologie de l'Egypte chrétienne, Leningrad, Leipzig, 1901; W. E. Crum, Coptic Monuments, Catalogue général des antiquités égyptiennes, Cairo, 1902; A. Gayet, L'art copte, Paris, 1902; J. Strzygowski, Seidenstoffe aus Ägypten im Kaiser Friedrich Museum, Jhb. der preussischen Kunstsamml., XXIV, 1903, p. 147 ff.; J. Strzygowski, Koptische Kunst, Catalogue général du Musée du Caire, Vienna, 1904; J. Clédat, Le monastère et la nécropole de Baouit, Cairo, 1904–06; A. Baumstark, Die Ausgrabungen am Menasheiligtum in der Mareotischen Wüste, Römische Quartalschrift, XXV, 1907, p. 7 ff.; T. Schreiber, Die Nekropole von Kôm-esch-Schugafa, Leipzig, 1908; J. E. Quibell, Excavations at Saqqara, 1906–07, Service des antiquités de l'Egypte, Cairo, 1908–10; O. Wulff, Altchristliche und mittelalterliche Bildwerke, I, Berlin, 1909; K. M. Kaufmann, Die Menasstadt, Leipzig, 1910; E. Chassinat, Fouilles à Bawit, Mémoires, Institut français d'archéologie orientale, XIII, 1911; O. M. Dalton, Byzantine Art and Archaeology, Oxford, 1911; S. Clarke, Christian Antiquities in the Nile Valley, Oxford, 1912; J. E. Quibell, The Monastery of St. Jeremias at Saqqara, Cairo, 1912; Johann Georg Herzog zu Sachsen, Streifzüge durch die Kirchen und Klöster Ägyptens, Leipzig, 1914; C. R. Morey, East Christian Paintings in the Freer Collection, University of Michigan Studies, Humanistic Series, XII, New York, 1914; O. Wulff, Altchristliche und byzantinische Kunst, Berlin, Neubabelsberg, 1914; W. Dennison, A Byzantine Treasure from Egypt, AJA, series II, XIV, 1916, p. 79 ff.; I. Errera, Collection d'anciennes étoffes égyptiennes, Brussels, 1916; S. Poglayen-Neuwall, Eine koptische Pyxis mit den Frauen am Grabe, Monatshefte für Kunstwissenschaft, XII, 1919, p. 81 ff.; A. F. Kendrick, Catalogue of Textiles from Burying Grounds, I, London, 1920; W. de Grüneisen, Les caractéristiques de l'art copte, Florence, 1922; G. Patricolo and U. Monneret de Villard, The Church of Sitt Burbâra in Old Cairo, Florence, 1922; U. Monneret de Villard, Saggio di una bibliografia dell'arte cristiana in Egitto, RIASA, I, 1922, p. 20 ff.; U. Monneret de Villard, La scultura ad Ahnâs, Milan, 1923; O. Wulff and W. F. Volbach, Die altchristlichen und mittelalterlichen Bildwerke, Ergänzungsband, Berlin, Leipzig, 1923; V. Berstl, Indocoptische Kunst, Jbh.

der asiatischen Kunst, 1924, p. 165 ff.; M. Dimand, Die Ornamentik der ägyptischen Wollwirkereien, Leipzig, 1924; O. M. Dalton, East Christian Art, Oxford, 1925; U. Monneret de Villard, Una pittura del Deir el-Abiad, Raccolta di scritti in onore di G. Lombroso, Milan, 1925; U. Monneret de Villard, Les couvents près de Sohâg, Milan, 1925; H. Ranke, Koptische Friedhöfe bei Karrara, Berlin, Leipzig, 1926; W. F. Volbach and E. Kühnel, Late Antique, Coptic and Islamic Textiles of Egypt, New York, 1926; H. Winlock, W. E. Crum, and H. G. Evelyn-White, The Monastery of Epiphanus at Thebes, New York, 1926; O. Wulff and W. F. Volbach, Spätantike und koptische Stoffe, Berlin, 1926; H. G. Evelyn-White and W. Hauser, The Monasteries of the Wadi'n Natrûn, 3 vols., New York, 1926–33; F. Morris, A Group of Early Silks, B. of the Metropolitan Museum of Art, 1927, p. 118; A. L. Schmitz, Das weisse und das rote Kloster, Die Antike, 1927, p. 326 ff.; U. Monneret de Villard, S. Simeone presso Aswan, Milan, 1927; R. Pfister, La décoration des étoffes d'Antinoë, Revue des Arts Asiatiques, V, 1928, p. 1 ff.; N. Toll, Tessuti copti, Prague, 1928; U. Monneret de Villard, Les églises du monastère des Syriens au Vadi-en-Natrûn, Milan, 1928; C. K. Wilkinson, Early Christian Paintings in the Oasis of Khargeh, B. of the Metropolitan Museum of Art, II, 1928, p. 29 ff.; C. Boreux, La salle de Baouit, B. des Musées de France, X, 1929, p. 240 ff.; A. Tulli, Le stele copte, Rivista di Archeologia Cristiana, 1929, p. 127 ff.; W. F. Volbach, Sculptures en bois coptes, CahArt, 1929, p. 193 ff.; W. F. Volbach, Neuerworbene koptische Holzschnitzereien, Mainzer Z., 1929, p. 41 ff.; M. S. Dimand, Coptic Tunics in the Metropolitan Museum of Art, Metropolitan Museum Studies, 1930, p. 239 ff.; R. Pfister, Gobelins sassanides du Musée de Lyon, Revue des Arts Asiatiques, 1930; E. M. Sawyer, The First Monasteries, Antiquity, IV, 1930, p. 316 ff.; W. F. Volbach, Spätantike und frühmittelalterliche Elfenbeinarbeiten aus dem Rheinland und ihre Beziehungen zu Ägypten, Festschrift Schumacher, Mainz, 1930; E. Weigand, Zur spätantiken Elfenbeinskulptur (R. Delbrueck, Die Consulardiptychen und verwandte Denkmäler), Kritische Berichte zur Kunstgeschichte und Literatur, III, IV, 1930–31, 1931–32; R. Delbrueck, Porphyr, Studien zur spätantiken Kunstgeschichte, VI, Berlin, 1931; G. Duthuit, La sculpture copte, Paris, 1931; W. F. Volbach, Arte copta, EI, s.v.; D. Zuntz, Koptische Grabstelen, Mitteilungen des deutschen Instituts für ägyptische Altertumskunde in Kairo, II, 1931, p. 22 ff.; A. Apostolaki, Coptic Textiles in the Museum for Decorative Arts in Athens (in Greek), Athens, 1932; E. Breccia, Le Musée greco-romain, 1925–31, Bergamo, 1932; E. Breccia, Le antichità cristiane del deserto maerotico, Actes du III$^{e}$ Congrès international d'études byzantines, Athens, 1932, p. 224 ff.; R. Pfister, Les débuts du vêtement copte, Etudes d'orientalisme publiées par le Musée Guimet, II, 1932, p. 433 ff.; R. Pfister, Les premières soies sassanides, Etudes d'orientalisme publiées par le Musée Guimet, 1932, p. 461 ff.; C. Schmidt, Das Kloster des Apa Menas, Ägyptische Z., 1932, p. 60 ff.; W. F. Volbach, Spätantike Stoffe, Katalog 10 des Römisch-Germanischen Zentralmuseums, Mainz, 1932; W. F. Volbach, Das christliche Kunstgewerbe der Spätantike und des frühen Mittelalters in H. T. Bossert, Geschichte des Kunstgewerbe, V, Berlin, 1932, p. 46 ff.; H. Peirce and R. Tyler, L'art byzantin, Paris, 1932–34; W. F. Volbach, G. Salles, and G. Duthuit, Art byzantin, Paris, 1933; L. M. Wilson, Ancient Textiles from Egypt in the University of Michigan, Ann Arbor, 1933; D. Zuntz, Koptische Malerei, Forschungen und Fortschritte, IX, 1933, p. 226 ff.; R. Pfister, Textiles de Palmyre, Paris, 1934; J. Sauer, Koptische Kunst, Lexicon für Theologie und Kirche, VI, Freiburg im Breisgau, 1934, p. 196 ff.; B. de la Société d'archéologie copte, 1935; C. Martin, Les monastères de Vadi'n Natrûn, Nouvelle Revue Théologique, XLVII, 1935, p. 113; A. M. Murray, Coptic Painted Pottery, Ancient Egypt, 1935, p. 1 ff.; J. Simon, Le monastère de Samuel de Kalamon, Orientalia Christiana Periodica I, 1935, p. 46 ff.; A. Westholm, Stylistic Features of Coptic Sculpture, ActaA, V, 1935, p. 215 ff.; D. Zuntz, The Two Styles of Coptic Painting, J. of Egyptian Archaeology, XXI, 1935, p. 63 ff.; C. Cecchelli, La Cattedra di Massimiano ed altri avori romano-orientali, 7 fasc., Rome, 1936 ff.; E. Drioton, L'art copte au Musée du Louvre, B. de l'Association des amis de l'art copte, II, 1936, p. 1 ff.; O. von Falke, Decorative Silks, 3d ed., London, 1936; R. Kautzsch, Kapitellstudien, Berlin, Leipzig, 1936; W. von Bissing, Die Kirche von Abd El Gadir bei Wadi Halfa und ihre Wandmalereien, Mitteilungen des deutschen Instituts für ägyptische Altertumskunde, 1937; E. Drioton, Art syrien et art copte, B. de l'Association des amis de l'art copte, III, 1937, p. 29 ff.; E. Kitzinger, Notes on Early Coptic Sculpture, Archaeologia, LXXXVII, 1937, p. 181 ff.; R. Pfister, Nouveaux textiles de Palmyre, Paris, 1937; Worcester Art Museum, The Dark Ages (cat.), Worcester, Mass., 1937; E. Breccia, Le prime ricerche italiane a Antinoe, Aegyptus, XVIII, 1938, p. 285 ff.; E. Kühnel, La tradition copte dans les tissus musulmans, B. de la Société d'archéologie copte, IV, 1938, p. 79 ff.; W. Holmqvist, Kunstprobleme der Merovingerzeit, Stockholm, 1939, p. 29 ff.; L. T. Lefort, Les premiers monastères pakhomiens, Muséon, LIII, 1939, p. 1 ff.; H. Schlunk, Kunst der Spätantike im Mittelmeerraum, Austellung, Berlin, 1939; U. Monneret de Villard, Per la storia del portale romanico, Medieval Studies in Memory of A. Kingsley Porter, I, 1939, p. 113 ff.; O. Wulff, Bibliographisch-kritischer Nachtrag zu Altchristliche und byzantinische Kunst, Potsdam, [1939]; R. Pfister, Textiles de Palmyre, III, Paris, 1940; S. Poglayen-Neuwall, Eine koptische Elfenbeinschnitzerei mit Anbetungsscene aus der Sammlung Trivulzio, Orientalia Christiana Periodica, VI, 1940, p. 523 ff.; U. Monneret de Villard, Le chiese della Mesopotamia, Rome, 1940; D. N. Willer, The Coptic Frescoes of Saint Menas and Medinet Habu, AB, XXII, 1940, p. 86; U. Monneret de Villard, Gli studi sull'archeologia cristiana d'Egitto, 1920–40, Orientalia Christiana Periodica, VII, 1941, p. 274 ff.; J. Drescher, St. Menas' Camels Once More, B. de la Société d'archéologie copte, VII, 1942, p. 19 ff.; E. Drioton, Un bas-relief copte des troix Hebreux dans la fournaise, B. de la Société d'art copte, VIII, 1942, p. 1 ff,; E. Drioton, Les sculptures coptes du nilomètre de Rodah, Cairo, 1942, p. 1 ff.; G. H. Myers, The Dating of Coptic Textiles in the Light of Excavations at Dura-Europos, Ars Islamica, IX, 1942, p. 156 ff.; G. H. Myers, Pagan and Christian Egypt: An Exhibition, Ars Islamica, IX, 1942, p. 150 ff.; W. F. Volbach, I tessuti, Catalogo del Museo sacro, III, 1, Vatican City, 1942, K. Weitzmann, An Early Copto-Arabic Miniature in Leningrad, Ars Islamica, X, 1943, p. 119; K. Wessel, Ägyptische Elfenbeinschnitzerschulen des 5. und 6. Jahrhunderts, Diss., Berlin, 1943; Late Egyptian and Coptic Art: An Introduction to the Collections in the Brooklyn Museum, New York, 1943; A. Grabar, Martyrium, 3 vols., Paris 1943–46; N. Åberg, The Occident and the Orient in the Art of the 7th Century, 3 vols., Kungliga Vitterhets Histoire och Antikvitets Akademiens Handlingar 56, Stockholm, 1943–47; Le Caire, Exposition d'art copte, Cairo, 1944; Coptic Egypt, Symposium held at the Brooklyn Museum, Brooklyn, 1944 (M. S. Dimand, Classification of Coptic Textiles in Coptic Egypt, p. 51 ff.; D. Dunham, Romano-Coptic Egypt and the Culture of Meroë in Coptic Egypt, p. 31 ff.; S. Der Nersessian, Some Aspects of Coptic Painting, p. 43 ff.); P. Friedländer, Documents of Dying Paganism, Berkeley, Los Angeles, 1945; U. Monneret de Villard, La basilica cristiana in Egitto, Atti del IV Congresso di archeologia cristiana, I, 1945, p. 291 ff.; E. Kitzinger, The Horse and Lion Tapestry, Dumbarton Oaks Papers, III, 1946, p. 1 ff.; F. Salvoni, Bollettino bibliografico copto, Aevum, XX, 1946, p. 131 ff.; A. Badawy, Les premières églises d'Egypte jusqu'au siècle de Saint Cyrille, Kyrilliana, 1947, p. 319 ff.; Baltimore, The Walters Art Gallery, Early Christian and Byzantine Art (exhibition cat.), Baltimore, 1947; A. Fakhry, The Monastery of Kalamoun, Annales du Service d'antiquité de l'Egypte, XLVI, 1947, p. 63 ff.; H. Zaloscer, Quelques considérations sur les rapports entre l'art copte et les Indes, Annales du Service d'antiquité de l'Egypte, sup. 6, 1947; Ghali Bey and Mirrit Boutros, Note sur la découverte du monastère de Phoebammon dans la montagne thébaine, Cairo, 1948; A. Badawy, L'art copte: Les influences égyptiennes, Cairo, 1949; J. Doresse, Monastères coptes aux environs d'Arment en Thébaïde, Mél. Peeters, I, Analecta Bollandiana, LXVII, 1949, p. 327 ff.; J. Simon, Bibliographie copte, Orientalia, XVIII, 1949, p. 227 ff.; E. Stein, Histoire du Bas-Empire, II, Paris, Brussels, 1949; J. B. Ward Perkins, The Shrine of St. Menas, Papers of the British School at Rome, XVII, 1949, p. 26; E. Drioton, De Philae à Baouit, Coptic Studies in Honor of W. E. Crum, Boston, 1950, p. 443 ff.; E. Riefstahl, A Coptic Roundel, Brooklyn Museum, Coptic Studies in Honor of W. E. Crum, Boston, 1950, p. 532 ff.; U. Monneret de Villard, Una chiesa di tipo georgiano nella necropoli tebana, Coptic Studies in Honor of W. E. Crum, Boston, 1950, p. 495 ff.; T. Whittemore, An Epiphaneia of Dionysos, Coptic Studies in Honor of W. E. Crum, Boston, 1950, p. 541 ff.; C. Bachatly, A Coptic Monastery near Thebes, Archaeology, 1951; J. Doresse, Nouvelles études sur l'art copte: Les monastères de Saint-Antoine et de Saint-Paul, Comptes rendus de l'Académie des inscriptions et belles lettres, 1951, p. 268 ff.; A. Fakhry, The Necropolis of Bagaouat in Khârga Oasis, Cairo, 1951; P. Labib, Abu Mena, B. de l'Institut d'Egypte, 1951–52; J. Doresse, Deux monastères coptes oubliés, Saint-Antoine et Saint-Paul, RArts, II, 1952, p. 3 ff.; J. Doresse, Recherches d'archéologie copte: Les monastères de Moyenne-Egypte, Comptes rendus de l'Académie des inscriptions et belles lettres, 1952, p. 390 ff.; W. F. Volbach, Elfenbeinarbeiten der Spätantike und des frühen Mittelalters, Katalog 7. des Römisch-Germanischen Zentralmuseums, Mainz 1952; A. Badawy, Guide de l'Egypte chrétienne, Cairo, 1953; C. R. Morey, Early Christian Art, 2d ed., Princeton, 1953; E. Kitzinger, Early Medieval Art in the British Museum, London, 1955;Coptic Textiles from Burying Grounds in Egypt in the Collection of the Kanegafuchi Spinning Company, ed. K. Akashi, Kyoto, 1955; Handbook of the Dumbarton Oaks Collection, Harvard University, Washington, 1955; A. Apostolaki, Woollen Embroidery of the 4th–9th Centuries from the Egyptian Tombs (in Greek), Athens, 1956; P. Labib, The Coptic Museum at Old Cairo, Cairo, 1956; G. Millet, Doura et El-Bagawat, Cahiers d'Archéologie, VIII, 1956, p. 1 ff.; P. du Bourguet, Les découvertes d'ordre paléochrétien effectuées en Egypte, Acts du V$^{e}$ Congrès international d'archéologie chrétienne, Vatican City, Paris, 1957, p. 83 ff.; P. du Bourguet, Certains groupes de tissus... coptes et datés du VII$^{e}$ siècle, Actes du V$^{e}$ Congrès international d'archéologie chrétienne, Vatican City, Paris, 1957, p. 505 ff.; Cabrol-Leclercq, Antinoë, Bagaouat, Baouït, Chaqqara; A. Hermann, Der Nil und die Christen, Jhb. für Antike und Christentum, II, 1959, pp. 30-69.

W. Friedrich VOLBACH

Illustrations: PLS. 445–458; 3 figs. in text.

**COROT**, JEAN-BAPTISTE-CAMILLE. A major French landscape artist of the 19th century, Corot was born July 16, 1796, in Paris. His father was Louis-Jacques Corot, a cloth merchant; his mother, born Marie-Françoise Oberson, was a modiste. He attended school at Rouen from 1807 to 1812 and at Passy until 1814, with little distinction. To please his parents he worked from 1817 with dealers in textiles. His father ultimately gave him an annual stipend, and from 1822 on he was able to devote himself to the study of painting. He studied first with Achille Etna Michallon, until the latter's untimely death, and then with Jean-Victor Bertin, a painter in the classical landscape tradition derived from Poussin.

In the fall of 1825 Corot made his first trip to Italy, where he remained for three years, until the fall of 1828, visiting Rome, Naples, and Venice. In Rome he received encouragement from Caruelle d'Aligny, a painter of classical landscapes with romantic overtones; Corot always considered Aligny his real teacher. He exhibited at the Salon for the first time in 1827, presenting two paintings: a *Roman Campagna* (now

destroyed), and the *Bridge at Narni* (Ottawa, Nat. Gall. of Canada). In the 1833 Salon he won a medal (second class) with his *Ford in the Forest of Fontainebleau*.

Corot returned to Italy in the spring of 1834. Traveling with the painter Grandjean, he went via Lyons and Marseilles to Genoa. After almost three weeks there, he went on to Tuscany and to Venice and the nearby lakes. In 1835 he was at Fontainebleau almost continuously; in 1836 he was in Auvergne, where he met Auguste Ravier, and in the environs of Avignon, where he painted with Marilhat.

In 1840, during one of his customary stays at Rosny with Abel Osmond (in the collection of letters from Corot to this friend those from Italy are of especial interest), he painted a *Flight into Egypt* (Rosny, church), which was exhibited at the Salon together with a *Little Shepherd* (Metz, Mus. B.A.) and a *Monk Reading* (Louvre). The *Little Shepherd* was the first of his works to be purchased by the state; the second was the *Italian View* (Avignon, Mus. Calvet) exhibited at the Salon of 1842. In the same year he went to Switzerland, where he was to return frequently. At the home of M. Robert at Mantes he decorated a bathroom with six Italian views (Louvre). His *Destruction of Sodom*, refused by the jury of the 1843 Salon, was accepted the following year; it was retouched and presented again in 1857.

In May, 1843, Corot made his third trip to Italy, spending all his time in and around Rome. He was commissioned in 1845 to paint a baptism of Christ for the Church of Saint-Nicolas-du-Chardonnet in Paris. A regular exhibitor at the Salons, in 1845 he presented *Homer and the Shepherds* (Saint-Lô, Mus.). The Legion of Honor was conferred on him in 1846. In 1847 he met the painter and engraver Constant Dutilleux, who became one of his most devoted friends; it was in Dutilleux's studio, at Arras, that Corot tried his hand at engraving. Also during 1847, which was the year of his father's death, Corot worked on decorations in the family property at Ville d'Avray. On Mar. 14 of this year Eugène Delacroix records in his *Journal* a visit to Corot in his studio; he notes, in addition to his impressions, Corot's advice on his *Orpheus*.

In 1848 Corot was elected by the artists to the jury of admission of the Salon. However, he received fewer votes than the academicians, even though his reputation was beginning to be established and he already had many students and imitators. In 1849 he exhibited, among other works, a *View of the Colosseum* (Louvre), painted during his first trip to Italy, and *Christ in the Garden of Olives* (Langres, Mus.). In 1851, after his first trip to Arras, he painted an important series of landscapes at La Rochelle; among these was the *Port of La Rochelle* (New York, Stephen C. Clark Coll.), exhibited at the Salon the following year. While he was at Crémieu in the Dauphiné in 1852, he met Daubigny, who became a very close friend. In 1854 he made a brief trip to Holland with Dutilleux.

The Exposition Universelle of 1855, where he presented six canvases, was a triumph for Corot: he won a medal (first class), and Napoleon III bought his *La Charrette: Souvenir de Marcoussis* (Louvre). From this point on, there was an enormous demand for Corot's works. He painted for the church at Rosny, as a sign of his gratitude to Osmond, the *Fourteen Stations of the Cross*, inspired by a series of popular prints of this subject. In the little church at Ville d'Avray he painted, with the assistance of Jules Richomme, a series of religious murals in which landscape predominated. While at the Château de Gruyères in Switzerland, visiting Antoine Bovy and his brother Daniel, a painter and one of Corot's favorite pupils, Corot painted some decorative panels with landscapes, and a still life (glass of water and pipe). In Paris, pursuing his interest in music, he frequented concert halls and the Opéra, where he made notes and sketches for figure compositions, to which he was giving more and more attention. When, on Apr. 11, 1858, Corot allowed 38 of his works to be sold at auction, the profits were so much greater than he had anticipated that he actually suspected some trickery.

In 1860 Dutilleux left his studio in Arras and moved to Paris; the communication that the two friends had maintained thus came to an end. Corot continued his travels with various colleagues, especially with Daubigny. He frequently visited Ville d'Avray, where his sister, Mme Sennegon, took up residence after she became ill. Among the young people who followed him there were the Morisot sisters. In 1862 he spent a week in London, where he was well received; three studies were executed there. He met Courbet at the home of the art patron E. Baudry at Port-Berteau in Saintonge. Of the three paintings exibited at the Salon of 1863, two studies from nature, *Study of Méry* and *Study of Ville d'Avray*, had great critical success.

Corot was a member of the jury of admission of the 1864 Salon and showed, among other works, the famous *Souvenir de Mortefontaine* (Louvre). His *L'Etoile du Berger* was acquired by the Musée des Augustins in Toulouse; Henry Walters, the first American collector to show interest in Corot, had wanted to buy this painting. *La Solitude* (1866), which was acquired by Napoleon III for 18,000 francs, was painted after the death of Dutilleux. At the Exposition Universelle of 1867 Corot exhibited seven important canvases, but he received only one, and that a second-class, medal. In compensation, the Emperor bestowed on him the rank of officer of the Legion of Honor. During 1867 Corot's health kept him from traveling, but in 1868 he visited Daubigny in his house at Auvers, on one wall of which Daumier had frescoed a *Don Quixote*. Corot painted a counterpart to this and, with Daubigny's son Karl, decorated the whole house. In 1869, while visiting the Robert family at Mantes, he painted an important series of views.

During the reorganization of the Salon of 1870 Daubigny tried without marked success to involve Corot in the struggle in behalf of the younger painters. When the unexpected outbreak of the Franco-Prussian War drove almost everyone from Paris, Corot, leaving his house in Ville d'Avray, stayed in the capital, selling most of his paintings to raise money to help those in need. When the Commune was established, he went to Arras and then to Douai — where he painted his famous *Belfry of Douai* (Louvre) — with Alfred Robaut, who recorded Corot's activities day by day in these last years. By now the demand for his work by private collectors and dealers was unremitting. The most persistent were Brame, Tedesco, Beugniet, Breysse, Weyl, Audrey, and Durand-Ruel. In Durand-Ruel's catalogue of 300 pieces the largest group by one artist was 28 paintings by Corot.

Corot's generosity is well known; he helped Louis-Adolphe Hervier, Henri-Joseph Harpignies, and Eugène Lavieille, and he bought a house in Auvers for Daumier when he grew old and blind. He assisted Aligny's widow, and when he heard that Millet, for whom he had never had much liking, had died leaving his family indigent, he presented them with 10,000 francs. Out of kindheartedness he even signed, after retouching them, canvases by needy students or works acquired by imprudent buyers. Such deeds made him known as the "St. Vincent de Paul of painting," but the epithet cost him dear. In order to get away from his too numerous clients, he had a studio built at Coubron.

At the Salon of 1874 Corot again suffered the affront of losing the medal of honor, this time to Jean-Léon Gérome. A group of his friends got together, however, to present him with a medal. During the summer of 1874 he went to Sens, where he painted his last landscapes from nature and the *Interior of the Cathedral of Sens* (Louvre). Corot died on Feb. 22, 1875, in his studio on the Rue Paradis-Poissonnière in Paris.

Robaut was never able to finish the monumental book on Corot's life and works for which he had collected information so painstakingly. It was published by Etienne Moreau-Nélaton in 1905, on the thirtieth anniversary of the artist's death. It lists 2,460 paintings (almost all reproduced photographically after the paintings themselves or after sketches of them by Robaut), 100 prints, and 761 drawings. Robaut's unused material was deposited in the Bibliothèque Nationale; it has been studied by Germain Bazin and systematically reexamined by André Schoeller and Jean Diéterle.

Analysis of the studies from nature by neoclassic landscape painters, beginning with Valenciennes, makes possible a more accurate understanding of Corot's early work. In paintings

he did before the first trip to Italy (*Sennegon's Cottage at Bois-Guillaume*; *Entrance to the Park at Saint-Cloud*; *The Old Bridge of St. Michel*; *Interior of a Court*; *Forest of Fontainebleau*; *The Dock at Honfleur*) the thick impasto and dense, humid greens already indicate that Corot's feeling for nature was more intimate than that of his first neoclassic masters, Michallon and Bertin, even in their more informal sketches. Nevertheless, in choice of subject, precision of drawing, and accurate definition of local color he was influenced by their teachings. In his conversations with Robaut, Corot may have minimized their importance in the formation of his style in order to lay greater stress on the educational value of the direct study of nature. It is true that in his early years he did not disdain exercises in academic composition inspired by Poussin, such as the study *Dance of the Nymphs* (copy after a Michallon; now in the Louvre).

If Corot's attitude was always antirevolutionary, still his instinct led him to revive spontaneity in painting. Aligny was the first to recognize Corot's superiority to his colleagues Léopold Robert, Victor Schnetz, Louis-Auguste Lapito, and Léon Fleury, who also came to Rome to study landscape. The solemn harmony in the Roman Campagna between the heavy skies and the clear masses of the landscape impelled Corot to abandon the dry neoclassic technique for a far richer one. With dense, thick brush strokes he preserved an immediate record of the plastic values his eye perceived, translating them directly into harmonious tonal masses. In a letter of this period, Corot complains of the difficulty of rendering a landscape in which the air is too rarefied and the sun so bright that the shadows are sharp to excess. To obtain tonal harmony in works from nature he restricted his range of color; he would work out the exact "physiognomy" of his subject in quiet grays, pale greens, ochers, pinks, and the soft white of whitewashed walls touched by the sun. Thus in the early period Corot already used the technique referred to by Robaut, that of mixing white lead with other colors to create an impression of uniform density while avoiding the transparencies and chiaroscuro effects produced through glazing. By this method, he obtained a luminosity so brilliant that one senses the weight of the atmosphere pressing on the volumes and feels the tangibility of the vision created. Among the works of this happy creative phase are *The Colosseum* (formerly Paris, private coll.) and *The Aqueduct of Claudius in the Roman Campagna* (Zurich, private coll.), dated December, 1825, *The Tiber at the Acqua Acetosa*, also called *La Promenade du Poussin* (Louvre), *The Colosseum from the Arch of the Basilica* (Paris, Mus. des Arts Décoratifs), *The Island of S. Bartolomeo* (PL. 464), *The Town of Castel Sant'Elia* (Northampton, Mass., Smith College Mus.), *The Basilica of Constantine* and *The Aqueduct in the Roman Campagna* (London, Lord Berners Coll.), *Trinità dei Monti* (Geneva, Mus. d'Art et d'Histoire). These paintings are fundamental examples of Corot's ability to capture the emotional qualities of landscape through soft gradations of tone and an "affectionate adherence" (Venturi) to the subject without recourse to the literary allusions deemed essential by the neoclassicists. Working in the studio with sketches made from nature, he did, however, construct traditional ideal landscapes, literarily suggestive and Vergilian in mood. This method is abundantly documented by the paintings he prepared for the Salons. A comparison of the study for the *Bridge at Narni* (Louvre; PL. 459) with the completed work shown in the Salon of 1827, now in Ottawa (Nat. Gall. of Canada), is revealing. The natural effects of brilliant light on a dramatic ruin to be seen in the study are transformed in the painting into subtle transparencies and carefully composed passages that conjure up an unreal and idyllic world.

Some of the figure studies that Corot painted before he went to Italy for the first time, although they were carried out almost in secret and received little attention during his lifetime, are considered as interesting as his landscapes. The self-portrait (Louvre) given to his parents just before his departure already showed a capacity for very personal interpretations. The *Girl from Albano* (Baden, Sidney W. Brown Coll.), the *Seated Italian Girl* (Louvre), the *Italian Girl with a Jug* (Switzerland, private coll.), the *Melancholy Italian Girl* (Merion, Pa., Barnes Foundation), the *Italian Girl with a Mandolin* (Paris,

private coll.), prototype of *The Atelier* (PL. 461), so often repeated in the artist's later years, reveal, in the same way as the landscapes, his ability to translate pure contemplation into a poetic image without literal description or psychological devices. The precise relations between volumes and colors, the disdain for pictorial refinements, create the profound though detached vitality with which Corot's figures, particularly his portraits, are imbued. Among the portraits done shortly after he returned to France are Abel Osmond (New York, A. Lewisohn Coll.) and his nieces, daughters of Mme Sennegon (Louvre).

In 1830, during a trip to Chartres with the architect P. A. Poirot, Corot painted the famous *Chartres Cathedral* (PL. 460), retouched, after the artist's custom, in 1872. He also did two rather detailed studies of the portals. The same precision, animated by a more poetic feeling, is to be seen in the paintings done for M. Henry in 1833 in the environs of Soissons (Otterlo, Netherlands, Rijksmuseum Kröller-Müller, and private coll.).

When painting compositions for exhibition Corot assembled studies, previously made around Rome and in the forest of Fontainebleau, of rocks, trees, and roots. While in studies of this sort he equaled and sometimes surpassed the painters of the Barbizon school, he did not reach in the completed paintings that penetrating perception of the quality of material that Courbet achieved in the same years. Nevertheless, the *Ford in the Forest of Fontainebleau*, a painting worked up from such studies, was judged the most complete landscape in the Salon of 1833 by Charles Lenormant, the critic on *Le Temps*, and from this time on praise from the critics, who knew Corot only through his finished paintings, became frequent. In the *Ford* one finds a certain relation to the "picturesque" quality of Constable, whose treatment of a similar subject, exhibited in Paris nine years before, had greatly interested not only Delacroix but all those among the French landscapists who were trying to break away from the restrictions of neoclassicism. But the underlying drama of an esthetic like that of Constable was in fact ill-suited to the tonal equilibrium that Corot achieved instinctively in his studies and attempted to achieve in his studio paintings.

At the Salon of 1834 Corot presented the *Mercantile Piers at Rouen* (formerly Paris, private coll.), a simple reworking of the very beautiful studies made in Normandy the year before; the same silvery light and transparencies are found in the famous *View of Florence from the Boboli Gardens* (Louvre), a reworking of a study made during the second trip to Italy. However, the two views of Volterra (Louvre and private coll.) show his former solidity of form, and the studies of Venice, Como, and Riva del Garda are among the most perceptive interpretations of misty, silvery atmosphere that Corot ever did. A *View at Riva* (formerly Paris, private coll.) was presented at the Salon of 1835, together with the extremely Poussinesque *Hagar in the Wilderness* (New York, Met. Mus.), which was engraved by Célestin Nanteuil for *Charivari*. It was praised by Lenormant for its classical qualities, but in the years that followed E.-J. Delécluze did not hesitate to reproach Corot for having, in violation of his true temperament, adopted a tradition alien to his feelings. Gustave Planche very severely criticized the *St. Jerome* of 1837 (Ville d'Avray, church) and the *Silenus* of 1838 (St. Paul, Minn., Hill Coll.) for the lack of accord between the landscape studied from nature and the mannered figures. Planche was so severe precisely because by this time a more intensely personal expression was expected from Corot — the kind of work he had proved himself capable of in the *Fort of Avignon* (London, Tate Gall.), painted in 1836 during his trip with Marilhat. It is on the basis of this painting that Bazin accepts the similar *View of St. André, Villeneuve-lès-Avignon* (Reims, Mus. B.A.), although it is not cited by Robaut among the works of Corot.

One of the fantastic landscapes Corot was painting in increasing numbers, composed from sketches collected on his frequent peregrinations in Italy — sketches of trees, ponds, flashes of light — inspired Théophile Gautier's poem "Le Soir," which appeared in the Apr. 27, 1839, edition of *La Presse*. These works, though little varied, are often exquisitely harmonious. And in them appears, more clearly than in the neo-

classic exercises, Corot's ingenuous conception of a romantically melancholy, idyllic world: in them the desire for poetry creates a wistful sentimentality.

Corot's artistic ambivalence, which was accentuated by the formulation of the frank naturalism of the Barbizon painters, became a subject of discussion among critics. Planche and Delécluze praised the works that do not rely on the usual idyllic themes, such as the *Flight into Egypt* in the Rosny church. The handling there, although classical, even Carraccesque, is without doubt more authentic than the scenic presentation and Vergilian tone of the famous *Homer and the Shepherds* (Saint-Lô, Mus.) of 1845. L. Legrange was to return in 1861 to Corot's ingenuous "Vergilianism," as did later, and more acutely, Paul Valéry. But T. Thoré, the discoverer of Vermeer and future defender of the impressionists, realized that Corot's studies were far superior to his carefully finished paintings. Champfleury and Baudelaire (after 1845), perhaps because of their trained literary sensibilities, recognized that the distance between Corot and his imitators was due to the quality of his lyricism as well as to the high standard of his painting even when he repeated themes in an almost uniform manner.

During his third trip to Italy Corot went to the Sistine Chapel for the first time; it was, as he said, "a courtesy call." He depicted Tivoli, Genzano, and Nemi in the style of his *Souvenirs*, as if to test by reality his powers of evocation. In Rome, as a guest of his friend and follower Jean-Achille Benouville, he painted *Marietta, l'Odalisque romaine* (Paris, Mus. B.A. de la Ville). Though considered by some an exercise à la Ingres, it is more probably a study for his free adaptations of 16th-century compositions of figures in landscape; certainly it is not a study of plein-air effects such as those (of which the *Reclining Nymph* of about 1855 is an example) that Corot carried out in later years.

It is significant that Corot exhibited at the Salon of 1849 a *View of the Colosseum* (Louvre) painted in 1826 — the most scenic of the works done during his first trip to Italy. By this time he evidently regarded some of his studies from nature as finished works of art. During this period, and still more at the end of his life, it became natural for him, even when painting a scene directly, to compose the elements of reality in the manner of his ideal landscapes. Nevertheless, these were years in which his perception of the poetic quality of light and atmosphere at certain moments was extremely sensitive — sharpened perhaps by his working with Daubigny, as happened frequently from 1852 on.

Of the very beautiful series of landscapes painted in 1851 at La Rochelle, the *Port of La Rochelle* (New York, Stephen C. Clark Coll.) exhibited in the Salon of 1852 is considered the first study from nature sent to an official exhibition. The painting, unusually diaphanous in effect as compared with more straightforward versions (in the Louvre and other museums), presents a subtle play of volumes in pale blue light. Corot thought this work one of his most successful; he called it "cette jolie personne en bleu"; it was in fact one of the most complete realizations of his ideal of transparent atmosphere.

On the trip to Holland with Dutilleux in 1854, Corot expressed enthusiasm for Rembrandt but was somewhat disappointed by Paulus Potter and Van der Helst. As Fierens has shown, it does not seem possible that the two friends were able to see the work of Vermeer, in whom it is customary to find an ideal parallel to Corot. The hypothesis of an influence of Rembrandt on Corot's late figure compositions is tenable, but that of an affinity with Delacroix (maintained by Meier-Graefe) is more persuasive. Certainly Corot's style was as much indebted to the old masters — Rembrandt together with Leonardo, Raphael, and the Venetians — as it was profoundly new. *The Woman with a Pearl* (1868–70; Louvre) was inspired by the *Mona Lisa* of Leonardo, the two busts in the Metropolitan Museum (New York) by Raphael, the Venuses in landscapes and the theme of the toilette by the Venetians. *The Woman with the Rose, The Monk with a Cello* (Hamburg, Kunsthalle), and the many figures in Oriental costume could depend on recollections of Rembrandt, but they are more closely related, in the taste for sumptuous ornaments and rich color, to the works of Delacroix. Nevertheless, in the search for personal

compositions and carefully controlled color harmonies, Corot's efforts remain unique and are to be distinguished, moreover, from the new realistic movement. Oddly enough, Corot was able to derive some suggestions from Courbet's work; he was never actually in direct controversy with Courbet, but his protest against the entire order of values embodied in Courbet's painting is implicit both in his own work — especially after the meeting of the two artists at Saintes — and in his sometimes violent reaction against those among his own followers who showed interest in the new luminary. His complete opposition to Pissarro, when the latter pursued a new adherence to local color, was symptomatic.

At the very time when Corot was enjoying his greatest financial and critical success, his painting was attacked from two contradictory points of view. The critics of the early phases of impressionism (e.g., F. de Lasteyrie, *Review of the Salon*, 1864) saw in him the prototype of facile, cursory work that did not demand a knowledge of either drawing or painting. The impressionists found him lacking in that full participation in reality so essential to their artistic goals. Moreover, his apparent indifference to the new social interests in which some artists were passionately involved must have made him seem detached. Millet expressed his disapproval, in the form of a severe esthetic judgment, of Corot's seeming lack of concern for the condition of mankind. For his part, Corot responded halfheartedly when Daubigny asked him to help the younger painters in their quest for official recognition, every time the two artists succeeded in gaining control of the jury of admission to the Salon. The Salon was usually fiercely guarded by the academicians — always the most blind to Corot's merit even when his paintings began to be sought after by collectors throughout the world.

In 1863 the *Study of Méry* and the *Study of Ville d'Avray* were great successes, receiving unreserved praise from even the most severe of his critics, such as Thoré and J.-A. Castagnary. In the 1864 Salon Corot exhibited the *Gust of Wind*, frequently repeated (by forgers as well), and *Souvenir de Mortefontaine* (Louvre), the masterpiece of his studio paintings, recalling his studies of trees and water in a delicate equilibrium of luminous reflections. The expressive intensity that Corot achieved in his fantasy compositions (*Souvenir of Castelgandolfo, Souvenir of Mortefontaine, Souvenir of Capri*, at the Louvre; *The Lake* and *Ville d'Avray* in New York, Frick Coll., and in Reims, Mus. B.A.; *Capraio* and *Arleux-Palluel: The Bridge of Trysts* in Chicago, Art. Inst.; other works in Philadelphia, Boston, Geneva, Hamburg, etc.) make them almost equal in value to the studies he made directly from nature. He expressed the same elegiac harmony, in the late romantic sense, in such paintings done from nature as *The Tower of Montlhéry, The Church of Marissel, The Road at Sèvres* (Louvre); *M. Wallet's Park at Vosinlieu* (Switzerland, Werner Herold Coll.); *The Cathedral of Mantes* (Reims, Mus. B.A.); *The Boatman of Mortefontaine* (New York, Frick Coll.); *The Road at Sin-le-Noble* (Louvre); *The Street of the Station at Ville d'Avray* (Washington, Nat. Gall.); *The Windmill of St. Nicolas-lès-Arras* (Louvre). But Corot reached the peak of his ability to compose and to adjust color within a rigorously limited tonal range in the last years of his life. Parallel to figure compositions such as *The Woman in Blue* (Louvre; PL. 462) were landscapes such as *The Peasants' Courtyard, The Ramparts of Arras* (Louvre); *The Port of Dunkirk* (New York, Paul Rosenberg Coll.); *Etretat: The Beach*, (St. Louis, Mo., City Art Mus.); the very famous *Belfry of Douai* and the *Interior of the Cathedral of Sens* (Louvre). In these, as in much earlier pictures, solid volumes determine the density of the atmosphere instead of being absorbed into a uniform, flickering luminosity.

Although the construction of images through the relation of color values found in Corot was important for the formulation of impressionism, the difference between his and the later style cannot be mistaken. His desire to follow older traditions is indicated not by his adoption of a few classical motifs but by the composition of his paintings, as well as of the studies, in which the image is completed within the frame and thereby within an absolute limit of time and space. Between Corot's

almost religious contemplation of nature and the impressionists' active participation in reality, there is a break in the history of esthetic conceptions — a break, however, that does not imply a difference in artistic value.

The enormous quantities of forgeries found on the market (more than 2,000 in one collection alone) were not without importance in the shift of interest in Corot several decades after his death. Some of these forgeries, but very few, are the paintings of poor students which Corot agreed to sign so that they would bring better prices.

Corot's methods are well known. He advocated thorough study of the subject as a means of gaining complete control of all the forms to be represented. The forms themselves were to be built in terms of tonal harmonies, with the differentiation between hues subordinated to their tonal relations. At the end of his life, to prepare canvases for the studio he would indicate from nature the points of greatest depth and prominence, marking them with little squares and circles. From youth he took pleasure in repainting old canvases daubed with gaudy, discordant tints, bringing the colors into balance through tonal gradations. Between maximums of dark and light he showed how as many as twenty intermediate tones could be identified. Among his always beautiful drawings, certain ones sketched with extreme rapidity from memory demonstrate in the clarity of their atmospheric unity the perfect balance with which the vision was formulated in Corot's mind. Through them we glimpse the immediacy and intensity with which he was able to capture the forms that he wanted to portray, the forms that seemed to him to express his feeling for nature.

BIBLIOG. *Books*: T. Silvestre, Histoire des artistes français vivants et étrangers, 3d ed., Paris, 1855, pp. 85–104; P. Burty, Exposition de l'œuvre de Corot, Ecole des Beaux-Arts, Paris, 1875; H. Dumesnil, Corot: Souvenirs intimes, I, Paris, 1875; J. Claretie, Peintres et sculpteurs contemporains, I, Paris, 1882, pp. 97–120; J. Rousseau, Camille Corot, Paris, 1884; J. W. Mollet, The Painters of Barbizon, II, London, 1890, pp. 1–117; L. Roger-Miles, Corot, Paris, 1891; L. Roger-Miles, Album classique des chefs-d'œuvre de Corot, Paris, 1895; A. Robaut, Corot, 3d ed., Paris, 1899; T. Brice and I. Lanoë, Histoire de l'école française de paysage, 2 vols., Paris, 1901; M. Hamel, Corot et son œuvre, Paris, 1905; J. Meier-Graefe, Corot und Courbet, Leipzig, 1905; E. Michel, Corot, Paris, 1905; A. Robaut, L'œuvre de Corot: Catalogue raisonné et illustré, précédé de l'histoire de Corot et de son œuvre par E. Moreau-Nélaton, 4 vols., Paris, 1905; W. Gensel, Corot und Troyon, Bielefeld, 1906; E. Meynell, Corot and His Friends, London, 1908; L. Delteil, Le peintre graveur illustré, V, Paris, 1910; P. Cornu, Corot, Paris, 1911; E. Moreau-Nélaton, Corot, Paris, 1913; E. Moreau-Nélaton, Le roman de Corot, Paris, 1914; L. Rosenthal, Du romantisme au réalisme, Paris, 1914; J. E. Blanche, De David à Degas, Paris, 1919; A. Fontainas, Histoire de la peinture française au XIXᵉ et XXᵉ siècles, Paris, 1922; A. Lhote, Corot, Paris, 1923; D. Baud-Bovy, Les séjours de Corot en Suisse, Actes du Congrès d'Histoire de l'Art de 1921, Paris, III, 1923–24; Camille Corot: Briefe aus Italien, ed. H. Graber, Leipzig, 1924; G. Geffroy, Corot, Paris, 1924; E. Moreau-Nélaton, Corot raconté par lui-même, 2 vols., Paris, 1924; P. Dorbec, L'art du paysage en France, Paris, 1925; L. Hourticq, Etudes et catalogue (Le paysage français de Poussin à Corot, au Petit Palais), Paris, 1925; M. Lafargue, Corot, Paris, 1925 (Eng. trans. by L. Wellington); C.-E. Oppo, Corot, Rome, Paris, 1925; F. Focillon, La peinture au XIXᵉ siècle, I, Paris, 1927; E. Faure, Catalogue de l'exposition de la Galerie Rosenberg, Paris, 1928; J. Magnin, Le paysage français des enlumineurs à Corot, Paris, 1928; C. Corot: The Paintings and Drawings of J. B. C. Corot in the Artist's Own Collection, New York, 1929; G. Bernheim de Villers, Corot, peintre de figures, Paris, 1930; Corot and Daumier: Exhibition, Museum of Modern Art, New York, 1930; E. Faure, Corot, Paris, 1930; E. Faure, Catalogue de l'exposition de la Galerie Rosenberg, Paris, 1930; F. Fosca (G. Traz), Corot, Paris, 1930; C. Holme, Corot and Millet, New York, 1930; C. Mauclair, Corot, Paris, 1930; J. Meier-Graefe, Corot, Berlin, 1930; J. Cain, P.-A. Lemoisne, and J. Laran, Exposition des estampes et dessins de Corot, Bibliothèque Nationale, Paris, 1931; René-Jean, Corot, Paris, 1931; P. Valéry, Pièces sur l'art, Paris, 1931; W. Wartmann, Catalogue de l'exposition des œuvres de Corot, Kunsthaus, Zurich, 1934; M. Alpatov, Corot, Moscow, 1936; E. Faure, Corot, Paris, 1936; P. Jamot, Catalogue de l'exposition des oeuvres de Corot, Musée de l'Orangerie, Paris, 1936; P. Jamot, Corot, Paris, 1936; M. Serullaz, Corot: Quatorze dessins, Musée du Louvre, Paris, 1939; P. du Colombier, Corot, Paris, Geneva, 1940; L. Venturi, Peintres du XIXᵉ siècle, Paris, 1941; G. Bazin, Corot, Paris, 1942 (2d ed., 1951); J. Combe, Peintures de Corot, Paris, 1944; G. Nicodemi, Corot, Milan, 1944; A. M. Brizio, Ottocento e Novecento, Turin, 1945; H. Marceau and L. Venturi, Catalogue of Corot Exhibition, Philadelphia Museum of Art, 1946; G. Rosa, La foresta incantata, Milan, 1946; P. Cailler, Corot, raconté par lui-même et par ses amis, Geneva, 1946–47; F. Fosca (G. Traz), Corot, Milan, 1948; A. Schoeller and J. Diéterle, Corot: Premier supplément à "l'Oeuvre de Corot" par A. Robaut et E. Moreau-Nélaton, Paris, 1948; M. Raynal, History of Modern Painting, trans. S. Gilbert, Geneva, 1949; J. Maret, Corot: Catalogue de l'exposition de la Galerie Daber, Paris, 1951; M. Raynal, The 17th Century: New Sources of Emotion, from Goya to Gauguin, trans. J. Emmos, Geneva, 1951; M. Serullaz, Corot, Paris, 1951; J. Alazard, Corot,

Paris, 1952; V. Gilardoni, Corot, Milan, 1952; F. Fosca (G. Traz), La peinture française au XIXᵉ siècle, 1800–1870, Paris, 1956; D. Baud-Bovy, Corot, Geneva, 1957; A. Schoeller and J. Diéterle, Corot, Paris, 1958. *Periodicals*: H. Heilbuth, Figurenbilder von Corot, Kunst und Künstler, III, 1904–05, pp. 93–106· H. Franz, The Torny Thiery Collection of Paintings, The Studio, 1905, no, 149, p. 193, no. 151, p. 300 ff.; E. G. Halton, The Collection of Mr. A. Young, I, The Corots, The Studio, 1906, no. 163, pp. 3–20; P. Goujon, Corot, peintre de figures, GBA, LI, 1909, pp. 469–79; P. Korb, Corot, Delacroix und Courbet, Der Cicerone, III, 1911, pp. 161–69; C. Gebhardt, Die neue Erwerbungen französischer Malerei im Städelschen Kunstinstitut zu Frankfurt a. M., Der Cicerone, IV, 1912, pp. 761–69; G. Biermann, Die Kunst auf dem internationalen Markt, Der Cicerone, V, 1913, pp. 309–26, 359–74; A. Dubuisson, Some Personal Reminiscences of Corot, The Studio, V, 1913, pp. 209–14; A. Karr, Eine Corot-Anekdote, Kunst und Künstler, XI, 1913, pp. 625–27; V. Pica, Raccolte d'Arte, La Collezione Rouart, Emporium, 370, Jan., 1913, pp. 42–60; R. Fry, Recent Acquisitions for Public Collections, BM, XXXIV, 1919, pp. 15–23, 1920, pp. 152–61; R. Fry, Modern Paintings in a Collection of Ancient Art, BM, 1920, pp. 303–09; P. Jamot, La Cathédrale de Sens par Corot, Revue d'Art Ancien et Moderne, XXIV, 1, 1920, pp. 305–06; A. Fontainas, J. B. C. Corot, Amour de l'Art, 1922, pp. 122–28; P. Jamot, Ravier et Corot, Revue de l'Art Ancien et Moderne, XXVII, 2, 1923, pp. 321–22; T. Bodkin, Exhibition of French Landscapes in Paris, I, Poussin to Corot, BM, XLVII, 1925, pp. 3–9; P. Jamot, Corot. portraitiste au Musée du Louvre, Revue de l'Art Ancien et Moderne, XXX, 1, 1926, pp. 273–81; A. Lhote, Art Vivant, Paris, 1928, p. 551; H. G. Fells, Corot in America, The Connoisseur, II, 1934, pp. 283–88; R. Fry, A New Corot at the National Gallery, BM, XLV, 1934. p. 53; M. B. Wehle, Hagar in the Wilderness, Met. Mus. of Art B., XXXIII, 1938, pp. 246–49; M. R. Rogers, Girl with a Mandolin, St. Louis City Art Mus. B., XXIV, 1939, pp. 25–27; J. Rewald, Corot Sources: The Camera Tells; His Italian Landscapes Seen in Photographs of a Century Later, AN, XLI, Nov., 1942, pp. 11–13; J. S. Held, Corot in Castel Sant'Elia. GBA, LXXXV, 1943, pp. 183–86; B. Tarkington, Ville-d'Avray: Woodland Path Bordering the Pond, John Herron Art Inst. B., XXX, 1943, pp. 1–4; H. Marceau and F. C. Watkins, Beneath the Paint and Varnish, Mag. of Art, XXXVII, 1944, pp. 128–34; Two Paintings by Corot: "Thatched Village" and "Road at Ville-d'Avry," Baltimore Mus. News, XII, 1948, pp. 1–4; F. Arcangeli, Corot e Soutine a Venezia, Paragone, XXXIII, 1952, p. 58 ff.; P. Fierens, Le voyage de Corot en Belgique et aux Pays-Bas, GBA, XL, 1952, pp. 123–28; Sele-Arte, Antologia per Corot, 1952, pp. 32–37; N. Wallis, Diversity of Corot, The Connoisseur, CXXXII. 1953. p. 103; C. Doria, Corot et le Baptême du Christ, GBA, XLIII, 1954, pp. 317–44; G. Bazin, Le problème de l'authenticité dans l'œuvre de Corot, Revue des Arts, sup. 1, June, 1956, pp. 18–48; R. M. Coates, Loan Exhibition at the Rosenberg, New Yorker, XXXII, Nov. 17, 1956, p. 231; Special Vision of Corot, Loan Exhibition at the Paul Rosenberg Galleries, Arts, XXXI, 1956, pp. 28–29; Notable Works of Art Now on the Market, BM, XCIX (sup. 7), 1957; A. T. Schoener, Portrait of Captain Faulte du Puyparlier, Cincinnati Mus. B., V, 1957, pp. 6–7; R. S. Davis, Collections of James J. Hill, Minneapolis Inst. B., XLVII, 1958, pp. 15–27.

Renata CIPRIANI

Illustrations: PLS. 459–464.

**CORREGGIO.** Antonio Allegri, called "Correggio," the son of Pellegrino Alegris and Bernardina Ormani, was born (ca. 1489) in Correggio, where he died about Mar. 15, 1534. According to Vasari he was of modest origin; but local men of learning have maintained, although without verification, that the family was quite wealthy and even aristocratic. Indications in Vasari's text concerning the date of his birth have lately been under discussion. The statement that Correggio died at the age of forty would place his birth date in 1494. But A. Luzio (*La galleria dei Gongaza venduta all'Inghilterra nel 1627–28*, Milan, 1913) reached a different conclusion by examining the contract for the altarpiece of the *Madonna of St. Francis*, which was ordered in 1514. Luzio remarks that, merely because his father appears as an assistant, one cannot conclude that the artist was a minor when the contract was made, but only that he was still living with his family. Furthermore, according to the statutes of Correggio, one came of age not at twenty-one but at twenty-five. Finally, the absence of the judge required by the statutes to be present for contracts involving minors leads to the assumption that Correggio had already reached his twenty-fifth year when the contract was made. Luzio, therefore, fixed upon 1489 as the birth year. This hypothesis has been ably contested by L. Testi ("Quando nacque Correggio," *Archivio storico per le provincie parmensi*, 1922) among others, but was supported by A. Venturi (*Il Correggio*, Rome, 1926) and by C. Ricci ("La data di nascita del Correggio," *Aurea Parma*, XVI, 1932, pp. 83–85), and is now generally accepted, since it agrees with the development of the artist's style as it is now understood.

The most important documentary evidence concerning Correggio's activity is as follows: On Aug. 30, 1514, he made a contract with the Franciscans of the monastery in Correggio for the *Madonna of St. Francis* altarpiece (now in Dresden). The contract for the frame, which was to be gilded on the raised parts of the relief and painted blue on the background, was made on Oct. 4 of the same year. On Apr. 4, 1515, he received the payment agreed upon, 100 ducats. From the content of a letter of May 12, 1517, from the archpriest of Albinea to Alessandro Malaguzzi, it may be inferred that at that time Correggio was engaged on the altarpiece for the Church of S. Prospero in Albinea (Reggio Emilia): "prego . . . che scrivate una lettera a quello majstro de l'anchona che per più durezza sel po che la faza secondo me dicisseve . . . sel non èl tanto inanze che non la possa lassarla." ("I beg you to write a letter to that master of the altarpiece [saying] that for greater durability, if he can, he should make it as he told me he would, if it is not so far advanced that he cannot leave it"). The payments for the altarpiece, which represented the Madonna and Child between the Magdalen and St. Lucy, were completed on Oct. 14, 1519 (G. Saccani, *La storia di un capolavoro*, Reggio Emilia, 1915). It was removed from Albinea in 1647 by Francesco I of Modena and today is known only through copies, the best of which is preserved in Parma (Gall. Naz.). On July 14, 1517, Correggio, together with one Melchiorre Fassi, is recorded as witness to a deed of the notary Francesco Alfonso Bottoni. Fassi, in December of the same year, named the Church of S. Quirino in Correggio as heir of all his worldly goods, on condition that a chapel be built "cum una anchona cum quattuor sanctis, S. Leonardus, S. Marta, S. Petrus Apostolus, et S. Maria Magdalena." The chapel was not constructed, and in the end Fassi left his worldly goods to the Church of S. Maria della Misericordia in Correggio. But there is in existence an altarpiece, showing the four saints named, that came from that church and passed from the collection of Lord Ashburton in London into the Metropolitan Museum, New York. The style of the painting indicates this phase of Correggio's activity, and it is likely that it is, in fact, the one referred to in the earlier of Fassi's bequests. There follow, from July 6, 1520, to Jan. 23, 1524, the payments (published by Ricci and Venturi) for the decoration of the Church of S. Giovanni Evangelista in Parma. The dome came first, then the half dome of the apse. The latter was demolished in 1587 to enlarge the choir, and Correggio's fresco was copied in the new apse by Cesare Aretusi (d. 1612). Correggio then frescoed the underarches of the dome. Finally, he provided drawings for the nave frieze, subsequently used by Francesco Maria Rondani (1490–ca. 1548) and others, and evidently executed a small section of it himself (S. Zamboni, review of A. E. Popham, *Correggio's Drawings*, London, 1957, in *Arte antica e moderna*, I, 1958, p. 194).

Correggio's son, Pomponio Quirino, later a mediocre painter, was born Sept. 3, 1521. Correggio had married in 1519, if the dates given by L. Pungileoni are correct. His bride was the sixteen-year-old Girolama Merlini, daughter of the deceased armiger Bartolomeo. The dowry of 257 ducats was agreed upon July 26, 1521. Besides Pomponio, Correggio had two daughters: Francesca Letizia, born Dec. 6, 1524, and Anna Geria, born Oct. 3, 1527.

On Oct. 14, 1522, Correggio was employed with Alberto Pratoneri to execute a "Natività del Sire nostro" for the chapel of the nobility in S. Prospero in Reggio Emilia. For this he presented a sketch, which many be the one in sanguine, ink, sepia, and watercolor in the L. C. G. Clark Collection in Cambridge, England. The payment was to be "libre duecento otto di moneta vecchia reggiana," of which he received "libre quaranta di moneta vecchia" in advance. The contract, with the receipt signed by Correggio, was published by G. Campori ("Relazione di un autografo del Correggio rinvenuto nell'Archivio Palatino di Modena," *Atti e memorie della RR. deputazioni di storia patria per le provincie modenesi e parmensi*, Modena, 1863) and reproduced in facsimile by C. Pini and G. Milanesi (*La scrittura di artisti italiani secolo XIV–XVII riprodotta con la fotografia, e corredata di notizie*, Florence, 1876, pl. 115). The work in question is the famous "Notte"

(PL. 475). It was removed from the church in 1640 by Francesco I of Modena and entered the Gemäldegalerie, Dresden, in 1746 with the 100 masterpieces from the Este picture gallery that were sold by Duke Francesco III to the King of Poland, Augustus III. The work must have been finished in 1530, the year in which the chapel was dedicated, according to the inscription on the right pier. On Nov. 3, 1522, Correggio signed a contract for the decoration of the choir and dome of the Cathedral of Parma. From two payment receipts, dated respectively Sept. 29, 1526, and Nov. 17, 1530, we may conclude that the artist was occupied with the decoration of the dome (including the squinches and underarches) in the period indicated. The decoration of the apse was executed after Correggio's death, by Girolamo Mazzola Bedoli (ca. 1500–1569). In the spring of 1523, according to Pungileoni, Correggio moved with his family to Parma, where he took lodgings near S. Giovanni Evangelista (borgo Pescara). A record in the archives of the Monastery of St. Anthony in Parma, mentioned by G. Tiraboschi, states that in 1523 Donna Briseida Colla entrusted the artist with the execution of the panel representing the Madonna between St. Jerome and the Magdalen (the famous *Madonna of St. Jerome*, PL. 474; Parma, Gall. Naz.). The painting was placed in the Colla family chapel in the Church of S. Antonio in 1528 (Pungileoni, I, p. 185). In 1524 a certain Cristoforo Bandini bequeathed a sum for the altarpiece of the Church of the Sto Sepolcro in Parma. This was the "Madonna della Scodella" (PL. 468; Parma, Gall. Naz.), which, however, was executed later, for the date June 2, 1530, is legible on the frame (C. Ricci, "La Madonna della Scodella," *Per l'arte*, Parma, June, 1894).

On Feb. 15, 1525, Correggio witnessed a deed signed in the presence of Veronica Gambara and Manfredo, lord of Correggio. On Aug. 26, 1525, he was engaged, with 15 other artists, to study means to remedy the instability of the Church of the Steccata in Parma. The construction of this church had begun in 1521, on a plan by Giovanni Francesco Zaccagni (1491–1543), which had previously been approved by a commission of 11 artists. Correggio does not appear among these last, and four architectural drawings, identified by A. E. Popham (1957) on the reverses of preparatory studies for the frescoes in S. Giovanni Evangelista, indicate that the artist failed to participate because he was involved in the competition for the design of the building. That Correggio's range of interests included architectural problems is proved by the fact that in 1525, when it became apparent that the altar would have to be moved, he was engaged, with Filippo Gonzate and Marcantonio Zucchi (1469–ca. 1531), to prepare drawings for a new altar, constructed later by Gianfranco D'Agrate.

On Sept. 3, 1528, Veronica Gambara, in a letter from Correggio, gave to Isabella d'Este "qualche notizia intorno al capo d'opera di pittura che il nostro Mr. Antonio Allegri ha hor hora terminato . . ." ("some news about the masterpiece of painting that our Master Antonio Allegri has just finished . . ."). This refers to a Magdalen of which the writer gives a description, adding: "In quest'opera ha espresso tutto il sublimo dell'arte della quale è gran maestro" ("In this work he has expressed all that is sublime in the art of which he is a great master"). The Magdalen in question cannot be identified with any known painting. Although the letter was published by Pungileoni (*Elogio storico di G. Santi*, Urbino, 1822, pp. 108 ff.), its authenticity has been disputed. In 1530 there is record of a payment made to Correggio by the Duke of Mantua. If, as Venturi suggests, the date 1531, which Dirochers recorded in making his engraving of the *Danae*, is correct, it may have been in 1530 that the Duke of Mantua commissioned a series of the Loves of the Gods intended as a gift for the Emperor Charles V. On Mar. 5, 1534, the painter died in Correggio and was buried modestly in the Chiesa dei Francescani. A little later, on June 15, the artist's father returned to Dr. Alberto Panciroli, of Reggio, the 25 gold scudi advanced for an altarpiece for the Church of S. Agostino, a painting that had barely been begun. Between Sept. 12 and Oct. 24, 1534, the Duke of Mantua asked the governor of Parma to return either the prepayment or the cartoons for the Loves of Jupiter and

the canvases which the artist had begun. The governor there-upon announced that everything belonging to Correggio had been removed to his native city.

It is evident that factual information relating to the first decade of Correggio's activity is quite scarce. The only work known from the period before 1518 (the approximate date of the lost *Madonna di Albinea*) is the *Madonna of St. Francis* (1514–15). Venturi examined the copy by Gian Battista Spaccini of the Modenese *Cronaca* of Jacopino and Tommaso Lancilotto, and discovered, in the brief excursus on the painters of Modena under the date 1543, mention of Correggio as a pupil of Francesco de' Bianchi Ferrari (ca. 1460–1510) (*Il Correggio*, Rome, 1926). But criticism has been influenced less by this hint, and by the other that associates him with the narrowest local and family circle (Antonio Bartolotti, called "Tognino," and his uncle Lorenzo Allegri), than by that furnished by Padre Ippolito Donesmondi, author of a *Storia ecclesiastica di Modena* (1613). This records Correggio working in Mantua, in the Mantegna family chapel in S. Andrea, where he is said to have painted "negli angoli della cuba i quattro Evangelisti" ("the four Evangelists in the corners of the square," i.e., on the pendentives). The attribution of two *tondi* in the atrium of the same church (*Madonna and Child with St. Joseph, St. Elizabeth, and the Infant John the Baptist; Entombment of Christ*) now appears to be confirmed by a fragment of a cartoon for the *Entombment* in the Pierpont Morgan Library, New York. It seems legitimate, therefore, to look for Correggio's beginnings in the sphere of Andrea Mantegna's classicism or of the Mantuan culture of the first decade of the century. The paintings associated with the young Correggio which most clearly recall Mantegna may be ascribed to this period (ca. 1510–14). To mention only the most noted, and omit the additions proposed by Longhi (1958), these include: the *Madonna and Child* (London, Barrymore Coll.); *Madonna and Child with St. Elizabeth and the Youthful St. John* (Philadelphia, Mus. of Art, Johnson Coll.); *Mystic Marriage of St. Catherine* (Detroit, Institute of Arts); *Virgin and Child* with angel musicians (Florence, Uffizi; PL. 473); *Mystic Marriage of St. Catherine* (Washington, D.C., Nat. Gall., formerly Coll. Frizzoni); *Judith* (Strasbourg, Musée des Beaux-Arts); *Nativity* (Milan, Brera, formerly Coll. Crespi); and the *Madonna of St. Francis*, signed Antonius de Allegris (Dresden, Gemäldegal.).

In this group, of which the masterpiece is the *Nativity* in the Brera and the culmination the Dresden altarpiece, Correggio keeps faithful in the main to Mantegna's classicism, and only softens its "gemlike intaglio" by means of a "more delicate and depth-enhancing chiaroscuro," Leonardesque only by virtue of a "twilight or even nocturnal flavor" (Longhi). His vision, presently to become more naturalistic. is here still limited by a style of knotted and convoluted strokes. Of the two, the Brera *Nativity* is the work of greater breadth; the *Madonna of St. Francis* in Dresden has a more impressive monumentality, but is less successful formally. The derivations in this altarpiece, which mark a critical moment in Correggio's development, have been listed repeatedly. Thus, in addition to the Mantegnesque and Mantuan elements, such as the placing of the Virgin, which repeats Mantegna's *Madonna della Vittoria* (Verona, S. Zeno), painted 20 years before, there are to be felt, in the more tender spirit and the more atmospheric handling of some portions, stimuli from later sources, such as the *Sistine Madonna* of Raphael, if it is true that it was already in Piacenza in 1513. This orientation of Correggio toward atmospheric forms is apparent in his landscapes with their glades of trees rising like oversize bushes and in the glimpses of castles and villages in the distant haze. It is also seen, more fluidly articulated, in forms of Venetian-Ferrarese origin connected with the protomannerism that circulated in Emilia. This mannerism is found in the works of Amico Aspertini (ca. 1475–1552), Dosso Dossi (d. ca. 1542), and Benvenuto Tisi ("Il Garofalo"; 1481–1559), and even touched Mantua lightly, as evidenced by the paintings of Lorenzo Leonbruno (1489–1537?). Correggio's feeling for the atmospheric is thus most pronounced in works that Longhi, in clarifying the artist's development, placed in the second

phase of his youthful activity, between the Dresden altarpiece and the Albinea, which is known only through copies (1517).

The most widely recognized and impressive of these works include a *Holy Family* (Milan, Orombelli Coll.) whose Mantegnesque composition is softened by the luminosity of the landscape. Longhi has perspicaciously set the Brera (Milan) *Adoration of the Magi* apart from the Mantegnesque *Holy Family* because of the tortuous movement of its figures and its "uneasy and tense" composition. Besides indicating the influence of Dossi, these features show the inspiration of northern models and of Emilian protomannerism. In this group of works we may also cite the *Madonna and Child* (Vienna, Kunsthist. Mus.), a Voss attribution; *La Zingarella* (Naples, Capodimonte); the *Madonna and Child with the Youthful John the Baptist* called the "Madonna Bolognini" (Milan, Castello Sforzesco); *St. Anthony Abbot* (Naples, Capodimonte), a Venturi attribution; *St. Jerome* (Madrid, Acad. de S. Fernando), a Longhi attribution; *Christ Taking Leave of His Mother* (London, Nat. Gall., formerly R. H. Benson Coll.), a work in which the artist used a Dürer print as a means to discovering a modest simplicity of his own and an intimate and consuming pathos; the *Madonna Campori* (Modena, Gall. Estense); *Four Saints* (New York, Met. Mus.), the only work among those mentioned to which we can even indirectly assign a date (1517); the *Portrait of a Lady* (perhaps Veronica Gambara; Leningrad, Hermitage), formerly attributed to Lorenzo Lotto and reclaimed for Correggio by Longhi. The Leningrad portrait bears the signature Anton[ius] Laet[us], a latinized signature that, as the copies testify, appeared first in the Albinea altarpiece. (The Dresden altarpiece is signed Antonius de Alegris.)

From 1517 to 1520, when Correggio signed the contract for the frescoes in S. Giovanni Evangelista, there are no known works that can be dated on the basis of documents. But the contrast between the *Madonna di Albinea* and the frescoes of the dome is so great, and the efforts through which these last took form so exacting, as to make it more than likely that for Correggio these were years of intense spiritual growth. Indeed, it is believed that at this time occurred an event of the greatest importance for Correggio's development: a journey to Rome. The direct influence of Raphael and Michelangelo would have enabled Correggio to outgrow the retardataire culture of the centers in which his development had so far taken place. It was formerly maintained that Correggio's genius was completely provincial, solitary, autochthonous. But despite the absence of documentary evidence, Venturi's studies and the searching analyses of Longhi, emphasizing the significance of a Roman journey, have made it clear that his art can be understood only as a product of genius and culture together. Rome and the contact with the more naturalistic works of Raphael and Michelangelo must have spelled the end of the petrified classicism of Mantegna and its academic aftermath and inspired in him a rebirth of the classicistic ideal, which meant a revived Hellenism. This classicism, however, was not pompous and literary but, rather, wholly naturalistic in temper and precisely what he instinctively sought, in a typically Lombard, or even (leaving Vasari's geographical notions for the moment), typically Emilian fashion. It must have been in the Roman ambient that the superb fantasies which took form on the vault of the Camera di S. Paolo were matured — even before Correggio's conversations with the Abbess Giovanna Piacenza (one of the most intelligent women of her time), and before his brilliant achievement of the dome of S. Giovanni Evangelista (Parma).

Long disregarded and forgotten, the Camera di S. Paolo was rediscovered in the second half of the 18th century. By common agreement it is dated, for reasons of style, in the period between the *Madonna di Albinea* and the dome of S. Giovanni Evangelista. The idea of the vault (PL. 465) — a network of reeds carrying festoons of fruit and punctuated by ovals through which putti, against a luminous sky, glance downward — and the shells of the base of the dome, with their delightful collection of antiquarian rarities, are still largely Mantegnesque. Indeed, it may have been suggested to Correggio by the little dome of the Chapel of Innocent VIII in the Vatican, frescoed in 1490 by Mantegna. The description of this

dome by Giovanni Pietro Chattard (*Nuova descrizione del Vaticano*, Rome, 1762–66) suggests that its motifs were not very different from those we see at Parma. The contrast between these frescoes and Correggio's preceding works could not be more emphatic. Even though they recall motifs of Raphael or Michelangelo, the relation between the soft flesh tones and the luminous opening of the sky behind them, the vibrant and fluid handling of the little monochrome mythological figures, the frieze of emblems that carries the lunettes, and the figure of Diana moving across the great hood of the chimney, assume the character of Correggio's Hellenic sensuousness in the effect of a "rose blush on the soft glow of mother-of-pearl" (Venturi) or in the piquant contrasts of lighting. Here a new humanity takes form and life: the unique humanity of Correggio, expressed in a series of subsequent masterpieces.

In the frescoes of the Church of S. Giovanni Evangelista (1520–23), the connections with the culture of Rome, and with the works of Raphael and Michelangelo in particular, became increasingly urgent and imperative. Correggio's imagination soared freely, in a flight that carried him beyond his time. Anton Raphael Mengs (1728–79) remarked that the dome of S. Giovanni Evangelista (PL. 470) was "the most beautiful of all that were painted before and after him." Analogies with the figures of Raphael's *Stanze* and Michelangelo's Sistine Chapel ceiling are to be found not only in Correggio's preparatory studies for these decorations, but also in the Biblical figures on the underarches of the dome, in the Evangelists and Doctors of the Church on the spandrels, and in the apostles and other figures on the dome. But as these comparisons were made long ago, it is not worth insisting on them here. More important is the overpowering impression created by Correggio's imagination, which, in response to his sensitive feeling for nature, freed the decoration from any suggestion of architectural support and thrust the nubile figures, transformed as in an apocalyptic vision, into a luminous abyss. Separated by only half a century from Mantegna's Camera degli Sposi in the Castello Gonzaga in Mantua, Correggio, with the audacity of genius, succeeded in enclosing in this dome the bright infinity of the sky and thus provided a precedent of the greatest importance for the baroque period. The decoration of the tribune followed that of the dome. Of this there remain in Parma (Gall. Naz.), the *Coronation of the Virgin*, which originally stood out against a background of tree architecture; in the National Gallery in London, three angels' heads from the glory that surrounded the central part; and in the Boston Museum of Fine Arts, a fourth head. But in the church there is still preserved, in the lunette over the door of the transept, the inspired figure of the Evangelist, one of Correggio's most harmonious images. Of the 13 sections of the nave frieze — which, as the drawings attest, the artist studied lovingly and at length — the one with a representation of a sibyl has survived, as correctly noted by Zamboni (*Arte antica e moderna*, I, 1958, p. 194). In the Del Bono Chapel (from which come the two canvases in the Parma Galleria discussed below) there remain the frescoes of the underarches either executed by the artist himself, as Popham proposes, or after his drawings, as documented by the preparatory studies at Chatsworth.

Evidently the winter of 1522 prevented continuation of the work in S. Giovanni Evangelista, for early in November of that year Correggio was employed to decorate the tribune and the dome of the Cathedral of Parma. This task must have been carried out, as far as the dome is concerned, between 1526 and 1530. For reasons of style, however, we must assign several works to the interval between the Camera di S. Paolo and the dome of the Cathedral, though none of them bears a date and those about which the facts are known were completed and installed much later.

Among these are the *Madonna and Child with the Infant St. John* (Madrid, Prado); *Rest on the Flight into Egypt* (Florence, Uffizi); *Marriage of St. Catherine* (Naples, Capodimonte); *Noli me Tangere* (Madrid, Prado); *Madonna della Scala* (detached fresco; Parma, Gall. Naz.); *Madonna Adoring the Christ Child* (Florence, Uffizi); *Christ in the Garden of Gethsemane* (London, Vict. and Alb. Mus.); *Ecce Homo* (London, Nat. Gall.); *Madonna del latte* (Budapest, Nat. Mus.); *Madonna della Cesta* or *Holy Family* (London, Nat. Gall.); *Mystic Marriage of St. Catherine* (Paris, Louvre; PL. 466); *Annunciation* (detached fresco; Parma, Gall. Naz.). The following great altarpieces belong to the same period: the *Deposition* (Parma, Gall. Naz.); *Martyrdom of SS. Placidus and Flavia* (Parma, Gall. Naz.; PL. 469); *Madonna of St. Sebastian* (Dresden, Gemäldegal.).

In some of these works Correggio's earlier themes and motifs reappear, but the shimmer of gold flecks gives the landscapes a more varied modulation of light and a livelier sparkle of colors than is found earlier, and the compositions and forms have a more deliberate rhythm, as well as a shy grace that almost amounts to affectation. At this point, where his psychological penetration was keenest, Correggio's works became strongly significant for Ludovico Carracci, and prefigured — for example, in the Virgin of the *Ecce Homo* — the mystic exaltations, even the ecstasies, of the baroque. The two great canvases in the Galleria Nazionale, Parma, the *Deposition* and the *Martyrdom of SS. Placidus and Flavia*, come from the fifth chapel on the right in the Church of S. Giovanni Evangelista (the Del Bono Chapel), and have experienced the same vicissitudes. Unless they reflect an adjustment made in the course of installation, the half figures at the margins are altogether exceptional in Renaissance taste and again attest the freedom of Correggio's imagination, ever pregnant with suggestions for the future. [It is true that a drawing in the Louvre gives the entire scene, at least for the *Martyrdom of SS. Placidus and Flavia*; but the copy by Lelio Orsi (probably 1511–87), executed about twenty years later, contains the same marginal half figures: for illustration, see *Arte antica e moderna*, April–June, 1958.] In both pictures, the figures are disposed on diagonals and both, in their accentuated drama, draw upon the crepuscular melancholy that is the most intimate sign of the spirituality of the artist; note the more violent expressionism, the more subtle cruelty of the Lelio Orsi copy. In the great altarpiece in Dresden, which is more joyous and exultant, the children astride the clouds echo motifs from the dome of S. Giovanni Evangelista.

The dome of the Cathedral of Parma marks the culmination of Correggio's career (PLS. 471, 472). If the artist continued to use the ideas of the preceding decorations (Camera di S. Paolo and dome of S. Giovanni Evangelista), it was either because they still stimulated the same rich imaginative vein or because he wanted to probe deeper. Actually the work moves with a more unified and animated rhythm and energes more airily and harmoniously blended in color. Here we see not merely the sky opening into the church, to fill it with its lights and colors but, according to Francesco Scannelli (*Il microcosmo della pittura . . .*, Cesena, 1651), Paradise itself with its "inexpressible gladness" and its "laughter." From the immense valves of the open shells on the spandrels arise the grandiose figures of the patron saints of the city (Thomas, Ilarius, Bernard, and John the Baptist) on soft masses of clouds, gray infused with violet, amidst the exultation and festive capers of the angels. In the underarches are sinuous youths, whose vague smiles and forms perfect as Greek marbles, are revealed in the mysterious light. This is the exciting preface to the supreme frolic of the angels who accompany the Virgin in the luminous and brilliant sky of the dome, a scene intensified and given a greater illusion of spaciousness by the use of the drum for the representation of a low octagonal wall. In front of the wall are the immense figures of the apostles, and behind it, above these, are the nude, rosy youths, who are shown in daring poses burning perfumed essences in the projecting tripods. The effect of the immense, airy scene is deliberately heightened by the energetic movement of the figures, by the rapidity of their unexpected foreshortenings and impromptu intertwinings and the fluidity of their sudden flights in the great vortex of light. In this work Correggio's imagination surged like a river in flood. The piling up of figures not only inspired such artists as Giulio Romano (1492–1546) and Francesco Primaticcio (1504–70), but surpassed even the Michelangelo of the Sistine Chapel ceiling in the masterful drawing and the audacity of movement. Yet this does not seem to have

satisfied the officials of the Cathedral, for one of them, evidently voicing the complaints of the rest, spoke of the decoration as a "frogs' leg stew." However that may be, the artist stopped working at the Cathedral and, as the documents seem to show, withdrew to his native Correggio, where he continued in fervent activity for the remaining four years of his life.

During the period of his work on the Cathedral decorations, Correggio finished several altarpieces, besides the mythological and allegorical paintings which will be discussed below. The altarpieces, according to the contracts which are known, had already been agreed upon in the preceding years. They are all paintings whose stylistic connections with the frescoes allow us, lacking external evidence, to assign them approximate dates.

The series opens with the *Madonna of St. Jerome* ("Il Giorno;" Parma, Gall. Naz.; PL. 474), ordered by Donna Briseida Colla in 1523, but apparently not installed in her family chapel in S. Antonio in Parma until 1528. From the next year, as is seen from the inscription DIE. VI. IVLI. MDXXVIIII, are two canvases portraying St. Joseph and a worshiper. These are to be regarded as a single composition, even if each figure is arranged separately in its own niche. The paintings were rediscovered after a long period of neglect and are preserved in the Capodimonte in Naples. F. Bologna (1957) suggests, with suitable caution, that the worshiper might be identified as Count Guido da Correggio, the same person who is represented, a little younger, in the stylistically related portrait (formerly, Lee of Fareham Coll., now Courtauld Inst., London). Belonging to 1530, to accept the dates that are legible, respectively, on a pilaster of the chapel and on the frame, are the *Adoration of the Shepherds* (PL. 475), formerly in the Pratoneri Chapel in the Church of S. Prospero in Reggio Emilia (now, Dresden, Gemäldegal.), and the so-called "Madonna della Scodella," formerly in the Church of the Sto Sepolcro in Parma (now, Parma, Gall. Naz.; PL. 468). The *St. Catherine Reading* (Hampton Court, Royal Colls.) must also have been painted at this time. About a year later is the *Madonna of St. George* [PL. 467; formerly in the Oratorio of S. Pietro Martire, Modena, whence it was withdrawn by the duke in 1649 to be copied by Giovanni Francesco Barbieri ("Il Guercino"; 1591–1666)]. It is now in the Gemäldegalerie, Dresden, with other paintings sold to the King of Poland.

The close connection between these works and the frescoes of the Cathedral of Parma is a matter not only of chronology but also of style. In the *Madonna of St. Jerome*, for example, the analogy with the figures of the dome is not limited to the figure of St. Jerome, which is akin to the enormous apostles of the drum. It also concerns the compositional order, in which the figures are banked on an ascending plane, with the group gathered in the shadow of the red hanging set in contrast with the open countryside that recedes, brilliantly lighted, into the remote distance. The whole composition, here as in the Cathedral frescoes, is fused by a golden atmosphere and pervaded by a subtle, disquieting charm; its tone recalls Tasso rather than Bernini, from the angel's smile to the rapt expression of the Madonna. Vivid color contrasts again occur in the "Madonna della Scodella," which the artist has organized on the diagonal according to a favorite scheme of his. The St. Joseph, who gives one hand to the Child while he grasps at a palm branch with the other, has the somewhat melodramatic air of a hero in Tasso; but he also provides a pretext for the splendid articulation of the great folds of the cloak, while the angels wheel in flight on the clouds, as on the squinches below the dome of the Cathedral. The painting is sumptuous, largely as a result of the luminosity of the colors, set against the depth of the landscape. The counterpart of this St. Joseph is the one in the rediscovered composition in Naples, as large as he is bashful. Here the color, as Bologna has acutely observed, "fades and equalizes the truth of appearances . . . in a subdued monochrome" and also strongly emphasizes the unforgettable figure of the worshiper. A capacity to infuse the substance of the painting with the breath of inner life characterizes the few known portraits by Correggio, and it is for this that one is inclined to include in the brief series the obviously earlier one in the Castello Sforzesco in Milan, which has been insistently attributed to him by Longhi. Just as the *Madonna of St. Jerome*, because of the great light that shines on the landscape, is called "Il Giorno," so the *Adoration of the Shepherds* (Dresden, Gemäldegal.), because of the light that emanates from the Child to dispel the shadows and illuminate the whole scene, is called "La Notte" (PL. 475). This is one of the most fascinating, most admired, and most widely imitated of Correggio's pictures. The link with the *Madonna of St. Jerome*, of which this is a nighttime variant, is also apparent in some of the figures, for example, the shepherd in the foreground, and in the composition itself. A recollection of the Cathedral dome is to be found in the group of angels on the illuminated and light-reflecting clouds, suspended in flight over the rough crib.

The *Madonna of St. George* revives an earlier compositional scheme and amplifies it with a series of motifs that were to become the delight of the mannerists of Parma. Here Correggio epitomizes his favorite themes; but in doing so he pushes the movements of the figures to the extreme of ambiguity, causing them to reveal themselves one by one and binding them to the center by means of restless, nervous gestures. The quality that has long been called Correggio's *grazia* borders on affectation, and that point is almost reached in this painting.

In the last years of his life Correggio executed a series of canvases with mythological and allegorical subjects. He had already painted pictures of this kind, in addition to the lost painting of *Apollo and Marsyas*, engraved in 1562 by Giulio Santo. Among those which have been attributed to him, it is worth at least mentioning the *Education of Cupid* (London, Nat. Gall.) and *Antiope* (Paris, Louvre), which were probably executed a little after his return from Rome, at the time of the dome of S. Giovanni Evangelista, and were recorded in 1627 in the inventory of the Gonzagas. It was then that Correggio must have begun the series of canvases on the Loves of Jupiter mentioned earlier. Vasari, documenting the series, mentions the *Danae* and the *Leda*. Probably the artist began the paintings immediately when he interrupted work on the Cathedral and retired to his native city. Besides the *Danae* and the *Leda*, which are respectively in the Borghese Gallery in Rome and the Staatliche Museen, Berlin, the series includes the two canvases *Io* and *The Rape of Ganymede* (PL. 476) in the Kunsthistorisches Museum, Vienna. Of the *Danae* and the *Leda* we may first remark [although the *Leda* is restored in many places and the head of the central figure was repainted by Jacob Schlesinger (1792–1855)] that in these works Correggio seems to have been primarily concerned with beauty of form. Of the *Danae*, we may recall what Mengs wrote about the *Madonna of St. Jerome*, namely, that the colors seem as if they had been melted together like wax over a fire, rather than applied with a brush. The main image is isolated by the pale golden tones that stand forth between the whiteness of the bed linen and the darkness of the background, like an ancient marble miraculously given warmth and life.

*Io* and *The Rape of Ganymede* are among Correggio's boldest inventions. In the figure of Io the theme of the *Danae* is revived, but the rain of gold turns into a cloud that bears down on the figure and encloses it in its mysterious embrace, revealing the complete nudity of the body, which is seen from behind. The figure of Ganymede, with the vanishing landscape seen from above, echoes the angel in the middle of the shell with St. Bernard in one of the squinches of the Cathedral dome. The upward-flying drapery, in that celestial light in which we seem to hear the fading howl of the dog, furnishes the clearest possible evidence of the artist's supreme decorative gift; and the angel, so easily transformed into Ganymede, the most obvious proof of the secular character of his imagination. That imagination vitalized Christian themes with the breath of a revived Hellenism, or projected them into the remote world inhabited by his soul: an undefiled and timeless dream. It is for this that, on the one hand, Correggio stands aloof from Italian Renaissance painting in general, while on the other hand he becomes completely contemporary during the course of the 18th century.

In the correspondence between the Duke of Mantua and the governor of Parma at the time of Correggio's death, there

is mention of what seems to have been a second Loves of Jupiter series. Evidently differing from the first, this series was left in the form of sketches. It is probable that the projected canvases (or tapestries, as Ricci prefers to think) were to have been installed in the Ducal Palace at Mantua in a special room to be finished off with a cupola decorated with a representation of Olympus, a sketch for which has survived in a small painting in Christ Church College, Oxford. Apparently this concerns an extremely interesting decorative project, in which Correggio exceeded his previous conquests to the point of anticipating not merely Primaticcio but even Pellegrino Tibaldi (1527–96).

In conjunction with the mythological paintings the allegorical ones should be mentioned. These are represented by the two temperas *Virtue* (PL. 468) and *Vice*, both in the Louvre, which Isabella d'Este placed at either side of the door of the *studiolo* decorated with paintings by Mantegna, Lorenzo Costa (d. 1535), and Pietro Perugino (ca. 1450–1523). A copy of the *Virtue* is preserved in an unfinished canvas in the Galleria Doria Pamphili in Rome. G. Morelli considered this to be modern, while Ricci thought it had been started by Correggio and abandoned because of a mistake in the measurements, which would have prevented its being installed in the place for which it was intended. These paintings have the decorative character of tapestries and wonderful pictorial qualities as well; but they also have a sententiousness and a complexity of form that would not have displeased the mannerists. Among the paintings for the *studiolo*, Perugino's *Contest between Sensuality and Chastity* does not seem to have met with Isabella d'Este's favor. It is not improbable that Correggio was employed to provide a substitute for it, of which, according to Popham, there remains a trace in a drawing in the Musée Bonnat in Bayonne.

Among the paintings attributed to Correggio, in addition to those already mentioned, it is worth citing the following: a youthful *Holy Family* in a Lombard private collection (Longhi); a *Nativity* with two saints, formerly in Rome in the possession of Fr. Rossi (Longhi); *St. Helen with Four Saints* in a private collection in Brescia (Longhi); a *Deposition* formerly in the Coccapani Collection, Modena (Longhi). A *John the Baptist* that was formerly in the Robinson Collection, London, is held by Ricci and Venturi to be part (the left wing) of a triptych of *The Humanity of Christ* that used to be in the Oratorio della Misericordia in Correggio. Of the right wing (*St. Bartholomew*) there is no record; of the central part (*Christ in Glory*), on the other hand, there is a copy in the style of the Carracci preserved in the Vatican Museums.

Any discussion of the work of Correggio implicitly involves the historiographical vicissitudes that have accompanied him through the centuries. Thus an attempt to clarify these may increase our own understanding.

Except for the youthful sojourn in Mantua, Correggio's activity was divided between his native city and Parma, and only a brief journey to Rome may have interrupted its laborious course. Though ruled by princes who delighted in enhancing the prestige of their courts by encouraging culture and the arts, his surroundings were yet remote and provincial. This explains why, in his own time, Correggio's fame was limited to his native province, to which his presence and his art later brought a place in history. The scarcity of sources is counterbalanced by the interest of Vasari, who was in Parma a few years after the artist's death (1542) and collected on the spot the materials for his biography. With Vasari's *Lives* the critical fortunes of Correggio's work began; in it can be found the themes that fed the literature on Correggio for a long time to come. Some of these—the anecdotal and strictly biographical ones—have by now lost all interest. Others still survive and provide, either negatively or positively, a point of departure for an interpretation of the artist.

Vasari is the great exponent of the Florentine art tradition and of the culture based upon it that gained the ascendency in Rome when, in the early 16th century, the latter emerged as the more important art center. Vasari's judgment was obviously influenced by his preferences. He recognized Correggio's genius, but his appreciation was limited because he saw in Correggio's art a lack of that quality of *disegno* which

for him lay at the root of all art, and, in a more general sense, a lack of contact with Roman-Tuscan culture. If only Correggio had been in Rome — this is Vasari's evident conclusion — he would have worked miracles.

This evaluation sets Correggio aside from the great highway along which culture moves, despite his place as a genius among the promoters of the revival of Lombard painting. The myth that Correggio was a solitary and autochthonous genius was developed on this basis, assisted by a dash of provincial pride. This was true also in the time of Ludovico Antonio Muratori (1672–1750), when the attempt was made to give that myth a solid basis in historical research and rational explanation (Affò, Tiraboschi, Antonioli, and others). The idea of Correggio's contacts with Roman culture was first broached by Roger de Piles at the end of the 17th century. That of an actual journey to Rome was put forward at the beginning of the next century by Padre Sebastiano Resta (*Parnasso dei Pittori*, Perugia, 1707). He tried by this means to confirm the attribution to Correggio of certain drawings related to the Vatican Logge. It was suggested again in the second half of the century, this time with an enlightened historical awareness, by Mengs (*Opere*, ed. d'Azara, Parma, 1780, passim), who saw in the culture of Rome the key to an understanding of such a work as the rediscovered Camera di S. Paolo. And it is the path followed by the most up-to-date and sensitive contemporary criticism, from Venturi to Longhi.

Mengs' high estimation of Correggio's works, whose most intimate problems he studied, from the peculiarities of drawing to the "ideal beauty of the chiaroscuro," seems to have been conditioned less by his theoretical assumptions than by his painter's experience and sensitivity. This enabled him to perceive in the work of Correggio (the Correggio who had rediscovered the Greek spirit in classicism) the most stimulating tendencies of his time. Mengs' sensitivity as an artist sharpened his critical investigations, resolving in the only way possible the controversy about *grazia*, *regola*, and *disegno*, in which the criticism of the time seems to have been entangled. In a different climate of taste this controversy restated the limitations established by Vasari and made Daniel Webb exclaim, in the mid-18th century: "Correggio has baffled criticism."

The romantics did not reject the fascination of Correggio; rather they based their evaluation on his most ambiguous and elusive qualities. But in the 19th-century accounts, which drew upon the ample researches of Pungileoni, the predominant themes are still those touched on by Mengs. It was only Pre-Raphaelitism that began to weaken these attitudes, hinting at limitations of a moral order. The decorator, the innovator of the great baroque tradition, and the subtle technician began to take precedence over the painter (Kugler, Burckhardt, Springer, Strzygowski, etc.). The series of great monographs based on a foundation of historism opened with that of J. Meyer (1871) and continued, to mention only the most important, with those of C. Ricci (1896, repr. 1930) and H. Thode (1898). But the premises of the main critical tradition were taken up again, first by A. Venturi in special studies and in his monograph (1926) and then by R. Longhi, whose essay on the Camera di S. Paolo (1956) is fundamental for the understanding of the whole of Correggio's work, as well as for the related attitudes of historiography.

SOURCES. In the brief list of sources, the main item is Vasari's biography (ed. L. Torrentino, Florence, 1550; amplified, ed. I. Giunta, 1568; Am. ed., trans. E. H. and E. W. Blashfield and A. A. Hopkins, 4 vols., New York, 1913). Documents include: G. Tiraboschi, Notizie de' pittori, scultori, incisori e architetti natii degli stati del serenissimo duca di Modena, Modena, 1786, pp. 22–92; I. Affò, Ragionamento sopra una stanza dipinta dal celeberrimo pittore Antonio Allegri da Correggio nel Monastero di S. Paolo in Parma, Parma, 1794 (the first extensive illustration of the famous work, dated by Affò 1518–20): L. Pungileoni, Memorie istoriche di Antonio Allegri detto il Correggio, Parma, 1817–21 (although chaotic, the most comprehensive collection of records on Correggio); G. Campori, Lettere artistiche inedite, Modena, 1866; Q. Bigi, Notizie di Antonio Allegri, di Antonio Bartolotti suo maestro e di altri pittori ed artisti correggesi, Modena, 1873; Q. Bigi, Della vita e delle opere certe e incerte di Antonio Allegri detto il Correggio, Modena, 1881; A. Venturi, Quadri del Correggio per Albinea, Archivio storico dell'arte, I, 1888 (with letter of the archpriest of Albinea mentioned above); G. Tiraboschi, Lettere al padre Ireneo Affò, ed. C. Frati, Modena, 1895.

BIBLIOG. The literature on Correggio up to 1934 is collected in S. de Vito Battaglia, Correggio, Rome, 1934 (a fundamental list). Among subsequent books and articles, the following deserve mention: A. O. Quintavalle, C. Brandi, G. Copertini, and G. Masi, Mostra del Correggio: Catalogo, Parma, 1935; Manifestazioni parmensi nel IV centenario della morte del Correggio, Parma, 1936; E. Bodmer, Il Correggio e gli emiliani, Novara, 1943; A. Ros-Theier, Antonio da Correggio, Bildnisse, Zurich, 1947; P. Bianconi, Tutta la pittura del Correggio, Milan, 1953; R. Longhi, Il Correggio e la Camera di San Paolo a Parma, Genoa, 1956; F. Bologna, Ritrovamento di due tele del Correggio, Paragone, 91, 1957, pp. 9–25; A. E. Popham, Correggio's Drawings, London, 1957; R. Longhi, Le fasi del Correggio giovine e l'esigenza del suo viaggio romano, Paragone, 101, 1958, pp. 34–53; L. Volpi, Una copia da Correggio di Lelio Orsi, Arte Antica e Moderna, 2, 1958, p. 178, pl. 64.

Stefano BOTTARI

Illustrations: PLS. 465–476.

## COSMATI

COSMATI. By a generally accepted convention the marble-workers active in Rome and its vicinity from the beginning of the 12th to the end of the 13th century are collectively known as "the Cosmati," from the name Cosma, which occurs repeatedly in several families of marbleworkers. Cosmati work represents an important aspect of medieval art in Italy (see ROMANESQUE ART).

SUMMARY. Cosmati decoration (col. 829). Families of Cosmati workers (col. 830): *The Vassallettos*. Individual masters and unattributed works (col. 833). Architectural work (col. 834). Pictorial and sculptural trends (col. 834).

COSMATI DECORATION. What the Cosmati have in common are certain stylistic characteristics; despite individual differences, their works constitute one style and one school. Even when working as architects they remained essentially decorators; they were interested not in constructional or spatial problems but in surfaces. Their characteristic ornamental system lies within these limits of surface decoration. It consisted in the use at first of tesserae of marble and other hard stone such as porphyry, serpentine, fine white marble, and *giallo antico*, and later of glass and gold cubes. Sometimes panels of mosaic were framed with white marble bands; sometimes the tesserae themselves would surround roundels or rectangular fields of pure serpentine or porphyry. But the colored areas were always framed by white bands that acted as rhythmic caesurae, or intervals of quiet and repose. This ornamental system extends to all planar surfaces, from the pavement of a basilica to the panels of chancel barriers and ambos; it covers thrones, ciboriums, altar frontals, the lintels and cornices of doorways, and, finally, the shafts of those spiral columns that reveal the first hint of the Gothic. Sculptural decoration, whether figured or foliate, is rare in the Roman region, its place being taken by colored marble mosaic.

Among the possible sources of this unusual type of decoration, local tradition may be the most important. In Rome there are early medieval pavements of polychrome marble composed of more or less small fragments (S. Marco and S. Maria Antiqua) and pavements with minute designs resembling mosaic (S. Clemente, S. Maria in Aracoeli); patterns of disks and twisted ribbons appear as simulated marble wall decoration (S. Crisogono; Temple of Fortuna Virilis).

If all this shows a special predilection of the Roman marble craftsmen for polychrome decoration, it does not necessarily follow that the entire known Cosmati repertory developed out of the ornamental motifs used in this formative stage. Indeed the Cosmati seem to have more in common with Byzantine modes. Aside from various literary accounts, there exist in Hagia Sophia, in the Basilica of St. John in Studion, and in the Church of the Pantokrator (all in Istanbul) remains of pavements, perhaps of the 11th to 12th century, that reveal, in the great porphyry or serpentine roundels, in the intertwined bands of mosaics and white, and in the rectangular panels bordered with mosaic or marble strips, the closest analogy with the Cosmati repertory. The diffusion of such motifs is attested by pavements from the Monastery of Iviron on Mount Athos, from St. Mark's in Venice, and from the Palatine Chapel in Palermo, whose Norman rulers maintained close relations with the Byzantine capital. Another center of diffusion was the Abbey of Montecassino in southern Italy. The artisans who came together there at the time of Abbot Desiderius (1058–87) executed the floor of the basilica, which, before the recent discovery of its actual remains, was known to us from a print. Disks, squares, strips, and interlaces form a carpet of intense color which, although executed in a somewhat summary manner with rather large tesserae, contains a number of the motifs common in the repertory of the Cosmati.

However, to speak of a strict derivation of the Cosmati style from Byzantine sources and thus implicitly to deny originality to the Roman marbleworkers would not be just; distinct differences from Byzantine models can be noted — technically, in the motifs, and in the sense of composition. Especially in the regular intervals created by the white panels between the more colorful zones, it would seem as if a trace of classical balance had been transmitted to these marbleworkers.

The Islamic East also exerted an influence on the Roman marbleworkers, although it is not apparent in the earliest work. This influence was transmitted through the marbleworkers of Campania and perhaps also in part by way of Byzantium. The use by the Cosmati of glass cubes for vertical surfaces was derived from Early Christian models, but the heightened effects of light and color of the Roman work owe something also to the influence of Campanian craftsmen.

A direct influence from Campania is clearly visible in the Cosmati works of the late 13th century, in which the white intervals become attenuated almost to the point of disappearance, giving place to triangles, hexagons, and stars, occasionally with borders of white glass cubes, arranged in carpetlike patterns. There is definite south Italian influence in the small broken patterns of the ornamentation in the cloister of St. John Lateran in Rome, in the triangular patterns on panels from the dismantled chancel barrier and throne in the Cathedral of Anagni, and again in the combination of sculptured motifs and mosaic seen in the altar frontals of S. Maria Maggiore and SS. Nereo e Achilleo in Rome. Finally, this southern influence is confirmed by the presence of figured elements next to the geometric, as in the panels, now lost, from S. Maria Maggiore and S. Lorenzo fuori le Mura and in the great altar frontal of S. Cesareo (all in Rome). The appearance of heraldic shields in the friezes of porticoes, the altar frontal now at Vico in Latium, the figured mosaic of the door of S. Tommaso in Formis (Rome), the lunettes of late 13th-century tombs, show that the marbleworkers even attempted to compete with pictorial mosaicists.

The activity of the marbleworkers was not limited to Rome, where they reigned unrivaled, but extended throughout the Roman region, reaching, at the end of the 12th century, the district around Viterbo and also southern Latium (there, however, merging with Campanian work); it even reached the Abruzzi and spread through Umbria. As to the chronological limits of the style, while the first Cosmati works go back to the beginning of the 12th century, the style continued past the end of the 13th century. Thus, when after the interruption caused by the Western schism and the transference of the papal seat to Avignon the restoration of churches was resumed, it was the Cosmati tradition that was followed. However, the intensity of color was lessened, as the pavement with the arms of Martin V in St. John Lateran attests. Toward the middle of the 15th century the floor of the Chapel of the Crucifixion in S. Maria in Aracoeli was inlaid with mosaic; though the panels are still done in the manner of the Cosmati, the design here is of a labyrinth.

FAMILIES OF COSMATI WORKERS. The art of the Roman marble craftsmen, transmitted from father to son, is classified by families. The attribution of specific works is based chiefly on inscriptions. Many of these are present *in situ*; others, now lost, are preserved in old collections of inscriptions. Attributions on the basis of style alone can be made only for the more outstanding personalities; in such cases grouping around works of certain authorship is feasible. A great number of works

are of unknown authorship and are likely to remain so because of the difficulty of making attributions solely on stylistic evidence.

The oldest recorded family descends from a certain Paolo, a Roman master who worked between 1108 and 1110 in the Cathedral of Ferentino. He left his name on a chancel barrier inlaid with compact patterns of squares and triangles in porphyry and serpentine. Certain panels of the chancel barrier in S. Maria in Cosmedin (Rome), with 8th-century plaitwork reliefs on one side, are decorated on the reverse with marble inlay similar to that in Ferentino; though the general character of these panels suggests an attribution to the Cosmati, there is no documentary evidence to support it. Paolo had four sons, Giovanni, Pietro, Angelo, and Sasso, working in Rome. Together they signed the ciborium of S. Lorenzo fuori le Mura, dated 1148; the four are again found together in the ciborium of S. Marco, and probably they were also responsible for the now lost ciboriums of SS. Cosma e Damiano and SS. Apostoli. The ciborium of Sta Croce in Gerusalemme was the work of three of the brothers, Giovanni, Angelo, and Sasso. Paolo and his sons were especially concerned with church furnishings; in general, their works lack the color found in some later Cosmati works.

Angelo had a son, Niccolò, whose activity is documented in S. Bartolomeo all'Isola (Rome), in the portico of the principal façade of St. John Lateran, and in the lower part of the Campanile of Gaeta. Later, with his son Jacopo, Niccolò d'Angelo worked on the high altar of the Cathedral of Sutri, and he worked with Pietro Vassalletto on the Paschal candlestick of S. Paolo fuori le Mura (PL. 477); whether he worked at Narni is uncertain. The only absolutely sure chronological reference to Niccolò's activity is in the inscription, dated 1170, at Sutri; the portico of St. John Lateran is assigned to the pontificate of Alexander III (1159–81). The candlestick in S. Paolo, of which possibly only the base is attributable to Nicco ò's collaborator, is an unusual monument of the Romanesque period; it reflects the artist's study of Early Christian sarcophagi and indicates his interest in sculpture. However, the ambo of the Cathedral of Gaeta, now in a fragmentary state, cannot be attributed to Niccolò because the scenes of Jonah and the tight, small-scale composition clearly indicate a Campanian origin; still less can we attribute to Niccolò the historiated candelabrum from Gaeta, which is later.

The identification of the son of Niccolò as Jacopo is based on a stone inscription formerly in the Church of SS. Giovanni e Paolo in Rome; we do not know to what work this inscription refers. The Giovanni di Niccolò who signed the ambo of S. Pietro at Fondi cannot be identified as a son of Niccolò for the simple reason that his home was in southern Latium; in all probability he belongs to another family.

Another family group is headed by Rainerio, who with his sons Nicola and Pietro left his name in a now lost inscription from the Church of S. Silvestro in Capite in Rome. (The Cosmatesque fragments formerly in the same church and now in SS. Nereo e Achilleo cannot be connected with these craftsmen because they are definitely 13th-century.) There may be an error of transcription in the name of the head of the family, since in other sources Pietro and Nicola are spoken of as the sons of Ranuccio, or, despite the similarity of the two names, it may be that the three craftsmen working at S. Silvestro constitute an independent group. Pietro di Ranuccio left his name on the architrave of the main portal of S. Maria di Castello, dated 1143 (PL. 478). Nicola, with his sons Giovanni and Guittone, signed the ciborium in the Church of S. Andrea in Flumine at Ponzano Romano; Giovanni and Guittone then worked in Tarquinia, where, in S. Maria di Castello, they signed the ciborium dated 1164 (?); Giovanni may be identifiable with the author of the ambo of Fondi, but the southern character of the work seems to argue against this supposition. Guittone's son Giovanni left a clear inscription on the ambo of S. Maria di Castello and also in S. Andrea in Flumine, on an ambo dated 1209; thus in both churches the decoration was carried on at two successive periods. As for the Giovanni who, with his associate Andrea, executed the ambos of S. Pietro

at Massa d'Albe in the Abruzzi and the other Cosmati furnishings of the same church, his family is unknown.

The work of the family of marble craftsmen whose head is Tebaldo has a different orientation; records begin with his son Lorenzo, who seems to have inscribed the date 1162 on the altar of S. Stefano del Cacco in Rome. If the date is genuine, we have here a first work of the craftsman who afterward was active, with his son Jacopo, on the door of the Sacro Speco of Subiaco, on the central portal of the Cathedral of Civita Castellana, and on the door of S. Maria at Falleri; father and son also worked on the ambo of S. Maria in Aracoeli, now reassembled from scattered components, and on two lost productions, a ciborium in the Church of SS. Apostoli and an ambo for Old St. Peter's, later worked on but left unfinished by one of the Vassallettos. Along with the simple intarsia work in S. Maria in Aracoeli — we can no longer judge the form of the ambos — the portals of Falleri and of Civita Castellana attest, better than the door of S. Maria di Castello by Pietro di Ranuccio, the deep penetration by the Lombard style and its fusion with the local polychrome decoration.

Lorenzo's son Jacopo alone signed the door of S. Saba (Rome), the iconostasis of S. Alessio (Rome), of which only a few fragments remain, and the right transept door of the Cathedral of Civita Castellana (PL. 478), and he began the cloister of S. Scolastica at Subiaco. With his son Cosma, Jacopo signed the façade of the Cathedral of Civita Castellana, in 1210; they also left an inscription on the portal of the Hospital of S. Tommaso in Formis (Rome), a work that exhibits a profound assimilation of the forms of classical antiquity. Civita Castellana is especially noteworthy. As if in anticipation of the Renaissance study of the antique, the artist has incorporated an imposing triumphal arch into the impressive structure of the portico, which is reminiscent of the portico that Niccolò d'Angelo had designed earlier for St. John Lateran.

Cosma worked alone from the year 1231 in the Cathedral of Anagni, where later he was joined by his sons, Luca and Jacopo. Together they signed the pavement of the crypt and that of the church itself. Still with his sons' collaboration, at the time of Abbot Lando, Cosma completed the cloister of S. Scolastica at Subiaco. Later Luca, in a secondary position, signed with Drudo de Trivio the truly sumptuous panels of the Cathedral of Civita Castellana. The activity of Drudo has been fairly well established, as he signed the ciborium of the Cathedral of Ferentino; the altar under the ciborium is decorated with two very large roundels of porphyry encircled with bands of white. He also executed a lavabo, carved with a sure and expressive economy, now in the Palazzo Venezia in Rome. Perhaps his last work was the now lost ciborium of the parish church of Lanuvio, dated 1240, which he signed together with his son Angelo.

A family that continued into later times begins with one Pietro Mellini, of whom however we have no reliable records. His son Cosmato is mentioned in documents between 1264 and 1279. Cosmato's only signed work was the Chapel of the Sancta Sanctorum in Rome, which he reconstructed in Gothicizing style between 1278 and 1282. Giovanni, son of Cosmato, signed three similar funerary monuments in Rome: the De Surdis tomb in S. Balbina, the Durante tomb in S. Maria sopra Minerva, and the Rodriguez tomb in S. Maria Maggiore (PL. 479). These already reflect the Gothicizing architecture of Arnolfo di Cambio (q.v.) and the pictorial style of Cavallini (q.v.). Various other works, including the Acquasparta tomb in S. Maria in Aracoeli, the ciborium of the Magdalen in St. John Lateran, and tombs at Anagni, Assisi, etc., are attributed to Giovanni di Cosma. His brother Deodato signed the ciborium in S. Maria in Cosmedin (PL. 479) and another in St. John Lateran, of which only fragments remain. There are traces of Deodato's activity at S. Pietro in Tivoli and at S. Giacomo alla Lungara in Rome, where he worked jointly with one Jacopo, not otherwise identified. Finally, he executed the portal of the Cathedral of Teramo, dated 1322. A third son of Cosmato, Jacopo, was, according to documents, the chief stonemason at the Cathedral of Orvieto in 1293, but cannot be identified with the Jacopo who was working with

Deodato in S. Giacomo alla Lungara because the inscription connects only Deodato with the father's name.

*The Vassallettos.* Another family whose activities have been carefully studied and reconstructed is that of the Vassallettos. They descended from one Bassallicto or Basiletto, who is mentioned in a document of 1130 from the archives of S. Prassede in Rome and who signed the now lost tomb (formerly in the Church of SS. Cosma e Damiano) of Cardinal Guido (d. 1154); to him also belongs the signed lion of SS. Apostoli in Rome. Pietro Vassalletto, who may have been Bassallicto's son, is known from an inscription, dated 1185, once in the Cathedral of Segni. He collaborated with Niccolò d'Angelo and about 1190 began the ambo of Old St. Peter's, which Lorenzo Cosmati later finished with his son Jacopo. He then executed the choir enclosure of S. Saba and began work on the cloisters of S. Paolo (PL. 480) and St. John Lateran; both were completed by his son Vassalletto the Younger. Pietro Vassalletto's work in these cloisters is in the style which had been slowly developing to the highest pitch of compositional balance. Its perfect fusion of decoration and architecture constitutes the finest expression of the art of the Roman marble craftsmen. The younger Vassalletto, who finished the cloister of St. John Lateran between 1232 and 1236, was more open to southern influence. This is reflected in the later parts of the cloisters and in the episcopal throne of Anagni, where crouching animal supports are integrated into the architectural structure in an orderly, simple, and vigorous way. An outstanding characteristic of the Vassallettos was their skill in carving, which the other marbleworkers generally lacked. This ability is revealed in sculptured animals and small figures, as in the cornice of the cloister of St. John Lateran with its frieze of grotesque heads. It is seen again in the forechurch of S. Lorenzo fuori le Mura as well as in the portico with its classicizing antae; indeed it is this characteristic that leads to attribution to the Vassallettos.

INDIVIDUAL MASTERS AND UNATTRIBUTED WORKS. Certain isolated marble craftsmen are known to us, such as Pietro de Maria, who signed and dated (1229) the cloister of the Abbey of Sassovivo near Foligno; a Roman, Andrea, who signed the iconostasis of S. Pietro at Massa d'Albe; Pasquale, whose name appears on a sphinx in the Museo Civico of Viterbo and on the candelabrum of S. Maria in Cosmedin; and Pietro d'Oderisio, who signed the tomb of Clement IV, now in S. Francesco in Viterbo, and those of Edward the Confessor and Henry III in Westminster Abbey (1269). Pietro may also have executed the pavement of the Chapel of St. Thomas in Canterbury Cathedral and the tomb of Adrian V in S. Francesco in Viterbo. He is further to be identified with the "associate Pietro" whose name appears with that of Arnolfo in the tabernacle of S. Paolo fuori le Mura; they may also have collaborated on other works.

As has been pointed out, there are a large number of Cosmati works from the 12th and 13th centuries which must remain unattributed. The pavement of S. Maria in Cosmedin in Rome (like the early-12th-century work of Paolo at Ferentino and perhaps in S. Maria in Cosmedin) and that of S. Clemente, consecrated in 1128 (PL. 477), as well as that of S. Benedetto in Piscinula (Rome), also clearly of an early date, all show the complete maturity of the Cosmati ornamental repertory from the first decades of the 12th century. By that time there were fixed norms for ambos, thrones, ciboriums, and tombs. Except for variations in chromatic richness, these ecclesiastical furnishings did not change in form until the second half of the 13th century, when Gothic influence began to be perceptible. Among the works of uncertain attribution it will suffice to note a few pieces remarkable for their richness of color. At S. Lorenzo fuori le Mura one of the two ambos seems very close in style to Drudo de Trivio; the throne recalls in its ornamentation the episcopal throne of S. Balbina (PL. 477); the panels of the chancel barrier, derived from Civita Castellana, along with the Vassallettian examples of S. Saba and those of SS. Nereo e Achilleo (PL. 481) and of S. Cesareo, are among the most noteworthy of all for the expanse of the colored areas and their chromatic intensity. In contrast to simpler

ambos, that of S. Cesareo (PL. 482) is unusual in its sculptural decoration in south Italian taste. It might well be compared with the work of the last Vassalletto. Finally we must note, in addition to the altars decorated with the usual geometric interlaces, others in which sculptured pilasters, cornices, and triangular or curvilinear pediments form an architectonic framework for areas almost entirely occupied by inlay panels. Very rich is the example, in the style of Pietro d'Oderisio, in the Chapel of the Nativity in S. Maria Maggiore. Another, with an even more vigorous architectonic framework, is in SS. Nereo e Achilleo.

But perhaps the most superbly decorative piece of the whole Cosmati production in this kind of church furnishing is the altar (now damaged) of the Church of S. Cesareo. It is 11 ft., $1^7/_8$ in. wide — an exceptional size. There is an unwonted abundance of mosaic representation of animals, sometimes drawn from the Early Christian repertory but more often — in the case of some of the intarsia panels also — deriving from the work of Campanian marble craftsmen. The relation of this altar, of the second half of the 13th century, to the other decorative work in S. Cesareo is analogous to that of the pavement of the Cathedral of Terracina (PL. 483). In the latter at least an echo of the Cosmati manner is blended with the Campanian influences that otherwise dominate all mosaics and intarsia work. However, in southern Latium the line of demarcation is not always clear; for example, Campanian influences prevail in the altar frontal of S. Maria at Sermoneta, where rock crystals are included in the small decorative patterns (a technique foreign to Rome), but at Fondi the ambo, by a Roman master, is rectangular and ornamented in the Campanian style. Even Niccolò d'Angelo, unless the attribution to him of the lower part of the Campanile of Gaeta is mistaken, employed squared dressed stone and pointed arches over columns without distinct bases, in the Campanian manner, thus departing from the methods he used in the Lateran portico.

ARCHITECTURAL WORK. Although in Niccolò d'Angelo and the Vassallettos we have examples of Cosmati who were architects as well as marble craftsmen, it does not seem logical to include in the Cosmati orbit all the numerous campaniles and portals of the Romanesque period, as some have done. The families mentioned in the records were certainly primarily decorative marble craftsmen and they engaged in actual construction only when the part of the decorator was major, as on the façade of Civita Castellana. On the other hand, the series of Roman cloisters may be considered as part of Cosmati activity: in them the work of the marble craftsmen is a determining and preponderant factor, for while the Cosmati play the role of architects, they are not concerned with spatial problems and therefore remain decorators. The development of cloister decoration may be traced from the simple examples of S. Cecilia and SS. Quattro Coronati in Rome to Subiaco and finally to the two examples of the Lateran and S. Paolo, in which the mature talent of the Vassallettos blends a rhythmic harmony and a strong color sense with elements derived from classical antiquity.

The portals by Lorenzo Cosmati at Falleri and at Civita Castellana show a Romanesque vigor in the treatment of masses. The more sculptural Lombard scheme, with grouped columns on the jambs, appears influential to an even greater degree at Civita Castellana. In Rome itself, on the contrary, portals as a rule follow the classical framing format, with quiet, flat profiles and wide bands decorated with mosaics. Contact with the Romanesque modes dominant around Rome encouraged the marbleworkers to find eclectic solutions occasionally both original and felicitous.

PICTORIAL AND SCULPTURAL TRENDS. The lunettes of portals, shrines, tabernacles (such as the two no longer extant 13th-century examples from the nave of S. Maria Maggiore), and certain late-13th-century tombs gave various marbleworkers the opportunity to function as pictorial mosaicists. In the early phase they worked in a local Byzantinizing manner; later the pictorial style became freer and more popular, as in the

altar now in the parish church of Vico in Latium but originally in S. Maria Maggiore. The final phase was marked by an ever increasing tendency toward the Cavallinesque. However the Cosmati arrived at a pictorial art in their mosaics, their pictorial work shows a graceful and unpretentious interweaving with motifs from their decorative repertory.

During the 12th century the Cosmati were sculptors only on occasion, as in the case of the candlestick of S. Paolo and in some animal figures — lions and sphinxes — supporting portals in the Lombard manner. The study of classical work gave the Vassallettos a superior capacity to carve; this ability is exhibited in their decorative capitals (such as the one with the lizard and the frog in S. Lorenzo fuori le Mura), in the friezes of the portico of the same church, and in the cornice of the cloister of St. John Lateran.

Only Pietro d'Oderisio and Giovanni di Cosma included the human figure in their repertory; they may both be considered distant followers of Arnolfo di Cambio. It is possible that Arnolfo's innovation of giving an active colored background to low relief was suggested by Cosmatesque work; it was then imitated by Giovanni di Cosma in the relief of the Magdalen in St. John Lateran. Although there are Campanian works with reliefs against mosaic backgrounds, these do not seem to have exercised any influence.

The Cosmati were typical medieval craft workmen, functioning in family units and handing down the techniques of their art from father to son. Since training took place within the family circle, clear preferences for particular types of church furnishings or for certain designs emerged as the hallmarks of individual lineal groups.

Bibliog. K. White, Über di Cosmaten, eine römische Künstler-Familie des XIII. Jahrhunderts, Kunst-Blatt, 1825, no. 41, pp. 161–63, no. 42, pp. 165–68, no. 43, pp. 171–72, no. 44, pp. 174–76, no. 45, pp. 178–80, no. 46, pp. 182–84; C. Promis, Notizie epigrafiche degli artefici marmorari romani, Turin, 1836; C. Boito, Architettura cosmatesca, Milan, 1860; J. P. Richter, Die Cosmaten-Familien, ZfBk, XII, 1877, pp. 337–38; C. Boito, L'architettura del medioevo in Italia: I Cosmati, Milan, 1880: K. Frey, Genealogie der Cosmati, JhbPreussKSamml, 1885, pp. 125–27; G. Clausse, Les Cosmati et l'église de S. Maria à Civita Castellana, Revue de l'Art Chrétien, 1897, pp. 271–79; G. Clausse, Les marbriers romains et le mobilier presbytéral, Paris, 1897; A. Melam, I cosiddetti Cosmati, Arte e Storia, XVIII, 1899, pp. 26–27; G. Giovannoni, I monasteri sublacensi, I, Rome, 1904, p. 313 ff.; G. Giovannoni, Note sui marmorari romani, Archivio della Società Romana di Storia Patria, 1904, p. 5 ff.; A. Frothingham, The Monuments of Christian Rome, New York, 1908; G. Giovannoni, Opere dei Vassalletto, L'Arte, 1908, p. 26 ff.; A. Muñoz, La decorazione e gli amboni cosmateschi della basilica di S. Pancrazio fuori le mura, L'Arte, XIV, 1911, pp. 97–106; F. Grossi Gondi, La confessio dell'altar maggiore e la cattedra papale a S. Lorenzo in Lucina, Studi Romani, I, 1913, pp. 53–62; R. Jullian, Le candélabre pascal de St. Paul, Mél., XLV, 1928, pp. 75–99; F. Hermanin, L'arte a Roma del secolo VIII al XIV, Bologna, 1945, p. 59 ff.; E. Hutton, The Cosmati, London, 1950; G. Bendinelli, Intorno all'origine e per una nuova denominazione dei mosaici "cosmateschi," Studies Presented to David Moore Robinson, I, St. Louis, 1951, pp. 13–28; G. Matthiae, Componimenti del gusto decorativo cosmatesco, RIASA, 1952, p. 249 ff.; A. Piazzesi, V. Mancini, and L. Benevolo, Una statistica sul repertorio geometrico dei Cosmati, Quaderni dell'Istituto di Storia dell'Architettura, 5, 1954, pp. 11–19; Toesca, Md, p. 582 ff.; Venturi, III, p. 771 ff.

Guglielmo Matthiae

Illustrations: pls. 477–483.

## COSMOLOGY AND CARTOGRAPHY.

The world may be represented realistically as consisting of immediately visible objects: animals and plants (see ZOOMORPHIC AND PLANT REPRESENTATIONS), landscapes (see LANDSCAPE IN ART), the starry heavens (see ASTRONOMY AND ASTROLOGY), etc. — by images, that is, which despite their vastness are limited by the sensory experience of the human observer and which can never be more than parts of a greater whole. But from earliest times attempts have also been made to reconstruct, by an extension of this perceptible reality, a deeper, more integrated, and more complete cosmic reality which could be attained only through a conceptual process. By its very nature this reality was at first connected with religious ideas and was expressed through symbols or allusive forms; but it was later conceived rather as a concrete reconstruction, on a scientific basis, of the actual shape of the earth and of its surface. In every civilization cosmology provided a broad basis of inspiration for artistic phenomena, in the realms of architecture and artistic iconography. This inspiration is found in motifs dealing with the origin, order, and form of the universe, along with the relevant myths, and also in the broader symbolism of the "universal power," considered as a prerogative not only of divinity but also of royalty.

Cartography, on the other hand, is a graphic mode of expression which is by its very nature largely independent of esthetic goals; and yet during the long development that leads from the earliest sketches of primitive itineraries through portolanos to precise modern maps and charts, one finds a series of representations which in their elegant execution, their draftsmanship, and the inventiveness of their accessory ornament are related to painting. As a matter of fact, great artists contributed to some of these works, and it is apparent that artistic problems are involved in the study of this subject.

Summary. Cosmological ideas and allusive and symbolic images of the world (col. 836): Antiquity; The Occident; The Orient; Primitive cultures. Representation of the earth's surface as an artistic motif (col. 851): Primitive cultures; Ancient Near East; Antiquity; China; Korea; Japan; The Occident.

COSMOLOGICAL IDEAS AND ALLUSIVE AND SYMBOLIC IMAGES OF THE WORLD. The problem of the relationship between cosmology and art is especially apparent in primitive cultures. It has been studied particularly in connection with the Near and Far East, but it has also emerged as one of the most interesting problems of Renaissance and medieval art history. Although at present it is impossible to provide a clear and broad synthesis of a problem so complex and varied, one may remark that this relationship has three main aspects. The first is purely symbolic: a building, especially if dedicated to worship or if funerary in purpose (see ESCHATOLOGY), imitates the presumed principles of proportion of the universe and so strives toward a mystical assimilation into it. According to the Bible (I Kings 6), this was true of the Temple of Solomon; and in general the influence of this principle is seen in every monument which displays a marked search for proportion, for symmetry, or for a correspondence among its parts. The second aspect may be called allegorical: the structure is an attempt at a compendium or synthesis of cosmological elements which are clearly recognizable and are point for point associated with individual architectonic elements: the corners or sides are meant to represent the four parts of the earth, the column recalls the terrestrial axis, the square or circular plan stands for the earth or the sky as in the well-known temples in Peking, and so on, even to an extremely complex system of relationships such as we find in the long Syriac description of the Hagia Sophia at Edessa (Grabar, 1947). The third and perhaps most interesting aspect is purely imitative and therefore may be observed in painting as well as in architecture. The work of art (e.g., the archaic stupa) is intended to be a precise reproduction of the shape of the universe. In many unrelated cultures we find similarities in form and emblem which suggest a common cosmic implication: for example, the dome, either with or without a central opening; the pyramid; the tower; the mound or staircase; the canopy (which imitates the vault of the heavens); the egg or gilded ball, frequently an attribute of imperial power; the crown, etc. The greatest difficulty in the study of such forms arises from the amalgam of cultures present everywhere, as a result of which archaic cosmological concepts survive alongside other concepts either of a later period or foreign in origin.

Another aspect of the relationship between cosmology and the representational arts has been less studied although it is equally remarkable. It concerns the effect that a given stylistic trend may have on the astronomical conception of the earth found among the scientists of the period. A mind trained to seek a precise order will tend to attribute an analogously exact structure to the universe, producing a similarity of effect often highly significant. In the modern world it is instructive to contrast the ideas of Galileo — as they have been studied by Panofsky (1954) in their relationship to the visual arts — with the animistic concepts of Giordano Bruno, which are closer to the baroque taste. Such a line of inquiry may be conducted at least as far

back as Plato. In general, however, cosmological concepts are dominated by ideas of law and of order; and consequently they are reflected in plans for perfect cities formulated by utopians through the centuries and already realized, according to Herodotus, in ancient Persian cities.

*Antiquity.* The absence of cosmographic representations in the prehistoric and protohistoric periods in Europe can be explained in several ways. These cultures seldom expressed themselves in terms of abstract, speculative concepts. In their preurban societies, they lacked any true organization on the level of the state, but were governed rather by a tribal or clan organization in which a vision that systematized the world according to a complex hierarchical order had no place; moreover, they had no priestly caste sufficiently developed to be able to impose the theocratic concepts necessary to the creation of an integrated image of the universe.

\* \*

In Egypt the complex process by which religious concepts evolved makes it difficult to give a precise account of cosmological ideas. Nevertheless, we can distinguish certain basic elements common to various religious currents, as they emerge from a comparison of their respective iconographical representations. The gods, including those who personified elements of the cosmos, were not considered eternal, but were believed to have originated from the primeval ocean, Nun, defined as "the old one who first had origin." From Nun, the first creator god was born. According to the widespread Heliopolitan theological system, the creator sun god Atum gave birth to Shu (air god) and Tefnut (moisture goddess). Their children were Nut (sky goddess) and Geb (earth god). The latter two were united at birth but were separated by Shu to form sky and earth: the classic representation of the cosmos, which is found in drawings on papyrus (PL. 487), is composed of three anthropomorphic divinities — Nut above, her body arched, Geb reclining at the bottom, and Shu standing in the center supporting Nut. According to other conceptions, the celestial goddess is represented as a mammoth cow, or the sky is shown as an enormous ceiling resting on four supports. It was believed that the earth, with the Nile running through its central part, was surrounded by the ocean.

The most important element of the cosmos was the sun, personified as the divinity Ra (Rē'). According to a widespread belief, also represented in drawings on papyrus, every morning the solar disk was born of the sky goddess and undertook his celestial crossing in the diurnal bark accompanied by a cortege of minor divinities. Every evening the sun entered the subterranean world, a cavernous region traversed by a river similar to the Nile, which he crossed in the nocturnal bark in the midst of the acclamations of the spirits of the dead. Ra was opposed during his journey by the powers of darkness, headed by the serpent Apophis (see DEMONOLOGY). The iconography and nomenclature of the sun god vary in different theological currents: generally he appears as anthropomorphic and hawk-headed (Ra, Horus, Horakhte) or as simply anthropomorphic (Atum); sometimes he assumes the appearance of a scarab (Khepri) and at other times, of a golden calf, while during the nocturnal journey he has the head of a ram on a human body.

In the hierarchy of cosmic elements personified as divinities, the moon god I'oh (or Aah, masculine form of "moon" in Egyptian) occupied a position of little importance. The most important star, because its heliacal elevation coincided with the annual flooding of the Nile, was Sirius (Sothis), represented sometimes as the goddess Isis, sometimes as a cow. Orion (Sah), represented as a running man looking backward, also found a place among the major astral divinities; and finally, the four winds were considered divine beings: the north wind appears as a bull, the east wind as a hawk, the south wind as a lion, and the west wind as a serpent.

Sergio Bosticco

In the Near East the cosmological conceptions indicate an evolution from a predominantly mythical phase to a more conscious, meditative one. Such an evolution is naturally accompanied by a variety of interpretations. The Sumerians conceived of an original chaos that produced sky and earth, united at first in the primordial, cosmic mountain, suggested in the structure of the ziggurat (PL. 485). Such a concept is probably behind the epithet *kur-gal* ("the great mountain") given to Enlil, the god of air, who divided the two elements sky and earth.

The most complete exposition of Mesopotamiam cosmology is found in the initial verses of the Babylonian "Epic of Creation" (*Enuma elish*), which in its extant form, however, presents certain inconsistencies owing to substitutions such as that of Marduk for Enlil, the god originally celebrated. According to the *Enuma elish*, original chaos consisted of the sweet waters (Apsu), the sea (personified by the female monster Ti'amat), and a third element, Mummu, which is not clearly identified. The first creative act consisted of the separation of the fresh and the salt waters (one notes the appropriateness of this to the geographic conditions of Mesopotamia), which occurred with the creation of the divine couple Lahmu and Lahamu. In consequence of this separation the boundaries of the sky and the earth were defined, personified by the divine couple Anshar and Kishar. The couple An-Ki, that is the sky and the earth, must originally have derived from this union; but the Babylonian theologians, wishing to exalt Enki (god of the earth), father of Marduk, made Anu the son of Anshar and Kishar and the father of Nudimmut (another name for Enki). Like their progenitors, both Anu and Nudimmut were elements having the form of a disk. The final phase of the cosmogony is found in the fourth book of the same poem, where Marduk (being substituted for Enlil), after having conquered and killed Ti'amat, cuts her in two and covers the sky with one of the halves. The world, therefore, appears to be composed of the two vast superimposed disks (the earth and the sky), held apart by the air (or by a mountain) and surrounded by the sea. In other texts the creation of the world appears as the work of a divinity (Anu, Enki), and the universe is seen as a sphere with a series of superimposed heavens, the last of which is that of Anu.

These ideas derived from literature have little in the way of iconographic equivalents. The symbolic representations of the world hitherto known in Mesopotamian art are limited to illustrations of some partial aspect of the cosmos (PL. 487). The representations of the foreparts of bulls (some with human heads), united at the backs, are frequently found in the minor arts, especially in carved gems, and symbolize the mountains in the midst of which the god of the sun, Utu or Shamash, arose. The freshwater ocean, or Apsu, is sometimes represented as a gigantic nude man in a horizontal position, sometimes as a river with human heads at the two ends. The sky appears as supported by figures of animals stretched upward; among these the scorpion and the man-scorpion predominate. In regions subject to Egyptian cultural influence, however indirect, the sky appears as a winged disk (Horus). In Anatolia and Mitanni it is at first supported by one or more pillars, in accordance with an old Indo-European concept; later, local influences transformed the pillar into a "tree of life" (see GEMS AND GLYPTICS). In Assyria the winged disk seems to be supported by a genius or man-scorpion. The sun god in a boat is a fairly frequent subject on seals; it is not clear, however, whether the daily voyage across the sky is represented, or rather the nocturnal voyage from west to east on the ocean, as suggested by the presence of the boat.

Giovanni Garbini

Some 18th- and 19th-century scholars believed that a cosmological symbolism was present and operative in the monuments of the classical world, but this belief was a result of projecting Egyptian and Near Eastern cultures on the classical and was not based on fact. The determining influence was rather that of the application of geometrical laws. In the antique world geometry was, in fact, a required branch of study for every cultured person and hence for every artist. This requirement accounts for an artistic vision of the external world that proceeded from the laws of optics (see OPTICAL CONCEPTS) or perspective (q.v.) or, when referring to man, from the canons of

proportion (q.v.) based on the human figure (q.v.). The measurement of the earth led to the measurement of the cosmos, and man's dimensions were seen as a yardstick for the universe.

Geometry, which evaluates every measurement of the earth in terms of theoretical schemes, relates to the laws of symmetry, by means of which a single unit of measure is established for a variety of aspects of nature; these laws, in turn, point toward that eurythmy which reconciles many symmetries in a harmonious whole and thus leads to the concept of the classical (see CLASSIC ART). Cosmology and cartography play a part in these rhythms, or space-time relationships, because they coordinate the earth and the space surrounding it in a harmonious whole, the universe. The sole point of contact for these two realms lies in their relation to a lowest common denominator, the plane; and this fact accounts for the representation of the earth and space as a great surface containing a central nucleus, the earth, and a band that circumscribes it, the cosmos.

It was discovered that natural and man-made objects having elevation — mountains, cities, constructions — could be represented in profile against the plane surface of a map with those "multiple perspectives" traditionally held to have been invented by Kimon of Kleonai about the end of the 6th century B.C. and transferred from maps to the figure-adorned monuments of other times and cultures. An example is the Antonine Column, in Rome, on which a group of soldiers, seen in profile, hasten in boats — those too in profile — to cross a river seen in a cartographic perspective, that is, from above.

During the Alexandrian period one finds in the Mediterranean area architectural phenomena that bear the marks of astrological and cosmological symbolisms perhaps deriving from the Orient. Certain architectural elements such as the great perforated dome of the Pantheon have obvious parallels in Oriental buildings almost certainly invested with cosmological meanings. Similarly the no longer extant Septizonium, a kind of architectural screen on the Palatine in Rome, which was to be seen from the Appian Way, is believed by some scholars to have alluded, in its division into seven stories, to the seven spheres of the planets. There are frequent instances (see ASTRONOMY AND ASTROLOGY) of astral and celestial symbols in various decorations often expressive of the purpose of the building involved and of its religious program (as perhaps in the Temple of the Sun at Baalbek).

Of particular importance for the subsequent development in the Byzantine and medieval periods were cosmological allusions in the decoration of imperial palaces and in symbols of power, such as the throne, the canopy, the scepter, and the crown (see SYMBOLISM AND ALLEGORY). There can be no doubt of the bond between these conceptions and the symbolisms of the Near East.

* *

In ancient Iran cosmological symbolism occurred in the arts and architecture: witness the city of Ecbatana (Herodotus, I, 98) with its seven surrounding walls of different colors, probably meant to correspond to the seven planetary spheres; their diminishing height from the center to the periphery presents an obvious parallel to the great towers of Babylonia and Assyria. Apparently within the innermost circle, which was of gold and corresponded to that of the sun, was the dwelling of the king, who, seated at the center of his cosmos, identified himself in that manner with the divinity. The Parthian Darabgerd and the Sassanian fortress of Firuzabad are examples of cities with circular plans that were probably inspired by analogous symbolisms.

One of the most remarkable monuments in the Sassanian epoch was the throne of Khosrau II. According to the Arab Tha'ālibī of Nishapur, the throne room was surmounted by a dome in gold and lapis lazuli in which were represented the movements of the heavens, the stars, the signs of the zodiac, and the seven planets. According to an independent description of this room found in Theophanes and alluded to by Cedrenus, the ceiling of the dome of the royal chamber bore a representation of Khosrau seated on his throne and surrounded by the sun, moon, and stars. Another text, the *Martyrologium*

of St. Adus, who died in 870 (Migne, *Patrologia Latina*, vol. 123, col. 356), replaces the movement of the stars and planets with the movement of the throne room itself, which is said to have rotated on its axis by means of horses. The fact that according to Hesychius the royal chamber was actually called "heaven" by the Persians (οὐρανός; cf. Hesychius, s.v.) indicates that a cosmic symbolism of this sort must have been common in Sassanian royal palaces.

In the minor arts, this range of ideas is reflected by the so-called "Cup of Khosrau" in the Cabinet des Médailles in Paris (PL. 490). The center of this cup is a sort of clipeus in which a Sassanian king is shown seated on a throne supported by two horses (alluding to the sun?). Over the ruler's head is placed a crescent supporting a sphere (the earth?), symbols associated with Sassanian royalty. The insets that surround the central clipeus represent the stars. Similar symbolic themes appear in the Sassanian silver plate found at Kazvin, now in the Archaeological Museum, Teheran, and in another silver plate found at Klimova, now in The Hermitage, Leningrad (PL. 490).

Raniero GNOLI

*The Occident.* Under the influence of Christianity the West saw a great flowering of cosmological iconography. This was a consequence of the persistence of antique custom, the taste for metaphor seen in many writers and theologians, and the wide absorption of the Hebraic symbolic tradition. As E. B. Smith (1950) has pointed out, "Between the 4th and 7th centuries... churchmen were formulating a mystical conception of the architectural House of God as a symbol and manifestation of divine Presence... Many of them accepted literally the ideas running through the Book of Isaiah, where God is presented as builder of the world. For the most part they based their imaginative concept of the universe on the statement: 'He that established heaven as a vaulted chamber and stretched it out as a tent to dwell in' (40:22). Furthermore, to such late antique men, accustomed to visualize an earthly kosmokrator as enthroned beneath his celestial baldachin, there was the specific implication of a vaulted covering in the words of the prophet: 'The heaven is my throne, and the earth is my footstool: where is the house ye build unto me?' (Isa. 66:1)."

Domes, except for those in baptisteries, were primarily a feature of Eastern Christian architecture. And not only does the dome have celestial implications, but the entire church building is conceived as a microcosm in accordance with the concept transmitted to us by Cosmas Indicopleustes. Clear proof of this has been found in a Syriac hymn describing the Church of Hagia Sophia in Edessa. The "Essence," it says, resides in the Holy Temple and "it is something truly admirable that its smallness should be similar to the vast world." The dome is comparable to the "Heaven of Heavens" and is decorated "with mosaics of gold like the firmament with brilliant stars." The four arches represent the four sides of the world, the three façades the Trinity, the light from three windows the mystery of the Trinity, the five doors the five virgins, the columns the apostles, the nine steps leading to the throne of Christ the nine choirs of angels. A. Grabar (1947) holds that the form of this and of other Byzantine churches was actually determined by their iconography and their inherent symbolism. E. B. Smith (1950), though he believes that meaning has not necessarily created form, does maintain that ideas and not structural interests occasioned the use of the dome in Byzantine architecture.

In those churches for which the dome was the determinant factor, it also became the form-giving element creating vast interior spaces; one would be tempted to conclude that these buildings were conceived as a coherent and organic entity were it not known that the plan of Hagia Sophia in Istanbul (II, FIG. 774) conforms closely to that of the Basilica of Maxentius in Rome. The existence of this prototype proves, on the one hand, the overwhelming importance of the great dome (not present in the basilica) and, on the other, disproves the idea that the entire church was a replica in miniature of the universe. The cosmological themes, in fact, appear to be limited to a few structural elements and to the decorative scheme. In Hagia

Sophia the pendentives of the dome and the four arches (alluding to the four sides of the earth) produce a curved shape resembling a four-sided tent pegged down at the corners, on which there rests the celestial dome, pierced by windows (I, PLS. 378, 379; II, PLS. 427, 428).

Another richly developed theme was that of the Heavenly Jerusalem, described by St. John in the Book of Revelation and greatly eleborated by St. Augustine. One of the reasons that some contemporary scholars have interpreted religious buildings as images of the Heavenly Jerusalem is that it can be proved that antique basilicas imitated in abbreviated form the cities in which they were erected. But while it is true that the basilica was eventually connected with the Heavenly Jerusalem, the derivation of its shape from this symbolism is not proved (FIG. 842).

Sedlmayr (1950) advanced the hypothesis that for the Middle Ages the cathedral also represented the Heavenly Castle, symbolized explicitly during the Romanesque period in the many towers of the churches. According to E. B. Smith (1956), however, the towers owe their origin to a survival of Roman imperial symbolism. There is no doubt, however, that the medieval church is rich in symbolic motifs, at least in the orientation of some of its architectural elements (columns, windows, episcopal throne, etc.) and in the decoration, which E. Mâle (I, II) long ago interpreted as a true encyclopedia of all knowledge. Furthermore, the orientation to the four cardinal points and to the four sides of the world reveals an intention to relate the building to the cosmos. The starry vaults may have represented the heavens, and perhaps men still understood the labyrinths on pavements in mosaic and other media as the earth and the underworld (PL. 486). The rose window (I, PL. 397) had already become a cosmic symbol in the early Middle Ages, as had many other motifs popular from Carolingian times on. There is at least one concrete example of derivation from the City of God in the Book of Revelation. This is the plan of an ideal city described by Eximeniç (Eiximenez) in his *Crestia*.

The relation between architecture and cosmological ideas was even closer, or at least better documented, in the Renaissance, when an imitation of the cosmos was attempted which was concrete as well as symbolic. Naturally the conceptions behind the representations of buildings of the time are not always the same, so that the general picture is at once rich and confused. In general, medieval ideas persisted; many great architects continued to base their plans on traditional schemes, particularly Filarete and Leonardo. In his architectural treatise Filarete offered a plan of the town Sforzinda, consisting of two squares superimposed to form a star shape inscribed in a circle (PL. 484). This is an antique motif found in Roman mosaic pavements, on church façades, and in manuscripts. Today its significance would be lost were it not that writers of the Middle Ages had clearly interpreted it as a cosmic symbol. This is attested by illustrations in medieval codices in which the seasons of the year, the four elements, the four winds, and the four corners of the world are arranged in just such a scheme of two superimposed squares. Sometimes the actual words and names are inscribed in circles. In other instances figures symbolic of these conceptions are arranged in the same fashion. This scheme alludes to the world and to the universe. The *Hypnerotomachia Poliphili* makes it clear that this idea was still held valid in the Renaissance, and a 17th-century commentator on Sacrobosco's *Sphere* used the same two superimposed squares to represent the cosmos. Filarete's Sforzinda was widely imitated in the "ideal cities" of the Renaissance; they sometimes had a symbolic meaning, and some of the patterns were actually put into execution by military engineers.

A. Chastel has pointed out that there is no literary evidence for cosmological influences on Leonardo's architecture. One drawing by the artist is of particular importance in this respect, however. It is an interlace which, according to Heydenreich (1954), was probably the point of departure for projects for St. Peter's by Bramante and others. A similar interlace can be found on the ciborium in S. Ambrogio, Milan, in a decoration on the throne of Solomon in an illustrated copy of the *Hortus deliciarum* of Herrad von Landsberg (now destroyed), and in

chancel barrier panels. All these parallels occur on sacred objects and must therefore have more than just a decorative significance. Ultimately these motifs go back to antiquity; a simple interlace is found in a mosaic floor of Roman Britain, where it is combined with the meander motif, a theme analogous to the labyrinth. Leonardo's most intricate interlace designs are his famous knots with the inscription "Academia Leonardo da Vinci" and the much-restored frescoes in the Sala delle Asse in the Castello Sforzesco, Milan. Coomaraswamy (1944) has called these knots "a map of the universe in the precise terms of Dante's lines in *Paradise*, XXIX, 31–36." There is, furthermore, in Piacenza Cathedral a medieval labyrinth which is compared to the universe in an inscription beside it. It seems impossible, therefore, that Leonardo had used this scheme for the plan of a church without knowing its traditional symbolic

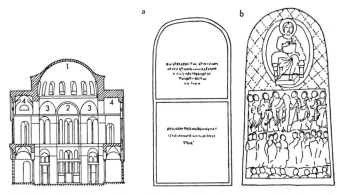

*Left*: St. Luke in Phocis, Greece, interior of church, ca. 1000. The Heavenly Jerusalem according to the architectural and mosaic layout of Byzantine churches: (1) Christ and the angels; (2) the Virgin; (3) evangelical scenes; (4) saints. *Center and right*: Illustrations from a treatise on cosmography by Cosmas Indicopleustes, 6th cent. (*a*) Schematic image of the world; (*b*) the same scheme showing the positions of God, angels, and men (*from Symbolisme cosmique et monuments religieux, 1953*).

meaning. We also have two plans by Leonardo, one of which occurs again in Serlio, for a central-plan church with circular chapels surrounding it on all sides (PL. 485). Curiously, these patterns have an antecedent in a Cosmatesque pavement mosaic in Westminster Abbey. The same pattern is found in a 10th-century manuscript at Göttingen (Universitätsbib., Theol. fol. 231), in which the four elements inscribed in circles are attached to a central circle containing the Year with busts of the Sun and the Moon in his hands. The whole is surrounded by the series of the twelve months, forming once more an abbreviated version of the universe. This latter plan is found again in G. B. Montano's 16th-century publication, *Scielta di varii tempietti antichi*. As we have seen, Leonardo left no written statement of his intention to create an image of the universe in his churches.

At about the same time, however, Francesco di Giorgio Martini, whose treatises Leonardo knew, provides some evidence in this respect. For him, man was a microcosm closely related to the macrocosm. Consequently, he wanted buildings to follow the measurements and proportions of the human body, so that they too would be images of the universe. Actually, Leonardo also shared this theory. His famous drawing of the Vitruvian man within the square and the circle, incorporated by Cesare Cesariano in his edition of Vitruvius, was proclaimed the perfect proportional measurement by Luca Pacioli, a friend of Leonardo. Nonetheless, Leonardo seems somewhat bound to medieval ideas, and by comparison Alberti, who lived earlier, seems more "modern" and directly anticipates Palladio. Alberti and Palladio followed Platonic and Neoplatonic conceptions of the universe. They tried to imitate not a presumed shape of the cosmos but its inherent order. Alberti was primarily concerned with religious buildings. Palladio, on the other hand, applied his geometrical principles and harmonic proportions chiefly to villas, perhaps in connection with that cult of the countryside typical of Venetian culture. We have his

statement, "The little temples we make ought to resemble the very great one which by His immense goodness was perfectly completed by one word of His" (*I Quattro libri dell'architettura*, Venice, 1570, Book IV, preface).

During the Renaissance the ancient symbolism of the dome as the heavens reemerged. Palladio says of the Pantheon that it "contains in itself the figure of the world," and when Vasari speaks of the Cathedral of Florence and its domical crossing, he calls it a "universal church." Michelangelo intended to create in the Medici Chapel in Florence an abbreviated image of the universe with its spheres arranged hierarchically one above the other. The lowest zone with tombs is the realm of Hades; the intermediate one with its rich architectural decoration represents the terrestrial sphere; the light-filled zone of lunettes and dome alludes to the celestial sphere. In realizing this program Michelangelo found it necessary to employ sculpture. Other artists similarly achieved their symbolic expression by recourse to a synthesis of the various arts. As in the Middle Ages, sculpture and pictorial decoration often served to clarify the cosmological significance of a building, which might not be apparent from its plan or elevation alone. The constellations in the dome of the Old Sacristy of S. Lorenzo, Florence, for example, allude to the date of the end of the schism between the Greek and Roman churches. The astrological decoration in the Ottoheinrichsbau in Heidelberg lends the building a cosmological significance, and there are other similar examples. The frescoed ceiling of the Farnesina in Rome is famous. Less well known are the representations of the planets on the ceiling of the Town Hall in Posen (Poznań). A late survival of such ideas, which are perhaps more astrological than cosmological, is seen in the Chapel of the Imperial Monastery of the Dominicans on the island of Hispaniola.

After the Renaissance and particularly during the baroque period, man's changed view of the universe led to a break with traditional symbolism and iconography. Nevertheless, the old conceptions often reemerged, as in the Città del Sole of Campanella.

In the 17th and 18th centuries, although the taste for circular forms survived, usually in consequence of the persistent revival of classical antiquity (e.g., in C. N. Ledoux and A. L. T. Vaudoyer, who designed a circular "House of the Cosmopolitan"), symbolic schemes that represented cosmological concepts by then obsolete became empty and meaningless. During the baroque period, however, the new sense of space, which seemed to reflect Bruno's limitless and centerless infinities, found expression in religious architecture. And as Chastel has pointed out, the great decorative devices (catafalques, table ornaments, etc.) still had close ties with cosmology. He also notes that not even in the 20th century has cosmological meaning ceased to be applied to architecture. Just as Hadrian re-created all the wonders of the Roman Empire at his villa, so does modern man, in his various world exhibitions, attempt to encompass the growing world in a small territory.

Frank Lloyd Wright's project for the Golden Triangle in Pittsburgh shows a relatively superficial sense of cosmic symbolism, and a similarly questionable intention is evident in Rudolf Steiner's Goetheanum at Dornach, Germany. For 20th-century architects the desire to re-create the universe seems for the most part unconscious and involuntary. Yet there is no evidence of a genuine disappearance of this theme, to which architecture may well owe its original concern with monumentality and its abiding attempt at representation.

Susanne LANG

In addition to the direct representations of the earth in cartography, and the symbolic and allegorical allusions to the universe in a variety of forms and at different epochs in architecture, there are many other links between the arts and man's conceptions of the universe. If we limit ourselves to iconographical evidence and avoid the uncertain ground of the relationships between space and time (see SPACE AND TIME), we must recognize the importance attached in the Renaissance and later times to the representation of sacred or political subjects against a backdrop of open skies or landscapes that frequently contain heavenly or demonic apparitions or else are charged with a dramatic pathos. The poetic effect of Giorgione's painting is in large part a result of the twilight or nocturnal setting, the representation of which forms an essential part of the composition. Leonardo da Vinci, as is well known, attempted to accompany his battle scenes with backgrounds showing corresponding movement and convolution, also relating them to the cartographic and geological investigations he himself had undertaken. Later, while the Counter Reformation was condemning astrological representations, great popularity attached to the motif of celestial glory against a luminous background: in this connection particular mention should be made of Tintoretto's *Paradise* in the Doges' Palace in Venice. The great baroque allegorical frescoes of Pietro da Cortona and Andrea Pozzo and all of German rococo developed an increasingly explicit cosmological allusiveness marked by the personification of the elements, the areas of the earth, etc. Meanwhile northern European painting (e.g., Elsheimer's famous nocturne in Munich with the Flight into Egypt, and certain turbulent landscapes by Ruisdael) had pioneered a new taste for the rendering of nature in a highly evocative manner that calls to mind the great scientific illustrations for the treatises of Kircher (PL. 489) and others, which often seek almost unconsciously to emphasize the uncertainty of the human condition amid a virtually Lucretian battle of the elements. This is a theme which was to pervade the poetry, literature, and painting of the romantic period (note in this connection Géricault's *Raft of the Medusa*, Louvre, VI, PL. 118), which was not without reason deeply interested in the baroque.

In modern times topographical and cosmological iconography has declined, at least as a stimulus to the artistic imagination. In recent years, however, and especially in the realm of nonobjective painting, there has been much concern with this matter. Some modern movements, such as vorticism and spatialism consciously assume a cosmological orientation; many works and artists could be cited in illustration. We shall limit ourselves to mentioning Mondrian (q.v.), whose writings show his conscious intention of expressing the forces controlling the universe, in a nonobjective mode, by means of a system of spatial and proportional balances. That to this end he should have had recourse to a checkerboard structure which had already had a cosmic and magical significance to a variety of civilizations is another indication of the vitality of the symbol (PL. 486).

Eugenio BATTISTI

*The Orient.* Notwithstanding the religious and cultural differences due to the strains of Brahmanism (Hinduism), Jainism, and Buddhism, Indian cosmological concepts appear sufficiently unified to be treated under a single heading. The world was seen as having the shape of a sphere or an egg, and it was thought to consist of two equal halves, as is seen clearly from Vedic and post-Vedic texts, in which it is called "Brahmanda" or "Egg of Brahma." On the basis of the customary geometrical schematization, it was further thought that the disk of the earth, surrounded by the ocean, was situated at the center beneath the luminous vault of the heavens and was divided into quadrants in accordance with the four principal directions. Originally, however, the earth was thought of as a single and undivided disk. It was only later, with the acceptance of the earth's curvature, that an immense central mountain was conceived as dominating the earth disk; around it the stars were thought to revolve in concentric orbits. (A Western parallel for this conception is seen in the Byzantine manuscript of Cosmas Indicopleustes in the Vatican Library, Vat. gr. 699.) The "King of the Mountains," Himavant (Himalaya), was probably originally considered that central part of the earth and was later replaced by Sumeru or Meru — etymologically the name is still uncertain — in that role in all three systems. Brahmans and Buddhists conceived of it as of four different colors corresponding to the four principal directions, following a color symbolism dominant in central and eastern Asia, which penetrated deeply into Indian iconography as well.

On the basis of these primitive developments, the Indian cosmos was destined to have a dualistic aspect. The upper and lower worlds were in an opposition similar to that between light and darkness. The world of the sky, the realm of the stars and light, was the home of the gods and the final resting place of the "innocent," that is, of the pure victims, the heroes, and of the ascetics free of passions. The subterranean world, on the other hand, the abyss and the realm of darkness, was not only the home of the demonic spirits, but also a place of punishment for the wicked.

This primitive image of the world developed with the passage of time and became populated with imaginary personages. Two numbers enjoyed roles of particular prominence in the organization of the world: first the number three and later the number seven. The predominance of the number three is attested by many passages in Vedic and post-Vedic literature as well as by Jain texts, which speak of three worlds, the celestial, terrestrial, and infernal, each of which is subdivided into three parts, with three heavens, three continents, and three subterranean worlds. It is possible but not certain that the number seven, which gained prominence later, was related to the knowledge of the seven planets. The Brahmans conceived of the world as being of seven layers of increasing thickness from bottom to top. In the realm of the terrestrial world it was held that the central continent, Jambudvīpa, was divided into seven regions by six parallel mountain ranges. In the lower world, at first the Brahman system recognized seven Patalas, which were legendary areas located in layers one above another and were the habitations of demonic divinities, with their respective colors recalling their Babylonian prototypes. Later these were replaced by infernal regions in the lists of whose names the number seven is almost always conspicuous.

The same observation may be made with respect to the Jain system as well. The three heavens found in the primitive mythology were increased in number, and the same was true of the rings of oceans and continents. The division of Jambudvīpa into seven zones by mountain ranges was, however, adopted. And although for the most part the number three was dominant in connection with the mythical realms of the lower world, the number seven prevailed among the infernal regions lying beneath these regions.

Even in the most ancient of the canonical Buddhist texts we find the concept of seven celestial regions and seven corresponding infernal regions. Yet speculation concerning the possibility of new heavens or at least of new categories of gods finally brought to eight the number of the infernal regions; and the same happened with respect to the parts of the earth.

The final phase of the development of Indian cosmography prior to the rise of modern natural sciences remained basically restricted to astronomical treatises and consequently had no influence on the religious systems, which continued to be based on the concepts found in the sacred writings.

One may conclude that it is virtually impossible to speak of cosmographic and cartographic representations in ancient India based on actual experience. It is true that the geographical treatises in the Purāṇas and in other works provide lists of peoples that were probably real; but we do not as yet know of any cartographic reproductions corresponding to these lists. Manuscript miniatures such as those found in the *Lokaprakāśa* (Florence, Bib. Naz., Ms. Indiano 625) or the *Trailokyadīpikā* (Poona, Deccan College, Ms. 603, Collection VIII of 1875–76), or larger drawings, prints, and the like are in fact limited to representing mythical illustrations of the earth and its inhabitants. There is a possible exception in the drawings of Bhāratāvarṣa (i.e., India), conceived as being on the southern border of Jambudvīpa, which bear indications of Indian rivers, and occasionally in those of the city of Ajodhya (Ayodhya).

Willibald KIRFEL

In Serindia, the region north of India including the Pamir Mountains and the Chinese province of Sinkiang, the prevalent cosmological concepts were those of the major religious currents, especially Buddhism. One is confronted with symbolic forms ranging from astral ones on corridor ceilings to those associated with the image of the Buddha identifying him with the axis of the universe about which the major heavenly luminaries move. In these representations Iranian influences are particularly evident, although at times they may extend no further than the symbolic use of color. The decoration of domes — false domes, that is to say, for this is an architecture in stone — is also connected with cosmological ideas; and the dome itself is representative of the vault of the heavens in its concavity.

An interesting development in Buddhist architecture in Central Asia is the construction that A. von Le Coq has termed the lantern roof. This is formed by a series of diminishing squares in which the corners of a smaller square rest on the midpoints of the sides of the larger that lies immediately beneath it. When reduced to a purely decorative role, this motif also appears in pictorial ornament and sometimes dominates the center of flat or slightly concave ceilings in grottoes, recalling an architectural structure that originally consisted of wooden beams, which are in some cases meticulously traced in the rock. This structural element occurs throughout an immense area including most of Inner Asia, China (in various periods), Kashmir, Tibet, and even the Caucasus and Armenia. It is found in a certain type of house, consisting often of a single room with a central opening designed as an outlet for smoke, which sometimes serves as an entrance reserved for the men, while women and children have a secondary, half-subterranean entrance. The upper opening represents the point of passage between the celestial and phenomenal worlds, in accordance with a conception that the three worlds (celestial, phenomenal, and infernal) are placed one above the other and are in direct communication with one another, for those who are able to descend or ascend freely from one to another (such as the shaman). Extremely varied legends, as well as the rites of shamanism, allude to this possibility. When Buddhism came into contact with these currents of thought, it assimilated them, despite a certain early hesitation; and thus it is that one finds grottoes dug into the rock with the lantern roof, which was by then purely symbolic.

The tents of the nomads and Siberian constructions in wood also represent the contrast between earth and heaven or — from the religious point of view — the contact and integration of earth and heaven. Functional requirements, easily met in a variety of ways, are not inherently extraneous to a symbolic structure. Thus there has persisted to the present day the custom, which goes back to the Han dynasty, of grouping the rooms of a square house around a central court known as the "well of heaven" (*t'ien-tsin*). The result is a sort of magic square formed by eight smaller houses arranged about a ninth in the center, as one sees already in the perspective drawings of the Sung dynasty (cf. the reconstruction in the *San-li-t'u* of the so-called "House of the Calendar": Ming T'ang). R. Stein has demonstrated that it is in this central court, where the waters flow together, that one enters into contact with the divinity of the soil and that at the same time one is in communication with the heavens. The Han house, the traditional ordinary Chinese house, has a precedent in the double habitation from the Chou dynasty which consisted of a group of raised rooms resting on a partially or entirely subterranean nucleus. The tomb in China may also be interpreted as both a house and a model of the earth. This is proved by the symbolism of the Shang tombs which have their entrances from the south, like Chinese capital cities, and have a hole containing a dog (the dog as psychopomp) at the center beneath the bier. Further proof is the tomb of Emperor Ch'in Shih Huang-ti (late 3d cent. B.C.), which attempted to achieve a complete image of the universe. Similarly in Korean tombs, such as those of the Koguryo dynasty on the Yalu (5th–6th cent.), the terraced ceiling, a variant of the lantern roof, symbolized the heavens and has paintings of signs of the zodiac.

The Chinese scheme is dependent upon the notion of a space consisting of the four cardinal points surrounding a central point. At the same time the idea of the multiple superimposition of worlds was translated into the architectural form of the tower (pagoda). This form was probably adopted from Buddhism, which in China and in the countries under Chinese influence

abandoned the classical form of the stupa and replaced it with the tower containing a square or octagonal base (referring to the points of the compass). The clearest artistic development of Chinese cosmological concepts is to be found in the Temple of Heaven at Peking (FIG. 847). In a vast spatial organization defined by enclosing walls, various units are arranged along the longitudinal axis: the sacrificial area; the pavilion which holds the tablet of the sky and is the seat of the divinity; and another construction enclosed within a square walled area with entrances at the four points of the compass. The sacrificial area with its circular plan rises on three concentric platforms linked to one another by three stairs at each of the four compass points. Each flight of stairs consists of nine steps and corresponds to the nine heavenly ranks. The pavilion is covered with blue tiles symbolizing the sky and is supported by eight piers which correspond to the eight directions. A similar structure is located at Hué in Vietnam (FIG. 847) in the area set apart for the triennial

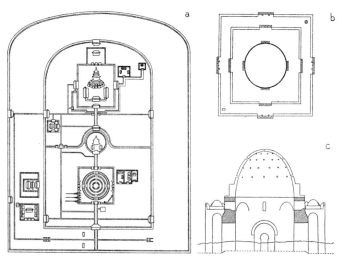

Cosmic symbolism in architectural forms. *Left:* (a) Peking, Temple of Heaven, schematic plan (*from drawing by De Groot*). *Right:* (b) Hué, Vietnam, area of the triennial sacrifice to heaven, earth, and ancestors; (c) Ctesifon, Iran, Qasr-i-Shīrīn, section of the main domed building (*reconstruction by O. Reuter, SPA, I*).

sacrifice to heaven, earth, and ancestors. Here a square yellow elevation (since the earth was thought of as square and yellow) holds a further circular elevation covered with a blue awning symbolizing the sky. The scheme relating a square base and a circular elevation is found elsewhere, for example in the stupa (as at Borobudur, PL. 485), although this latter is not a representation of the cosmos but of the cosmic mountain, the axis of the universe. A similar scheme is found in the mandalas (literally, "circles"), which as Tucci points out are "psycho-cosmograms" in that they symbolize the structure of the universe and, by means of the symbolic values of the various figures, induce the spirit of the meditator to unite itself with the primal essence of the cosmos symbolized in the center. The mandala was especially popular in Tibetan Tantric Buddhism (PL. 486).

Returning to Central Asia, we find the circular city of Koy-krylgan Kale in Khwarizm, which derived perhaps from the military encampments of the Assyrians (PL. 484) and which must have had similar symbolic associations. In the legendary plan of the city of Ecbatana the different colors of the seven encompassing walls (Herodotus, I, 98) were apparently meant to correspond to certain astral configurations. Such correspondences are found in India as well, and from them is derived some of the typical color symbolism in the representational arts. The best-known example, of Babylonian origin, is perhaps lapis lazuli (Skr., *vaidurya*), which symbolizes the vault of the sky.

Mario BUSSAGLI

When Indian cosmological concepts penetrated into the countries of southeast Asia, they found there an exceptionally

fertile ground where they could be expressed in architectural forms of a completeness and grandeur that surpassed anything found in India itself. The Indian conception of space, and by extension of the cosmos, is expressed less by philosophic systems than by the popular religious sentiment flourishing in Tantric currents. Space and time are the two great expressions of divine power, which is conceived as a center of light from which the circle comprehending all directions radiates. The divinity — whether Buddha, Śiva, or Viṣṇu — stands at the center with the devout soul, which enters into communion with him. The temple, as a sacred place, is thus always a center around which the various parts of the cosmos are arranged. In contrast, the profane space is more or less consciously perceived as disorder and chaos. During the rite both the space chosen by the devout soul and also his body itself assume a cosmic value. In many mystical schools in India the ritual is preceded by a true "universalization" or "cosmic transformation" of the body, onto which are projected, by means of certain ceremonies, all the spaces of the external world; these spaces are represented in their turn by the mandala and by the temple. Not infrequently this is a reciprocal process; so that if the temple reproduces the structure of the cosmos, the cosmos may be thought of and meditated upon as a temple, within one's own body.

In the cosmology of southeast Asia, as in that of India, the world sphere is bisected along its diameter by a flat plane which represents the actual earth. The center of this circle is occupied by the mountain Meru — the home of the gods or, more precisely, of their terrestrial epiphanies — in the form of a gigantic golden lingam which has the earth as its pedestal (*pīṭha*). It is surrounded concentrically by seven continents separated by a corresponding number of seas. The two halves of the sphere are occupied by lower and upper worlds of varying number and character according to the various schools.

Such a cosmological conception is at the basis of the architectural structures of Cambodia and Indonesia. In the temple of Phnom Bakheng (Angkor, Cambodia), constructed about 900, the central tower with seven levels represents Meru. About it are 108 towers, which represent the length of a cosmic period. By a trick of perspective the number of towers visible from each cardinal point is only 33, and this is the number of the gods inhabiting the mountain Meru. In the temples of Angkor Wat and of Neak Pean at Angkor, circular or quadrangular canals arranged around the temple represent the oceans that separate the various continents surrounding Meru. In the Bayon of Angkor Thom, the axis of Mt. Meru is continued beneath the earth, by a well. The central cell, access to which is denied to the public, was occupied during certain astronomical recurrences by the king, who identified himself with the divinity by placing himself in this way at the center of the cosmos. The Buddhist temple at Borobudur in Java (PL. 485), on the other hand, is a gigantic mandala (which at the same time reproduces the cosmic mountain in immense proportions). Through the various zones of the cosmos, represented by the parts of the building, the devout reach the circular terrace at the top and return to the point of origin of all things. In the architectural motifs of the building the spiritual itinerary of the faithful is repeated. After having passed through the various planes of samsara (the world of birth and death), they arrive with a sudden leap at the plane of the unconditioned (for which there is no preparation), at nirvana, to which there is an allusion of sorts in the bareness of the central terrace. A curious fact is that the images of the infernal worlds, artistically highly accomplished, were probably intended to remain permanently buried beneath the earth.

Raniero GNOLI

*Primitive cultures.* Most primitive peoples have explored in nearly parallel fashion the traditional great divisions of the universe and the problem of their origin. Sky maps, zodiacs, calendars, images of the universe, and systems of correspondences between the elements making up the universe have been represented both by constructions of fixed proportions and by symbolic figures and decoration.

In Oceania art is generally associated with important theo-

gonic myths. In spite of the diversity of the individual societies and the physical distance between the island cultures, some common characteristics can be pointed out. On bark paintings executed by the Australian natives of Arnhemland, C. P. Mountford has noted many representations of stars and constellations closely related to myths. The native constellations of the Crab (the head of Hydra) and the Scorpions (in Lynx), Orion, the Pleiades, the Magellanic Cloud, the Southern Cross, and the Milky Way are found in feminine form when in conjunction with the sun and in masculine form when in conjunction with the moon. They are anthropomorphous or zoomorphic and are always related to some cosmogonic myth. According to W. Schmidt, the sun and moon are frequently represented on objects belonging to the secret societies of the Bismarck Archipelago. M. Mauss has pointed out the microcosmic significance of the tiki of the Maori, known through many representations, phallic and anthropomorphous, sculptural and pictorial.

With respect to pre-Columbian America, H. Lehmann (1953) has noted that the fire serpents which decorate the interior of the cosmic temple of Mexico City represent the visible course of the sun, and that the 365 niches of the pyramid of Tajín stand for the 365 days of the year (PL. 485). The great porphyry disk of Tenochtitlán (now Mexico City), incorrectly called a calendar, gives the hieroglyphs of the 20 days that surround the face of the sun god who presides over the present world (II, PL. 19). The various Mexican codices carry no text, but their illustrations can be interpreted through the explanations given to the first Spanish chroniclers by the Aztecs. Some leaves of the Codex Cospianus (Bologna, Italy, Univ. Lib.) represent calendar systems in which the signs relative to the days of the liturgical year are combined with figures of the gods corresponding to the cardinal points. Other drawings from the Codex Borgia symbolize the Milky Way, the stars of the Northern and Southern Hemispheres, the planet Venus, the sun, and the moon. On a page of the Codex Fejarvery-Mayer (Liverpool, Free Public Mus., Ms. 12014) we see the present world at the center and the four preceding worlds at the four ends of the cross. On another sheet the world is shown subdivided into five parts, the center and the four cardinal points. An analogous symbolism is found among present-day primitive peoples in America.

The architecture of the ceremonial chambers (kivas) of the Pueblo is dominated by cosmic symbolism: some elements record the passage of mythical ancestors from the underworld to the surface of the earth. The plan of the "village of the great kiva" shows the ancient development of this type of religious architecture. In the same way the complex structure of Bororo villages (Brazil) "reflects a cosmic and metaphysical system," according to Lévi-Strauss (1936). They are divided into eight clans, each including three sections, and their plan recalls that of ancient Cuzco. Among the Hopi (southwest United States) the Seleko Mana katchina (anthropomorpous figure of cult character) "contains in his person such meteorological phenomena as clouds, the rainbow, rain, etc." The *salimobra* masks of the Zuñi "are painted in colors which refer to the elements, seasons, and cardinal points." The altar of the *newekwe* confraternity of the Zuñi "has on its upper part a long band of carved and painted wood which represents the Milky Way as a girder of the sky. The circular figure in the center is the sun surrounded by the seven stars of Ursa Major. The black and white semicircles as well as the inverted green pyramids are clouds. At the end of these hang bats, which announce rain, while 'birds of the zenith' surmount the whole."

The archaeological evidence from central and southern Africa testifies to an advanced cultural level. The terra cottas of Nok, the monumental architecture of Zimbabwe, now attributed to the ancient Bantu, the bronzes of Ife and Benin, and the clay statuettes of Chad, the Cameroons, and the Sudan all pose problems for the archaeologist and historian. In most cases, the absence of texts permits only hypotheses on the symbolic value of the representations. We must note, however, the carving of a wooden plate found in a cave not far from Zimbabwe, which represents in a crude fashion the signs of the zodiac, the sun, the moon, a group of stars, a triangle,

and four plaques with triangular dotting (II, PL. 19). L. Frobenius (1936) identified "the cosmic mountain and the four supports of the sky" in the royal "chairs" of wood from Dahomey and Togo, while on the carved wooden disks of Merca in Somaliland (IV, PL. 86) he found "the image of the sun at the center surrounded by a double band representing the ocean, and an exterior crown divided into four parts according to the cardinal points." Furthermore, he attributed a similar symbolic significance to the bronze disks from Benin and to the wooden plates from Ife which were used by diviners. The pictorial and sculptural arts and the architecture of the various peoples of the Sudan have as their primary purpose the expression in concrete terms of a series of symbols, and it is perfectly clear to the eyes of initiates that they refer to cosmology. In every aspect of their form and color and in every detail of their execution (period, instruments, materials used) and of their generally ritual functions, they relate to mythical events.

Pictorial art occupies a privileged position. For the Sudanese the world was created through the mental act of a single god and was made manifest in symbols before its material realization. Among the Dogon such signs and symbols present four successive phases. The first series is made up of 266 fundamental ideograms, called *bummo*, of fundamentally abstract character, in which the symbolic value of numbers, an essential element in Sudanese cosmology, intervenes. Each *bummo* is made up of segments corresponding to the four basic, indispensable elements of life — fire, air, earth, and water. The second series, *yala*, is made up of dotted sketches of the object or creature represented. It is the basis for the subsequent series, called *tonu*, diagrammatic forms leading to the final category, called *toy* or *toyum*, which represents objects and beings in their realistic aspect. The various series evolved from these fundamental elements include several thousand pictograms and consist of 24 parallel categories which provide a systematic classification of all the constituent parts of the universe. The execution of the pictograms is connected with ritual occasions. They are used on the walls of caverns prepared for initiation rites, on the façades and interiors of dwellings, and for various ceremonies.

A comparable study can be made of statuary. For example, in sculpture representing mythical figures, the anatomical details indicated are related to events in the cosmological myths in which these personages participate. Similarly, a basket woven in a spiral pattern reproduces an image of the internal vibration animating the "seed" from which the universe emerged, and is its "sign" or "symbol." The bands of cotton used in the manufacture of clothing — for which the number of component parts is also fixed — have designs and colors symbolic of the wearer's position. Among the Bambara a *koso wala* ("picture blanket"), consisting of alternate squares of indigo and white with polychrome motifs placed irregularly but according to a precise order, represents a complex system of stars, constellations, and such meteorological phenomena as rain, thunderbolts, rainbows, etc. (PL. 486).

The architecture, too, is entirely permeated with cosmological concepts. The "great family house" of the Dogon is a complex made up of several sections placed around a central space; its plan symbolically represents the mythical creator lying on his right side in the act of procreation. The structure is inscribed in an oval representing the "placenta" issued from the creator seed, from which in the course of time everything contained in the universe has come. In the house of the supreme chief of the Dogon, the Hogon of Arou, as in the family houses, rectangular niches on the façade are symbolically related to the cultivation of rectangular plots of land. On the chief's house are two rows of eight rectangular niches adorned with black, white, and red geometric paintings. Each niche is dedicated to one of the 16 kinds of grain given to men by the creator in mythical times. Over the door are representations of the sun, the moon, the stars, and the imprints of the "sandals" of the chief on the ground he possessed but might not tread barefoot. Like the paintings in totemic sanctuaries, these are repainted every year with the necessary variations.

Comparable paintings are executed during the septennial rite in the Malinke sanctuary of Kangaba, which is called the

"vestibule of the Mande (Mandingo)" and is considered the prototype of all Sudanese totemic sanctuaries. It is dedicated to the silurus, the first and most important animal connected with totemic taboo. The circular building is constructed in the image of the first "seed of the world," which God realized in accordance with the "signs," and from which the universe emerged. It is covered by a straw roof which represents the unwinding spiral of the initial vibration by which this "seed" was animated. The paintings represent stars, ancestors, grains, and primordial fields.

In Dia four sculptured doors have been found, associated with the four directions of space. The zoomorphic sculptures in low relief are based on a symbolism of both number and position, and they reflect the categories and the whole familial organization and social structure of the people "born of the Mande" (PL. 488).

A carved, painted, or woven object such as a mask may reflect a series of meanings, all equally valid. Thus the *kanaga* of the Dogon, which to the uninitiate is simply a bird, for the initiate means "the gesture of God creating the heavens and the earth." At the same time it represents the vanquished enemy of the sacrificial hero, as well as the fox dying of thirst and lying on its back with raised paws begging the pardon of its creator. The function of the mask is to exhibit these meanings simultaneously.

In its symbolic and dynamic character, the present-day Negro art of central Africa faithfully reflects a system of the world that is both theoretical and empirical. Certain details concerning mythical cartography, ornamental symbols in architecture as well as in representatve objects, and the "long calendar" of these peoples (connected with the heliacal rising of Sirius) pose problems of the historical links between the African world and the Mediterranean, particularly ancient Egypt.

On the occasion of the exibition of prehistoric rock paintings collected by H. Lhote at Tassili (Algeria), a Fulah, Amadou Hampaté Ba, recognized in the frescoes of the bovid period the principal themes of the initiation of Fulah shepherds; he maintained that most of the scenes had a cosmological function.

Germaine DIETERLEN

REPRESENTATION OF THE EARTH'S SURFACE AS AN ARTISTIC MOTIF. It is virtually impossible to trace in all its complexity the gradual evolution from a symbolic to a realistic representation of the universe and the earth. Certain bonds may be detected, however, between the objective of realistic description and the employment of symbolism. Topographic maps often aspired to artistic value and were executed in precious materials (even during the Middle Ages and the Renaissance); they were displayed in places with a religious or other exalted function; in brief, they had an unquestionably esoteric character. Recourse to symbolism was a preliminary condition of cartographic representation, which, until the adoption of a bird's-eye perspective, common from the 16th to the 19th century, was essentially two-dimensional and therefore unable to represent topography except by means of an allusive technique.

The importance of "realistic" cartography as an artistic phenomenon naturally varies with the times, according to the interest in geographical exploration on the part of the political and cultural elite and according to the adaptability of a given pictorial style to such a theme. Particularly felicitous instances are seen in pre-Columbian America in the use of lively pictograms and fantastic conventions; in the "symbolic" views of medieval cities, which have a clearly magical feeling; in Leonardo's forceful sketches; in the admirable Renaissance and baroque perspective views; and in modern graphic art, where one finds — albeit for the promotion of tourism — a free use of forms and colors with undeniably decorative effects. The many fantastic insertions in the marginal illustrations of medieval manuscripts almost deserve to be placed in a separate category; but it may be mentioned that in nearly all cases the artist has been inspired almost exclusively by literary and mythological sources and above all by traditional astrological and cosmological motifs. This fact provides further evidence of the link between the symbolic and the realistic methods of representing the universe, a link which is never wholly destroyed.

*Primitive cultures.* Primitive peoples use any available means and materials in making maps. They draw diagrams in snow, sand, and earth and inscribe bark, wood, and skins.

In the nautical relief maps in the Marshall Islands (Micronesia), already in use in precolonial times, knots or shells represent the position of the islands in the archipelago, and the lines joining them represent marine currents (PL. 499). The rigorously geometrical form of some of these maps, the veneration in which they were held, and the unwillingness of the natives to discuss their significance all tend to confirm the theory of J. Wanamaker (1919) that they were primarily objects worshiped as the symbols of an occult science. Rudimentary topographical representations are found on certain Australian message sticks: circles and ovals in white indicate lagoons and shallow lakes, while the courses of rivers, points, trees, etc., are traced in carving.

In pre-Columbian Mexican civilizations, graphic records of journeys by land or water were required of merchants, whom Aztec authorities considered the official explorers. The reports of the Conquistadores show that these ancient maps were detailed and reliable. They were for the most part painted on a fabric made of agave fiber. The painted maps executed by natives after the Conquest may provide some idea of their nature: a handsome example is the Metlaltoyuca (Puebla, Mexico) map (London, Br. Mus.). The boundaries of districts and cities are represented along three sides by a narrow black line, on which are painted the hieroglyphs of cities and mountains; at the top border is a broad roadway, which runs from right to left as shown by the footprints that appear there. The Aztec indicated roads by means of yellow or purple bands, with footprints along their entire length; cities were represented by the symbol for their name, and if, as was usual, they were on top of a mountain, by its symbol as well. In the Metlaltoyuca map one may observe at the right a river with three tributaries, represented by a blue stripe within which black lines mark the current of the water. The map is completed by various hills, the symbol of a temple, family genealogies, and various date formulas, which are obscure to us.

The Tepetlaoxtoc map (PL. 494) is surely of the colonial period: it is part of the manuscript of the same name at the British Museum and was painted on European paper perhaps toward the middle of the 16th century. Tepetlaoxtoc signifies "cavern in the rocks," and the usual hieroglyph indicating the city is a huge open mouth placed on rocks or on a straw mat resting on a rocky layer. In the map in question, however, the symbol is somewhat different. It is a hill with an open mouth almost at the peak. It is not known whether this was meant to indicate Tepetlaoxtoc or a neighboring city. The mountain chain covered with forests is probably part of the Anáhuac, which includes the Valley of Mexico. Other details are a torrential river that rises in the mountains and flows to the left in a straight line, and streets, hills, rocks, and a "temple."

A manuscript in Basel (PL. 492) includes another important Mexican map, in the Mixtec style. It is the plan of a city, as yet unidentified, accompanied by a series of genealogical figures.

In a class by itself is the great topographic map on rock found at Sayhuit, near Abancay in Peru; lines and zoomorphic figures are cut into it: the former represent the rivers, and the latter indicate symbolically the regional topography — monkeys for the forests, llamas for the plains, condors for the mountains.

The pictographic ivory carvings of the Alaskan Eskimos also attempt to represent landscape, with hills indicated by wavy lines and plains and the surface of the sea by straight lines (see ESKIMO CULTURES). An Aivilik Eskimo of Canada could trace the outline of the coast from the Churchill River to Lancaster Sound, that is, for a tract of over 900 miles. The nautical maps of the Angmagssalik Eskimos of eastern Greenland (Copenhagen, Nationalmuseet) are sculptured in wood.

Very little has survived from protohistoric Europe. Two stone inscriptions of Valcamonica, Italy, seem to reproduce a section of the cultivated valley according to a rigorously planimetric representation, in the most ancient of the styles of Val-

camonica and Monte Bego carvings (similar maps, but in a re-duced and schematic form, are found in both these groups); they probably date from the first half of the 2d millennium B.C. The group of houses and human and animal figures in vertical projection on one of the two maps are an addition from a some-what later period, as is shown by their different manner of execution.

An alternation between planimetric views and vertical projections in cartographic representations seems to have taken place in the Near East: witness the large painted vase of Tepe Gawra, Iraq, and the incised silver cup of Maikop, U.S.S.R.

\* \*

*Ancient Near East.* The oldest existing map of a region is inscribed on a Babylonian clay tablet (ca. 2400 B.C.) and repre-sents a river valley, possibly the Euphrates, with mountains drawn in a fish-scale pattern on either side. Directions are in-scribed in circles. The accurate cadastral surveys made in the Tigris-Euphrates and Nile river valleys are important for the history of cartography. An early survey of this kind was con-ducted in Babylonia during the reign of Sargon I (ca. 2300 B.C.). The practical importance of maps in Babylonian life is indicated by the hundreds of surviving clay tablets containing plans of districts, towns, town walls, estates, temples, houses, and military camps. An example is a plan dating from about 1200 B.C., which shows the fields and canals near Nippur. Six townships are indicated. Probably the most interesting of such tablets is the plan of Nippur unearthed during excavations conducted by the University of Pennsylvania (PL. 493). The accurate measurements of this carefully drawn plan guided the archaeologists in excavating Nippur and in identifying structures.

Cadastral surveys were conducted at a fairly early time also in Egypt. A great survey conducted by Ramses II (ca. 1250 B.C.) located boundaries of estates. A papyrus in the Museo Egi-zio in Turin, dated about 1320 B.C., shows a rather detailed dia-gram of an Egyptian mine. Another papyrus in the Turin mu-seum depicts the triumphal return of Seti I (ca. 1300 B.C.) from Syria and shows the road from Pelusium to Heroopolis and a canal with crocodiles and fish.

The oldest existing map of the world (PL. 493) is a clay tablet in the British Museum, dated about 500 B.C. The cuneiform inscriptions locate Babylon in the center with the Euphrates River running through the city. The islands refer to neighbor-ing cities. Neighboring countries are also indicated, and sur-rounding them is the circular ocean known as the "Bitter River." Beyond it are triangles, which may represent the seven climates or foreign countries.

*Antiquity.* Shortly after the opening of the great age of Greek colonization in the 8th century B.C., the Greeks began to make maps of the territories they had discovered. Strabo attributes to Eratosthenes a statement that Anaximander of Miletos, pupil of Thales, was the first to publish a geographical map. In his *History* (V, 49), Herodotus recounts that during an Ionian revolt against Persia, Aristagoras, tyrant of Miletos, gave Kleomenes, king of Sparta, a bronze tablet on which was engraved "the whole earth, with all its seas and rivers."

During the Alexandrian period, Eratosthenes (ca. 220 B.C.) was able to produce a map based on astronomical principles by using the recorded observations of Pytheas, a Greek navigator, and others. Hipparchus, the greatest astronomer and mathema-tician of ancient Greece, also made significant contributions to cartography; he criticized Eratosthenes' map and proposed as a more scientific basis for cartography accurate astronomical observations for determining latitude and longitude according to a division of the earth's surface into 360 degrees.

Because they controlled a vast empire, the Romans naturally developed an interest in maps. Consequently, we have plans of military camps and battle formations, of highways and routes used in campaigns; greater still was the Romans' activity in compiling maps of the colonies and municipal property registers. References to maps are numerous in early Latin literature: Augustus directed Marcus Agrippa to map the entire empire,

a project that required more than 20 years to complete. In 7 B.C., five years after Agrippa's death, a marble copy of his map was erected in Rome and became the source of innumerable other maps and itineraries. It is usually believed that the so-called "Peutinger Map" (PL. 493), probably executed in the 3d century, is derived from the map of Agrippa. The Peutin-ger Map is in the form of a parchment roll 21 ft. long and 1 ft. wide, obviously designed to be folded or rolled in a portfolio. Because of its dimensions the world is flattened out, and countries are distorted almost beyond recognition. It traces the course of over 50,000 miles of paved highways from Britain and Spain to China. The map contains 534 illustrations; 311 of these refer to Europe, 62 to Africa, and 161 to Asia. Rivers, including the Nile, run east and west; the Adriatic, the Mediterranean, and the Black Sea resemble canals, and some areas, such as the Nile delta, receive especially detailed treatment for administrative reasons. The distances recorded between places are fairly ac-curate. Eleven segments of the map have survived, but that with the British Isles and the Iberian peninsula has been lost.

Cartography, like other branches of Greek science, reached its culmination at Alexandria late in the Hellenistic age. Ptol-emy's *Geography* (ca. A.D. 150) was considered an authorita-tive book for the compilation of maps. In world maps known to be inspired by this book, the size of the Mediterranean is grossly overestimated, Scotland is placed almost at right angles to England, the Black Sea is too far north, the Caspian Sea has a horizontal rather than vertical position, India does not have a triangular shape, Ceylon is fourteen times too large, and the Indian Ocean is enclosed by a great land mass extending from eastern Asia to the African continent.

Ptolemy's *Geography*, despite its inaccuracies and misconcep-tions, had a good effect upon medieval geography. Wherever it was circulated and translated, as among the Arabs, it raised the level of cartographic studies. Geographers in western Eu-rope, however, generally followed Latin encyclopedic traditions instead of Ptolemy, and it was in geography that Latin encyclo-pedic science was most deficient.

In the early Middle Ages Biblical authority was frequently used to refute the theories of a spherical earth and human habitations in the antipodes. It produced fantastic theories such as the Orientalizing one of Cosmas of Alexandria, known as Cosmas Indicopleustes, a merchant of the 6th century who sailed on the Red Sea and the Indian Ocean; he later retired to become a monk and wrote a work entitled *Christian Topography*. Such theories as his provoked interesting attempts at stylistic translation, as, for example, in architecture.

William H. STAHL

*China.* Chinese cartography, which is of fundamental im-portance to the Asiatic world, may be divided into five periods: (1) ancient, until the end of the Chin dynasty (A.D. 1234); (2) Mongol or Yüan (1234–1368); (3) Ming (1368–1644); (4) Westernized, chiefly as a result of the activity of Jesuit geogra-phers (1600–1842); (5) modern, since 1842.

The earliest examples of Chinese cartography are based pri-marily on cosmogonic concepts. The five cosmic elements — metal, wood, water, fire, and earth — are represented by means of trigrams deriving from the *I-ching*, or *Book of Changes* (ca. 175 B.C.). The simplified and diagrammatic representations of heaven, earth, wind, fire, water, thunder, mountains, and rivers contributed to the development of geographic maps (*t'u*). The oldest world map (*shan-hai yü-ti-t'u*) of Chinese origin is a square map of China surrounded by the four seas (*ssŭ-hai*), according to the cosmological concept of Tsou Yen (ca. 336–280 B.C.). The pictorial character of Chinese cartography is immediately apparent.

In ancient China, landscape painting and map drawing be-longed to the same class of art, as was also true for many cen-turies in the West. Chinese cartography may be formally traced to 227 B.C., when Ching K'o made a map of China for the prince of the kingdom of Yen. It is known that in 99 B.C. an itinerary map of western China was in the possession of General Li Ling. There are many evidences of map making during the Han

dynasty (206 B.C.–A.D. 221) and the subsequent centuries. The most prominent early cartographer of China was Chia Tan (730–805), who compiled a general map of China and her neighbors in 801. The brothers Li Chi-fu and Li Tê-yü made a political map of China (806–20), and in 821 Yüan Chen compiled two maps of the northern part of the Chinese empire. At the beginning of the 11th century Cheng Tu offered Emperor Chen-tsung his two newly made maps of China, and in the same century Shên Kua invented the relief map. A map of China and adjacent countries, a kind of world map perhaps printed from wood blocks, was in existence about 1043. The earliest extant maps of China, however, are those engraved on stone by Yü Ch'ih (1137 and 1142). A third map, compiled in 1193 by Huang Shang, was engraved in 1247.

During the Mongol period China was influenced by Persian, Arabian, and, through those sources, Byzantine geographic knowledge. With his map of China compiled in 1320, in this period, Chu Ssǔ-pên exerted an important influence on Chinese geographic tradition up to the introduction of modern European science in the 19th century. His "terrestrial map" (yü-t'u) was revised and made into an atlas by Lo Hung-hsien in 1541 and was published again in 1555, 1558, 1561, 1566, 1572, 1579, and 1799, under the title of Kuang-yü -t'u (PL. 498). The 1579 edition had a wide influence on European studies, especially through the work of the Jesuit missionaries Matteo Ricci (d. 1610), Martino Martini (d. 1661), Michael Boym (d. 1658), and others. The original of the first world map of Li Tse-min (ca. 1330) is lost, but the Korean version of 1402 is preserved.

The Ming (1368–1644) and Ch'ing (1644–1912) dynasties are conspicuous for their geographical literature including the great Ming Gazetteer (ca. 1461) and the Ch'ing Gazetteer. The Ming atlas of 1564 contained two world maps. These were later reprinted in 1595 together with a general map of the world in the descriptive geography and atlas, Kuang-yü-k'ao, by Wang Tso-chou. Also famous was the 24-volume description of the Chinese empire, the Kuang-yü-chi, of Lu Ying-yang, published in 1600 and again in 1686.

The first 16 volumes of the great Ming encyclopedia, published between 1607 and 1610 (San-ts'ai t'u-hui), show the influence of Jesuit teaching, in particular that of Matteo Ricci, who published his famous Chinese world map in 1584. It was reprinted in 1596 and had several later editions. Copies after this map by Giulio Aleni are in the Bibliothèque Nationale, Paris, and the Ambrosian Library, Milan (PL. 498).

Until the 19th century, two schools, one traditional, the other Westernized, existed simultaneously in China. To the Westernization of Chinese knowledge in the 17th century the following men contributed: P'an Kuang-tzu; Chu Kuo-ta, Lo Chung-min, and Ch'ien Wei-ch'i; Ch'ên Tzǔ-lung and Wu Kuo-fu; Fêng Ying-chin, a friend of Ricci; Chu Mou-wei; Ch'êng Yu-yü; and, particularly, Chiao Hung and Li Pên-ku, disciples of Ricci and authors of a very important work, the Fang-yü shêng-lüeh, a combination of geographic text and atlas, full of geographical, statistical, and economic data. Among the Europeans, in addition to Aleni, were Ferdinand Verbiest (d. 1688) and Joachim Bouvet (d. 1730). The first important geographical measurements were undertaken by order of Emperor K'ang-hsi (1662–1722) and led to the compilation of an atlas of China. The measurements were also used for the Description de l'empire de la Chine, a European atlas of China in four volumes published in Paris in 1735. With the suppression of the Jesuits in China in 1773, there was an arrest in the development of scientific knowledge. The 18th century is characterized by local geographical dictionaries and illustrated topographical reports.

In the 19th century the important figures are the geographers Wei Yüan and Hsü Chi-yu and the compiler and editor Ch'ên Li, initiator of modern Chinese cartography and cosmography. Credit should be given also to the missionaries whose translations and compilations founded contemporary Chinese cosmography and geography.

*Korea.* After the 11th century cosmography and cartography were introduced from China into Korea. The Korean version of the world map of Li Tse-min (ca. 1330) dates from 1402 and was prepared by Ch'üan Chin, who corrected the maps of Korea and added Japan. Another map of China, by Ch'ing-jui (1328–92), was brought to Korea in 1399. These two maps were combined into a new one, of which there exists a colored copy from about 1500 (ca. 5 ft., 4 in. × 4 ft., 6 in.).

The traditional Korean atlases, containing 13 maps, were compiled from the 15th to the 17th century; we have faithful copies in manuscripts from the 18th and early 19th centuries. It was customary also in the Buddhist monasteries to have maps pasted on screens as decorations; usually these were world maps or general maps of Korea. The earliest atlas and description of the Korean peninsula was compiled in 1481 by the king of Korea, Cheng-tsong. In the 16th century several atlases were block-printed. Among the preserved manuscript maps, which are of little scientific value, are several world maps, Chinese in origin and limited in their scope to continental Asia (including Persia). A world map of Buddhist character is included in an illustrated Korean encyclopedia compiled between 1562 and 1577. The first scientific and modern maps of Korea appeared only after its annexation by Japan in 1910.

*Japan.* Until Japanese cartographers underwent Western influence in the 17th century, they followed Chinese models exclusively. The first known attempt at map making dates from the reign of Emperor Kōtoku (A.D. 646–54). Cadastral maps were compiled during the Nara period (710–84). There also exist four gazetteer-reports called *fudoki*, which were executed throughout Japan at the order of Empress Gemmei (708–23). A regional map dates from 738.

The appearance of wood-block-printed maps should be associated with the beginning of printing in Japan in 770. The first general map of Japan is perhaps that compiled in 784. A sketch map of Japan from the end of the 8th century is known through a copy of 805. A map of the Buddhist world (*Go tenjiku zu*, or the "Map of the Five Indies") was brought from China to Japan in the middle of the 9th century. We also have a 19th-century copy of a map of Kyoto made in 1200, a map of the Buddhist world drawn by the priest Zukai in 1365, and a copy, made in 1806, of a map of Edo (Tokyo) from about 1457. A map of Japan was printed in 1595. Maps of the Western world and of Japan, painted on screens, appeared about the same year. In 1605 there was in the Imperial Palace a copy of the world map (ed. 1600) of Matteo Ricci.

With the beginning of Western relations and especially with the Jesuit missions, Western maps and atlases were imported to Japan, and the influence of the Dutch and English was felt through their sojourns at Hirado and Deshima. Western influence was superimposed on the traditional cartography of the Chinese type. Printed atlases of Japan appeared in the second half of the 17th century. In 1789 an *Atlas of the Western World* was published in Edo in 15 volumes. In 1790 the most prominent of the scholars under Western influence, Shiba Kokan, published his *Account of Travels in the West* in five volumes, and in 1792, his world map, the first copper-engraved world map in Japan. In 1796 a new and complete map of the Western world was published at Edo. From the second half of the 19th century Japanese cartography was identified with that of the West, although traditional examples persist.

In addition to those on screens, plans and maps (principally road maps or water-route maps) were also executed on hanging or horizontal scrolls or in accordion-folded volumes. Maps in Japan, however, always have had a more esthetic than utilitarian character. The Buddhist type of map belongs to the religious iconography. Until the middle of the 19th century, the maps were printed from wood blocks in color.

In a category by themselves are the landscape views published in voluminous works such as *Views of Prominent Places on the Tōkaidō* (6 vols., 1795) and *Noted Places in Kyoto* (11 vols., 1780–87).

Boleslav SZCZEŚNIAK

*The Occident.* Cosmographic representation of the earth had little importance throughout the earlier Middle Ages. The medieval world maps were developed on the basis of antique

COSMOLOGY AND CARTOGRAPHY

copies after Martianus Capella, Macrobius, Isidore of Seville, and others whose works contained representations of the earth; they were gradually perfected with the aid of direct experience.

The clergy were among the first to produce these maps; as is well known, Pope Zacharias (741–52) had one painted in the Lateran in Rome. The cosmography found in the *Historiae* of Paulus Orosius (completed in 418) generally served as a model. The world map in the *Commentaries on the Apocalypse* compiled by Beatus of Liebana (d. 798) and known through numerous illustrated copies is also of particular importance. Other noteworthy maps are those by Heinrich of Mainz (1110), Guido of Brussels (1119), and Lambert of Saint-Omer (1120–25); the map in Hereford Cathedral by Richard of Haldingham (ca. 1280; PL. 494), which shows Jerusalem at the center of the world, in the form of a wind rose with eight points, and contains a representation of the Last Judgment; the great planisphere formerly in the Ebstorf monastery, probably painted by Belmont in Lüneburg in 1284 (PL. 494); the Psalter map painted in England in the 13th century; and the map of the world which Ranulf Higden (d. 1364) included in his history of the world.

Familiarity with the Holy Land was of great importance for European Christians; and maps of Jerusalem, Bethlehem, and other cities, as well as of Constantinople, were drawn as early as 700 by St. Adamnan, the Abbot of Iona (Scotland). The mosaic map of Palestine in the church in Madaba, an episcopal see from the 4th through the 7th century, is of great importance (PL. 494). After 1300 the maps of the Holy Land became more numerous as a result of the frequent journeys to Palestine. In his *Holy Land*, published in Mainz in 1486, Bernhard of Breydenbach included a woodcut by Erhard Reuwich representing Palestine from Sidon to Alexandria and Damascus, with Mecca and the pyramids in the background. Later there appeared an essentially archaeological type of representation showing Palestine with its holy places as they are described in the Bible (*Liber chronicarum* by H. Schedel in 1493 with three woodcuts of Jerusalem; maps by Hans Asper of 1525, J. Ziegler of 1532, G. Mercator of 1537, Oronce Finaeus and Tilemann Stella of 1552–57). Peter Laickstein visited Palestine in 1556 and compiled a map published by C. Sgrooten in 1570 in his *Terra Sancta*. The Old Testament type of map survived for some time, as, for example, in the *Speculum orbis terrae* by Cornelius de Judaeis (1593) and in the *Atlas major* (1629) by Willem Janszoon Blaeu. Eighteenth-century heirs to this convention are the *Terra Sancta* of M. Seutter, the *Atlas minor* of Tobias K. Lotter, and the *Terra Sancta* of J. B. Homann, as well as the maps published by M. Seutter in his *Deserta Aegypti, Thebaidis, Arabiae, Syriae*. An extensive map of Jerusalem and of the Church of the Holy Sepulcher was published in 1722 by De Pierre, *Eques SS. Sepulchri* (Bamberg, Staatliche Bibliothek, Atl. ggr. 12, no. 83–84).

Even before 1300, mariners were using the compass along with maps and portolano charts. There were Italian portolano charts, limited to the Mediterranean and the western coasts of Spain and France, and Catalan charts which included all of the world as it was then known. In the oldest nautical maps, as in the so-called "Pisan Chart," only the coasts and names of coastal towns were indicated; later the cities and regions were indicated by means of crests, as in the chart by the priest Johannes (Giovanni di Carignano), of Genoa, which dates from about 1310. There is much detail in the nautical maps by Angelino Dulceti of 1339 and Mecia de Viladestes of 1336 and in the *Catalan Atlas* of 1375. The so-called "Borgia Planisphere" in the Vatican Museums dating from the first half of the 15th century is of inlaid enamel on a great plate of colored copper; in its original condition it was further adorned with semiprecious stones. The navigational map by Grazioso Benincasa (Ancona, 1482) is decorated with boats, some with oars and some with sails; unfortunately it has survived only in fragmentary form.

After 1500 navigational maps became maps of the world. Notable examples are the map of Juan de la Cosa of 1500, which includes the earth from America to Asia; the world map of Diego Ribero e Sevilla of 1527; and the map of Domingo Olives of 1568. The transition from navigational to more conventional maps may be seen in the *Carta marina* of Martin Waldseemüller of 1516 and in the map of Europe by John Rotz of 1542. Particular mention should be made of the *Carta marina et descriptio septentrionalium terrarum ac mirabilium rerum in eis contentarum diligentissime elaborata* by Olaus Magnus (1539) and the handsome navigational map of Giorgio Calapoda (1552; PL. 500).

Noteworthy examples of the period of transition between medieval and modern maps may be seen in the world maps of Fra' Mauro of Murano (d. 1460) and of his collaborators (Venice, Biblioteca Marciana; PLS. 491, 495).

The world map in the form of a globe, devised by Johannes Stabius, decorated and carved in wood by Dürer in 1515, does not contain the numerous confusing inscriptions in the maps of Mauro. A woodcut in the *Novus orbis* of Simon Grynaeus (Basel, 1532) shows a terrestrial sphere projected in an oval form. The stylistic quality of this planisphere, together with the fact of its publication at Basel during the period when Hans Holbein the Younger was living there, permits the hypothesis that it is a product of the latter's circle.

Certain other world maps should be mentioned: the copperplate published at Venice about 1560, *Totius orbis descriptio*; the *Cosmographia universalis et exactissima iuxta postremam neotericorum traditionem* published at Venice in 1581 by Giovan Francesco Camocio; the *Theatrum orbis terrarum* of Abraham Ortelius (1570).

L. J. Waghenaer published *Dess Spiegels der Seefahrt, von Navigation des occidentalischen Meers* at Amsterdam in 1589. The *Geographia Blaviana*, or *Atlas major*, of Willem Janszoon Blaeu and Jan Blaeu of 1641–47 is distinguished for its handsome frontispieces to the various volumes. Of particular note is the *Nova totius terrarum orbis geographica ac hydrographica tabula*, with the seven planets and the seven wonders of the world represented at its upper border.

There were maps of cities as early as the time of Charlemagne. These include the square plate containing a map of Constantinople and the round plate with a map of Rome, both of which are mentioned in Einhard's biography of Charlemagne.

The oldest city maps extant include one of Florence, from 1472; a bird's-eye view of Rome made between 1490 and 1538; one published by Michele Tramezini (1561) and one of Florence by Lorenzo Benvenuto della Volpaia (ca. 1560). There is a view of Venice by Leon Battista Alberti (1472); a 16th-century bird's-eye view of Venice is in the Vatican (PL. 497).

There are maps and views of the major German cities in the *Liber chronicarum* of H. Schedel (1493), in the *Cosmographiae libri VI* of S. Münster (1550), and later in the *Civitates orbis terrarum* of G. Braun and F. Hogenberg. Georg Seld designed a large map of Augsburg, of which many woodcut copies were made (1521). A large round map of Nuremberg was made about 1510 by Georg Glockendon; and there is a large view of the same city, *Das ist Nurenberck* by Hans Wurm (1559). Individual squares and streets were engraved on copper in 1599 by Lorenz Strauch and in 1715–25 by J. Adam Delsenbach. J. Murer made a handsome map of the vicinity of Zurich in 1566, and in 1576 he designed a bird's-eye view of the city that was engraved by Fryg. Many cities appeared in the *Topographia Germaniae* of Matthias Merian in 1642.

The house of G. Braun and F. Hogenberg published a great atlas, *Civitates orbis terrarum* (Cologne, 1576–1618). It was compiled with the collaboration of Joris Hoefnagel of Antwerp, who had traveled throughout Europe from 1560 on, drawing whatever seemed to him worth noticing, and of the painters Hendrick van Steenwyck (1576), Lucas van Valkenborgh (before 1593), Nicola Aginelli (1566), Alexander Colyns and Lodewyk Toeput (before 1590), Gerd Hane (1588), Egidius van der Rye (before 1617), and Pieter Bruegel (before 1617), who drew the Strait of Messina with Etna in the background. On the commission of Count H. Rantzau, Daniel Frese depicted the cities of Heide, Meldorf, Bardewick, Plön, Odense, Copenhagen, and the island of Hven with the observatories and instruments of the Danish astronomer Tycho Brahe. The atlas is incomplete; it includes only cities of special interest and cities for which there was a commission. The favorite illustrations were those by Hoefnagel, which were

COSMOLOGY AND CARTOGRAPHY

very picturesque (views of Cádiz; Seville; Poitiers; Tivoli with its waterfalls; the Roman Campagna; Naples with Vesuvius; the antiquities of Rome and Ostia; Venice with St. Mark's, the Campanile, the Clock Tower, the Piazza, and the burning of the Doges' Palace in 1577; and, finally, Antwerp).

A true monument of cartography is the *Liber chronicarum* (*Nuremberg Chronicle*) of H. Schedel (Nuremberg, 1493), with woodcuts of famous cities and places, frequently fantastic ones. There are also faithful reproductions, however, such as that of Bamberg, which probably derives from H. W. Katzheimer's painting *The Dispersion of the Apostles*. There are also noteworthy views of Florence, Regensburg, Nuremberg, Strasbourg, Salzburg, Ulm, Passau, Munich, Basel, Venice, and Rome.

Also important are the six books of the *Cosmographia universalis* by Sebastian Münster (Basel, 1550), which contain maps of Rome, Florence, Venice, and Constantinople. Münster also commissioned views or maps of other cities from the Masters WS, HHF, and HSD, during the years 1548–49.

Of note among battle maps are the circular woodcuts executed in Nuremberg by Nicolaus Meldemann at the time of the siege of Vienna by the Turks in 1529. These woodcuts show the siege as it was seen from the top of the tower of St. Stephen's. Other examples of the genre are the *Warhafftige Contrafactur der löblichen und weitberühmten Hauptstadt Wien* in the Germanisches National-Museum in Nuremberg; a woodcut showing the siege of Ofen (1541); the map by Johannes Stab of the expedition of Charles V against the Turks; the engraving (1634) by W. Hondius of the siege of Smolensk. The number of battle maps increased greatly in the 18th century, when particular importance came to be attached to the "theaters of war." These appeared in many of the maps in the *Grosser Atlas über di gantze Welt* of J. B. Homann (Nuremberg, 1737), with many sheets dedicated to the art of war. The atlas also contains many views and maps of cities, castles, and quarries. In 1738–52 the publishing firm of Homann published 11 maps of Silesia with 73 views of cities and castles. In 1748 the astronomer Tobias Mayer designed a map of the county of Glatz containing 21 different symbols for churches, hamlets, post offices, etc., which anticipate modern map conventions.

Even at the time modern maps began to evolve, dropping unnecessary details in favor of more precise and useful information, maps of imaginary regions were in vogue. At the end of the vast Homann atlas is the map *Accurata Utopiae tabula*, which treats the traditional theme of the land of milk and honey, with inscriptions pointing to specific localities. Of similar type is the map *The Kingdom of Love* of 1777.

In 1722 there was published in London a handsome colored map of the island of Barbados, containing the picture of a plantation with Negroes at work. The engraving by J. Schnitzer of Armsheim from a drawing of J. Senex was published in the *Map of Barbados* of W. Mayo.

The custom of making geographical maps in the shape of animals or plants should be mentioned. Giovan Battista Guicci (1549) published a map of the world in the form of a two-headed eagle; in the same period Hieronymus Gourmont designed another showing the head of a fool; A. Thevet (1583) devised a map in the form of a lily; and C. Visscher (ca. 1650) published a map of Belgium (*Leo Belgicus*) in the shape of a lion, bordered with portraits of princes.

Important mural maps include the one in the Palazzo Venezia in Rome, perhaps by Girolamo Bellavista, and those by Jacopo Gastaldi (Castaldi) in the Doges' Palace in Venice (1549 and 1553), which were later replaced by eight maps by Grisellini. In 1563–67 Cosimo de' Medici commissioned in the Palazzo Vecchio in Florence a wardrobe room with "maps of Ptolemy on the doors"; these, the work of Ignazio Danti, have been accurately described by Vasari. It was this same Danti who later designed the maps in the Palazzo del Podestà in Bologna and those of Italy (1580–83) for the Galleria delle Carte Geografiche in the Vatican, which were restored in 1635 by Lucas Holstenius.

Maps frequently provided subject matter for tapestries: the Jesuit Schall von Bell commissioned a map of the world in silk in 1628. In England there was such a demand for Gob-elin tapestries with geographic maps that they were also produced locally.

The terrestrial globe is an outstanding instance of an adaptation of geographic data to an *objet d'art*. The oldest globe of this kind is in the Germanisches National-Museum in Nuremberg (1492). The *Erdapfel* ("terrestrial apple") of Behaim was decorated by Georg Glockendon with the signs of the zodiac, banners, crests and images of princes, saints, ships, animals, etc. The much smaller Laon globe, of gilded copper, shows those countries known before the discovery of America. After the discovery there were many requests for globes showing the new continent (e.g., the correspondence between Thomas Dainer, the secretary of the Papal Ambassador to the Hungarian court, and Duke Ercole of Ferrara). Examples of these globes are preserved in the Vatican Library. Worthy of mention, too, are the brass globes now in Budapest, where they were brought from Nuremberg, probably by Celtis; the Lenox globe in gilded copper, with a diameter of $4^7/_8$ in., and the Jagellon globe of $2^3/_4$ in. diameter; the globe made in 1530 by Robert de Bailly, $5^1/_2$ in. in diameter, noted for its handsome support and details; the fine terrestrial globe supported by a dolphin, by C. Schniepp (Augsburg, ca. 1530), now in the Bibliothèque Nationale in Paris; the gilded globe in the shape of a cup, by C. Heiden (Nuremberg, ca. 1560), and the similar one in the Adler Planetarium in Chicago, formerly in the Mensing Collection (no. 16); and the elaborate globes of Joachim Praetorius, now in the Germanisches National-Museum in Nuremberg.

Others who made globes were Francesco Basso of Milan (globe of 1570 in Turin, Bib. Naz.) and J. Reinhold and Georg Roll of Augsburg, who from 1586 to 1588 made gilded celestial spheres with mechanisms (Dresden, Mathematisch-Physikalischer Salon; Paris, Mus. du Conservatoire Nat.; Vienna, Kunsthistorisches Mus.; Greenwich, Nat. Maritime Mus.). Philip V, count of Hanau-Lichtenberg, executed a handsome terrestrial globe and celestial sphere in gilded copper. Also of interest is the terrestrial globe supported by Atlas, by Christoph Schissler. The 17th-century French terrestrial globe at Doorn (Netherlands) is of silver, with a handsome support in gilded copper. About 1660 partly gilded silver globes were made in southern Germany. An example is the finely carved parallactic globe now in the Adler Planetarium in Chicago (Mensing Coll., no. 15). In the 18th century Waechtler made silver terrestrial and celestial globes in Fürth.

Terrestrial globes cut along the horizontal line of the equator were made chiefly in Switzerland and were used as cups. The oldest is perhaps that of the Musée Historique Lorrain in Nancy, of about 1530 (PL. 500); similar globes are those made by J. Stampfer in 1539 and that perhaps by Abraham Gester, from about 1600. The handsome globe-goblet in gilded copper from the Airthrey Treasures, sold at auction in 1937 by Sotheby's in London, dates from about 1555–65. C. Heiden constructed a fine terrestrial globe of $2^3/_4$ in. diameter, in gilded brass, resting on three dolphins, in the interior of which is found a silvered celestial globe. In Nuremberg J. Hauer engraved (1620) the globe-goblet of silver made by Jeremias Ritter (Stockholm, Statens Sjöhistoriska Mus.). In 1552 the watchmaker Jacques de la Garde constructed a sounding clock contained in a gilded terrestrial ball (Greenwich, Nat. Maritime Mus.).

The Musée des Beaux-Arts et de Céramique in Rouen possesses a terrestrial and celestal globe on a base supported by lions, executed in faïence from Rouen; and the Germanisches National-Museum in Nuremberg has a terrestrial and celestial globe supported by Hercules, in Meissen porcelain, dating from about 1740–50. Most terrestrial globes, however, are of wood or papier-mâché, covered with paper or parchment on which the continents are drawn or printed. In 1575–77 Philipp Apian designed a map of the world for a terrestrial globe $31^1/_2$ in. in diameter, painted by Hans Donauer (PL. 500). Of papier-mâché, too, is the great terrestrial globe known to have been executed in 1595 in Saint Gallen (Zurich, Schweizerisches Landesmus.). The large terrestrial and celestial globes in the Wolfenbüttel library are of the same period; later examples are seen in the remarkable terrestrial globe of Jodocus Hondius (1600) and that of Willem Janszoon Blaeu (1622). In Italy

globes were produced by Matteus Greuter (1638), Domenico Rossi (1695), Silvester Amantius Moroncelli (1672), and P. Vincenzo Coronelli (1693). Examples of 18th-century globes are the simple and pleasing ones by G. and L. Valk, M. Seutter (1710), J. G. Doppelmayr (1728), Pietro Rosini (1762), Nathaniel Hill (1754), and Giovan Maria Cassini (1790).

Ernst ZINNER

BIBLIOG. *Cosmology. a. Prehistory*: R. Battaglia, Ricerche etnografiche su petroglifi della cerchia alpina, SEtr, VIII, 1934, p. 11 ff., PL. 15; E. Anati, Rock Engravings in the Italian Alps, Archaeology, XI, 1, 1958, p. 30 ff.; S. Ferri, La corografia protostorica e le leggi della Mimesis, RendLinc, series VIII, vol. XIII, fasc. 5–6, 1958, p. 190 ff. *b. The ancient world.* (1) *Egypt*: H. Haas, Bilderatlas zur Religionsgeschichte, fasc. 2–4, Leipzig, 1924, figs. 1–23. (2) *Middle East*: P. Jensen, Die Kosmologie der Babylonier, Strasbourg, 1890; A. Jeremias, Handbuch der altorientalischen Geisteskultur, Leipzig, 1913, pp. 20–129; B. Meissner, Babylonien und Assyrien, II, Heidelberg, 1925, pp. 102–50; E. Ebeling and M. Ebert, Reallexikon der Vorgeschichte, VII, Berlin, 1926, pp. 54–55; H. Frankfort and others, Before Philosophy, Harmondsworth, 1949, pp. 182–87; P. Amiet, Problèmes d'iconographie mésopotamienne, Revue d'Assyriologie, 1953, pp. 183–85; M. T. Barrelet, Taureaux et symbolique solaire, Revue d'Assyriologie, 1954, pp. 16–27; P. Amiet, Le symbolisme cosmique du répertoire animalier en Mésopotamie, Revue d'Assyriologie, 1956, pp. 113–26; B. Segal, Notes on the Iconography of Cosmic Kingship, AB, XXXVIII, 1956, pp. 75–80; R. Largement, Histoire des religions (publiée sous la direction de M. Brillant et R. Aigrain), IV, Tournai, n.d., pp. 153-57. *c. The classical world*: R. Eisler, Weltenmantel und Himmelzeit, Munich, 1910; F. Cumont, Les religions orientales dans l'Empire romain, Paris, 1929; F. Cumont, L'Egypte des astrologues, Brussels, 1937; J. Bayet, L'immortalité astrale d'Auguste, REL, 1939, p. 141 ff.; H. P. L'Orange, Domus Aurea, Der Sonnenpalast, Serta Eitremenia, sup. XI, SymbOsl, 1942, pp. 68–101 (rev. of A. Boethius, Eranos, 1946, p. 442 ff.; of J. Guey, Note sur le Septizonium du Palatin, Mélanges de la Société Toulousaine d'Etudes Classiques, Toulouse, 1946, p. 147 ff.; of J. Toynbee, JRS, 1948, p. 160 ff.; of M. P. Charlesworth, JRS, 1950, p. 69 ff.); R. Bloch, Antiquité classique: Grèce, Etrurie et Rome: Symbolisme cosmique et monuments religieux, Paris, 1953, pp. 19–29. *d. The West*: T. Campanella, Città del Sole, 1623; A. Averlino (Il Filarete), Trattato di architettura, ed. W. von Oettingen, Quellenschriften für Kunstgeschichte, N.S., III, Vienna, 1890; A. Muñoz and M. Lazzaroni, Filarete scultore e architetto del sec. XV, Rome, 1908; H. Wispler, Über die Stuckbilder an den Gewölben des Posener Rathauses, Lissa (Poland), 1912; E. Panofsky, Die Entwicklung der Proportionslehre als Abbild der Stilentwicklung, Monatshefte für Kunstwissenschaft, XIV, 1921, pp. 188–219 (Eng. trans. in E. Panofsky, Meaning in the Visual Arts, New York, 1955, pp. 55–107); J. Sauer, Symbolik des Kirchengebäudes und seiner Ausstattung in der Auffassung des Mittelalters, 2d ed., Freiburg im Breisgau, 1924; Mâle, II; Mâle, I; G. Munter, Die Geschichte der Idealstadt, Städtebau, XXV, 1929; A. Warburg, Gesammelte Schriften, Leipzig, 1932; K. Greiner, Der astronomische Figurenfries am Hirsauer Turm, Calw, 1934; J. F. Puig i Cadafalch, Idees teoriques sobre urbanisme en el segle XIV, un fragment d'Eiximenez, Homenatge a Antoni Rubio i Lluch, I, Barcelona, 1936; J. Baltrusaitis, Quelques survivances de symboles solaires dans l'art du Moyen Age, GBA, XVII, 1937; J. Baltrusaitis, L'image du monde céleste du IX^e au XII^e siècle, GBA, XVIII, 1938; J. Baltrusaitis, Roses des vents et roses de personnages à l'époque romaine, GBA, XIX, 1938; L. Kitschelt, Die frühchristliche Basilika als Darstellung des himmlischen Jerusalems, Munich, 1938 (reviewed by J. Kollwitz in Byzantinische Z., XLII, 1943–49, p. 273); J. Baltrusaitis, Cercles astrologiques et cosmographiques à la fin du Moyen Age, GBA, XXI, 1939; W. Born, Spiral Towers in Europe and Their Oriental Prototypes, GBA, XXIV, 1943; A. Coomaraswamy, The Iconography of Dürer's Knots and Leonardo's Concatenation, AQ, VII, 1944; K. Lehmann, The Dome of Heaven, AB, XXVII, 1945; R. Papini, Francesco di Giorgio Martini, architetto, Florence, 1946; A. Grabar, Le témoignage d'une hymne syriaque sur l'architecture de la cathédrale d'Edesse au VI^e siècle, CahA, II, 1947; C. de Tolnay, The Medici Chapel, Princeton, 1948; H. Sedlmayr, Die Entstehung der Kathedrale, Zurich, 1950; A. Stange, Das frühchristliche Kirchengebäude als Bild des Himmels, Cologne, 1950; E. B. Smith, The Dome, Princeton, 1950; E. W. Palm, A Vault with Cosmotheological Representations at the Imperial Monastery of the Dominicans on the Island of Hispaniola, AB, XXXII, 1950; G. Bandmann, Mittelalterliche Architektur als Bedeutungsträger, Berlin, 1951; R. Wittkower, Architectural Principles in the Age of Humanism, 2d ed., London, 1952; S. Lang, The Ideal City from Plato to Howard, Architectural Review, CXII, 1952; E. Beer, Die Rose der Kathedrale von Lausanne und der Kosmologische Bilderkreis des Mittelalters, Bern, 1952; G. F. Hartlaub, Zur Symbolik des Skulpturenschmucks am Ottheinrichsbau, Wallraf-Richartz Jhb., XIV, 1952; M. Brion, Leonardo da Vinci, Paris, 1952 (Eng. trans., London, 1954); R. Wittkower, Systems of Proportions, Architects Yearbook, V, 1953; M. Brion, Les nœuds de Léonard de Vinci et leur signification, l'art et la pensée de Léonard de Vinci, Paris, 1953; C. de Tolnay, Music of the Universe, J. of the Walters Art Gallery, IV, 1953; Symbolisme cosmique et monuments religieux, Musée Guimet, Paris, 1953 (see especially the articles of A. Chastel); S. Lang, A Few Suggestions towards a New Solution of the Origin of the Early Christian Basilica, RACr, XXX, 1954; L. Hautecœur, Mystique et architecture, Paris, 1954; L. H. Heydenreich, Leonardo da Vinci, London, 1954; E. Panofsky, Galileo as a Critic of the Arts, The Hague, 1954; E. B. Smith, Architectural Symbolism of Imperial Rome and the Middle Ages, Princeton, 1956; E. Panofsky, Gothic Architecture and Scholasticism, New York, 1957; F. Saxl, Lectures, London, 1957 (with a general bibliog. of his writings); Le symbolisme cosmique des monuments religieux, Série Orientale, XIV, IsMEO, Rome, 1957; H. Foramitti, En quoi le développement de l'architecture moderne a été influencé par l'évolution de la conception scientifique du monde, Archivio di Filosofia, La Filosofia dell'Arte Sacra, Padua, 1957; H. J. Dow, The Rose-window, Warburg, XX, 1957; O. Reutersvärd, Klotpalats och Pyramidtempel, Byggmästaren, A: Arkitektur, XXXVII, 1958, pp. 132–35. *e. Asia: India and Southest Asia*: W. Kirfel, Die Kosmographie der Inder, Bonn, Leipzig, 1920; W. Kirfel, Bharatavarsa (Indien), textgeschichtliche Darstellung zweier geographischen Purāna-Texte, Beiträge zur indischen Sprachwissenschaft und Religionsgeschichte, Heft 67, Stuttgart, 1931; A. C. Soper, "The Dome of Heaven" in Asia, AB, XXIX, 1947, p. 227 ff.; G. Tucci, Teoria e pratica della mandala, Rome, 1949; R. Shafer, Ethnography of Ancient India, Wiesbaden, 1954; W. Kirfel, Das Purāna vom Weltgebäude, Bonn, 1954; R. Stein, L'habitat, le monde et le corps humain en Extrême-Orient et en Haute Asie, JA, 1957, pp. 37–74. *f. Primitive cultures*: F. H. Cushing, Outlines of Zuñi Creation Myths, 13th Annual Report of the Bureau of American Ethnology (1891–92), Washington, 1896; L. Frobenius, Kulturgeschichte Afrikas, Vienna, 1933; C. Lévi-Strauss, Contribution à l'étude de l'organisation chez les Indiens Bororo, JSA, XXXIV, 1936; M. Griaule, Masques Dogons, Travaux et mémoires de l'Institut d'Ethnologie de Paris, XXXIII, 1938; J. Soustelle, La pensée cosmologique des anciens Mexicains, Paris, 1940; M. Griaule, Dieu d'eau, Paris, 1948; M. Griaule, L'image du monde au Soudan français, JSA, XIX, 1949; G. Dieterlen, Les correspondances cosmobiologiques chez les Soudanais, J. de Psychologie Normale et Pathologique, 1950; G. Dieterlen, Essai sur la religion Bambara, Paris, 1951; M. Griaule, Le savoir des Dogon, JSA, 1952; M. Griaule and G. Dieterlen, Signes graphiques soudanais, Paris, 1952; H. Lehmann, Les civilisations précolombiennes, Paris, 1953; H. Lehmann, Amérique: Symbolisme cosmique et monuments religieux, Musée Guimet, Paris, 1953; G. Dieterlen, Mythe et organisation sociale au Soudan français, JSA, XXV, 1955; M. Griaule, Rôle du silure "Clarias senegalensis" dans la procréation au Soudan français, Deutsche Akademie der Wissenschaften zu Berlin, Institut für Orientforschung, Afrikanische Studien, Berlin, 1955; A. and J. P. Lebeuf, Monuments symboliques du palais royal de Logone-Birni (Nord-Cameroun), JSA, XXV, 1955; G. Dieterlen, Parenté et mariage chez les Dogon, Africa, XXVI, 1956; C. P. Mountford, Art, Myth and Symbolism, Records of the American-Australian Scientific Expedition to Arnhem Land, I, Melbourne, 1956; J. Eberhardt, La notion de la vie, base de la structure sociale Venda, JSA, XXVII, 1957; C. Lévi-Strauss, Le serpent au corps rempli de poissons, Anthropologie structurale, Paris, 1958; H. Lhote, The Search for the Tassili Frescoes, New York, 1959.

*Cartography. a. Prehistory and primitive cultures*: W. J. Hoffman, The Graphic Art of the Eskimos, Washington, 1897; J. Wanamaker, A Marshall Islands Chart, The Museum J., Philadelphia, 1919; E. Guzman, The Art of Map-making among the Ancient Mexicans, Imago Mundi, III, London, 1939. *b. The classical world*: E. H. Bunbury, A History of Ancient Geography among the Greeks and Romans, 2 vols., London, 1879; A. E. Nordenskiöld, Facsimile-atlas to the Early History of Cartography, Stockholm, 1889 (trans. from the Swedish by J. A. Ekelöf and C. R. Markham); K. Miller, Mappae mundi: Die ältesten Weltkarten, 6 vols., Stuttgart, 1895–98; A. E. Nordenskiöld, Periplus: An Essay on the Early History of Charts and Sailing Directions (trans. from the Swedish by F. A. Bather), Stockholm, 1897; C. R. Beazley, Dawn of Modern Geography, I, London, 1897; E. H. Berger, Geschichte der wissenschaftlichen Erdkunde der Griechen, 2d ed., Leipzig, 1903; B. F. Adler, Maps of Primitive Peoples, St. Petersburg, 1910 (résumé from the Russian in the B. of the American Geographical Society, 1911, pp. 669–79); M. Cary and E. Warmington, The Ancient Explorers, London, 1929; H. F. Tozer, A History of Ancient Geography, 2d ed., Cambridge, England, 1935; J. O. Thomson, History of Ancient Geography, Cambridge, England, 1948. *c. Far East.* (1) *China*: J. B. Du Halde, Description géographique, historique, chronologique, politique et physique de l'empire de la Chine et de la Tartarie chinoise, 4 vols., Paris, 1735 (for the translations of Du Halde's work, see H. Cordier, Bibliotheca Sinica, Paris, 1904–24, I, cols. 45–52); E. Chavannes, Les deux plus anciens spécimens de la cartographie chinoise, BEFEO, Apr., 1903, pp. 214–47; L. Richard, Comprehensive Geography of the Chinese Empire and Dependencies, Shanghai, 1905, 1908; F. S. Couvrer, Géographie Ancienne et moderne de la Chine, Hien Hien, 1917; A. Vacca, Sull'opera geografica di Giulio Aleni, missionario in Cina nel secolo XVII, Atti X Congresso Geografico Italiano, Milan, 1927, pp. 366–68; W. E. Soothill, The Two Oldest Maps of China Extant, GJ, LXIX, 1927, pp. 532–55; Wang Yung, Collection of Source Material Relating to the History of Chinese Maps, B. of the National Library of Peiping, VI, 1932, pp. 559–600; Quarterly B. of Chinese Bibliog., Peiping, from 1934; Ti-li hsüehpao (Geographical Society of China), Nanking, from 1934; W. Fuchs, Materialien zur Kartographie der Mandju-Zeit, Monumenta Serica, I, 1935, pp. 386–427; H. Bernard, Les étapes de la cartographie scientifique pour la Chine et les pays voisins depuis le XVI^e jusqu'à la fine du XVIII^e siècle, Monumenta Serica, I, 1935, pp. 428–77; R. Joüon, Géographie commerciale de la Chine, Shanghai, 1937; P. M. D'Elia, Il mappamondo cinese del P. Matteo Ricci, S.J., Vatican City, 1938; A. Wylie, Notes on Chinese Literature, Peiping, 1939, pp. 34–54; K. Ch'en, Matteo Ricci's Contribution to and Influence on Geographical Knowledge in China, JAOS, LIX, 1939, pp. 325–59; K. Ch'en, The Early Expansion of Chinese Geographical Knowledge, Tien Hsia Monthly, XI, 1940, pp. 52–62; W. Fuchs, The Mongol Atlas of China by Chu Ssŭ-pen and the Kuang-yü-t'u, Peiping, 1946; Fung Yu-lan, A History of Chinese Philosophy (trans. Derk Bodde with introduction, notes, bibliog., and index), 2 vols., Princeton, 1952–53; B. Szcześniak, Matteo Ricci's Maps of China, Imago Mundi, XI, 1954, pp. 127–36; J. V. Mills, Chinese Coastal Maps, Imago Mundi, XI, 1954, pp. 151–68; B. Szcześniak, The Seventeenth Century Maps of China, Imago Mundi, XIII, 1956, pp. 116–36; M. J. Meijer, A Map of the Great Wall of China, Imago Mundi, XIII, 1956, pp. 110–15; Mai-mai Sze, The Tao of Painting, 2 vols., New York, 1956. (2) *Japan*: K. Toda, Descriptive Catalogue of Japanese and Chinese Illustrated Books in the Ryerson Library of the Art Institute of Chicago, Chicago, 1931; M. Ramming, The Evolution of Cartography in Japan, Imago Mundi, II, 1937, pp. 17–21; H. Nakamura, Les

cartes du Japon qui servaient de modèle aux cartographes européens au début des relations de l'Occident avec le Japon, Monumenta Nipponica, II, 1939, pp. 100–23; G. Kish, Some Aspects of the Missionary Cartography of Japan during the Sixteenth Century, Imago Mundi, IV, 1940, pp. 39–46; G, H. Beans, A List of Japanese Maps of the Tokugawa Era, 2 vols., Jenkintown, Pa., 1951–55; S. Ayusawa, The Types of World Map Made in Japan's Age of National Isolation, Imago Mundi, X, 1953, pp. 123–27; B. Szcześniak, The Antoine Gaubil Maps of the Ryukyu and Southern Japan, Imago Mundi, XII, 1955, pp. 141–49; R. B. Hall and Foshio Noh, Japanese Geography: A Guide to Japanese Reference and Research Materials, Ann Arbor, 1956. (3) *Korea*: M. Courant, Bibliographie coréenne, tableau littéraire de la Corée contenant la nomenclature des ouvrages publiés dans ce pays jusqu'en 1890, 3 vols., Paris, 1894–96, sup., 1899; H. Cordier, Description d'un atlas sino-coréen manuscrit du British Museum, Paris, 1896; H. Nakamura, Old Chinese World Maps Preserved by the Koreans, Imago Mundi, IV, 1947, pp. 3–22. *d. The West*: Vasari; E. F. Jomard, Les monuments de la géographie, Paris, 1842–62; C. Fomard, Lettere di Tommaso Dainero ad Ercole Duce de Ferraria (1501–02), Budapest, 1881; F. Ongania, Raccolta di mappamondi e carte nautiche dal XIII al XVI secolo, Venice, 1881; J. Del Badia, Egnazio Danti cosmografo e matematico, Florence, 1882; L. Gallois, De Orontio Finaeo geographo, Paris, 1890; F. Denza, Globi celesti della Specola Vaticana, Pubblicazioni della Specola Vaticana, IV, Turin, 1894, pp. xvii–xxiii; Remarkable Maps of the XV, XVI and XVII Centuries, Amsterdam, 1894–97; K. Miller, Die ältesten Weltkarten, 6 vols., Stuttgart, 1895–98, II, pls. 1–2, III, pl. 4, figs. 14, 16; G. Marcel, Choix de cartes et de mappemondes des XIVᵉ et XVᵉ siècles, Paris, 1896; A. E. Nordenskiöld, Periplus: An Essay on the Early History of Charts and Sailing Directions (trans. from the Swedish by F. A. Bather), Stockholm, 1897, pls. 8–9, 11–14, 25, 51; M. Fiorini, Sfere terrestri e celesti, Rome, 1899; E. von Bassermann-Jordan, Die dekorative Malerei der Renaissance am bayerischen Hof, Munich, 1900; V. Hantzsch, Die ältesten gedruckten Karten der sächsisch-thüringischen Länder (1550–93), Dresden, 1905, pls. 3, 7; S. Lönborg, Swedish Maps, Gothenburg, 1906; F. G. Ravenstein, Martin Behaim: His Life and His Globe, London, 1908; P. Philipps, A List of Geographical Atlases in the Library of Congress, Washington, 1909–20; A. Anthiaume, Cartes marines, Paris, 1916; E. L. Stevenson, Terrestrial and Celestial Globes: Their History and Construction, 2 vols., New Haven, 1921; M. Engelmann, Sammlung. Mensing: Altteissenschaftliche Instrumente (cat.), Amsterdam, 1924; F. C. Wieder, Monumenta cartographica, The Hague, 1925–30; A. L. Humphrey, Old Decorative Maps and Charts, London, 1926 (2d ed., R. A. Shelton, Decorative Printed Maps, London, New York, 1952, pls. 27, 841); H. G. Fordham, Maps: Their History, 2d ed., Cambridge, England, 1927; O. Hartig, Die Globen in der Bayerischen Staatsbibliothek und ihre Münchner Meister, Kultur des Handwerks, Munich, 1927, pp. 242–48, pl. 6; L. Bagrow, A. Ortelii Catalogus cartographarum, Gotha, 1928–30, II, p. 44; R. Almagià, Monumenta Italiae cartographica, Florence, 1929; E. Buron, Ymago mundi de Pierre d'Ailly, I–III, Paris, 1930; A. Cortesão, Cartografia e cartógrafos portugueses dos séculos XV e XVI, Lisbon, 1935; E. Lehmann, Alte deutsche Landkarten, Leipzig 1935; Sotheby and Co., Catalogue of the Airthrey Renaissance Gold Globe Cup, London, 1937 (sales cat.); Cristoforo Colombo e la scuola cartografica genovese, Genoa, 1937; A. Herrmann, Die ältesten Karten von Deutschland, Leipzig, 1940, pl. 17; P. Leemann van Elck, Die Offizin Froschauer, Zurich, 1940, fig. 28; O. Muris, Der Behaim-Globus zu Nürnberg: Eine Faksimile-Wiedergabe in 92 Einzelbildern, Ibero-Amerikanisches Archiv, XVII, Berlin, 1943, fasc. 1–2; E. Armao, Vincenzo Coronelli, Florence, 1944; P. J. Dahlgren and H. Richter, Sveriges sjökarta, Stockholm, 1944; H. Krüger, Ein Jubilaeum Nürnberger Kartographie, Mitteilungen des Vereins für Geschichte der Stadt Nürnberg, 1944, p. 127; R. Almagià, Monumenti cartografici vaticani, I: Planisferi, carte nautiche e affini dal secolo XIV al XVII esistenti nella Biblioteca Vaticana, Vatican City, 1944, II: Carte geografiche a stampa di particolare pregio o rarità dei secoli XVI e XVII esistenti nella Biblioteca Vaticana, Vatican City, 1948, III: Le pitture murali della Galleria delle Carte Geografiche, Vatican City, 1952, IV: Le pitture geografiche delle Loggie di Raffaello, Vatican City, n.d.; L. A. Brown, The Story of Maps, Boston, 1949; R. V. Tooley, Maps and Map-makers, London, 1949; L. Bagrow, Rüst's and Sporer's World Maps, Imago, VII, Stockholm, 1950, pp. 32–36; L. Bagrow, Die Geschichte der Kartographie, Berlin, 1951; W. Matthey, Sebastian Münsters Deutschlandkarte von 1525 auf einem Messingastrolabium, Germanisches National-Museum, Nürnberg, 96. Jahresbericht, 1951, pp. 42–51; F. Bonasera, Terrestrial and Celestial Globes by Vincenzo Coronelli, Imago, X, Leiden, 1953, p. 79; G. R. Crone, Maps and Their Makers, London, (1953); Raccolta di carte e documenti esposti alla Mostra tenuta in Palazzo Vecchio a Firenze nel XV centenario della nascita di Amerigo Vespucci, Florence, 1954–55; H. Child, Decorative Maps, London, 1956; E. Zinner, Deutsche und niederländische astronomische Instrumente des 11.–18. Jahrhunderts, Munich, 1956, pls. 60, 68; R. Oehme, Alte Globen aus dem Besitz der Universität, in K. Bauch, Kunstwerke aus dem Besitz der Universität Freiburg im Breisgau (1457–1957), pp. 61–64; A. Berendsen, Samenspel der eeuwen, Amsterdam, n.d.

Illustrations: PLS 484–500; 2 figs. in text.

PLATES

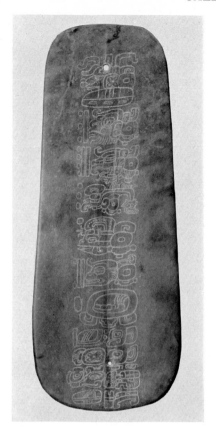

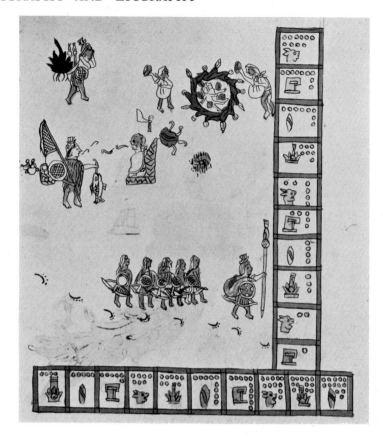

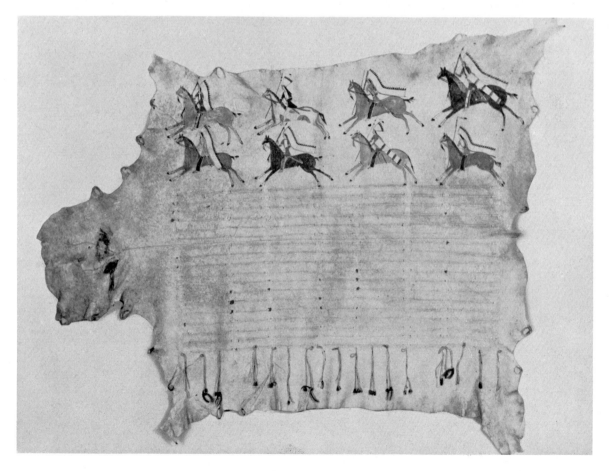

Pl. 1. *Above, left*: Mayan calendar inscription, "the Leiden Plate," from Tikal, Guatemala, A.D. 320. Jade. Leiden, Rijksmuseum voor Volkenkunde. *Right*: Aztec hieroglyphs framing a military scene, from the Codex Telleriano-Remensis (fol. 81), colonial period. Rome, Vatican Library. *Below*: Cheyenne mnemonic pictograph. Skin. Denver, Art Museum.

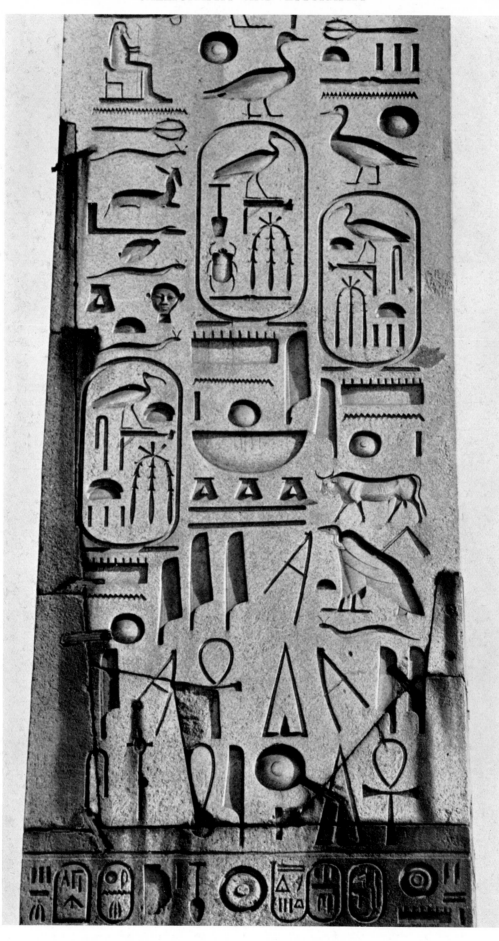

Pl. 2. Egyptian hieroglyphs, detail of the obelisk of Thutmosis III, 15th cent. B.C. Red granite. Rome, Piazza S. Giovanni in Laterano.

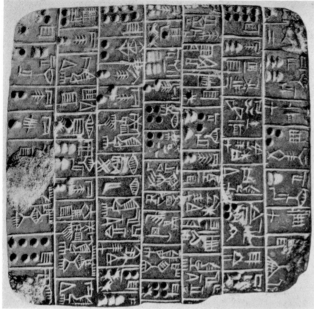

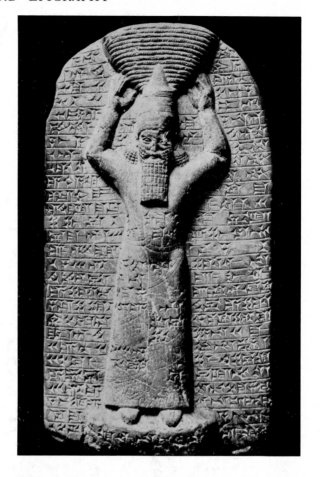

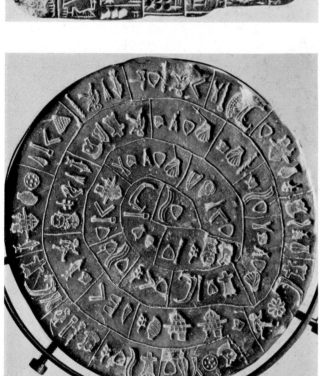

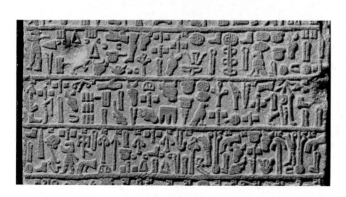

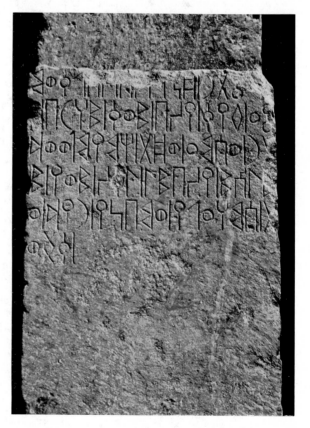

Pl. 3. *Left, above*: Sumerian ideographic inscription, from Lagash, early 3d millennium B.C. Stone, ht., 5¹/₈ in. Philadelphia, University Museum. *Center*: Disk, from Phaestos, with ideographic inscription, ca. 1700 B.C. Clay, diam., ca. 6¹/₄ in. Heraklion, Crete, Archaeological Museum. *Below*: Hittite hieroglyphs, from Carchemish, ca. mid-2d millennium B.C. Stone. Ankara, Archaeological Museum. *Right, above*: Neo-Assyrian cuneiform on a stele of Ashurbanipal, ca. 668–626 B.C. Sandstone, ht., 16¹/₂ in. London, British Museum. *Below*: Arabian pre-Islamic inscription. Stone. Marib, Yemen.

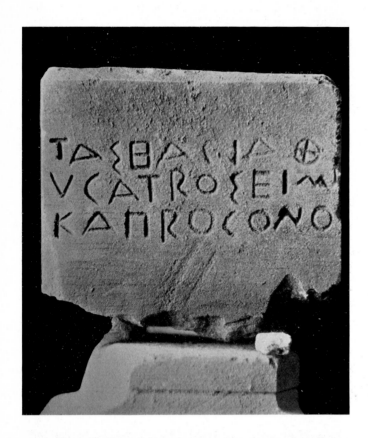

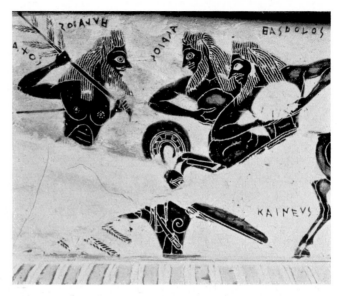

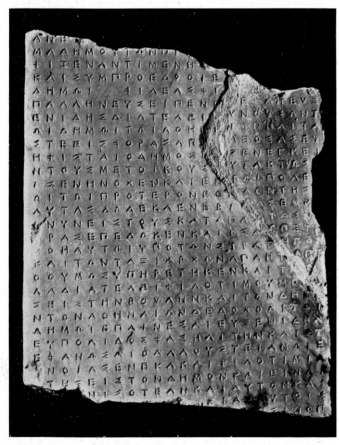

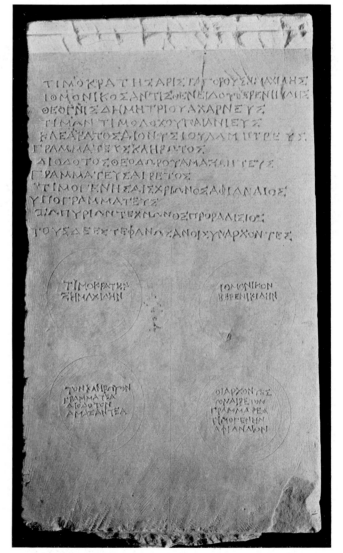

Pl. 4. *Above, left*: Archaic Greek inscription, from Megara Hyblaea, Sicily, late 7th cent. B.C. Limestone. *Right*: Detail of the François Vase, with labels, mid-6th cent. B.C. Florence, Museo Archeologico. *Below, left*: Fragment of an Attic decree with *stoichedon* inscription, 306–305 B.C. Marble. *Right*: Attic stele, mid-2d cent. B.C. Marble. Last two, Athens, National Museum.

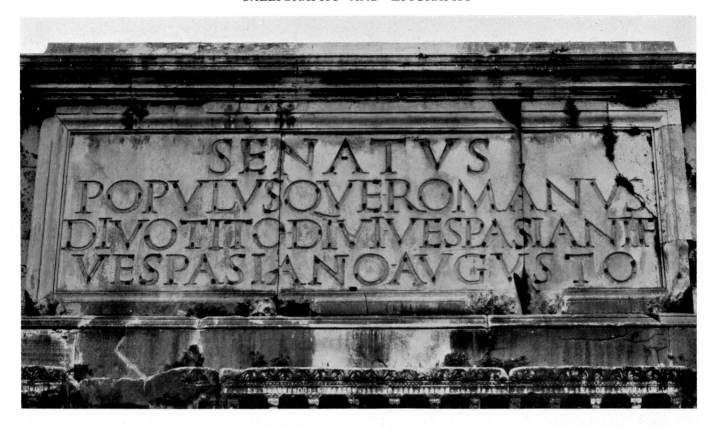

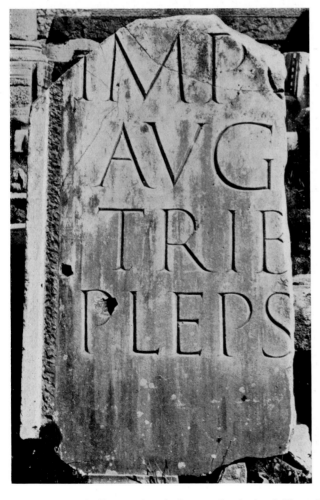

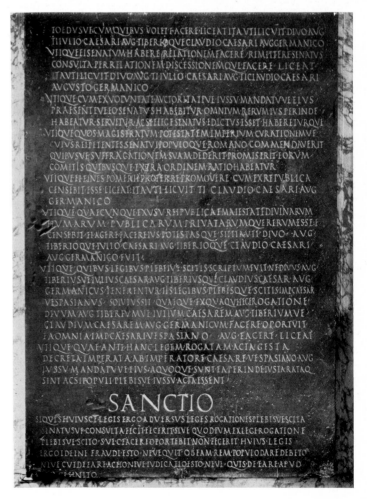

Pl. 5. *Above*: Dedicatory inscription on the Arch of Titus, last quarter of 1st cent. Marble. *Below, left*: Fragment of a dedicatory inscription of Augustus, 2 B. C. Marble. Both, Rome, Roman Forum. *Right*: Bronze tablet with the concession of imperial power by the Senate to Vespasian, A. D. 69. Rome, Capitoline Museum.

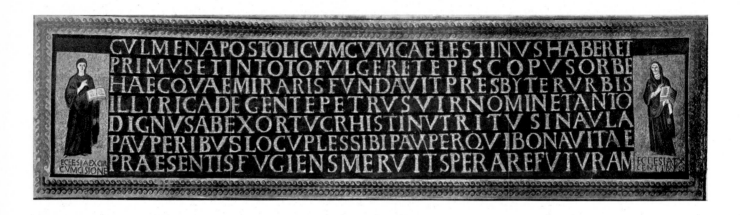

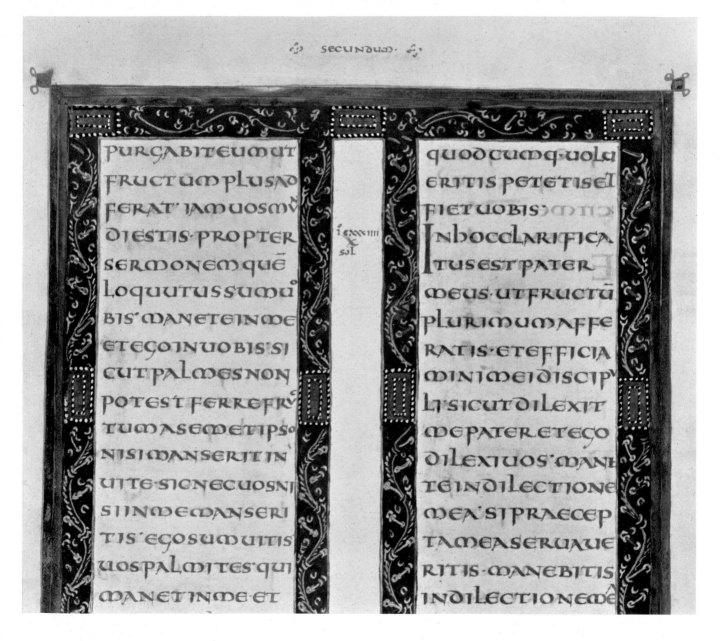

Pl. 6. *Above*: Mosaic inscription inside the façade of S. Sabina, Rome, 5th cent. *Below*: Carolingian minuscule, Lorsch Gospels, 9th cent. Rome, Vatican Library (Pal. lat. 50, fol. 103v, detail).

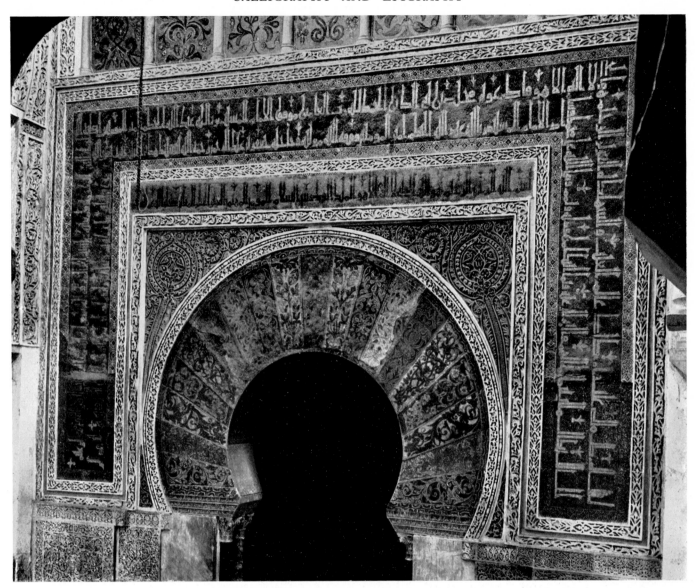

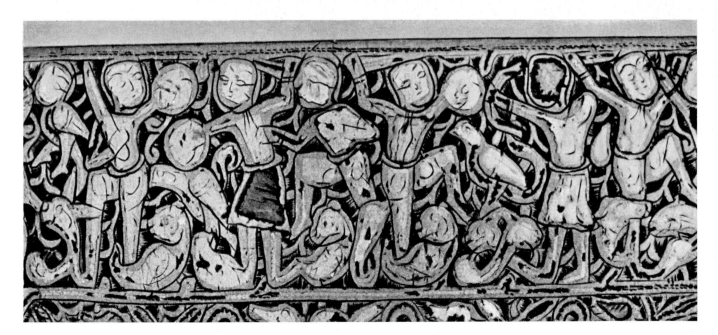

Pl. 7. *Above*: Mosaic frieze with Islamic inscription, 964–65. Cordova, Spain, Mosque, detail of the mihrab. *Below*: Anthropomorphous Islamic inscription, detail of the Wade Cup, Persian, 13th cent. Brass, inlaid with silver; full diam., 6³/₄ in. Cleveland, Museum of Art.

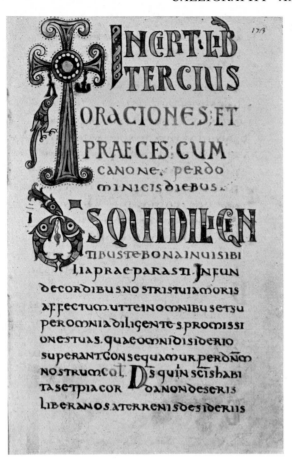

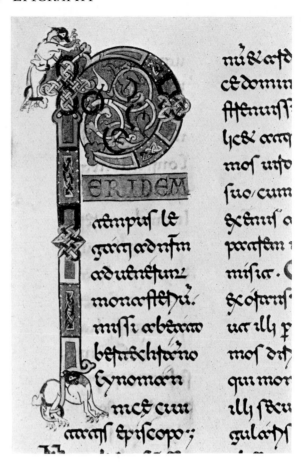

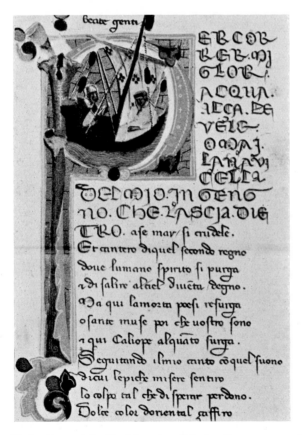

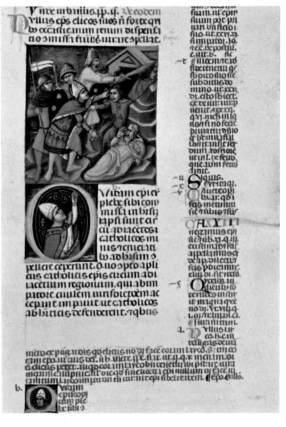

Pl. 8. *Above, left*: Uncial script, Gelasian Sacramentary, 8th cent. (?). Rome, Vatican Library (Reg. lat. 316, fol. 173r). *Right*: Beneventan minuscule script, Lectionary of SS. Benedict and Maurice, 11th cent. Rome, Vatican Library (Cod. Vat. lat. 1202, fol. 128r). *Below, left*: Italian chancery script, *The Divine Comedy*, 14th cent. Milan, Biblioteca Ambrosiana (Cod. Trivulziano 1080). *Right*: Gothic minuscule, Decretum Gratiani, Bologna, 14th cent. Rome, Vatican Library (Urb. 161, fol. 222r).

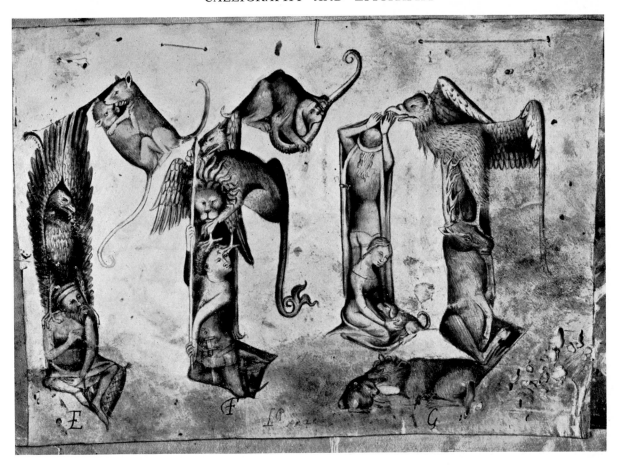

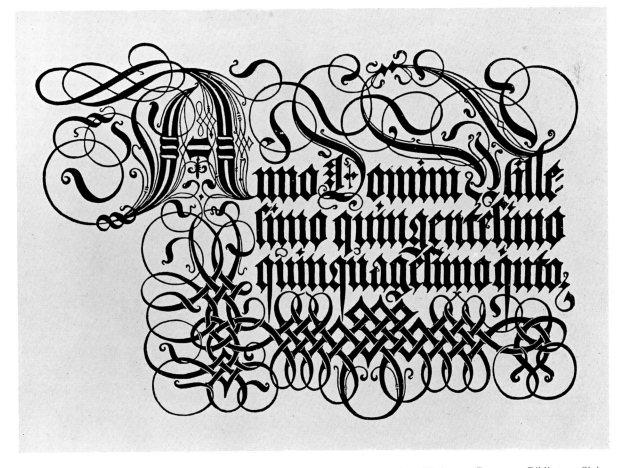

Pl. 9. *Above*: Giovannino de' Grassi, notebook page with figured letters e, f, g. Miniature. Bergamo, Biblioteca Civica.
*Below*: U. Wyss, letters and ornamentation, from *Ein neu Fundamentenbuch*, Zurich, 1562.

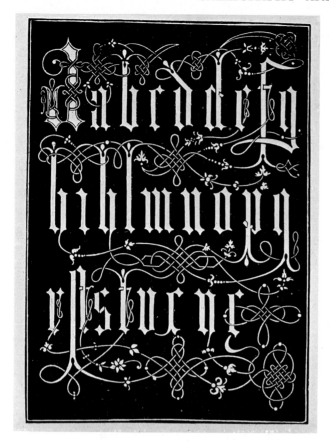

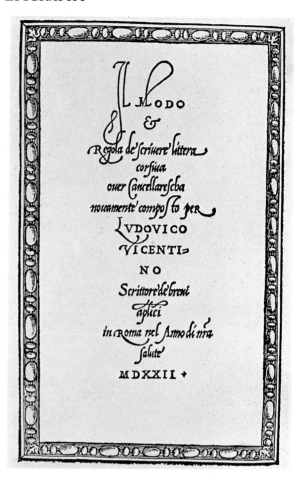

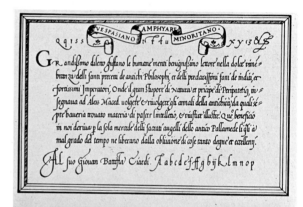

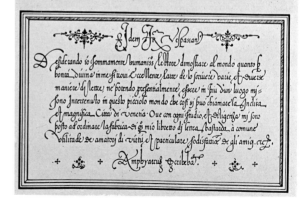

Pl. 10. *Above, left*: G. A. Tagliente, decorated page, from . . . *La vera Arte de lo excellente scrivere* . . . , Venice, 1524. *Right*: L. Vicentino (Arrighi), title page of *Il modo e Regola de scrivere littera corsiva over Cancelleresca*, Rome, 1522. *Below, left*: G. B. Palatino, page from *Libro modo d'imparare e scrivere* . . . , Rome, 1540. *Right*: V. Amfiareo, page from *Opera* . . . *nel quale s'insegna a scrivere varie sorti di littere*, Venice, 1544.

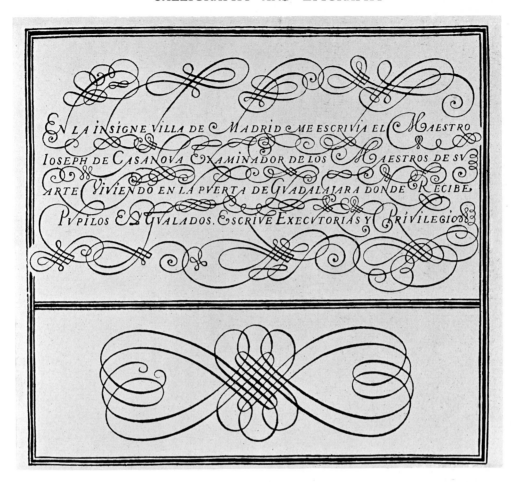

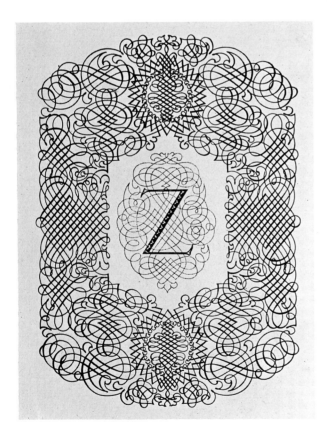

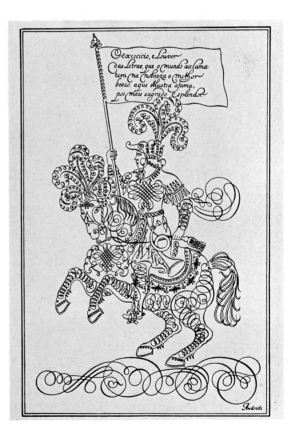

Pl. 11. *Above*: J. de Casanova, page from *Primera parte del Arte de escrivir . . .*, Madrid, 1650. *Below, left*: J. G. Schwandner, page from *. . . Dissertatio epistolaris de Calligraphiae nomendatione . . .*, Vienna, 1756. *Right*: M. Andrade de Figueiredo, calligraphic drawing in *Nova escola para aprender a ler, escriver . . .*, Lisbon, 1622.

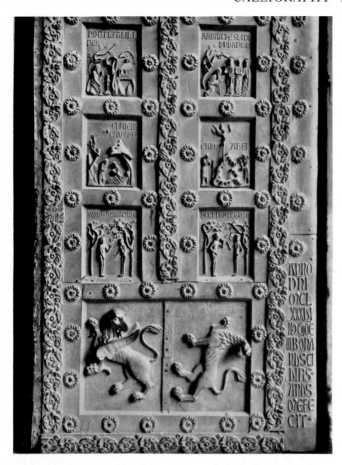

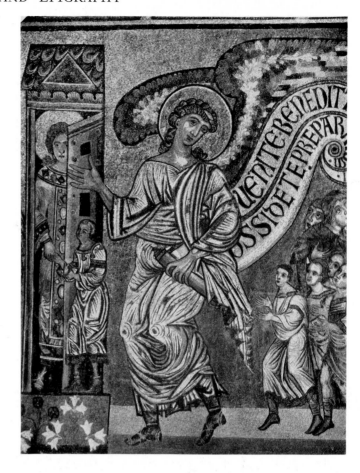

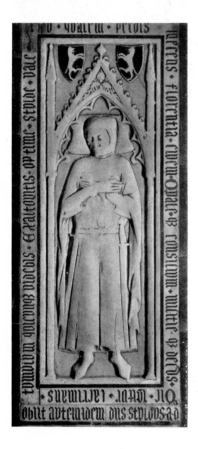

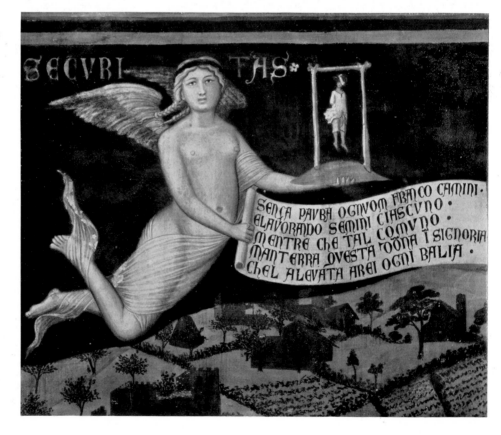

Pl. 12. Medieval monumental inscriptions. *Above, left*: Bonannus of Pisa, door with inscriptions and reliefs, detail, 1186. Bronze. Monreale, Sicily, Cathedral. *Right*: The elect led by an angel to the gates of Paradise, 13th cent. Mosaic. Florence, Baptistery, detail of the interior of the dome. *Below, left*: Tombstone of Stoldo Altoviti, 1392. Marble. Florence, SS. Apostoli. *Right*: A. Lorenzetti, Good Government, detail, 1338–40. Fresco. Siena, Palazzo Pubblico.

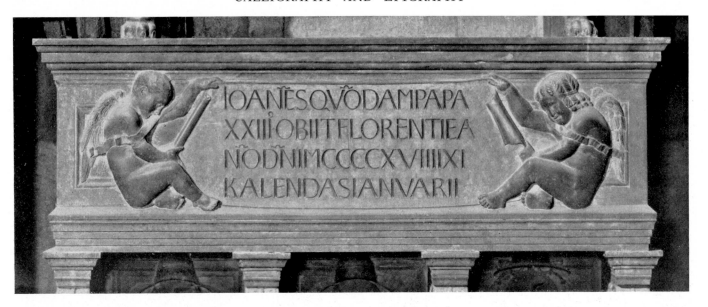

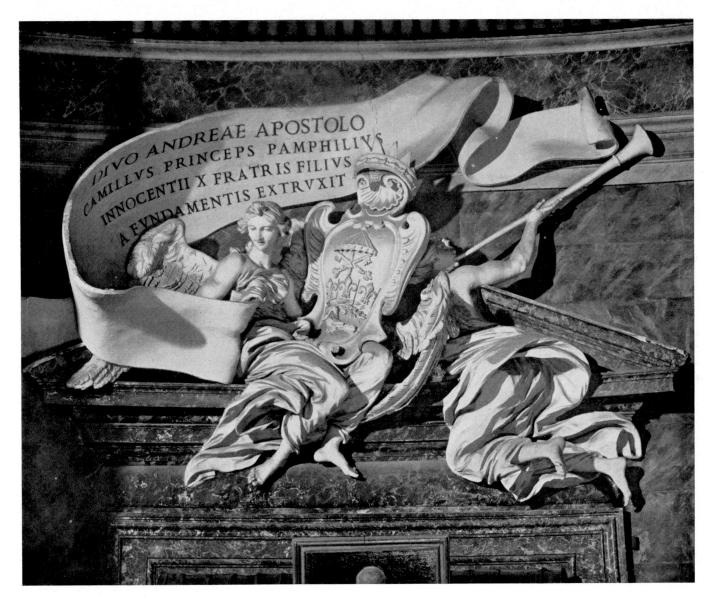

Pl. 13. Renaissance and baroque monumental inscriptions. *Above*: Donatello and Michelozzo, tomb of the anti-Pope John XXIII (d. 1419), detail. Marble. Florence, Baptistery. *Below*: Workshop of Bernini, angels with the Pamphilij coat of arms and dedicatory inscription. Stucco. Rome, S. Andrea al Quirinale.

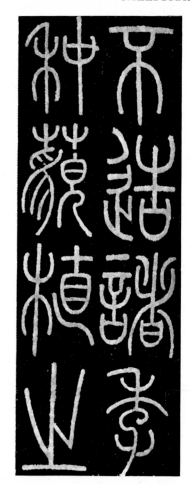

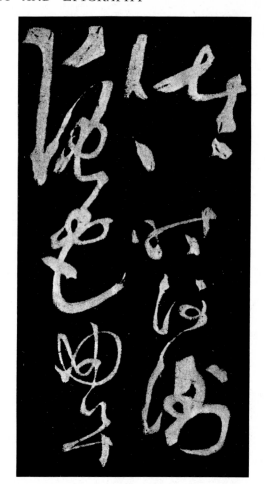

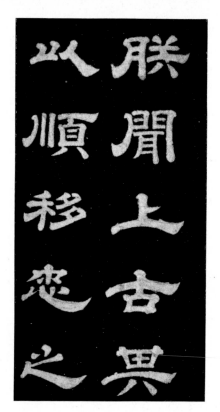

郎琅邪顔真卿書
朝散大夫撿校尚書
都官郎中東海徐浩
題額粵妙法蓮華諸

朕聞上古其
以順移戀之

Pl. 14. Chinese scripts, T'ang dynasty, 618–906. *Above, left*: Li Yang-ping (ca. 750), inscribed seal. Rubbing, ht., 8⁵/₈ in. *Right*: Chang Hsü (ca. 700), sample of draft script. Rubbing, ht., 7⁷/₈ in. *Below, left*: Yen Chêng-ch'ing (709–84), sample of regular script. Rubbing, ht., 10¹/₄ in. *Right*: Emperor T'ang Hsüan-tsung (712–56), sample of chancery script. Rubbing, ht., 8⁵/₈ in.

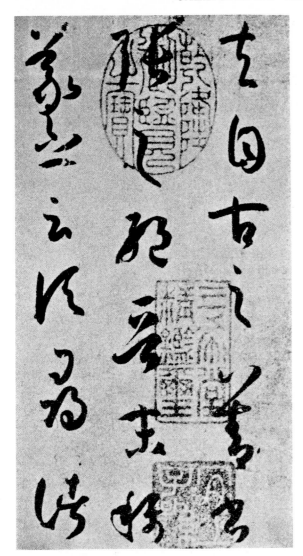

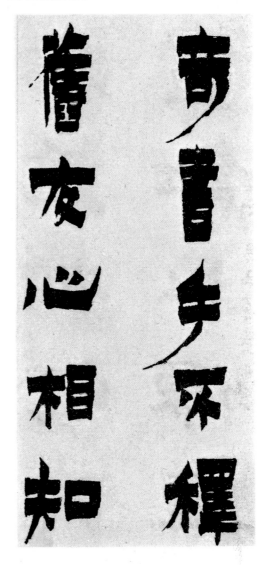

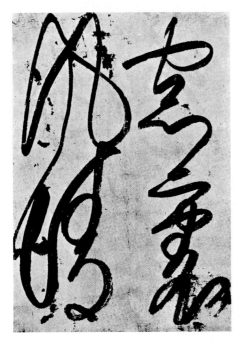

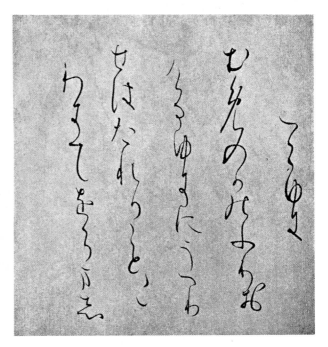

Pl. 15. *Above*: Chinese scripts. *Left*: Sun Kuo-t'ing, sample of draft script, T'ang dynasty, 618–906. Ht., 6³/₄ in. Formerly, Peking, Palace Coll. *Right*: Chin Nung (1687–1764), a couplet, Ch'ing dynasty, 1644–1912. Ht., 31¹/₂ in. *Below*: Japanese scripts. *Left*: Emperor Daigo (893–930), four characters. Ht., 11 in. Tokyo, Japanese Palace Coll. *Right*: Kino Tsurayuki (?; 883–946), poem. Ht., 5⁵/₈ in. Tokyo, Coll. Baron Masuda.

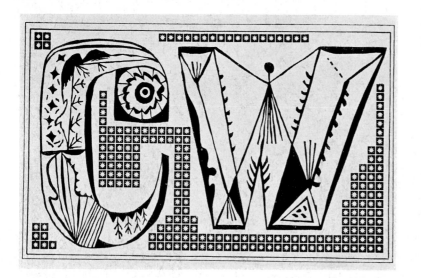

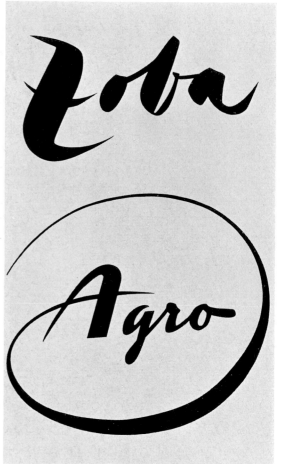

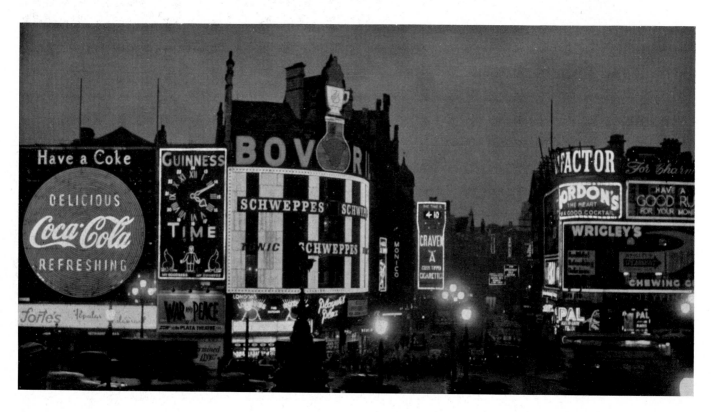

Pl. 16. Modern scripts. *Left, above*: A. Fischl, Art nouveau alphabet, Viennese Sezession. *Center*: I. Reiner, cover device for catalogue of Chatto & Windus, London. *Right*: H. and G. Troost, manufacturers' trademarks for the firms of Bayer and Milly. *Below*: Advertising scripts in lights, Picadilly Circus, London.

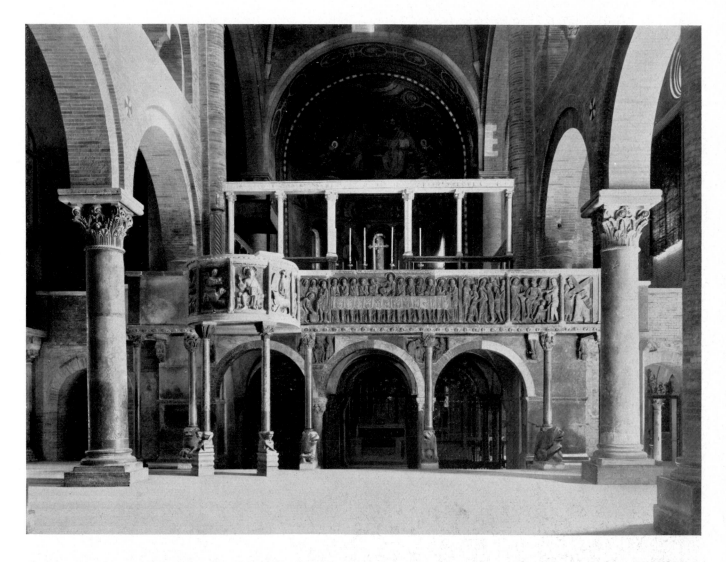

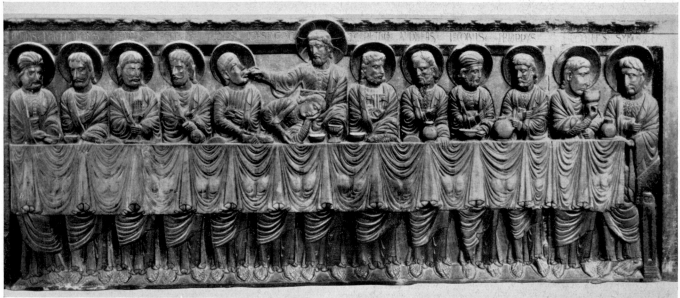

Pl. 17. Pontile of the Cathedral in Modena, Italy, by Anselmo da Campione and workshop, with (*below*) the bas-relief of the Last Supper, late 12th cent. Stone.

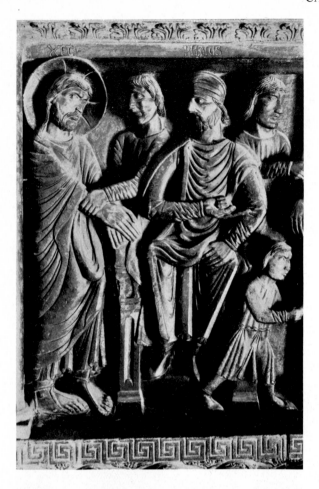
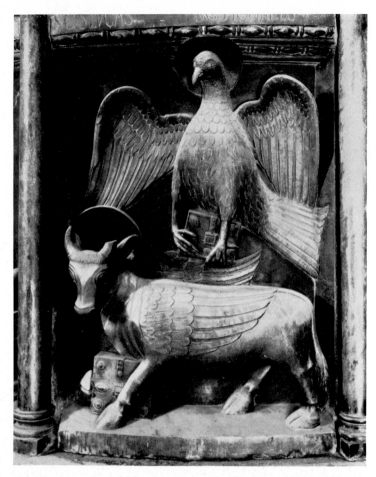
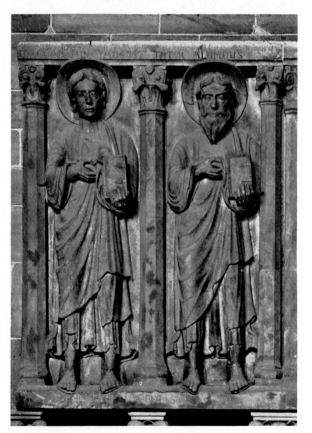
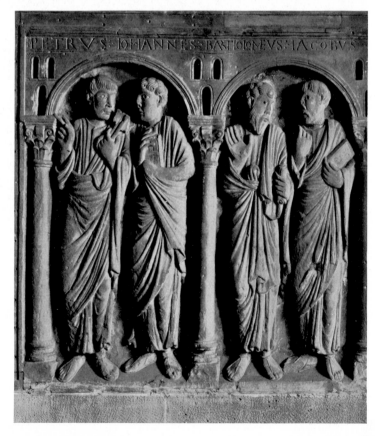

Pl. 18. *Above*: Bas-reliefs of the pontile shown in PL. 17, Christ before Pilate, detail (*left*), and symbols of the Evangelists John and Luke (*right*). *Below, left*: Apostles, ca. 1185–87. Marble. Milan, Cathedral. *Right*: Apostles, late 12th cent. Stone. Basel, Switzerland, Cathedral.

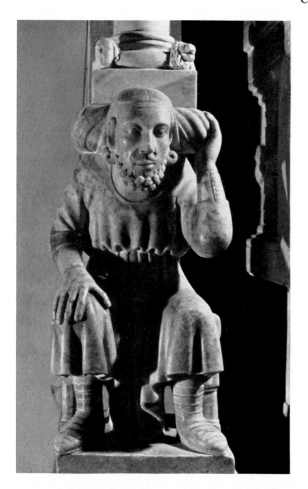
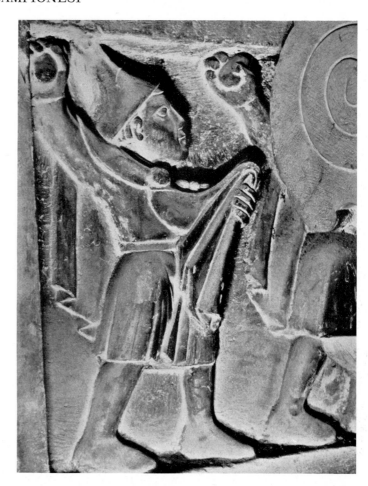
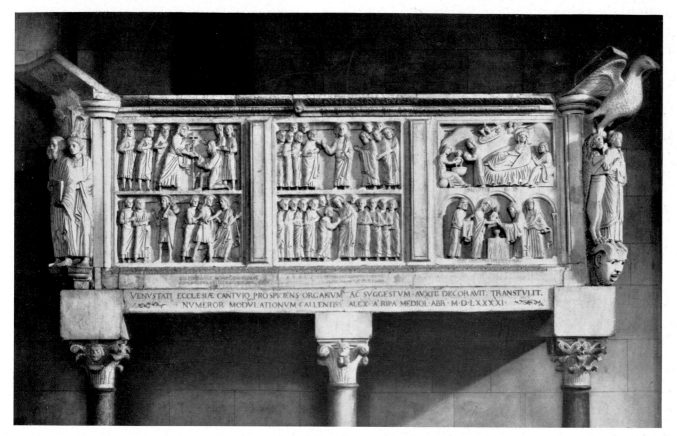

Pl. 19. *Above, left*: Tomb of Guglielmo Longhi, left telamon, attributed to Ugo da Campione, after 1319. Marble. Bergamo, Italy, S. Maria Maggiore. *Right*: The Stoning of St. Stephen (?), detail, from the workshop of Adamo d'Arogno, 13th cent. Stone. Trent, Italy, Cathedral, left apsidiole. *Below*: Pulpit by Guido Bigarelli da Como, 1250. Marble. Pistoia, Italy, S. Bartolomeo in Pantano.

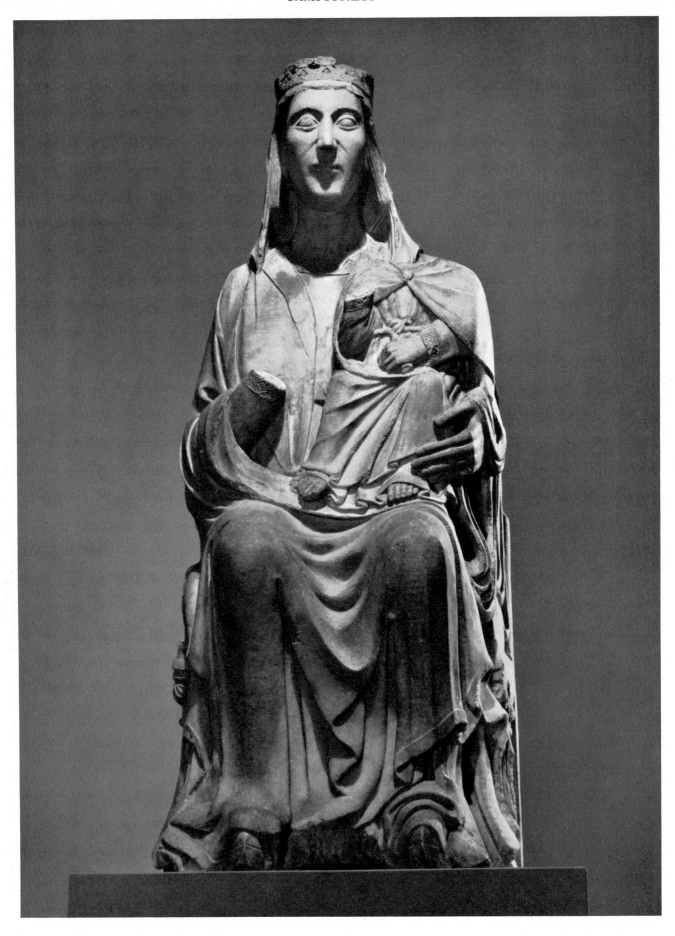

Pl. 20. The Virgin and Child, early 14th cent. Marble, ht., 46¹/₂ in. Chicago, Art Institute.

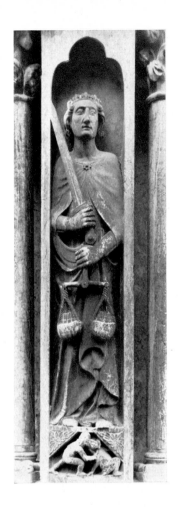

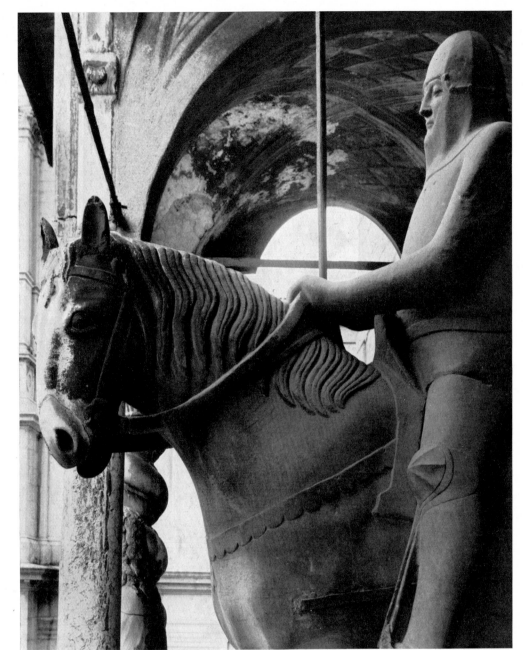

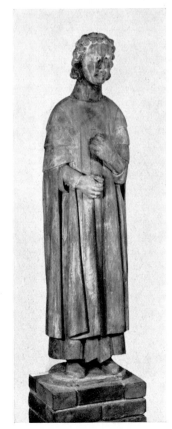

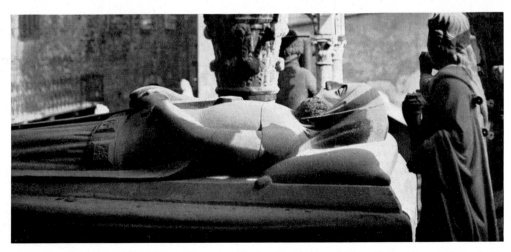

Pl. 21. *Above, left*: Justice, by Giovanni da Campione, 1340. Stone. Bergamo, Italy, Baptistery. *Right*: Equestrian statue of St. Alexander, detail, by Giovanni da Campione, 1353. Stone. Bergamo, Italy, S. Maria Maggiore. *Below, left*: St. Stephen, 1316–30. Stone. Milan, Loggia degli Osii. *Right*: Tomb of Cansignorio, detail, by Bonino da Campione, ca. 1376. Marble. Verona, Italy, Tombs of the Scaligeri.

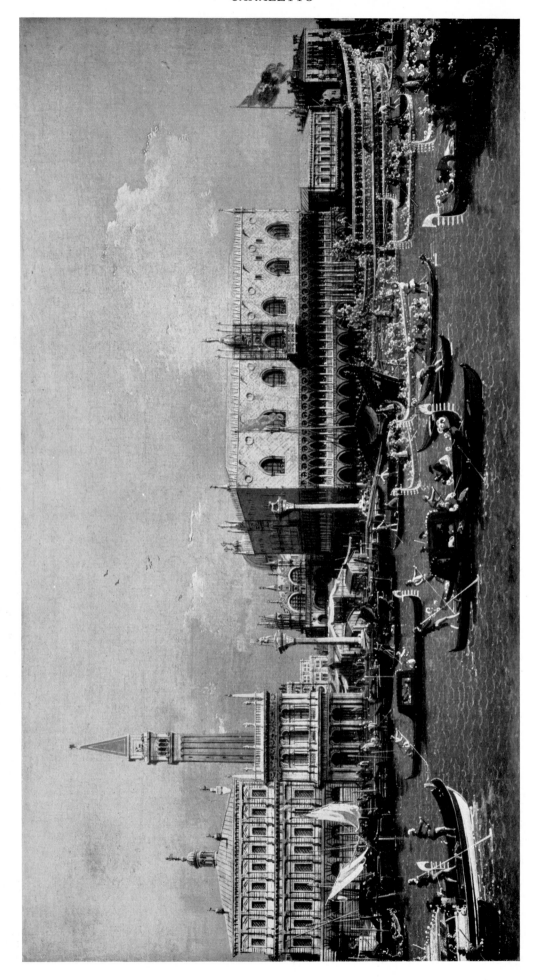

Pl. 22. The Bucentoro at the Molo in Venice during the Festival of the Ascension. Canvas, 22×39 in. London, Dulwich College Gallery.

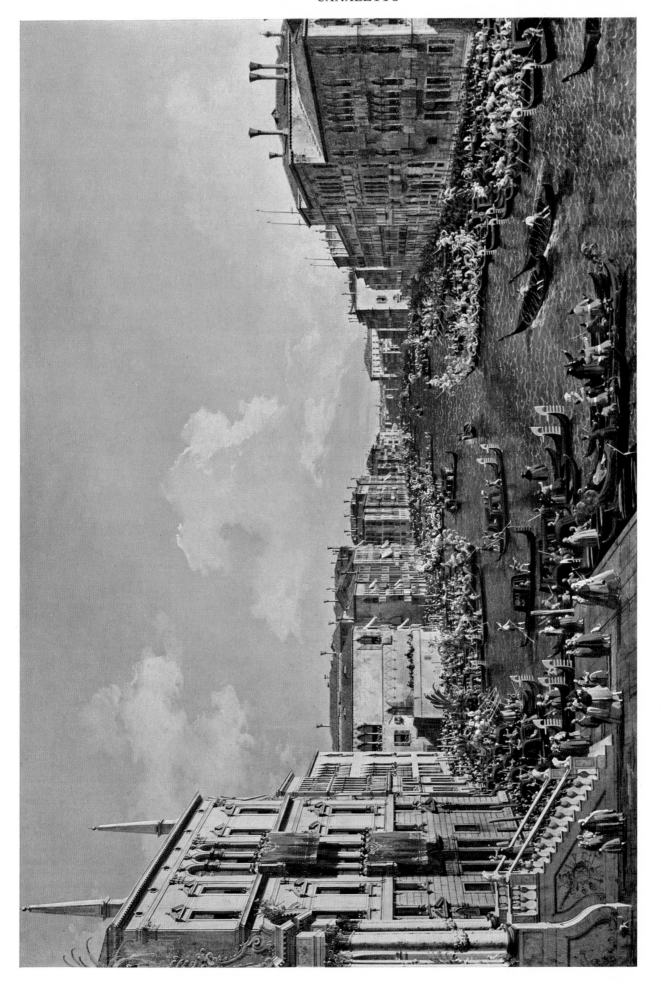

Pl. 23. Regatta on the Grand Canal. Canvas, 4 ft. × 5 ft., 11⅝ in. London, National Gallery.

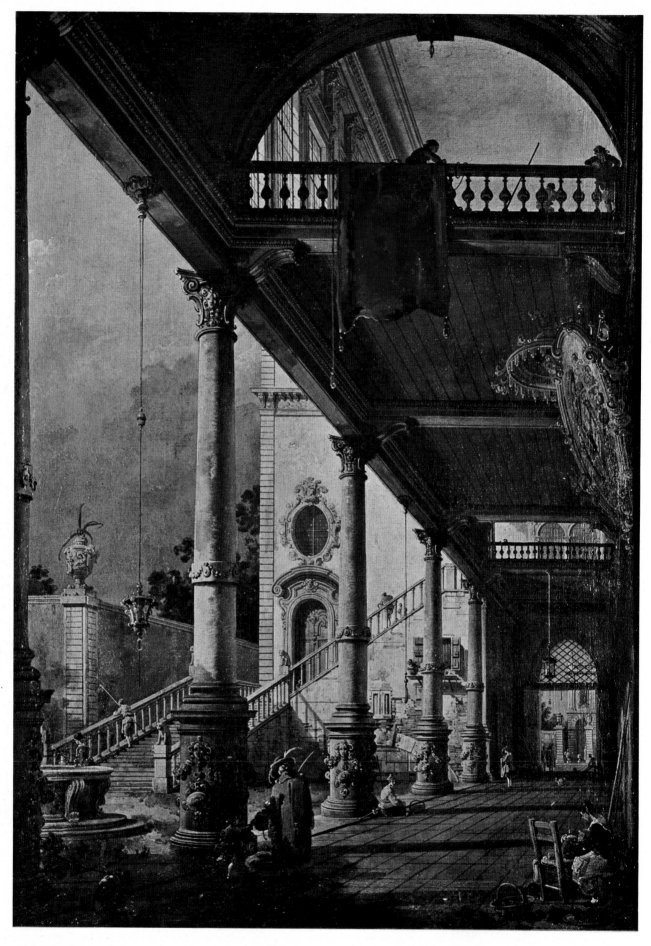

Pl. 24. Capriccio, with the portico of a palace. Canvas, $50^{3}/_{4} \times 36^{5}/_{8}$ in. Venice, Accademia.

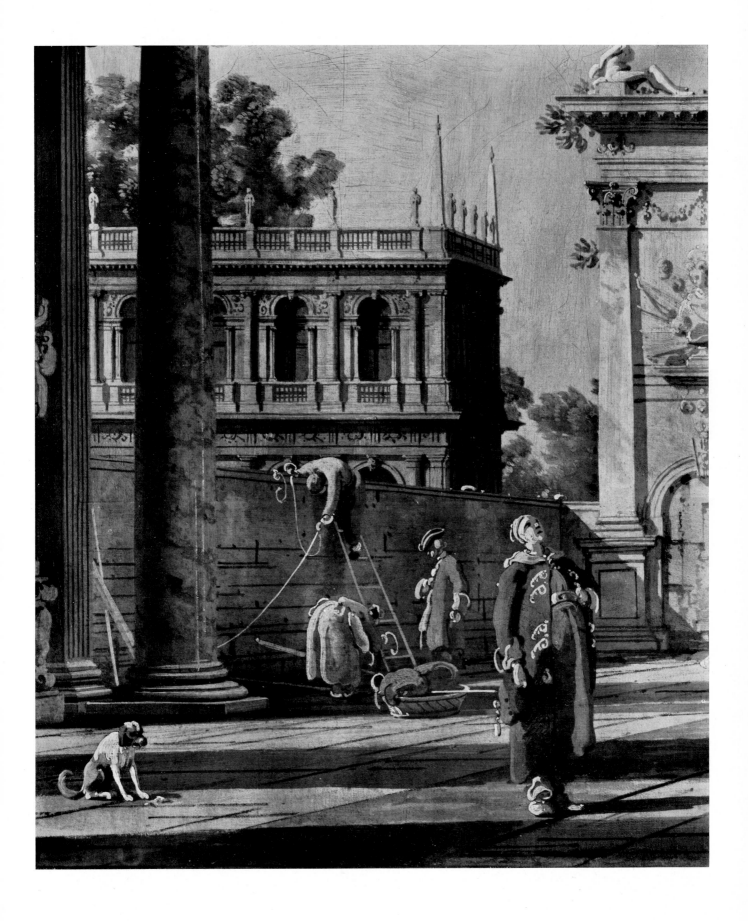

Pl. 25. Capriccio, with buildings seen from a portico, detail. Canvas, full size, 11³/₄×9⁷/₈ in. Arundel Castle, Sussex, England, Duke of Norfolk Coll.

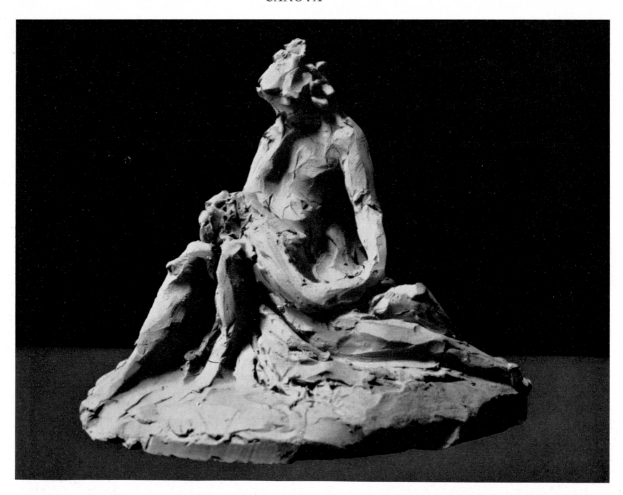

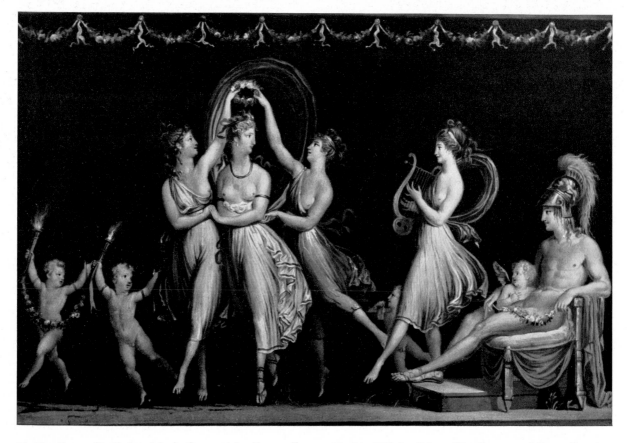

Pl. 26. *Above*: Study for Adonis Crowned by Venus. Terra cotta, ht., 11 3/4 in. *Below*: The Graces and Venus Dancing before Mars. Tempera, 9 7/8 × 15 3/8 in. Both, Possagno, Italy, Museo Canoviano.

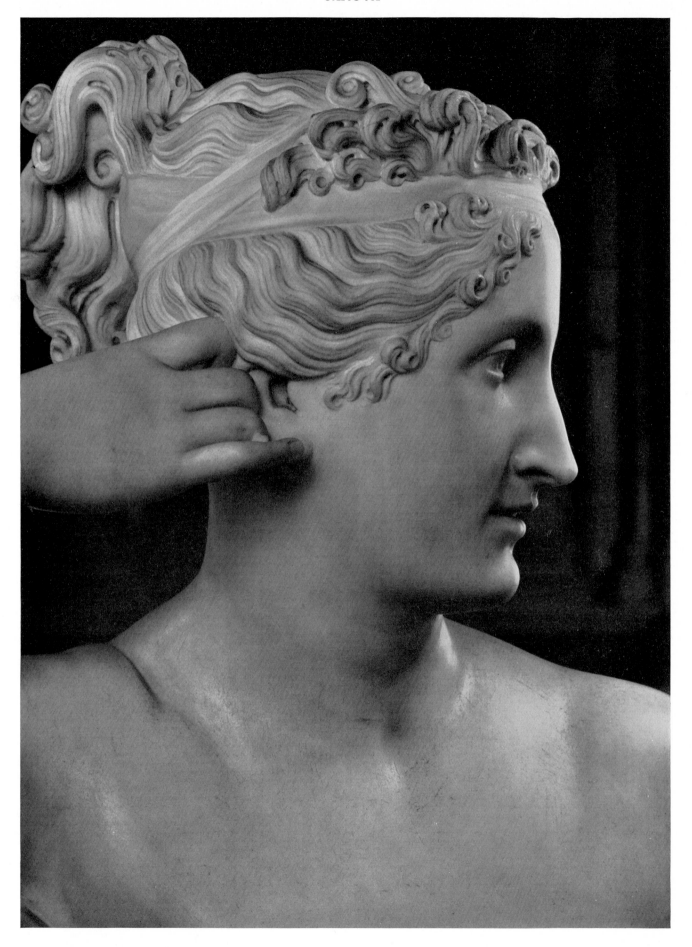

Pl. 27. Pauline Borghese, detail. Marble. Rome, Galleria Borghese.

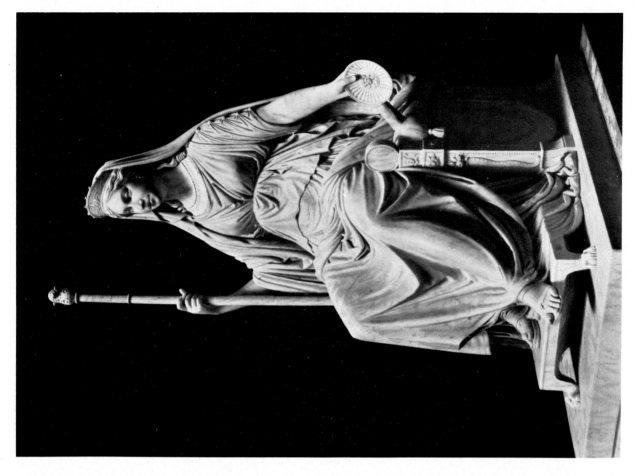

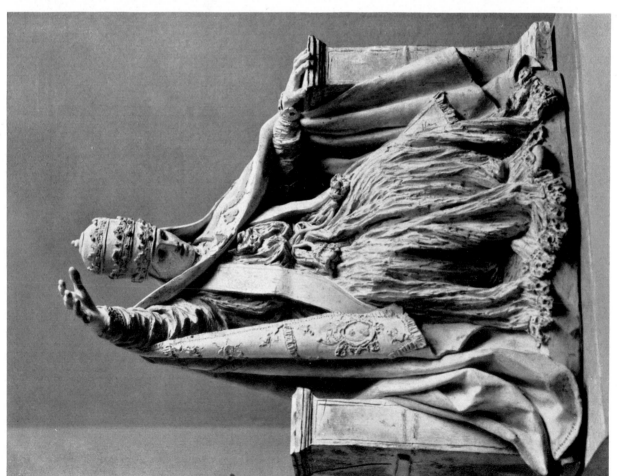

Pl. 28. *Left*: Study for the monument to Clement XIV. Terra cotta, 18¹/₂×16¹/₈ in. Possagno, Italy, Museo Canoviano. *Right*: Marie Louise as Concordia. Marble. Parma, Italy, Galleria Nazionale.

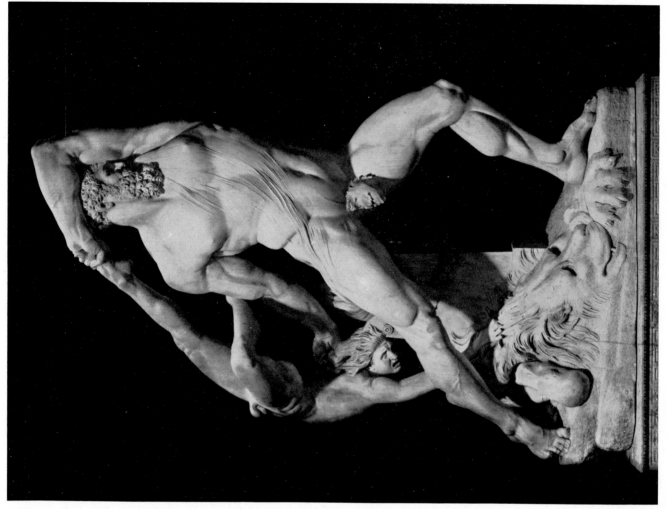

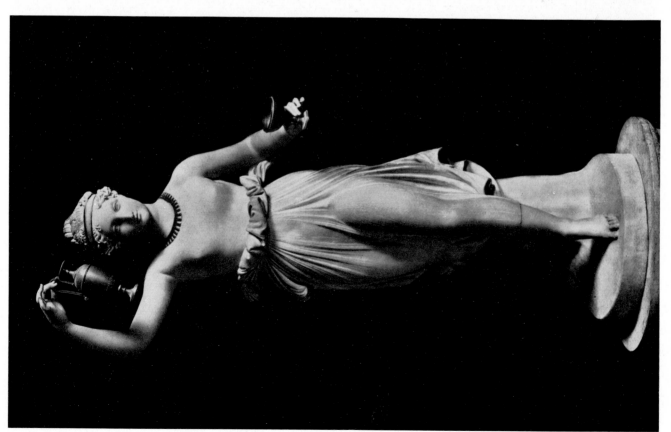

Pl. 29. *Left*: Hebe. Marble. Forlì, Italy, Pinacoteca e Musei Comunali. *Right*: Hercules and Lichas. Marble. Rome, Galleria Nazionale d'Arte Moderna.

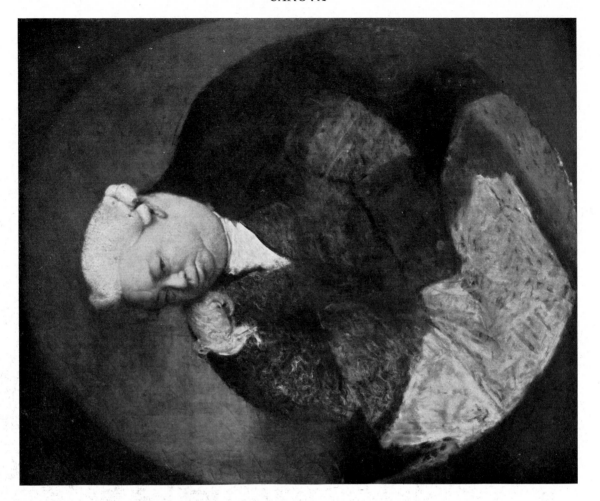

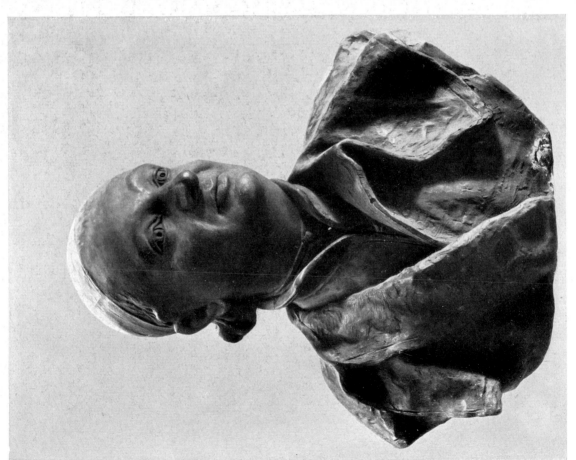

Pl. 30. *Left*: Gian Matteo Amadei. Terra cotta. Venice, Seminario Patriarcale. *Right*: Amedeo Svajer. Canvas, 42¹/₈×34¹/₄ in. Venice, Museo Correr.

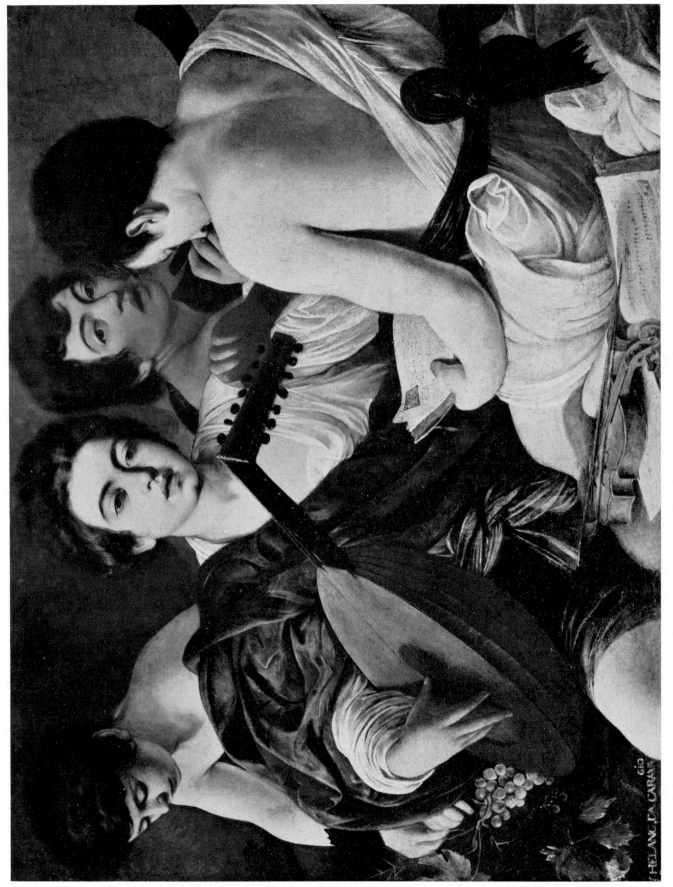

Pl. 31. The Musical Party. Canvas, 36¹/₄×46¹/₂ in. New York, Metropolitan Museum.

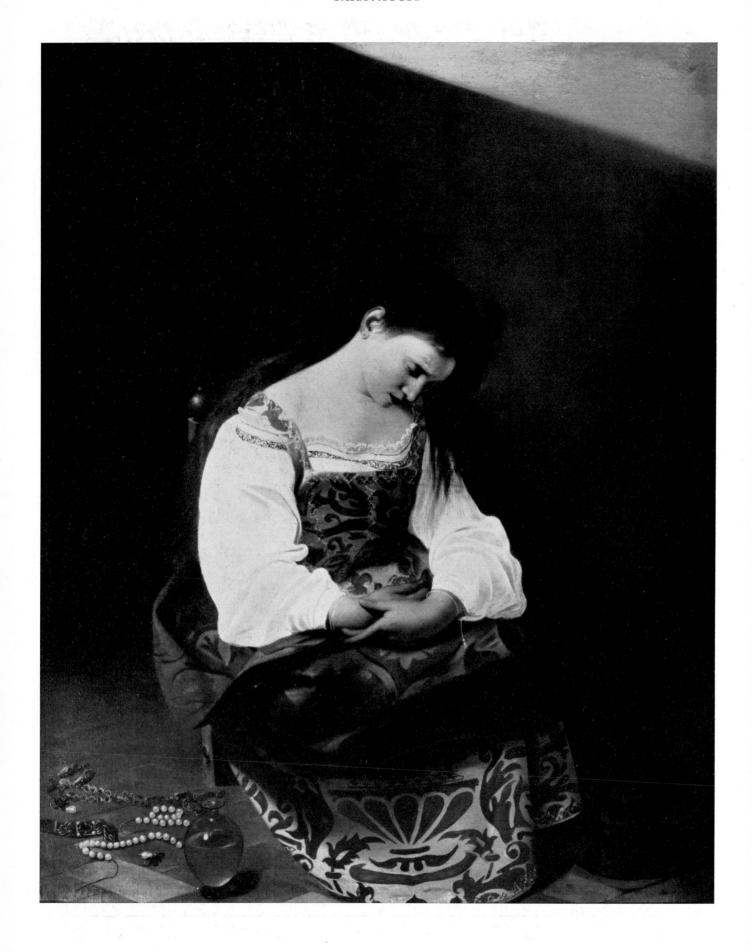

Pl. 32. The Magdalen. Canvas, 41³/₄×38¹/₄ in. Rome, Galleria Doria Pamphili.

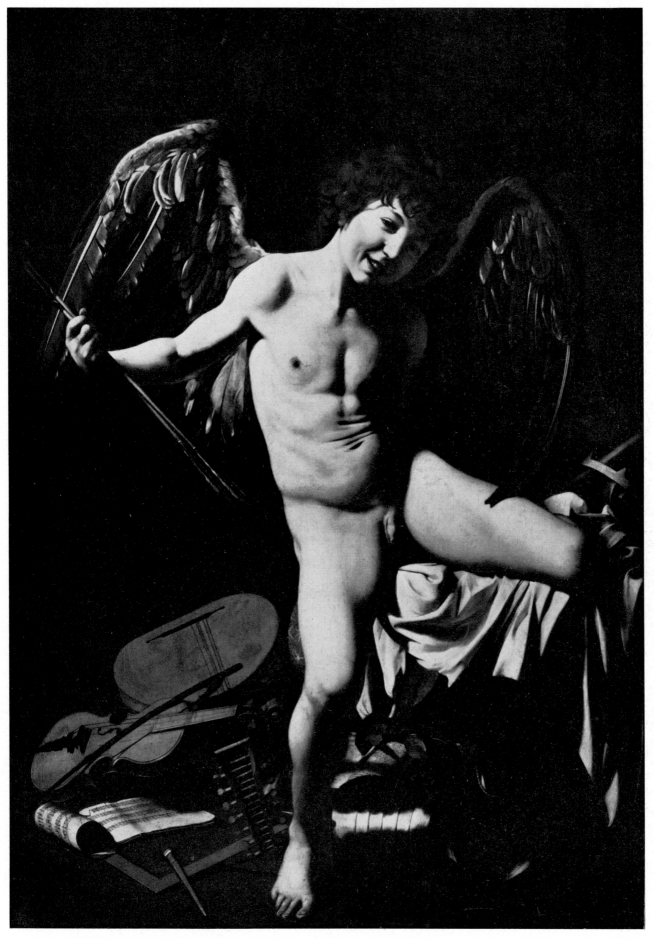

Pl. 33. Amor Victorious. Canvas, 5 ft., $^5/_8$ in. × 3 ft., $7^1/_4$ in. Berlin, Staatliche Museen.

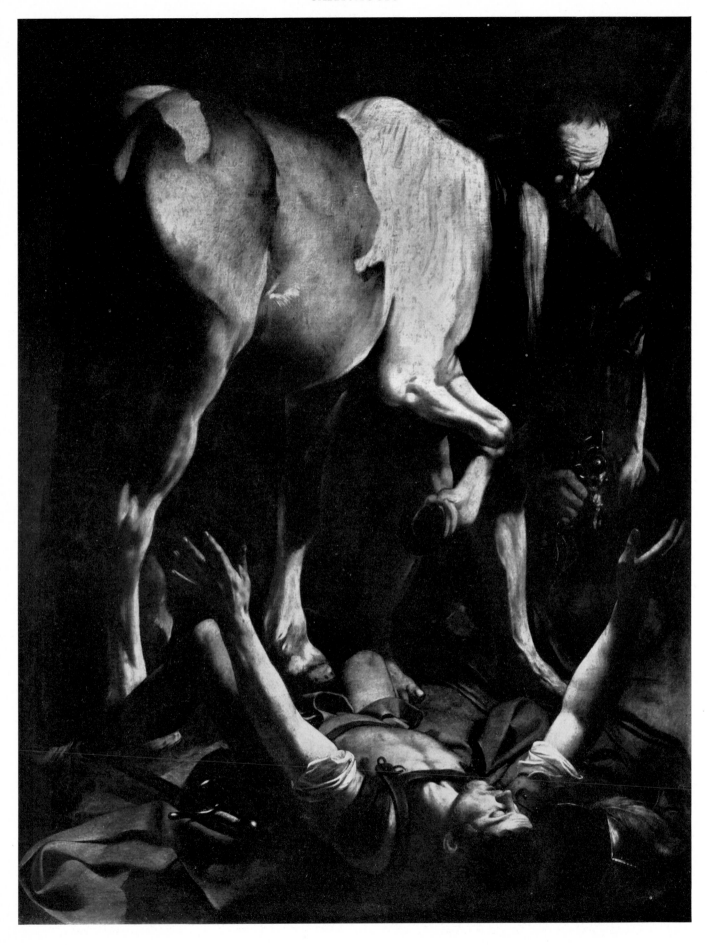

Pl. 34. The Conversion of St. Paul. Canvas, 7 ft., 6¹/₂ in. × 5 ft., 8⁷/₈ in. Rome, S. Maria del Popolo.

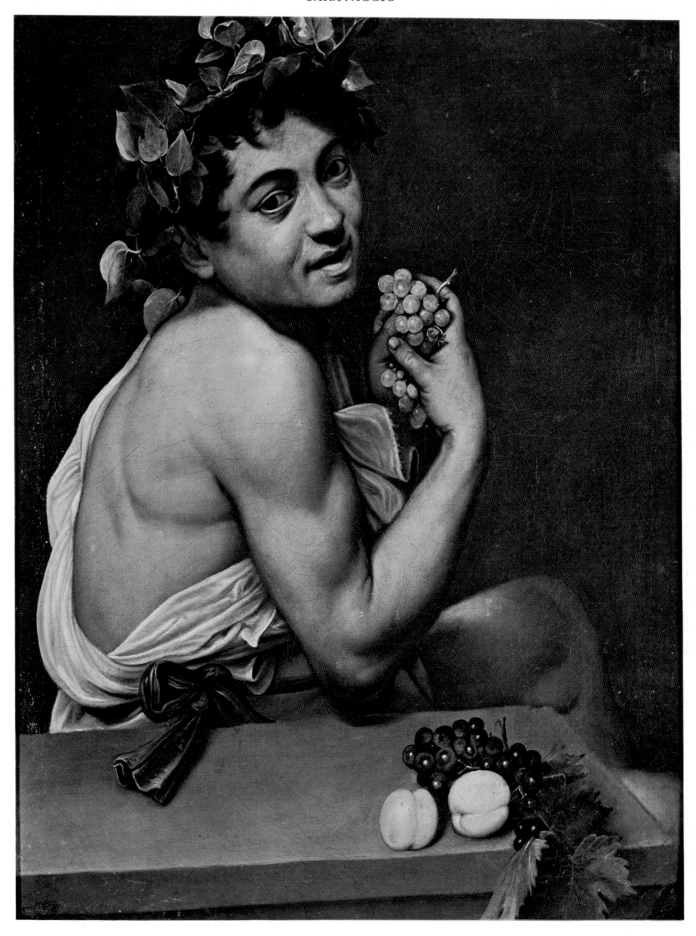

Pl. 35.  Boy with Fruit, or "Bacchino Malato." Canvas, $26 \times 20^{1}/_{2}$ in. Rome, Galleria Borghese.

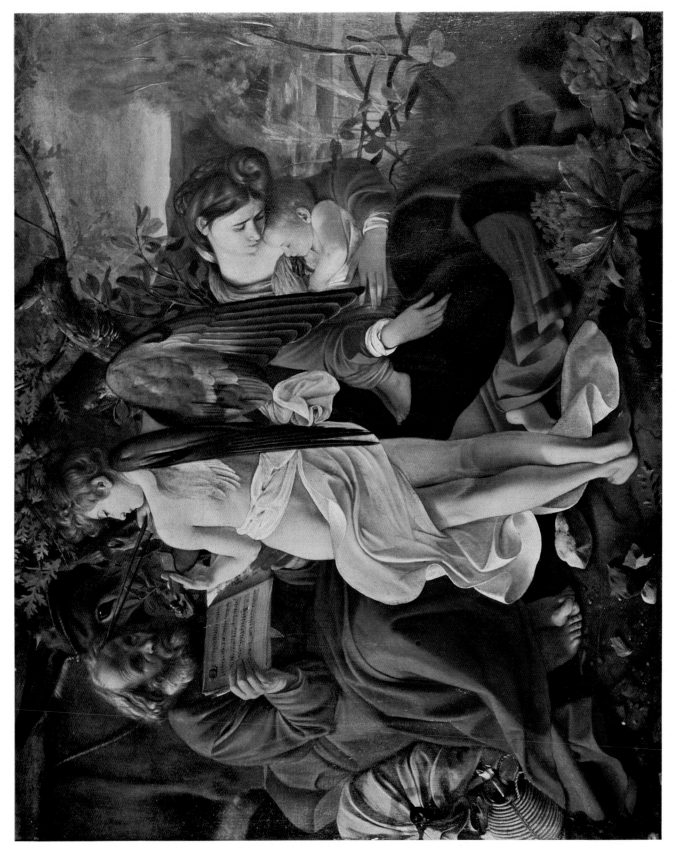

Pl. 36. Rest on the Flight into Egypt. Canvas, 4 ft., 3¹/₈ in. × 5 ft., 3 in. Rome, Galleria Doria Pamphili.

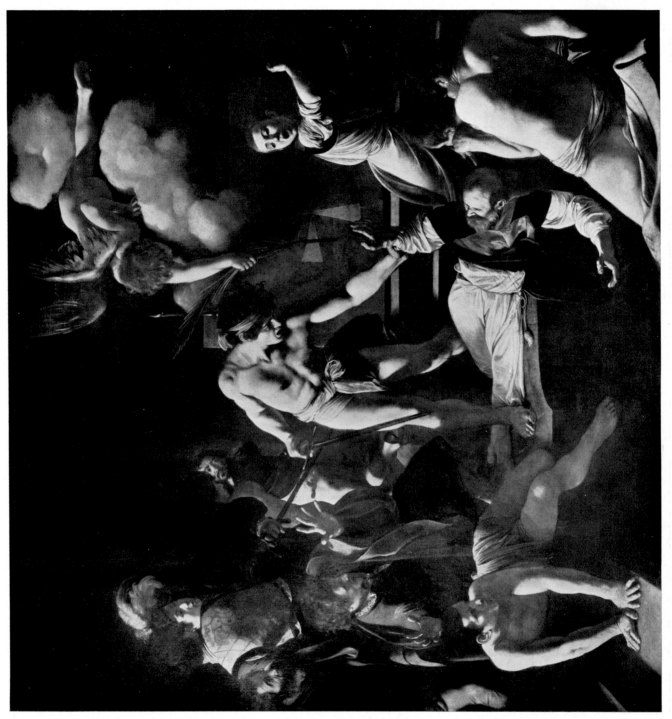

Pl. 37. The Martyrdom of St. Matthew. Canvas, 10 ft., 9 1/8 in. × 11 ft., 5 in. Rome, S. Luigi dei Francesi.

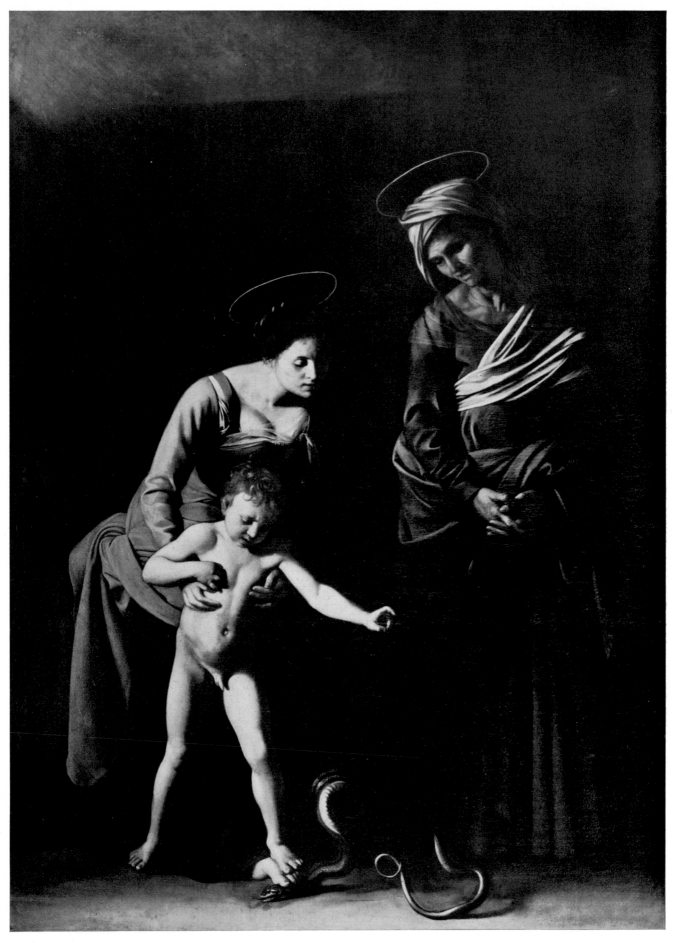

Pl. 38.  The Virgin and Child with St. Anne. Canvas, 9 ft., 7 in. × 6 ft., 11 in. Rome, Galleria Borghese.

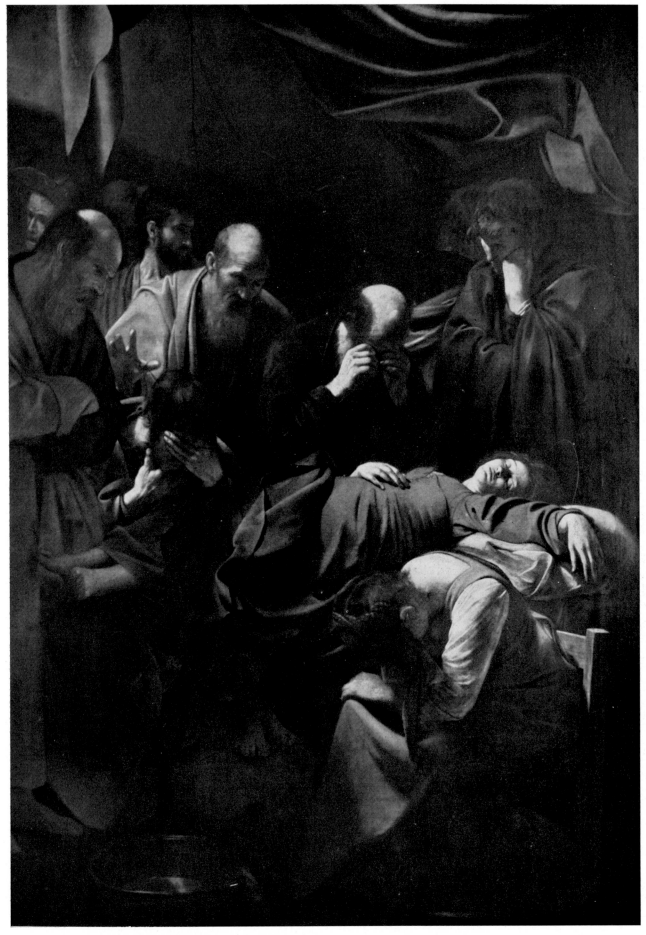

Pl. 39. Death of the Virgin, detail. Canvas; full size, 12 ft., 1¹/₄ in. × 8 ft., ¹/₂ in. Paris, Louvre.

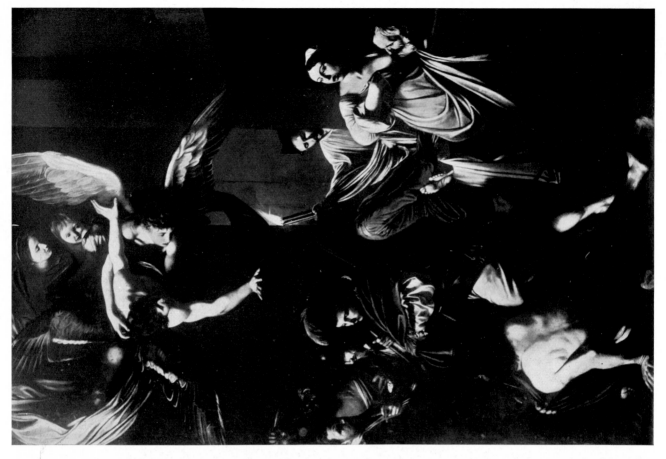

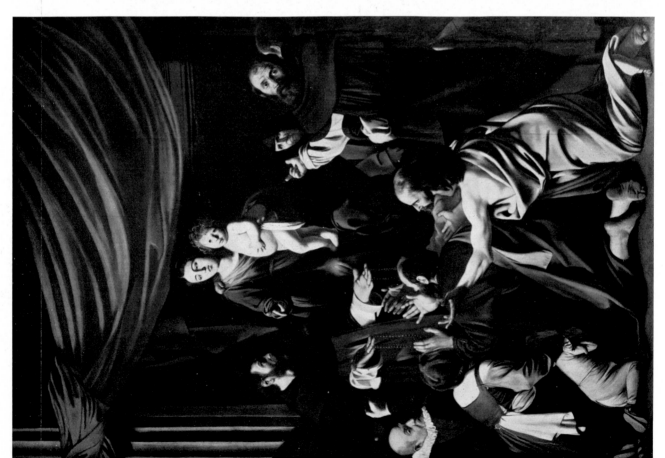

Pl. 40. *Left*: The Madonna of the Rosary. Canvas, 11 ft., 11¼ in. × 8 ft., 2 in. Vienna, Kunsthistorisches Museum. *Right*: The Seven Works of Mercy. Canvas, 12 ft., 9½ in. × 8 ft., 6⅜ in. Naples, Pio Monte della Misericordia.

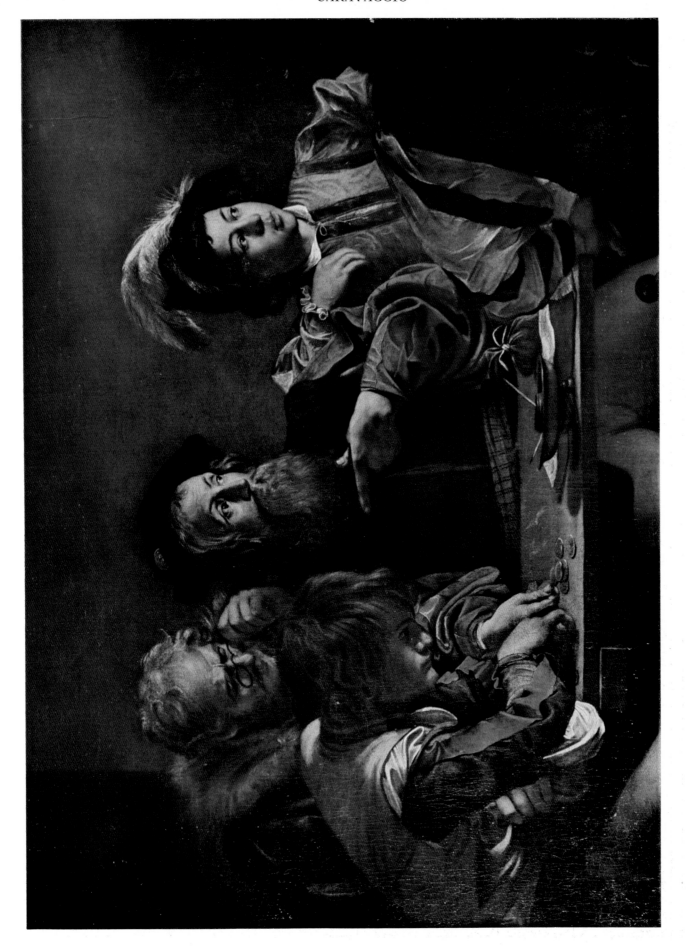

Pl. 41. The Calling of St. Matthew, detail. Canvas; full size, 10 ft, 9 in. × 11 ft, 5 in. Rome, S. Luigi dei Francesi.

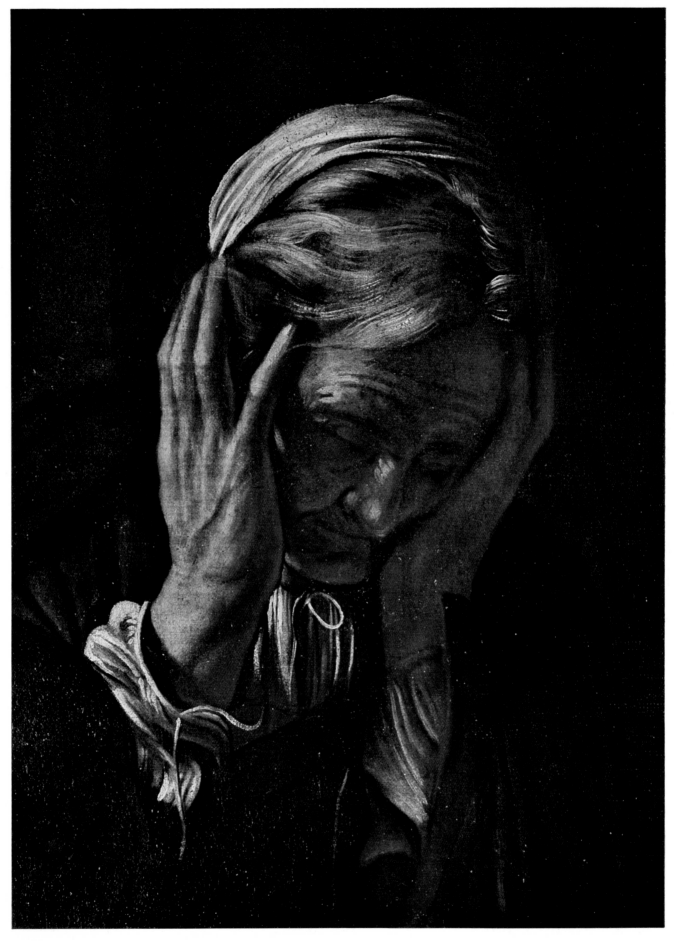

Pl. 42. The Beheading of John the Baptist, detail. Canvas; full size, 11 ft., 10 in. × 17 ft., ³/₄ in. Valletta, Malta, Cathedral.

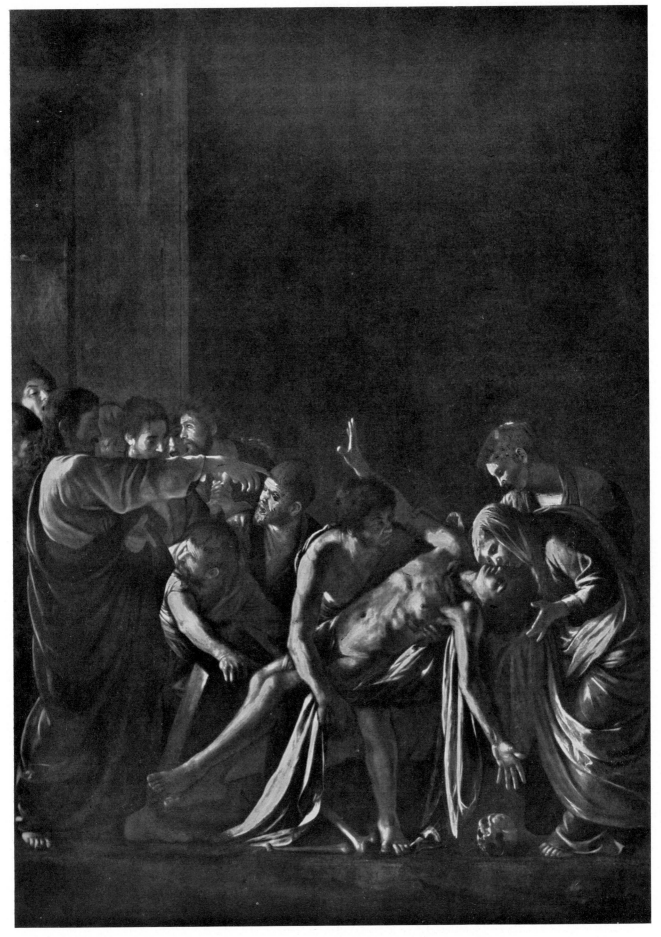

Pl. 43. The Raising of Lazarus. Canvas, 12 ft., 5⁵/₈ in. × 9 ft., ¹/₄ in. Messina, Sicily, Museo Nazionale.

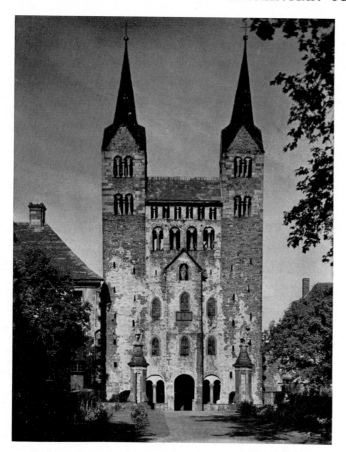
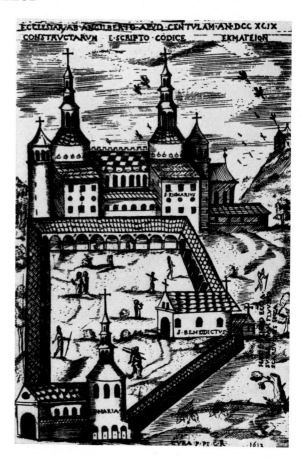

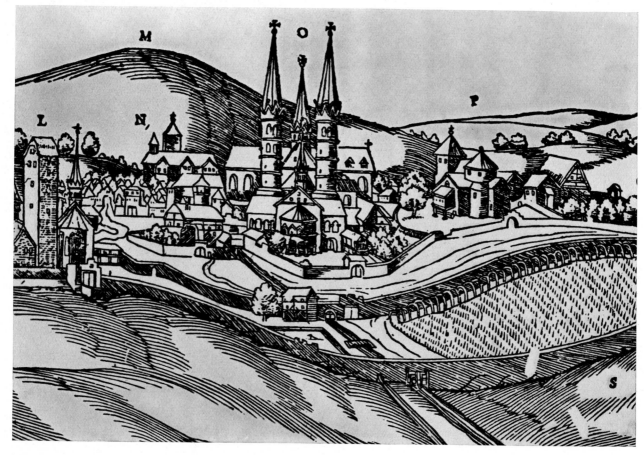

Pl. 44. *Above, left*: Corvey, Lower Saxony, Germany, the *Westwerk* of the church of the Benedictine abbey, 873–85, with later additions. *Right*: Saint-Riquier (anc. Centula), Somme, France, abbey church, 790–99. Engraving of 1612. *Below*: View of Fulda, Hesse, Germany, showing the abbey church of 819 in the center. Woodcut of 1550.

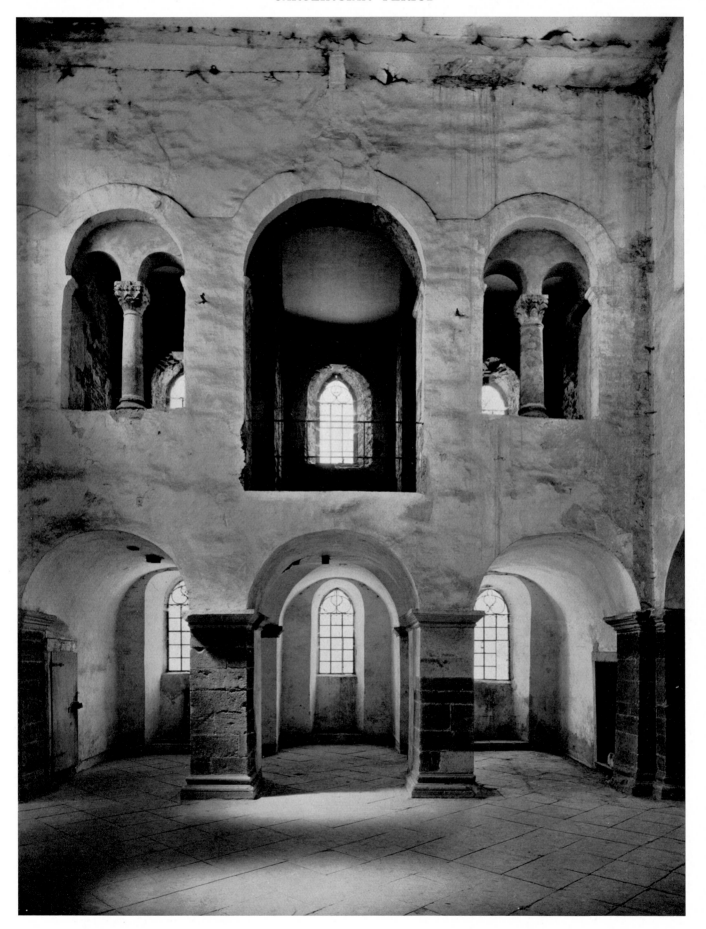

Pl. 45. Corvey, Lower Saxony, Germany, church of the Benedictine abbey, interior of the upper level of the *Westwerk*, showing the imperial box, 873–85.

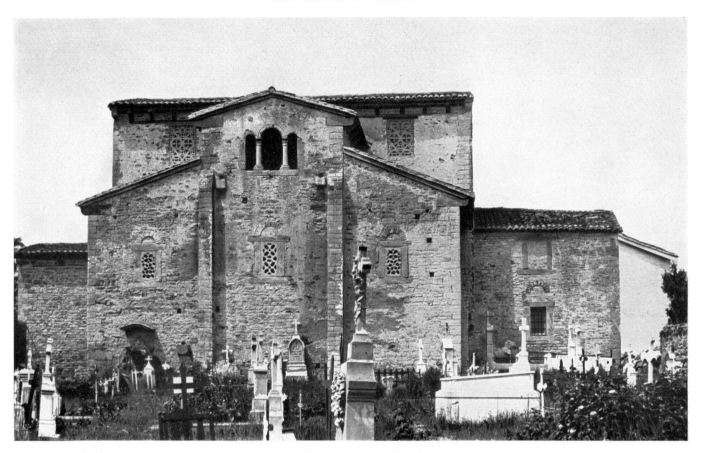

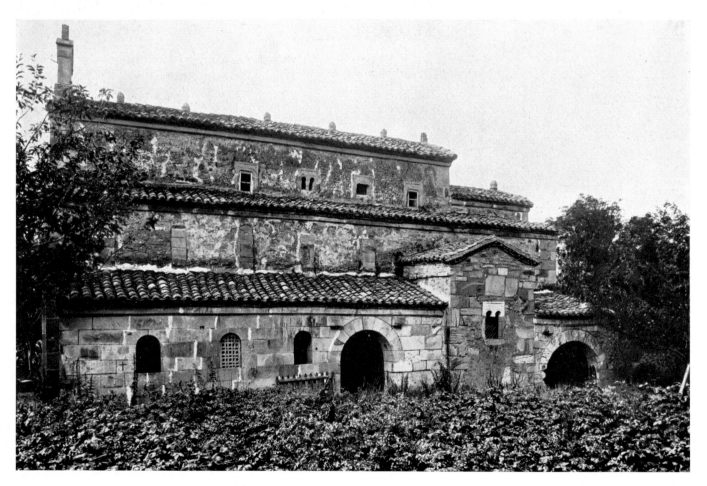

Pl. 46. Oviedo, Asturias, Spain. *Above*: S. Julián de los Prados, east view, 812–42. *Below*: S. Salvador de Val de Dios, view of flank, 893.

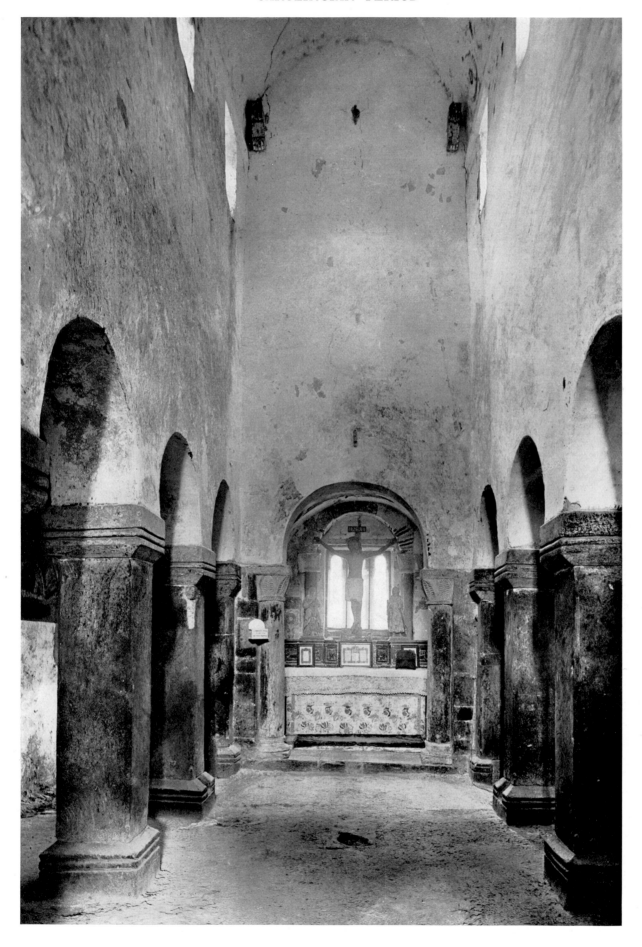

Pl. 47. Oviedo, Asturias, Spain, S. Salvador de Val de Dios, interior, 893.

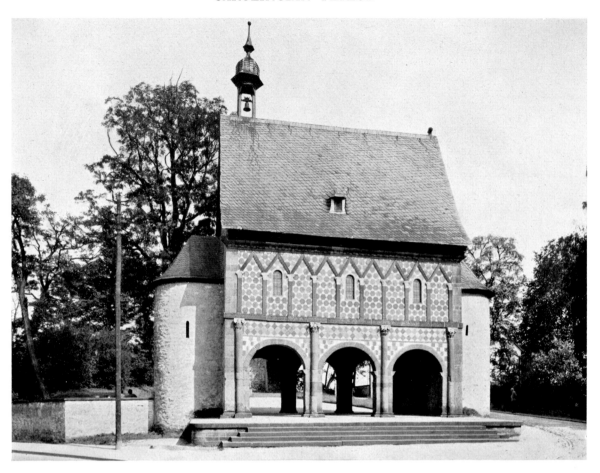

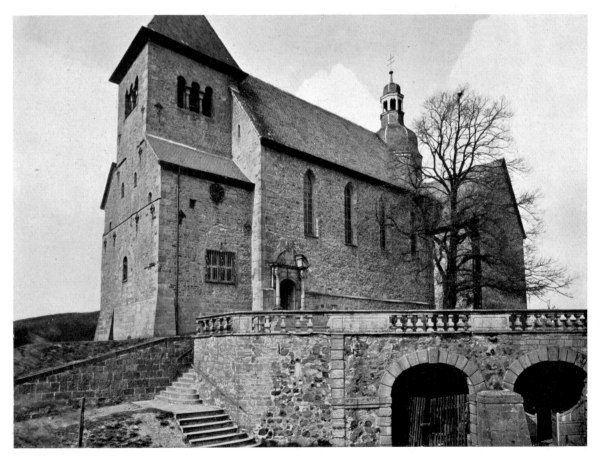

Pl. 48. *Above*: Lorsch, Hesse, Germany, gateway (*Torhalle*) of the imperial abbey, 768–74. *Below*: Fulda, Hesse, Germany, abbey church of St. Peter on the Petersberg, 9th cent.

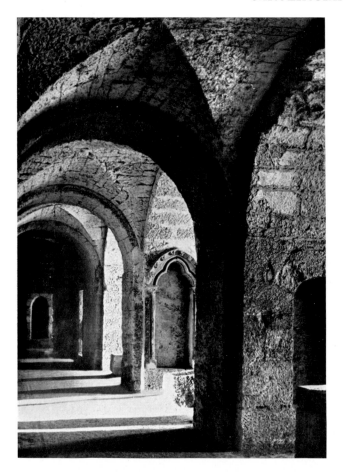

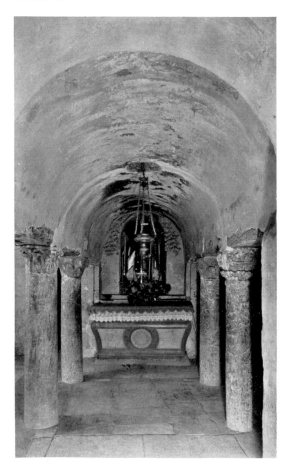

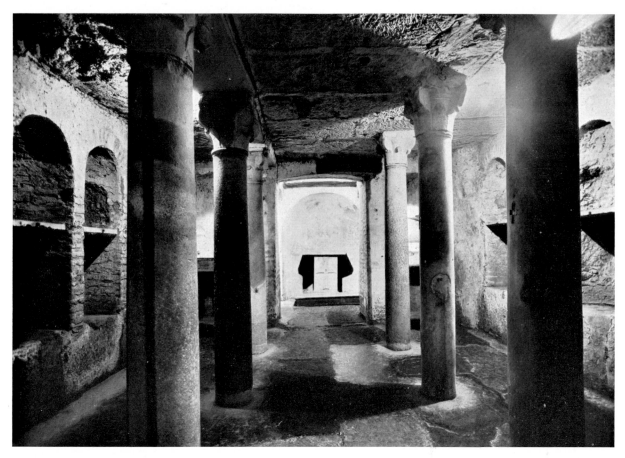

Pl. 49. *Above, left*: Soissons, Aisne, France, St. Médard, crypt, 817–41. *Right*: Auxerre, Yonne, France, St. Germain, crypt, ca. 832. *Below*: Rome, S. Maria in Cosmedin, crypt, 772–95.

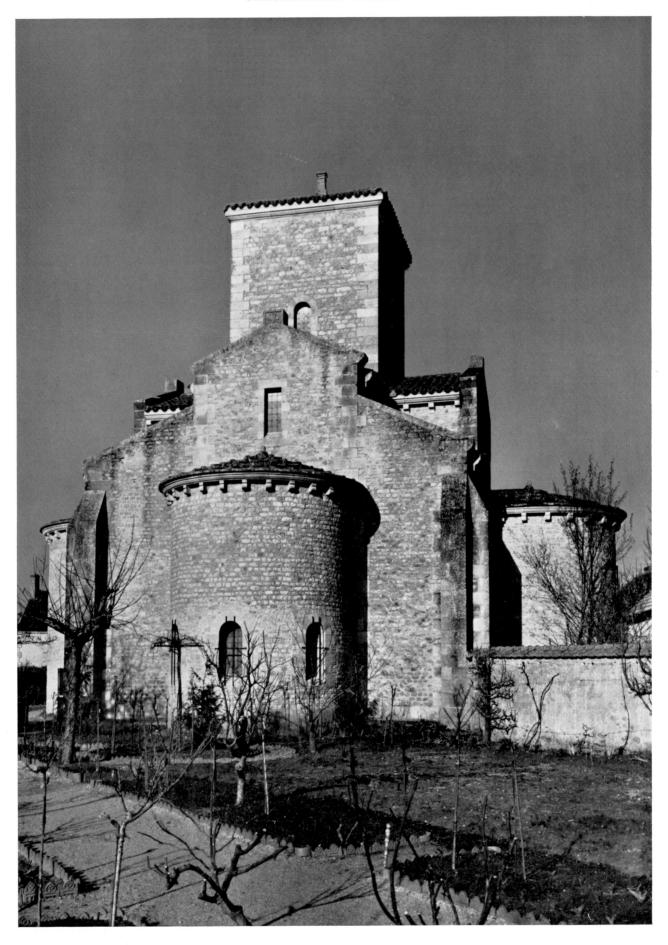

Pl. 50. Germigny-des-Prés, Loiret, France, oratory, view showing the apse, ca. 806.

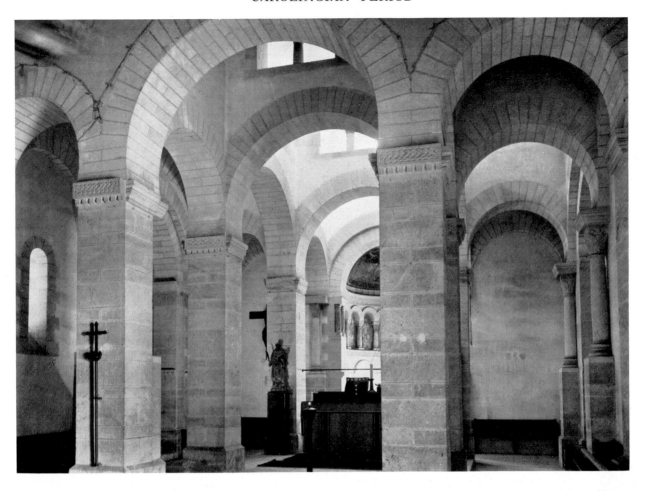

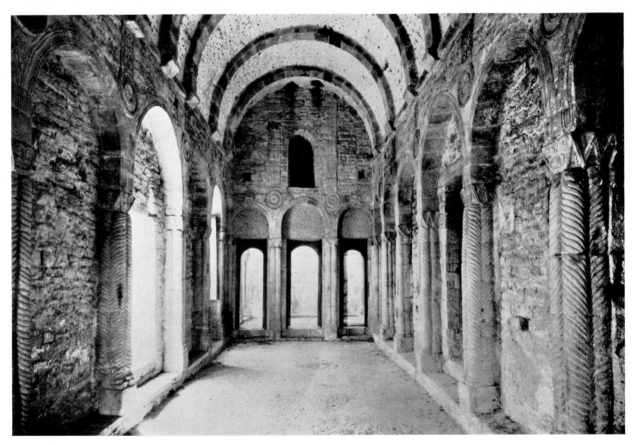

Pl. 51. *Above*: Germigny-des-Prés, Loiret, France, interior of the oratory, ca. 806. *Below*: Naranco, Asturias, Spain, S. Maria, interior, mid-9th cent.

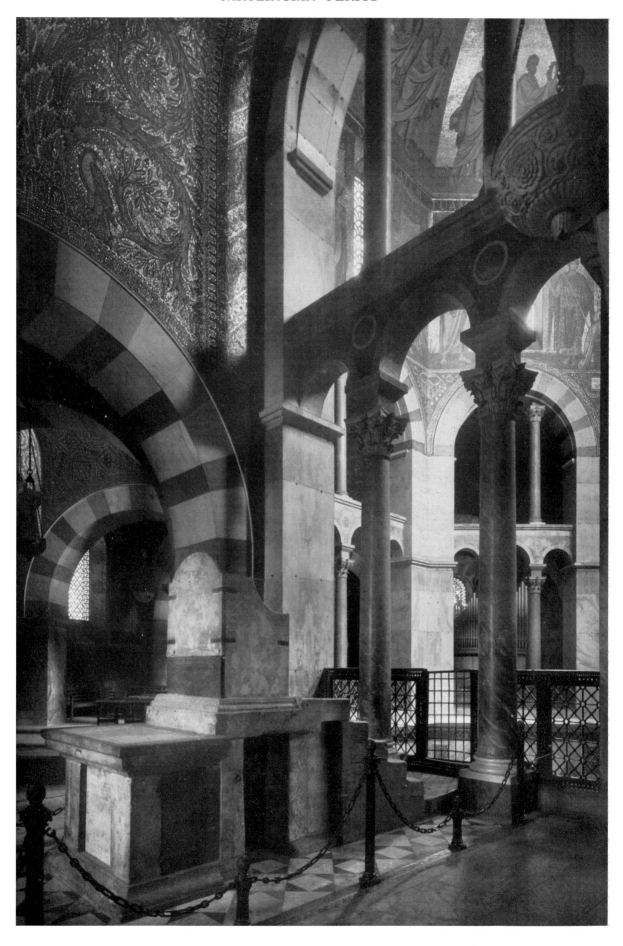

Pl. 52. Aachen, Germany, Palatine Chapel, interior, 805.

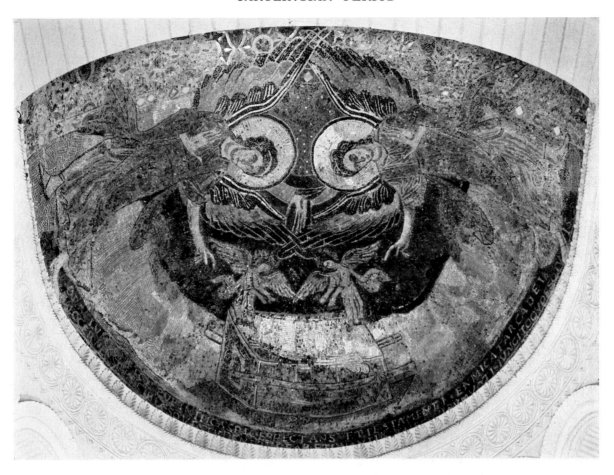

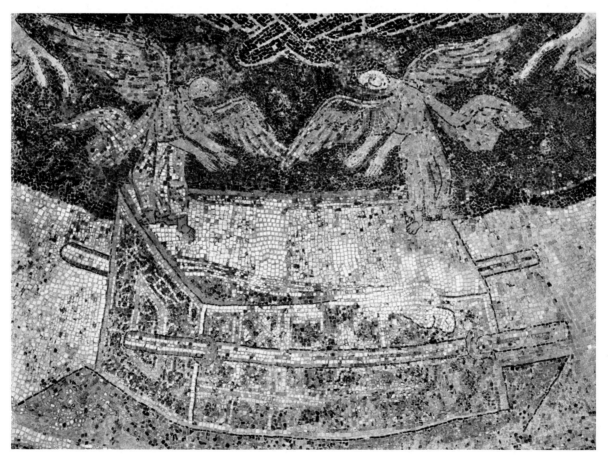

Pl. 53. The Ark of the Covenant, whole and detail, mosaic in the apse of the oratory at Germigny-des-Prés, Loiret, France, 9th cent.

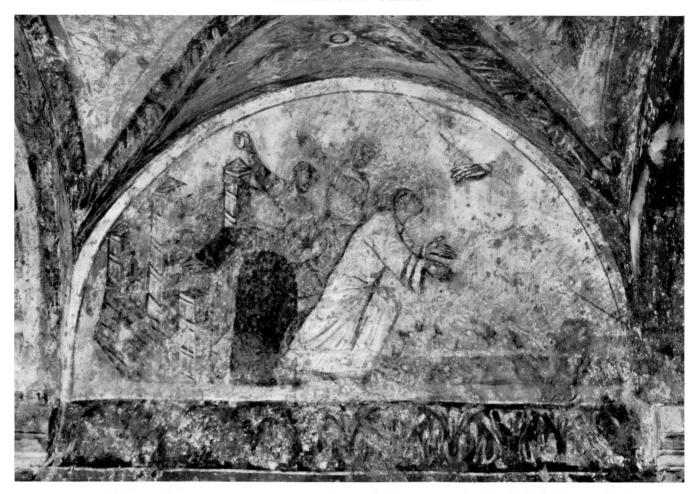

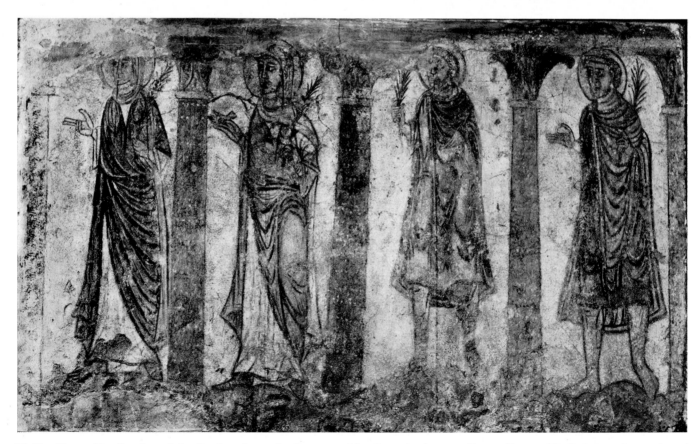

Pl. 54. *Above*: The Stoning of St. Stephen, fresco in the crypt of St. Germain, Auxerre, Yonne, France, 841–61. *Below*: Procession of martyrs, fresco from the crypt of St. Maximin, Trier, Rhineland Palatinate, Germany, late 9th cent. Trier, Landesmuseum.

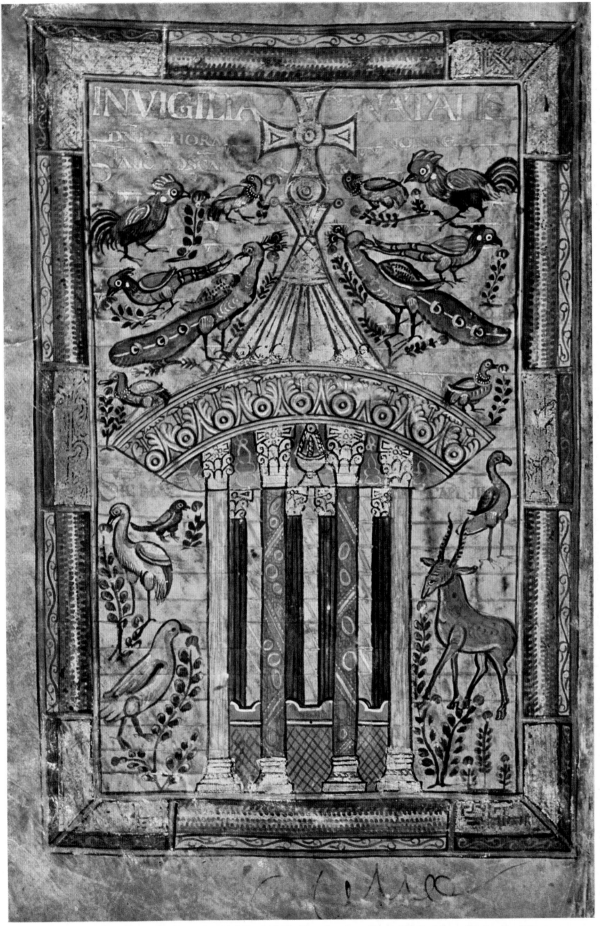

Pl. 55. Godescalc Gospels. The Fountain of Life, 781–83. Illumination. Paris, Bibliothèque Nationale (Ms. nouv. acq. lat. 1203, fol. 3v).

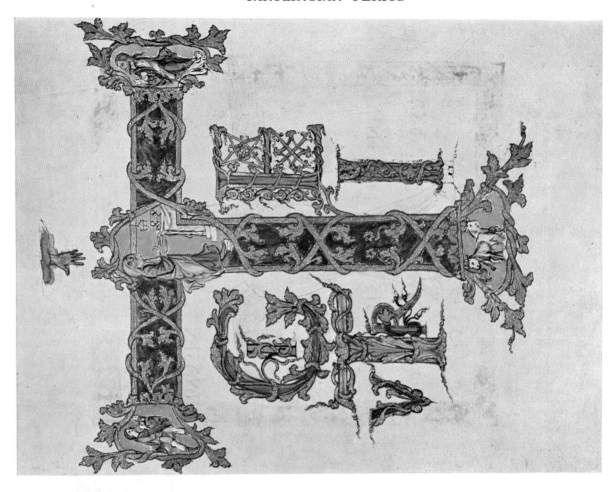

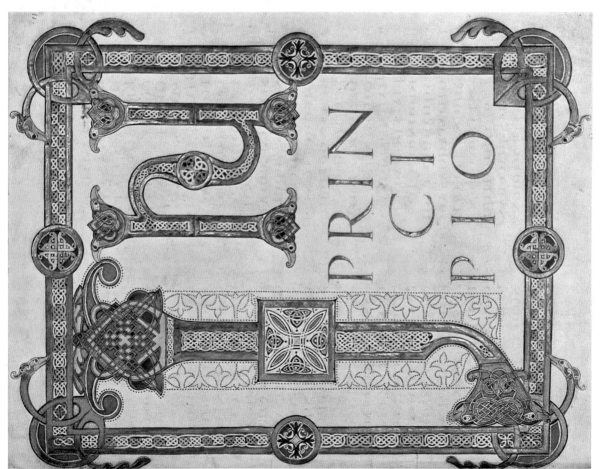

Pl. 56. *Left*: Second Bible of Charles the Bald. Illuminated initial, 871–77. Paris, Bibliothèque Nationale (Ms. lat. 2, fol. 11). *Right*: Drogo Sacramentary. Illuminated initial, 826–55. Paris, Bibliothèque Nationale (Ms. lat. 9428, fol. 15v).

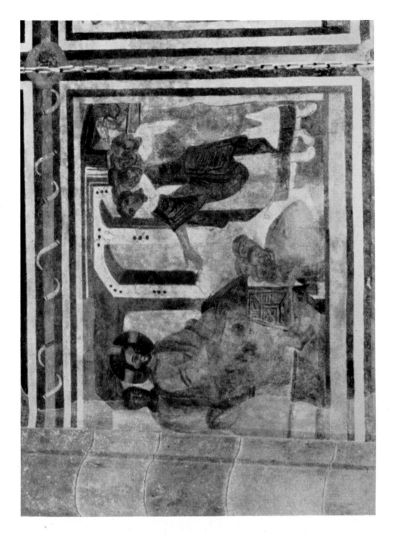

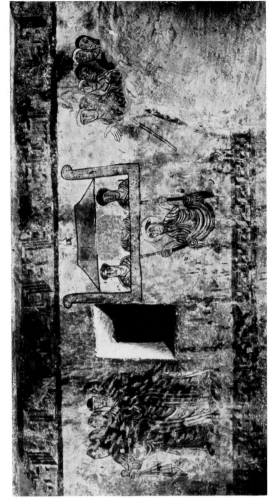

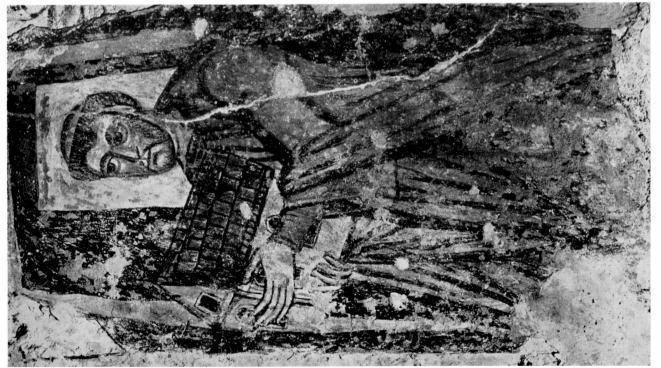

Pl. 57. *Left*: A founder, fresco in S. Benedetto, Malles, Val Venosta, Italy, before 881. *Right, above*: Christ and the apostles, fresco in the nave of St. Johann, Münster, Grisons, Switzerland, late 8th cent. *Below*: Scenes from the life of St. Paul, detail, fresco in the nave of S. Procolo, Naturno, Italy, 9th cent. (?).

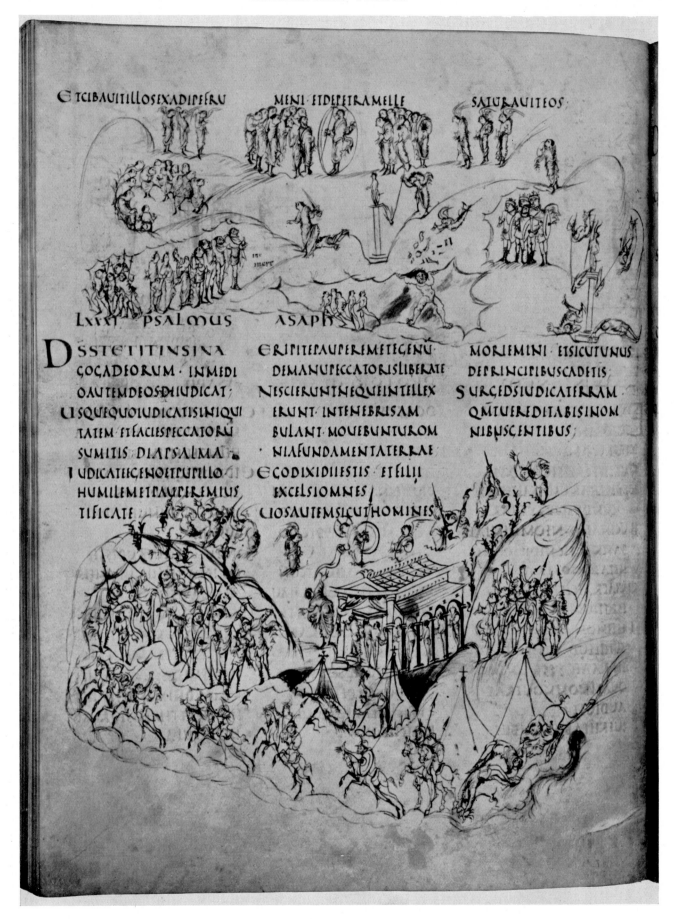

Pl. 58. Utrecht Psalter, 9th cent. Illumination. The Last Judgment (upper scene). The angels of the Lord smiting the enemies of the Israelites (lower scene). Utrecht, Netherlands, University Library (Script. eccl. 484, fol. 48v).

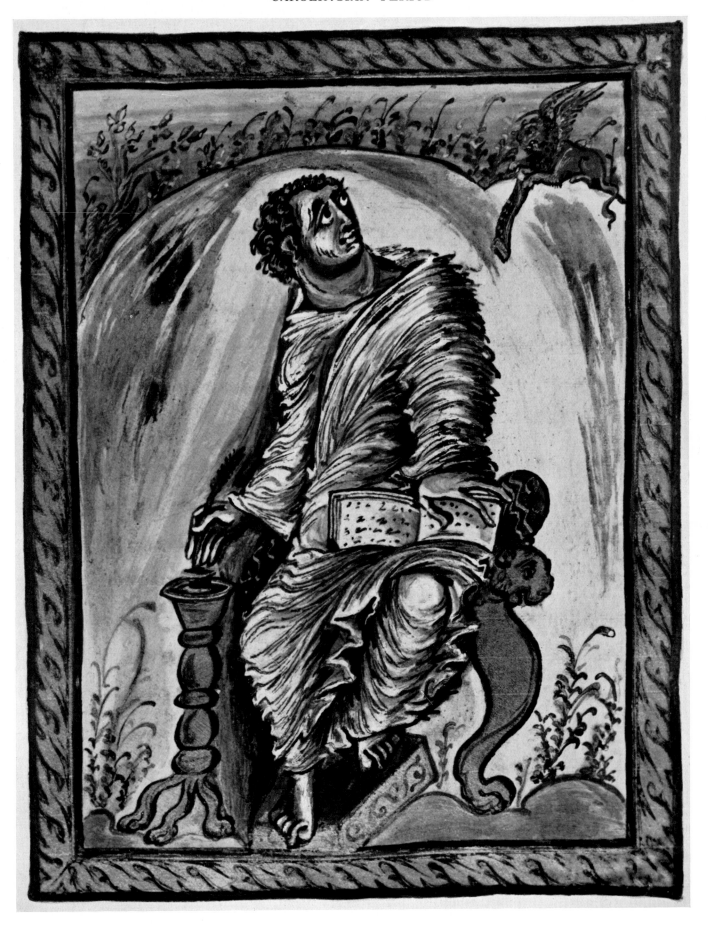

Pl. 59. Ebbo Gospels. Mark the Evangelist, 816–35. Illumination. Epernay, Marne, France, Bibliothèque Municipale (Ms. 1, fol. 60v).

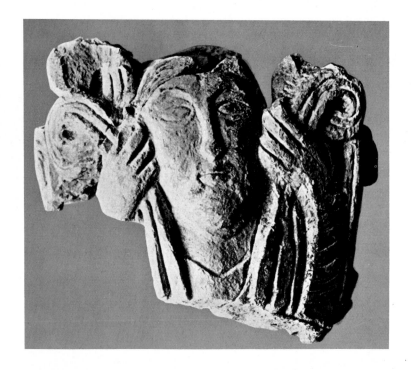

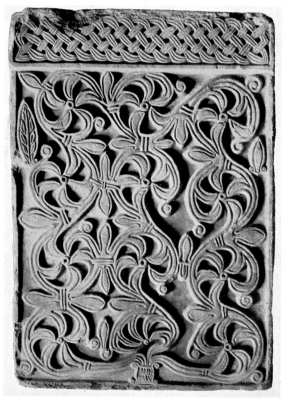

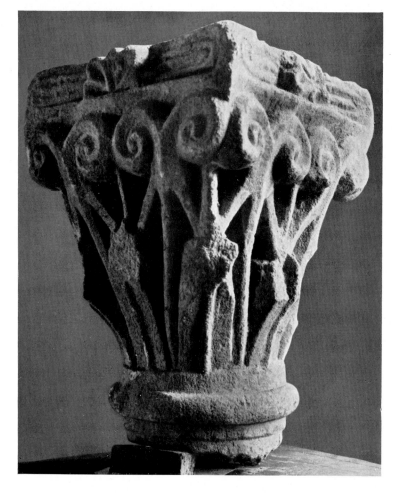

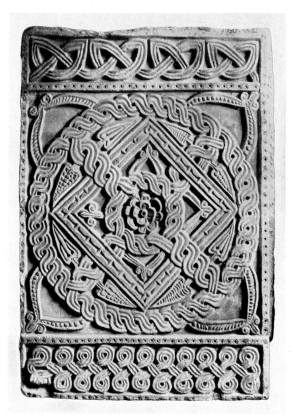

Pl. 60. *Left, above*: Fragment of a capital, 9th cent. Stucco. Malles, Val Venosta, Italy, S. Benedetto. *Below*: Capital from the abbey church of Fulda, Hesse, Germany, 9th cent. Stone. Marburg, Germany, Universitätsmuseum. *Right, above and below*: Slabs from a chancel barrier, originally in the church at Schänis, Switzerland, 8th cent. Stucco. Zurich, Switzerland, Schweizerisches Landesmuseum.

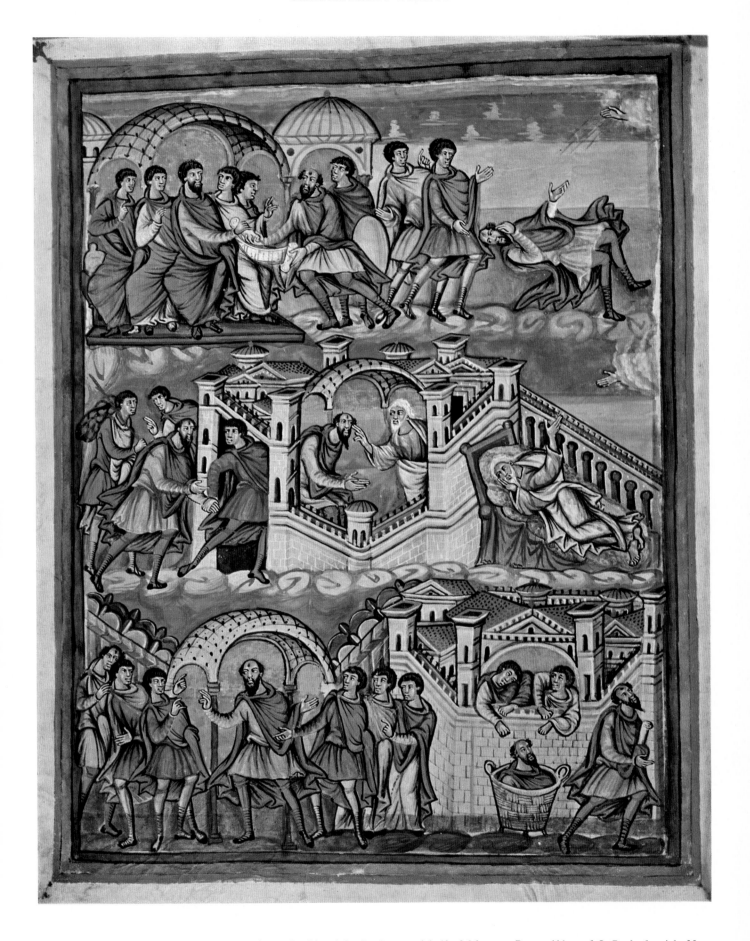

Pl. 61. Bible of Charles the Bald. Scenes from the life of St. Paul, second half of 9th cent. Rome, Abbey of S. Paolo fuori le Mura (fol. CCCVIIv).

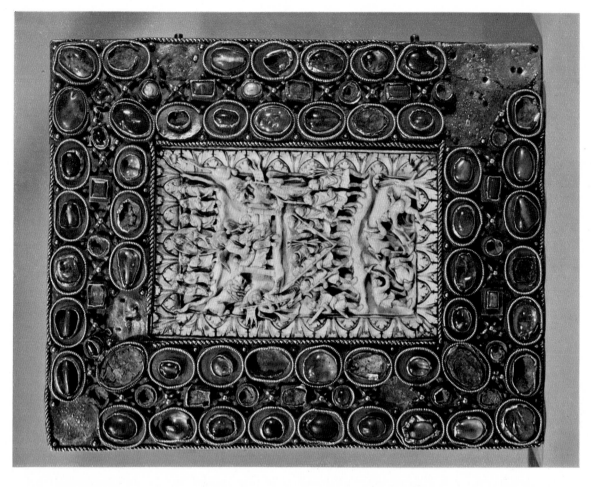

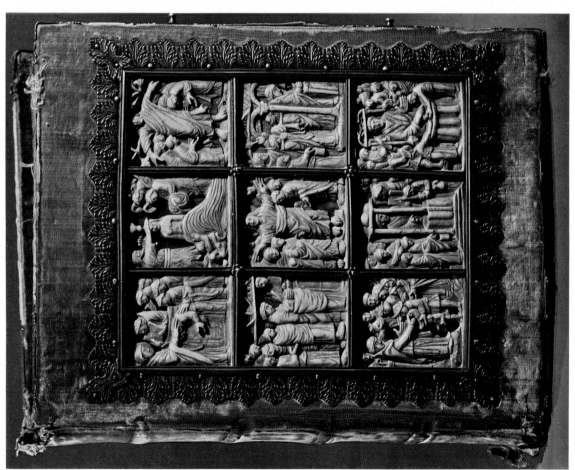

Pl. 62. *Left*: Cover of the Drogo Sacramentary, 826–55. Ivory and silver. Paris, Bibliothèque Nationale (Ms. lat. 9428). *Right*: Cover of the Psalter of Charles the Bald, 860–70. Ivory, copper, and precious stones. Paris, Bibliothèque Nationale (Ms. lat. 1152).

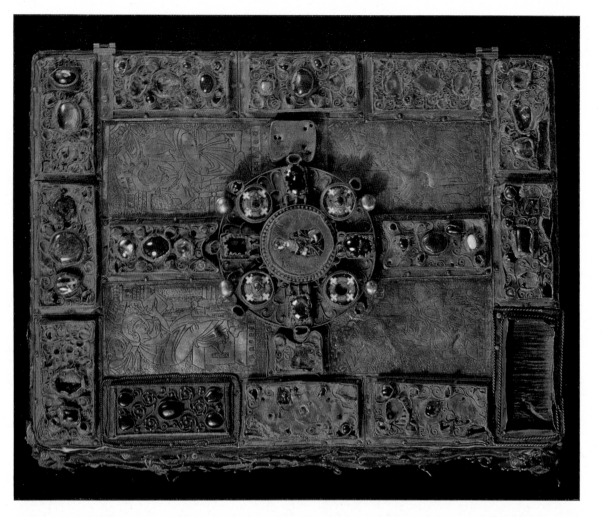

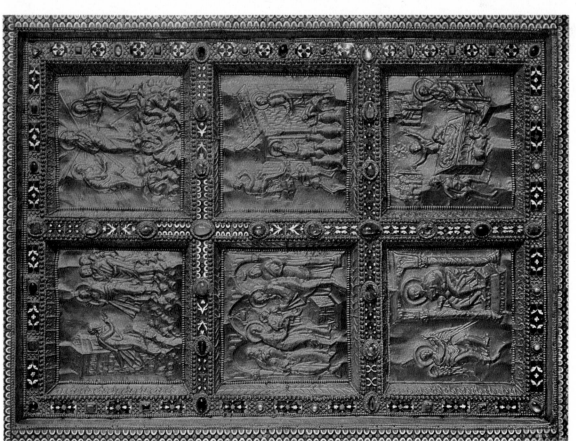

Pl. 63. *Left*: Golden altar of S. Ambrogio, detail of the front, with scenes from the Gospels, 824–59. Gold, enamel, and precious stones. Milan, S. Ambrogio. *Right*: Cover of the Gospels of St. Gauzelin, 807–34. Precious metals and stones with enamel. Nancy, France, Cathedral.

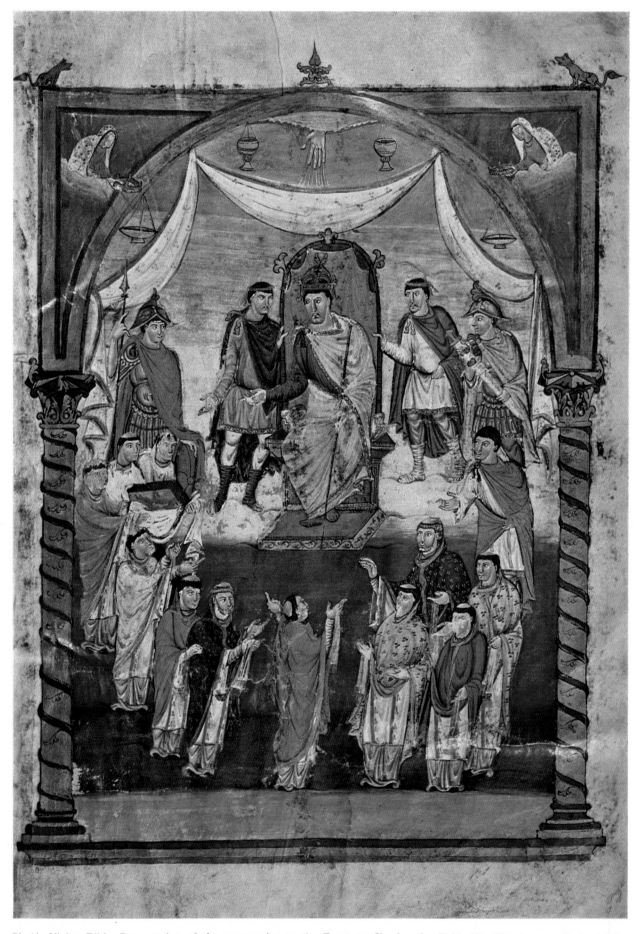

Pl. 64. Vivian Bible. Presentation of the manuscript to the Emperor Charles the Bald, 846. Illumination. Paris, Biblio-thèque Nationale (Ms. lat. 1, fol. 423).

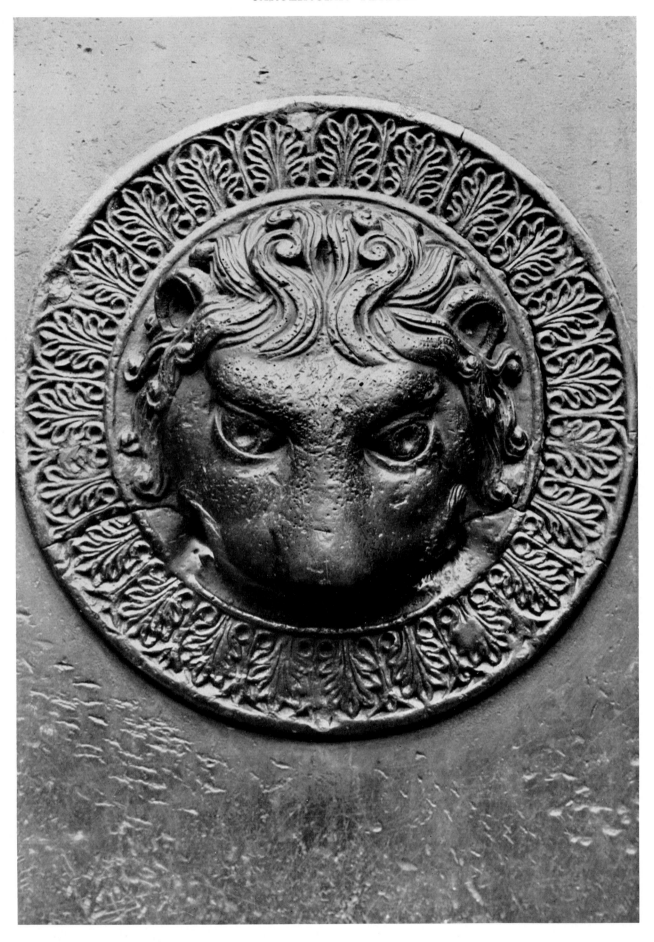

Pl. 65. Aachen, Germany, Palatine Chapel, detail of the right door of the main portal, 9th cent. Bronze.

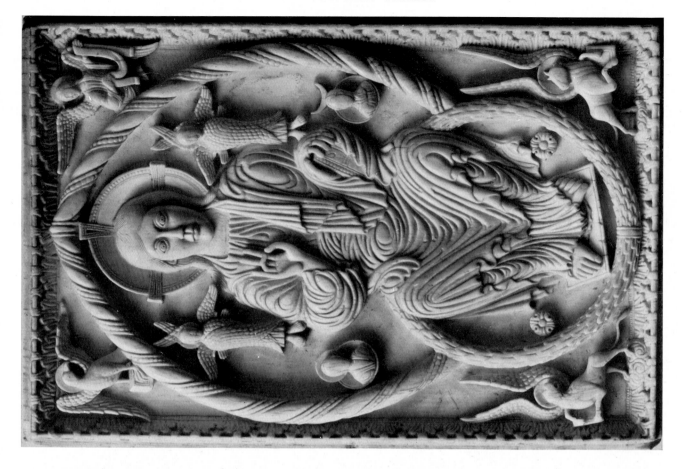

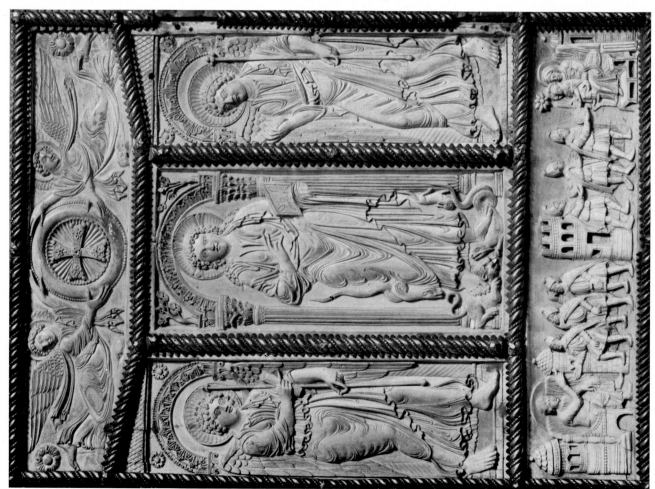

Pl. 66. *Left*: Cover of the Lorsch Gospels, first half of 9th cent. Ivory. Rome, Vatican, Museo Sacro. *Right*: Christ in Majesty, 10th cent. Ivory, 7¹⁄₂×5¹⁄₈ in. Berlin, Staatliche Museen.

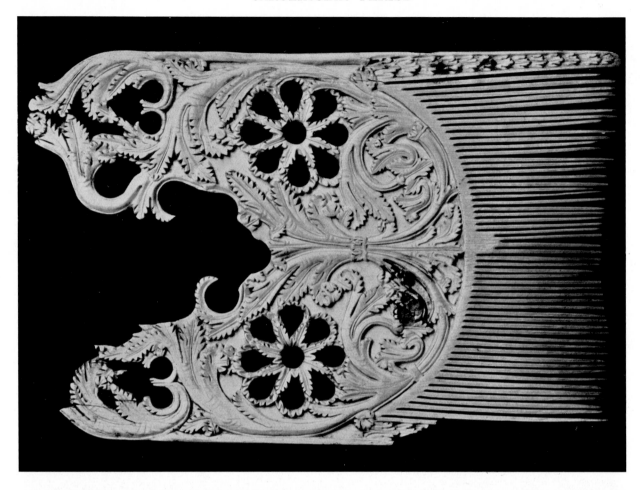

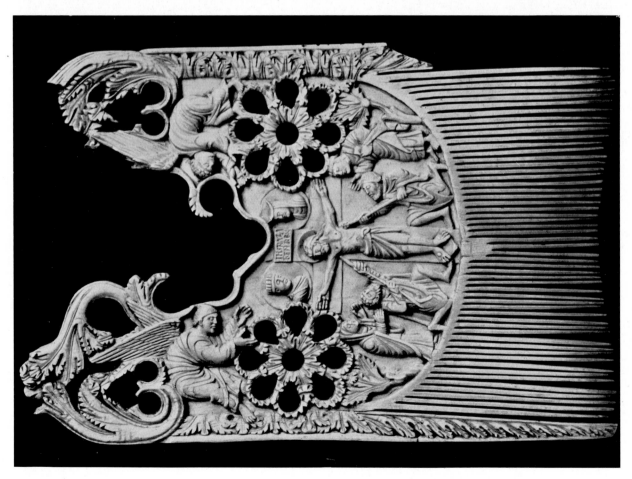

Pl. 67. The Comb of St. Heribert, front and back, late 9th cent. Ivory, $7^5/_8 \times 4^7/_8$ in. Cologne, Germany, Schnütgen-Museum.

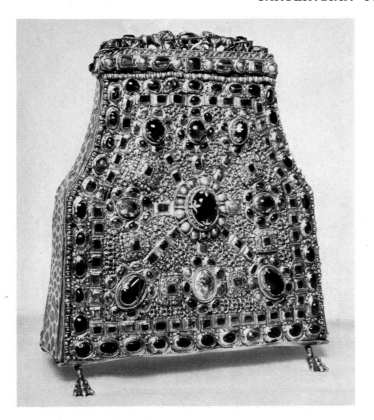

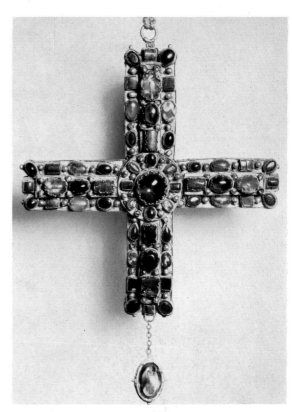

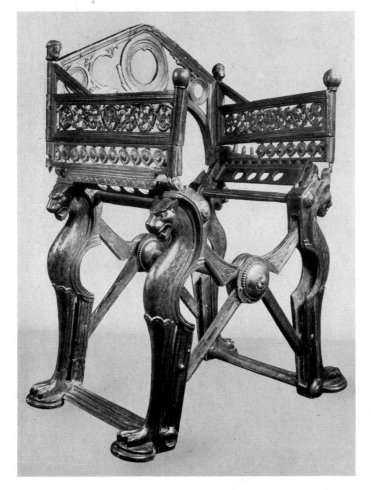

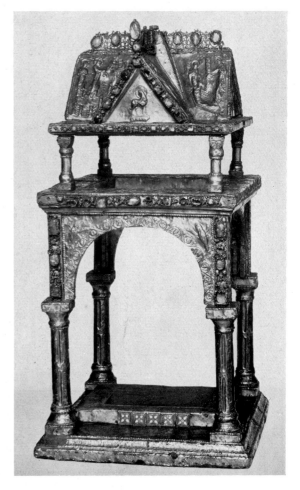

Pl. 68. *Above, left*: Tooth reliquary, late 9th cent. Gold and precious stones, ht., 9¼ in. *Right*: Cross of Berengar I, 888–924. Gold and precious stones, 9½×9½ in. Both, Monza, Italy, Cathedral Treasury. *Below, left*: The so-called "Throne of Dagobert," early 9th cent. (?). Bronze. Paris, Louvre. *Right*: Portable altar of Arnulf of Carinthia, late 9th cent. Gold, precious stones, and enamel, 23¼×12¼ in. Munich, Residenzmuseum.

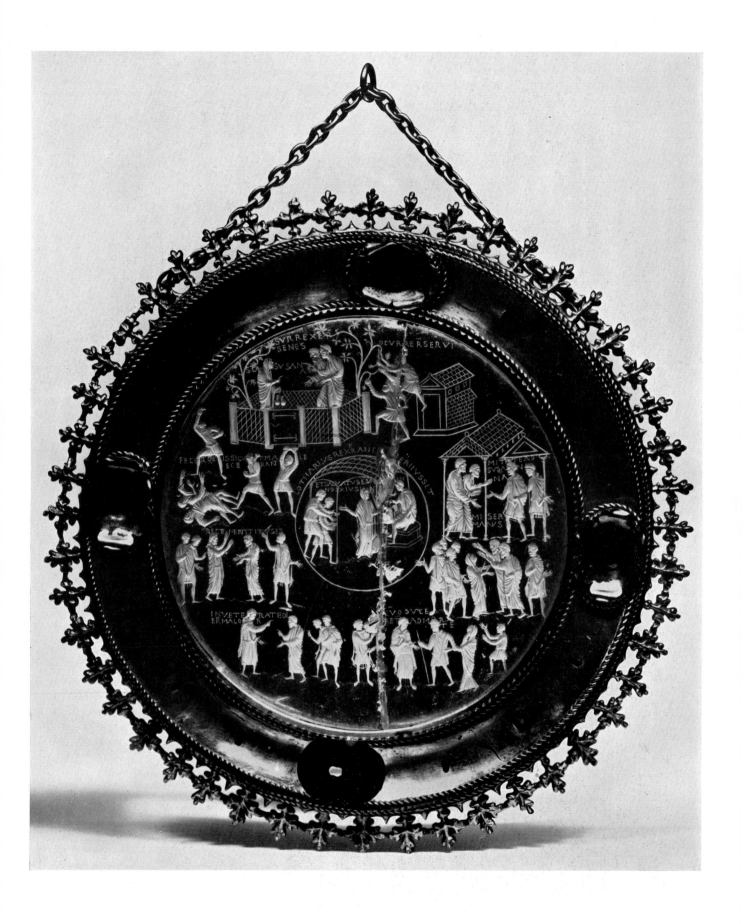

Pl. 69. The Lothair Crystal, with scenes from the story of Susanna, 9th cent. Rock crystal, diam., 4¹/₂ in. London, British Museum.

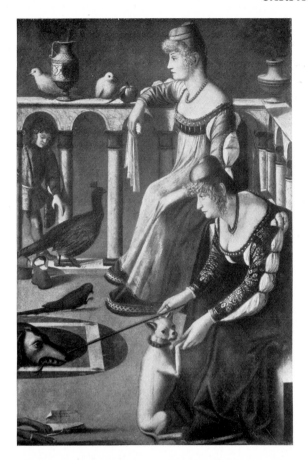

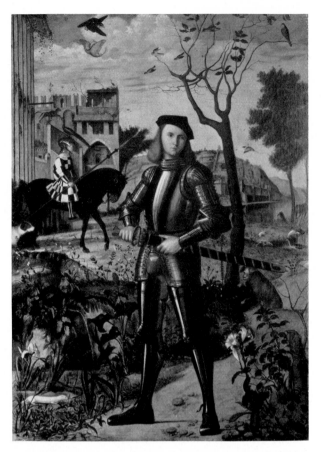

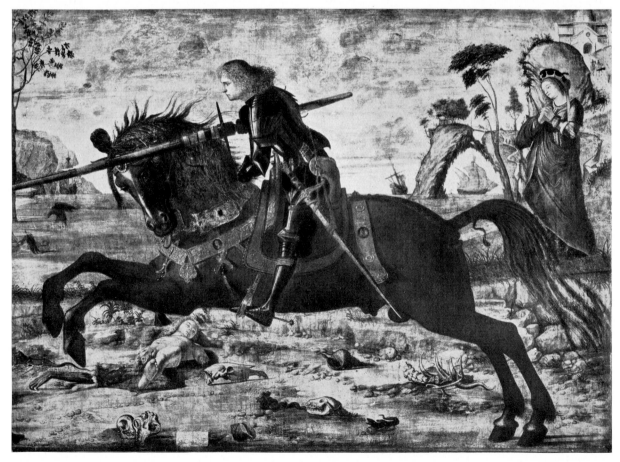

Pl. 70. *Above, left*: The so-called "Courtesans." Canvas, possibly now incomplete, 37×25¹/₄ in. Venice, Museo Correr. *Right*: Knight in a Landscape. Canvas, 7 ft., 1⁷/₈ in. × 4 ft., 7⁷/₈ in. Lugano, Switzerland, Thyssen-Bornemisza Coll. *Below*: St. George and the Dragon, detail. Canvas; full size, 4 ft., 5¹/₂ in. × 11 ft., 7³/₈ in. Venice, Scuola di S. Giorgio degli Schiavoni.

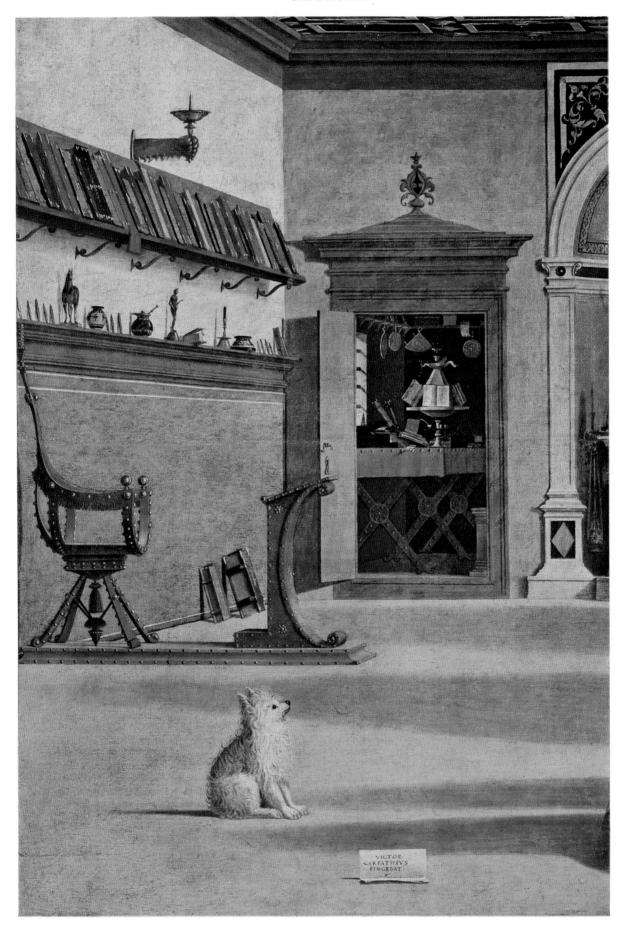

Pl. 71. St. Jerome in His Study, detail. Canvas; full size, 4 ft., 8³/₄ in. × 6 ft., 10 in. Venice, Scuola di S. Giorgio degli Schiavoni.

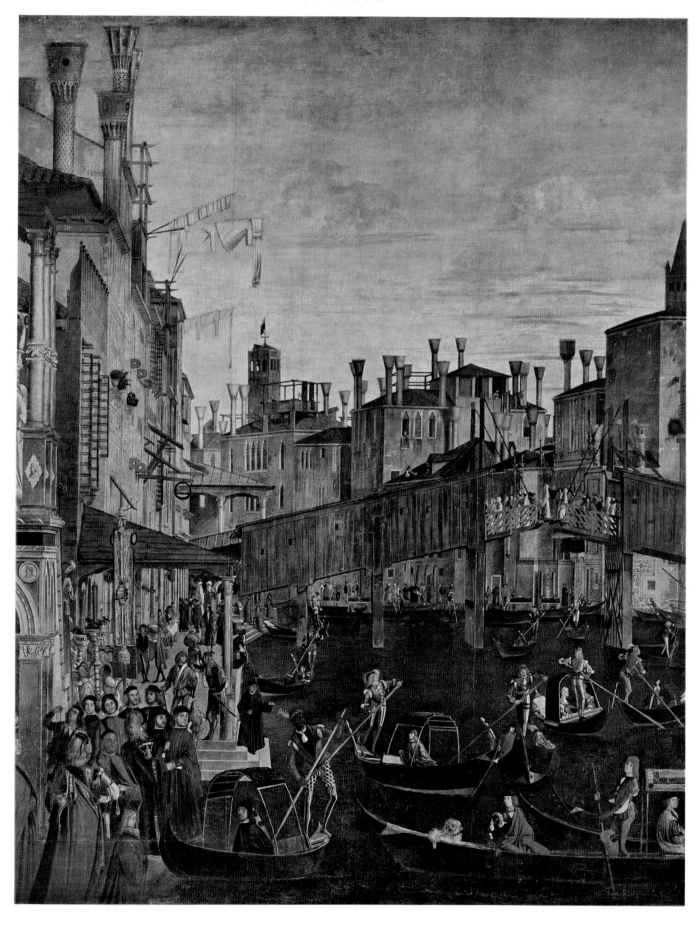

Pl. 72. The Healing of the Madman, detail. Canvas; full size, 11 ft., 11³/₄ in. × 12 ft., 9 in. Venice, Accademia.

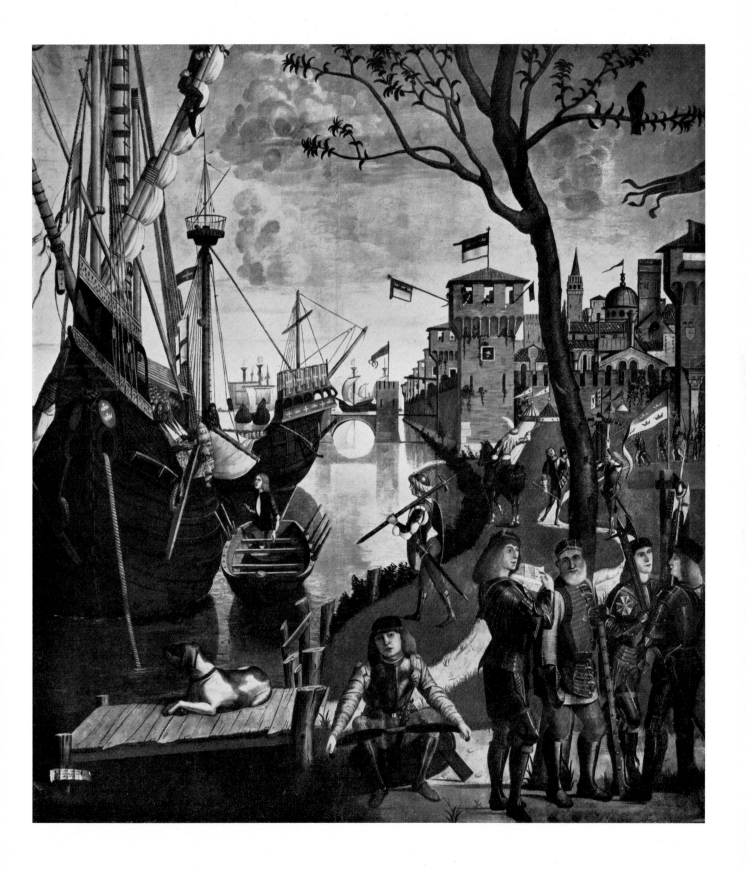

Pl. 73. The Arrival of St. Ursula at Cologne. Canvas, 9 ft., 1 in. × 8 ft., 4³/₈ in. Venice, Accademia.

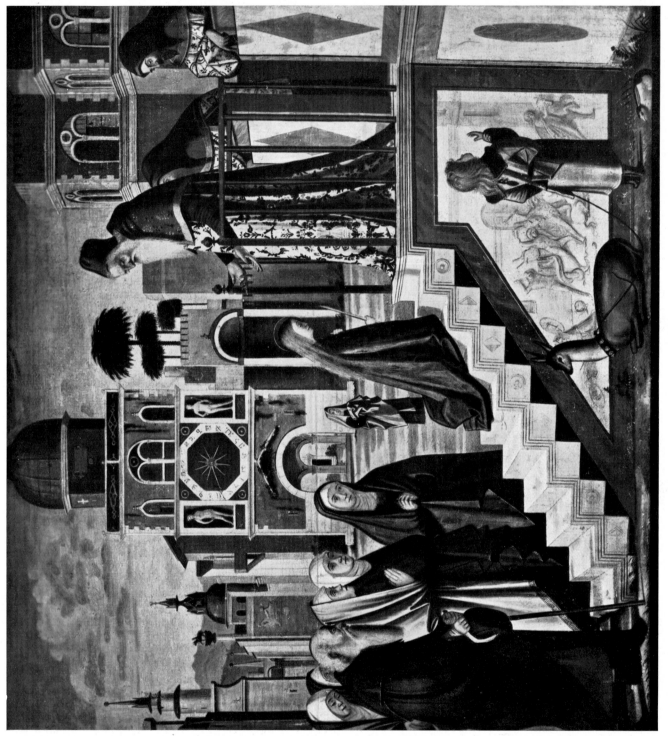

Pl. 74.  The Presentation of the Virgin in the Temple. Canvas, 4 ft., 3¹/₈ in. × 4 ft., 6 in. Milan, Brera.

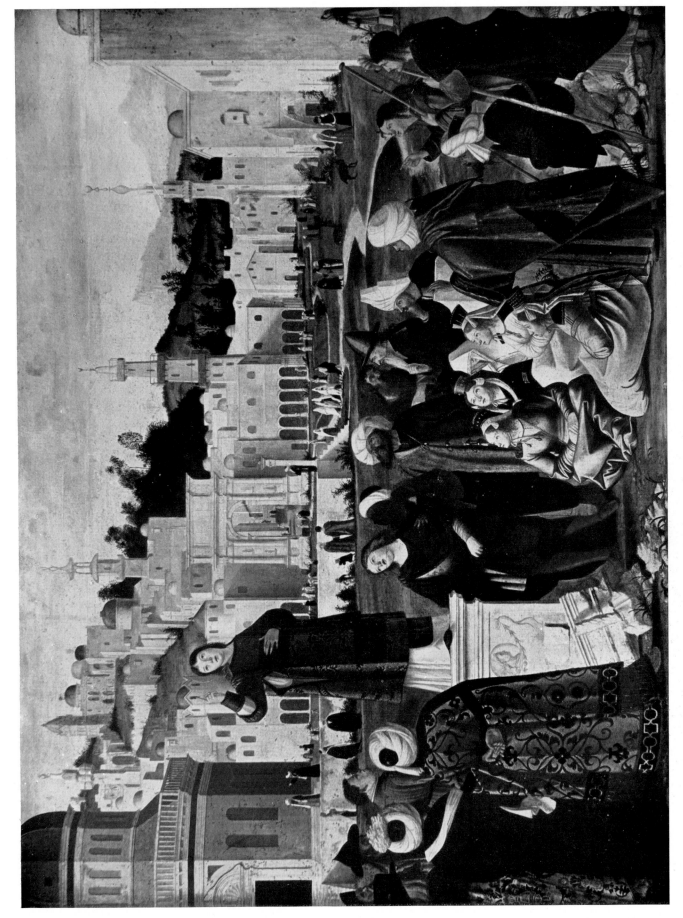

Pl. 75. St. Stephen Preaching. Canvas, 4 ft., 11⁷/₈ in. × 6 ft., 4³/₄ in. Paris, Louvre.

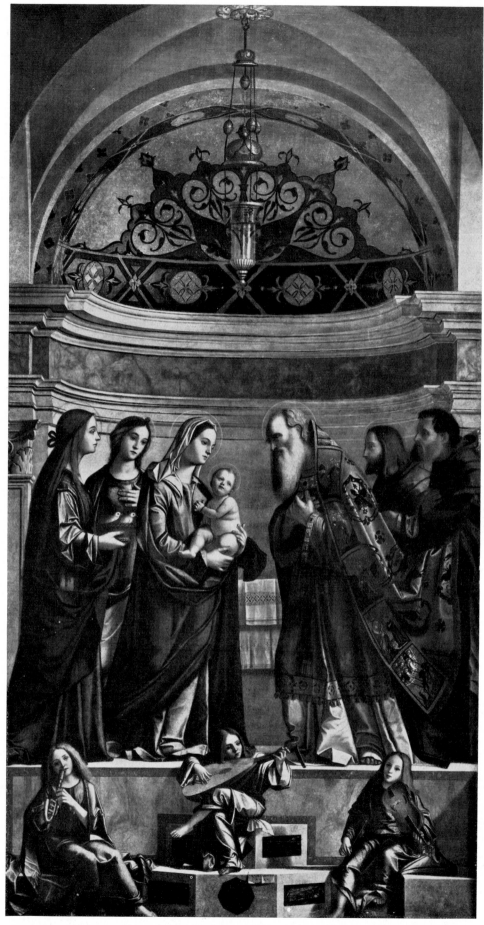

Pl. 76. The Presentation of Christ in the Temple. Canvas, 13 ft., 9³/₄ in. × 7 ft., 8⁷/₈ in. Venice, Accademia.

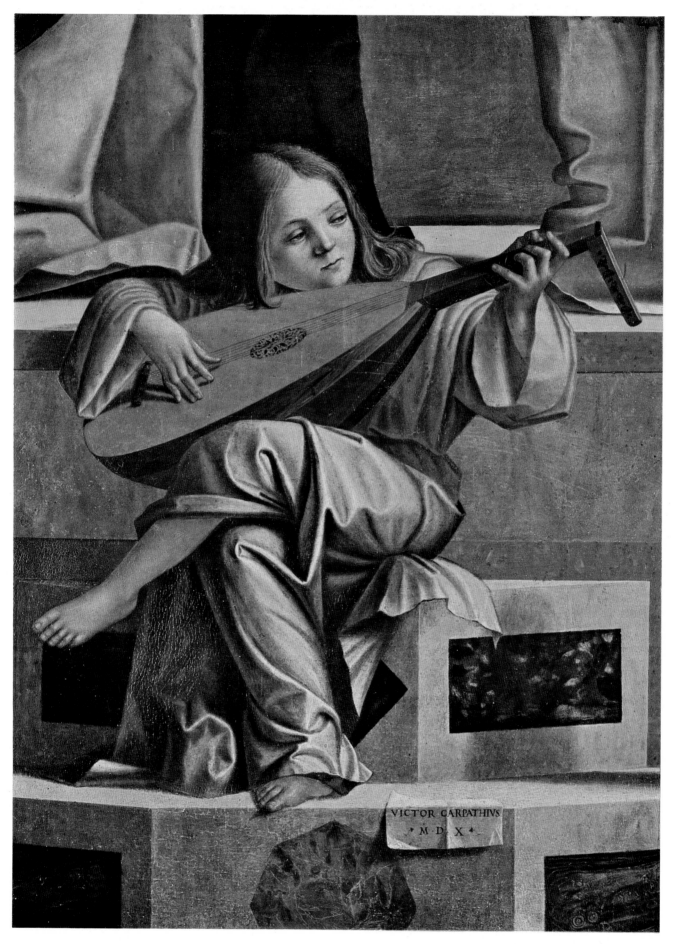

Pl. 77. Detail of PL. 76.

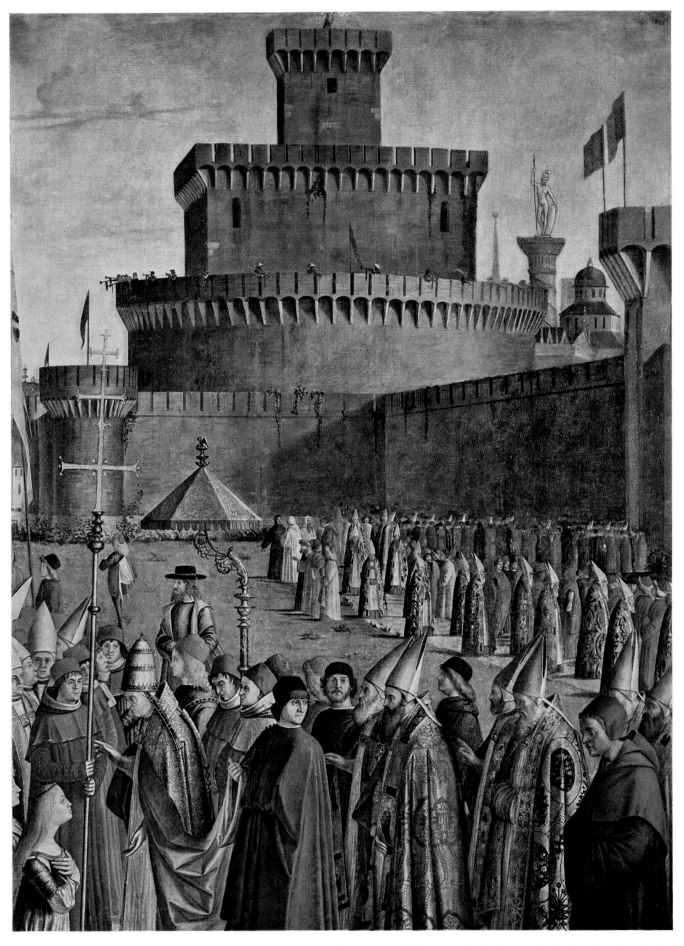

Pl. 78. The Meeting of St. Ursula and the Pope in Rome, detail. Canvas; full size, 9 ft., 9³/₈ in. × 10 ft. Venice, Accademia.

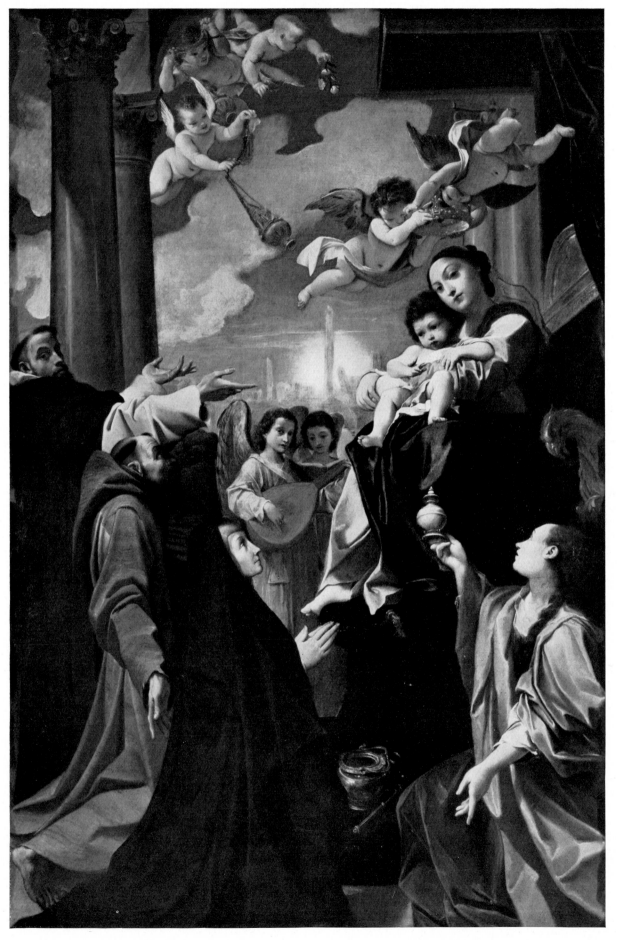

Pl. 79. L. Carracci, The Bargellini Madonna. Canvas, 9 ft., 3 in. × 6 ft., 2 in. Bologna, Pinacoteca Nazionale.

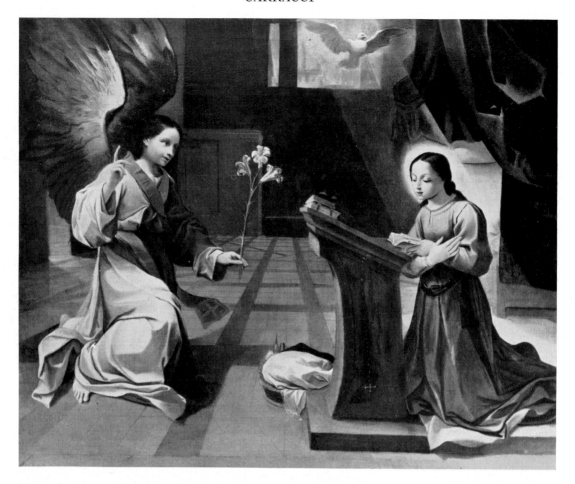

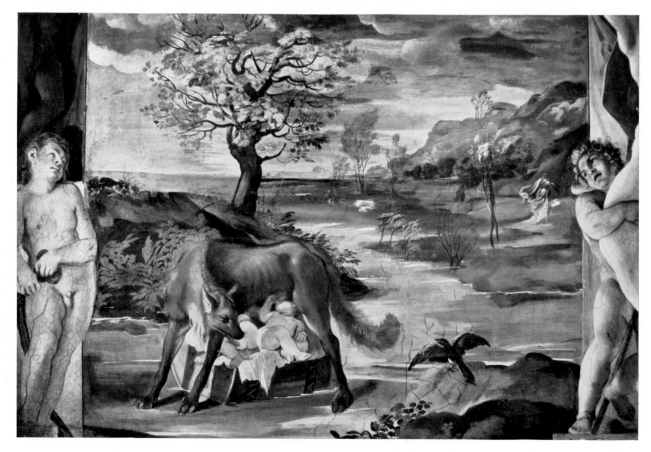

Pl. 80. L. Carracci. *Above*: The Annunciation. Canvas, 6 ft., 10⅝ in. × 7 ft., 6½ in. Bologna, Pinacoteca Nazionale. *Below*: The She-wolf. Fresco. Bologna, Palazzo Magnani (Palazzo Salem).

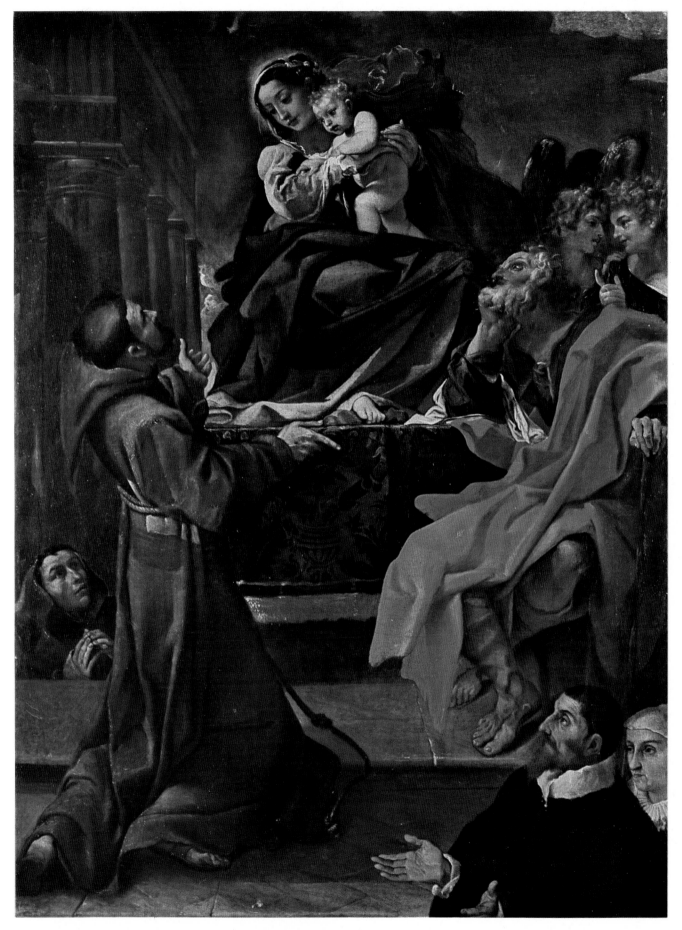

Pl. 81.  L. Carracci, The Holy Family with St. Francis and donors. Canvas, 7 ft., 4⅝ in. × 5 ft., 5⅜ in. Cento, Italy, Pinacoteca
Civica.

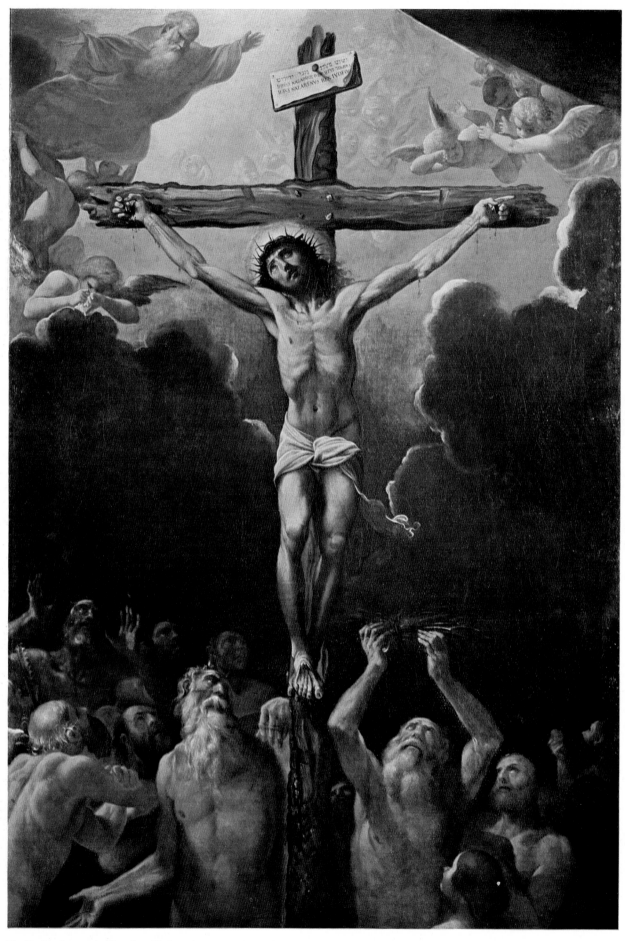

Pl. 82.  L. Carracci, The Crucifixion. Canvas, 9 ft., 2¹/₄ in. × 6 ft., 3⁵/₈ in. Ferrara, Italy, S. Francesca Romana.

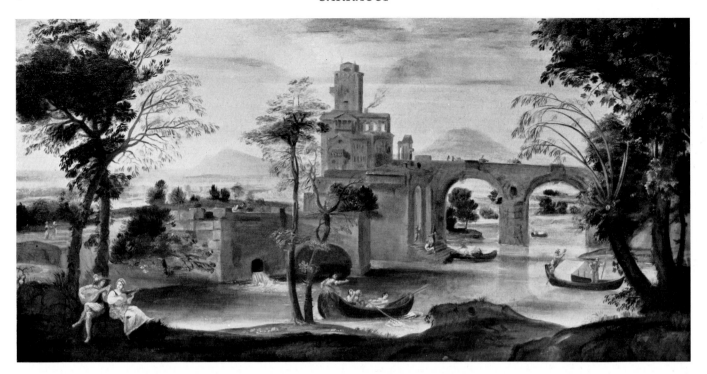

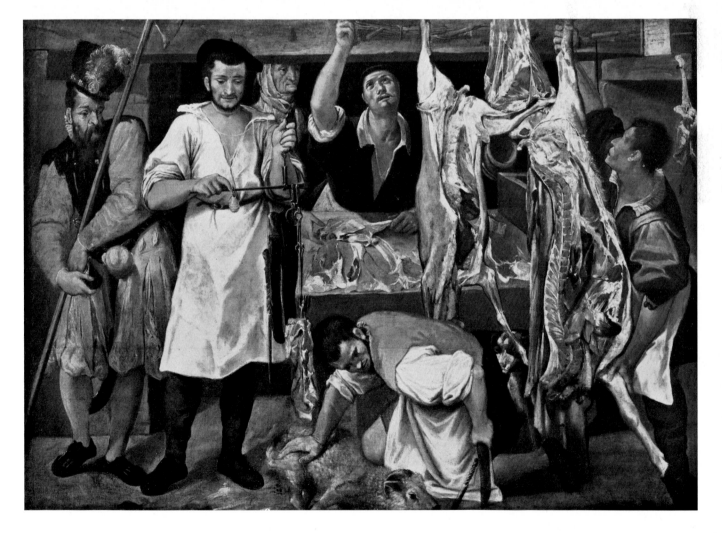

Pl. 83. Annibale Carracci. *Above*: Landscape. Canvas, 2 ft., 7¹/₂ in. × 4 ft., 8¹/₄ in. Berlin, Staatliche Museen. *Below*: The Butcher's Shop. Canvas, 6 ft., ⁷/₈ in. × 8 ft., 8³/₄ in. Oxford, Christ Church.

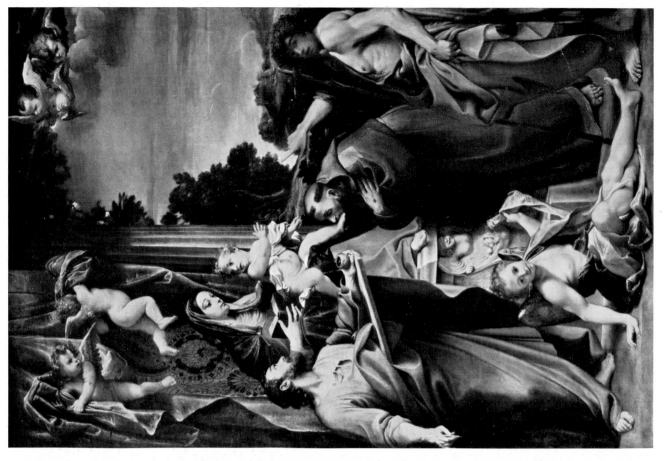

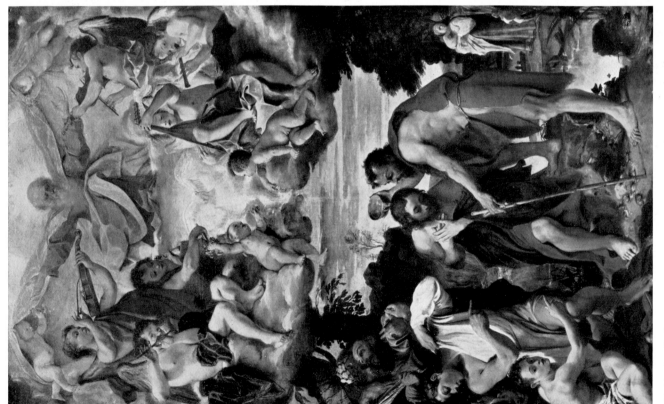

Pl. 84. Annibale Carracci. *Left*: The Baptism of Christ. Canvas, 8 ft., 8³/₄ in. × 6 ft., ⁷/₈ in. Bologna, S. Gregorio. *Right*: The Virgin and Child with SS. Matthew, Francis, and John the Baptist. Canvas, 12 ft., 7¹/₈ in. × 8 ft., 4³/₈ in. Dresden, Gemäldegalerie.

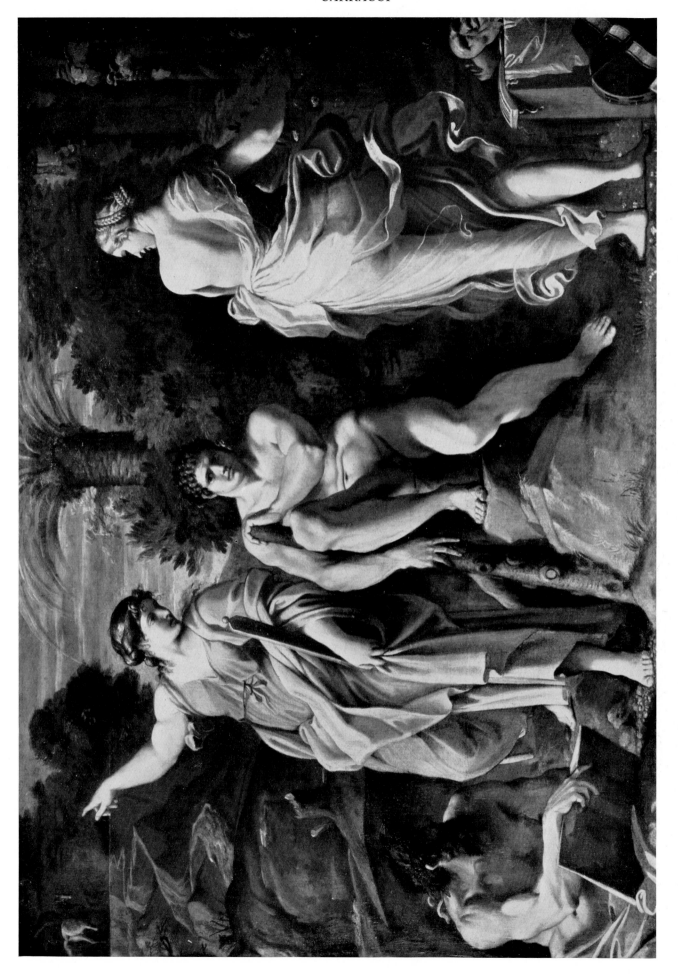

Pl. 85. Annibale Carracci, Hercules at the Crossroads. Canvas, 5 ft., 5³/₄ in. × 7 ft., 9¹/₄ in. Naples, Museo di Capodimonte.

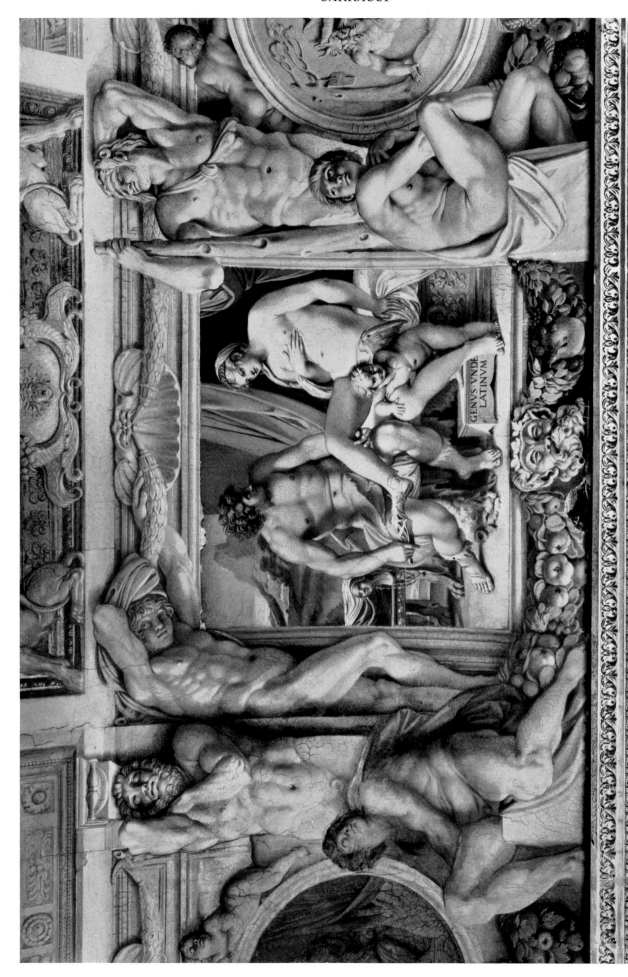

GENVS VNDE
LATINVM

Pl. 86. Annibale Carracci, Venus and Anchises, detail of the frescoes in the Galleria Farnese. Rome, Palazzo Farnese.

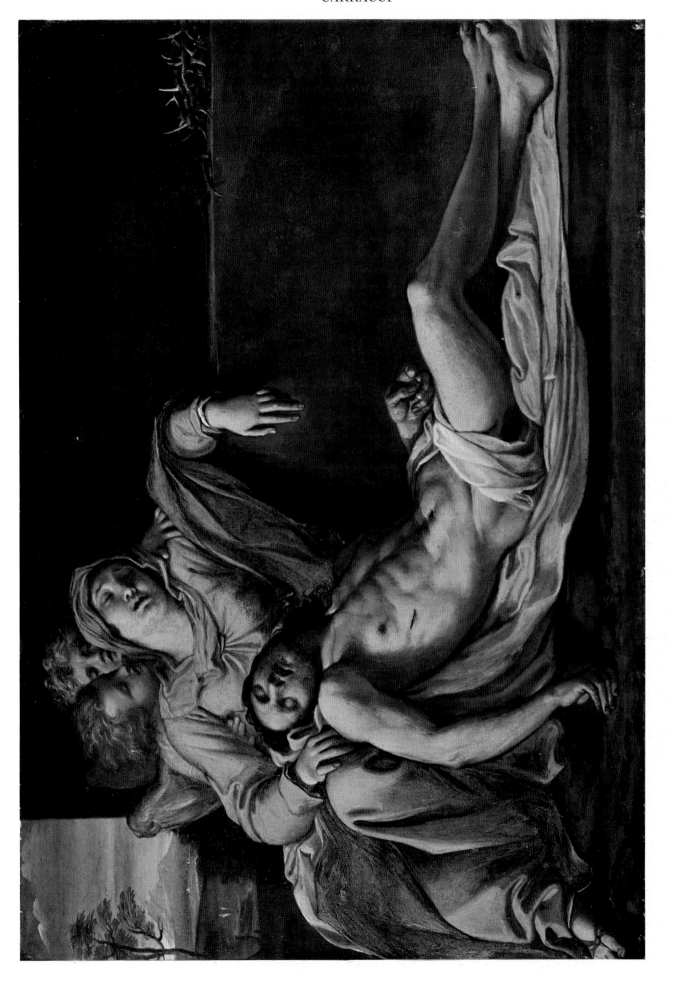

Pl. 87. Annibale Carracci, Pietà. Copper, 16⁷/₈×24³/₈ in. Vienna, Kunsthistorisches Museum.

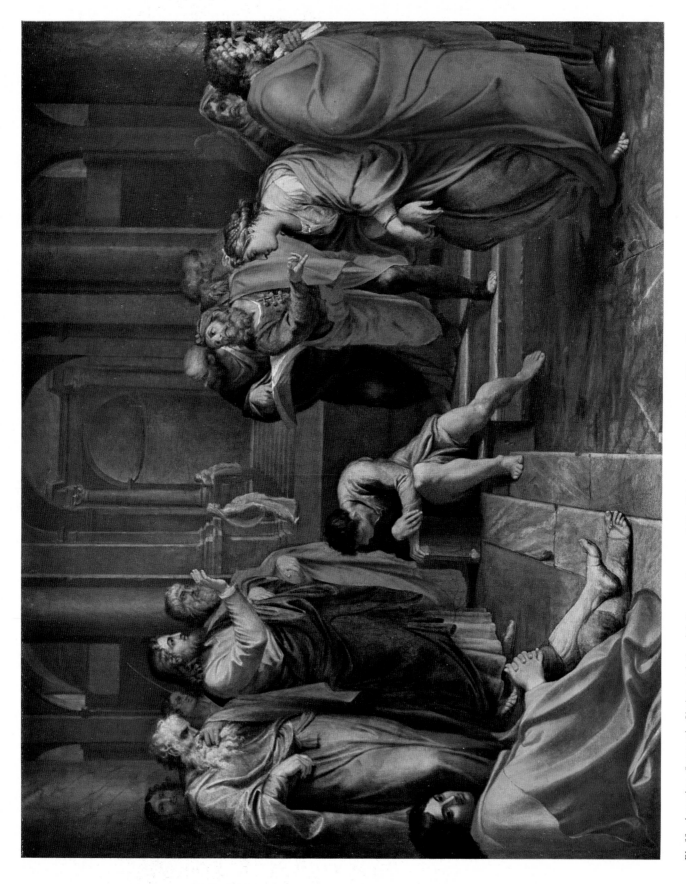

Pl. 88. Agostino Carracci, Christ and the Adulteress. Canvas, 5 ft, 6⅞ in. × 7 ft, 4⅝ in. Milan, Brera.

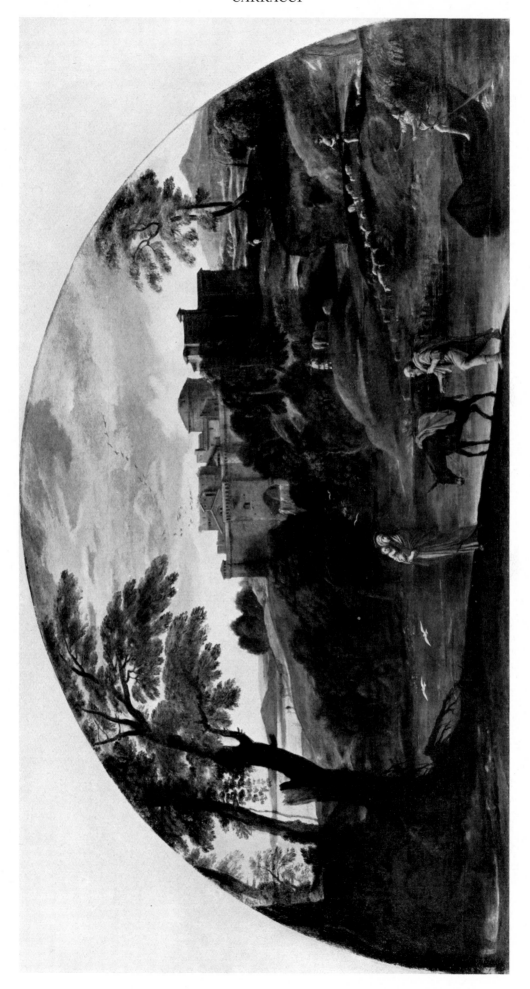

Pl. 89. Annibale Carracci, The Flight into Egypt. Canvas, 4 ft. × 7 ft., 6½ in. Rome, Galleria Doria Pamphili.

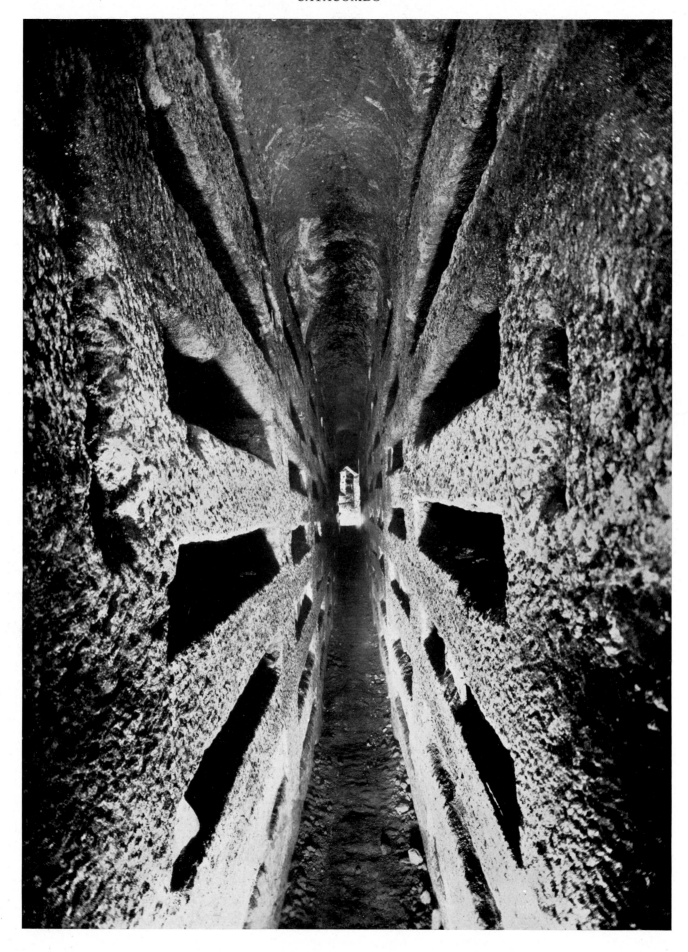

Pl. 90.  Rome, Catacomb of Pamphilus, one of the galleries.

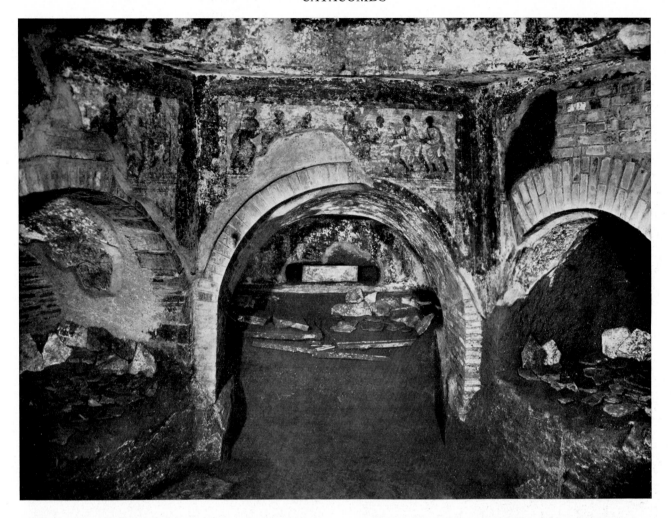

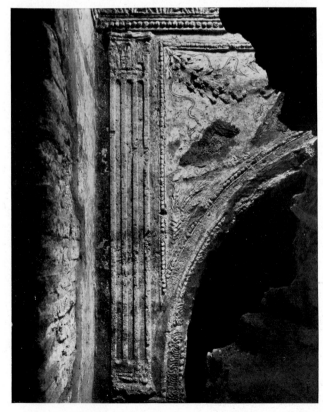

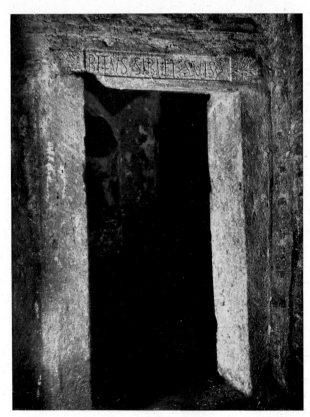

Pl. 91. *Above*: Rome, Catacomb of Domitilla, the so-called "Cubiculum of the Six Saints," 4th cent. *Below, left*: Stucco decoration in the tomb of St. Quirinus, 4th cent. Rome, Catacomb of St. Sebastian. *Right*: Doorway with inscription, 4th cent. Rome, Catacomb of Callixtus, region of SS. Mark and Marcellianus.

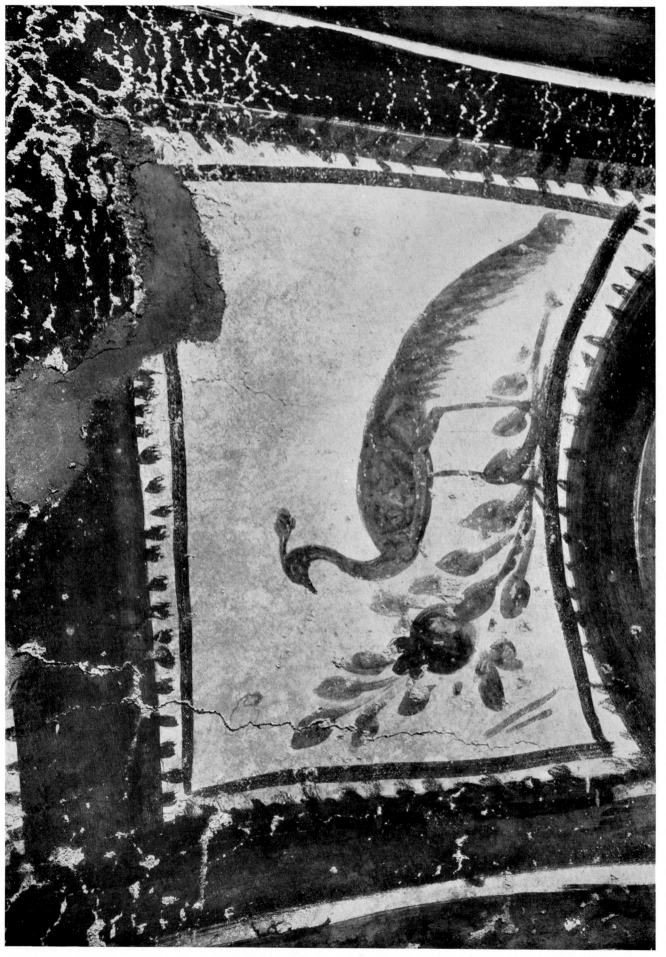

Pl. 92. Wall painting of a peacock, 3d cent. Rome, Catacomb of Pamphilus.

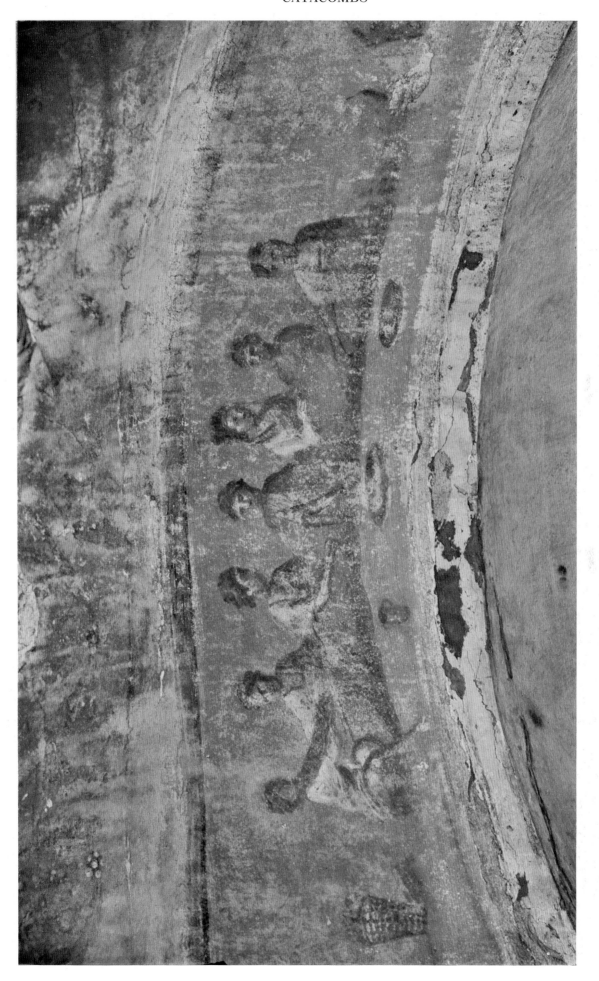

Pl. 93. Fractio panis (the Breaking of Bread), late 2d cent. (?). Wall painting in the so-called "Greek Chapel." Rome, Catacomb of Priscilla.

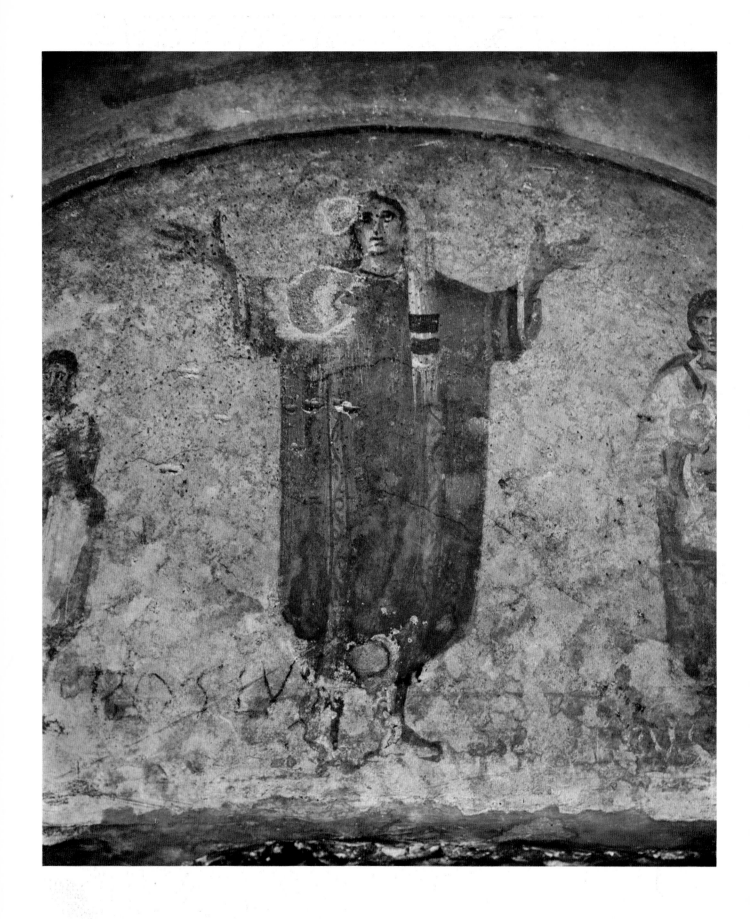

Pl. 94.  Veiled orant, ca. 220–40. Wall painting. Rome, Catacomb of Priscilla.

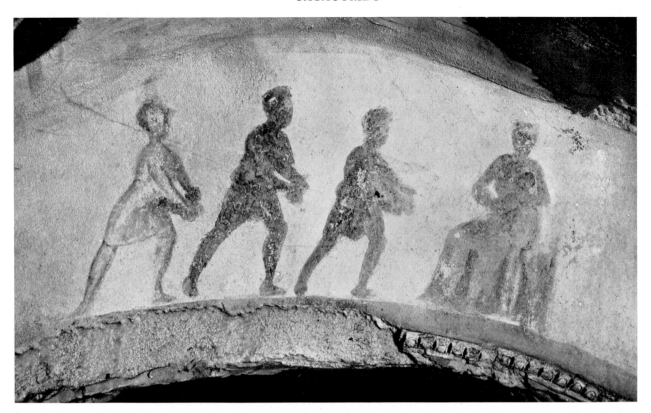

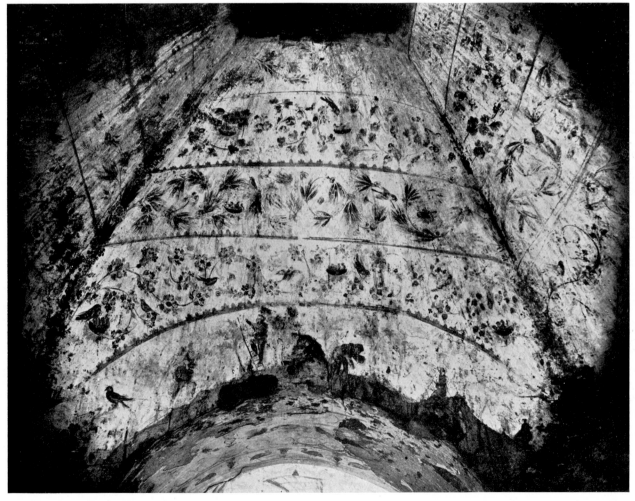

Pl. 95. *Above*: Adoration of the Magi, second half of 2d cent. Wall painting in the so-called "Greek Chapel." Rome, Catacomb of Priscilla. *Below*: Olive harvest, detail of decoration representing the four seasons, late 2d cent. Vault painting. Rome, Catacomb of Praetextatus.

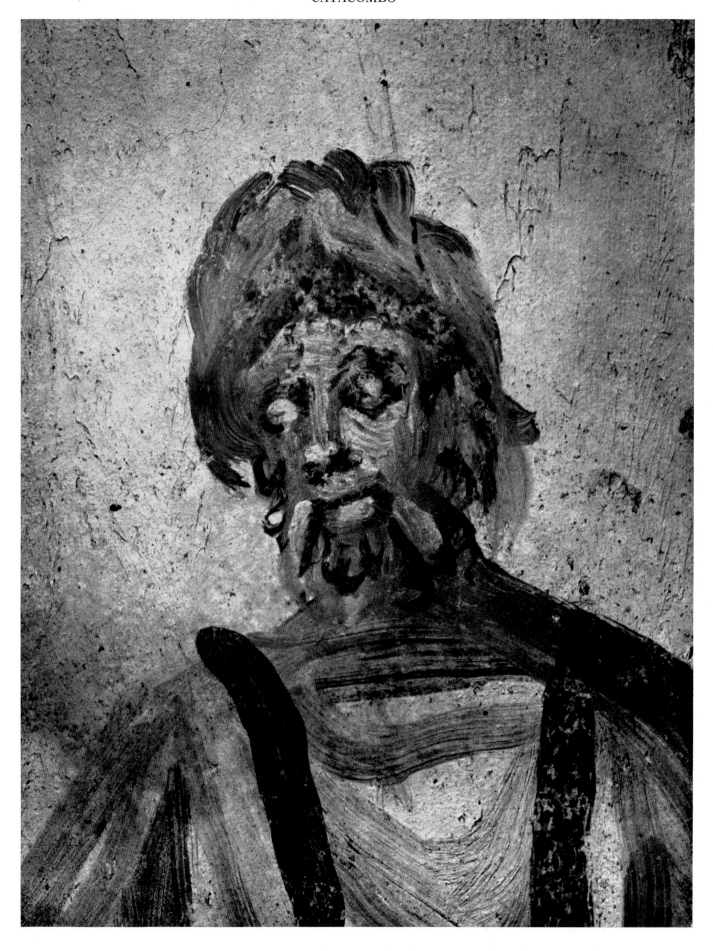

Pl. 96. Head of Moses, detail of a wall painting, second half of 3d cent. Rome, Catacomb of SS. Peter and Marcellinus.

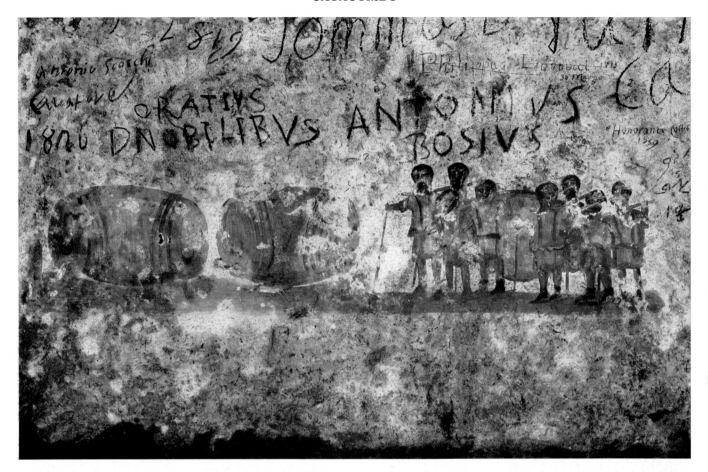

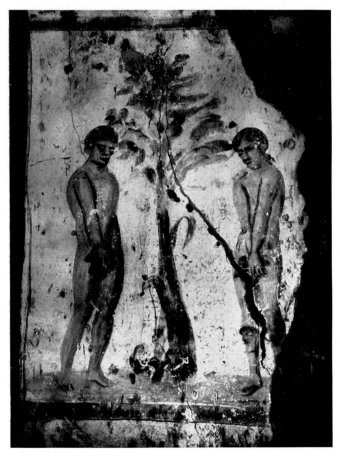

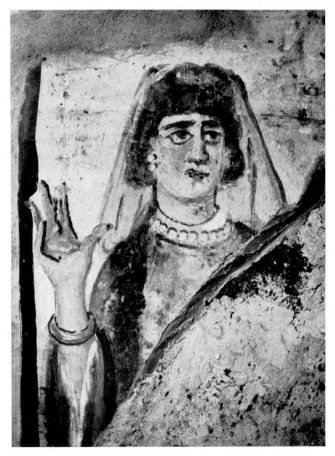

Pl. 97. *Above*: Wall painting in the so-called "Cubiculum of the Coopers," early 4th cent. Rome, Catacomb of Priscilla. *Below, left*: Adam and Eve, early 4th cent. Wall painting. Rome, Catacomb of SS. Peter and Marcellinus. *Right*: Woman wearing a veil, detail of a wall painting, 4th cent. Rome, Catacomb of Thraso.

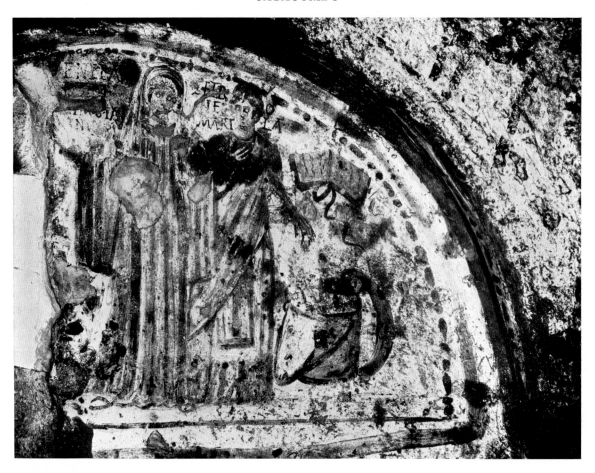

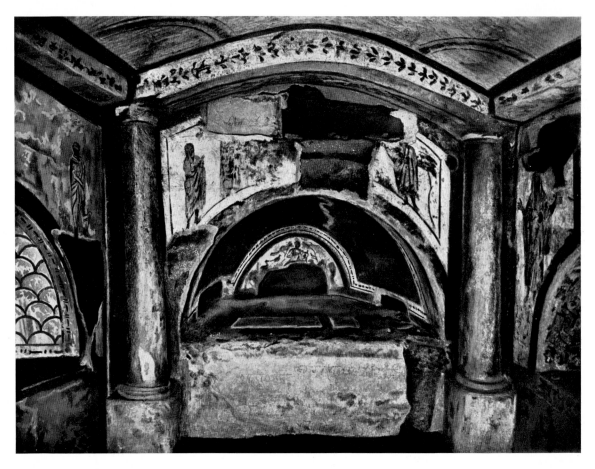

Pl. 98. Rome, Catacomb of Domitilla. *Above*: Veneranda and the martyr Petronilla, second half of 4th cent. Wall painting. *Below*: Wall paintings in the so-called "Cubiculum of Orpheus," 4th cent.

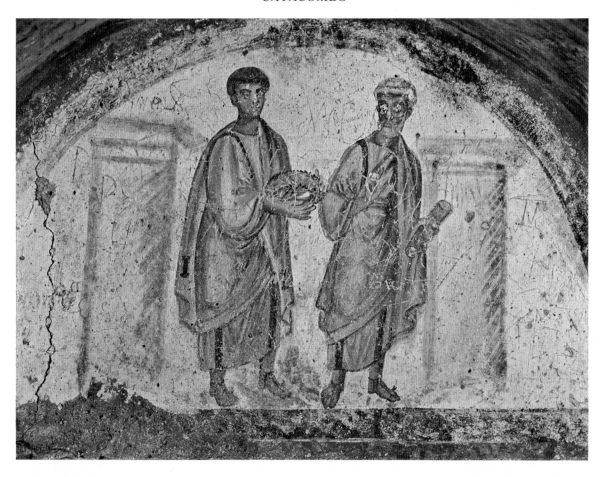

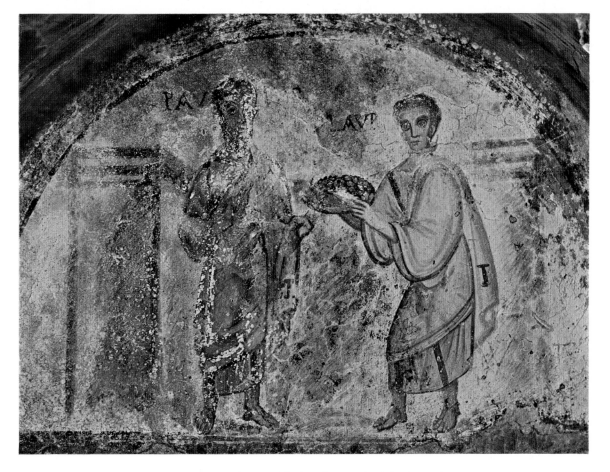

Pl. 99. Figures of saints, 5th cent. Wall paintings. Naples, Catacomb of St. Januarius.

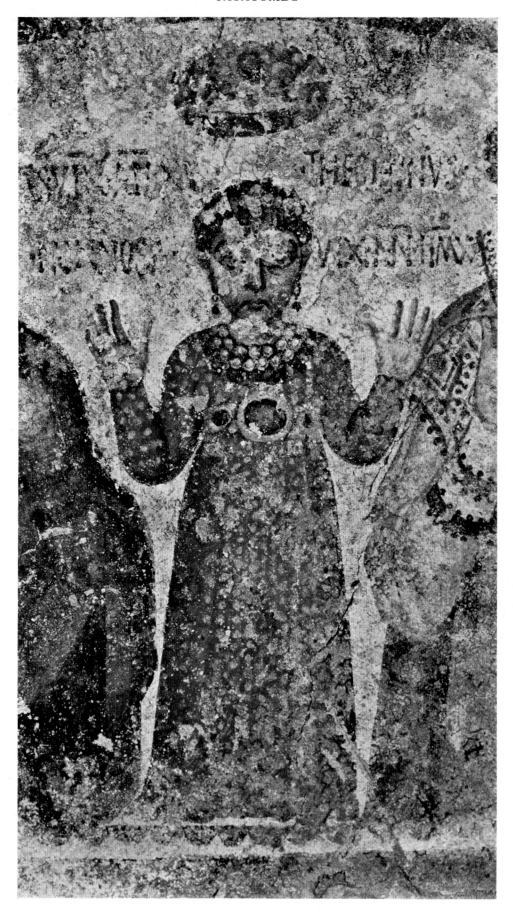

Pl. 100. The child Nonnosa depicted as deceased, detail of the wall painting on the lunette, which shows also the parents, Ilaritas and Theotecnus, 5th cent. Naples, Catacomb of St. Januarius, main gallery.

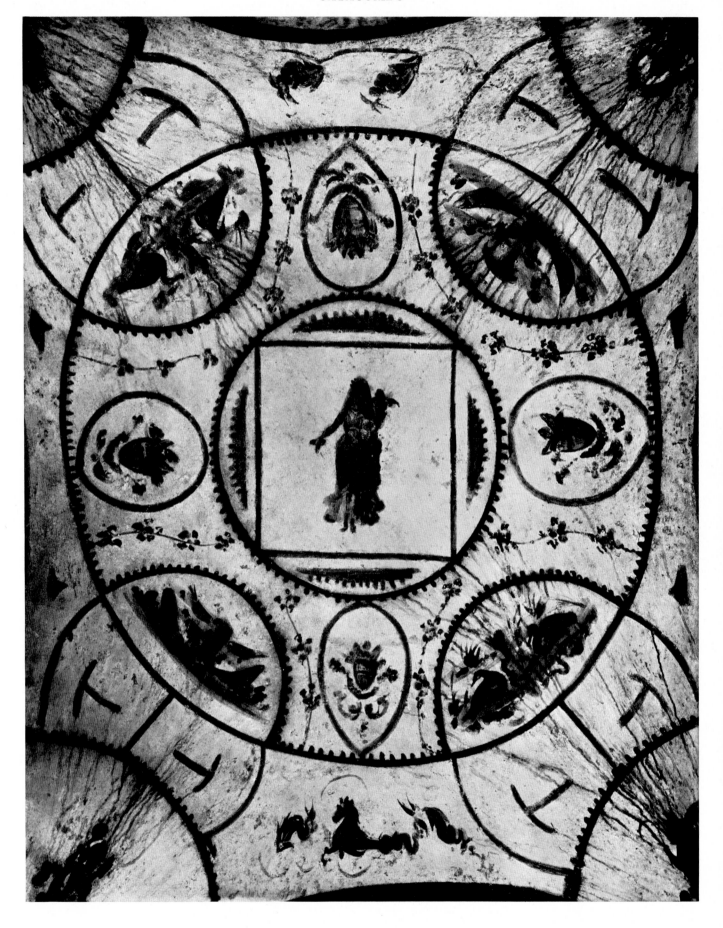

Pl. 101. Ceiling painting. Rome, Jewish Catacomb of Vigna Rondanini.

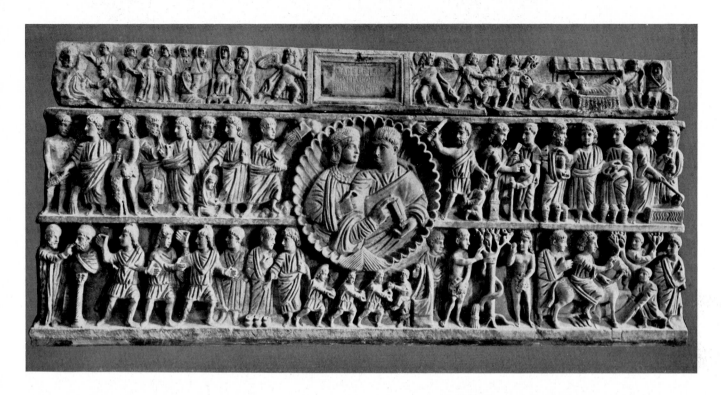

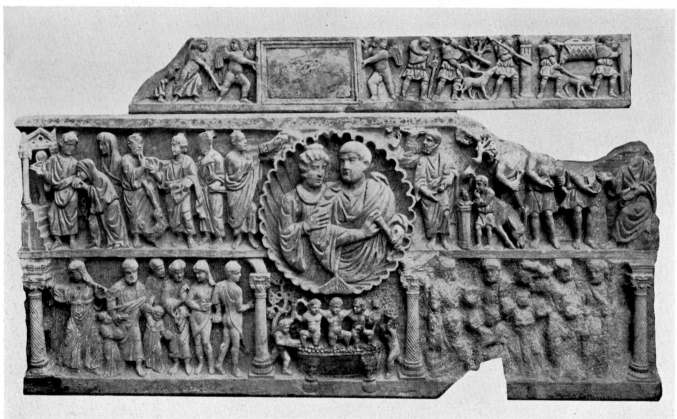

Pl. 102. *Above*: Sarcophagus of Adelfia, 340–50. Marble. Syracuse, Sicily, Museo Archeologico. *Below*: Sarcophagus of Lot, ca. 350–60. Marble. Rome, Catacomb of St. Sebastian.

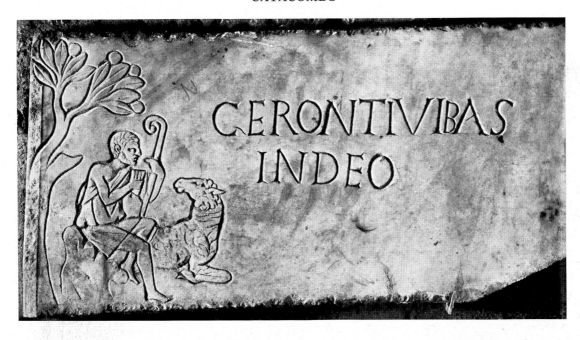

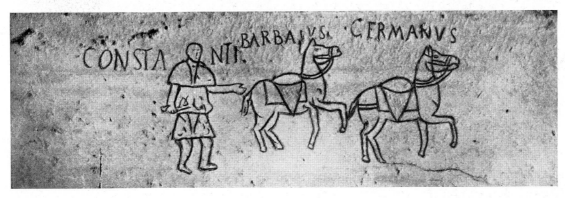

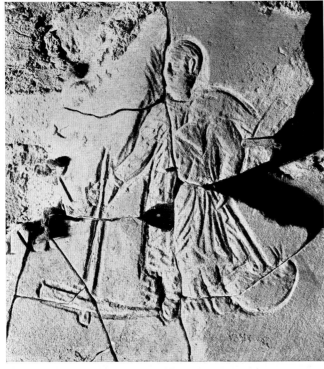

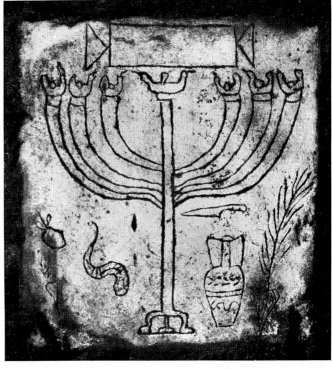

Pl. 103. Marble graffiti. *Above*: The epitaph of Gerontius, 3d cent. *Center*: Graffito referring to the groom Constantius, 4th cent. Both, Rome, Catacomb of Domitilla. *Below, left*: Fossor, 4th cent. Rome, Catacomb of Callixtus, region of SS. Mark and Marcellianus. *Right*: Seven-branched candlestick and other symbols. Rome, Jewish Catacomb of Vigna Rondanini.

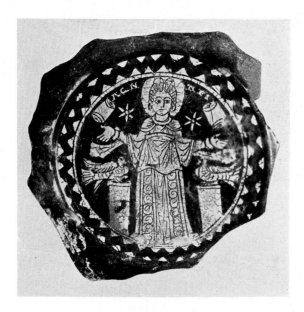

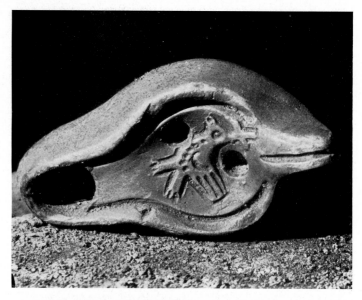

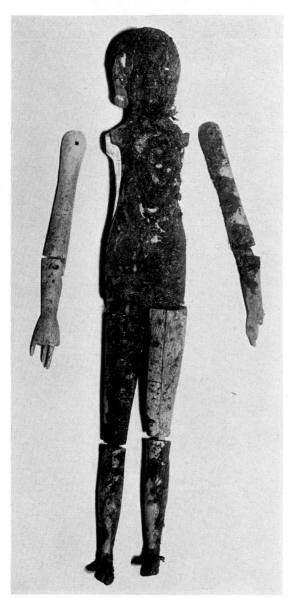

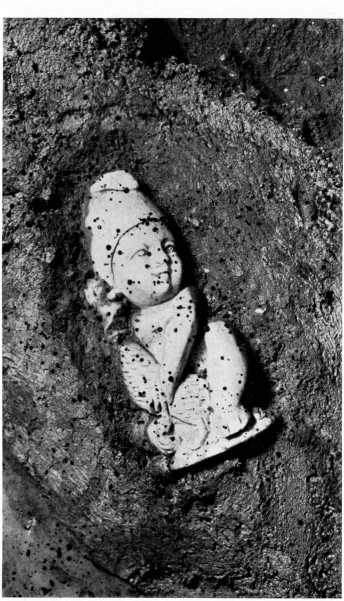

Pl. 104. *Above, left*: Gold glass, with representation of St. Agnes, 4th cent. Rome, Catacomb of Pamphilus. *Right*: Lamp with Christian symbol. Rome, Catacomb of Commodilla. *Below, left*: Doll. Bone. Rome, from Catacomb of St. Sebastian. *Right*: Figurine of a child, embedded in the masonry seal of a loculus, from Catacomb of Pamphilus, Rome, 3d–4th cent. Ivory. Now, Rome, Vatican, Museo Sacro.

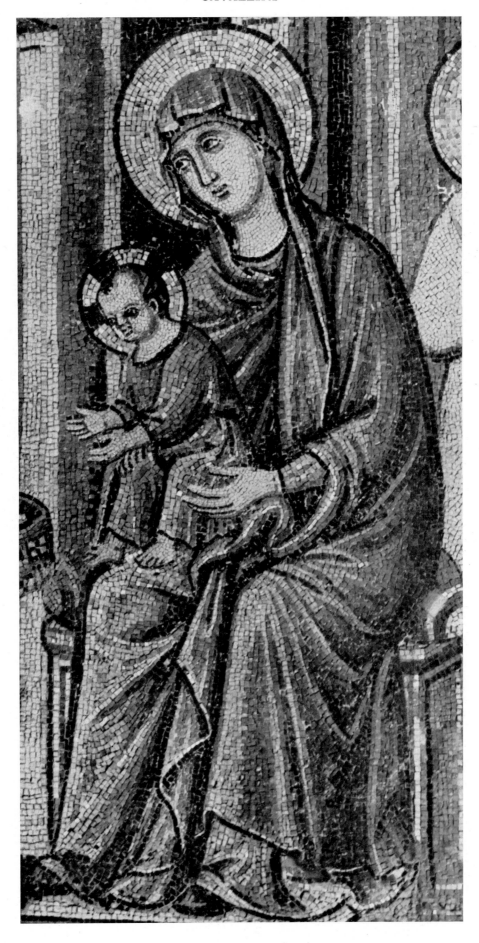

Pl. 105. Adoration of the Magi, detail. Mosaic. Rome, S. Maria in Trastevere.

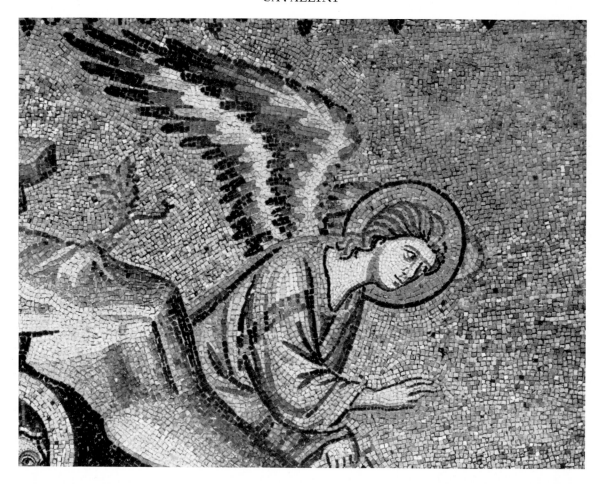

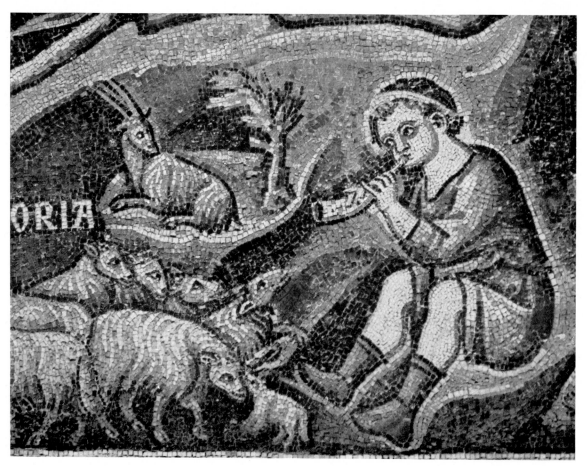

Pl. 106. The Nativity, two details. Mosaic. Rome, S. Maria in Trastevere.

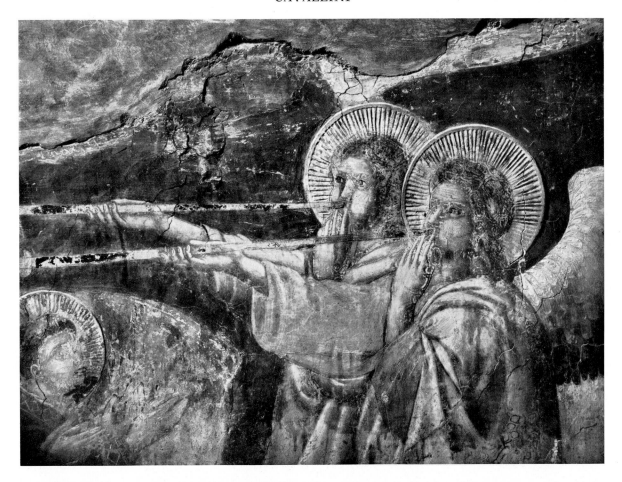

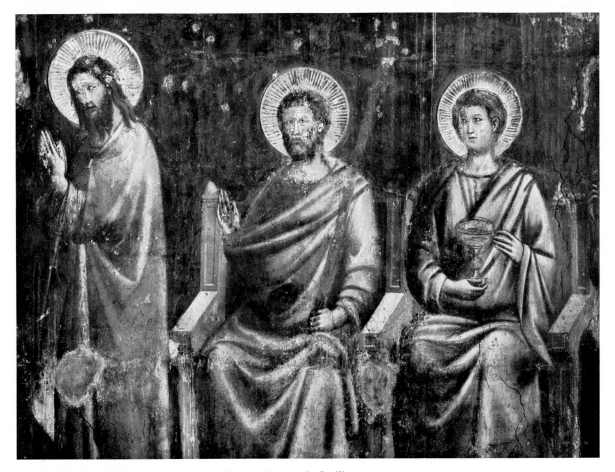

Pl. 107. The Last Judgment, two details. Fresco. Rome, S. Cecilia.

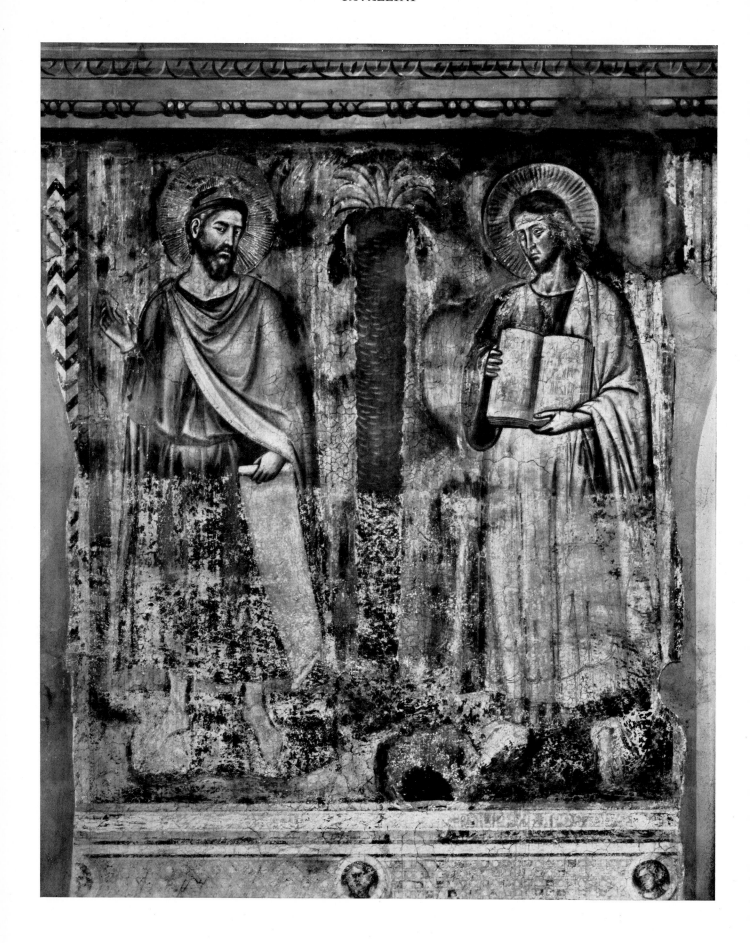

Pl. 108. Two Apostles. Fresco. Naples, S. Maria Donnaregina.

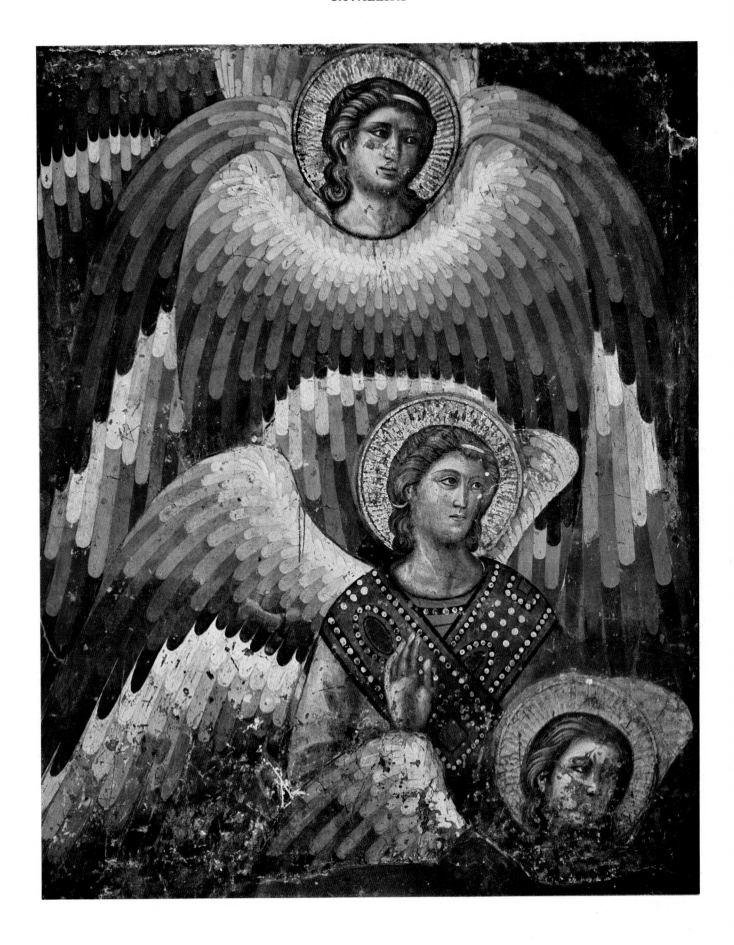

Pl. 109. The Last Judgment, detail. Fresco. Rome, S. Cecilia in Trastevere.

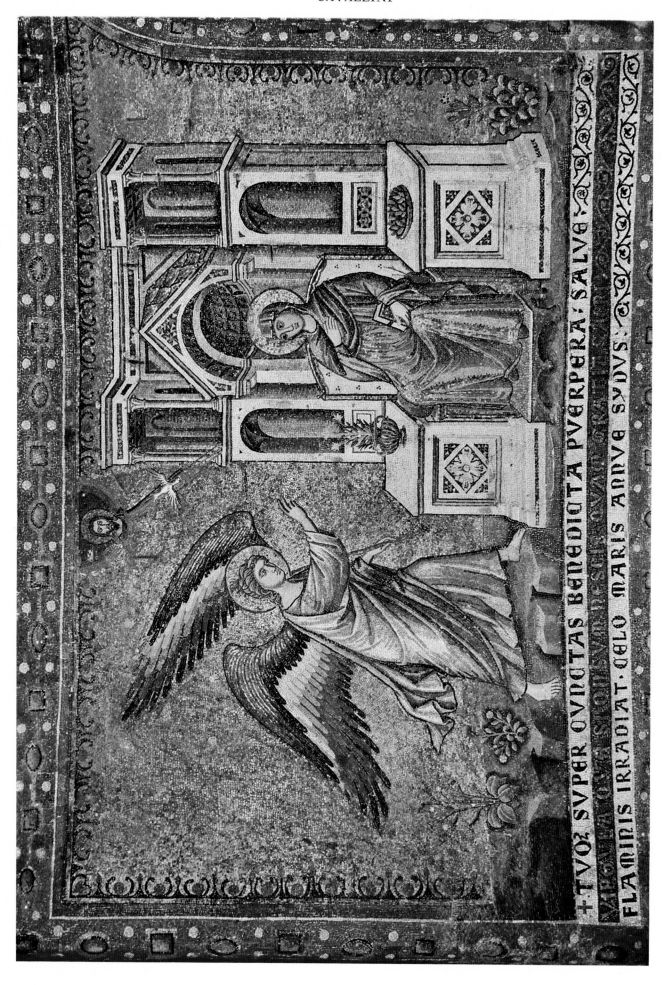

Pl. 110. The Annunciation. Mosaic. Rome, S. Maria in Trastevere.

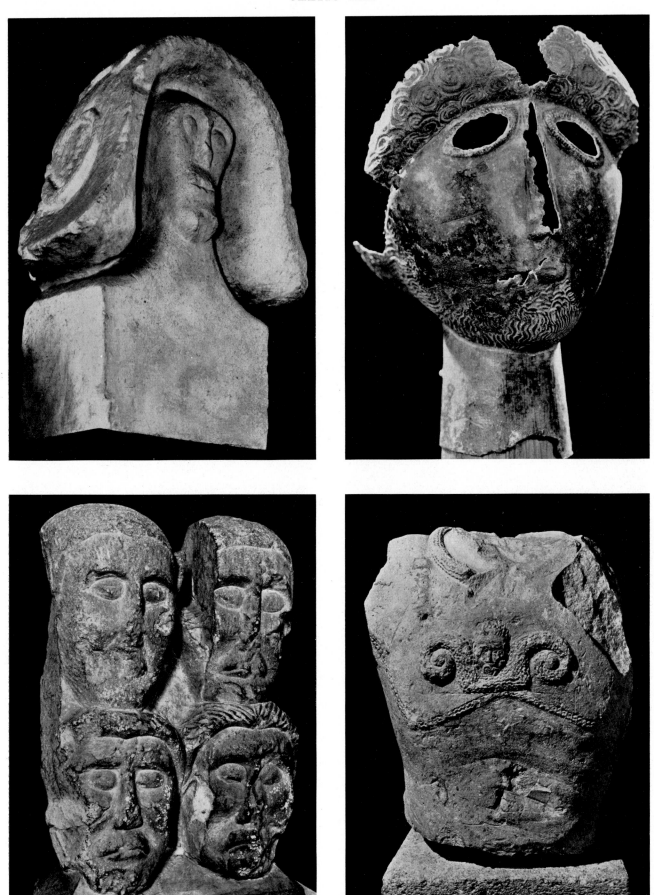

Pl. 111. *Above, left*: Limestone head, from Sainte-Anastasie, Gard, France, 3d–2d cent. B.C. Ht., 22 in. Nîmes, France, Musée Archéologique. *Right*: Bronze head, from Tarbes, Hautes-Pyrénées, France, 3d cent. B.C. Ht., 6³/₄ in. Tarbes, Musée Massey. *Below, left*: Group of *têtes coupées*, from Entremont, Bouches-du-Rhône, France, 3d cent. B.C. Limestone, ht., 16⁷/₈ in. *Right*: Torso of a warrior, from Entremont, 3d–2d cent. B.C. Limestone, ht., 16³/₄ in. Last two, Aix-en-Provence, France, Musée Granet.

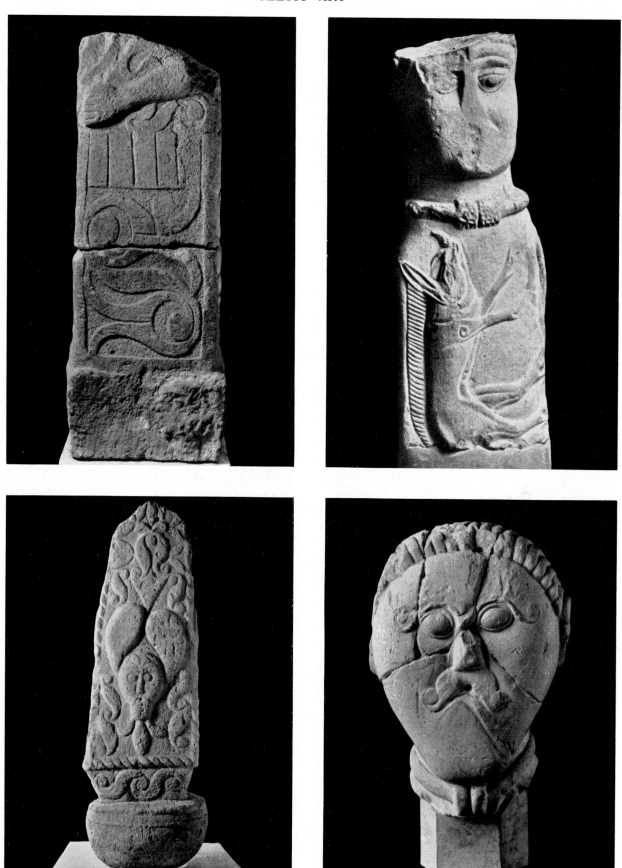

Pl. 112. *Left*: Carved sandstone pillars. *Above*: Pillar from Waldenbuch, Württemberg, Germany, late 4th cent. B.C. Ht., 4 ft., 1¼ in. Stuttgart, Landesmuseum. *Below*: Pillar from Pfalzfeld, Rhineland, Germany, 3d cent. B.C. Ht., 4 ft., 10¼ in. Bonn, Rheinisches Landesmuseum. *Right, above*: God with boar, from Euffigneix, Haute-Marne, France, 3d cent. B.C. Limestone, ht., 10¼ in. Chaumont, France, Musée d'Art et d'Histoire. *Below*: Head from Mšecké-Žehrovice, near Prague, ca. end of 1st cent. B.C. (?). Limestone, ht., 9½ in. Prague, National Museum. Last two, photographed from casts in Musée des Antiquités Nationales, Saint-Germain-en-Laye, France.

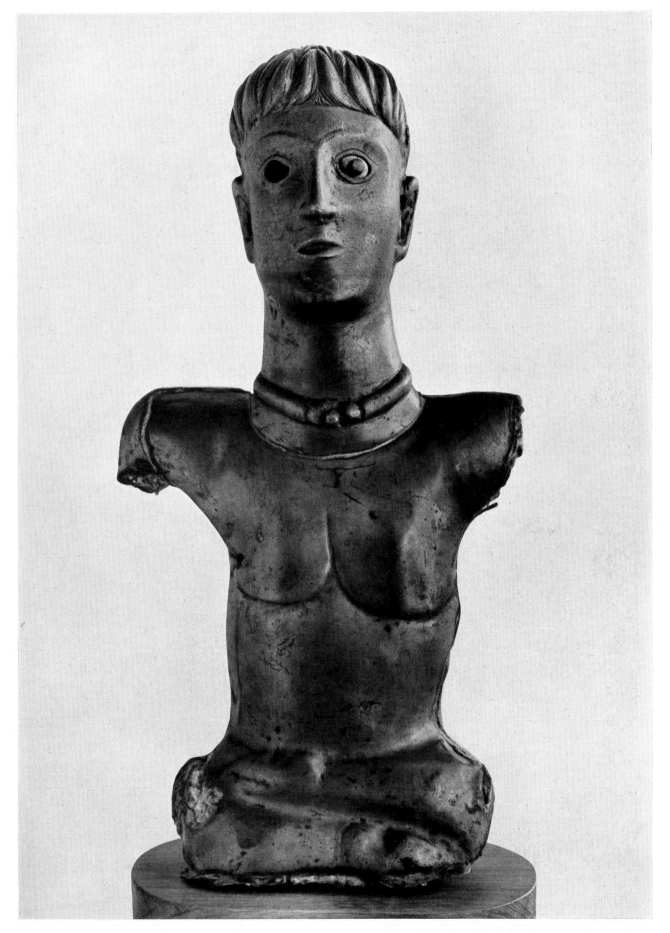

Pl. 113.  Seated god, from Bouray, Seine-et-Oise, France, 3d–1st cent. B.C. Bronze, ht., 17³/₄ in. Saint-Germain-en-Laye, France, Musée des Antiquités Nationales.

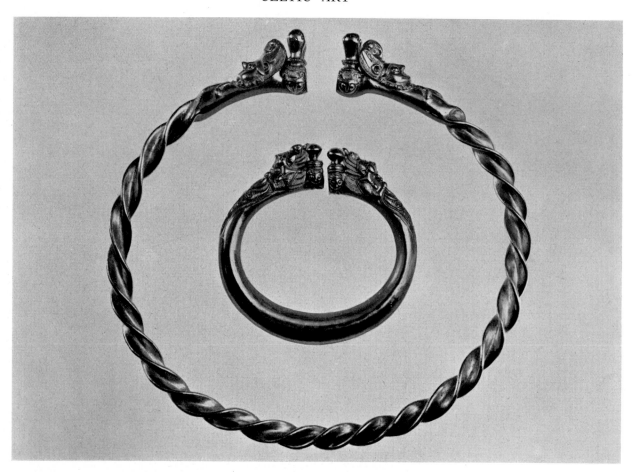

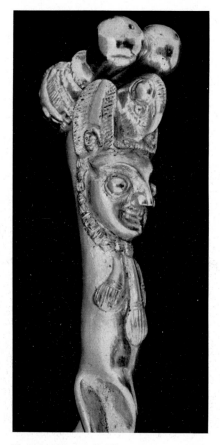

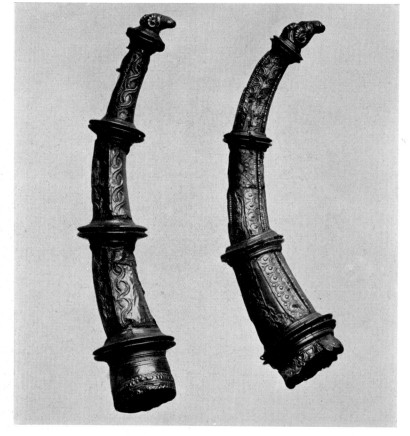

Pl. 114. *Above*: Gold torque and bracelet, from Reinheim, Saarland, Germany, 5th cent. B.C. Diam., 6³/₄ in. and 3³/₈ in. Saarbrücken, Saarlandmuseum. *Below, left*: Detail of the Reinheim torque. *Right*: Small gold horns (mounts for oxhorns?), from Klein-Aspergle, Germany, second half of 5th cent. B.C. Length, 5³/₄ in. and 6⁷/₈ in. Stuttgart, Landesmuseum.

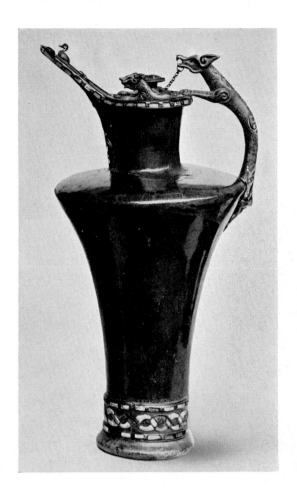

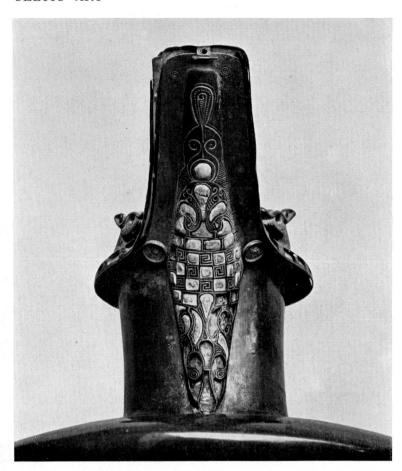

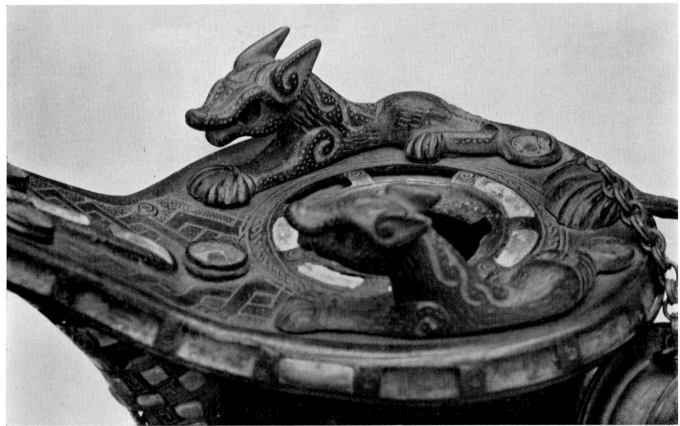

Pl. 115. Beaked flagon, from Basse-Yutz, Moselle, France, whole and two details, ca. mid-4th cent. B.C. Bronze and coral, ht., ca. 15³/₄ in. London, British Museum.

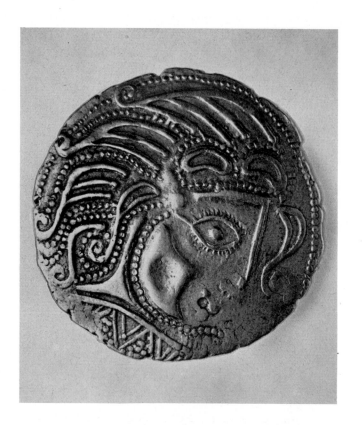

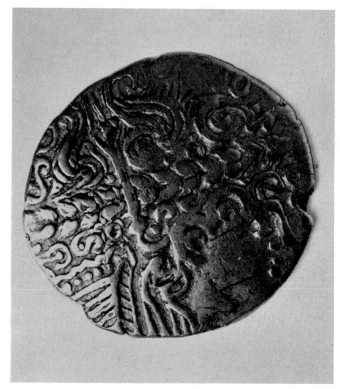

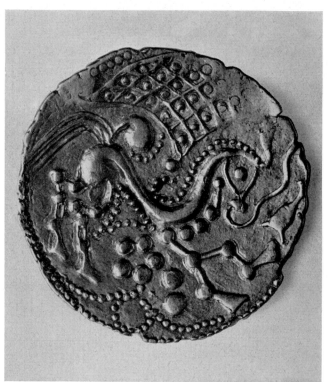

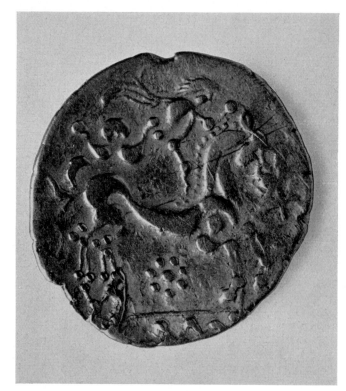

Pl. 116. Gold coins, 1st cent. B.C. *Left, above and below*: Stater of the Parisii, obverse and reverse. Diam., ca. 1 in. *Right*: Stater of the Bellovaci, obverse and reverse. Diam., ca. ¹¹/₁₆ in. Both, Paris, Cabinet des Médailles.

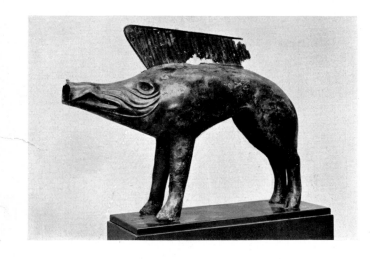

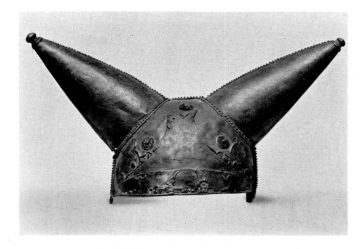

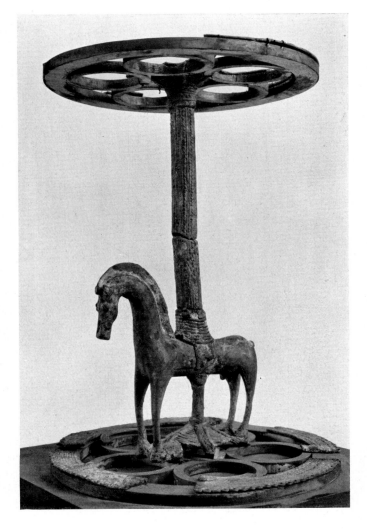

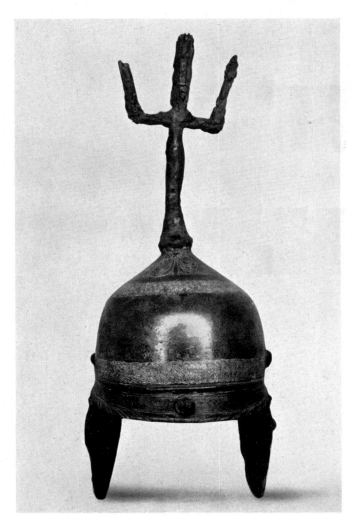

Pl. 117. *Above, left*: Boar, from Neuvy-en-Sullias, Loiret, France, 3d–2d cent. B.C. (?). Bronze, ht., 9⁷/₈ in. Orléans, Musée Historique de l'Orléanais. *Right*: Helmet, 1st cent., found in the Thames at London. Bronze; ht. of casque, 6¹/₄ in. London, British Museum. *Below, left*: Horse, incorporated in an object of uncertain use, from Calaceite, Teruel, Spain, 5th cent. B.C. Bronze, ht., 12¹/₈ in. Madrid, Museo Arqueológico Nacional. *Right*: Helmet, from Filottrano, near Ancona, 4th cent. B.C. Bronze; ht. of casque, 6¹/₄ in. Ancona, Italy, Museo Nazionale.

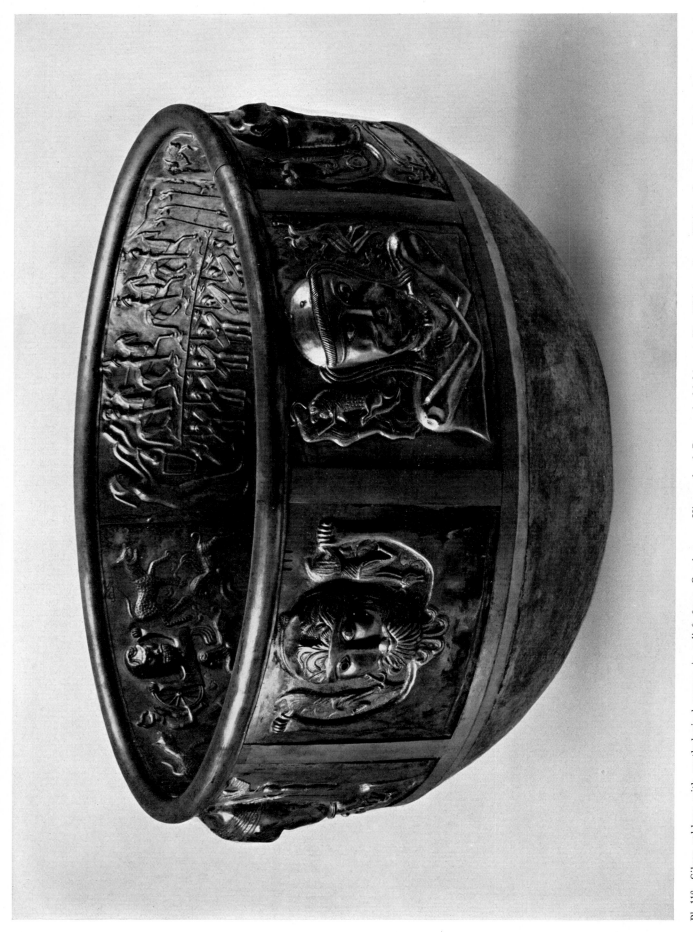

Pl. 118. Silver caldron with mythological scenes in relief, from Gundestrup, Himmerland, Denmark, 2d-3d cent. Ht., 16⅞ in., diam., 27⅛ in. Copenhagen, Nationalmuseet; photographed from a cast in Musée des Antiquités Nationales, Saint-Germain-en-Laye, France.

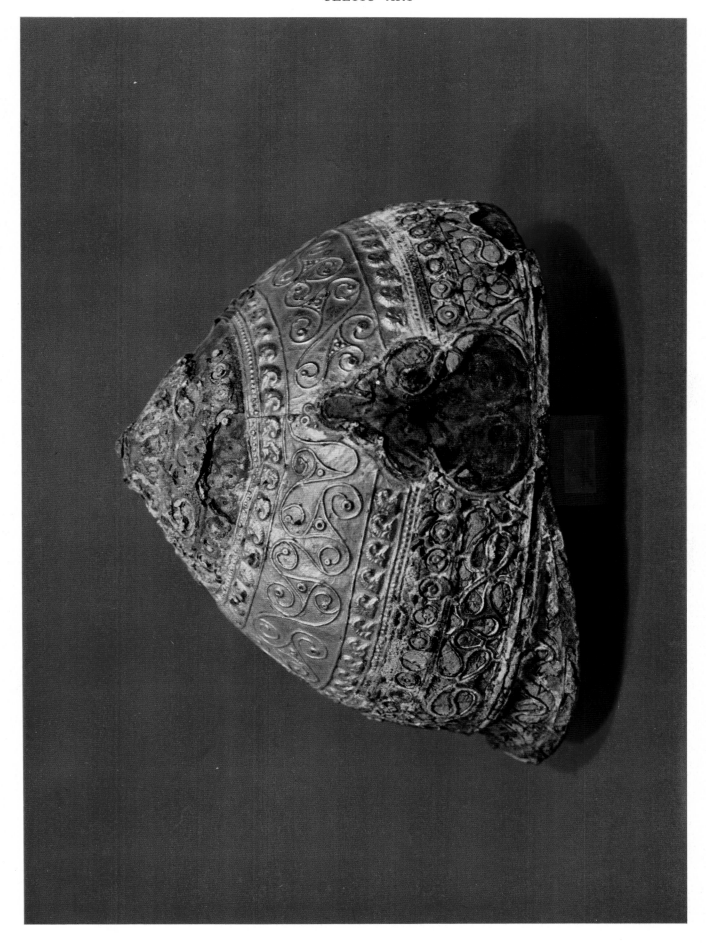

Pl. 119. Helmet, from Amfreville, Eure, France, ca. mid-4th cent. B.C. Copper, iron, and gold; ht, 6⅝ in. Paris, Louvre.

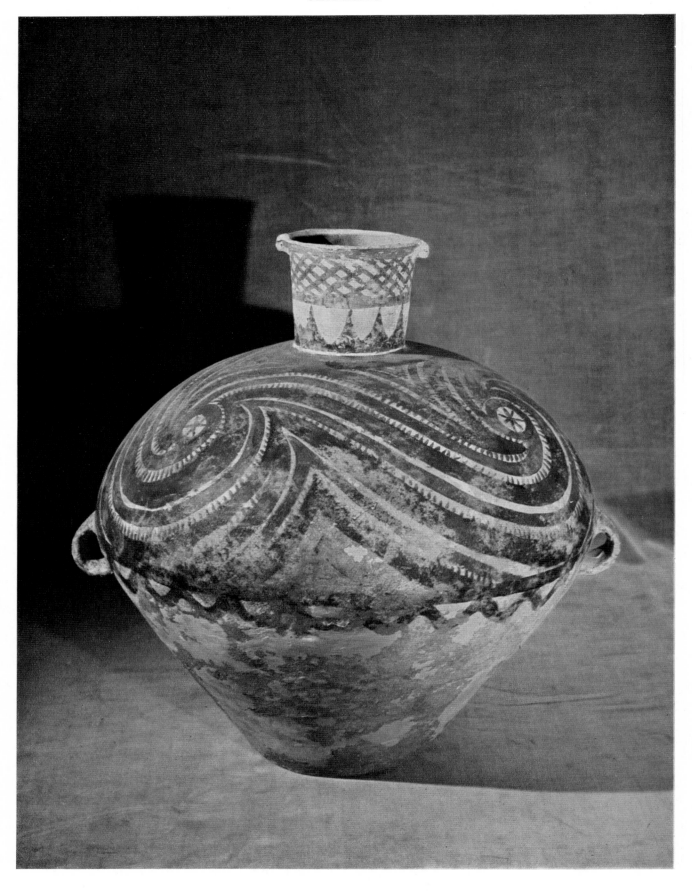

Pl. 120. Neolithic vessel, from Pan Shan, Kansu, China, 2d millennium B.C. Ht., 18¹/₂ in. Paris, Musée Cernuschi.

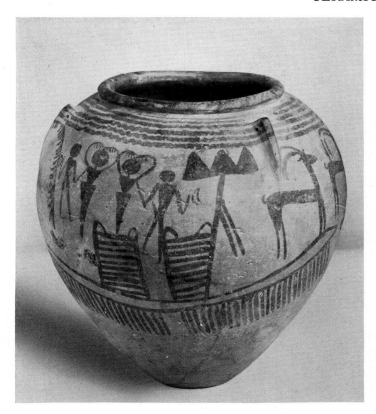

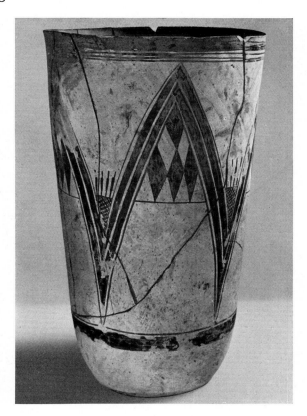

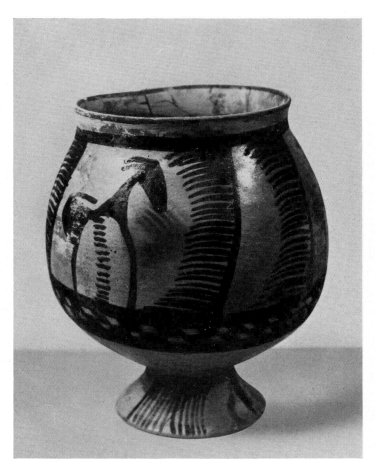

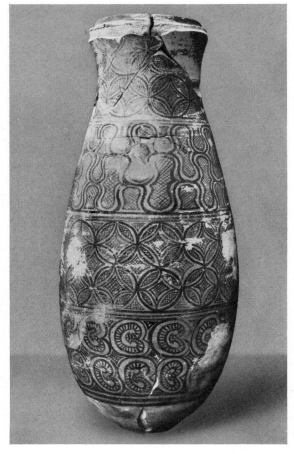

Pl. 121. *Above, left*: Egyptian jar, predynastic period, 4th millennium B.C. Ht., 8³/₄ in. Hanover, Kestner-Museum. *Right*: Goblet, from Susa, Iran, Style I, late 4th millennium B.C. Rome, Museo Pigorini. *Below, left*: Cup, from Tepe Hissar, near Damghan, Iran, Period III, second half of 3d millennium B.C. Ht., 7¹/₄ in. Teheran, Archaeological Museum. *Right*: Jar, from Mohenjo-daro, Pakistan, 3d–2d millennium B.C. New Delhi, Museum of Central Asian Antiquities.

# CERAMICS

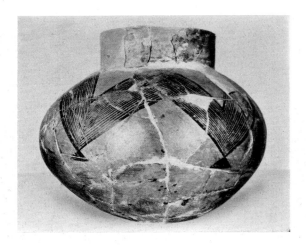

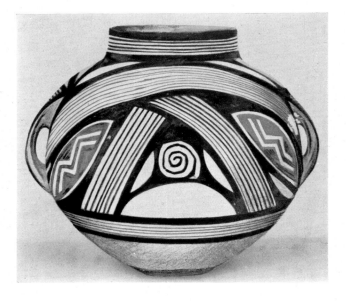

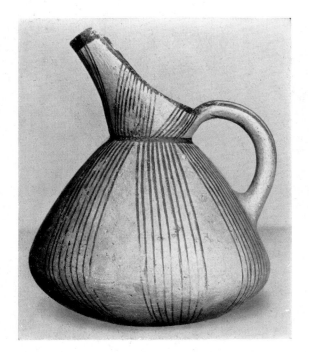

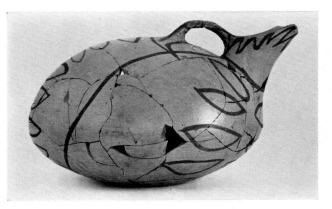

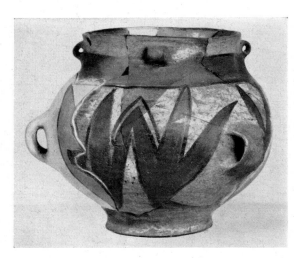

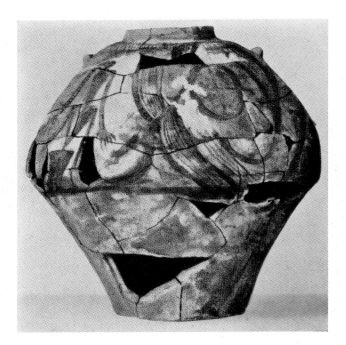

Pl. 122. *Above, left*: Vessel of Sesklo type, from Chaironeia, Greece, 4th millennium B.C. Athens, National Museum. *Right*: Vessel of Dimini type, Greece, first half of 3d millennium B.C. (reproduced from a water-color rendering). Location unknown. *Center, left*: Pitcher, from Hagios Onouphrios, Crete, subneolithic phase of Minoan culture, 3d millennium B.C. Heraklion, Crete, Archaeological Museum. *Right*: Proto-Helladic pitcher, from Lerna, Greece, 3d millennium B.C. Athens, National Museum. *Below, left*: Vessel in Capri style, from the island of Lipari, Italy, early 3d millennium B.C. Lipari, Museo Eoliano. *Right*: Vessel of the Tripolje culture, from Petreny, southern Russia, 3d–2d millennium B.C. Location unknown.